Sabiston & Spencer Surgery of the Chest, Volume I

Seventh Edition

Editor-in-Chief

Frank W. Sellke, M.D.
Johnson and Johnson Professor of Surgery
Harvard Medical School
Chief, Division of Cardiothoracic Surgery
Beth Israel Deaconess Medical Center
Boston, Massachusetts

Editors:

Pedro J. del Nido, M.D.
Professor of Surgery
Harvard Medical School
Chairman, Department of Cardiac Surgery
Children's Hospital Boston
Boston, Massachusetts

Scott J. Swanson, M.D.
Chief, Division of Thoracic Surgery
The Eugene W. Friedman Professor of Surgical Oncology
Mount Sinai School of Medicine
New York, New York

ELSEVIER
SAUNDERS

ELSEVIER
SAUNDERS
An Affiliate of Elsevier

The Curtis Center
Independence Square West
Philadelphia, Pennsylvania 19106-3399

Notice

Surgery is an ever-changing field. Standard safety precautions must be followed, but as new research and clinical experience broaden our knowledge, changes in treatment and drug therapy may become necessary or appropriate. Readers are advised to check the most current product information provided by the manufacturer of each drug to be administered to verify the recommended dose, the method and duration of administration, and contraindications. It is the responsibility of the treating physician, relying on experience and knowledge of the patient, to determine dosages and the best treatment for each individual patient. Neither the Publisher nor the author assumes any liability for any injury and/or damage to persons or property arising from this publication.

The Publisher

Library of Congress Cataloging-in-Publication Data

Sabiston & Spencer surgery of the chest.–7th ed./editor-in-chief, Frank W. Sellke; editors, Pedro J. Del Nido, Scott J. Swanson.
   p. ; cm.
   Rev ed. of: Surgery of the chest/[edited by] David C. Sabiston, Jr., Frank C. Spencer. 6th ed. c1995.
   Includes bibliographical references and index.
   ISBN 0-7216-0092-1 (set)
   1. Chest–Surgery. 2. Heart–Surgery. I. Title: Sabiston and Spencer surgery of the chest. II. Title: Surgery of the chest. III. Sellke, Frank W. IV. Del Nido, Pedro J. V. Swanson, Scott J. VL Sabiston, David C., VII. Spencer, Frank Cole. VIII. Surgery of the chest.
   [DNLM: 1. Thoracic Surgical Procedures–methods. WF 980 S116 2005]
RD536.S236 2005
617.5'4059–dc22

2004059212

Publisher: Anne Lenehan
Editorial Assistant: Vera Ginsbergs

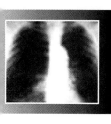

Dedication

This book is dedicated to my loving wife, Amy, who gives me unwavering support, inspiration, and love in all of my endeavors, and our children, Michelle, Eric, Nick, and Amanda. They provide us with limitless pleasure and humor and give us our purpose in life.

Frank W. Sellke

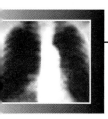

Contributors

Brian G. Abbott, M.D.
Assistant Professor of Medicine (Cardiology);
Associate Director, Cardiology Fellowship Training
Program, Yale University School of Medicine,
Section of Cardiovascular Medicine; Chief,
Cardiology Clinics, Veterans Administration Connecticut
Healthcare System, West Haven, Connecticut
*Nuclear Cardiology and Positron Emission
Tomography in the Assessment of Patients with
Cardiovascular Disease*

David H. Adams, M.D.
Marie-Josée and Henry R. Kravis Professor,
Department of Cardiothoracic Surgery, Mount Sinai
School of Medicine; Chairman,
Department of Cardiothoracic Surgery,
Mount Sinai Medical Center, New York, New York
*Acquired Disease of the Mitral Valve; Ischemic Mitral
Regurgitation*

Arvind K. Agnihotri, M.D.
Assistant Professor of Surgery, Department of Cardiac
Surgery, Harvard Medical School; Attending Surgeon,
Department of Cardiac Surgery, Massachusetts General
Hospital, Boston, Massachusetts
Postinfarction Ventricular Septal Defect

Lishan Aklog, M.D.
Associate Chief, Cardiac Surgery, Department of
Cardiothoracic Surgery, Mount Sinai Medical Center, New
York, New York
*Acquired Disease of the Mitral Valve; Ischemic Mitral
Regurgitation*

Mark S. Allen, M.D.
Professor of Surgery; Chair, Division of General Thoracic
Surgery, Mayo School of Medicine, Rochester, Minnesota
Chest Wall Reconstruction

Nikki Allmendinger, M.D.
Surgical Research Fellow, Department of Surgery, Harvard
University; Surgical Research Fellow, Department of
Surgery, Children's Hospital Boston, Boston,
Massachusetts
Congenital Diaphragmatic Hernia

Nasser Altorki, M.D.
Professor of Cardiothoracic Surgery, Department of
Cardiothoracic Surgery, Weill Medical College of Cornell
University, New York, New York
Screening for Lung Cancer

Robert H. Anderson, B.Sc., M.D., F.R.C.Path.
Joseph Levy Professor of Paediatric Cardiac Morphology,
Cardiac Unit, Institute of Child Health, University
College; Great Ormond Street Hospital for Children
National Health Service Trust, Cardiac Services, London,
United Kingdom
Surgical Anatomy of the Heart

David A. Ashburn, M.D.
Research Fellow, Congenital Heart Surgeons Society Data
Center and Division of Cardiovascular Surgery, Hospital
for Sick Children, Toronto, Ontario, Canada; Senior
Administrative Resident in Surgery, Department of
Surgery, Wake Forest University School of Medicine,
Winston-Salem, North Carolina
Adult Congenital Cardiac Surgery

Simon K. Ashiku, M.D.
Instructor in Surgery, Department of Surgery,
Harvard Medical School; Division of Cardiothoracic
Surgery, Beth Israel Deaconess Medical Center, Boston,
Massachusetts
Tracheal Lesions

Louis I. Astra, M.D.
Fellow, Department of Cardiothoracic Surgery,
Ohio State University Medical Center, Columbus, Ohio
Surgical Treatment of Cardiac Arrhythmias

Erle H. Austin, III, M.D.
Professor of Surgery, Department of Surgery,
University of Louisville; Chief, Department of Pediatric
Cardiac Surgery, Kosair Children's Hospital, Louisville,
Kentucky
Pulmonary Atresia with Intact Ventricular Septum

Eric H. Awtry, M.D., F.A.C.C.
Assistant Professor of Medicine, Boston University
School of Medicine; Director, Education, Division of
Cardiology, Boston Medical Center, Boston,
Massachusetts
The Pharmacological Management of Heart Failure

Leon Axel, Ph.D., M.D.
Professor of Cardiac Imaging; Director, Cardiac Imaging,
Department of Radiology, New York University School of
Medicine, New York, New York
Ventricular Mechanics

Emile A. Bacha, M.D.
Assistant Professor of Surgery and Pediatrics; Director, Pediatric Cardiac Surgery, Department of Cardiothoracic Surgery,
The University of Chicago Children's Hospital, Chicago, Illinois
Ventricular Septal Defect and Double-Outlet Right Ventricle

Carl Lewis Backer, M.D.
Professor of Surgery, Department of Surgery, Northwestern University Feinberg School of Medicine; A.C. Buehler Professor of Surgery, Division of Cardiovascular–Thoracic Surgery, Children's Memorial Hospital, Chicago, Illinois
Congenital Tracheal Disease; Surgery for Arrhythmias and Pacemakers in Children

Donald S. Baim, M.D.
Professor of Medicine, Harvard Medical School; Director, Center for Integration of Medicine and Innovative Technology, Brigham and Women's Hospital, Boston, Massachusetts
Nonatherosclerotic Coronary Heart Disease

Leora B. Balsam, M.D.
Research Fellow and Resident in Surgery, Department of Cardiothoracic Surgery, Stanford University School of Medicine; Stanford, California
Heart Transplantation

Michael K. Banbury, M.D.
Cardiothoracic Surgeon, Department of Cardiothoracic Surgery, The Cleveland Clinic Foundation Cleveland, Ohio
Acquired Aortic Valve Disease

Hendrick B. Barner, M.D.
Clinical Professor of Surgery, Department of Surgery, Washington University School of Medicine; Staff Surgeon, Department of Surgery, Forest Part Hospital, St. Louis, Missouri
Bypass Conduit Options

David J. Barron, M.D., M.R.C.P. (U.K.), F.R.C.S.(C.T.)
Consultant Cardiac Surgeon, Birmingham Children's Hospital, Birmingham, United Kingdom
Surgery for Congenitally Corrected Transposition of the Great Arteries

Céline Liu Bauwens, M.A.Sc.
Postdoctoral Student, Institute of Biomaterials and Biomedical Engineering, Department of Chemical Engineering and Applied Chemistry, University of Toronto, Toronto, Ontario, Canada
Tissue Regeneration

David P. Bichell, M.D.
Director, Department of Cardiovascular Surgery; Director, Children's Heart Institute; Children's Hospital and Health Center, San Diego, California
Atrial Septal Defect and Cor Triatriatum

Edward L. Bove, M.D.
Professor of Cardiac Surgery; Head, Section of Cardiac Surgery, Department of Surgery, University of Michigan, Ann Arbor, Michigan
Truncus Arteriosus and Aortopulmonary Window

William J. Brawn, F.R.C.S., F.R.C.T.
Cardiac Surgeon, Birmingham Children's Hospital, Birmingham, United Kingdom
Surgery for Congenitally Corrected Transposition of the Great Arteries

Christian P. Brizard, M.D.
Director, Cardiac Surgery Unit, Royal Children's Hospital, Melbourne, Victoria, Australia
Congenital Anomalies of the Mitral Valve

Malcolm V. Brock, M.D.
Assistant Professor of Surgery, Department of Surgery, Johns Hopkins University School of Medicine; Johns Hopkins Hospital, Baltimore, Maryland
Thoracic Trauma

Kelli R. Brooks, M.D.
Resident, Department of Surgery, Duke University Medical Center, Durham, North Carolina
Combined Modality Therapy for Esophageal Cancer

Redmond P. Burke, M.D.
Chief Cardiac Surgeon, Department of Cardiac Surgery, Miami Children's Hospital, Miami, Florida
Patent Ductus Arteriosus and Vascular Rings

Harold M. Burkhart, M.D.
Assistant Professor of Cardiothoracic Surgery, Department of Cardiothoracic Surgery, University of Iowa Hospitals and Clinics, Iowa City, Iowa
Congenital Lung Diseases

Whitney M. Burrows, M.D.
Assistant Professor of Surgery, Division of Thoracic Surgery, Department of Surgery, University of Maryland, Baltimore, Maryland
Staging Techniques for Carcinoma of the Esophagus

Christopher A. Caldarone, M.D.
Associate Professor of Cardiovascular Surgery, Department of Cardiovascular Surgery, The University of Toronto; Staff Surgeon, Department of Cardiovascular Surgery, The Hospital for Sick Children; Associate Scientist, Research Institute, The Hospital for Sick Children, Toronto, Ontario, Canada
Surgical Considerations in Pulmonary Vein Anomalies

Robert M. Califf, M.D.
Associate Vice Chancellor for Clinical Research, Director, Duke Clinical Research Institute; Professor of Medicine, Department of Medicine, Division of Cardiology, Duke University Medical Center, Durham, North Carolina
Medical Management of Acute Coronary Syndromes

David N. Campbell, M.D.
Professor of Surgery, Department of Surgery, Section of
Cardiovascular Surgery, University of Colorado Health
Sciences Center; Surgical Director, Pediatric Cardiac
Transplantation, The Children's Hospital, Denver,
Colorado
*Thrombosis and Thromboembolism of Prosthetic Cardiac
Valves and Extracardiac Prostheses*

Justine M. Carr, M.D.
Assistant Professor of Surgery, Department of Surgery,
Harvard Medical School; Director, Clinical Resource
Management, Department of Health Care Quality,
Beth Israel Deaconess Medical Center, Boston,
Massachusetts
Clinical Quality and Cardiac Surgery

Joseph P. Carrozza, Jr., M.D.
Associate Professor of Medicine, Harvard Medical School;
Chief, Section of Interventional Cardiology, Beth Israel
Deaconess Medical Center, Boston, Massachusetts
Interventional Cardiology

Robert J. Cerfolio, M.D.
Chief, Thoracic Surgery; Associate Professor of Surgery,
Department of Surgery, University of Alabama at
Birmingham; Chief, Thoracic Surgery, Birmingham
Veterans Administration Hospital, Birmingham, Alabama
Benign Lesions of the Lung

A. Alfred Chahine, M.D.
Assistant Professor of Surgery and Pediatrics,
Department of Surgery and Pediatrics, The George
Washington University School of Medicine; Chief,
Department of Pediatric Surgery, Georgetown University
Medical Center; Attending Surgeon, Department of
Pediatric Surgery, Children's National Medical Center,
Washington, D.C.
Surgery for Congenital Lesions of the Esophagus

Dharmender Chandhok, M.B.B.S.
Assistant Professor of Anesthesia and Critical Care;
Director, Cardiac Anesthesia and Perioperative
Echocardiography; Director, Ancillary Service;
Assistant Clinical Director, Department of Anesthesia
and Critical Care, St. Louis University Hospital,
St. Louis, Missouri
Adult Cardiac Anesthesia

W. Randolph Chitwood, Jr., M.D.
Professor of Surgery; Chairman, Department of Surgery,
East Carolina University, Brody School of Medicine,
Greenville, North Carolina
Robotic and Novel Visualization Systems

Neil A. Christie, M.D., F.R.C.S.(C.)
Assistant Professor of Surgery, University of Pittsburgh;
Attending Surgeon, Division of Thoracic and Foregut
Surgery, University of Pittsburgh Medical Center,
Pittsburgh, Pennsylvania
Innovative Therapy and Technology

Andrew D. Cochrane, M.B.B.S., F.R.A.C.S.,
F.R.C.S.(C.Th.), M.P.H.
Consultant Cardiac Surgeon, Department of
Pediatric Cardiac Surgery, Royal Children's Hospital;
Consultant Cardiac Surgeon, Department of
Cardiothoracic Surgery, Monash Medical Centre;
Cardiothoracic Surgeon, Heart and Lung Transplant
Service, Alfred Hospital, Melbourne, Victoria,
Australia
*Surgery for Congenital Anomalies of the Coronary
Arteries*

Herbert E. Cohn, M.D.
Anthony E. Narducci Professor of Surgery; Interim
Chairman, Department of Surgery, Thomas Jefferson
University, Philadelphia, Pennsylvania
Secondary Lung Tumors

William E. Cohn, M.D.
Associate Professor of Surgery, Department of
Surgery, Transplant and Assist Devices, Baylor
College of Medicine; Direct, Minimally Invasive
Surgical Technology, Department of Transplant,
Texas Heart Institute at St. Luke's Episcopal Hospital,
Houston, Texas
*Alternative Approaches to Surgical Coronary Artery
Bypass Grafting*

Yolonda L. Colson, M.D., Ph.D.
Assistant Professor of Surgery; Assistant Professor of
Medicine; Thoracic Surgeon, Department of Surgery,
Brigham and Women's Hospital; Thoracic Surgeon,
Department of Thoracic Oncology, Dana-Farber Cancer
Institute, Boston, Massachusetts
Interstitial Lung Diseases

Wilson S. Colucci, M.D., F.A.C.C., F.A.H.A.
Thomas J. Ryan Professor of Medicine; Director,
Myocardial Biology Unit, Boston University School of
Medicine; Chief, Cardiovascular Medicine Section,
Boston University Medical Center, Boston,
Massachusetts
The Pharmacological Management of Heart Failure

Andrew C. Cook, B.Sc., Ph.D.
British Heart Foundation Lecturer, Cardiac Unit, Institute
of Child Health, London, United Kingdom
Surgical Anatomy of the Heart

Joel D. Cooper, M.D.
Evarts A. Graham Professor of Surgery; Chief, Division of
Cardiothoracic Surgery, Washington University School
of Medicine; Barnes-Jewish Hospital, St. Louis,
Missouri
Surgery for Emphysema

Robert M. Cortina, M.D.
Attending Thoracic Surgeon, Department of Surgery,
New Hanover Regional Medical Center, Wilmington,
North Carolina
Chylothorax

x

Sabine H. Daebritz, M.D.
Professor of Surgery, Department of Cardiac Surgery,
Ludwig Maximilians University; Ludwig Maximilians
University Hospital Grosshadern, Munich, Germany
Atrioventricular Canal Defects

Thomas A. D'Amico, M.D.
Associate Professor of Surgery, Division of Thoracic
Surgery, Department of Surgery; Director, Clinical
Oncology, Duke Comprehensive Cancer Center, Duke
University Medical Center, Durham, North Carolina
Lung Cancer: Minimally Invasive Approaches

Thomas M. Daniel, M.D.
Professor of Surgery; Section Chief, Department of
Thoracic and Cardiovascular Surgery, University of
Virginia Health System, Charlottesville, Virginia
Mediastinal Anatomy and Mediastinoscopy

Gordon K. Danielson, M.D.
Professor of Surgery, Division of Thoracic and
Cardiovascular Surgery, Mayo Clinic School of Medicine,
Rochester, Minnesota
Ebstein's Anomaly

Philippe G. Dartevelle, M.D.
Professor of Thoracic and Vascular Surgery and
Heart–Lung Transplantation, Paris Sud University, Paris;
Chairman, Department of Thoracic and Vascular Surgery
and Heart–Lung Transplantation, Marie Lannelongue
Hospital, Le Plessis Robinson, France
Anterior Approach to Pancoast Tumors

Tirone E. David, M.D.
Professor of Surgery, University of Toronto; Chief, Cardiac
Surgery, Toronto General Hospital, Toronto, Ontario,
Canada
Surgery of the Aortic Root and Ascending Aorta

Jonathan D'Cunha, M.D., Ph.D.
Cardiovascular and Thoracic Surgery Fellow, Department
of Surgery, University of Minnesota; Fairview–University
Medical Center, Minneapolis, Minnesota
The Use of Genetic Science in Thoracic Disease

Barbara J. Deal, M.D.
M. E. Wodika Professor of Pediatrics, Northwestern
University Feinberg School of Medicine; Director,
Electrophysiology Services, Department of Cardiology,
Children's Memorial Hospital, Chicago, Illinois
Surgery for Arrhythmias and Pacemakers in Children

Joseph A. Dearani, M.D.
Associate Professor of Surgery, Division of Cardiovascular
Surgery, Mayo Clinic, Rochester, Minnesota
Ebstein's Anomaly

Daniel T. DeArmond, M.D.
Thoracic Surgery Resident, Department of Cardiothoracic
Surgery, University of Iowa Hospitals and Clinics, Iowa
City, Iowa
Congenital Lung Diseases

Malcolm M. DeCamp, M.D.
Chief, Section of Thoracic Surgery, Beth Israel
Deaconess Medical Center; Associate Professor of
Surgery, Harvard Medical School, Boston,
Massachusetts
Lung Cancer: Multimodal Therapy

Ralph De La Torre, M.D.
Chief, Section of Cardiac Surgery, Beth Israel Deaconess
Medical Center; Instructor in Surgery, Harvard Medical
School, Boston, Massachusetts
*Occlusive Disease of the Supraaortic Trunk and
Management of Simultaneous Surgical Carotid/Coronary
Disease; Valve Replacement Therapy: History, Options,
and Valve Types*

Marc R. de Leval, M.D., F.R.C.S.
Professor of Cardiothoracic Surgery, Cardiothoracic Unit,
University of London; Professor of Cardiothoracic Surgery,
Cardiothoracic Unit, Great Ormond Street Hospital for
Children National Health Service Trust, London, United
Kingdom
*Management of Single Ventricle and Cavopulmonary
Connections*

Pedro J. del Nido, M.D.
Professor of Surgery, Harvard Medical School; Chairman,
Department of Cardiac Surgery, Children's Hospital
Boston, Boston, Massachusetts
*Surgical Approaches and Cardiopulmonary Bypass in
Pediatric Cardiac Surgery; Atrioventricular Canal Defects;
Transposition of the Great Arteries (Complex Forms)*

Tom R. DeMeester, M.D.
Chairman, Department of Surgery, Keck School of
Medicine, University of Southern California; Chief,
Department of Surgery, University of Southern California
University Hospital; University of Southern California Los
Angeles County Hospital; Norris Cancer Center, Los
Angeles, California
Esophageal Anatomy and Function

Philippe Demers, M.D., M.Sc.
Postdoctoral Research Fellow, Department of
Cardiovascular Surgery, Stanford University School of
Medicine, Stanford, California
*Postpneumonectomy Empyema and Bronchopleural
Fistula; Type A Aortic Dissection; Type B Aortic
Dissection*

Todd L. Demmy, M.D.
Associate Professor of Surgery, Department of Surgery,
University of Buffalo; Chair, Department of Thoracic
Surgery, Department of Surgery, Roswell Park Cancer
Institute, Buffalo, New York
Malignant Pleural and Pericardial Effusions

Jean Deslauriers, M.D., F.R.C.S.(C.)
Professor of Surgery, Division of Thoracic Surgery, Laval
University, Centre de Pneumologie de l'Hôpital Laval,
Sante-Foy, Quebec, Canada
Postpneumonectomy Empyema and Bronchopleural Fistula

Eric J. Devaney, M.D.
Assistant Professor of Surgery, Department of
Cardiac Surgery, University of Michigan, Ann Arbor,
Michigan
Truncus Arteriosus and Aortopulmonary Window

Elisabeth U. Dexter, M.D.
Assistant Professor of Thoracic Surgery, Department
of Surgery, State University of New York, Upstate
Medical University; Chief, Thoracic Surgery, Syracuse
Veterans Administration Medical Center, Syracuse,
New York
*Perioperative Care of Patients Undergoing Thoracic
Surgery*

Paul L. DiGiorgi, M.D.
Cardiothoracic Surgery Research Fellow, Division of
Cardiothoracic Surgery, Columbia University, New York,
New York
Left Ventricular Assist Devices

Abdul R. Doughan, M.D.
Internal Medicine Resident, Department of Internal
Medicine, Emory University School of Medicine; Emory
University Hospital, Atlanta, Georgia
Physiology of the Coronary Circulation

Robert D. Dowling, M.D.
Professor of Surgery, Department of Surgery,
University of Louisville; Attending Surgeon,
Department of Surgery, Jewish Hospital; Attending
Surgeon, Department of Surgery, Norton's Hospital;
Attending Surgeon, Department of Surgery, University
Hospital, Louisville, Kentucky
Total Artificial Heart

Brian W. Duncan, M.D.
Associate Staff, Department of Pediatric and Congenital
Heart Surgery, The Children's Hospital at The Cleveland
Clinic, Cleveland, Ohio
Tetralogy of Fallot with Pulmonary Stenosis

Carlos M. G. Duran, M.D., Ph.D.
Professor and Chair, Department of Cardiovascular
Sciences, The University of Montana; Cardiovascular and
Thoracic Surgeon; President and CEO, The International
Heart Institute of Montana, St. Patrick Hospital, Missoula,
Montana
Acquired Disease of the Tricuspid Valve

Jeremy J. Erasmus, M.D.
Associate Professor of Radiology,
Department of Radiology, University of Texas–Houston;
University of Texas M. D. Anderson Cancer Center,
Houston, Texas
Imaging the Thorax

Dario O. Fauza, M.D.
Assistant Professor of Surgery, Department of Surgery,
Harvard Medical School; Associate, Department of
Surgery, Children's Hospital Boston, Boston,
Massachusetts
Congenital Diaphragmatic Hernia

Paul W. M. Fedak, M.D., Ph.D.
Clinical and Research Assistant; Professor of Surgery;
Toronto General Hospital, University of Toronto, Toronto,
Ontario, Canada
Cell Transplantation for Cardiovascular Disease

Hiran C. Fernando, F.R.C.S., F.R.C.S.Ed., F.A.C.S.
Assistant Professor of Surgery; Attending Surgeon,
Division of Thoracic and Foregut Surgery, University of
Pittsburgh Medical Center; Attending Surgeon,
Department of Surgery, Veterans Administration Medical
Center, Pittsburgh, Pennsylvania
*Endoscopic Therapies for the Airway and the Esophagus;
Innovative Therapy and Technology*

Farzan Filsoufi, M.D.
Assistant Professor of Surgery; Director, Cardiac Valve
Center, Department of Cardiothoracic Surgery, Mount
Sinai Medical Center, New York, New York
*Acquired Disease of the Mitral Valve; Ischemic Mitral
Regurgitation*

Mitchell P. Fink, M.D.
Professor and Chair, Department of Critical Care
Medicine, University of Pittsburgh School of Medicine;
Chairman, Department of Critical Care Medicine,
University of Pittsburgh Medical Center Presbyterian
Hospital, Pittsburgh, Pennsylvania
Shock and Sepsis

Rosario Freeman, M.D., M.S.
Assistant Professor of Internal Medicine, Division
of Cardiology, University of Washington, Seattle, Washington
Diagnostic Echocardiography

Joseph S. Friedberg, M.D., FACS
Chief, Division of Thoracic Surgery, Department of
Surgery, University of Pennsylvania Medical Center,
Presbyterian, Philadelphia, Pennsylvania
Secondary Lung Tumors

Willard A. Fry, M.D.
Professor Emeritus of Clinical Surgery, Northwestern
University Feinberg School of Medicine; Former Chief,
Section of Thoracic Surgery, Evanston Northwestern
Healthcare, Evanston, Illinois
Spontaneous Pneumothorax

David A. Fullerton, M.D.
Professor of Surgery, University of Colorado Health
Sciences Center; Chief, Division of Cardiothoracic
Surgery, Denver, Colorado
Prosthetic Valve Endocarditis

Lawrence A. Garcia, M.D., F.A.C.C., F.A.H.A.
Assistant Professor of Medicine, Harvard Medical School;
Director, Peripheral Cardiovascular Program and
Peripheral Interventions; Director, Interventional
Cardiology Fellowship Program, Beth Israel Deaconess
Medical Center, Boston, Massachusetts
*Coronary Angiography, Valve and Hemodynamic
Assessment; Peripheral Angiography and Percutaneous
Intervention*

xii

J. William Gaynor, M.D.
Associate Professor of Surgery, Department of
Surgery, University of Pennsylvania; Associate Professor
of Surgery, Department of Cardiac Surgery, The
Children's Hospital of Philadelphia, Philadelphia,
Pennsylvania
*Coarctation of the Aorta, Aortopulmonary Shunts, and
Aortopulmonary Collaterals*

Tal Geva, M.D.
Associate Professor of Pediatrics, Department of
Pediatrics, Harvard Medical School; Senior Associate;
Director, Cardiovascular Magnetic Resonance Imaging
Program, Department of Cardiology, Children's Hospital
Boston, Boston, Massachusetts
*Diagnostic Imaging: Echocardiography and Magnetic
Resonance Imaging*

Sébastien Gilbert, M.D., F.R.C.S.C.
Clinical Instructor, Division of Cardiothoracic Surgery,
University of Pittsburgh; Chief Resident, Division of
Cardiothoracic Surgery, University of Pittsburgh Medical
Center, Pittsburgh, Pennsylvania
Endoscopic Therapies for the Airway and the Esophagus

A. Marc Gillinov, M.D.
Staff Surgeon, Department of Thoracic and
Cardiovascular Surgery; Surgical Director, Center for
Atrial Fibrillation, The Cleveland Clinic Foundation,
Cleveland, Ohio
Tumors of the Heart

Robert J. Ginsberg, M.D., F.R.C.S.C.[†]
Professor of Surgery, Department of Surgery, University of
Toronto, Toronto, Ontario, Canada
Lung Cancer: Surgical Treatment

Donald D. Glower, M.D.
Professor of Surgery; Associate Professor of Biomedical
Engineering, Duke University Medical Center, Durham,
North Carolina
Pericardium and Constrictive Pericarditis

Sean C. Grondin, M.D., M.P.H., F.R.C.S.C.
Associate Professor of Surgery, Department of Surgery,
University of Calgary; Attending Thoracic Surgeon,
Department of Thoracic Surgery, Foothills Medical
Centre, Calgary, Alberta, Canada
Spontaneous Pneumothorax

Frederick L. Grover, M.D.
Professor and Chairman, Department of Surgery,
University of Colorado Health Sciences Center;
Surgeon-in-Chief, Department of Surgery, University
of Colorado Hospital, Denver, Colorado
*Prosthetic Valve Endocarditis; Thrombosis and
Thromboembolism of Prosthetic Cardiac Valves and
Extracardiac Prostheses*

Kyle J. Gunnerson, M.D.
Chief Fellow, Critical Care Medicine, University of
Pittsburgh School of Medicine, Pittsburgh, Pennsylvania
Shock and Sepsis

Constanza J. Gutierrez, M.D.
Associate, Capital Imaging Association, Austin, Texas
Imaging the Thorax

John R. Guyton, M.D.
Associate Professor of Medicine, Department of Medicine;
Assistant Professor of Pathology, Duke University Medical
Center, Durham, North Carolina
*The Coronary Circulation: Dietary and Pharmacological
Management of Atherosclerosis*

Zane T. Hammoud, M.D.
Assistant Professor of Surgery, Division of Thoracic
Surgery, Northwestern University Feinberg School of
Medicine; Evanston Northwestern Healthcare,
Department of Thoracic Surgery, Evanston, Illinois
Middle Mediastinum

David H. Harpole, Jr., M.D.
Professor of Surgery, Division of Thoracic Surgery; Thoracic
Surgeon; Director, Cardiothoracic Surgical Intensive Care
Unit, Duke University Medical Center; Chief,
Cardiothoracic Surgery, Department of Surgery, Durham
Veterans Affairs Medical Center, Durham, North Carolina
Combined Modality Therapy for Esophageal Cancer

David G. Harrison, M.D.
Director, Division of Cardiology, Department of Medicine,
Emory University; Professor of Medicine, Department of
Cardiology, Emory Hospital and The Emory Clinic;
Professor of Medicine, Department of Cardiology, Atlanta
Veterans Administration Medical Center, Atlanta, Georgia
Physiology of the Coronary Circulation

Chuong D. Hoang, M.D.
General Surgery Resident, Department of Surgery,
University of Minnesota; General Surgery Resident,
Department of Surgery, Fairview–University Medical
Center, Minneapolis, Minnesota
The Use of Genetic Science in Thoracic Disease

Katherine J. Hoercher, R.N.
Director of Research, Kaufman Center for Heart Failure,
The Cleveland Clinic Foundation, Cleveland, Ohio
*Left Ventricular Reconstruction and the Surgical
Treatment of the Failing Heart*

Lauren D. Holinger, M.D.
Head, Division of Otolaryngology and Department of
Communicative Disorders; Paul H. Holinger Professor;
Professor of Otolaryngology, Head, and Neck Surgery,
Northwestern University Feinberg School of Medicine;
Head, Division of Pediatric Otolaryngology; Medical
Director, Department of Communicative Disorders,
Children's Memorial Hospital and Medical Center,
Chicago, Illinois
Congenital Tracheal Diseases

†Deceased.

Keith A. Horvath, M.D.
Chief, Cardiothoracic Surgery Branch, National Institutes of Health, Bethesda, Maryland
Transmyocardial Laser Revascularization

Michael T. Jaklitsch, M.D.
Assistant Professor of Surgery, Department of Surgery, Harvard Medical School; Thoracic Surgeon, Division of Thoracic Surgery; Surgical Director, Lung Transplant Program, Brigham and Women's Hospital, Boston, Massachusetts
Surgery of the Diaphragm: A Deductive Approach

Stuart W. Jamieson, M.B., F.R.C.S., F.A.C.S.
Professor of Cardiothoracic Surgery; Head, Department of Cardiothoracic Surgery, University of California, San Diego School of Medicine, San Diego, California
Surgery for Pulmonary Embolism

Doraid Jarrar, M.D.
Chief Resident, Department of Surgery, University of Alabama at Birmingham, Birmingham, Alabama
Benign Lesions of the Lung

David W. Johnstone, M.D.
Associate Professor of Surgery and Oncology, Division of Cardiothoracic Surgery, University of Rochester Medical Center, Rochester, New York
Chylothorax

Mark E. Josephson, M.D.
Professor of Medicine; Chairman, Cardiovascular Division, Beth Israel Deaconess Medical Center, Boston, Massachusetts
Catheter Ablation of Arrhythmias

Lilian P. Joventino, M.D.
Cardiologist; Electrophysiologist, New England Heart Institute, Catholic Medical Center, Manchester, New Hampshire
Cardiac Devices for the Treatment of Bradyarrhythmias and Tachyarrhythmias

Amy L. Juraszek, M.D.
Instructor in Pathology, Department of Pathology, Harvard Medical School; Medical Director, Cardiac Registry, Department of Pathology; Assistant in Cardiology, Department of Cardiology, Children's Hospital Boston, Boston, Massachusetts
Cardiac Embryology and Genetics

Larry R. Kaiser, M.D.
The John Rhea Barton Professor and Chairman, Department of Surgery, University of Pennsylvania; Chief of Surgery, Hospital of the University of Pennsylvania, Philadelphia, Pennsylvania
The Posterior Mediastinum

Steven M. Keller, M.D.
Professor of Cardiothoracic Surgery, Albert Einstein College of Medicine; Chief, Thoracic Surgery, Department of Cardiothoracic Surgery, Montefiore Medical Center, Bronx, New York
Surgical Treatment of Hyperhidrosis

Kemp H. Kernstine, M.D., Ph.D.
Professor and Director, Department of Thoracic Surgery; Director, Lung Cancer Program, City of Hope National Medical Center, Duarte, California
Congenital Lung Diseases

Shaf Keshavjee, M.D., M.Sc., F.R.S.C.S., F.A.C.S.
Professor of Surgery, Department of Surgery, University of Toronto; Head, Division of Thoracic Surgery; Director, Thoracic Surgery Research, Toronto General Hospital, University of Toronto, Toronto, Ontario, Canada
Lung Cancer: Surgical Treatment

Leslie J. Kohman, M.D.
Professor of Surgery, Department of Surgery, State University of New York Upstate Medical University; University Hospital, Syracuse, New York
Perioperative Care of Patients Undergoing Thoracic Surgery

Robert J. Korst, M.D.
Associate Professor of Cardiothoracic Surgery, Department of Cardiothoracic Surgery, Weill Medical College of Cornell University; Attending Cardiothoracic Surgeon, Department of Cardiothoracic Surgery, New York Presbyterian Hospital—Cornell Campus, New York, New York
Screening for Lung Cancer

Peter C. Kouretas, M.D., Ph.D.
Cardiopulmonary Transplant Fellow, Department of Cardiothoracic Surgery, Stanford University, Stanford, California
Heart–Lung Transplantation

Mark J. Krasna, M.D.
Professor of Surgery; Chief, Thoracic Surgery, University of Maryland Medical School; Associate Director, Echocardiography Laboratory, Greenebaum Cancer Center, Baltimore, Maryland
Staging Techniques for Carcinoma of the Esophagus

Judy Krempin, M.S.
Clinical Data Manager, Department of Cardiac Surgery, Beth Israel Deaconess Medical Center, Boston, Massachusetts
Clinical Quality and Cardiac Surgery

John C. Kucharczuk, M.D.
Assistant Professor of Surgery, Section of General Thoracic Surgery, University of Pennsylvania School of Medicine; Chief, Thoracic Surgical Section, Philadelphia Veterans Affairs Administration Medical Center, Philadelphia, Pennsylvania
Anterior Mediastinal Masses

Eugene L. Kukuy, M.D.
Cardiothoracic Surgery Resident, Department of Cardiothoracic Surgery, Weill Medical College of Cornell University; New York Presbyterian Hospital—Cornell Campus, New York, New York
Left Ventricular Assist Devices

xiv

Alan P. Kypson, M.D.
Assistant Professor of Surgery, Division of Cardiothoracic Surgery, East Carolina University, Brody School of Medicine, Greenville, North Carolina
Robotic and Novel Visualization Systems

Roger J. Laham, M.D.
Associate Professor of Medicine, Department of Medicine; Director, Angiogenesis Research Center and Basic Angioplasty Research, Department of Cardiology, Beth Israel Deaconess Medical Center, Harvard Medical School, Boston, Massachusetts
Nonatherosclerotic Coronary Heart Disease

Peter Lang, M.D.
Associate Professor of Pediatrics, Harvard Medical School; Senior Associate in Cardiology, Children's Hospital Boston, Boston, Massachusetts
Cardiac Catheterization

Christine L. Lau, M.D.
Fellow, Lung Transplantation, Division of Cardiothoracic Surgery, Washington University School of Medicine, St. Louis, Missouri
Lung Transplantation

Peter C. Laussen, M.B.B.S.
Associate Professor of Anaesthesia, Department of Anaesthesia, Harvard Medical School; Director, Cardiac Intensive Care Unit, Department of Cardiology, Children's Hospital Boston, Boston, Massachusetts
Mechanical Circulatory Support; Pediatric Anesthesia and Critical Care

Richard Lee, M.D., M.B.A.
Assistant Professor of Surgery, Department of Surgery, St. Louis University; Active Staff, Department of Cardiothoracic Surgery, St. Louis University Hospital, St. Louis, Missouri
Left Ventricular Reconstruction and the Surgical Treatment of the Failing Heart

Robert B. Lee, M.D., F.A.C.S.
Associate Clinical Professor of Cardiac and Thoracic Surgery, Department of General Surgery, University of Mississippi Medical Center; Chief, Surgery, Central Mississippi Medical Center, Jackson, Mississippi
Empyema Thoracis

Sidney Levitsky, M.D.
David W. and David Cheever Professor of Surgery, Department of Surgery, Division of Cardiothoracic Surgery, Harvard Medical School; Director, Cardiothoracic Surgery, CareGroup; Senior Vice Chairman, Department of Surgery, Beth Israel Deaconess Medical Center, Boston, Massachusetts
Myocardial Protection

Ren-Ke Li, M.D., Ph.D.
Professor of Surgery, Division of Cardiac Surgery, Department of Surgery, University of Toronto; Senior Scientist, Toronto General Research Institute, Toronto General Hospital, Toronto, Ontario, Canada
Cell Transplantation for Cardiovascular Disease

John Liddicoat, M.D., M.B.A.
Assistant Professor of Surgery, Department of Surgery, Harvard Medical School; Division of Cardiothoracic Surgery, Beth Israel Deaconess Medical Center, Boston, Massachusetts
Tumors of the Heart

Chien-Chih Lin, M.D.
Assistant Professor of Surgery, Department of Thoracic Surgery, KaoHsiung Medical University; Assistant Professor of Surgery, Department of Thoracic Surgery, KaoHsiung Medical University Attached Chung-Ho Memorial Teaching Hospital, KaoHsiung, Taiwan
Surgical Treatment of Hyperhidrosis

Philip A. Linden, M.D.
Instructor in Surgery, Harvard Medical School; Staff Surgeon, Division of Thoracic Surgery, Brigham and Women's Hospital, Boston, Massachusetts
Pleural Tumors; Esophageal Resection and Replacement

John C. Lipham, M.D.
Assistant Professor of Surgery, Department of Surgery, Keck School of Medicine; University of Southern California University Hospital; University of Southern California Los Angeles County Hospital; Norris Cancer Center, Los Angeles, California
Esophageal Anatomy and Function

Michael J. Liptay, M.D., F.A.C.S.
Assistant Professor of Surgery, Northwestern University Feinstein School of Medicine; Chief, Division of Cardiothoracic Surgery, Department of Surgery, Evanston Northwestern Healthcare, Evanston, Illinois
Middle Mediastinum

Andrew J. Lodge, M.D.
Assistant Professor of Surgery, Department of Surgery, Duke University Medical Center, Durham, North Carolina
Transposition of the Great Arteries

Gary K. Lofland, M.D.
Professor of Surgery, University of Missouri–Kansas City School of Medicine; Joseph Boon Gregg Chair, Section of Cardiac Surgery, Children's Mercy Hospital, Kansas City, Missouri
Interrupted Aortic Arch

James D. Luketich, M.D.
Associate Professor of Surgery, Department of Thoracic Surgery, University of Pittsburgh; Chief, Division of Thoracic and Foregut Surgery; Department of Thoracic Surgery, University of Pittsburgh Medical Center Health System, Presbyterian University Hospital; Shadyside Hospital; St. Margaret Hospital; Pittsburgh, Pennsylvania
Endoscopic Therapies for the Airway and the Esophagus; Innovative Therapy and Technology

Bruce W. Lytle, M.D.
Staff Surgeon, Department of Cardiovascular Surgery, The Cleveland Clinic Foundation, Cleveland, Ohio
Redo Coronary Artery Bypass Surgery

Michael A. Maddaus, M.D.
Professor of Surgery, Department of Surgery, University of Minnesota; Fairview–University Medical Center, Minneapolis, Minnesota
The Use of Genetic Science in Thoracic Disease

Feroze Mahmood, M.D.
Instructor in Anesthesia, Department of Anesthesia and Critical Care, Harvard Medical School; Director, Division of Thoracic Anesthesia, Department of Anesthesia and Critical Care, Beth Israel Deaconess Medical Center, Boston, Massachusetts
Adult Cardiac Anesthesia

Abeel A. Mangi, M.D.
Fellow, Department of Cardiac Surgery, Columbia Presbyterian Medical Center, New York, New York
Postinfarction Ventricular Septal Defect

Warren J. Manning, M.D.
Professor of Medicine and Radiology, Harvard Medical School; Section Chief, Noninvasive Cardiac Imaging, Cardiovascular Division, Beth Israel Deaconess Medical Center, Boston, Massachusetts
Cardiovascular Magnetic Resonance in Cardiovascular Diagnosis

Edith M. Marom, M.D.
Associate Professor of Radiology, Department of Radiology, University of Texas–Houston; University of Texas M. D. Anderson Cancer Center, Houston, Texas
Imaging the Thorax

Audrey C. Marshall, M.D.
Instructor of Pediatrics, Harvard Medical School; Assistant in Cardiology, Department of Cardiology, Children's Hospital Boston, Boston, Massachusetts
Catheter-Based Interventions

David P. Mason, M.D.
Assistant Professor of Surgery, Division of Thoracic Surgery, Johns Hopkins University School of Medicine, Baltimore, Maryland
Thoracic Trauma

Douglas J. Mathisen, M.D.
Hermes C. Grillo Professor of Surgery, Harvard Medical School; Chief Emeritus, General Thoracic Surgery Unit, Department of Thoracic Surgery, Massachusetts General Hospital, Boston, Massachusetts
Tracheal Lesions

Constantine Mavroudis, M.D.
Professor of Surgery, Department of Surgery, Northwestern University Feinberg School of Medicine; Willis J. Potts Professor of Surgery, Division of Cardiovascular–Thoracic Surgery, Children's Memorial Hospital, Chicago, Illinois
Congenital Tracheal Disease; Surgery for Arrhythmias and Pacemakers in Children

Patrick M. McCarthy, M.D.
Professor of Surgery, Department of Surgery, Northwestern University Feinberg School of Medicine; Chief, Cardiothoracic Surgery; Co-Director, Northwestern Cardiovascular Institute, Northwestern Medical Faculty Foundation, Inc., Chicago, Illinois
Left Ventricular Reconstruction and the Surgical Treatment of the Failing Heart

James D. McCully, Ph.D.
Associate Professor of Surgery, Department of Surgery, Harvard Medical School, Division of Cardiothoracic Surgery, Beth Israel Deaconess Medical Center, Boston, Massachusetts
Myocardial Protection

Edwin C. McGee, Jr., M.D.
Assistant Professor of Surgery, Department of Surgery, Northwestern University Feinberg School of Medicine; Northwestern Memorial Hospital, Chicago, Illinois
Valve Replacement Therapy: History, Options, and Valve Types

Francis X. McGowan, Jr., M.D.
Professor of Anesthesia, Department of Anesthesia (Pediatrics), Harvard Medical School; Chief, Division of Cardiac Anesthesia, Department of Anesthesiology, Children's Hospital Boston; Director, Anesthesia/Critical Care Medicine Research Laboratory, Children's Hospital Boston, Harvard Medical School, Boston, Massachusetts
Surgical Approaches and Cardiopulmonary Bypass in Pediatric Cardiac Surgery

Roger B.B. Mee, M.B., Ch.B., F.R.A.C.S.
Chairman, Department of Pediatric and Congenital Heart Surgery, The Children's Hospital at The Cleveland Clinic, Cleveland, Ohio
Tetralogy of Fallot with Pulmonary Stenosis

Bryan F. Meyers, M.D.
Associate Professor of Surgery, Department of Surgery, Washington University School of Medicine; Attending Physician, Barnes-Jewish Hospital, St. Louis, Missouri
Surgery for Emphysema

Robert E. Michler, M.D.
John G. and Jeanne B. McCoy Chair, Department of Cardiothoracic Surgery; Associate Director, Davis Heart and Lung Institute, The Ohio State University; Chief, Cardiothoracic Surgery and Transplantation, The Ohio State University Medical Center, Columbus, Ohio
Surgical Treatment of Cardiac Arrhythmias

Carmelo A. Milano, M.D.
Assistant Professor of Surgery, Department of Surgery, Duke University; Director of Surgical Cardiac Transplantation, Department of Surgery, Duke University Medical Center, Durham, North Carolina
Critical Care for the Adult Cardiac Patient

D. Craig Miller, M.D.
Thelma and Henry Doelger Professor of Cardiovascular Surgery, Department of Cardiothoracic Surgery, Stanford University School of Medicine; Medical Staff of Cardiovascular Surgery, Department of Cardiothoracic Surgery, Stanford University Hospitals and Clinics, Stanford, California
Type A Aortic Dissection; Type B Aortic Dissection

John D. Mitchell, M.D.
Chief, Section of General Thoracic Surgery, Division of Cardiothoracic Surgery, University of Colorado Health Sciences Center; University of Colorado Hospital; Consulting Surgeon, National Jewish Medical and Research Center, Denver, Colorado
Infectious Lung Diseases

R. Scott Mitchell, M.D.
Professor, Department of Cardiovascular Surgery, Stanford University School of Medicine, Stanford, California
Endovascular Therapy for the Treatment of Thoracic Aortic Aneurysms and Dissections

Susan D. Moffatt-Bruce, M.D., Ph.D.
Assistant Professor of Surgery, Department of Cardiovascular Surgery, University of British Columbia, Vancouver, British Columbia, Canada
Endovascular Therapy for the Treatment of Thoracic Aortic Aneurysms and Dissections

Bassem N. Mora, M.D.
Instructor in Surgery, Harvard Medical School; Assistant in Cardiac Surgery, Department of Cardiac Surgery, Children's Hospital Boston, Boston, Massachusetts
Atrioventricular Canal Defects

Ivan P. Moskowitz M.D., Ph.D.
Instructor in Pathology, Department of Pathology, Harvard Medical School; Scientific Director, Cardiac Registry, Department of Pathology, Children's Hospital Boston, Boston, Massachusetts
Cardiac Embryology and Genetics

Nabil A. Munfakh, M.D.
Associate Professor of Surgery, Department of Cardiothoracic Surgery, Washington University School of Medicine; Chief, Cardiothoracic Surgery, Christian Hospital, St. Louis, Missouri
Bypass Conduit Options

Sudish C. Murthy, M.D., Ph.D.
Staff Surgeon, Department of Thoracic and Cardiovascular Surgery, The Cleveland Clinic Foundation, Cleveland, Ohio
Lung Cancer: Multimodal Therapy; Surgical Treatment of Benign Esophageal Diseases

Sacha Mussot, M.D.
Fellow, Department of Thoracic and Vascular Surgery and Heart–Lung Transplantation, Paris-Sud University, Paris; Thoracic Surgery Fellow, Department of Thoracic and Vascular Surgery and Heart–Lung Transplantation, Marie-Lannelongue Hospital, Le Plessis Robinson, France
Anterior Approach to Pancoast Tumors

Yoshifumi Naka, M.D., Ph.D.
Herbert Irving Assistant Professor of Surgery, Department of Cardiothoracic Surgery, Columbia University, College of Physicians and Surgeons, New York, New York
Left Ventricular Assist Devices

Siyamek Neragi-Miandoab, M.D.
Division of Thoracic Surgery, Brigham and Women's Hospital, Boston, Massachusetts
Pleural Tumors

Kurt D. Newman, M.D.
Professor of Surgery, Department of Surgery and Pediatrics, George Washington University School of Medicine; Executive Director, Center for Surgical Care, Children's National Medical Center, Washington, D.C.
Surgery for Congenital Lesions of the Esophagus

L. Wiley Nifong, M.D.
Assistant Professor of Cardiothoracic Surgery, Department of Surgery, East Carolina University, Brody School of Medicine; University Health Systems of Eastern Carolina, Greenville, North Carolina
Robotic and Novel Visualization Systems

Chukwumere Nwogu, M.D.
Assistant Professor of Surgery, Department of Surgery, University at Buffalo; Attending, Department of Thoracic Surgery, Roswell Park Cancer Center, Buffalo, New York
Malignant Pleural and Pericardial Effusions

James E. O'Brien, Jr., M.D.
Assistant Professor of Surgery, University of Missouri–Kansas City School of Medicine; Attending Surgeon, Section of Cardiac Surgery, Children's Mercy Hospital, Kansas City, Missouri
Interrupted Aortic Arch

Kirsten C. Odegard, M.D.
Assistant Professor of Medicine, Harvard Medical School; Senior Associate in Anesthesia, Department of Anesthesia, Children's Hospital Boston, Boston, Massachusetts
Pediatric Anesthesia and Critical Care

Richard G. Ohye, M.D.
Assistant Professor of Surgery, Department of Surgery, University of Michigan, Ann Arbor, Michigan
Truncus Arteriosus and Aortopulmonary Window

William C. Oliver, Jr., M.D.
Associate Professor of Anesthesiology, Department of Anesthesiology, Mayo Clinic College of Medicine, Rochester, Minnesota
Blood Coagulation, Transfusion, and Conservation

Mark Onaitis, M.D.
Resident, Thoracic Surgery, Department of Surgery, Duke University Medical Center, Durham, North Carolina
Lung Cancer: Minimally Invasive Approaches

Catherine M. Otto, M.D.
Professor of Medicine; Director, Cardiology Fellowship
Programs, Division of Cardiology, Department of
Medicine, University of Washington; Associate Director,
Echocardiography Laboratory; Co-Director, Adult
Congenital Heart Disease Clinic, University of Washington
Medical Center, Seattle, Washington
Diagnostic Echocardiography

Mehmet C. Oz, M.D., F.A.C.S.
Professor of Surgery, Department of Cardiothoracic
Surgery, Columbia University; Director, Cardiovascular
Institute; Vice Chairman, Cardiovascular Services,
Department of Cardiovascular Surgery, New York
Presbyterian Hospital—Columbia University, New York,
New York
Left Ventricular Assist Devices

Peter C. Pairolero, M.D.
Chair, Department of Surgery, Mayo Clinic College of
Medicine, Rochester, Minnesota
Chest Wall Tumors

Bernard J. Park, M.D.
Clinical Assistant Surgeon, Thoracic Service,
Department of Surgery, Memorial Sloan-Kettering
Cancer Center; Cornell University Medical College,
New York, New York
Lung Cancer Workup and Staging

Kyung W. Park, M.D.
Associate Professor of Anesthesia, Department of
Anesthesia, Harvard Medical School; Department of
Anesthesia, Critical Care, and Pain Medicine, Beth Israel
Deaconess Medical Center, Boston, Massachusetts
Adult Cardiac Anesthesia

Amit N. Patel
Department of Surgery, University of Texas Southwestern
Medical School, Dallas, Texas
Thoracic Outlet Syndrome and Dorsal Sympathectomy

G. Alexander Patterson, M.D.
Joseph C. Bancroft Professor of Surgery; Chief, General
Thoracic Surgery, Division of Cardiothoracic Surgery,
Washington University School of Medicine, St. Louis,
Missouri
Lung Transplantation

Edward F. Patz, Jr., M.D.
James and Alice Chen Professor of Radiology; Professor of
Pharmacology and Cancer Biology; Professor of Pathology,
Department of Radiology, Duke University Medical
Center, Durham, North Carolina
Imaging the Thorax

Subroto Paul, M.D.
Chief Resident, General Surgery, Department of
Surgery, Brigham and Women's Hospital, Boston,
Massachusetts
Interstitial Lung Diseases

Glenn Pelletier, M.D.
Assistant Professor, Department of Cardiovascular Surgery,
Drexel University College of Medicine; Department of
Cardiothoracic Surgery, St. Christopher's Hospital for
Children, Philadelphia, Pennsylvania
Atrial Septal Defect and Cor Triatriatum

Frank A. Pigula, M.D.
Assistant Professor of Surgery, Department of Surgery,
University of Pittsburgh School of Medicine; Director,
Department of Pediatric Cardiothoracic Surgery,
Children's Hospital of Pittsburgh, Pittsburgh,
Pennsylvania
*Surgery for Congenital Anomalies of the Aortic Valve and
Root; Hypoplastic Left Heart Syndrome*

Duane S. Pinto, M.D.
Instructor in Medicine, Harvard Medical School;
Co-Director, Cardiology Fellowship Training
Program, Division of Cardiology, Interventional Section,
Beth Israel Deaconess Medical Center, Boston,
Massachusetts
Interventional Cardiology

Marvin Pomerantz, M.D.
Professor of Surgery, Division of Cardiothoracic
Surgery, University of Colorado Health Sciences Center;
University of Colorado Hospital; Consulting Surgeon,
National Jewish Medical and Research Center, Denver,
Colorado
Infectious Lung Diseases

Jeffrey L. Port, M.D.
Assistant Professor of Cardiothoracic Surgery, Department
of Cardiothoracic Surgery, Weill Medical College of
Cornell University; Assistant Attending Cardiothoracic
Surgeon, Department of Cardiothoracic Surgery, New
York Presbyterian Hospital—Cornell Campus, New York,
New York
Screening for Lung Cancer

D. Dean Potter, Jr., M.D.
Research Fellow, Division of Cardiovascular Surgery, Mayo
Clinic, Rochester, Minnesota
Blood Coagulation, Transfusion, and Conservation

Harry Rakowski, M.D., F.R.C.P.C., F.A.S.E.
Professor of Medicine, Department of Medicine,
University of Toronto; Director, Hypertrophic
Cardiomyopathy Clinic, Department of Medicine,
Toronto General Hospital, University Health Network,
Toronto, Ontario, Canada
Surgical Management of Hypertrophic Cardiomyopathy

Anthony C. Ralph-Edwards, B.Sc., M.D.
Lecturer, Department of Surgery, University of
Toronto; Staff Surgeon, Department of Cardiovascular
Surgery, Toronto General Hospital, Toronto, Ontario,
Canada
Surgical Management of Hypertrophic Cardiomyopathy

xviii

Daniel P. Raymond, M.D.
Surgical Resident, Department of Surgery, University of
Virginia Health System, Charlottesville, Virginia
Mediastinal Anatomy and Mediastinoscopy

Brian L. Reemtsen, M.D.
Resident, Department of Cardiothoracic Surgery,
University of Washington, Seattle, Washington
Endoscopic Diagnosis of Thoracic Disease

John J. Reilly, Jr., M.D.
Associate Professor of Medicine, Department of Medicine,
Harvard Medical School; Clinical Director, Pulmonary and
Critical Care Medicine, Department of Medicine, Brigham
and Women's Hospital, Boston, Massachusetts
*Preoperative Assessment of Patients Undergoing Thoracic
Surgery*

Bruce A. Reitz, M.D.
The Norman E. Shumway Professor, Department
of Cardiothoracic Surgery, Stanford University School
of Medicine, Stanford, California
Heart–Lung Transplantation

Thomas W. Rice, M.D.
Head, Section of General Thoracic Surgery, The Cleveland
Clinic Foundation, Cleveland, Ohio
*Lung Cancer: Multimodal Therapy; Surgical Treatment
of Benign Esophageal Diseases*

John R. Roberts, M.D., M.B.A.
Co-Director, Thoracic Oncology, Department of Thoracic
Surgery, Sarah Cannon Cancer Center; Oncology Thoracic
Surgeon, Centennial Medical Center, Baptist Hospital,
Nashville, Tennessee
Other Primary Tumors of the Lung

Robert C. Robbins, M.D.
Associate Professor of Cardiothoracic Surgery, Department
of Cardiothoracic Surgery, Stanford University; Stanford
University School of Medicine, Stanford, California
Heart Transplantation

Evelio Rodriguez, M.D.
Cardiothoracic Surgery Fellow, Department of Surgery,
Division of Cardiothoracic Surgery, Thomas Jefferson
University, Philadelphia, Pennsylvania
Secondary Lung Tumors

Audrey Rosinberg, M.D.
Postdoctoral Fellow, Department of Surgery, Columbia
University Medical Center; New York Presbyterian
Hospital, New York, New York
*Nonatherosclerotic Coronary Heart Disease; Alternative
Approaches to Surgical Coronary Artery Bypass Grafting*

Stephen J. Roth, M.D., M.P.H.
Associate Professor of Pediatrics, Department of
Pediatrics, Stanford University School of Medicine;
Director, Cardiovascular Intensive Care Unit, Division of
Pediatric Cardiology, Lucile Packard Children's Hospital,
Palo Alto, California
Mechanical Circulatory Support in Children

Fraser D. Rubens, M.D., M.Sc., F.R.C.S.(C.)
Associate Professor of Surgery, Department of Cardiac
Surgery, University of Ottawa Heart Institute, Ottawa,
Ontario, Canada
Cardiopulmonary Bypass: Technique and Pathophysiology

Marc Ruel, M.D., M.P.H.
Cardiac Surgeon; Assistant Professor of Surgery; Director,
Cardiac Surgery Laboratory Research, Division of Cardiac
Surgery, Cross-Appointed to the Department of
Epidemiology, University of Ottawa Heart Institute,
Ottawa, Ontario, Canada
*Coronary Artery Bypass Grafting; Therapeutic
Angiogenesis*

Valerie W. Rusch, M.D.
Chief, Thoracic Service, Department of Surgery; William
G. Cahan Chair of Surgery, Memorial Sloan-Kettering
Cancer Center; Professor of Surgery, Cornell University
Medical College, New York, New York
Lung Cancer Workup and Staging

Sacha P. Salzberg, M.D.
Research Fellow, Department of Cardiothoracic Surgery,
Mount Sinai Medical Center, New York, New York
Acquired Disease of the Mitral Valve

Hartzell V. Schaff, M.D.
Stuart W. Harrington Professor of Surgery; Chair, Division
of Cardiovascular Surgery, Mayo Clinic,
Rochester, Minnesota
Blood Coagulation, Transfusion, and Conservation

Jess M. Schultz, M.D.
Senior Resident, Department of Surgery, Oregon Health
and Science University, Portland, Oregon
Right Ventricle-to-Pulmonary Artery Conduits

Frank W. Sellke, M.D.
Johnson and Johnson Professor of Surgery, Harvard
Medical School; Chief, Division of Cardiothoracic Surgery,
Beth Israel Deaconess Medical Center, Boston,
Massachusetts
*Physiology of the Coronary Circulation; Coronary Artery
Bypass Grafting; Therapeutic Angiogenesis*

Michael V. Sefton, Sc.D.
University Professor and Director, Institute of Biomaterials
and Biomedical Engineering, University of Toronto,
Toronto, Ontario, Canada
Tissue Regeneration

Rohit Shahani, M.D.
Chief Resident, Department of Cardiothoracic Surgery,
Mount Sinai Medical Center, New York, New York
Anatomy of the Thorax

Robert C. Shamberger, M.D.
Robert E. Gross Professor of Surgery, Department
of Surgery, Harvard Medical School; Chief, Department
of Surgery, Children's Hospital Boston, Boston,
Massachusetts
Congenital Chest Wall Deformities

Irving Shen, M.D.
Associate Professor of Surgery, Division of Pediatric
Cardiac Surgery, Doernbecher Children's Hospital,
Oregon Health and Science University, Portland,
Oregon
Right Ventricle-to-Pulmonary Artery Conduits

Joseph B. Shrager, M.D.
Assistant Professor of Surgery, Department of Surgery,
University of Pennsylvania School of Medicine; Chief,
Section of General Thoracic Surgery, Hospital of the
University of Pennsylvania; Director, Department of
General Thoracic Surgery, Pennsylvania Hospital,
Philadelphia, Pennsylvania
Anterior Mediastinal Masses

Dhruv Singhal, M.D.
Surgery Resident, Department of Surgery, Brigham and
Women's Hospital, Boston, Massachusetts
The Posterior Mediastinum

Peter K. Smith, M.D.
Professor and Chief, Department of General Thoracic
Surgery, Duke University Medical Center, Durham,
North Carolina
Critical Care for the Adult Cardiac Patient

R. John Solaro, Ph.D.
University Professor and Head, Department of Physiology
and Biophysics, University of Illinois at Chicago, Chicago,
Illinois
Physiology of the Myocardium

Thomas L. Spray, M.D.
Professor of Surgery, Department of Surgery, University of
Pennsylvania; Alice Langdon Warner Endowed Chair in
Pediatric Cardiothoracic Surgery, Department of Surgery,
Children's Hospital of Philadelphia, Philadelphia,
Pennsylvania
Transposition of the Great Arteries

William Stanford, M.D.
Professor of Radiology, Department of Radiology,
University of Iowa Hospitals and Clinics, Iowa City, Iowa
*Applications of Computed Tomography in Cardiovascular
Disease*

William L. Stanford, Ph.D.
Assistant Professor, Institute of Biomaterials and
Biomedical Engineering, University of Toronto; Associate
Scientist, Samuel Lunenfeld Research Institute, Mount
Sinai Hospital, Toronto, Ontario, Canada
Tissue Regeneration

Michael Straznicka, M.D.
Instructor in Surgery, Department of Thoracic and
Cardiovascular Surgery, University of Texas M. D.
Anderson Cancer Center, Houston, Texas; Surgeon,
Department of Thoracic Surgery, John Muir Medical
Center, Walnut Creek, California; Surgeon, Department of
Thoracic Surgery, Mount Diablo Medical Center, Concord,
California
*Lung Cancer: Surgical Strategies for Tumors Invading the
Chest Wall*

David J. Sugarbaker, M.D.
Richard E. Wilson Professor of Surgical Oncology,
Department of Surgery, Harvard Medical School; Chief,
Division of Thoracic Surgery, Department of Surgery,
Brigham and Women's Hospital, Boston, Massachusetts
Pleural Tumors

Lars G. Svensson, M.D., Ph.D.
Director, Center for Aortic Surgery, Marfan Syndrome,
and Connective Tissue Disorder Clinic, The Cleveland
Clinic Foundation, Cleveland, Ohio
*Surgery of the Aortic Arch; Descending Thoracic and
Thoracoabdominal Aortic Surgery*

Scott J. Swanson, M.D.
Chief, Division of Cardiothoracic Surgery, Mount Sinai
School of Medicine; Eugene W. Friedman Professor of
Surgical Oncology, Mount Sinai Hospital, New York,
New York
Esophageal Resection and Replacement

Patricia A. Thistlethwaite, M.D., Ph.D.
Associate Professor of Surgery, Division of Cardiothoracic
Surgery; Professor and Head, Division of Cardiothoracic
Surgery, University of California, San Diego, San Diego,
California
Surgery for Pulmonary Embolization

David F. Torchiana, M.D.
Associate Professor of Surgery, Department of Surgery,
Harvard Medical School; CEO and Chairman, Massachusetts
General Physical Organization, Boston, Massachusetts
Postinfarction Ventricular Septal Defect

Ross M. Ungerleider, M.D.
Professor of Surgery; Chief, Pediatric Cardiac Surgery,
Doernbecher Children's Hospital, Oregon Health and
Science University, Portland, Oregon
Right Ventricle-to-Pulmonary Artery Conduits

Harold C. Urschel, Jr., M.D., L.L.D.(Hon.), D.S.(Hon.)
Clinical Professor of Cardiovascular and Thoracic Surgery,
University of Texas Southwestern Medical School; Chair,
Cardiovascular and Thoracic Surgical Research, Education,
and Clinical Excellence, Baylor University Medical Center,
Dallas, Texas
Thoracic Outlet Syndrome and Dorsal Sympathectomy

Glen S. Van Arsdell, M.D.
Associate Professor of Surgery, Department of Surgery,
University of Toronto; Head, Division of Cardiac Surgery,
CIT Chair, Cardiovascular Surgery, Department of Surgery,
Hospital for Sick Children, Toronto, Ontario, Canada
*Pulmonary Atresia and Ventricular Septal Defect; Adult
Congenital Cardiac Surgery*

Carin van Doorn, M.D. F.R.C.S.(C./Th.)
Senior Lecturer in Cardiothoracic Surgery, Cardiothoracic
Unit, Institute of Child Health; Honorary Consultant
Cardiothoracic Surgeon, Cardiothoracic Unit, Great
Ormond Street Hospital for Children National Health
Service Trust, London, United Kingdom
*Management of Single Ventricle and Cavopulmonary
Connections*

Timothy L. Van Natta, M.D.
Assistant Professor of Surgery, Department of Surgery,
University of Iowa Hospitals and Clinics, Iowa City, Iowa
Congenital Lung Diseases

Richard Van Praagh, M.D.
Professor Emeritus of Pathology, Department of
Pathology, Harvard Medical School; Director Emeritus,
Cardiac Registry, Departments of Pathology, Cardiology,
and Cardiac Surgery, Children's Hospital Boston, Boston,
Massachusetts
Segmental Anatomy

Jeffrey S. Veluz, M.D.
Chief Resident, Division of Cardiothoracic Surgery, Beth
Israel Deaconess Hospital; Harvard Medical School,
Boston, Massachusetts
*Occlusive Disease of the Supraaortic Trunk and
Management of Simultaneous Surgical Carotid/Coronary
Disease*

Gus J. Vlahakes, M.D.
Professor of Surgery, Department of Surgery,
Harvard Medical School; Chief, Division of Cardiac
Surgery, Massachusetts General Hospital, Boston,
Massachusetts
*Valve Replacement Therapy: History, Options, and Valve
Types*

Garrett L. Walsh, M.D.
Professor of Surgery, Department of Thoracic and
Cardiovascular Surgery, University of Texas M. D.
Anderson Cancer Center, Houston, Texas
*Lung Cancer: Surgical Strategies for Tumors Invading the
Chest Wall*

Thomas J. Watson, M.D.
Associate Professor of Surgery, Division of Thoracic
and Foregut Surgery, University of Rochester School of
Medicine and Dentistry; Attending Physician, Strong
Memorial Hospital, Rochester, Minnesota
Fibrothorax and Decortication of the Lung

Ronald M. Weintraub, M.D.
David S. Ginsburg Associate Professor of
Surgery, Harvard Medical School; Chief Emeritus,
Division of Cardiothoracic Surgery, Beth Israel
Deaconess Medical Center; Chief, Surgery, Department
of Surgery, Cambridge Health Alliance, Boston,
Massachusetts
Clinical Quality and Cardiac Surgery

Richard D. Weisel, M.D., F.R.C.S.C.
Professor and Chairman, Division of Cardiac Surgery,
University of Toronto; Surgeon, Division of Cardiovascular
Surgery, Toronto General Hospital, Toronto, Ontario,
Canada
Cell Transplantation for Cardiovascular Disease

Margaret V. Westfall, Ph.D.
Assistant Professor of Surgery, Department of Surgery,
University of Michigan, Ann Arbor, Michigan
Physiology of the Myocardium

Daniel C. Wiener, M.D.
Resident, Department of General Surgery, Dartmouth
Hitchcock Medical Center, Lebanon, New Hampshire;
Research Fellow, Department of Adult Oncology, Dana-
Farber Cancer Institute, Boston, Massachusetts
Surgery of the Diaphragm: A Deductive Approach

Dennis A. Wigle M.D., Ph.D.
Resident in Thoracic Surgery, Department of Surgery,
University of Toronto, Toronto, Ontario, Canada
Lung Cancer: Surgical Treatment

Ernest D. Wigle, M.D.
Professor Emeritus of Medicine, Department of Medicine,
University of Toronto; Staff Physician, Department of
Medicine (Cardiology), Toronto General Hospital, Toronto,
Ontario, Canada
Surgical Management of Hypertrophic Cardiomyopathy

Benson R. Wilcox, M.D.
Professor of Surgery, Department of Cardiothoracic
Surgery, University of North Carolina, Chapel Hill, North
Carolina
Surgical Anatomy of the Heart

William G. Williams, M.D., F.R.S.C.(C.)
Cardiac Surgeon, Department of Cardiac Surgery, Toronto
General Hospital, Toronto, Ontario, Canada
*Surgical Management of Hypertrophic Cardiomyopathy;
Adult Congenital Cardiac Surgery*

Jay M. Wilson, M.D.
Associate Professor of Surgery, Department of Surgery,
Harvard Medical School; Senior Associate in Surgery,
Department of Surgery, Children's Hospital Boston,
Boston, Massachusetts
Congenital Diaphragmatic Hernia

Douglas E. Wood, M.D.
Professor and Chief, Section of General Thoracic Surgery,
University of Washington, Seattle, Washington
Endoscopic Diagnosis of Thoracic Disease

David Wrobleski, M.D.
Staff Electrophysiologist, Department of Cardiology, St.
Vincent Hospital, Indianapolis, Indiana
Catheter Ablation of Arrhythmias

Stephen C. Yang, M.D., F.A.C.S., F.C.C.P.
Chief, Thoracic Surgery; Associate Professor of Surgery
and Oncology, Department of Surgery, The Johns Hopkins
Medical Institutions; Chief, Thoracic Surgery, Department
of Surgery, The Johns Hopkins Bayview Medical Center,
Baltimore, Maryland
Thoracic Trauma

Susan B. Yeon, M.D., J.D.
Instructor in Medicine, Harvard Medical School;
Department of Medicine, Cardiovascular Division, Cardiac
Magnetic Resonance Center, Beth Israel Deaconess
Medical Center, Boston, Massachusetts
*Cardiovascular Magnetic Resonance in Cardiovascular
Diagnosis*

Peter Zandstra, Ph.D.
Associate Professor, Institute of Biomaterials and
Biomedical Engineering, University of Toronto; Canada
Research Chair in Stem Cell Bioengineering, Toronto,
Ontario, Canada
Tissue Regeneration

Barry L. Zaret, M.D.
Robert W. Berliner Professor of Medicine; Chief, Section
of Cardiovascular Medicine, Department of Internal
Medicine, Yale University School of Medicine, New
Haven, Connecticut
*Nuclear Cardiology and Positron Emission Tomography in
the Assessment of Patients with Cardiovascular Disease*

Peter J. Zimetbaum, M.D.
Assistant Professor of Medicine, Harvard Medical School;
Director, Clinical Arrhythmia Service, Department of
Medicine, Division of Cardiology, Beth Israel Deaconess
Medical Center, Boston, Massachusetts
*Cardiac Devices for the Treatment of Bradyarrhythmias
and Tachyarrhythmias*

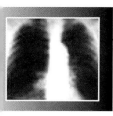

Preface

When first asked to be editor of the 7th Edition of *Sabiston and Spencer Surgery of the Chest*, I considered it a great honor and privilege, since this textbook is widely regarded as one of the premier resources in cardiothoracic surgery. Drs. David Sabiston and Frank Spencer have been regarded as leaders in the field of surgery for nearly the past half century. When asking some of my esteemed colleagues if they would be willing to contribute a chapter to this new edition, they almost universally said yes, but in a few cases their initial reply was, "In these days of electronic publishing and web based information gathering, why do we need another printed textbook?" While much information can be obtained from the web, including the contents of most peer-reviewed journals, I believe that the most efficient, authoritative method to obtain clinical information remains reading the textbook. This can be in the traditional hard copy, printed form, or an electronic version. Considering that the sales of cardiothoracic surgery textbooks has not diminished recently, I can say that most of my surgical colleagues would agree with this assertion.

Despite being one of the best regarded textbooks in the field, the other editors and I felt that the next edition should be totally rewritten. This is, in fact, what we did. The format has been reorganized to better reflect the modern practice of cardiothoracic surgery. Virtually all authors contributing chapters in the 7th Edition are new. In fact, none of the authors were given the related chapter from the previous book. The content was changed to reflect recent major changes in adult and pediatric cardiac surgery and general thoracic surgery. Even when a chapter was thought to be acceptable in the previous edition, it was usually re-assigned to a new author to revitalize and modernize the book. The content of several previous chapters was eliminated, and many new chapters were added, again reflecting these recent changes in the field. Chapters were included covering most areas of basic science that the editors believed should be in the knowledge base of practicing cardiac and thoracic surgeons. These chapters include those covering coronary physiology, myocardial contractile function, congenital and adult cardiac anatomy, and pulmonary and esophageal physiology. In addition, new chapters that overlap with the surgical treatment of cardiothoracic diseases were added. These chapters include catheter-based treatment of cardiac disease, electrophysiology, cell-based treatment of cardiac disease, and multimodality treatment of thoracic malignancies. Not to lessen the impact or importance of these chapters dealing with "peripheral or supporting information," the chapters dealing with the "heart" of cardiothoracic surgery are certainly the major thrust of the current edition. We are very pleased to have recruited those who we believe to be internationally recognized experts in their respective subspecialties. One of the strengths of this book is that all areas of cardiothoracic surgery are covered in one edition: adult and pediatric cardiac surgery and general thoracic surgery. Almost everything that needs to be known for practice, with the exception of basic operative techniques and clinical judgment, is included. This ranges from basic science to medically-based approaches to cardiac and thoracic disease. As the boundary between the classical medical and surgical treatments of many disorders seems to be disappearing, we feel that it is critical that surgeons are aware of a broad range of treatment options.

As with most textbooks, one of the main jobs of the editors was to hound delinquent authors for their contributions. We hope that these authors will not hold a grudge and apologize if we were too abrupt at times. We hope most will consider contributing to the next edition.

I wish to express my sincere thanks and gratitude to my co-editors, Drs. Pedro del Nido and Scott Swanson. Their knowledge of the field and perseverance made this book the success that it is. Finally, I would like to thank the staff at Elsevier for their unwavering support of this book. Despite some of the not unexpected initial inconveniences, they were always available for the duration of the project and especially when problems occurred, and I cannot thank them enough for all of their hard work. My assistant, Mrs. Susan Lerman, was a tremendous asset with organization and loyalty and provided comic relief, not just in regard to this book.

Frank W. Sellke
Pedro J. del Nido
Scott J. Swanson

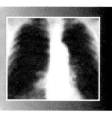

Table of Contents

Sabiston & Spencer Surgery of the Chest

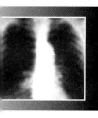

Color Plates

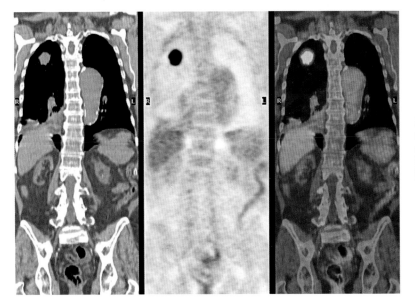

Figure 2-8 Non-small-cell lung cancer. Coronal CT, PET, and fused CT-PET images show small nodule in right upper lobe with increased uptake of [18F]fluorodeoxyglucose, which is consistent with malignancy.

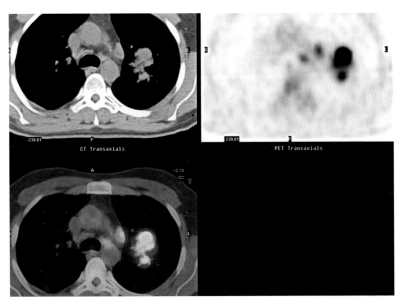

Figure 2-10 Non-small-cell lung cancer. Axial CT, PET, and fused CT-PET images show left upper lobe lung malignancy with increased [18F]fluorodeoxyglucose uptake consistent with a malignancy. Enlarged prevascular and normal sized left lower paratracheal nodes show increased FDG uptake compared with uptake in mediastinum confirmed to be metastases. Note absence of FDG uptake in right lower paratracheal nodes indicative of absence of nodal metastases.

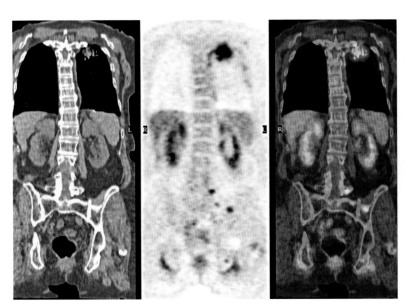

Figure 2-11 Non-small-cell lung cancer. Coronal CT, PET, and fused CT-PET images show left upper lobe lung malignancy with increased [18F]fluorodeoxyglucose. Note focal increased FDG uptake in lumbar spine and pelvis due to metastases.

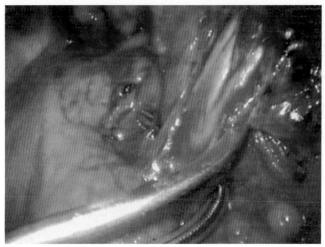

Figure 18-1 Left superior pulmonary vein, encircled with curved clamp.

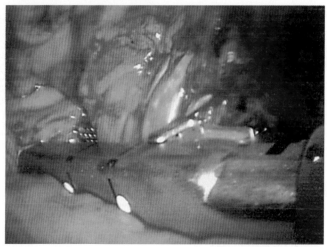

Figure 18-2 Left superior pulmonary vein, just prior to division with stapler.

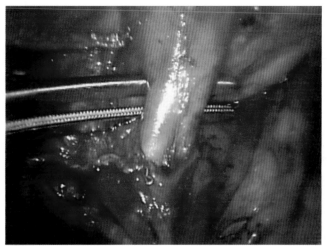

Figure 18-3 Apical anterior branches of left pulmonary artery.

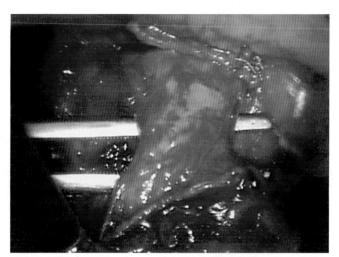

Figure 18-4 Left upper lobe bronchus, encircled with a curved clamp.

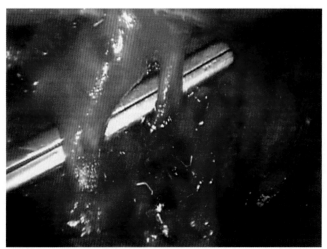

Figure 18-5 Posterior and lingular branches of left pulmonary artery.

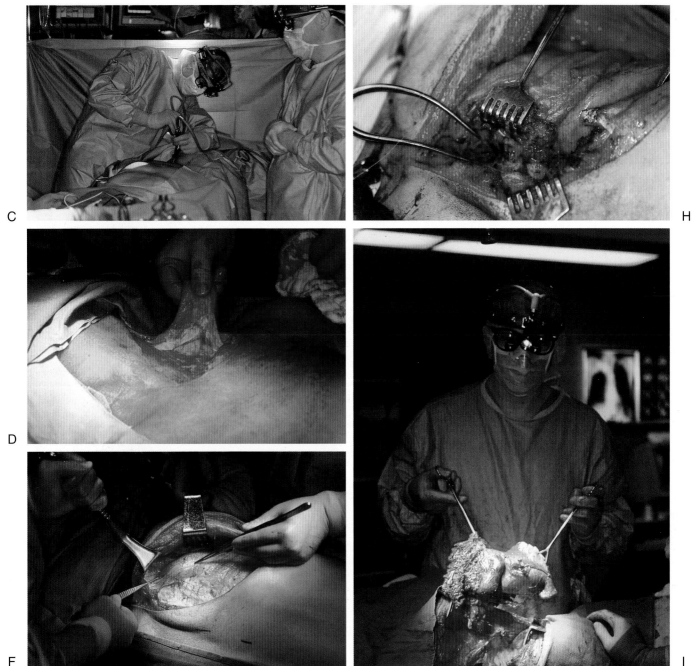

Figure 20-2 C, A mediastinoscopy is performed routinely to rule out N_2 or N_3 nodal involvement before proceeding with the extensive lung and chest wall resection. **D,** An initial supraclavicular neck dissection is performed to dissect the subclavian vessels and brachial plexus. This is the initial hockey-stick skin incision along the anterior border of the sternocleidomastoid muscle and along the clavicle. **F,** The patient is repositioned. The initial dissection is through a posterolateral thoracotomy with elevation of the scapula after division of the latissimus dorsi muscle and reflection of the serratus anterior muscle. The tumor bulge into the interspaces of the chest wall can be appreciated. There is no gross tumor involvement of the external surface of the chest wall, however. **H,** The posterior elevation of the paraspinous muscles and disarticulation of the posterior ribs from the transverse processes and vertebral bodies. **I,** Complete en bloc removal of the chest wall (ribs one to five) and the right upper lobe.

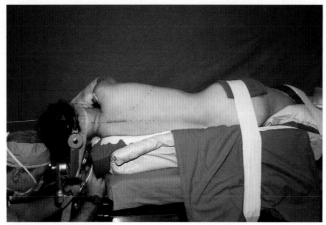

Figure 20-4 B, Operative positioning of the patient with the head in cervical tongs to immobilize it and to maintain the alignment of the cervical and thoracic spines. The patient is additionally secured on a beanbag and taped with the appropriate padding of the anterior superior iliac spine.

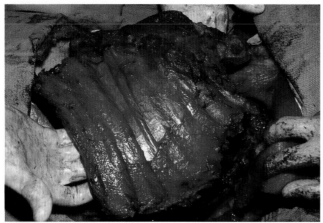

Figure 20-5 C, Operative photo demonstrating extensive chest wall resection of seven ribs with en bloc left upper lobe attached.

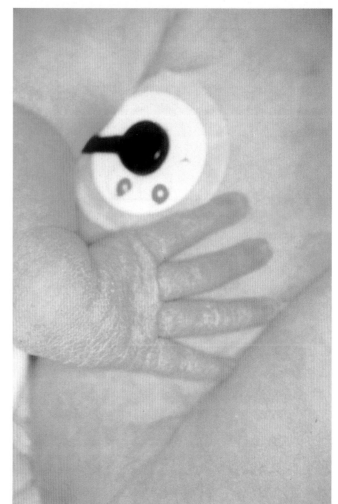

Figure 34-2 Radial aplasia, one component of the VATER association.
(Courtesy of Dr. R. Ricketts, Emory University Medical Center.)

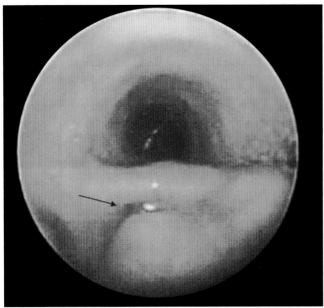

Figure 34-7 Bronchoscopic appearance of a tracheoesophageal fistula in the membranous portion of the trachea proximal to the carina.

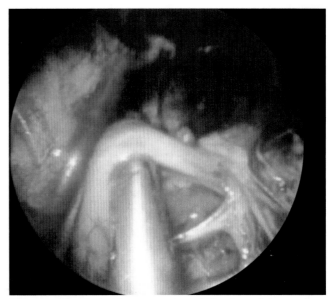

Figure 34-11 A, Thoracoscopic mobilization of the tracheoesophageal fistula.
(Courtesy of Dr. C. Albanese, Stanford University Medical Center.)

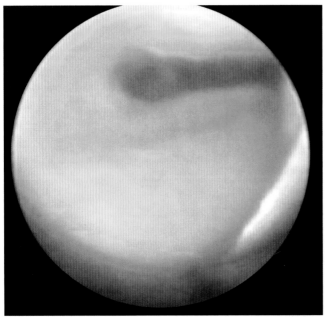

Figure 34-12 A, Bronchoscopic appearance of tracheomalacia in a patient with esophageal atresia with tracheoesophageal fistula. Note that the anterior and posterior walls of the trachea are almost touching.
(Courtesy of Dr. D. Powell, Children's National Medical Center.)

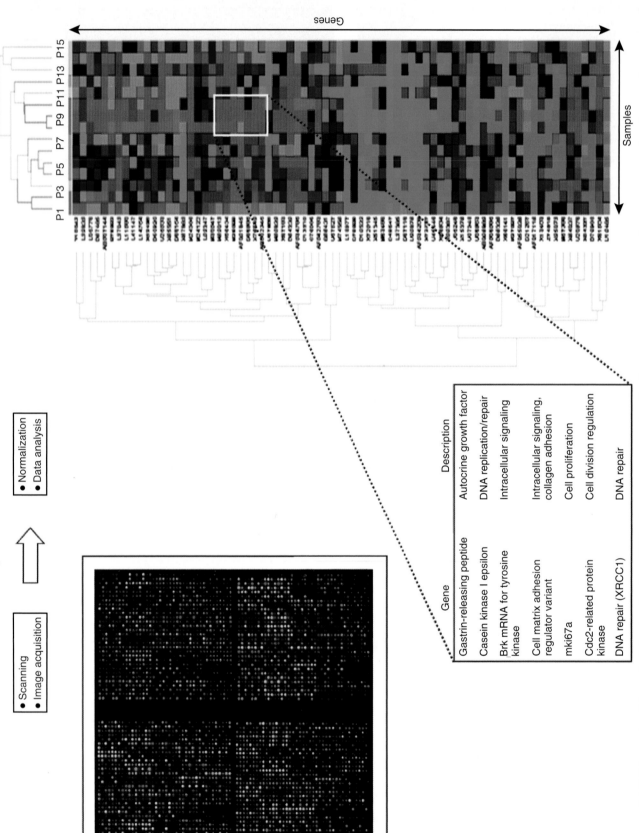

| Scanning | Normalization |
| Image acquisition | Data analysis |

Gene	Description
Gastrin-releasing peptide	Autocrine growth factor
Casein kinase I epsilon	DNA replication/repair
Brk mRNA for tyrosine kinase	Intracellular signaling
Cell matrix adhesion regulator variant	Intracellular signaling, collagen adhesion
mki67a	Cell proliferation
Cdc2-related protein kinase	Cell division regulation
DNA repair (XRCC1)	DNA repair

Figure 44-3 Schematic of the principles involved in cDNA microarray processing. B, The main steps in microarray data acquisition and analysis are shown. For cDNA microarrays, dual-channel fluorescence for each gene spotted onto the microarray is detected by a confocal scanning microscope. Computer software merges and converts this data into a graphical image. Gene expression data are analyzed with sophisticated algorithms. Shown is an example of a two-dimensional hierarchical cluster analysis. Gene expression ratios are color coded (red, overexpression; green, underexpression; and black, no change) to reflect relative mRNA transcript abundance. Further details are provided in the text.

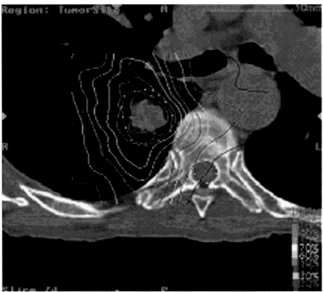

Figure 45-7 Radiation plan generated with CyberKnife radiation delivery system with radiation doses superimposed on the image of the tumor.

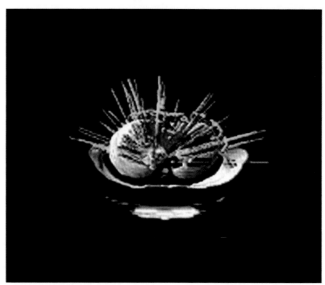

Figure 45-8 Radiation paths used to administer the radiation plan.

Figure 46-1 The heart is shown as seen by the surgeon through a median sternotomy. The pericardial cavity has been opened and is between the fibrous pericardium and the epicardium. The "compass" shows the orientation.
(Copyright in the original illustration from which this figure was prepared belongs to Robert H. Anderson, Benson R. Wilcox, and Andrew C. Cook.)

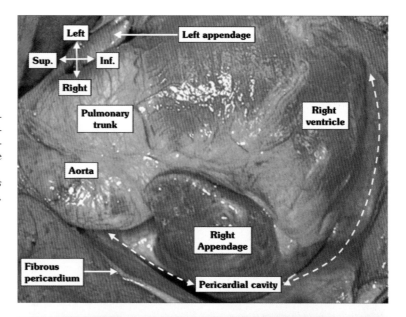

Figure 46-2 With the pericardium opened in the operating room, the surgical clamp has been passed through the transverse sinus of the pericardium, which is between the back of the arterial trunks and the front of the atrial chambers.
(Copyright in the original illustration from which this figure was prepared belongs to Robert H. Anderson, Benson R. Wilcox, and Andrew C. Cook.)

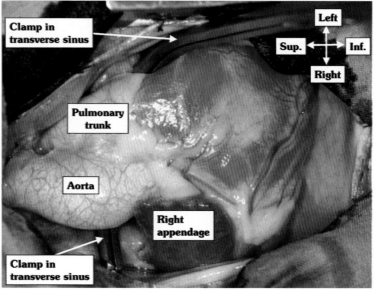

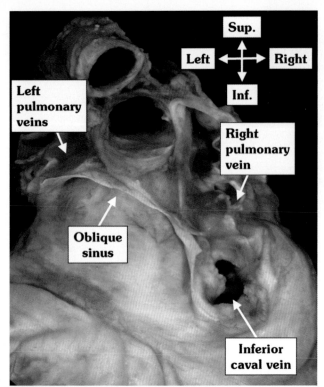

Figure 46-3 This anatomical specimen has been removed from the body and is viewed from behind, with the apex pointing down. The oblique sinus of the pericardium is seen between the pericardial reflections around the pulmonary veins and the inferior caval vein. *(Copyright in the original illustration from which this figure was prepared belongs to Robert H. Anderson, Benson R. Wilcox, and Andrew C. Cook.)*

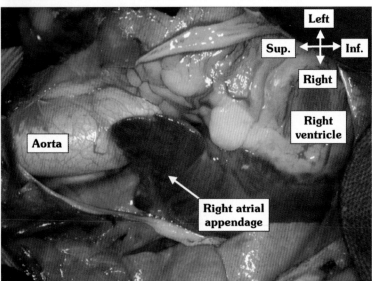

Figure 46-4 This picture of the heart, as seen in the operating room through a median sternotomy, shows the typical triangular appearance of the morphologically right atrial appendage. *(Copyright in the original illustration from which this figure was prepared belongs to Robert H. Anderson, Benson R. Wilcox, and Andrew C. Cook.)*

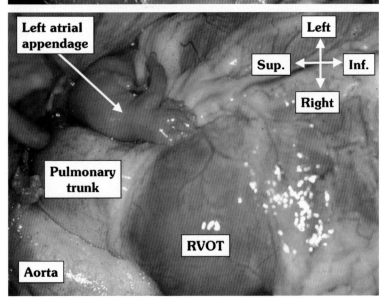

Figure 46-5 In this picture, with the pericardium opened through a median sternotomy, the heart has been rotated slightly to show the typical tubular configuration of the morphologically left atrial appendage. RVOT, right ventricular outflow tract. *(Copyright in the original illustration from which this figure was prepared belongs to Robert H. Anderson, Benson R. Wilcox, and Andrew C. Cook.)*

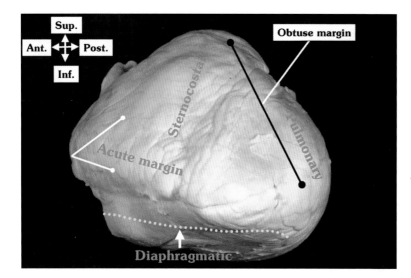

Figure 46-7 This heart has been removed from the thorax, and is viewed from the apex, looking toward the base of the ventricular mass. It shows the surfaces of the ventricular mass and the locations of the acute and obtuse margins.
(Copyright in the original illustration from which this figure was prepared belongs to Robert H. Anderson, Benson R. Wilcox, and Andrew C. Cook.)

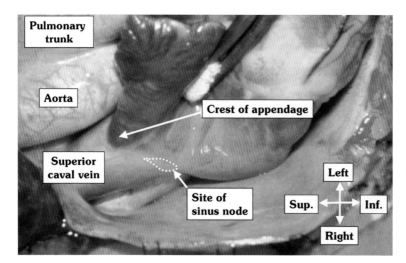

Figure 46-8 In this picture, taken in the operating room, the surgeon has reflected the atrial appendage to show the location of the terminal groove and the crest of the appendage. Note the site of the sinus node, which is shown by the *dotted lines.*
(Copyright in the original illustration from which this figure was prepared belongs to Robert H. Anderson, Benson R. Wilcox, and Andrew C. Cook.)

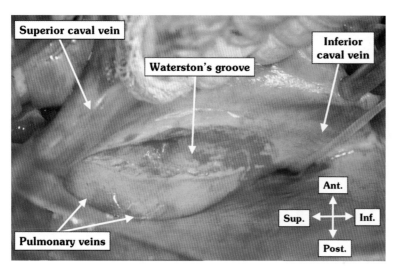

Figure 46-9 In this picture, showing the view through a median sternotomy, the surgeon has incised through the epicardium covering Waterston's groove, showing the base of the deep fold between the systemic venous tributaries and the right pulmonary veins.
(Copyright in the original illustration from which this figure was prepared belongs to Robert H. Anderson, Benson R. Wilcox, and Andrew C. Cook.)

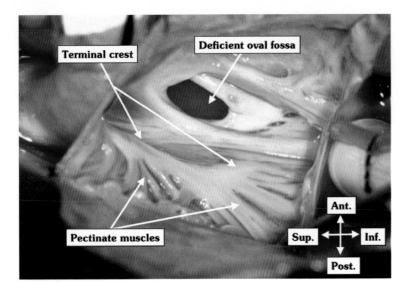

Figure 46-10 Opening the right atrial appendage in this patient with a defect within the oval fossa reveals the markedly different configuration of the endocardial surfaces of the pectinated appendage as opposed to the smooth-walled systemic venous sinus. The pectinate muscles originate from the terminal crest, marked externally by the terminal groove (see Figure 46-7).
(Copyright in the original illustration from which this figure was prepared belongs to Robert H. Anderson, Benson R. Wilcox, and Andrew C. Cook.)

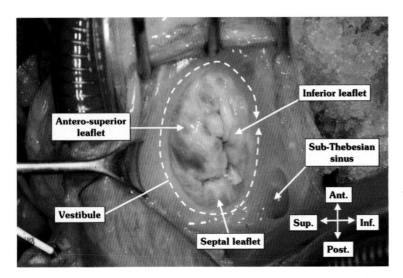

Figure 46-11 The right atrium has been opened to show the smooth vestibule of the tricuspid valve. Note that the three leaflets of the valve are positioned septally, anterosuperiorly, and inferiorly. Note also the extensive subthebesian sinus, often described as subeustachian when the heart is viewed in attitudinally incorrect fashion.
(Copyright in the original illustration from which this figure was prepared belongs to Robert H. Anderson, Benson R. Wilcox, and Andrew C. Cook.)

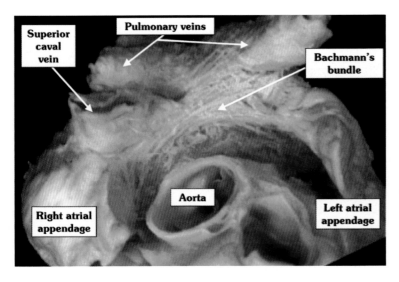

Figure 46-12 The heart has been photographed from in front, having removed the epicardium from the surface of the anterosuperior interatrial groove. Note the broad sweep of parallel fibers that extend from the crest of the atrial appendage in front of the superior caval vein toward the left atrial appendage. This is Bachmann's bundle.
(Copyright in the original illustration from which this figure was prepared belongs to Robert H. Anderson, Benson R. Wilcox, and Andrew C. Cook.)

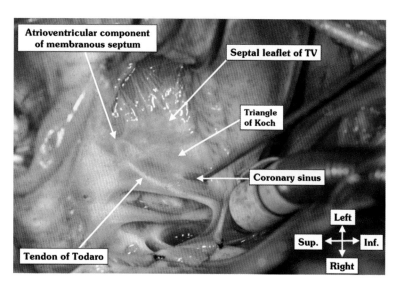

Figure 46-14 The right atrium has been opened via a median sternotomy to show the landmarks of the triangle of Koch. In this patient, the continuation of the eustachian valve through the tendon of Todaro is clearly seen, with the tendon inserting into the atrioventricular component of the central fibrous body.
(Copyright in the original illustration from which this figure was prepared belongs to Robert H. Anderson, Benson R. Wilcox, and Andrew C. Cook.)

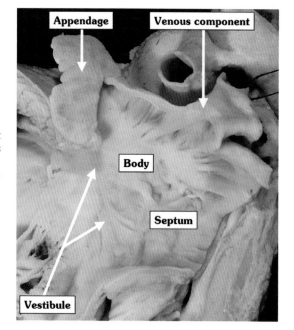

Figure 46-16 The morphological left atrium is photographed from its left side to show the component parts. Note the extensive body, which also receives the septal aspect of the chamber.
(Copyright in the original illustration from which this figure was prepared belongs to Robert H. Anderson, Benson R. Wilcox, and Andrew C. Cook.)

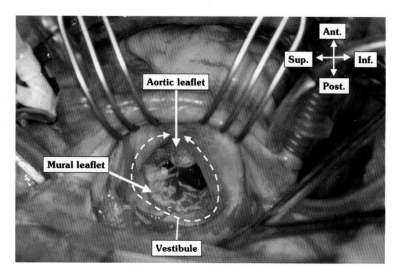

Figure 46-17 The left atrium is photographed in the operating room through an incision made in the dome. Note the vestibule of the mitral valve, which has aortic and mural leaflets.
(Copyright in the original illustration from which this figure was prepared belongs to Robert H. Anderson, Benson R. Wilcox, and Andrew C. Cook.)

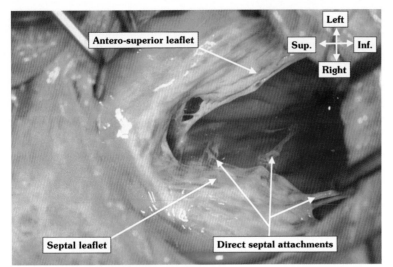

Figure 46-19 The tricuspid valve is seen through the right atrium in the operating room. Note the tendinous cords that attach the septal leaflet directly to the septum. This is the most characteristic morphologic feature of the tricuspid valve.
(Copyright in the original illustration from which this figure was prepared belongs to Robert H. Anderson, Benson R. Wilcox, and Andrew C. Cook.)

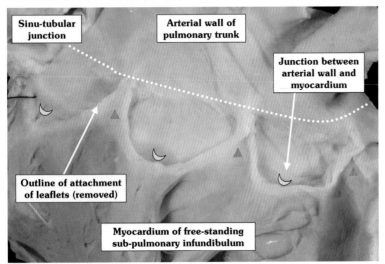

Figure 46-20 The pulmonary outflow tract has been opened and the leaflets of the pulmonary valve removed, showing their initial semilunar attachment. Note that the most distal attachment is to the sinotubular junction *(dotted line)*, and proximally, the hinge point incorporates right ventricular musculature into the base of each pulmonary valvar sinus *(gray crescents)*. Fibrous triangles made up of the wall of the pulmonary trunk *(red triangles)* are incorporated within the ventricular outflow tract.
(Copyright in the original illustration from which this figure was prepared belongs to Robert H. Anderson, Benson R. Wilcox, and Andrew C. Cook.)

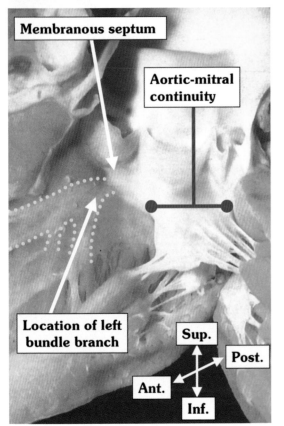

Figure 46-26 The specimen is opened through the left ventricular outflow tract, showing the relationship of the left bundle branch to the membranous septum and the aortic root. Note also the region of aortic to mitral valvar fibrous continuity.
(Copyright in the original illustration from which this figure was prepared belongs to Robert H. Anderson, Benson R. Wilcox, and Andrew C. Cook.)

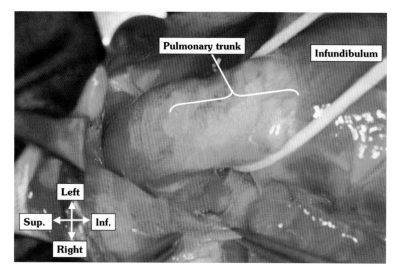

Figure 46-29 This view of the heart through a median sternotomy shows the extent of the pulmonary trunk, the surgeon having encircled the trunk with a tape. Note the circular ventriculoarterial junction.
(Copyright in the original illustration from which this figure was prepared belongs to Robert H. Anderson, Benson R. Wilcox, and Andrew C. Cook.)

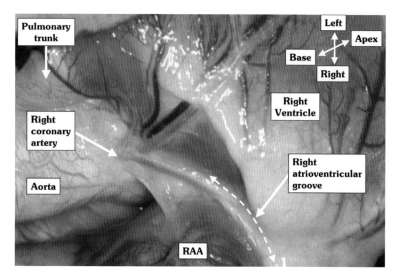

Figure 46-32 This picture, taken in the operating room through a median sternotomy, shows the aortic origin of the right coronary artery.
(Copyright in the original illustration from which this figure was prepared belongs to Robert H. Anderson, Benson R. Wilcox, and Andrew C. Cook.)

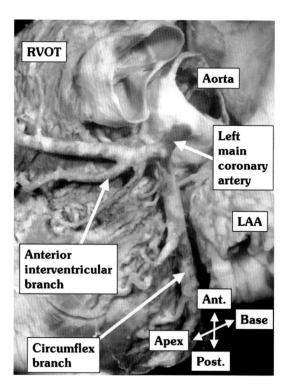

Figure 46-34 This dissection, with the heart positioned in anatomical position and photographed from the left side, shows the branches of the main stem of the left coronary artery. RVOT, right ventricular outflow tract; LAA, left atrial appendage.
(Copyright in the original illustration from which this figure was prepared belongs to Robert H. Anderson, Benson R. Wilcox, and Andrew C. Cook.)

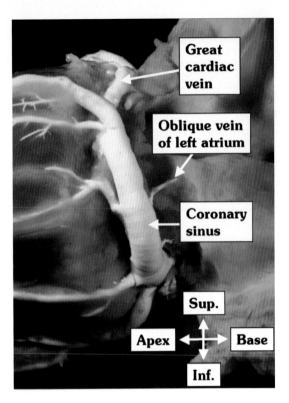

Figure 46-36 This specimen has been prepared by filling the coronary sinus with Silastic. The heart is positioned to show its diaphragmatic aspect. The coronary sinus is formed at the union of the great cardiac vein with the oblique vein of the left atrium.
(Copyright in the original illustration from which this figure was prepared belongs to Robert H. Anderson, Benson R. Wilcox, and Andrew C. Cook.)

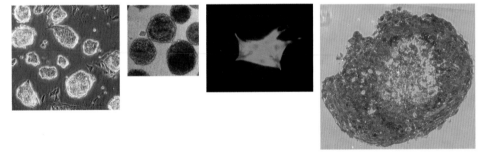

Figure 51-5 The bioreactor mediated generation of purified cardiac cells from embryonic stem cells. Embryonic stem cells are transduced with an appropriate selection cassette and grown in scalable stirred suspension bioreactors as embryoid bodies. Once cardiac commitment has begun, a selectable agent is added to the bioreactor to eliminate noncardiac cells. After selection, the purified cardiac cells can be used in tissue engineering or cardiac transplantation studies.

Sabiston & Spencer Surgery of the Chest

Thoracic

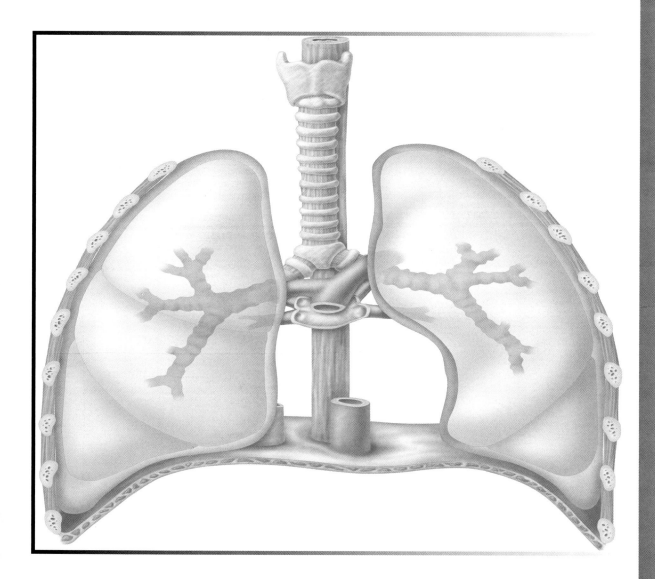

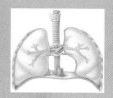

Evaluation and Care

Anatomy of the Thorax

Rohit Shahani

▶ INTRODUCTION

The thorax is the upper part of the trunk, bounded by the 12 thoracic vertebrae, ribs, and sternum (thorax = breastplate in Greek). The presence of the rib cage distinguishes the thorax, and in air-breathing mammals its primary function is respiratory. The mediastinum with the heart and great vessels partitions the thoracic cavity and separates the two pleural cavities. The trachea and esophagus gain access to the thorax through the narrow superior thoracic aperture. The inferior aperture is wide and irregular and is separated from the abdominal viscera by the diaphragm.

▶ THORACIC APERTURES

The bony thorax has two apertures or openings: the superior thoracic aperture, often referred to as the thoracic inlet, and the inferior thoracic aperture (Figure 1-1). The head and neck and the upper limbs communicate with the thoracic cavity through the thoracic inlet. This aperture is limited by the body of the first thoracic vertebra posteriorly, the first pair of ribs and their costal cartilages anterolaterally, and the superior end of the manubrium sternum anteriorly. Though this kidney-shaped opening is relatively small (about 5 cm anteroposteriorly and 11 cm transversely), important structures pass through it. The trachea and esophagus fill the midline space while the great arteries and veins that supply and drain the head, neck, and upper extremities fill the space laterally. The main muscles of this region are the sternocleidomastoid and scalene muscles, and the main nerves include the brachial plexus while the phrenic and vagus nerves also pass through this aperture.

As the margin of the aperture slopes inferoanteriorly, the apex of each lung and its covering pleura (pleural cupola) projects superiorly through the lateral parts of the thoracic inlet and is covered by a piece of cervical fascia, the suprapleural membrane (Sibson's fascia).

The inferior thoracic aperture separates the thoracic cavity from the abdominal cavity by the musculotendinous thoracic diaphragm. The inferior thoracic aperture, which slopes inferoposteriorly, is limited by the twelfth thoracic vertebra posteriorly, the twelfth pair of ribs and costal margins anterolaterally, and the xiphisternal joint anteriorly. The thoracic outlet is uneven and much larger than the superior thoracic aperture and most structures that pass through it go through openings in the diaphragm.

The inferior vena cava penetrates the diaphragm somewhat anteriorly and to the right of the midline, within the region of the central tendon, at the level of T8 vertebra. The right phrenic nerve often goes through the same diaphragmatic opening while the left phrenic nerve penetrates the muscular region of the diaphragm, at the level of T8 laterally through its own specific aperture. The esophageal aperture is at the level of vertebra T10 and the right and left vagal trunks that adhere to it enter the abdomen along with the esophagus.

The aortic aperture at the T12 vertebral level is formed by the interdigitating fibers (median arcuate ligament) of the right and left diaphragmatic crurae. The azygos and hemiazygos veins and the thoracic duct also pass through this opening.

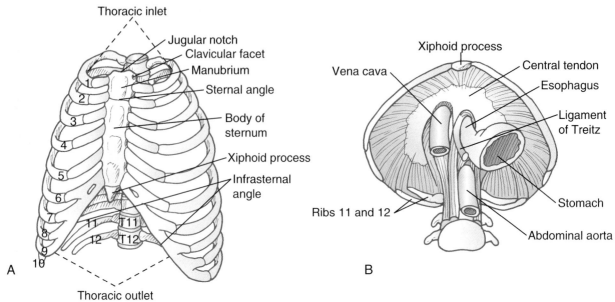

Figure 1–1 Bony thorax and its boundaries. A, Anterior view of the rib cage and prominent surface structures. **B,** Inferior view showing the inferior thoracic aperture and the openings in the diaphragm.

The greater and lesser splanchnic nerves gain access to the abdominal cavity via two small apertures within each of the crura, and musculophrenic branches of the internal mammary artery penetrate the diaphragm through small apertures near its connection with the costal cartilages of ribs 7–9.

▶ SURFACE ANATOMY

An understanding of surface anatomy enables identification of bony and prominent structures and hence the position of deeply related structures. The chest radiograph is an extension of the routine physical examination (Figure 1-2).

The midline sternum is entirely subcutaneous and is made up of the manubrium, the body, and the xiphisternum from above downward. The suprasternal notch on the superior aspect of the manubrium is palpable between the prominent medial ends of the clavicle and it lies opposite the lower border of the body of the second thoracic vertebra. The sternal angle of Louis forms an important landmark for the description of structures inside the chest and is the junction of the manubrium with the body of the sternum. At this level the

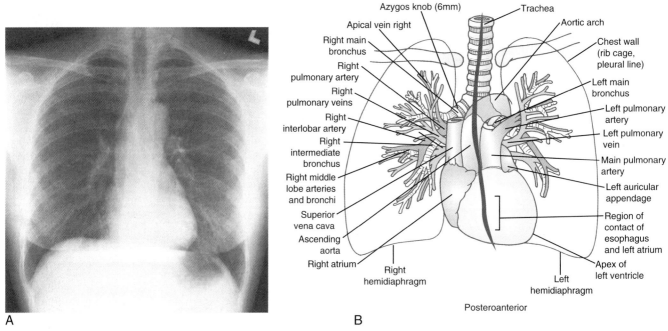

Figure 1–2 A, Chest Radiograph. Posteroanterior radiograph of the chest in a normal adult male. Surface projection of intrathoracic structures (schematic) on a normal chest X-ray. **B,** Schematic representation of the surface projection of intrathoracic structures seen on a normal chest X-ray.
(From Butler P, Mitchell AWM, and Ellis H: Applied Radiological Anatomy. Cambridge University Press, 1999.)

second costal cartilage joins the lateral margin of the sternum. The sternal angle lies opposite the lower border of the fourth thoracic vertebral body. All other ribs are counted from this point, as the first rib is not palpable. The xiphisternum is covered by the rectus abdominus muscles and is less easily palpable and can be of variable length. The xiphisternal joint lies opposite the body of the ninth thoracic vertebra.

The clavicle is entirely subcutaneous and laterally it articulates with the acromion process of the scapula. The costal margin is the lower boundary of the bony thorax and is formed by the cartilages of the seventh, eighth, ninth, and tenth ribs and the ends of the eleventh and twelfth cartilages. The lowest part of the margin is the tenth rib and it lies at the level of the third lumbar vertebra. The lower border of the pectoralis major muscle forms the anterior axillary fold. The tendon of the latissimus dorsi forms the posterior axillary fold as it passes around the lower border of the teres major muscle.

Posteriorly the thoracic cage is covered by muscles (trapezius, latissimus dorsi, and erector spinae) and is obscured by the scapula, but there are a few useful landmarks to the rib levels. The superior angle of the scapula lies opposite the spine of the second thoracic vertebra. The transversely running spine of the scapula is easily felt and lies at the level of the third thoracic vertebra. The lower angle of the scapula overlies the seventh rib.

The first prominent spinous process in the low midline of the neck posteriorly is that of the seventh cervical vertebra, the vertebrae prominens. The tip of a spinous process of a thoracic vertebra lies posterior to the body of the next vertebra below.

The apex of the pleura extends about 3 cm above the medial third of the clavicle and then passes downward and medially behind the sternoclavicular joints. The left pleura, at the level of the fourth costal cartilage, deviates laterally for a variable distance from the cardiac notch. Both pleurae lie at the level of the eighth rib in the midclavicular line, at the level of the tenth rib in the mid-axillary line and at the level of the twelfth rib at the paravertebral level posteriorly.

The lower border of the lung has an excursion of 5–8 cm in the extremes of respiration but in the neutral position it lies about two rib breadths above the corresponding lower border of the parietal pleura, thus creating the lateral recesses.

The more constant right oblique fissure of the lung follows the course of the fifth rib from the midline posteriorly, more toward its lower border. Anteriorly it ends at the costochondral junction at the level of the sixth rib. The left oblique fissure has a more variable origin from the third to the fifth rib level, however, anteriorly it follows a more predictable course along the fifth rib.

The transverse or horizontal fissure presents only on the right side is marked by a horizontal line that runs backward from the fourth costal cartilage to reach the oblique fissure at the mid-axillary line at the level of the fifth rib.

The trachea extends from the lower border of the cricoid cartilage in the neck to the level of the sternal angle in the chest. It is easily palpable at the suprasternal notch

▶ THE STERNUM

The sternum or breastbone is made of cancellous bone and filled with hemopoietic marrow throughout life. The main

parts, the manubrium and body, are connected by a secondary cartilaginous joint that normally never ossifies and contributes to movement of the ribs.

Up to puberty the six segments, or sternebrae, are held together by hyaline cartilage. The central four fuse to form the body of the sternum between 14 and 21 years of age. Superiorly the manubrium sterni and inferiorly the xiphoid process remain separate.

The manubrium receives the sternal ends of the clavicles in a shallow concave facet. The widest portion of the manubrium has bilateral costal incisurae that articulate with the first costal cartilage to form a primary cartilaginous joint. The second costal cartilage articulates with both the lower lateral ends of the manubrium and the body of the sternum, forming separate synovial joints. The muscular attachments of the manubrium include the sternocleidomastoid muscle, the sternohyoid and the sternothyroid superiorly, and anterolaterally the pectoralis major muscle. Most of the posterior surface is bare bone and may be in contact with the brachiocephalic vein, unless thymic remnants lie between.

The gladiolus, or body of the sternum, is slanted at a steeper angle than the manubrium; hence its articulation with that bone forms an angle called the sternal angle. Ossification of this joint, synchrondrosis, in adult life may limit the normal movement at this joint. The articular facets for ribs two to seven lie along the lateral border of the body of the sternum. These make single synovial joints with the costal cartilages. The facets for the sixth and seventh costal cartilages may coalesce especially in the female. The lateral border gives attachment to the anterior intercostal membrane and the internal intercostal muscles while the pectoralis major arises anteriorly. Weak sternopericardial ligaments pass into the fibrous pericardium.

The cartilaginous xiphoid may be bifid or perforated, of variable length, and usually ossifies in the fourth decade. The costoxiphoid ligaments prevent its displacement during diaphragmatic contractions.

▶ THE RIBS

The 12 pairs of ribs are divided into the upper seven, which that are called true ribs or vertebrosternal ribs because they form complete loops between the vertebrae and the sternum, and the lower five ribs, which fail to reach the sternum and are considered false ribs. The eighth, ninth, and tenth ribs are called vertebrocostal because each of their costal cartilages articulates with the adjacent rib cartilage. Ribs 11 and 12 are free floating or vertebral ribs because their only articulation is with their vertebrae.

Ribs 3–9 are classified as typical ribs and have a head, neck, and a shaft. The head has an upper and a lower articular facet divided by a crest for articulation with two adjacent vertebrae in synovial costovertebral joints, the lower facet articulating with the upper border of its own vertebra. The neck is flattened, with the upper border curling up into a prominent ridge, the crest. A tubercle projects posteriorly from the end of the neck and marks the junction of the neck and the body (Figure 1-3).

The medial facet on the tubercle is covered with hyaline cartilage and makes a synovial joint with the transverse process of its own vertebra. The lateral facet receives the costotransverse ligament from the tip of its own transverse

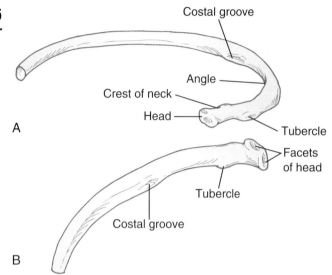

A

B

Figure 1–3 A typical right rib, as viewed from (A) the macposterior aspect and (B) the inner aspect of the rib.

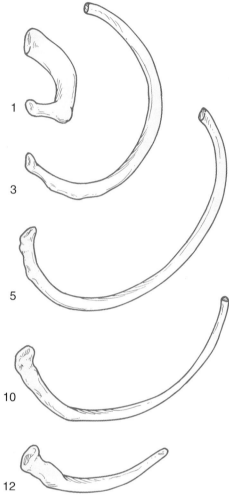

Figure 1–4 The atypical (right) ribs as seen from the superior aspect.

process. The shaft slopes downward and laterally for about 5–8 cm to an angle and then curves forward. Lateral to the angle, the lower border projects down as a sharp ridge sheltering a costal groove. The angles of the ribs also correspond to the lateral extent of the erector spinae muscles of the back. The upper six ribs are bent into a tight curve so that the shaft has turned parallel with the neck of the rib. The lower six ribs have an opening out of the curve, which is completed by the long costal cartilages at the front of the chest. The fused cartilages of ribs 7–10 course diagonally upward to the lower end of the sternum to form the sub-costal angle. The anterior ends of the ribs have a concave fossa that is plugged by the costal cartilage in an immovable primary cartilaginous joint.

The first rib is exceptionally broad and short and most highly curved. The head is small and has a single facet for the synovial joint it makes with the upper part of the body of the T1 vertebra. The prominent tubercle is a fusion of the tubercle and the angle and its medial facet forms a synovial joint with the first transverse process. The lateral prominent part of the tubercle receives the lateral costotransverse ligament and the costalis and longissimus parts of the erector spinae. Near the middle of the shaft, the sulci for the subclavian vessels are identified by the scalene tubercle, a spur that attaches the scalenus anterior muscle.

The second rib is larger than the first rib and its head has the typical two facets for articulation with the adjacent vertebrae. It is distinguished by the tuberosity of the serratus anterior muscle and a smaller more posterior "bump" for the attachment of the scalenus posterior. The costal groove is present but poorly developed.

Usually the heads of the tenth, eleventh, and twelfth ribs bear only one articular facet for their corresponding vertebrae. Ribs 11 and 12 have absent necks, angles, and costal grooves and do not articulate with their transverse processes (Figure 1-4).

Variations in human rib structure can be clinically significant. The incidence of cervical rib is between 0.5 and 1%. Occasionally the eighth rib may reach the sternum on one or

both sides. A lumbar rib has no clinical significance except that identification of vertebral levels may be inaccurate when counting ribs from below. An absent or small and non-palpable twelfth rib can cause the same confusion.

Knowledge of the basic anatomy of the ribs, costovertebral joints (between the head of the rib and the vertebral body), and costotransverse joints (between the tubercle and the transverse process) is a prerequisite to understanding the two types of respiratory movements. Thoracic dimensions enlarge in all dimensions during inspiration.

In the lower ribs the tubercular facets and the articular facets of their transverse processes are flat; hence movement here only causes the tubercle to ride up and down rather than roll. The axis of this passes through the joint of the rib head and the appropriate sternocostal or intercostal joint. Because of the angulation of the ribs, seen predominantly in ribs 7–10, elevation causes each unit to move upward and laterally, akin to lifting a bucket handle. This increase in transverse diameter is best appreciated by placing the hands on the sides of the lower chest.

The forward and upward movement of the sternum is known as the pump handle movement. The tubercle of the rib rolls downward in the fixed, deep, cup-shaped synovial joint, the axis of which is along a line drawn through the head, neck, and tubercle of each rib. Most of the movement

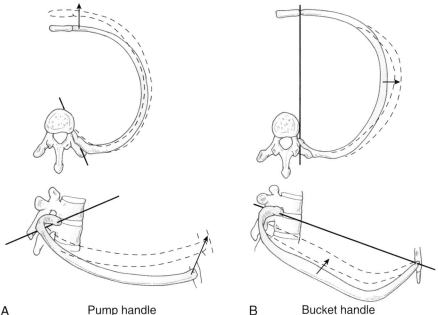

Figure 1–5 Respiratory movements. Pump handle (**A**) and bucket handle (**B**). The dotted lines represent inspiration and the solid line indicates the axes of movements.

A   Pump handle   B   Bucket handle

occurs in the upper ribs, with maximum movement occurring at the level of the longest ribs 5–7. There is no movement over the back where the relatively fixed rib neck is allowed to roll only (Figure 1-5).

MUSCLES OF THE THORACIC WALL

As in other regions of the trunk, during development the thoracic myotomes split into epimeres and hypomeres. The deep back muscles are derived from the epimeres (dorsal part of the myotome). The hypomeres give rise to the anterolateral muscles of the body wall, namely, the intercostals and abdominal muscles. An intermediate group, developmentally related to the anterolateral muscles of the trunk, includes the serratus posterior superior and the serratus posterior inferior muscles. By definition, hypomeric muscles are innervated by the primary ventral ramus of a spinal nerve. The appendicular muscles of the thoracic wall develop from migrating somatic myoblasts (Box 1-1 and Table 1-1).

Each hypomere on each side splits into four major parts, three anterolateral muscular sheets and one anteromedial component, the rectus abdominus. A thoracic rectus muscle also known as the sternalis usually does not persist and is present in only 0.5% of individuals. The remainder of the hypomere forms the intercostal muscles.

INTERCOSTAL MUSCLES

Fibers of the intercostalis externi muscle arise from the sharp lower border of the rib above and course inferomedially (i.e., the direction of the fingers when the hands are put into the front pocket of one's trousers) to the smooth upper border of the rib below. Anteriorly it is replaced by the anterior intercostal membrane. Between the bony ribs is muscle; between the costal cartilages is membrane. In the lower

Box 1–1. Appendicular Muscles.

Trapezius
Levator scapula
Rhomboid major and minor
Teres major and minor
Deltoid
Supraspinatus
Infraspinatus
Subscapularis
Latissimus dorsi
Serratus anterior
Pectoralis major and minor

spaces the muscle interdigitates with the fibers of the external oblique (Figure 1-6).

The intercostalis interni muscle runs from the lower costal groove of ribs 1–11 to the upper surfaces of ribs 2–12 downward and backward. Anteriorly they extend up to the sternum but posteriorly only up to the angles of the rib. Beyond that they are replaced by the internal intercostal membrane, which attaches to the tubercle of each rib and vertebra.

The innermost or transverses layer is broken up into three groups: the innermost intercostals (anterolateral), subcostal (posterior), and transversus thoracis (anteromedial) muscles.

The fibers run downward and backward, similar to the internal intercostal muscles. The subcostal muscles lie in the paravertebral gutter, are better developed inferiorly, and cross more than one space.

The transversus thoracis was formally called the sternocostalis, a more appropriate name. Digitations arise from the sternum bilaterally to the costal cartilages of ribs 2–6.

The intercostalis intimi muscles also traverse more than one space and are better developed in the lower lateral spaces.

Table 1–1

Attachments and Innervation of the Muscles of the Thoracic Wall

Muscle	*Proximal attachments*	*Distal attachments*	*Innervation*
Pectoralis major sternocostal head	Half of sternum, costal cartilages 1–6, aponeurosis of external obliquus muscle	Lateral lip of intertubercular sulcus of humerus	Medial pectoral nerve (C8–T1)
Pectoralis major clavicular head	Medial half of clavicle	Lateral lip of intertubercular sulcus of humerus	Lateral pectoral nerve (C5, 6, 7)
Pectoralis minor	Ribs 3–5	Coracoid process of scapula	Medial pectoral nerve
Subclavius	First rib	Medial clavicle	Nerve to subclavius (C5–6)
Deltoid	Lateral third of clavicle, acromion, and spine of scapula	Deltoid tuberosity of humerus	Axillary nerve (C5–6)
Serratus anterior	Angles of superior 10 ribs	Medial border of scapula	Long thoracic muscle nerve (C5, 6, 7)
Supraspinatus	Supraspinous fossa of the scapula, fascia of trapezius	Greater tubercle of the humerus	Suprascapular nerve (C5)
Infraspinatus	Infraspinous fossa	Greater tubercle of the humerus	Suprascapular nerve
Subscapularis	Costal surface of the scapula	Lesser tubercle of the humerus and its crest	Upper (C5–6) and lower (C5, 6, 7) subscapular nerve
Latissimus dorsi	Spinous processes of T7–12, L1–5, S1–3 vertebrae, posterior part of iliac crest, lower 3–4 ribs	Crest of the lesser tubercle and floor of the intertubercular groove of the humerus	Thoracodorsal nerve (C6–7)
Serratus posterior inferior	Spines of C6–T2 vertebrae	Angles of ribs 2–5	Segmental intercostal nerves
Serratus posterior superior	Spine of T11–L2 vertebrae	Lower border of ribs 9–12	Segmental intercostal nerves
Trapezius	Ligamentum nuchae, external occipital protuberance, thoracic vertebral spinous processes	Lateral one third of clavicle, acromion process along spine of scapula	Spinal accessory nerve
Levator scapulae	Transverse process of C1, 2, 3, 4 cervical vertebrae	Medial border of scapula, superior angle to base of scapular spine	Dorsal scapular nerve (C5)
Rhomboid major and minor	Spinous processes of C7–T5 and supraspinous ligaments	Medial border of scapula up to the inferior angle	Dorsal scapular nerve (C5)
Teres major	Lower lateral border of the scapula	Crest of the lesser tubercle of the humerus	Lower subscapular nerve (C5, 6, 7)
Teres minor	Mid to upper lateral border of the scapula	Greater tubercle of the humerus	Axillary nerve (C5–6)

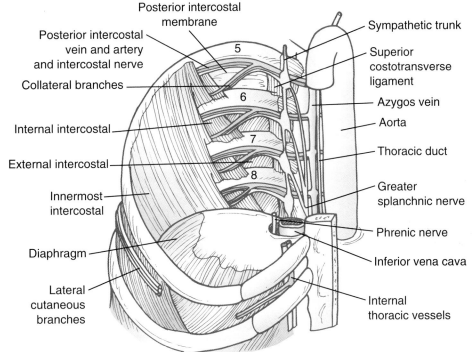

Figure 1–6 Spatial organization of the thoracic wall on the right side.

Posterior intercostal membrane

Posterior intercostal vein and artery and intercostal nerve

Collateral branches

Internal intercostal

External intercostal

Innermost intercostal

Diaphragm

Lateral cutaneous branches

Sympathetic trunk

Superior costotransverse ligament

Azygos vein

Aorta

Thoracic duct

Greater splanchnic nerve

Phrenic nerve

Inferior vena cava

Internal thoracic vessels

▶ **THE INTERCOSTAL SPACE: ORGANIZATION, NERVES, ARTERIES, AND VEINS**

The intercostal spaces between the ribs are filled by muscles of the three layers described above. In the plane between the innermost and outer two layers runs the neurovascular bundle. From above downward the order is vein, artery, and nerve (VAN). Beyond the angle of the rib posteriorly they are protected by the downward projection of the lower border of the rib. Hence for a thoracotomy, the periosteum is stripped off the upper half of the rib avoiding the lower border and the neurovascular bundle (Figure 1-7).

As in the rest of the body the mixed spinal nerve is formed from a dorsal and a ventral root, the dorsal root being sensory and the ventral root containing somatic motor neurons. As it emerges from the intervertebral foramina it branches into a dorsal and a ventral ramus. The dorsal ramus of the thoracic spinal nerve supplies the paravertebral back muscles and skin of the back. The ventral ramus communicates with the sympathetic chains via white rami communicantes (postganglionic fibers). Beyond this point, the true intercostal nerve lies just superficial to the parietal pleura within the endothoracic fascia. It gains the costal groove between the innermost intercostal and the internal intercostal muscles near the angle of the rib, where a collateral branch is given off. This small branch supplies the muscles of the space, the parietal pleura, and the periosteum of the rib. The main nerve itself has muscular branches, a lateral cutaneous branch, and a terminal anterior cutaneous branch. The lateral cutaneous branch given off along the mid-axillary line gives off anterior and posterior branches to supply the skin over that space. Just lateral to the sternal margin the terminal anterior cutaneous branches of the upper six nerves pierce the internal intercostal muscles, the external intercostal membrane, and the pectoralis major to reach skin. The lower five intercostal

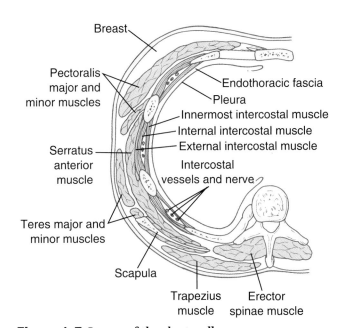

Breast

Pectoralis major and minor muscles

Serratus anterior muscle

Teres major and minor muscles

Scapula

Trapezius muscle

Erector spinae muscle

Endothoracic fascia

Pleura

Innermost intercostal muscle

Internal intercostal muscle

External intercostal muscle

Intercostal vessels and nerve

Figure 1–7 Layers of the chest wall.

nerves slope downward behind the costal margin into the neurovascular plane of the abdominal wall. The subcostal or twelfth thoracic nerve leaves the thorax by passing behind the lateral arcuate ligament, the subcostal artery, and vein (Figure 1-8). The cutaneous branches of each dermatome tend to overlap considerably; hence anesthesia after thoracic incisions is quite rare unless multiple intercostal nerves have been damaged. Note also that the first intercostal nerve is very small and supplies no skin, lacking both lateral and anterior cutaneous branches.

Two sets of intercostal arteries, the posterior and the anterior, are responsible for supplying the intercostal spaces.

10

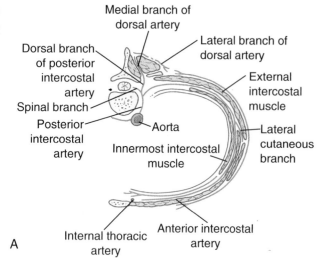

A

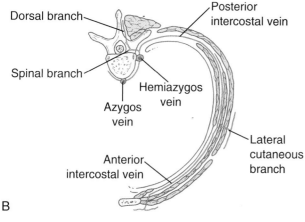

B

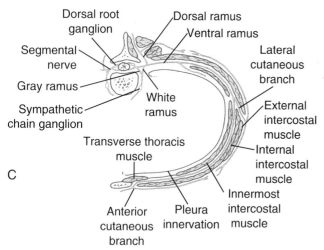

C

Figure 1–8 Organization of the intercostals space and the relationship of the arteries (A), veins (B), and nerves (C) to the muscle layers.

Their course and branching pattern closely conform to those of the intercostal nerves.

The posterior intercostal arteries are branches of the descending thoracic aorta except in the first two spaces where they are branches of the supreme intercostal artery, given off by the costocervical trunk of the second part of the

subclavian artery. The aortic branches lie on the left side of the mediastinum; consequently the right posterior intercostal arteries are longer, can be easily dissected in the left chest, and are seen best while operating on descending thoracic aortic aneurysms.

The roots of all 12 pairs of posterior intercostal arteries give rise to a dorsal branch that supplies the vertebrae, spinal cord, and deep muscles of the back. Similar to the nerve the intercostal artery gives off a collateral branch, the largest muscular branch that runs along the upper border of the rib below the space. After gaining the costal groove, near the mid-axillary line, it gives off the lateral cutaneous branch. The subcostal artery or the twelfth thoracic posterior intercostal artery follows a similar course but has no collateral branch.

The anterior intercostal arteries are branches of the internal thoracic arteries from the first part of the subclavian artery. The internal thoracic artery runs anterior to the transversus thoracis and on the internal surface of the costal cartilages and the internal intercostal muscles. About a finger's breadth from the border of the sternum running vertically downward it gives off two anterior intercostal arteries in each space. At the costal margin, below the sixth costal cartilage it divides into the superior epigastric and musculophrenic arteries.

The anterior intercostal arteries are smaller than the posterior intercostal arteries with which they anastomose and run predominantly along the lower border of each costal cartilage in the same fascial neurovascular plane. In the lower spaces they are branches of the musculophrenic artery. There are no true anterior intercostal arteries in the last two spaces.

The internal thoracic arteries also give branches to the mediastinum, the thymus, the pericardium, and the sternum, and especially large perforating branches in the second to fourth space, the predominant supply to the lactating breast in females.

In each space there is one posterior and two anterior intercostal veins, designated by names identical to the arteries that they accompany. They lie above the nerve and the artery throughout their course (VAN) in the intercostal space. The anterior veins drain into the musculophrenic and internal thoracic veins. The vein of the first space or the supreme intercostal vein, posteriorly, may be a tributary of the brachiocephalic, vertebral, or superior intercostal vein. The superior intercostal vein is formed by the posterior intercostal veins of the second, third, and sometimes the fourth spaces. This drains into the azygos vein on the right side and on the left side arches over the aorta, superficial to the vagus and deep to the phrenic to open into the left brachiocephalic veins. Subcostal veins join the ascending lumbar veins and ascend on the left side as the hemiazygos and on the right side as the azygos vein draining the lower eight spaces. The blood within the hemiazygos vein drains across the midline, through median anastomoses into the azygos vein.

The internal thoracic vessels are part of the anastomotic chain that links the subclavian artery and brachiocephalic veins to the external iliac vessels. The intercostal vessels in turn connect to the descending aorta and azygos system of veins. In the presence of obstruction to flow, these anastomoses provide alternative channels for arterial and venous blood flow.

LYMPHATIC DRAINAGE AND THORACIC DUCT

There are three upgoing lymph channels on each side of the thoracic cavity, and they freely communicate with each other. They are the right and left parasternal, and broncho-mediastinal trunks (alongside the trachea), the thoracic duct, and the right lymphatic duct.

The somatic paraaortic nodes extend laterally into the posterior intercostal spaces where they are known as the posterior intercostal nodes. Anteriorly the spaces drain into the parasternal nodes, also known as the internal mammary nodes. The anterior diaphragmatic nodes between the xiphisternum and pericardium are members of the parasternal group. The posterior diaphragmatic nodes are the lower thoracic paraaortic nodes. The middle diaphragmatic group lies on the dome of the diaphragm and on the right side drains the bare area of the liver. Upper intercostal spaces drain into the thoracic duct while the lower spaces are tributaries to the cisterna chyli via the descending intercostal trunk that passes through the aortic opening in the diaphragm.

Lymphatics of the superficial tissues of the thorax including the breast drain primarily into the axillary lymph nodes.

The thoracic duct is the upward continuation of the cisterna chyli at the level of the T12 vertebra. It enters the thorax through the aortic hiatus of the diaphragm and ascends in the posterior mediastinum on the vertebral bodies, lying between the aorta and the azygos vein. From behind the right crus it passes to the right of the aorta to lie against the right of the esophagus. It arches to the left around the T4 to T5 vertebrae behind the esophagus and leaves the thorax behind the left subclavian artery to join the left innominate vein, arching forward over the dome of the left pleura. There are many valves within the duct system except in its terminal inch or two. The thoracic duct receives tributaries from most of the lymph nodes in the mediastinum and ultimately from most of the body itself.

A corresponding trunk on the right side, the right lymphatic duct, drains the posterior right thoracic wall. The right subclavian trunk drains the right upper extremity while the right jugular lymph trunk drains the right side of the head and neck. These trunks may join together or open separately into the great veins on the right side, jugular, and subclavian.

Thus it can be seen that the thoracic duct drains all the lymph in the body except that from the right half of the thorax and the head and neck.

THORACIC ESOPHAGUS

Measured from the incisor teeth to the cardia of the stomach, the esophagus is 38–40 cm in men and generally 2 cm shorter in women. From the cricopharyngeus muscle to the cardia the range is 23–30 cm with an average of 25 cm. Hence the esophagus is predominantly a thoracic organ. Endoscopic examination reveals the cricopharyngeus at 15 cm, while the bifurcation of the trachea and the indentation of the aortic arch ranges between 24 and 26 cm from the incisor teeth. Avoiding interference from the aortic arch is the primary concern while choosing the side of the thoracotomy, left or right, and these useful landmarks serve as consistent reference points for the same.

Slightly to the left in the cervical portion, the esophagus enters the thoracic inlet in the midline in front of the body of the T1 vertebra and is intimately related to the posterior wall of the trachea up to its bifurcation. A notch indentation is often seen in its left lateral wall on a barium swallow radiograph as the esophagus passes to the right of the aorta at the level of the tracheal bifurcation. The left mainstem bronchus may indent it slightly as it passes over the esophagus. From there down it inclines forward and passes in front of the descending thoracic aorta and to its right side is in contact with the pericardium of the left atrium to pierce the diaphragm 1 inch to the left of the midline, opposite the body of the T10 vertebra. The fibers of the right crus surround the esophageal opening in a sling-like loop.

At the level of the T8 vertebra, the left lateral wall of the esophagus that was covered by the aorta is in contact with the parietal pleura as the aorta goes directly behind it and is a common site of perforation in Boerhaave's syndrome. The right lateral surface of the esophagus is completely covered by parietal pleura except where the vena azygos crosses it at the level of the T4 vertebra. The thoracic duct is intimately related to the esophagus as previously described.

The blood supply of the thoracic esophagus is from the esophageal branches of the aorta and the bronchial arteries. Most individuals have one right-sided and one or two left-sided bronchial arterial branches. The upper aortic esophageal branch usually is shorter and originates at the T6 or T7 vertebral level while the lower larger branch originates at the level of the eighth or ninth thoracic vertebrae.

The cervical esophagus is supplied by branches of the inferior thyroid artery, while the abdominal esophagus receives its supply from branches of the left gastric and inferior phrenic arteries.

Within the wall of the esophagus there is an extensive longitudinal anastomotic network in the muscular and submucosal layers, a basis for portasystemic anastomoses. The venous drainage follows the arterial supply. A submucosal plexus drains into a periesophageal venous plexus from which the veins originate and empty into the inferior thyroid, bronchial, azygos, and left gastric veins.

Two large interconnecting networks that course longitudinally form the lymphatic network of the esophagus. The mucosal network extends into the submucosal network, and flow is predominantly (6:1) longitudinal rather than segmental. These pierce the muscular wall, and ultimately lymph channels follow the arterial supply. The cervical esophagus drains into the deep cervical nodes alongside the inferior thyroid vessels, while the abdominal portion drains to the preaortic group of the celiac nodes along the left gastric artery. The thoracic esophagus drains into the tracheobronchial nodes superiorly and the subcarinal and paraesophageal nodes inferiorly.

After giving off their recurrent laryngeal branches, which supply the cricopharyngeal sphincter and cervical esophagus, the vagus nerves descend onto the anterior wall of the esophagus and form a complex vagal esophageal plexus, a network of interconnecting fibers that forms the preganglionic parasympathetic supply to the esophagus. These connect to the enteric ganglia in the myenteric and submucosal plexuses that are located in the wall of the esophagus.

12 A little above the diaphragm, the plexus usually gives rise to two nerve trunks, the anterior and posterior vagal trunks.

The anterior trunk contains predominantly left vagal fibers and the posterior contains mainly right with considerable contribution from each other.

Cervical and thoracic sympathetic ganglia contribute visceral branches to the esophagus, and a few branches from the splanchnic nerves also reach the esophagus. Their effect on the esophageal muscle is unknown. The vagus nerve is the motor supply to both the esophageal muscle and secretomotor to the esophageal glands. Afferent pain fibers appear to run in both the vagal and vasomotor sympathetic supply; hence esophageal pain can be referred to the neck, arm, and thoracic wall.

The mucosal lining of the esophagus is composed of nonkeratinized, stratified squamous epithelium supported by a lamina propria and a thick muscularis mucosa. The mucous membrane is thick and in the collapsed state is thrown into longitudinal folds. Mucosal glands in the submucosa are mainly found at the upper and lower ends of the esophagus. The muscular wall consists of an inner circular and an outer longitudinal layer that is visceral smooth muscle in the lower two thirds and skeletal striated muscle in the upper third. Except for the short intraabdominal segment, the lack of a serosa in the rest of the esophagus accounts for the difficulty in suturing the esophagus.

The upper esophageal sphincter, cricopharyngeus, is 15 cm from the incisor teeth. Although there is no anatomic or histologic thickening of the lower end of the esophagus, the lower 5 cm of the esophagus acts as a physiological sphincter to prevent regurgitation of gastric contents into the esophagus.

▶ THORACIC TRACHEA

The trachea is a continuation of the larynx and begins in the neck at the infracricoid level at the level of the C6 vertebra and averages 11.8 cm in length to its termination at the carinal spur. It has approximately 17–21 incomplete cartilaginous rings 4 mm wide and 1 mm thick that maintain its elliptical shape in the adult while it is more circular in children. With flexion of the neck the trachea becomes almost completely an intrathoracic organ coursing backward and downward from a subcutaneous position to rest ultimately on the esophagus and vertebral column at the level of the carina. Bearing a common embryological origin with the esophagus, these two structures remain in intimate contact with one another with the posterior muscular membranous wall of the trachea resting on the esophagus. Anterior relations in the neck include the thyroid and in the mediastinum include the thymus and parts of some of the great vessels.

The innominate artery crosses the mid-trachea obliquely from right to left while the arch of the aorta indents the esophagus slightly and appears to shift the trachea toward the right, away from its midline position. Lateral relations on the right side are predominantly venous structures and include the superior vena cava, azygos, and right brachiocephalic veins; lateral arterial structures on the left side include as above the arch of the aorta and the left common carotid artery. Both right and left vagi, along with their recurrent laryngeal nerves and right and left sympathetic trunks, are also lateral relations of the trachea.

Segmental blood supply to the trachea is from the inferior thyroid arteries and the bronchial arteries that form anastomotic networks in the tracheal wall. Lymph drains to the posterior inferior group of deep cervical nodes and to paratracheal nodes.

▶ LUNG LOBES AND FISSURES AND BRONCHOPULMONARY SEGMENT ANATOMY

To conserve healthy tissue and to perform operations safely on the lung, the thoracic surgeon must have a thorough knowledge of the segmental bronchopulmonary anatomy. Developing as outpouchings of the foregut, the ventral lung buds undergo repeated branching, to yield approximately 20 generations from the principal bronchi to the terminal alveolar sacs. With the bronchus at the center, each bronchopulmonary segment functions as an individual unit with its own pulmonary arterial and venous supply. Importantly the pulmonary veins run in the intersegmental plane and do not accompany the bronchus and the pulmonary artery to each unit.

The larger right lung has three lobes—upper, middle, and lower—and is composed of 10 bronchopulmonary segments. The left lung has two lobes and 8 segments. The lingula on the left side is the anatomical equivalent of the middle lobe and is incorporated into the upper lobe. However, in approximately 8% of the population the horizontal fissure may be well developed on the left side, but is never complete, also giving the impression of three lobes on the left side.

Conversely the horizontal or minor fissure may be absent on the right side in 10% of the population and is complete in only one third of the individuals.

The oblique fissure on each side separates the lower lobe from the rest of the lung. Anomalous fissures of varying depth may be seen along any of the segments but are most commonly seen separating the superior segment of the lower lobe. Rarely the apical segment of the right upper lobe may be a true tracheal lobe with its bronchus arising directly from the trachea. The azygos lobe is not a true segment but is formed by the azygos vein cutting into the pleura and apex of the lung.

The terminology proposed by Jackson and Huber for the pulmonary segments and the branches supplying them has been universally adopted. The apparent discrepancy of only eight segments on the left side is explained by the fact that the apical and posterior segmental bronchi of the left upper lobe and the anterior and medial segmental bronchi of the left lower lobe originate from a common stem bronchus (Figure 1-9 and Table 1-2).

▶ EXTERNAL ANATOMY

The lungs are cone shaped and conform to the shape of the cavity that contains it. The costal surface is convex while the diaphragmatic surface is concave and is separated from the costal and medial surfaces by a sharp inferior border. The apex of the cone extends above the first rib to fit into the cupola of the pleura and is an extension of the rounded posterior border of the lung that sits in the paravertebral gutter. The anterior border of the lung is thin and

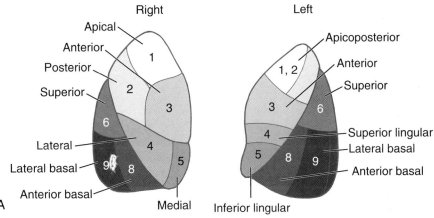

Figure 1–9 The bronchopulmonary segments: **(A)** lateral surface, **(B)** medial surface, and **(C)** diaphragmatic surface.

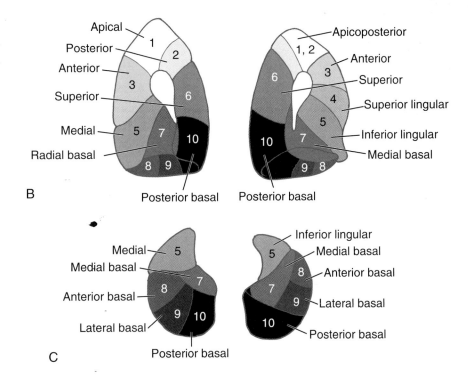

sharp and separates the costal and medial surfaces of the lung. The lower part of this border is deeply concave on the left to form the cardiac notch (Figures 1-10 and 1-11).

The medial or mediastinal surfaces of each lung differ somewhat and are contoured with the impressions of organs that protrude from the lateral walls of the mediastinum. Besides the cardiac notch, the aortic arch and the ascending aorta make a deep groove around the hilum on the left sides and above these are the vertical impressions of the subclavian artery and the esophagus. On the right side the cardiac impression is small and consists of the right auricle, while the impressions of the vena cava, the arch of the azygos vein, the trachea, and the esophagus are more prominent.

The region where the lung is connected to the mediastinum, largely by the bronchus and pulmonary vessels, is the root of the lung, and the region where these structures enter or leave the lung is the hilum.

The pulmonary ligament and reflected pleura covering each lung root enclose the following structures: principal bronchi, pulmonary arteries and veins, bronchial arteries and veins, autonomic and visceral nerve fibers, lymphatic vessels and bronchopulmonary lymph nodes, and connective tissue.

TRACHEOBRONCHIAL ANATOMY

The trachea bifurcates into the right and left principal bronchi. The right principal bronchus arises in a more direct line with the trachea at an angle of about 25° and passes behind the superior vena cava to reach the hilum of the lung. The left principal bronchus is slightly smaller, leaves the trachea more obliquely at an angle of about 45°, passes below the arch of the aorta and the left pulmonary artery, and is almost twice as long as the right main bronchus (about 4–6 cm).

The right upper lobe bronchus, also known as the eparterial bronchus, branches from the lateral wall of the right principal bronchus about 1.2 cm distal to the trachea. The

14

Table 1–2	
Pulmonary Segmental Classification	
Right	*Left*
Upper lobe	Upper lobe
1. Apical	1 and 2. Apical posterior
2. Posterior	3. Anterior
3. Anterior	
Middle lobe	Lingula
4. Lateral	4. Superior lingula
5. Medial	5. Inferior lingula
Lower lobe	Lower lobe
6. Superior	6. Superior
7. Medial basal	7 and 8. Anteromedial basal
8. Anterior basal	
9. Lateral basal	9. Lateral basal
10. Posterior basal	10. Posterior basal

and bifurcates into lateral and medial branches. The superior segmental bronchus to the lower lobe arises from the posterior wall of the bronchus intermedius as it terminates into the basal stem bronchus that sends off segmental bronchi to the medial, anterior, lateral, and posterior basal segments. The medial basal segment arises anteromedially while the lateral basal and posterior basal most often arise as a common stem.

The longer left principal bronchus appears to bifurcate into the upper lobe bronchus that arises anterolaterally and the lower lobe bronchus continues posteromedially. The upper lobe bronchus divides into the superior and inferior divisions that supply the upper lobe and lingula, respectively. The superior division branches into an apical posterior segmental bronchus and an anterior segmental bronchus. The inferior or lingual bronchus is the equivalent of a middle lobe bronchus on the right, is 1–2 cm in length, and divides into the superior and inferior divisions.

The lower lobe bronchus, on the right side, gives off the superior segmental bronchus as its first branch before the basal trunk continues for about 1.5 cm as a single trunk. This then bifurcates into an anteromedial basal segmental bronchus and a common bronchial stem for the remaining basal segments.

Anatomical variations usually involve segmental bronchi arising as a common stem. Occasionally additional bronchi may arise from the mainstem and distribute to a segment that has its own bronchus, for example, a subsuperior bronchus that distributes to a portion of the superior and posterior basal segments of the lower lobe, seen more commonly on the left side.

upper lobe bronchus about 1 cm in length gives off three segmental bronchi as it makes almost a 90° angle with the right main bronchus and the bronchus intermedius. After a distance of approximately 1.5–2 cm the middle lobe bronchus arises from the anterior surface of the bronchus intermedius. The middle lobe bronchus is 1.5–2.2 cm long

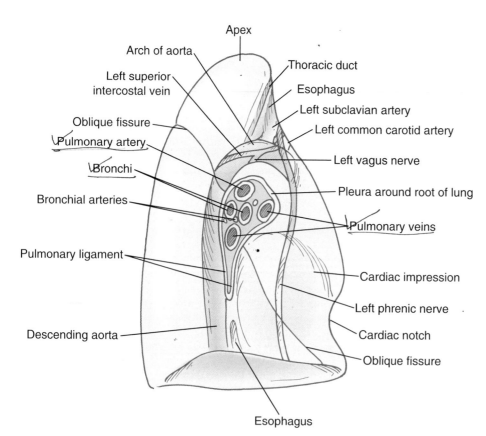

Figure 1–10 The medial surface of the left lung.

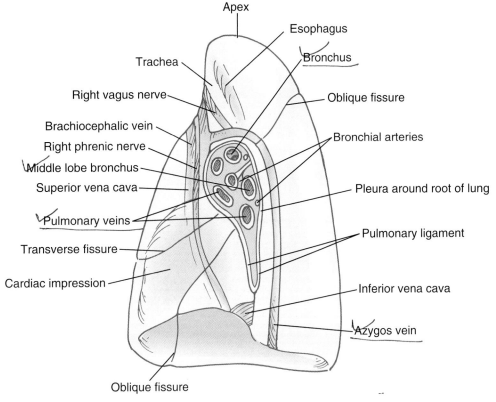

Figure 1–11 The medial surface of the right lung.

PULMONARY ARTERIAL AND VENOUS ANATOMY

The position of the pulmonary artery is somewhat different on the two sides. On the left, the artery lies anterior and superior to the bronchus and runs in a slightly posterior direction before curving around and behind the left upper lobe bronchus. The right mainstem bronchus is the most superior and posterior of the right hilar structures and the artery though slightly anterior is inferior to the bronchus. The azygos vein on the right side and the aortic arch on the left form a vascular arch roofing the hila on either side. The superior pulmonary veins are inferior and anterior to the pulmonary arteries, and the inferior pulmonary veins are even more inferior and posterior to the superior veins.

The segmental branches of the pulmonary arteries usually lie on the superior or lateral surfaces of the segmental bronchi that they accompany and with which they branch. The venous tributaries occupy an intersegmental position, do not bear as close a relationship to the segmental bronchi, and tend to lie on their medial or inferior surfaces. Variations from the usual pattern are common and as a general rule veins vary more than arteries and arteries vary more than bronchi.

The main pulmonary artery arises to the left of the aorta and passes superiorly and to the left, anterior to the left mainstem bronchus where it divides into the right and left main pulmonary arteries.

The right pulmonary artery passes to the right behind the ascending aorta and forms the superior border of the transverse sinus. It then passes posterior to the superior vena cava and forms the superior border of the postcaval recess of Allison while the right superior pulmonary vein forms the inferior border of the recess. The first branch is

the truncus anterior (rarely intrapericardial); it arises superolaterally and supplies the upper lobe before the pulmonary artery enters the lung hilum. The interlobar portion crosses over the bronchus intermedius and gives off the posterior ascending artery to the posterior segment of the upper lobe.

Opposite this branch the middle lobe artery arises anteromedially, usually at the junction of the horizontal and oblique fissures. The arterial branch to the superior segment of the lower lobe arises posteriorly and opposite the middle lobe artery at the same level or slightly distal to it. Beyond the superior segmental artery, the common basal trunk continues in the fissure to give rise to the medial basal segmental artery, occasionally as a common branch with the anterior basal branch. The terminal branches supply the lateral and posterior basal segments.

The left pulmonary artery passes more posteriorly and superiorly from the right and has a longer length before giving off its first branch. Commonly there are four branches to the left upper lobe, but this may vary from two to seven. The first branch arises from the anterior portion of the artery and is quite short and often its branches appear as separate vessels arising from the main artery. The second branch usually arises posterosuperiorly as the main artery passes over the left upper lobe bronchus and into the interlobar fissure where more ascending upper lobe branches may originate. As it enters the interlobar fissure it gives off a branch to the superior segment of the left lower lobe and the lingular artery. Beyond the lingular branch, the common basal trunk divides into two major branches. The anterior branch supplies the anteromedial basal segments and the posterior branch supplies the lateral basal segments.

16

Among the common variations of the pulmonary arterial supply it is important to remember that the first anterior trunk on the left may be the major supply to the lingular segments while on the right side two major arteries may arise from the truncus anterior. These are designated as the truncus anterior superior and the truncus anterior inferior.

The left superior pulmonary vein receives all the tributaries from the left upper lobe. It is closely applied to the anteroinferior portion of the pulmonary artery and makes dissection of the anterior branches quite hazardous. Its three main tributaries are apical posterior, anterior, and lingular. Occasionally the superior and inferior lingular veins may be separate. A common anomaly is drainage of the inferior lingular vein into the inferior pulmonary vein. The inferior pulmonary vein lying more posteriorly and inferiorly drains the entire lower lobe via two principal tributaries, the superior segmental and common basal veins. The right superior pulmonary vein is usually made up of four branches: the apical anterior, anterior–inferior, and posterior branches that drain the upper lobe and the inferior branch that drains the middle lobe. Occasionally the middle lobe vein may drain into the atrium as a separate vessel and very rarely if may become a tributary of the inferior pulmonary vein.

The right inferior pulmonary vein is similar to the one on the left and is made up of two trunks. The common basal vein is made up of the superior basal and inferior basal tributaries while the superior segmental vein drains the superior segment of the lower lobe.

The superior and inferior pulmonary veins on the right most often enter the left atrium separately. In contrast, on the left, the two veins form a common trunk in more than 25% of the population.

PULMONARY LYMPHATICS AND NODAL STATIONS

Lymphatic drainage channels run towards the hilum from subpleural vessels along the bronchi and pulmonary arteries. This flow is interrupted by multiple lymph nodes along the way, mostly situated at forking points of the bronchi. Each nodal station has a number assigned to it and is the basis of the most recent staging system for primary bronchogenic carcinoma as proposed by Mountain and Dressler in 1997.

The most peripheral pulmonary nodes include subsegmental lymph nodes (14) and segmental (13), lobar (12), and interlobar (11) in the fissures and are reliably removed during a lobectomy. The hilar lymph nodes (10), also known as bronchopulmonary nodes, are at the root of the lung and can be accessed via thoracoscopy or thoracotomy. The inferior pulmonary ligament nodes (9) lie within the inferior pulmonary ligament on the left and the right and the paraesophageal nodes (8) lie dorsal to the posterior wall of the trachea and inferior to the carina, to the right or left of the midline esophagus.

From then on drainage is to the central mediastinal and tracheobronchial nodes and upward via mediastinal lymph trunks to the brachiocephalic veins.

The right and left paratracheal (2R and 2L) and the lower paratracheal at the tracheobronchial angle (4R and 4L) and the subcarinal (level 7) lymph nodes can be identified and sampled via a standard cervical mediastinoscopy. The

Chamberlain procedure gives access to the subaortic (5) and paraaortic (6) lymph nodes. The Delphian lymph nodes or the highest mediastinal, pretracheal lymph node is classified as level 1.

Thus levels 1 through 9 are considered mediastinal lymph nodes and metastases are classified as N2 if ipsilateral and N3 if contralateral spread of cancer is present in these lymph node stations. Nodes 11 through 14 are intrapulmonary with hilar (10) being the transition point.

Anomalies of this ipsilateral centrally directed drainage pattern are quite common and are more likely on the left side, especially with lower lobe tumors. Up to 50% of left lower lobe tumors and 35% of left upper lobe tumors have positive contralateral (N3) mediastinal nodes while only 42% of right lower lobe tumors and 18% of right upper lobe tumors have contralateral metastasis.

Instead of draining to hilar nodes the left upper lobe tumors may follow an alternate path to the subaortic, periaortic, and anterior mediastinal nodes in up to one third of patients.

BRONCHIAL CIRCULATION

The systemic circulation of the lung tissues is derived from the bronchial arteries that supply the bronchi from the carina to their terminal bronchioles and also nourish the connective tissue and visceral pleura. A single right bronchial artery usually branches from the third posterior intercostal artery, and two left bronchial arteries usually branch from the dorsal aorta, one near vertebra T5 and one inferior to the left principal bronchus. Although variations are known, most bronchial arteries arise from the anterolateral aspect of the aorta or its branches within 2–3 cm of the origin of the left subclavian artery and come to lie on the membranous portion of the principal bronchi. The bronchial arteries usually give off branches to the esophagus and then follow the bronchi into the lung, also giving off branches along the interalveolar connective tissue septae to the visceral pleura. There is a rich anastomosis with the pulmonary arterial supply, which is important after pulmonary transplantation.

The bronchial veins have a superficial system with two bronchial veins on each side draining from the hilar region and visceral pleura into the azygos vein on the right and the accessory hemiazygos vein on the left. Most of the venous drainage from the deeper lung substance drains into the pulmonary venous system, accounting for the less than 100% saturation of the blood in the left atrium.

NERVE SUPPLY TO THE LUNG

The vagus nerve and the sympathetic plexus contribute to the poorly developed anterior pulmonary plexus around the main pulmonary arteries and the well-developed posterior plexus of nerves around the bronchi.

The vagus carries all the afferent innervation from the bronchial mucosa, sensing stretch in the alveoli and pleura, pressure in the pulmonary veins, and mediating pain. Efferent fibers in the vagus constrict the bronchi, while the sympathetic efferents are vasoconstricting to the pulmonary vessels and secretomotor to the bronchial plexus.

BIBLIOGRAPHY

Agur AMR, Lee MJ: Grant's Atlas of Anatomy, 10th ed. Philadelphia: Lippincott Williams & Wilkins, 1999.

Bannister LH, Berry MM, Collins P, et al: Gray's Anatomy: The Anatomical Basis of Medicine and Surgery, 38th ed. New York: Churchill Livingstone, 1995.

Brock RC: The Anatomy of the Bronchial Tree: With Special Reference to the Surgery of Lung Abcsess, 2nd ed. London: Oxford University Press, 1954.

Butler J: The Bronchial Circulation; Lung Biology in Health and Disease, Vol. 57. New York: Marcel Dekker, 1992.

Butler P, Mitchell AWM, and Ellis H: Applied Radiological Anatomy. Cambridge University Press, 1999.

Clemente CD: Gray's Anatomy, 30th American Edition. Philadelphia: Lea & Febiger, 1985.

Conley DM, Rosse C: The digital anatomist: The interactive atlas of thoracic viscera (CD-ROM). Seattle: University of Washington School of Medicine, 1996.

Funatsu T, Yoshito M, Hatakenoka R, et al: The role of mediastinoscopic biopsy in preoperative assessment of lung cancer. J Thorac Cardiovasc Surg 104:1688, 1992.

Jackson CL, Huber JF: Correlated applied anatomy of the bronchial tree and lungs with a system of nomenclature. Dis Chest 9:319, 1943.

Kubik S, Healy JE: Surgical Anatomy of the Thorax. Philadelphia: W.B. Saunders, 1970.

Liebow AA: Patterns of origin and distribution of the major bronchial arteries in man. Am J Anat 117:19, 1965.

Mountain CF, Dressler CM: Regional lymph node classification for lung cancer staging. Chest 111:1718, 1997.

Netter FM: The Ciba Collection of Medical Illustrations, Vol. 7. Summit, NJ: Ciba-Geigy Corporation, 1996.

Riquet M, Manach D, Dupont P, et al: Anatomic basis of lymphatic spread of lung carcinoma to the mediastinum: Anatomo-clinical correlations. Surg Radiol Anat 16:229, 1994.

Roussos C: The Thorax; Lung Biology in Health and Disease, Vol. 85. New York: Marcel Dekker, 1995.

Rosse C, Rosse PG: Hollinshead's Textbook of Anatomy, 5th ed. Philadelphia: Lippincott-Raven, 1997.

Wragg LE, Milloy FJ, Anson BJ: Surgical aspects of the pulmonary artery supply to the middle lobe and lower lobes of the lungs. Surg Gynecol Obstet 127:531, 1968.

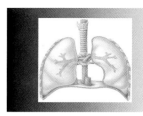

Imaging the Thorax

Constanza J. Gutierrez, Edith M. Marom, Jeremy J. Erasmus, and Edward F. Patz, Jr.

CHAPTER 2

▶ INTRODUCTION

Over the past decade advances in imaging including digital chest radiographs, multidetector spiral computed tomography (CT), and the transition of positron emission tomography (PET) from experimental to routine clinical use have improved diagnostic accuracy and patient management. Additionally digital images have allowed electronic distribution of studies throughout the hospital and clinics via a Picture Archiving and Communication System (PACS) resulting in improvements in communication.

This chapter is a general overview of thoracic imaging with a focus on radiological evaluation of the surgical patient. Topics reviewed include a spectrum of lung, mediastinal, pleural, and chest wall abnormalities commonly encountered by thoracic surgeons where imaging is important in diagnosis and management.

▶ MEDIASTINAL ABNORMALITIES

Mediastinal abnormalities are due to a wide variety of etiologies including congenital malformations, infections, trauma, and neoplasms. Clinical history and evaluation of prior chest radiographs or CT are often sufficient to determine the etiology and the necessity for further evaluation. In the absence of prior radiological studies, a chest radiograph, CT, and or magnetic resonance (MR) imaging may be required to establish a diagnosis.[85]

Aortic Dissection

Spiral CT is the modality of choice for aortic dissection with nearly 100% sensitivity and specificity, and accuracy superior to angiography.[2,86] CT is used not only to confirm the diagnosis, but also to determine the type and extent of the dissection for management decisions. The primary diagnostic finding on CT is an intimal flap separating the true from false lumen. Type A dissections involve the ascending aorta and typically originate just above the aortic valve plane, and thus are usually considered for surgical repair (Figure 2-1). Type B dissections, however, usually originate just below the level of the ligamentum arteriosum, and spiral down the descending aorta. These patients are often hypertensive and are managed medically.

In patients with a contraindication to iodinated contrast, MR imaging or transesophageal echo (TEE) can be used to diagnosis and determine the type of dissection. An advantage of MR is its multiplanar capabilities and its ability to evaluate the heart and great vessels at the same time.[86] However, these imaging modalities are more optimal for reevaluation of the patient in the nonacute setting.

Trauma

Patients suspected of traumatic injury to the mediastinum usually require immediate radiological evaluation, and the type of study depends on the mechanism of injury and structures potentially involved. The chest radiograph is typically the first study as it rapidly provides a tremendous amount of information, and usually indicates whether additional studies are warranted.

The chest radiographic findings in patients with suspected traumatic aortic injury (TAI) may show an indistinct aortic arch or descending aorta, left apical cap, tracheal displacement to the right, displacement of the nasogastric tube to the right of the T-4 spinous process, mediastinal widening, and inferior displacement of the left main-stem bronchus[14,84,88] (Figure 2-2). Less specific findings include a left pleural effusion and widened of the paravertebral stripe.[58] These features, however, are only suggestive, not indicative of an aortic injury. In contradistinction, the

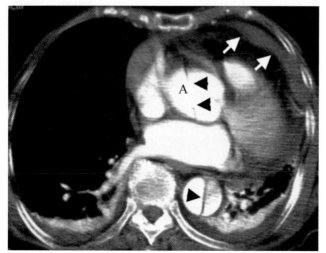

Figure 2–1 Ruptured type A aortic dissection. Axial contrast-enhanced chest CT shows pericardial fluid (*arrows*) surrounding dilated ascending aorta (A) with an intimal flap extending from the value plane into the descending aorta (*arrowheads*). There are small pleural effusions and basilar atelectasis.

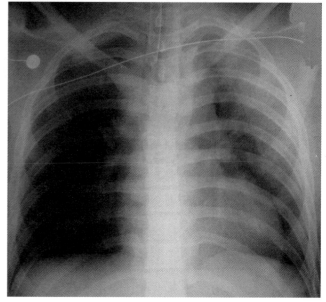

Figure 2–2 Traumatic aortic injury. Portable chest radiograph shows indistinct descending aorta, left apical cap, tracheal displacement to the right, and inferior displacement of the left mainstem bronchus.

negative predictive value of a normal chest radiograph for an aortic injury is 94–96%.[59,102]

Recent advances in multidetector spiral CT with thin sections and three-dimensional (3-D) reconstruction have become the primary imaging method for the diagnosis of TAI if the chest radiograph is abnormal. The sensitivity for this technique is 100%, and the specificity ranges from 83–99.7%[10,11,16,24,60] (Figure 2-3). The absence of a periaortic abnormality and normal appearing aorta on a spiral CT excludes TAI, and the negative predictive value is 100%.[24,60] Additional thoracic injuries can also be identified at the same time, thus limiting investigation of the trauma patient to one study.[11]

Indirect signs of TAI, most notably a periaortic hematoma, are found in 91% of patients with surgically proven TAI.[11] If this finding is present, further evaluation with an aortogram is required. Aortography is safe and accurate with a negative predictive value for TAI approaching 100%. Direct signs for TAI include a linear intraluminal filling defect, pseudoaneurysm formation, abrupt caliber change, and active contrast extravasation.[11,26,27]

In select cases distinction between TAI and nontraumatic aortic entities such as ductus diverticulum, prominent origin of a bronchial artery, and atherosclerosis may be difficult. In this minority of cases, aortography, and sometimes TEE may help define the aortic abnormality.

Trauma—Airways and Esophagus

Tracheal and esophageal injuries are uncommon but are typically found following acceleration–deceleration and penetrating trauma. Many of these injuries are not recognized initially because of subtle or nonspecific clinical and radiological findings. Delayed or missed diagnosis can result in death or severe complications such as ventilatory failure, mediastinitis, sepsis, airway stenosis, bronchiectasis, recur-

rent pulmonary infections, and permanent pulmonary function impairment.[45]

Chest radiographic findings of tracheobronchial and esophageal injury are nonspecific but include pneumomediastinum, pneumothorax, and progressive subcutaneous emphysema.[21,45] If the diagnosis is entertained additional studies should be performed. CT is the imaging modality of choice for visualization of the airways, and all patients with tracheal rupture have some form of abnormal air collection and occasionally demonstrate air within the soft tissues of the neck.[9] Direct tracheal injury was seen in 71% of patients as a wall defect or deformity (Figure 2-4). CT overall sensitivity for detecting tracheal injury was 85%.

CT also provides information about the esophagus, although if pneumomediastinum with or without mediastinal fluid is found on plain films or CT following trauma, a barium swallow, or endoscopy is recommended to exclude an esophageal tear.

Evaluation of Airways—Nontrauma

Focal or diffuse lesions of the central airways are produced by a variety of diseases, including infection, malignancy, trauma, aspiration, collagen vascular disease, and idiopathic entities such as sarcoidosis or amyloidosis. Even though patients may present with significant symptoms, airway abnormalities are frequently not apparent or overlooked on chest radiographs. If there is a clinical suspicion of tracheobronchial abnormality, further evaluation by CT is warranted.[46,64] Helical CT is preferred as it produces excellent axial images of tracheobronchial anatomy. Thin slices are preferred (1–3 mm) as web-like stenosis can easily be missed or underestimated with thicker sections (Figure 2-5).[64]

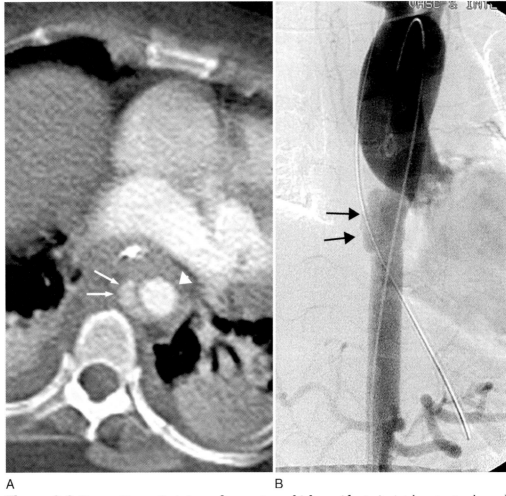

A   B

Figure 2–3 **Traumatic aortic injury after motor vehicle accident. A,** Axial contrast-enhanced chest CT demonstrates contrast located in a pouch *(arrows)* beside the descending aorta *(arrowhead)* consistent with traumatic injury and pseudoaneurysm. **B,** Aortogram confirms CT finding of aortic transection *(arrows).*

Figure 2–4 **Tracheal rupture after motor vehicle accident in a patient with no respiratory symptoms and a chest radiograph demonstrating pneumomediastinum.** Coronal reformations of CT (2.5-mm collimation) show pneumomediastinum and discontinuation of the trachea *(arrows).*

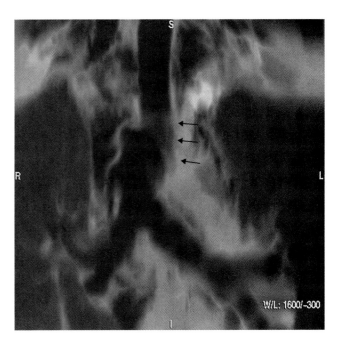

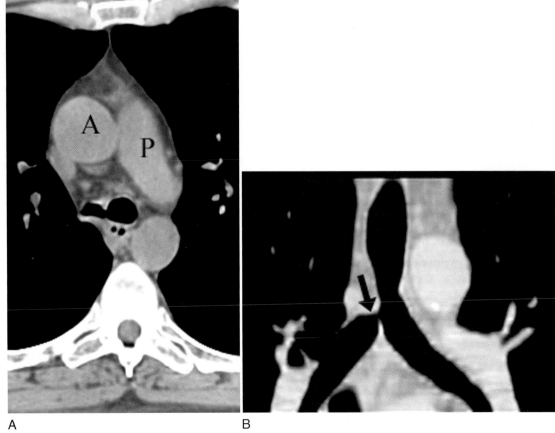

A   B

Figure 2–5 **Focal stenosis of the right mainstem bronchus from invasive aspergillosis. A,** Axial CT shows normal caliber of left main bronchus and marked concentric narrowing of right main bronchus. A, ascending aorta; P, pulmonary artery. **B,** Coronal reconstruction shows right main bronchus stenosis involves short focal segment (*arrow*).

Mediastinal Tumors

Mediastinal tumors, a large, diverse group of neoplasms, have historically been described radiographically according to their localization within anterior, middle, and posterior compartments. This description facilitates differential diagnosis and can aid in treatment planning.

Tumors that occur primarily in the anterior mediastinum include hemangiomas, lymphatic malformations, thymic lesions (cysts, thymolipoma, thymoma, thymic carcinoma), parathyroid adenomas, germ cell tumors, and lymphoma (Figure 2-6). CT and MR imaging are particularly useful in showing local soft tissue and vascular invasion of thymomas, local invasion and early dissemination to regional lymph nodes of thymic carcinomas and, because of the varying composition of soft tissue, fat, calcium, and hemorrhage in teratomas, can occasionally differentiate these tumors from thymomas and lymphomas.[7,44,61,95,105]

Tumors that occur primarily in the middle mediastinum are foregut duplication cysts, pericardial cysts, and neoplasms arising from the esophagus and trachea. Bronchogenic cysts are the most common mediastinal foregut cysts and are typically located in the subcarinal or right paratracheal region. They typically manifest on CT as round or spherical masses of water attenuation, although many have increased attenuation from proteinaceous debris or blood.[3,43,51] Esophageal tumors can manifest as middle mediastinal masses, although esophageal carcinoma more frequently manifests as diffuse thickening of the esophagus. Endoscopy and endoscopic-directed ultrasound biopsy are usually used to evaluate locoregional extent and nodal metastases. CT is useful in showing the extent of involvement of adjacent structures such as the airways, aorta, pericardium, and spine, and distant nodal metastases (celiac, gastrohepatic ligament).

Tumors that occur primarily in the posterior compartment are neurogenic tumors. In fact 20% of all adult and 35% of all pediatric mediastinal neoplasms are due to neurogenic tumors and most are located in the posterior mediastinum.[1,15] Neurogenic tumors are classified as tumors of peripheral nerves (neurofibromas, schwannomas, malignant tumors of nerve sheath origin) or sympathetic ganglia (ganglioneuromas, ganglioneuroblastomas, neuroblastomas) and are optimally assessed by MR imaging. MR imaging is the preferred modality for evaluating neurogenic tumors as it can simultaneously assess (1) intraspinal extension, (2) spinal cord abnormalities, (3) longitudinal extent of tumor, and (4) extradural extension.

► LUNG ABNORMALITIES

Thoracic imaging is essential in the workup of pulmonary abnormalities including lung nodules, intrathoracic malig-

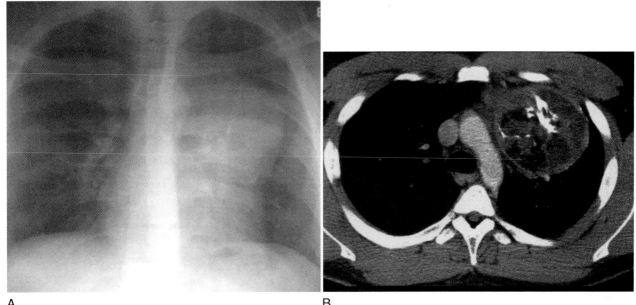

A   B

Figure 2–6 Anterior mediastinal mass. A, PA chest radiograph demonstrates a smoothly marginated left-sided anterior mediastinal mass. **B,** Axial CT image confirms the mass with mixed heterogeneous components including fat, soft tissue, fluid, and calcification. These findings are diagnostic of a teratoma.

nancies, diffuse interstitial lung disease, and infection. Imaging studies provide exquisite detail in characterizing pulmonary abnormalities and in determining the anatomical extent of disease for possible biopsy or resection.

Solitary Pulmonary Opacities

Solitary pulmonary opacities are a common incidental radiological finding and are usually benign, but because of the concern for lung cancer further evaluation is often suggested. The goal is to differentiate the malignancies from benign lesions so that those patients who require surgery are correctly identified. Although morphological features may be used to suggest whether a nodule is benign or malignant there is considerable overlap and at least 20% of malignant nodules will have a benign appearance.[35,81,107] Detection of specific patterns of calcification and stability in size for 2 years have historically been the only reliable findings useful in determining benignity. More recently, the ability to distinguish benign and malignant opacities has improved with assessment of perfusion and metabolism using contrast-enhanced CT and PET using a d-glucose analog, ^{18}F-labeled 2-deoxy-D-glucose (FDG), respectively.

Contrast-enhanced CT can be used to differentiate between benign and malignant nodules because the intensity of enhancement is directly related to the vascularity of the nodule and to the likelihood of malignancy.[90,106] Typically, malignant nodules enhance more than 20 Hounsfield units (HU), while benign nodules enhance less than 15 HU[90] (Figure 2-7).

PET imaging also allows differentiation of malignant and benign nodules that are indeterminate after conventional imaging (Figure 2-8). A meta-analysis of the accuracy of FDG–PET reports a sensitivity of 96.8% and specificity of 77.8% when used in the evaluation of 10-mm or larger nodules.[32]

Staging Lung Cancer

Treatment and prognosis of patients with non–small cell lung cancer (NSCLC) are currently dependent on the anatomical extent of disease, and staging typically includes CT and occasionally PET to assess the primary tumor, regional lymph nodes, and presence of metastases.[62] CT is usually used to define chest wall or mediastinal invasion but is inaccurate in differentiating between anatomic contiguity and subtle invasion.[42b,47,52,72,103] Although MR has superior soft-tissue contrast resolution compared to CT, it has the same limitations as CT in assessing local disease[42b,54,98,99] (Figure 2-9).

The presence of nodal metastases and their location are important in determining management and prognosis.[62,63] CT is most commonly used to assess the size of nodes (>10 mm in short-axis diameter) and is the only criterion used to suggest nodal metastases.[28] The accuracy of CT (62–88%) is suboptimal, although more recently,* PET using [^{18}F]fluorodeoxyglucose (FDG–PET) has improved noninvasive accuracy (81–96%)[20,93,96] (Figure 2-10).

The adrenal glands, liver, brain, bones, and lymph nodes are the most common sites of metastatic disease at presentation; however, the role of imaging these areas at presentation still remains controversial.[42,69,71] Routine imaging of the upper abdomen is performed in most patients with NSCLC. If an adrenal mass contains fat or has an attenuation value of less than 10 HU on a noncontrast CT scan, the mass can be considered benign.[5] Lesions with attenuation values more than 10 HU can be further evaluated with MR imaging using chemical shift analysis and dynamic gadolinium enhancement to determine whether they are malignant or benign.[50]

Routine CT or MR imaging of the central nervous system has also been advocated because up to 18% of patients with NSCLC have brain metastases at presentation and

*References 42b, 53, 70, 82, 87, 99.

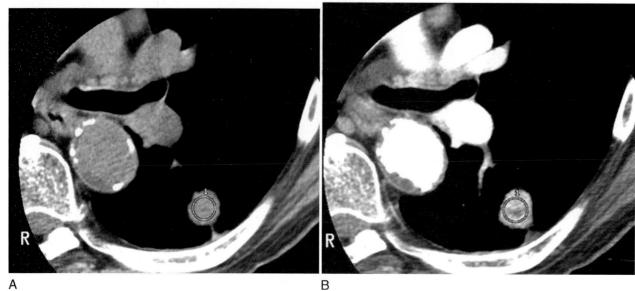

A   B

Figure 2–7 Non-small-cell cancer. A, Noncontrast CT shows left lung nodule with attenuation value of 24 HU. **B,** Contrast CT shows nodule enhancement of 70 HU and central necrosis. Enhancement more than 20 HU is suggestive of malignancy and resection revealed non-small-cell cancer.
(Courtesy of Tom Hartman, M.D., Mayo Clinic, Rochester, MN; reprinted with permission from Haaga.)

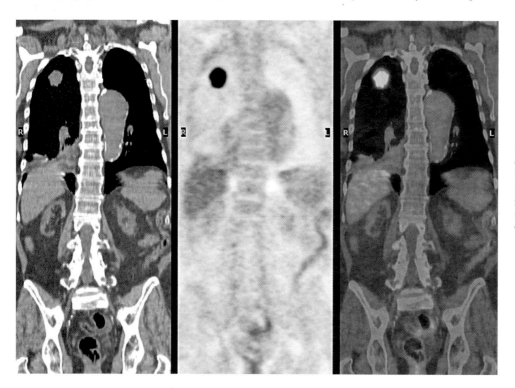

Figure 2–8 Non-small-cell lung cancer. Coronal CT, PET, and fused CT-PET images show small nodule in the right upper lobe with increased uptake of [18F]fluorodeoxyglucose, which is consistent with malignancy. (See color insert.)

10% of these patients will have no associated neurological symptoms.* Because imaging rarely reveals occult skeletal metastases in an asymptomatic patient, bone radiographs, 99mTc-labeled methylene diphosphonate bone scintigraphy, and MR imaging are generally performed only if the patient has focal bone pain or an elevated alkaline phosphatase level.[56,79,83]

Because clinical staging of NSCLC is often inaccurate, whole body imaging with PET can be performed to improve the accuracy. PET has a higher sensitivity and specificity than CT in detecting metastases to the adrenal glands, bones, and extrathoracic lymph nodes, thus the addition of PET to conventional workup (radiographs, CT, MR imaging) improves the selection of patients for surgically curable resection in one out of five patients* (Figure 2-11). Additionally, whole-body PET stages intrathoracic and extrathoracic disease with a single study and has been shown to alter management in up to 40% of patients.†

*References 12, 13, 38, 57, 65, 83.

*References 8, 22b, 48, 67, 94, 100.
†References 17, 20, 67, 91, 94, 100.

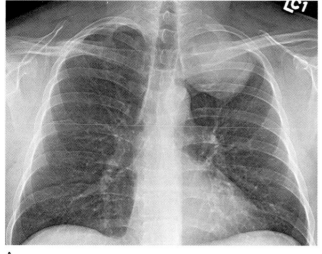

A

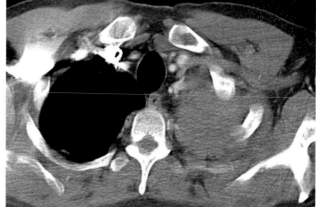

B

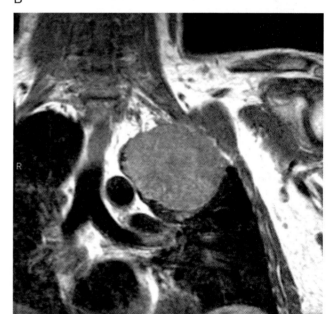

C

Figure 2–9 Non–small-cell lung cancer. A, Posteroanterior chest radiograph shows large left upper lobe lung mass. **B,** CT confirms a large, well-circumscribed mass in the apex of the left thorax. Note difficulty in evaluation of local invasion on axial image. **C,** Coronal T1-weighted image shows preservation of adjacent soft tissue planes, a finding consistent with absence of mediastinal, chest wall, and brachial plexus invasion.

Interstitial Lung Disease and Pulmonary Abscesses

Imaging studies are essential in suggesting the diagnosis in patients with pulmonary symptoms and focal or diffuse lung disease. If the diagnosis is uncertain after clinical and imaging evaluation, surgical biopsies may be requested before therapy is initiated. Radiological studies are often very useful in guiding the biopsy and therapeutic intervention as needed (Figure 2-12).

Lung abscesses, usually caused by aspiration of anaerobic bacteria, typically occur in patients with altered levels of consciousness, gastroesophageal dysmotility, and poor dental hygiene. Medical therapy (systemic antibiotics, postural drainage) is the initial treatment of choice and is curative in most patients. However, lung abscesses in children less than 7 years of age typically do not drain spontaneously and are less likely to respond to medical management. Surgical or percutaneous drainage is required in the 11–21% of patients

with lung abscesses who fail to respond to medical therapy. Drainage of an abscess is recommended when (1) the patient has persistent sepsis 5 to 7 days after initiation of antibiotic therapy, (2) the abscess is larger than 4 cm, or (3) the abscess increases in size while the patient is on medical therapy.

Percutaneous CT-guided catheter drainage has less morbidity and mortality than surgical resection and in most cases clinical and radiological improvement usually occurs rapidly after catheter drainage. Although the mean time to abscess resolution is 10–15 days, marked improvement of sepsis (fever, leukocytosis) usually occurs within 48 h of drainage. Failure of percutaneous drainage can occur when the abscess (1) contains viscous, organized tissue, (2) is multiloculated, or (3) has a thick noncollapsible wall. Potential complications of lung abscesses drainage include bleeding, bronchopleural fistula, and empyema.[22a,42a]

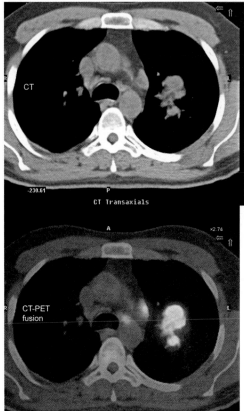

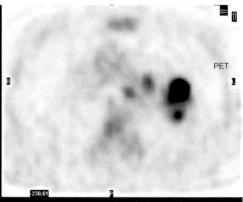

Figure 2–10 Non–small-cell lung cancer. Axial CT, PET, and fused CT-PET, images show left upper lobe lung malignancy with increased [18F]fluorodeoxyglucose uptake consistent with a malignancy. Enlarged prevascular and normal sized left lower paratracheal nodes show increased FDG uptake compared with uptake in mediastinum confirmed to be metastases. Note absence of FDG uptake in right lower paratracheal nodes indicative of absence of nodal metastases. (See color plate.)

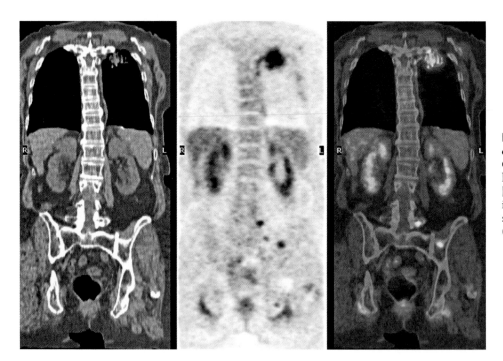

Figure 2–11 Non–small-cell lung cancer. Coronal CT, PET, and fused CT-PET images show left upper lobe lung malignancy with increased [18F]fluorodeoxyglucose. Note focal increased FDG uptake in lumbar spine and pelvis due to metastases. (See color plate.)

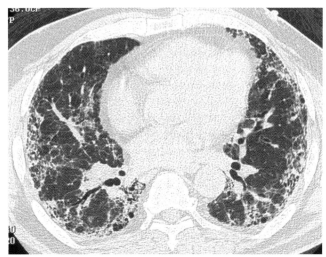

Figure 2–12 Usual interstitial pneumonitis (UIP). Axial high resolution CT image through the bases demonstrates diffuse lung disease with area of predominantly peripheral ground glass opacities, architectural distortion, and cystic spaces consistent with pulmonary fibrosis. Lung biopsy confirmed UIP.

PLEURAL AND CHEST WALL ABNORMALITIES

Malignant Pleural Mesothelioma

Malignant pleural mesothelioma (MPM) is an uncommon tumor that arises from mesothelial cells of the pleura and less commonly of the pericardium or peritoneum. There are approximately 2000 new cases diagnosed in the United States each year, the majority of which are associated with prior asbestos exposure.[76] Treatment options depend on stage at presentation with an increasing tendency to perform surgical resection in limited disease.[97,104] Primarily in an attempt to distinguish patients who are potentially resectable, the New International Staging System for MPM emphasizes criteria used to determine local tumor extension and regional lymph nodes status in a traditional TMN system.[66,77] In a recent study, MR and CT imaging were performed in 65 patients with MPM and were found to be of nearly equivalent diagnostic accuracy (50–65%).[37] Determination of mediastinal nodal disease by both modalities was approximately 50%, although significant differences between CT and MR imaging were seen in two categories: invasion of the diaphragm (CT accuracy 55%, MR 82%, $p = .01$) and invasion of endothoracic fascia or a single chest wall focus (CT accuracy 46%, MR 69%, $p = .05$). PET imaging has been used to evaluate patients with MPM but the role in the staging remains unclear. In one small series comparing PET imaging to CT evaluation, PET detected occult metastases in two patients being considered for surgical resection[80] (Figure 2-13).

Pleural Collections

Fluid collections in the pleural space are caused by a variety of diseases including infection, trauma, inflammation, and neoplasm. Although some patients can be managed conservatively, interventional procedures such as pleural fluid aspiration with or without placement of a drainage catheter or pleural biopsies are frequently performed for either diagnostic or therapeutic purposes. The type of intervention depends on a spectrum of clinical and imaging features including symptoms, extent of disease, and etiology of the pleural abnormality. Imaging studies most frequently with CT can delineate the extent and complexity of the pleural collection.

Chest Wall Disease

Abnormalities of the chest wall are unusual, but are most commonly due to soft tissue tumors, metastatic disease, infections, iatrogenic causes, trauma, and congenital lesions. Imaging this spectrum of diseases often depends on the suspected etiology, but CT is usually the study of choice. It can provide the requisite diagnostic information and will accurately define the anatomical extent of disease with multiplanar capabilities for surgical planning.

POSTOPERATIVE IMAGING

Chest radiographs commonly demonstrate abnormalities in patients following cardiothoracic procedures. An increase in heart size may be due to perioperative myocardial infarction or hypervolemia, although most frequently it is the result of fluid in the pericardial sac or mediastinal fat. In some cases the mediastinal contours appear normal on chest radiographs even though a significant amount of bleeding has occurred.[40] In other cases the mediastinum may appear enlarged but is normal and is due to magnification effects on the supine, expiratory radiograph.[36]

Early awareness of surgical complications is important, as timely management is associated with a decrease in mortality.[6,10,78] Some entities such as postoperative mediastinitis is primarily a clinical diagnosis. Radiographs are both insensitive and nonspecific, with mediastinal widening and air collections typically found in all patients following sternotomy. CT cannot clearly distinguish mediastinitis from the early normal, noninfected postoperative mediastinum. During the first 3 weeks following surgery, CT will exhibit infiltration and indistinctness of the mediastinal fat, fluid collections, small air bubbles, air fluid levels, and a thickened pericardium.[29–31,39,41] A negative CT may direct attention elsewhere for the source of sepsis; a positive CT, although nondiagnostic, may be used for guidance in sampling a fluid collection in a febrile patient.

Pulmonary Embolism

Clinical signs and symptoms of pulmonary embolism (PE) are neither sensitive nor specific as patients can present with chest pain, shortness of breath, or oxygen desaturation. Initial imaging with chest radiographs is useful to search for other causes that can clinically mimic PE such as pleural effusions, pneumothorax, pneumonia, or congestive heart failure. The chest radiographic findings in patients with PE are nonspecific chest film findings including consolidation, atelectasis, pleural effusion, peripheral wedge-shaped opacities, enlarged pulmonary artery, and focal oligemia. Eight percent of patients with PE, however, have a normal chest film.[89]

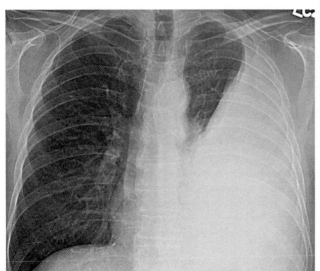

A

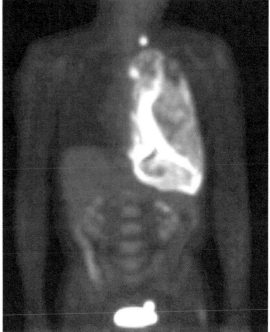

C

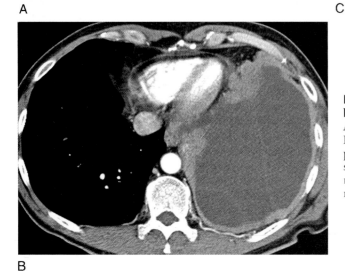

B

Figure 2–13 Malignant pleural mesothelioma in a patient being evaluated for extrapleural pneumonectomy. **A,** Posteroanterior chest radiograph shows large left pleural effusion. **B,** Contrast-enhanced CT shows large left effusion and a diffuse pleural mass encasing the left hemithorax. **C,** Coronal whole body PET scan shows diffuse pleural increased [18F]fluorodeoxyglucose uptake in mass and focal uptake in the neck. Biopsy of left lower neck node revealed metastatic mesothelioma, precluding resection.

If the diagnosis of PE is suspected, and the chest film does not suggest a reasonable alternative diagnosis, other imaging modalities are always employed. This typically includes CT angiography (CTA), pulmonary angiography, ventilation–perfusion (V̇/&Q̇) scans, venography, and/or ultrasound. Although pulmonary angiography has traditionally been the gold standard in establishing the diagnosis, spiral CTA has become the study of choice. CTA is noninvasive and permits direct visualization of a clot within the pulmonary artery seen as a low-density intravascular filling defect, either completely or partially occluding the vessel (Figure 2-14). CT has virtually 100% accuracy for central pulmonary emboli,[73] although it appears to be inferior to pulmonary angiography for subsegmental clots, but these smaller emboli are of uncertain clinical significance. Early results suggest that patients with a negative CT studies do well, with less than 5% having a documented PE within 3 months of the initial evaluation. Large randomized and con-

trolled collaborative studies are planned to further evaluate CTA in the diagnosis of PE.

CT has also proven superior to V̇/&Q̇ scanning, and early CT trials report sensitivities of 75–92% and specificities of 90–95% as compared to sensitivities of 36–65% and specificities of 74–94% by V̇/&Q̇ scan.[18,49,73,92] With progressive decrease in slice collimation and speed, recent series have found the negative predictive value for helical CT in the diagnosis of PE approaches 99–100%.[25,74]

Some patients, however, still benefit from a V̇/&Q̇ study, eliminating the need for iodinated contrast. Those patients with a normal chest film and a normal V̇/&Q̇ scan have an extremely low probability of pulmonary embolus.[25,76] No further evaluation for PE is required. Patients with a high pretest probability of PE and a high probability scan will most likely have pulmonary embolism and treatment is often initiated. Unfortunately, the majority of patients suspected of PE have an abnormal chest radiograph and an

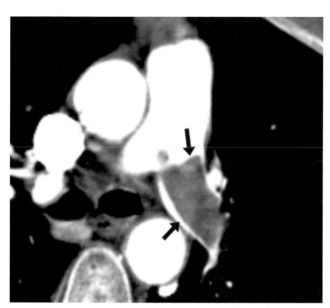

Figure 2–14 Pulmonary embolism. Axial contrast-enhanced spiral CT (1.25 mm collimation) shows filling defect surrounded by contrast medium in left main pulmonary artery (arrows) consistent with acute pulmonary embolism.

indeterminate $\dot{V}/\&\dot{Q}$, which then results in additional diagnostic studies. It should be noted that CT provides greater interobserver agreement than $\dot{V}/\&\dot{Q}$ scans for the diagnosis of PE and provides more alternative diagnoses (e.g., pneumonia, pulmonary edema) than $\dot{V}/\&\dot{Q}$ scan does, 93 vs. 51%, respectively.[92]

Patients with contraindications to iodinated contrast most commonly have a $\dot{V}/\&\dot{Q}$ scan, or, alternatively, MR angiography, which allows excellent evaluation of the aorta and pulmonary vessels. MR imaging detection of a pulmonary embolus has been reported to have a sensitivity of 90–100% and a specificity of 62–77%.[23,34] However, these studies were limited to larger vessels as MR has not been successful in detecting peripheral emboli beyond the subsegmental artery branch level, even with administration of contrast.[34,55] Another limitation of MR is that the study may be technically challenging, especially in the acute setting, postoperative, or intensive care unit patient. MR studies can be lengthy and require special nonferrous equipment to continue physiological support and monitoring.[4,19,75]

▶ SUMMARY

Imaging plays a crucial role in the diagnosis and follow-up in patients with pulmonary diseases. Recent advances in imaging technologies have revolutionized evaluation of thoracic disease with improvements in patient management. Careful selection of the appropriate imaging studies improves diagnostic accuracy, limits the number of tests performed, and decreases unnecessary surgery. It is anticipated that further improvement of existing modalities and continued development of novel imaging technologies will improve diagnostic imaging strategies and patient's outcomes in the future.

REFERENCES

1. Azarow KS, Pearl RH, Zurcher R, et al: Primary mediastinal masses. A comparison of adult and pediatric populations. J Thorac Cardiovasc Surg 106(1):67–72, 1993.
2. Bansal RC, Chandrasekaran K, Ayala K, et al: Frequency and explanation of false negative diagnosis of aortic dissection by aortography and transesophageal echocardiography. J Am Coll Cardiol 25(6):1393–1401, 1995.
3. Barakos JA, Brown JJ, Brescia RJ, et al: High signal intensity lesions of the chest in MR imaging. J Comput Assist Tomogr 13(5):797–802, 1989.
4. Barnett GH, Ropper AH, Johnson KA: Physiological support and monitoring of critically ill patients during magnetic resonance imaging. J Neurosurg 68(2):246–250, 1988.
5. Boland GW, Lee MJ, Gazelle GS, et al: Characterization of adrenal masses using unenhanced CT: An analysis of the CT literature. AJR Am J Roentgenol 171:201–204, 1998.
6. Breyer RH, Mills SA, Hudspeth AS, et al: A prospective study of sternal wound complications. Ann Thorac Surg 37(5):412–416, 1984.
7. Brown LR, Aughenbaugh GL: Masses of the anterior mediastinum: CT and MR imaging. AJR Am J Roentgenol 157(6):1171–1180, 1991.
8. Bury T, Barreto A, Daenen F, et al: Fluorine-18 deoxyglucose positron emission tomography for the detection of bone metastases in patients with non-small cell lung cancer. Eur J Nucl Med 25(9):1244–1247, 1998.
9. Chen JD, Shanmuganathan K, Mirvis SE, et al: Using CT to diagnose tracheal rupture. AJR Am J Roentgenol 176(5):1273–1280, 2001.
10. Cheung EH, Craver JM, Jones EL, et al: Mediastinitis after cardiac valve operations. Impact upon survival. J Thorac Cardiovasc Surg 90(4):517–522, 1985.
11. Cleverley JR, Barrie JR, Raymond GS, et al: Direct findings of aortic injury on contrast-enhanced CT in surgically proven traumatic aortic injury: A multi-centre review. Clin Radiol 57(4):281–286, 2002.
12. Colice GL: Detecting lung cancer as a cause of hemoptysis in patients with a normal chest radiograph. Chest 111:877–884, 1997.
13. Colice GL, Birkmeyer JD, Black WC, et al: Cost-effectiveness of head CT in patients with lung cancer without clinical evidence of metastases. Chest 108:1264–1271, 1995.
14. Creasy JD, Chiles C, Routh WD, et al: Overview of traumatic injury of the thoracic aorta. Radiographics 17(1):27–45, 1997.
15. Davis RD Jr, Oldham HN Jr, Sabiston DC Jr: Primary cysts and neoplasms of the mediastinum: Recent changes in clinical presentation, methods of diagnosis, management, and results. Ann Thorac Surg 44(3):229–237, 1987.
16. Demetriades D, Gomez H, Velmahos GC, et al: Routine helical computed tomographic evaluation of the mediastinum in high-risk blunt trauma patients. Arch Surg 133(10):1084–1088, 1998.
17. Dietlein M, Weber K, Gandjour A, et al: Cost-effectiveness of FDG-PET for the management of solitary pulmonary nodules: A decision analysis based on cost reimbursement in Germany. Eur J Nucl Med 27(10):1441–1456, 2000.
18. Diffin DC, Leyendecker JR, Johnson SP, et al: Effect of anatomic distribution of pulmonary emboli on interobserver agreement in the interpretation of pulmonary angiography. AJR Am J Roentgenol 171(4):1085–1089, 1998.
19. Dunn V, Coffman CE, McGowan JE, et al: Mechanical ventilation during magnetic resonance imaging. Magn Reson Imaging 3(2):169–172, 1985.
20. Dwamena BA, Sonnad SS, Angobaldo JO, Wahl RL: Metastases from non-small cell lung cancer: Mediastinal

30

staging in the 1990's: Meta-analytic comparison of PET and CT. Radiology 213:530–536, 1999.

21. Eijgelaar A, Homan van der Heide JN: A reliable early symptom of bronchial or tracheal rupture. Thorax 25(1):120–125, 1970.

22a. Erasmus JJ, McAdams HP, Rossi S, Kelley MJ: Percutaneous management of intrapulmonary air and fluid collections. Radiol Clin N Am 38(2): 385–393.

22b. Erasmus JJ, Patz EF, McAdams HP, et al: Evaluation of adrenal masses in patients with bronchogenic carcinoma by using 18F-fluorodeoxyglucose positron emission tomography. AJR Am J Roentgenol 168:1357–1360, 1997.

23. Erdman WA, Peshock RM, Redman HC, et al: Pulmonary embolism: Comparison of MR images with radionuclide and angiographic studies. Radiology 190(2):499–508, 1994.

24. Fabian TC, Davis KA, Gavant ML, et al: Prospective study of blunt aortic injury: Helical CT is diagnostic and antihypertensive therapy reduces rupture. Ann Surg 227(5):666–676; discussion 676–677, 1998.

25. Garg K, Sieler H, Welsh CH, et al: Clinical validity of helical CT being interpreted as negative for pulmonary embolism: Implications for patient treatment. AJR Am J Roentgenol 172(6):1627–1631, 1999.

26. Gavant ML, Flick P, Menke P, et al: CT aortography of thoracic aortic rupture. AJR Am J Roentgenol 166(4):955–961, 1996.

27. Gavant ML, Menke PG, Fabian T, et al: Blunt traumatic aortic rupture: Detection with helical CT of the chest. Radiology 197(1):125–133, 1995.

28. Glazer GM, Gross BH, Quint LE, et al: Normal mediastinal lymph nodes: Number and size according to American Thoracic Society Mapping. AJR Am J Roentgenol 144: 261–265, 1985.

29. Goodman LR: Imaging after cardiac surgery. In Goodman LR, Putman CE, editors: Critical Care Imaging. Philadelphia: Saunders, 1992, p. 83.

30. Goodman LR, Teplick SK: Computed tomography in acute cardiopulmonary disease. Radiol Clin North Am 21(4): 741–758, 1983.

31. Goodman LR, Kay HR, Teplick SK, et al: Complications of median sternotomy: Computed tomographic evaluation. AJR Am J Roentgenol 141(2):225–230, 1983.

32. Gould MK, Maclean CC, Kuschner WG, et al: Accuracy of positron emission tomography for diagnosis of pulmonary nodules and mass lesions: A meta-analysis. JAMA 285(7):914–924, 2001.

33. Grist TM, Sostman HD, MacFall JR, et al: Pulmonary angiography with MR imaging: Preliminary clinical experience. Radiology 189(2):523–530, 1993.

34. Gupta A, Frazer CK, Ferguson JM, et al: Acute pulmonary embolism: Diagnosis with MR angiography. Radiology 210(2):353–359, 1999.

35. Gurney JW, Lyddon DM, McKay JA: Determining the likelihood of malignancy in solitary pulmonary nodules with Bayesian analysis. Part II. Application. Radiology 186:415–422, 1993.

36. Harris RS: The pre-operative chest film in relation to postoperative management—some effects of different projection, posture and lung inflation. Br J Radiol 53(627):196–204, 1980.

37. Heelan RT, Rusch VW, Begg CB, et al: Staging of malignant pleural mesothelioma: Comparison of CT and MR imaging. AJR Am J Roentgenol 172(4):1039–1047, 1999.

38. Hooper RG, Tenholder MF, Underwood GH, et al: Computed tomographic scanning of the brain in initial staging of bronchogenic carcinoma. Chest 85:774–776, 1984.

39. Jolles H, Henry DA, Roberson JP, et al: Mediastinitis following median sternotomy: CT findings. Radiology 201(2): 463–466, 1996.

40. Katzberg RW, Whitehouse GH, deWeese JA: The early radiologic findings in the adult chest after cardiopulmonary bypass surgery. Cardiovasc Radiol 1(4):205–215, 1978.

41. Kay HR, Goodman LR, Teplick SK, et al: Use of computed tomography to assess mediastinal complications after median sternotomy. Ann Thorac Surg 36(6):706–714, 1983.

42a. Klein JS, Schultz S, Heffner JE, Am J Roent 164(3):581–588.

42b. Klein JS, Webb WR: The radiologic staging of lung cancer. J Thorac Imaging 7:29–47, 1991.

43. LeBlanc J, Guttentag AR, Shepard JA, et al: Imaging of mediastinal foregut cysts. Can Assoc Radiol J 45(5):381–386, 1994.

44. Lee JD, Choe KO, Kim SJ, et al: CT findings in primary thymic carcinoma. J Comput Assist Tomogr 15(3):429–433, 1991.

45. Lee RB: Traumatic injury of the cervicothoracic trachea and major bronchi. Chest Surg Clin N Am 7(2):285–304, 1997.

46. Marom EM, Goodman PC, McAdams HP: Focal abnormalities of the trachea and main bronchi. AJR Am J Roentgenol 176(3):707–711, 2001.

47. Martini N, Heelan R, Westcott J, et al: Comparative merits of conventional, computed tomographic, and magnetic resonance imaging in assessing mediastinal involvement in surgically confirmed lung carcinoma. Journal of Thoracic and Cardiovascular Surgery 90:639–648, 1985.

48. Maurea S, Mainolfi C, Bazzicalupo L, et al: Imaging of adrenal tumors using FDG PET: Comparison of benign and malignant lesions. AJR Am J Roentgenol 173:25–29, 1999.

49. Mayo JR, Remy-Jardin M, Muller NL, et al: Pulmonary embolism: Prospective comparison of spiral CT with ventilation-perfusion scintigraphy. Radiology 205(2):447–452, 1997.

50. Mayo-Smith WW, Boland GW, Noto RB, et al: State-of-the-art adrenal imaging. Radiographics 21(5):995–1012, 2001.

51. McAdams HP, Kirejczyk WM, Rosado-de-Christenson ML, et al: Bronchogenic cyst: Imaging features with clinical and histopathologic correlation. Radiology 217(2):441–446, 2000.

52. McLoud TC: CT of bronchogenic carcinoma: Indeterminate mediastinal invasion. Radiology 173:15–16, 1989.

53. McLoud TC, Bourgouin PM, Greenberg RW, et al: Bronchogenic carcinoma: Analysis of staging in the mediastinum with CT by correlative lymph node mapping and sampling. Radiology 182:319–323, 1992.

54. McLoud TC, Filion RB, Edelman RR, et al: MR imaging of superior sulcus carcinoma. J Comput Assist Tomogr 13:233–239, 1989.

55. Meaney JF, Weg JG, Chenevert TL, et al: Diagnosis of pulmonary embolism with magnetic resonance angiography. N Engl J Med 336(20):1422–1427, 1997.

56. Michel F, Soler M, Imhof E, Perruchoud AP: Initial staging of non-small cell lung cancer: Value of routine radioisotope bone scanning. Thorax 46:469–473, 1991.

57. Mintz BJ, Tuhrim S, Alexander S, et al: Intracranial metastases in the initial staging of bronchogenic carcinoma. Chest 86:850–853, 1984.

58. Mirvis SE, Bidwell JK, Buddemeyer EU, et al: Imaging diagnosis of traumatic aortic rupture. A review and experience at a major trauma center. Invest Radiol 22(3):187–196, 1987.

59. Mirvis SE, Bidwell JK, Buddemeyer EU, et al: Value of chest radiography in excluding traumatic aortic rupture. Radiology 163(2):487–493, 1987.

60. Mirvis SE, Shanmuganathan K, Buell J, et al: Use of spiral computed tomography for the assessment of blunt trauma patients with potential aortic injury. J Trauma 45(5):922–930, 1998.

61. Moeller KH, Rosado-de-Christenson ML, Templeton PA: Mediastinal mature teratoma: Imaging features. AJR Am J Roentgenol 169(4):985–990, 1997.

62. Mountain CF: Revisions in the international system for staging lung cancer. Chest 111:1710–1717, 1997.

63. Mountain CF, Dresler CM: Regional lymph node classification for lung cancer staging. Chest 111:1718–1723, 1997.

64. Naidich DP, Gruden JF, McGuinness G, et al: Volumetric (helical/spiral) CT (VCT) of the airways. J Thorac Imaging 12(1):11–28, 1997.

65. Newman SJ, Hansen HH: Proceedings: Frequency, diagnosis, and treatment of brain metastases in 247 consecutive patients with bronchogenic carcinoma. Cancer 33(2):492–496, 1974.

66. Patz EF Jr, Rusch VW, Heelan R: The proposed new international TNM staging system for malignant pleural mesothelioma: Application to imaging. AJR Am J Roentgenol 166(2):323–327, 1996.

67. Pieterman RM, van Putten JW, Meuzelaar JJ, et al: Preoperative staging of non-small-cell lung cancer with positron-emission tomography. N Engl J Med 343(4):254–261, 2000.

68. Price B: Analysis of current trends in United States mesothelioma incidence. Am J Epidemiol 145(3):211–218, 1997.

69. Quint LE, Francis IR: Radiologic staging of lung cancer. J Thorac Imaging 14(4):235–246, 1999.

70. Quint LE, Francis IR, Wahl RL, et al: Preoperative staging of non-small-cell carcinoma of the lung: imaging methods. AJR Am J Roentgenol 164:1349–1359, 1995.

71. Quint LE, Tummala S, Brisson LJ, et al: Distribution of distant metastases from newly diagnosed non-small cell lung cancer. Ann Thorac Surg 62:246–250, 1996.

72. Ratto GB, Piacenza G, Frola C, et al: Chest wall involvement by lung cancer: Computed tomographic detection and results of operation. Ann Thorac Surg 51:182–188, 1991.

73. Remy-Jardin M, Remy J, Deschildre F, et al: Diagnosis of pulmonary embolism with spiral CT: Comparison with pulmonary angiography and scintigraphy. Radiology 200(3):699–706, 1996.

74. Remy-Jardin M, Tillie-Leblond I, Szapiro D, et al: CT angiography of pulmonary embolism in patients with underlying respiratory disease: Impact of multislice CT on image quality and negative predictive value. Eur Radiol 12(8):1971–1978, 2002.

75. Rotello LC, Radin EJ, Jastremski MS, et al: MRI protocol for critically ill patients. Am J Crit Care 3(3):187–190, 1994.

76. Royal HD: Radionuclide imaging of the lung. Curr Opin Radiol 1(4):446–459, 1989.

77. Rusch VW: A proposed new international TNM staging system for malignant pleural mesothelioma. From the International Mesothelioma Interest Group. Chest 108(4):1122–1128, 1995.

78. Rutledge R, Applebaum RE, Kim BJ: Mediastinal infection after open heart surgery. Surgery 97(1):88–92, 1985.

79. Salvatierra A, Baamonde C, Llamas JM, et al: Extrathoracic staging of bronchogenic carcinoma. Chest 97:1052–1058, 1990.

80. Schneider DB, Clary-Macy C, Challa S, et al: Positron emission tomography with f18-fluorodeoxyglucose in the staging and preoperative evaluation of malignant pleural mesothelioma. J Thorac Cardiovasc Surg 120(1):128–133, 2000.

81. Seemann MD, Staebler A, Beinert T, et al: Usefulness of morphological characteristics for the differentiation of benign from malignant solitary pulmonary lesions using HRCT. Eur Radiol 9(3):409–417, 1999.

82. Shimoyama K, Murata K, Takahashi M, et al: Pulmonary hilar lymph node metastases from lung cancer: Evaluation based on morphology at thin-section, incremental, dynamic CT. Radiology 203:187–195, 1997.

83. Silvestri GA, Littenberg B, Colice GL: The clinical evaluation for detecting metastatic lung cancer. American Journal of Respiratory and Crit Care Med 152:225–230, 1995.

84. Simeone JF, Deren MM, Cagle F: The value of the left apical cap in the diagnosis of aortic rupture: A prospective and retrospective study. Radiology 139(1):35–37, 1981.

85. Slater EE, DeSanctis RW: The clinical recognition of dissecting aortic aneurysm. Am J Med 60(5):625–633, 1976.

86. Sommer T, Fehske W, Holzknecht N, et al: Aortic dissection: A comparative study of diagnosis with spiral CT, multiplanar transesophageal echocardiography, and MR imaging. Radiology 199(2):347–352, 1996.

87. Staples CA, Moller NL, Miller RR, et al: Mediastinal nodes in bronchogenic carcinoma: Comparison between CT and mediastinoscopy. Radiology 167:367–372, 1988.

88. Stark P, Cook M, Vincent A, et al: Traumatic rupture of the thoracic aorta. A review of 49 cases. Radiologe 27(9):402–406, 1987.

89. Stein PD, Alavi A, Gottschalk A, et al: Usefulness of noninvasive diagnostic tools for diagnosis of acute pulmonary embolism in patients with a normal chest radiograph. Am J Cardiol 67(13):1117–1120, 1991.

90. Swensen SJ, Brown LR, Colby TV, et al: Pulmonary nodules: CT evaluation of enhancement with iodinated contrast material. Radiology 194:393–398, 1995.

91. Valk PE, Pounds TR, Tesa RD, et al: Cost-effectiveness of PET imaging in clinical oncology. Nucl Med Biol 23:737–743, 1996.

92. van Rossum AB, Pattynama PM, Mallens WM, et al: Can helical CT replace scintigraphy in the diagnostic process in suspected pulmonary embolism? A retrolective-prolective cohort study focusing on total diagnostic yield. Eur Radiol 8(1):90–96, 1998.

93. Vansteenkiste JF, Stroobants SG, De Leyn PR, et al: Lymph node staging in non-small-cell lung cancer with FDG-PET scan: A prospective study on 690 lymph node stations from 68 patients. J Clin Oncol 16:2142–2149, 1998.

94. van Tinteren H, Hoekstra OS, Smit EF, et al: Effectiveness of positron emission tomography in the preoperative assessment of patients with suspected non-small-cell lung cancer: The PLUS multicentre randomised trial. Lancet 359(9315):1388–1393, 2002.

95. Verstandig AG, Epstein DM, Miller WT Jr, et al: Thymoma—report of 71 cases and a review. Crit Rev Diagn Imag 33(3):201–230, 1992.

96. von Haag DW, Follette DM, Roberts PF, et al: Advantages of positron emission tomography over computed tomography in mediastinal staging of non-small cell lung cancer. J Surg Res 103(2):160–164, 2002.

97. Waller DA: The role of surgery in diagnosis and treatment of malignant pleural mesothelioma. Curr Opin Oncol 15(2):139–143, 2003.

98. Webb WR, Sostman HD: MR imaging of thoracic disease: Clinical uses. Radiology 182:621–630, 1992.

99. Webb WR, Gatsonis C, Zerhouni EA, et al: CT and MR imaging in staging non-small cell bronchogenic carcinoma: Report of the Radiologic Diagnostic Oncology Group. Radiology 178:705–713, 1991.

100. Weder W, Schmid RA, Bruchhaus H, et al: Detection of extrathoracic metastases by positron emission tomography in lung cancer. Ann Thorac Surg 66:886–893, 1998.

101. Wicky S, Capasso P, Meuli R, et al: Spiral CT aortography: An efficient technique for the diagnosis of traumatic aortic injury. Eur Radiol 8(5):828–833, 1998.

102. Woodring JH, King JG: The potential effects of radiographic criteria to exclude aortography in patients with blunt chest trauma. Results of a study of 32 patients with proved aortic or brachiocephalic arterial injury. J Thorac Cardiovasc Surg 97(3):456–460, 1989.

103. Yokoi K, Mori K, Miyazawa N, et al: Tumor invasion of the chest wall and mediastinum in lung cancer: Evaluation with pneumothorax. Radiology 181:147–152, 1991.

32

104. Zellos L, Sugarbaker DJ: Current surgical management of malignant pleural mesothelioma. Curr Oncol Rep 4(4): 354–360, 2002.

105. Zerhouni EA, Scott WW Jr, Baker RR, et al: Invasive thymomas: Diagnosis and evaluation by computed tomography. J Comput Assist Tomogr 6(1):92–100, 1982.

106. Zhang M, Kono M: Solitary pulmonary nodules: Evaluation of blood flow patterns with dynamic CT. Radiology 205(2):471–478, 1997.

107. Zwirewich CV, Vedal S, Miller RR, et al: Solitary pulmonary nodule: High-resolution CT and radiologic-pathologic correlation. Radiology 179:469–476,

Preoperative Assessment of Patients Undergoing Thoracic Surgery

John J. Reilly, Jr.

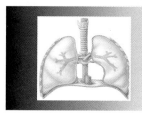

CHAPTER 3

▶ INTRODUCTION

The decision to proceed with any surgical procedure involves a careful consideration of the anticipated benefits of surgery and an assessment of the risks associated with the surgical procedure. An important component of estimating the benefit of surgery is knowledge of the natural history of the condition in question in the absence of surgery.

A popular, and inaccurate, conception of preoperative evaluation is that the evaluating physician "clears" the patient for surgery. Implicit in this terminology is the assumption that a cleared patient has a low risk for perioperative morbidity. As discussed in this chapter, it is more accurate to view the role of preoperative evaluation as meeting two goals: more accurately defining the morbidity and risks of surgery, both short term and long term, and identifying specific factors or conditions in patients that can be addressed to modify the patient's risk of morbidity. The formulation of an approach to accomplish these goals requires a knowledge of the effects of thoracic surgery on patients.

▶ PHYSIOLOGICAL EFFECTS OF THORACIC SURGERY

Surgical procedures and the anesthesia administered to allow such procedures have significant impact on respiratory physiology that contributes to the development of postoperative pulmonary complications. Given that the incidence of pulmonary complications is directly related to the proximity of the planned procedure to the diaphragms, patients undergoing pulmonary, esophageal, or other thoracic surgical procedures fall into the category of patients at high risk for postoperative respiratory complications.[34]

Intraoperatively, the use of inhaled volatile agents can affect gas exchange by altering diaphragmatic and chest wall function. These changes occur without corresponding alterations in blood flow, resulting in the creation of low ventilation–perfusion areas, resulting in the widening of the alveolar–arterial gradient for oxygen.

In the postoperative period, a variety of factors contribute to the development of complications. These include an alteration in breathing pattern to one of rapid shallow breaths with the absence of periodic deep breaths (sighs) and abnormal diaphragmatic function. These result both from pain and from diaphragmatic dysfunction resulting from splanchnic efferent neural impulses arising from the manipulation of abdominal contents. This has the effect of reducing the functional residual capacity (FRC), the resting volume of the respiratory system. The FRC declines by an average of 35% after thoracotomy and lung resection and by ~30% after upper abdominal operations.[1,12,21] If the FRC declines sufficiently to approach closing volume, the volume at which small airway closure begins to occur, patients develop atelectasis and are predisposed to infectious complications. Closing volume is elevated in patients with underlying lung disease.

The alterations in lung volumes that occur result in a reduction in both the inspiratory capacity (the maximal inhalation volume attained starting from a given lung volume) and the expiratory reserve volume (the maximal exhalation volume from a given lung volume), contribute to a decline in the effectiveness of cough, and result in increased difficulty in clearing pulmonary secretions.

▶ PATIENT POPULATION UNDERGOING THORACIC SURGERY

Many patients undergoing a noncardiac thoracic surgical procedure do so because of known or suspected lung or esophageal cancer. These diseases share the common risk

34

factor of a significant and prolonged exposure to cigarette smoking. The combination of age and prolonged cigarette smoking results in a patient population with a significant incidence of comorbid factors in addition to the primary diagnosis. Several reports use the Charlson Comorbidity Index as an indicator of comorbid conditions and predictor of postoperative complications. This index generates a score based on the presence of comorbid conditions and has been demonstrated to stratify risk of postoperative complications in thoracic surgery patients.[5,11]

In a recent study, the mean age of patients undergoing esophagectomy was 58.1 years, with 45% of patients being greater than 60 years of age.[20] In another, the median age was 62.3 years, and 88% were male.[16] In a recent study comparing transhiatal esophagectomy to transthoracic esophagectomy, the mean ages of the patients were 69 and 64 years, with patients up to age 79 included in the study.[18] In a recent review, 28–32% of patients undergoing esophagectomy in the United States were over 75 years of age, and 40% had a Charlson score >3.[6]

Similarly, patients with lung cancer tend to be older and have comorbid conditions. In a series of 344 patients, 36% were over the age of 70 years and 95% had a significant history of smoking.[26] A recent review of Medicare patients undergoing thoracic surgery in the United States showed that in patients undergoing lobectomy, 32–35% were over the age of 75 years (44% women), and 32% had a Charlson score > 3.[6] In the same series, 21–26% of patients undergoing pneumonectomy were over 75 years of age (28% women), and 56% had a Charlson score >3.

A significant source of comorbidity in the population of patients with lung cancer is the presence of chronic obstructive pulmonary disease (COPD). The diagnosis of COPD is an independent risk factor, controlling for cigarette smoke exposure, for the development of lung cancer.[33,37]

Thus, the patient population presenting for major thoracic surgical procedures tends to be older, has a high incidence of comorbid conditions, and contains a disproportionate number of patients with obstructive lung disease. The combination of these factors, plus the magnitude of the surgical procedures, presents a challenge to the clinicians evaluating such patients. The potential for perioperative morbidity and mortality is substantial but, at the same time, the lack of effective alternative therapy for the patient's malignancy means that the consequences of not being a surgical candidate are almost certain death. This quandary has led Gass and Olsen to ask "What is an acceptable surgical mortality in a disease with 100% mortality?"[15]

▶ MOST COMMON COMPLICATIONS AFTER THORACIC SURGERY

These are discussed in more detail elsewhere in this book. In general, the most frequent complications after major thoracic procedures fall into the categories of respiratory and cardiovascular. Although the exact frequency varies from series to series, pneumonia, atelectasis, arrhythmias (particularly atrial fibrillation), and congestive heart failure are the most common. Myocardial infarction, prolonged air leak, empyema, and bronchopleural fistula also occur at a significant frequency.[4,19,26] It follows, therefore, that particular attention to pulmonary and cardiac reserve and risk factors should be a major component of the preoperative evaluation.

▶ GOALS OF THE PREOPERATIVE EVALUATION

The clinicians evaluating a patient for a major thoracic surgical procedure have several goals for the evaluation process. The most obvious of these goals is to provide all parties with an assessment of the risks, both short and long term, of morbidity and mortality from the procedure in a given patient, as well as simultaneously identifying factors that can be addressed to reduce the possibility of adverse events. Less obvious is the fact that the comprehensive evaluation of a patient as part of the preoperative assessment allows the identification of risk factors and health issues independent of the planned surgery and facilitates the institution of interventions indicated regardless of plans for surgery.

▶ HISTORY AND PHYSICAL EXAMINATION

History

Although the field of thoracic surgery has been dramatically altered by the development of new technologies, both in imaging and therapeutics, the history and physical examination remain the most important components of the preoperative evaluation. There is no substitute for a careful history and examination by an experienced clinician.

Table 3-1 highlights the important components of the patient history. Although many of the elements of the history are self-explanatory, several bear some further exposition. A critical component of the preoperative evaluation is the assessment of a patient's functional status. Functional status is an important component of the decision algorithm for both the pulmonary and cardiac elements of the preoperative evaluation. A variety of approaches have been taken to determine functional capacity. These include questionnaires, tests of locomotion such as the 6-min walk or stair climbing, and cardiopulmonary exercise testing (discussed below). One convenient approach to use is the Duke Activity Status Index (see Table 3-2), which can be administered during an interview or can be a self-administered questionnaire.[17]

There is a rough correlation between the score on the Duke Activity Status Index (DASI), which ranges from 0 to 58.2, and maximal oxygen uptake. In addition, the answers to this questionnaire can be used to estimate the functional capacity of the patient in metabolic equivalents (METS), as described in the section on cardiac assessment.

In addition to these considerations, patients should be asked about signs or symptoms suggesting the presence of metastatic disease. These include new headaches, focal neurological signs or symptoms, new onset seizure disorder, bone pain, or recent fractures. Patients should also be questioned about symptoms related to paraneoplastic syndromes. These can range from the relatively subtle symptoms of hypercalcemia to more dramatic neurological symptoms.

Table 3–1
Important Components of History in Preoperative Evaluation
Presenting symptoms and/or circumstances of diagnosis
Prior diagnosis of pulmonary or cardiac disease
Comorbid conditions: diabetes mellitus, liver disease, renal disease
Prior experiences with general anesthesia and surgery
Cigarette smoking: never, current, ex-smoker (if ex-, when did patient stop?)
Inventory of functional capacity of patient (e.g., Duke Activity Status Index)
Medications/allergies
Alcohol use, including prior history of withdrawal syndromes

Physical Examination

The examination of the patient should include an assessment of general overall appearance, including signs of wasting. Respiratory rate and the use of accessory muscles of respiration should be noted. Examination of the head and neck should include assessment of adenopathy and focal neurological deficits or signs, particularly Horner's syndrome in patients with a lung mass. The pulmonary examination should include an assessment of diaphragmatic motion (by percussion) and note any paradoxical respiratory pattern in the recumbent position. The relative duration of exhalation, as well as the presence or absence of wheezing, should be noted. The presence of rales should raise the possibility of pneumonia, heart failure, or pulmonary fibrosis. The cardiac examination should include assessment of a third heart sound to suggest left ventricular failure, murmurs to suggest valvular lesions, or an accentuated pulmonic component of the second heart sound suggesting pulmonary hypertension. The heart rhythm and the absence or presence of any irregular heart beats should be noted. The abdominal examination should note liver size, presence or absence of palpable masses or adenopathy, and any tenderness. The examination of extremities should note any edema, cyanosis, or clubbing. The presence of clubbing should not be attributed to COPD and raises the possibility of intrathoracic malignancy or congenital heart disease. The patient's gait should be observed, both as an assessment of neurological function as well as a confirmation of the patient's ability to participate in postoperative mobilization.

Laboratory Studies

It is reasonable practice to check electrolytes, renal function, clotting parameters, and a complete blood count as part of the preoperative assessment. In patients with known or suspected malignancy, liver function tests and serum calcium should also be checked.

IMAGING STUDIES

This issue is covered in detail in Chapter 2. For patients undergoing pulmonary parenchymal resection, review of images is essential to estimate the amount of lung that will be removed in surgery. In this setting, patients usually have a computed tomography (CT) scan of the chest. In addition to the pathology for which the patient has been referred, the scan should be reviewed for the presence of signs of emphysema or pulmonary fibrosis. In general, review of imaging is an important component of surgical planning and determination of the extent of resection, which in turn influences the process of patient evaluation.

PULMONARY FUNCTION TESTING

The utility of preoperative pulmonary function testing in part depends on the type of operative procedure being planned. For patients undergoing mediastinoscopy, drainage of pleural effusions, or pleural biopsy and who have no prior history of lung disease or unexplained dyspnea, preoperative pulmonary function testing is unlikely to contribute to the preoperative evaluation.

For patients being considered for pulmonary parenchymal resection, preoperative pulmonary function testing should be performed. Although a variety of pulmonary function tests have been examined in this setting, the two that have emerged as being predictive of postoperative complications are the *forced expiratory volume in 1 s* (FEV_1) measured during spirometry and the *diffusing capacity for carbon monoxide* (DL_{CO}). Both of these values can be used to provide a rough estimate of the risk of operative morbidity and mortality.[32] In addition, they are used to calculate the *predicted postoperative* values for FEV_1 and DL_{CO} (ppo-FEV_1 and ppo-DL_{CO}, respectively).

For patients under consideration for esophageal surgery, the FEV_1 and DL_{CO} have also been demonstrated to have value for risk stratification. There is no clear cut-off of "acceptable" lung function for esophageal surgery, however, and measured lung function should be used as one component of the decision process in these patients.

PREDICTION OF POSTOPERATIVE LUNG FUNCTION

Predicted postoperative lung function after lung resection has been demonstrated to be an important predictor of operative risk. In general, the available methods for calculating postoperative lung function result in an underestimate of actual measured lung function once the patient has recovered from surgery. There are two commonly used approaches for calculating postoperative lung function: simple

Table 3–2

Duke Activity Status Index [17]

Question	Activity: can you	Yes	No
1	Take care of yourself, that is, eating, dressing, bathing, or using the toilet?	2.75	0
2	Walk indoors, such as around your house?	1.75	0
3	Walk a block or two on level ground?	2.75	0
4	Climb a flight of stairs or walk up a hill?	5.50	0
5	Run a short distance?	8.00	0
6	Do light work around the house like dusting or washing dishes?	2.70	0
7	Do moderate work around the house like vacuuming, sweeping floors, or carrying in groceries?	3.50	0
8	Do heavy work around the house like scrubbing floors or lifting or moving heavy furniture?	8.00	0
9	Do yard work like raking leaves, weeding, or pushing a power mower?	4.50	0
10	Have sexual relations?	5.25	0
11	Participate in moderate recreational activities like golf, bowling, dancing, doubles tennis, or throwing a baseball or football?	6.00	0
12	Participate in strenuous sports like swimming, singles tennis, football, basketball, or skiing?	7.50	0

calculation and the use of a regional assessment of lung function.

Simple calculation is based on the assumption of homogeneously distributed lung function and requires knowledge of the number of segments to be resected and the preoperative value. For FEV_1, the formula is ppo – FEV_1 = FEV_1 [1– (number of segments resected × 0.0526)]. A similar calculation is done for DL_{CO}. For the majority of patients, this approach to calculation is sufficient and, as mentioned above, results in a postoperative predicted value that is somewhat less than what is measured after recovery.

In certain situations, simple calculation is inaccurate in predicting postoperative lung function. The clinical situations in which regional assessment of lung function is indicated are summarized in Table 3-3. A variety of approaches have been used to attempt to assess the regional distribution of lung function, including lateral position testing, bronchospirometry, quantitative radionuclide ventilation–perfusion scanning, and quantitative CT scanning. Although quantitative CT scanning holds promise in this regard, the current standard test is radionuclide scanning.[30] Typically, the data from quantitative radionuclide ventilation–perfusion scans are reported as the percentage of function contributed by six lung regions: upper one third, middle one third, and lower one third of each hemithorax. These data, combined with the knowledge of the preoperative lung function value and the location and planned extent of resection, allow the calculation of a predicted postoperative value.

Table 3–3
Indications for Preoperative Assessment of the Regional Distribution of Lung Function

Significant airflow obstruction on spirometry (FEV_1 <65% predicted and FEV_1/FVC <0.70)

Significant pleural disease

Known or suspected endobronchial obstruction

Central lung mass

History of prior lung resection

ASSESSMENT OF FUNCTIONAL CAPACITY

For patients undergoing pulmonary resection, functional capacity is an important predictor of postoperative morbidity and mortality. In addition to the role of functional capacity in determining the appropriate cardiac evaluation prior to surgery (Figure 3-1), functional capacity has predictive value for postoperative complications independent of that derived from pulmonary function testing.

In clinical practice, there are two common approaches to assessment of functional capacity: symptom limited maximal cardiopulmonary exercise testing with expired gas analysis and threshold testing requiring patients to attain a certain functional goal. Among the latter, the most commonly employed test is stair climbing. Published data on stair climb testing suggest that patients with the ability to climb more than three flights (54 steps) are at acceptable risk for lobectomy and greater than 4.6–5 flights are at acceptable risk for pneumonectomy.[23–35]

Maximal symptom limited cardiopulmonary testing has been studied as a mode of assessment of functional capacity. The most commonly reported result of such testing is the maximal oxygen uptake ($M\dot{V}O_2$) normalized for body mass, expressed as ml/kg/min. Alternatively, the data are reported as a percentage of predicted value. There is good agreement that patients with an $M\dot{V}O_2$ >15–20 ml/kg/min are at low or "acceptable" risk for perioperative complications and mortality.[22,36,38] Conversely, patients with an $M\dot{V}O_2$ <10–12 ml/kg/min are at high risk for thoracic surgery.[2,9,31,38] In addition to these applications, the preoperative $M\dot{V}O_2$ can also be used in concert with a regional assessment of lung function to calculate a predicted

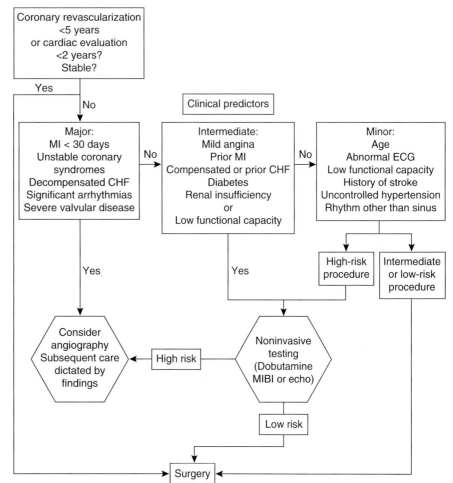

Figure 3–1 Cardiac evaluation algorithm.
(*Adapted from the American College of Cardiology/American Heart Association Task Force on Practice Guidelines.*[13])

38 postoperative $M\dot{V}O_2$ (ppo-$M\dot{V}O_2$), in a manner analogous to that described for lung function parameters.[9] The ppo-$M\dot{V}O_2$ can then be used to stratify perioperative risk.

Currently available data suggest that patients with a ppo-FEV_1 or DL_{CO} of <40% predicted should have additional risk stratification with a test of functional capacity. An alternative sequence of evaluation has been assessed by Bolliger and Perruchoud, who advocate functional assessment in all patients with an FEV_1 or DL_{CO} <80% predicted and reserve regional assessment of lung function for patients with a maximal oxygen uptake of 10–20 ml/kg/min or 40–75% of predicted.[8] A synthesis of current recommendations for preoperative evaluation for pulmonary resection is presented in Figure 3-2.

Arterial Blood Gas Measurements

Commonly measured preoperatively, arterial blood gases have been used to attempt to stratify risk of perioperative complications. Resting hypoxemia has not been established as a predictor for perioperative risk. Common clinical dogma is that patients with a resting pCO_2 >45 mm Hg are at increased risk.[22,28] Several studies, however, have demonstrated that resection may be safely undertaken in patients with resting hypercarbia in the absence of other contraindications to surgery.[7,19,22]

Pulmonary Hemodynamics

Measurements of resting pulmonary hemodynamics, pulmonary artery occlusion, or exercise hemodynamics have all been studied as preoperative assessments. The data generated are contradictory and generally do not add substantially to information obtained from functional assessment and pulmonary function testing.[29]

Age

Although age has been confirmed in many series as a risk factor for perioperative complications, much of the additional risk from age results from comorbid factors. When studies control for comorbidities, patients are at mildly (~2-fold) increased risk because of age.[35] Current consensus is that age alone, particularly in the presence of a good functional capacity, is not a contraindication to surgery.[32]

▶ CARDIAC ASSESSMENT OF PATIENTS UNDER CONSIDERATION FOR THORACIC SURGICAL PROCEDURES

The basic philosophy of cardiac assessment for surgical procedures has changed in recent years, as reflected in

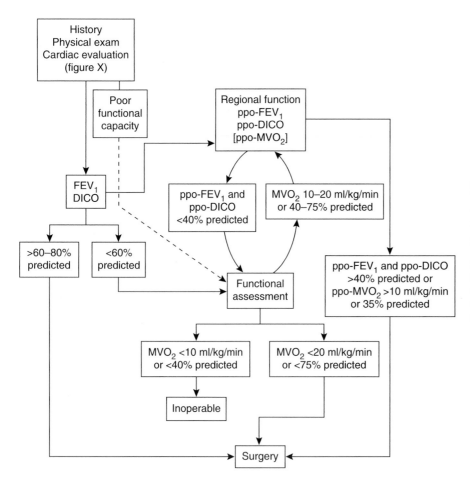

Figure 3–2 Recommended evaluation for patients considered for lung surgery. This figure illustrates one approach to evaluation of surgical candidates. Recommendations concerning cardiac evaluation are presented in Figure 3-1. The choice between proceeding to functional assessment or regional assessment of lung function as the next step in patients with abnormal spirometry or diffusing capacity depends on clinician preference and locally available resources.

the recent guidelines jointly formulated by the American College of Cardiology and the American Heart Association.[13] The preoperative evaluation is now viewed as an opportunity to do a general cardiac assessment and initiate risk factor modification/management rather than a specific intervention centered on surgery. The practice is to institute medical management as indicated by the patient's condition, rather than specific preoperative recommendations. In keeping with this approach, current concepts are that coronary revascularization, by either catheter approach or bypass grafting, is rarely indicated solely to reduce operative risk in a particular patient.

The preoperative cardiac evaluation incorporates consideration of both the cardiac risks associated with the operation under consideration as well as the specific risk factors of the particular patient under consideration. In general, thoracic surgical procedures fall into the high (cardiac risk >5%, operations with an anticipated long procedure time, major fluid shifts and/or blood loss) or intermediate (1%> cardiac risk <5%, intrathoracic surgery) risk categories.

As with the evaluation in general, the cornerstone of preoperative cardiac evaluation is a careful history and physical examination. In addition to inquiries directed at cardiac risk factors such as family history, smoking history, history of hypercholesterolemia, history of diabetes mellitus or hypertension, and history of prior cardiac disease, special attention should be directed to questions to assess the patient's functional capacity. One common way is to classify a patients functional capacity in terms of metabolic equivalents or METS. Four METS are the energy expenditure required to climb a flight of stairs, walk up a hill or briskly on level ground, or to run a short distance (Items 3–5 on the DASI). One to four METS are required to perform self-care, ambulate on level ground within a residence, and perform light housework (Items 1, 2, 3, and 6 on the DASI).

Clinical predictors in increased perioperative cardiovascular risk are stratified into three classes:

1. *Major:* unstable coronary syndromes, including recent myocardial infarction (MI; defined as <30 days); unstable or severe angina, decompensated congestive heart failure; severe valvular disease; *significant* arrhythmias, including high degree atrioventricular block, symptomatic ventricular arrhythmias in setting of underlying heart disease, or supraventricular arrhythmias with an uncontrolled ventricular response.
2. *Intermediate:* mild angina; prior MI or electrocardiogram (ECG) evidence of same; compensated or history of prior heart failure; diabetes mellitus; renal insufficiency.
3. *Minor:* advanced age; abnormal ECG; rhythm other than sinus; low functional capacity; history of stroke; uncontrolled systemic hypertension.

The combination of the classification of clinical predictors, the patient's functional capacity, and the risk of surgery then determines the approach to preoperative evaluation. Current guidelines recommend a stepwise approach to the

evaluation after a comprehensive history, physical examination, and review of the ECG. A suggested implementation of these guidelines for the thoracic surgery population is illustrated in Figure 3-2. If a patient has had coronary revascularization within the past 5 years and has not had a clinical change since then, or if the patient has had a cardiac evaluation within the past 2 years that did not demonstrate the patient to be at high risk, further testing is usually not indicated. If neither of these considerations apply, then the next step is to classify patients according to their clinical predictors.

For patients with major clinical predictors, delay of the procedure should be considered for all but emergency procedures. Such patients should have medical risk factor management and modification initiated and consideration should be given to performing coronary angiography.

For patients with intermediate clinical predictors who either have a poor functional capacity (<4 METs) or are contemplating a high-risk procedure, noninvasive testing should be performed. Should such testing demonstrate high risk, coronary angiography should be considered. If noninvasive testing indicates a low risk, the patient may proceed to surgery. Patients with moderate or excellent functional capacity scheduled for intermediate or low-risk surgical procedures may proceed with surgery without further evaluation.

For patients with minor or no clinical predictors and low functional capacity considering a high-risk surgical procedure, noninvasive testing is recommended. In others with minor or no clinical predictors scheduled for procedures of lesser risk and in patients with moderate or excellent functional capacity, no further preoperative evaluation is needed.

For all patients, any long-term issues meriting consideration of risk factor modification and/or therapy should be addressed in the postoperative period and appropriate therapy instituted when the patient is stable enough to tolerate it.

► SUGGESTED EVALUATION ALGORITHM

A suggested approach to patients undergoing lung surgery in illustrated in Figure 3-2. Patients currently smoking should be advised to cease cigarette smoking 6–8 weeks prior to surgery, if possible, and offered pharmacological therapy to increase their chances of successful smoking cessation.[14] Given the lack of current consensus about the optimal approach to evaluating patients with impaired lung function, options are shown for starting such an evaluation with either an assessment of functional capacity or regional distribution of lung function. Parameters stratifying surgical risk are presented in Table 3-4.

For both lung surgery and other thoracic surgical procedures, the mainstay of preoperative evaluation remains the history and physical examination, followed by integration of available data by an experienced clinician. It is easier to determine whether a patient is a good candidate for surgery than it is to determine whether a patient is at prohibitive risk.

Table 3–4

Risk Assessment for Pulmonary Surgery

Higher risk	*Lower risk*
Age >70	FEV_1 >2 liters for pneumonectomy,[10,39] >1 liter for lobectomy, >0.6 liters for segmentectomy
Higher extent of resection (pneumonectomy > lobectomy > wedge resection)	Predicted postoperative FEV_1 >30–40% predicted
Poor exercise performance	Stair climbing > five flights for pneumonectomy; three flights for lobectomy
Low predicted postoperative predicted FEV_1	Cycle ergometry >83 W^3
Low predicted postoperative DL_{CO}	Predicted postoperative DL_{CO} >40% predicted
High pco_2 (controversial)	Maximal oxygen uptake >15–20 ml/kg/min
Prolonged operative time	

REFERENCES

1. Ali J, Weisel RD, Layug AB, et al: Consequences of postoperative alterations in respiratory mechanics. Am J Surg 128:376–382, 1974.
2. Bechard D, Wetstein L: Assessment of exercise oxygen consumption as preoperative criterion for lung resection. Ann Thorac Surg 44:344–349, 1987.
3. Berggren H, Ekroth R, Malmberg R, et al: Hospital mortality and long-term survival in relation to preoperative function in elderly patients with bronchogenic carcinoma. Ann Thorac Surg 38:633–636, 1984.
4. Bernard A, Ferrand L, Hagry O, et al: Identification of prognostic factors determining risk groups for lung resection. Ann Thorac Surg 70:1161–1167, 2000.
5. Birim O, Maat AP, Kappetein AP, et al: Validation of the Charlson comorbidity index in patients with operated primary non-small cell lung cancer. Eur J Cardiothorac Surg 23:30–34, 2003.
6. Birkmeyer JD, Siewers AE, Finlayson EV, et al: Hospital volume and surgical mortality in the United States. N Engl J Med 346:1128–1137, 2002.
7. Bolliger CT: Pre-operative assessment of the lung cancer patient. S Afr Med J 91:120–123, 2001.
8. Bolliger CT, Perruchoud AP: Functional evaluation of the lung resection candidate. Eur Respir J 11:198–212, 1998.
9. Bolliger CT, Wyser C, Roser H, et al: Lung scanning and exercise testing for the prediction of postoperative performance in lung resection candidates at increased risk for complications. Chest 108(2):341–348, 1995.
10. Boushy SF, Billig DM, North LB, Helgason AH: Clinical course related to preoperative and postoperative pulmonary function in patients with bronchogenic carcinoma. Chest 59:383–391, 1971.
11. Charlson ME, Pompei P, Ales KL, MacKenzie CR: A new method of classifying prognostic comorbidity in longitudinal studies: Development and validation. J Chronic Dis 40:373–383, 1987.
12. Craig DB: Postoperative recovery of pulmonary function. Anesth Analg 60:46–52, 1981.
13. Eagle KA, Berger PB, Calkins H, et al: ACC/AHA guideline update for perioperative cardiovascular evaluation for noncardiac surgery—executive summary: A report of the American College of Cardiology/American Heart Association Task Force on Practice Guidelines (Committee to Update the 1996 Guidelines on Perioperative Cardiovascular Evaluation for Noncardiac Surgery). J Am Coll Cardiol 39:542–553, 2002.
14. Fiore M: Treating Tobacco Use and Dependence, Vol. 2000. U.S. Department of Health and Human Services, 2000.
15. Gass GD, Olsen GN: Preoperative pulmonary function testing to predict postoperative morbidity and mortality. Chest 89:127–135, 1986.
16. Gomi K, Oguchi M, Hirokawa Y, et al: Process and preliminary outcome of a patterns-of-care study of esophageal cancer in Japan: Patients treated with surgery and radiotherapy. Int J Radiat Oncol Biol Phys 56:813–822, 2003.
17. Hlatky MA, Boineau RE, Higginbotham MB, et al: A brief self-administered questionnaire to determine functional capacity (the Duke Activity Status Index). Am J Cardiol 64:651–654, 1989.
18. Hulscher JB, van Sandick JW, de Boer AG, et al: Extended transthoracic resection compared with limited transhiatal resection for adenocarcinoma of the esophagus. N Engl J Med 347:1662–1669, 2002.
19. Kearney DJ, Lee TH, Reilly JJ, et al: Assessment of operative risk in patients undergoing lung resection: Importance of predicted pulmonary function. Chest 105:753–759, 1994.
20. Mariette C, Finzi L, Fabre S, et al: Factors predictive of complete resection of operable esophageal cancer: A prospective study. Ann Thorac Surg 75:1720–1726, 2003.
21. Meyers JR, Lembeck L, O'Kane H, Baue AE: Changes in functional residual capacity of the lung after operation. Arch Surg 110:576–583, 1975.

22. Morice RC, Peters EJ, Ryan MB, et al: Exercise testing in the evaluation of patients at high risk for complications from lung resection. Chest 101:356–361, 1992.

23. Olsen GN, Bolton JW, Weiman DS, Hornung CA: Stair climbing as an exercise test to predict the postoperative complications of lung resection. Two years' experience. Chest 99:587–590, 1991.

24. Olsen GN, Bolton JW, Weiman DS, Hornung CA: Stair climbing as an exercise test to predict the postoperative complications of lung resection. Two years' experience. Chest 99:587-590, 1991.

25. Pate P, Tenholder MF, Griffin JP, et al: Preoperative assessment of the high-risk patient for lung resection. Ann Thorac Surg 61:1494–1500, 1996.

26. Ploeg AJ, Kappetein AP, van Tongeren RB, et al: Factors associated with perioperative complications and long-term results after pulmonary resection for primary carcinoma of the lung. Eur J Cardiothorac Surg 23:26–29, 2003.

27. Pollock M, Roa J, Benditt J, Celli B. Estimation of ventilatory reserve by stair climbing. A study in patients with chronic airflow obstruction. Chest 104:1378–1383, 1993.

28. Preoperative pulmonary function testing. American College of Physicians [comment]. Ann Intern Med 112:793–794, 1990.

29. Reilly JJ: Preparing for pulmonary resection: Preoperative evaluation of patients. Chest 112:206S–208S, 1997.

30. Reilly JJ Jr: Evidence-based preoperative evaluation of candidates for thoracotomy. Chest 116:474S–476S, 1999.

31. Richter Larsen K, Svendsen UG, et al: Exercise testing in the preoperative evaluation of patients with bronchogenic carcinoma. Eur Respir J 10:1559–1565, 1997.

32. Schuurmans MM, Diacon AH, Bolliger CT: Functional evaluation before lung resection. Clin Chest Med 23:159–172, 2002.

33. Skillrud DM, Offord KP, Miller RD: Higher risk of lung cancer in chronic obstructive pulmonary disease. A prospective, matched, controlled study. Ann Intern Med 105:503–507, 1986.

34. Smetana GW. Preoperative pulmonary evaluation. N Engl J Med 340:937–944, 1999.

35. Smetana GW: Preoperative pulmonary assessment of the older adult. Clin Geriatr Med 19:35–55, 2003.

36. Smith TP, Kinasewitz GT, Tucker WY, et al: Exercise capacity as a predictor of post-thoracotomy morbidity. Am Rev Respir Dis 129:730–734, 1984.

37. Tockman MS, Anthonisen NR, Wright EC, Donithan MG: Airways obstruction and the risk for lung cancer. Ann Intern Med 106:512–518, 1987.

38. Wang JS, Abboud RT, Evans KG, et al: Role of CO diffusing capacity during exercise in the preoperative evaluation for lung resection. Am J Respir Crit Care Med 162:1435–1444, 2000.

39. Wernly JA, DeMeester TR, Kirchner PT, et al: Clinical value of quantitative ventilation-perfusion lung scans in the surgical management of bronchogenic carcinoma. J Thorac Cardiovasc Surg 80:535–543, 1980.

Perioperative Care of Patients Undergoing Thoracic Surgery

Elisabeth U. Dexter and Leslie J. Kohman

Elisabeth U. Dexter and Leslie J. Kohman

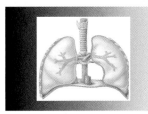

CHAPTER 4

▶ INTRODUCTION

Thoracic surgical patients require careful attention in the perioperative period. Often these patients are elderly, have baseline abnormalities of lung function, and have other comorbid diseases. Postoperatively, factors that impact patient recovery include removal of all or a portion of a lung, painful incision(s), change in the shape and mechanics of the thoracic cage, and/or reconfiguration of gastrointestinal continuity causing suboptimal pulmonary function, decreased appetite, decreased mobility and strength, and increased risk of aspiration.

Perioperative care of the thoracic surgical patient requires a team approach. The surgeon is uniquely qualified to be the captain of the team because he or she is aware of the patient's functional status preoperatively, operative findings and events, and the postoperative anatomy that will dictate each patient's needs and restrictions. Members of the team include the surgeon, anesthesiologist, pain management specialist, nurse, respiratory therapist, physical therapist, occupational therapist, speech pathologist, dietician, and social worker.

▶ PREOPERATIVE PREPARATION

An in-depth review of preoperative assessment is covered in Chapter 3. Medical optimization for thoracotomy patients includes adjustment of medications for chronic obstructive

44 pulmonary disease (COPD) including administration of bronchodilators and steroids and treatment of acute bronchitis or pneumonia.[15] Total resolution may not be possible if the pneumonia is due to a postobstructive process secondary to lung mass or chronic aspiration from gastroesophageal reflux disease. Patients with borderline pulmonary function benefit from pulmonary rehabilitation that increases their exercise tolerance and respiratory muscular strength prior to resection.[73,100] Smoking cessation is of great importance. Support groups, counseling, nicotine replacement therapy, and wellbutrin therapy are available and successful.[59] If there is no smoking cessation program associated with the provider's hospital, programs can be located by calling the local American Lung Association. Timing of smoking cessation is just as important as cessation itself. Recently, Vaporciyan et al showed that patients who quit smoking 4 weeks or more prior to operation had a lower incidence of pulmonary complications compared with patients who continued to smoke or quit less than 4 weeks prior to pneumonectomy.[97] Historically, 6 weeks of smoking cessation prior to surgery is recommended to avoid the copious bronchorrhea that accompanies regeneration of the cilia that clear mucus between 2 and 4 weeks after smoking cessation.[23]

Additional comorbid diseases that need to be managed include coronary artery disease, diabetes mellitus, failure to thrive/malnutrition, and myasthenia gravis.[15,62] The goal of preoperative preparation of patients with myasthenia gravis is to reduce the risk of myasthenic crisis, which is acute respiratory muscle malfunction leading to respiratory failure. Doses of steroids and cholinesterase medications should be tailored to the patient's symptoms. More aggressive and rapid therapies include infusion of intravenous (IV) immune globulin and plasmapheresis.[62,93] Plasmapheresis usually requires multiple exchanges and is recommended for patients with a vital capacity <2.0 liters.

Prophylaxis

Atrial Fibrillation

The incidence of postoperative atrial fibrillation ranges between 20 and 40% in thoracic surgical patients. It increases the risk of stroke and prolongs postoperative length of stay.[31] The only consistent risk factor in surgical patients is age >60 years.[2] Numerous studies on the prevention and treatment of postoperative atrial fibrillation exist, but the majority were performed for cardiac surgical patients. There is no superior regimen for preventing postoperative atrial fibrillation in thoracic surgical patients. Meta-analysis shows that β-blocker, d-sotalol, and amiodarone are all effective in lowering the incidence of postoperative atrial fibrillation. Only amiodarone had a significant decrease in length of stay by 0.9 days.[32] There have been reports of acute pulmonary toxicity from amiodarone therapy in postoperative cardiothoracic surgery patients, but no randomized trial has been done to study this phenomenon.[5,82] Digoxin has been tried for prophylaxis, but is not effective.[45] Intravenous diltiazem was studied specifically in thoracic surgical patients and almost halved the incidence of postoperative atrial fibrillation (15 vs. 25% for placebo patients).[2] Studies of magnesium for prophylaxis and therapy of postoperative atrial fibrillation have mixed results.[16,40,78] For atrial fibrillation with rapid ventricular response, rate control is the main priority. Conversion back to normal sinus rhythm is a secondary, but not immediate goal. It is our recommendation that prophylaxis for atrial fibrillation for patients over age 60 years be incorporated into each institution's clinical pathway using one of the known effective agents (see Table 4-1).

Deep Venous Thrombosis

A majority of thoracic surgery patients are slow to move postoperatively secondary to pain, respiratory distress, and age. A recent review of multiple studies estimated a 10–30% incidence of deep venous thrombosis in medical and surgical intensive care patients.[6] The current recommendations for deep venous thrombosis prophylaxis from the American College of Chest Physicians vary depending upon patient risk (Tables 4-2, 4-3, and 4-4).[48] Low-dose unfractionated heparin use does not interfere with epidural catheter placement or removal. However, low-molecular-weight heparin should be held for 12–24 h prior to epidural placement or removal to decrease the risk of hematoma formation.

Stress Ulceration and Gastritis

Stress ulceration or gastritis can lead to gastrointestinal bleeding, nausea, vomiting, and poor appetite. There are several strategies for stress ulcer prophylaxis. Sucralfate decreases the risk of nosocomial pneumonia compared to the other agents.[30] There is no intravenous formulation of sucralfate, so it can be given only to patients who can have oral or intragastric medications and it must be given four times a day.[13] Histamine-2 (H_2) blockers can be given orally or intravenously. A recent randomized study of ranitidine showed that it decreased the number of gastroesophageal reflux episodes versus placebo for patients in the lateral decubitus position.[1] With the prevention of gastroesophageal reflux, the incidence of postoperative pneumonia from aspiration may also be diminished, although there are no data to definitively prove this. H_2 blockers interfere with the metabolism of medications that pass through the P-450 pathway, and dosage of other medications may need to be adjusted.[13,42] Proton pump inhibitors work well to reduce acid and have fewer side effects/interactions than sucralfate and H_2 blockers.[42] Eating, or if that is not possible, enteral feeding is also helpful for prevention of stress ulcers postoperatively. However, data suggest that enteral intake alone is not sufficient prophylaxis in critically ill patients. It should be used in conjunction with drug therapy.[65]

Antimicrobial

A properly timed dose of a first-generation cephalosporin is efficacious in preventing wound infections from skin pathogens.[75] However, use of a second-generation cephalosporin with continuation for 48 h has been shown to decrease the incidence of empyemas and bronchopneumonia postoperatively and to provide wound infection prophylaxis to thoracic surgical patients and is our recommendation.[12,41] Duration of postoperative administration of antibiotics is controversial. Some surgeons prefer to use a

Table 4–1				
Prophylaxis for Atrial Fibrillation[a]				
Agent	*Dose*	*Route*	*Frequency*	*Duration*
Propranolol[71]	10 mg	PO	Q 6 h	Start 1–2 weeks preop to attain HR of 60–70 bpm
Sotalol[51]	80–120 mg	PO	BID	Start 48 h preop; D/C on POD 4
Amiodarone[34]	200 mg then 200 mg	PO PO	TID QD	Start 7 days preop; while hospitalized, D/C on day of discharge
Diltiazem[2]	0.25 mg/kg over 30 min then 0.1 mg/kg/h for 24 h then 120 mg SR	IV PO	 QD	Start in recovery room D/C 14 days postop
Magnesium[40]	96 meq over first 24 h then 72 meq over next 72 h	IV	Continuous infusion in IVF	Start immediately postoperatively; D/C after 4 days

[a]PO, orally; IV, intravenous; Q, every; BID, twice a day; TID, three times a day; QD, every day; IVF, intravenous fluid; HR, heart rate; D/C, discontinue; POD, postoperative day.

first-generation cephalosporin as long as thoracostomy tubes are in place, but there is no evidence that there is decreased wound infection or empyema with this practice and it should be abandoned.[56,75]

Miscellaneous

Bowel preparation may be desired prior to complicated gastroesophageal operations during which colon interposition may be needed. Blood products are reserved for patients who have anemia due to preoperative chemotherapy, chronic disease, phlebotomy, or bleeding. If a surgery is 4–6 weeks in the future, erythropoietin is efficacious in increasing hemoglobin level and decreasing the amount of blood transfusion required.[64] Warfarin therapy for patients with prosthetic heart valves, low ejection fractions, and/or arrhythmias should be stopped 4–5 days ahead of surgery and subcutaneous low-molecular-weight heparin substituted up to 12 h prior to operation.

Nothing is more frustrating than having an operation delayed because of poor planning and unavailability of needed equipment. Often hospitals have certain pieces of equipment that are used by several different services. It is prudent to reserve ahead of time to ensure the necessary equipment is available and is functioning properly. Examples include laparoscopes/thoracoscopes, video equipment, lasers, harmonic scalpel, robots, and retractors.

INTRAOPERATIVE CARE

Good communication with the anesthesiologist or anesthetist is key. Airway management should be discussed beforehand if there are special circumstances. The whole operative team should know the plan of the operation including (1) position and position changes, (2) instrument, equipment, and medication needs, i.e., harmonic scalpel, drainage tubes, local anesthetic, (3) general length of the operation, and (4) postoperative disposition, i.e., extubation versus postoperative ventilation. Single lung ventilation during thoracotomy or thoracoscopy is accomplished by a double lumen tube, bronchial blocker, or Univent tube.[22]

Monitoring

Different operations will require different levels of monitoring.[15] Electrocardiogram (ECG) monitoring and continuous pulse oximetry are necessary in all cases. An arterial line is placed if there is a need for multiple blood draws. Continuous arterial pressure monitoring is useful during procedures involving mediastinal dissection such as transhiatal esophagectomy to gauge cardiac or great vessel compression.

Intravenous access should be appropriate for the level of the procedure. Anticipated blood loss is rarely enough to justify the need of large bore central lines. However, adequate access is necessary before the procedure starts since the arms, chest, and groins are often inaccessible for line placement during operation. In emergency situations, placement of a large bore line in the operative field into the subclavian vein, superior vena cava, inferior vena cava, or azygous vein can be performed.

Body Temperature

Mild hypothermia has been shown to increase wound infection, blood loss and transfusion requirements, and cardiac events including ventricular tachycardia, cardiac arrest, and

Table 4–2

Additional Risk Factors for Deep Venous Thrombosis[a]

Increasing age

Prolonged immobility, stroke, or paralysis

Previous deep venous thrombosis

Cancer and cancer therapy

Major surgery especially involving the abdomen, pelvis, and lower extremities

Trauma especially with fractures of the hip, pelvis, or leg

Obesity

Varicose veins

Cardiac dysfunction

Indwelling central venous catheter

Inflammatory bowel disease

Nephrotic syndrome

Pregnancy or estrogen use

Thrombophilic disorders

[a]From the Sixth American College of Chest Physicians Consensus Conference on Antithrombotic Therapy.

myocardial infarction.[44,63,87] Heat loss through thoracotomy, sternotomy, and/or laparotomy incisions can be lessened by keeping the room temperature greater than 21° C, using airway heating and humidification devices, covering portions of the patient not in the operative field, and using forced-air warming blankets. Warm saline lavage intrapleurally and intraperitoneally can also be performed. Rarely are intravenous fluid warmers needed.

Positioning

Careful positioning of the patient is of utmost importance in the operating room. The surgeon needs to ensure adequate access for the planned operation as well as any possible need for counterincisions or chest wall resection. Use of muscle flaps often requires planning ahead to protect vascular sup-

ply and leave adequate skin coverage. Padding to prevent neuropathy includes use of an axillary roll for the decubitus position and padding of both arms. Stability of the patient during the operation can be achieved using a deflatable beanbag, sand bags, laminectomy rolls, and security straps or tapes. Lithotomy position also requires careful positioning to prevent postoperative neuropathy.[69]

Drainage

If the planned operation is scheduled to take longer than 3 h and/or an epidural catheter is used, a bladder catheter should be placed. Orogastric and/or nasogastric tube drainage is important for decompression during esophageal and gastric operations. The semirigid tube can be helpful for localization during reoperations or within radiated fields with abundant scar tissue or fibrous reaction.

The viscosity of the substance being drained dictates the size/shape necessary for adequate drainage of the pleural space. Smaller anterior tubes are used to drain air. Larger, posterior tubes, including preformed 90° angled tubes, are useful for dependent drainage along the diaphragm of blood, pus, chyle, or exudative fluid. One pleural tube is adequate drainage after routine lobar resection if it is positioned posterior and to the apex of the pleural cavity to drain both fluid and air. Additional chest tubes are used for empyema or hemothorax drainage, expected large air leakage from friable parenchyma, or fistula drainage. Use of a drainage tube after pneumonectomy is controversial. Reasons cited for leaving a chest tube after pneumonectomy include ability to monitor bleeding and ability to manipulate intrapleural pressure and adjust mediastinal shifting by instilling or removing air. These are removed intraoperatively after the patient is placed supine, in the recovery room, or on the first postoperative day. Many surgeons leave no drainage tube after pneumonectomy and encounter no increased morbidity. It is our recommendation that no drainage tube be left after pneumonectomy unless bleeding is of significant concern. We question the sterility and advisability of adding or removing air from the postpneumonectomy pleural space.

A gastrostomy tube is useful if prolonged stomach drainage is needed. This may decrease the risk of aspiration that is theoretically present from having a tube traversing and stenting the upper esophagus or neoesophageal conduit open. A gastrostomy tube is more comfortable for the patient than an indwelling nasoenteral tube. A jejunostomy tube is placed as access for nutrition and medicine administration if failure to thrive or a prolonged period of nothing by mouth (NPO) status is anticipated.

If flaps are created, drains to prevent seroma formation are placed. If there is concern of leakage of the gastrointestinal tract, bronchopleural fistula, empyema, or chylothorax, good drainage can prevent systemic infection and allow time for healing and nutritional support.

Miscellaneous

The surgeon must also ensure that sample and specimen collection is done properly. Careful labeling and delivery of frozen sections are paramount in determining resection margins and operative resectability and/or staging. Intraoperative communication with the pathologist per-

Table 4–3

Risk Groups for Deep Venous Thrombosis[a]

Low risk	Moderate risk	High risk	Highest risk
Minor surgery, age <40 years, no additional risks	Minor surgery, additional risks	Minor surgery, age >60 years, or additional risks	Major surgery, age >40 years with prior deep venous thrombosis or hypercoaguable state
	or	or	or
	Minor surgery, age 40–60 years, no additional risks	Major surgery, age >40 years, or additional risks	Hip or knee arthroplasty, hip fracture surgery
	or		or
	Major surgery, age ≤40 years, or additional risks		Major trauma
			or
			Spinal cord injury

[a]From the Sixth American College of Chest Physicians Consensus Conference on Antithrombotic Therapy.

forming frozen section may be necessary prior to proceeding with the next portion of an operation. If possible, orienting the specimen and viewing the frozen section with the pathologist are recommended. Cultures for bacterial, fungal, and acid-fast bacilli need to be processed and collected in the correct specimen containers/mediums.

▶ POSTOPERATIVE CARE

As in many other specialties, clinical pathways serve to improve quality of care. They have the added benefit of reducing cost.[79,102,105] Almost all thoracic surgical patients can be transferred from the recovery room to a step-down unit or surgical ward instead of an intensive care unit. For thymectomy, segmentectomy, lobectomy, pneumonectomy, lung volume reduction, and esophagectomy patients, telemetry and continuous pulse oximetry are recommended. The arterial line placed during surgery is transduced until the day after operation.

Fluid Management

Fluid administration for lung resection patients must be determined on an individual basis. Vasodilatation secondary to use of local anesthetic in epidural catheters and/or use of antihypertensive medications justify careful administration of fluid to maintain blood pressure and adequate end-organ perfusion. In a review of published reports of postoperative pulmonary edema, Slinger found that multiple factors were

likely contributors to the formation of the edema.[91] The review gives guidelines regarding postoperative fluid management: (1) a maximum of 20 ml/kg fluid be given intravenously for the first 24 postoperative hours, (2) acceptance of average urine output of 0.5 ml/kg/h the first 24 h, and (3) use of vasopressors if tissue perfusion is inadequate and the 20 ml/kg maximum of fluid administration has already been given. Other manipulations such as lowering the dose of the epidural infusion or removing the local anesthetic component of the epidural infusion and leaving only narcotic may decrease sympathetic blockade and vascular vasodilatation. There are no randomized trials that show a benefit of colloid administration versus crystalloid administration for fluid boluses.[86]

Blood Administration

There is no threshold hemoglobin or hematocrit that has been documented for recommendation for transfusion. In critically ill patients with cardiovascular disease, a hemoglobin level of 7.0–9.0 g/dl is well tolerated.[54] Although intuition argues that a higher hemoglobin level provides better oxygen delivery, the increased oxygen extraction by most organs and tissues when stressed negates the need for a higher hemoglobin level. This is not true for the heart, which extracts most of the oxygen delivered under nonstressed physiological conditions and requires increases in blood flow to increase oxygen delivery with physiological stress. For critically ill patients with *acute* cardiac ischemia, increased mortality was found with a restrictive transfusion protocol.[55]

Table 4–4

Recommendations for Prophylaxis[a]

Risk	Recommendation
Low	Aggressive mobilization
Moderate	Heparin 5000 U SQ 1–2 h preop and then Q 12 h
	Enoxaparin 20 mg SQ 1–2 h preop and then Q 24 h
	Dalteparin 2500 U SQ 1–2 h preop and then Q 24 h
	Graded elastic hose
	Sequential compression devices
High	Heparin 5000 U SQ 1–2 h preop and then Q 8 h
	Enoxaparin 40 mg SQ 1–2 h preop and then Q 24 h
	Dalteparin 5000 U SQ 8–12 h preop and then Q 24 h
	Sequential compression devices
Highest	Graded elastic hose and sequential compression devices and enoxaparin or heparin SQ

[a]From the Sixth American College of Chest Physicians Consensus Conference on Antithrombotic Therapy.

Medications

Each patient's preoperative medications should be reviewed prior to restarting them postoperatively. Often antihypertensive medications will need to be held for several doses until fluid shifting and reequilibrium are attained to prevent continued hypotension. We recommend restarting β-blocker therapy as soon as possible after the operation to prevent rebound tachycardia from withdrawal. This also decreases the occurrence of atrial fibrillation and of rapid ventricular response should postoperative atrial fibrillation occur. Administration of postoperative antibiotics for more than 48 h has not been proven definitively to decrease the amount of pneumonia or wound infection in thoracic surgical patients.[56]

Many patients suffer from nausea after general anesthesia and/or postoperative pain medications. Antiemetics such as metoclopramide, ondansetron, promethazine, trimethobenzamide, and prochlorperazine can help. Stress ulcer prophylaxis is started preoperatively and used postoperatively. These agents in combination with enteral intake maximize protection. For low-risk patients, stopping the pharmacological agent once consistent oral intake is established is likely to be safe. For higher risk patients (see Table 4-5)[42] medications should be continued even after intake is started.[65] Esophagectomy patients have a high risk of reflux.[53,67] Histamine-2 receptor blockers or proton pump inhibitors should be continued in those patients who demonstrate reflux on barium swallow tests postoperatively, have symptoms of heartburn, or have a history of Barrett's disease. Vagotomized patients may benefit from the prokinetic effects of erythromycin or metoclopramide. However, erythromycin may cause gastrointestinal upset and metoclopramide can produce extrapyramidal symptoms. Use of low-molecular-weight heparin, low-dose unfractionated heparin, or sequential compression devices continues until the patient is reliably walking at least 4 times a day for patients with a low risk for deep venous thrombosis. In higher risk patients, a combination of pharmacological and mechanical prophylaxis should be used until the same ambulatory criteria.[48] The constipating effects of narcotic medications and decreased motility dictate the need for an aggressive bowel management protocol.

Analgesia

Pain control is one of the most important aspects of postoperative care for thoracic surgery patients. Studies have shown the benefit of continuous and patient-controlled

Table 4–5

Risk Factors for Development of Stress Ulcers[a,b]

Burns >35% BSA	Major surgery
Shock	Multisystem organ failure
Anoxia	High-dose vasopressor
Hypotension	Mechanical ventilation
Sepsis	Peritonitis
Multiple trauma	Malignancy
Brain injury GCS <7	Lengthy ICU stay
Coagulopathy	Poor nutrition

[a]From Flannery and Tucker.[42]
[b]BSA, body surface area; GCS, Glasgow Coma scale; ICU, intensive care unit.

epidural analgesia on pain control and the potential benefit on pulmonary function.[19,72,89] Patient-controlled intravenous analgesia is also effective for postthoracotomy and laparotomy pain.[92] Nonsteroidal antiinflammatory agents such as ketorolac have been effective adjuncts with either epidural or patient-controlled intravenous analgesia.[39,80,90] Perhaps studies in the future will support use of COX-2 inhibitors, which may have fewer antiplatelet and gastrointestinal side effects. Other methods of pain relief that have mixed reports with small study size include intercostal blocks,[46,83] phrenic nerve infiltration,[85] transcutaneous electrical nerve stimulation,[11] and intrapleural or extrapleural nerve block.[7,29] Cryoanalgesia of the intercostal nerves resulted in paresthesias and is not recommended.[18,58,84]

Nutrition

Adequate nutrition is paramount in the postoperative period.[20,74] Most lung resection patients can be started on clear liquids the evening of surgery. A more cautious approach may be necessary if there is concern about a difficult airway or a higher risk of respiratory failure. Nausea and vomiting are fairly common after general anesthesia, and narcotic medications may magnify the problem. If liquids are tolerated, the patient's diet can be advanced starting the day after surgery. After uneventful laparoscopic fundoplication, clear liquids can be given the evening of surgery. These patients need to be counseled preoperatively and/or postoperatively about taking most of their fluid between meals, eating smaller portions more frequently during the day, and avoiding foods such as dry bread, raw vegetables, large chunks of meat, and foods/fluids that increase gas production in the immediate postoperative period. A list of eating tips and foods to avoid for patients to take home with them at discharge is recommended. Dysphagia due to swelling of a complete wrap may occur after the operation. This can lead to inability to advance the diet beyond liquids for several days to weeks.[101] If this persists past several weeks and the patient is losing weight, the need for dilatation or investigation for a complication such as a slipped wrap, stricture, or previously undiagnosed motility disorder must be considered and investigated.

Oral intake after esophagectomy is started after a confirmatory test for leakage and blockage such as a barium swallow test or grape juice test is passed.[95] Most surgeons wait 5–7 days postoperatively.[50,105] Surgeon preference, problems encountered during the operation, and neoadjuvant therapy will influence when the study is obtained, although recent data showed no evidence of increased anastomotic leakage when neoadjuvant treatment was given.[36] If the test results are favorable, clear liquids are started and the diet is advanced as tolerated. Counseling about expected changes in eating habits, dietary intake, jejunostomy tube feeding, and weight stabilization is performed. Placement of a jejunostomy tube during esophagectomy allows feeding enterally 24–48 h after operation. Tube feedings are generally started at a low rate such as 20 ml/h and advanced to a goal rate to provide total caloric and protein needs over the next 48 h. If a jejunostomy tube is not placed, total parenteral nutrition administration until oral intake is tolerated can be considered.

Respiratory Therapy

The most common complications after thoracic surgery are related to the pulmonary system. Vigilant pulmonary care postoperatively decreases the incidence of complications.[41,43,50] Incentive spirometry, chest physiotherapy including clapping, postural drainage, and vibratory therapy aid in mobilizing mucous secretions and allowing patients to clear their own secretions. Cough can be stimulated and secretions suctioned by placing a soft suction catheter through the nose and into the trachea. Studies have advocated placement of a minitracheostomy in high-risk patients and have shown favorable results in reducing pulmonary complications.[14,98] Ambulation is an excellent method of decreasing atelectasis. Nebulized albuterol is very helpful in curtailing or preventing bronchospastic episodes. If a patient has had multiple manipulations of the upper airway and there is concern about edema and stridor, intravenous and aerosolized steroids and aerosolized racemic epinephrine are effective in reducing edema.[76]

Wound Care

Incision care usually is routine if the skin is closed. Open wounds historically are packed with gauze moistened with saline, dilute antibiotic solution, sodium hypochlorite (Dakin's) solution, acetic acid solution, or dilute Betadine solution. Newer dressings including silicone-impregnated dressings, thin polyurethane films, hydrocolloids, alginates, polyurethane foams, and hydrogels are available.[24] Assessment of the features of the dressing needed such as absorbency of fluid, debriding qualities, and frequency of dressing change will help determine which type of dressing to use. Vacuum dressings can be placed in clean wounds and

50 speed the healing process.[4] Open chests for bronchopleural fistula are packed with gauze soaked in antibiotic solution.[35,49] If muscle or skin flaps are raised and there is potential for seroma formation, drains may be left and binders or ace bandages can be considered. Depending upon the muscle rotation used and the tautness of the closure, restriction of range of motion may be required to prevent tension and dislodgement or compromise of flap vascular supply for several days. When tracheal resection with primary anastomosis with release procedures are done, a sturdy skin stitch from the chin to the anterior chest will remind the patient to keep the head flexed to allow healing of the tracheal anastomosis with less tension.[52] For wounds that are difficult to heal such as those within previous radiation fields, hyperbaric oxygen therapy can be considered.[99] A minimum oxygen concentration must be achieved for any benefit of this cumbersome and costly wound care alternative. No randomized, blinded studies have shown definite benefit of hyperbaric oxygen therapy for wound healing except for osteoradionecrosis.

Management of Drainage Tubes

Placement and removal of chest tubes should be standardized by protocol after lung resection. Tubes are left in while any air leak remains, but recent studies indicate that earlier transition from water suction to water seal is not harmful and may promote quicker resolution of parenchymal air leakage.[26,27,66] Fluid drainage of 300–400 ml or less per 24 h is acceptable for chest tube removal after lung resection.[26] Chest tube removal after pleurodesis for malignant pleural effusion needs a stricter volume requirement as these patients are known to have problems absorbing pleural fluid normally. Chest tube removal after drainage of chylothorax or empyema must be tailored to a particular patient's course. If there is any concern about anastomotic leak in the chest or mediastinum after esophageal resection or tracheal reconstruction, tubes should be left until resolution of the leakage. Mediastinal tubes are left after median sternotomy is done for removal of bilateral lung tumors, lung reduction surgery, or mediastinal mass resection.

A nasogastric tube is left after esophagectomy and for complicated benign esophageal operations. The tube is removed when drainage from the gastrointestinal tract is less that 300–500 ml/24 h and there is no concern of anastomotic leak.

Bladder catheters are placed for drainage and as a measure of adequate end-organ perfusion in patients having operations longer than 3 h. Patients, especially elderly men, who have an epidural catheter often have difficulty voiding and usually will require the bladder catheter until the epidural is discontinued.

Physical Therapy

Exercise therapy after lung resection benefits the patients by decreasing pulmonary complications, restoring mobility and independence, and decreasing the potential for deep venous thrombosis. Pulmonary rehabilitation is designed specifically to help patients clear secretions, strengthen respiratory muscles, and provide cardiopulmonary exercise.[28,41,73,100] A patient who requires continuous chest tube suction can exercise on a stationary bicycle brought to the hospital room.

► MANAGEMENT OF COMPLICATIONS

Early Complications

Respiratory Failure

Atelectasis/Pneumonia

The most common complication after a thoracic operation is respiratory failure. When complications are due to atelectasis and retained secretions, treatment with aggressive pulmonary toilet, postural drainage, incentive spirometry, nasotracheal suction, ambulation, and nebulizer treatments will aid in avoidance of developing pneumonia. If pneumonia is suspected, empiric treatment with a second-generation cephalosporin is justified as radiographic changes of pneumonia may lag temporally.[41] Ferdinand and Shennib[41] advocate using bronchoscopy with lavage and/or protected brush for diagnosis of postthoracotomy pneumonia. Antibiotic therapy can be adjusted after culture results return. The worsening spiral of need for intubation can sometimes be avoided with bronchoscopy to remove thick tenacious secretions or retained clot. The benefits of mini-tracheostomy have already been mentioned.[14,98]

Pulmonary Edema

Pulmonary edema in lobectomy patients is serious, but can usually be treated with diuresis. Postpneumonctomy pulmonary edema may be fatal. Aggressive respiratory care including intubation may be necessary to manage a patient with postpneumonectomy pulmonary edema, which has a mortality rate of >50%.[91] Postpneumonectomy pulmonary edema should always be considered, and avoidance of excessive fluid administration is important.[91] Urine output should be accepted at 0.5 ml/kg/h the night of surgery and excess fluid administration should be avoided. Measures to keep pulmonary artery pressures low should be instituted. The patient should be given adequate fraction of inspired oxygen (FIO_2), and hypercarbia and pain causing splinting and atelectasis need to be avoided.[91] Routine administration of diuretic starting in the recovery room can be considered.

Acute Respiratory Distress Syndrome

Acute respiratory distress syndrome (ARDS) is a dreaded complication after thoracic surgery and is due to multiple etiologies. Aggressive support with reintubation if necessary and administration of positive end-expiratory pressure (PEEP) and adequate FIO_2 to support the patient while the lung recovers is important. There is no proven medication that helps ARDS at this time. Steroids can be tried and given for a short course.[70] Prostaglandins and prone positioning improve arterial oxygenation, but no randomized controlled studies to show increased survival with these treatments have been performed.[47,57,68] Treatment of underlying pneumonia helps. Careful attention to other organ systems and nutritional support give the patient's lungs time to recover. The mortality rate for ARDS with no other organ system affected remains 60%.

If a patient displays signs of hypoxia and the etiologies mentioned above are not the cause, pulmonary embolism, myocardial ischemia, arrhythmia, and heart failure need to be investigated.

Cardiac Complications

Myocardial Infarction

Myocardial infarction should be treated with oxygen therapy, ECG monitoring, morphine, and aspirin if bleeding is not a large concern. Inotropic or pressor support may be needed in the immediate postoperative period. If there is evidence of continued ischemia and an adequate blood pressure, nitroglycerin is recommended. If the patient's blood pressure cannot be adequately supported with medications, intraaortic balloon pump placement should be considered. Patients with continuing ischemia and hemodynamic instability should be taken for cardiac catheterization. Anticoagulants such as heparin and/or GIIb/IIIa platelet inhibitors are recommended for unstable angina, but recent surgery and risk of bleeding may preclude their use. The surgeon must use his or her judgment regarding the risks and benefits of these drug interventions after surgery.[9] Arrhythmias should be treated per ACLS protocol if the patient is hemodynamically unstable.[33]

Atrial Fibrillation

The immediate goal of treatment of postoperative atrial fibrillation is rate control (see Table 4-6). When atrial fibrillation occurs while a patient is on β-blocker, d-sotalol,

amiodarone, magnesium, or diltiazem prophylaxis, ventricular response rate is significantly lower than that of placebo.[2,16,32] If the patient is on one of the above agents and continues with a rapid ventricular response, combination therapy may be necessary for rate control and/or cardioversion. Careful monitoring of the ECG is necessary if drug combinations are used. The shortest acting β-blocker available is esmolol. It requires a loading dose and administration by continuous infusion because of its short half-life. It is more costly than other β-blockers, but can be more easily titrated, and its effects dissipate quickly if discontinued should the patient develop hypotension. Digoxin can be given for rate control, but a load must be given in multiple doses over several hours to achieve an adequate serum level. It is inexpensive and has no negative inotropic or vasodilating effects. Of the calcium channel blockers, diltiazem has become favored for rate control of atrial fibrillation because it causes less vasodilatation leading to hypotension.

Amiodarone has a long half-life and variable solubility and uptake when given orally. Onset of action is about 0.5–3 h after an intravenous load. Oral loading can be done if started preoperatively. Magnesium is poorly absorbed orally and is usually given intravenously perioperatively. Sotalol can be given orally or intravenously for atrial fibrillation. The d-enantiomer works as a class III agent, not as a β-blocker. All of the oral agents are safe to start as an outpatient if there is time preoperatively. Monitoring of pulmonary function is needed with amiodarone because of reported acute and chronic pulmonary toxicity. Sotalol may need to be

---

Table 4–6

Drug Treatment for Atrial Fibrillation/Flutter[a]

Agent	Dose	Route	Frequency	Duration
Digoxin	0.25 mg	IV	Q 4 h	4 doses
	then 0.25 mg	PO	QD	2 months
Diltiazem	0.25–0.35 mg/kg	IV	Q 10 min × 2 doses	Over 3 min
	then 5–20 mg/h	IV	Continuous	24 h
	then 120–360 mg SR	PO	QD	2 months
Esmolol	500 µg/kg then	IV	Loading dose	
	50–200 µg/h	IV	Continuous	Convert to other β-blocker when taking PO
Metoprolol	2.5–5.0 mg then	IV	Q 6 h	
	25–100 mg	PO	QD	When taking PO
Amiodarone	150 mg then	IV	Once	Over 20 min
	1 mg/min	IV	Continuous	For 8 h
	then 0.5 mg/min	IV	Continuous	For 16 h
	then 400 mg then	PO	BID	3 days
	200 mg	PO	QD	3 months
Sotalol	40–80 mg	PO	BID	3 months

[a]IV, Intravenous; PO, orally; Q, every; QD, every day; BID, twice a day.

52

withdrawn because of bradycardia and hypotension. Fortunately, new onset postoperative atrial fibrillation needs to be treated for only 6–12 weeks postoperatively. Anticoagulation will need to be instituted if the patient remains in atrial fibrillation, or in and out of atrial fibrillation for more than 48 h, to prevent thrombus formation and stroke. Rarely will cardioversion be necessary, but if it has been more than 48 h since the onset of atrial fibrillation, echocardiography should be performed to check for atrial thrombus. If present, cardioversion should not be performed.

Bleeding

Postoperative bleeding is monitored by chest tube output. Sudden occurrence of large volume, bloody drainage requires immediate reexploration to find and stop the source of bleeding. Less rapid bleeding of more than 100 ml/h for 2 h in a row is also excessive after thoracic surgery. Prothrombin time, partial thromboplastin time, platelet count, and if the patient has been on aspirin, bleeding time should be measured. If a coagulopathy exists, expeditious administration of deficient factors and keeping the patient normothermic should help slow or stop bleeding. If bleeding persists after correction of deficient factors, exploration for a bleeding source should be performed. If there is no coagulopathy or if hematoma causes significant mediastinal or lung compression, reexploration is necessary. Transfusion of packed red blood cells should be considered depending on the hemoglobin and hemodynamic condition of the patient.

Late Complications

Pulmonary Complications

A prolonged air leak is defined as one that lasts longer than 7 days postoperatively. If the patient has an emphysematous lung and the leak is small, several manipulations can be performed to encourage the leak to stop. If a pneumothorax or residual space still exists, placing the chest tube on higher suction by raising the water level in the suction chamber or closing the air vent to the suction chamber and controlling the amount of suction pressure from the wall source can be tried. Pressures above 40–60 mm Hg are not recommended. Placement of another chest tube may help fully reexpand the lung if the air leak is substantial. If no residual space exists, placement of the chest tube to water seal or on a Heimlich valve can encourage the leak to seal. A Heimlich valve may allow the patient to leave the hospital sooner. If the tube happens to be lying against a bleb or a raw surface of the lung, pulling the tube back several centimeters if it is possible to still leave the last side hole within the pleural cavity and twisting the tube 180° can be helpful. A blood patch can be attempted by injecting approximately 50 ml of the patient's own blood through the chest tube.[3,21] This has been shown to be effective in both partially and fully expanded lungs, but may need to be repeated several times and may increase the risk of empyema. Talc sclerosis through the chest tube can be performed, although this will cause pleural fusion making it difficult to reenter the chest cavity in the future.[27] If none of these works, the patient may need to be taken back to the operating room for leak closure. Air leak from the lung parenchyma can be trouble-

some because of friable lung tissue. Direct suturing with or without pledgets, use of fibrin sealants and glue,[10] and stapling of a leak with pericardial or polytetrafluoroethylene strips can be attempted.

Bronchial Fistula

Bronchopleural Fistula

If air is leaking from the bronchial stump, adequate chest tube drainage to prevent and/or drain empyema is important.[35,49] Bronchoscopy should be performed to look at the stump. If no large opening is seen, selective bronchography can be performed with 5–10 ml of propyliodone diluted 1:1 with saline.[103] Treatment may consist of operative closure or endobronchial closure. Fibrin glue has been used to seal leaks 4 mm in diameter or less endobronchially.[10,103] Special catheters are necessary to administer the separate components of the glue through the bronchoscope to the site of the leak. Coughing must be avoided for several hours after the glue is placed to allow the clot to set within the bronchus and prevent plug displacement. Absolute alcohol injection has also been reported to stop air leakage by causing swelling and sclerosis.[94] Redo thoracotomy and operative closure of the leaking bronchial stump may be needed.

The standard approach of Deschamps and colleagues includes trimming a long bronchial stump or debriding a poorly vascularized stump and then covering the stump with an extraskeletal muscle flap, i.e., serratus anterior or latissimus dorsi.[35] If there is no adequate vascularized tissue to primarily close a bronchopleural fistula, the extraskeletal muscle is sewn circumferentially to the stump for closure. Wide drainage to prevent unilateral empyema and contralateral soiling should be performed. This may include reopening the whole thoracotomy and performing open packing in the operating room every several days or under conscious sedation in the patient's room for several days to weeks until the cavity is clean. An Eloesser flap can be performed to facilitate open packing. Once clean, instillation of dilute antibiotic solution and airtight chest closure is performed. Mobilization of the remaining chest wall musculature and additional rib resection may be necessary to allow chest wall closure without tension. This alleviates a lifetime of packing an open chest, which predisposes to failure to thrive and recurrent bronchitis and pneumonia, and limits the patient's daily activities and lifestyle. Gharagozloo et al advocate a more aggressive approach. Pleural irrigation, intravenous antibiotics, and nutritional support are instituted. Instillation of dilute antibiotic solution (gentamicin 80 mg/liter, neomycin 500 mg/liter, polymyxin B 100 mg/liter) and airtight thoracotomy closure without drainage should be instituted when pleural cultures are negative.[49]

A persistent pleural space after lung resection can be prevented with a pleural tent if anticipated at the time of operation.[17,81] The apical portion of the parietal pleura is dissected from the chest wall and tacked to the upper intercostal muscle of the thoracotomy. The chest tubes are placed within the pleural tent. The pleura will adhere to the surface of the remaining lung and help seal over any leaking areas as well as decrease the volume of space that the remaining lung needs to fill. Either the space on top of the pleural tent in the apex will fill with serous fluid as after a pneumonectomy or the lung will expand to fill the whole space. This is also aided by elevation of the hemidiaphragm. Encouraging the diaphragm to rise can be accomplished by pneumoperitoneum.[81] Air can be instilled across the diaphragm with a needle during thoracotomy. Care not to damage the liver, spleen, or stomach must be taken. Injection of the phrenic nerve with local anesthetic causes a temporary paralysis that will also encourage the hemidiaphragm to rise. No respiratory compromise due to this practice has been reported. Filling of a residual space with healthy living tissue such as muscle or omentum can also be performed, although these are generally not done during resection because of the unlikely need for such extreme measures. Lastly, thoracoplasty can be performed, but is rarely used.

Bronchovascular Fistula

Bronchovascular fistula is a rare complication that needs to be considered after bronchoplastic procedures are performed.[61] Fistulas sometimes present with a herald bleed followed by massive hemoptysis. Salvage after a major bleed is rare and the best treatment is to decrease the chance of fistula formation by placing vascularized tissue such as intercostal or extraskeletal muscle, pleura, pericardium, or omentum between the pulmonary artery and the sutured bronchus. If massive hemoptysis does occur, an attempt at placing a double lumen tube to isolate the nonaffected lung from blood spillage may allow enough time for the chest to be opened and the bleeding controlled. More often, the patient dies of exsanguination or suffocation.

Postpneumonectomy Syndrome

Postpneumonectomy syndrome is torsion or compression of the trachea, bronchus, or pulmonary vasculature due to mediastinal shift after pneumonectomy. Tissue expander placement into the postpneumonectomy space is reported to reverse some of the mediastinal shift and its consequences.[38,96]

Wound Infection and Empyema

Wound infection after thoracotomy is very rare. The wound should be opened to allow adequate drainage. If the patient also has an empyema, tube drainage of the pleural cavity through a separate site can be attempted along with opening of the wound. If the infection goes through and through, it is better to take the patient back to the operating room for a thorough drainage, irrigation, debridement, and decortication. Strong consideration for leaving the skin open after redo thoracotomy should be given. If the cause of empyema is a bronchopleural fistula, the infection should be cleared and then definitive treatment of the bronchopleural fistula is undertaken as mentioned above.

Postthoracotomy Pain

Postthoracotomy pain remains a devastating and debilitating result after thoracotomy. This may occur because of nerve irritation or reflex sympathetic dystrophy. Typically medications such as narcotics and antiinflammatory drugs are not effective in relieving this pain syndrome. Transcutaneous electrical nerve stimulation (TENS), nerve block, and medications such as gabapentin can be helpful. Assistance from anesthesiology pain specialists can be invaluable, but these patients may require chronic therapy to relieve or attenuate their pain.

Complications after Esophageal Surgery

Many of the complications encountered after thoracotomy or lung resection, particularly the respiratory complications, also occur after esophageal surgery. In addition, esophageal surgery has its own unique complications.

Dysphagia

Difficulty swallowing is one of the most frequent complications after any esophageal surgery. At times it is self-limited and due to recent surgery. However, persistence of dysphagia after fundoplication, myotomy, or esophageal resection should be investigated. Workup usually includes barium swallow, motility studies, and/or esophagogastroduodenoscopy. Anatomical or functional abnormalities such as too tight a fundoplication, slipped fundoplication, recurrent herniation, motility disorder, and ulceration may be found. Treatment will depend on the cause of the dysphagia, but may range from simple observation to dilatation to medical treatment to need for reoperation.

Anastomotic Leak

Anastomotic leak or perforation occurs because of ischemia, distention of conduit and pressure at suture lines, poor nutrition, anastomotic tension, or technical problems.[60,77] The location and size of the leak determine the treatment. If a neck anastomosis is leaking, the neck wound is opened to allow drainage and healing over time. Stricture may form and require dilatation, but that is usually not incapacitating. The patient should generally be kept NPO during that time to reduce the amount of pressure and fluid draining past the hole. Antibiotics are not necessary if the hold is adequately drained. If the leak is more than a quarter of the circumference of the anastomosis, debriding unhealthy tissue and primary reclosure of the anastomosis should be considered.

If the anastomosis is within the chest, a leak may be contained in the space around the conduit, into the pleural cavity, or into the mediastinum. A leak into the pleural cavity can be drained with chest tubes. The patient is made NPO. Antibiotics should be administered unless the patient has no fever or leukocytosis and there is a well-formed drainage tract to the tube. Drainage into the mediastinum can be fatal and if the patient is toxic, reoperation for adequate drainage will have to be performed to prevent mediastinitis and sepsis. If there is adequate healthy tissue after debridement and the patient is not toxic at that time, reanastomosis can be considered. If ischemia or soiling with unhealthy tissue exists, wide debridement with esophageal exclusion may be needed. If a significant amount of the stomach needs to be resected, closure of the hiatus to prevent herniation will need to be done.

Chylothorax

The incidence of chylothorax is 0.4–0.8% after esophagectomy. It usually manifests several days after the operation when tube feedings or oral intake is started. Drainage of moderate to large volumes of milky whitish fluid from the chest tube or with thoracentesis is almost always diagnostic. Analysis of the fluid for lipids with a triglyceride/cholesterol ratio of greater than 1 or a triglyceride level greater than 110 g/dl confirms the diagnosis. The thoracic duct may be torn or transected while mobilizing the lower thoracic esophagus and leakage is usually into the right chest. Conservative measures such as a low fat or medium chain triglyceride diet can be tried, but if the drainage does not decrease after several days, full NPO status and total parenteral nutrition should be instituted. Chyle contains abundant proteins and patients can become nutritionally depleted quickly. Some surgeons prefer not to wait more than 5 days prior to taking the patient back to the operating room for thoracic duct ligation just above the right hemidiaphragm. Lymphangiography is generally not helpful in localizing the leak, and most radiologists are not trained in this method anymore. Feeding the patient cream or a fat-laden food several hours prior to surgery can elucidate the leaking portion of the duct. The leaking point is ligated and the duct is also ligated at multiple other points just above the diaphragm. Chest tube output should decrease drastically and the patient can be fed again.

Motility Disorders

Dumping syndrome occurs because of high osmotic load from the stomach into the small bowel because of lack of antral control after the vagus nerves are divided.[67,104] This can occur approximately 20 min after a meal or several hours after a meal. Dietary adjustments need to be made so that high carbohydrate foods are limited. Delayed gastric emptying also occurs after esophagectomy because of division of the vagus nerves and decreased stomach motility. Most surgeons perform a drainage procedure at the pylorus to prevent gastric outlet obstruction. At times, dilation of the pylorus or the anastomosis will need to be performed.

Gas-bloat syndrome occurs after fundoplication. Patients complain of feeling full of gas and being unable to belch for relief. Dietary changes and time usually relieve the symptoms of this syndrome.

Reflux

Gastroesophageal reflux is a common occurrence after esophagectomy and gastric pull-up. The stomach is now subjected to negative intrathoracic pressures and the lower esophageal sphincter no longer exists. The more cephalad the anastomosis, the less chance there is for reflux to occur. If patients have a history of Barrett's esophagus or symptoms or findings of esophagitis after pull-up, they should be on antireflux medication. They need to be counseled to eat and drink in the upright position and remain upright for at least 2 h after eating. The head of the bed should be elevated 30° to avoid nighttime reflux. Avoiding damage to the recurrent laryngeal nerves will help diminish the risk of aspiration when reflux occurs.

Stricture

Stricture after esophageal surgery can occur at an anastomosis, at the diaphragmatic hiatus, above, below, or within a fundoplication, at the pylorus, or at the site of previous myotomy. Stricture may be secondary to technical problems, ischemia, leak, or ulceration, and may be multifactorial. Short length strictures often can be treated with dilatation. Dilatation may be attempted for longer strictures, but reoperation may be needed.

Conduit Ischemia

Conduit ischemia can be avoided by careful assessment of blood supply prior to operation if the patient has had previous gastric or colonic operations. Angiogram of the mesenteric arteries may be desired prior to use of the colon as conduit. Continuous knowledge of the position of the right gastroepiploic artery as the greater curvature dissection is performed prevents inadvertent ligation or damage to the main vascular pedicle used during gastric pull-up. Leaving the right gastric artery intact provides a dual blood supply to ensure adequate blood flow to the stomach as it is transposed into the chest or neck.

Recurrent Laryngeal Nerve Damage

Damage to the recurrent laryngeal nerve is more common after transhiatal resection or three hole resection because of the dissection and retraction in the neck where the recurrent nerves are exposed in the tracheoesophageal groove. Careful avoidance of metal retractors deep in the neck wound and visualization of the nerve lower the incidence of this complication. In addition to hoarseness, recurrent laryngeal nerve damage causes incoordination of swallowing and predilection for aspiration.

Miscellaneous

Myasthenic crisis is respiratory muscle weakness causing respiratory failure after thymectomy for myasthenia gravis. Positive pressure mask breathing or ventilation should be used to support the patient through the acute crisis. Mestinon is usually not effective during crisis. If steroids and intravenous immune globulin do not provide enough symptom relief, plasmapheresis may be needed to clear the circulating antibodies.[5,62,93] Cholinergic crisis results from overtreatment with anticholinesterase medications. The patient may have symptoms related to muscarinic receptor activity (e.g., excessive salivation, sweating, abdominal cramping, urinary urgency, and bradycardia). Nicotinic receptor symptoms include fasciculations and muscle weakness. Cholinergic crisis does not respond to neostigmine. Treatment includes respiratory support, atropine, and cessation of anticholinesterase medications.[8]

Cerebrospinal fluid leak is a rare complication seen when tumor is resected near the spine. Assistance of a neurosurgeon is recommended and primary closure if possible should be done. Coverage with fat or pleura can also be used to help seal the leak. Other treatments involve placing lumbar drains to decrease the amount of cerebrospinal fluid and pressure to allow the leak to seal on its own. The symptoms include leakage of clear fluid and development of intractable headache after resection close to the spine or involving the vertebrae.[37,88]

DISCHARGE PLANNING

Discharge needs should be assessed preoperatively or soon postoperatively. The surgeon can often predict what services a certain patient will need according to their preoperative health and family support network. The patient and family are made active participants in plans for timely discharge. Team meetings with the social workers, nurses, physical therapists, and respiratory therapists about each patient's needs are helpful for planning. Occupational therapists and physical medicine physicians can indicate what level of rehabilitation patients will need after discharge. A list of home going medications, their purpose, and dosage schedule should be explained to the patient and their caregivers prior to discharge. Often the medications have changed and they need to be reminded which of their preoperative medications to take and if the schedule or dosage has changed. Activity level and home going exercises should be reviewed and demonstrated by patients to the therapist prior to leaving to ensure they are doing the exercises correctly. Driving and lifting are limited for 2–3 weeks postoperatively. There is no prohibition for showering or stair climbing. Outpatient pulmonary rehabilitation programs should be contracted and set up prior to discharge. The goal is to return the patient to a normal lifestyle as soon as possible. Visiting nurses can be invaluable in helping patients once home. They allow patients to be discharged who need help for only several minutes a day or for administration of antibiotics or blood draws and wound checks. The follow-up appointment and any laboratory studies or radiology studies that need to be obtained before the appointment should be arranged prior to the patient's discharge. Appropriate contact phone numbers should be provided should the patient have difficulty after discharge.

REFERENCES

1. Agnew NM, Kendall JB, Akrofi M, et al: Gastroesophageal reflux and tracheal aspiration in the thoracotomy position: Should ranitidine premedication be routine? Anesth Analg 95:1645–1649, 2002.
2. Amar D, Roistacher N, Rusch VW, et al: Effects of diltiazem prophylaxis on the incidence and clinical outcome of atrial arrhythmias after thoracic surgery. J Thorac Cardiovasc Surg 120:790–798, 2000.
3. Ando M, Yamamoto M, Kitagawa C, et al: Autologous blood-patch pleurodesis for secondary spontaneous pneumothorax with persistent air leak. Respir Med 93(6):432–434, 1999.
4. Argenta LC, Morykwas MJ: Vacuum-assisted closure: A new method for wound control and treatment: Clinical experience. Ann Plast Surg 38:563–577, 1997.
5. Asharafian H, Davey P: Is amiodarone an underrecognized cause of acute respiratory failure in the ICU? Chest 120:275–282, 2001.
6. Attia J, Ray JG, Cook DJ, et al: Deep vein thrombosis and its prevention in critically ill adults. Arch Int Med 161(10):1268–1279, 2001.
7. Baker JW, Tribble CG: Pleural anesthetics given through an epidural catheter secured inside a chest tube. Ann Thorac Surg 51(1):138–139, 1991.
8. Baraka A: Anesthesia and critical care of thymectomy for myasthenia gravis. Chest Surg Clin North Am 11(2):337–361, 2001.
9. Bates ER: Treatment of acute myocardial infarction: A cardiologist's perspective. Int Anesth Clin 30:237–250, 1992.
10. Bayfield MS, Spotnitz WD: Fibrin sealant in thoracic surgery. Chest Surg Clin North Am 6:567–583, 1996.
11. Benedetti F, Amanzio M, Casadio C, et al: Control of postoperative pain by transcutaneous electrical nerve stimulation after thoracic operations. Ann Thorac Surg 63(3):773–776, 1997.
12. Bernard A, Pillet M, Goudet P, Viard H: Antibiotic prophylaxis in pulmonary surgery. A prospective randomized double-blind trial of flash cefuroxime versus forty-eight-hour cefuroxime. J Thorac Cardiovasc Surg 107(3):896–900, 1994.
13. Bobek MB, Arroliga AC: Stress ulcer prophylaxis: The case for a selective approach. Cleveland Clin J Med 64(10):533–542, 1997.
14. Bonde P, Papachristos I, McCraith A, et al: Sputum retention after lung operation: Prospective, randomized trial shows superiority of prophylactic minitracheostomy in high-risk patients. Ann Thorac Surg 74(1):196–202, 2002.
15. Boysen PG: Perioperative management of the thoracotomy patient. Clin Chest Med 14(2):321–333, 1993.
16. Brodsky MA, Orlov MV, Capparelli EV, et al: Magnesium therapy in new-onset atrial fibrillation. Am J Cardiol 73:1227–1229, 1994.
17. Brunelli A, Refai MA, Muti M, et al: Pleural tent after upper lobectomy: A prospective randomized study. Ann Thorac Surg 69:1722–1724, 2000.
18. Brynitz S, Schroder M: Intraoperative cryolysis of intercostal nerves in thoracic surgery. Scand J Thor Cardiovasc Surg 20(1):85–87, 1986.
19. Burgess FW, Anderson DM, Colonna D, Cavanaugh DG: Thoracic epidural analgesia with bupivicaine and fentanyl for postoperative thoracotomy pain. J Cardiothorac Vasc Anesth 8:420–424, 1994.
20. Burns HJG: Nutritional support in the perioperative period. Br Med Bull 44:357–373, 1988.
21. Cagirici U, Sahin B, Cakan A, et al: Autologous blood patch pleurodesis in spontaneous pneumothorax with persistent air leak. Scan Cardiovasc J 32:75–78, 1998.
22. Campos JH: Lung isolation techniques. Anesthesiol Clin North Am 19(3):455–474, 2001.
23. Camu F, Beckers S: The anesthetic risk of tobacco smoking. Acta Anaesthesiol Belg 42:45–56, 1991.
24. Cerfolio RJ, Bryant A, Thruber J, et al: Intraoperative solumedrol® helps prevent postoperative post-pneumonectomy edema. Presented at the 39th Annual STS, 2003.
25. Cerfolio RJ, Pickens A, Bass C, Katholi C: Fast tracking pulmonary resections. J Thor Cardiovasc Surg 122:318–324, 2001.
26. Cerfolio RJ, Tummala RP, Holman WL, et al: A prospective algorithm for the management of air leaks after pulmonary resection. Ann Thorac Surg 66(5):1726–1731, 1998.
27. Cimprich B, Gaydos D, Langan R: A preoperative teaching program for the thoracotomy patient. Cancer Nurs 1(1):35–39, 1978.
28. Cole AF: Intrapleural-another approach to sensory phrenic nerve block. Anesth Analg 94(3):764–765, 2002.
29. Cook DJ: Stress ulcer prophylaxis: Gastrointestinal bleeding and nosocomial pneumonia. Best evidence synthesis. Scand J Gastroenterol Suppl 210:48–52, 1995.
30. Cresswell LL, Schuessler RB, Rosenbloom M, Cox JL: Hazards of postoperative atrial arrhythmias. Ann Thorac Surg 56:539–549, 1993.
31. Crystal E, Connolly SJ, Sleik K, et al: Interventions on prevention of postoperative atrial fibrillation in patients undergoing heart surgery: A meta-analysis. Circulation 106(1):75–80, 2002.
32. Cummins RO, editor: ACLS Provider Manual. American Heart Association, 2000.

33. Daoud EG, Strickberger SA, Man KC, et al: Preoperative amiodarone as prophylaxis against atrial fibrillation after heart surgery. N Engl J Med 337:1785–1791, 1997.

34. Deschamps C, Allen MS, Miller DL, et al: Management of postpneumonectomy empyema and bronchopleural fistula. Semin Thorac Cardiovasc Surg 13(1):13–19, 2001.

35. Donington JS, Miller DL, Rowland CC, et al: Morbidity and mortality after neoadjuvant chemoradiation and esophagectomy. Ann Thorac Surg (in press).

36. Doss NW, Ambrish M, Ipe J, et al: Epidural blood patch after thoracotomy for treatment of headache caused by surgical tear of dura. Anesth Analg 91(6):1372–1374, 2000.

37. Downey RJ, Trastek VF, Clay RP: Right pneumonectomy syndrome: Surgical correction with expandable implants. J Thorac Cardiovasc Surg 107:953–955, 1994.

38. Etches RC, Gammer T, Cornish R: Patient-controlled epidural analgesia after thoracotomy: A comparison of meperidine with and without bupivicaine. Anesth Analg 83(1):81–86, 1996.

39. Fanning WJ, Thomas CS Jr, Roach A, et al: Prophylaxis of atrial fibrillation with magnesium sulfate after coronary artery bypass grafting. Ann Thorac Surg 52:529–533, 1991.

40. Ferdinand B, Shennib H: Postoperative pneumonia. Chest Surg Clin North Am 8(3):529–539, 1998.

41. Flannery J, Tucker DA: Pharmacologic prophylaxis and treatment of stress ulcers in critically ill patients. Crit Care Nurs Clin North Am 14(1):39–51, 2002.

42. Forshag MS, Cooper AD: Postoperative care of the thoracotomy patient. Clin Chest Med 13:33–45, 1992.

43. Frank SM, Fleisher LA, Breslow MJ, et al: Perioperative maintenance of normothermia reduces the incidence of morbid cardiac events. JAMA 277:1127–1134, 1997.

44. Frost L, Molgaard H, Christiansen EH, et al: Atrial fibrillation and flutter after coronary artery bypass surgery: Epidemiology, risk factors and preventive trials. Int J Cardiol 36:253–261, 1992.

45. Galway JE, Caves PK, Dundee JW: Effect of intercostal nerve blockade during operation on lung function and the relief of pain following thoracotomy. Br J Anaesthesial 47(6):730–735, 1975.

46. Gattinoni L, Tognoni G, Pesenti A, et al: Effect of prone positioning on the survival of patients with acute respiratory failure. N Engl J Med 345:568–573, 2001.

47. Geerts WH, Heit JA, Clagett GP, et al: Prevention of venous thromboembolism. Chest 119(1 Suppl):132S–175S, 2001.

48. Gharagozloo F, Trachiotis G, Wolfe A, et al: Pleural space irrigation and modified Clagett procedure for the treatment of early postpneumonectomy empyema. J Thorac Cardiovasc Surg 116(6):943–948, 1998.

49. Gillinov AM, Heitmiller RF: Strategies to reduce pulmonary complications after transhiatal esophagectomy. Dis Esophagus 11(1):43–47, 1998.

50. Gomes JA, Ip J, Santoni-Rugiu F, et al: Oral d,1 sotalol reduces the incidence of postoperative atrial fibrillation in coronary artery bypass surgery patients: A randomized, double-blind, placebo-controlled study. J Am Coll Cardiol 34(2):334–339, 1999.

51. Grillo HC, Donahue DM: Post-intubation tracheal stenosis. Semin Thorac Cardiovasc Surg 8(4):370–380, 1996.

52. Headrick JR, Nichols FC 3rd, Miller DL, et al: High-grade esophageal dysplasia: Long-term survival and quality of life after esophagectomy. Ann Thorac Surg 73(6):1697–1702, 2002.

53. Hebert PC, Wells G, Blajchman MA, et al: A multicenter, randomized, controlled clinical trial of transfusion requirements in critical care. N Engl J Med 340:409–417, 1999.

54. Hebert PC, Yetisir E, Martin C, et al: Is a low transfusion threshold safe in critically ill patients with cardiovascular diseases? Crit Care Med 29(9):227–234, 2001.

55. Hopkins CC: Antibiotic prophylaxis in clean surgery: Peripheral vascular surgery, noncardiovascular thoracic surgery, herniorrhaphy, and mastectomy. RID 13(Suppl 10):S869–873, 1991.

56. Jorg M, Theilmeier G, Van Aken H, et al: Inhaled prostaglandin E1 for treatment of acute lung injury in severe multiple organ failure. Anesth Analg 86:753–758, 1998.

57. Joucken K, Michel L, Schoevaerdts JC, et al: Cryoanalgesia for post-thoracotomy pain relief. Acta Anaesthesiol Belg 38(2):179–183, 1987.

58. Karnath B: Smoking cessation. Am J Med 112:399–405, 2002.

59. Katariya K, Harvey JC, Pina E, Beattie EJ: Complications of transhiatal esophagectomy. J Surg Oncol 57:157–163, 1994.

60. Kawahara K, Akamine S, Takahashi T, et al: Management of anastomotic complications after sleeve lobectomy for lung cancer. Ann Thorac Surg 57:1529–1533, 1994.

61. Krucylak PE, Naunheim KS: Preoperative preparation and anesthetic management of patients with myasthenia gravis. Semin Thorac Cardiovasc Surg 11(1):47–53, 1999.

62. Kurz A, Sessler DI, Lenhardt R: Perioperative normothermia to reduce the incidence of surgical wound infection and shorten hospitalization. N Engl J Med 334:1209–1215, 1996.

63. Langer CJ, Choy H, Glaspy JA, Colowick A: Standards of care for anemia management in oncology: Focus on lung carcinoma. Cancer 95(3):613–623, 2002.

64. MacLaren R, Jarvis CL, Fish DN: Use of enteral nutrition for stress ulcer prophylaxis. Ann Pharmacother 35(12): 1614–1623, 2001.

65. Marshall MB, Deeb ME, Bleier JIS, et al: Suction versus water seal after pulmonary resection. Chest 121:831–835, 2002.

66. McLarty AJ, Deschamps C, Trastek VF, et al: Esophageal resection for cancer of the esophagus. Long term function and quality of life. Ann Thorac Surg 63:1568–1572, 1997.

67. Michaels AJ, Wanek S, Dreifuss BA, et al: A protocolized approach to pulmonary failure and the role of intermittent prone positioning. J Trauma 52:1037–1047, 2002.

68. Miller RD, editor: Anesthesia, 5th ed. New York: Churchill Livingston, 2000, pp. 1019–1020.

69. Modig J: Adult respiratory distress syndrome. Acta Chir Scand 152:241–249, 1986.

70. Mohr R, Smolinsky A, Goor DA: Prevention of supraventricular tachyarrhythmias with low-dose propranolol after coronary bypass. J Thorac Cardiovasc Surg 81:840–845, 1981.

71. Moon MR, Luchette FA, Gibson SW, et al: Prospective, randomized comparison of epidural versus parenteral opioid analgesia in thoracic trauma. Ann Surg 229(5): 684–692, 1999.

72. Nomori H, Kobayashi R, Fuyuno G, et al: Preoperative respiratory muscle training. Assessment in thoracic surgery patients with special reference to postoperative pulmonary complications. Chest 105(6):1782–1788, 1994.

73. Nwiloh J, Freeman H, McCord C: Malnutrition: An important determinant of fatal outcome in surgically treated pulmonary suppurative disease. J Natl Med Assoc 81(5): 525–529, 1989.

74. Olak J, Jeyasingham K, Forrester-Wood C, et al: Randomized trial of one-dose versus si-dose cefazolin prophylaxis in elective general thoracic surgery. Ann Thorac Surg 51:956–958, 1991.

75. Orlicek S: Management of acute laryngotracheobronchitis. Pediatr Infect Dis J 17:1164–1165, 1998.

76. Orringer MB, Marshall B, Iannettoni MD: Transhiatal esophagectomy: Clinical experience and refinements. Ann Surg 230:392–403, 1999.

77. Parikka H, Toivonen L, Pellinen T, et al: The influence of intravenous magnesium sulfate on the occurrence of atrial fibrillation after coronary artery by-pass operation. Eur Heart J 14:251–258, 1993.

78. Patton MD, Scaerf R: Thoracotomy, critical pathway, and clinical outcomes. Cancer Pract 3:286–294, 1995.

79. Power I, Bowler GMR, Pugh GC, Chambers WA: Ketorolac as a component of balanced analgesia after thoracotomy. Br J Anaesthesiol 72:224–226, 1994.

80. Rainer WG, Newby JP: Prevention of residual space problems after pulmonary resection. Am J Surg 114:744–747, 1967.

81. Retz JL, Martin WJ II: Amiodarone pulmonary toxicity. Intens Care Med 18:388–390, 1992.

82. Roviaro GC, Varoli F, Fascianella A, et al: Intrathoracic intercostal nerve block with phenol in open chest surgery. A randomized study with statistical evaluation of respiratory parameters. Chest 90(1):64–67, 1986.

83. Roxburgh JC, Markland CG, Ross BA, Kerr WF: Role of cryoanalgesia in the control of pain after thoracotomy. Thorax 42(4):292–295, 1987.

84. Scawn ND, Pennefather SH, Soorae A, et al: Ipsilateral shoulder pain after thoracotomy with epidural analgesia: The influence of phrenic nerve infiltration with lidocaine. Anesth Analg 93(2):260–264, 2001.

85. Schierhout G, Roberts I: Fluid Resuscitation with colloid or crystalloid solutions in critically ill patients: A systematic review of randomized trials. Br Med J 316:961–964, 1998.

86. Schmied H, Kurz A, Sessler DI, et al: Mild hypothermia increases blood loss and transfusion requirements during total hip arthroplasty. Lancet 347:289–292, 1996.

87. Sganzerla EP, Tisi E, Lucarini C, et al: Acute pneumocephalus: An unusual complication of thoracotomy. J Neurosurg Sci 41(3):309–312, 1997.

88. Simpson T, Wahl G, DeTraglia M, et al: The effects of epidural versus parenteral opioid analgesia on postoperative pain and pulmonary function in adults who have undergone thoracic and abdominal surgery: A critique of research. Heart Lung 21(2):125–138, 1992.

89. Singh H, Bossard RF, White PF, Yeatts RW: Effects of ketorolac versus bupivacaine coadministration during patient-controlled hydromorphone epidural analgesia after thoracotomy procedures. Anesth Analg 84(3):564–569, 1997.

90. Slinger PD: Perioperative fluid management for thoracic surgery: The puzzle of postpneumonectomy pulmonary edema. J Cardiothorac Vasc Anesthesiol 9(4):442–451, 1995.

91. Smythe M: Patient-controlled analgesia: A review. Pharmacotherapy 12(2):132–143, 1992.

92. Spring PJ, Spies JM: Myasthenia gravis: Options and timing of immunomodulatory treatment. Biodrugs 15(3):173–183, 2001.

93. Takaoka K, Inoue S, Ohira S: Central bronchopleural fistulas closed by bronchoscopic injection of absolute ethanol. Chest 122:374–378, 2002.

94. Tanomkiat W, Galassi W: Barium sulfate as contrast medium for evaluation of postoperative anastomotic leaks. Acta Radiol 41(5):482–485, 2000.

95. Tsunezuka Y, Sato H, Watanabe S, et al: Improved expandable prosthesis in postpneumonectomy syndrome with deformed thorax. J Thorac Cardiovasc Surg 116:526–528, 1998.

96. Vaporciyan AA, Merriman KW, Ece F, et al: Incidence of major pulmonary morbidity after pneumonectomy: Association with timing of smoking cessation. Ann Thorac Surg 73:420–426, 2002.

97. Wain JC, Wilson DJ, Mathisen DJ: Clinical experience with minitracheostomy. Ann Thorac Surg 49:881–886, 1990.

98. Wattel F, Mathieu D, Coget J-M, Billard V: Hyperbaric oxygen therapy in chronic vascular wound management. Angiology 9:59–65, 1990.

99. Weiner P, Man A, Weiner M, et al: The effect of incentive spirometry and inspiratory muscle training on pulmonary function after lung resection. Thorac Cardiovasc Surg 113(3):552–557, 1997.

100. Wills VL, Hunt DR: Dysphagia after anti-reflux surgery. Br J Surg 88(4):486–499, 2001.

101. Wright CD, Wain JC, Grillo HC, et al: Pulmonary lobectomy patient care pathway: A model to control cost and maintain quality. Ann Thorac Surg 64:299–302, 1997.

102. York EL, Lewall DB, Hirji M, et al: Endoscopic diagnosis and treatment of postoperative bronchopleural fistula. Chest 97:1390–1392, 1990.

103. Young MM, Deschamps C, Allen MS, et al: Esophageal reconstruction for benign disease: Self-assessment of functional outcome and quality of life. Ann Thorac Surg 70(6):1799–1802, 2000.

104. Zehr KJ, Dawson PB, Yang SC, Heitmiller RF: Standardized clinical care pathways for major thoracic cases reduce hospital costs. Ann Thorac Surg 66(3):914–919, 1998.

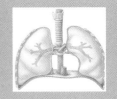

Endoscopy

Endoscopic Diagnosis of Thoracic Disease

CHAPTER **5**

Brian L. Reemtsen and Douglas E. Wood

▶ **INTRODUCTION**

The armamentarium of the thoracic surgeon is plentiful, but two procedures, bronchoscopy and esophagoscopy, allow minimal invasiveness with maximal effectiveness in diagnosis as well as therapeutic intervention. Although many clinicians may perform endoscopy, thoracic surgeons in particular should be facile with these procedures, and not count upon others to help diagnose or stage thoracic pathology. Many times these procedures may be performed in combination on certain patients, but we will discuss them separately.

▶ **ESOPHAGOSCOPY**

History

The history of endoscopy started with Kassmaul, who in 1868 intubated a sword swallower's stomach via the esophagus with a 13-mm hollow metal tube. This maneuver proved that the oral cavity, esophagus, and stomach could be simultaneously intubated with one rigid instrument. Mikulicz added one crucial aspect to the tube, distal light to illuminate the esophagus and stomach, and he was able to visualize gastric motility and view probable malignancies. The fiberoptic endoscope was introduced in 1958. This instrument allowed more patient comfort as well as greater therapeutic possibilities in the distal stomach and proximal small intestine. Although the scope itself has not changed greatly, the adjunctive instruments have dramatically changed the way many disease states can be treated.[7]

Indications

The indications for esophageal endoscopy are many, but for the thoracic surgeon symptoms of dysphasia or odynophagia are two of the most common. Others include reflux, abnormal esophagogram, trauma, screening, or staging of gastrointestinal (GI) or adjacent masses including tracheoesophageal fistulas. Upper GI bleeding is another very common indication for endoscopy and has become the first line in management of this clinical scenario (Table 5-1).

Dysphagia can arise from a number of pathological processes. Many causes can be distinguished with a proper history recording the duration and persistence of symptoms as well as accompanying constitutional symptoms. Endoscopy provides the surgeon with the ability to access the possibility of malignancy versus benign causes of dysphagia, thereby guiding therapy.

Reflux is another indication for upper endoscopy. The thoracic surgeon is searching for any long-term sequelae associated with chronic gastroesophageal reflux disease (GERD) such as Barrett's esophagus. Esophagoscopy is crucial in the surveillance of known Barrett's esophagus because of the link with the development of adenocarcinoma. It is still unclear at what interval these patients should be followed.

Upper gastrointestinal bleeding is another indication for endoscopy and is the most common potentially therapeutic procedure performed with an endoscope. The most common esophageal bleeding point is variceal bleeding. Although a difficult problem, it can be palliated with banding or sclerotherapy.

Table 5–1
Current ASGE Indications for Upper Endoscopy
Persistent nausea and vomiting
Upper abdominal pain, heartburn, or acid reflux symptoms (an acid or burning sensation in the throat or chest)
Gastrointestinal (GI) bleeding (vomiting blood or blood found in the stool)
Difficulty swallowing; food/liquids getting stuck in the esophagus
Abnormal or unclear findings on an upper GI X-ray
Removal of a foreign body
Follow-up on previously found polyps (growths), tumors, or ulcers

The most common indication for a thoracic surgeon to perform upper endoscopy is the visualization and biopsy of esophageal and proximal stomach masses. Biopsy has a sensitivity of 66–96% in esophageal cancers.[5,15] The number of biopsies is usually 7–10, throughout the area of the lesion or randomly in the setting of Barrett's esophagitis. If the lesion presents with a tight stricture two different solutions may help the surgeon. First a smaller diameter scope may allow passage or brushings have been shown to increase the yield of tissue in the face of stricture.[15,17] Finally the role of endoscopic ultrasound in the diagnosis and staging of esophageal disease will be discussed later.

Other mediastinal masses and malignancies may cause esophageal obstructive symptoms and upper endoscopy can play a role in the assessment of these processes. At endoscopy it may be ascertained whether the lesion is causing mass effect or actual erosion through the wall of the esophagus potentially with or without development of a fistula.

Two other scenarios where upper endoscopy is critical are trauma, whether it be blunt, penetrating, or caustic, and foreign body retrieval. A frequent thoracic surgery consult involves the documentation and management of iatrogenic trauma to the esophagus via instrumentation. Although the mainstay for the diagnosis of perforation is the esophagogram, the utility of endoscopy for the diagnosis and documentation of the extent of injury should not be understated. Corrosive ingestion is another indication for early (with in 36 h) endoscopic inspection.[3] This modality helps to identify transmural involvement and subsequent development of strictures. Foreign body diagnosis and treatment may be performed with upper endoscopy. Foreign bodies lodged in the esophagus should alert the surgeon to the potential for intraesophageal lesions being responsible for the nonpassage of material.

Preprocedure

The overwhelming majority of endoscopies can and should be performed on an outpatient basis with conscious sedation. Patients should be nothing by mouth (NPO) after midnight for a morning examination, and those with obstructive symptoms should be placed on a clear liquid diet for 24–48 h prior to the examination.

Upon arrival a peripheral intravenous line should be placed and electrocardiogram (ECG) monitors placed. Because of the respiratory depression caused by the common sedatives given, constant ECG, pulse oximetry, and frequent blood pressure measurements should be obtained during the procedure. Once the monitors are in place, the sedation should be given to ensure a cooperative, comfortable patient. Local anesthesia can be used, and minimizes the degree of conscious sedation required.

Technique

Flexible Esophagoscopy

The most common position for the examination of the outpatient is the left lateral decubitus, with the head flexed. A bite block is placed into the mouth to protect the endoscope from the teeth, and the endoscope is introduced under direct vision. The epiglottis and larynx should be seen and advanced over until the piriform sinuses become apparent. If the vocal cords are visualized, any abnormalities should be documented. Gentle pressure against the upper esophageal sphincter at the cricopharyngeus while the patient is instructed to swallow usually results in successful and atraumatic esophageal intubation.

There are four normal endoluminal landmarks in the human esophagus. First, the upper esophageal sphincter is at the cricopharyngeus at 15–18 cm from the incisors. The next indentation that is normally evident is the aortic arch, which appears on the left anterolateral wall. The left atrium may be seen in the distal esophagus as wave-like pulsations of the anterior wall of the esophagus. Lastly, the lower esophageal sphincter, which in reality is just a physiological sphincter, can be demonstrated by asking the patient to perform a Valsalva maneuver and noting the pinching off of the lumen. The esophagus is generally easy to assess, and takes very little air insufflation to view its entire course.

Once the gastroesophageal junction has been passed it is easy to advance into the stomach. The stomach should be insufflated with enough air to flatten out the rugae and allow visualization of the entire mucosal surface. The pylorus is visualized and the scope can be advanced beyond the sphincter when it is relaxed. The duodenum should be inspected to the third portion. Once this has been performed satisfactorily, the scope should be removed slowly to see any potentially missed pathology. In the stomach, retroflexion of the scope will allow the visualization of the body and cardia of the stomach. Insufflated air should be suctioned before leaving the confines of the stomach. During withdrawal the scope should be slowly pulled back to more carefully assess the esophagus, then removal of the endoscope and continued monitoring of the patient occur.

Rigid Esophagoscopy

Rigid esophagoscopy is a rarely used modality, usually reserved for three instances: trauma, removal of impacted food, and removal of foreign bodies. The current method of examination was championed by Chevalier-Jackson. The scope is held in the examiner's right hand while the left hand keeps the mouth open with the left thumb protecting the upper dentition. During the insertion of the scope the head is initially held forward, in the "sniffing position" used for tracheal intubation; once the cricopharyngeus is passed the head is extended to eliminate the angle of the mouth and the pharynx. The scope can then be carefully advanced throughout the length of the esophagus and proximal stomach; manipulating the head and cervical spine at the areas of narrowing allows less traumatic passage.

Complications

Complications are rare after flexible upper endoscopy. Morbidity rates of 0.13–0.092% include cardiovascular reactions to premedication, perforation, and bleeding specific to the procedure. Mortality rates are exceedingly rare, quoted at 0.018–0.004%.[2,11]

► ENDOSCOPIC ULTRASOUND

A relatively new adjunctive procedure that has expanded the examination of the esophagus and the periesophageal tissues uses a small ultrasonic transducer placed at the end of the endoscope. This examination should never be the initial procedure but is indicated when a previous esophagoscopy has been performed and pathology has been located and evaluated. Indications for esophageal ultrasound range from benign to malignant esophageal disease or evaluation of periesophageal pathology, usually bronchogenic carcinoma (Table 5-2). The most common indication for esophageal ultrasound (EUS) is the evaluation of esophageal malignancy. The stage of the lesion, as defined by the depth of invasion and nodal involvement, is the best predictor of surgical resection and therefore possible cure.

The normal esophagus is represented by five distinct alternating layers of differing echogenicity. The first layer, which is the most hyperechoic (white), represents the epithelium and lamina propria. The second layer, which is hypoechoic (black), represents the muscularis mucosa. The third layer, which is again hyperechoic, represents the submucosa. The fourth hypoechoic layer represents the muscularis propria. The last thick hyperechoic layer represents the paraesophageal tissue. The T stage is determined by the invasion of the layers characterized. Accumulating data suggest that EUS is the most accurate imaging modality for staging esophageal malignancies. Preoperative accuracy of 80–92% sensitivity has been demonstrated when compared with surgical pathology specimens.[1] The main advantage of EUS over conventional radiology (computed tomography [CT] scan) is the differentiation of the T stage, especially between the T3 and T4 stages, which may influence the decision to offer an operation to the patient.[16] Staging regional lymph node metastasis has been in the range of 70–80%, which is also much more accurate than CT or magnetic resonance imaging (MRI).[16] The regional lymph nodes and distant metastasis are characterized by their presence or absence on examination. Accuracy is dramatically improved with fine needle sampling, which can be performed on nodal tissue or distant organ metastasis in direct contact with the esophageal wall.[10] After the examination of the three different TNM tissues the patient can be preoperatively staged. EUS is fast becoming the standard of care in the evaluation of esophageal malignancies.

► TRACHEOBRONCHOSCOPY

The inspection of the tracheobronchial tree is the most common procedure performed by thoracic surgeons. The inspection may be performed with a flexible or rigid instrument. The procedure, which can be both diagnostic and therapeutic, is indispensable for the thoracic surgeon for proper preoperative diagnosis and staging, as well as intraoperative decision making about the ability or extent of resection therapy to benefit a given patient.

History

The first reported use of bronchoscopy was therapeutic, in which Killian was able to successfully remove a foreign body (bone) from the right main stem bronchus of a patient. The modern era of flexible bronchoscopy was ushered in about the same time as esophagoscopy, once the problem of flexible fiber orientation was solved. Ikeda was the first to report the use of a flexible fiberoptic bronchoscope in a patient.[14] Since that time the caliber and resolution have been declining and improving, respectively. The addition of instrument ports has made the procurement of tissue for diagnosis and other therapeutic interventions possible.

Indications

Evaluation of signs or symptoms such as cough, wheezing, or stridor, radiological findings, and assessment of nearby

---

Table 5–2
Indications for Endoscopic Ultrasound

Esophagus
  Staging esophageal cancer
  Evaluating esophageal submucosal lesions
  Evaluation of high-grade dysplasia arising within Barrett's
    esophagus
  Evaluation of response of esophageal cancer after
    chemotherapy
  Differentiating achalasia from pseudoachalasia
  Evaluation for periesophageal varices

Mediastinum
  Nodal staging of lung cancer
  Evaluation of selected mediastinal masses
  Evaluating posterior mediastinal lymphadenopathy

62 pathology are the most frequent indications for bronchoscopy. The most common indication for a thoracic surgeon is the preoperative diagnosis and staging of thoracic malignancies, usually bronchopulmonary carcinoma. After physical examination, routine radiographs, and sputum studies suggest the presence of malignancy, the first line of invasive procedure is usually bronchoscopy. Bronchoscopy can be helpful in the determination of the extent and pathology of the tumor.[4] Other possible benefits of preoperative bronchoscopy include the exclusion of synchronous or metastatic disease that would drastically alter the surgical plan, and the evaluation of the tracheobronchial anatomy to better optimize the surgical approach.

Hemoptysis can be both diagnosed as well as palliated with the bronchoscope. Individuals presenting with pulmonary abscess should have an airway evaluation to ensure no obstructive lesion is responsible. Workup of patients with tracheoesophageal fistula, lobar collapse, hydropneumothorax, and bronchopleural fistulas usually mandate bronchoscopy. Adjacent tumors of the esophagus and mediastinum may benefit from tracheobronchoscopy to rule out invasion of the esophagus, to further delineate the extent of the mass, or for transbronchial biopsy. Pulmonary infections with poor pulmonary toilet can also be an indication for bronchoscopy, for both specimen procurement and therapeutic airway suctioning.

Patients with metastatic cancers who have physical signs such as minor hemoptysis, chronic cough, or unexplained atelectasis on a chest film benefit from diagnostic bronchoscopy. Malignancies that have been demonstrated to have a high occurrence of airway metastasis are colorectal cancer, breast cancer, and genitourinary cancers[12] (Table 5-3).

Technique

Flexible Bronchoscopy

With few exceptions most diagnostic bronchoscopy procedures can and should be done with an awake patient with topical anesthesia. In some instances the patient may already be intubated or need general anesthesia for a combined procedure, which obviates the need for local anesthesia. In the outpatient setting the room should be equipped with monitors for the readings of pulse, blood pressure, and a continuous pulse oximetry.

Bronchoscopes come in many sizes and calibers, with the usage usually dependent on the size of the patient and the need for larger working channels if endobronchial intervention is anticipated. The field of vision is generally 80° with the angle of deflection usually 160–180°. The light source is connected with a flexible light cord and the transmission of light and the resultant resolution are based upon the number of flexible fiberoptic bundles. More light, however, will result in larger caliber scopes.

Essential equipment consists of the bronchoscope, light source, camera, biopsy tools, suction and irrigation, as well as a sputum trap available. After informed consent has been obtained, the patient should be positioned in a sitting position where topical anesthesia and gentle sedation can be administered. Either a transnasal or transoral approach may be used in the awake patient; intubated patients are generally examined through the endotracheal tube. The

Table 5–3	
Indications for Flexible Bronchoscopy	
Diagnostic	*Therapeutic*
Lung cancer	Mucous plugs
Positive sputum cytology	Acute lobar collapse
Paralyzed vocal cord	Difficult intubation
Localized wheeze	Foreign body removal
Unexplained pleural effusion	Hemoptysis
Hemoptysis	Brachytherapy
Cough	Laser ablation
Diffuse interstitial infiltrates	Electrocautery
Immunocompromised patient with pulmonary infiltrates	Stent placement
Ventilator-associated pneumonia	Balloon dilation
Endotracheal tube position/ patency	
Atelectasis	
Tracheal esophageal fistula	
Acute inhalation injury	
Bronchography	

transnasal approach in the awake patient has the advantage of viewing the nasal and upper airway.[6] Manipulation of these scopes begins with the user holding the scope in the dominate hand, with views either from an eyepiece or video screen. After insertion the trachea is examined searching for luminal irregularities. The first landmark is the carina, which should be a sharp bifurcation; any fullness in this area should alert the operator to subcarinal adenopathy or mass involvement of the proximal airway. The operator should then systematically examine all airways to the segmental and subsegmental bronchus level. All pathology should be documented with detailed written descriptions or pictures of the actual findings. Depending on the findings the surgeon has the option of further investigation using tools for washings, lavage, brushings, and biopsy, which will be discussed later in this chapter. Once extracted the bronchoscope should be irrigated with sterile solution and sent for disinfection.

Rigid Bronchoscopy

This procedure is performed less often than flexible bronchoscopy, because of the need for general anesthesia, as well as the difficulty of becoming facile with this instrument. This method of viewing the upper airway is indispensable to the thoracic surgeon, and provides a conduit in which to help palliate certain disease processes with dilation and or stents.

Despite the increase in technical difficulty, the rigid scope has several distinct advantages over the flexible scope. First, the rigid scope allows more accurate definition of central airway lesions, as well as the ability to palliate these lesions. Second, the rigid scope allows for ventilation through the lumen of the scope, providing direct control of the airway in the setting of airway disease. Third, instrumentation and suctioning capabilities are larger and more effective than the small instruments developed for use through the working channel of the flexible scope. Because of this the rigid scope has been proven to be more helpful in managing hemoptysis as well as foreign body removal.

Massive hemoptysis, defined as 600 ml over 24 h, mandates urgent rigid bronchoscopy. Once introduced the airway is controlled, the point of bleeding is investigated, and intervention can be attempted. Use of a proximal eyepiece allows visualization without compromising ventilation. Rigid bronchoscopy does not obviate the use of the flexible scope; flexible bronchoscopy may be utilized through the lumen of the rigid scope to further help in the examination and possible intervention of the airway disease.

Foreign body extraction is usually technically easier through the rigid scope because of the large caliber of the instrument. Again airway control is established and the foreign body can be extracted with forceps, or on some occasions with a balloon catheter should the offending mass be lodged in the airway.

Shortcomings of the rigid method include poor visualization of the terminal bronchi, the inability to perform instrumentation and suction with excellent vision, and the incumbent need for general anesthesia.

Contraindications

There are very few absolute contraindications for bronchoscopy. Most are relative contraindications and deal with coagulopathy, recent myocardial ischemia, or the risk of increasing intracranial pressure in patients who are in high-risk situations. All of these problems can be addressed and with replacement of any clotting deficiencies, as well as judicious use of local anesthesia and sedation, these relative contraindications can usually be overcome. The main risk during bronchoscopy is compromising the airway of the patient. When dealing with difficult situations such as tracheal stenosis or tumor, the bronchoscopist must ensure an airway before proceeding with the examination, reverting to rigid bronchoscopy if necessary.

Complications

Although rare, complications of bronchoscopy do happen. Crucial steps before the procedure should include workup of any comorbid cardiac disease or coagulopathy, and careful consideration of the underlying pathology and the possible consequences of bronchoscopic intervention. An essential step to any procedure should involve informed consent with detailed education of the patient of the possible complications and the probable effect on the patient.

Most large series on flexible bronchoscopy quote morbidity from 0.0.5 to 0.1% and mortality around 0.01%.[13] Morbidity was generally defined as respiratory compromise, symptomatic bradycardia, hypotension, syncope, or arrhythmias. Although manipulation of the instrument may be responsible for some of these manifestations, most agree that the majority of morbidity lies in the administration and reactivity to the premedication and local anesthesia.

This risk of rigid bronchoscopy is much more significant, with the largest series quoting a morbidity of 5.1% with 1.1% being construed as major.[9] The main contradistinction between rigid and flexible bronchoscopy lies in the fact that the majority of the increase of morbidity is due to selection of more complex patients and more complex pathology with the likelihood of interventional procedures. This morbidity reflects the increased ability of palliative procedures using the rigid scope and the increased risk of subsequent complications. The mortality rate of most large series on rigid bronchoscopy parallels that of flexible bronchoscopy.

Specimen Procurement

One of the most potentially helpful diagnostic tools of bronchoscopy is the procurement of tissues or secretions from the tracheobronchial tree or adjacent structures. Specimens are usually characterized as washings, brushings, biopsies, or needle aspiration.

Washings fall into two different categories. First, routine washings are performed by simply administering sterile saline though the irrigation port, usually in 10-ml volumes. This fluid is then aspirated into a sterile specimen and sent for both cytology and culture. The second form of washing is termed bronchoalveolar lavage (BAL). The main contradistinction between BAL and simple washings is that larger volumes of saline are used in more terminal bronchioles during lavage. The advantage is that more cellular and noncellular material is retrieved for examination. After the flexible scope is wedged into the fourth or fifth terminal bronchioles, sterile saline is instilled in increments of 50 ml, then aspirated into a specimen trap. The aim is a total aspirate of 150–200 ml. The first aspirations contain mostly airway cells, whereas later aspirations can contain alveolar samples. The specimens are handled identically to simple washings, but also absolute cell counts are useful in the workup of inflammatory, allergic, and autoimmune lung disease. Certain infections, such as *Mycobacterium tuberculosis*, atypical tuberculosis, *Pneumocystis carinii*, histoplasmosis, and mycoplasma, are readily diagnosed by BAL.[8]

Bronchial brushings are obtained by inserting a small brush in the working port of the scope and abrading the surface of the airway or identified lesion. The brush is then wiped on a slide that is immediately fixed with spray or liquid to avoid structural distortion for subsequent examination.

Endobronchial biopsies can be readily obtained by both rigid and flexible bronchoscopy. Larger size biopsies can be obtained for more central lesions by rigid bronchoscopy; more distal lesions may be accessible only by flexible bronchoscopy. Usually biopsy site bleeding can be stopped with simple pressure or irrigation. For the unlikely situation of difficult bleeding, epinephrine irrigation or electrocautery can be used.

Needle aspirations may be utilized for intrabronchial or transbronchial sampling of tissue. Once obtained the specimen should be ejected to a slide and immediately fixed. If a core needle is used it should be handled like a regular biopsy. For all biopsies that are questionable a pathologist should be consulted for tissue procurement and storage for optimal beneficial results.

REFERENCES

1. Botet JF, Lightdale CJ, Zauber AG, et al: Preoperative staging of esophageal cancer: Comparison of endoscopic US and dynamic CT. Radiology 181(2):419–425, 1991.
2. Enns R, Branch MS: Management of esophageal perforation after therapeutic upper gastrointestinal endoscopy. Gastrointest Endosc 47(3):318–320, 1998.
3. Ferguson MK, Migliore M, Staszak VM, Little AG: Early evaluation and therapy for caustic esophageal injury. Am J Surg 157(1):116–120, 1989.
4. Fulkerson WJ: Fiberoptic bronchoscopy. N Engl J Med 311:511–515, 1984.
5. Graham D, Schwartz J, Cain G, Gyorkey F: Prospective evaluation of biopsy number in the diagnosis of esophageal and gastric carcinoma. Gastroenterology 82:228–231, 1982.
6. Harrell JH: Transnasal approach for fiberoptic bronchoscopy. Chest 73:704–706, 1978.
7. Linder TE, Simmen D, Stool SE: The history of endoscopy. Arch Otolaryngol Head Neck Surg 123:1161–1163, 1997.
8. Lloveras JJ, Lecuyer I, Dider A: Benefits of bronchoscopy and bronchoalveolar lavage in the diagnosis of pneumonitis is transplant recipients. Transplant Proc 25:2293, 1993.
9. Lukonsky GI, Ovchinnikov AA, Bilal A: Complications of bronchoscopy. Chest 79:316, 1981.
10. Parmar KS, Zwischenberger JB, Reeves AL, Waxman I: Clinical impact of endoscopic ultrasound-guided fine needle aspiration of celiac axis lymph nodes (M1a disease) in esophageal cancer. Ann Thorac Surg 73(3):916–920, 2002.
11. Pasricha PJ, Fleischer DE, Kalloo AN: Endoscopic perforations of the upper digestive tract: A review of their pathogenesis, prevention, and management. Gastroenterology 106(3): 787–802, 1994.
12. Poe RH, Ortiz C, Israel RH: Sensitivity, specificity, and predictive values of bronchoscopy in neoplasm metastatic to the lung. Chest. 88:84–88, 1985.
13. Pue CA, Pacht ER: Complications of fiberoptic bronchoscopy at a university hospital. Chest 107:430–432, 1995.
14. Sackner MA: Bronchofiberoscopy. Am Rev Respir Dis 111:62–88, 1975.
15. Winawer S, Sherlock P, Belladonna J, et al: Endoscopic brush cytology in esophageal cancer. JAMA 232:1358, 1975.
16. Wu LF, Wang BZ, Feng JL, et al: Preoperative TN staging of esophageal cancer: Comparison of miniprobe ultrasonography, spiral CT and MRI. World J Gastroenterol 9(2):219–224, 2003.
17. Zargar S, Khuroo M, Jan G, et al: Prospective comparison of the value of brushings before and after biopsy in the endoscopic diagnosis of gastroesophageal malignancy. Acta Cytol 35:549–552, 1991.

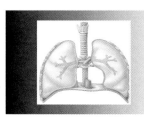

Endoscopic Therapies for the Airway and the Esophagus

Sébastien Gilbert, James D. Luketich, and Hiran C. Fernando

CHAPTER **6**

INTRODUCTION

The first recorded bronchoscopic intervention is attributed to Gustav Killian, who, in 1897, removed a piece of pork bone from the right mainstem bronchus using an esophagoscope.[7] A few decades later, Chevalier Jackson pioneered the field of rigid endoscopy of the airway and esophagus. Jackson held tenure at the University of Pittsburgh from 1912 to 1916.[7] Advancement of endoscopic technology has led to the development of improved tools, which provide a minimally invasive alternative to surgery in some cases. This chapter will focus on endoscopic techniques specific to the airway and esophagus. Established therapies will be discussed including photodynamic therapy, stenting, laser ablation, and brachytherapy. In addition, evolving endoscopic procedures for benign esophageal disorders including transoral endoscopic stapling for Zenker's diverticulum and newer endoscopic therapies for gastroesophageal reflux disease will also be reviewed.

PHOTODYNAMIC THERAPY

Definition and Mechanism of Action

The basic principle of photodynamic therapy (PDT) is the accumulation in target cells of a photosensitizing substance that, when activated by light of a specific spectrum, causes selective tissue destruction. Photosensitizers relevant to the surgeon include purified hematoporphyrin derivatives (porfimer sodium or Photofrin, Axcan Scandipharm, Birmingham, AL), chlorines [temoporfin or *m*-tetrahydroxyphenyl chlorin (*m*-THPC)], and 5-aminolevulinic acid (5-ALA). The optimal wavelengths of light absorption are 630 nm for porfimer sodium and 5-ALA and 652 nm for *m*-THPC.

Photosensitizers accumulate in all cells of the body. However, after 1–4 days, higher concentrations are found within tumor cells and their interstitium. Altered lymphatic drainage, neovascularization, and increased cellular proliferation are some of the mechanisms hypothesized to be responsible for this phenomenon. Laser light delivered directly to cancer cells harboring the photosensitizer triggers a series of events culminating in cell destruction. When cells are bombarded with photons of a wavelength specific to the photosensitizer, the absorbed energy acts as a catalyst in the formation of highly reactive oxygen species (e.g., superoxide anions, peroxide anions, singlet oxygen). The

66 primary targets of photodamage are cellular membranes, amino acids, and nucleosides.

Technique and General Considerations

The first step in PDT is the administration of the photosensitizer. Porfimer sodium (1.5–2.0 mg/kg) and m-THPC (0.15 mg/kg) are injected intravenously while 5-ALA (60 mg/kg) is given orally. Despite an improved side effect profile and increased tumor specificity, 5-ALA has limited applications in thoracic surgery since it produces necrosis only to a depth of 1 mm using current dosing regimens.[53,70] Higher doses of 5-ALA cannot be used because of severe side effects including nausea, vomiting, and transient elevation of liver enzymes. The chemical agent m-THPC is more photoactive than other agents and has a shorter elimination half-life than porfimer sodium, but is not yet approved for clinical use in the United States.

PDT is considered effective and indicated for tumors with a significant endoluminal component in the airway or esophagus. The most commonly used photosensitizer is Photofrin, which has a depth of penetration of approximately 5 mm. It can be given in the outpatient setting, 1–4 days prior to endoscopic light application. Patient education is essential to minimize complications related to photosensitivity. All bright light and sunlight exposure must be avoided initially. Patients remain photosensitive for a period of 4–8 weeks, after which they can be gradually reexposed to sunlight.

Our preference has been to use conscious sedation and flexible endoscopy in most cases. A cylindrical diffuser fiber is used to deliver light therapy to the tumor. The fiber sizes include 1, 2.5, and 5 cm (Figure 6-1). The diffuser fiber is placed endoluminally alongside the tumor. If this is not possible because of occlusion of the lumen, the tumor can be impaled with the probe. Multiple light illumination cycles may be needed depending on the length of the tumor relative to the length of the probe. The diffuser must be positioned so as to minimize light delivery to normal tissues. Repeat endoscopy is performed at 48 h and, sometimes, on a third setting another 48 h later. During the repeat endoscopic procedures necrotic debris is removed using irrigation, suction, and balloon dilation. Frequently, additional light treatments are delivered to the tumor at the time of repeat endoscopy.

In many cases, PDT can be performed in the outpatient setting. However, caution should be exercised when treating the central airways. Perioperative edema and necrotic tissue may temporarily worsen obstruction. We frequently begin the procedure by debulking the tumor using a rigid bronchoscope to "core out" the tumor. It has been our preference to treat such tumors in the inpatient setting. For obstructing esophageal tumors, the patient may be admitted to hospital depending on the degree of obstruction and the presence of malnutrition and/or dehydration.

Contraindications

Contraindications to PDT include porphyria or allergies to porphyrins. PDT is contraindicated in the presence of an esophagorespiratory fistula or in tumors eroding into a major blood vessel. PDT is not recommended for the treatment of obstruction caused primarily by extraluminal compression.

Lung Cancer

Curative Intent; Airway

PDT may be used for the treatment of small, proximal endobronchial tumors. These small central tumors are rare, although some centers with active early screening programs such as sputum cytology or light-induced fluorescence bronchoscopy (LIFE) may encounter these more frequently.[92] The results of PDT for small lesions should be compared to the results of surgical resection. In many cases, resection of these proximal tumors may require complex airway reconstruction because of their central location. PDT is attractive because of its potential to replace extended pulmonary resections with an outpatient endoscopic procedure.

Superficially spreading tumors (<3 cm²) and small endobronchial tumors (<1 cm) that are not amenable to surgical resection are good candidates for PDT. Initial complete response can be expected in 65% (<3 cm²) to 85% (<1 cm²) of superficial neoplasms, and in 30% (>0.5 cm) to 92% (<0.5 cm) of nodular endobronchial tumors.[21,28] Long-term response rates (i.e., >1 year) vary between 30 and 70%.[15,28,89–91] At 5 years of follow-up, local recurrences have been reported in over 50% of patients.[15]

In one North American study, 21 patients who were considered surgical candidates had small airway tumors treated initially with PDT. At 1 year, bronchoscopy revealed that 52% (11/21) were free of tumor.[15] The remaining patients failed curative PDT and were offered surgery. Of the 11 responders, 9 (9/21; 43%) did not require surgery (mean follow-up = 68 months), and 2 were operated for second primary lung cancer. It is noteworthy that in patients who eventually underwent resection, 30% were found to have N1 disease. Since these patients had superficial cancers at the time of PDT, it is possible that nodal spread occurred following PDT failure, thereby emphasizing the importance of surgical resection whenever possible. Pulmonary resection should remain the preferred treatment for these small cancers. We reserve PDT for patients who have significant comorbidity and for those who refuse pulmonary resection.

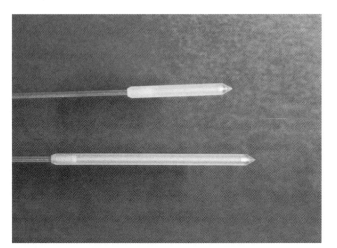

Figure 6–1 PDT diffuser fibers 2.5 and 5 cm.

In this group of patients, PDT offers a reasonable alternative to surgery with an expected 1-year survival of 80%.[47] In a prospective series of nonsurgical candidates, 93% were alive at 5 years of follow-up.[90] Our initial experience with 10 superficial cancers yielded a complete response in 70% of patients at 30 months of follow-up.[90]

Palliative Intent; Airway

A relatively small number of patients will have central airway tumors that are amenable to curative PDT. A much larger group of patients with advanced lung cancers will be candidates for palliative PDT. In this situation, the therapeutic goal should be symptomatic relief, preservation of quality of life, and improvement in functional status. Most of these patients who are candidates for endobronchial PDT have symptoms of dyspnea or hemoptysis related to central airway involvement.

In a large prospective study, 175 patients with endobronchial non-small-cell lung cancer (NSCLC) were palliated with PDT.[12] Most patients had squamous cell carcinoma (89.3%), and 73.1% had failed treatment by conventional modalities, such as chemotherapy, radiotherapy, laser ablation, or surgery. The mean number of PDT courses was 2.8 per patient. Poor performance status (i.e., Karnofsky Performance Status [KPS] <50) had a negative impact on outcome only in advanced-stage tumors (IIIa–IV). However, patients with a low KPS (<50) secondary to pulmonary symptoms benefited from PDT. In fact, of the 44 patients with stage IV disease, 21% survived 12 months or longer. The median survival for all stages was 7 months.

We have used palliative PDT for airway obstruction and hemoptysis in 44 patients with primary NSCLC.[48] Patients with mild, persistent hemoptysis were treated with PDT, whereas those with massive hemoptysis were treated with other modalities. There were no fatalities, and 82% of treatments were performed without complications. At a mean of 2.3 months, 13 patients (30%) required a second treatment course for recurrent symptoms. Hemoptysis was effectively palliated in 90% of cases. Obstruction was successfully palliated in 59%. In our patients with endobronchial metastases from nonpulmonary malignancies, PDT provided effective palliation in 95%.[41] Figures 6-2 through 6-6 provide radiographic and endoscopic illustrations of an obstructing airway lesion before and after PDT.

In a randomized prospective trial, PDT was compared to neodymium–yttrium–aluminum–garnet laser (Nd-YAG) for inoperable NSCLC with endobronchial obstruction.[18] The bronchoscopic response (PDT = 38.5%; laser = 23.5%) and symptomatic improvement at 1 month were equivalent in both groups. PDT resulted in significantly longer relief of symptoms (50 versus 38 days) and median survival (265 versus 95 days) when compared to Nd-YAG. However, the survival benefit may be explained in part by the lower proportion of stage III–IV tumors in the PDT group.

Complications

PDT is well tolerated with minimal morbidity. In our experience, complications included respiratory failure (7.8%),

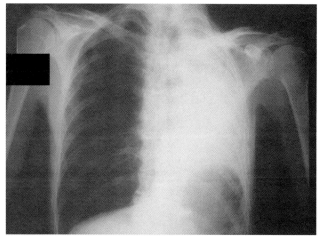

Figure 6–2 Radiographic picture of Patient A with lung cancer obstructing the left mainstem bronchus prior to PDT.

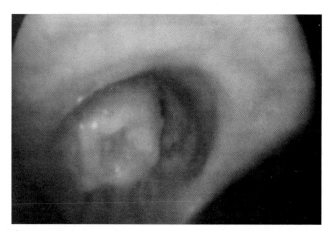

Figure 6–3 Bronchoscopic picture of Patient A before PDT.

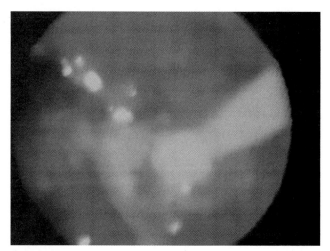

Figure 6–4 Bronchoscopic picture of Patient A during PDT.

68

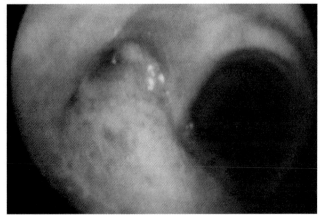

Figure 6–5 Bronchoscopic picture of Patient A after PDT.

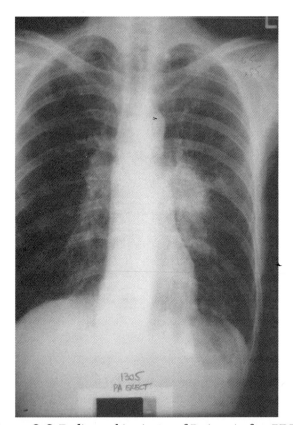

Figure 6–6 Radiographic picture of Patient A after PDT.

pleural effusion (1.3%), and sunburn (5.2%). Respiratory failure occurs since many patients have central airway tumors, and often present with respiratory distress.[45,57] Direct sunlight exposure has been reported to cause first and second-degree burns in up to 10% of cases in some series.[16] The immediate postprocedure mortality after PDT for endobronchial obstruction ranges from 4 to 7.1%.[18,56]

Barrett's Esophagus and Esophageal Cancer

Curative Intent; Esophagus

The management of high-grade dysplasia (HGD) associated with Barrett's esophagus is controversial. Most surgeons advocate esophagectomy because of the risk (~40%) of missing an occult cancer.[94] On the other hand, concerns over the morbidity and mortality of esophagectomy have led some clinicians to advocate alternative approaches, such as surveillance endoscopy or mucosal ablation.[20] In our experience, we have reported good results using a minimally invasive method for esophagectomy in patients with HGD.[24,63]

Mucosal ablative methods include laser ablation, argon plasma coagulation electrocoagulation, endoscopic mucosal resection, and PDT.[30,55,74,87] All these techniques attempt to eradicate Barrett's epithelium with the hope that it will be replaced by squamous epithelium. Unfortunately islands of columnar epithelium may recur under the squamous layer.[3] PDT is arguably the most established of these ablative techniques. In the largest study to date, PDT was combined with Nd-YAG laser to treat 73 patients with HGD and 14 with low-grade dysplasia (LGD).[69] All patients were followed endoscopically for 12 months. Regression to LGD or no dysplasia was reported in 88% of HGD and 93% of LGD cases. Complete eradication of Barrett's occurred in 9% of patients following PDT alone. When there was a focus on the PDT-treated mucosa, a 49% eradication rate was reported. The addition of laser ablation to residual areas of Barrett's increased the response rate to 87%. This group used a transparent centering balloon to facilitate uniform delivery of PDT to the esophageal mucosa. The centering balloon is not yet approved by the Food and Drug Administration (FDA) for general use.

PDT can also be used to treat early-stage esophageal tumors (T1–T2) in patients who refuse or are not candidates for surgical resection. In a group of patients that included mostly T1 tumors (12/13), regression to Barrett's with LGD or without dysplasia was observed in 77% (10/13).[69] At our center, PDT with curative intent is reserved for high-operative-risk patients. All others undergo minimally invasive esophagectomy.[24] In our initial experience of 14 high-risk patients with either HGD or early stage cancer, four patients died of tumor progression, one died from a postprocedure cardiovascular accident, and two developed recurrent disease. At a median follow-up of 20 months, 70% were alive, but only 7 (50%) had an excellent outcome without evidence of recurrent disease.[46] Although these results may be acceptable for high-risk patients, they are inferior to the results of esophagectomy for HGD. In a cohort of 28 patients who underwent minimally invasive esophagectomy, there was only one postoperative death.[24] All 27 patients discharged from the hospital were free of disease a median follow-up of 13 months, supporting the role of esophagectomy for these patients.

Other endoscopic techniques, such as endoscopic mucosal resection (EMR), have been used to remove Barrett's mucosa and superficial cancers. One of the EMR techniques involves submucosal injection of epinephrine solution and subsequent resection of the mucosa using cautery. EMR has been used to remove small cancers with a recurrence rate of 14% at 12 months.[22] In another series including 17 patients with superficial cancers or Barrett's with HGD, there was no recurrence at a median follow-up of 10 months.[64] In contrast to PDT, this approach provides tissue samples for pathological analysis. In one study, review of EMR specimens led to revision of the diagnosis made with routine endoscopic biopsy samples in over 40% of patients.[64]

Complications

Minor side effects include nausea, regurgitation, constipation, odynophagia, dysphagia, weight loss (average 6 kg), and noncardiac chest pain.[32,68] Other complications include stricture, tumor growth below the PDT-induced scarring, Barrett's, and tumor recurrence.[50] In our experience, approximately 30% of patients with high-grade dysplasia undergoing PDT will develop an esophageal stricture.[46] In Overholt's series of 87 patients with Barrett's treated with PDT the stricture rate was 34%.[69] Strictures frequently respond to dilations but in cases of multiple stricture recurrences, we have had to use expandable metal stents.

Palliative Intent; Esophagus

Stenting of the esophagus is probably the most commonly used modality to palliate dysphagia.[11] However, PDT offers some advantages in certain clinical situations. For instance, PDT can prevent further bleeding from the tumor along with relieving obstruction. It may also prevent the globus sensation associated with stents in the proximal esophagus, and the reflux symptoms observed with stenting of the gastroesophageal junction. PDT is an excellent alternative to stenting for endoluminal cancers in both of these locations. Moreover, it has been compared to laser ablation in a prospective randomized trial.[40] Although relief of dysphagia was equivalent in both groups, PDT was associated with a lower risk of acute perforation than laser ablation (PDT = 1%; laser = 7%).

We have reviewed our results in 215 patients with obstructing esophageal cancer who underwent palliative PDT.[43] The most common disease was adenocarcinoma (83%). The distal esophagus was involved in 71% of cases. Dysphagia improved in 85% of patients and bleeding was successfully controlled in 90%. Stenting was subsequently required in 24% of patients because of disease progression. As expected, median survival was poor at 4.9 months; however, effective palliation was provided to these unfortunate patients. In another prospective series of 77 patients who failed conventional therapy or were deemed unfit for surgery, investigators reported a median survival of 6.3 months following PDT.[57] Photosensitivity appears to be an acceptable trade-off in these patients. In a study utilizing satisfaction questionnaires, patients reported that the ability to swallow food was more important than the limitations of photosensitivity.[32] In most cases, the potential benefits of PDT far outweigh the risk of complications.

Complications

In patients with obstructing aerodigestive tumors, PDT carries a risk of adverse consequences. Esophageal strictures (4.8–5.2%), perforation (0–9.1%), and esophagorespiratory fistulas (0–5.2%) are among the most serious PDT-related complications.[15,49,51,53,57] Esophageal perforations and fistu-

las are probably best treated by esophageal stenting. In PDT for malignant esophageal obstruction, the immediate post-procedure mortality ranges from 1.3 to 3.9%.[45,57] Other factors contributing to the mortality rate and risk of esophageal perforation include the frequently end-stage performance status of this group of patients and the fact that some patients with obstructing tumors commonly receive concurrent radiation therapy and chemotherapy.

▶ STENTS

General Considerations and Insertion

Malignant endoluminal obstruction and extraluminal compression by enlarged lymph nodes or tumor are common indications for stenting of the airway or esophagus. The two major types of stents used in thoracic surgery are expandable metal stents and silicone-based stents.

Expandable Metal Stents

Expandable metal stents (EMS) are constructed using either cobalt alloys (Wallstent, Schneider, Minneapolis, MN), stainless steel (Gianturco, Cook, Bloomington, IN), or a nickel–titanium alloy referred to as nitinol (Esophacoil, Medtronic, Minneapolis, MN; Ultraflex, Microvasive, Natick, MA). These materials are resistant to corrosion and biologically inert. The wire stents can be woven (Wallstent), knitted (Ultraflex), or bent into a zigzag (Gianturco) or coil (Esophacoil) configuration. The stent design influences its retraction (i.e., shortening) properties. Retraction percentage is highest with the coil and lowest with the zigzag configuration. The shape memory characteristics of the materials allow the stent to reexpand to its original tubular shape, even when compressed into a delivery system. The available systems can deploy stents from the proximal end, the center, or the distal end. Proximal delivery is better suited for proximal strictures, and distal delivery is best for strictures of the gastroesophageal junction. EMS can also be partially covered with polyurethane or silicone. Covered designs help reduce tumor ingrowth, but they also increase the risk of migration.[2] The wide range of available diameters and lengths allows EMS to fit most upper aerodigestive strictures.

EMS placement can be performed with patient under conscious sedation or under general anesthesia. The stricture is identified endoscopically and measured. Esophageal stents are available in a wide range of lengths (60–150 mm) but, in contrast to airway stents, most have a similar maximal internal diameter (17–23 mm). Larger diameters are available from some manufacturers. If the opening of the stricture is too small to accept the endoscope, the lumen may require dilation, and or laser ablation before length can be assessed accurately. Fluoroscopy is then used to mark the location of the stricture, on the patient's skin. This is done by using two radiopaque markers (e.g., small stylets, paper clips), which are taped to the skin at points corresponding to the proximal and distal edges of the stricture. Alternatively, some clinicians prefer to inject the submucosa at the proximal and distal ends of the tumor with a radiopaque liquid (Conray). Once the measurement of the tumor length is completed, the proper stent is selected. In general, we use an 18- to

70 23-mm-diameter stent that is 1–2 cm longer than the stricture to avoid crimping and infolding of the proximal and distal ends. A guide wire is passed through the stricture and the endoscope is withdrawn. Under fluoroscopic control, the delivery system is inserted over the guide wire through the stricture and aligned with the skin or mucosal markers. The stent is deployed and expands within the lumen. Proper positioning and deployment are confirmed fluoroscopically and endoscopically. Minor adjustments are possible immediately postdeployment by grasping the proximal or distal end of the stent with endoscopic grasping forceps. A postprocedure chest radiograph (in all cases) and barium esophagogram (in esophageal cases) are obtained to assess patency and serve as a reference for later assessment of position in the clinic. EMS are popular, as they are easier to insert than their silicone counterpart, and do not require expertise in rigid endoscopy. Silicone stents are more challenging to place but are preferable for patients with benign strictures.

Silicone Stents

Silicons stents are made of Silastic rubber (Silatic, Dow Corning, Midland, MI), a ubiquitous component of industrial, household, and medical equipment. The Celestin esophageal tubes have fallen out of favor because of the need for an open gastrotomy for anchoring and the higher complication rate in comparison to EMS.[37] Flanged (Hood, Hood Laboratories, Pembroke, MA) or studded (Dumon, Bryan Corp., Woburn, MA) cylindrical silicons stents are used in the trachea or bronchi. T-, Y-, and T-Y-shaped silicone stents are also available to treat tracheal and proximal tracheobronchial strictures. If a silicone stent has to be shortened to fit the patient's airway, the manufacturer can provide a customized replacement upon request.

Unless the patient has a tracheal stoma, rigid bronchoscopy is required to insert a silicon-based stent. A large-bore-diameter chest tube, cut to size, and the stent are passed over a rigid scope in sequence. The chest tube serves as a pusher to deliver the stent over the rigid scope. For Y-shaped stents, the right mainstem bronchus limb is invaginated and the rigid scope passed through the left mainstem bronchus limb. After it is positioned, the scope is pulled back within the tracheal limb and biopsy forceps are used to push out the right-sided limb. An alternative technique is to guide the ride-sided limb into the right mainstem bronchus using a Fogarty catheter positioned endoscopically. A complete technical description of rigid endoscopic stent insertion has been previously published by our group.[26] Table 6-1 compares some of the features of silicone and metal stents.

Airway Stents

The recommended definitive treatment of benign airway strictures is surgical resection. Stenting is indicated for strictured or malacic airways not amenable to resection, or for nonsurgical candidates in whom dilatation and/or laser resection have failed. Stenting may be used as a bridge to surgery in patients needing time for their general condition to improve. In this situation, silicone stents are preferable as these are easily removed at the time of operation. Malignant airway strictures and esophagorespiratory fistulas can also be managed by stenting.

Benign Airway Strictures

Stenting of benign airway strictures should be regarded as second-line therapy, reserved for situations in which surgi-

---

Table 6–1

Characteristics of Silicone and Expandable Metal Stents

Stent type	Description	Method of insertion	Pros	Cons
Silicon-based Internal	Made of silastic rubber Straight or Y-shaped Studded (Dumon) Flanged (Hood)	Rigid bronchoscopy	Resistance to lateral compression Prevents ingrowth Easy to remove	Eliminates mucociliary clearance Propensity for mucous plugging Propensity for dislodgement Cosmesis
External	T- or T-Y-shaped	Rigid bronchoscopy and/or peritracheal stoma	Maintains tracheal stoma Tracheal port allows suction Prolong relief of dyspnea in nonoperative candidates Custom-fitted	Regular maintenance (irrigation, suction)
Expandable metal Ultraflex Wallstent Gianturco	Nickel–titanium Cobalt–steel Steel	Flexible bronchoscopy	Easy to insert Adapt to irregularly shaped stricture	Relatively weaker expansile force Granulation Allow ingrowth of tumor Very difficult to remove

cal resection in not possible. It should be clear that stenting of benign strictures is suboptimal therapy, as up to 40% of patients will need reintervention.[14] In comparison to the shorter survival expected with malignant strictures, patients with benign strictures live longer and will require further intervention over time. For this reason, silicone stents are recommended for benign strictures. Previous experiences with silicone stents for benign strictures in nonoperative candidates have been relatively good.[14,29] Out of 112 patients with T-stents, only five (4.5%) required removal for obstructive problems, and 85% were managed successfully for periods of 3 months to over 5 years.[29] In another more recent series, 94% of patients with benign strictures were successfully palliated with silicone stents.[14] Only 5.6% of these stents needed removal or replacement for migration or compression. There were no procedure-related deaths, and late mortality (10.4%) was not related to stenting. Other studies involving smaller numbers of patients (n = 6–22) reported symptomatic and spirometric improvement after stenting.[19,31,62]

Our unpublished experience supports the use of silicon-based stents over EMS for benign stricture. In a cohort of 36 patients, reintervention was necessary in 61% of patients at a mean of 6 months. Nd-YAG lasering was required to ablate granulation in a significantly higher number of patients with metal stents. Other investigators have described the common finding of stent-related granulation (up to 80% of patients), and this problem may ultimately lead to stent removal.[62] Twenty percent of our EMS have had to be removed for complications. Extirpation required thoracotomy in one third of these cases.

Life-threatening complications, such as stent dislocation and rupture, leading to acute airway obstruction and aorto-bronchial fistula have been previously described.[13,73] Despite their relative ease of insertion, EMS should probably be avoided in nonsurgical candidates with benign airway strictures. The lung transplant patient with a benign stricture is a noteworthy exception. Although restenosis related to fibrosis occurs commonly, with appropriate reintervention, prolonged airway patency and improvement in pulmonary function can be achieved.[66]

Malignant Airway Strictures

To successfully alleviate malignant airway obstruction, the surgeon should be familiar with a variety of interventional techniques, including rigid endoscopy and debridement, dilation, PDT, endoscopic lasering, and stent insertion. Additionally the surgeon should be familiar with the indications and limitations of external beam radiotherapy and brachytherapy. Familiarity with all options will lead to selection of the optimal course of action and best combination of the various techniques, when necessary. For example, the patient with a central airway tumor who is becoming symptomatic, but is not yet obstructed, may benefit from external beam radiotherapy with excellent results. If the obstruction is more acute or if the patient has recurred after external beam radiotherapy, the surgeon needs to perform bronchoscopy and determine which endoscopic therapy is best suited to the needs of the individual patient. If obstruction is almost complete, it may be difficult to assess the distal lumen for patency. This is a crucial step in the evaluation

since aggressive proximal therapy with a stent or laser is doomed to failure if the distal airways are blocked with tumor. On then other hand, patients with proximal extrinsic compression and patent distal airways are ideal candidates for stents.

Since most patients with malignant airway involvement have a limited survival, the type of stent used is of lesser importance. Surgeons familiar with silicone stents have reported relief of dyspnea in up to 87–94% of patients.[78,82] Complications, including migration and occlusion, were reported in 12.5–23.1% of stents placed. Over 30% of patients were alive at a mean interval of 7.6 months.[78] Polyurethane-covered EMS can also provide significant improvement in dyspnea and Karnofsky score.[5] However, up to 55.6% of patients experience complications, including stent migration in 22.2%.[5] Although covered stents prevent tumor ingrowth, migration may occur if the stent is not well seated against the wall of the airway.

In malignant airway obstruction, stenting should be considered in the context of a multidisciplinary approach to palliation. In most of the studies discussed above, patients had already received chemotherapy and/or radiation prior to referral for endoscopic palliation. The importance of initial chemotherapy and/or radiation therapy has been highlighted in a prospective trial.[93] In 22 patients with tracheobronchial strictures treated by stenting, 50% eventually had their stent removed following appropriate radiation and/or chemotherapy regimens. Thus, early intervention with chemoradiotherapy may delay or avoid the need for aggressive endoluminal therapy in selected cases.

We recently reviewed 53 cases in which expandable stents were used to treat tracheobronchial obstruction.[42] Concurrent interventions included balloon dilation (29%), Nd-YAG laser (29%), photodynamic therapy (23%), rigid bronchoscopy with debridement (15%), and brachytherapy (2%). Bronchoscopic patency was achieved in 92% of patients. Radiographic improvement was noted in 46% of patients with lung collapse. Reintervention was required in 19 patients (36%) for obstruction by mucus plugging or granulation tissue. The median poststenting survival was relatively short at 41 days.

Esophageal Stents

Benign Esophageal Strictures

The routine use of stents for benign esophageal strictures cannot be recommended in light of a 41% rate of stent-induced restenosis, and almost uniform (91%) recurrence of dysphagia.[60,75] However, in select cases, silicon-based stents may play a role for short-term use and occasionally EMS are chosen when other options, such as definitive surgical resection, are not feasible.

Malignant Esophageal Strictures

Depending on the referral pattern, up to 50% of malignant esophageal tumors will be inoperable at the time of diagnosis. Endoscopic palliation with laser or stents assumes an important role in providing relief from dysphagia to many of these patients. Over the past decade, advances in expandable stent technology have led to smaller, more flexible delivery systems, which are easier to manipulate than their silicone equivalent. These attributes often allow successful deployment without exposing the patient to the risks of mechanical dilation.

Both silicon-based and mesh wire stents are susceptible to tumor growth above and below the stent, leading to recurrence of esophageal obstruction. Additionally, tumor ingrowth through stent interstices can occur with uncovered metal stents. In the absence of an esophagorespiratory fistula, the decision to use a covered stent is influenced by the potential for recurrent obstruction by tumor ingrowth and the likelihood of stent migration. When tumor overgrowth or ingrowth occurs, therapeutic modalities including PDT, laser, or further stenting (i.e., placing a stent within a stent) may be of additional palliative benefit.[35]

A few prospective randomized trials have compared silicone and metal stents for malignant esophageal obstruction.[37,77] Both trials, which included comparable groups of patients, reported that technical success (95–100%), improvement in dysphagia (91–100%), and the need for reintervention were similar regardless of stent type. However, the use of silicone stents was associated with a higher rate of complications (silicone = 43–47%; metal = 0–16%) and a prolonged hospital stay (silicone = 6–12 days; metal = 4–5 days).[37,77] Even though poststent survival was not statistically different (silicone = 29%; metal = 14%), death as a result of stent insertion occurred only in the silicone stent group.[37] Despite a higher purchase price, EMS were found to be more cost-effective because of shorter hospital stays and lower complication rates.[37]

At the University of Pittsburgh, a review of 100 stented patients demonstrated relief of dysphagia in 85% with a low perforation rate (0.8%) and no fatalities.[11] Reasons for initial stent failure were the inability to resume an oral diet, intractable reflux and pain, bulky tumors resulting in inadequate stent expansion, and stent malposition. Sixteen stents were placed in patients undergoing neoadjuvant therapy for possible later esophagectomy. Supplemental enteral or intravenous nutrition was not necessary in 88% (n = 14) of these patients. At the time of esophagectomy, dissection of the periesophageal planes was more difficult but no operative complications could be directly attributed to preoperative stenting. Patients receiving chemotherapy and/or radiation following placement of EMS may be prone to later perforation or fistulization, so alternatives to stenting should be sought in this subgroup of patients.[6,11,52] In other large series of patients undergoing stenting (>100 patients), successful placement and improvement of dysphagia were achieved in 90–100% of patients.[17,67,72,79,80] Procedure-related mortality was low (0–2.5%). The above findings lend support to the use of stents as a relatively safe and effective method of palliation for obstructing esophageal cancer.

▶ THERMAL LASER ABLATION OF ENDOLUMINAL TUMORS

Although carbon dioxide, argon, potassium-tetanyl-phosphate, and diode lasers are available, the most commonly used laser in thoracic surgery is the Nd-YAG. The latter can be delivered through a small-caliber fiberoptic conduit, thus making it ideal for use with the flexible bronchoscope or esophagoscope. Adjustments in power level allow for a combination of coagulation (low power, defocused beam) and vaporization (high power, focused beam) of tissue. The maximum depth of penetration when firing the Nd-YAG laser is approximately 4 mm. Airway and esophageal Nd-YAG laser procedures can be performed safely using sedation alone. Communication between the surgeon, anesthesiologist, and the rest of the operating team is essential to minimize the risk to the patient and to the staff. Experienced centers have published simple rules to increase the safety of endobronchial lasering. These rules are also applicable to the esophagus. Other investigators have contributed mnemonics to remember favorable lesion characteristics, power and pulse settings, as well as the techniques used to optimize results from lasering the airway.[39] Lesions of the central airways less than 4 cm in length, localized to one wall, and protruding through the lumen (e.g., exophytic, pedunculated) without complete obstruction are ideal for laser ablation.[39] Candidates for laser therapy include patients with minimal extrinsic compression and a primarily endoluminal tumor burden with distal patent lumen. This assessment may require rigid bronchoscopy with a "core out" technique using the end of the rigid scope. Other options include proximal laser therapy, to a point at which the distal lumen can be assessed.

Airway

Symptomatic relief from cough, dyspnea, hemoptysis, postobstructive pneumonia, and accelerated weaning from mechanical ventilation can be achieved in approximately 80% of patients with malignant airway obstruction.[69] In a series of over 1800 patients treated with Nd-YAG laser, 93% had improvement in symptoms and quality of life.[10] Even in patients with advanced tumors who had failed radiotherapy and chemotherapy, laser photoresection provided symptomatic relief in 64%.[33] Nd-YAG lasering is successful in controlling hemoptysis in 60% of patients. However, recurrence of symptoms is frequently seen within 30 days of treatment.[35] At least 50% of these patients can be extubated immediately following laser treatment.[39] There is no difference in response between primary and metastatic airway lesions. Success rate decreases from 90 to 60% when the tumor is located in the central airways.[9]

The overall major complication rate of endobronchial laser therapy varies between 3 and 4%.[10] Serious complications include perforation of vascular structures and endobronchial fire. The latter usually involves the endotracheal tube, the flexible bronchoscope sheath, or suction catheters. Ignition can be avoided by keeping the fraction of inspired oxygen less than 40%, using nonflammable anesthetic agents, and keeping the scope and field as clean as possible. Hemorrhage of the tumor, pneumothorax, and pneumomediastinum are other recognized complications of airway lasering.

Esophagus

Malignant tumors of the esophagus are also amenable to treatment with Nd-YAG laser. Depending on the size of the tumor, several weekly treatments may be necessary to provide significant relief from obstruction. Lasering can also be used to recanalize a tumor in preparation for stenting. The best candidates for laser therapy are patients with small

(<5-cm) exophytic tumors located in the middle third of the esophagus, at the site of a previous esophagogastric anastomosis, or above a stent. The incidence of laser-related esophageal perforation varies between 0 and 6%.[4,8] Recurrence of dysphagia can be expected within 4–6 weeks of treatment. The combination of laser with radiotherapy has resulted in prolongation of the dysphagia-free interval in patients with malignant obstruction.[76] However, it should be emphasized again that endoscopic Nd-YAG laser is associated with a higher risk of acute perforation than PDT.[40]

BRACHYTHERAPY

Brachytherapy can be defined as the placement of interstitial or intracavitary radioactive sources to facilitate the safe delivery of high radiation doses with relative sparing of normal surrounding tissues. High-dose rate brachytherapy (HDR-Br) allows the delivery of high doses of radiation to the airway over a short period of time with minimal effect to surrounding tissue. There are numerous technical approaches to these patients, depending on the location of the brachytherapy device and the choice of the interventionalist. In our center, we typically perform airway brachytherapy by initially performing bronchoscopy to directly view the problem area. A blind-ended 6F afterloading catheter is passed through the working channel of a bronchoscope and dummy seeds placed within the catheter to confirm its position by fluoroscopy. We typically place radiopaque markers on the skin to correspond to the proximal and distal extents of the endobronchial tumor. Again, attention to the presence of a patent distal lumen is important. The catheter is taped securely and the patient transferred to the radiation suite. Radiation seeds (iridium-192) are placed in the afterloading catheter. Typically, three treatments are given at weekly intervals each requiring only 10–15 min of radiation exposure. An advantage of brachytherapy over Nd-YAG laser is the greater depth of penetration (0.5–2 cm), making it more suitable for tumors with some degree of extraluminal involvement. A disadvantage is that symptomatic improvement will be slower to occur than with PDT or Nd-YAG. On longer follow-up, bronchitis with stricturing (9–13%) or hemoptysis (7%) may develop as a result of brachytherapy.[39,81] The latter two complications are more commonly encountered with high radiation doses to the central airways. Symptomatic improvement following brachytherapy occurs in 72–94% of cases.[39,58] Endobronchial tumor regression is observed in 54–94% of patients.[39] For stage I and II lung cancer, a 72% complete histological response has been documented.[85] Finally, there is prospective randomized evidence suggesting that the combination of brachytherapy with external beam radiation therapy leads to additive improvement in symptom-free interval and quality of life.[82]

COMPARISON OF PALLIATIVE ENDOSCOPIC THERAPIES

We have described a number of different approaches to palliate obstruction or bleeding from endoluminal tumors. Typically, these patients have a short survival, and the goal of therapy is to improve symptoms and quality of life while min-

imizing morbidity and hospital stay. The perception among physicians that palliative treatment modalities are complementary rather than alternative has been a major obstacle to patient accrual for randomized trials.[59] It is our opinion that the thoracic surgeon should be familiar with all these modalities, as certain clinical situations will be better handled by one approach compared to another. The ability to combine these approaches is likely to result in better outcomes. An example is given in our approach to palliation of obstructing lung cancer (Figure 6-7). The relative merits of each of these treatment modalities are summarized in Table 6-2.

EVOLVING ENDOSCOPIC TREATMENT MODALITIES FOR BENIGN ESOPHAGEAL DISEASES

Zenker's Diverticulum

Traditionally, a Zenker's diverticulum is repaired using open surgical techniques, with the primary goal being division of the cricopharyngeus muscle and the secondary goal, resection or pexy of the diverticulum. Surgical approaches to this problem have been uniformly excellent. Alternative methods using endoscopic stapling have been slow to gain popularity with surgeons.[12] For stapling to be successful, the diverticulum must be at least 3 cm in size. The technique is performed with patients under general anesthesia and the diverticulum is assessed with the flexible endoscope. Rigid esophagoscopy is then performed using the Weerdascope (Karl Storz, Tuttlingen, Germany). One jaw of the scope is placed in the esophagus and the other in the diverticulum. Expansion of the jaws allows clear visualization of the diverticulum and the common septum formed by the cricopharyngeus muscle. We have modified the technique to include the placement of a traction suture on the common septum using the US Surgical Endostitch (Norwalk, CT). The suture provides traction to facilitate application of a modified Endo-GIA 30 stapler (US Surgical, Norwalk, CT) across the septum (Figure 6-8). The septum is divided with the stapler down to the base of the diverticulum, thereby dividing the cricopharyngeus muscle and creating a common channel between the diverticulum and esophageal lumen. A barium swallow is obtained on the first postoperative day, and if the results are satisfactory, the patient is started on a liquid diet.

In our preliminary series, the procedure was completed successfully in 91% of patients.[25] There were no procedure-related complications, and dysphagia scores were significantly improved at a median interval of 7 months. Several other groups have published retrospective reviews of their experience with endoscopic stapled diverticulotomy.° The number of patients varied between 14 and 102. The success rate in completing the endoscopic procedure was 79–100%. The only major complication was a postoperative fatal myocardial infarction.[65] In one study, minor complications included pneumomediastinum (10%) and respiratory or urinary tract infections (10%).[88] Hospital stay was between 1 and 7 days with a mean of 4 days.[61,65,71,88] Complete relief of dysphagia was reported in 76–100% of

---

°References 1, 16, 44, 61, 65, 71, 83, 88.

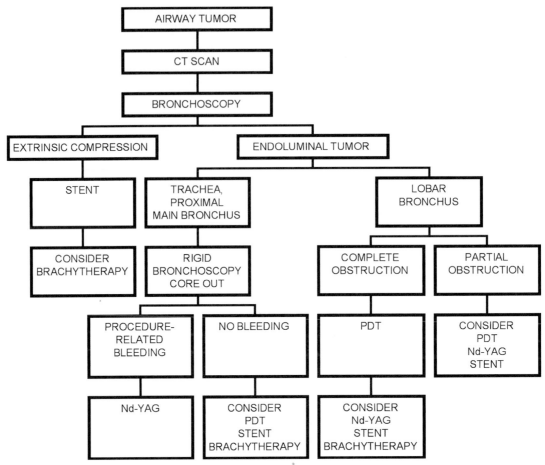

Figure 6–7 Approach to malignant obstruction of the airway.

patients. On long-term follow-up (5 years), 19% of patients required a second endoscopic procedure.[16] Endoluminal stapling appears to be a safe and effective approach to treat Zenker's diverticula suitable for selected patients.

Gastroesophageal Reflux Disease

Recently, endoscopic approaches to treat gastroesophageal reflux disease (GERD) have been described. Three approaches, which are gaining in popularity, are endoscopic suturing, radiofrequency ablation, and submucosal injection of the gastroesophageal junction.

Endoluminal Gastroplication

Endoluminal gastroplication (ELGP) is performed with patients under conscious sedation, using an esophageal overtube because multiple reinsertions of the endoscope are necessary. At least three sutures are placed on the proximal aspect of the lesser curve of the stomach in either a linear or helicoidal pattern in order to change the configuration of the angle of His and to tighten the gastroesophageal junction. A special endoscopic suturing device is used (Endocinch, Bard, Billerica, MA).

Initial results of ELGP in a cohort of 102 patients treated over a period of 4 years were reported.[84] Follow-up pH and manometry were completed in 49% of patients. Significant reductions in DeMeester score and esophageal acid expo-

sure were documented along with an increase in lower esophageal sphincter (LES) pressure. In a prospective multicenter cohort study with 6 months follow-up, heartburn frequency, heartburn severity, and regurgitation scores significantly improved at 3 and 6 months.[27] However, only 45% of patients completed the postprocedure testing. A repeat procedure was performed in 17% of patients for suboptimal results, as subjectively determined by the investigators. The authors also found that the type of ELGP configuration did not have a significant impact on outcome.

Radiofrequency Ablation

Radiofrequency ablation (RFA) relies on the delivery of radiofrequency energy to the muscular layer of the distal esophagus and gastroesophageal junction (GEJ). The healing response induces thickening of the GEJ musculature and augmentation of the LES pressure. Damage to the vagal nerve afferents reduces the frequency of transient LES relaxation. The delivery catheter is a bougie tip balloon with four 5.5-mm retractable electrodes (22 gauge) (Stretta, Curon Medical, Sunnyvale, CA). Between 15 and 25 lesions are created at 45° angles from 1 cm above to 2 cm below the z-line.

In a study involving 118 patients, heartburn frequency score improved from 4 to 1 at 12 months.[86] At 6 months, esophageal acid exposure decreased from 10.2 to 6.4%. DeMeester scores also decreased significantly from 40.0 to 26.3. Requirement for proton pump inhibitors went from

Table 6–2

Relative Attributes of Endoscopic Therapies

	PDT	*Stent*	*Nd-YAG*	*Brachytherapy*
Local anesthesia	Yes	Yes	Yes	Yes
Effective for intraluminal tumor	Yes	Yes	Yes	Yes
Effective for extrinsic compression	No	Yes	No	Yes
Effective for complete obstruction	Yes	No	Occasionally	No
Effective for bleeding	Yes	No	Yes	Yes (not acutely)
Depth of penetration	0.5 cm	N/A	N/A	0.5–2 cm
Onset of effect	Rapid	Immediate	Rapid	Slow
Photosensitivity	Yes	No	No	No
Late hemoptysis (non-tumor-related)	No	No	No	Yes
Late stricture/dysphagia (non-tumor-related)	Yes (if normal tissue treated)	Yes (migration)	No	Yes (radiation bronchitis)

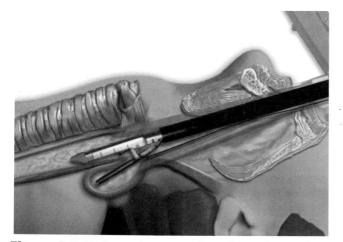

Figure 6–8 Endoscopic transoral stapling of a Zenker's diverticulum.

88.1 to 30.0%. Chest pain (1.7%) and transient dysphagia (0.8%) were reported following treatment. Self-limited fever (1.7%) and superficial mucosal injury (2.5%) related to the probe were also documented. In another study involving 41 patients, there was only one minor complication.[34] At 6-month follow-up, 65% were off proton pump inhibitors (PPI), which is less than would be expected with fundoplication.

Submucosal Injection

This treatment modality shares similarities with endoscopic sclerotherapy for esophageal varices. A non-biodegradable polymer with a radiopaque marker is initially dissolved in a liquid solvent (Enteryx, Boston Scientific, Natick, MA). Using the sclerotherapy injection needle, the deep submucosal or muscular layer of each quadrant of the GEJ is injected with 4–8 ml of solution. A multicenter prospective cohort study involving 170 patients with GERD symptoms controlled by PPI has been published.[36] At 6 months, the median heartburn-related quality of life (HRQL) score was significantly improved. In addition, 74% of patients no longer needed PPI and 10%

76

had reduced their PPI regimen by 50%. LES length was also increased significantly from a median of 2 to 3 cm. Most patients reported transient (1–7 days) mild to moderate chest pain after the procedure but there were no serious complications. This technique appears to have a favorable safety and efficacy profile, but longer follow-up data are necessary to assess durability.

Evidence

The prospective trials of ELGP and RFA were industry sponsored and included patients with symptomatic reflux, esophagitis grade 0–2, and more than 4% esophageal acid exposure time.[27,86] Patients with dysphagia, severe esophagitis, Barrett's metaplasia, previous esophageal or gastric surgery, or a type I hiatal hernia greater than 2 cm were excluded. Subjects were either self-referred or, in the RFA trial, selected by the investigators from their clinical practice. The process leading to the selection of the experimental group was not described in the ELGP trial. In light of the potential for selection bias and the lack of a control group, these nonoperative approaches cannot be considered superior to antireflux surgery. Until additional data become available, their use should be reserved for the nonsurgical candidate or in the setting of a clinical trial. However, these truly minimally invasive techniques will potentially become attractive to patients because of their reduced morbidity and invasiveness. It is important therefore that surgeons become familiar with and critically evaluate new therapeutic modalities as they are introduced into clinical practice.

REFERENCES

1. Adams J, Sheppard B, Andersen P, et al: Zenker's diverticulostomy with cricopharyngeal myotomy: The endoscopic approach. Surg Endosc 15(1):34–37, 2001.
2. Angueira CE, Kadakia SC: Esophageal stents for inoperable esophageal cancer: Which to use? J. Gastroenterol 92(3):373–376, 1997.
3. Biddlestone LR, Barham CP, Wilkinson SP, et al: The histopathology of treated Barrett's esophagus: Squamous reepithelialization after acid suppression and laser and photodynamic therapy. Am J Surg Pathol 22(2):239–245, 1998.
4. Bisgaard T, Wojdemann M, Heindorff H, Svendsen LB: Nonsurgical treatment of esophageal perforations after endoscopic palliation in advanced esophageal cancer. Endoscopy 29(3):155–159, 1997.
5. Bolliger CT, Heitz M, Hauser R, et al: An airway Wallstent for the treatment of tracheobronchial malignancies. Thorax 51(11):1127–1129, 1996.
6. Boulis NM, Armstrong WS, Chandler WF, Orringer MB: Epidural abscess: A delayed complication of esophageal stenting for benign stricture. Ann Thorac Surg 68(2):568–570, 1999.
7. Boyd AD: Chevalier Jackson: The father of American bronchoesophagoscopy. Ann Thorac Surg 57(2):502–505, 1994.
8. Casale V, Lapenta R, Gigliozzi A, Villotti G: Endoscopic palliative therapy in neoplastic diseases of the esophagus. J Exp Clin Cancer Res 18(1):63–67, 1999.
9. Cavaliere S, Foccoli P, Farina PL: Nd:YAG laser bronchoscopy. A five-year experience with 1,396 applications in 1,000 patients. Chest 94(1):15–21, 1988.
10. Cavaliere S, Venuta F, Foccoli P, et al: Endoscopic treatment of malignant airway obstructions in 2,008 patients. Chest

11. Christie NA, Buenaventura PO, Fernando HC, et al: Results of expandable metal stents for malignant esophageal obstruction in 100 patients: Short-term and long-term follow-up. Ann Thorac Surg 71(6):1797–1801, 2001.
12. Collard JM, Otte JB, Kestens PJ: Endoscopic stapling technique of esophagodiverticulostomy for Zenker's diverticulum. Ann Thorac Surg 56(3):573–576, 1993.
13. Cook CH, Bhattacharyya N, King DR: Aortobronchial fistula after expandable metal stent insertion for pediatric bronchomalacia. J Pediatr Surg 33(8):1306–1308, 1998.
14. Cooper JD, Pearson FG, Patterson GA, et al: Use of silicone stents in the management of airway problems. Ann Thorac Surg 47(3):371–378, 1989.
15. Cortese DA, Edell ES, Kinsey JH: Photodynamic therapy for early stage squamous cell carcinoma of the lung. Mayo Clinic Proc 72(7):595–602, 1997.
16. Counter PR, Hilton ML, Baldwin DL: Long-term follow-up of endoscopic stapled diverticulotomy. Ann R Coll Surgeons Engl 84(2):89–92, 2002.
17. Cwikiel W, Tranberg KG, Cwikiel M, Lillo-Gil R: Malignant dysphagia: Palliation with esophageal stents—long-term results in 100 patients. Radiology 207(2):513–518, 1998.
18. Diaz-Jimenez JP, Martinez-Ballarin JE, Llunell A, et al: Efficacy and safety of photodynamic therapy versus Nd-YAG laser resection in NSCLC with airway obstruction. Eur Respir J 14(4):800–805, 1999.
19. Ducic Y, Khalafi RS: Use of endoscopically placed expandable nitinol tracheal stents in the treatment of tracheal stenosis. Laryngoscope 109(7: Pt 1):t-3, 1999.
20. Dumon JF, Reboud E, Garbe L, et al: Treatment of tracheobronchial lesions by laser photoresection. Chest 81(3): 278–284, 1982.
21. Edell ES, Cortese DA: Bronchoscopic phototherapy with hematoporphyrin derivative for treatment of localized bronchogenic carcinoma: A 5-year experience. Mayo Clinic Proc 62(1):8–14, 1987.
22. Ell C, May A, Gossner L, et al: Endoscopic mucosal resection of early cancer and high-grade dysplasia in Barrett's esophagus. Gastroenterology 118(4):670–677, 2000.
23. Falk GW: Gastroesophageal reflux disease and Barrett's esophagus. Endoscopy 33(2):109–118, 2001.
24. Fernando HC, Luketich JD, Buenaventura PO, et al: Outcomes of minimally invasive esophagectomy (MIE) for high-grade dysplasia of the esophagus. Eur J Cardio-Thorac Surg 22(1):1–6, 2002.
25. Fernando HC, Ferson PF, Buenaventura PO, et al: Preliminary experience with endoscopic trans-oral stapling of Zenker's diverticulum. Western Thoracic Surgical Association Meeting, 2002, Big Sky, MO (abstract).
26. Ferson PF, Landreneau RJ, Keenan RL, et al: Interventional Bronchoscopy. Minimal Access Cardiothroacic Surgery. Philadelphia: W.B. Saunders, 2000, pp. 363–378.
27. Filipi CJ, Lehman GA, Rothstein RI, et al: Transoral, flexible endoscopic suturing for treatment of GERD: A multicenter trial. Gastrointest Endosc 53(4):416–422, 2001.
28. Furuse K, Fukuoka M, Kato H, et al: A prospective phase II study on photodynamic therapy with photofrin II for centrally located early-stage lung cancer. The Japan Lung Cancer Photodynamic Therapy Study Group. J Clin Oncol 11(10): 1852–1857, 1993.
29. Gaissert HA, Grillo HC, Mathisen DJ, Wain JC: Temporary and permanent restoration of airway continuity with the tracheal T-tube. J Thorac Cardiovasc Surg 107(2):600–606, 1994.
30. Gossner L, Stolte M, Sroka R, et al: Photodynamic ablation of high-grade dysplasia and early cancer in Barrett's esophagus by means of 5-aminolevulinic acid. Gastroenterology 114(3): 448–455, 1998.

110(6):1536–1542, 1996 [erratum of serious dosage error appears in Chest 111(5):1476, 1997].

31. Gotway MB, Golden JA, LaBerge JM, et al: Benign tracheobronchial stenoses: Changes in short-term and long-term pulmonary function testing after expandable metallic stent placement. J Comput Assist Tomogr 26(4):564–572, 2002.

32. Hemminger LL, Wolfsen HC: Photodynamic therapy for Barrett's esophagus and high grade dysplasia: Results of a patient satisfaction survey. Gastroenterol Nurs 25(4):139–141, 2002.

33. Hetzel MR, Nixon C, Edmondstone WM, et al: Laser therapy in 100 tracheobronchial tumours. Thorax 40(5):341–345, 1985.

34. Houston H, Khaitan L, Holzman M, Richards WO: First year experience of patients undergoing the Stretta procedure. Surg Endosc 17(3):401–404, 2003.

35. Jain PR, Dedhia HV, Lapp NL, et al: Nd:YAG laser followed by radiation for treatment of malignant airway lesions. Lasers Surg Med 5(1):47–53, 1985.

36. Johnson DA, Gans R, Aisenberg J, et al: Endoscopic, deep mural implantation of enteryx for the treatment of GERD: 6-month follow-up of a multicenter trial. Am J Gastroenterol 98(2):250–258.

37. Knyrim K, Wagner HJ, Bethge N, et al: A controlled trial of an expansile metal stent for palliation of esophageal obstruction due to inoperable cancer. N Engl J Med 329(18):1302–1307, 1993.

38. Langendijk H, de Jong J, Tjwa M, et al: External irradiation versus external irradiation plus endobronchial brachytherapy in inoperable non-small cell lung cancer: A prospective randomized study. Radiother Oncol 58(3):257–268, 2001.

39. Lee P, Kupeli E, Mehta AC: Therapeutic bronchoscopy in lung cancer. Laser therapy, electrocautery, brachytherapy, stents, and photodynamic therapy. Clinics Chest Med 23(1):241–256, 2002.

40. Lightdale CJ, Heier SK, Marcon NE, et al: Photodynamic therapy with porfimer sodium versus thermal ablation therapy with Nd: YAG laser for palliation of esophageal cancer: A multicenter randomized trial. Gastrointest Endosc 42(6):507–512, 1995.

41. Litle VA, Christie NA, Buenaventura PO, et al: Photodynamic therapy for endobronchial metastases from non-bronchogenic primaries. Society of Surgical Oncology Meeting, 2001 (abstract).

42. Litle VA, Fernando HC, Christie NA, et al: Expandable metal stents for malignant tracheobronchial obstruction. Society of Surgical Oncology Annual Meeting, 2002 (abstract).

43. Litle VA, Luketich JD, Christie NA, et al: Photodynamic therapy as palliation for esophageal cancer: Experience in 215 patients. Annual Meeting of the Society of Thoracic Surgeons, 2003 (abstract).

44. Luscher MS, Johansen LV: Zenker's diverticulum treated by the endoscopic stapling technique. Acta Oto-Laryngol Suppl 543:235–238, 2000.

45. Luketich JD, Christie NA, Buenaventura PO, et al: Endoscopic photodynamic therapy for obstructing esophageal cancer: 77 cases over a 2-year period. Surg Endosc 14(7): 653–657, 2000.

46. Luketich JD, Christie NA, Lovas KE, Weigel TL: Photodynamic therapy: Results of curative intent for esophageal cancer and Barrett's with high-grade dysplasia in high-risk patients. International Biomedical Optics Symposium SPIE—The International Society for Optical Engineering, 2000 (abstract).

47. Luketich JD, Fernando HC, Christie NA, et al: Optical methods for tumor treatment and detection: Mechanisms and techniques in photodynamic therapy X. Proc SPIE 4248:28–33, 2001.

48. Luketich JD, Fernando HC, Christie NA, et al: Photodynamic therapy in thoracic oncology: A single institution experience. Proc SPIE 4248:28–33, 2001.

49. Luketich JD, Westkaemper J, Sommers KE, et al: Bronchoesophagopleural fistula after photodynamic therapy for malignant mesothelioma. Ann Thorac Surg 62(1):283–284, 1996.

50. Luketich JD, Wong HY, Buenaventura PO, Christie NA: Photodynamic therapy: Results of curative intent for esophageal cancer and Barrett's with high-grade dysplasia in high-risk patients. International Organization for Statistical Studies on Disease of the Esophagus (OESO). Paris, France. Abstract. Aug. 1, 2000.

51. Maier A, Anegg U, Fell B, et al: Hyperbaric oxygen and photodynamic therapy in the treatment of advanced carcinoma of the cardia and the esophagus. Lasers Surg Med 26(3):308–315, 2000.

52. Maier A, Pinter H, Friehs GB, et al: Self-expandable coated stent after intraluminal treatment of esophageal cancer: A risky procedure? Ann Thorac Surg 67(3):781–784, 1999.

53. Maier A, Tomaselli F, Gebhard F, et al: Palliation of advanced esophageal carcinoma by photodynamic therapy and irradiation. Ann Thorac Surg 69(4):1006–1009, 2000.

54. Maier A, Tomaselli F, Matzi V, et al: Photosensitization with hematoporphyrin derivative compared to 5-aminolaevulinic acid for photodynamic therapy of esophageal carcinoma. Ann Thorac Surg 72(4):1136–1140, 2001.

55. May A, Gossner L, Pech O, et al: Local endoscopic therapy for intraepithelial high-grade neoplasia and early adenocarcinoma in Barrett's oesophagus: Acute-phase and intermediate results of a new treatment approach. Eur J Gastroenterol Hepatol 14(10):1085–1091, 2002.

56. McCaughan JS Jr, Williams TE: Photodynamic therapy for endobronchial malignant disease: A prospective fourteen-year study. J Thorac Cardiovasc Surg 114(6):940–946, 1997.

57. McCaughan JS Jr, Ellison EC, Guy JT, et al: Photodynamic therapy for esophageal malignancy: A prospective twelve-year study. Ann Thorac Surg 62(4):1005–1009, 1996.

58. Mehrishi S, Raoof S, Mehta AC: Therapeutic flexible bronchoscopy. Chest Surg Clinics North Am 11(4):657–690, 2001.

59. Moghissi K, Bond MG, Sambrook RJ, et al: Treatment of endotracheal or endobronchial obstruction by non-small cell lung cancer: Lack of patients in an MRC randomized trial leaves key questions unanswered. Medical Research Council Lung Cancer Working Party. Clin Oncol (R Coll Radiol) 11(3):179–183, 1999. [erratum appears in Clin Oncol (R Coll Radiol) 11(5):365, 1999].

60. Morgan RM, Adam AF: Use of metallic stents and balloons in the esophagus and gastrointestinal tract. J Vasc Intervent Radiol 12(3):283–297, 2001.

61. Narne S, Cutrone C, Bonavina L, et al: Endoscopic diverticulotomy for the treatment of Zenker's diverticulum: Results in 102 patients with staple-assisted endoscopy. Ann Otol Rhinol Laryngol 108(8):810–815, 1999.

62. Nashef SA, Dromer C, Velly JF, et al: Expanding wire stents in benign tracheobronchial disease: Indications and complications. Ann Thorac Surg 54(5):937–940, 1992.

63. Nguyen NT, Schauer P, Luketich JD: Minimally invasive esophagectomy for Barrett's esophagus with high-grade dysplasia. Surgery 127(3):284–290, 2000.

64. Nijhawan PK, Wang KK: Endoscopic mucosal resection for lesions with endoscopic features suggestive of malignancy and high-grade dysplasia within Barrett's esophagus. Gastrointest Endosc 52(3):328–332, 2000.

65. Omote K, Feussner H, Stein HJ, et al: Endoscopic stapling diverticulostomy for Zenker's diverticulum. Surg Endosc 13(5):535–538, 1999.

66. Orons PD, Amesur NB, Dauber JH, et al: Balloon dilation and endobronchial stent placement for bronchial strictures after lung transplantation. J Vasc Intervent Radiol 11(1):89–99, 2000.

78

67. O'Sullivan GJ, Grundy A: Palliation of malignant dysphagia with expanding metallic stents. J Vasc Intervent Radiol 10(3):346–351, 1999.

68. Overholt BF, Panjehpour M, Ayres M: Photodynamic therapy for Barrett's esophagus: Cardiac effects. Lasers Surg Med 21(4):317–320, 1997.

69. Overholt BF, Panjehpour M, Haydek JM: Photodynamic therapy for Barrett's esophagus: Follow-up in 100 patients. Gastrointest Endosc 49(1):1–7, 1999.

70. Peng Q, Warloe T, Berg K, et al: 5-Aminolevulinic acid-based photodynamic therapy. Clinical research and future challenges. Cancer 79(12):2282–2308, 1997.

71. Philippsen LP, Weisberger EC, Whiteman TS, Schmidt JL: Endoscopic stapled diverticulotomy: Treatment of choice for Zenker's diverticulum. Laryngoscope 110(8):1283–1286, 2000.

72. Raijman I, Siddique I, Ajani J, Lynch P: Palliation of malignant dysphagia and fistulae with coated expandable metal stents: Experience with 101 patients. Gastrointest Endosc 48(2):172–179, 1998.

73. Rousseau H, Dahan M, Lauque D, et al: Self-expandable prostheses in the tracheobronchial tree. Radiology 188(1):199–203, 1993.

74. Sampliner RE, Fennerty B, Garewal HS: Reversal of Barrett's esophagus with acid suppression and multipolar electrocoagulation: Preliminary results. Gastrointest Endosc 44(5):532–535, 1996.

75. Sandha GS, Marcon NE: Expandable metal stents for benign esophageal obstruction. Gastrointest Endosc Clinics North Am 9(3):437–446, 1999.

76. Sargeant IR, Tobias JS, Blackman G, et al: Radiotherapy enhances laser palliation of malignant dysphagia: A randomised study. Gut 40(3):362–369, 1997.

77. Siersema PD, Hop WC, Dees J, et al: Coated self-expanding metal stents versus latex prostheses for esophagogastric cancer with special reference to prior radiation and chemotherapy: A controlled, prospective study. Gastrointest Endosc 47(2):113–120, 1998.

78. Sonett JR, Keenan RJ, Ferson PF, et al: Endobronchial management of benign, malignant, and lung transplantation airway stenoses. Ann Thorac Surg 59(6):1417–1422, 1995.

79. Song HY, Do YS, Han YM, et al: Covered, expandable esophageal metallic stent tubes: Experiences in 119 patients. Radiology 193(3):689–695, 1994.

80. Song HY, Lee DH, Seo TS, et al: Retrievable covered nitinol stents: Experiences in 108 patients with malignant esophageal strictures. J Vasc Intervent Radiology 13(3):285–293, 2002.

81. Speiser BL, Spratling L: Radiation bronchitis and stenosis secondary to high dose rate endobronchial irradiation. Int. J Radiat Oncol Biol Phys 25(4):589–597, 1993.

82. Stephens KE Jr, Wood DE: Bronchoscopic management of central airway obstruction. J Thorac Cardiovasc Surg 119(2):289–296, 2000.

83. Stoeckli SJ, Schmid S: Endoscopic stapler-assisted diverticuloesophagostomy for Zenker's diverticulum: Patient satisfaction and subjective relief of symptoms. Surgery 131(2):158–162, 2002.

84. Swain P, Park P-O, Kjellin T, Gong F: Endoscopic gastroplasty for gastro-esophageal reflux disease. Gastrointest Endosc 51(4):AB14, 2000.

85. Tredaniel J, Hennequin C, Zalcman G, et al: Prolonged survival after high-dose rate endobronchial radiation for malignant airway obstruction. Chest 105(3):767–772, 1994.

86. Triadafilopoulos G, DiBaise JK, Nostrant TT, et al: The Stretta procedure for the treatment of GERD: 6 and 12 month follow-up of the U.S. open label trial. Gastrointest Endosc 55(2):149–156, 2002.

87. Van Laethem JL, Cremer M, Peny MO, et al: Eradication of Barrett's mucosa with argon plasma coagulation and acid suppression: Immediate and mid term results. Gut 43(6):747–751, 1998.

88. Von Doersten PG, Byl FM: Endoscopic Zenker's diverticulotomy (Dohlman procedure): Forty cases reviewed. Otolaryngol Head Neck Surg. 116(2):209–212, 1997.

89. Weigel TL, Kosco PJ, Luketich JD: Photodynamic therapy for endobronchial lesions. In: Esophageal Surgery, 2nd ed. New York: Harcourt, 2002, pp. 901–905.

90. Weigel TLM, Kosco PJR, Christie NAM, et al: Photodynamic therapy for early non-small cell lung carcinoma in high-risk patients. Chest 118(4):90S, 2000 (abstract).

91. Weigel TL, Keenan RL, Christie NA, et al: Photodynamic therapy: A curative approach to early non-small cell lung carcinomas in high-risk patients. International Biomedical Optics Symposium SPIE—The International Society for Optical Engineering, 2000 (abstract).

92. Weigel TL, Kosco PJ, Dacic S, et al: Postoperative fluorescence bronchoscopic surveillance in non-small cell lung cancer patients. Ann Thorac Surg 71(3):967–970, 2001.

93. Witt C, Dinges S, Schmidt B, et al: Temporary tracheobronchial stenting in malignant stenoses. Eur J Cancer 33(2):204–208, 1997.

94. Zaninotto G, Parenti AR, Ruol A, et al: Oesophageal resection for high-grade dysplasia in Barrett's oesophagus. Br J Surg 87(8):1102–1105, 2000.

Trauma

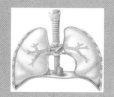

Thoracic Trauma

Malcolm V. Brock, David P. Mason, and Stephen C. Yang

▶ INTRODUCTION

The earliest recorded reference to thoracic trauma is found in the *Edwin Smith Surgical Papyrus* written around 3000 BC.[18] In this report of 58 cases, three were related to the chest: a penetrating injury to the cervical esophagus, a stab wound to the sternum, and blunt trauma resulting in rib fractures. Through the eras of Hippocrates and Galen, open packing and local treatment with common ingredients (e.g., red meat, honey, lint) were the mainstay of treatment, until the thirteenth century, when wound débridement and closure was advocated. However, wound closure became a topic of great debate somewhat clarified by Paré in 1514. He advocated immediate closure of wounds that had either no blood or a small amount of blood in the chest; enlarging small wounds if better drainage of blood was required; and delaying wound closure until blood drainage had ceased (usually 2–4 days).[78] During the next century, various cannulas were developed to irrigate infected wounds and empyemas, which eventually evolved into the closed drainage systems used during World War II.

Also during World War II, thoracotomy became commonplace as the most effective method not only to drain retained blood and infected debris, but also to remove the peel from the hemothorax that formed over the lung. As thoracic surgical principles developed, so did advances in endotracheal intubation, mechanical ventilators, and thoracic pain control, which became pivotal in the management of most thoracic injuries over the next several decades.

As a result, mortality from chest wounds had progressively decreased from a wartime high of 80% to 90% as reported by Billings during the Civil War[14] to 4% to 7% in recent civilian experience. Nevertheless, thoracic trauma accounts for 25% of all trauma deaths, representing approximately 160,000 deaths annually.[64] Over 70% of thoracic injuries result from blunt trauma, most of which are caused by automobile accidents. One in four cases with cardiothoracic trauma, regardless of etiology, requires hospital admission.

Age of the patient plays an important role in the severity of injuries. In the pediatric patient, in whom the immature chest wall is elastic and flexible, fractures are rare, but intrathoracic injuries are more significant. In the elderly patient, the fragile bony thorax is highly susceptible to even low-impact forces and offers poor protection for the underlying viscera; mortality is high even with minor injuries.

Penetrating injuries are uncommon in either elderly or pediatric patients, but they remain one of the most common causes of death from trauma in persons up to 40 years of age. Low-velocity handguns, seen primarily in the civilian population, transmit very little damage to surrounding tissues. Conversely, much more damage and energy is conducted along the path of high-velocity missiles, usually associated with the military, but now often seen in violent assaults as well.

▶ THE PRIMARY SURVEY

Rapid and thorough performance of the "ABCs" cannot be overemphasized. This begins with traditional resuscitation as outlined by the American College of Surgeons in the Advanced Trauma Life Support guidelines. The airway must be controlled and breathing assessed and established immediately if necessary. Circulation must be supported through rapid establishment of reliable, large-bore venous access and the initiation of fluid resuscitation. The patient's neurological disabilities are quickly assessed, and the entire body is exposed to note significant deformities or penetrating injuries. The primary survey is performed to search for immediate life-threatening injuries that could account for ventilation or hemodynamic instabilities, which, if left uncorrected, could cause the acute demise of the patient. These life-threatening injuries are listed in Table 7-1.

Generally speaking, some form of intervention is needed as an "urgent" life-saving measure. The preferred treatment measures also are included in Table 7-1. Although many diagnostic modalities are currently available, these problems always should be kept in suspect at all times during the resuscitative phase of every trauma patient. The mechanism of injury also should influence the index of suspicion for these injuries. For blunt trauma, aortic rupture, diaphragm hernias, and tracheobronchial injuries are considered; for penetrating injuries, cardiac tamponade and massive intrathoracic hemorrhage are considered; finally, pneumothorax is a common result of all types of trauma.

▶ DIAGNOSTIC TESTS

Approximately one third of all deaths from thoracic trauma occur immediately or shortly thereafter when the patient is transported to a treatment facility. Diagnostic and emergency management modalities are essential to fully evaluate and predict the potential for uncontrolled bleeding or ventilation inadequacies.

Table 7–1

Potentially Acutely Lethal Injuries of the Chest and Their Management

Injury	Management
Tension pneumothorax	Tube thoracostomy
Massive intrathoracic hemorrhage	Tube thoracostomy, operative repair
Cardiac tamponade	Pericardiocentesis, operative repair
Deceleration aortic injury	Operative repair
Massive flail chest with pulmonary contusion	Intubation, pain control, fluid restriction
Upper and lower airway obstruction	Intubation, airway, bronchoscopy
Tracheobronchial rupture	Bronchoscopy, operative repair
Diaphragmatic rupture with visceral herniation	Operative repair
Esophageal perforation	Operative repair

Chest Radiography

The chest X-ray remains paramount in every trauma victim and should be the central focus from which potential life-threatening thoracic problems are suspected. A systematic review of the film should reveal suspected and unsuspected injuries, and the presence of any foreign bodies. Fractures of the bony thorax, including the ribs, clavicles, spine, and scapulae, should be excluded. The lung fields should be examined for pneumothorax, hemothorax, or pulmonary contusion. Along the mediastinum, widening, pneumomediastinum, or shifting is highly suspect for aortic transection, tracheobronchial or esophageal injuries, or tension pneumothorax or hemothorax, respectively. The soft tissues may reveal subtle subcutaneous air or foreign bodies. Finally, the width of the cardiac silhouette may raise the suspicion of tamponade.

Computerized tomography (CT) is not essential for every patient with chest trauma and should not be performed in the severely hemodynamically unstable patient or in the presence of life-threatening injuries. However, it can be done rapidly and may reveal injuries not seen clearly on plain radiographs, such as aortic disruption, pneumothorax, pneumomediastinum, and hemothorax. It may be useful to screen all patients with blunt trauma and evaluate unusual or abnormal findings on initial chest X-ray (e.g., diaphragmatic injuries).

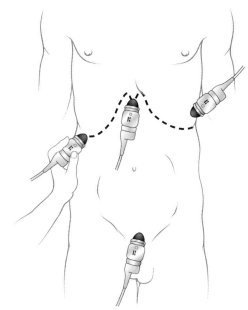

Figure 7–1 The *focused assessment* for the *sonographic evaluation* of the *trauma patient*, or *FAST examination*, using four standard viewing ports: right upper quadrant, left upper quadrant, pelvis, and subxiphoid. *(Modified from Rozycki GS, Feliciano DV, Schmidt JA, et al: The role of surgeon-performed ultrasound in patients with possible cardiac wounds. Ann Surg 223:737–746, 1996.)*

Echocardiography

Ultrasonography has now become fairly common in the early evaluation of the abdomen and pericardium.[86] Termed as the *focused assessment for the sonographic evaluation of the trauma patient, or FAST examination,* four standard viewing ports are used to quickly access abnormal fluid collection: right upper quadrant, left upper quadrant, pelvis, and subxiphoid (Figure 7-1). Although not as precise as an ultrasound performed by a board-certified radiologist or cardiologist, it is able to detect fluid collections that might influence the need for urgent operative intervention. Of the four views, the subxiphoid view is the most accurate in the hands of surgeons in detecting abnormalities in the trauma setting.[86] It has the advantages of being safe, expeditious, repeatable, and effective even in the hands of surgeons from different specialties.[90]

Transesophageal echocardiography (TEE) has found an increasing indication over the past decade.[27,88] Unlike transthoracic echo or the FAST examination, results and interpretation from TEE are extremely user dependent, and the expertise requires an understanding of the anatomical structures and the sensitivity levels of the machine. Its usefulness may eventually lie in its ability to detect and follow small intimal tears not seen on angiography and the evaluation of patients too unstable to transport to the angiography suite. Although the primary focus of its use centers on aortic injuries and the evaluation for transaction, it also is used to estimate cardiac function, search for intracardiac injuries (particularly after penetrating trauma), and distinguish pericardial fluid. It has, however, variable diagnostic accuracy for injuries to the brachiocephalic vessels.

For the diagnosis of aortic transection, TEE has been reported to have sensitivities as high as 90%, but specificities of only 50%. Despite the numerous studies, most trauma surgeons still hesitate to use an operative repair of the descending thoracic aorta based on a positive TEE alone and use angiography as the gold standard.

Angiography

Angiography remains the gold standard in the diagnosis of aortic transection or injuries to the great vessels.[81] It is useful to determine the angiographic abnormalities in order to help plan the operative thoracic incision. Retrograde femoral arteriography is the preferred method—the risk is low when passing the angiocatheter by the potential site of rupture. Box 7-1 lists the commonly accepted indications for angiographic study of the thoracic aorta and great vessels based on thoracic injuries.

In aortic transection, the classic aortographic image displays a pseudoaneurysm near the site of the isthmus (Figure 7-2). Partial or complete interruption of the aortic contour may be seen when the aortic wall has retracted, or if debris of the wall prolapses into the lumen. Occasionally, a ductus diverticulum is a normal finding at the site of the uninterrupted intimal surface at the site of the ligamentum arteriosum.[71]

▶ EMERGENCY DEPARTMENT THORACOTOMY

The indications for emergency department (ED) thoracotomy have been widely debated. ED thoracotomy clearly plays a role in penetrating thoracic trauma, particularly in the setting of trauma patients with cardiac tamponade from

Box 7–1. Indications for Angiographic Studies for Potential Thoracic Injuries.

High-speed deceleration injuries
Chest X-ray findings:
    Widened mediastinum
    Loss of aortic knob shadow
    Tracheal or esophageal deviation to the right
    Widening of paraspinal stripe and/or apical capping
    Downward displacement of left mainstem bronchus
    Obliteration of the aortopulmonary window
Fractured first rib, sternum, or scapula
Multiple rib fractures or flail chest
Massive hemothorax
Upper extremity hypertension
Unexplained hypotension
Pulse deficits or asymmetry
Systolic murmur

Box 7–2. Indications and Contraindications for Emergency Room Thoracotomy.

Accepted Indications

Unresponsive hypotension (SBP <60 mm Hg)
Rapid exsanguination from indwelling chest tube (>1500 ml)
Traumatic arrest with previously witnessed cardiac activity (prehospital or in-hospital) after penetrating thoracic injuries
Persistent hypotension (SBP <60 mm Hg) with diagnosed cardiac tamponade, air embolism

Relative Indications

Traumatic arrest with previous witnessed cardiac activity (prehospital or in-hospital) after blunt trauma
Traumatic arrest without previously witnessed cardiac activity (prehospital or in-hospital) after penetrating chest injuries
Prehospital cardiopulmonary resuscitation less than 10 minutes in intubated patient, 5 minutes in nonintubated patient

Contraindications

Blunt thoracic injuries with no previously witnessed cardiac activity
Multiple blunt trauma
Severe head injury

SBP, Systolic blood pressure.

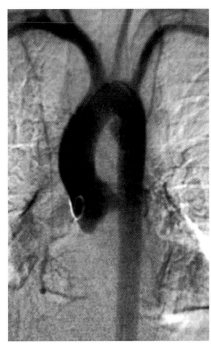

Figure 7–2 Angiogram demonstrating aortic transection injury just distal to the left subclavian artery.

penetrating chest injuries.[62] Thoracotomy allows relief of the tamponade, the ability to perform open cardiac massage, and the ability to control ongoing intrathoracic hemorrhage, as well as limit intraabdominal hemorrhage and the ability to cross-clamp the aorta to improve cerebral and coronary perfusion in the setting of exsanguinating hemorrhage. Patients with penetrating cardiac stab wounds, as well as other penetrating cardiac injuries, are the most likely patient population to survive resuscitation with ED thoracotomy. The likelihood of patient survival depends on patient down time, the patient's age and comorbidities, and signs of life on arrival to the ED. General guidelines have been recommended for ED thoracotomies in the setting of thoracic trauma and are listed in Box 7-2.

Although these general guidelines have been debated, most physicians agree that the best results occur in patients with penetrating cardiac trauma and in whom there is a good likelihood for cerebral activity. Even with an experienced team and established protocols, results are still poor. The length of time of prehospital cardiopulmonary resuscitation (CPR) has become one of the determinants whether to perform ED thoracotomy. In one report, there were no survivors from ED thoracotomy when prehospital CPR had been in progress in an intubated patient for more than 10 minutes, or more than 5 minutes in an nonintubated patient.[32] Another relatively poor marker of outcome is refractory metabolic acidosis monitored during the initial resuscitation efforts, with a pH of less than 6.8 or severe base deficits restraining the use of ED thoracotomy.

The surgical approach is a left fourth interspace anterolateral thoracotomy. This approach can be performed with the patient lying prone or preferably with a few folded blankets placed under the patient's left side to elevate it and allow the incision to be opened more posteriorly if necessary. The incision also may be carried across the sternum into the right side of the chest, if necessary, to further improve exposure or to evaluate the right side for injury. The pectoralis muscle is divided with a large scalpel, and the intercostal muscles are divided widely using a curved mayo scissors. The sternum is transected with an oscillating saw, a Lebsche knife, a Gigli saw, and even (if nothing else is available) a good pair of trauma scissors. The mammary vessels are divided as they are crossed, and ligated once the patient is more stable. The pericardium is opened widely in a cranial, caudal direction, staying anterior and avoiding the phrenic nerve. A large pericardiotomy allows easier evacuation of clot, visualization of the heart, and the ability to perform more efficient open heart massage. Cross-clamping the descending aorta requires opening the overlying parietal pleura and then getting around it bluntly using digital dissection. Care should be taken not to avulse any intercostal vessels. At this point a vascular aortic cross-clamp can be placed across it. Aortic cross-clamp time should be kept to the minimal amount of time (less than 30 minutes) required to resuscitate the patient to avoid the sequelae of spinal cord ischemia and lactic acidosis caused by distal hypoperfusion. When the patient is stable enough, he or she should be taken immediately to the operating room to definitively manage any injuries and to provide a sterile chest washout with antibiotic irrigation and formal closure of the thoracotomy with wide chest tube drainage.

BLUNT TRAUMA

As mentioned previously, blunt trauma to the chest in the United States is far more common than penetrating injury. A 2002 report by the National Safety Council reported that of all blunt trauma deaths, 25% were caused by thoracic trauma. The high-speed deceleration and crush injuries involved in automobile accidents have become increasingly prevalent since the 1950s and account for the majority of incidents of blunt thoracic trauma. Falls, sports injuries, assaults, and blast injuries are other leading causes. The damage from a powerful blast can be particularly severe because the blast pressure wave imparts a large amount of kinetic energy to a small area. Blast kinetic energy especially affects gas-containing organs, such as the lungs, resulting in pulmonary hemorrhage, hypoxia, and shock.

Chest Wall

Optimal mechanical properties of the chest wall are important determinants for effective functioning of the entire respiratory system. Blunt trauma to the chest wall can disrupt respiratory mechanics, leading to poor pulmonary toilet and significant morbidity. Chest wall trauma alone occurs in only 16% of cases[91] and is more often a marker of more ominous visceral injury inside the thoracic cage or below the diaphragm. Because the chest wall provides a protective bony skeleton around the vital organs of the chest, composed of the ribs, sternum, clavicles, and scapulae, the impact of fracturing each of these bones is considered.

Rib Fractures

Fracture of the ribs is the most common blunt thoracic injury, occurring in an estimated 300,000 people in the United States during the year 2000, or 39% of patients admitted to major trauma centers.[57,92] Rib fractures represent an important indicator of trauma severity. In general, the greater the number of ribs fractured, the higher the patient's morbidity and mortality. The number of ribs fractured has been significantly correlated with the presence of hemothorax or pneumothorax, with 81% of patients having either condition if two or more ribs were fractured.[63] Fractures of the fourth through the ninth rib are associated with injuries to the lung, bronchus, pleura, and heart, whereas fractures below the ninth rib are indicative of spleen, hepatic, or renal injuries.

The main symptoms include pain, exquisite tenderness, and possibly crepitus. Only an upright chest X-ray performed as a routine part of the trauma series is advocated unless special documentation of a crime, such as child abuse, is needed, in which case rib detail films are performed. Careless dismissal of a simple rib fracture and underestimating its pathophysiological potential, especially in the elderly patient, is a common management pitfall. After adjusting for severity of injury, comorbidity, and presence of multiple rib fractures, elderly patients (>65 years old) with simple rib fractures still were five times more likely to die compared with patients under age 65.[10] First rib fracture has particular significance because of the great force required for it to occur and the likelihood that intrathoracic visceral injury also has taken place. The two most common sites of first rib fracture are at the subclavian sulcus and in the neck of the first rib posteriorly. Subclavian artery and/or aortic arch arteriography are indicated if the first rib fracture is displaced posteriorly, if the subclavian groove is fractured anteriorly, if there is widened mediastinum on chest X-ray, or if there is an upper-extremity pulse deficit, a concomitant brachial plexus injury, or an expanding hematoma.[1]

Although binders, cumbersome rib belts, and taping were advocated in the past, the modern approach to treatment emphasizes relief of pain, prevention of atelectasis, and optimization of pulmonary toilet. A recent prospective case series at a Level 1 trauma center found that patients with isolated, simple rib fractures suffered an average of over 50 days of disability and lost work or usual activity because of pain.[57] Interventions favored for short-term pain relief include epidural analgesia, intercostal rib blocks, intrapleural instillation of anesthesia, and intravenously giving opiates and oral nonsteroidal antiinflammatory drugs (NSAIDs).[40,46,57,103] Chronic pain control invariably is necessary, usually with oral narcotics, NSAIDs, and transdermal patches. Patients must be reminded to practice adequate pulmonary toilet after discharge by using an incentive spirometer, deep breathing, coughing, and ambulation. Patients should be counseled that their pain will likely continue for weeks and that sustained need for oral analgesics during this time is not uncommon. In addition to chronic pain, other long-term sequelae include chest wall deformities, persistent dyspnea, and neurological deficits. A relatively uncommon but potential long-term complication of severe blunt trauma is a thoracic lung hernia. Because these entities pose a constant threat of incarceration, pneumothorax, or strangulation, they should be repaired.[19]

Flail Chest

During the primary survey of a patient who has suffered blunt trauma, careful observation for the presence of a flail chest is imperative. This injury usually results with the fracture of four or more ribs at two sites either unilaterally or bilaterally, promoting enough instability that the thoracic cage exhibits paradoxical motion locally. This impairs respiratory mechanics, resulting in hypoventilation, poor pulmonary drainage, and atelectasis. Patients with flail chest are distinct from those with multiple rib fractures because they are at a higher risk of respiratory compromise and often require early intubation.[98] Endotracheal intubation is necessary in more than two thirds of patients with flail chest and

84 is indicated for a respiratory rate over 40 breaths per minute, or a Po_2 of less than 60 mmHg despite 60% face mask oxygen. Relative indications for intubation include shallow respirations, depressed consciousness, preexisting chronic lung disease, and/or the presence of associated injuries. In fact, in the presence of multiple injuries, intubation of the patient with a flail chest is almost unavoidable, and early controlled intervention often obviates sudden respiratory decompensation and its subsequent morbidity.[98]

A flail chest invariably is due to high kinetic energy absorption by the thoracic cage and thus is an important marker for significant intrathoracic injury in the blunt trauma patient. It is highly associated with pulmonary contusion, which occurs in about 45% of patients.[25] Pneumothorax and/or hemothorax are common acute sequelae, whereas acute respiratory distress syndrome occurs in as many as one third of patients, resulting in mortality rates as high as 33%.[25]

Conservative therapy, with emphasis on pain relief, with thoracic epidural analgesia is the mainstay of therapy in most trauma centers. In a minority of cases, however, patients require chest wall stabilization (Figure 7-3).[22,77] These usually are intubated patients with no possibility of being weaned from the ventilator because of a large unstable flail segment of chest wall.

Sternal Fractures

Isolated fractures of the sternum are seen with increasing frequency in motor vehicle accidents, particularly since the passing of the mandatory seatbelt legislation. Point tenderness, edema, and obvious deformity occasionally are detected on physical examination, but lateral chest X-ray is diagnostic in the majority of patients.

Morbidity and mortality from isolated sternal fractures is low. Bar and associates[6] suggest that patients with isolated sternal fractures, a normal echocardiogram, and no elevation of cardiac enzymes in the early hours of injury will have a benign course. They advocate discharging these patients home within 24 hours of arrival in the ED. Surgical repair of a sternum is very uncommon (<2%) and is indicated usually for either persistent pain or cosmesis. Surgical management options include metal plates with or without autologous bone grafts.[12,59] Although an isolated sternal fracture carries a favorable prognosis, other life-threatening concomitant injuries occur in up to one third of patients, necessitating careful evaluation and clinical vigilance.

Clavicular Fractures

Because the clavicles are thin and exposed, the midclavicular shaft, in particular, is often fractured, occurring in three out of four patients with clavicular fractures.[75] One out of four patients fractures the acromial part of the clavicle. Right and left clavicles tend to be fractured with equal frequency. Clinical examination reveals tenderness, deformity, crepitus, and occasional upper extremity neurovascular injury. Routine chest X-rays often demonstrate the diagnosis. Conservative treatment for pain control using closed reduction and figure of eight slings heals 95% of patients. Surgical techniques include placement of steel reconstruction plates and cannulated bone screws. Late sequelae of

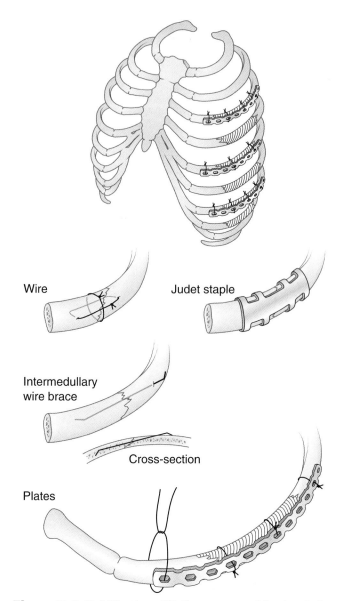

Figure 7–3 Stabilization of flail segments with wire, Judet staple, intermedullary wire brace, and periosteal plates. (*Modified from Trunkey DD: Chest wall injuries. In Blaisdel FW, Trunkey DD, editors: Cervicothoracic Trauma, 2nd ed. New York: Thieme Medical Publishers, 1994.*)

clavicular fractures include painful nonunions, altered shoulder mechanics, neurogenic thoracic outlet syndrome, vascular abnormalities, and brachial plexus injuries. Contributing factors to nonunion include severe initial trauma, open fracture, marked initial displacement and shortening, soft tissue interposition, primary open reduction and internal fixation, refracture, multiple trauma, and inadequate initial mobilization.[52]

Scapular Fracture

Because the scapula is thick and well protected, scapular fractures are relatively rare and occur usually only after high-kinetic energy impacts. Still, they should always be in the differential diagnosis in any patient who complains of shoulder pain or violent muscular contractions of the shoulder after blunt trauma. Most fractures occur in the neck and body, with glenoid, acromion, and coracoid process injuries being less frequent. As is the case with other thoracic cage trauma caused by severe blunt trauma, associated pulmonary contusions and rib fractures are common. Diagnosis often is difficult on physical examination, occasionally identified by localized tenderness, swelling, and hematoma formation over the fracture site. Scapular fractures often are overlooked on supine chest X-rays, and the three-view trauma series of the shoulder often is necessary to reveal the fracture. Chest CT scans are not recommended. Immobilization in a sling with pain relief and early range-of-motion exercises usually is all that is needed for recovery of good glenohumeral function. Open surgical reduction is rare. Brachial plexus injuries sustained are often chronic and lead to long-term disability, including loss of shoulder mobility. In these patients, a severely debilitated, insensate extremity occasionally may require amputation.

Traumatic Asphyxia

Traumatic asphyxia is an uncommon clinical syndrome usually occurring after a severe crushing or compression-related injury to the chest. Symptoms and associated physical findings include subconjunctival hemorrhage, cervicofacial cyanosis resulting in a purplish blue neck and face discoloration, facial edema, vascular engorgement of the head, mucosal petechiae, and multiple ecchymotic hemorrhages of the face, neck, and upper chest. Cerebral hypoxia resulting from hypoventilation is an ever-present danger, resulting in varying degrees of cerebral dysfunction. Sore throat, hoarseness, dizziness, numbness, and headaches are common. Pitting lower-extremity edema, hemoptysis, hemotympanum, hematuria, rectal bleeding, and transient visual loss also may be evident.[104] The diagnosis is made primarily from the patient history and physical examination, with chest X-rays being largely normal.

Prompt establishment of the ABCs of trauma management is critical, with special attention paid to reestablishing oxygenation and perfusion to ensure a successful outcome. Head elevation should be maintained at 30°. If a patient survives the initial insult, the prognosis is excellent. Skin discoloration resolves within 3 weeks, but complete resolution of subconjunctival hemorrhage can take up to 1 month.

Pulmonary Contusion

The lung parenchyma fills a large portion of the chest cavity and lies very close to the bony thorax, making it vulnerable to contusion. In fact, pulmonary contusion is the most common injury in blunt chest trauma. The mechanism of injury usually involves a sudden deceleration injury, such as in a motor vehicle accident with the chest hitting the steering wheel, or in a blast injury or a fall from a great height. Although pulmonary contusions generally are associated with concomitant thoracic cage damage and other visceral injuries, they can occur in isolation, without evidence of rib fracture. Wagner and associates[99] have suggested that the pathophysiology of a pulmonary contusion is based on hemorrhage into adjacent alveolar spaces rather than injury to the alveolar capillary wall itself.

Classic symptoms include dyspnea, tachypnea, hemoptysis, cyanosis, and hypotension. Physical examination can demonstrate inspiratory rales and decreased breath sounds on the affected side. CT scan is the study of choice and has been found to be more sensitive than radiography in detecting a pulmonary contusion. All patients with a pulmonary contusion should be observed on supplementary oxygen in a hospital setting because their ventilatory status tends to deteriorate rapidly. By standard Advanced Trauma Life Support (ATLS) protocol, patients with significant hypoxia with PaO_2 <65 mmHg and SaO_2 <90% should be intubated and ventilated within 1 hour after injury (ATLS protocol). If large volumes of fluid are necessary for resuscitation of associated extrathoracic injuries, a pulmonary artery catheter should be placed.

As mentioned, patients with pulmonary contusions are at high risk of respiratory insufficiency and secondary pneumonia because of the parenchymal damage and large systemic inflammatory response that accompanies this injury. The formation of a pulmonary contusion, along with an Injury Severity Score below 65, have been identified as risk factors that have the greatest contribution to the development of acute respiratory distress syndrome (ARDS).[70] The mortality rate from an isolated pulmonary contusion is low, but when combined with other severe injuries, it rises to as high as 50%.[74] Clinical factors predisposing to mortality after a pulmonary contusion include patient's age, resuscitation volume, and severity of the pulmonary parenchymal injury as measured by PaO_2/FiO_2 at 24 and 48 hours after injury.[60]

Laryngeal Injuries

The larynx enjoys a position of relative protection in the neck shielded laterally by the sternocleidomastoid, posteriorly by the cervical spine, and from the front and above by the mandible. Blunt trauma to the larynx is therefore rare, but has a mortality rate reaching as high as 40%. Death is due primarily to asphyxia from laryngospasm, hemorrhage from an associated major vascular laceration, or laryngeal concussion. Laryngeal trauma is suspected after motor vehicle accidents, hanging attempts, sporting blows such as in karate or soccer, and severe falls.

Signs and symptoms after laryngeal blunt trauma include hoarseness, pain, skin contusions, cervical emphysema, cervical neck crepitus, dysphagia, and upper airway obstruction. Subtle signs of dysphonia, including easy fatigue during phonation, marked difficulty with high-pitched and singing voice, and decreased phonation time, also can occur. Diagnosis requires a high index of suspicion because many patients remain asymptomatic at an early stage of injury and minor symptoms may belie serious abnormalities. Furthermore, patients may be unable to supply critical aspects of the history and physical because of aphonia or intubation. Early diagnosis and appropriate therapy have a significant impact on the patient's condition later, especially regarding scar formation, ease of breathing, and voice quality.

After securing a patent and stable airway, transnasal flexible laryngoscopy is used for definitive diagnosis. Because the risk for laryngospasm and sudden airway obstruction is increased in the presence of a laryngeal lesion, preparations for emergency intubation or tracheostomy should be readied before performing endoscopy. Flexible laryngoscopy involves inspection for vocal cord mobility, mucosal edema, hematomas, tears, and arytenoid cartilage luxation. CT scan is a sensitive diagnostic test for laryngotracheal injury and

86 may be indicated despite normal flexible laryngoscopy. The status of the laryngeal skeleton can be determined more precisely via high-resolution CT scanning.

The decision to repair or observe laryngeal trauma is based primarily on the patient's respiratory distress and associated injuries. The presence of laryngeal fractures, air in the soft tissues, and extravasation of contrast material in the neck are helpful in assessing the extent of the injuries before surgical intervention. Immediate initial surgery is aimed at stabilizing the cartilaginous framework of the larynx and repairing the mucosa. Early and low tracheostomy is recommended for patients with endoluminal disruption of the larynx, and immediate surgical exploration with anatomical repair is performed for all laryngeal injuries. Suboptimal results are found in patients with bilateral vocal cord paralysis, displaced cricoid fracture, and arytenoid subluxation.

Tracheobronchial Injuries

Tracheobronchial injuries are uncommon, but usually occur after high-energy impact and are associated with trauma to other vital organs. According to Kiser and associates,[58] who did an extensive review of all published tracheobronchial injuries since 1873, 59% of these injuries are due to motor vehicle accidents, 76% occur within 2 cm of the main carina, and 43% are located within 2 cm of the right main bronchus. Three potential mechanisms of blunt tracheobronchial disruption have been identified. The first and most common is due to a forceful anteroposterior compression of the thoracic cage, the so-called dashboard injury, in which an unrestrained automobile occupant hyperextends and strikes his or her neck on the dashboard or steering wheel, producing a crushing injury of the cervical trachea. The second mechanism is a consequence of high airway pressures, whereas the third is due to rapid deceleration. The typical clinical features include respiratory distress, dyspnea, and air leak. Hoarseness or dysphonia also is common, occurring in up to 45% in some series. Persistence of an undiagnosed air leak is life threatening and may lead to hypoventilation and, ultimately, respiratory insufficiency. On physical examination, the most common diagnostic signs are subcutaneous emphysema (35% to 85%), pneumothorax (20% to 50%), and hemoptysis (14% to 25%).

The definitive diagnostic study of choice is a flexible bronchoscopy. A careful bronchoscopic examination includes an inspection of the tracheobronchial tree documenting the site and extent of injury, including a withdrawal of the endotracheal tube in an intubated patient to diagnose proximal tracheal tears. A high level of suspicion is imperative for diagnosis because occasionally patients with tracheobronchial injuries may have normal clinical appearance and negative endoscopic findings. In fact, diagnoses of tracheobronchial injuries often are delayed, with repairs being performed months and even years after the initial injury.[58] No statistically significant association was found between delay in treatment and successful repair of the injury, with 90% of patients undergoing successful surgical reconstruction more than 1 year after initial injury. Effective airway management consists of bypassing the lesion with endobronchial intubation to the healthy bronchus using a single-lumen or double-lumen endotracheal tube. Primary surgical repair of the injured airway often is necessary, with the decision to intervene based on the size of the lesion and the respiratory status of the patient. Simple, clean lacerations without much devitalized tissue can be repaired primarily with simple, interrupted 4-0 Vicryl sutures (Ethicon, Cincinnati, OH). More severe injury may even require lobectomy or pneumonectomy. The proximal one half to two thirds of the trachea is best seen via a low cervical collar incision, whereas the distal third of the trachea, the carina, and both the proximal right and left mainstem bronchi should be approached through a right thoracotomy. Prompt diagnosis and treatment generally lead to good functional recovery, but if tracheobronchial injuries remain undetected and untreated, late complications such as bronchial stenosis, recurrent pneumonia, and bronchiectasis can develop.

Great Vessels

The thoracic great vessels consist of the aorta and its major intrathoracic branches, the pulmonary arteries and veins, the vena cavae, and the azygous vein. By far the most lethal of these is the descending aortic injury, which accounts for as many as 40% of fatalities after blunt thoracic trauma. Most of these deaths are due to free intrapleural aortic rupture before surgical repair. The site of injury usually is the medial descending aorta at the ligamentum arteriosum, where shear forces resulting from rapid deceleration cause a tear at this point of fixation of the vasculature. Again, a high index of suspicion in a patient who has suffered a high-speed collision is critical because about half of the patients with contained aortic rupture have no external signs of trauma.[68]

A plain chest film has a 95% negative predictive value for identifying blunt traumatic aortic lesions, and thus represents an adequate diagnostic screening study.[102] The classic signs on plain chest X-ray (Figure 7-4) as described by Kirsch and Sloan include a widened mediastinum (>10 cm), loss of aortic knob contour, shift of the endotracheal tube and the trachea to the right, elevation of the left mainstem bronchus, depression of the right mainstem bronchus, shift of the nasogastric tube to the left, apical capping, first rib fracture, acute left-sided hemothorax, and a retrocardiac

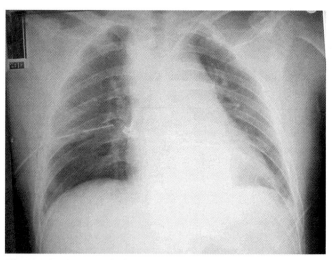

Figure 7–4 Typical chest X-ray with widened mediastinum suggestive of aortic transection from decelerating blunt chest injury.

density. Of these, the finding that most reliably correlates with an aortic tear is loss of aortic knob contour. Spiral CT scanning with angiography, which has 96.2% sensitivity and 99.8% specificity for blunt traumatic aortic abnormalities, as well as wide availability, has become the next preferred study in the algorithm of blunt aortic injury for hemodynamically stable trauma patients. Unstable patients can undergo TEE. Biplane contrast aortography remains the gold standard, however, and should be considered despite previous negative studies if the clinical suspicion remains high. Feliciano[34] suggested that 2% of patients with great vessel injuries have this scenario.

Once contained, aortic rupture is diagnosed and urgent management is required. Specifically, invasive monitoring and careful blood pressure and heart rate control with intravenous nitroprusside and beta blockade is indicated as a first step. A thorough neurological examination to document any preoperative deficits is vital. If other life-threatening injuries such as intraabdominal bleeding are detected in the primary or secondary survey, these are repaired first, before the thoracic aorta. If there is little time for preoperative studies, a TEE can even be performed during laparotomy to identify signs of blunt traumatic aortic injury. In the last decade or so, the four most dramatic changes in management of these patients have been nonoperative management, delay of definitive treatment, use of endovascular stenting for repair, and the increasing use of left-sided heart bypass via centrifugal pumps in the operating room.[34]

A subset of patients with contained aortic rupture, including those with severe central nervous system injury, extensive burns, hemodynamic instability from other traumatic injuries, respiratory failure, or small intimal defects is appropriately managed either nonoperatively or with a delayed operation. Mean arterial pressure should be maintained near 60–70 mm Hg in a manner similar to patients who have suffered an acute dissection of the descending thoracic aorta.[34] Although the length of time necessary for rigorous antihypertensive therapy is unknown, Kepros and associates[56] reported, in a small series of patients followed serially by TEE, that complete resolution of small injuries (<20 mm) occurs in about 9 days (range, 3–19 days).

Since 1991, when the first endovascular stenting of the aorta was performed for an abdominal aortic aneurysm, interest in stent grafting as an alternative to traditional aortic surgery has surged. Preliminary experience of percutaneous positioning of endovascular stent grafts under angiographic guidance for blunt traumatic aortic lesions is now accumulating.[28,76] Although the patients stented so far are carefully selected and only few in number, reported mortality rates with the endovascular approach range from 0% to 9% versus 15% to 30% observed with open surgical repair.[76] As the technology progresses and the grafts, as well as their delivery systems, become easier to employ, long-term studies evaluating the durability and efficacy of this approach are warranted.

The open surgical approach is via a fourth interspace left posterolateral thoracotomy. Proximal and distal control is obtained, with care taken to avoid injury of the recurrent laryngeal and vagus nerves, as well as the thoracic duct. There has been considerable controversy over more than 2 decades between proponents of the use of "clamp and sew" techniques versus unloading the heart proximally and shunting the blood distally. Traditional arguments against the use of left-sided heart bypass via passive shunts included the need to heparinize a trauma patient with associated injuries and the lack of data showing decreased neurological injury with passive shunting. Convincing evidence is accumulating, however, demonstrating the benefits of left atrial to femoral shunting via a centrifugal pump. Many of these systems do not require heparin, and there is a growing recent literature demonstrating low rates of paraplegia and mortality.[9,23,37] Although prolonged clamp times and the increasing complexity of the repair are associated with rising paraplegia rates, another important predictor of paraplegia has been the occurrence of upper body hypotension during surgery. Left atrial to femoral shunting during and immediately after clamping of the aorta allows strict control of upper body blood pressure. In fact, Cardarelli and associates,[23] reporting on a 30-year experience of blunt traumatic aortic rupture, remark on the gradual evolution in clinical surgical technique in their institution from "clamp-and-sew" to "passive shunt" to "heparin-less partial bypass."

Blunt Cardiac Injuries

For decades, the term *cardiac contusion* has been used to describe a wide clinical spectrum of conditions thought to be associated with blunt injury, ranging from elevation of cardiac enzymes to complex intracardiac defects or rupture. This term should now be omitted entirely because of its inconsistent clinical descriptions and because it offers little in therapy or predicting outcomes.[67] In keeping with the system of assigning trauma scores in the acutely injured patient, a new classification for blunt cardiac injury has been developed and currently is being used at major trauma centers (Table 7-2).[2]

Although frequently highlighted in the literature, only a few patients require management for blunt cardiac injuries. These injuries usually are a result of high-speed motor vehicle accidents, falls from heights, crushing and blast injuries, and direct violent assaults. Most motor vehicle–related deaths, however, are related to blunt injuries of the heart and great vessels. Mechanisms of decelerating cardiac trauma include compression by the sternum, impingement between the sternum and vertebral bodies, and increased venous return from crushing lower extremities injuries, resulting in rupture of the cardiac chambers from overdistention. Although it was once thought that sternal fractures were associated with a high incidence of blunt cardiac injuries, ironically, there has been no proven association between the two. The incidence of these injuries, however, ranges from 10% to 70%, depending upon the diagnostic modality and criteria used.

Clinically, there are few signs and symptoms that are specific for blunt cardiac injuries. Sternal or rib abnormalities may or may not be present. Chest pain is common, usually related to external injuries, and occasionally patients will describe anginal-type pain, which is not relieved with nitrates. Surgeons rely on the mechanism of injury, external chest trauma, and a high index of suspicion to determine whether a more aggressive workup of cardiac trauma is warranted. With more significant blunt injuries, hemopericardium is associated with hypotension and elevated central

Table 7-2

Blunt Cardiac Injury Terminology and Scoring System

Blunt cardiac injury with	Trauma score
No ECG, physiological or abnormality	1
Minor ECG abnormality	1
Major ECG abnormality	1
Cardiac enzyme elevation	1
Free wall hematoma	2
Septal hematoma	2
Septal defect	2
Valvular insufficiency	4
Free wall rupture	5
Cardiac herniation	5
Coronary artery injury	5

venous pressure (CVP). Auscultation may reveal decreased cardiac sounds or a murmur with septal and valvular defects.

To date, there is no diagnostic gold standard to make a diagnosis of blunt cardiac injury. Although no direct correlation exists, a diagnosis of blunt cardiac injury should be suspected when a sternal fracture is present. An electrocardiogram (ECG) should be performed on all patients in whom blunt cardiac injury is suspected, but practically all trauma victims eventually get an ECG on admission. New-onset tachyarrhythmias, especially sinus tachycardia, are the most common findings on initial ECG, and this initial ECG is the best indicator of blunt cardiac injury.[13,36] Otherwise, the ECG is unreliable unless ST elevation is present.

Levels of creatinine kinase-myocardial bands (CPK-MB) and troponin have become part of the standard laboratory evaluation tests, but, like the ECG, they are limited by the lack of a precise threshold for the diagnosis of a blunt cardiac injury. However, in the patient with musculoskeletal trauma, the CPK-MB level remains questionable. Recently, cardiac troponin I and T were found to be highly sensitive for myocardial injury and useful in the stratification of patients at risk for complications.[94] However, debate still exists about how the abnormal ECG, echocardiogram, and

enzyme levels determine myocardial injury, and how they affect therapy, decision making, and outcomes.[2]

Echocardiography, however, remains the best diagnostic tool for detecting injuries, wall motion abnormalities, effusions, valvular or septal defect, and particularly chamber rupture.[79] This should be performed in all patients who have an abnormal ECG or who are hemodynamically unstable. An attempt at transthoracic images should be made first, but if they are not optimal or yield little data, the transesophageal route should be done. Because of their anterior location, the right atrium and ventricle are the most frequent chambers injured, followed by the left atrium and left ventricle. Mortality from one chamber rupture is 60% and is universally fatal if two are involved.

Radionucleotide imaging can be helpful in documenting defects and predicting complications; however, it may not be practical in the acutely injured patient and cannot differentiate new injuries from chronic preexisting disease. However, in the presence of a normal echocardiogram, these tests add little to the management or predicting complications. Myocardial uptake gated (MUGA) scans are recommended, however, if the ECG is abnormal and there is evidence of ventricular failure.[55]

The recommended observation and treatment options also depend on suspicion of blunt cardiac injury, as well as any associated diagnostic test abnormalities. As stated previously, a sternal fracture does not predict the presence of a blunt cardiac injury, and thus monitoring is not necessarily indicated. Those patients with an abnormal ECG (arrhythmia, ischemia, heart block, or ST changes) should be admitted for continuous ECG monitoring for at least 48 hours. Conversely, a prolonged hospital stay with cardiac monitoring is no longer required if the initial ECG and echocardiogram are normal, and most patients are discharged after 12 hours. The younger patient rarely develops cardiac complications even when there are mild ECG, echocardiogram, and enzyme abnormalities. However, in the older patient who has known cardiac disease, hemodynamic instability, multisystem trauma, and ECG changes, and who is planning to undergo general anesthesia, appropriate cardiac monitoring is necessary, and consideration should be made to place a pulmonary artery catheter.

Operative intervention is required in 5% to 10% of patients who have nonpenetrating cardiac injuries. Chamber ruptures usually are isolated events. They should be repaired with simple cardiorrhaphy with a running suture, usually of 4-0 polypropylene; pledgets are required for right-and left-side ventricular repairs. Valvular injuries have been reported in the aortic, mitral, and pulmonary positions. Cardiopulmonary bypass is required for left-sided repairs. Occasionally, valve resuspension or cordae reattachment can be done, but most injuries require valvular replacement. Ventricular septal defects can present either acutely or after several days of progressively worsening congestive heart failure. Operative repair is required for larger defects and for those associated with a left ventricular aneurysm. Pericardial tears with associated cardiac herniation are uncommon and have been described in the left, right, and midline diaphragmatic locations. With small tears and complete herniation, death is almost immediate. Larger tears manifest as intermittent positional hypotension and usually are found at the time of exploration for other injuries. Direct suture closure is required. Patch closure rarely is needed. Finally, arteriovenous fistula or thrombosis is an uncommon complication with the coronary vessels. The diagnosis usually is made after the long-term sequelae occur: left ventricular pseudoaneurysm, cardiac failure, embolism, or arrhythmias. Surgery is directed at the specific complication.

Diaphragm

With the advent of modern high-speed transportation and traumatic diaphragmatic injury, there appears to be a disease in evolution. Injury to (or rupture of) the diaphragm as a result of blunt truncal trauma is seen with increasing frequency. In North American series, the prevalence of diaphragmatic rupture among blunt trauma victims ranges from 0.8% to 8%. Because of a greater awareness, routine use of chest roentgenograms in the initial evaluation of trauma patients, availability of minimally invasive techniques, and improved access to modern trauma care systems, surgeons increasingly are facing the diagnosis and management of diaphragmatic injuries.

Diaphragmatic injuries can be classified according to the mechanism of injury, side involved, unilateral or bilateral location, clinical sequelae after the onset of injury, and severity of the anatomical disruption. The latter has an important practical application in predicting outcome and associated visceral injury, because these patients with diaphragmatic injuries are at risk for severe multisystem trauma. Blunt diaphragmatic rupture occurs mainly from high-speed motor vehicle crashes when the rapid deceleration results in a nonuniform pressure load on the inflexible central tendon. In particular, lateral impact to the torso is three times more likely to rupture the diaphragm than that from a frontal direction. Because the diaphragm is buffered by the liver on the right side, 95% of injuries occur on the left side; bilateral injuries occur in less than 3% of all cases. Compared with the left side, patients with right hemidiaphragm ruptures tend to have worse increased multiorgan involvement, more hypovolemic shock, lower Glasgow coma scale scores, and higher mortality. Bilateral ruptures, including those involving the pericardium, are rare in patients who reach the hospital alive.

Diaphragmatic injury or rupture also can be classified by the time of presentation. Three clinical phases follow the onset of traumatic diaphragmatic injury: acute, latent, and obstructive phases. The acute phase begins with the original trauma and ends with the apparent recovery from other injuries, and thus may mask the diaphragm injury. Most patients (60%) have nonspecific pain in the left upper quadrant or lower thoracic or shoulder pain. Others have severe acute symptoms of dyspnea, hypotension, or cyanosis because of compression of the lung and mediastinal shift from the herniated organs.

In the latent or interval phase, symptoms are variable and nonspecific as the patient compensates for having intrathoracic abdominal contents. The symptoms are suggestive of other disorders such as peptic ulcer disease, gallbladder disorder, partial bowel obstruction, and chronic obstructive pulmonary disease. Symptoms of intermittent bowel obstruction aggravated by eating or lying on the left side are relieved by belching, vomiting, or flatus.

Finally, the obstructive phase may occur at any time when bowel obstruction occurs after incarceration of herniated viscera, leading to necrosis if diagnosis and treatment is further delayed. In one series, the onset of the obstructive phase ranged from 20 days to 28 years. However, 90% usually suffer from strangulation after 3 years. These patients have presenting symptoms consistent with slow progressive herniation of stomach and bowel contents into the chest cavity. These include nausea, vomiting, abdominal pain, and obstipation, finally leading to respiratory distress, shock, obstruction, strangulation, and signs of viscus perforation.

The diagnosis of acute diaphragm injury or rupture is a clinical challenge, especially in patients who do not have obvious indications for emergent exploration. Because diaphragmatic defects do not heal and can eventually lead to a latent visceral herniation, delayed diagnosis can be catastrophic. With previous blunt trauma, intermittent bowel obstruction without a previous abdominal incision should raise the possibility of diaphragm disruption. Findings on physical examination such as paradoxical motion of the left upper abdominal quadrant, decreased intercostal retraction, decreased breath sounds, or shifting of cardiac sounds should raise suspicion. Diagnosis in the latent phase also can be difficult, particularly with right-sided injuries, because of its vague symptoms. Often, patients may not recall any previous history of trauma, and physical examination may reveal bowel sounds over the chest.

Plain chest films are the initial screening test of choice, but up to 75% are nondiagnostic. Findings suggestive of a diaphragm defect include an indistinct costophrenic angle, elevated or indistinct hemidiaphragm, air fluid levels in the chest, and abnormal pleural densities (Figure 7-5). Right-side diaphragm injuries rarely are detected. CT and ultrasonography often are positive when there is frank visceral protrusion into the chest. Diagnostic peritoneal lavage may be helpful in the acute setting, but it carries a 25% to 34% false negative rate.

For left-sided ruptures, the diagnosis usually is made if a nasogastric tube passed into the stomach is seen in the hemithorax, or if an upper gastrointestinal contrast series reveals a narrowing of the obstructed stomach or bowel

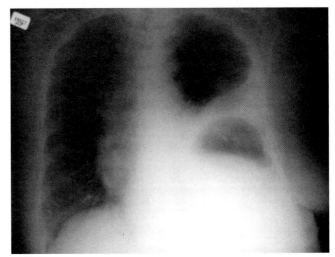

Figure 7–5 Chest X-ray after blunt thoracic trauma suggestive of left-side diaphragmatic rupture.

90 segment above the diaphragm (Figure 7-6). If an aortogram is performed for other reasons, the splenic or gastric vessels may be seen above the diaphragm. Although radionuclide scanning, fluoroscopy, and magnetic resonance imaging have high accuracy in the diagnosis of blunt diaphragmatic rupture, their use in unstable patients with multiple injuries is impractical. Right-sided ruptures may show a total or partial ("mushroom" projection) liver herniation with or without associated bowel contents.

Minimally invasive surgery for the evaluation of the diaphragm and other structures can be performed effectively while avoiding the morbidity of an open procedure. Routine laparoscopy is recommended to evaluate occult diaphragmatic injuries in stable patients with left thoracoabdominal penetrating injuries who otherwise have no other indication for an open operation. In patients with previous abdominal surgery, a video-assisted thoracic surgical approach may be preferred to evaluate the diaphragm once intraabdominal injuries have been ruled out.

The surgical approach to repair acute diaphragmatic injury or rupture depends on the mechanism of injury, condition of the patient, and time of presentation. Shock should be corrected, and a nasogastric tube should be in place to decompress the stomach. After immediate life-threatening injuries are addressed, the diaphragm can be thoroughly inspected for defects. Even the smallest of defects should be closed. Laparotomy can be first performed to explore the abdomen for other injuries, but diaphragmatic defects can be repaired from either the abdomen or chest. When both cavities need to be explored, separate incisions are favored over a continuous one because of the higher morbidity rate.

In patients who require emergent laparotomy for suspected intraabdominal injuries, thorough inspection of both hemidiaphragms is mandatory, regardless of the direction of the blunt impact. Diaphragmatic rupture resulting from blunt trauma should be approached through a laparotomy because of the high incidence of simultaneous intraabdominal solid organ injuries. Similarly, in hemodynamically stable patients whose diaphragm injury is confirmed by noninvasive imaging or by laparoscopy, laparotomy should be performed to rule out occult intraabdominal injuries.

In contrast to the acute presentation, many surgeons prefer a thoracotomy approach for those injuries and hernias that present in a delayed fashion. Although this approach provides excellent exposure to divide the adhesions between the trapped viscera and lung parenchyma, a transabdominal approach may be preferable for left hemidiaphragmatic hernias where segments of small or large bowel may have to be resected and anastomosed. However, a thoracotomy approach should be used for all right-sided diaphragmatic defects, regardless of the timing after initial injury.

The herniated viscera is first carefully reduced and returned to the abdominal cavity. The preferred method of closure of the diaphragmatic defect is by interrupted full-thickness nonabsorbable 0 or #1 sutures. Adhesions should be taken down, the lung should be decorticated, and, if necessary, the diaphragm should be loosened from the lower rib to take tension off the repair. For the chronic rupture, a splenectomy may need to be performed, followed by enlargement of the defect in order to facilitate repair. Finally, in the rare occasion where the tissue loss is extensive, closure of the defect can be achieved with fascia lata, biological material such as bovine pericardium, or synthetic material.

Mortality and morbidity in patients with acute diaphragmatic injuries differ considerably from those with a delayed presentation.[83] In the former, multiorgan trauma is usually present, and thus irreversible shock and head injury are most often cited as the causes of early death, approaching 40%. With strangulated bowel, the rate goes to 80%. When these injuries are isolated and repaired adequately, complications are rare and are usually pulmonary in nature. With the chronic type, sepsis and multisystem organ failure are the usual causes of mortality. In the presence of bowel strangulation and gangrene, a much higher postoperative mortality (66%) and morbidity (80%) rate is encountered compared with patients with an uncomplicated operative approach.

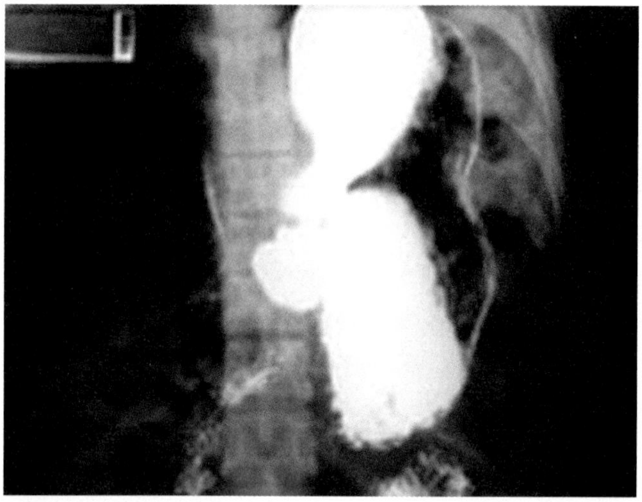

Esophagus

Blunt esophageal trauma is much rarer compared with penetrating injuries, but when it occurs, it happens more commonly as a result from a direct blow to the cervical region, such as hitting the steering wheel during decelerating motor vehicle accidents or even from padded objects such as boxing gloves. Simultaneous rupture of the esophageal wall and adjacent membranous trachea wall can occur if both are compressed between the sternum and vertebral body, resulting in fistula formation. It is estimated that one third of all tracheoesophageal fistula have this etiology, second only to iatrogenic causes. Other blunt force injuries include manual compression during cardiopulmonary resuscitation (up to 12% incidence found during autopsy) and the Heimlich maneuver, which can injure the intrathoracic esophagus.

A Boerhaave-like rupture injury can occur from increased intraluminal pressure with a closed glottis and increased intraabdominal pressure. This usually occurs just above the esophagogastric junction and into the left pleural space,

Figure 7–6 Upper gastrointestinal barium study delineating stomach and small bowel contents years after blunt decelerating injury.

where there is less protection by the pleural lining. Mortality is high not because of the severity of the injury, but rather from the delayed diagnosis and ensuing complications. Other etiologies of barotraumas include blast injuries and introduction of high-pressure gases (e.g., fire extinguisher discharges, eruption of carbonated drinks, gas ingestions from biting of inner tubes). Finally, localized wall or long segment necrosis has been described despite its rich blood supply, because the arterial inflow is torn away from severe blunt trauma.

Blunt esophageal injuries are often difficult to diagnose early because of the multisystem trauma issues and lack of recognition. Patients may show signs and symptoms of esophageal leak: subcutaneous air, pneumomediastinum, aspiration (from fistula formation), hypotension, tachycardia, and sepsis in the more advanced case. Diagnosis can be made from a contrast swallow study, but in the compromised trauma patient, this usually cannot be performed. In some cases a CT scan may detect small leaks into the neck or mediastinum not seen on contrast esophagography. Esophagoscopy is helpful and has been reported to have higher sensitivity than contrast studies.[8]

With free perforation or fistula formation, early surgical repair is advocated. Conservative medical therapy (broad spectrum antibiotics, close observation, parenteral nutritional support) is chosen only in selected patients when the leak is minimal and there are no signs of sepsis. Approaches are dictated by the level of involvement. Cervical incisions usually suffice for the defects in the neck, but may require exposure with an upper sternal split for the thoracic inlet. A right thoracotomy may be required for the upper thoracic third of the esophagus, whereas the left side is preferred for those just above the esophagogastric junction. The surgical principles are like those of other benign perforations of the esophagus: The edges are trimmed of devitalized tissue and closed in multiple layers. A tissue flap is added to buttress the repair. When a fistula is taken down, the esophageal and tracheal openings are closed primarily, and the suture lines must be separated by a tissue flap to prevent reformation. These flaps include intercostal muscle, strap muscles, mediastinal thymic fat, pericardium, and diaphragm. A tracheostomy has been advocated to help protect the tracheal suture line. Patients whose diagnosis was delayed and hemodynamically unstable may require esophageal diversion rather than primary repair.

Extensive necrosis of the esophagus is associated with a much higher mortality rate. When suspected, the diagnosis is made with endoscopy, noting the mucosal ischemic changes. In these circumstances, emergency esophagectomy and proximal diverting esophagostomy are necessary, with reconstruction of gastrointestinal continuity performed at a later date.

▶ PENETRATING TRAUMA

Stab Wounds Versus Firearm Injuries

The evaluation and management of penetrating trauma to the thorax is best broken down by anatomical distribution. This includes the chest wall, the great vessels and other major vascular structures, the trachea and major bronchi,

the lung parenchyma, the heart, the esophagus, and the diaphragm. Each of these structures can be injured individually, as well as in combination with other intrathoracic or extrathoracic structures. The evaluation of thoracic injury requires a systematic approach founded on anatomy to rapidly identify injury and initiate therapy. Penetrating injuries to the chest can be both subtle and dramatic in presentation. Paramount in the management is a rapid assessment and evaluation of the patient's severity of injury. Patients who appear "stable" can deteriorate rapidly and can become acutely moribund through tension pneumothorax or pericardial tamponade, as well as massive intrathoracic hemorrhage.

Once the initial primary survey has been performed, the patient's disability should be evaluated, specifically with determination of the location and mechanism of penetrating injury. Puncture wounds can be small and easily missed. The patient must be rolled and completely exposed with close inspection of critical areas such as the axilla. Central wounds and peripheral wounds have different implications. Lower thoracic versus upper thoracic wounds suggest potential injuries to neck structures and abdominal structures, respectively, in addition to a thoracic injury. Stab wounds differ from gunshot wounds in their potential depth of penetration and degree of damage to surrounding organs. Knife wounds are limited to the direct tract of the blade and impart only the kinetic energy transfer to surrounding tissue that is manually produced. Gunshot wounds, on the other hand, impart kinetic energy to the surrounding tissue produced by the mass and velocity of the bullet (kinetic energy = ½ mass × velocity ^{2}). In addition to injury along the direct wound path, radial injury is produced by the kinetic energy transferred to the surrounding tissue. Wounds can be classified as "low energy transfer" or "high energy transfer."[87] In general, handgun wounds produce low-energy transfer injuries and high-velocity rifles produce high-energy transfer injuries. All of these issues should be rapidly evaluated and considered in the primary survey.

Chest Wall Injury

The chest wall provides a rigid support and protection to the contents of the chest. Injuries that are limited to the chest wall itself rarely require surgical intervention. These injuries include intercostal vascular injuries, which can produce hemothorax, as well as injuries to the internal mammary artery. These usually are managed easily with ligation or electrocautery. Blast injuries usually caused by high-velocity missiles, or shotgun injuries, can result in major tissue loss of the chest wall, including both soft tissue and the bony thorax. These injuries can be covered initially with adhesive steridrapes or a soft Esmark covering with placements of chest tubes inside the thorax to achieve lung inflation and control any air leak. Definitive coverage of the defect using rotational flaps or free flaps of latissimus muscle, pectoralis major, serratus anterior, or omentum can be performed at a later time.

Tracheal and Bronchial Penetrating Injuries

Penetrating injuries to the trachea and major bronchi frequently are accompanied by respiratory distress. Airway

92 management and control of breathing with endotracheal intubation for adequate ventilation is the first role in management. The need to establish a surgical airway in more proximal laryngotracheal injuries should be anticipated and performed without hesitation should oral endotracheal intubation prove difficult or impossible. In one series, almost half of these injuries required surgical airway.[44] Cricothyroidotomy or tracheotomy is unlikely to provide any advantage over endotracheal intubation in more distal tracheal or bronchial injuries. Gunshot wounds are the most common cause of central airway injury, although stab wounds are also possible. Stab wounds that injure the airway are more likely to be in the neck.[24,49]

Signs of airway injury include subcutaneous emphysema, hemoptysis, and pneumothorax, as well as air leak upon chest tube insertion. Plain films may reveal pneumothorax, pneumomediastinum, atelectasis in an underinflated lung or lobe, and the "falling lung sign of Kumpe" if the lung has collapsed outward and downward (rather than inward and upward) from the hilum.[61] Adequate ventilation may prove challenging in the setting of a tracheal or hilar injury. Intrapleural injuries produce pneumothorax and should be treated with immediate chest tube insertion. Massive air leak should raise the suspicion of a major bronchial injury, but lack of air leak on the chest tube does not rule out the presence of injury. Bronchial edges may be approximated and seal a leak. A clot obstructing the bronchus may prevent air egress from in the area of injury. Intubation and bronchoscopy are the first steps in managing a suspected bronchial injury. Extrapleural or mediastinal injury may not manifest as pneumothorax but instead as massive mediastinal air or subcutaneous emphysema.

Flexible bronchoscopy should be performed and the complete tracheobronchial tree examined. If a proximal tracheal injury is suspected, the patient can be intubated over a bronchoscope to fully inspect the airway. Fiberoptic intubation can be performed awake and sedation and paralysis given after the airway has been established. Proximal tracheal injuries are best managed initially with intubation distal to the area of injury and control of the air leak. Injuries to the mainstem bronchi can be more challenging to manage initially. Bronchial blockers or Fogarty catheters are used to occlude the side of the injury and control massive air leak and prevent inadequate ventilation. Double-lumen endotracheal tubes should be used if possible for selective ventilation of the uninjured lung. Injuries to the airway can result in significant amounts of blood in the tracheobronchial tree and contribute to problems with ventilation. Aggressive toilet bronchoscopy must be performed with lavage of the airway until clear.

Surgical management of tracheal or bronchial injuries follows the same principles of tracheobronchial resection and repair used for neoplasms (Figure 7-7). Proximal tracheal injuries can be managed through a cervical collar incision or an upper sternal split. More distal tracheal injuries are best approached through a right posterolateral incision. Bronchial injuries are best approached through posterolateral thoracotomy to the side of the injury. Proximal left mainstem bronchial injuries and carinal injuries are best managed through a right posterolateral thoracotomy. On initial entry, control of the hilum with isolation of the pulmonary artery and veins is the initial goal. Unsuspected

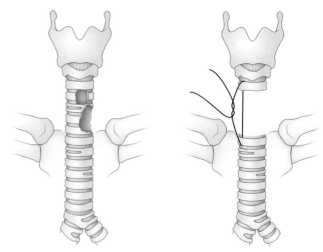

Figure 7–7 Resection and repair after gunshot wound to the cervical trachea.
(*Modified from Lee RB: Traumatic injury of the cervicothoracic trachea and bronchi. Chest Surg Clin N Am 7:300, 1997.*)

vascular injury may be present, and proximal control of these vessels is critical. We place umbilical tapes and loosely draped tourniquets around the vessels to enable rapid control of bleeding or potential air embolus. The airway is then dissected out and débrided and repaired using interrupted absorbable sutures in the standard manner of sleeve resection or bronchoplasty. Tension-free technique of airway repair should be performed. Mobilization of the airway should be adequate to decrease tension but not compromise blood supply. Large defects in the airway may require lung resection, although lung-sparing techniques should be attempted. Injury to a lobar bronchus might be best treated with standard or sleeve lobectomy. Pneumonectomy should be avoided at all costs given the extremely poor outcomes of patients requiring pneumonectomy for trauma.[17,54] Postoperative care should include aggressive pulmonary toilet and attempts to wean from positive pressure ventilation as quickly as possible. Aggressive bronchoscopy should be performed to keep the airway clear of secretions and prevent atelectasis. As in all thoracic surgery, early ambulation is critical.

Pulmonary Injuries and Hemothorax

Pulmonary injuries secondary to penetrating trauma can vary from small pleural or parenchymal lacerations from a stab wound to massive pulmonary injury secondary to a gunshot wound. The initial evaluation, in addition to the ABCs, should include a routine chest radiograph in the stable patient. Physical examination to detect hemothorax and hemopneumothorax can be unreliable, particularly in a patient who is stable with minimal symptoms. Asymptomatic patients with a normal chest X-ray can be safely observed and discharged after an appropriate time interval.[20] This time interval is a subject of debate, although a serial chest radiograph at 6 hours seems to be a reasonable time period to pick up a delayed hemothorax or pneumothorax. We do not recommend wound exploration and tractotomy of thoracic wounds because of the potential to cause a pneumothorax and contaminate the pleural space. Tube thoracostomy should be performed in all patients with a pneumothorax or findings of pleural fluid caused by penetrating trauma. We recommend this even if the pneumothorax is small or the fluid appears minimal. Tube thoracostomy allows monitoring of bleeding and any potential need for thoracotomy, should the bleeding prove to be significant. In addition, it prevents accumulation of clot that may later prove difficult to drain and require decortication. Patients with minimal chest tube output and no air leak can have the chest tube removed on the first hospital day and be discharged. Persistent bleeding mandates thoracotomy or thoracoscopy. Massive bleeding on chest tube insertion should be treated with emergent thoracotomy with no attempt to use thoracoscopic techniques.

Most pulmonary lacerations do not require surgery and can be treated by tube thoracostomy. In fact, in a series of 755 penetrating injuries to the chest, more than half of which were gunshot wounds, only 8% required thoracotomy.[50] Drainage of the pleural space with reestablishment of pleural apposition tamponades what is generally low-pressure venous bleeding and serves to seal an air leak. Even high-velocity, war-related injuries usually respond to conservative measures of chest tube drainage, antimicrobial therapy, and wound care.[80] Large air leaks on chest tube insertion should raise the concern for bronchial injury followed by prompt bronchoscopy and possible thoracotomy.

If thoracotomy is necessary, the general rule is to spare as much lung as possible and avoid anatomical resection. A posterolateral thoracotomy is performed to gain access to the hilum of the lung. Lung isolation is obtained expeditiously with a double-lumen tube or bronchial blocker. This serves to provide atelectasis to perform a tension-free repair or resection of the lung and to help prevent air embolus. As in all thoracotomies for penetrating thoracic trauma, the hilum and pulmonary vessels are controlled early with umbilical tapes or vessel loops to allow rapid vascular control, should an unsuspected central injury be present that was unnoticed. Nonanatomical resections are performed whenever possible. We use stapling devices with a generous margin around the area of injury to resect damaged tissue. Hematomas should be treated with a broad margin and vascular load to the stapler to achieve hemostasis. These staple lines can be oversewn to reinforce the region and support hemostasis if the staple line was not adequate to stop the bleeding. Persistent bleeding from deep missile injuries can be opened and exposed by inserting the anvil of the linear stapler into the tract and firing the device to perform a "tractotomy." If there is extensive tissue loss, anatomical resection of an injured lobe may be necessary. The literature shows that mortality increases with the level of complexity of the procedure.[53] Pneumonectomy is to be avoided and performed only if all other measures to salvage the lung have been exhausted. Anatomical resections require some form of bronchial stump coverage given the contamination of the pleural space and risk for subsequent infection and bronchopleural fistula.

The timing of thoracotomy for thoracic hemorrhage after trauma has been widely discussed. Recommendations have been made to perform thoracotomy if there is an initial chest tube output of greater than 1500 ml or if there is greater than 250 ml per hour of chest tube output for 3 consecutive hours after its placement.[66] Slightly differing amounts of chest tube outputs have been used as guidelines for operative intervention for ongoing bleeding. However, one recent multicenter trial showed that mortality linearly increased as the total amount of chest tube output increased and used 1500 ml of total chest tube output within the first 24 hours after injury as a recommendation to surgically intervene.[53]

Cardiac Injuries

Penetrating injuries to the heart are a significant challenge to manage. They are one of the leading causes of death in urban trauma, accounting for a high rate of prehospital death and in-hospital mortality. Most patients who sustain cardiac injuries die before reaching the hospital. Reported mortality for these injuries varies from one series to another. What is clear is that the mechanism of injury clearly influences survival. In general, these injuries are one of two types: either stab wounds or gunshot wounds. Penetrating cardiac injuries secondary to blunt trauma that produces fragments of fractured rib or sternum are rare. Gunshot wounds carry higher mortality than do knife wounds. The management of patients presenting in extremis or near extremis with penetrating injury to the heart consists of airway management with endotracheal intubation, the establishment of intravenous access capable of massive volume resuscitation, and immediate thoracotomy through a left anterolateral approach. This approach allows rapid exposure of the heart and the ability to relieve tamponade from hemorrhage. In addition, it allows the surgeon the ability to perform open heart massage, control cardiac injuries, cross-clamp the descending aorta to preferentially perfuse the brain and coronary arteries, and allow volume resuscitation in the setting of exsanguination and shock.

The patient's physiological condition at the time of presentation significantly affects the outcome. The clinical features of a patient who has a penetrating cardiac injury depend on the degree of pericardial tamponade and the amount of blood loss. Coronary artery injuries are rare but can cause ischemia, resulting in hemodynamic instability from myocardial dysfunction. One prospective study of 105 patients with penetrating cardiac injury showed that patients in physiological collapse on presentation who required emergent ED thoracotomy had a mortality rate of 86%, whereas those who were stable enough to be transported to the operating room for thoracotomy had a 26% mortality rate.[3] The need for aortic cross-clamping was a significant predictor of poor outcome (89% mortality), which was likely due to the poor physiological condition of these patients on presentation. The rate of survival from stab wounds (65%) in this study was significantly higher than that for gunshot wounds (16%).

All penetrating cardiac injuries have the potential for mortality, and it is not clear that the particular area of the heart that is wounded carries a worse prognosis. Ventricular injuries, particularly right ventricular injuries, seem to be more common given its more anterior location. The left and right atria are less commonly injured given their smaller size and more protected location. Intrapericardial great vessel injuries also are unusual. Although it is not possible to say

94 that one anatomical location of injury portends a worse outcome, it does appear that multichamber and complex cardiac wounds have a worse prognosis than a single-chamber injury.

Although many cardiac injuries are obvious on presentation as manifested by a hemodynamically unstable patient with a penetrating injury in proximity to the heart, diagnostic evaluation is necessary for other patients who are stable and may harbor occult cardiac injury. These injuries must be identified. Even small knife wounds to the heart are unlikely to seal spontaneously and eventually result in tamponade. The hole in the pericardium produced by the knife or projectile frequently seals with clot or pericardial fat. Blood from the heart accumulates and impinges on the filling of the atrium and ventricle. The incidence of occult injury has been reported to be as high as 20% in asymptomatic patients with penetrating stab wounds to the chest.[43] Workup is indicated in patients with penetrating precordial, right-sided, or left-sided chest wounds, as well as thoracoabdominal and abdominal wounds. Tachycardia is usually the earliest sign of hypovolemia and impending tamponade. As the pericardium fills with blood, elevated filling pressures are necessary to fill the heart. This results in the clinical findings of distended neck veins and pulsus paradoxus (decrease in systolic pressure with inspiration). These signs can be subtle and difficult to detect in a noisy ED or in a hypovolemic patient.

Several modalities can be used to evaluate occult cardiac injuries. Echocardiogram is sensitive in detecting pericardial fluid, and specific signs of tamponade can be demonstrated by echocardiogram before they become clinically evident, such as diastolic collapse of the atrium or ventricle. Cardiac ultrasound and echocardiography have been used with good reliability to evaluate penetrating intrapericardial injury.[1] Echocardiogram was found to be 97% specific and 90% sensitive in stable patients with precordial wounds.[51]

All patients with penetrating thoracic trauma and echocardiograms that are positive for free pericardial fluid or that suggest clotted lacerations should be explored surgically. This approach is based on poor outcomes in patients who are initially managed nonoperatively. One study showed that two out of three patients who were clinically stable with ultrasound, suggesting clotted laceration, subsequently became unstable, and only one of these patients survived.[47] Patients with echocardiographic evidence of even small amounts of pericardial effusion were found to have major intrapericardial injury at exploration.[16]

CT scan is another noninvasive modality used to evaluate cardiac injury, although it also may fail to pick up subtle injuries or small amounts of pericardial fluid. Although it is not sensitive for small amounts of fluid, it is an excellent means of identifying and localizing intrapericardial or intracardiac foreign bodies such as bullets and gunshot pellets. These should be removed in most circumstances to prevent embolization and infection. Because of a lack of sensitivity in imaging modalities, a high degree of clinical suspicion needs to be exercised when hemodynamic instability suggests cardiac injury despite a normal echocardiogram and more invasive measures must be taken. Minimally invasive evaluation has been recommended in selected stable patients using subxiphoid pericardial window (Figure 7-8), as well as a combined approach using subxiphoid window and laparoscopy.[43]

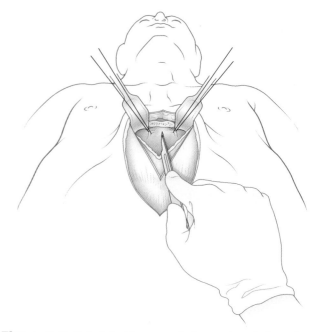

Figure 7–8 Subxiphoid approach for pericardial window. *(Modified from Brown J, Grover FL: Trauma to the heart. Chest Surg Clin N Am 7:325, 1997.)*

Management of penetrating injuries to the heart follows standard principles of cardiac surgery. If cardiac injury is suspected and time allows, transfer to the operating room with median sternotomy is performed. Otherwise, left anterolateral thoracotomy using a fourth interspace incision with extension across the sternum to the right side of the chest, if necessary, is performed. Minimally invasive procedures are not advocated in the setting of hemodynamic compromise and suspected cardiac injury. Unilateral thoracoscopy or laparoscopy is an option in the stable patient in whom diagnosis is unclear. Ventricular stab wounds should be repaired using mattress sutures with large, full-thickness bites across the injury. A 2-0 MH needle with Ethibond suture and Teflon pledgets is used to prevent tearing of the myocardium. Bleeding should be controlled using manual pressure or a sponge stick until sutures can be applied. In general, it is not advocated to use an inflated Foley balloon in a ventricular or atrial defect given the possible interference with the valvular apparatus of the tricuspid or mitral valve or obstruction of either the right or left ventricular outflow tract. Finally, the use of a Foley catheter increases the likelihood of pulmonary air embolus or stroke.

Atrial injuries using 4-0 proline suture with or without pledgets are used, depending on the quality of the atrial tissue and size of the defect. Autologous pericardium can be used to reconstruct larger defects. Bleeding can be massive, and cell saver should be used whenever possible, should a perfusionist be available. Coronary injuries present a particularly challenging injury and carry a high mortality rate. This is due to blood loss and early tamponade, as well as the resultant myocardial ischemia that can produce hemodynamic instability secondary to myocardial failure. Mattress sutures under the coronary artery that control bleeding but do not completely obstruct coronary flow should be attempted whenever possible (Figure 7-9).

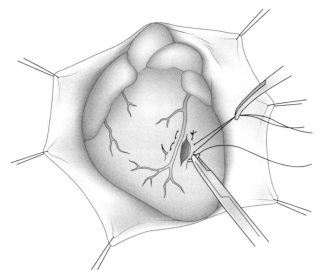

Figure 7–9 Suture repair of ventricular injuries positioned next to the coronary vessels.
(*Modified from Blaisdel FW, Trunkey DD, editors: Cervicothoracic Trauma, 2nd ed. New York: Thieme Medical Publishers, 1994.*)

Left main and anterior descending artery injuries likely produce the most catastrophic outcomes given the large territory of myocardium that the vessel supplies. Hemorrhage from coronary injuries can be temporarily controlled using a peanut to compress the artery both proximal and distal to the injury. Direct repair or coronary bypass on the beating heart is likely to be impractical, but might be considered if a cardiac surgeon with the equipment and experience is available. Ligation or oversewing of a major coronary artery should be undertaken only as a last option. If the hemodynamic instability is encountered after ligation, cardiopulmonary bypass should be considered and the performance of coronary bypass with standard aortic cross-clamping and saphenous vein grafting distal to the area of ligation.

Intrapericardial great vessel injuries are unusual because of their short segments but carry a high mortality. Intrapericardial aortic injuries were uniformly fatal in one series.[96] Lacerations to the intrapericardial aorta can be repaired using basic vascular technique, a side-biting vascular clamp, and oversewing using 3-0 proline suture. Temporary inflow occlusion of the inferior vena cava (IVC) and superior vena cava (SVC) can be used to try to minimize hemorrhage while performing the repair. Gunshot injuries producing a significant aortic disruption are usually fatal, but if cardiopulmonary bypass is available, aortic cross-clamping for repair and grafting is optimal.

SVC and IVC injuries also are difficult to control. Lifting or pulling on the heart to expose these injuries usually results in hemodynamic instability in the hypovolemic patient, so volume loading is critical. Side-biting vascular clamps can be used to control smaller, tangential injuries, but can result in iatrogenic injury if not placed carefully on fragile tissue. Shunts such as chest tubes and endotracheal tubes have been recommended to control hemorrhage but can be cumbersome to use, and care must be taken not to worsen the original injury. Cardiopulmonary bypass can be used for SVC or IVC drainage and allows for more controlled repairs of complex injuries. Cardiopulmonary

bypass, although not commonly used in emergent penetrating injuries to the heart, has been used with success if applied in a timely manner.[15,100] Outcomes for patients with penetrating wounds to the heart show that gunshot wounds have lower survival rates than stab wounds, and single-chamber injuries have lower survival rates than multiple-chamber injuries. Patients who have lower physiological status have lower survival rates than those with higher physiological status.[96]

Air Embolism & Bullet Embolism

Bullets and other missiles are not routinely removed from the chest if associated injuries are excluded. Foreign body embolism to the heart is rare. This occurs when missiles migrate intravascularly from sites of more peripheral injuries. Diagnosis is made by chest radiograph, CT scan, echocardiogram, or fluoroscopy. The management of intracardiac foreign bodies in asymptomatic patients has been debated and ranges from a philosophy of removing all intracardiac foreign bodies to expectant management. Most surgeons now recommend selective management.

The presence of an intracardiac foreign body must first be determined to be embolic and not resulting from direct thoracic injury. Direct injury resulting in an intracardiac foreign body clearly mandates sternotomy to evaluate a penetrating cardiac injury. However, if there is no thoracic injury, intracardiac missiles can be assumed to be embolic. Workup should include a chest CT scan and a two-dimensional echocardiogram.[85] The CT scan helps localize the foreign body. Echocardiogram confirms its presence and determines the exact location of the embolus in relation to other cardiac structures and whether there is any valvular dysfunction or septal defect. In addition, echocardiogram can determine whether the missile is fixed or mobile. Because of their embolic nature, these missiles generally are located on the right side of the heart. If these right-sided missiles appear to be stable and do not show any tumbling movement on echocardiogram, and if they appear to be lodged in a chamber or ventricular wall, they can be followed expectantly.[72,95] Some authors recommend intervention on larger missiles (>5 mm), irregularly shaped missiles, missiles proximal to an artery, and left-sided intracavitary or partially embedded missiles.[41]

In general, intracardiac embolic missiles should be removed if they are left-sided, mobile, large, or symptomatic with valvular incompetence. Anticoagulation or prophylactic antibiotics are not recommended for expectant management, but they are recommended for follow-up echocardiogram after 3 months, 6 months, and 1 year.

Systemic air embolus is a relatively uncommon but frequently unrecognized cause of death in patients with penetrating lung injury. It generally occurs in the setting of patients with a central lung injury. A missile or stab wound creates a fistula from the bronchus to the pulmonary veins, producing an air embolus in patients when they are placed on positive pressure ventilation. This is more likely to occur in the setting of high airway pressures. Cardiovascular collapse occurs when air enters the coronary arteries, causing myocardial ischemia and resulting in ventricular fibrillation or asystole. The hallmark of an air embolus is hemoptysis and bloody, frothy air leak from a lung injury. This can then

96 be confirmed intraoperatively by visualizing air in the coronary arteries.[33]

If air embolus is suspected, immediate thoracotomy should be performed to the side of the injury. The hilum of the lung should be clamped to prevent further sources of embolus from occurring, and the patient should be placed with his or her head down to prevent cerebral embolus from occurring. De-airing of a massive air embolus can then be performed using a large-gauge needle and a syringe through the left ventricular apex or through the roof of the left atrium as open cardiac massage is performed. The coronary arteries also can be de-aired using a syringe and a small-gauge needle. Outcomes for massive air embolus are poor, with only three out of nine patients surviving in the series by Estera. Prevention of this problem is paramount and should include lung isolation to prevent positive pressure on an injured lung until repair or resection is performed.[48] Management also has been described as using prompt institution of cardiopulmonary bypass to restore circulation while lung resection and cardiac de-airing are performed.[82]

Great Vessels

The thoracic great vessels include the ascending aorta, the aortic arch and descending aorta, the innominate artery and veins, the subclavian artery and veins, and the pulmonary artery and veins. Injuries to the great vessels are challenging to manage. Most patients die before reaching the hospital, and of those who reach the hospital, most require immediate ED thoracotomy.[29,30] Workup for major thoracic vascular injuries is frequently limited given the instability of these patients and the need for immediate thoracotomy. However, plain chest X-ray (CXR) may reveal hemothorax, hemopneumothorax, or mediastinal hematoma.

Further workup in the stable patient may include chest CT with intravenous contrast or aortography. This is particularly pertinent in the stable patient with a transmediastinal gunshot wound.[73,93] Given the improved sensitivity of the new generation of CT scanners and the increased speed with which a CT scan can generally be performed, we prefer this modality over angiography. In addition, CT scan allows the identification of other thoracic injuries. However, angiography is clearly an important modality to evaluate vascular injuries and is an important diagnostic and potentially therapeutic tool.

The initial management of major vascular thoracic penetrating injuries is prompt thoracotomy and manual tamponade of the injury or control with a vascular clamp. Subclavian injuries can be difficult to tamponade because of their location behind the clavicle. Foley balloon insertion into a neck wound and application of traction to tamponade the bleeding has been recommended until more definitive control can be achieved.[42]

Definitive management of thoracic vascular injuries follows the principles of vascular repair. Aortic injuries frequently are lethal. Rapid exposure of these injuries to establish control is critical, so the appropriate choice of incision cannot be overemphasized. Ascending aortic and aortic arch injuries are best approached through a median sternotomy. Manual pressure and/or control with side-biting vascular clamps may allow a primary repair. Cross-clamping the ascending aorta is not possible without cardiopulmonary bypass. Repair of complex vascular injuries has been described using cardiopulmonary bypass and deep hypothermic circulatory arrest.[39] Descending thoracic aortic injuries should be approached through a left thoracotomy. The descending aorta can be cross-clamped to achieve proximal and distal control and perform a primary repair or interposition graft.

Pulmonary artery or vein injuries are best approached through a posterolateral thoracotomy. Proximal control on the pulmonary artery should be achieved as a first step, and a tourniquet should be placed and cinched down to decrease blood loss and allow better visualization for vascular repair. Similar control can be achieved on the pulmonary veins. Primary repair should be attempted, and pneumonectomy should be avoided if at all possible.

Vena caval and innominate vein injuries also are repaired using standard vascular techniques. The intrapericardial SVC and IVC can be difficult to expose and repair. They can be approached through either a right thoracotomy or a median sternotomy. Ligation of either the SVC or IVC without shunting is not compatible with survival. Innominate vein injuries are best repaired through a sternotomy. The innominate vein can be ligated if repair is not possible, given the existence of adequate collateral venous drainage.

Subclavian injuries are the most frequent injuries of the thoracic great vessels, particularly given the subclavian vessels' exposure to injury through penetrating neck injury.[29] Surgical exposure for control of bleeding makes these injuries challenging. Many approaches have been recommended for control of the subclavian vessels. These approaches include a clavicular incision, clavicular incision combined with sternotomy (Figure 7-10), "trapdoor" or upper sternotomy combined with fourth interspace anterior thoracotomy (Figure 7-11), or a high anterior thoracotomy using a second or third interspace incision (Figure 7-12). Each of these techniques has its advantages, and the choice of incision should be based on the surgeon's familiarity with the approach, as well as whether the vascular injury is left or right sided or more proximal or distal. Left-sided subclavian injuries can be difficult to control through a sternotomy. In general, these injuries can be repaired primarily or, if necessary, with an interposition graft of autologous vein or prosthetic graft.[31]

Diaphragmatic Injuries

Diaphragmatic injuries in penetrating trauma can be difficult to diagnose, although once the diagnosis is made, their management is straightforward. Any penetrating injury at the nipple line or below should be considered to have the potential for both abdominal and thoracic injury and traversal of the diaphragm. The dilemma in management is how to diagnose the injury and inspect both the chest and diaphragm for injury. Injuries to the diaphragm may be slight, but repair is indicated because of the potential for associated abdominal injuries and the long-term sequelae of chronic diaphragmatic hernia with the potential for bowel incarceration. Noninvasive methods used to diagnose diaphragmatic injury are chest radiograph and chest CT scan. However, these methods can be unreliable for the diagnosis of diaphragmatic injury, with accuracy rates of only 50%.[69] Another, more invasive, method for diagnosing

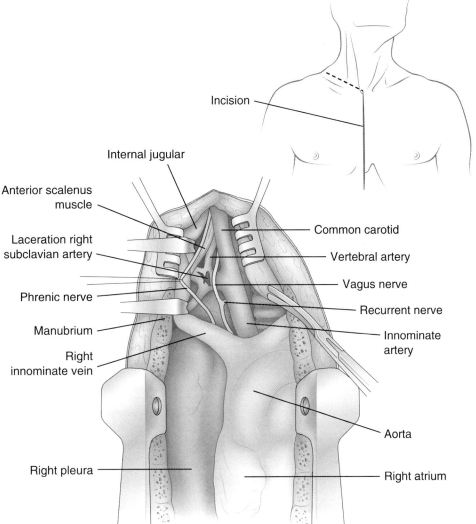

Figure 7–10 Clavicular incision and median sternotomy for exposure and control of the proximal innominate and right subclavian artery. *(Modified from Ravitch MR, Steichen FM, Schlossberg L: Atlas of General Thoracic Surgery, p. 147. Philadelphia: W.B. Saunders, 1988.)*

Incision

Internal jugular

Anterior scalenus muscle

Laceration right subclavian artery

Phrenic nerve

Manubrium

Right innominate vein

Right pleura

Common carotid

Vertebral artery

Vagus nerve

Recurrent nerve

Innominate artery

Aorta

Right atrium

penetrating diaphragmatic injury is the diagnostic peritoneal lavage (DPL), but this also can miss diaphragmatic injury. Therefore some surgeons have recommended exploratory laparotomy in patients with penetrating wounds inferior to the fourth intercostal space anteriorly, sixth interspace laterally, or eighth interspace posteriorly because of the contour and insertions of the diaphragm.[65] Laparoscopy and thoracoscopy have been used to improve diagnostic sensitivity in evaluating the diaphragm without resorting to laparotomy.

Video-assisted thoracic surgery (VATS) has proven to be an effective means of assessing the diaphragm. In one series of 171 patients with penetrating chest trauma, an algorithm was proposed to identify occult diaphragmatic injury. An initial chest radiograph was obtained, followed by chest tube placement should a pneumothorax or hemothorax be present. In addition, a DPL or abdominal CT scan was performed to assess abdominal injuries. If the DPL or abdominal CT scan suggested abdominal injury, or if the hemothorax was significant, the patient was taken to the operating room and the diaphragm evaluated via laparotomy or thoracotomy. In the setting of softer findings that do not mandate thoracotomy or laparotomy, the authors recommended VATS inspection of the diaphragm when two or

more of the following findings were present: abnormal CXR, associated abdominal injury, high-velocity injury, injury inferior to the nipple, or a right-sided wound.[38]

VATS has proven to be a safe and reliable method of evaluating the diaphragm and diagnosing and treating thoracoabdominal trauma.[97] Current recommendations incorporate concepts from these series. Clearly, any patient with indication for thoracotomy or laparotomy should have the diaphragm inspected at the time of surgery. For those patients without hard signs for surgery, VATS is a reasonable approach in the setting of an abnormal chest radiograph with an entry wound in the zone of insertion of the diaphragm, as well as in the setting of a high-velocity injury in the proximity of the diaphragm. Clearly a high degree of suspicion needs to be raised for diaphragmatic injury. Because the procedure is fast and simple with minimal morbidity, VATS should be used liberally when diagnosis is uncertain. Repair of the diaphragm can be performed using VATS coupled with standard suturing techniques and a running or interrupted method of repair. The diaphragm can be repaired transabdominally should laparotomy be required. An interrupted repair (of proline) rather than a continuous suture of the diaphragm should be used.

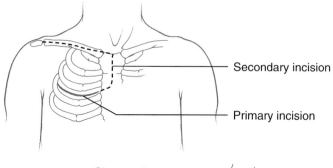

Secondary incision

Primary incision

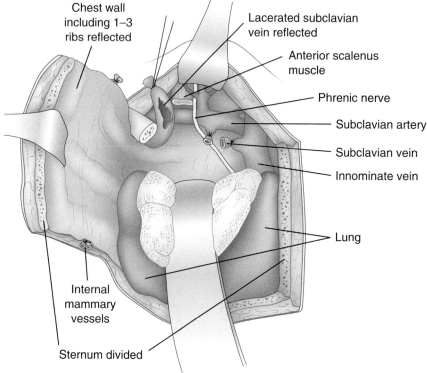

Chest wall including 1–3 ribs reflected

Lacerated subclavian vein reflected

Anterior scalenus muscle

Phrenic nerve

Subclavian artery

Subclavian vein

Innominate vein

Lung

Internal mammary vessels

Sternum divided

Figure 7–11 "Trapdoor" incision for exposure and control of the distal right subclavian artery injuries, which can be used for the left as well. *(Modified from Ravitch MR, Steichen FM, Schlossberg L: Atlas of General Thoracic Surgery, p. 155. Philadelphia: W.B. Saunders, 1988.)*

Esophageal Injuries

Injuries to the intrathoracic esophagus that result from penetrating injury are rare. The esophagus is more commonly injured in the neck, where it is most exposed. However, thoracic esophageal injuries carry high morbidity and mortality rates. The reasons are multiple. Given its central location in the chest, associated injuries are extremely common (98%) in one series.[4,101] In addition, these injuries can be missed unless specifically investigated. Finally, repair of the esophagus can be technically difficult and associated with morbid complications. A multicenter study of penetrating esophageal injuries showed that preoperative workup of esophageal injuries resulted in delay in surgery and poorer outcomes.[5] The authors concluded that if selective evaluation and management of injuries is performed, it should be done rapidly with the plan of expeditious transfer to the operating room. If this is not possible, they recommend proceeding to prompt surgical exploration.

Investigation for esophageal injuries depends on the stability of the patient. If the patient is stable with a mediastinal or transmediastinal gunshot wound, a CT scan of the chest should be done immediately with intravenous contrast

and injection of gastrographic contrast through a nasogastric tube. This can help the surgeon delineate associated injuries and the course of the bullet and choose a surgical approach. If the patient is not stable enough to undergo a CT scan and emergent operative exploration is necessary, intraoperative flexible bronchoscopy and esophagoscopy should be done first, followed by thoracotomy on the side in which the major associated injury is suspected. Thoracotomy should be performed on the left side if the injury is uncertain in order to have access to the descending aorta for cross-clamping should this prove necessary. Lung isolation through a double-lumen tube or bronchial blocker is preferred so as to provide atelectasis for better visualization and to optimize repair of injuries. Flexible endoscopy for the diagnosis of esophageal trauma has been shown to be an excellent diagnostic tool (100% sensitivity, 96% specificity with 97% accuracy in one study).[35] Intraoperative insufflation of air through the esophagoscope with the chest filled with saline can help identify a small injury. More proximal injuries are best explored through the right side of the chest through the fifth intercostal space, particularly if associated airway injury is suspected. Bronchoscopy is mandatory to

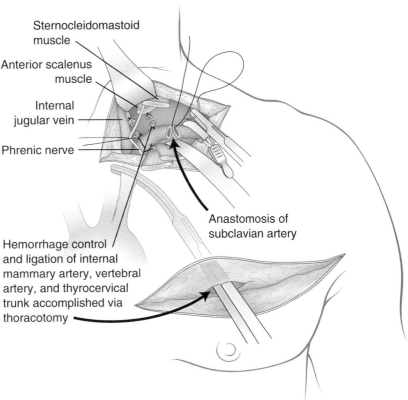

Sternocleidomastoid muscle

Anterior scalenus muscle

Internal jugular vein

Phrenic nerve

Anastomosis of subclavian artery

Hemorrhage control and ligation of internal mammary artery, vertebral artery, and thyrocervical trunk accomplished via thoracotomy

Figure 7–12 Clavicular incision for exposure and control of distal left subclavian artery injuries, and separate upper anterior thoracotomy for proximal control. *(Modified from Ravitch MR, Steichen FM, Schlossberg L: Atlas of General Thoracic Surgery, p. 150. Philadelphia: W.B. Saunders, 1988.)*

examine both the trachea and a more distal airway for injury. Distal esophageal injuries around the esophagogastric junction are best explored through a sixth interspace left thoracotomy.

Thoracic esophageal injuries should be repaired using primary closure with wide drainage. Prompt recognition of esophageal injury is critical, and it must be repaired. A missed diagnosis allows mediastinal soilage with ensuing sepsis in a patient who has already undergone one physiological insult. Nonoperative chest tube drainage alone has no place in the management of penetrating esophageal injuries. One series had a 50% mortality rate in this setting.[26]

The injured esophagus should be débrided back to clean, viable tissue. Like other esophageal repairs, a two-layer closure is performed with attention to a watertight mucosal closure using absorbable suture with an overlying second layer of nonabsorbable suture to close the muscular layer. The repair should be covered with an intercostal muscle flap or the fundus of the stomach if the injury is close to the gastroesophageal junction. Multiple chest tubes should be used to ensure complete drainage of the hemithorax and complete reexpansion of the lung to seal the pleura against the closure. In addition to chest tubes, soft, closed suction drains such as Jackson-Pratt or Blake drains should be left close to the area of injury. Therefore, should the repair prove to leak postoperatively, the chest tubes can be removed slowly and the patient eventually discharged from the hospital with the Jackson-Pratt drain in place controlling the leak until it seals. Gastric and jejunal feeding tubes should be considered and placed operatively either at the time of initial surgery or during a second operation to pro-vide access for long-term feeding should a postoperative leak preclude oral intake. Esophageal repairs are evaluated for leak with a barium esophagram on postoperative day 7.

COMPLICATIONS OF THORACIC TRAUMA

A complete discussion of complications after thoracic trauma is beyond the scope of this chapter, but the more common problems are listed in Box 7-3. Many complications and their therapies are similar to their counterparts found in non–trauma settings, and the reader is referred to those specific sections in this textbook. However, several issues specific to thoracic injuries are important to note.

Acute Lung Injury and Respiratory Distress Syndrome

Up to 20% of cases of ARDS in the United States have thoracic trauma as an etiology. Whether a direct injury to the lung parenchyma or sequelae of the critically injured patient, mortality rates from ARDS remain approximately 50%. Differentiation from acute lung injury (ALI) may be difficult, and although ALI and ARDS are sometimes included in the spectrum of diseases, both reflect the concept of acutely occurring nonhydrostatic pulmonary edema, infiltrates on chest X-ray, and hypoxemia, which are generally worse in ARDS.[11] With alterations in immune competence and production of proinflammatory cytokines, the systemic inflammatory response system (SIRS) can develop and can progress to septic shock and ARDS with a proven infection source.[7] Irrespective of the

100

Box 7–3. Complications of Thoracic Trauma.

Pulmonary

Atelectasis
Acute respiratory distress syndrome/acute lung injury
Pneumonia
Infarction
Lung abscess
Arteriovenous fistula
Bronchial stenosis
Tracheoesophageal fistula

Pleural Space

Empyema
Bronchopleural fistula
Organized hemothorax
Chylothorax
Fibrothorax
Diaphragmatic hernias

Vascular

Thromboembolism
Air embolism
Pseudoaneurysm
Great vessel fistula

Chest Wall

Hernias
Persistent pain

Mediastinum

Mediastinitis
Pericarditis

etiology, the development of ARDS is difficult to predict, but there are several factors that increase the risk of ARDS in these patients (Box 7-4).

Therapy for ALI and ARDS is mainly supportive, directed at correcting the possible underlying etiology that precipitated the pulmonary problem. Other therapies include mechanical ventilatory support, adequate nutritional status, minimization of fluid requirements, and constant rotation of position to redistribute pulmonary edema. Pharmacological therapy includes inhaled nitric oxide,

Box 7–4. ARDS Risk Factors.

Pneumonia /aspiration
Pulmonary contusion /penetrating injury
Closed head injuries
Orthopedic injuries
Sepsis/infections
Multiple transfusions
Pancreatitis
Coagulopathies
Inhalation injury
Burns

exogenous or aerosolized surfactant, corticosteroids, and the use of mediator-directed therapy such as NSAIDs and monoclonal antibodies directed against endotoxins. Although most mediators have not shown vast improvement in a prospective fashion, these unconventional therapies still hold great promise.

Pneumonia

Pneumonia remains the most common infectious complication after any multiple traumas, particularly those involving the thorax. The incidence increases with the duration of endotracheal intubation and is associated with up to 50% of deaths occurring after trauma. The etiology of nosocomially acquired pneumonias can be complex and is related to a number of factors, including underlying pulmonary conditions, associated injuries, multiple antibiotic therapies, colonization of the upper airway, aspiration at the time of initial injury, impairment of local defenses, and depression of the immune response.

Diagnosis often is difficult, with only one half of patients showing classic presenting symptoms such as fever, leukocytosis, respiratory distress, and an abnormal chest X-ray. Sputum sampling is essential; however, in the intubated patient, invasive testing is required, such as transtracheal or bronchoscopic aspiration with bronchoalveolar lavage. Pleural effusions can occur and are seen in 50% of patients with *Haemophilus influenzae* pneumonia.

Broad-spectrum antibiotic therapy is used initially, but narrowed once the offending organism and antibiotic sensitivities return. Other principles in therapy include good pulmonary care and toilet and the maintenance of nutritional function. Prophylaxis is paramount and includes effective infection control and prophylactic antibiotic and gastric bleeding measures.

Pleural Space Problems

The incidence of posttraumatic empyemas ranges from 2% to 6%, and has increased, with up to 26% of patients developing pleural space infections after chest tube insertion.[21] The management of these empyemas is the same as that resulting from parapneumonic processes, with similar goals of control of infection, evacuation of pus, obliteration of the pleural space, and restoration of complete lung reexpansion. However, these empyemas differ from their parapneumonic counterparts in several aspects. Posttraumatic empyemas usually have, in addition to gram-positive organisms, a mixture with gram-negative organisms; are usually the result of retained hemothorax; have an effusion that is often thick and of little volume; are not in the early or exudative phase; and require open thoracotomy, drainage, and aggressive decortication.[84]

Bronchopleural Fistula

Persistent bronchopleural fistula is a common problem that occurs after significant penetrating trauma to the lung parenchyma. Large massive air leaks, identified with loss of 30% to 50% of the tidal volume, are usually due to mainstem bronchial injuries and require immediate surgery. Fistula persisting more than 7–10 days is an indication for operative intervention. The use of sclerosing agents has been reported, but failure rates are high. If surgery is performed in the persistent parenchymal fistula, careful dissection and closure are advised because of the friability and fragility of the tissues, which are sometimes in the presence of ARDS inflammatory changes. The internal parenchymal injury should be exposed and major bronchioles oversewn. The parenchyma is closed in layers, and the visceral pleural lining is oversewn with a running suture to minimize air leaks. If not properly closed in layers, a parenchymal cavity persists, and acts as a nidus for a lung abscess. Anatomical resection rarely is needed, and, if required, wedge resection usually suffices.

Great Vessel Fistula

Nearly all traumatic arteriovenous fistulas result from penetrating injuries. Although a majority occurs in the cervicomediastinal areas, approximately 30% are found in the intrathoracic great vessels.[89] A trill is heard in only 20% of patients 1 week after the injury and goes to 100% after 2 weeks. After 12 weeks, 85% of patients have some type of significant clinical presentation.

Surgery is recommended once the fistula is documented, usually by angiography. There is no role for fistula "maturation" because venous hypertension can cause bleeding complications during and after the repair. Autogenous vein patch is suggested for peripheral vessels, whereas prosthetic grafts are reserved for the great vessels, aorta, and main pulmonary artery. Endovascular stenting and embolization have been reported; however, selective use of these methods is suggested for smaller vessels.

REFERENCES

1. Aaland MO, Bryan FC, Sherman R: Two-dimensional echocardiogram in hemodynamically stable victims of penetrating precordial trauma. Am Surg 60:412–415, 1994.
2. Adams JE 3rd, David-Roman VS, Bessey PQ, et al: Improved detection of cardiac contusion with cardiac troponin I. Am Heart J 131:308–312, 1996.
3. Asensio JA, Berne JD, Demetriades D, et al: One hundred five penetrating cardiac injuries: A 2-year prospective evaluation. J Trauma 44:1073–1082, 1998.
4. Asensio JA, Berne JD, Demetriades D, et al: Penetrating esophageal injuries: Time interval of safety for preoperative evaluation—how long is safe? J Trauma 43:319–324, 1997.
5. Asensio JA, Chahwan S, Forno W, et al: Penetrating esophageal injuries: Multicenter study of the American Association for the Surgery of Trauma. J Trauma 50:289–296, 2001.
6. Bar I, Friedman T, Rudis E, et al: Isolated sternal fracture: A benign condition? Isr Med Assoc J 5:105–106, 2003.
7. Bass TL, Miller PK, Campbell DB, et al: Traumatic adult respiratory distress syndrome. Chest Surg Clin N Am 7:429–440, 1997.
8. Bastos RBN, Graeber GM: Esophageal injuries. Chest Surg Clin N Am 7:357–371, 1997.
9. Benckart DH, Magovern GJ, Liebler GA, et al: Traumatic aortic transection: Repair using left atrial to femoral bypass. J Card Surg 4:43–49, 1989.
10. Bergeron E, Lavoie A, Clas D, et al: Elderly trauma patients with rib fractures are at greater risk of death and pneumonia. J Trauma 54:478, 2003.
11. Bernard GR, Artigas A, Brigham KL, et al: Report of the American-European Consensus conference on acute respiratory distress syndrome: Definitions, mechanisms, relevant outcomes, and clinical trial coordination. Consensus Committee. Am J Respir Crit Care Med 149:818–824, 1994.
12. Bertin KC, Rice RS, Doty DB, et al: Repair of transverse sternal nonunions using metal plates and autogenous bone graft. Ann Thorac Surg 73:1661–1662, 2002.
13. Biffl WL, Moore FA, Moore EE, et al: Cardiac enzymes are irrelevant in the patient with suspected myocardial contusion. Am J Surg 168:523–527, 1994.
14. Billings J: War of the Rebellion: Medical and Surgical History. Washington, DC: U.S. Printing Office, 1870.
15. Biocina B, Sutlic Z, Husedzinovic I, et al: Penetrating cardiothoracic war wounds. Eur J Cardiothorac Surg 11:399–405, 1997.
16. Bolton JW, Bynoe RP, Lazar HL, et al: Two-dimensional echocardiography in the evaluation of penetrating intrapericardial injuries. Ann Thorac Surg 56:506–509, 1993.
17. Bowling R, Marroudis C, Richardson JD, et al: Emergency pneumonectomy for penetrating and blunt trauma. Am Surg 51:136, 1985.
18. Breasted J: The Edwin Smith Surgical Papyrus, Vol. 1. Chicago: University of Chicago Press, 1930.
19. Brock MA, Heitmiller RF: Spontaneous anterior thoracic lung hernias. J Thorac Cardiovasc Surg 119:1046–1047, 2000.
20. Brown PF 3rd, Larsen CP, Symbas PN: Management of the asymptomatic patient with a stab wound to the chest. S Med J 84:591–593, 1991.
21. Caplan ES, Hoyt NJ, Rodriguez A, et al: Empyema occurring in the multiply traumatized patient. J Trauma 24:785–789, 1984.
22. Carbognani P, Cattelani L, Bellini G, et al: A technical proposal for the complex flail chest. Ann Thorac Surg 70:342–343, 2000.
23. Cardarelli MG, McLaughlin JS, Downing SW, et al: Management of traumatic aortic rupture: A 30-year experience. Ann Surg 236:465–469, 2002.
24. Cicala RS, Kudsk KA, Butts A, et al: Initial evaluation and management of upper airways in trauma patients. J Clin Anesth 3:88–90, 1991.
25. Ciraulo DL, Elliott D, Mitchell KA, et al: Flail chest as a marker for significant injuries. J Am Coll Surg 178:466–470, 1994.
26. Cohn HE, Hubbard A, Patton G: Management of esophageal injuries. Ann Thorac Surg 48:309–314, 1989.
27. Cohn SM, Burns GA, Jaffe C, et al: Exclusion of aortic tear in the unstable trauma patient: The utility of transesophageal echocardiography. J Trauma 39:1087–1090, 1995.
28. Dake MD, Miller DC, Semba CP, et al: Transluminal placement of endovascular stent-grafts for the treatment of descending thoracic aortic aneurysms. N Engl J Med 331:1729–1734, 1994.
29. Demetriades D, Asensio JA, Velhamos G: Complex problems in penetrating neck trauma. Surg Clin North Am 76:661–683, 1996.
30. Demetriades D, Rabinowitz ZE, Peziks A: Subclavian vascular injuries. Br J Surg 74:1001–1003, 1987.
31. Demetriades D: Penetrating injuries to the thoracic great vessels. J Card Surg 12:173–180, 1997.
32. Durham LA, Scalea T, Philips T, et al: Emergency center thoracotomy: Impact of prehospital resuscitation. J Trauma 32:775–779, 1992.
33. Estera AS, Pass LJ, Platt MR: Systemic arterial air embolus in penetrating lung injury. Ann Thorac Surg 50:257–261, 1990.
34. Feliciano D: Trauma to the aorta and major vessels. Chest Surg Clin N Am 7:305–323, 1997.
35. Flowers JL, Graham SM, Ugarte MA, et al: Flexible endoscopy for the diagnosis of esophageal trauma. J Trauma 40:261–266, 1996.

36. Foil MB, Mackersie RC, Furst SR, et al: The asymptomatic patient with suspected myocardial contusion. Am J Surg 160:638–642, 1990.

37. Forbes AD, Ashbaugh DG: Mechanical circulatory support during repair of thoracic aortic injuries improves morbidity and prevents spinal cord injury. Arch Surg 129:494–497, 1994.

38. Freeman RK, Al-dossari G, Hutcheson KA, et al: Indications for using video-assisted thoracoscopic surgery to diagnose penetrating chest trauma. Ann Thorac Surg 72:342–347, 2001.

39. Fulton JO, Brink JG: Complex thoracic vascular injury repair using deep hypothermia and circulatory arrest. Ann Thorac Surg 63:557–559, 1997.

40. Gabram SG, Schwartz RJ, Jacobs LM, et al: Clinical management of blunt trauma patients with unilateral rib fractures: A randomized trial. World J Surg 19:388–393, 1995.

41. Gandhi SK, Martz BG, Mistry BM, et al: Selective management of embolized intracardiac missiles. Ann Thorac Surg 62:290–292, 1996.

42. Gilroy D, Lakhoo M, Charalambides D: Control of life-threatening hemorrhage from the neck: A new indication for balloon tamponade. J Trauma 23:557–559, 1992.

43. Grewal H, Ivatury RR, Divakar M, et al: Evaluation of subxiphoid pericardial window used in the detection of occult cardiac injury. Injury 26:305–310, 1995.

44. Grewal H, Rao PM, Mukerji S, et al: Management of penetrating laryngotracheal injuries. Head Neck 17:494–502, 1995.

45. Gupta A, Jamshidi M, Rubin JR: Traumatic first rib fracture: Is angiography necessary? A review of 730 cases. Cardiovasc Surg 5:48–53, 1997.

46. Haenel JB, Moore FA, Moore EE, et al: Extrapleural bupivacaine for amelioration of multiple rib fracture pain. J Trauma 38:22–27, 1995.

47. Harris DG, Papagiannopoulos K, Pretorius J, et al: Current evaluation of cardiac stab wounds. Ann Thorac Surg 68:2119–2221, 1999.

48. Ho AM, Lee S, Tay BA, et al: Lung isolation for the prevention of air embolism in penetrating lung trauma. A case report. Can J Anaesth 47:1256–1258, 2000.

49. Huh J, Millikan JC, Chen JC: Management of tracheobronchial injuries following blunt and penetrating trauma. Am Surg 63:896–899, 1997.

50. Inci I, Ozcelic C, Tacyildiz I, et al: Penetrating chest injuries: unusually high incidence of high-velocity gunshot wounds in civilian practice. World J Surg 22:438–442, 1998.

51. Jimenez E, Martin M, Krukenkamp I, et al: Subxiphoid pericardiotomy versus echocardiography: A prospective evaluation of the diagnosis of occult penetrating cardiac injury. Surgery 108:676–680, 2001.

52. Jones GL, McCluskey GM, Curd DTJ: Nonunion of the fractured clavicle: Evaluation, etiology, and treatment. South Orthop Assoc 9:43–54, 2000.

53. Karmy-Jones R, Jurkowich GJ, Nathens AB, et al: Timing of urgent thoracotomy for hemorrhage after trauma: A multicenter study. 136:513–518, 2001.

54. Karmy-Jones R, Jurkowich GJ, Shatz DV, et al: Management of traumatic lung injury: A Western Trauma Association Multicenter review. J Trauma 51:1049–1053, 2001.

55. Keller KD, Shatney CH: Creatine phosphokinase-MB assays in patients with suspected myocardial contusion: Diagnostic test or test of diagnosis? J Trauma 28:58–63, 1988.

56. Kepros J, Angood P, Jaffe CC, et al: Aortic intimal injuries from blunt trauma: Resolution profile in nonoperative management. J Trauma 52:475–478, 2002.

57. Kerr-Valentic MA, Arthur M, Mullins RJ, et al: Rib fracture pain and disability: Can we do better? J Trauma 54:1058–1063, 2003.

58. Kiser AC, O'Brien SM, Detterbeck FC: Blunt tracheobronchial injuries: Treatment and outcomes. Ann Thorac Surg 71:2059–2065, 2001.

59. Kitchens J, Richardson JD: Open fixation of sternal fracture. Surg Gynecol Obstet 177:423–424, 1993.

60. Kollmorgen DR., Murray KA, Sullivan JJ, et al: Predictors of mortality in pulmonary contusion. Am J Surg 168:659–663, 1994.

61. Kumpe DA, Oh KS, Wyman SM: A characteristic pulmonary finding in unilateral complete bronchial transection. Am J Roentgenol 110:704–706, 1970.

62. Lewis G, Knottenbet JD: Should emergency room thoracotomy be reserved for cases of cardiac tamponade? Injury 22:5–6, 1991.

63. Liman ST, Kuzucu A, Tastepe AI, et al: Chest injury due to blunt trauma. J Cardiothorac Surg 23:374–378, 2003.

64. LoCicero J, Mattox KL: Epidemiology of chest trauma. Surg Clin North Am 69:15, 1989.

65. Madden MR, Paull DE, Finkelstein JL, et al: Occult diaphragmatic injury from stab wounds to the lower chest and abdomen. J Trauma 29:292–297, 1989.

66. Mansour MA, Moore EE, Moore FA, et al: Exigent postinjury thoracotomy analysis of blunt vs penetrating trauma. Surg Gynecol Obstet 175:97–101, 1992.

67. Mattox KL, Flint LE, Carrico CJ, et al: Blunt cardiac injury. J Trauma 33:649–650, 1992.

68. Mattox K: Approaches to trauma involving the major vessels of the thorax. Surg Clin North Am 69:77–91, 1989.

69. Miller L, Bennett EV, Root HD: Management of penetrating and blunt diaphragmatic injury. J Trauma 24:403–407, 1984.

70. Miller PR, Croce MA, Kilgo PD, et al: Acute respiratory distress syndrome in blunt trauma: Identification of independent risk factors. Am Surg 68:845–850, 2002.

71. Morse SS, Glickman MG, Greenwood LH, et al: Traumatic aortic rupture: False-positive aortographic diagnosis due to atypical ductus diverticulum. Am J Roentgenol 150:793–796, 1988.

72. Nagy KK, Massad M, Fildes J, et al: Missile embolization revisited: A rationale for selective management. Am Surg 60:975–979, 1994.

73. Nagy KK, Roberts RR, Smith RF, et al: Trans-mediastinal gunshot wounds: Are "stable" patients really stable? World J Surg 26:1247–1250, 2002.

74. Nelson L: Ventilatory support of the trauma patient with pulmonary contusion. Respir Care Clin N Am 2:425–447, 1996.

75. Nowak J, Mallmin H, Larsson S: The aetiology and epidemiology of clavicular fractures. A prospective study during a two-year period in Uppsala, Sweden. Injury 31:353–358, 2000.

76. Orford VP, Atkinson NR, Thomson K, et al: Blunt traumatic aortic transection: The endovascular experience. Ann Thorac Surg 75:106–111, 2003.

77. Oyarzun JR, Bush AP, McCormick JR, et al: Use of 3.5-mm acetabular reconstruction plates for internal fixation of flail chest injuries. Ann Thorac Surg 65:1471–1474, 1998.

78. Paré A: The Works of Ambrose Paré. Translated by Thomas Johnson. London, 1678.

79. Perchinsky MJ, Long WB, Hill JG: Blunt cardiac rupture. Arch Surg 130:852–857, 1995.

80. Petricevic A, Ilic N, Bacic A, et al: War injuries of the lungs. Eur J Cardiothorac Surg 11:843–847, 1997.

81. Pozzato C, Gedriga E, Donatelli F, et al: Acute posttraumatic rupture of the thoracic aorta: The role of angiography in a 7-year review. CV Intervent Radiol 14:338–341, 1991.

82. Rawlins R, Momin A, Platts D, et al: Traumatic cardiogenic shock due to massive air embolism. A possible role for cardiopulmonary bypass. Eur J Cardiothorac Surg 22:845–846, 2002.

83. Reber PU, Schmied B, Seiler CA, et al: Missed diaphragmatic injuries and their long-term sequelae. J Trauma 44:183–188, 1998.

84. Richardson JD, Carrillo E: Thoracic infection after trauma. Chest Surg Clin N Am 7:401–427, 1997.

85. Robinson RJ, Brown JE, Caldwell R, et al: Management of asymptomatic intracardiac missiles using echocardiography. J Trauma 28:1402–1403, 1988.

86. Rozycki GS, Feliciano DV., Schmidt JA, et al: The role of surgeon-performed ultrasound in patients with possible cardiac wounds. Ann Surg 223:737–746, 1996.

87. Ryan JM, Rich NM, Dale RF, et al: Biophysics and pathophysiology of penetrating injury. In Ballistic Trauma: Clinical Relevance in Peace and War. Oxford, UK: Oxford University Press, 1997.

88. Saletta S, Lederman E, Fein S, et al: Transesophageal echocardiography for the initial evaluation of the widened mediastinum in trauma patients. J Trauma 39:137–142, 1995.

89. Sebastian MW, Wolfe WG: Traumatic thoracic fistula. Chest Surg Clin N Am 7:385–400, 1997.

90. Shackford S: Focused ultrasound examination by surgeons: The time is now. J Trauma 35:181, 1993 (editorial).

91. Shorr RM, Crittenden M, Indeck M, et al: Blunt thoracic trauma. Analysis of 515 patients. Ann Surg 206:200–205, 1987.

92. Sirmali M, Turut H, Topcu S, et al: A comprehensive analysis of traumatic rib fractures: Morbidity, mortality and management. Eur J Cardiothorac Surg 24:133–138, 2003.

93. Stassen NA, Lukan JK, Spain DA, et al: Reevaluation of diagnostic procedures for transmediasinal gunshot wounds. J Trauma 53:635–638, 2002.

94. Sybrandy KC, Cramer MJ, Burgersdijk C: Diagnosing cardiac contusion: Old wisdom and new insights. Heart 89:485–489, 2003.

95. Symbas PN, Picone AL, Hatcher CR, et al: Cardiac missiles. Ann Surg 211:639–648, 1990.

96. Tyburski JG, Astra L, Wilson RF, et al: Factors affecting prognosis with penetrating wounds of the heart. J Trauma 48:587–590, 2000.

97. Uribe RA, Pachon CE, Frame SB, et al: A prospective evaluation of thoracoscopy for the diagnosis of penetrating thoracoabdominal trauma. J Trauma 37:650–654, 1994.

98. Velmahos GC, Vassiliu P, Chan LS, et al: Influence of flail chest on outcome among patients with severe thoracic cage trauma. Int Surg 87:240–244, 2002.

99. Wagner RB, Crawford WO, Schimpf PP, et al: Quantitation and pattern of parenchymal lung injury in blunt chest trauma. Diagnostic and therapeutic implications. J Comput Tomogr 12:270–281, 1988.

100. Webb DP, Ramsey JJ, Dignan RJ, et al: Penetrating injury to the heart requiring cardiopulmonary bypass: A case study. J Extra Corpor Technol 33:249–251, 2001.

101. Weiman DS, Walker WA, Brosnan KM, et al: Noniatrogenic esophageal trauma. Ann Thorac Surg 59:845–850, 1995.

102. Wintermark M, Wickey S, Schnyder P: Imaging of acute traumatic injuries of the thoracic aorta. Eur Radiol 12:431–442, 2002.

103. Wu CL, Jani ND, Perkins FM, et al: Thoracic epidural analgesia versus intravenous patient-controlled analgesia for the treatment of rib fracture pain after motor vehicle crash. J Trauma 47:564–567, 1999.

104. Yeong EK, Chen MT, Chu SH: Traumatic asphyxia. Plast Reconstr Surg 93:739–744, 1994.

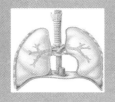

Tracheal Lesions

CHAPTER 8

Simon K. Ashiku and Douglas J. Mathisen

▶ INTRODUCTION

A wide range of neoplastic and inflammatory lesions develop within the trachea. The relative rarity of these lesions and the nonspecific nature of presenting symptoms, such as wheezing and dyspnea, often lead to the erroneous diagnosis of asthma and delay in treatment. Diagnosis is usually made when the tracheal air column is carefully viewed or a diagnostic flexible bronchoscopy is performed. Advances in surgical and anesthetic techniques have allowed for the safe and effective resection of many of these lesions with primary reconstruction. Perioperative complications have been minimized and outcomes are generally excellent. For tracheal lesions whose extent precludes primary resection and reconstruction there remains no universally definitive treatment.

This chapter focuses on surgically correctable lesions of the trachea, including those that involve the lower larynx. Carinal lesions are not discussed. Preoperative assessment, operative strategies, and postoperative care are discussed in detail.

▶ ANATOMY

The trachea averages 11 cm in length from the lower border of the cricoid cartilage to the carinal spur, with an additional 1.5–2 cm of subglottic intralaryngeal airway. The structural support comes from 18–22 cartilaginous C-rings, with about two rings per centimeter.[8] The cricoid is the only complete cartilaginous ring in the normal airway. Most of the trachea lies within the thoracic inlet and the chest. Cervical hyperextension brings up to half of the trachea into the neck, and flexion devolves the trachea almost entirely into the mediastinum.[9,18,20]

The blood supply to the trachea is from multiple small terminal end arteries. The upper trachea is supplied principally by branches of the inferior thyroid artery, and the lower trachea by branches of the bronchial arteries (Figure 8-1). These vessels enter the trachea via very fine lateral pedicles that lack collateralization[23] (Figure 8-2). The pretracheal plane and the plane between the esophagus and trachea are avascular.

The recurrent laryngeal nerves ascend in the tracheoesophageal grooves bilaterally and pass medial to the inferior cornua of the thyroid cartilage. The nerve on the left runs along the entire length of the trachea, while the nerve on the the right runs along the upper few centimeters only. They enter the larynx at its junction with the cricoid posteriorly, adjacent to the cricoarytenoid joints (Figure 8-3).

▶ TRACHEAL LESIONS

Many disease processes result in pathological lesions of the trachea. The resultant lesions may be diffuse or discrete and can involve any portion of the trachea from the larynx to the carina. The most common lesions amenable to a surgical solution are the result of traumatic, neoplastic, and idiopathic processes.

Iatrogenic injuries resulting from tracheal intubation have long been the most common traumatic lesion. Postintubation tracheal stenosis occurs following prolonged intubation and develops principally at the level of the endotracheal tube or tracheostomy tube cuffs. The radial pressure exerted from the cuff causes circumferential pressure necrosis, which results in cicatricial scaring stenosis[2,3] (Figure 8-4). Cuff stenosis resulted formerly from high-pressure cuffs and, more recently, from overinflated low-pressure cuffs.

Stomal stenosis occurs with tracheostomies. Excessive leverage applied to the tracheostomy tube from unsupported ventilatory tubing can erode the anterior and lateral

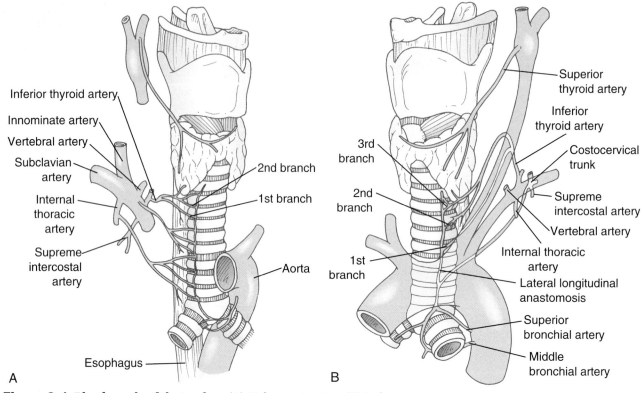

Figure 8–1 **Blood supply of the trachea.** (**A**) Right anterior view. (**B**) Left anterior view.
(*From Salassa JR, Pearson BW, Payne WS: Gross and microscopical blood supply of the trachea. Ann Thorac Surg 24:100–107, 1977. Reprinted with permission from the Society of Thoracic Surgeons.*)

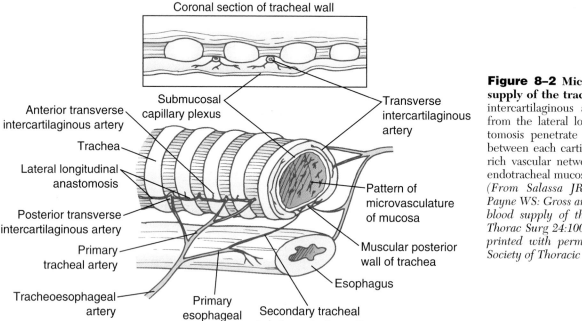

Figure 8–2 **Microscopic blood supply of the trachea.** Transverse intercartilaginous arteries derived from the lateral longitudinal anastomosis penetrate the soft tissues between each cartilage to supply a rich vascular network beneath the endotracheal mucosa.
(*From Salassa JR, Pearson BW, Payne WS: Gross and microscopical blood supply of the trachea. Ann Thorac Surg 24:100–107, 1977. Reprinted with permission from the Society of Thoracic Surgeons.*)

tracheal walls at the level of the stoma. Cicatricial healing creates an A-shaped stenosis as viewed bronchoscopically (Figure 8-5). Traction on the tracheostomy tube may cause varying degrees of destruction of the cartilaginous rings between the stoma and point of cuff stenosis, resulting in a complex lesion with areas of tracheal malacia mixed with areas of tracheal stenosis.[15]

Stenosis in the subglottic region may occur as a result of prolonged intubation with endotracheal tubes, following cricothyroidotomy, or following high placement of a tracheostomy where the tube erodes through the cricoid cartilage.[25] Prolonged endotracheal intubation combined with a nasogastric tube may lead to tracheoesophageal fistula (Figure 8-6). Pressure necrosis of tissue develops between a

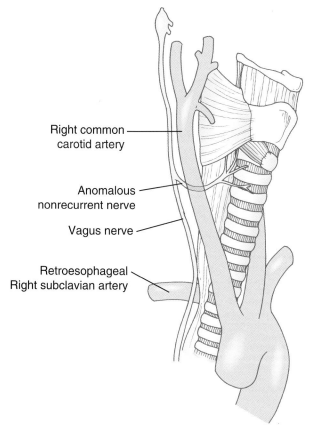

Figure 8–3 Position of the recurrent laryngeal nerves in relation to the trachea and larynx.
(From Pearson FG et al: Thoracic Surgery, 1st ed. Philadelphia: W.B. Saunders, p. 278. Reprinted with permission from W.B. Saunders Company.)

Right common carotid artery

Anomalous nonrecurrent nerve

Vagus nerve

Retroesophageal Right subclavian artery

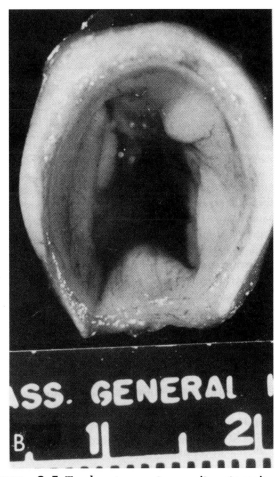

Figure 8–5 Tracheostomy stoma site stenosis. The characteristic "A"-shaped lumen is evident and results from a primarily anterior and lateral cicatricial process.
(From Sabiston DC Jr, Spencer FC: Surgery of the Chest, 6th ed. Philadelphia: W.B. Saunders, 1996, p. 413. Reprinted with permission from W.B. Saunders Company.)

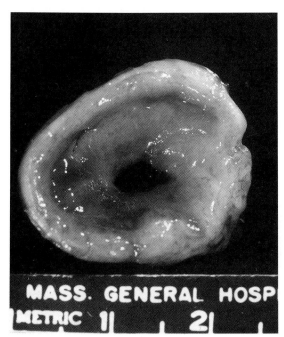

Figure 8–4 Cuff level stenosis. The stenosis here is circumferential and the remaining lumen round.
(From Sabiston DC Jr, Spencer FC: Surgery of the Chest, 6th ed. Philadelphia: W.B. Saunders, 1996, p. 413. Reprinted with permission from W.B. Saunders Company.)

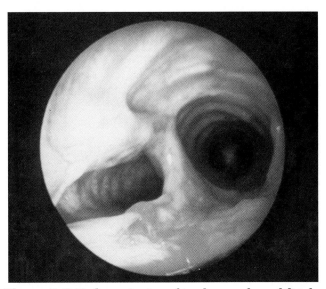

Figure 8–6 Endoscopic view of tracheoesophageal fistula.

108 nasogastric tube in the esophagus and an inflated balloon cuff in the trachea. A tracheal-innominate artery fistula may arise either from a tracheostomy tube placed too low in the thoracic trachea or from an innominate artery lying high at the sternal notch. The tracheostomy tube can erode into the vessel at the inferior margin of the stoma.

Direct external trauma, blunt or penetrating, may result in a tear or complete disruption of the trachea at any level. Inhalational burns are usually maximal in the proximal subglottic region and diminish in the more distal airway. In most cases, the tracheal rings are not destroyed.[5]

Primary tracheal tumors are rare with an estimated incidence of 2.7 cases per million per year. Most are malignant. Squamous cell carcinoma and adenoid cystic carcinoma are the two most common malignant primary tracheal neoplasms. Squamous cell carcinoma occurs primarily in smokers in their sixth and seventh decade and may present confined to the trachea or invading into adjacent mediastinal structures (Figure 8-7). Adenoid cystic carcinoma is an exophytic intratracheal lesion that involves the tracheal wall to variable extents. This mass may compress mediastinal structures without invading them initially. Lymph node metastases occur, but less commonly than in squamous cell carcinoma. A characteristic feature of adenoid cystic carcinoma is its proclivity for extending long distances submucosally and perineurally.[12,22]

Secondary neoplasms may involve the trachea through direct extension. Thyroid carcinomas typically invade the trachea at the second and third rings where the thyroid isthmus is adherent to the trachea.[14] Both bronchogenic and midesophageal carcinomas may erode into the carina.

The most common idiopathic lesion involves the upper trachea and lower larynx and is termed idiopathic laryngotracheal stenosis. It occurs predominantly in young and middle-aged women. Histologically, the lesions are characterized by circumferential keloidal type fibrosis with thickening of the lamina propria without cartilaginous destruction.[1,11]

SIGNS AND SYMPTOMS

Most lesions of the trachea result in a slow, progressive airway obstruction. Initially, this manifests as dyspnea on exertion, then at rest, and finally as wheezing and/or stridor. It generally takes 1–6 weeks following extubation for postintubation lesions to become symptomatic. While patients with pure stenosis tend to have stridor on inspiration those with malacia have a characteristic barking cough with an expiratory wheeze. Cough and hemoptysis are more characteristic of malignancies. Extensive extratracheal extension may result in hoarseness or dysphagia.

DIAGNOSTIC EVALUATION

A standard posteroanterior chest radiograph, centered high on the trachea, will reveal most tracheal stenoses. Detailed information about the location of the lesion, its longitudinal extent, and the amount of normal trachea available for reconstruction is best demonstrated by longitudinal tomograms of the entire airway (Figure 8-8). The addition of fluoroscopy can, on occasion, be helpful in evaluating the functional state of the glottis and in demonstrating areas of malacia.[4,24] Computerized tomograms (CTs) have been supplemental in evaluating tumors. They are useful in identifying extraluminal extension and enlarged mediastinal lymph nodes. Recently, the use of high-speed helical CT scanners to acquire images combined with the powerful three-dimensional-image software has created impressive two- and three-dimensional airway reconstructions that will likely supplant plain films in the near future (Figure 8-9).

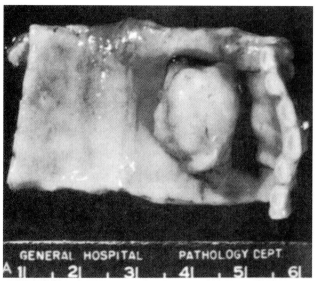

Figure 8–7 An exophytic squamous cell carcinoma of the trachea.
(From Sabiston DC Jr, Spencer FC: Surgery of the Chest, 6th ed. Philadelphia: W.B. Saunders, 1996, p. 407. Reprinted with permission from W.B. Saunders company.)

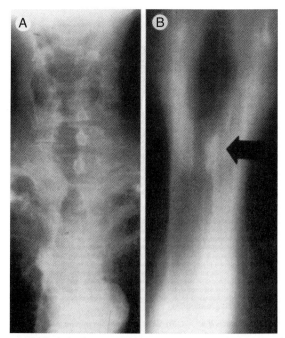

Figure 8–8 (**A**) Plain posteroanterior chest radiograph of cuff stenosis. (**B**) A typical tomographic view of the same lesion.
(From Sabiston DC Jr: Textbook of Surgery, 15th ed. Philadelphia: W.B. Saunders, p. 1819. Reprinted with permission from W.B. Saunders Company.)

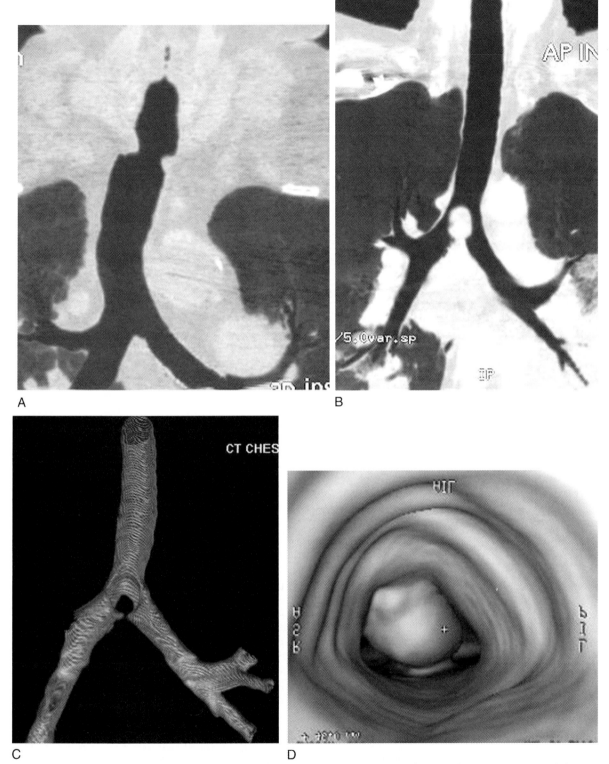

Figure 8–9 (**A**) Reformatted computed tomography two-dimensional image of posttracheostomy stenosis. (**B**) Two-dimensional image of an adenoid cystic carcinoma of the carina. (**C**) Three-dimensional image of a tracheal airway column showing the endobronchial component of the same carinal mass. (**D**) The same carinal mass as viewed endobronchially by three-dimensional image virtual computed tomography bronchoscopy.

For these images to be useful, the studies must be performed without an indwelling tracheostomy tube. In cases where a tracheostomy tube has been in place chronically and must be removed for the examinations, there must be a physician competent in tube replacement present in the event the airway is lost.

▶ BRONCHOSCOPY

Bronchoscopic evaluation is necessary to confirm the diagnosis, design an operative strategy, and treat impending airway obstruction. Measurements taken bronchoscopically determine the amount of normal trachea proximal and distal available for reconstruction. Under the best of circumstances up to 50% of the trachea can be resected and a primary anastomosis performed. Many factors such as age, body habitus, amount of cervical trachea, prior surgery, and lesion location influence the amount of trachea that can be safely resected. With benign strictures, special attention must be given to assessing the state of the mucosa. Indwelling stents or T-tubes must be removed and the mucosa assessed. If extensive mucosal inflammation or ulceration exists, definitive repair should be delayed until mucosal healing occurs. This may require a short period of decannulation or change to a smaller T-tube. Often, patients with idiopathic laryngotracheal stenosis have active inflammation extending into the subglottis. These patients should be dilated and the operation delayed while the inflammation subsides. Patients taking corticosteroids should be weaned from them and be off for at least a month before an operative repair.

Expertise with the techniques of interventional bronchoscopy is essential to safely dilate a benign stenosis or "core out" an obstructing tumor. This allows evaluation of the distal airway, safe passage of an endotracheal tube, or temporary establishment of a patent airway to allow delay in operation. Dilating a narrow, fibrotic stricture, such as postintubation stenosis, is challenging and can result in airway rupture, complete obstruction, or excessive destruction of tracheal mucosa. Progressively larger Jackson dilators passed through the rigid bronchoscope can be used to effectively dilate the stenosis. An assortment of pediatric rigid bronchoscopes and adult rigid bronchoscopes can then be used with increasing sizes using a gentle corkscrew motion.[15]

Obstructing tracheal tumors are managed first by "core out" using the rigid bronchoscope, forceps, and suction.[16] Using the tip of the bronchoscope in a corkscrew motion, most tumors can be easily "cored out." Forceps are then used to remove tumor fragments. If bleeding ensues, the bronchoscope is advanced distal to the lesion and used to tamponade the bleeding. Direct application of epinephrine-soaked pledgets can stop persistent oozing.

Patients with critical airway stenosis should be endoscoped in the operating room where rigid bronchoscopy is available and ready for use. Flexible bronchoscopes can precipitate airway obstruction in patients with critical airway stenosis (<4 mm) by inducing secretions, edema, and bleeding. Without the ability to dilate and control the airway with rigid bronchoscopy, death may result. Tracheostomies may be useful in some patients as the only way to secure an airway. When possible, they should be placed through the stenosis, preserving the uninvolved trachea for future reconstruction.[15]

▶ ANESTHESIA

Replacement of spontaneous breathing with positive pressure ventilation can convert a partially obstructing lesion into a complete obstruction. When maintenance of the airway is a concern, a breathe down with an inhalation agent is employed and paralytics given once the airway is secured.[26] Anesthesia is maintained with total intravenous anesthesia (TIVA) using short acting agents such as Remifentanyl and Propafol. This allows immediate extubation at the completion of the procedure and maintains continuous anesthesia during periods when inhalational agents are interrupted by the procedure. For lower tracheal and carinal resections, endotracheal intubation is accomplished with an extralong, armored endotracheal tube. Its flexibility allows bronchoscopic placement into one of the mainstem bronchi. After transecting the airway, the orotracheal tube is pulled back into the trachea and intermittent ventilation is performed with sterile cross-field equipment. The orotracheal tube is again advanced once the anastomosis is completed.

▶ SIMPLE TRACHEAL RESECTION

The technique for uncomplicated resections of the middle and upper trachea is described. Rigid bronchoscopy with dilation is performed at the time of planned operation to assess the resectability of the lesion.

The patient is positioned supine with an inflatable airbag beneath the shoulders and the neck extended. The inflatable bag facilitates exposure by extending the neck during dissection and allows for cervical flexion when deflated just prior to tying the anastomosis. The head is supported in a foam ring and the arms are tucked at the sides.

A low collar incision is adequate for most tracheal resections that involve the upper trachea. When the lesion involves the middle to lower trachea, vertical extension with a partial sternal split facilitates exposure (Figure 8-10A). Dissection is carried through the platysma, and subplatysmal flaps are elevated superiorly to the level of the cricoid and inferiorly to the level of the sternal notch. The strap muscles are separated in the midline, and a plane of dissection is established very close to the tracheal wall to avoid injury to the recurrent laryngeal nerves (Figure 8-10B). The pretracheal plane is dissected to the level of the carina. The investing fascia of the innominate artery and the adjacent mediastinal fat are left intact to guard against postoperative tracheoinnominate fistulization. Retraction on the innominate artery is kept to a minimum to avoid impeding cerebral blood flow.

The area of involved trachea is transilluminated with a flexible bronchoscope allowing the assistant to mark the distal extent. The trachea is sharply dissected circumferentially at the most distal extent of the lesion, with the dissection plane maintained on the tracheal wall. The endotracheal tube is withdrawn into the upper trachea, the trachea is divided at the most distal extent of the lesion, and bilateral

2-0 Vicryl traction sutures are placed. A cuffed, wire-wound endotracheal tube is promptly passed into the distal tracheal segment, attached to the sterile connecting tubing, and cross table ventilation is commenced (Figure 8-10C). The diseased segment of trachea is sharply dissected from the esophagus and amputated at the most proximal extent of the lesion.

The patient's neck is then flexed and the anastomosis tested for tension. If the limits of flexion and safe dissection have been reached and anastomotic tension exists, then one proceeds with release procedures. When the surgeon is satisfied that the anastomosis will not be under tension, interrupted, 4-0 Vicryl anastomotic sutures are placed such that the knots will be on the outside, beginning posteriorly in the midline and proceeding around either side to the front (Figure 8-10D). The sutures are placed 5–6 mm from the cut edge of the trachea and 4 mm apart. They should encircle a tracheal ring on either side of the anastomosis to help prevent dehiscence. Frequently, the endotracheal tube must be withdrawn for short periods to allow accurate placement of the more difficult sutures or for suctioning blood from the distal airway. Before placing the anterior sutures, the endotracheal tube is permanently removed from the distal tracheal segment and the translaryngeal endotracheal tube advanced carefully beyond the anastomosis. Prior to tying down the anastomotic sutures, the inflatable airbag

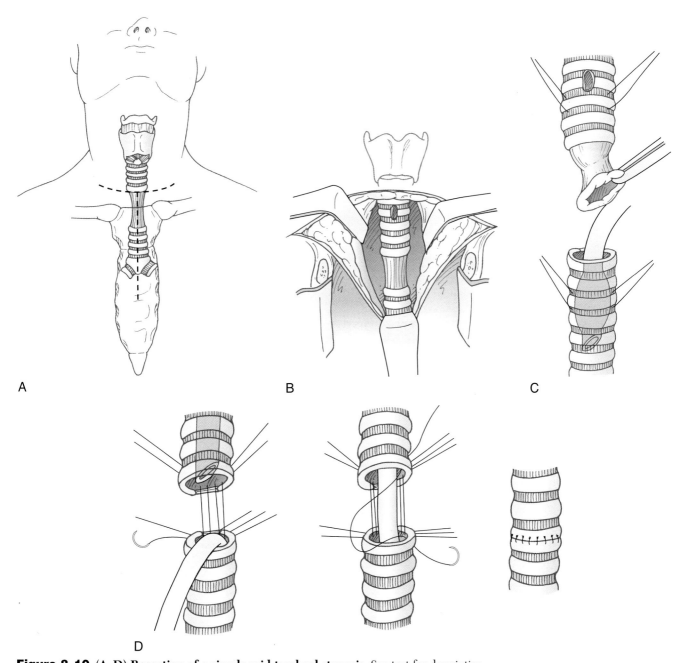

Figure 8–10 (A–D) Resection of a simple mid-tracheal stenosis. See text for description.
(From Grillo HC: Surgery of the trachea. Current problems in surgery. Ann Thorac Surg 7:3–59, 1970. Reprinted with permission from Mosby, Inc.)

112 beneath the shoulders is deflated, the 2-0 traction sutures are tied, and any last few degrees of neck flexion that may be required are instituted. The anastomotic sutures are then tied from anterior to posterior. The integrity of the suture line is tested under saline with the cuff deflated or placed proximal to the anastomosis. If the field has not been irradiated, we do not employ tissue flaps to cover the anastomosis. A closed suction drain is left in the pretracheal space.

A chin-to-chest suture is placed to prevent cervical hyperextension. This suture is tied without slack to prevent neck extension for the first 5–7 postoperative days. Patients are extubated in the operating room. In situations in which postoperative intubation is thought to be necessary, a small endotracheal tube is left in place, a stitch is placed at least two rings below the anastomosis to mark the site for possible future tracheostomy, and the thyroid gland or strap muscles are interposed to protect the anastomosis. This allows limited dissection and accurate placement in a reoperative field. It is best to wait a few days before placing a tracheostomy to allow skin flaps and other tissue layers to seal before exposing them to airway secretions. This also allows postsurgical airway edema to resolve, possibly obviating the need for a tracheostomy.

For tumors, the approach is modified. Considerable experience is required to judge whether a tumor can be safely resected with sufficient tissue to provide a clear margin and yet allow successful primary reconstruction of the airway. This can be particularly difficult in patients with adenoid cystic carcinoma in whom frozen sections may show microscopic tumor at grossly clear resection margins. The plane of dissection in tumor cases must be kept away from the involved portion of trachea to ensure an adequate radial margin. This endangers the recurrent laryngeal nerves more than in resections for benign disease. If a recurrent nerve is involved by tumor, the nerve is sacrificed. Adjacent paratracheal lymph nodes are removed en bloc with the specimen, but extensive lymph node dissection should not be done to prevent devascularizing the tracheal anastomosis. Postoperative radiation therapy is recommended in all cases of bronchogenic or adenoid cystic carcinoma, unless contraindicated by performance status or anastomotic complications.[12]

▶ LARYNGOTRACHEAL RESECTION

In cases in which an upper tracheal lesion involves the cricoid, occurring most commonly in idiopathic laryngotracheal stenosis, trauma, or tumor, a laryngotracheal resection will be necessary. In idiopathic laryngotracheal stenosis the lesion typically involves the cricoid on its anterior and lateral luminal surface. The operative procedure must be tailored to address the particular anatomical involvement encountered (Figure 8-11). The recurrent laryngeal nerves are protected by bevelling off the cricoid anteriorly and laterally while preserving the posterior plate.[6,13] The extent of anterior cricoid resection ranges from complete, with a line of transection through the cricothyroid membrane, to none at all, depending on the extent of involvement. Tracheal resection depends on the distal extent of the lesion (Figure 8-12A and B). The

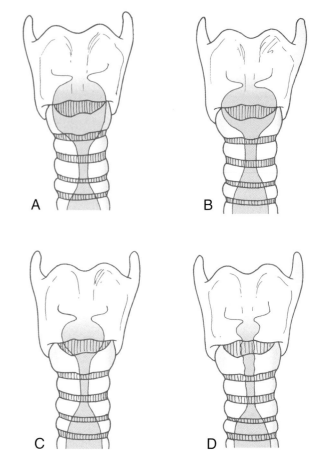

Figure 8–11 Upper airway stenosis. (**A**) High tracheal stenosis, easily treated by segmental resection and tracheotracheal anastomosis. (**B**) Stenosis that reaches to the lower border of the cricoid cartilage. (**C**) Stenosis of the lower subglottic larynx and upper trachea. The extent of the lesion anteriorly is so great that correction requires removal of the anterior portion of the cricoid cartilage. (**D**) Stenosis that reaches to the glottis. There is no subglottic space to which an effective anastomosis can be made. *(From Grillo HC: Reconstruction after subglottic laryngeal and upper tracheal stenosis resection. Ann Thorac Surg 33:3–18, 1982. Reprinted with permission from the Society of Thoracic Surgeons.)*

trachea is appropriately tailored so that the proximal trachea coapts well with the cut edge of the larynx (Figure 8-12C and D). 2.0 Vicryl "traction sutures" are placed in the mid-lateral position both proximally and distally. Interrupted 4-0 Vicryl sutures were used to fashion the anastomosis. The midline of the thyroid cartilage is approximated to the midline of the tracheal "prow." 2-0 Vicryl traction sutures are tied followed by individual 4-0 Vicryl anastomotic sutures (Figure 8-12E and F).

When the lesion involves the posterior cricoid, the line of mucosal division is performed high on the posterior cricoid plate to excise involved mucosa and submucosa (Figure 8-13). Mucosal resection stops short of the superior border of the cricoid plate, immediately below the arytenoid cartilages. A posterior broad-based flap of membranous wall is created and advanced to resurface the posterior cricoid plate. The posterior portion of the anastomosis is made with interrupted 4-0 Vicryl sutures placed only through the full

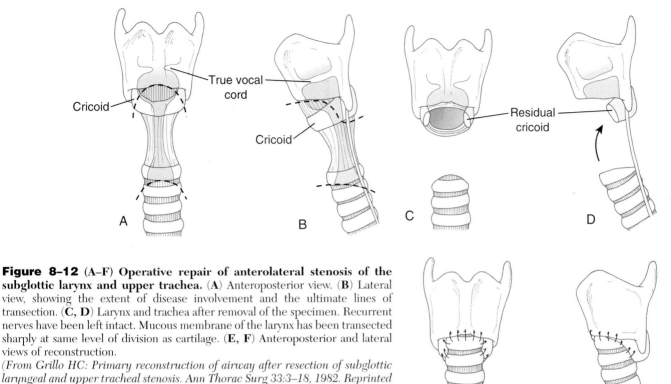

Figure 8–12 (**A–F**) **Operative repair of anterolateral stenosis of the subglottic larynx and upper trachea.** (**A**) Anteroposterior view. (**B**) Lateral view, showing the extent of disease involvement and the ultimate lines of transection. (**C, D**) Larynx and trachea after removal of the specimen. Recurrent nerves have been left intact. Mucous membrane of the larynx has been transected sharply at same level of division as cartilage. (**E, F**) Anteroposterior and lateral views of reconstruction.
(From Grillo HC: Primary reconstruction of airway after resection of subglottic laryngeal and upper tracheal stenosis. Ann Thorac Surg 33:3–18, 1982. Reprinted with permission from the Society of Thoracic Surgeons.)

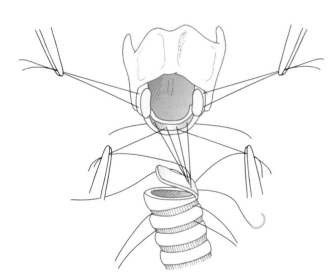

Figure 8–13 Techniques of posterior membranous tracheal wall flap with cricoid resurfacing.
(From Grillo HC: Laryngotracheal resection and reconstruction for subglottic stenosis. Ann Thorac Surg 53:54–63, 1992. Reprinted with permission from the Society of Thoracic Surgeons.)

thickness of mucosa and submucosa of the posterior wall of the larynx, then through the full thickness of the membranous wall of the trachea. They are inverted so that the suture knots lay external to the lumen. Four sutures are placed through the cartilaginous portion of the inferior margin of the cricoid plate and the outer portion of the membranous wall of the trachea below the proximal edge of the flap in order to fix the membranous wall to the inferior edge of the cricoid plate.[6,13]

▶ RELEASE PROCEDURES

Dissection of the pretracheal plane combined with cervical flexion produces sufficient airway mobility to allow tracheal resection and primary reconstruction in most patients. When extensive resections are performed, further mobilization with "release" procedures is often required to allow a tension-free anastomosis. This has been shown to be necessary in 8.3% of patients undergoing resections for postintubation stenosis and 15% of patients undergoing resections for tumors.[15] Certain release maneuvers are more effective for achieving additional mobility of the cervical trachea, whereas others are more effective for freeing the intrathoracic trachea.

When an upper trachea resection is performed, an additional 1.5 cm of length may be gained by releasing the larynx with a Montgomery suprahyoid release.[19] This is performed by dividing the muscles that insert on the superior aspect of the central part of the hyoid bone. The hyoid itself is then divided just medial to its lesser cornua on either side, and the stylohyoid tendons are divided (Figure 8-14). While laryngeal release maneuvers may predispose patients to postoperative aspiration, in time, this problem has resolved in most patients.

For intrathoracic tracheal resections, additional length is best achieved by hilar release.[21] Mobilization of the right hilum should be done first along with division of the inferior pulmonary ligament. A U-shaped incision is then made in the pericardium below the inferior pulmonary vein. The pericardium can be incised 360° around the hilus for additional mobility. In this event, the vascular and lymphatic

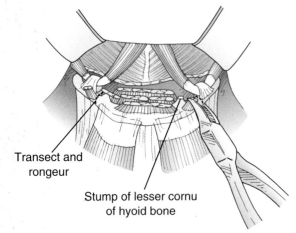

Transect and
rongeur

Stump of lesser cornu
of hyoid bone

Figure 8–14 The dotted lines indicate the point where the hyoid bone is divided, separating its body from the greater horn on each side.
(From Montgomery WW: Suprahyoid release for tracheal anostomosis. Arch Otolaryngol 99:255–260, 1974. Reprinted with permission from the American Medical Association.)

pedicle to the mainstem bronchus is left preserved behind the pericardium. If further mobility is needed, the left hilum may be similarly mobilized (Figure 8-15). This can be accomplished easily only through a median sternotomy by opening the pericardium anteriorly, or bilateral thoracotomies, or an extended clamshell incision. As with most airway surgery, neck flexion is helpful. However, laryngeal release has not been shown to produce meaningful mobility at the level of the carina.[7]

▶ REPAIR OF TRACHEOINNOMINATE AND TRACHEOESOPHAGEAL FISTULAS

Tracheoinnominate fistulas most often result from a stoma placed too low, allowing the tracheostomy cannula to erode into the artery. Less often, it is caused by an overinflated cuff

or the tip of a tracheostomy tube. It presents as either massive airway bleeding or episodic hemoptysis. Significant bleeding from around or through a tracheostomy should be evaluated in the controlled environment of the operating room. The surgeon should be prepared to manage massive airway bleeding before removing the tracheostomy cannula. The patient is then decannulated and a bronchoscopy performed. In the event of massive hemorrhage, control can usually be obtained by finger compression through the stoma, pushing forward against the sternum at the site of bleeding. A small endotracheal tube is slipped into the airway beyond the finger and the cuff firmly inflated to ventilate and protect the lungs from aspiration of blood. If the fistula lies beyond reach, hemorrhage may be controlled by placing an inflated endotracheal tube cuff over the bleed vessel.

Exposure is obtained through a collar incision at the level of the stoma along with a vertical extension for sternotomy. With the finger continuing to maintain hemostasis, the vessel is dissected to obtain proximal and distal control. The involved segment of artery is resected and the proximal and distal ends oversewn. The stumps are buried under surrounding healthy tissue.

Innominate division usually does not result in neurological sequelae. Depending on the degree of airway destruction, a concomitant tracheal resection may be necessary. A new tracheal stoma is created at a higher level and a tracheostomy tube long enough to pass beyond the previous stoma is employed. Strap muscle is sutured over the original stoma to hasten its healing.

Acquired, nonmalignant tracheoesophageal fistulas often present while the patient remains ventilatory dependent. The fistula develops at the level of the cuff and is usually associated with a circumferential tracheal injury.[17] Temporizing measures are taken to allow weaning from the ventilator before repair is undertaken. The tube is positioned with the occluding balloon below the fistula to prevent contamination of the tracheobronchial tree. Gastrostomy and jejunostomy tubes are placed for drainage and feeding, while the esophagus is kept free of tubes and cuff overinflation is assiduously avoided.

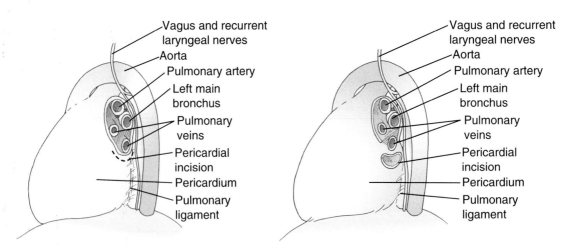

Vagus and recurrent
laryngeal nerves
Aorta
Pulmonary artery
Left main
bronchus
Pulmonary
veins
Pericardial
incision
Pericardium
Pulmonary
ligament

Vagus and recurrent
laryngeal nerves
Aorta
Pulmonary artery
Left main
bronchus
Pulmonary
veins
Pericardial
incision
Pericardium
Pulmonary
ligament

Figure 8–15 The left-side intrapericardial hilar release technique shows the U-shaped pericardial incision allowing 1–2 cm of upward hilar mobility to facilitate the creation of a tension-free anastomosis.
(From Newton JR, Grillo HC, Mothisen DJ: Main bronchial sleeve resection with pulmonary conservation. Ann Thorac Surg 52:1272–1280, 1991. Reprinted with permission from the Society of Thoracic Surgeons.)

A collar incision is performed that circumscribes the stoma (Figure 8-16). As described previously, the trachea is dissected and divided distal to the fistula. As the posterior wall of the trachea is dissected from inferior to superior, the fistulous connection is isolated circumferentially and detached from the esophagus with a small rim of normal esophageal tissue (Figure 8-17). After removal of the specimen, the esophagus is closed longitudinally with two layers of 4-0 silk (Figure 8-18). A strap muscle is used to buttress the esophageal closure and as interposed healthy tissue between the esophageal and tracheal suture lines (Figure 8-19). An end-to-end tracheal anastomosis is then performed. On occasion, it is necessary to partially repair the defect in the posterior membranous wall with a vertical suture line to limit the amount of tracheal resection needed to treat a large fistula. Rarely, there is no significant damage to the trachea and tracheal resection is unnecessary. A simple esophageal and tracheal repair, with a muscle buttress, is performed.

POSTOPERATIVE ISSUES

The goals of both intraoperative and postoperative care are the promotion of anastomotic healing and the maintenance of good pulmonary toilet. Ideally, patients should be extubated in the operating room. The need for postoperative ventilation is a relative contraindication to tracheal resection. Patients with marginal lung function need careful

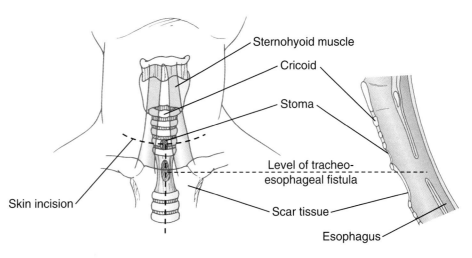

Figure 8–16 Exposure for most tracheoesophageal fistulas is through a low collar incision. Occasionally, a partial upper sternotomy is required for more distal exposure of the trachea.
(From Mathisen DJ, Grillo HC, Wain JC: Management of acquired nonmalignant tracheoesophageal fistula. Ann Thorac Surg 52:759–765, 1991. Reprinted with permission from the Society of Thoracic Surgeons.)

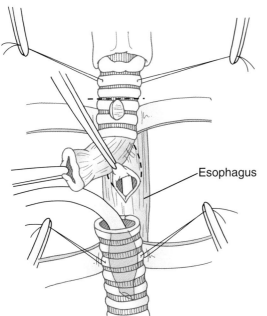
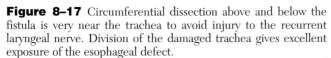

Figure 8–17 Circumferential dissection above and below the fistula is very near the trachea to avoid injury to the recurrent laryngeal nerve. Division of the damaged trachea gives excellent exposure of the esophageal defect.
(From Mathisen DJ, Grillo HC, Wain JC: Management of acquired nonmalignant tracheoesophageal fistula. Ann Thorac Surg 52:759–765, 1991. Reprinted with permission from the Society of Thoracic Surgeons.)

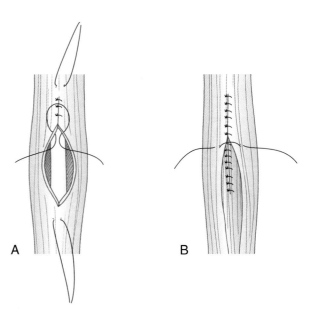

Figure 8–18 The esophageal defect is closed in layers. (A) The first layer closes the esophagus. (**B**) The esophageal muscle is closed over the first layer.
(From Mathisen DJ, Grillo HC, Wain JC: Management of acquired nonmalignant tracheoesophageal fistula. Ann Thorac Surg 52:759–765, 1991. Reprinted with permission from the Society of Thoracic Surgeons.)

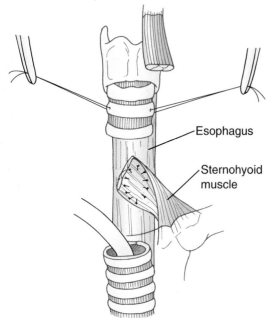

Figure 8–19 A local strap muscle is used to buttress the esophageal closure and separate it from the suture line. *(From Mathisen DJ, Grillo HC, Wain JC: Management of acquired nonmalignant tracheoesophageal fistula. Ann Thorac Surg 52:759–765, 1991. Reprinted with permission from the Society of Thoracic Surgeons.)*

management during the operation to help avoid the need for postoperative ventilation. During the procedure secretions and blood are kept from running distally into the lungs and volume overload is avoided. Postoperatively, fluids are minimized, elevating the head of the bed and administering racemic epinephrine to help prevent laryngeal edema. Rarely, an especially high laryngotracheal resection will cause enough laryngeal edema to necessitate one or two doses of steroids to avoid impending reintubation and/or tracheostomy. Heliox, with its low viscosity, is sometimes useful in these circumstances since it can occasionally gain enough time for the other maneuvers to take effect. The patient is cautioned against unnecessary speech during this period, as it can contribute to the laryngeal edema. Postoperatively, patients are supplied with humidity by face mask to facilitate clearance of secretions. Most patients are able to clear their airway by coughing. Frequently, therapeutic flexible bronchoscopy is performed to suction secretions under direct vision. Cervical flexion is maintained with the chin-to-chest suture for 5–7 days, after which the patient is advised not to extend the neck for another week. Before removing the chin-to-chest suture, we routinely examine the anastomosis with a flexible bronchoscope or obtain tracheal tomograms to ensure normal healing. Oral alimentation is begun cautiously in the first few postoperative days.

▶ RESULTS AND COMPLICATIONS

For resections of postintubation stenoses, including the earliest cases and reoperations, of 503 patients there were 12

deaths and 18 failures.[10] Four hundred and forty (87%) had good and 31 (6%) satisfactory results. Of 80 patients undergoing laryngotracheal resections for all causes of subglottic stenosis, there was one postoperative death.[13] Results were excellent in 18 (22%), good in 52 (65%), and satisfactory in 8 (10%). In only two patients was there failure to achieve a functional airway.

The results of single-staged laryngotracheal resection for idiopathic laryngotracheal stenosis, (ILTS) have recently been reported in a series of 73 patients.[1] The majority were women (71/73) with a mean age of 46 (range 13–74); 28/73 (38%) had undergone a previous procedure with laser, dilation, laryngeal, or tracheostomy procedures. Following laryngotracheal resection, the majority of patients (67/73) were extubated in the operating room and seven required temporary tracheostomies, with only one in the last 30 cases. All were successfully decannulated. There was no perioperative mortality. Principal morbidity was alteration in voice quality, which improved with time. Of patients 67/73 (91%) required no further intervention for their ILTS. Six patients required at least one bronchoscopy for granulation tissue and/or dilatation. Progression of disease was observed in only one patient.

The results from the repair of tracheoesophageal fistulas were reported in a series of 38 patients in whom 41 operations were performed.[17] Simple division and closure of the fistula were done in nine patients. Tracheal resection and reconstruction were combined with esophageal repair in the remainder. The esophageal defect was closed in two layers, and a viable strap muscle was interposed between the airway and esophageal suture lines in all cases. There were four deaths (10.9%). Three patients developed recurrent fistulas and one patient suffered a delayed tracheal stenosis. All were successfully managed with reoperation. Of the 34 survivors, 33 can swallow normally and 32 breathe without the need for a tracheal appliance.

For the oncological results of primary tumors of the trachea, 208 patients were evaluated in a retrospective multicenter study.[22] Histological types included 94 squamous cell carcinomas, 4 adenocarcinomas, 65 adenoid cystic carcinomas, and 45 miscellaneous tumors. The procedures performed consisted of 19 laryngotracheal, 165 simple tracheal, and 24 carinal resections. Operative mortality was 10.5%. As expected, long-term survival was significantly better for adenoid cystic carcinoma over squamous cell carcinoma, with 73% versus 47% at 5 years and 57% versus 36% at 10 years, respectively. Lymph node and margin status do not appear to significantly affect survival.[7,12,22] Postoperative radiation therapy is recommended in all cases of adenoid cystic or bronchogenic carcinoma, unless contraindicated by performance status or anastomotic complications. The role of chemotherapy has not been established.

Secondary cancers arising in the thyroid and invading the trachea have also been resected with good results. Of 27 patients undergoing resection and reconstruction of the trachea for thyroid cancer invading the airway, including patients with both simple and complex laryngotracheal reconstructions, two died in the postoperative period, one had a short segment tracheal necrosis requiring reresection, and all others were provided with an adequate airway by their initial operation. Only two patients experienced an airway recurrence.[14]

▶ SUMMARY

Some of the most challenging problems facing thoracic surgeons include benign strictures arising from postintubation stenosis or idiopathic laryngotracheal stenosis, fistulas from the trachea to the esophagus or innominate artery, and primary or secondary tumors of the trachea. Linear tomography and bronchoscopy are essential to diagnosis and preoperative planning. If critical airway stenosis is suspected, flexible bronchoscopy should be performed only in an operative suite where a rigid bronchoscope is available in case the airway needs to be reestablished. An anesthesia team familiar with the techniques of cross-table ventilation and capable of an interactive team approach is essential.

All patients with tracheal lesions, from benign strictures to malignant tumors, deserve serious consideration for definitive resection. Nonsurgical methods such as dilation, ablation, or stenting are palliative and should be used only as temporizing maneuvers or in nonsurgical candidates. Deciding on whether a lesion is resectable requires mature surgical judgment. Postoperative radiation should be given to all patients with resected squamous cell or adenoid cystic carcinomas. Patients with thyroid cancer secondarily invading the trachea should be considered for tracheal resection, even with advanced disease, to avoid fatal loss of the airway. With an experienced team, most patients can be successfully treated by a single-staged tracheal resection with low morbidity and mortality and excellent long-term results.

REFERENCES

1. Ashiku SK, Kuzucu A, Grillo HC, et al: Idiopathic laryngotracheal stenosis: Effective definitive treatment by laryngotracheal resection. J Thorac Cardiovasc Surg 2002 (in press).
2. Cooper JD, Grillo HC: The evolution of tracheal injury due to ventilatory assistance through cuffed tubes: A pathologic study. Ann Surg 169:334–348, 1969.
3. Cooper JD, Grillo HC: Experimental production and prevention of injury due to cuffed tracheal tubes. Surg Gynecol Obstet 129:1235–1241, 1969.
4. Felson B, Wiott JF, editors: The trachea. Semin Roentgenol 18:1–64, 1983.
5. Gaissert HA, Lofgren RH, Grillo HC: Upper airway compromise after inmation injury: Complex strictures of larynx and trachea and their management. Ann Surg 218:672–678, 1993.
6. Grillo HC: Primary reconstruction of the airway after resection of subglottic and upper tracheal stenosis. Ann Thorac Surg 33:39–58, 1982.
7. Grillo HC: Carinal neoplasia. In Grillo HC, Austen WG, Wilkins EW, et al, editors: Current Therapy in Cardiothoracic Surgery. Ontario: B.C. Decker, 1989, p. 134.
8. Grillo HC, Bendixon HH, Gephart T: Resection of carina and lower trachea. Ann Surg 158:889–893, 1963.
9. Grillo HC, Dignam EF, Miura T: Extensive resection and reconstruction of the mediastinal trachea without prosthesis or graft: An anatomical study in man. J Thorac Cardiovasc Surg 48:741–750, 1964.
10. Grillo HC, Donahue DM, Mathisen DJ: Postintubation tracheal stenosis: Treatment and results. J Thorac Cardiovasc Surg 109:486–493, 1995.
11. Grillo HC, Mark EJ, Mathisen DJ, Wain JC: Idiopathic laryngotracheal stenosis and its management. Ann Thorac Surg 56:80–87, 1993.
12. Grillo HC, Mathisen DJ: Primary tracheal tumors: Treatment and results. Ann Thorac Surg 49:69–77, 1990.
13. Grillo HC, Mathisen DJ, Wain JC: Laryngotracheal resection and reconstruction for subglottic stenosis. Ann Thorac Surg 53:54–63, 1992.
14. Grillo HC, Suen HC, Mathisen DJ, Wain JC: Resectional management of thyroid carcinoma invading the airway. Ann Thorac Surg 54:3–9, 1992.
15. Mathisen DJ: Surgery of the trachea. Curr Probl Surg 35:455–542, 1998.
16. Mathisen DJ, Grillo HC: Endoscopic relief of malignant airway obstruction. Ann Thorac Surg 48:469–475, 1989.
17. Mathisen DJ, Grillo HC, Wain JC, Hilgenberg AD: Management of acquired nonmalignant tracheoesophageal fistula. Ann Thorac Surg 52:759–765, 1991.
18. Michelson E, Solomon R, Miura T: Experiments in tracheal reconstruction. J Thorac Cardiovasc Surg 41:748–759, 1961.
19. Montgomery WW: Suprahyoid release for tracheal anastomosis. Arch Otolaryngol 99:255–260, 1974.
20. Mulliken J, Grillo HC: The limits of tracheal resection with primary anastomosis: Further anatomical studies in man. J Thorac Cardiovasc Surg 48:741–750, 1964.
21. Newton JR, Grillo HC, Mathisen DJ: Main bronchial sleeve resection with pulmonary conservation. Ann Thorac Surg 52:1272–1280, 1991.
22. Regnard JF, Fourquier P, Levasseur P, et al: Results and prognostic factors in resections of primary tracheal tumors: A multicenter retrospective study. J Thorac Cardiovasc Surg 111:808–814, 1996.
23. Salassa JR, Pearson BW, Payne WS: Gross and microscopical blood supply of the trachea. Ann Thorac Surg 24:100–107, 1977.
24. Weber AL, editor: Symposium on the larynx and trachea. Radiol Clin North Am 16:227–309, 1978.
25. Whited R-E: A prospective study of laryngotracheal sequelae in long-term intubation. Laryngoscope 94:367–377, 1984.
26. Wilson RS: Tracheal resection. In Marshall BE, Longnecker DE, Fairley HB, editors: Anesthesia for Thoracic Procedures. Boston: Blackwell Scientific, 1988, pp. 415–432.

Benign Lung Disease

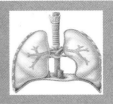

Congenital Lung Diseases

Kemp H. Kernstine, Timothy L. Van Natta, Harold M. Burkhart, and Daniel T. DeArmond

▶ INTRODUCTION

There are many congenital abnormalities involving the pulmonary system. A number of these result in arrested development and stillbirth. Some infants survive delivery only to die shortly thereafter. Neonates with severe anomalies typically display dyspnea and cyanosis at birth. Older children with less critical anomalies may have feeding problems, respiratory infections, developmental delays, or activity limitations. For neonates who are in respiratory distress, speed of diagnosis and treatment are critical. Intubation may be life saving. Examination of the nasooropharynx, neck, and chest, along with an emergent radiograph, allows rapid diagnosis in most cases. Quality computed tomography (CT) may be necessary to delineate the anomaly. Other important adjuncts that may enhance diagnostic speed and accuracy include echocardiography, magnetic resonance imaging (MRI), and endoscopy.

Over the last decade there have been improvements in prenatal diagnosis,[117] even allowing intrauterine repair of some defects.[87] With non–life-sustaining defects such as an anencephaly or renal agenesis, parents may opt for pregnancy termination. For potentially correctable lesions, the pregnant mother can be transferred to a tertiary medical center. Advanced supportive and surgical techniques have led to improved survival in these infants.

▶ HISTORY

The first report of a congenital lung defect was by Fontanus in 1639,[49a] describing an infant with a lung cyst. In 1777 Huber[77] described intralobar sequestration, with blood supply from the thoracic aorta. In the mid-1800s, extralobar (Rokitansky's lobe) sequestration was reported. The neonatal prevalence of lung infections in the 1900s was so high

120

that it was difficult to formulate concepts of congenital lung disease, let alone correct such defects. In 1917 Gladstone and Cockayne theorized on the formation of sequestrations, and in 1925 Koontz reviewed congenital pulmonary cystic diseases. The first surgical correction of a congenital lung anomaly was performed by Reinhoff in 1933,[123a] that being local lung cyst excision in a 3-year-old boy.[123] Gross and Lewis[61] performed the first pediatric lobectomy in a child with congenital lobar emphysema. Cystic disease in the right upper and right middle lobes was resected by lobectomy in 1943.[48] In 1946 Gross[60a] performed a pneumonectomy in a 3-year-old with cystic lung disease. Potts performed the first neonatal lobectomy in 1949. Lewis later reported the death of a child upon whom a lobectomy was being performed for intralobar sequestration, citing exsanguination after lost control of the systemic feeding artery. With development of advanced supportive, anesthetic, vascular, and bypass techniques, mortality rate for children at high-risk for congenital lesions has significantly improved.

▶ EMBRYOLOGY

Lung development occurs both prenatally and postnatally, continuing into adulthood. Intrauterine pulmonary development is divided into the following four phases: (1) embryonic, the first 5 weeks; (2) pseudoglandular, weeks 5–16; (3) canalicular, weeks 16–26; and (4) terminal sac, weeks 26 to birth.[26,125] The foregut begins to develop from the embryonic endoderm on day 9. On day 22 the median pharyngeal groove develops from the foregut. Then, when the embryo is approximately 4 weeks old, there is a 3-mm outpouching from the ventral wall of the embryonic foregut. This respiratory diverticulum (lung bud) is surrounded by splanchnic mesenchyme, later to become the visceral pleura. Concurrently, the lung separates from the esophagus as the lateral mesoderm grows to form the tracheoesophageal septum. The lung bud forms the trachea and then two bronchial buds. These two buds enlarge to form the right and left main bronchi at the start of the fifth week. The individual five lobes become evident over the next few weeks.

In the pseudoglandular stage (weeks 5–16), the bronchial tree develops, including the cuboidal and columnar epithelial layers and cartilaginous rings. The pulmonary vasculature develops in tandem with the airways. By the sixteenth week the bronchial tree and the pulmonary arteries are fully formed, and the common pulmonary vein drains into the sinoatrial region of the heart.

In the canalicular phase (weeks 16–26), bronchioles divide into respiratory bronchioles. These subsequently divide to form alveolar ducts. By the twenty-fifth week, the pulmonary venous drainage has completely developed.

In the terminal sac period (weeks 26–40), there is proliferation of primitive alveoli that become intimately involved with the surrounding capillaries. The adult form of alveoli has developed by the thirtieth to the thirty-sixth week. Type II pneumocytes produce surfactant in preparation for delivery.

Lung development continues postnatally. Airways are nearly fully developed before term. After birth, acinar length increases. Alveoli are fairly thick walled and number about 20 million, less than 10% of their eventual number. Acinar development continues to the eighth year of life, but the rate

of development diminishes after the second to fourth years. By the end of the eighth year there are approximately 300 million acini. After the tenth year of life, alveoli enlarge rather than increase in number. The lung–environmental interface increases from 3–4 m² at birth to 75 m² in adults. From birth to age 5, airway diameter increases. The proximal airway grows at a faster rate than the more distal airways after age 5. Initially the trachea is funnel-like, becoming more cylindrical by age 4. Pulmonary vessel length and diameter rapidly increase until 18 months of age.

Normal airway and vascular development depends on a variety of factors. These include cell-to-cell interactions, local and systemic hormones and growth factors, central and peripheral neural influences, and chest wall effects. The latter involve contact influences of the bony and muscular structures. Alterations in normal development may result from defects in any of these factors. Viral infection, hypoxia, starvation, and teratogens also may disrupt normal lung development. In utero airway obstruction may produce a variety of lesions.[94] Eighty-four percent of these patients have additional nonpulmonary anomalies.[102]

Patients with tracheal agenesis may present in utero with maternal polyhydramnios and premature birth. This defect is apparent immediately at birth with respiratory distress, cyanosis, and lack of an audible cry. These infants may be very difficult to ventilate because an endotracheal tube cannot be placed below the level of the vocal cords. Unless there is an esophageal communication allowing ventilation with esophageal intubation, the abnormality is uniformly fatal.

Lung resection in neonates and children is fairly well tolerated. Anatomy is easily defined because there is less mediastinal and hilar fat, adenopathy, and scarring from "chronic" disease compared with adults. Outcomes after pediatric lung resection are good. Children under 5 years of age develop new alveoli after resection. In those over 5–10 years, the alveoli enlarge, although they no longer increase in number. In an infant pneumonectomy model, lung function returns to normal within 9–12 months.[99] Emphysematous changes do occur, as in adults. After lung resection in children in whom the remaining lung is normal, the child appears to grow, develop, and perform normally with maximal exercise.[96,120] The diffusion capacity for carbon monoxide is reduced, and pulmonary artery pressure increases with exercise, but pulmonary vascular resistance is normal after resection.[52]

▶ TRACHEAL ABNORMALITIES

Tracheal Agenesis and Atresia

Payne[119] first described congenital absence of the trachea in 1900. There have been fewer than 100 cases reported. It represents a partial or complete absence of the trachea below the level of the normal larynx. This abnormality is incompatible with life if there is no connection of trachea or bronchi to the esophagus.[33] Floyd and others[49,88] suggested three distinct types of tracheal agenesis (Figure 9-1). In type I the trachea originates from the esophagus, and the distal trachea, including the carina, is fairly normal. It comprises 10–13% of the total number of tracheal agenesis cases. In type II the trachea and carina are fused to the esophagus, and there is no residual trachea. This is 59–62% of the total. In type III the left and right main stem bronchi originate from the esophagus, and there is no carina. This comprises 22–31% of the total. Male incidence predominates in a 2:1 ratio. In 90% of the cases there are other congenital lesions.[44] Tracheal agenesis may be associated with VACTERL (vertebral, anal, cardiac, tracheal, esophageal, renal, and limb patterns of congenital anomalies)[111] or with complex congenital heart defects, as well as with upper extremity defects and duodenal atresia (referred to as TACRD).[45] It is believed that tracheal agenesis is the result of developmental failure of the laryngeal tracheal bud at the third to sixth week of development. The laryngeal tracheal groove fails to develop normally.

Survivors are rare. Those who are successfully managed are endoesophageally intubated, with a nasogastric tube alongside the endotracheal tube for gastric decompression. Once stabilized, patients are examined for other life-threatening defects that may require correction, such as neural and cardiac anomalies. Extracorporeal membrane oxygenation (ECMO) may temporize.° Long-term success has been reported.[64,74]

Congenital Tracheal Stenosis

Congenital tracheal stenosis (Figure 9-2) is rare. Cantrell and Guild[23] described three forms of stenosis. Type I is stenosis of the full length of the trachea. Type II is a funnel-shaped stenosis of the upper, lower, or entire trachea. Type III is a segmental stenosis of the lower trachea. This classi-

°References 10, 11, 19, 93, 153, 154.

fication assists in identifying patients who are more likely to have associated anomalies and in planning treatment. Stenotic regions have complete cartilaginous rings, the number of which is variable, anywhere from 2 to 18. This rare anomaly is associated with pulmonary vascular sling or vascular ring in 50% of cases.[98]

These patients usually have exertional wheezing or stridor after birth. The types II and III abnormalities are associated with anomalous location of one more bronchi, most likely associated with a left pulmonary artery sling. All three types are associated with pulmonary agenesis. CT provides enough detail to assess the tracheobronchial abnormality and any associated anomalies. Bronchoscopy aids in diagnosis, treatment planning, and evaluating the surgical repair intraoperatively and postoperatively. Echocardiography is helpful to assess for cardiac and vascular anomalies. Patients should be aggressively treated, because they are at high risk for sudden death without surgical correction.[34] Partial tracheal resection is the most frequently performed operation. The neonatal trachea does not tolerate tension well compared with the adult.[56] Up to 50% of the infant trachea can be resected with primary reanastomosis. The repair is much more difficult if more than 50% of the trachea or the carina is involved.

Reconstruction has been performed with pericardium,[42] aortic homograft,[25] costochondral graft,[152] slide tracheoplasty (Figure 9-3),[57,58] and tracheal autograft.[7] Complete repair of the tracheal stenosis and any vascular ring or sling requires cardiopulmonary bypass and potential circulatory arrest. Backer et al[8] reviewed their 18-year experience in 50 patients, comparing four tracheal stenosis repair techniques: pericardial patch, primary resection, tracheal autograft, and slide tracheoplasty. They concluded that when eight or fewer rings are involved, primary resection is preferable. For stenosis longer than eight rings, an autograft was better. Vascular endothelial growth factor application has the potential of improving the results of tracheal autograft.[39] In

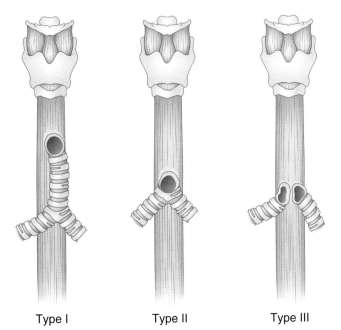

Type I   Type II   Type III

Figure 9–1 Tracheal agenesis classification. There are three types of tracheal agenesis: Type I, the trachea originates from the esophagus rather than from the larynx; Type II, no trachea is present and the carina originates from the esophagus; and Type III, each main stem bronchus originates from the esophagus. *(Modified from Haben CM, Rappaport JM, Clarke KD: Tracheal agenesis. J Am Coll Surg 194:217–222, 2002.)*

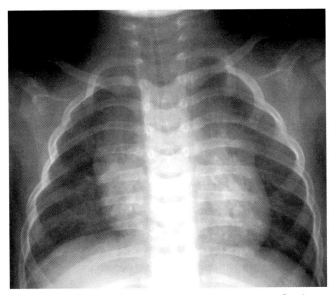

Figure 9–2 Tracheal stenosis (stovepipe trachea) in 20-month-old boy with stridor since birth. Frontal chest radiograph shows a diffusely narrowed trachea faintly outlined by water-soluble contrast medium. *(Courtesy Simon C. Kao MD, Iowa City, Iowa.)*

122 contrast, Muraji et al[115] demonstrated that the slide tracheoplasty technique allowed early extubation and an excellent long-term result in one case. ECMO may be necessary to support the neonate postoperatively.[152] Long-term outcome after resection appears to result in normal growth and development.[68] For patients who are considered surgically uncorrectable, palliative maneuvers include balloon dilation and split posterior tracheoplasty,[22,109] stenting, local steroid injection, electroresection, and cryotherapy.

Tracheomalacia

In tracheomalacia the weakened cartilage collapses on expiration. With inspiration there is sufficient suspension of the tracheal wall to maintain patency. Pathologically the most common finding is oval rather than round cartilaginous rings. There is a congenital and an acquired form of tracheomalacia. The congenital form can be diffuse and both proximal and distal, involving the main stem bronchi. It is associated with tracheoesophageal fistula.[124,131] The more common acquired form results from degeneration of the cartilaginous support, usually from vascular compression such as from a vascular ring or sling, an adjacent inflammatory process, tumor, or chest wall deformity (e.g., pectus excavatum).

Tracheomalacia is not usually manifest at birth. It worsens as the child grows, usually after several weeks of life. Coughing, respiratory distress, severe dyspnea, stridor, and cyanosis may occur. Acute apnea, referred to as "dying spells," is the most severe presentation. Dyspnea worsens with agitation or respiratory tract infections. These severe symptoms should prompt further investigation.

One fourth of all esophageal atresia patients have tracheomalacia. Tracheoscopy, bronchoscopy, esophagoscopy, and esophagram may be necessary for complete evaluation. CT and MRI provide additional information. The differen-

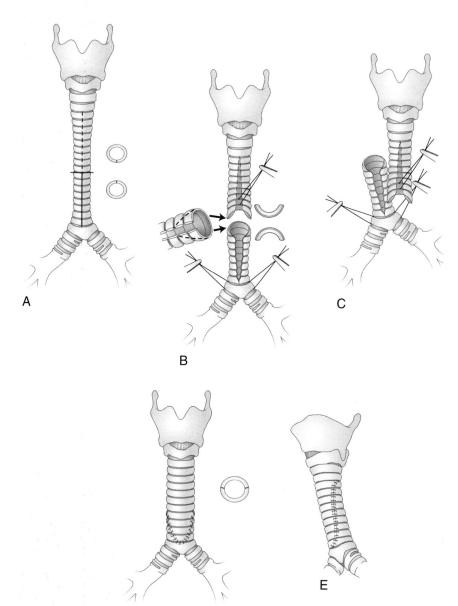

Figure 9–3 Congenital tracheal stenosis. A, After identifying the area of stenosis, the midportion of the stenosis is transected, leaving two halves of the trachea disconnected. **B,** Then, a longitudinal tracheal incision is made in each half, the full length of the stenosis; the upper half, posterior and in the lower half, anterior. The corners are trimmed to allow for an even, un-crimped anastomosis. **C,** Stay sutures help in retracting and alignment. **D** and **E,** The anastomosis results in an oblique suture line. The resultant cross sectional area is quadrupled.
(Modified from the Society of Thoracic Surgeons: Ann Thorac Surg 58:613-621, 1994.)

tial includes normal pulsatile collapse, bronchial webs, and tracheal tumors. Many patients suspected of having tracheomalacia may instead have gastroesophageal reflux disease, or reflux disease in addition to tracheomalacia. This may warrant either a trial of a proton pump inhibitor and prokinetic agent or a formal evaluation for reflux.[29]

Tracheomalacia improves with age in most cases. "Dying spells," inability to wean from the ventilator, and failure to thrive are indications for more aggressive therapy. If tracheomalacia is mild, the infant should be supported and observed, because infants usually outgrow their tracheomalacia within the next 2 years. In more severe forms, mortality is as high as 80% with conservative management. Stents have been used with varying success to allow for cartilage maturation, usually taking several months.[32,47] Tracheostomy also has been used, but is associated with some complications.[55] Aortopexy (Figure 9-4), by itself or with tracheal resection or stenting, has been performed through a left submammary thoracotomy through the third interspace. The thymus is preserved. After exposing the ascending aorta, three to four nonabsorbable sutures are placed through the aortic adventitia above and below the innominate artery take-off. These sutures are attached to the periosteum. Finally, the endotracheal result is visualized by intraoperative bronchoscopy. Eighty percent of the patients are extubated by 4 weeks, and the long-term results are good.[129] The acquired form is treated similarly to the congenital form. Longer segment lesions without vascular compression often require tracheostomy and mechanical ventilation for a period. Bronchomalacia may require both aortopexy and pulmonary artery pexy.[84]

▶ BRONCHIAL BRANCHING ABNORMALITIES

Bronchial branching abnormalities are rarely symptomatic. There are case reports of bronchi crossing the mediastinum to supply the opposite lung.[4] Accessory bronchi can originate off the trachea or main stem bronchi and may be attached to rudimentary lung. They are usually incidental findings at autopsy. Cervical diverticula present in utero may regress before birth. The most frequent tracheal bronchus is to the right upper lobe. These abnormalities may be isolated or associated with other tracheopulmonary anomalies. They can be associated with wheezing, stridor, pneumonia, bronchiectasis, and hemoptysis. Accessory bronchi and associated abnormal pulmonary tissue should be resected if symptomatic.[108] Chest radiograph and high-resolution CT are helpful in defining the anomaly.[133]

The following are anomalies that are more frequently symptomatic, potentially life threatening, and potentially treatable.

Bronchial Atresia

Bronchial atresia, first described by Ramsay in 1953,[121] is the second most common abnormality of the airway after tracheoesophageal fistula. A lobar or segmental bronchus ends blindly in the lung tissue. Lung tissue distal to the bronchial atresia expands and becomes emphysematous as a result of air entering through the pores of Kohn.[112] Beyond the atretic segment, but proximal to the hyperinflated lung, the terminal airway is mucus filled. It is believed that the bronchial bud somehow separates distally from the proximal bronchial bud and continues to develop. Another potential explanation is that there is a vascular insult of the airway in the atretic segment. In either case, the distal airway continues to develop normally.

Infants usually develop respiratory distress 4–5 days to several weeks after birth. They may have wheezing, stridor, and repeated pulmonary infections. The most common location is in the left upper lobe; then the left lower lobe, followed by the right upper lobe. A segmental bronchus rather than a lobar bronchus is atretic, most frequently presenting as a lung mass on the first chest X-ray of the newborn. Fetal lung fluid slowly absorbs, becoming a localized translucency with an opaque circular oval density at the hilum. Patients rarely mature to adulthood without investigation.

For better assessment of this abnormality, a CT scan should be performed.[80,107] The differential diagnosis includes acquired bronchial stenosis (which may occur as a result of long-term intubation), bronchial adenoma, sequestration, mucoid impaction, vascular compression syndrome, Swyer–James syndrome, and atypical bronchogenic cyst.

Indications for resection in bronchial atresia include a recurrent and possibly serious pulmonary infection, and increasing size of the translucent lung.[66] Some resect the

Figure 9–4 Tracheomalacia and aortopexy. In patients with severe tracheomalacia and aortopexy, suturing the proximal transverse-ascending aorta to the anterior chest wall or sternum may significantly improve the obstructive symptoms.
(Modified from Weber TR, Keller MS, Fiore A: Aortic suspension (aortopexy) for severe tracheomalacia in infants and children. Am J Surg 184:573-577, 2002.)

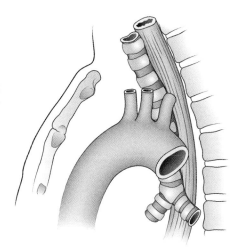
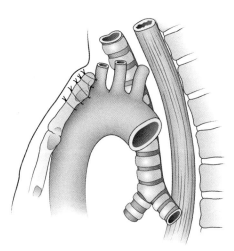

124 abnormal tissue to prevent infection. Segmentectomy is possible, but usually lobectomy is required.

Congenital Bronchiectasis

Bronchiectasis is an abnormal dilation of the bronchi or bronchioles. It is believed to be secondary to failure of the mesenchyme to differentiate into cartilage and muscle.[83] It results in a chronic, mildly productive cough with recurrent pneumonia. CT usually achieves the diagnosis,[91] and bronchoscopy typically is unnecessary. Bronchography also is unnecessary, given the detail provided by CT. Patients who have localized congenital symptomatic bronchiectasis may require a segmentectomy, lobectomy, or possibly pneumonectomy. Treatment and prognosis depend on the number of segments or lobes involved. Patients are provided with humidity, chest physiotherapy, and oxygen as necessary. Therapeutic bronchoscopy is performed for suspected mucoid obstruction or bleeding. Initially bleeding is controlled by embolization, topical epinephrine, or intravenous pitressin. Oral, intravenous, and nebulized antibiotics may be helpful in controlling symptoms.[159]

Tracheobronchomegaly (Mounier-Kuhn Syndrome)

Tracheobronchomegaly (TBM) was first described in 1932 by Mounier-Kuhn.[113] It is characterized by excessive dilation of the trachea and main bronchi (Figure 9-5).[157] This dilatation is the result of atrophy of the elastic tissue and smooth muscle of the trachea and main stem airways.[86] Airway dilatation continues to third-order subdivisions. Over the course of the disease, mucosal herniations develop between tracheal rings, creating a diverticulosis pattern. Associated conditions include cutis laxa, Ehlers–Danlos syndrome, Marfan's syndrome, Kenny–Caffey syndrome, ataxia–telangiectasia, ankylosing spondylitis, Brachmann–de Lange syndrome, and light chain deposition disease. When an isolated process occurs, there is recessive inheritance.[81] TBM also may result from severe pulmonary fibrosis with increased traction on the tracheal wall.[14,156] As these diverticula develop, there is mucus retention with resultant development of bronchiectasis and fibrosis. Patients eventually are unable to clear secretions and succumb to chronic infection and respiratory failure.

The patients are usually men in their third to fourth decades of life. Fifty percent of TBM patients have no symptoms until their third decade. Usually they have recurrent lower respiratory tract infections. Asymptomatic patients may be identified in that their tracheas are three standard deviations larger than normal; for adults it exceeds 3 cm.[15]

TBM patients frequently have recurrent respiratory tract infections and persistent cough. Plain chest X-ray demonstrates an enlarged trachea and main stem airways that may be ectatic. CT more clearly demonstrates changes, and tracheal dimensions for adults[18] and children[59] are helpful in making the diagnosis. Bronchography may be necessary to differentiate it from acquired bronchiectasis. Bronchoscopy generally is unrewarding, with inadequate visualization of the airway lumen as a result of multiple tracheal wall diverticula.

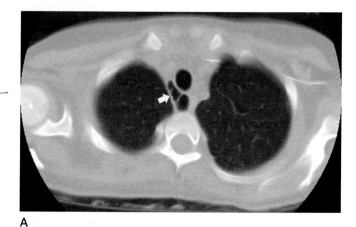

A

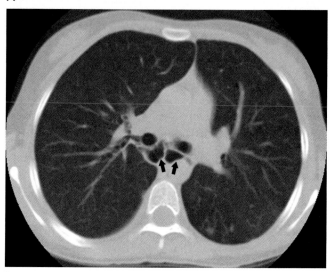

B

Figure 9–5 **Tracheobronchomegaly (Mounier-Kuhn syndrome) in a 13-year-old girl with chronic cough and bronchiectasis.** CT scan at levels of the trachea (**A**) and main stem bronchi (**B**) shows air-filled saccules (*arrows*) around the airway from chronic inflammation destroying the normal elastic properties of the tracheobronchial tree and its smooth muscles. (*Courtesy of Simon C. Kao, MD, Iowa City, Iowa.*)

There is no surgical role in the treatment of TBM. Managing secretions helps minimize the symptoms. Stenting and T-tubes[51,134] may provide significant palliation.

Laryngotracheoesophageal Cleft

Laryngotracheoesophageal cleft is a rare congenital abnormality resulting from failure of the esophagus to separate from the laryngotrachea.[27] Infants have a toneless cry and choke with feeding. On an attempt to pass a nasogastric tube, a communication with the airway is seen. A barium study or endoscopy can demonstrate the fistula. One half to over three fourths of reported patients survive.[78,100] With late detection, mortality is high. Patients are first treated with a gastrostomy. Then, through a cervical approach, the fistula is divided, the esophagus and larynx are repaired, and a muscle flap is placed between them to reduce likelihood for recurrence. A nasogastric stent is left in place for a period. For large defects, a combined cervical and thoracic approach may be necessary.[40]

Tracheobronchial Esophageal Fistula

Tracheobronchial esophageal fistula (TEF) is the most common abnormality of the trachea, occurring in 2.4 per 10,000 births.[67] A frequently used anatomical classification system for TEF is the one proposed by Gross[60]: type A, esophageal atresia without TEF; type B, esophageal atresia with proximal TEF; type C, atresia with distal TEF; type D, atresia with both proximal and distal TEF; type E, TEF without esophageal atresia (H-type). Type C is the most common, accounting for 87% of the anomalies, followed by type A (8%), type E (4%), type B (1%), and type D (1%).

Patients have presenting symptoms of feeding difficulty, excessive salivation, bouts of cyanosis, or tracheobronchial infections. Diagnosis of the most common form is suspected when a large amount of air is seen in the esophagus, stomach, and small bowel. Failure nasogastric tube passage and its position on plain X-ray or contrast fluoroscopy can confirm the fistula. Patients are treated by division of the fistula and repair of the defect via right extrapleural thoracotomy. For the H-type fistula, a right neck incision is made, thereby avoiding the thoracic duct. The sternocleidomastoid muscle and carotid sheath contents are retracted laterally. The recurrent laryngeal nerve is identified and protected, and the fistula is divided and oversewn. An interposition muscle flap reduces the likelihood of recurrence.

Bronchobiliary Fistula

Bronchobiliary fistula is a very rare congenital abnormality, with perhaps fewer than 25 cases reported (Figure 9-6).[37] The fistula tract is composed of bronchial and biliary-type tissue from its origin in the airway to the liver. Patients have productive green sputum, as well as associated dyspnea and chronic cough. Females are more commonly affected. The right middle lobe and right main stem airways are most fre-

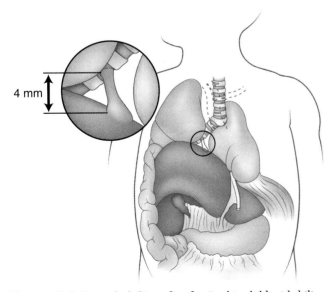

Figure 9–6 Bronchobiliary fistula. In this child with bilious sputum and a congenital diaphragmatic defect, a fistula was found between the right main stem bronchus and the biliary tree. *(Modified from DiFiore JW, Alexander F: Congenital bronchobiliary fistula in association with right-sided congenital diaphragmatic hernia. J Pediatr Surg 37:1208–1209, 2002.)*

quently involved and usually drain to the left hepatic ductal system. Diagnosis is made by bronchoscopy wherein a catheter is passed into the fistula for a contrast study.[126] Bronchography may be helpful as well. Diagnosis also has been achieved with a nuclear biliary scan.[43] These patients are treated by dividing the fistula, transecting it as close to the airway as possible. For those with biliary sepsis, a left hepatic lobectomy is performed.[46]

Bronchopulmonary Foregut Malformations

Bronchopulmonary foregut malformations represent another category of congenital lung diseases. The classification includes sequestrations (intralobar and extralobar), bronchogenic cysts, and other less common entities.

Bronchopulmonary foregut malformations are an abnormal communication between normal lung and esophagus or stomach and represent the second most frequent abnormal communication between the airway and intestinal tract, tracheoesophageal fistula being most common. Right and left lower lobes are equally and most commonly affected. The fistula rarely involves the gastric fundus or mid-esophagus, almost always tracking to the lower esophagus. It is associated with extralobar sequestrations, more often on the left side. Diagnosis is usually made in the first few months of life up to 18 years of age. The most useful diagnostic test is an esophagram. These malformations are associated with other anomalies such as diaphragmatic hernia or cardiac, gastrointestinal, or vertebral anomalies. Because of chronic infection, lobectomy is usually necessary, and the fistulous communication must be divided and the esophageal defect repaired. If there is no evidence of infection, lung tissue may be preserved.

Sequestrations

Sequestrations are lung defects that have systematic arterial blood supply and abnormal bronchial connections. Blood supply most commonly enters the anomalous lung away from the hilum. They are invariably located in the base of the lung. Males are more frequently affected, with a 3:1 ratio. Intralobar sequestrations (ILS) (Figure 9-7) are cystic abnormalities located within the visceral pleural covering of the lung, whereas extralobar sequestrations (ELS) (Rokitansky's lobe) (Figure 9-8) are mass lesions that have their own separate visceral covering. ILS comprise 75% of all sequestrations. As a group, ILS receive vascular blood supply from the thoracic aorta 74% of the time, from the abdominal aorta in 19% of cases, and from the intercostals in 3% of cases. Multiple sources are present in 20% of patients. Venous drainage is usually via pulmonary veins, but may be systemic.

ELS are rounded, smooth, soft masses that usually lie just above the dome of the diaphragm, with 90% occurring at the base of the left lung. They most frequently drain into the systemic circulation, either to azygos or hemiazygos systems. Twenty percent do drain into the pulmonary veins. Microscopically, all lung structures are present in ELS, including alveoli, bronchi, and cartilage. ILS and ELS are both derived from foregut tissue and thus may possess an esophageal fistula. ILS may present in utero as polyhydramnios or may become symptomatic in adolescents or

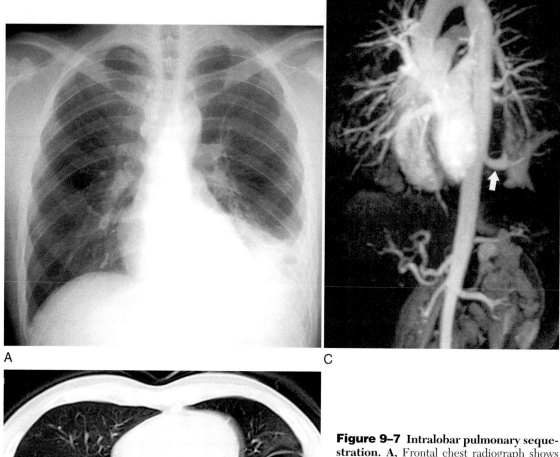

A

C

B

Figure 9–7 Intralobar pulmonary seque-stration. A, Frontal chest radiograph shows consolidation of the left lower lobe. **B,** CT image of lung base shows opacification of the left posterior lower lobe. **C,** Contrast-enhanced magnetic resonance angiography shows that a large arterial branch *(arrow)* arising from the low thoracic aorta supplies this region.
(Courtesy Koji Takahashi, MD, Asahikawa Medical College, Asahikawa, Japan.)

young adults. Repeated bouts of pulmonary infection and hemoptysis are the most common symptoms. ILS are most frequently found within the posterior segment of the left lower lobe and is rarely associated with other congenital anomalies.

In contrast, ELS are associated with other anomalies, especially congenital diaphragmatic hernias. ELS may be found within either the pericardium or the diaphragm or beneath the diaphragm retroperitoneally. Malignancies have been reportedly found within ELS, and a simultaneous dis-covery of congenital cystic adenomatoid malformations has been reported, as have other anomalies such as pericardial cysts, esophageal achalasia, and cardiac defects.

CT is quite sensitive and specific to identify either ILS or ELS. MRI may be helpful.[28] Bronchography and bron-choscopy are less likely to provide additional information. Barium esophagram may be necessary to demonstrate an esophageal communication. Angiogram is seldom necessary because noninvasive studies generally demonstrate the feeding systemic vessels.

Many lesions are discovered prenatally, and careful follow-up is recommended. If hydropic changes are noted, delivery is indicated.[12,75] In infants, cysts that are large or cause hemodynamic compromise may be temporarily drained by needle aspiration or tube thoracostomy to allow for adequate induction of anesthesia. If no infection is

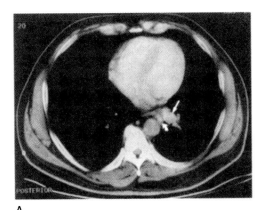

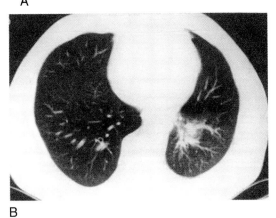

Figure 9–8 Extralobar sequestration. Extralobar sequestration is most frequently found in the lower left chest with its own pleural investment and systemic venous drainage. CT scan beneficial in better identifying the anatomical details of the defect.
(From Singh SP, Nath H: A 53-year-old man with hemoptysis. Chest 120:298–301, 2001.)

involved, the cyst alone, or possibly a segment, may be removed. In most cases, however, lobectomy is required. Early identification of the aberrant arterial blood supply is critical and helps avoid disastrous bleeding. Most of the arteries are less than 1 mm in diameter, but some have been reported to be as large as 2.5 mm. Atherosclerotic changes in the systemic artery may make it difficult to manipulate during surgery. A communication with the gastrointestinal tract should be thoroughly searched for at the time of surgery. Venous drainage also may be aberrant, and it should be ascertained before resection if possible. Extralobar sequestrations may be potentially resected by minimally invasive techniques. The outcomes after resection are excellent.[9,63]

Azygos Lobe

An azygos lobe (Figure 9-9) is present on 0.5% of routine chest X-rays. It is found as an abnormal lobation where the azygos vein creates an additional sulcus separating two portions of the upper lobe. The azygos vein lies within the substance of the right lung, producing an azygos lobe that is not a true anatomical lobe, because it does not have a separate segmental bronchus. Separate lobations also may be found. They appear more frequently in the lingula or in the right and left superior segments. These abnormal lobations are

not associated with any other congenital anomaly, nor do they increase the likelihood for any future pathological or developmental abnormality. They require no treatment.

Horseshoe Lung

In this rare, recently reviewed pulmonary anomaly,[151] right and left lung bases are fused by common tissue extending through the posterior mediastinum anterior to the aorta but posterior to the heart and esophagus. The clinical relevance lies in its association with recurrent pulmonary infections and pulmonary hypertension. Scimitar syndrome accompanies horseshoe lung in up to 80% of cases.[141] Horseshoe lung also should be suspected in patients with the VACTERL constellation and in patients with other bronchopulmonary foregut anomalies.[151]

Bronchogenic Cysts

Bronchogenic cysts result from abnormal budding from the perimeter of the trachea after it has differentiated from the foregut. They are the most frequent cysts of the mediastinum, accounting for approximately 60%. Their usual location is along the right paratracheal area. They may be attached to the carina, frequently anterior to the esophagus, or they may be hilar, attached to a lobar bronchus. Occasionally they are intrapulmonary. Furthermore, they may be situated below the diaphragm or in the peristernal subcutaneous tissue, skin, or pericardium. Men are more frequently affected than women. The cyst's inner lining is composed of ciliated pseudostratified respiratory epithelium interspersed with goblet cells. Bronchial communication is rare.[138] The cysts are unilocular and usually measure from 2–10 cm. They may contain normal bronchial elements, including cartilage and smooth muscle. Cartilaginous elements differentiate a bronchogenic cyst from an enteric cyst. Noninfected cysts may contain mucus, blood, and/or milky material. Symptoms may relate to pulmonary artery compression and possibly paroxysmal atrial fibrillation.[150,158]

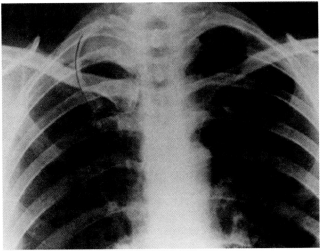

Figure 9–9 Azygous lobe. An additional fissure is found in this chest radiograph. The azygous vein creates a separate division within the right upper lobe.

128 They most commonly present as an incidental finding on chest radiograph, usually seen as an air-filled cyst with or without an air–fluid level (Figure 9-10). Serial radiographs may demonstrate rapid expansion. Intraparenchymal cysts more frequently have infectious presenting symptoms (90%) compared with the mediastinal cysts (36%).[135]

Differential diagnosis includes lymphadenopathy, pulmonary sequestrations, teratoma, hemangioma, lipoma, hamartoma, neurogenic tumors, foregut and pericardial cysts, and lung abscesses. CT is helpful, and a low Hounsfield unit (less than 20) is characteristic. MRI may provide additional information. In contrast, enteric cysts are usually present in the posterior mediastinum and are associated with the esophagus. Bronchopulmonary foregut malformations are usually multilocular and are more frequently associated with recur-

rent cough, pneumonia, and hemoptysis. Endoscopic ultrasound (EUS) may be beneficial, but EUS-directed fine-needle aspiration (FNA) may be hazardous.[155]

Bronchogenic cysts should be excised completely if possible with repair of any associated communication. Needle aspiration alone is likely to result in recurrence. Mediastinoscopic unroofing has been performed and has been diagnostic. Asymptomatic cysts should be removed to achieve a diagnosis and to reduce complications, including perforation, hemorrhage, enlargement and infection, or potentially retaining malignant tissue. In children the airways are pliable and much more susceptible to life-threatening compression by an enlarging cyst.[65] Malignant degeneration has been reported,[17,122,142] including an adenocarcinoma in an 8½-year-old girl.[138] Typically the bron-

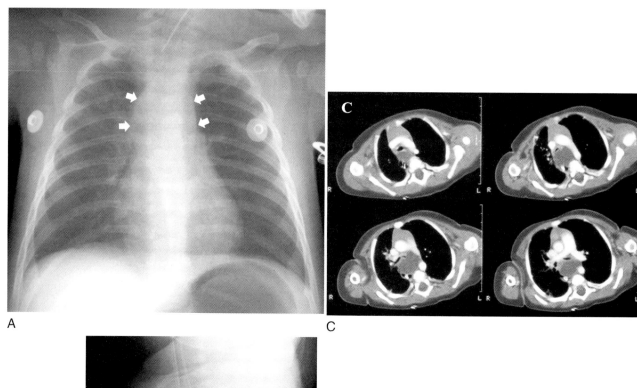

Figure 9–10 Bronchogenic cyst in a 4-month-old boy with cough. Anteroposterior (**A**) and lateral (**B**) chest radiographs show a central mediastinal mass (*arrows*) displacing the esophagus (outlined by nasogastric tube, *arrows*) posteriorly. **C,** Four contiguous axial CT image of the chest shows a retrotracheal and subcarinal mass with low-density contents. Excision of the mass and pathological examination shows bronchogenic cyst.

(*Courtesy Simon C. Kao, MD, Iowa City, Iowa.*)

chogenic cyst can be enucleated from the mediastinum. If there is a stalk, it is ligated and the bronchial defect repaired. Long-term results are excellent. Video-assisted removal has become increasingly popular,[69] but pericystic adhesions, tracheal or bronchial communications, and the possibility of malignancy should be considered as indications for thoracotomy.

► LUNG BUD ANOMALIES

Pulmonary Agenesis, Aplasia, and Hypoplasia

Pulmonary agenesis is the complete absence of the carina, as well as the main stem bronchus, the lung, and the pulmonary vasculature on the affected side. First described by Morgagni, there are fewer than 10 reported cases. Cardiac anomalies are usually associated when pulmonary agenesis is bilateral. Unilateral cases have cardiac anomalies in 50% and are more frequently associated with right-sided agenesis.[128] The sex distribution is fairly equal. Right and left agenesis is also equally distributed. There is some evidence of a chromosomal abnormality.[127]

When the carina and bronchus are present, but the vessels and parenchyma are absent, the defect is referred to as pulmonary aplasia. There is a rudimentary bronchial stump, and the carina appears to be normal. Aplasia may be present in a single lobe or in a combination of lobes. It is most frequently unilobar. The right upper and right middle lobes are the most frequently involved. The heart may be displaced by the reduced lung volume.

Agenesis and aplasia may be asymptomatic when a single lobe is involved or when unilateral. Patients may have tachypnea, dyspnea, and/or cyanosis. Older patients may have wheezing. Men are more commonly affected than women. When congenital cardiac anomalies are present, cyanosis and respiratory distress are evident at birth.

Chest radiograph shows a shift in the mediastinum toward the area of agenesis and aplasia (Figure 9-11). A pulmonary angiogram shows absence of a pulmonary artery. Bronchoscopy may be helpful to evaluate for presence of a rudimentary bronchial stump in patients with aplasia. CT and esophagram are a helpful part of the evaluation to differentiate agenesis or aplasia from sequestration and atelectasis.

Bilateral agenesis is incompatible with life. Survival periods for up to 6 years in right-sided lesions and up to 16 years in left-sided lesions have been reported.[103] Of patients, 30% usually die within the first year, and 50% die within the first 5 years.[106]

In pulmonary hypoplasia, the bronchus and the bronchial tissue are poorly formed and there is a reduced number of alveoli. Lung weight is at least one standard deviation below the mean.[118] Most cases of hypoplasia are the result of another defect that prevents normal lung development, such as a chest wall abnormality or diaphragmatic hernia, bone dysplasia, or muscular dystrophy. Primary pulmonary hypoplasia is rare and is frequently associated with Down syndrome.[31] It is frequently fatal and is the result of hypertrophy of the pulmonary artery smooth muscle and resultant pulmonary artery hypertension. The associated congenital abnormalities reduce the life expectancy of these patients.[116]

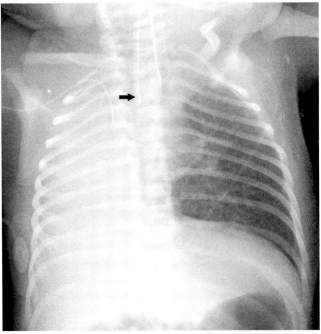

Figure 9-11 Right pulmonary agenesis. Frontal chest radiograph in a newborn with respiratory distress. Note complete opacification of the right hemithorax with mediastinal shift toward the same side. The patient also has esophageal atresia (nasogastric tube lodged in the dilated proximal esophageal pouch, *arrow*) with distal tracheoesophageal fistula (note presence of air in the stomach).
(Courtesy Simon C. Kao, MD, Iowa City, Iowa.)

In pulmonary aplasia, removal of the rudimentary stump may be necessary if recurrently infected. There is no specific surgical therapy for pulmonary hypoplasia, except to treat the cardiac and chest wall abnormalities. The severity of the pulmonary artery hypertrophy may result in persistent fetal circulation. At delivery, patients may be hypoxemic, acidotic, and hypercarbic. Hypoplasia patients are treated with sedation, paralysis, high-frequency ventilation, vasodilators, respiratory alkalosis, and, if necessary, ECMO. Survival has improved with ECMO.[93,153,154] Another means to treat these patients is with high-frequency oscillatory ventilation.[110] Half of the patients with congenital diaphragmatic hernias require ECMO, and 70% of those patients who require ECMO survive. In patients with anomalies such as congenital diaphragmatic hernia, it is unnecessary to resect the underdeveloped lung at the time of the repair. There should be no attempt to aggressively inflate the lung. Lung transplantation has been performed for hypoplasia.[95]

Congenital Lobar Emphysema

Congenital lobar emphysema comprises 50% of all congenital lung anomalies. It is the result of an obstruction of a lobar bronchus, usually an upper airway, resulting in overexpansion of alveolar air spaces but lacking parenchymal destruction, as in the adult form. The vasculature to the affected lobe is normal. Expanded lung frequently compresses adjacent lung and in some cases shifts the mediastinum away from the emphysematous lobe. Other

130 descriptive terms include infantile lobar emphysema, congenital segmental bronchomalacia, congenital lobar overinflation, and emphysema of infancy or childhood. A cartilaginous defect obstructs the lobar bronchus in 25% of cases.[13,16,70,97] Other potential causes of intrinsic obstruction include mucous plugging and granulations within the airway. Extrinsic obstruction may result from cardiac or vascular anomalies such as tetralogy of Fallot, pulmonary stenosis, anomalies of pulmonary venous return, adenopathy, mediastinal tumors, and bronchogenic or enteric duplication cysts.[130] In over 50% of cases there is no identifiable etiological factor.[143]

Patients with congenital lobar emphysema are asymptomatic at birth. Within several days they can develop wheezing, dyspnea, or cough.[34] The left upper lobe is most frequently involved, followed by the right upper lobe, right middle lobe, and finally the lower lobes.[71] It can present bilaterally. When it does, it is usually the left upper lobe or right middle lobe that is affected. There is a 3:1 male to female ratio of involvement. Of those affected, 80% are symptomatic by 6 months of age. Fourteen percent of patients have an associated cardiac malformation. Rib and thoracic cage abnormalities also are common. Once congenital lobar emphysema is symptomatic and if untreated, the mortality is 50% within the first week, and an additional 30–40% of patients will die over the next month.

In the newborn with severe respiratory distress, a chest radiograph usually suffices for diagnosis (Figure 9-12). The combination of an enlarged, hyperlucent lobe with fairly normal vasculature, coupled with compression of adjacent lung tissue and contralateral mediastinal deviation, is diagnostic. For mild to moderate symptoms, a CT scan (see Figure 9-12) may be necessary to rule out mediastinal masses or vascular anomalies. In older children, bronchoscopy may be helpful to assess for mucous plugs or foreign bodies. Bronchography is unlikely to be helpful. Ventilation-perfusion scan also has been used to assess these patients.[104] Respiratory distress in the newborn must be differentiated from other lung abnormalities, such as pneumothorax, congenital diaphragmatic hernia, parenchymal lung cysts with a ball valve mechanism, cystic adenomatoid malformation, and ELS. Acquired lobar emphysema is yet a different disease entity, a complication of respiratory distress syndrome and long-term intubation and is usually present in the right upper lobe. In acquired childhood emphysema, lung scans demonstrate low flow to the affected lung, in contrast to normal flow in the congenital form.[30] For the congenital form, echocardiography and additional tests (e.g., magnetic resonance angiography) may be required to evaluate for associated cardiac or vascular anomalies.

There is no indication for surgical resection in asymptomatic or mildly symptomatic patients. Pulmonary function is likely to remain stable. Half of the patients will normalize during infancy. For patients who are symptomatic, all emphysematous tissue should be resected. Lobectomy frequently is required. Operative mortality is as high as 7% in some series. The greatest risk appears to be at the time of anesthesia induction. Selective intubation has been used to prevent overinflation of the emphysematous lobe, with resulting cardiovascular collapse.[62] High-frequency ventilation also has been employed to prevent mediastinal shift

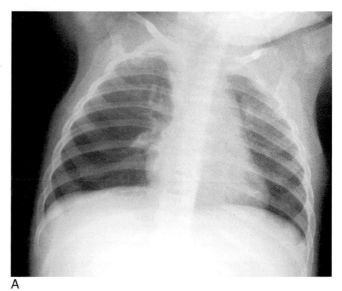

A

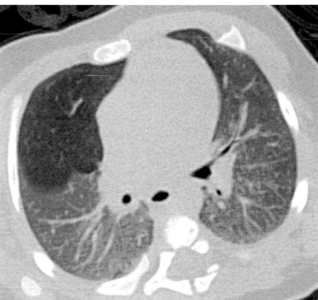

B

Figure 9-12 Congenital lobar emphysema. A, Chest radiograph of a 1-month-old boy shows hyperlucency in the right lower lung field. **B,** CT image of the lungs just below the carinal bifurcation shows right middle lobe emphysema with paucity of blood vessels and decreased attenuation. *(Courtesy Simon C. Kao, MD, Iowa City, Iowa.)*

and hemodynamic compromise.[54] Needle aspiration has been performed as necessary.[89] The surgeon should be prepared for immediate thoracotomy soon after induction. Once the chest is open, the emphysematous lobe almost pops out of the chest. Typically it remains inflated after the lobe has been removed. The hilar anatomy is usually normal, and the goal should be to resect all of the emphysematous tissue, preserving the adjacent normal lung. Lung function is compromised after resection,[35,143] but the child's development is normal.[132] In contrast to patients with congenital lobar emphysema, those with acquired lobar emphysema progress to further respiratory difficulties after lung resection.[5] Balloon dilatation of airway stenosis has been used successfully.[79]

Congenital Parenchymal Cysts

Congenital parenchymal cysts are rare and may present as a unilocular cyst within the parenchyma, usually in the left lower lobe and supplied by an aberrant systemic artery. The cyst is lined with pseudostratified columnar epithelium that secretes mucus. Usually the cyst communicates with a bronchus. This condition may represent a variant of cystic adenomatoid malformation. It may result from entrapped lung blood, with subsequent air trapping after the blood has absorbed. The infant has presenting symptoms of chronic cough and possibly even sepsis. Other anomalies are frequently associated with congenital parenchymal cysts. Respiratory distress is common within the first few days of life, and the cyst usually becomes infected by the first few weeks of age. The air trapping may shift the mediastinum.

It is difficult to differentiate the cyst from an intraparenchymal abscess. Presence of a systemic artery feeding the cyst is diagnostic. Failure of the cyst to completely collapse with tube drainage also is helpful in making the diagnosis. Other anomalies that appear similar include congenital diaphragmatic hernia and postpneumonic staphylococcal pneumatoceles.

Once discovered, congenital parenchymal cysts can be observed unless they become infected, expand, or are otherwise symptomatic. If present for more than a year, they are unlikely to resolve. Once infected, the cyst is best treated with antibiotics first, followed by resection once sepsis subsides. Lobectomy is usually necessary, although cyst resection can suffice. A pneumonectomy occasionally may be necessary for definitive treatment.

Congenital Cystic Adenomatoid Malformation

Congenital cystic adenomatoid malformation (CCAM) was first described by Ch'in and Tang in 1949.[24] It is a mass of excessive proliferation of bronchi without the normal alveolar development. Composed of cartilage, smooth muscle, bronchial glands, and columnar and cuboidal epithelial cells, it comprises 25% of all congenital lung anomalies, second only to congenital lobar emphysema. There is normal vascular development, and the affected area communicates with a normal airway. Usually only one lobe is affected, and lesions are usually single.

The abnormality may be identified in the fetus whose mother has polyhydramnios by the twenty-third week of gestation. Up to one third of those identified in utero resolved before birth.[1,105,140] It presents as neonatal acute respiratory distress and must be differentiated from congenital diaphragmatic hernia, because both entities show multiple air fluid levels within the affected chest. The initial chest radiograph shows a solid mass. Over time, the fetal fluid is resorbed and the cysts become filled with air (Figure 9-13). CT may be helpful in achieving a diagnosis. The most commonly associated anomaly is pectus excavatum, and there can be cardiac and pulmonary vessel malformations as well. Bale[9a] attempted to classify the CCAM to for treatment planning and prognosis.[136] The Stocker classification assists in treatment planning.[137] Type I lesions are large, widely spaced, irregular cystic structures that exceed 1 cm. Affected patients usually reach term, but occasionally are stillborn. It is rare to have polyhydramnios or other anom-

alies associated with a type I lesion. Of these patients, 75% have mediastinal shifting with some associated cyanosis and grunting. The prognosis generally is good. Half of the patients develop pneumonia in infancy or early childhood. In type II CCAM, 40% of cases, the cysts are smaller than 1 cm and have an appearance of dilated bronchioles. The patients are more frequently premature or stillborn. Mediastinal shift is less often seen, and there appears to be more bronchiolar proliferation. Type III lesions are very small cysts, less than 0.5 cm. They comprise 10% of all of cases. The mass is much more firm, appearing to surround the entire affected lobe, most often the left lower lobe. Prognosis is very poor, and patients usually expire within a few hours of birth.

Asymptomatic CCAM patients may be observed for the first 4–6 months. Repeated CT at 6 months is performed to

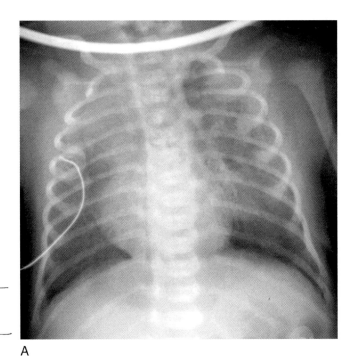

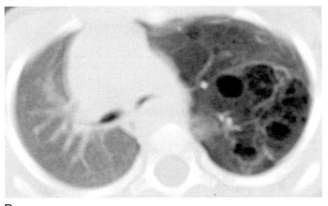

Figure 9–13 Cystic adenomatoid malformation. A, Chest radiograph of a newborn with ill-defined lesions in the mid-left lung field. **B,** CT image of the chest shows multicystic lesions in the same region. Excision and histological examination shows cystical adenomatoid malformation.
(Courtesy Simon C. Kao, MD, Iowa City, Iowa.)

132 assess for CCAM enlargement or malignant degeneration. Delayed intervention allows the child to mature, reducing the operative morbidity. Symptomatic lesions after birth should be resected, and lobectomy is the treatment of choice. Remaining unaffected lung tissue should be preserved. Once the lesion is resected, prognosis is excellent. In utero cysts may be aspirated.[21] Any lesion that decreases in size but has not completely regressed should be observed until it has completely resolved.

Infantile Pulmonary Emphysema

Infantile pulmonary emphysema is uncommon and accounts for approximately 2% of congenital anomalies. It usually occurs in the lower lobes and is frequently associated with other anomalies. It presents as gas surrounding the bronchovascular structures and may evolve to pneumomediastinum and/or pneumothorax. It may occur in 20% of patients with respiratory distress syndrome and 40% of patients who require positive end-expiratory pressure. It presents as a diffuse multicystic abnormality within all lobes.[145] It must be differentiated from congenital cystic adenomatoid malformation and congenital diaphragmatic hernia. Once the diagnosis is made, fewer than 2% of patients require surgical resection; most improve with supportive measures alone. Atelectasis, ventilator dependence, and recurrent or persistent infections are indications for surgery. Thoracentesis or thoracostomy is necessary to treat pneumothorax and respiratory embarrassment. Resection of affected tissues with preservation of relatively healthy parenchyma is the objective of surgical intervention.

Polyalveolar Lobe

Polyalveolar lobe is a significant increase in the number of alveoli compared with the bronchi. It was first described in 1970 and was thought to be congenital lobar emphysema.[73] It is differentiated from lobar emphysema in that there is little trapped air without true emphysematous changes. Radiographic translucency in this condition is the result of a reduction in vasculature to amount of lung, unlike congenital lobar emphysema.[73,114] In older children, bronchoscopy should be performed to evaluate for obstructive emphysema

from foreign bodies or bronchial obstructive inflammation. Diagnosis is usually made by a high-resolution CT scan. Resection is performed as necessary for symptomatic patients.

Pulmonary Lymphangiectasia

Pulmonary lymphangiectasia (Figure 9-14) was first described by Virchow as diffuse cystic lymphatic duct dilation in infancy.[76,149] There are primary and secondary forms. The primary form involves dilated lymphatic channels within the lung, and the secondary form results from pulmonary venous obstruction. Both forms are symptomatic in neonates, with respiratory distress and cyanosis. Half of these patients have associated cardiac anomalies, usually involving venous return. Their chest radiographs demonstrate a "soap bubble" appearance with ground glass opacification. The prognosis is poor if lymphangiectasia is present bilaterally. Survival beyond infancy is rare. There is no specific treatment.

▶ VASCULAR ABNORMALITIES

Unilateral Absence of a Main Pulmonary Artery

Absence of a main pulmonary artery is exceedingly rare. The pulmonary vein is normal, and a systemic artery, which usually is adjacent to the trachea, supplies the affected lung. The patients develop recurrent respiratory infections and dyspnea in later childhood. These lesions are associated with cardiac anomalies. Hemoptysis is the most serious complication and may be associated with bronchiectasis. Pulmonary infection warrants surgical resection.

Idiopathic, Hyperlucent Lung Syndrome (Swyer–James or Macleod's Syndrome)

Hyperlucent lung syndrome is defined as a small or normal-sized lung with few pulmonary vessels and associated air trapping. It is a very rare anomaly with a prevalence of 0.01% in routine chest radiographs.[50] It was first described by Swyer and James,[139] and later by Macleod.[101] It is felt to result from chronic childhood lower respiratory tract infec-

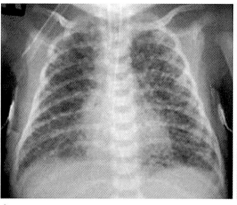
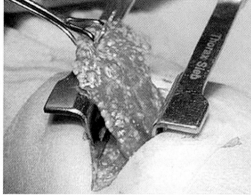

| A | B |

Figure 9–14 Pulmonary lymphangiectasia. The chest radiograph demonstrates the bilateral "soap bubble" appearance of lymphangiectasia. Gross findings at surgery demonstrate the cystic nature of the disease.

tions, potentially caused by bronchiolitis obliterans. From the chronic infections arise pulmonary vascular changes and bronchiectasis.

Patients are usually asymptomatic. The finding of a small or normal-sized lobe that is hyperlucent is incidentally discovered by chest radiography. The infants may have a mildly productive cough or dyspnea. CT and bronchoscopy are helpful in evaluating these patients. Agenesis or hypoplasia of the pulmonary artery can be associated with hyperlucent lung, but air trapping is absent, an important finding in this syndrome. A dynamic inspiratory and expiratory CT scan is performed to assess for trapping. The pulmonary vessels are markedly diminished. Hyperlucent lung usually requires no treatment, although surgical resection has been reported.[90]

Pulmonary Artery Sling

Pulmonary artery sling relates to an anomalous origin of the left pulmonary artery. It arises from the right pulmonary artery anteriorly and then passes over the right main stem bronchus behind the trachea and in front of the esophagus. It may be associated with tracheal stenosis secondary to complete cartilage tracheal rings. Symptoms include respiratory distress, choking, cyanosis, and stridor. The chest radiograph demonstrates hyperinflation. A bronchoscopy should be performed to rule out complete tracheal rings.[6] An esophagram and CT scan (Figure 9-15) may be helpful to assess the anatomy.

To correct the anomaly, the pulmonary artery is transected via median sternotomy with the use of extracorporeal circulation. The left pulmonary artery is transected and reanastomosed to the main pulmonary artery anterior to the trachea.[105] If tracheal stenosis is present, it may be treated at the same time. Others have reported an alternate procedure in which the trachea is divided and the left pulmonary artery is moved anterior to the trachea before the trachea repair is performed.[82,147] Backer and Mavroudis[7a] report no operative mortality in 27 patients who underwent repair of pulmonary artery sling via a median sternotomy.

Isolated Pulmonary Artery Aneurysm

Pulmonary artery aneurysm is a rare vascular anomaly. It was first described in 1947 by Deterling and Clagett.[36] The aneurysms are either fusiform or saccular. Approximately 40–50% of isolated aneurysms are congenital, and a familial pattern has been described.[2] Other causes include those resulting from trauma (e.g., penetrating stab wounds), prior chest tube placement, and pulmonary artery catheter–related injury with vessel wall laceration but contained bleeding. It also has been associated with infection from syphilis, tuberculosis (Rasmussen's aneurysms), or, more frequently, fungus.[41] Isolated pulmonary aneurysms also may be associated with a pulmonary vasculitis in giant cell arteritis or Behçet's syndrome. Behçet's syndrome usually has presenting symptoms of oral and genital ulcers and uveitis. It is a widespread vasculitis in which 5% of patients have pulmonary artery aneurysms from inflammatory destruction of the vasa vasorum. Hughes–Stovin syndrome may be a subset of Behçet's syndrome without the oral or genital ulcers, but with associated peripheral venous thrombosis.

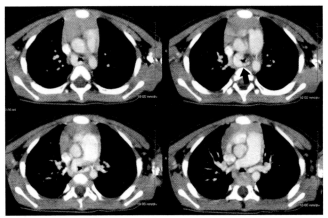

Figure 9–15 Pulmonary sling (aberrant left pulmonary artery). Four contiguous enhanced CT images at the level of aortopulmonary window show that the left pulmonary artery (*arrow*) arises from the right pulmonary artery. (*Courtesy Koji Takahashi, MD, Asahikawa Medical College, Asahikawa, Japan.*)

Patients with isolated pulmonary artery aneurysms are usually asymptomatic, and these lesions appear as a mass on a chest radiograph. They may rupture and cause uncontrollable hemoptysis or hemothorax. These aneurysms may occur in the main pulmonary artery, lobar artery, or segmental artery. They are further evaluated using high-resolution CT scan, MRI angiogram, or, classically, pulmonary artery angiogram. Transesophageal echo may be helpful to assess for any associated thrombosis.

Aneurysms that are enlarging or symptomatic should be treated.[148] If the lesions are fairly peripheral, embolization may be performed.[92] In patients who have Behçet's or Hughes–Stovin syndrome, immunosuppressive agents may be helpful in reducing the associated symptoms. Anticoagulation is used cautiously. Resection of the lung, primary resection of the pulmonary artery with reanastomosis, and/or patch repair has been performed. In the case of vasculitis there is a 25% recurrence.[144] The perioperative medical treatment with steroids and immunosuppressive drugs may help reduce this recurrence rate.

Pulmonary Varix

The pulmonary varix is an aneurysmal dilatation of a pulmonary vein. It may be seen in any area of the lung, and it is a very rare anomaly; as of 1988 only 71 cases had been reported.[146] It is believed that varying combinations of two processes may be important for the development of a varix: pulmonary venous hypertension and inflammatory changes in the area of the affected pulmonary vein. It has been described with bronchiectasis, tuberculosis, mitral valve disease, and also congenital cardiac anomalies. Single lesions are usually asymptomatic. The age range of presentation is between 7 and 82 years, and most patients have presenting symptoms in their fourth to seventh decades of life.[85] There is an equal gender distribution, and the symptoms usually are from the cardiopulmonary abnormality, not from the varix. Pulmonary varix has been described as a surprise discovery at cervical mediastinoscopy.[3] It also may have

134 presenting symptoms of cerebral embolism or hemoptysis from spontaneous rupture into a bronchus. In patients who have a varix from mitral valve disease, it is more frequently found in the right lung. If a varix is found, the patient should be evaluated for cardiac disease. On pulmonary angiogram, a Mueller maneuver (post-expiratory–inspiratory effort against a closed glottis) increases the size of the varix, whereas a Valsalva maneuver decreases its size. CT scan or dynamic CT may be helpful. There are three anatomical forms: saccular, tortuous, and confluent. The confluent form is that in which there is a dilation of the confluence of veins, and it is more frequently associated with mitral and left-sided heart disease.[146] If asymptomatic, and if there is no cardiac anomaly or infectious process, the patient may be observed and the prognosis is good.[72] If there is a cardiac anomaly, it should be repaired and the varix will frequently regress thereafter.

Pulmonary Arteriovenous Malformations

As the name implies, there is a direct connection between branches of a pulmonary artery and vein in pulmonary arteriovenous malformations (PAVMs). They may be acquired lesions from trauma, schistosomiasis, cancer, or actinomycosis. There is an association with pregnancy. One third of patients have hereditary hemorrhagic telangiectasia (HHT

or Osler–Weber–Rendu syndrome). Sixty-five percent are single lesions. The more diffuse lesions are frequently symptomatic in children and are associated with cyanosis and congestive failure. They also may have presenting symptoms of hemoptysis, chest pain, epistaxis, and/or palpitations. Over 50% are less than 1 cm in size, and they are rarely larger than 5 cm. They are frequently subpleural. Complications include hemoptysis, cerebral thrombosis, brain abscesses, and pneumothorax. The chest radiograph may demonstrate a noncalcified mass; dynamic CT scan may be helpful in achieving a diagnosis (Figure 9-16). When identified, the patient should be evaluated for any family history, recurrent epistaxis, skin lesions, or hematuria (HHT). HHT is a rare autosomal dominant abnormality that is associated with mucocutaneous and visceral telangiectasias. Between 7 and 15% of patients with HHT have PAVMs. When PAVMs are present, patients have an increased likelihood for complications.[38] The patients may have hemoptysis, polycythemia, epistaxis, cerebral bleeding, or brain abscesses. A contrast transthoracic echocardiogram has been helpful in assessing patients with PAVMs, with a sensitivity of 94%.

If the patient has HHT or is symptomatic, if the lesion is large, or if the diagnosis is questionable, surgical resection may be necessary. In the case of HHT, one half of patients left untreated progress to brain abscess and stroke.[53] If resected, proximal vessel control is advisable. When telang-

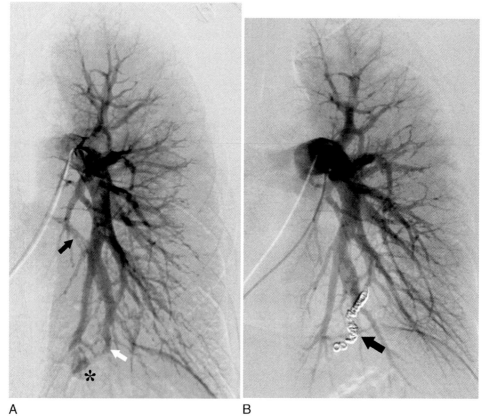

A   B

Figure 9–16 Pulmonary arteriovenous malformation. Selective left pulmonary arteriogram and coil embolization in a 14-year-old girl. **A,** Left pulmonary arteriogram shows a tangle of vessels (°) at left lung base with arterial supply *(white arrow)* from a basal branch of left lower lobe artery and early pulmonary venous opacification *(black arrow)*. **B,** After embolization of coils *(arrow)* using superselective catheterization, the malformation is occluded.
(Courtesy Simon C. Kao, MD, Iowa City, Iowa.)

iectasias are found, only symptomatic or enlarging lesions should be treated. When telangiectasias are present on the lung surface, it is unnecessary to resect them unless they are unusually large.

One other congenital anomaly of note is scimitar syndrome (Figure 9-17). In this condition the venous drainage from either part of the right lung or the entire right lung enters the inferior vena cava rather than the left atrium. Right lung arterial supply also may be anomalous with associated pulmonary sequestration and/or pulmonary hypertension. Left-to-right shunting may be so significant, akin to

an atrial septal defect, that surgical repair may be necessary. Surgical options recently have been reviewed.[20]

135

CONCLUSION

This chapter reviews the wide range of congenital lung diseases. Abnormalities may involve the tracheobronchial tree, lung parenchyma, and/or pulmonary vasculature. Defects may be so severe as to result in stillbirth or profound neonatal respiratory distress with cyanosis. Other manifestations assume a more insidious course. Knowledge of pulmonary embryology and historical contributions relating to these disorders allows a logical diagnostic and therapeutic approach in most instances. Advances in technology, neonatal surgery, and antenatal diagnosis and treatment have led to a markedly improved outlook for patients with congenital lung diseases.

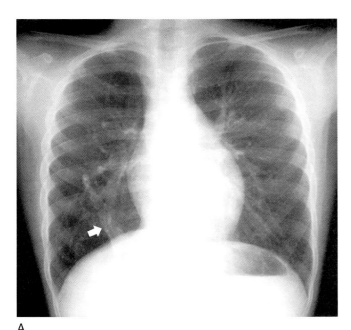

A

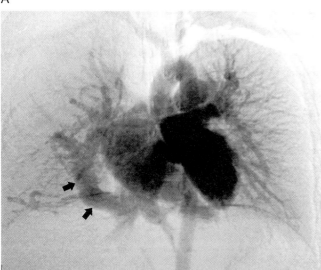

B

Figure 9–17 **Scimitar syndrome. A,** Frontal chest radiograph shows a curvilinear band–like shadow *(arrow)* parallel to right heart border with broadening toward the right hemidiaphragm. **B,** Digital subtraction angiogram shows anomalous right pulmonary venous drainage *(arrows)* to the junction between the hepatic venous confluence and the inferior vena cava.
(Courtesy Koji Takahashi, MD, Asahikawa Medical College, Asahikawa, Japan.)

REFERENCES

1. Adzick NS, Harrison MR, Crombleholme TM, et al: Fetal lung lesions: Management and outcome. Am J Obstet Gynecol 179:884–889, 1998.
2. Aoyagi S, Hiratsuka R, Takaseya T, Yokose S: Pulmonary artery aneurysm developed in a family. J Cardiovasc Surg (Torino) 43:661–663, 2002.
3. Arnett JC, Patton RM: Pulmonary varix. Thorax 31:107–112, 1976.
4. Atwell SW: Major anomalies of the tracheobronchial tree with a list of minor anomalies. Dis Chest 52:611, 1967.
5. Azizkhan RG, Grimmer DL, Askin FB: Acquired lobar emphysema (overinflation): Clinical and pathological evaluation of infants requiring lobectomy. J Pediatr Surg 27:1145, 1992.
6. Backer CL, Mavroudis C: Vascular rings and pulmonary artery sling. In Mavroudis C, Backer CL, editors: Pediatric Cardiac Surgery, 3rd ed. Philadelphia: Mosby, 2004.
7. Backer CL, Mavroudis C, Dunham ME, et al: Repair of congenital tracheal stenosis with a free tracheal autograft. J Thorac Cardiovasc Surg 115:869–874, 1998.
7a. Backer CL, Mavroudis C, Dunham ME, Holinger LD: Pulmonary artery sling: Results with median sternotomy, cardiopulmonary bypass, and reimplantation. Ann Thorac Surg 67:1738–1745, 1999.
8. Backer CL, Mavroudis C, Gerber ME, Holinger LD: Tracheal surgery in children: An 18-year review of four techniques. Eur J Cardiothorac Surg 19:777–784, 2001.
9. Bailey PV, Tracy T, Connors RH, et al: Congenital bronchopulmonary malformations. J Thorac Cardiovasc Surg 99:597–603, 1990.
9a. Bale PM: Congenital cystic malformation of the lung. A form of congenital bronchiolar ("adenomatoid") malformation. Am J Clin Pathol 71:411–420, 1979.
10. Bartlett RH, Toomasian J, Roloff D, et al: Extracorporeal membrane oxygenation (ECMO) in neonatal respiratory failure. Ann Surg 204:236, 1987.
11. Beals DA, Schloo BL, Vacanti JP, et al: Pulmonary growth and remodeling in infants with high-risk congenital diaphragmatic hernia. J Pediatr Surg 27:997–1002, 1992.
12. Becmeur F, Horta-Geraud P, Donato L, et al: Pulmonary sequestrations: prenatal ultrasound diagnosis, treatment and outcome. J Pediatr Surg 33:492–496, 1998.

136

13. Berlinger NT, Porto DP, Thompson TR: Infantile lobar emphysema. Ann Otol Rhinol Laryngol 96:106, 1987.

14. Bhutani VK, Ritchie WG, Schaffer TH: Acquired tracheomegaly in very preterm neonates. Am J Dis Child 140:449–452, 1986.

15. Blake MA, Chaoui AS, Barish MA: Thoracic case of the day: Mounier-Kuhn syndrome (tracheobronchomegaly). AJR Am J Roentgenol 173:822,824–825, 1999.

16. Boland RB, Schneider AF, Boggs J: Infantile lobar emphysema. Arch Pathol 61:289, 1956.

17. Bolton JWR, Shahian DM: Asymptomatic bronchogenic cysts: What is the best management? Ann Thorac Surg 53:1134–1137, 1992.

18. Breatnach E, Abbott GC: Dimensions of the normal human trachea. AJR Am J Roentgenol 142:903–906, 1984.

19. Breaux CW, Rouse TM, Cain WS, Georgeson KE: Congenital diaphragmatic hernia in an era of delayed repair after medical and/or extracorporeal membrane oxygenation stabilization: A prognostic and management classification. J Pediatr Surg 27:1192–1196, 1992.

20. Brown JW, Ruzmetov M, Minnich DJ, et al: Surgical management of scimitar syndrome: An alternative approach. J Thorac Cardiovasc Surg 125:238–245, 2003.

21. Brown MF, Lewis D, Brouillette RM, et al: Successful prenatal management of hydrops, caused by congenital cystic adenomatoid malformation, using serial aspirations. J Pediatr Surg 30:1098–1099, 1995.

22. Brown SB, Hedlund GL, Glasier CM, et al: Tracheobronchial stenosis in infants: Successful balloon dilation therapy. Radiology 164:475, 1987.

23. Cantrell JP, Guild HG: Congenital stenosis of the trachea. Am J Surg 108:297, 1964.

24. Ch'in KY, Tang MY: Congenital adenomatoid malformation of one lobe of a lung with general anasarca. Arch Pathol 48:221, 1949.

25. Chahine AA, Tam V, Ricketts RR: Use of the aortic homograft in the reconstruction of complex tracheobronchial tree injuries. J Pediatr Surg 34:891–894, 1999.

26. Chinoy MR: Lung growth and development. Front Biosci 8:d392–415, 2003.

27. Chitkara AE, Tadros M, Kim HJ, et al: Complete laryngotracheoesophageal cleft: Complicated management issues. Laryngoscope 113:1314–1320, 2003.

28. Cohen MD, Scales RL, Eigen H, et al: Evaluation of pulmonary parenchymal disease by magnetic resonance imaging. Br J Radiol 60:223, 1987.

29. Contencin P, Narcy P: Gastroesophageal reflux in infants and children: A pharyngeal pH monitoring study. Arch Otolaryngol Head Neck Surg 118:1028–1030, 1992.

30. Cooney DR, Minke JA, Allen JE: "Acquired" lobar emphysema: A complication of respiratory distress in premature infants. J Pediatr Surg 12:897, 1977.

31. Cooney DR, Thurlbeck WM: Pulmonary hypoplasia in Down's syndrome. N Engl J Med 307:1170–, 1982.

32. Davies MR, Cywes S: The flaccid trachea and tracheoesophageal congenital anomalies. J Pediatr Surg 13:363, 1978.

33. De Jose Maria B, Durdi R, Monclus E, et al: Management of tracheal agenesis. Paediatr Anaesth 10:441, 2000.

34. DeLorimer AA: Congenital malformations and neonatal problems of the respiratory tract. In Welch KJ, Randolph JG, Ravitch MM, et al, editors: Pediatric Surgery, 4th ed., Vol. 1, p. 631. Chicago: Mosby Year Book, 1986.

35. DeMuth GI, Sloan H: Congenital lobar emphysema: Long term effects and sequelae in treated cases. Surgery 59:601, 1966.

36. Deterling RA, Clagett DT: Aneurysms of the pulmonary artery: Review of the literature and report of a case. Am Heart J 34:471–498, 1947.

37. DiFiore JW, Alexander F: Congenital bronchobiliary fistula in association with right-sided congenital diaphragmatic hernia. J Pediatr Surg. 37:1208–1209, 2002.

38. Dines DE, Arms RA, Bernatz PE, et al: Pulmonary arteriovenous fistulas. Mayo Clin Proc 49:461, 1974.

39. Dodge-Khatami A, Backer CL, Holinger LD, et al: Healing of a free tracheal autograft is enhanced by topical vascular endothelial growth factor in an experimental rabbit model. J Thorac Cardiovasc Surg 122(3): 554–561, 2001.

40. Donahoe P, Gee PE: Complete laryngotracheal cleft; management and repair. J Pediatr Surg 19:143, 1984.

41. Dransfield MT, Johnson JE: A mycotic pulmonary artery aneurysm presenting as an endobronchial mass. Chest 124:1610–1612, 2003.

42. Dykes EH, Bahoric A, Smith C, et al: Reduced tracheal growth after reconstruction with pericardium. J Pediatr Surg 25:25–29, 1990.

43. Egrari S, Krishnamoorthy M, Yee CA, et al: Congenital bronchobiliary fistula: Diagnosis and postoperative surveillance with HIDA scan. J Pediatr Surg 31:785–786, 1996.

44. Evans JA, Greenberg CR, Erdile L: Tracheal agenesis revisited: Analysis of associated anomalies. Am J Med Genet 82:415, 1999.

45. Evans JA, Reggin J, Greenberg C: Tracheal agenesis and associated malformations: A comparison with tracheoesophageal fistula and the VACTERL association. Am J Med Genet 21:21–38, 1985.

46. Ferkol T, McDowell KM, Gauderer MW, et al: Sinopulmonary manifestations of congenital bronchobiliary fistula. Clin Pediatr (Phila) 33:181–184, 1994.

47. Filler RM, Forte V, deFraga JC, et al: The use of expandable metallic airway stents for tracheobronchial obstruction in children. J Pediatr Surg 30:1050–1056, 1995.

48. Fisher CC, Tropea F Jr, Barley CP: Congenital pulmonary cysts. J Pediatr 23:219, 1943.

49. Floyd J, Campbell DC, Dominy DE: Agenesis of the trachea. Am Rev Respir Dis 86:557, 1962.

49a. Fontano N: Responsionum and curationum medicinalium. Typis IO Annis IanssonII anno m. DC XXXIX, 1639.

50. Gaensler EA: Unilateral hyperlucent lung. In Simon M, Potchen EJ, LeMay M, editors: Frontiers of Pulmonary Radiology, pp. 312–359. New York: Grune & Stratton, 1969.

51. Gaissert HA, Grillo HC, Mathisen DJ, et al: Temporary and permanent restoration of airway continuity with the tracheal T-tube. J Thorac Cardiovasc Surg 107:600–606, 1994.

52. Giammona ST, Mandelbaum I, Battersby JS, et al: The later cardiopulmonary effects of childhood pneumonectomy. Pediatrics 37:79–88, 1966.

53. Gossage JR, Kanj G: Pulmonary arteriovenous malformations: A state of the art review. Am J Respir Crit Care Med 158:643–661, 1998.

54. Goto H, Boozalis ST, Benson KT, et al: High-frequency jet ventilation for resection of congenital lobar emphysema. Anesth Analg 66:684, 1987.

55. Greenholz SK, Karrer FM, Lilly JR: Contemporary surgery of tracheomalacia. J Pediatr Surg 21:511, 1986.

56. Grillo HC: Tracheal surgery. Scand J Thorac 17:67, 1983.

57. Grillo HC: Slide tracheoplasty for long-segment congenital tracheal stenosis. Ann Thorac Surg 58:613–619, 1994.

58. Grillo HC, Wright CD, Vlahakes GJ, et al: Management of congenital tracheal stenosis by means of slide tracheoplasty or resection and reconstruction, with long-term follow-up of growth after slide tracheoplasty. J Thorac Cardiovasc Surg 123:145–152, 2002.

59. Griscom NT, Wohl MEB: Dimensions of the growing trachea related to age and gender. AJR Am J Roentgenol 146: 233–237, 1985.

60. Gross RE: The Surgery of Infancy and Childhood. Philadelphia: W.B. Saunders, 1953.

60a. Gross RE: Congenital cystic lung: Successful pneumonectomy in a 3-week-old baby. Ann Surg 123:229–237, 1946.

61. Gross RE, Lewis JE Jr: Defect of the anterior mediastinum: Successful surgical repair. Surg Gynecol Obstet 80:549, 1945.

62. Gupta R, Singhal SK, Rattan KN, et al: Management of congenital lobar emphysema with endobronchial intubation and controlled ventilation. Anesth Analg 86:71–73, 1998.

63. Gustafson RA, Murray EF, Warden HE, et al: Intralobar sequestration: A missed diagnosis. Ann Thorac Surg 47:841–847, 1989.

64. Haben CM, Rappaport JM, Clarke KD: Tracheal agenesis. J Am Coll Surg 194:217–222, 2002.

65. Haller JA Jr, Golladay ES, Pickard LR: Surgical management of lung bud anomalies: Lobar emphysema, bronchogenic cyst, cystic adenomatoid malformation, and intralobar pulmonary sequestration. Ann Thorac Surg 28:33–44, 1979.

66. Haller JA Jr, Tepas JJ 3rd, White JJ, et al: The natural history of bronchial atresia. Serial observations of a case from birth to operative correction. J Thorac Cardiovasc Surg 79:868–872, 1980.

67. Harmon CM, Coran AG: Congenital anomalies of the esophagus. In O'Neill JA, Rowe MI, Grosfeld JL, et al, editors: Pediatric Surgery, 5th ed. St Louis: Mosby, 1998.

68. Harrison MR, Heldt GD, Brosch RC, et al: Resection of distal tracheal stenosis in a baby with agenesis of the lung. J Pediatr Surg 15:938, 1980.

69. Hazelrigg SR, Landreneau RJ, Mack MJ, et al: Thoracoscopic resection of mediastinal cyst. Ann Thorac Surg 56:659–660, 1993.

70. Hendren WH: Repair of laryngotracheoesophageal cleft using interposition of a strap muscle. J Pediatr Surg 11:425–429, 1976.

71. Hendren WH, McKee DM: Lobar emphysema of infancy. J Pediatr Surg 1:24, 1966.

72. Hipona FA, Jamshidi A: Observations on the natural history of varicosity of pulmonary veins. Circulation 35:471-75, 1967.

73. Hislop A, Reid L: New pathological findings in emphysema of childhood: I. Polyalveolar lobe with emphysema. Thorax 25:682, 1970.

74. Hiyama E, Yokayama T, Ichikawa T, et al: Surgical management of tracheal agenesis. J Thorac Cardiovasc Surg 108:830–833, 1994.

75. Hubbard AM, Crombleholme TM: Anomalies and malformations affecting the fetal/neonatal chest. Semin Roentgenol 33:117, 1998.

76. Huber A, Schranz D, Blaha I, et al: Congenital pulmonary lymphangiectasia. Pediatr Pulmonol 10:310–313, 1991.

77. Huber JJ: Observations aliquot de arteria singulari pulmoni concessa. Acta Helvet 9:85, 1777.

78. Hugh-Jones P, Whimster W: The etiology and management of disabling emphysema. Am Rev Respir Dis 117:343–378, 1978.

79. Jaffe RB: Balloon dilation of congenital and acquired stenosis of the trachea and bronchi. Radiology 203:405, 1997.

80. Jederlinic PJ, Sicilian LS, Baigelman W, et al: Congenital bronchial atresia. Medicine 66:73, 1987.

81. Johnson FR, Green FA: Tracheobronchomegaly: Report of five cases and demonstration of familial occurrence. Am Rev Respir Dis 91:35–50, 1965.

82. Jonas RA, Spevak PJ, McGill T, et al: Pulmonary artery sling: Primary repair by tracheal resection in infancy. J Thorac Cardiovasc Surg 97:548, 1989.

83. Jones VF, Eid NS, Franco SM, et al: Familial congenital bronchiectasis: Williams-Campbell syndrome. Pediatr Pulmonol 16:263–267, 1993.

84. Kamata S, Usui W, Sawai T, et al: Pexis of the great vessels for patients with tracheobronchomalacia in infancy. J Pediatr Surg 35:454–457, 2000.

85. Katagiri S, Itoh T: A case highly suspected of pulmonary varix. Nippon Kyobu Rinsho 36:537–540, 1977.

86. Katz I, Levine M, Herman P: Tracheobronchomegaly (Mounier-Kuhn syndrome): CT diagnosis. AJR Am J Roentgenol 88:1084–1094, 1962.

87. Kitano Y, Adzick NS: New developments in fetal lung surgery. Curr Opin Pulm Med 5:792, 1999.

88. Koltai PJ, Quiney R: Tracheal agenesis. Ann Otol Rhinol Laryngol 101:560–566, 1992.

89. Korngold HW, Baker JM: Nonsurgical treatment of unilobar obstructive emphysema of the newborn. J Pediatr 14:206, 1954.

90. Koyama T, Osada H, Kitanaka Y, et al: Surgically treated Swyer-James syndrome. Jpn J Thorac Cardiovasc Surg 49(11):671–674, 2001.

91. Kuhn JP, Brody AS: High-resolution CT of pediatric lung disease. Radiol Clin North Am 40:89–110, 2002.

92. Lacombe P, Frija G, Parlier H, et al: Transcatheter embolization of multiple pulmonary artery aneurysms in Behçet's syndrome: Report of a case. Acta Radiol Diagn (Stockh) 26:251–253, 1985.

93. Lally KP, Paranka MS, Roden J, et al: Congenital diaphragmatic hernia. Stabilization and repair on ECMO. Ann Surg 216:569–573, 1992.

94. Langston C: New concepts in the pathology of congenital lung malformations. Semin Pediatr Surg 12(1):17–37, 2003.

95. Lee R, Mendeloff EN, Huddleston C, et al: Bilateral lung transplantation for pulmonary hypoplasia caused by congenital diaphragmatic hernia. J Thorac Cardiovasc Surg 126:295–297, 2003.

96. Lester CW, Cournand A, Riley RL: Pulmonary function after pneumonectomy in children. J Thorac Surg 11:529, 1942.

97. Lincoln JC, Stark J, Subramanian S, et al: Congenital lobar emphysema. Ann Surg 173:55–62, 1971.

98. Loeff DS, Filler RM, Vinograd I, et al: Congenital tracheal stenosis: A review of 22 patients from 1965 to 1985. J Pediatr Surg 23:744–748, 1988.

99. Longacre JJ, Carter BN, Quill LM: An experimental study of some of the physiological changes following total pneumonectomy. J Thorac Surg 6:237, 1937.

100. MacArthur AM, Fountain SW: Intracavitary suction and drainage in the treatment of emphysematous bullae. Thorax 32:668–672, 1977.

101. Macleod WM: Abnormal transradiancy of one lung. Thorax 9:147–153, 1954.

102. Manschot HJ, Van Den Anker JN, Tibboel D: Tracheal agenesis. Anesthesia 49:788, 1994.

103. Mardini MK, Nyhan WL: Agenesis of the lung. Report of four patients with unusual anomalies. Chest 87:522, 1985.

104. Markowitz RI, Mercurio MR, Vahjen GA, et al: Congenital lobar emphysema: The roles of CT and V/Q scan. Clin Pediatr (Phila) 28:19, 1989.

105. Mashiach R, Hod M, Friedman S, et al: Antenatal ultrasound diagnosis of congenital cystic adenomatoid malformation of the lung: Spontaneous resolution in utero. J Clin Ultrasound 21:453–457, 1993.

106. Massumi R, Taleghani M, Ellis I: Cardiorespiratory studies in congenital absence of one lung. J Thorac Cardiovasc Surg 51:561, 1966.

107. Matsushima H, Takayanagi N, Satoh M, et al: Congenital bronchial atresia: Radiologic findings in nine patients. J Comput Assist Tomogr 36:860–864, 2002.

108. McLaughlin FJ, Strieder DJ, Harris GB, et al: Tracheal bronchus: Association with respiratory morbidity in children. J Pediatr 106:751–755, 1985.

109. Messineo A, Forte V, Joseph T, et al: The balloon posterior tracheal split: A technique for managing tracheal stenosis in the premature infant. J Pediatr Surg 27:1142–1144, 1992b.

110. Miguet D, Claris O, Lapillonne A, et al: Preoperative stabilization using high-frequency oscillatory ventilation in the management of congenital diaphragmatic hernia. Crit Care Med 22(suppl 9):S77–S82, 1994.

111. Milstein JM, Lau M, Bickers RG: Tracheal agenesis in infants with VATER syndrome. Am J Dis Child 139:77, 1985.

112. Mori M, Kidogawa H, Moritaka T, et al: Bronchial atresia: Report of a case and review of the literature. Surg Today 23:449–454, 1993.

113. Mounier-Kuhn P: Dilatation de la trachee: Constatations, radiographiques et bronchoscopies. Lyon Med 150:106–109, 1932.

114. Munnell ER, Lambird PA, Austin RL: Polyalveolar lobe causing lobar emphysema in infancy. Ann Thorac Surg 16:624, 1973.

115. Muraji T, Satoh S, Tsugawa C, et al: Slide tracheoplasty: A case report of successful concomitant reconstruction of extensive congenital tracheal stenosis and pulmonary artery sling. J Pediatr Surg 33:1658, 1998.

116. Nelson CS, McMillar IKR, Bharucha RK: Tracheal stenosis, pulmonary agenesis and patent ductus arteriosus. Thorax 22:7, 1967.

117. Olutoye OO, Coleman BG, Hubbard AM, et al: Prenatal diagnosis and management of congenital lobar emphysema. J Pediatr Surg 35:792–795, 2000.

118. Page DV, Stocker JT: Anomalies associated with pulmonary hypoplasia. Am Rev Respir Dis 125:861–870, 1982.

119. Payne WA: Congenital absence of the trachea. Brooklyn Med J 14:568, 1900.

120. Peters RM, Roos A, Black H, et al: Respiratory and circulatory studies after pneumonectomy in childhood. J Thorac Surg 20:484–493, 1950.

121. Ramsay G, Beatty H: Mucocele, congenital bronchiectasis, and bronchiogenic cyst. J Thor Surg 25:21–30, 1953.

122. Ribet ME, Copin MC, Gosselin B: Bronchogenic cysts of the mediastinum. J Thorac Cardiovasc Surg 109:1003–1010, 1995.

123. Ricinhoff WF Jr, Reichert FL, Heuer GJ: Compensatory changes in the remaining lung following total pneumonectomy. Bull Johns Hopkins Hosp 57:373, 1935.

123a. Rienhoff WF, Jr.: Pneumonectomy; Preliminary report of operative technique in 2 successful cases. Bulletin Johns Hopkins Hospital 53:390–393, 1933.

124. Rideout DT, Hayashi AH, Gillis DA, et al: The absence of clinically significant tracheomalacia in patients having esophageal atresia without tracheoesophageal fistula. J Pediatr Surg 26:1303–1305, 1991.

125. Sadler TW: Respiratory system. In Sadler TW, editor: Langman's Medical Embryology, 9th ed. Philadelphia: Lippincott Williams & Wilkins, 2004.

126. Sane SM, Sieber WK, Girdany BR: Congenital bronchobiliary fistula. Surgery 69:599, 1971.

127. Say B, Carpenter NJ, Giacola G, et al: Agenesis of the lung associated with a chromosome abnormality. J Med Genet 17:477–478, 1980.

128. Sbokos CG, McMillan IK: Agenesis of the lung. Br J Dis Chest 71:183, 1977.

129. Schwartz MZ, Filler RM: Tracheal compression as a cause of apnea following repair of tracheoesophageal fistula treatment by aortopexy. J Pediatr Surg 15:842–848, 1980.

130. Scully RE, Mark EJ, McNeely WF, et al: Case records of the Massachusetts General Hospital: Case 30-1997. N Engl J Med 337:916–924, 1997.

131. Slany E, Holzki J, Holschneider AM, et al: Flaccid trachea in tracheoesophageal malformations. Z Kinderchir 45:78–85, 1990.

132. Sloan H: Lobar obstruction emphysema in infancy treated by lobectomy. J Thorac Surg 26:1, 1953.

133. Sotile SC, Brady MB, Brogdon BG: Accessory cardiac bronchus: demonstration by computed tomography. J Comput Tomogr 12:144, 1988.

134. Stern Y, Willging JP, Cotton RT: Use of Montgomery T-tube in laryngotracheal reconstruction in children: Is it safe? Ann Otol Rhinol Laryngol 107:1006–1009, 1998.

135. St-Georges R, Deslauriers J, Duranceau A, et al: Clinical spectrum of bronchogenic cysts of the mediastinum and lung in the adult. Ann Thorac Surg 52:6–13, 1991.

136. Stocker JT, Madewell JE: Persistent interstitial pulmonary emphysema: Another complication of the respiratory distress syndrome. Pediatrics 59:847, 1977.

137. Stocker JT, Madewell JE, Drake RM: Congenital cystic adenomatoid malformation of the lung. Classification and morphologic spectrum. Hum Pathol 8:155–171, 1977.

138. Suen HC, Mathisen DJ, Grillo HC, et al: Surgical management and radiological characteristics of bronchogenic cysts. Ann Thorac Surg 55:476–481, 1993.

139. Swyer P, James G: A case of unilateral pulmonary emphysema. Thorax 8:133–136, 1953.

140. Taguchi T, Suita S, Yamanouchi T, et al: Antenatal diagnosis and surgical management of congenital cystic adenomatoid malformation of the lung. Fetal Diagn Ther 10:400–407, 1995.

141. Takahashi M, Murata K, Yamori M, et al: Horseshoe lung: Demonstration by electron-beam CT. Br J Radiol 70:964, 1997.

142. Tanita M, Kikuchi-Numagami K, Ogoshi K, et al: Malignant melanoma arising from cutaneous bronchogenic cyst of the scapular area. J Am Acad Dermatol 46(suppl case reports 2):S19–S21, 2002.

143. Tapper D, Schuster S, McBride J, et al: Polyalveolar lobe: Anatomic and physiologic parameters and their relationship to congenital lobar emphysema. J Pediatr Surg 15:931, 1980.

144. Tuzun H, Hamuryudan V, Yildirim S, et al: Surgical therapy of pulmonary arterial aneurysms in Behçet's syndrome. Ann Thorac Surg 61:733–735, 1996.

145. Unger JM, England DM, Bogus G: Interstitial emphysema in adults: Recognition and prognostic implications. J Thorac Imaging 4:86–94, 1989.

146. Uyama T, Monden Y, Harada K, et al: Pulmonary varices: A case report and review of the literature. Jpn J Surg 18:359–362, 1988.

147. van Son JAM, Hambsch J, Haas GS, et al: Pulmonary artery sling: Reimplantation versus antetracheal translocation. Ann Thorac Surg 68:989, 1999.

148. Veldtman GR, Dearnai JA, Warnes CA: Low pressure giant pulmonary artery aneurysms in the adult: Natural history and management. Heart 89:1067–1070, 2003.

149. Verlaat CW, Peters HM, Semmekrot BA, et al: Congenital pulmonary lymphangiectasis presenting as a unilateral hyperlucent lung. Eur J Pediatr 153:202–205, 1994.

150. Volpi A, Cavalli A, Maggioni AP, et al: Left atrial compression by a mediastinal bronchogenic cyst presenting with paroxysmal atrial fibrillation. Thorax 43:216–217, 1988.

151. Wales PW, Drab SA, Connolly B, et al: Horseshoe lung in association with other foregut anomalies: What is the significance? J Pediatr Surg 37:1205, 2002.

152. Walker LK, Wetzel RC, Haller JA: Extracorporeal membrane oxygenation for perioperative support during congen-

ital tracheal stenosis and repair. Anesth Analg 75:825–829, 1992.

153. Weber TR, Kountzman B, Dillon PA, et al: Improved survival in congenital diaphragmatic hernia with evolving therapeutic strategies. Arch Surg 133:498–502, 1998.

154. West KW, Bengston K, Rescorla FJ, et al: Delayed surgical repair and ECMO improves survival in congenital diaphragmatic hernia. Ann Surg 216:454–462, 1992.

155. Wildi SM, Hoda RS, Fickling W, et al: Diagnosis of benign cysts of the mediastinum: The role and risks of EUS and FNA. Gastrointest Endosc 58(3):362–368, 2003.

156. Woodring JH, Barrett PA, Rehm SR, et al: Acquired tracheomegaly in adults as a complication of diffuse pulmonary fibrosis. AJR Am J Roentgenol 152:743–747, 1989.

157. Woodring JH, Howard RS, Rehm SR: Congenital tracheobronchomegaly (Mounier-Kuhn syndrome): A report of 10 cases and review of the literature. J Thorac Imaging 6:1–10, 1991.

158. Worsnop CJ, Teichtahl H, Clarke CP: Bronchogenic cyst: A cause of pulmonary artery obstruction and breathlessness. Ann Thorac Surg 55:1254–1255, 1993.

159. Zamir O, Lernau OZ, Springer C, et al: Lung resection for bronchiectasis in children. Z Kinderchir 42:282–285, 1987.

Benign Lesions of the Lung

Doraid Jarrar and Robert J. Cerfolio

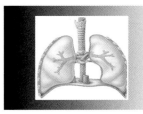

DEFINITION AND INCIDENCE

Benign lesions of the lung are rare. In one of the largest series reported, Martini and colleagues found that less than 1% of lung lesions resected at the Memorial Sloan-Kettering Cancer Center were benign.[16,25,26] A benign lung nodule is difficult to define and classify because some lesions that are called "benign" have malignant properties. However, the best definition of a benign lesion is one that is in the pulmonary parenchyma that does not metastasize and does not penetrate through surrounding tissue planes. When completely resected, a benign tumor lesion should not recur.[35] The controversy arises because some tumors often labeled as benign (such as pulmonary blastomas) have the potential to exhibit malignant properties, and thus clear-cut boundaries between malignant and benign often are blurred. Benign tumors of the lung can arise from all of the various cell types that are present in the lung. Box 10-1 lists the most common benign tumors based on their cells of origin.

Most times benign nodules are resected because of the inability to differentiate them from a malignant process. For this reason a benign lesion is identified after resection. Therefore the typical evaluation of a patient with an indeterminate pulmonary nodule is outlined first.

EVALUATION FOR AN INDETERMINATE PULMONARY NODULE

Probably the single most important test for a patient who arrives at the doctor's office with an indeterminate pulmonary nodule is the review of old chest X-rays (CXRs). If the nodule is new (not present on previous CXRs) or if the patient did not have a previous CXR, then chest computed tomography (CT) with or without intravenous contrast is helpful. If the nodule lacks calcification on chest CT, then it is indeterminate.[15,23] The radiogram should be interpreted in the context of the patient's medical history. Important factors include a history of a previous solid organ cancer and/or a history of smoking. The physical examination is typically unremarkable, without any neck adenopathy. Recently fluorodeoxyglucose-positron emission tomography (FDG-PET) scanning has become an important adjunct in the armamentarium of general thoracic surgeons in this text.[33,34,40] FDG-PET has helped physicians investigate an indeterminate pulmonary nodule that is larger than 6–8 mm (smaller nodules that are malignant can be missed by FDG-PET). If the nodule has glucose avidity and a standard unit value (SUV) of 2.5 or greater, it has a significant chance, above 90% in most series, of being malignant.[40] If the CT and/or FDG-PET scan is equivocal or positive, then resection is usually best if the patient's risks are acceptable. Needle biopsy, either by a transthoracic route or a transbronchial route, rarely changes the management of this type of nodule, especially if there is no lymphadenopathy. Definitive diagnosis is really only achieved by excisional biopsy, which can be performed via a video-assisted approach or an open technique, depending on many variables that are discussed elsewhere in this text.

In the remainder of this chapter we discuss the most common benign tumors of the lung and highlight the important clinical factors associated with each one. Each section is organized in the following fashion to help the reader find the pertinent points he or she is looking for: definition; incidence; any special history or physical examination findings; unique radiological characteristics; intraoperative tips for resection if indicated, pathological characteristics; and special postoperative care and/or follow-up care, including the risk of recurrence. Because some of these tumors are so rare, this format may be truncated to avoid redundancy.

HAMARTOMA

Hamartomas are the most common benign lung lesions and account for more than 70% of all nonmalignant tumors of the

142

Box 10–1. Common Benign Tumors of the Lung Based on Cells of Origin.

Tumors of epithelial origin

- Mucous gland adenoma
- Clara cell adenoma
- Mucous cystadenoma
- Pleomorphic adenoma

Tumors of mesenchymal origin

- Hamartoma
- Inflammatory pseudotumor
- Chondroma
- Fibroma
- Benign endobronchial fibrous histiocytoma
- Leiomyoma
- Lipoma
- Lymphatic lesions

Tumors of miscellaneous origin

- Nodular pulmonary amyloidosis
- Clear cell tumor (sugar tumor)
- Thymoma
- Granular cell tumor
- Teratoma
- Pulmonary paraganglioma

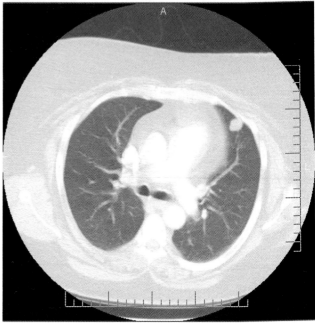

Figure 10–1 Computed tomography of the chest showing a chondroid hamartoma measuring 1.4 × 1.7 cm in the inferior lingual of the left lung. The patient was a 49-year-old female with a normal PET scan. Because her clinical presentation was suspicious for malignancy, a left upper lobe wedge resection was performed. Ninety percent of hamartomas are located in the periphery, and they account for about 4% of all solitary lung nodules.

lung.[3] They are mesenchymal tumors with a peak incidence in the sixth decade of life, and approximately 90% are asymptomatic. Men are affected twice as often as women. Ninety percent of these tumors present as solitary peripheral nodules and account for about 4% of all solitary pulmonary nodules (Figure 10-1). The 8–10% of hamartomas that have presenting symptoms such as cough, hemoptysis, and recurrent pulmonary infections are usually endobronchial lesions. Resection of these is usually needed even when a definitive biopsy has been performed on them, and they are proven to be benign because they cause local problems from airway obstruction. These problems include recurrent pneumonia, parapneumonic empyema, hemoptysis, and cough. Laser ablation can be used to help open the airway, but complete resection is preferred.

Cartilage is present in most lesions and is diagnostic of a hamartoma. Usually there are nests of cartilage surrounded by cellular fibrotic tissue. Mature fat cells are a frequent component, and their presence on CT scan (low Hounsfield units) is strong evidence for the diagnosis of a hamartoma.[19,24,36] Rarely, bone, vessels, bronchioles, and smooth muscle are found. On gross examination the bosselated appearance is typical for a hamartoma. The usual size is 1–3 cm, with the lesion being round and firm. They are easily shelled out from the surrounding lung tissue (Figure 10-2). As with any indeterminate pulmonary nodule, lung preserving techniques are best if possible.

Radiographically, as shown in Figure 10-3, hamartomas are peripheral lesions that are most often located in the lower lung fields and are well circumscribed. The majority are less than 4 cm in diameter, and calcifications can be appreciated on radiographs in 10–30% of cases (Figure 10-4). Calcifications are described as being "popcorn" like or

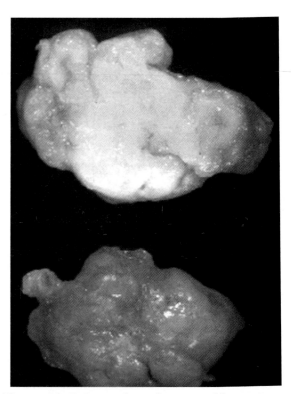

Figure 10–2 Cut surface of a resected hamartoma.

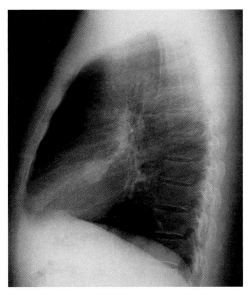

Figure 10–3 Lateral chest radiograph showing a round lesion consistent with a hamartoma.

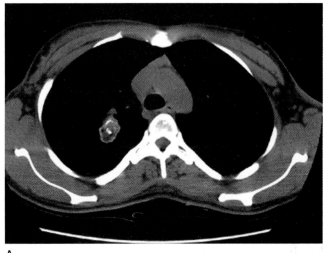

A

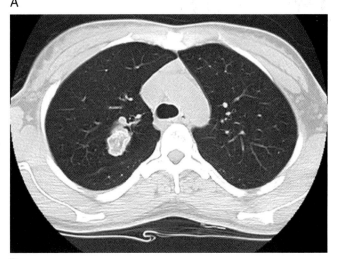

B

Figure 10–4 Right lung hamartoma. The lesion was resected, and benign pathology was confirmed. Lesions are most often located in the lower lung fields and are well circumscribed. The majority are less than 4 cm in diameter, and calcifications can be appreciated on radiographs in 10–30% of cases.

diffuse. Hamartomas display a slow growth rate (~3 mm/year) and are rarely multiple. Although only identifiable in half of the cases, fat density as identified by CT scan (low Hounsfield units) is strongly suggestive of a benign hamartoma.[1,9,28] Endobronchial lesions are not identifiable with radiographic examination, unless distal parenchymal changes have occurred (e.g., pneumonia or atelectasis).

Although percutaneous transthoracic needle aspiration yields a definitive diagnosis in up to 85% of cases, only a positive and specific result negates the need for excisional biopsy. Pending on the location, lesions might be amendable to video-assisted thoracoscopy (VATS) resection. Endobronchial lesions usually require a sleeve resection with lung preservation if possible. CO_2 or yttrium-aluminum-garnet (YAG) lasers, although effective at opening the airway, are rarely able to completely eradicate the offending lesion because of the lesion's depth of penetration.

Carney's triad is found infrequently and consists of a gastric epithelioid leiomyosarcoma, a functioning extraadrenal paraganglioma, and a pulmonary hamartoma.[9,28] Most commonly, the gastric lesion is the first cause, followed by the extraadrenal paraganglioma.

Although hamartomas are benign per se, several cases of malignancy arising at the resection site have been reported.[2] However, it appears that these synchronous or metachronous carcinomas are coincidental because the frequency is less than 7%. The etiology of these malignancies and their relationship to the hamartoma remain unknown.

► MUCOUS GLAND ADENOMA

Mucous gland adenoma is a rare, benign tumor arising from the mucous glands of the bronchus. The exact incidence is unknown, and several small series of case reports have been published. In order to be classified as a mucous gland adenoma, a tumor must contain cystic glands that are superfi-cial to the cartilaginous plate, it must be in the bronchus, and it must contain features of normal bronchial seromucous glands. Histologically, numerous small mucus-filled cysts lined by well-differentiated epithelium are observed (Figure 10-5).[1]

These benign lesions usually present because of hemoptysis, recurrent pneumonia, and persistent cough. The lesion itself does not have distinguishing radiographic features, but the chest radiograph may show obstructive pneumonitis. These tumors are evenly distributed between the left and right lung, with the major bronchi of the lower lobes being affected more often. They are soft, spherical, polypoid lesions that are usually less than 2 cm in diameter; however, lesions up to 6 cm have been reported.[22] They are noninvasive and well circumscribed. Although the lesions rarely have a stalk, stalks can be completely removed endoscopically by curettage, cryotherapy, or laser ablation. Surgical resection is only indicated if the distal lung tissue is destroyed or chronically infected.

144

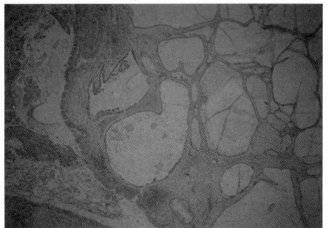

Figure 10–5 Photomicrograph of a mucous gland adenoma.

► INTRAPULMONARY FIBROUS TUMOR

Intrapulmonary fibrous tumors are contiguous with the visceral pleura and are identical to localized fibrous tumors of the pleura. Terms such as intraparenchymal localized fibrous mesotheliomas, intrapulmonary fibrous mesotheliomas, localized fibrous tumor of the pleura, and inverted fibrous tumor of the pleura have been used and are essentially interchangeable. The visceral pleura is the most common location of these tumors, but they also have been found in the retroperitoneum, mediastinum, and parietal surfaces of the intraabdominal viscera. The tumors are round to oval and contain a smooth cover of visceral pleura (Figure 10-6). Most lesions are less than 10 cm in diameter, and histological examinations show spindle cells with oval nuclei, diffuse fine chromatin, and positive staining for vimentin and the surface receptor CD 34.[8] In most cases the tissue of origin is the mesenchymal layer of the visceral pleura. No distinctive radiographic features are known for these lesions, although the radiologist often includes a malignant mesothelioma in the differential diagnosis. The obtuse angle

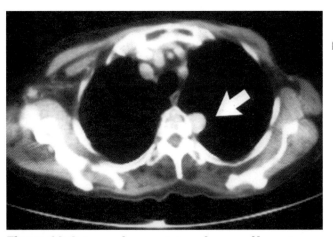

Figure 10–6 Arrow shows an intrapulmonary fibrous tumor. Lesions are contiguous with the visceral pleura. Tumors are round to oval and are usually less than 10 cm in diameter.

that these tumors make with the chest wall strongly suggests that the tumor is arising from the pleura and not from the lung. Unlike diffuse mesotheliomas, intrapulmonary fibrous tumors are not related to asbestos exposure. Surgical resection is usually performed via VATS, which usually offers complete resection because these lesions are often on a stalk and easy to remove. Resection is curative.[5]

► BENIGN ENDOBRONCHIAL FIBROUS HISTIOCYTOMA

A fibrous histiocytoma is a benign lung tumor that is composed of collagen and inflammatory and mesenchymal cells. These are rare endobronchial lesions that occur most often in either children or young adults.[13] Because they are so rare, their exact incidence is unknown. No specific radiographic findings distinguish these lesions from others. Depending on the location or the extent of bronchial involvement, surgical therapy might entail a lobectomy or sleeve lobectomy. Bueno and co-workers[6] described bronchoplastic resections of five endobronchial fibrous histiocytomas.

► GRANULAR CELL TUMOR

Granular cell tumors, also called granular cell myoblastomas, are another type of rare, benign tumor. They initially were thought to derive from skeletal muscle. However, evidence now suggests that these lesions originate from Schwann cells, as Deavers and associates[10] described in 20 cases. In half of the patients the lesion was an incidental finding. In the other half, symptoms were caused by obstruction, including postobstructive pneumonia and atelectasis. The lesions were solitary in 75% of the cases. Chest radiographs showed lobar infiltrates, coin lesions, and atelectasis. Tumors usually are located in a large bronchus and can protrude into the bronchial lumen, but they also can be found in the pulmonary parenchyma. Tumors usually are circumscribed but not encapsulated and range in size from 0.3–5.0 cm. Complete resection is curative, although recurrences have been described.[10] Epstein and Mohsenifar[14] reported the use of neodymium:YAG laser to treat obstructing lesions.

► INFLAMMATORY PSEUDOTUMOR

Inflammatory pseudotumors are usually asymptomatic solitary nodules that are found on routine CXR or CT scan.[7] However, they can be large or also be primarily of the airway (as shown in Figure 10-7). Because these tumors go by many other names, such as plasma cell granuloma–histiocytoma complex, plasma cell granuloma, histiocytoma, xanthofibroma, and xanthoma, there is often confusion. Inflammatory pseudotumors usually are well circumscribed, nonencapsulated, firm, white or yellow masses. Two major groups have been identified: fibrohistiocytic and plasma cell granulomas. In both groups the histological examinations reveal a mixture of inflammatory cells, including plasma cells; lymphocytes; and macrophages. Some reports have shown that there may be two types of inflammatory pseudo-

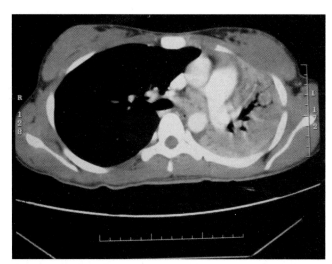

Figure 10–7 Inflammatory pseudotumor of the left main stem bronchus involving the carina. Patient has been treated successfully in the past with steroids. However, she has recently become afflicted with multiple pneumonias, and radiographic studies suggest that she has obstruction of the main stem bronchus. Patient did undergo left main stem bronchial sleeve resection.

tumors.[7] One type is invasive, large, and more difficult to resect as opposed to the other, which is characterized by a small, easily wedged mass without evidence of local tissue invasion. The mechanism for these two types is unclear, although microscopically it appears to depend on the degree of inflammatory cells present. A clinicopathological series from the Massachusetts General Hospital provided evidence that organizing pneumonia may be the nidus for the formation of inflammatory pseudotumors. Excision of these lesions usually is both diagnostic and curative. In patients with multiple lesions not amendable to excision, radiation or corticosteroid therapy are other options.

These unusual tumors can occur at any age, and there is no predilection for men or women. Although primary lung tumors are infrequent in childhood, plasma cell granuloma is the most common lung lesion in the preadolescent age category. Serial chest radiographs usually show the nodule to be unchanged in size, and in some patients it may even shrink without treatment. Slow growth occurs in less than 10% of cases.[27] On CT these lesions appear as a well-marginated, lobulated mass with some heterogenous attention.

▶ SQUAMOUS PAPILLOMA

Squamous papilloma is a benign epithelial neoplasm formed by squamous epithelium. Papillomas of the endobronchial tree have been classified into two main groups: multiple squamous papillomas and solitary papillomas.[11] Drennan and co-workers[12] also distinguished a third class, inflammatory polyps. Multiple squamous papillomas usually are seen in children with laryngeal papillomatosis, usually caused by human papillomavirus. Children can become infected during vaginal childbirth because their oropharynges and respiratory systems are exposed during the delivery. Serotypes 16 and 18 may act as promoters in carcinogenesis. On gross

examination the papillomas can be exophytic and have a component outside the bronchial wall and endophytic and obstruct part of the airway. There may be distal bronchiectasis with atelectasis or consolidation of the surrounding lung. Papillomas have a connective tissue stroma that often is heavily infiltrated with lymphocytes and covered completely with cuboidal or squamous epithelium.

Solitary squamous papillomas are rare and affect men, most commonly smokers, in their fifth to seventh decades of life. Productive cough, hemoptysis, wheezing, and dyspnea are common complaints as a result of obstruction by the lesion. Histologically they have a thin central fibrovascular core that is covered by stratified squamous epithelium, and they form multiple papillary fronds. CXR may show a lesion or atelectasis. The papillomas usually are located in segmental or more proximal bronchi. The human papillomavirus is the most common cause of these lesions.

Fibrous polyps are the third group and can be found solitary or in multiple locations. Usually they arise from the bronchial mucosa, have a fibrous stalk, and are covered by ciliated columnar epithelium. The stalk usually is composed of loose connective tissue with an infiltrate of plasma cells, lymphocytes, and eosinophils. These polyps are always benign and may be secondary to chronic inflammatory processes. Photodynamic therapy and laser or endoscopic removal are some of the options available to treat these lesions. Bronchotomy or sleeve resection usually are not needed. All three of these types of squamous papillomas can be associated with dysplasia, carcinoma in situ, and/or foci of invasive squamous cell carcinoma. Close surveillance and repeated biopsies are sometimes necessary when following these patients.

▶ NODULAR AMYLOID LESION

Nodular amyloid lesions represent a focal collection of amyloid deposition in the lung. They are most frequently found in the lower lobes. They are sometimes referred to as amyloidomas. They can occur as either a solitary nodule or multiple nodules. The following three types have been described: (1) tracheobronchial, (2) nodular pulmonary, and (3) diffuse pulmonary. Although nodular amyloid lesions are not associated with primary systemic amyloidosis, multiple myeloma should be ruled out. Patients usually are asymptomatic, and lesions are discovered incidentally on CXR. Patients should be followed up long-term because of the association with macroglobulinemia and malignant lymphoma. Surgical resection usually is curative.

▶ CHONDROMA

Chondromas are defined as benign cartilaginous tissue that can occur in the lung parenchyma or in the cartilaginous airways. Endobronchial lesions can cause obstructive symptoms, whereas parenchymal tumors are asymptomatic.[9] Histological examination of chondromas shows benign cartilaginous tissue. Some patients with this unusual lesion may have Carney's triad. This is made up of pulmonary chondroma, multiple gastric smooth muscle tumors, and extraadrenal paragangliomas.[9] The lesions may contain

146

metaplastic bone, mature cartilage, and myxoid stroma. Single lesions are most commonly resected for diagnosis and have an excellent prognosis. When patients have multiple lesions, a tissue diagnosis, often using a minimal invasive approach with a needle biopsy, usually is sufficient to make the diagnosis.

MYOEPITHELIOMA

Myoepitheliomas are rare, benign tumors arising from myoepithelial cells that lie between the epithelial cells of a gland and the basement membrane. Although these lesions are more commonly found in salivary glands and the breast, rare cases have been reported in the lung parenchyma. Strickler and associates[37] reported on two patients in whom these lesions were found. Both had a mass on chest radiograph. Immunostaining for S-100 was positive, which is consistent with the diagnosis of a myoepithelioma. These patients were followed up for several years, and no recurrence was observed. Surgery appears to be curative. Because these lesions are so rare, pathognomonic radiographic and clinical signs have not been described.

MUCINOUS CYSTADENOMA

Mucinous cystadenoma is a unilocular cystic lesion whose fibrous wall is lined by well-differentiated, benign columnar mucinous epithelium.[32] These lesions occur usually in the fifth and sixth decades of life in patients who smoke. However, their exact incidence is unknown. Most patients with this tumor are asymptomatic, and they represent an incidental finding on chest radiography. The lesions usually are located more toward the periphery. Once excised, the lesion appears as a unilocular cyst filled with gelatinous material. Sometimes the mucin extravasates into the surrounding lung parenchyma. Because these cysts may harbor adenocarcinoma, they should be completely excised. Microscopically these lesions may look similar to a bronchogenic cyst, as well as a bronchoalveolar carcinoma.

ALVEOLAR ADENOMA

Alveolar adenomas are proliferations of alveolar epithelium and septal mesenchyme. These lesions are extremely rare. Yousem and Hochholzer[41] reported one of the largest series with six patients, most of them women. Other smaller reports also have been published.[4] Lesions usually were identified on routine chest radiographs as an indeterminate nodule in the middle lung field. Excision appears to be curative.

LEIOMYOMA

Leiomyomas are benign lesions of the lung that can occur in the trachea, bronchus, or the pulmonary parenchyma itself. They account for about 2% of all benign lung lesions. Vera-Roman and co-workers[38] reviewed the literature and found

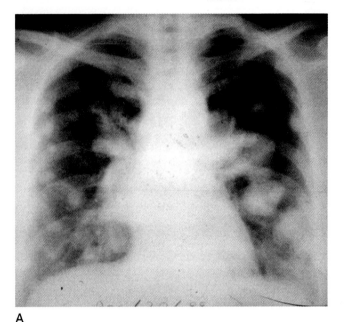

A

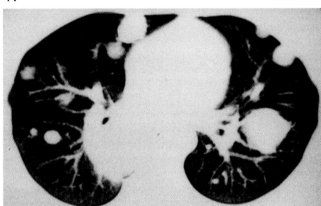

B

Figure 10–8 Benign metastasizing leiomyoma. These lesions occur in young women and are associated with leiomyomas of the uterus.

a female to male ratio of 1.5:1 (Figure 10-8). There are no discrete findings on physical examination. Some patients have hemoptysis if it is an endobronchial lesion, whereas in others, the tumor is an incidental finding on chest radiograph. It appears that the distribution between tracheobronchial and parenchymal lesions is equal. Histologically, smooth muscle differentiation is found. Some of these lesions stain for estrogen and progesterone receptors.[38] They may be dependent on a certain hormonal milieu, and this may explain why some of these lesions occasionally disappear during pregnancy.[21] Surgical treatment consists of excision and is the treatment of choice. Endobronchial lesions sometimes can be treated with laser ablation. Otherwise, sleeve bronchoplasty is needed. Benign metastasizing leiomyomas occur in young women and are associated with leiomyomas of the uterus.[31] Treatment consists of surgery, hormonal manipulation, and chemotherapy. Although labeled as a benign condition, these lesions can metastasize and cause death.

Lymphangiomyomatosis (LAM) is a rare disease primarily found in women of childbearing age and was first described in the medical literature by von Stossel in 1937.[30] It is characterized by progressive proliferation of spindle cells, resembling immature smooth muscle in the lung parenchyma and along lymphatic vessels in the chest and abdomen. The proliferation of spindle cells along the bronchioles leads to air trapping and eventually to the development of thin-walled cysts. Pneumothorax can be a complication when these cysts rupture. The proliferation of spindle cells also can affect the lymphatics and result occasionally in a chylous pleural effusion. Main symptoms stem from either a chylous pleural effusion (up to 80%) or a pneumothorax (30–50%). In both cases, dyspnea is the lead symptom.[20]

Radiographic presentation of LAM includes reticular, reticulonodular, miliary, and honeycomb patterns on plain X ray. CT scan usually shows multiple thin-walled lung cysts within normal lung parenchyma. The usual diameter of these cyst is between 0.2–5 cm. The disease pattern does not spare any lung zones and is distributed diffusely throughout the lungs. Hilar and mediastinal adenopathy are not uncommon. Diagnostic workup includes plain radiographs, chest CT scan, and lung biopsy. Biopsies can be obtained by either thoracoscopy or transbronchial biopsy. Unfortunately, most patients die within 10 years of the onset of symptoms. Although no definitive evidence has linked the disease to the estrogen levels, oophorectomy is an accepted treatment modality. Moreover, for LAM patients with severe disease, lung transplantation is an established therapy. The National Institutes of Health (NIH) currently conducts phase II trials using octreotide in patients with LAM to reduce symptoms from chylous effusions and/or ascites and peripheral lymphedema.

CLEAR CELL TUMOR (SUGAR TUMOR)

Clear cell tumor is a benign lesion of the lung of unknown tissue origin. Recent evidence suggests it originates from either Clara cells (nonciliated bronchiolar epithelium) or epithelial serous cells. More detailed examination of these tumors showed some neuroendocrine differentiation and positive staining for human melanin black or melanosome-associated protein and S-100. Radiographically the lesions are often peripheral and range in size from 1.5–3 cm.[17,18] Excision is curative. The differential diagnosis includes clear cell carcinoma and carcinoid, as well as renal cell carcinoma.

PRIMARY PULMONARY THYMOMA

A primary pulmonary thymoma is a tumor that is present in the lung in a patient with a normal mediastinal thymus gland. Pulmonary thymomas are quite rare, and their exact incidence is unknown. They can occur either peripherally or centrally. By definition the tumor must be within the visceral pleura, because ectopic mediastinal thymic tissue can be found in the aortopulmonary window, as well as in the aortocaval grove. No distinctive radiological features are known. Recent studies have used immunohistochemistry to confirm the diagnosis. Thymic T-lymphocytes must

be differentiated from lymphoepithelial-like carcinoma of the lung and from primary lymphomas.[39] Surgical resection usually is curative. However, in rare cases, when the tumor is extensive and complete resection is difficult, neoadjuvant therapy using radiation has been described (Figure 10-9).[29]

There are several tumors that are often called benign but that really represent a type of low-grade malignancy.

▶ CONCLUSION

Benign lesions of the lung are extremely rare and often are diagnosed only after complete surgical resection. If a nodule

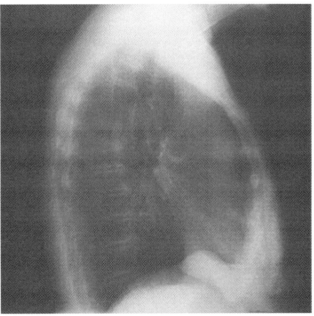

A

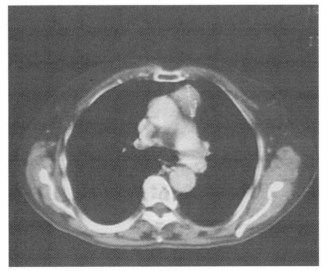

B

Figure 10–9 **Primary pulmonary thymoma.** In rare cases, when the tumor is extensive, radiation therapy may be a good alternative.

148 remains indeterminate after a thorough evaluation as described in the preceding sections, then resection is best if the patient's risk is acceptable. If surgery is not chosen, then careful follow-up is needed to ensure that a malignancy is not missed and is removed before it spreads. The solitary pulmonary nodule is a common radiological finding that can require an extensive evaluation to establish a benign or malignant diagnosis. Morphological evaluation of the size, margins, and contour with conventional imaging techniques alone often is not satisfactory. CT, PET, and PET-CT scans have added to the noninvasive armamentarium available to the general thoracic surgeon. However, careful interpretation of these tests are needed, and none supplant the need for tissue biopsy or, in some cases, complete excision. A negative needle biopsy does not exclude a malignant process. VATS, which offers minimal morbidity, allows for complete excisional biopsy. Even if the nodule is benign, this procedure offers peace of mind to the patient and obviates the need for repeated, expensive, time-consuming radiological tests. Benign lesions of the lung are most commonly a diagnosis of exclusion during the evaluation of an indeterminate pulmonary nodule. Benign lesions can have worrisome clinical presenting symptoms such as recurrent pneumonia, hemoptysis, and atelectasis. Although rare, the general thoracic surgeon should be familiar with the different types of benign lesions in order to counsel his or her patients and provide a differential diagnosis. The surgeon must be able to interpret the radiograms and also the disease, which often is equivocal in these lesions.

REFERENCES

1. Allen MS Jr., Marsh WL Jr., Geissinger WT: Mucus gland adenoma of the bronchus. J Thorac Cardiovasc Surg 67:966–968, 1974.
2. Altiner M, Paksoy N, Ozturk H: Large cell carcinoma of the lung with unilateral hamartoma. Pathologica 88:311–312, 1996.
3. Arrigoni MG, Woolner LB, Bernatz PE, et al: Benign tumors of the lung. A ten-year surgical experience. J Thorac Cardiovasc Surg 60:589–599, 1970.
4. Bohm J, Fellbaum C, Bautz W, et al: Pulmonary nodule caused by an alveolar adenoma of the lung. Virchows Arch 430:181–184, 1997.
5. Brunelli A, Sabbatini A, Catalini G, et al: Intrapulmonary benign fibrous tumor of the pleura. J Thorac Cardiovasc Surg 111:1292–1293, 1996.
6. Bueno R, Wain JC, Wright CD, et al: Bronchoplasty in the management of low-grade airway neoplasms and benign bronchial stenoses. Ann Thorac Surg 62:824–828, 1996.
7. Cerfolio RJ, Allen MS, Nascimento AG, et al: Inflammatory pseudotumors of the lung. Ann Thorac Surg 67:933–936, 1999.
8. Chang YL, Lee YC, Wu CT: Thoracic solitary fibrous tumor: Clinical and pathological diversity. Lung Cancer 23:53–60, 1999.
9. Dajee A, Dajee H, Hinrichs S, et al: Pulmonary chondroma, extra-adrenal paraganglioma, and gastric leiomyosarcoma: Carney's triad. J Thorac Cardiovasc Surg 84:377–381, 1982.
10. Deavers M, Guinee D, Koss MN, et al: Granular cell tumors of the lung. Clinicopathologic study of 20 cases. Am J Surg Pathol 19:627–635, 1995.
11. Dedo HH, Yu KC: CO_2 laser treatment in 244 patients with respiratory papillomas. Laryngoscope 111:1639–1644, 2001.
12. Drennan J, Douglas A: Solitary papilloma of a bronchus. J Clin Pathol 18:401, 1965.
13. Duncan JD, Greenberg SD, Mattox KL, et al: Benign fibrous histiocytoma: A rare endobronchial neoplasm. Int Surg 71:110–111, 1986.
14. Epstein LJ, Mohsenifar Z: Use of Nd:YAG laser in endobronchial granular cell myoblastoma. Chest 104:958–960, 1993.
15. Erasmus JJ, McAdams HP, Connolly JE: Solitary pulmonary nodules: Part II. Evaluation of the indeterminate nodule. Radiographics 20:59–66, 2000.
16. Flehinger BJ, Melamed MR, Zaman MB, et al: Early lung cancer detection: Results of the initial (prevalence) radiologic and cytologic screening in the Memorial Sloan-Kettering study. Am Rev Respir Dis 130:555–560, 1984.
17. Gaffey MJ, Mills SE, Askin FB, et al: Clear cell tumor of the lung. A clinicopathologic, immunohistochemical, and ultrastructural study of eight cases. Am J Surg Pathol 14:248–259, 1990.
18. Gaffey MJ, Mills SE, Ritter JH: Clear cell tumors of the lower respiratory tract. Semin Diagn Pathol 14:222–232, 1997.
19. Hamper UM, Khouri NF, Stitik FP, et al: Pulmonary hamartoma: Diagnosis by transthoracic needle-aspiration biopsy. Radiology 155:15–18, 1985.
20. Hancock E, Osborne J: Lymphangioleiomyomatosis: A review of the literature. Respir Med 96:1–6, 2002.
21. Horstmann JP, Pietra GG, Harman JA, et al: Spontaneous regression of pulmonary leiomyomas during pregnancy. Cancer 39:314–321, 1977.
22. Key BM, Pritchett PS: Mucous gland adenoma of the bronchus. South Med J 72:83–85, 1979.
23. Khouri NF, Meziane MA, Zerhouni EA, et al: The solitary pulmonary nodule. Assessment, diagnosis, and management. Chest 91:128–133, 1987.
24. Ledor K, Fish B, Chaise L, et al: CT diagnosis of pulmonary hamartomas. J Comput Tomogr 5:343–344, 1981.
25. Martini N: Results of Memorial Sloan-Kettering lung project. Recent Results Cancer Res 82:174–178, 1982.
26. Martini N: Surgical treatment of lung cancer. Semin Oncol 17:9–10, 1990.
27. Matsubara O, Tan-Liu NS, Kenney RM, et al: Inflammatory pseudotumors of the lung: Progression from organizing pneumonia to fibrous histiocytoma or to plasma cell granuloma in 32 cases. Hum Pathol 19:807–814, 1988.
28. McLaughlin SJ, Dodge EA, Ashworth J, et al: Carney's triad. Aust N Z J Surg 58:679–681, 1988.
29. Moiseenko V, Craig T, Bezjak A, et al: Dose-volume analysis of lung complications in the radiation treatment of malignant thymoma: A retrospective review. Radiother Oncol 67:265–274, 2003.
30. Pacheco-Rodriguez G, Kristof AS, Stevens LA, et al: Filley Lecture. Genetics and gene expression in lymphangioleiomyomatosis. Chest 121:56S–60S, 2002.
31. Parenti DJ, Morley TF, Giudice JC: Benign metastasizing leiomyoma. A case report and review of the literature. Respiration 59:347–350, 1992.
32. Roux FJ, Lantuejoul S, Brambilla E, et al: Mucinous cystadenoma of the lung. Cancer 76:1540–1544, 1995.
33. Sarinas PS, Chitkara RK: PET and SPECT in the management of lung cancer. Curr Opin Pulm Med 8:257–264, 2002.
34. Scott WJ: Positron emission tomography (PET) and combined imaging modalities for staging lung cancer. Surg Clin North Am 82:477–495, 2002.
35. Scott WJ: Surgical treatment of other bronchial tumors. Chest Surg Clin N Am 13:111–128, 2003.

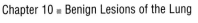
36. Siegelman SS, Khouri NF, Scott WW Jr., et al: Pulmonary hamartoma: CT findings. Radiology 160:313–317, 1986.

37. Strickler JG, Hegstrom J, Thomas MJ, et al: Myoepithelioma of the lung. Arch Pathol Lab Med 111:1082–1085, 1987.

38. Vera-Roman JM, Sobonya RE, Gomez-Garcia JL, et al: Leiomyoma of the lung. Literature review and case report. Cancer 52:936–941, 1983.

39. Veynovich B, Masetti P, Kaplan PD, et al: Primary pulmonary thymoma. Ann Thorac Surg 64:1471–1473, 1997.

40. Wong WL, Campbell H, Saunders M: Positron emission tomography (PET)—evaluation of 'indeterminate pulmonary lesions'. Clin Oncol (R Coll Radiol) 14:123–128, 2002.

41. Yousem SA, Hochholzer L: Alveolar adenoma. Hum Pathol 17:1066–1071, 1986.

Interstitial Lung Diseases

Subroto Paul and Yolonda L. Colson

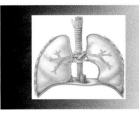

INTRODUCTION

Despite the common name, interstitial lung disease (ILD) is actually a group of over 200 individual clinical entities that is manifest by chronic, progressive, diffuse inflammation of the pulmonary interstitium. This inflammatory process may result from a primary pulmonary process, or may be the result of a systemic illness, such as a connective tissue disease (CTD). By definition, ILD does not include inflammatory responses secondary to known malignant or infectious etiologies and for the purposes of this chapter, will not include adult respiratory distress syndrome. However, these entities may present with very similar clinical and radiographic findings and, as such, are certainly in the clinical differential of immunological disease of the lung.

The interstitium includes the alveoli, epithelial and capillary cells within the alveolar wall, the septal tissues, and the connective tissues that surround the vascular, bronchial, and lymphatic structures within the lung parenchyma. Any or all of these structures may be involved in the inflammatory response. The pathological response to the resulting immunological insult permits a clinically useful, although not strict, categorization of ILD into those entities characterized by alveolitic and diffuse interstitial inflammation and those that result in a predominantly granulomatous pattern of disease (Box 11-1).

Either immunological response may progress from injury to fibrosis and thus all of these entities manifest themselves clinically as progressive dyspnea on exertion and/or a persistent nonproductive typically paroxysmal cough in the setting of radiographic evidence of interstitial opacities. Symptoms are usually chronic, increasing over years. However, presentation may be acute as in allergic responses seen with hypersensitivity pneumonitis, eosinophilic pneumonia, drug-induced alveolitis, or acute interstitial pneumonia or subacute as with sarcoidosis, alveolar hemorrhage syndromes, cryptogenic organizing pneumonia, and some of the CTDs.

Fatigue and weight loss are common. Wheezing, hemoptysis, or pleuritic chest pain may be present but are relatively rare as presenting symptoms in ILDs. In fact, the sudden onset or a marked increase in chest pain in the setting of these diseases is more suggestive of spontaneous pneumothorax, which occurs with increased frequency in histiocytosis X (pulmonary Langerhans cell histiocytosis), tuberous sclerosis, lymphangiomyomatosis (LAM), and neurofibromatosis. Hemoptysis is associated with diffuse alveolar hemorrhage (DAH) syndromes and the granulomatous vasculitides. Disease manifestation in other organ systems is helpful in the diagnosis of Wegener's granulomatosis or Goodpasture's syndrome. Age; gender; past medical, family, and smoking history; and occupational/environmental exposure all figure prominently in the development of a differential diagnosis for a particular patient. Physical examination usually reveals bibasilar end-inspiratory "Velcro" crackles but is less common in the granulomatous diseases. Baseline tachycardia is common. Cyanosis and clubbing can occur with advanced disease.

GRANULOMATOUS PATTERNS OF INTERSTITIAL LUNG DISEASE

Granulomas in their simplest form consist of activated immune cells, typically macrophages, encircling a particle that is not recognized by the antigen-specific, or adaptive immune system. The particle can be a foreign body or an

152

intrinsic protein antigen that results in the activation of the innate immune system. Innate immunity results in a non-antigen-specific means by which the body provides a first line of defense against foreign pathogens, such as inhaled irritants. These particles induce macrophage activation directly, without any need for prior exposure or antigen processing as is required for an adaptive T and B cell-dependent response. Activated macrophages mature to form epithelioid cells around the foreign material and thereby form a granuloma.[69] Both macrophage activation and the innate immune responses are directly influenced by specific signals generated by other cells of the immune system that may be triggered in an antigen-specific manner by the foreign particle.

Through this indirect pathway, the protein is processed by antigen-presenting cells, such as dendritic cells, and these protein antigen fragments are displayed on the cell surface in the context of the host major histocompatibility complex (MHC). Antigen-specific CD4+ T helper cells are activated in the context of MHC class II presentation whereas CD8+ effector T cells traditionally require the MHC class I complex. These activated T cells produce various cytokines, which subsequently lead to the activation of antigen-specific and nonspecific cellular subsets. It has been shown that activated Th1 subsets of CD4+ helper cells produce interferon-gamma (IFN-γ) and interleukin-2 (IL-2) leading to primarily macrophage activation. The Th2 subset of T cells, on the other hand, once activated, produce interleukin-4 (IL-4) and interleukin-5 (IL-5), which result in eosinophil production and activation.[3,68,69] Other T cells subsets, such as CD8+ effector cells, are also recruited to help "clear" the protein antigen and thus help regulate the immune system. This inflammatory process, once activated, results in the recruitment of other immune cells, complement, and growth factors to form discrete granulomas or may "spread" to the alveolar spaces and walls leading to alveolitic changes, as described later in this section. The process of granuloma formation is illustrated in Figure 11-1. Granulomatous mechanisms are involved in a variety of pulmonary diseases, yet they all share this fundamental pathophysiological mechanism. The clinical presentations and findings of these individual disease entities are described below.

► FOREIGN BODY/INORGANIC DUST

Patients who have inhaled foreign bodies are typically asymptomatic at the time of initial exposure unless the particle is large enough to occlude the tracheobronchial tree. In such cases, as often seen in children, the diagnosis is made by history and confirmed by chest radiography and, if needed, diagnosed as well as treated via bronchoscopy. Prolonged exposure to smaller foreign particles, whether organic or inorganic, can lead to a spectrum of pulmonary disease processes. Chronic exposure to metal dusts, such as beryllium, aluminum, and zirconium, where the foreign particle cannot be cleared by the mucociliary system or broken down by the pulmonary macrophages, is associated with a marked interstitial granulomatous disease pattern.[55] In contrast, continuous exposure to small organic particles in susceptible individuals can lead to hypersensitivity pneumonitis with both alveolitic and granulomatous responses.

► HYPERSENSITIVITY PNEUMONITIS

Hypersensitivity pneumonitis, also known as extrinsic alveolitis, describes a pulmonary disease process characterized by immunologically induced injury of the lung parenchyma with granuloma formation, alveolitis, and an antibody response, as the result of repeated exposure to inhaled protein antigen.[9,36,61] Numerous antigens have been implicated, from aspergillus and fish meal dust to male rat urine, leading to various interesting occupation-associated disease names (Table 11-1). Initial exposure to the antigen induces neutrophil and macrophage extravasation to the distal bronchi-

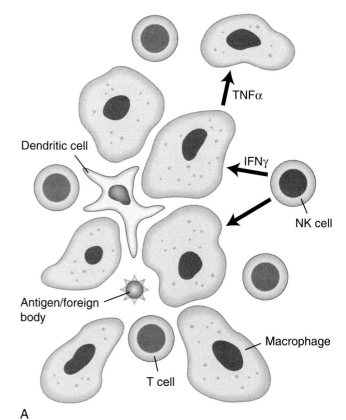

A

Figure 11–1 Granuloma formation and maturation. A, Early accumulation of macrophages around antigen/foreign body. Release of proinflammatory cytokines tumor necrosis (TNF)-α and IFN-γ, and chemokines such as MIP-1α results in activation of macrophages and recruitment of other immune cells.

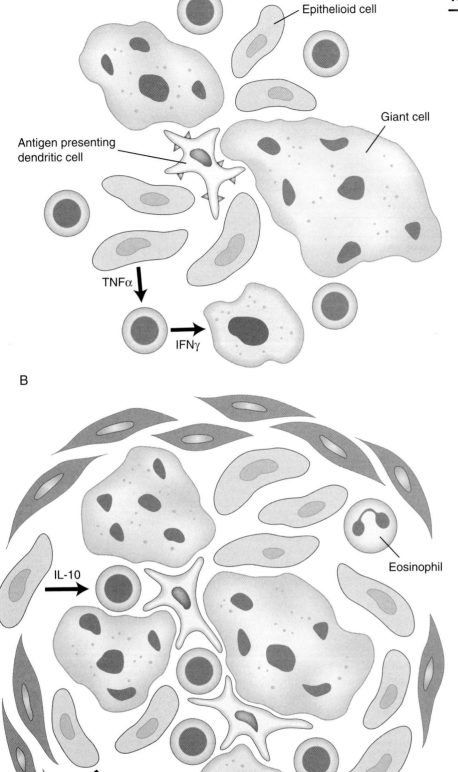

Figure 11–1 cont'd B, Antigen presentation by dendritic cells and macrophages to incoming T cells results in further activation with development of epithelioid and giant cells. It is at this stage that fibroblasts become activated resulting in focal areas of fibrosis. **C,** As the granuloma matures the structure becomes more compact with giant cells and T cells at the core. The initial Th1 response leads to the release of Th2 cytokines as well, with IL-5 recruitment of eosinophils.

Table 11–1

Selected Hypersensitivity Pneumonitis Syndromes

Syndrome	Antigen
Bagassosis	*Actinomycetes* species from sugar cane
Cheese washer's lung	*Penicillium casei* from moldy cheese
Compost lung	*Aspergillus* species from compost
Furrier's lung	Animal fur dust
Hot tub lung	Mold on ceilings
Laboratory worker's lung	Rat urine
Fish meal worker's lung	Fish meal dust
Woodworker's lung	Wood dust

oles and alveoli, thus leading to early alveolitis. Patients may present acutely with cough, fever, and chills several hours after exposure. With continued antigen exposure, patients develop a persistent cough with worsening dyspnea secondary to granuloma formation within the pulmonary parenchyma and progressive interstitial disease.[9,61] The diagnosis lies in careful history taking, especially where a known occupational exposure is suspected. Chest radiographs have no diagnostic pattern and may show a reticular nodular pattern consistent with "interstitial" lung disease. Chest computed tomography (CT) is typically nondiagnostic as well.[36,61] Bronchoalveolar lavage (BAL) may be helpful, showing an increase in CD4$^+$ T cells acutely and CD8$^+$ T cells chronically. However, this narrows the spectrum only marginally, as this is characteristic of nearly all granulomatous disease processes. Serum tests looking for antibodies to the suspected antigen are often required to make a diagnosis. Lung biopsy, either transbronchially or through video-assisted thorascopy (VATS) techniques or open thoracotomy, may be necessary to make a diagnosis in those patients for which other evidence is lacking; even this, however, may be ineffective in late stages of diseases where the acute granulomatous and alveolitic changes are replaced by interstitial fibrosis. Treatment consists of removing exposure to the suspected antigen and steroids for patients with the severe acute form of the disease or with chronic persistent fibrosis.[36,61]

▶ INFECTIONS

Pulmonary infection with *Myobacterium tuberculosis* is probably the most common cause of granulomatous lung disease worldwide.[3,12] Local as well as disseminated miliary

disease leads to granuloma formation in the infected field. Other infectious organisms such as *Aspergillus* and certain helminths can also lead to pulmonary granulomatous disease.[3] The clinical pathogenesis, presentation, course, and treatment of pulmonary infections are discussed elsewhere in this book, and are not included in this discussion of ILD.

▶ SARCOIDOSIS

Sarcoidosis is a chronic systemic disorder that, although common, is still poorly understood. Affected individuals often have other organ systems affected by granulomatous disease and patients may or may not manifest pulmonary involvement.[34,40,49] The exact incidence of sarcoidosis varies with the population studied. The incidence in Western populations is estimated to be 10–20 per 100,000 population with a higher rate in females and those of African ancestry.[71] Sarcoidosis is uncommon in Asian populations. Although, the disease can manifest at any age, most patient present between the ages of 20 and 40.[31,34,40,70]

The etiology of sarcoidosis is unknown. Environmental, infectious, hereditary, and immunological factors have been postulated, with variable evidence to support each hypothesis.[70] The interstitial granulomatous disease that results from inhalation of metal dusts is pathologically identical to sarcoidosis, suggesting that an unknown environmental exposure may be responsible.[17,30,55] Supporters of an infectious etiology argue that the causative agent must be inhaled as 80% of affected individuals have pulmonary and mediastinal lymph node involvement. In fact, BAL of individuals with extrapulmonary sarcoid contains inflammatory cells even without evidence of pulmonary disease. The causative agent is suspected by some to be *Mycobacterium tuberculosis* or other nontuberculosis mycobacteria. Genetic analyses of affected tissue by polymerase chain reaction (PCR) as well as antibody analysis of afflicted individuals have been inconclusive. Other agents implicated have been *Yersinia enterocolitica* and *Borrelia burgdorferi*. The evidence linking these agents to sarcoidosis, however, is even less well established. There is familial clustering of the disease and sarcoidosis has been linked in white individuals to human leukocyte antigens (HLA) A1 and B8, suggesting that hereditary and genetic factors play an important role in this disease. Non-MHC immunological factors are probably also involved, as patients with sarcoidosis have numerous abnormalities of the immune system, including altered T cell ratios, poorly responsive CD4$^+$ T cell subsets, hyperactive B cell lines, and altered production of the inflammatory cytokines, IFN-γ and RANTES by macrophages.[15,16,29,41,73]

Symptoms of sarcoidosis are variable and fluctuate with time. Most patients identified to have the disease by routine chest radiography are asymptomatic. Others may present with the acute onset of constitutional symptoms such as fever, chills, fatigue, and weight loss. Afflicted individuals often have associated CTD, such as rheumatoid arthritis, systemic lupus erythematosus, and progressive systemic sclerosis. Pulmonary symptoms include dyspnea and a dry cough.[31] Diagnosis is typically made radiographically with chest radiographs showing bilateral hilar and mediastinal lymph node enlargement with or without an accompanying reticulonodular pulmonary pattern indicative of interstitial disease. Consolidation and a ground glass pattern may also be evident, particularly on chest CT (Figure 11-2). Fibrosis is seen in later stages of the disease. Serum abnormalities may include an increase in levels of angiotensin-converting enzyme (ACE) levels, presumably produced by the activated macrophages within the granulomas. A preponderance of lymphocytes in the BAL suggests an alveolitic process with granulomatous changes. Diagnosis, however, is most often made by mediastinal lymph node biopsy if adenopathy is present.[5,18,31] In rare cases, transbronchial or VATS biopsy may be needed to establish the diagnosis.

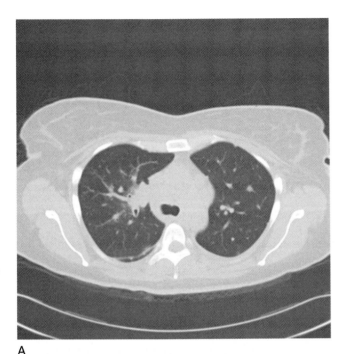

A

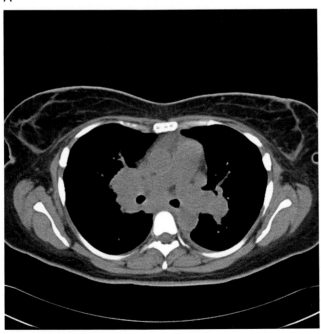

B

Figure 11–2 **(A, B) Computed tomography from a patient subsequently found to have noncaseating, nonnecrotizing granulomata within the mediastinal lymph nodes on cervical mediastinoscopy.** These findings are consistent with the diagnosis of sarcoidosis.

Histological findings of affected pulmonary tissue show noncaseating granulomas with high tissue ACE levels. Treatment consists mainly of steroids in symptomatic patients.[31] For advanced disease isolated to the lungs, lung transplantation is an option in select cases.

155

▶ GRANULOMATOUS VASCULITIDES: WEGENER'S GRANULOMATOSIS AND CHURG-STRAUSS SYNDROME

Wegener's granulomatosis is another systemic disorder, like sarcoidosis, which is characterized by granuloma formation and which may involve multiple organ systems. Wegener's is a rare disease with an incidence that varies between 1 and 3 in 100,000. Affected individuals typically present between the ages of 40 and 60.[2]

Wegener's granulomatosis is characterized in its most extreme form by necrotizing granulomatous involvement of the pulmonary parenchyma, as well as both pulmonary and renal vasculature.* Disease expressions is variable and the disease may be limited to the pulmonary system. Numerous etiologies have been suggested including infectious organisms such as parvovirus B19 and other respiratory agents, inhaled environmental agents such as silica, and genetic factors linked to the HLA alleles DR1, DR2, and DR12. Although all of these possible etiologies have some evidence to validate them, no explanation is conclusive. The sera of individuals afflicted with the disease contain antibodies to antineutrophil cystoplasmic antibodies (ANCA). Specifically, 90% of those with Wegener's granulomatosis have c-ANCA, which chiefly binds to the PR3 plasmic serine proteinase in neutrophils, as opposed to p-ANCA, which are antibodies to a perinuclear myeloperoxidase enzyme.[23,25,30] The exact role of c-ANCA in the pathogenesis of Wegener's granulomatosis is unclear and, unfortunately, ANCAs are also found in other disease states, such as systemic lupus erythematosus, in which ILD may develop.†

Individuals afflicted with Wegener's granulomatosis may present with fulminant disease, massive hemoptysis, and renal failure secondary to extensive necrotizing granulomatous lesions, or with the more subtle findings of fever, malaise, weight loss, and progressive dyspnea, which can lead to hemoptysis as the disease progresses. Neurological or ocular symptoms may also be present. Diagnosis relies not only on the history, but laboratory measures such as c-ANCA serologies and other associated systemic abnormalities.[23,30,53] Chest imaging shows a reticulonodular pattern consistent with "interstitial" disease or discrete nodules in only 50% of affected individuals. Central necrosis within these nodules can give the appearance of cavitary lesions (Figure 11-3). BAL from patients with Wegener's granulomatosis contains neutrophils and eosinophils. Biopsy of pulmonary and/or renal lesions may be necessary to establish or confirm the diagnosis. Pathology typically shows granulomas with neutrophils, macrophages, and eosinophils. Treatment options vary with the severity of the disease and include steroids and immunosuppressive agents, such as cyclophosphamide.[53]

156

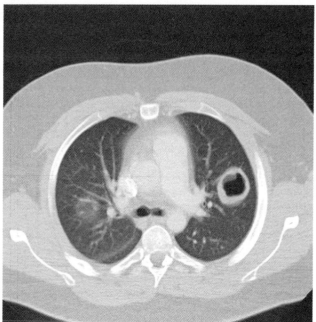

Figure 11–3 Computed tomography from a young male with Wegener's granulomatosis. Central necrosis within the granulomatous lesion gives the appearance of a cavitary lesion. Many other lesions were present throughout the lung parenchyma.

Churg–Strauss syndrome is a rare systemic disorder characterized by eosinophila, vasculitis, and pulmonary parenchymal granuloma formation. Many view this disease as part of a spectrum of disease that includes Wegener's granulomatosis and other CTD.[25,30,44] The true incidence is unknown because of the difficulty in establishing a diagnosis, but is estimated at 1–2 per 1 million people and affects individuals between the ages of 20 and 50.[19,30] Like Wegener's granulomatosis and sarcoidosis, multiple etiologies have been suggested including pigeon exposure, helminth infection, and cocaine use. Recently, Churg–Strauss syndrome has been associated with the weaning of steroids in asthma patients placed on leukotriene antagonists.[30,38,44,75]

Afflicted individuals typically have a history of asthma or allergic symptoms and present with fever, cough, and occasionally hemoptysis. Gastrointestinal bleeding or neuropathy may also be present. Diagnosis rests on clinical suspicion, and the combination of symptomology, laboratory studies, and pathological findings. Chest radiographs typically reveal patchy consolidation throughout the lung fields. Elevated immunoglobin E and p-ANCA levels may be present. As expected, the BAL shows large numbers of eosinophils.[5,18] Lung biopsy is usually required for diagnosis and demonstrates vasculitis and parenchymal granulomas with eosinophils. Treatment consists of steroid therapy. Prognosis for those diagnosed with the syndrome is poor with a mortality of 50–60% at 5 years.[25,44]

▶ EOSINOPHILIC PNEUMONIAS

Eosinophilic pneumonia is part of a spectrum of pulmonary processes that is distinguished by the accumulation of eosinophils in parenchymal tissue. Eosinophilic pulmonary diseases with known etiologies include those caused by helminth infections, such as *Strongyloides stercoralis* and *Ancylostoma duodenale* and drug allergies, which cause peripheral blood eosinophila and can have systemic effects, as well as those conditions associated with the granulomatous vasculitides discussed above in which the etiology is unclear.[33,65] All of these disease states can have pulmonary involvement. Diagnosis is made by history, blood eosinophil counts, blood serologies, and occasionally lung biopsy.

Idiopathic eosinophilic pneumonias can be divided into simple, acute, and chronic forms. Simple eosinophilic pneumonia, also known as Löffler's syndrome, is rare and is characterized pathologically by interstitial edema with abundant eosinophils. Patients typically present with few or no symptoms. Chest radiographs show patchy parenchymal consolidation, and the diagnosis rests on the demonstration of peripheral blood eosinophilia in patients with a history of asthma or atopy. The disease usually resolves spontaneously, and, therefore, biopsy or BAL is rarely indicated to make a diagnosis. Patients with symptoms or those with prolonged symptoms may benefit from steroid therapy.[33,65]

Acute eosinophilic pneumonia is a rare disorder that presents as an acute illness with severe respiratory distress that may require ventilatory assistance. Its etiology is unclear, but is thought to be secondary to an eosinophil-mediated immune response toward an unknown allergen. Patients present with severe shortness of breath and pleuritic symptoms. Chest radiography show reticular opacities similar to the pattern found with interstitial pulmonary edema. BAL samples from patients with this syndrome contain a high number of eosinophils, up to 80%, and are characteristic of this disease. Steroids are the mainstay of treatment, but a high relapse rate is associated with this disease.[33,65]

Chronic eosinophilic pneumonia has a similar histological, and in most cases, radiographic appearance. Diagnosis, again, relies on the demonstration of peripheral blood eosinophilia in patients with a history of asthma or atopy. However, affected patients have chronic symptoms that do not resolve overtime, and therefore eosinophilia on BAL and/or tissue biopsy is often needed to make the diagnosis.[18,65] Steroid treatment usually results in rapid disease regression.[33,65]

▶ HISTIOCYTOSIS X

Histiocytosis X, also known as eosinophilic granuloma, pulmonary Langerhan's cell histiocytosis, or Langerhan's cell granulomatosis, is a rare disorder characterized by the peribronchial accumulation of specialized antigen-presenting cells known as Langerhan's cells. Letter–Siwe and Hand–Schüller–Christian diseases are variants typically found in children and may or may not have pulmonary involvement.[6,32] The adult form, eosinophilic granuloma, is characterized by pulmonary and skeletal system involvement. Although rare, histiocytosis X predominantly occurs in whites and females. Viral infection with Epstein–Barr virus or other members of the herpes virus family has been suggested as a possible etiology for this disease.[6,32] Chest radiographs in the early stages of the disease show bilateral nodular opacities. With progression of disease, a reticulonodular pattern is noted. Patients are typically asymptomatic at the time of diagnosis in young adulthood. Diagnosis is commonly made by routine chest radiography. Symptomatic patients present with a dry cough and shortness of breath. BAL can be useful as Langerhan's cells are abundant in the fluid.[5,18,32] Lung biopsy will confirm clinical suspicions in unclear cases, since the demonstration of Langerhan's cells infiltrating the pulmonary bronchioles is pathognomonic of this disease. Despite its name, granulomas are not formed in the strict sense since the chief cellular component in these lesions is Langerhan's cells and not macrophages. Long standing disease leads to interstitial fibrosis. Remission may occur spontaneously and can often be aided with steroid therapy.[78]

ALVEOLITIC PATTERNS OF INTERSTITIAL LUNG DISEASE

When immunological injury is primarily directed toward the alveolar epithelial surface, inflammation of the alveolar wall and air spaces results in a histopathological pattern of alveolitis. Cellular as well as "humoral" components of the immune system are involved in these alveolitic changes in the lung. Alveolitic mechanisms are involved in a variety of pulmonary diseases (Box 11-1).[79]

Activated macrophages, T cells, and inflammatory cytokines discussed earlier can lead to B cell activation and antibody production. These antibodies form complexes with the antigen and are deposited within the lung parenchyma,

leading to the activation of complement. Although the formation of the membrane attack complex is an attempt to "destroy" the antigen, injury to the surrounding lung tissue may be significant if this inflammatory reaction is not regulated. Chemotactic peptides produced by the complement pathways, such as C5a and C3b, recruit other components of the cellular immune system. Neutrophils and macrophages thus destroy the pathogen and cause further parenchymal destruction. Activated macrophages and other immune cells produce additional cytokines, such as tumor necrosis factor and interleukin-1, which, together with immune complex deposition and complement activation, lead to direct injury to the lung parenchyma and surrounding vasculature. A basic diagram of this cascade is illustrated in Figure 11-4.[79] Numerous other cytokines and inflammatory modulators, such as prostaglandins, may also play important roles in the pathophysiology of ILDs. If the immune process continues unmitigated, the acute inflammatory response present within the lung parenchyma in the early phase of the disease is replaced by increasing degrees of fibrosis as more and more fibroblasts are recruited into the area of injury to repair the damage. Fibrosis is the final common pathway for both the alveolitic and granulomatous immune responses, making it often impossible to differentiate these two disease processes in the late stages of ILD. Irreversible scarring and fibrosis of the alveolar–endothelial interface and surrounding parenchyma result in significant impairment in gas exchange and are consistent with end-stage ILD. The clinical presentations and findings of

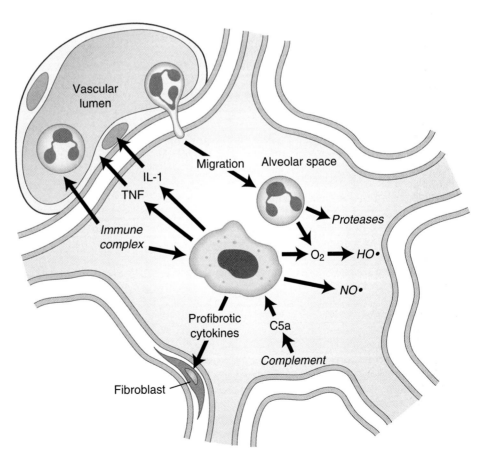

Figure 11-4 Pathogenesis of alveolitic injury. Activation of alveolar macrophages and polymorphonuclear leukocytes by complement, immune complex deposition, and subsequent cytokine/chemokine release triggers a cascade of responses that results in acute lung injury to the surrounding alveolar membrane and interstitium.

158 diseases characterized by a predominantly alveolitic pattern of ILD are described below.

▶ DRUG-ASSOCIATED INJURY

Whether directly toxic or immune mediated, drug-associated injury to the lung results in an alveolitic pattern of damage. Chronic concomitant damage often leads to irreversible fibrosis. As numerous drugs have been implicated in pulmonary injury, only key drugs and their mechanisms will be discussed. Direct toxic effects can result from radiation, bleomycin, nitrofurantoin, and prolonged exposure to high oxygen concentrations.[57] Injury in these cases is principally the result of free oxygen radical production. Acute changes are predominantly alveolitic followed by progressive fibrosis as the lungs recover from the initial insult. BAL specimens from patients during the acute phase contain numerous neutrophils and/or eosinophils.[5,18]

Amiodarone, a potent antiarrhythmic agent, has the ability to induce direct as well as immune-mediated injury. Direct amiodarone toxicity probably results from the generation of free oxygen radical species. However, the large numbers of lymphocytes in the BAL, particularly CD8+ T cells, suggest that immune-mediated mechanisms are also involved.[57,77] A fulminant form of amiodarone pulmonary toxicity has been described, especially in patients undergoing lung surgery, and that is probably an idiosyncratic immune response.[77] Chest radiographs in drug-associated ILD demonstrate an interstitial disease pattern. As fibrosis intervenes, the BAL specimen becomes acellular and the chest radiograph shows a more prominent reticulonodular pattern.[5,18] Diagnosis rests on the realization of prior drug exposure. Lung biopsy, if done in late stages, may show only fibrotic change.

▶ GOODPASTURE'S SYNDROME

Goodpasture's syndrome is characterized by the presence of pulmonary hemorrhage and glomerulonephritis. Its incidence is rare, predominantly affects males 15–25 years in age, and is linked to the HLA-DR2 MHC allele. Other immunological and hereditary factors as well as an association with free-base cocaine use have all been implicated.[35] The pathogenesis of alveolitis, pulmonary hemorrhage, and glomerulonephritis is due to the presence of antibodies directed against a collagen protein in the alveolar and glomerular membranes. These antibodies, as a result of complement activation and cell-mediated injury, result in immune complex-mediated injury to both lung and renal parenchyma.[4,8,29]

In most cases, patients present with hemoptysis and occasionally hematuria. Diagnosis is based on clinical symptomatology and the characteristic linear staining of the basement membrane with anti-IgG antibodies present on renal biopsy.[8,29] Chest radiographs demonstrate patchy consolidation secondary to hemorrhage. BAL is nondiagnostic and lung biopsy is rarely needed to make a diagnosis.[5,18] Therapy consists of plasmapheresis to remove the antibody and immunosuppressive therapy.

Idiopathic pulmonary hemorrhage is similar to Goodpasture's syndrome in terms of its pulmonary manifestations. However, this disease predominantly affects children less than 10 years of age and does not have any renal involvement. Patients present with hemoptysis and weakness secondary to iron deficiency. The radiographic appearance is similar to Goodpasture's syndrome, but the absence of anti-basement membrane antibodies in lung and renal biopsies differentiates the diagnosis. Prognosis is variable, and treatment consists of plasmapheresis and immunosuppressive therapy.[29]

▶ IDIOPATHIC INTERSTITIAL PNEUMONIAS

Idiopathic interstitial pneumonias are a spectrum of pulmonary disorders characterized by the infiltration of immune cells into the pulmonary interstitium and the resultant alveolitic changes. Unabated inflammation leads to fibrosis of the lung parenchyma. Multiple terms have been given to the various forms of this disease, including Hamman–Rich disease, idiopathic pulmonary fibrosis, usual interstitial pneumonitis, and diffuse pulmonary alveolar fibrosis, leading to much diagnostic confusion about this disease entity. A useful subclassification scheme based on the respective pathology has been proposed by Averill Liebow and a modification of this scheme is presented in Box 11-2. Many argue that even this classification scheme is arbitrary and that the diseases categorized are merely different manifestations of the same disease.[26,45,46] Nonetheless, many of these terms are in clinical use and therefore, even brief familiarity with the various terms and the histological findings is important (Table 11-2).

Usual Interstitial Pneumonia (UIP)/Idiopathic Pulmonary Fibrosis (IPF)

Usual interstitial pneumonia (UIP) refers to the "usual" pathological findings of thickened fibrotic alveolar interstitium infiltrated by inflammatory cells, such as lymphocytes and plasma cells. Histological analysis in the acute phase of the disease demonstrates alveolitis with an interstitium overrun with inflammatory cells and areas of patchy fibrotic changes.[26] Patients with "interstitial" lung disease on chest radiography and pathological evidence of UIP on lung biopsy are given the clinical diagnosis of idiopathic pulmonary fibrosis (IPF) when other causes of "interstitial disease" such as sarcoidosis, hypersensitivity pneumonitis,

---

Box 11–2. Idiopathic Interstitial Pneumonias.

Usual interstitial pneumonia (UIP)/idiopathic pulmonary fibrosis (IPF)
Desquamative interstitial pneumonia (DIP)
Nonspecific interstitial pneumonia (NIP)
Acute interstitial pneumonia (AIP)
Respiratory bronchiolitis-associated interstitial lung disease (RB-ILD)
Cryptogenic organizing pneumonia (COP)
Lymphocytic interstitial pneumonia (LIP)

Table 11–2

Summary of Histological Findings for Immunological Lung Diseases

Disease	Histology
Granulomatous	
Foreign body/inorganic dust	Simple granuloma
Hypersensitivity pneumonitis	Granulomas with CD4+/CD8+ T cells; interstitial edema; fibrosis in later stages
Infections	
Tuberculosis	Caseating granulomas
Sarcoidosis	Noncaseating granulomas
Granulomatous vasculitides	
Wegener's granulomatosis	Necrotizing granulomas involving vasculature
Churg–Strauss syndrome	Necrotizing granulomas involving vasculature
Eosinophilic pneumonias	Granulomas with eosinophilic predominance; interstitial edema
Histiocytosis X	Granulomas with Langerhan's cells
Alveolitic	
Drug-associated injury	Interstitial edema with inflammatory cells
Goodpasture's syndrome	Linear staining of basement membrane with anti-IgG antibodies typically seen on renal biopsy; interstitial edema with inflammatory cells
Idiopathic interstitial pneumonias	
Usual interstitial pneumonia (UIP)/idiopathic pulmonary fibrosis (IPF)	Interstitial edema and/or fibrosis with inflammatory cells; patchy fibrotic change
Desquamative interstitial pneumonia (DIP)	Interstitial edema with sparse inflammatory cells; mild diffuse fibrotic change
Nonspecific interstitial pneumonia (NIP)	Thickened interstitium with inflammatory cells; some patchy fibrosis
Acute interstitial pneumonia (AIP)	Diffuse alveolar damage with thickened fibrotic interstitium; proliferating fibroblasts
Respiratory bronchiolitis-associated interstitial lung disease (RB-ILD)	Macrophages infiltrating distal bronchioles
Cryptogenic organizing pneumonia (COP)	Chronically inflamed alveoli with granulation tissue in bronchioles and macrophages within alveoli
Lymphocytic interstitial pneumonia (LIP)	Diffuse lymphocytic and plasma cell infiltration; minimal alveolar injury

hystiocytosis X, or infection have been excluded. It is important to realize that the pathological finding of UIP and the clinical diagnosis of IPF are often used interchangeably in clinical practice.°

IPF occurs with an estimated incidence of 5–20 per 100,000 persons with a slightly male predominance.[19,20,28] The etiology of IPF is unknown. Heavy metal dusts, solvents, Epstein–Barr virus, and hepatitis C virus have all been named as possible mediators of the initial lung injury in susceptible individuals, but there has been no definitive proof for any of these theories.[18] Cigarette smoking has been implicated in some case–control studies. IPF has been linked to HLA-B15, HLA-B8, and HLA-B12 loci and a familial form of IPF has been described, suggesting a hereditary/immunological component to this disease.[7,24] Further evidence for an immunological basis lies in the fact that individuals afflicted with CTD, such as rheumatoid arthritis, systemic lupus erythematosus, and progressive systemic sclerosis, have a high incidence of interstitial inflammation and fibrosis that is clinically and pathologically indistinguishable from IPF.

Individuals with IPF present with progressive shortness of breath, weight loss, and a nonproductive cough. In 80% of individuals, the chest radiograph reveals linear opacities in a diffuse reticulonodular pattern. The lower lung zones may be preferentially involved. Chest CT expands on these findings by showing a reticular pattern with honeycombing cysts and ground glass opacities (Figure 11-5).[62,63] Mediastinal lymph node enlargement is common. BAL typically shows large numbers of neutrophils, eosinophils, and/or lymphocytes.[5,18,28] Patients with high levels of lymphocytes in their BAL fluid have been shown to have a better response to steroid therapy and an improved prognosis in some studies.[50,51] Transbronchial biopsy yields inadequate tissue to

°References 26, 28, 42, 48, 60, 66.

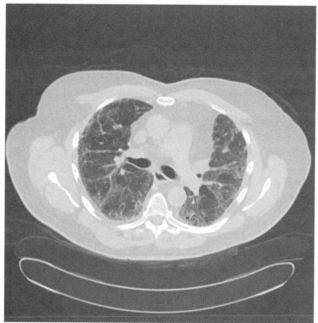

Figure 11–5 Computed tomography from a patient with idiopathic pulmonary fibrosis prior to undergoing single lung transplant.

make a diagnosis of IPF.[28] The principal role for lung biopsy is to exclude other etiologies of "interstitial" lung disease, which may alter the therapeutic plan or prognosis.

The mainstay of treatment for IPF is steroid and/or other immunosuppressive therapies, including methotrexate, penicillamine, colchicine, and cyclosporine. All have variable response rates. Lung transplant is indicated for those patients who deteriorate despite maximum medical therapy.[56,67] In general, single lung transplantation is the procedure of choice for patients with IPF or other end-stage ILDs that fail medical management.[27,28,54,59,76] The basic criteria for lung transplantation in this setting are as follows: (1) progressive dyspnea/hypoxia despite maximal medical therapy, (2) a vital capacity ≤60–70% predicted and/or a diffusing capacity ≤50–60% predicted, and (3) an age of 60 or less for double lung transplant or 65 or less for single lung transplant.[58] Diagnosis and treatment of pulmonary fibrosis associated with CTD are similar to that for IPF.[27,54,59] However, pulmonary symptoms typically wax and wane with the disease and often respond to treatment of the primary disease.[28] Lung transplant, as stated in the criteria above, is indicated in those patients with stable connective tissue disease and progressive pulmonary symptoms refractory to medical therapy.[58] Although the 5-year survival is only 50–60% following transplantation for IPF, this is a significant improvement over the 28-month median survival reported for medically treated IPF.[72]

Desquamative Interstitial Pneumonia (DIP)

Desquamative interstitial pneumonia (DIP) tends to be more uniform in appearance in histological section than UIP/IPF, and the interstitium is only mildly thickened with a sparse infiltrate of inflammatory cells and mild fibrosis. The inci-

dence of DIP is low and it affects smokers usually aged 40–50.[11,19,20,26,28]

Patients present with dyspnea and fatigue and the chest radiograph reveals characteristic bilateral ground glass opacities, which may be linear depending upon the degree of fibrosis. Chest CT further highlights these ground glass abnormalities. BAL specimens typically have less inflammatory cells than those from patients with IPF.[5,11,18,28] Lung biopsy, as for IPF, may be indicated to exclude other etiologies of "interstitial lung disease." However, the diffuse changes present throughout the lung in DIP may be seen focally in IPF, making it difficult to distinguish IPF from DIP by this means. Patients may respond to steroid therapy, but the disease is typically progressive. Lung transplant is indicated in end-stage disease.[11]

Nonspecific Interstitial Pneumonia (NIP)

Lung biopsy specimens from patients with nonspecific interstitial pneumonia (NIP) reveal a mildly thickened interstitium with an infiltrate of inflammatory cells and some fibrosis.[26,28,45,47] The incidence of NIP is rare with no gender predominance unlike UIP/IPF. Clinical presentation and radiological features of the disease are similar to UIP/IPF. However, NIP has a much better clinical response to steroid and immunosuppressive therapy and is associated with improved overall survival.[28,45,47]

Acute Interstitial Pneumonitis (AIP)

Acute interstitial pneumonia is rapidly progressive and clinically similar to acute lung injury and acute respiratory distress syndrome (ARDS), with the exception that there is no preceding trauma, sepsis, or known source of injury. Clinical presentation is one of rapid onset with progressive dyspnea, respiratory failure, and death usually within a year. Pathological examination of lung biopsy tissue consists of diffuse alveolar damage with a thickened fibrotic interstitium infiltrated by proliferating fibroblasts.[26,28] In very acute fulminant cases, the fibrosis can be replaced with an exudative interstitial edema similar to that found in diffuse alveolar damage (DAD), suggesting that AIP may be a point on the spectrum of disease between IPF and DAD. Radiologically, AIP is similar to ARDS in that chest radiographs and chest CT demonstrate characteristic bilateral patchy air-space disease and ground glass opacities. Prognosis for those afflicted with AIP, as for ARDS, is poor.[28]

Respiratory Bronchiolitis-Associated Interstitial Lung Disease (RB-ILD)

Respiratory bronchiolitis-associated interstitial lung disease (RB-ILD) is pathologically distinct in that it is characterized by the infiltration of macrophages surrounding the distal bronchioles.[39] Its incidence is rare and chiefly affects men aged 40–50 with a prior history of smoking.[28,39] Chest radiographs demonstrate a diffuse reticulonodular pattern. BAL samples are characteristic with abundant macrophages.[5,18] Biopsy is essentially to distinguish the disease from eosinophilic granuloma and histiocytosis X.[39] Treatment consists of steroid therapy.

Cryptogenic Organizing Pneumonia (COP)

Cryptogenic organizing pneumonitis (COP) or idiopathic bronchiolitis obliterans organizing pneumonia (BOOP) is an alveotic pulmonary disease characterized by chronic inflammation of the alveoli, the production of granulation tissue in the bronchioles and alveoli, and the accumulation of macrophages within the alveoli.[14,16,22,39,43] The incidence and etiology of COP are unknown, although an association with antibodies to nuclear proteins suggests an immune etiology.[13] Patients with this rare disorder present with weight loss and a nonproductive cough. Chest radiographs demonstrate bilateral diffuse opacities. Chest CT shows air-space disease with ground glass opacities, similar to other peribronchial processes, such as RB-ILD and histiocytosis X.[62,63] BAL fluid analysis reveals high levels of immune cells including lymphocytes, eosinophils, macrophages, and neutrophils. However, the definitive diagnosis is dependent upon lung biopsy.[14,16,22,39,43] Treatment consists of steroid therapy with a typically rapid response and resolution of the disease. Relapses do occur and are treated with steroids or other immunosuppressive regimens.

Lymphocytic Interstitial Pneumonia (LIP)

Lymphocytic interstitial pneumonia (LIP) is a lymphoproliferative disorder characterized by the infiltration of lymphocytes and plasma cells within the lung parenchyma.[7,52] There is minimal to no alveolar injury. It is included, however, in the differential diagnosis of "interstitial" lung disease and a lung biopsy may be required to exclude this disorder in some patients. LIP is a rare disorder predominantly seen in children, immunosuppressed patients, and women between the ages of 40 and 80 years. As with the vast majority of the ILDs discussed previously, the etiology is unknown. Afflicted individuals present with the nonspecific symptoms of fever, fatigue, and weight loss. Chest radiography and chest CT illustrate a reticulonodular pattern and sporadic ground glass opacities (Figure 11-6). BAL shows a large number of lymphocytes but lung biopsy is usually required to make the diagnosis in susceptible patient populations.[5,18] Progression to lymphoma has been documented, but initial treatment of LIP consists of steroid therapy.[10,52]

▶ PATIENT EVALUATION

In approaching patients with suspected ILD, a thorough history and physical examination are critical (Figure 11-7). The diagnosis may be suggested by a history of environmental/occupational exposures, CTD, or genetic diseases. A similar clinical picture can also be seen when intraparenchymal lymphatics are involved by malignant disease, and therefore a history or evidence of malignancy must be sought.[64] Laboratory studies are utilized to look for various antibodies to suggest a CTD, serum precipitins, or elevated angiotensin-converting enzyme.

Pulmonary function tests are utilized to measure the extent of pulmonary dysfunction. ILDs are usually characterized by restrictive pulmonary physiology with a reduced total lung capacity (TLC), functional residual capacity, and

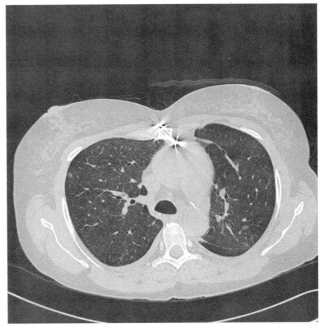

Figure 11–6 Computed tomography from a patient with progressive dyspnea in the setting of a connective tissue disorder. Open lung biopsy revealed a predominant T and B cell lymphocytic infiltrate with subsequent immunoperoxidase staining consistent with lymphocytic interstitial pneumonitis.

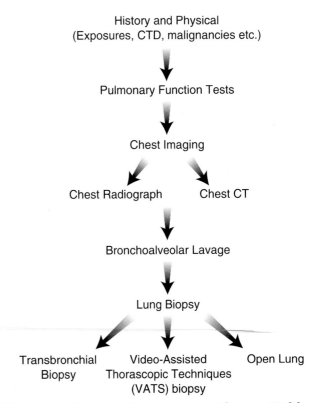

Figure 11–7 Approach to a patient with interstitial lung disease.

residual volume. The forced expiratory volume in 1 s (FEV_1) and forced vital capacity (FVC) are often decreased as a result of the decrease in TLC. The diffusing capacity for carbon monoxide (DL_{CO}) is impaired secondary to the reduced compliance of the lung parenchyma, and thus reflects the degree of resulting ventilation–perfusion ($\dot{V}/\dot{Q}$) mismatch, more so than the stage of disease. Arterial blood gases may be normal but can reveal hypoxemia as a result of significant $\dot{V}/\dot{Q}$ mismatch, particularly during exercise or sleep. Hypercarbia is usually indicative of end-stage disease. Chest imaging by plain film radiography and chest CT is helpful in separating "interstitial" disease patterns from consolidative patterns with their associated disease.[21] Chest radiography findings are often nonspecific with bibasilar reticular markings and may include nodular opacities, particularly in the upper lung fields in sarcoidosis, hypersensitivity pneumonitis, silicosis, berylliosis, and some of the CTD. High-resolution chest CT provides information as to the extent and distribution of disease and is particularly useful in the investigation of early disease when the chest radiograph may appear normal, and in the evaluation of coexisting adenopathy, malignancy, or emphysema, which impact subsequent treatment. In general, the radiographic appearance may not directly correlate with the histopathological stage of the disease or the degree of clinical impairment. However, the presence of classic radiographic findings on chest CT may be sufficient for diagnosis to obvi-

ate the need for tissue diagnosis. Furthermore, evidence of honeycombing and extensive fibrosis is indicative of a poor prognosis.

BAL can be useful in the identification of diseases with a large inflammatory component, such as Wegener's granulomatosis, or in the detection of α particular cellular subset as seen in eosinophilic pneumonias or histiocytosis X (Langerhan's cells), but is nonspecific in most forms of ILD.[5,18] Therefore in many cases, lung biopsy by transbronchial, open, or VATS is required to make a definitive diagnosis.[60] Transbronchial biopsy is usually attempted first, particularly if sarcoidosis, Goodpasture's syndrome, or eosinophilic pneumonia is a likely diagnosis, or to rule out lymphangitic carcinomatosis (Figure 11-8) or an infectious etiology. If definitive diagnosis is not possible, surgical biopsy of two distinct disease sites, preferably on two different lobes, is warranted and provides the most effective means of establishing a diagnosis and prognosis. If biopsy is performed early in the disease course prior to treatment and adequate-sized representative biopsies are obtained, avoiding areas of honeycombing that reveal only nonspecific fibrosis, the diagnostic accuracy approaches 90%.[37] Biopsy may not be necessary if the clinical and radiographic find-

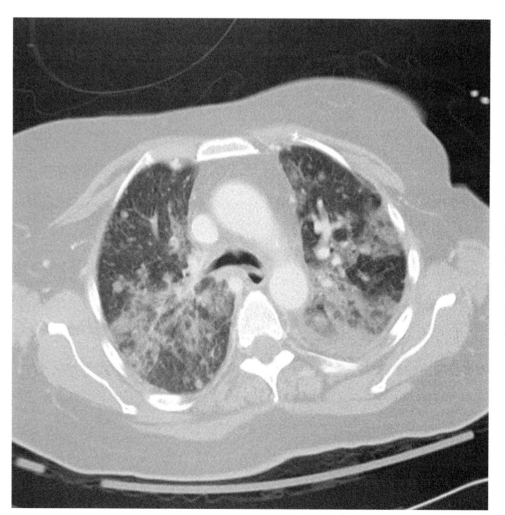

Figure 11–8 Computed tomography from a patient with a prior history of breast cancer and rapidly progressive bilateral ground glass opacities. Lung biopsy revealed metastatic adenocarcinoma. There was a desmoplastic reaction around the tumor in some areas leading to focal areas of interstitial fibrosis as well.

ings, i.e., extensive honeycombing, suggest that the patient is a high-operative risk or that there is little benefit given the extent or prognosis of the disease.

▶ TREATMENT

There is currently no known therapy that effectively reverses pulmonary fibrosis once it has occurred. Therefore treatment of hypoxemia with supplemental oxygen and early intervention to limit injury and prevent progression of the granulomatous or alveolitic process toward fibrosis is the primary goal. Unless a causative agent is identified that can be removed or specifically treated, success is low. Glucocorticoids, usually prednisone at 0.5–1.0 mg/kg/day for 4–12 weeks, is the cornerstone of medical therapy and is recommended for all symptomatic patients diagnosed with idiopathic, interstitial, eosinophilic, or cryptogenic organizing pneumonias, CTD, sarcoid, radiation, dust, or drug-induced ILDs. A slow taper over several months is attempted if symptoms are improved, as a rapid wean can be associated with recurrent disease. Only approximately 20% of patients with IPF will respond to steroids and this failure has led to treatment attempts with cyclophosphamide, aza-thioprine, methotrexate, and cyclosporine, with variable and inconsistent results. Although recent evidence suggests that IFN-γ may be helpful through its ability to modulate cytokines and the inflammatory response, the only currently available treatment option for the significant number of patients that are medical failures is that of lung transplantation.[1,46] If patients do not die awaiting a donor lung allograft and are successfully transplanted, the 5-year survival approaches 50–60%, significantly better than the median survival of 28.2 months seen with IPF.[72]

Diagnosis often does not affect treatment, as many of these diseases are treated by steroid or immunosuppressive therapy. It does, however, play a critical role in ruling out other diseases with vastly different treatments such as cancer and infection and in defining the overall prognosis of these patients and the potential therapeutic options available for treatment. It also allays patient and physician anxiety about diagnostic uncertainty later in the disease course if there is no response to therapy. End-stage therapy consists of lung transplantation. Early diagnosis permits close follow-up and is imperative to ensure "transplant listing" in sufficient time to allow survival until a donor organ is available.

REFERENCES

1. American Thoracic Society/European Respiratory Society International Multidisciplinary Consensus Classification of the Idiopathic Interstitial Pneumonias. This joint statement of the American Thoracic Society (ATS), and the European Respiratory Society (ERS) was adopted by the ATS board of directors, June 2001 and by the ERS Executive Committee, June 2001. Am J Respir Crit Care Med 165:277–304, 2002.
2. Aberle DR, Gamsu G, Lynch D: Thoracic manifestations of Wegener granulomatosis: Diagnosis and course. Radiology 174:703–709, 1990.
3. Adams DO: The granulomatous inflammatory response. A review. Am J Pathol 84:164–191, 1976.
4. Ball JA, Young KR Jr: Pulmonary manifestations of Goodpasture's syndrome. Antiglomerular basement membrane disease and related disorders. Clin Chest Med 19:777–791, 1998.
5. Baughman RP, Drent M: Role of bronchoalveolar lavage in interstitial lung disease. Clin Chest Med 22:331–341, 2001.
6. Ben-Ezra J, Bailey A, Azumi N, et al: Malignant histiocytosis X. A distinct clinicopathologic entity. Cancer 68:1050–1060, 1991.
7. Bitterman PB, Rennard SI, Keogh BA, et al: Familial idiopathic pulmonary fibrosis. Evidence of lung inflammation in unaffected family members. N Engl J Med 314:1343–1347, 1986.
8. Bolton WK: Goodpasture's syndrome. Kidney Int 50: 1753–1766, 1996.
9. Bourke SJ, Dalphin JC, Boyd G, et al: Hypersensitivity pneumonitis: Current concepts. Eur Respir J Suppl 32:81s–92s, 2001.
10. Bragg DG, Chor PJ, Murray KA, et al: Lymphoproliferative disorders of the lung: Histopathology, clinical manifestations, and imaging features. AJR Am J Roentgenol 163:273–281, 1994.
11. Carrington CB, Gaensler EA, Coutu RE, et al: Natural history and treated course of usual and desquamative interstitial pneumonia. N Engl J Med 298:801–809, 1978.
12. Chan ED, Iseman MD: Current medical treatment for tuberculosis. Br Med J 325:1282–1286, 2002.
13. Chapman JR, Charles PJ, Venables PJ, et al: Definition and clinical relevance of antibodies to nuclear ribonucleoprotein and other nuclear antigens in patients with cryptogenic fibrosing alveolitis. Am Rev Respir Dis 130:439–443, 1984.
14. Colby TV: Bronchiolitis. Pathologic considerations. Am J Clin Pathol 109:101–109, 1998.
15. Conron M, Du Bois RM: Immunological mechanisms in sarcoidosis. Clin Exp Allergy 31:543–554, 2001.
16. Cordier JF, Loire R, Brune J: Idiopathic bronchiolitis obliterans organizing pneumonia. Definition of characteristic clinical profiles in a series of 16 patients. Chest 96:999–1004, 1989.
17. Costabel U, Teschler H: Biochemical changes in sarcoidosis. Clin Chest Med 18:827–842, 1997.
18. Costabel U, Guzman J: Bronchoalveolar lavage in interstitial lung disease. Curr Opin Pulmon Med 7:255–261, 2001.
19. Coultas DB, Gong H Jr, Grad R, et al: Respiratory diseases in minorities of the United States. Am J Respir Crit Care Med 149:S93–131, 1994.
20. Demedts M, Wells AU, Anto JM, et al: Interstitial lung diseases: An epidemiological overview. Eur Respir J Suppl 32:2s–16s, 2001.
21. Dick JA, Morgan WK, Muir DF, et al: The significance of irregular opacities on the chest roentgenogram. Chest 102:251–260, 1992.
22. Epler GR, Colby TV, McLoud TC, et al: Bronchiolitis obliterans organizing pneumonia. N Engl J Med 312:152–158, 1985.
23. Falk RJ, Jennette JC: ANCA small-vessel vasculitis. J Am Soc Nephrol 8:314–322, 1997.
24. Fan K, D'Orsogna DE: Diffuse pulmonary interstitial fibrosis. Evidence of humoral antibody mediated pathogenesis. Chest 85:150–155, 1984.
25. Faul JL, Kuschner WG: Wegener's granulomatosis and the Churg-Strauss syndrome. Clin Rev Allergy Immunol 21:17–26, 2001.
26. Fleming MV, Travis WD: Interstitial lung disease. Pathology (Phila) 4:1–21, 1996.
27. Fraser RS, Colman, N, Muller, N, Pare PD: Connective tissue disorders. In Fraser and Pare's Diagnosis of Diseases of the Chest. Philadelphia: W.B. Saunders, 1999, pp. 1421–1487.
28. Fraser RS, Colman, N, Muller, N, Pare PD: Interstitial pneumonitis and fibrosis. In Fraser and Pare's Diagnosis of

Diseases of the Chest. Philadelphia: W.B. Saunders, 1999, pp. 1584–1626.

29. Fraser RS, Colman, N, Muller, N, Pare PD: Goodpasture's syndrome and idiopathic pulmonary hemorrhage. In Fraser and Pare's Diagnosis of Diseases of the Chest. Philadelphia: W.B. Saunders, 1999, pp. 1757–1769.

30. Fraser RS, Colman, N, Muller, N, Pare PD: Vasculitis. In Fraser and Pare's Diagnosis of Diseases of the Chest. Philadelphia: W.B. Saunders, 1999, pp. 1489–1532.

31. Fraser RS, Colman, N, Muller, N, Pare PD: Sarcoidosis. In Fraser and Pare's Diagnosis of Diseases of the Chest. Philadelphia: W.B. Saunders, 1999, pp. 1533–1583.

32. Fraser RS, Colman, N, Muller, N, Pare PD: Langerhan's cell histiocytosis. In Fraser and Pare's Diagnosis of Diseases of the Chest. Philadelphia: W.B. Saunders, 1999, pp. 1627–1640.

33. Fraser RS, Colman, N, Muller, N, Pare PD: Eosinophilic lung disease. In Fraser and Pare's Diagnosis of Diseases of the Chest. Philadelphia: W.B. Saunders, 1999, pp. 1743–1756.

34. Gal AA, Koss MN: The pathology of sarcoidosis. Curr Opin Pulmon Med 8:445–451, 2002.

35. Garcia-Rostan y Perez GM, Garcia Bragado F, Puras Gil AM: Pulmonary hemorrhage and antiglomerular basement membrane antibody-mediated glomerulonephritis after exposure to smoked cocaine (crack): A case report and review of the literature. Pathol Int 47:692–697, 1997.

36. Glazer CS, Rose CS, Lynch DA: Clinical and radiologic manifestations of hypersensitivity pneumonitis. J Thorac Imaging 17:261–272, 2002.

37. Green FH: Overview of pulmonary fibrosis. Chest 122:334S–339S, 2002.

38. Gross WL: Churg-Strauss syndrome: Update on recent developments. Curr Opin Rheumatol 14:11–14, 2002.

39. Guerry-Force ML, Muller NL, Wright JL, et al: A comparison of bronchiolitis obliterans with organizing pneumonia, usual interstitial pneumonia, and small airways disease. Am Rev Respir Dis 135:705–712, 1987.

40. Hunninghake G, Gadek J, Weinberger S, et al: Comparison of the alveolitis of sarcoidosis and idiopathic pulmonary fibrosis. Chest 75:266–267, 1979.

41. Hunninghake GW, Crystal RG: Pulmonary sarcoidosis: A disorder mediated by excess helper T-lymphocyte activity at sites of disease activity. N Engl J Med 305:429–434, 1981.

42. Hunninghake GW, Zimmerman MB, Schwartz DA, et al: Utility of a lung biopsy for the diagnosis of idiopathic pulmonary fibrosis. Am J Respir Crit Care Med 164:193–196, 2001.

43. Izumi T, Kitaichi M, Nishimura K, et al: Bronchiolitis obliterans organizing pneumonia. Clinical features and differential diagnosis. Chest 102:715–719, 1992.

44. Jennette JC, Falk RJ: Small-vessel vasculitis. N Engl J Med 337:1512–1523, 1997.

45. Katzenstein AL, Fiorelli RF: Nonspecific interstitial pneumonia/fibrosis. Histologic features and clinical significance. Am J Surg Pathol 18:136–147, 1994.

46. Katzenstein AL, Myers JL: Idiopathic pulmonary fibrosis: Clinical relevance of pathologic classification. Am J Respir Crit Care Med 157:1301–1315, 1998.

47. Katzenstein AL, Myers JL: Nonspecific interstitial pneumonia and the other idiopathic interstitial pneumonias: Classification and diagnostic criteria. Am J Surg Pathol 24:1–3, 2000.

48. Katzenstein AL, Myers JL: Idiopathic pulmonary fibrosis: To biopsy or not to biopsy. Am J Respir Crit Care Med 164:185–186, 2001.

49. Keogh BA, Hunninghake GW, Line BR, et al: The alveolitis of pulmonary sarcoidosis. Evaluation of natural history and alveolitis-dependent changes in lung function. Am Rev Respir Dis 128:256–265, 1983.

50. King TE Jr, Tooze JA, Schwarz MI, et al: Predicting survival in idiopathic pulmonary fibrosis: Scoring system and survival model. Am J Respir Crit Care Med 164:1171–1181, 2001.

51. King TE, Jr., Schwarz MI, Brown K, et al: Idiopathic pulmonary fibrosis: Relationship between histopathologic features and mortality. Am J Respir Crit Care Med 164:1025–1032, 2001.

52. Koss MN, Hochholzer L, Langloss JM, et al: Lymphoid interstitial pneumonia: Clinicopathological and immunopathological findings in 18 cases. Pathology 19:178–185, 1987.

53. Leavitt RY, Fauci AS: Wegener's granulomatosis. Curr Opin Rheumatol 3:8–14, 1991.

54. Lynch JP 3rd, Hunninghake GW: Pulmonary complications of collagen vascular disease. Annu Rev Med 43:17–35, 1992.

55. Maier LA: Clinical approach to chronic beryllium disease and other nonpneumoconiotic interstitial lung diseases. J Thorac Imaging 17:273–284, 2002.

56. Mapel DW, Samet JM, Coultas DB: Corticosteroids and the treatment of idiopathic pulmonary fibrosis. Past, present, and future. Chest 110:1058–1067, 1996.

57. Martin W: Injury from drugs. In Crystal R, West J, Barnes P (editors): The Lung: Scientific Foundations. Philadelphia: Lippincott-Raven, 1997, pp. 2465–2473.

58. Maurer JR, Frost AE, Estenne M, et al: International guidelines for the selection of lung transplant candidates. The International Society for Heart and Lung Transplantation, the American Thoracic Society, the American Society of Transplant Physicians, the European Respiratory Society. Transplantation 66:951–956, 1998.

59. Mayberry JP, Primack SL, Muller NL: Thoracic manifestations of systemic autoimmune diseases: Radiographic and high-resolution CT findings. Radiographics 20:1623–1635, 2000.

60. Miller JD, Urschel JD, Cox G, et al: A randomized, controlled trial comparing thoracoscopy and limited thoracotomy for lung biopsy in interstitial lung disease. Ann Thorac Surg 70:1647–1650, 2000.

61. Moran JV, Greenberger PA, Patterson R: Long-term evaluation of hypersensitivity pneumonitis: A case study follow-up and literature review. Allergy Asthma Proc 23:265–270, 2002.

62. Muller NL, Guerry-Force ML, Staples CA, et al: Differential diagnosis of bronchiolitis obliterans with organizing pneumonia and usual interstitial pneumonia: Clinical, functional, and radiologic findings. Radiology 162:151–156, 1987.

63. Nagai S, Kitaichi M, Itoh H, et al: Idiopathic nonspecific interstitial pneumonia/fibrosis: Comparison with idiopathic pulmonary fibrosis and BOOP. Eur Respir J 12:1010–1019, 1998.

64. Nanki N, Fujita J, Yamaji Y, et al: Nonspecific interstitial pneumonia/fibrosis completely recovered by adding cyclophosphamide to corticosteroids. Intern Med 41:867–870, 2002.

65. Pope-Harman AL, Davis WB, Allen ED, et al: Acute eosinophilic pneumonia. A summary of 15 cases and review of the literature. Medicine (Baltimore) 75:334–342, 1996.

66. Ravini M, Ferraro G, Barbieri B, et al: Changing strategies of lung biopsies in diffuse lung diseases: The impact of video-assisted thoracoscopy. Eur Respir J 11:99–103, 1998.

67. Rennard SI, Bitterman PB, Ozaki T, et al: Colchicine suppresses the release of fibroblast growth factors from alveolar macrophages in vitro. The basis of a possible therapeutic approach to the fibrotic disorders. Am Rev Respir Dis 137:181–185, 1988.

68. Reynolds HY, Huck JL: Immunologic responses in the lung. Respiration 57:221–228, 1990.

69. Robinson D, Richeldi L, Saltini C, du Bois R: Granulomatous processes. In Crystal R, West, J, Barnes P (editors): The Lung: Scientific Foundations. Philadelphia: Lippincott-Raven, 1997, pp. 2395–2409.

70. Rybicki BA, Maliarik MJ, Major M, et al: Genetics of sarcoidosis. Clin Chest Med 18:707–717, 1997.

71. Rybicki BA, Major M, Popovich J Jr, et al: Racial differences in sarcoidosis incidence: A 5-year study in a health maintenance organization. Am J Epidemiol 145:234–241, 1997.

72. Schwartz DA, Helmers RA, Galvin JR, et al: Determinants of survival in idiopathic pulmonary fibrosis. Am J Respir Crit Care Med 149:450–454, 1994.

73. Sharma OP: Sarcoidosis and other autoimmune disorders. Curr Opin Pulmon Med 8:452–456, 2002.

74. Sneller MC, Fauci AS: Pathogenesis of vasculitis syndromes. Med Clin North Am 81:221–242, 1997.

75. Stoloff S, Stempel DA: Churg-Strauss syndrome: Is there an association with leukotriene modifiers? Chest 118:1515–1516, 2000.

76. Sulica R, Teirstein A, Padilla ML: Lung transplantation in interstitial lung disease. Curr Opin Pulmon Med 7:314–322, 2001.

77. Van Mieghem W, Coolen L, Malysse I, et al: Amiodarone and the development of ARDS after lung surgery. Chest 105:1642–1645, 1994.

78. Vassallo R, Ryu JH, Schroeder DR, et al: Clinical outcomes of pulmonary Langerhans'-cell histiocytosis in adults. N Engl J Med 346:484–490, 2002.

79. Warren JaW P: Immunoglobulin- and complement-mediated immune injury. In Crystal R, West J, Barnes P (editors): The Lung: Scientific Foundations. Philadelphia: Lippincott-Raven, 1997, pp. 2411–2419.

Infectious Lung Diseases

John D. Mitchell and Marvin Pomerantz

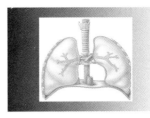

INTRODUCTION

The development of techniques to treat complications of infectious lung disease formed the cornerstone of modern thoracic surgery, dominating the specialty until about 1960. Although advances in critical care, antibiotic therapy, and other alternative treatments have lessened the impact of many lung infections in the practice of today's cardiothoracic surgeon, current evidence suggests other categories of pulmonary infection are on the rise. There are several reasons for this change: the use of broad-spectrum antimicrobial agents, selecting out resistant organisms; the emergence of new, opportunistic organisms, freshly minted as human pathogens; the widespread application of transplant techniques, accompanied by the ubiquitous immunosuppression protocols; and importantly, the failure of preventive medicine and public hygiene measures to reduce the rate of community-acquired infection. If anything, the infectious challenges facing the cardiothoracic surgeon today are more daunting than they were 40 years ago. In this chapter, we review the more common causes of pulmonary infection and their treatment.

BACTERIAL LUNG INFECTIONS

Community-Acquired Pneumonia

The term *pneumonia* refers to infection of the lower respiratory tract, involving the respiratory bronchioles to the distal alveoli. These illnesses have been subclassified based on the mode and timing of presentation and the existing comorbidities of the affected patient. These distinctions are often useful when considering empiric antibiotic therapy. The terms *typical* and *atypical pneumonias*, which refer to the causative organism, are outdated but still occasionally useful when considering this subject. Pneumonias due to so-called atypical organisms (including *Mycoplasma pneumoniae*, *legionella* species, and *Chlamydia pneumoniae*) can comprise up to 40% of cases, but are rarely distinguishable from typical bacterial pneumonias at clinical presentation.[22] Thus, the initial therapy chosen should consider both typical and atypical pathogens.

Community-acquired pneumonia (CAP) describes an acute bacterial or viral respiratory infection, contracted outside the confines of the hospital or long-term care facility setting.[5] It remains a common illness, with an estimated incidence between 5 and 6 million cases resulting in over 1 million hospitalizations annually.[56,57] Because CAP is not a reportable illness, these figures likely underestimate the actual magnitude of the problem. The aggregate cost for treating these patients approaches $9 billion a year,[57] almost all due to the costs associated with inpatient management. The length of hospitalization has been shown to be the key factor in determining the cost of treatment.[24] Pneumonia remains the sixth leading cause of death in the United States. The mortality rate associated with the development of pneumonia ranges from 1 to 5% for ambulatory patients without comorbidities to close to 40% for those requiring intensive care unit (ICU) admission.[25]

The most common pathogens responsible for CAP are listed in Box 12-1. *S. pneumoniae* has remained the most commonly identified organism, followed by *Haemophilus influenzae*, *Staphylococcus aureus*, enteric gram-negative bacilli, *Legionella* species, *M. pneumoniae*, *C. pneumoniae*, and respiratory viruses.[6,56] In up to 50% of cases, a causative organism is not identified. The likelihood of finding a particular pathogen often depends on the population studied (see Box 12-1) and the diagnostic tests used. For example, the use of sputum culture favors pneumococcus as the most

168 frequently identified organism, whereas *M. pneumoniae* is seen more commonly when serological tests are used. The presence of a "mixed" infection involving atypical and typical organisms can approach 40%,[44] although it is uncertain whether the atypical organisms when present represent an actual coinfection, a preceding infection, or simple colonization. However, empiric antibiotic regimens that cover both typical and atypical organisms have been associated with improved survival and shorter hospitalizations in several large retrospective studies.[28,35,71]

Certain risk factors may predispose patients to infection with particular organisms. For example, pneumonia due to drug-resistant pneumococcus has been associated with advanced age (>65 years), alcoholism, immune-suppressive illness or therapy, recent β-lactam therapy, and other significant comorbidities. Enteric gram-negative infections are seen more frequently in nursing home patients, those with other significant medical conditions including cardiopulmonary disease, and recent antibiotic therapy. Pseudomonal infections are more likely to arise in those with structural lung disease, malnutrition, or in the presence of immune suppressive or broad-spectrum antibiotic therapy.[56] *H. influenzae* infections occur more frequently in smokers than nonsmokers.

Clinical Presentation of CAP

Patients with CAP typically present with cough (90%), dyspnea (66%), sputum production (66%), and pleuritic chest pain (50%). Nonrespiratory symptoms such as malaise, headache, nausea, myalgias, arthralgias, abdominal pain, and mental confusion are seen in 10–30% of patients. Elderly patients often have fewer or less severe symptoms than younger patients. Presenting signs on physical exam include fever (80%), tachypnea, tachycardia, and a generalized toxic state. Crackles on auscultation are common (80%), with indications of consolidation in up to 30% of patients.[48]

Evaluation with chest radiography should be undertaken in all patients who present with symptoms and signs suggestive of pneumonia.[45] Standard posterior-anterior (PA) and lateral films classically reveal a segmental (Figure 12-1) or lobar infiltrate, often with evidence of a parapneumonic effusion. Chest films also help distinguish pneumonia from other disorders that may present with similar symptoms, and can help assess the severity (e.g., multi-lobar involvement) of the illness. Contributing or causative factors such as bronchial obstruction, lung abscess, or tuberculosis can also be seen. The addition of computed tomography may occasionally be helpful in difficult cases, but there is little data to support its routine use in the initial evaluation of patients with CAP.

Routine collection of laboratory studies in ambulatory patients is rarely necessary, but may occasionally steer the clinician toward hospital admission in equivocal cases. Laboratory studies in hospitalized patients should include complete blood count, electrolytes and glucose, renal and liver function tests, and assessment of oxygen saturation. Patients aged 15–54 should undergo HIV testing with informed consent.[45] Tests used to identify an etiologic agent (including blood cultures and sputum gram stain and culture) should be performed on all patients admitted with pneumonia, although some have questioned the utility of blood cultures in low-risk patients.[53] Viral cultures have not been shown to be useful in the initial evaluation of patients with CAP and should not be routinely performed.[7] Every attempt should be made to obtain these cultures prior to initiation of therapy, but not at the expense of unnecessary delays in treatment. Culture data should be correlated with

---

Box 12–1. Community-Acquired Pneumonia: Likely Pathogens.

Outpatients without Comorbidities*	Outpatients with comorbidities	Hospitalized Patients without Comorbidities	Hospitalized Patients Requiring ICU Admission
S. pneumoniae	*S. pneumoniae*	*S. pneumoniae*	*S. pneumoniae*
M. pneumoniae	*M. pneumoniae*	*H. influenzae*	Legionella spp.
C. pneumoniae	*C. pneumoniae*	*M. pneumoniae*	*H. influenzae*
H. influenzae	Mixed infection†	*C. pneumoniae*	Enteric gram-negative bacilli
Respiratory viruses	*H. influenzae*	Mixed infection	*S. aureus*
Legionella spp.	Enteric gram-negative bacilli	Enteric gram-negative bacilli	*M. pneumoniae*
M. tuberculosis	Respiratory viruses	Aspiration (Anaerobes)	Legionella spp.
Endemic fungi	*M. catarrhalis*	Respiratory viruses	Respiratory viruses
	Legionella spp.	Legionella spp.	*C. pneumoniae*
	Aspiration (Anaerobes)	*M. tuberculosis*	*M. pneumoniae*
	M. tuberculosis	Endemic fungi	Endemic fungi plus
	Endemic fungi	*P. carinii*	*P. aeruginosa*

*COPD, congestive heart disease, diabetes mellitus.
†Often a polymicrobial infection of *typical* and *atypical* organisms.
Modified from Niederman MS, Mandell LA, Anzueto A, et al: Guidelines for the management of adults with community-acquired pneumonia. Diagnosis, assessment of severity, antimicrobial therapy, and prevention. Am J Respir Crit Care Med 163:1730–1754, 2001.

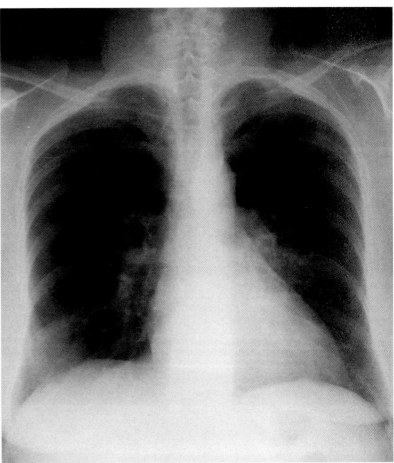

Figure 12–1 Posteroanterior (A) and

A

the gram stain result prior to narrowing antibiotic therapy. Significant pleural effusions should be tapped and sent for laboratory and culture studies. Routine serological and cold agglutinin testing is generally not recommended in the initial evaluation of patients with CAP,[56] but may prove useful in select cases. A pneumococcal urinary antigen assay recently approved by the FDA may be used to augment the standard diagnostic methods detailed above, with the advantage of rapid results similar to the gram stain. Sensitivity and specificity rates of 80–90% have been reported.[14]

Patients with pneumonia due to *mycoplasma* species often present with signs and symptoms reminiscent of a mild viral illness, with a more gradual onset and less intense nature. These infections, as with other "atypical" infections, occur more frequently in younger patients. Headache, malaise, sore throat, low-grade fever, and rhinorrhea are common. Cough, when present, is frequently nonproductive and spasmodic in character. Extrapulmonary manifestations may predominate, with rash, arthralgias, and neurological abnormalities present. The physical exam of the chest may yield minimal findings, although a wheeze and crackles can sometimes be appreciated. Radiological findings include nodular or peribronchial infiltrates, an interstitial pattern of disease (Figure 12-2), and occasional consolida-

tion. Pleural effusions occur frequently. Although the white cell count is often normal, anemia can be seen because of hemolytic anemia associated with a positive Coomb's test. Serological diagnosis may be obtained through measurement of IgM or IgG titer using a complement fixation test.

Pneumonia due to *Legionella* (*Legionella pneumophila*) remains problematic since the initial recognized outbreak of the disease at an American Legion convention in Philadelphia in 1976. The organism is identified in 1–5% of patients hospitalized with pneumonia, with considerable variation in detection due to geographical patterns and difficulties in accurate diagnosis. Culture may still be the best way of identifying *Legionella*, along with a urinary antigen assay.[45] However, the latter test can remain positive months after the acute infection.[61] Symptoms suggestive of pneumonia predominate (high fever, chills, dyspnea, cough), but extrapulmonary manifestations (gastrointestinal complaints, malaise, myalgias) are not uncommon. Radiographs usually reveal either patchy or diffuse interstitial infiltrates, and occasionally consolidation (Figure 12-3).

Pulmonary infection with *Chlamydia* organisms such as *C. pneumoniae* present in similar fashion to other "atypical" pneumonias. Infection with this organism has also been associated with chronic diseases such as atherosclerotic

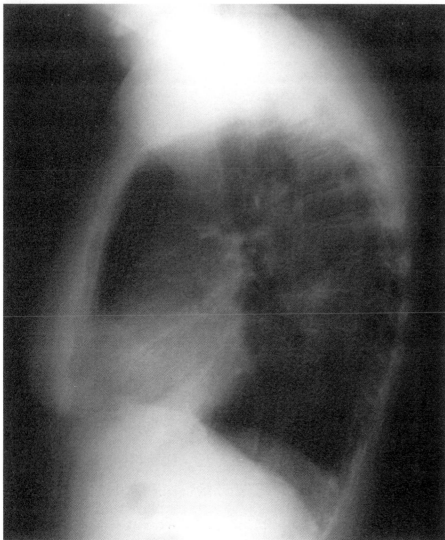

Figure 12–1 cont'd (B) lateral chest radiographs demonstrating segmental pneumonia involving the superior segment of the left lower lobe.

B

coronary disease. Diagnostic tests used to identify this organism include direct tissue culture (sputum smear and culture are not helpful) and display of a four-fold increase in IgG titer or a IgM titer of ≥1:16 using a microimmunofluorescence test.

Determination of CAP Severity

One of the key decisions made in the initial evaluation of CAP, beyond establishing a presumptive diagnosis, pertains to the need for inpatient therapy. Many of the patients afflicted with CAP are elderly with significant comorbidities for whom the progressive pulmonary infection is clearly life-threatening. On the other hand, improper admission for CAP therapy taxes the health care system billions of dollars annually, as noted previously. As a result, various guidelines have been developed to assist clinicians in the assessment of severity of illness at presentation. One such system, termed the Pneumonia Severity Index (PSI), was validated with

data from almost 2300 patients in the Pneumonia Patient Outcomes Research Team (PORT) cohort study.[23] Based on clinical parameters obtained at initial presentation, a risk score or class is determined (Figure 12-4). Patients with a risk class of I–III had a low mortality rate (<1%) and were felt to be at low risk, thus amenable to outpatient management. Patients with a risk class of IV or V were associated with higher mortality rates (9.3 and 27.0%, respectively) and were felt to be appropriate candidates for hospitalization. The PSI has since been recommended in several recent articles[18,31,54] and is endorsed by the Infectious Diseases Society of America (ISDA).[45] The ISDA recommends a three-step process in determining the initial site of treatment, based on (1) assessment of factors that compromise the safety of home care; (2) the PSI score; and (3) clinical judgment.

In contrast, the American Thoracic Society[56] still feels the admission decision is an "art of medicine" decision, where such tools as the PSI may be used to assist, but not

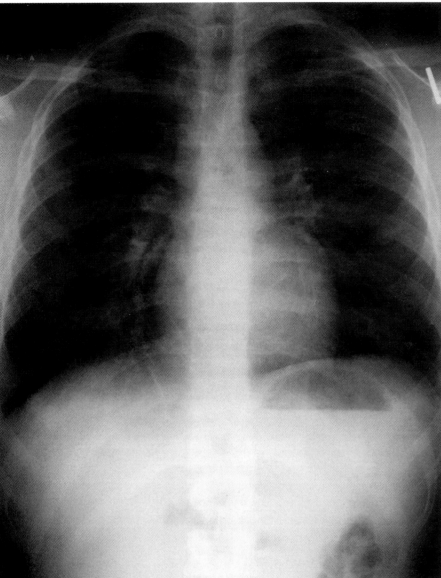

Figure 12–2 Posteroanterior chest radiograph demonstrating a fine interstitial pattern due to *Mycoplasma* pneumonia.

replace, this process. Prediction rules such as the PSI tend to oversimplify the decision-making process and often inappropriately favors certain factors at the expense of others. Further, tools such as the PSI limit input such as patient preference, which may favor outpatient care in the low-risk setting.[10] The ATS also endorses a report by Ewig and colleagues[19] that examines the criteria for severe CAP requiring admission to the ICU. In this retrospective study, the need for ICU admission could be defined by the presence of one of two major criteria (need for mechanical ventilation or septic shock) or two of three minor criteria (systolic blood pressure ≤90 mm Hg, multilobar disease, and/or PaO_2/FiO_2 ratio <250). Using these criteria the need for ICU admission could be predicted with a sensitivity of 78%, a specificity of 94%, a positive predictive value of 75%, and a negative predictive value of 94%.

Treatment of CAP

The treatment of CAP at initial presentation is outlined in Figure 12-5, as described by the ISDA.[45] The ATS has published similar guidelines, stratified by the presence or absence of modifying factors, comorbidities, and site of initial treatment.[56] Data from published reports support the use of the published guidelines, leading to better outcomes.[27,28] It should be reinforced that the timing of therapy is important, with the first dose of antibiotic given 4–8 hours after initial presentation. Prompt administration of therapy has been associated with improved survival.[50] The use of the published guidelines facilitates prompt delivery of appropriate therapy. Further, although it is desirable to narrow the spectrum of administered antibiotic agents, this is not possible in up to 50% of cases because of a lack of an identifiable organism. In addition, a significant proportion of cases rep-

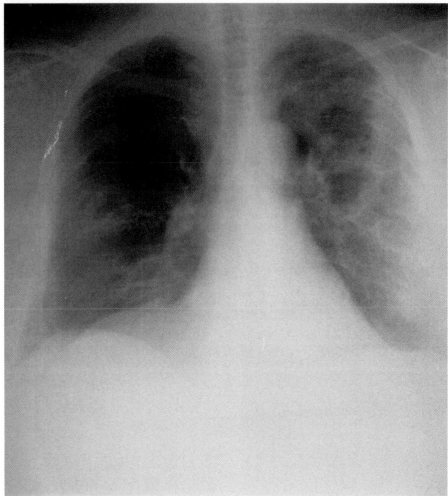

Figure 12–3 Posteroanterior (A) and

A

resent mixed polymicrobial infections. The use of these guidelines employing broad spectrum therapy allows for appropriate treatment in these patients.

Clinical decisions regarding duration of therapy are poorly supported in the literature. In general, most treatment regimens last 7–14 days; the severity of the presenting illness, the response to therapy, and the underlying comorbidities should all be considered when addressing duration of treatment. Most bacterial infections, including those due to *S. pneumoniae*, are treated for 7–10 days provided a good clinical response is seen. *Mycoplasma, Chlamydia*, and *Legionella* infections should be treated for 10–14 days and perhaps longer if significant comorbidity exists.

Successful response to therapy in a patient with CAP usually follows a predictable course. Stabilization of clinical parameters often occurs by 72 hours, with gradual improvement noted thereafter. The severity of the presenting illness and underlying patient disease understandably play a role in the response to therapy. The febrile response and leukocytosis typically resolve by day 4–5, with the radiological findings lagging behind. In fact, it has been documented that the initial radiographic abnormalities may actually worsen before improvement. Only 15% of chest films are clear at

discharge, and many take 2–3 months to return to normal. With a successful response to treatment, consideration should be given to conversion to oral therapy. The ATS describes four criteria that should be met prior to switching to oral therapy: improvement in cough and dyspnea; afebrile (<100°F) at two consecutive assessments 8 hours apart; resolving leukocytosis; and a functioning gastrointestinal tract with oral intake.[56] Obviously, some leeway may be allowed in these criteria given the clinical situation. Compliance can be an issue with oral therapy, and consideration of drug dosing schedules and side effects should be taken into account when selecting an oral regimen.[9]

Clinicians should resist the urge to switch antibiotic therapy within the first 72 hours, unless marked clinical deterioration occurs. Failure to respond to initial therapy does occur in up to 10% of patients for a variety of factors. The presence of a drug-resistant or unusual pathogen may be the cause, which may be remedied by further diagnostic tests for the etiologic agent, broadening the antibiotic therapy, or both. A complication of the initial pneumonia may be present, either at a local (e.g., lung abscess, empyema) or at a distant (e.g., meningitis, endocarditis, septic arthritis) site. Selected imaging such as computed tomography and

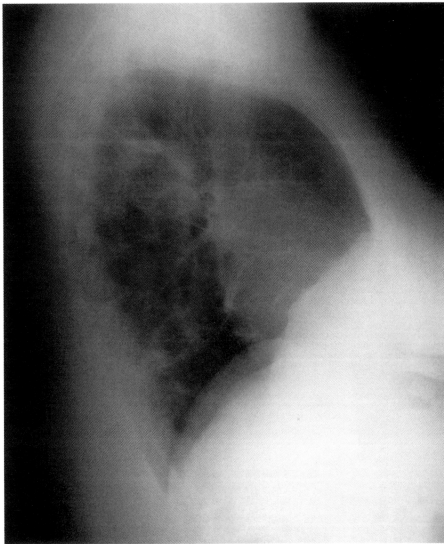

Figure 12–3 cont'd (B) lateral chest radiographs demonstrating diffuse infiltrates with cavitation due to *Legionella* infection.

B

echocardiography as well as sampling of fluid collections based on these studies and physical exam, can often reveal the source of the persistent infection. Finally, several noninfectious illnesses can mimic pneumonia and should be ruled out. This group of disease states is extensive and includes bronchogenic cancer, lymphoma, and a variety of inflammatory and interstitial lung diseases.

Nosocomial Pneumonia

Nosocomial pneumonia refers to pulmonary infection that occurs within 48–72 hours of admission to an acute care facility, or in intubated patients. It is the second most common nosocomial infection and has the highest mortality,[46] with crude mortality rates of 30% previously reported.[43] Risk factors for nosocomial pneumonia have been described and include the extremes of age, chronic lung disease, pre-

vious abdominal or thoracic surgery, endotracheal intubation, and duration of mechanical ventilation.[26]

Two factors occur that predispose patients to nosocomial pneumonia: the colonization of the aerodigestive tract with bacteria and aspiration of the contaminated secretions into the lower respiratory system.[12] Several of the preventative strategies described are aimed at interrupting these two processes.

Ventilator-Associated Pneumonia

Ventilator-associated pneumonia (VAP) is a nosocomial pulmonary infection developing in patients receiving mechanical ventilation. VAP that occurs early, within 48–72 hours after intubation, is typically caused by bacteria responsive to antibiotic therapy (e.g., pansensitive *S. aureus*, *H. influenzae*, and *S. pneumococcus*) and frequently results from

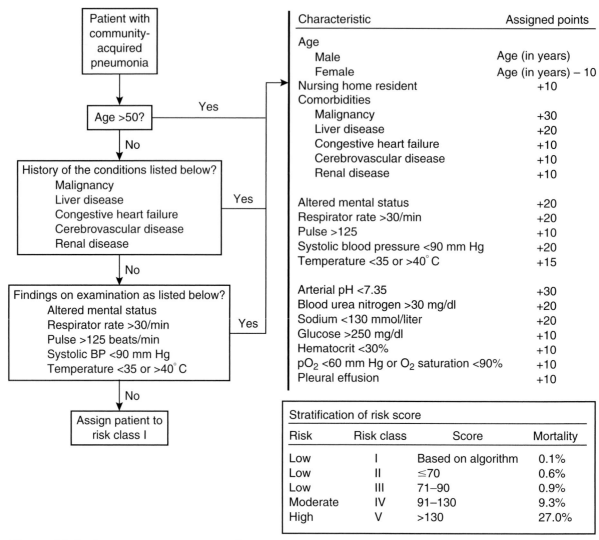

Figure 12–4 The Pneumonia Severity Index.
(Modified from Fine MJ, Auble TE, Yealy DM, et al: A prediction rule to identify low-risk patients with community-acquired pneumonia. N Engl J Med 336:243–250, 1997.)

aspiration complicating the intubation process. In contrast, late-onset ventilator-associated pneumonia is often caused by antibiotic resistant organisms (e.g., MRSA, *P. aeruginosa*, Acinetobacter and Enterobacter species).[40] Risk factors for VAP include the duration of mechanical ventilation,[42] the need for reintubation,[65] and gastric aspiration.[33,75] The incidence of VAP is significantly higher in surgical ICUs as opposed to medical ICUs, according to the Centers for Disease Control.[55]

Some controversy exists in the literature regarding optimal diagnosis of VAP.[20] To date, there seems to be little evidence supporting the use of invasive (bronchoscopic) techniques for diagnosis compared with quantitative tracheobronchial aspirates.[67,69] Bronchoscopy may be of use in patients who fail to respond to initial therapy.[59] The treatment of VAP consists of general supportive care and the administration of empiric broad-spectrum antibiotics, guided by the severity of the illness.[21] The adequacy of ini-

tial antibiotic therapy appears to be the most important factor determinant of outcome.[40,51] Numerous studies have examined preventive measures to limit the development of VAP. The use of semirecumbent positioning, sucralfate instead of H2-antagonists for stress ulcer prophylaxis, and selective digestive tract decontamination were found to have the strongest support in the literature.[11]

Aspiration Pneumonia

Aspiration refers to the inhalation of oropharyngeal or gastric contents into the tracheobronchial tree. This usually results in either a *pneumonitis* caused by a chemical injury from contact with sterile, acidic gastric contents, or a *pneumonia* due to inhalation of infected material. Rarely, aspiration can lead to airway obstruction, lung abscess, and other findings. Aspiration pneumonia is a common problem, accounting for 5–15% of CAP and is frequently seen in

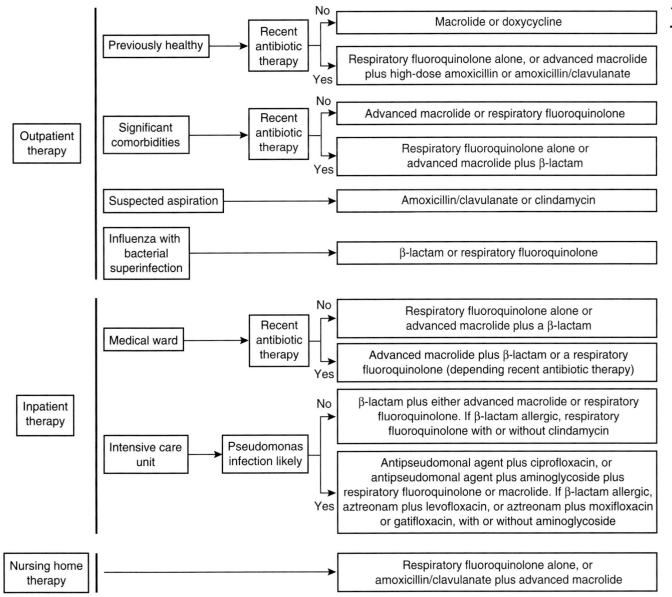

Figure 12–5 Empiric therapy for community-acquired pneumonia (CAP).
(*Adapted from Mandell LA, Bartlett JG, Dowell SF, et al: Update of practice guidelines for the management of community-acquired pneumonia in adults. Clin Infect Dis 37:1405–1433, 2003.*)

nursing home residents, in those with swallowing disorders, and in patients with altered mental states. It is also a recognized complication of general anesthesia, occurring in about 1 in 3000 operations and accounting for 10–30% of deaths related to anesthesia.[77]

The acute lung injury or pneumonitis from gastric aspiration, termed *Mendelson's syndrome*,[52] appears directly related to the acidity and volume of aspirated material. In general, a pH <2.5 and a volume in excess of 0.3 ml/kg (about 21 ml in a 70-kg adult) are required to initiate lung injury. The injury follows a biphasic pattern, with the initial insult caused by direct damage of the acid on the delicate capillary and alveolar cells, followed several hours later by the rapid accumulation of inflammatory cells and mediators

resulting in a local and systemic inflammatory response. Progression to acute respiratory distress syndrome and multiorgan system failure may ensue. Because the gastric contents are sterile because of the acidity, infection is usually not an initial feature in these cases, but may become prominent later in the course of the illness with secondary infection of the damaged lung parenchyma. Efforts to modify the gastric pH may lead to gastric colonization with gram-negative bacteria as well as other organisms, leading to infection early following the aspiration episode. Treatment is largely supportive in nature. Particularly if the aspiration is witnessed, bronchoscopy is indicated to remove any residual fluid or debris from the airway. The use of corticosteroids in the treatment of aspiration pneumonitis has not been shown to be of benefit. Although it is common practice to initiate antibiotic therapy in these patients, this often overtreats simple pneumonitis that may resolve with supportive measures only. Further, early use of antibiotics may encourage development of resistant organisms. Antibiotic therapy should be considered early in those thought to have gastric colonization and in those patients who do not improve within 48 hours of the inciting event, with evidence of ongoing lung injury, infection, or infiltrate.[47] Empiric coverage with broad-spectrum agents is recommended.

Aspiration pneumonia commonly arises from inhalation of colonized oropharyngeal bacteria, causing the signs, symptoms, and radiographic changes of pneumonia. About half of normal adults aspirate while asleep,[29] and for infection to occur the normal protective mechanisms must either fail or be overwhelmed by the volume or bacterial burden of the aspirate. In supine patients, the dependent lung segments (posterior aspects of upper lobes, superior segments of lower lobes) are affected most frequently. In upright individuals, the basilar segments, particularly on the right side, are at greatest risk of infection. The aspiration episode in patients developing pneumonia is frequently not observed, and the diagnosis is derived from the clinical picture and characteristic radiographic changes in individuals known to be at risk. Treatment with antimicrobial therapy is appropriate. Use of antibiotics with anaerobic coverage is probably overdone, but appropriate in select cases in which severe periodontal disease, alcoholism, and other disorders predominate. In hospitalized patients, coverage of gram-negative bacteria is essential.

Bronchiectasis

Bronchiectasis was first described in 1819 by Laennec. It is defined by the permanent dilation of the bronchi,[64] caused by a recurrent process of transmural infection and inflammation. The disease process is characterized by the pathological or radiographic appearance of the airways. Cylindrical or tubular bronchiectasis results in dilated, slightly tapered airways; varicose bronchiectasis resembles the chronic venous state of the same name, with areas of dilation and constriction; and saccular or cystic bronchiectasis, where progressive dilation of the airway can end in saclike, cystic structures resembling a cluster of grapes. The cylindrical changes are frequently seen with tuberculosis infections, whereas the saccular or cystic type is more common after obstruction or bacterial infection. Thick, mucoid secretions are often noted pooled in the dilated airways, causing a chronic inflammatory state involving the airway walls. The lung parenchyma distal to the dilated, ectatic airways are often damaged as well, with fibrosis and emphysematous changes present. The accompanying bronchial arteries and lymph nodes are engorged and hypertrophied as well. The left lower lobe is the area most frequently involved, followed by the lingula and right middle lobe.

The causes and disease states associated with bronchiectasis are listed in Box 12-2. The common pathway for all these disorders is recurrent, transmural infection of the bronchial wall. Bacterial infections, particularly those involving potentially necrotizing agents such as *S. aureus*, *P. aeruginosa*, *S. pneumonia*, and various anaerobes, remain important causes of bronchiectasis, particularly when there is a delay in treatment or there are factors present to prevent eradication of the infection. Bronchiectasis in patients with allergic bronchopulmonary aspergillosis (ABPA) is due to an immune reaction to the fungal organism, with production of inflammatory mediators and subsequent direct airway invasion by the fungus. Viral infections can lead to bronchiectatic airways both through direct infection and through a reduction in host defenses. This latter theme is common when considering the pathophysiology of bronchiectasis. Primary ciliary dyskinesia and various immune deficiencies such as hypogammaglobulinemia are examples of congenital disorders in which there is impairment in host defense mechanisms. Cystic fibrosis is another important cause of bronchiectasis, with predilection for the upper lobes. Occasionally the appearance of bronchiectasis in middle age will be the presenting symptom in patients with milder forms of cystic fibrosis. Several autoimmune disorders, such as rheumatoid arthritis and inflammatory bowel disease, have been linked to the presence of recurrent pulmonary infections and the development of bronchiectasis.[2]

Both focal and diffuse forms of bronchiectasis are seen. The focal variety is often associated with an isolated abnormality causing relative or complete bronchial obstruction. An aspirated foreign body, slow-growing tumor, or broncholith are examples. Rarely bronchial compression (as seen with middle lobe syndrome) or angulation of the bronchus (following surgical lobectomy) produce obstruction leading to recurrent infection and the development of localized disease. Bronchiectasis due to postinfectious causes is more likely to be localized, whereas disease due to congenital

---

Box 12–2. Conditions Causing or Associated with Bronchiectasis.

Infection
  Bacterial
  Mycobacterial
  Aspergillus
  Viral (including HIV)
Congenital conditions
  Primary ciliary dyskinesia
  Alpha-1 antitrypsin deficiency
  Cystic fibrosis
  Tracheobronchomegaly (Mounier-Kuhn syndrome)
  Cartilage deficiency (Williams-Campbell syndrome)
  Pulmonary sequestration
  Marfan's syndrome
Immunodeficiency
  Hypogammaglobulinemia
  Secondary to disease states or therapy
Sequelae of toxic inhalation or aspiration
  Chlorine
  Foreign body
Rheumatic conditions
  Rheumatoid arthritis
  Systemic lupus erythematosus
  Sjögren's syndrome
  Relapsing polychondritis
Inflammatory bowel disease

Adapted from Barker AF: Bronchiectasis. N Engl J Med 346(18):1383–1393, 2002.

deficiencies is more likely to be diffuse. A recent study of stable patients with bronchiectasis revealed a 64% incidence of colonization with what were termed *potential pathogenic microorganisms,* or PPMs. The most frequently isolated PPMs were *H. influenzae, Pseudomonas* spp, and *S. pneumoniae.* Risk factors for PPM colonization included diagnosis of bronchiectasis before 14 years of age; an FEV1, 80% predicted; and the presence of varicose or saccular bronchiectasis.[4]

Patients with bronchiectasis present with recurrent pulmonary infections characterized by dyspnea and an unremitting chronic cough productive of thick, tenacious purulent sputum. Hemoptysis is common, and at times can be massive because of erosion into the enlarged bronchial vessels. Occasionally patients with bronchiectasis will describe a nonproductive cough, indicative of upper lobe involvement. Auscultation reveals crackles, wheeze, or rhonchi in the majority of patients.

The radiographical findings in bronchiectasis are understandably important in establishing the diagnosis. Standard radiographs are abnormal in the clear majority of cases, demonstrating focal areas of consolidation, atelectasis, evidence of thickened bronchi (best noted as ring shadows when seen on end) and in advanced cases, delineation of the dilated, cystic changes in the airway (Figure 12-6).

Computed tomography, particularly high-resolution images, are more sensitive and specific for the diagnosis of bronchiectasis. Evidence of airway dilation, changes consistent with saccules or varicosities of the airway, and lack of airway tapering toward the periphery are all consistent with bronchiectasis.[4] Upper lobe involvement suggests the diagnosis of cystic fibrosis or ABPA; middle lobe and lingular disease is more typical of environmental mycobacterial infection such as *Mycobacterium avium-intracellulare*; and lower lobe predominance suggests bacterial involvement.

Therapy for bronchiectasis involves treatment of the underlying disorder if possible, suppression of the bacterial load through appropriate use of antibiotics, encouragement of proper pulmonary hygiene including the routine use of bronchodilators, mucolytic agents and postural drainage, and surgery in select cases. The role of surgery is three-fold. First, patients with focal areas of disease causing unremitting symptoms and associated with localized lung parenchymal destruction are candidates for resection therapy, usually via a segmentectomy or lobectomy. Second, the rare patient who presents with massive hemoptysis should be considered for surgical therapy if less invasive maneuvers such as bronchial artery embolization are unsuccessful. Finally, some patients with end-stage bronchiectasis may be candidates for lung transplantation. As with other patients with

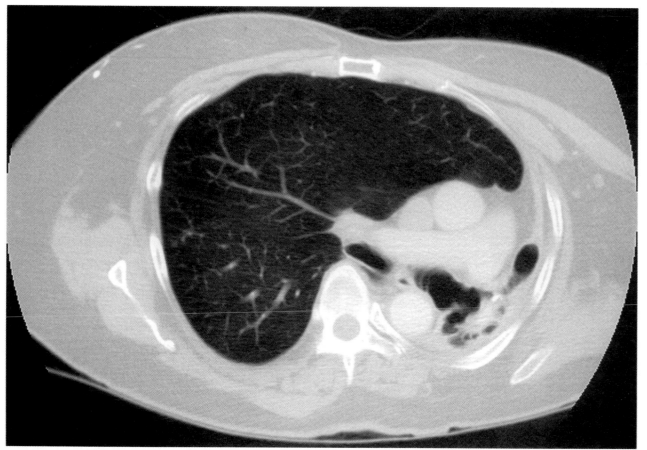

Figure 12–6 Computed tomography scan demonstrating end-stage bronchiectasis involving the left lung, with complete parenchymal destruction.

178 end-stage suppurative lung disease, sequential double lung transplantation is indicated to avoid contamination of the new lung grafts.

Lung Abscess

A lung abscess is a circumscribed cavity within the lung parenchyma filled with purulent material and air. The cavity may form as a result of a necrotizing infection, or may become secondarily infected. The abscess formation may be singular in nature, or multifocal depending on the etiology. The abscess is arbitrarily termed acute if present for 6 weeks or less, and chronic if it has been present for a greater length of time. Further classification comes from the underlying etiology, as noted above: a primary lung abscess arises from a necrotizing infection, whereas a secondary lung abscess forms as a result of another pathologic entity.

Box 12-3 lists the causes of lung abscess. The most common cause is inadvertent aspiration of infected oropharyngeal secretions, which can occur in the setting of impaired consciousness, in the presence of poor dental hygiene, and in association with gastroesophageal reflux disease or various dysphagia syndromes (strictures, Zenker's and other diverticula, dysmotility disorders, achalasia, and others). A lung abscess can occur as sequelae of necrotizing lung infections, particularly in the setting of an immunocompromised host. Bronchial obstruction, caused by tumor, foreign body, or external compression of the bronchus, can predispose to distal lung infection and subsequent abscess formation. A preexisting cavity within the lung parenchyma, as a result of a cavitating neoplasm, a resolving infarct, or even structural lung disease can lead to secondary infection and abscess. Direct extension of an adjacent abscess can occur. Finally, hematogenous seeding from another source can produce abscesses within the lung, often multifocal. Recognition of the secondary nature of the abscess can have direct therapeutic implications (e.g., an abscess resulting from a foreign body aspiration will likely respond poorly to treatment without removal of the offending item).

The location of lung abscesses is determined by the segmental anatomy of the tracheobronchial tree and the underlying cause. As aspiration is a major cause, the dependent segments—posterior segment of the right upper lobe and the superior segments of both lower lobes—tend to be involved frequently. The distribution roughly falls into: right upper lobe—25%; right middle lobe—10%; right lower lobe—33%; left upper lobe—12%; and left lower lobe—20%.[30]

The bacteriology of lung abscesses frequently falls in line with the underlying cause. Many ambulatory patients with lung abscess have gram-positive bacteria (e.g., α- and β-hemolytic streptococcus, *S. aureus*, *S. pneumoniae*, and *S. viridans*) as the source, whereas gram-negative organisms (e.g., *Proteus* spp., *Escherichia coli*, *P. aeruginosa*, *Enterobacter* and *Eikenella*) predominate in nosocomial infections. In lung abscess due to aspiration, mixed flora are often present and anaerobes play an important part. Aerobic gram-positive cocci and facultative gram-negative bacilli are commonly found, including *S. aureus*, *S. pyogenes*, *Klebsiella pneumoniae*, and *P. aeruginosa*.

Clinically, patients complain of cough, fever, malaise, weight loss, dyspnea, and occasionally pleuritic chest pain.

Box 12–3. Etiology of Lung Abscess.

Primary
  Aspiration
    Impaired consciousness
    Severe periodontal disease
    Dysphagia syndromes, esophageal reflux
  Necrotizing pneumonia
  Immunocompromised patient
Secondary
  Bronchial obstruction
    Neoplasm
    Foreign body
    Lymphadenopathy
  Cavitating lesions
    Neoplasm
    Pulmonary infarct
    Emphysema/bullous disease
  Direct extension
    Amebiasis (liver)
    Subphrenic abscess
  Hematogenous dissemination

Adapted from Hodder RV, Cameron R, Todd TRJ: Bacterial Infections. In: Pearson FG, Deslauriers J, Ginsberg RJ, et al, eds: Thoracic Surgery. New York: Churchill Livingstone, 1995, pp. 433–469.

The symptoms are reminiscent of pneumonia and may be insidious in onset. Hemoptysis may rarely be a complicating factor and can vary from blood streaks in the sputum to life-threatening hemorrhage. With cavitation and drainage into the tracheobronchial tree, patients will likely describe production of large volumes of foul-smelling sputum. The uninvolved lung can become soiled through a spill-over effect and produce respiratory failure. If large enough, the abscess can exert a mass effect on adjacent structures. Rupture into the pleural space is uncommon but can lead to empyema and fulminant sepsis.

A chest radiograph is likely to show a cavitary space within the lung, accompanied by an air-fluid level (Figure 12-7). In contrast with a hydropneumothorax, the abscesses are more likely to have equal air-fluid levels on both the PA and lateral films.[74] Features of a lung abscess may be difficult to appreciate on plain film exam and can be confused with alternative diagnoses. Computed tomography is helpful in these cases, delineating the exact anatomical features and location of the abscess and its relation to adjacent structures. For example, a cavitary neoplasm may be confused with an abscess. Compared with the thin, smooth walls of the abscess, cavitation secondary to tumor is usually associated with thick, irregular walls, features that do not respond to antibiotic therapy. An interlobar fluid collection or empyema may also be confused with a lung abscess. The presence of a lenticular shape, obtuse angle with the chest wall, compression of neighboring bronchovascular structures, and a "split pleura" sign signifies the presence of pleural fluid in these cases.[72] In addition to standard laboratory investigation, all patients should undergo bronchoscopy to assess for bronchial obstruction due to tumor or foreign body and possibly to obtain cultures. Accurate culture data

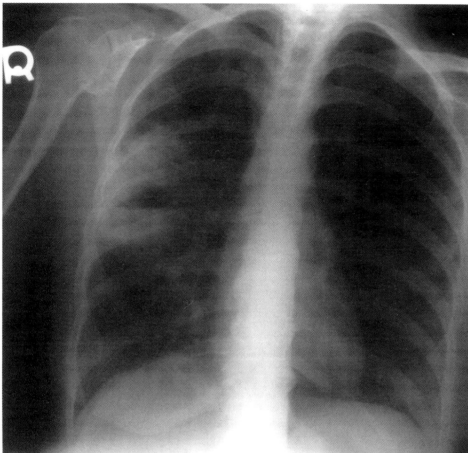

Figure 12–7 Posteroanterior chest radiograph demonstrating a lung abscess with air-fluid level.

may be best obtained through percutaneous fine needle aspiration (FNA). In a series reported by Yang and colleagues,[80] FNA yielded a 94% success rate in culturing pathogens, compared with 11% from sputum culture and only 3% from lavage. Attempted drainage via bronchoscopic means should be discouraged in most cases because of the risk of flooding the airways with purulent material.

The successful treatment of lung abscess centers around prolonged antimicrobial therapy targeted at the causative organism combined with establishment of adequate drainage. In most cases the drainage can be accomplished internally, aided by postural techniques and chest physiotherapy. If internal drainage is inadequate, percutaneous drainage may be done, usually with an excellent response (Figure 12-8). The complications of percutaneous drainage (empyema, pneumothorax, hemothorax) occur in less than 10% of cases, and even less so if pleural symphysis is present. The course of antibiotic therapy typically lasts 6–8 weeks, with radiographic resolution occurring by 4–5 months. Medical therapy for lung abscess is generally successful in 85–90% of cases.[79] Indications for surgical intervention would include empyema; development of a bronchopleural fistula; significant hemoptysis; persistence of the abscess despite adequate therapy; and suspicion of underlying malignancy. During surgical procedures for lung abscess special attention should be paid to protecting the

contralateral lung from spillage, usually through the use of a double-lumen tube. Resection of the involved segment of lung is usually performed, although in cases of rupture into the pleural space simple unroofing of the cavity, decortication and wide drainage will usually suffice.

MYCOBACTERIAL PULMONARY DISEASE

Mycobacterial pulmonary diseases include infections with mycobacterium tuberculosis and its more virulent form, multidrug resistant tuberculosis (MDR-TB). There are other mycobacterial infections that have gone through a series of name changes including atypical tuberculosis, non-tuberculosis mycobacterium (NTM), mycobacterium-other-than-tuberculosis (MOTT), and the more appropriately and recently named environmental mycobacterial (E.M.) infections.[37] While good epidemiology studies can be found for tuberculosis infections as well as MDRTB, poor epidemiology data exist for these E.M. infections. This is probably because E.M. infections are not transferable from person to person.

Annually there are currently 16,000 new cases of tuberculosis in the United States and 7–8 million new cases in the world with an estimated 2 and 3 million deaths.[16]

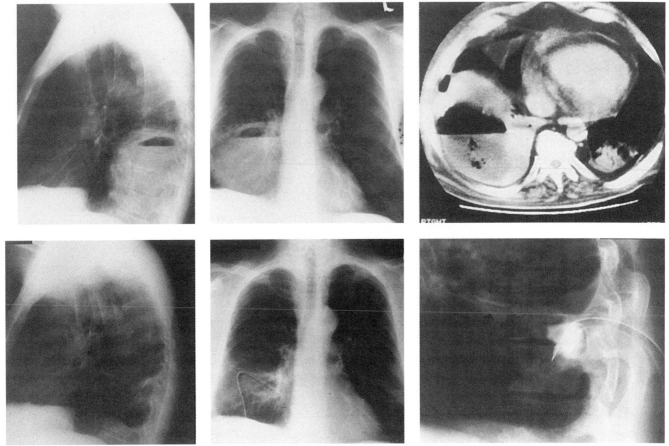

Figure 12–8 Computed tomography and chest radiographs demonstrating a large lung abscess *(upper panels)* with resolution after appropriate percutaneous drainage *(lower panels)*.
(Reproduced with permission from Darling G, Downey GP, Herridge MS: Bacterial infections of the lung. In: Pearson FG, Cooper JD, Deslauriers J, et al: Thoracic Surgery, 2nd ed. Philadelphia: Churchill Livingstone, 2002, pp. 521–651.)

Unfortunately, the majority of these cases are in countries where the health-care systems are in dire need of help. In India, nearly 500,000 people die from tuberculosis yearly. Fortunately, only 10–15% of those exposed to the tuberculosis organism acquire the clinical disease; however, this leaves a large number of individuals who make up a latent source for later activation with tuberculosis if their resistance breaks down because of disease or aging.

The early treatment of tuberculosis gave rise to the sanatoria system. It was felt that rest and fresh air were beneficial in the treatment of tuberculosis. However, it has never been well documented that this form of therapy produced any long-term benefit.

Surgery for tuberculosis began with collapse therapy. The tuberculosis organism is an obligate aerobe and it was reasoned that by preventing oxygen from entering the cavities this would be beneficial in the treatment of patients with cavitary pulmonary tuberculosis. Various forms of collapse therapy have been used including thoracoplasty, wax or lucite ball plombage, phrenic nerve crush or interruption, pneumoperitoneum, and induced pneumothorax. Collapse therapy continued to be the treatment of choice for tuberculosis infections until chemotherapy with streptomycin and para-aminosalicylic acid (PAS) was introduced in 1945. It

was not until the introduction of isoniazid in 1952 that prolonged cures could be obtained with antibiotic therapy.

Gradually resectional surgery replaced collapse therapy as the primary surgical approach to patients with tuberculosis infections having residual destroyed lung or cavitary disease. With the introduction of rifampin in 1966 the need for surgery was markedly reduced and the sanatoria system gradually became extinct. Drug-sensitive tuberculosis in almost all instances can be cured with antibiotic therapy alone. The standard treatment of drug-sensitive tuberculosis is with INH and rifampin and a short course of pyrazinamide. Patients with drug-sensitive tuberculosis who are treated appropriately as previously noted are only operated on for complications such as bronchostenosis; massive hemoptysis (>600 cc in 24 hours); bronchopleural fistula, to rule out the presence of cancer; and occasionally decortication of a trapped lung, which occurs when polymicrobial contamination occurs within the pleural cavity in tuberculosis patients who have had a pleural effusion. Patients having tuberculosis whose organism is resistant to both INH and rifampin are classified as having MDRTB and present a greater challenge to the surgeon. Often there is resistance to the three other first-line drugs; ethambutol, streptomycin, pyrazinamide, and many of these patients are also resistant to a number of the second-line drugs. Patients are operated on for the indications as previously noted for patients with drug-sensitive tuberculosis. However, they are also operated on for persistent cavitary disease, destroyed lobe, or destroyed lung with or without a positive sputum. In the United States today, patients with MDR-TB make up the largest group of patients operated on for pulmonary infections with tuberculosis.

Patients with E.M. infections present a different challenge. The most common E.M. infection is that of the Mycobacterium Avian complex. This includes both *Mycobacterium avian* and *M. intracellulare,* which are almost indistinguishable from each other on culture. Infections with the so-called rapid growers, such as *M. chelonae, M. abscessus,* and *M. fortuitum* seem to be increasing in the United States although accurate epidemiology is not available. These infections are more difficult to treat because good antibiotic coverage is not available. Some of these rapid grower infections are extremely virulent and may destroy an entire lung (Figures 12-9 and 12-10), and surgery offers the only hope to control the process along with continued use of any antibiotics available. Specific types of E.M. infection include infection of the middle lobe and lingula of women (Figure 12-11). This usually occurs in slender women with little or no body fat and is frequently associated with skeletal abnormalities such as scoliosis or pectus excavatum.[36,63] This syndrome has not been found in men, in our experience; however, if it does occur it is extremely rare.

Preparation for surgery is an important part of the therapeutic approach for patients with mycobacterial infections. The most important aspect of preparation is nutrition. Patients with albumin <3.0 g/dl are not operated upon. Nutritional supplementation is accomplished either orally or by gastrostomy or jejunostomy feeding tubes to improve the patient's anabolic state before surgery. The best available antibiotic therapy is given for approximately 3 months prior to surgery. This can be prolonged if bacterial counts are decreasing, and it can be shortened if the sputum becomes negative for acid-fast bacilli. In MDR-TB only about half the patients have negative sputum prior to surgery. Routine evaluation, as with other pulmonary surgery, includes pulmonary function tests, ventilation perfusion scans, and computed tomography.

Surgical principles include leaving enough viable lung tissue to have a functional postoperative patient. Double lumen tubes or bronchial-blockers are used in all operations. All grossly involved lung, which includes cavitary disease and destroyed lung should be removed, while nodular disease remaining in other parts of the lung can be left behind. Fluid administration during surgery is kept to below 1200 cc whenever possible and with pneumonectomies below 800 cc. The use of muscle flaps is controversial. However, it is our opinion that using muscle flaps to fill space following lobectomies is helpful. With muscle flaps we feel that the incidence of bronchopleural fistula has been decreased. Muscle flaps are used after pneumonectomy if there is a polymicrobial contamination or positive sputum at the time of surgery.[62] If there is massive contamination, the chest is left open and an omental flap is used. Omental flaps are also used to cover the bronchus in the absence of any muscle due to previous surgery or extreme cachexia. If the chest is left open (Eloesser procedure) it is packed with half strength Dakin's solution using Kerlix gauze and changed on a daily basis for 5–6 weeks. When the opening is closed, assuming the intrathoracic chest wall is clean, Claggets solution is left in the pleural cavity. Pleural tents have been suggested to help eliminate space and seal air leaks. This is not practical in mycobacterial surgery because most of the dissections over the upper lobe are done in extrapleural plane. The latissimus dorsi muscle is used whenever space problems are expected following lobectomy, and is also used to cover the bronchus and hilum. If only bronchial support is needed following a pneumonectomy, intercostal muscle can be used. Appropriate antibiotic therapy is continued for 12–24 months postoperatively with some of the injectable antibiotics being stopped prior to stopping the oral medications.

While tuberculosis infections can infect normal lung tissue, E.M. infections most frequently effect previously diseased lungs and have a much more indolent course than tuberculosis or MDR-TB. Lung damage can be due to previous infections such as tuberculosis, bronchiectasis, or chest wall irradiation. E.M. patients, in many instances, are also found to have genetic abnormalities such as heterozygous cystic fibrosis, alpha one antitrypsin deficiency, or cilia dysfunction. It is also of note that over 50% of the patients with E.M. infections have esophageal dysfunction. These patients often reflux at night causing contamination and damage to the lungs making them more susceptible to E.M. infections.

In the United States an abnormally high proportion of patients with E.M. are Caucasian. Additionally an overwhelming majority of E.M. patients are women (relative to men) and the reasons for these two findings are still not clear.

Operative mortality in experienced hands should be less than 5%.[62,63] Complications following mycobacterial surgery are high; in the 25–30% range (but with experience this can be brought down to less than 15%). Specific complications include bronchopleural fistula most often occurring after right pneumonectomy for E.M. infections. This may be as high as 20% without muscle or omental buttress. Wound infection after *M. chelonae* and abscessus are common and careful attention to wound closure is necessary. Other complications such as air leaks, bleeding, and post-pneumonectomy pulmonary edema are similar to other thoracic procedures for nonmycobacterial disease.

Results of surgery for tuberculosis or MDR-TB are gratifying whereas surgery for E.M. infections is less successful due to the long duration of indolent disease prior to surgical intervention. Earlier surgery in these patients should improve the results. Persistence in aggressively treating surgical complications is often necessary to obtain good results and requires dedicated thoracic surgeons experienced in these difficult cases.

With 33–40% of the world infected with tuberculosis and the presence of poverty, this disease will not go away. With the increasing number of E.M. infections, at least in the United States, surgery will continue to play a role in the therapy of these patients.

MAJOR MYCOTIC LUNG INFECTIONS

There are at least 100,000 species of fungi, but only 300 or so are associated with pulmonary disease. Fungal infection of the lung results from inhalation of the infectious agent.

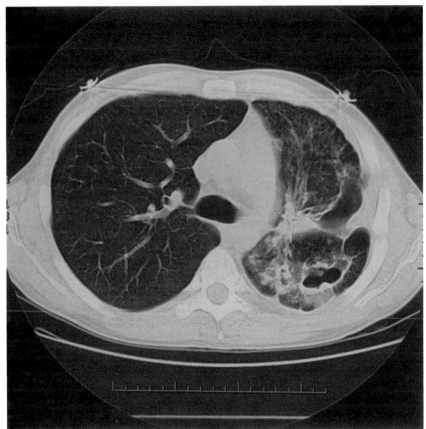

Figure 12–9 Computed tomography scan showing severe cavitary disease in a patient with *Mycobacterium chelonae* infection.

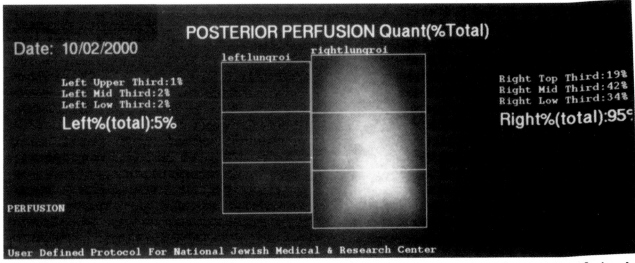

Figure 12–10 Perfusion scan of the same patient depicted in Figure 12–9, demonstrating absence of perfusion to the left lung.

Colonization or asymptomatic fungal infection is common in the United States: an estimated 30 million are infected with *Histoplasma capsulatum*, and another 10 million with *Coccidioides immitis*. Serious infection is rare, but is seen with increasing frequency in immunocompromised populations. The increasingly advanced use of chemotherapy for neoplasms, antibiotics for infections, immunosuppressive therapies for organ transplantation, and corticosteroids for various conditions has increased opportunistic infections by usually harmless saprophytes such as *Aspergillus, Candida,* and *Mucor.* Under these conditions, the formerly clear differentiation between so-called pathogenic and nonpathogenic fungi has become blurred.

In addition to detailing the medical conditions that predispose to infection, other areas of the patient history can yield important clues to the causative agent. The three major

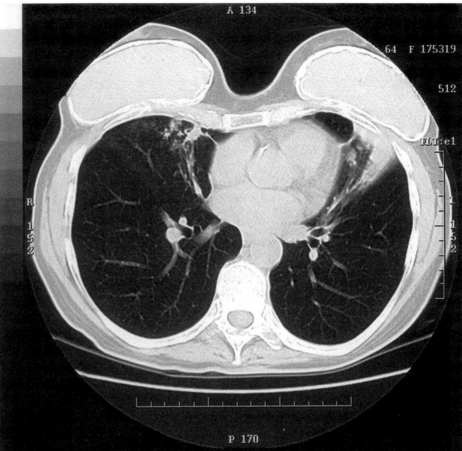

Figure 12–11 Computed tomography scan of a woman with MAC infection of the right middle lobe and lingula.

fungal infections seen in healthy populations—histoplasmosis, coccidioidomycosis, and blastomycosis—are recognized as endemic organisms in specific geographical areas of the United States. These organisms are dimorphic; they exist in nature as a mycelium (mold) that bears infectious spores, which later enter the host and develop into a yeastlike phase that is the tissue pathogen. These morphological differences occur in response to changes in temperature. The spores invade the host through an aerosolized form via the respiratory tract, resulting in a mild or asymptomatic infection. Chronic pulmonary or disseminated infection is uncommon, with the presence of an intact cell-mediated immune response critical to prevent serious illness. The more common opportunistic fungi—*Aspergillus, Cryptococcus, Mucor*—are ubiquitous and are located in the soil. Proximity to building or construction sites where aerosolization of these organisms can occur have been linked to an increased incidence of *Aspergillus, Histoplasmosis, Coccidioidomycosis,* and other infections.[73,78]

Fungal infection of the lung is best established by recovery of the infecting organism by culture, but recognition in smears or tissue sections may be enough for diagnosis. The best two stains for demonstration of fungi in tissue are periodic acid-Schiff and methenamine silver, but no one stain demonstrates all organisms. Specific immunological changes in the host response may provide a strong indication of the diagnosis and may often lead to therapy before actual isolation of the organism can be achieved.[68] All too often, how-

ever, it is not possible to find pathognomonic organisms in the stained specimens and only a presumptive diagnosis can be made. Cultures of fungi can be made from tissues, sputum, pleural fluid, and other clinical specimens. Induced sputum samples, obtained in the morning and at least six in number, are recommended.[68] Sabouraud's dextrose agar is an excellent general purpose culture medium. Prompt delivery of the specimens to the laboratory is essential. Because respiratory tract cultures may simply be the result of fungal colonization, the culture isolates from these sites, which are not sterile, may not correspond to infection. However, risk stratification of the host may aid in this matter. One study demonstrated a positive culture for *Aspergillus* in immunocompromised patients such as bone marrow transplant recipients was associated with invasive infection 50–70% of the time, while a positive culture in cystic fibrosis patients was rarely combined with invasive aspergillosis.[60] Serological tests for circulating fungal antigens (such as galactomannan in aspergillosis) and circulating antibodies to fungal antigen (histoplasmosis and coccidioidomycosis) can aid in diagnosis. Molecular diagnostic techniques using polymerase chain reaction technology are being developed for *Aspergillus, Candida,* and *Crytococcus.*[39,76]

Histoplasmosis

Histoplasmosis is a fungal infection caused by the dimorphic fungus *Histoplasma capsulatum*, which exists in mycelial

184 form in the soil, its natural habitat, and in yeast form at body temperature. It is endemic in the Mississippi and Ohio river valleys, where the incidence of positive skin reactions to the fungus exceeds 80%.[17] Further, the incidence of skin test reactivity probably underestimates the true incidence, because the skin test may revert to negative over a period of time.

The yeast phase of the organism is not contagious, and there is no danger of transmission through direct human contact. It is the microspores from the mycelial phase that act as the transmitted agent, inhaled into the distal air spaces in the lung. The critical inoculum is unknown. Within days the microspores germinate into yeast spores, attracting neutrophils and macrophages to the site of infection. Neutrophils are largely ineffective against the yeast spores, which are ingested by the macrophages. Infected macrophages transport the spores to other areas in the reticuloendothelial system, producing a subclinical disseminated infection. This process is poorly controlled in those with impaired T-cell immunity. The outcome of infection is determined by the development of a specific cell-mediated immune reaction within about 2 weeks. Granulomas form within the lungs and mediastinal lymph nodes to wall off residual organisms. As the epithelial cell granulomas age, caseating necrosis develops in the central areas and may calcify as the peripheral portions become fibrotic. Within these lesions, *H. capsulatum* organisms are usually found only in the caseous material, seen well with methenamine silver stain. The yeast is often found intracellularly in macrophages.

About half of the cases of acute pulmonary histoplasmosis are asymptomatic. The remaining patients have a flulike illness with chills, myalgias, headache, nonproductive cough, dyspnea, and pleuritic chest pain. The disease is self-limited, usually lasting a week or two, but frequently with fatigue lasting for several weeks. Occasionally patients will be troubled by pericarditis, persistent symptoms, or arthralgia and erythema nodosum.[66] These symptoms respond well to nonsteroidal antiinflammatory agents.

Progressive disseminated histoplasmosis develops rarely, usually seen in those with impaired cell-mediated immunity. The liver, spleen, lymphatic system, bone marrow, and adrenal glands are most frequently involved. Diffuse pulmonary infiltrates may appear and progress rapidly, at times accompanied by shock and disseminated intravascular coagulation.

Chronic cavitary pulmonary histoplasmosis occurs in about 10% of patients with symptomatic histoplasmosis. The majority has chronic obstructive pulmonary disease (COPD) and other structural defects in the lungs that predispose them to the illness. Clinically, the disease is similar to cavitary tuberculosis, except that the illness is less severe. The radiographic picture mimics that seen in TB, with fibronodular changes, often involving both pulmonary apices, cavities, and adjacent pulmonary pleural thickening.

Fibrosing mediastinitis represents excessive scarring from prior histoplasmosis infection. The symptoms are produced by gradual, relentless compression of mediastinal structures, including the superior vena cava, pulmonary vessels, esophagus, and tracheobronchial tree. The calcified nodes may actually erode into the latter two structures, presenting as a broncholith with airway obstruction and hemoptysis or with a localized esophageal leak and dysphagia (Figure 12-12). The progression is fatal in 10% to 20% of cases, and attempts to surgically bypass or remove the obstructing lesions are difficult and often unrewarding. Antifungal and steroid therapies are of limited use in fibrosing mediastinitis, and do not slow the progression of the disease.[49]

Histoplasmomas are the residua of healed primary histoplasmosis and are usually seen as asymptomatic coin lesions on routine chest films. Their significance lies in the fact that the lesions, if uncalcified, may be impossible to differentiate from neoplasm, and surgical excision may be indicated. Computed tomography may reveal central calcification or peripheral calcification with a "target" appearance indicating a benign diagnosis.

Definitive diagnosis of active histoplasmosis relies on isolation of the fungus in culture. Serological immunodiffusion tests detect antibodies to *H. capsulatum* in 24 to 48 hours, but may also be positive in those with a remote history of the disease. Further, the test is negative in up to 10% of patients with culture proven histoplasmosis, usually in immunocompromised patients.

Amphotericin B is the mainstay of significant histoplasmosis infections. The primary, self-limiting infection does not require therapy unless progression to severe illness is documented. Treatment is always indicated in the disseminated form of the disease and in immunocompromised populations. Chronic pulmonary histoplasmosis may alternatively be treated with ketoconazole or itraconazole. Surgical intervention in the chronic form of the disease is indicated only if the thick-walled cavities fail to respond to an adequate course of antimicrobial therapy, and pulmonary function permits.

Coccidioidomycosis

Coccidioidomycosis is the illness caused by the pathogenic fungus *Coccidioides immitis*. This dimorphic fungus is found in the soil as a mold and in tissues as an endosporulating spherule. Relatively hardy, it can withstand periods of high salinity and drought, but is intolerant of freezing temperatures. It is endemic in the desert southwest United States, and protection from infection in the endemic area is almost impossible. The infecting structures are termed arthroconidia, which is separated from the mold stalk by wind or other disturbances. The arthroconidia are transported through the air, resulting in inhalation into the distal air sacs of the lung and transformation into spherules. The spherules enlarge in the lung and become packed with endospores, which ultimately rupture, liberating the tiny endospores and perpetuating the invasive process. The severity of the clinical course after inhalation of the endospores is determined mainly by the host's ability to develop cell-mediated immunity against *C. immitis* to control infection. Children exposed are more likely to develop a mild or asymptomatic infection, whereas adults are more likely to have a severe primary infection with dissemination. African Americans are 12 times more likely to develop disseminated disease than Caucasians, with American Indian, Hispanic, and Filipino ethnic groups also at increased risk.[15] Men are at higher risk than women.

The most common clinical manifestations of primary pulmonary coccidioidomycosis, termed desert or valley fever, are cough, fever, fatigue, dyspnea, chest pain, and headache. The symptoms develop 1–4 weeks after exposure.

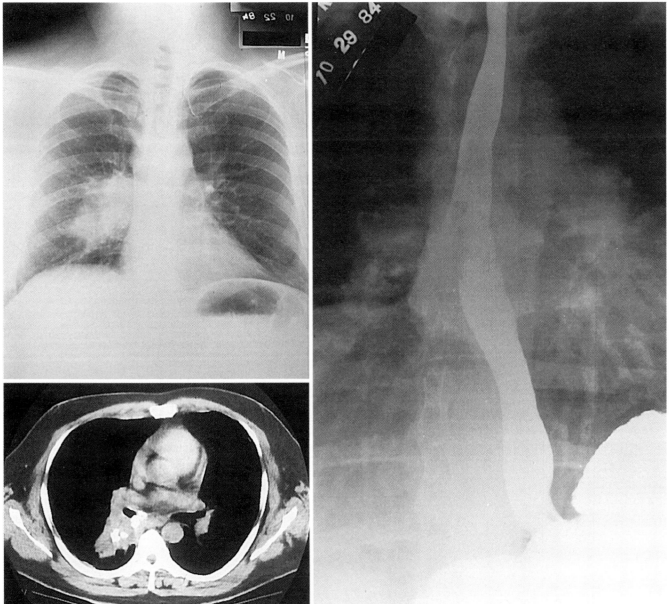

Figure 12–12 Computed tomography, contrast esophagography, and chest radiography demonstrating calcified mediastinal granulomatous disease secondary to *Histoplasmosis*, with erosion into the adjacent esophagus.
(Reproduced with permission from Darling G, Downey GP, Herridge MS: Bacterial infections of the lung. In: Pearson FG, Cooper JD, Deslauriers J, et al: Thoracic Surgery, 2nd ed. Philadelphia: Churchill Livingstone, 2002, pp. 521–651.)

Approximately 20% of patients will have erythema nodosum or erythema multiforme, indicating an excellent cell-mediated immune response and prognosis. In the majority of cases the disease is self-limiting and remits in a few days. More severe primary infections can be accompanied by high fever, cough, weight loss, and development of pulmonary infiltrates and may take weeks to resolve. If the symptoms persist for longer than 6 weeks with concomitant radiologic findings, treatment is usually started.

Patchy infiltrates are the most common radiographical finding in primary coccidioidomycosis, which range in size from subsegmental to lobar. Infiltrates may be single or multiple. Adenopathy can be present and be so dramatic as to resemble lymphoma. Subsequent necrosis of the infiltrate commonly occurs, resulting in cavitation or coalescence into a granulomatous nodule (Figure 12-13). The cavities are usually peripheral in location and may rupture into the pleural space, causing a pleural effusion, pneumothorax, bronchopleural fistula, and empyema. Secondary infection of the cavity and hemoptysis may also occur. The nodules that form within the lung parenchyma mimic bronchogenic carcinoma and often require resection to settle the issue.

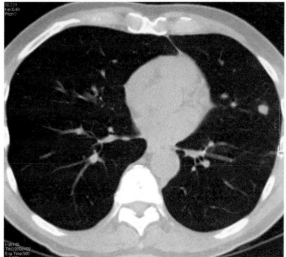

Figure 12–13 Computed tomography scan demonstrating a granuloma in the lingula due to *Coccidioidomycosis* infection.

Disseminated coccidioidomycosis may occur, typically as the result of hematogenous spread. The symptoms are insidious in onset several weeks after the primary infection. Skin and soft tissue lesions, bone and joint lesions, involvement of the genitourinary system, and meningitis may result.

The diagnosis of coccidioidomycosis depends on the identification of *C. immitis* within the body tissues or fluids. Detection by culture may take several weeks. Serum or cerebrospinal fluid may be tested to detect antibodies to *C. immitis* through an immunodiffusion method. This test usually becomes positive within 4 weeks after an initial infection and remains positive throughout the clinically active illness. Some individuals continue to produce detectable antibodies for up to 1 year after recovery. Negative serology does not exclude a diagnosis of coccidioidomycosis. A skin test is available that shows a reaction to coccidioidin, prepared from the mycelial phase of the organism. A positive test is highly correlated with protection and a favorable prognosis. Patients with disseminated disease often lose this measure of cell-mediated immunity, and a persistently negative skin test at the end of therapy suggests the possibility of relapse.

Most patients with coccidioidomycosis require no therapy. All patients with disseminated disease and those with extensive pulmonary disease should be treated. Amphotericin B is the treatment of choice. Meningeal involvement is treated with intrathecal therapy. Surgical intervention is indicated for resection of old granulomas suggestive of carcinoma, and for complications arising from cavitary disease.

Blastomycosis

Blastomycosis is a systemic mycotic infection caused by the dimorphic fungus *Blastomyces dermatitidis*. The fungus is a soil-dwelling organism endemic to the southeastern and central United States, although interestingly it has been cultured from soil only infrequently.[13] This fact, as well as the lack of a suitable skin test, has made precise definition of the endemic region problematic. The infecting microconidia are inhaled

to the level of the alveolus, where the organism converts to its parasitic yeastlike form. The yeast multiplies rapidly, attracting neutrophils and macrophages and later a T-cell mediated immune reaction. An area of pneumonitis forms, with involvement of the regional lymph nodes. As granuloma formation finally occurs, with the organisms walled off, healing begins with "rounding off" of the infiltrate and fibrosis. These produce the late coin lesions suggestive of carcinoma. Late calcification of these lesions is less common than with histoplasmosis or coccidioidomycosis. If delayed hypersensitivity does not develop, the fungus may disseminate throughout the body and involve the skin, bones, meninges, and prostate or adrenal glands, producing disseminated disease. In patients with cell-mediated immune deficiencies, blastomycosis can present as a rapidly progressive infection.[58]

The primary infection site is the lung, although the incidence of asymptomatic infection is difficult to determine. In symptomatic cases the disease may present acutely with fever, chills, myalgias, arthralgias, and a dry, hacking cough that becomes productive. Hemoptysis and pleuritic pain may occur. Most symptomatic patients recover within 2–3 weeks. Occasionally the symptoms will persist, resulting in chronic suppuration and cavitation. Patients who seem to have recovered may develop recurrent infection in areas remote from the primary site.

Radiological findings are variable. Single or multiple sites of infiltrate and or nodularity may occur, often with a lower lobe predilection. Pleural involvement may be seen, including thick, irregular pleural-based lesions.

B. dermatitidis is readily isolated from infected fluid or tissue, given proper care is given in the specimen processing. This round, thick-walled, single budding yeast measuring 8–15 fm in diameter may be seen reasonably well with routine H&E stains, although periodic acid-schiff and methenamine silver stains usually have many more organisms. Sputum or other fluids should be prepared with a 10% KOH solution and examined under a microscope using reduced illumination. A definitive diagnosis may be obtained within an hour. Identification by culture, in contrast, may take weeks. Serodiagnosis of blastomycosis has not been successful to date.

For subclinical disease, treatment may be deferred. In more severe but not life-threatening forms of the illness, itraconazole is used preferentially. Itraconazole may also be used as an adjunct following therapy with amphotericin B in disseminated cases, those with immune compromise, and in those with mild extrapulmonary disease. For life-threatening and diffuse disease, amphotericin B is the drug of choice. Meningeal involvement also mandates amphotericin B therapy. The role of surgery in blastomycosis is to help with diagnosis and rule out malignancy.

Aspergillosis

Aspergillus is a ubiquitous soil-dwelling organism which releases small conidiophores that are easily inhaled (Figure 12-14). It is inevitable that exposure occurs, and thus the development of active infection depends on other influences. Although more than 200 species of *Aspergillus* are known, only a few are thought to be pathogenic for humans. *A. fumigatus*, *A. flavus*, and *A. niger* are the most common, with *A. fumigatus* dominating in human disease. In patients

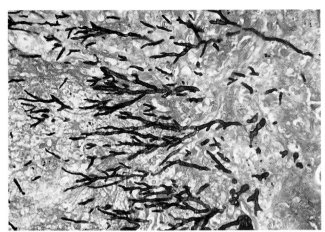

Figure 12–14 *Aspergillus fumigatus* infection, demonstrating the branching, septate hyphae of the organism. *(Reproduced with permission from Darling G, Downey GP, Herridge MS: Bacterial infections of the lung. In: Pearson FG, Cooper JD, Deslauriers J, et al: Thoracic Surgery, 2nd ed. Philadelphia: Churchill Livingstone, 2002, pp. 521–651.)*

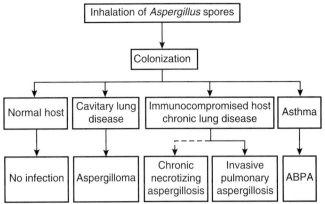

Figure 12–15 The spectrum of *Aspergillus* infection.

aspergillosis, or a hypersensitivity reaction to *Aspergillus*-causing illness. The spectrum of *Aspergillus* infection is detailed in Figure 12-15.

Aspergilloma

with normal immune function, no chronic or structural lung disease, and no hypersensitivity or allergic concerns, an infection is usually averted. In others, three main types of *Aspergillus* infection may occur, with considerable overlap. Patients may develop a noninvasive aspergilloma, invasive

Individuals with cavitary lung disease may develop an aspergilloma, a noninvasive infection characterized by a mass of fungal mycelia, inflammatory cells, mucus and tissue debris, all within a preformed lung cavity (Figure 12-16). The cavity classically has been attributed to a prior

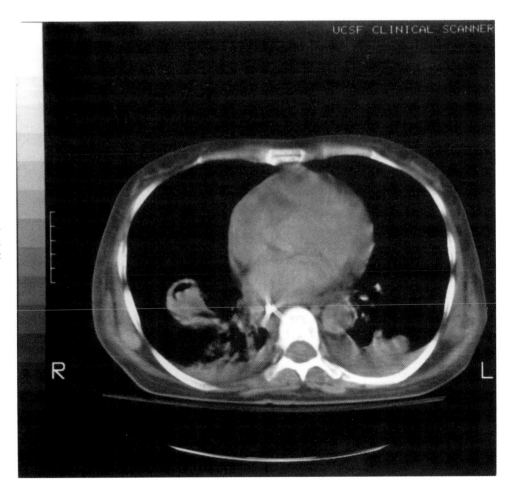

Figure 12–16 Computed tomography scan demonstrating an aspergilloma involving the right lower lobe.

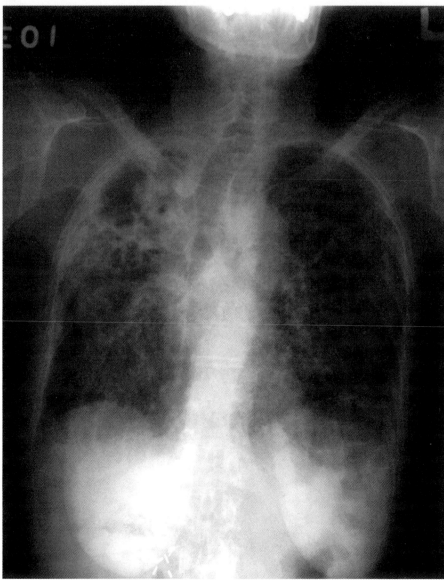

Figure 12–17 Posteroanterior (A) and

A

tubercular infection, although this is obviously not always the case. Other types of fungus may produce a fungal ball, yet *Aspergillus* is by far the most common.[38] The true incidence of aspergilloma is unknown. In a study of 544 patients with a preexisting lung cavity due to tuberculosis, 11% had radiographic evidence of aspergilloma.[3] Most aspergillomas remain asymptomatic, yet some may increase in size or cause hemoptysis requiring intervention. On the other hand, some resolve spontaneously. Invasion and dissemination from an aspergilloma rarely occur. In addition to hemoptysis, which is the most common presenting symptom, chronic cough and weight loss can occur. Rupture of the cavity into the pleural space with subsequent empyema and fistula has been reported.

Radiographic imaging reveals a thick-walled cavity, typically in the upper lobe, with a mass or "fungal ball" within the cavity. Movement of the mass inside the cavity with position change is variable and not a reliable diagnostic test, but remains an additional interesting finding (Figure 12-17). Differential diagnoses include cavitating hematoma, neoplasm, abscess, Wegner's granulomatosis, and hydatid cyst. It is important to note that aspergilloma may coexist with any of the above diagnoses. Culture of the sputum may yield *Aspergillus*, but is frequently negative. Serological testing will be helpful in the setting of a suspicious radiologic finding.

Systemic antimicrobial agents, including amphotericin B, have limited use in aspergilloma because of poor penetration into the cavity. Asymptomatic mycetomas should be left alone. Surgical resection is indicated if hemoptysis or other symptoms attributable to the lesion occurs, and adequate pulmonary reserve is present.

Invasive Aspergillosis

Acute invasive *Aspergillus* infection is a rare but dramatic occurrence in immunosuppressed and myelosuppressed

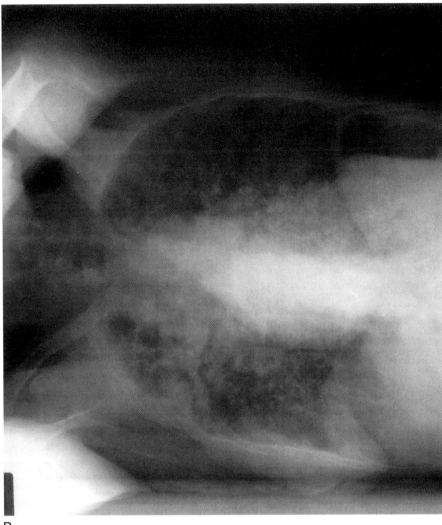

Figure 12–17 cont'd (B) chest radiographs demonstrating an aspergilloma within a right upper lobe cavity. The fungus ball "moves" with change in patient position.

B

patients. Myelosuppression appears to be the greatest risk factor for invasive pulmonary aspergillosis; patients with leukemia have an incidence 20 times higher than patients with lymphoma or patients with solid organ transplants.[8] Risk factors for invasive aspergillosis include prolonged neutropenia, corticosteroid therapy, transplantation (highest with lung and bone marrow), hematological malignancy, cytotoxic therapy, and AIDS.[70]

The lower respiratory tract is the focus of the invasive infection. As a result, respiratory symptoms predominate, including fever, cough, sputum production, and dyspnea. The presence of pleuritic chest pain (due to pulmonary infarction following vascular invasion) and hemoptysis, in the appropriate clinical setting, should alert the clinician to the possibility of the diagnosis.[1] With vascular invasion, the organism can spread to other organs, particularly the brain but also the heart and intraabdominal organs.

Radiological findings may be nonspecific. Rounded densities and peripheral, pleural-based infiltrates are suggestive of infarction. Typical computed tomography findings include multiple nodules, a halo sign (hemorrhage surrounding a nodule), and the air crescent sign (lucency in the region of the original nodule secondary to necrosis). The

presence of *Aspergillus* spp. in sputum samples could be due to colonization, although studies have shown positive cultures in patients who have leukemia or in those who have undergone bone marrow transplant and have a positive predictive value of 80–90%.[34] Bronchoalveolar lavage (BAL) is helpful in the diagnosis of invasive aspergillosis, particularly in patients with diffuse lung involvement. Transbronchial biopsies add little to the BAL testing except increased risk. Serological studies are not helpful in this setting. The use of lung biopsy remains the gold standard for diagnosis but should be reserved for equivocal cases.

The mortality for invasive aspergillosis remains high, and empiric therapy should be initiated as early as possible. The treatment of choice remains amphotericin B. Itraconazole and caspofungin are alternatives, and investigation is underway regarding combination therapy.

Allergic Bronchopulmonary Aspergillosis

Allergic bronchopulmonary aspergillosis (ABPA) is a hypersensitivity reaction to *Aspergillus* antigens, particularly *A. fumigatus*. It is typically seen in patients with long-standing asthma or cystic fibrosis. It is believed that IgE- and

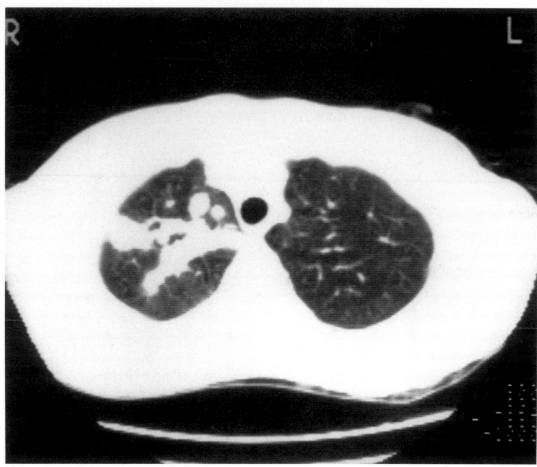

Figure 12–18 Computed tomography demonstrating allergic bronchopulmonary aspergillosis (ABPA) involving the right upper lobe.

IgG-mediated reactions play a central role in ABPA. The diagnosis is usually made on clinical grounds buttressed by radiological and serological testing. Patients present with wheezing, fever, and mucus plugging; radiological studies show pulmonary infiltrates that tend to be in the upper lobe and central in location. Volume loss secondary to mucus impaction may be seen, appearing as bandlike opacities emanating from the hilum with rounded distal margins (Figure 12-18). Treatment consists of oral corticosteroids to suppress the immunologic response to the *Aspergillus* antigens and the secondary inflammatory reaction. Concurrent itraconazole may be added to the regimen.

Cryptococcosis

Cryptococcus neoformans is an encapsulated yeast that is found worldwide as a soil organism. It is associated with bird (pigeon) droppings, although the birds do not serve as a vector or carrier for the microbe. The portal of entry in humans is the respiratory tract. As a result, pulmonary infection may be the first manifestation of disease, but is usually variable and nonspecific. Spontaneous remission usually occurs in most patients. In those with suppressed or impaired immune systems, disseminated disease can result. *C. neoformans* has a special predilection for the meninges, and lethal meningitis can occur.

Treatment of cryptococcosis involves amphotericin B and flucytosine. Cryptococcal infections usually come to the attention of the thoracic surgeon following resection of a pulmonary mass, which is found to be a chronic granulomatous reaction to a prior *C. neoformans* infection. Central necrosis and cavitation are not commonly seen, as in other major pulmonary mycotic infections. These lesions often involve the lower lobe and are solid. Up to 10% of patients with a resected pulmonary lesion develop cryptococcal meningitis after resection.[32] If incidental resection occurs, sampling of the spinal fluid should be performed. Evidence of extrapulmonary disease or residual pulmonary disease should prompt initiation of therapy.

Mucormycosis

Mucormycosis is a rare fungal infection, frequently fatal, caused by fungi of the subclass Zygomycetes. *Mucor* species are ubiquitous and are found in soil and decaying organic debris. Infection occurs by inhalation of spores and is commonly found in immunocompromised hosts. Risk factors for *Mucor* infection include neutropenia, acidosis, hyperglycemia, corticosteroid therapy, and deferoxamine therapy. This fungus grows best in acidic, hyperglycemic environments, thus accounting for the susceptibility of patients with diabetic ketoacidosis.

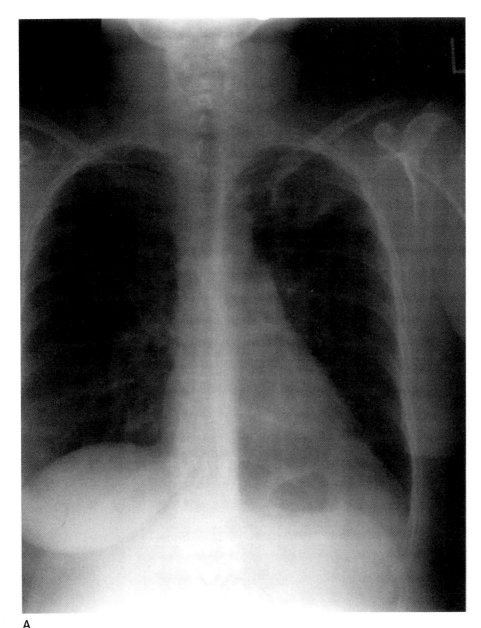

A

Figure 12–19 Posteroanterior (A) and

Mucor infections may involve several different areas of the body, including rhinocerebral, pulmonary, cutaneous, gastrointestinal, and the central nervous system. The rhinocerebral involvement is commonly seen in poorly controlled diabetics, and these patients may also have a pulmonary component. The pulmonary aspect typically presents with bronchopneumonia (Figure 12-19) and progresses to invade pulmonary vessels, causing infarction. The infection can directly invade the extrapulmonary tissues, including the chest wall and mediastinal structures.

The radiological findings are variable and contribute little to refining the diagnosis. Culture results are usually negative, but if positive, strongly suggest invasive disease. Direct pathological examination of infected tissue should reveal broad, usually nonseptate hyphae invading the tissue. The side branches are short and at a 90-degree angle.

The overall mortality rate for pulmonary mucormycosis exceeds 50%. Therapy consists of three components: correction of underlying abnormalities, such as the hyperglycemic acidotic state seen with diabetic ketoacidosis, and reversal of immunosuppression, if possible; early institution of high-dose amphotericin B therapy; and aggressive surgical resection of involved lung and soft tissue, when possible.

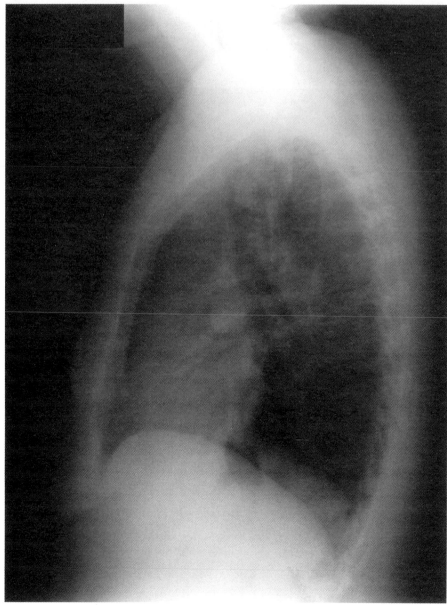

Figure 12–19 cont'd (B) lateral chest radiographs demonstrating *Mucormycosis* infection involving the left upper lobe.

B

REFERENCES

1. Albelda SM, Talbot GH, Gerson SL, et al: Pulmonary cavitation and massive hemoptysis in invasive pulmonary aspergillosis. Influence of bone marrow recovery in patients with acute leukemia. Am Rev Respir Dis 131:115–120, 1985.

2. Angrill J, Agusti C, de Celis R, et al: Bacterial colonization in patients with bronchiectasis: microbiological pattern and risk factors. Thorax 57:15–19, 2002.

3. Anonymous: Aspergilloma and residual tuberculous—the results of a resurvey. Tubercle 51:227–245, 1970.

4. Barker AF: Bronchiectasis. N Engl J Med 346:1383–1393, 2002.

5. Bartlett JG, Dowell SF, Mandell LA, et al: Practice guidelines for the management of community-acquired pneumonia in adults. Clin Infect Dis 31:347–82, 2000.

6. Bartlett JG, Mundy LM: Community-acquired pneumonia. N Engl J Med 333:1618–1624, 1995.

7. Bates JH, Campbell GD, Barron AL, et al: Microbial etiology of acute pneumonia in hospitalized patients. Chest 101:1005–12, 1992.

8. Burch PA, Karp JE, Merz WG, et al: Favorable outcome of invasive aspergillosis in patients with acute leukemia. J Clin Oncol 5:1985–1993, 1987.

9. Cockburn J, Gibberd RW, Reid AL, Sanson-Fisher RW: Determinants of non-compliance with short term antibiotic regimens. Br Med J (Clin Res Ed) 295:814–818, 1987.

10. Coley CM, Li YH, Medsger AR, et al: Preferences for home vs. hospital care among low-risk patients with community-acquired pneumonia. Arch Intern Med 156:1565–1571, 1996.

11. Collard HR, Saint S, Matthay MA: Prevention of ventilator-associated pneumonia: an evidence-based systematic review. Ann Intern Med 138:494–501, 2003.

12. Craven DE, Steger KA: Epidemiology of nosocomial pneumonia. New perspectives on an old disease. Chest 108:1S–16S, 1995.

13. Davies SF, Sarosi GA: Blastomycosis. In: Sarosi GA, Davies SF, eds: Fungal Diseases of the Lung. New York: Raven Press, 1993, pp. 51–64.

14. Dominguez J, Gali N, Blanco S, et al: Detection of Streptococcus pneumoniae antigen by a rapid immunochromatographic assay in urine samples. Chest119:243–249, 2001.

15. Drutz DJ, Catanzaro A: Coccidioidomycosis. Part II. Am Rev Respir Dis 117:727–771, 1978.

16. Dye CSS, Dolin P, Pathania V, Raviglione MC: Global burden of tuberculosis: estimated incidence, prevalence, and mortality by country. WHO Global Surveillance and Monitoring Project. JAMA282:677–686, 1999.

17. Edwards LB, Acquaviva FA, Livesay VT, et al: An atlas of sensitivity to tuberculin, PPD-B, and histoplasmin in the United States. Am Rev Respir Dis 99:Suppl:1–132, 1969.

18. Emergency Physicians A Co: Clinical policy for the management and risk stratification of community-acquired pneumonia in adults in the emergency department. Ann Emerg Med 38:107–113, 2001.

19. Ewig S, Ruiz M, Mensa J, et al: Severe community-acquired pneumonia. Assessment of severity criteria. Am J Respir Crit Care Med 158:1102–1108, 1998.

20. Ewig S, Torres A: Prevention and management of ventilator-associated pneumonia. Curr Opin Crit Care 8:58–69, 2002.

21. Fabian TC: Empiric therapy for pneumonia in the surgical intensive care unit. Am J Surg179:18S–23S, 2000; discussion 24S–25S.

22. Fang GD, Fine M, Orloff J, et al: New and emerging etiologies for community-acquired pneumonia with implications for therapy. A prospective multicenter study of 359 cases. Medicine 69:307–316, 1990.

23. Fine MJ, Auble TE, Yealy DM, et al: A prediction rule to identify low-risk patients with community-acquired pneumonia. N Engl J Med 336:243–250, 1997.

24. Fine MJ, Pratt HM, Obrosky DS, et al: Relation between length of hospital stay and costs of care for patients with community-acquired pneumonia. Am J Med 109:378–385, 2000.

25. Fine MJ, Smith MA, Carson CA, et al: Prognosis and outcomes of patients with community-acquired pneumonia. A meta-analysis. JAMA 275:134–141, 1996.

26. Fridkin SK, Welbel SF, Weinstein RA. Magnitude and prevention of nosocomial infections in the intensive care unit. Infect Dis Clin North Am. 11:479–496, 1997.

27. Gleason PP, Kapoor WN, Stone RA, et al: Medical outcomes and antimicrobial costs with the use of the American Thoracic Society guidelines for outpatients with community-acquired pneumonia. JAMA 278:32–39, 1997.

28. Gleason PP, Meehan TP, Fine JM, et al: Associations between initial antimicrobial therapy and medical outcomes for hospitalized elderly patients with pneumonia. Arch Intern Med 159:2562–2572, 1999.

29. Gleeson K, Eggli DF, Maxwell SL: Quantitative aspiration during sleep in normal subjects. Chest 111:1266–1272, 1997.

30. Hagan JL, Hardy JD: Lung abscess revisited. A survey of 184 cases. Ann Surg 197:755–762, 1983.

31. Halm EA, Teirstein AS: Management of community-acquired pneumonia. N Engl J Med 347:2039–2045, 2002.

32. Hatcher CR, Jr, Sehdeva J, Waters WC, 3rd, et al: Primary pulmonary cryptococcosis. J Thorac Cardiovasc Surg 61:39–49, 1971.

33. Heyland DK, Cook DJ, Griffith L, et al: The attributable morbidity and mortality of ventilator-associated pneumonia in the critically ill patient. The Canadian Critical Trials Group. Am J Respir Crit Care Med 159:1249–1256, 1999.

34. Horvath JA, Dummer S: The use of respiratory-tract cultures in the diagnosis of invasive pulmonary aspergillosis. Am J Med 100:171–178, 1996.

35. Houck PM, MacLehose RF, Niederman MS, Lowery JK: Empiric antibiotic therapy and mortality among Medicare pneumonia inpatients in 10 western states: 1993, 1995, and 1997. Chest 119:1420–1426, 2001.

36. Iseman MD, Buschman DL, Ackerson LM: Pectus excavatum and scoliosis. Thoracic anomalies associated with pulmonary disease caused by Mycobacterium avium complex. Am Rev Respir. Dis 144:914–6, 1991.

37. Iseman MD, Degroote M. Environmental mycobacterium infections. In: Gorbach SL, Bartlett JG, Blacklow NR, eds: Infectious Diseases. Baltimore: Lippincott Williams & Wilkins, 2004, pp. 1389–1410.

38. Joynson DH: Pulmonary aspergilloma. Br J Clin Pract 31:207–216,221, 1977.

39. Kami M, Fukui T, Ogawa S, et al: Use of real-time PCR on blood samples for diagnosis of invasive aspergillosis. Clin Infect Dis 33:1504–1512, 2001.

40. Kollef MH: Appropriate antibiotic therapy for ventilator-associated pneumonia and sepsis: a necessity, not an issue for debate. Intens Care Med 29:147–149, 2003.

41. Kollef MH: The prevention of ventilator-associated pneumonia. N Engl J Med 340:627–634, 1999.

42. Langer M, Mosconi P, Cigada M, Mandelli M: Long-term respiratory support and risk of pneumonia in critically ill patients. Intensive Care Unit Group of Infection Control. Am Rev Respir Dis 140:302–305, 1989.

43. Leu H, Kaiser D, Mori M, et al: Hospital-acquired pneumonia. Attributable mortality and morbidity. Am J Epidemiol 129:1258–1267, 1989.

44. Lieberman D, Schlaeffer F, Boldur I, et al: Multiple pathogens in adult patients admitted with community-acquired pneumonia: a one year prospective study of 346 consecutive patients. Thorax 51:179–184, 1996.

45. Mandell LA, Bartlett JG, Dowell SF, et al: Update of practice guidelines for the management of community-acquired pneumonia in immunocompetent adults. Clin Infect Dis 37:1405–1433, 2003.

46. Mandell LA, Campbell GD, Jr: Nosocomial pneumonia guidelines: an international perspective. Chest 113:188S–193S, 1998.

47. Marik PE: Aspiration pneumonitis and aspiration pneumonia. N Engl J Med 344:665–671, 2001.

48. Marrie TJ: Community-acquired pneumonia. Clin Infect Dis 18:501–513, 1994; quiz 514–515.

49. Mathisen DJ, Grillo HC: Clinical manifestation of mediastinal fibrosis and histoplasmosis. Ann Thorac Surg 54:1053–1057, 1992; discussion 1057–1058.

50. Meehan TP, Fine MJ, Krumholz HM, et al: Quality of care, process, and outcomes in elderly patients with pneumonia. JAMA 278:2080–2084, 1997.

51. Mehta R, Niederman MS: Adequate empirical therapy minimizes the impact of diagnostic methods in patients with ventilator-associated pneumonia. Crit Care Med 28:3092–3094, 2000.

52. Mendelson CL: The aspiration of stomach contents into the lungs during obstetric anesthesia. Am J Obstet Gynecol 52:191–205, 1946.

53. Metersky ML, Ma A, Bratzler DW, Houck PM: Predicting bacteremia in patients with community-acquired pneumonia. Am J Respir Crit Care Med 169:342–347, 2004.

54. Metlay JP, Fine MJ: Testing strategies in the initial management of patients with community-acquired pneumonia. Ann Intern Med 138:109–118, 2003.

55. Napolitano LM: Hospital-acquired and ventilator-associated pneumonia: what's new in diagnosis and treatment? Am J Surg 186:4S–14S, 2003; discussion 31S–34S.

56. Niederman MS, Mandell LA, Anzueto A, et al: Guidelines for the management of adults with community-acquired

194

pneumonia. Diagnosis, assessment of severity, antimicrobial therapy, and prevention. Am J Respir Crit Care Med 163:1730–1754, 2001.

57. Niederman MS, McCombs JS, Unger AN, et al: The cost of treating community-acquired pneumonia. Clin Ther 20:820–837, 1998.

58. Pappas PG, Threlkeld MG, Bedsole GD, et al: Blastomycosis in immunocompromised patients. Medicine 72:311–325, 1993.

59. Pereira Gomes JC, Pedreira WL, Jr, Araujo EM, et al. Impact of BAL in the management of pneumonia with treatment failure: positivity of BAL culture under antibiotic therapy. Chest 118:1739–1746, 2000.

60. Perfect JR, Cox GM, Lee JY, et al. The impact of culture isolation of Aspergillus species: a hospital-based survey of aspergillosis. Clin Infect Dis; 33:1824–1833, 2001.

61. Plouffe JF, File TM, Jr, Breiman RF, et al: Reevaluation of the definition of Legionnaires' disease: use of the urinary antigen assay. Community Based Pneumonia Incidence Study Group. Clin Infect Dis 20:1286–1291, 1995.

62. Pomerantz BJ, Cleveland JC, Olson HK, Pomerantz M: Pulmonary resection for multi-drug resistant tuberculosis. J Thorac Cardiovasc Surg 121:448–453, 2001.

63. Pomerantz M, Denton JR, Huitt GA, et al: Resection of the right middle lobe and lingula for mycobacterial infection. Ann Thorac Surg 62:990–993, 1996.

64. Reid LM: Reduction in bronchial subdivision in bronchiectasis. Thorax 5:233–247, 1950.

65. Rello J, Diaz E, Roque M, Valles J: Risk factors for developing pneumonia within 48 hours of intubation. Am J Respir. Crit Care Med 159:1742–1746, 1999.

66. Rosenthal J, Brandt KD, Wheat LJ, Slama TG: Rheumatologic manifestations of histoplasmosis in the recent Indianapolis epidemic. Arthritis Rheumat 26:1065–1070, 1983.

67. Ruiz M, Torres A, Ewig S, et al: Noninvasive versus invasive microbial investigation in ventilator-associated pneumonia: evaluation of outcome. Am J Respir Crit Care Med 162:119–125, 2000.

68. Seabury JH, Buechner HA, Busey JF: The diagnosis of pulmonary mycoses. Report of the Committee on Fungus Diseases and Subcommittee on Criteria for Clinical Diagnosis, American College of Chest Physicians. Chest 60:82–88, 1971.

69. Sole Violan J, Fernandez JA, Benitez AB, et al: Impact of quantitative invasive diagnostic techniques in the management and outcome of mechanically ventilated patients with suspected pneumonia. Crit Care Med 28:2737–2741, 2000.

70. Soubani AO, Chandrasekar PH: The clinical spectrum of pulmonary aspergillosis. Chest 121:1988–1999, 2002.

71. Stahl JE, Barza M, DesJardin J, et al: Effect of macrolides as part of initial empiric therapy on length of stay in patients hospitalized with community-acquired pneumonia. ArchIntern Med 159:2576–2580, 1999.

72. Stark DD, Federle MP, Goodman PC, et al: Differentiating lung abscess and empyema: radiography and computed tomography. Am J Roentgenol 141:163–167, 1983.

73. Storch G, Burford JG, George RB, et al: Acute histoplasmosis. Description of an outbreak in northern Louisiana. Chest 77:38–42, 1980.

74. Swensen SJ, Peters SG, LeRoy AJ, et al: Radiology in the intensive-care unit. Mayo Clin Proc 66:396–410, 1991.

75. Torres A, Aznar R, Gatell JM, et al: Incidence, risk, and prognosis factors of nosocomial pneumonia in mechanically ventilated patients. Am Rev Respir Dis 142:523–528, 1990.

76. Turin L, Riva F, Galbiati G, Cainelli T: Fast, simple and highly sensitive double-rounded polymerase chain reaction assay to detect medically relevant fungi in dermatological specimens. Eur J Clin Invest 30:511–518, 2000.

77. Warner MA, Warner ME, Weber JG: Clinical significance of pulmonary aspiration during the perioperative period. Anesthesiology 78:56–62, 1993.

78. Werner SB, Pappagianis D, Heindl I, Mickel A: An epidemic of coccidioidomycosis among archeology students in northern California. N Engl J Med 286:507–512, 1972.

79. Wiedemann HP, Rice TW: Lung abscess and empyema.[erratum appears in Semin Thorac Cardiovasc Surg 7(4):247, Oct 1995]. Semin Thorac Cardiovasc Surg 7:119–128, 1995.

80. Yang PC, Luh KT, Lee YC, et al: Lung abscesses: US examination and US-guided transthoracic aspiration. Radiology 180:171–175, 1991.

Surgery for Emphysema

Bryan F. Meyers and Joel D. Cooper

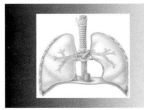

▶ INTRODUCTION

The debilitating symptoms of pulmonary emphysema have attracted the interest of surgeons throughout the history of our specialty. Many innovative and creative operations have been devised to treat the dyspnea caused by this disease. Costochondrectomy, phrenic crush, pneumoperitoneum, pleural abrasion, lung denervation, and thoracoplasty all proved to be dead ends in the evolution of surgical treatment for the hyperexpanded and poorly perfused emphysematous lung.[8] Only three surgical procedures have evolved to survive the test of time and withstand the close scrutiny of the medical community: bullectomy, lung transplantation, and lung volume reduction. Bullectomy has roots dating back to the first half of the last century when external drainage of the giant bulla was attempted to eliminate the space-occupying lesion by collapse rather than by resection. Although vestiges of this conservative approach remain in use for rare high-risk patients, the general approach has evolved to include resection of the bulla with sparing of all functional lung tissue. Lung transplantation was successfully performed in 1963 by Hardy et al,[17] and, after a prolonged period of incremental progress, the operation became clinically feasible in the early 1980s as heart–lung transplantation[36] and isolated lung transplantation.[42] Although lung transplantation was initially used as therapy for pulmonary fibrosis and pulmonary hypertension, the indications have evolved such that emphysema is the most common diagnosis leading to transplantation today. Lung volume reduction surgery (LVRS) was first proposed by Brantigan et al[5] in conjunction with lung denervation and was discarded after the initial experience; a mortality of 16% showed the oper-

ation to be too risky. Observations about the physiological behavior of emphysema patients during and after lung transplantation led the reconsideration of volume reduction by Cooper et al.[9]

The destruction of pulmonary parenchyma causes a decreased mass of functioning lung tissue and thus decreases the amount of gas exchange that can take place. As the lung tissue is destroyed, it loses elastic recoil and expands in volume. This leads to the typical hyperexpanded chest seen in emphysema patients with flattened diaphragms, widened intercostal spaces, and horizontal ribs. These anatomical changes result in the loss of mechanical advantages exploited in normal breathing and thus lead to increased work of breathing and dyspnea.[39] When the destruction and expansion occur in a nonuniform manner, the most affected lung tissue can expand to crowd the relatively spared lung tissue to impair ventilation of the functioning lung. Finally, there is obstruction in the small airways caused by a combination of reversible bronchospasm and irreversible loss of elastic recoil by adjacent lung parenchyma. The suitability of a given patient for surgical treatment of emphysema depends in part on the relative contributions of lung destruction, lung compression, and small airways obstruction to the overall physiological impairment of that patient.

▶ SELECTION OF PATIENTS FOR SURGICAL TREATMENT OF EMPHYSEMA

Bullectomy, lung transplantation, and lung volume reduction surgery are invasive procedures with risk of both morbidity and mortality to patients. Therefore, all three procedures are directed only at patients who remain symptomatic despite optimal medical therapy. This optimal medical treatment will include bronchodilators to eliminate any reversible component of airway obstruction. Smoking cessation is an absolute necessity and should be in effect for at least 6 months before considering surgical therapy. Participation in pulmonary rehabilitation has been shown to relieve subjective dyspnea, increase functional capabilities, and improve subjective quality of life.[35,37] All patients considered by the authors for surgical treatment of emphysema are enrolled in a supervised pulmonary rehabilitation program and their subsequent consideration for surgery is based in part on their compliance and progress with rehabilitation. Finally, since the operations carry an immediate risk of morbidity and mortality, and since none has been shown to reliably increase life expectancy, patients considering an operation must be willing to accept the risks of surgery in exchange for an anticipated relief from dyspnea and an uncertain effect on life expectancy.

▶ BULLECTOMY

Bullectomy is considered whenever a substantial air-filled bulla is detected on chest radiograph. Most patients considered for surgery are symptomatic with dyspnea, pain, or spontaneous pneumothorax. Other symptoms are rare but include bleeding and infection within the confines of the bulla. The natural history of bullae treated expectantly with observation is one of enlargement causing worsened dyspnea, but the lack of large series of patients treated without surgery makes prediction of the rate of expansion unreliable. Some asymptomatic patients with a single bulla encompassing more than half the volume of a pleural cavity would be considered surgical candidates, while patients with smaller lesions and no symptoms would be more controversial. Factors making surgery less appealing include the presence of multiple smaller bullae, advanced emphysema in the nonbullous adjacent lung, and notable comorbidities. The frequency with which bullectomy is performed is low, as demonstrated by a systematic review by Snider who cited 22 individual reports over a 39-year time period that included a total of 476 patients.[40]

The technique of operation is quite variable and depends on the anatomical details of the bulla as well as the preferred approach of the surgeon. A well-demarcated bulla with a clear pedicle can be excised with a stapler using a muscle-sparing thoracotomy or a video-assisted thoracoscopic approach. Numerous bullae, or bullae that merge indistinctly with the comparatively normal adjacent lung, will require a large, stapled wedge resection placed to maximize resection of destroyed lung while minimizing resection of spared parenchyma. It is unusual for a formal lobectomy to be necessary, but when a lobe is nearly completely destroyed and the fissures are complete, a lobectomy is an attractive option that might eliminate the possibility of a postoperative air leak and prolonged chest tube drainage. Many surgeons will combine a localized pleurectomy or a pleural tent with the bullectomy to help manage the pleural space and prevent a prolonged chest tube air leak.

The safety of bullectomy in well-selected patients is demonstrated by the 2.3% mortality reported by FitzGerald and colleagues over 30 years ago.[13] Our own modern results are similar with a single death in 43 operations (2.3%).[38] Since properly selected patients will have an increase in FEV_1 postoperatively, there is a very low rate of respiratory failure and the need for tracheostomy. Parenchymal air leaks are the biggest single postoperative complication and they are suitably managed with the surgeon's choice of buttressed stapled lines, pleural tent, pleurectomy, biological glues, or ambulatory Heimlich valves. In our recently reported series, 53% of patients experienced chest tube air leaks for more than 7 days.

There are few reports of long-term survival and functional changes after bullectomy and none of them is a prospective clinical trial. Our own clinical series demonstrated a 5-year survival of 91% with two late deaths attributed to pneumonia and one to pulmonary fibrosis. In general, the freedom from long-term return of dyspnea is proportional to the quality of the remaining lung after bullectomy. All patients with emphysema seem to experience a progressive decline in FEV_1 over time, so patients with near-normal underlying lung at the time of bullectomy will begin at a higher functional baseline than patients with moderate or severe emphysema in the remaining lung. Our experience demonstrated an improvement in the FEV_1 from 1.2 ± 0.6 liters preoperatively to 1.9 ± 0.9 liters at 6 months and 1 year postoperatively.[38] The persistence of a measurable airflow obstruction after bullectomy underscores the presence of residual emphysema in the remaining lung, regardless of the normal appearance it may have compared to the destroyed bullous regions.

▶ LUNG TRANSPLANTATION

Pulmonary emphysema was initially felt to be a contraindication for lung transplantation. In the era preceding bilateral lung transplantation (BLT), the perceived difficulty of ventilation–perfusion mismatching in the native and newly transplanted lung was felt to be an obstacle worth avoiding. For that reason, early isolated single lung transplants were directed at patients with pulmonary fibrosis, where the elevated pulmonary vascular resistance and poor compliance of the native lung created a situation in which the transplanted lung was both preferentially perfused and preferentially ventilated. After the initial success with single lung transplantation for emphysema was reported,[21] and after the development of techniques to allow safe, bilateral lung transplantation,[30,31] the application of lung transplantation for emphysema quickly increased. Management of the recipient of a single lung transplant for emphysema has proven not to be as complicated as feared. The main principles that lead to success are the avoidance of positive end expiratory pressure and the rapid weaning from mechanical ventilation.

Idiopathic emphysema and α_1-antitrypsin deficiency together have become the most common indication for pulmonary transplantation. These two diagnoses together account for 63% of the adult single lung transplants and 32% of the bilateral lung transplants reported in the 2003 Registry of the ISHLT as reported by Trulock and colleagues.[43]

The selection criteria for lung transplantation have been published elsewhere, but are chosen to identify patients with sufficient risk of death from their lung disease to make the risks of the transplant operation worth bearing. Unfortunately, the survival of emphysema patients has been notably hard to predict, leading to early listing and an excellent survival rate on the waiting list compared to patients with other diagnoses. Most emphysema patients have deteriorated to a point at which oxygen supplementation is required. In our own experience, the mean supplemental oxygen requirement is slightly in excess of 4 liters/min. The obstructive physiology in these patients results in a first second forced expiratory volume (FEV_1) of well under 1 liter, or approximately 15% of predicted normal values. Progressive elevation in pCO_2 has been observed in some patients, however, with several of these individuals undergoing transplantation with the pCO_2 in excess of 100 mm Hg.

The advantages of lung transplantation are obvious: a complete replacement of the diseased and nonfunctional lungs with a new and healthy donor lung. Initial and long-term function of patients with single or bilateral lung transplants for emphysema shows a dramatic improvement in pulmonary function and exercise tolerance with elimination of the need for supplementary oxygen. Figure 13-1 demonstrates the magnitude of change in the FEV_1 as a result of single lung transplantation, bilateral lung transplantation, and lung volume reduction surgery as reported by Gaissert et al.[14] Figure 13-2 shows a similar stratified analysis for exercise tolerance as measured by 6-min walking distances.

It can be seen that although the improvement in both outcome measures is greatest for BLT and least for LVRS, the absolute differences in exercise tolerance are much less than those seen in pulmonary function.

The disadvantages of lung transplant are well known but worth reviewing. First, the lack of available donor lungs has created a situation in which the waiting times for transplant recipients in programs such as ours can routinely exceed 2 years. Once lungs become available, the initial morbidity and mortality of lung transplant are higher than that reported for lung volume reduction, with mortality variously described as 5–15% for the first 30 days and somewhat higher by the end of the first year. For the survivors, the presence of allograft lungs creates the need for lifelong immunosuppression that carries with it higher medical costs to the individual and society as well as increased risk of neoplasm and infection when compared with nonimmunosuppressed patients. Finally, the risk of developing chronic allograft dysfunction, or bronchiolitis obliterans syndrome, increases with function of time since transplant reaches 50–60% by 5 years after transplant. The cumulative 5-year survival of our lung transplant experience is 50%, a fact that clearly demonstrates the imperfect solution that transplant offers to emphysema patients.

A controversial aspect of lung transplantation is the question of whether it conveys a survival benefit to the recipient.

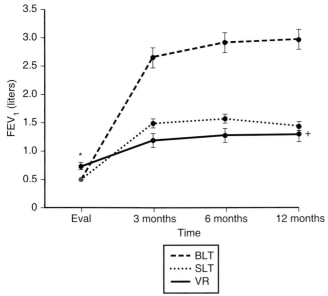

Figure 13–1 Changes observed in first second expired volumes in patients after bilateral lung transplantation, single-lung transplantation, and lung volume reduction surgery.

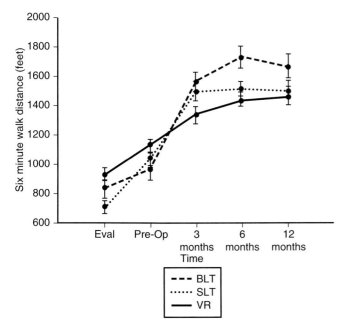

Figure 13–2 Changes observed in 6-min walk test results after single-lung transplantation, bilateral lung transplantation, and lung volume reduction surgery.

Box 13–1. Indications and Contraindications for Lung Volume Reduction Surgery and Lung Transplantation.

Indications common to both procedures
    Emphysema with destruction and hyperinflation
    Marked impairment (first second expired volume
       <35% predicted)
    Marked restriction in activities of daily living
    Failure of maximal medical treatment to correct symptoms
Contraindications to both procedures
    Abnormal body weight (<70% or >130% of ideal)
    Coexisting major medical problems increasing surgical risk
    Inability or unwillingness to participate in pulmonary
       rehabilitation
    Unwillingness to accept the risk of morbidity and mortality
       of surgery
    Tobacco use within the past 6 months
    Recent or current diagnosis of malignancy
    Increasing age (>65 for transplant, >70 for volume
       reduction)
    Psychological instability such as depression or anxiety
       disorder
Discriminating conditions favoring lung volume reduction
    surgery
    Marked thoracic distention
    Heterogeneous disease with obvious apical target areas
    FEV_1 greater than 20% predicted
    Age between 60 and 70 years
Discriminating conditions favoring lung transplantation
    Diffuse disease without target areas
    FEV_1 less than 20% predicted
    Hypercarbia with $PaCO_2$ >55 mm Hg
    Pulmonary hypertension
    Age less than 60 years
    α_1-Antitrypsin deficiency

There have been no prospective randomized trials in which lung transplantation has been directly compared to medical therapy as a treatment for advanced lung disease. As a result, the analysis of this question has been limited to the use of Cox regression analysis with the transplant procedure entered into the model as a time-dependent covariable. In essence, the patient's time spent on the waiting list is used as the medical "arm" of the trial, and the survival after transplantation is used as the surgical "arm." One such analysis by Hosenpud and colleagues showed the surprising finding that lung transplantation did not reduce the risk of death compared to the risk faced by remaining on the waiting list.[18] This finding is graphically depicted in Figure 13-3. One explanation for this finding is the stable survival of emphysema patients on the waiting list and the unique situ-

ation in the United States that allows for listing patients for transplantation long before they were considered truly ready for such an operation. Other Cox regression models looking at this exact question have shown clear survival benefit for emphysema patients undergoing lung transplantation.[12] More work in this field has been done, but it has been applied to lung transplantation in general and not to emphysema transplant recipients specifically.[1,16,34]

The choice of bilateral or unilateral transplantation for emphysema patients is controversial. In general, for younger patients, particularly those with α_1-antitrypsin deficiency, we prefer bilateral sequential single-lung transplantation (SLT). The bilateral option is also more attractive in larger recipients who might never obtain a sufficiently large single-lung allograft. On the other hand, for smaller recipients, single-

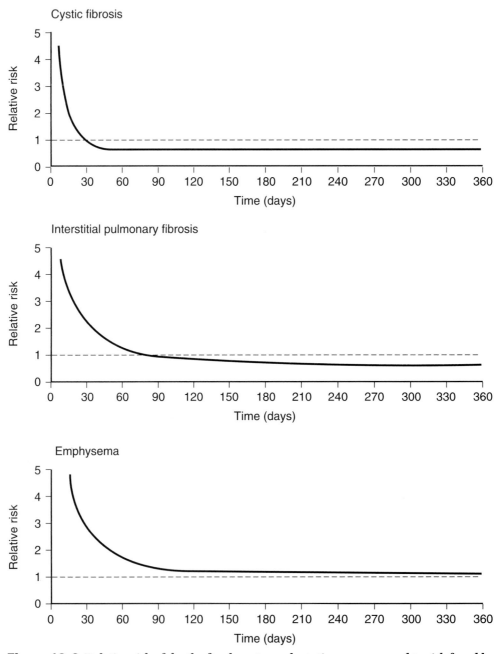

Figure 13-3 Relative risk of death after lung transplantation as compared to risk faced by remaining on the waiting list, stratified by underlying diagnosis leading to transplantation.

lung transplantation offers a suitable option, particularly when an oversized donor lung can be grafted. The earliest reports on the efficacy of lung transplant for pulmonary emphysema compared the merits and risks of BLT versus SLT for these patients. The authors of these reports demonstrated a higher perioperative risk of the bilateral operation without a demonstrable functional benefit to the bilateral recipients.[22,32] As a result, the SLT quickly became the preferred operation for obstructive lung disease.

Our group recently reported a retrospective analysis of outcomes after lung transplantation in patients with chronic obstructive pulmonary disease (COPD).[6] This report included 306 patients, 86 of whom received a single-lung transplant and 220 of whom received a bilateral transplant. In contrast to earlier reports from our institution, the morbidity and mortality were comparable for the two groups with an overall hospital mortality of 6.2%. There were no differences in hospital stay, ICU stay, or duration of mechanical ventilation. There was, however, a difference in long-term survival as the 5-year survival (Figure 13-4) of the bilateral transplant recipients was 66.7%, whereas the survival of the single-lung recipients was 44.9%. The International Society for Heart and Lung Transplantation (ISHLT) has reported a similar finding, but neither analyses adjusted for other factors that might bias such a result.[43] There is a likelihood that patients receiving single-lung transplants for emphysema might have a disproportionate share of risk factors such as advanced recipient age and other comorbidities. Box 13-1 shows the survival data for all lung transplants performed by our group. As demonstrated, COPD and α_1-antitrypsin deficiency emphysema make up over half of our total recipients. It can also be seen that emphysema patients enjoy a better survival than all other groups of patients, though the differences are not statistically significant. As a group, these COPD patients experience the best early outcomes after transplantation in most programs: the ISHLT database cites a statistically significant 1.65 odds ratio of death in the first year after transplant for patients with non-COPD diagnoses compared to those with COPD.[43]

Techniques

Our current approach to a bilateral sequential transplant involves bilateral anterior thoracotomies in the fourth or fifth interspace. The patient is positioned supine with all extremities padded and the arms tucked in at the patient's side. Typically, the fourth intercostal space is entered and the internal mammary artery is ligated and divided bilaterally. The fourth rib is shingled anteriorly by resecting 1 cm of the costal cartilage at the sternal border. More mobility is obtained by dividing the intercostal muscle from within the pleural space back as far as the posterior axillary line. Should additional access to the thorax become necessary during the conduct of the operation, the sternum is easily divided transversely at the fourth interspace and the entire chest is clamshelled open. The least functional lung, as determined by preoperative quantitative ventilation and perfusion scans, is resected and replaced first. When numerous adhesions of the visceral and parietal pleura are encountered because of previous pleural sepsis or thoracotomy, care is taken to avoid injuring the lung parenchyma during the first of the two sequential pneumonectomies. Preliminary dissection of both lungs shortens the time that the first implanted lung is

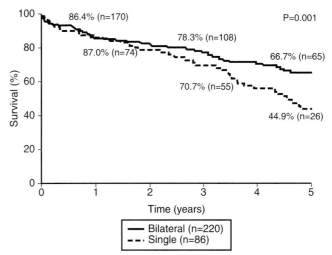

Figure 13–4 Survival curves for bilateral and single-lung transplant recipients at Washington University from 1988 to 2002.

exposed to the entire cardiac output and thus lessens the likelihood of reperfusion edema.

The pulmonary arteries and pulmonary veins are dissected beyond their primary bifurcations to preserve the length of the main trunks. The right pulmonary artery is usually transected between firings of a vascular stapling device 1 cm beyond the ligated first branch to the right upper lobe. The left pulmonary artery is kept longer and transected between staple lines beyond the second branch to the left upper lobe. The vein branches are usually not stapled; rather they are double ligated and divided at their secondary branch points to save length for the future recipient atrial cuff. The arterial and venous dissection and division are accomplished prior to the bronchial division to avoid prolonged contamination of the operative field by the open distal airway. The bronchus is transected between cartilaginous rings, and the posterior bundle of lymphatics and bronchial arteries is exposed to facilitate ligation and subsequent division. The pulmonary artery stump is mobilized centrally, then grasped with a clamp and retracted anteriorly to afford better access to the posterior bronchus. The pulmonary vein stumps are then grasped and retracted anteriorly and laterally to permit circumferential opening of the pericardium. With the pericardium freed, the vein stumps are then retracted and temporarily fixed anteriorly. This provides an excellent view of the bronchus that is then mobilized well into the mediastinum and divided. Meticulous hemostasis in the mediastinum is achieved at this point, with the knowledge that reaching this portion of the operative field after implantation of the graft lung will be extremely difficult.

Meanwhile, the donor lung is prepared on the back table. The donor bronchus is divided two rings proximal to the upper lobe orifice. Care is taken to minimize dissection of the donor bronchus to preserve collateral flow through the peribronchial nodal tissue. The pulmonary artery and left atrial cuffs are freed from any pericardial attachments that may cause kinking after the anastomosis is completed.

Once the native lung is removed, the atelectatic graft lung is placed into the chest and kept cold with iced saline and slush. We conduct the anastomoses from posterior to anterior in the following sequence: bronchus, artery, and atrium. The first stitch is a running 4-0 PDS that unites the peribronchial tissue and lymphatics of the graft to peribronchial tissue surrounding the recipient bronchus. The back wall of this suture is performed just before the bronchial anastomosis, and the front wall is performed immediately after the bronchus is closed. The next stitches are also 4-0 PDS, and they are placed at the two corners of the bronchial anastomosis at the medial and lateral junction of the membranous and cartilaginous airway. These sutures are tied, and one end is used to join the donor and recipient membranous airways in a continuous suture. The cartilaginous rings of the donor and recipient are joined with interrupted figure-of-eight 4-0 PDS sutures. This process can usually be accomplished with only five such sutures. The anastomosis is finished with the completion of the anterior half of the peribronchial tissue layer.

The second anastomosis is the pulmonary artery. The pulmonary artery, by now, has already been extensively and circumferentially dissected into the mediastinum. The pulmonary artery is then clamped centrally with a Satinsky clamp with care taken to avoid including the Swan–Ganz catheter in the jaws of the clamp. The clamp is sewn to the wound edge to immobilize it and to render it less likely to spring open prematurely. The vascular staple line is resected at a location that matches the size of the donor and recipient artery. A larger recipient artery can be divided beyond the first ligated branch to match a smaller donor artery, while a smaller recipient artery is divided proximal to the first branch, or through it, to maximize circumference. The donor pulmonary artery is trimmed to an appropriate length and the anastomosis is created with running 5-0 Prolene suture. This anastomosis must be made with precise, small suture bites to avoid any anastomotic stricture.

The atrial anastomosis is performed last. A Satinsky clamp is placed centrally on the atrium. Placing this clamp too centrally can reduce venous drainage from the contralateral lung and decrease cardiac output, while placing the clamp too peripherally will compromise the recipient atrial cuff. Once the clamp is placed, an umbilical tape is used to tie the clamp closed to minimize the likelihood of dislodgement during subsequent lateral retraction of the clamp. The ties are then cut off the recipient vein stumps and the bridge of atrium between vein stumps is divided to create the atrial cuff. The anastomosis is performed with 4-0 Prolene suture and the last few sutures are left intentionally loose to allow flushing and deairing of the graft and the recipient atrium. For this maneuver, the lung is partially inflated and the pulmonary artery clamp is loosened momentarily. The lung is flushed with the atrial clamp still in place to force out the residual pulmonary perfusate solution. The pulmonary artery clamp is then reapplied, and the atrial clamp is opened momentarily to completely deair the atrium. The atrial sutures are then secured and the clamps removed. All suture lines are then checked for hemostasis as ventilation and perfusion are restored. An identical procedure is then conducted on the opposite side.

► VOLUME REDUCTION

The concept of LVRS was first explored by Brantigan many decades ago, but it failed to be widely adopted as a result of a high mortality rate in his reported case series.[5] The idea is con-

ceptually an extension of the bullectomy operation in which destroyed and functionless lung is resected and the result is better function of the remaining lung that is relatively spared from emphysematous destruction. In contrast to bullectomy where the bulla being resected is truly only an air-filled cavity, the lung tissue resected in LVRS is diseased but does not represent a macroscopic bulla. The advantages of lung volume reduction for suitable candidates are numerous, including the relief of dyspnea and improvement of functional capabilities without the cost and adverse side effects of organ transplantation. There is no built-in waiting time as with transplantation; as soon as a candidate can reach the pulmonary rehabilitation exercise goals they are ready for the procedure. The early and late mortality for lung volume reduction are lower than those seen for transplantation. Because LVRS liberates the patient and the physician from the concern about the distribution of a scarce commodity such as donor lungs, lung volume reduction can be offered with slightly less rigid adherence to selection criteria. For example, a 72-year-old patient who is otherwise an ideal volume reduction candidate would be considered for the procedure, whereas such a patient would be unlikely to be added to a transplant waiting list. Box 13-1 reviews the differences and similarities in the indications and contraindications for lung transplantation and LVRS.

The drawback of volume reduction is that it is quite dependent on stringent anatomical and pathological characteristics in the patient's lungs. Early work has shown that the lack of specific target areas and, to a lesser extent, the absence of apical target areas in particular will decrease the likelihood of a good result. Figure 13-5 shows a perfusion scintigram that demonstrates the absence of apical perfusion often seen in ideal candidates for LVRS. Our own results have shown a less dramatic and less durable improvement in FEV_1 when LVRS is applied to patients with lower lobe predominant emphysema.[7]

Many groups have reported preliminary results for LVRS, and these results have consistently shown benefit to the recipient with acceptable mortality and varying morbidity.[*] The remarkable finding is that these fairly uniform results have been obtained despite the use of a wide array of surgical strategies including bilateral and unilateral approaches; open and thoracoscopic operations, and buttressed or unbuttressed staplers. The consistent theme among reports of successful lung volume reduction programs has been meticulous patient selection (Box 13-2), methodical patient preparation with reduction of risk factors, and attentive postoperative care. Most groups have reported operating on patients with a mean age of 65 years and a preoperative FEV_1 of 600–800 ml. The typical postoperative hospitalization described is 8–14 days with somewhat less than half the patients being detained because of persistent air leaks from the stapled lung resection. Mortality has been described ranging from 0 to 7% for the initial hospitalization. The expected benefits of the operation vary according to whether a unilateral or bilateral approach has been utilized, but gains of 20–35% in the FEV_1 have been reported for unilateral operations and gains of 40–80% are seen with bilateral operations. Most authors also report substantial gains in exercise tolerance, freedom from oxygen use, freedom from steroid use, and subjective quality of life.

*References 2, 4, 10, 14, 23, 26.

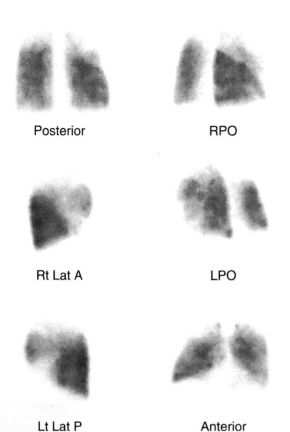

Posterior	RPO
Rt Lat A	LPO
Lt Lat P	Anterior

Figure 13–5 Pulmonary perfusion scintigraphy demonstrating typical upper lobe predominant emphysema that is viewed as the most suitable morphology for lung volume reduction surgery.

Box 13–2. Selection Criteria for LVRS.

Inclusion criteria	Exclusion criteria
General	
Disability despite maximal rehabilitation	Inability to participate in rehabilitation
Cessation of tobacco use >6 months	Continued use of tobacco
Patient expectation of goals reasonable	Significant comorbidity
	Previous pleurodesis or thoracotomy
	Underweight, overweight
Anatomical radiographic evaluation	
Marked emphysema	Bronchiectasis
Heterogeneously distributed emphysema	Minimal radiographic emphysema
	Homogeneously distributed emphysema
Target zones of poorly perfused lung	No target zones
Areas with better preserved lung	No preserved lung tissue
Marked thoracic hyperinflation	Chest wall or thoracic cage abnormalities
Physiological evaluation	
Marked airflow obstruction	Minimal to moderate airflow obstruction
Marked hyperinflation	Minimal to moderate thoracic hyperinflation
Alveolar gas exchange	Markedly disordered alveolar gas exchange
$DL_{CO} <50\%ss$	$DL_{CO} <10\%$
Cardiovascular function	$PaCO_2 >60$ mm Hg
Essentially normal ejection fraction	Cardiovascular function
	Mean pulmonary artery pressure >35 mm Hg
	Left ventricular ejection fraction <40%
	Significant coronary artery disease

Ciccone et al, working with us, reported long-term results in 250 bilateral LVRS recipients.[7] After a median follow-up of 4.4 years, the 5-year survival was estimated to be 68%. Eighteen of the 250 patients in that report had gone on to lung transplantation after a median interval of 4.3 years. Five years after surgery the mean change in FEV_1 was a 7% increase with 53% of patients demonstrating persistence in benefit over preoperative FEV_1 values. This finding takes on greater importance when one considers the relentless progression in functional impairment seen in the medical arms of the randomized trials described below.

After the initial wave of single institution case series, there has been a handful of reports describing prospective, randomized trials comparing lung reduction surgery to best medical care.[11,15,27–29,33] The results of these trials have been controversial in that they have failed to duplicate the physiological and functional gains reported in many case series. Furthermore, the mortality and morbidity in the prospective, randomized trials exceeded that seen in most retrospective case series. Part of the discordance between the case series reports and the controlled trials stems from the more liberal selection criteria of the randomized trials as compared to individual case series. The inclusion of patients with severe, diffuse emphysema has altered the generalizability of the results by including patients previously felt by many to be contraindicated for the procedure.[15,28,29]

In 2003, the National Emphysema Treatment Trial (NETT) reported the main results of a 5-year effort. This trial included 1218 patients randomized between LVRS and medical therapy between January 1998 and July 2002.[29] This multicenter trial reported a 90-day surgical mortality of 7.9%, which did not differ according to surgical approach [sternotomy versus video-assisted thoracoscopic surgery (VATS)] or specific center. A survival benefit (Figure 13-6) was seen in the surgical arm for upper-lobe predominant emphysema patients with low baseline exercise capacity, whereas a survival benefit was seen in the medical arm for non-upper-lobe predominant emphysema patients with high baseline exercise capacity. A previous interim report by the study group identified a subset of patients at high risk for death after surgery, specifically those with either a very low FEV_1 and homogeneous emphysema or those with very low FEV_1 and very low diffusing capacity for carbon monoxide (DL_{CO}).[28] Our own group has refrained from offering LVRS to patients with homogeneous emphysema from the outset of our experience, but our results in the latter high-risk group are different that that suggested by the NETT report. Our patients with FEV_1 and DL_{CO} both less than 20% predicted experienced a perioperative mortality of

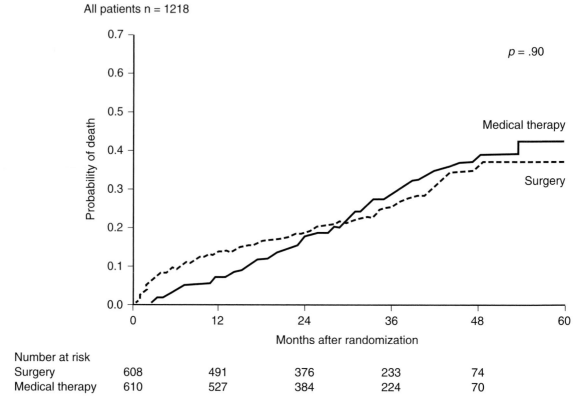

A

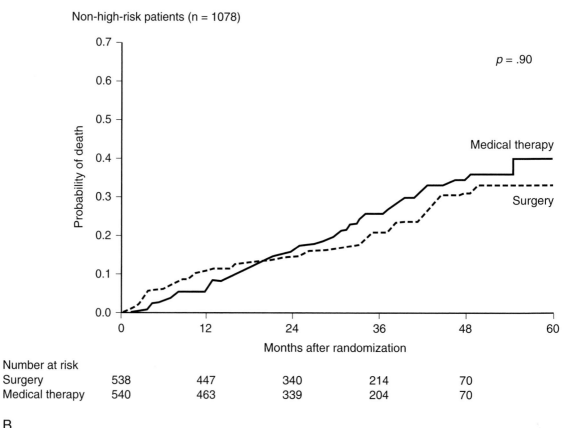

B

Figure 13–6 NETT survival curves.

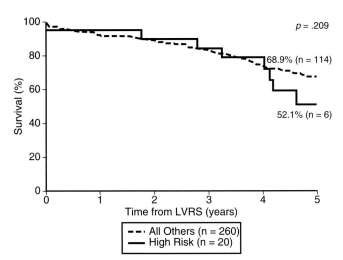

Figure 13–7 Kaplan–Meier survival graph after bilateral LVRS.

5% and durability of benefit that was not different than that experienced by the rest of the LVRS cohort.[25] The survival curves from that study are shown in Figure 13-7.

Techniques

We continue to favor the median sternotomy approach for bilateral lung volume reduction procedures because of the exposure and flexibility that it provides with a minimum of morbidity. With this exposure there is no injury to chest wall muscles or to intercostal nerves either from the operative approach, or even from the chest tubes, which are brought out below the costal arch. Similar results have been obtained using a bilateral VATS approach.

Many patients with severe emphysema have a significant element of chronic bronchitis with increased sputum production. Following induction of anesthesia, a single lumen tube is placed and flexible bronchoscopy is carried out to suction secretions and obtain a specimen for culture and for stat gram stain. If thick, tenacious secretions are encountered, a minitracheostomy may be inserted at the end of the operative procedure to facilitate postoperative pulmonary toilet. Following bronchoscopy, the endotracheal tube is replaced with a left-sided double lumen tube.

Before sternal division, ventilation to both lungs is briefly suspended. A rolled sponge held in a long curved sponge forceps is advanced upward behind the sternum from the subxiphoid position to sweep the pleura away from the retrosternal area on either side. This keeps the mediastinal pleura intact on either side as the sternum is divided. With ventilation suspended the sternum is divided with a sternal saw. The right mediastinal pleura is incised sharply taking care to visualize and avoid injury to the phrenic nerve near the apex of the chest. Ventilation is maintained to the right lung until just before entrance into the pleural space, as this facilitates assessment of the degree of emphysematous damage in various portions of the lung. Demarcation of the fissures, or lack thereof, is also seen best when the lung is inflated. Ventilation

to the right lung is then suspended while ventilation to the left lung is continued. Care is taken by the anesthesiologist to avoid overinflation of the left lung and airway pressures are generally restricted to the range of 15–20 cm H_2O pressure. Hypercapnia may well occur, but this is usually well tolerated.

The majority of candidates for this procedure have upper lobe predominant disease. Several minutes after ventilation is suspended to the right lung, the right middle and lower lobes are usually well deflated and become progressively atelectatic. At that stage the pulmonary ligament is divided. Dense adhesions are not commonly present, but may be a problem if there have been prior episodes of pneumonia. Adhesions are taken down under direct vision, occasionally utilizing an extrapleural dissection if necessary to avoid injury to the lung.

For upper lobe disease, 70–80% of the right upper lobe is excised with multiple applications of a linear stapler buttressed with strips of bovine pericardium. It is often easier to apply the stapler to the deflated lung and this can rapidly be accomplished by using the cautery to fenestrate the apex of the right upper lobe. The marked collateral ventilation leads to prompt collapse. A long, straight intestinal clamp can be applied to the lung to create a linear "crush" mark prior to application of the linear stapler. We initially tailored the upper lobe staple line in the form of an inverted "U," but we now go straight across the upper lobe beginning medially just above the hilum and ending up just above the upper extent of the oblique fissure. Care should be taken to avoid crossing the fissure as this may damage the lower lobe. Such a practice may also tether the apex of the superior segment to the remaining upper lobe and prevent the superior segment from filling the apex of the chest.

After the first two applications of the linear stapler, it is occasionally awkward to insert the stapler into the chest again for completion of the excision. In this case an endoscopic stapler, fitted with pericardial strips, can be used to reach deeply into the chest to complete the excision. We prefer to use a single line of excision to remove most of the right upper lobe rather than the use of multiple excisions, remembering that the goal is to adequately reduce volume, not to remove all of the badly diseased lung.

Occasionally the apex of the upper lobe will be densely adherent to the apex of the chest and to the superior mediastinum. In such cases, it may be easier to first transect the upper lobe as described above before attempting to dissect the apical and mediastinal adhesions. Once the transection has been accomplished, then the specimen can be more easily detached from the chest wall and mediastinum using blunt or sharp dissection, cautery, or even a linear stapler leaving a small remnant of the lung attached to the mediastinum if necessary, to avoid injury to the phrenic nerve.

Following upper lobe resection, the chest is filled with warm saline and the lung is gently inflated. Ordinarily there are no air leaks present at this time. It is not uncommon to find that the reexpanded, remaining lung does not completely fill the apex of the chest. We have explored the use of a pleural tent in this situation but now reserve it for only rare instances, in particular when the remaining lung remains tethered in the chest by virtue of adhesions to the chest wall or diaphragm. It has not been our practice to do pleurodesis either by abrasion or by talc, even if the patient is not a potential candidate for subsequent lung transplantation.

Two chest tubes are placed in the pleural space and brought out near the midline through small subcostal stab wounds. The posterior tube is brought across the dome of the diaphragm and halfway up the posterior chest. The anterior tube is brought to the apex of the chest near the mediastinum.

Ventilation is shifted from the left lung to the right lung and the mediastinal pleura is then opened on the left side. Particular care should be taken to visualize the phrenic nerve and avoid injury to it when opening the upper portion of the mediastinal pleura since the anatomic location of the left phrenic nerve makes it more vulnerable to injury then the right phrenic nerve. With upper lobe predominant disease, the goal is to excise the superior subdivision of the left upper lobe leaving the lingula intact, as this is usually much less diseased. The pulmonary ligament on the left side is divided if possible, but this requires displacement of the heart and the ligament may be difficult to visualize. In such case, the ligament is left undivided though any adhesions between the left lower lobe and the diaphragm are taken down. Unlike the anatomical situation on the right side, the superior segment of the left lower lobe usually reaches easily to the apex of the chest even without division of the pulmonary ligament.

The upper half to two thirds of the left upper lobe is excised with multiple applications of the linear GIA stapler. This may be facilitated by cautery puncture of the apex of the left upper lobe allowing it to deflate. The long straight intestinal clamp is often useful in helping to identify and demarcate the proposed line of excision. The line of excision is usually parallel to the oblique fissure separating the upper and lower lobes. As on the right side care is taken to avoid stapling across the fissure into the superior segment of the left upper lobe.

Following left upper lobe excision, the lung is reinflated and inspected for air leaks. Two chest tubes are placed as on the right, one to the base and one to the apex. The mediastinal pleura is closed on either side. Several centimeters are left open inferiorly to allow drainage of any mediastinal fluid collection into the pleural spaces. No mediastinal chest tube is placed.

Because many volume reduction patients are on prednisone prior to the operation, and this might interfere with healing of the sternotomy, we use overlapping figure-of-eight stainless-steel wire closure of the sternum for added security. Following completion of the operation the double lumen tube is removed in the operating room. If a minitracheostomy is thought to be necessary on the basis of the initial bronchoscopy, this is placed immediately following removal of the double lumen tube, generally using a 4-mm diameter minitracheostomy.

▶ ## COMBINATIONS OF LUNG TRANSPLANTATION AND LUNG VOLUME REDUCTION

There are several permutations in which lung transplantation and lung volume reduction can be combined to optimize treatment for patients with emphysema. These combinations have been reported in anecdotal clusters of patients. The combined approaches can be summarized as follows: volume reduction as a bridge to transplant, simultaneous single-lung transplant and unilateral volume reduction to prevent native lung hyperexpansion, early posttransplant unilateral volume reduction to treat acute native lung hyperexpansion, and late unilateral volume reduction to treat chronic native lung hyperexpansion. Todd et al[41] reported the Toronto experience with simultaneous

unilateral volume reduction to prospectively improve overall lung function after a single-lung transplant. They experienced no postoperative problems, and the pulmonary function at 3 months was better than expected based on historic controls receiving a single lung for emphysema.

Yonan and colleagues retrospectively analyzed 27 patients who received 31 single-lung transplants for emphysema.[44] They identified 12 patients who experienced early or late native lung hyperexpansion and they performed two early lung volume reduction operations to address this problem. Their analysis included an assessment of risk factors and they concluded that lower pretransplant FEV_1, higher residual volume, and pulmonary hypertension were all associated with a higher risk for native lung hyperexpansion. They did not perform, nor did they advocate, volume reduction surgery simultaneous with a single-lung transplant for emphysema.

The use of volume reduction as a bridge to transplant is the form of combined procedures that has been most frequently attempted. The concept was introduced to the medical literature by Zenati and colleagues in 1995 when they reported two patients who received single-lung transplants 17 months and 4 months after laser ablation of emphysematous bullae.[45] One group has prospectively performed reduction in patients felt to be also eligible for transplantation.[3] This center found 31 patients eligible for both procedures while, at the same time, they identified 20 patients who were suitable for LVRS alone and 139 who were felt to be transplant candidates only. Twenty-four patients had successful LVRS while 7 (including one death) were considered LVRS failures. Follow-up was too short at the time of the report to know how frequently late transplants would be performed. The authors' results with LVRS in transplant-eligible patients were recently reported.[24] We identified 99 of 200 patients who underwent bilateral LVRS and who were felt to have been transplant eligible. With a median follow-up of 5.1 years, 32 of the 99 had been listed for transplant and 15 had undergone transplantation. The Kaplan–Meier curve depicting freedom from listing and freedom from transplantation is shown in Figure 13-8. The only preoperative or operative factor that was predictive for the subsequent need for transplantation was a lower lobe rather than upper lobe LVRS procedure. Many of our patients have had LVRS as a functional bridge to transplant. This has occurred in most cases not as part of an a priori plan to bridge them, as it was a stepwise treatment for crippling dyspnea that was not improved sufficiently either by degree or by duration of effect after lung volume reduction. The concept is attractive on the surface: patients get volume reduction initially and continue to accrue waiting time toward lung transplantation. One potential benefit for the patient successfully completing volume reduction surgery is the possibility that a transplant might be avoided altogether by an excellent response to volume reduction. A second possibility is that transplant is delayed by several years and the patient is transplanted with a later cohort with the possibility of improved techniques, better immunosuppression, and overall better survival. Finally, since the hazard rate of death after lung transplantation is higher than the hazard rate of death after LVRS, anything that can safely delay entry onto the steeper survival curve seems worth pursuing.

The logic of the potential benefits of LVRS as a bridge to transplant weakens when faced with some aspects of reality.

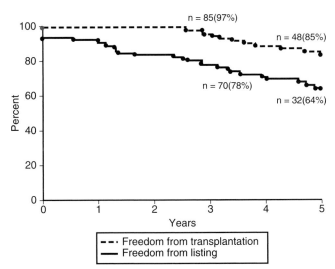

Figure 13–8 Freedom from listing and freedom from transplant in 99 patients felt to be eligible for either LVRS or transplantation at the time of bilateral LVRS operation.

pulmonary emphysema, they are unique in their ideal selection criteria and in their expected outcomes. We favor a meticulous selection process in which all options are considered and the best option is selected for a given patient. Patients referred with a functionless, space-occupying bulla that compresses relatively normal adjacent lung will be offered thoracoscopic or open bullectomy. Patients with ideal circumstances for LVRS—hyperinflation, heterogeneous distribution of disease, FEV_1 of greater than 20%, and a normal pCO_2—are offered LVRS. Finally, patients with diffuse disease, lower FEV_1, hypercapnia, and associated pulmonary hypertension are directed toward transplant. LVRS has not been a satisfactory option for patients with α_1-antitrypsin deficiency and we prefer to transplant in these cases. With strict adherence to these criteria, we find that very few emphysema patients are serious candidates for any surgical procedures. Combinations of lung volume reduction and lung transplantation, either simultaneously or sequentially, are possible but rarely necessary.

First, the anatomical and physiological criteria that require heterogeneous destruction for volume reduction are much more restrictive than the criteria for transplantation, so it is unlikely that a large fraction of emphysema transplant candidates could be safely and successfully treated with volume reduction. Also, the dilemma remains as to how to treat a patient near the upper age limit for transplantation. It is quite possible that a patient who is acceptable for both procedures at age 62 might receive volume reduction as a bridge, not to transplantation, but to ineligibility for future lung transplantation several years later. Our own results have confirmed this suspicion: of the 15 patients that have been transplanted after bilateral LVRS, only one was older than 60 years of age at the time of LVRS evaluation. The next oldest was 58 and the mean age for the group of LVRS-transplant recipients was 54 years.[24]

The use of LVRS for late native lung hyperexpansion after single-lung transplantation can be described as rare and anecdotal. Kroshus and colleagues reported three patients who were treated with unilateral LVRS for native lung hyperinflation and posttransplant dyspnea that was not attributable to infection or rejection. The patients represented a small fraction of the 66 single-lung transplants performed at that center for emphysema. The volume reduction operations were performed 12, 17, and 42 months after the initial lung transplantation and all patients experienced a substantial relief in dyspnea with an improvement in exercise tolerance and an improvement in the appearance of the chest radiograph.[19] A similar report by Le Pimpec-Barthes et al describes successful treatment of symptomatic native lung hyperexpansion by volume reduction of the native side in the form of a right upper lobectomy.[20]

SUMMARY

Although bullectomy, LVRS, and lung transplantation are similar in that each represents a surgical procedure aimed at

REFERENCES

1. Anyanwu AC, McGuire A, et al: An economic evaluation of lung transplantation. J Thorac Cardiovasc Surg 123(3):411–418; discussion 418–420, 2002.
2. Argenziano M, Moazami N, et al: Extended indications for volume reduction pneumoplasty in advanced emphysema. Ann Thorac Surg 62:1588–1597, 1996.
3. Bavaria JE, Pochettino A, et al: Effect of volume reduction on lung transplant timing and selection for chronic obstructive pulmonary disease. J Thorac Cardiovasc Surg 115(1):9–18, 1998.
4. Bissinger R, Zollinger A, et al: Bilateral volume reduction surgery for difuse pulmonary emphysema by video-assisted thoracoscopy. J Thorac Cardiovasc Surg 112:875–882, 1996.
5. Brantigan OC, Mueller E, et al: A surgical approach to pulmonary emphysema. Am Rev Respir Dis 80:194–202, 1959.
6. Cassivi SD, Meyers BF, et al: Thirteen-year experience in lung transplantation for emphysema. Ann Thorac Surg 74(5):1663–1669, 2002.
7. Ciccone AM, Meyers BF, et al: Long-term outcome of bilateral lung volume reduction in 250 consecutive patients with emphysema. J Thorac Cardiovasc Surg 125(3):513–525, 2003.
8. Cooper JD: The history of surgical procedures for emphysema. Ann Thorac Surg 63:312–319, 1997.
9. Cooper JD, Trulock EP, et al: Bilateral pneumectomy (volume reduction) for chronic obstructive pulmonary disease. J Thorac Cardiovasc Surg 109(1):106–116, 1995.
10. Cooper JD, Patterson GA, et al: Results of 150 consecutive bilateral lung volume reduction procedures in patients with severe emphysema. J Thorac Cardiovasc Surg 112:1319–1330, 1996.
11. Criner GJ, Cordova FC, et al: Prospective randomized trial comparing bilateral lung volume reduction surgery to pulmonary rehabilitation in severe chronic obstructive pulmonary disease. Am J Respir Crit Care Med 160(6):2018–2027, 1999.
12. De Meester J, Smits JM, et al: Listing for lung transplantation: Life expectancy and transplant effect, stratified by type of end-stage lung disease, the Eurotransplant experience. J Heart Lung Transplant 20(5):518–524, 2001.
13. FitzGerald MX, Keelan PJ, et al: Surgery for bullous emphysema. Respiration 30:187, 1973.

14. Gaissert HA, Trulock EP, et al: Comparison of early functional results after volume reduction or lung transplantation for chronic obstructive pulmonary disease. J Thorac Cardiovasc Surg 111:296–307, 1996.

15. Geddes D, Davies M, et al: Effect of lung-volume-reduction surgery in patients with severe emphysema. N Engl J Med 343:239–245, 2000.

16. Geertsma A, TenVergert EM, et al: Does lung transplantation prolong life? A comparison of survival with and without transplantation. J Heart Lung Transplant 17:511–516, 1998.

17. Hardy JD, Webb WR, et al: Lung homotransplantation in man. JAMA 186(12):1065–1074, 1963.

18. Hosenpud JD, Bennett LE, et al: Effect of diagnosis on survival benefit of lung transplantation for end-stage lung disease. Lancet 351(9095):24–27, 1998.

19. Kroshus TJ, Bolman RM, et al: Unilateral volume reduction after single-lung transplantation for emphysema. Ann Thorac Surg 62:363–368, 1996.

20. Le Pimpec-Barthes F, Debrosse D, et al: Late contralateral lobectomy after single-lung transplantation for emphysema. Ann Thorac Surg 61:231–234, 1996.

21. Mal H, Andreasian B, et al: Unilateral lung transplantation in end stage pulmonary emphysema. Am Rev Respir Dis 140:797–802, 1989.

22. Mal H, Sleiman C, et al: Functional results of single-lung transplantation for chronic obstructive lung disease. Am J Respir Crit Care Med 149:1476–1481, 1994.

23. McKenna RJ, Brenner M, et al: Should lung volume reduction for emphysema be unilateral or bilateral? J Thorac Cardiovasc Surg 112:1331–1339, 1996.

24. Meyers BF, Yusen RD, et al: Outcome of lung volume reduction surgery in emphysema patients eligible for lung transplant. J Thorac Cardiovasc Surg 122(1):10–17, 2001.

25. Meyers BF, Yusen RD, et al: Results of lung volume reduction surgery in patients meeting a NETT high risk criterion. J Thorac Cardiovasc Surg 127(3):829–835, 2004.

26. Naunheim KS, Keller CA, et al: Unilateral video-assisted thoracic surgical lung reduction. Ann Thorac Surg 61:1092–1098, 1996.

27. NETT Research Group: Rationale and design of the national emphysema treatment trial (NETT): A prospective randomized trial of lung volume reduction surgery. J Thorac Cardiovasc Surg 118:518–528, 1999.

28. NETT Research Group: Patients at high risk of death after lung-volume-reduction surgery. N Engl J Med 345:1075–1083, 2001.

29. NETT Research Group: A randomized trial comparing lung-volume-reduction surgery with medical therapy for severe emphysema. N Engl J Med 348(21):2059–2073, 2003.

30. Pasque MK, Cooper JD, et al: An improved technique for bilateral lung transplantation: Rationale and initial clinical experience. Ann Thorac Surg 49:785–791, 1990.

31. Patterson GA, Cooper JD, et al: Technique of successful clinical double-lung transplantation. Ann Thorac Surg 45(6):626–633, 1988.

32. Patterson GA, Maurer JA, et al: Comparison of outcomes of double and single lung transplantation for obstructive lung disease. J Thorac Cardiovasc Surg 101:623–632, 1991.

33. Pompeo E, Marino M, et al: Reduction pneumoplasty versus respiratory rehabilitation in severe emphysema: A randomized study. Ann Thorac Surg 70:948–953, 2000.

34. Ramsey SD, Patrick DL, et al: The cost-effectiveness of lung transplantation: A pilot study. Chest 108(6):1594–1601, 1995.

35. Reardon J, Awad E, et al: The effect of comprehensive outpatient pulmonary rehabilitation on dyspnea. Chest 105:1046–1052, 1994.

36. Reitz B, Wallwork J, et al: Heart-lung transplantation: Successful therapy for patients with pulmonary vascular disease. N Engl J Med 306:557–564, 1982.

37. Ries AL, Ellis B, et al: Upper extremity exercise training in chronic obstructive pulmonary disease. Chest 93:688–692, 1988.

38. Schipper PH, Meyers BF, et al: Outcomes following resection of giant emphysematous bullae. Ann Thorac Surg (in press), 2004.

39. Shrager JB, Kim D-K, et al: Lung volume reduction surgery restores the normal diaphragmatic length-tension relationship in emphysematous rats. J Thorac Cardiovasc Surg 121:217–224, 2001.

40. Snider GL: Reduction pneumoplasty for giant bullous emphysema—implications for surgical treatment of non-bullous emphysema. Chest 1996(109):540–548, 1996.

41. Todd TR, Perron J, et al: Simultaneous single-lung transplantation and lung volume reduction. Ann Thorac Surg 63:1468–1470, 1997.

42. Toronto Lung Transplantation Group: Unilateral lung transplantation for pulmonary fibrosis. N Engl J Med 314:1140–1145, 1986.

43. Trulock EP, Edwards LJ, et al: The registry of the International Society for Heart and Lung Transplantation: Twentieth Official Adult Lung and Heart-Lung Transplant Report-2003. J Heart Lung Transplant 22(6):625–635, 2003.

44. Yonan NA, El-Gamel A, et al: Single lung transplantation for emphysema: Predictors for native-lung hyperinflation. J Heart Lung Transplant 17(2):192–201, 1998.

45. Zenati M, Keenan RJ, et al: Lung reduction as a bridge to lung transplantation in pulmonary emphysema. Ann Thorac Surg 59:1581–1583, 1995.

Lung Transplantation

Christine L. Lau and G. Alexander Patterson

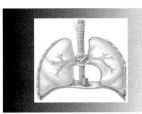

INTRODUCTION

The first successful human lung transplant was performed in 1983, by the Toronto Lung Transplant Group.[172] Two decades have passed since this landmark procedure, and in the interim almost 15,000 lung transplants have been performed.[75] Lung transplantation currently is the preferred treatment option for a variety of end-stage pulmonary diseases. Remarkable progress has occurred through refinement in technique and improved understanding of transplant immunology and microbiology. Despite these improvements donor shortages and chronic lung allograft rejection continue to plague the field and prevent it from reaching its full potential. Attempts have been made to address these issues. Marginal donors,[165] living-lobar donors,[160] split-lung donor techniques,[37] and the use of non-heart-beating donors[163] have been used clinically, while xenotransplantation has remained in the research realm. Chronic rejection of the lung allograft is currently the major hurdle limiting long-term survival. To date, prevention of known risk factors and treatment strategies have not lessened the devastating toll this process has on lung transplant survival. It may only be through the promotion of immune tolerance that chronic rejection may be abolished.

HISTORICAL ASPECTS

In 1947, Vladimir Demikhov performed the first lung transplantation in a dog.[46,47,95] The animal survived 7 days, dying from complications of bronchial dehiscence. Dr. James D. Hardy performed the first human lung transplantation in 1963.[74] The patient was a 58-year-old male prisoner with lung cancer, and the donor was a male who had died from a massive myocardial infarction. Notably the recipient was blood group A yet the donor was blood group B. Succumbing to renal failure the recipient survived 18 days. Over the next 20 years approximately 40 lung transplants were attempted with none achieving long-term success.[192] Most recipients died in the first 2 weeks after transplantation from respiratory failure secondary to rejection, infection, or both. After 14 days the majority of deaths could be attributed to bronchial dehiscence. Derom and colleagues[48] reported 10-month survival in a 23-year-old male with silicosis following right lung transplantation. Eight of the 10 months were spent hospitalized. The patient was eventually released but died shortly thereafter from chronic rejection and sepsis. This patient was the only recipient to leave the hospital alive during these attempts at lung transplantation. The Toronto Lung Transplant Group's initial attempt at lung transplantation was in 1978, ending with the patient dying following a bronchial dehiscence.[123] On the basis of this patient and the poor results of lung transplantation reported, this group began experimental studies into the causes of lung transplant failure. Through these investigations they discovered that perioperative steroid usage contributed significantly to poor bronchial anastomotic healing.[103] Wrapping an omental pedicle around the bronchus resulted in restoration of blood supply and protection from dehiscence.[104] Additionally recognizing that most of the early attempts had been in acutely ill often ventilator-dependent patients,

208

recipient selection issues were addressed. On November 7, 1983 the first successful isolated lung transplant was performed in a 58-year-old man with pulmonary fibrosis.[172] Subsequently this patient returned to work. In subsequent analysis it appears to be the attention to detail that this group practiced that led to long term transplant success as the use of the omental flap and the concept of withholding steroids perioperatively have now been largely abandoned.

Following this success, Patterson and colleagues expanded the use of lung transplantation to patients with septic lung diseases and emphysema with the en-bloc double lung transplant technique.[136] As for the single lung technique this procedure was initially perfected in the laboratory prior to attempts in humans.[39] The en-bloc double lung transplant, however, had several drawbacks: it was technically difficult requiring cardiopulmonary bypass, tracheal anastomotic ischemic complications occurred frequently, cardiac denervation occurred, and bleeding into the posterior mediastinum was common because of poor operative exposure. In an effort to avoid these problems, Pasque and colleagues[133] devised the technique of bilateral sequential pulmonary transplantation. Exposure by a transverse thoracosternotomy provided excellent visualization of the mediastinum and both pleural spaces but sternal wound complications occurred frequently and recently this incision has been modified to avoid sternal division.[116]

Initially it was felt patients with emphysema would not be good candidates for single lung transplantation, because the overly compliant native lung would be prone to hyperinflation resulting in mediastinal shift and compression of the transplanted lung. Despite this concern, successful single lung transplantation for emphysema was reported in 1989 by Mal and colleagues.[109] Fremes and colleagues[59] reported the first single lung transplantation and closure of patent ductus arteriosus in a patient with Eisenmenger's syndrome. Pasque and colleagues[134] reported success with single-lung transplantation for patients with pulmonary hypertension. The first applications of living related lobar transplants were reported by Starnes and colleagues.[160] Split-lung techniques have been developed allowing a large left donor lung to be bipartitioned and the individual lobes transplanted bilaterally.[37] Furthermore the use of lungs from non-heart-beating donors has moved from the research realm to clinical reality.[163]

▶ RECIPIENT SELECTION

International guidelines for selection of lung transplant candidates have been proposed.[112] As these are general guidelines, they may be relaxed at times depending on the specifics of individual cases. The presence of declining end-stage lung disease with a life expectancy of less than 24–48 months despite optimal medical therapy and the potential for improvement in survival and/or quality of life with transplantation are absolute criteria. Abstinence from smoking for at least 6 months is another absolute requirement. Recipient age has been shown to be a significant predictor of adverse outcome.[75] In general, we do not transplant patients older than 65. Medical management of the patient's pulmonary disease needs to be maximized and other possible options considered (for example, lung volume reduction

surgery for patients with chronic obstructive pulmonary disease [COPD]; epoprostenol for primary pulmonary hypertension [PPH]) before lung transplant listing.

Potential transplant recipients should be without significant comorbid diseases. Clinically relevant coronary artery disease that cannot be revascularized, systemic vascular diseases, poorly controlled insulin-dependent diabetes mellitus, symptomatic osteoporosis, or end-staged hepatic or renal failure usually contraindicates isolated lung transplantation. The steroid requirements after transplantation can exacerbate osteoporosis[5] and insulin-dependent diabetes. Additionally, attempts are made to wean steroids preoperatively in patients who require them to doses <20 mg/day of prednisone in order to minimize the complications related to their use. On occasion combined lung and liver or kidney transplants have been performed. Treatable coronary disease can be addressed and if resolved does not prevent listing for lung transplantation.

Adequate nutrition is particularly important. Patients with an ideal body weight <70% or >130% predicted are not considered for transplantation. Patients with cystic fibrosis and COPD are particularly prone to cachexia.[63] Dietary consultation and oral supplements may suffice, but the placement of a percutaneous endoscopic gastrostomy tube for tube feedings prior to transplantation may also prove useful. Morbid obesity is most commonly seen in patients with idiopathic pulmonary fibrosis (IPF), pulmonary hypertension, and sarcoidosis. Weight reduction via a supervised diet and routine exercise to the degree possible given physiological constraints of the disease (particularly pulmonary hypertension) are undertaken in these patients prior to transplant listing.

Noncutaneous malignancy unless greater than 5 years from diagnosis and curative treatment remain a contraindication. Prior thoracic surgery may increase the technical difficulty with greater risk of hemorrhage and nerve injury but is not a contraindication to lung transplantation. Active infection outside the thorax is a contraindication to transplantation.

After initial evaluation, patients with end-stage lung disease who are being considered for lung transplantation undergo extensive preoperative testing to assess their overall medical condition as well as the severity of their lung disease. At our center the transplant evaluation consists of the tests shown in Box 14-1. Laboratory tests consisting of general blood work, blood typing, and immunological determination of preformed antibodies are done. Excluding patients with pulmonary vascular diseases, potential recipients are required to complete pulmonary rehabilitation in order to improve cardiac conditioning prior to transplantation. Consults with nutrition and social work are obtained and financial issues are addressed.

▶ DISEASE-SPECIFIC GUIDELINES

Before being considered for pulmonary transplantation, patients with COPD should have maximization of medical therapy consisting of bronchodilator therapies and oxygen therapy. Consideration should be given to lung volume reduction surgery (LVRS) in ideal patients (hyperinflation, heterogeneous distribution of disease, forced expiratory

Box 14–1. Tests and Consults Obtained at Lung Transplant Evaluation.

Complete blood work
Pulmonary function testing and room-air arterial blood gas
Pulmonary rehabilitation consult with 6-min walk test
Electrocardiogram
Chest radiograph
High-resolution chest computed tomography (CT) (majority)
Quantitative ventilation–perfusion scan
Right and left coronary catheterization (<40 years old just right side)
DEXA (dual–energy X-ray absorptiometry) bone scan (not everyone but especially if on steroids)
Social work consult
Dietary consult
Financial consult
Psychiatric consult (only as needed)

volume in 1 s (FEV_1) of more than 20%, and normal pco_2).[118] We have not found LVRS to be an ideal option in patients with α_1-antitrypsin deficiency as in general these patients have diffuse disease.[118] Preliminary LVRS does not jeopardize subsequent successful lung transplantation.[121] Generally, in patients with COPD, the FEV_1 should be less than or equal to 25% predicted and not reversible, although most patients actually have FEV_1 of <20% predicted at the time of transplantation. Progressive deterioration as evidenced by hypercarbia ($Pa_{co}2 \geq 55$ mm Hg), increasing oxygen requirement (resting $Pa_o2 <55$ mm Hg), the development of secondary pulmonary hypertension, rapid decline of FEV_1, or frequent life-threatening infections indicate decreased survival, suggesting the need for transplantation.[112]

Recently debate has centered on whether bilateral lung transplants are preferred to single lung transplants in this population of patients.[114,166,189] According to the International Society for Heart and Lung Transplantation (ISHLT) registry a survival advantage is seen in COPD recipients who receive bilateral versus single-lung transplants.[75] This survival benefit, however, may not extend to older, less healthy recipients.[114] Our results have been consistent with the ISHLT data, and we have additionally reported improved lung function and exercise tolerance in bilateral lung patients.[166] For these reasons when possible we prefer to perform bilateral lung transplantation of patients with COPD.

Patients with septic lung diseases (cystic fibrosis, bronchiectasis) presenting with $FEV_1 \leq 30\%$ predicted or rapidly progressive disease despite optimal medical management should be evaluated for potential lung transplantation. Progressive disease is indicated by an increasing number of hospitalizations, rapid decline in FEV_1, massive hemoptysis, or increasing weight loss.[112] Young female cystic fibrotic patients have a tendency to do poorly and early consideration is appropriate.[50] Evidence of hypercarbia ($pco_2 >50$) or hypoxemia ($Pao_2 <55$ mm Hg) indicates the need for transplant evaluation.[112] Recently Liou and colleagues[106] have suggested that the use of a nine-parameter model to stratify pretransplant cystic fibrosis patients into five categories based on predicted survival (ranging from 30% to approaching 100%) would more accurately predict the group that would most benefit from lung transplantation. Bilateral transplantation is required for patients with septic lung diseases.

Patients with septic lung disease or those with significant sputum production are evaluated with frequent sputum cultures to assess bacterial sensitivities. Inhaled high-dose aminoglycosides or colistin are frequently used in this population. Patients with multidrug-resistant organisms, especially pan-resistant *Burkholderia cepacia*, are considered high risk, and many centers consider this a contraindication to transplantation. Early mortality in patients with cystic fibrosis (CF) infected with *B. cepacia* is significantly increased.[6,24] Successful transplantation in these patients often requires the use of multiple combinations of intravenous antibiotics using *in vitro* synergy testing to guide antibiotic selection. If no susceptible antibiotic regimen is found on synergy testing, we do not proceed with transplantation.

Patients with IPF should be evaluated for transplantation when they become symptomatic. IPF patients are associated with the highest mortality while waiting for transplantation.[81] For this reason potential recipients with pulmonary fibrosis in the United States are credited with 90 days waiting time at transplant listing.[178] Although initially helpful this added time no longer appears to be substantial enough to significantly alter waitlist mortality. Review of histological diagnosis is important because a minority of patients with IPF may have disease processes such as desquamative interstitial pneumonitis (DIP), which may be responsive to steroids preventing the need for transplantation.[176] In addition to symptomatic presentation, physiological parameters may be utilized, including a fall in vital capacity to below 60–70% predicted or a fall in diffusion capacity to below 50–60% predicted, as requirements for transplant evaluation. If the pulmonary fibrosis is part of a systemic disease process, the systemic symptoms should be under control and preferably in remission.[112] We prefer bilateral lung transplantation in this group, although a survival benefit has not been seen in bilateral verus single-lung transplant patients with IPF.[75,116]

Patients with pulmonary hypertension were previously considered for lung transplantation early in the course of their disease because of the poor outcome of this disease process. Recently, with the use of intravenous prostacyclin (Flolan) and other vasodilator therapies, an improvement in pulmonary artery pressures and relief of symptoms are seen in the majority of patients with PPH.[113] Transplantation may be delayed as long as patients remain clinically stable on vasodilatory therapy. For patients with pulmonary hypertension secondary to congenital heart defects or thromboembolic diseases consideration for surgical intervention for the primary diagnosis (atrial septostomy or thromboendarterectomy) should be given. Current indication for transplantation is progressive deterioration despite optimal therapy (i.e., NYHA class III or IV, mean pulmonary artery pressure >50, right atrial pressure > 10 mm Hg, cardiac index <2.5 liters/min/m², syncopal episodes).[112] With the widespread use of Flolan, patients with pulmonary hypertension often are in much worse medical condition with very shortened life spans by the time they require transplantation. We prefer bilateral lung transplantation in this group; however, a survival advantage with bilateral lung transplantation has not

210

been appreciated.[75] If the patient is to undergo single lung transplantation, we do not use a marginal donor lung as the bulk of the cardiac output will be through the transplanted lung. Patients with Eisenmenger's syndrome and secondary pulmonary hypertension have not shown an improvement in survival following lung transplantation.[26,45] Recently it has been suggested that heart–lung transplantation may preferable to isolated lung transplant in this group.[187]

▶ DONOR SELECTION

Despite aggressive measures including the use of marginal donors, efforts to boost organ donations, and use of lobar and non-heart-beating donors there remains a critical shortage of donor lungs. Further contributing to this shortage is the estimate that only 10–15% of multiorgan donors have lungs suitable for procurement.[164,167]

Careful donor selection is required (see Box 14-2). The donor's medical history is obtained, with particular emphasis and attention paid to the donor's age, cause of death, timing of death, smoking history, and prior thoracic procedures. Older donor age (greater than 60) is considered a significant risk factor for adverse outcome after pulmonary transplantation and in general donors younger than 55 are preferred.[75] Although a significant smoking history ($\geq$30 pack years) in the donor is a concern, it is not an absolute contraindication to the use of otherwise suitable donor lungs. ABO incompatibility between donor and recipient human immunodeficiency virus (HIV) positivity, active malignancies (outside CNS), and active hepatitis infections remain absolute contraindications to donor lung procurement. Histocompatibility antigen (HLA) matching currently is not usually performed between donor and recipient prior to transplantation unless the patient has an elevated panel reactive antibody or known HLA antibodies from prior sensitization.

Ideally the donor chest radiograph should be clear. Preferably both lung fields should be free of pulmonary contusions, pneumonia, or atelectasis. The presence of a radiological abnormality does not preclude further assessment by the harvest team, but it needs to be correlated with manual evaluation.[165] Size matching is primarily based on comparison of donor and recipient heights and sex. Donor lungs that are substantially larger than the recipient's chest

cavity but are otherwise usable should not preclude transplantation. Anatomical donor upper lobectomy is easily performed on the back table. In our experience this downsizing of donor lungs for smaller recipients can be done safely with minimal morbidity. We prefer this option to multiple wedge resections after implantation.[97]

Confirmation of satisfactory gas exchange, utilizing the standard gas exchange parameters of PaO_2 >300 mm Hg on FIO_2 of 100% and positive end-expiratory pressure (PEEP) of 5 cm H_2O, is obtained on the donor lungs. Additionally, lung parameters including mean airway pressures and compliance are evaluated. Mean airway pressures >30–32 mm Hg with standard volume ventilation are considered a relative contraindication for lung donation, unless a nonparenchymal explanation (i.e., a small endotracheal tube or morbid obesity) is evident.

Bronchoscopy is performed to assess the airways. The presence of mucopurulent secretions that are easily cleared are acceptable but the presence of frank pus, significant airway erythema, or evidence of aspiration contraindicates the use of the lung from which these findings arise (but not necessarily the contralateral lung). Median sternotomy provides adequate exposure for thorough gross inspection of both lungs. The presence of a mass, consolidation, or significant pulmonary contusions contraindicates the use of the lungs. Recipients without pulmonary hypertension receiving bilateral sequential lung transplants may tolerate one lung that has a small contusion when the other lung is free from injury. The noninjured lung is transplanted first if possible, followed by the slightly injured lung with a low threshold for utilizing cardiopulmonary bypass.

The primary reasons that lungs from a multiorgan donor are not suitable for transplantation are pulmonary contusions, pulmonary sepsis, and pulmonary edema.[58] Various techniques have been suggested to increase the recoverability of donor lungs including use of high-dose steroids early during the management of brain dead patients, maximization of pulmonary toilet, strict monitoring of ventilator support, and fluid administration.[38,58,164]

Living lobar transplantation using a lobe from two separate donors has been successfully employed in cystic fibrosis patients and other recipients.[91,159] This strategy was pioneered by the University of Southern California (USC) program.[34] They have reported impressive results in adults and children.[161] Furthermore since pediatric patients receiving living lobar transplants had less bronchiolitis obliterans syndrome and better pulmonary function than pediatric recipients receiving cadaveric donor lungs, this group believes living lobar transplantation is the preferred method for children.[161] Living lobar transplant has been conducted in other centers as well; however, the success of the USC program has been difficult to duplicate. Thus far there have been no reports of donor fatality, but a significant number of complications have been encountered.[12]

Two novel techniques to optimize donor usage have recently been introduced. The first is a split-lung technique that bipartitions the left lung of a large cadaveric donor and uses the two lobes to perform a bilateral lobar transplant in the smaller recipient.[37] It requires significant expertise in lung transplantation, but has been performed successfully with good outcomes at certain institutions.[8,37] The second technique is the use of non-heart-beating donors,[163] but it is

---

Box 14–2. Ideal Donor Criteria.[a]

Age <55 years
ABO compatibility
Clear chest radiograph
PaO_2 >300 on FIO_2 = 1.0, PEEP—5 cm H_2O
Tobacco history <20 pack years
Absence of chest trauma
No evidence of aspiration/sepsis
No prior cardiopulmonary surgery
Sputum gram stain—absence of organisms
Absence of purulent secretions at bronchoscopy

[a]Note these are ideal criteria and relaxation of individual requirements does not preclude successful transplantation if carefully evaluated.

doubtful to significantly increase donor supply as few donors meet the criteria. We have successfully used non-heart-beating donor lungs when the time from withdrawal of support to pronouncement of death was short (20 minutes). Unfortunately neither of these has the potential to substantially increase the number of available lungs. Xenotransplantation is one solution to overcoming the donor shortage with the potential for an unlimited supply. Unfortunately advances in this area have been hindered not only by the severe immune response of the recipient but also by apparent incompatibilities between the coagulation systems of different species.[61] It has therefore remained relegated to the research realm.

DONOR PROCUREMENT

If our initial evaluation (donor history, chest radiograph, bronchoscopy, and manual inspection) reveals no contraindications, we proceed with donor lung procurement. Our technique has previously been described.[167] Following median sternotomy and opening of the pleural spaces, the pericardium is opened and stay sutures are placed allowing exposure of the great vessels. The superior vena cava (SVC) is encircled caudal to the azygous vein with silk sutures. The inferior vena cava (IVC) is also encircled unless hemodynamic instability occurs on attempt to do so. The periadventitial tissue overlying the right pulmonary artery (PA) is dissected cleaning the plane between the artery and the SVC. The same is done to separate the right PA from the back of the ascending aorta.

The aortopulmonary artery window is dissected in preparation for placement of the aortic cross-clamp. The superior vena cava and the aorta are gently retracted laterally and the posterior pericardium is incised above the right pulmonary artery, allowing access to the trachea. The plane of the trachea is manually developed, and the trachea can be encircled with an umbilical tape. Following completion of the thoracic dissection, the donor is heparinized (250–300 units/kg). The ascending aorta is cannulated with a routine cardioplegia cannula for cardiac preservation. At the bifurcation of the main PA a Sarns (Ann Arbor, MI) 6.5-mm curved metal cannula is placed and secured with a purse-string suture. After placement of the cannulas, a bolus dose of prostaglandin E_1 (PGE_1) (500 μg) is given directly into the PA using a 16-gauge needle.

Immediately after the PGE_1 infusion, the SVC is ligated, and the IVC is divided, allowing the right heart to decompress. The aorta is cross-clamped and cardioplegia is initiated. The left atrial appendage is generously incised decompressing the left side of the heart. The pulmonary flush consisting of several liters (50–75 ml/kg) of cold (4° C) Perfadex is initiated (Figure 14-1). The chest cavity is cooled with ice-slush normal saline. Gentle ventilation is continued throughout to prevent hyperinflation or atelectasis and enhance the distribution of the flush solution.

After completion of the cardioplegia and the antegrade pulmonary flush, the cannulas are removed. The heart is then extracted. The IVC is freed posteriorly and dissected up to the level of the right atrium. Division of the left atrium proceeds with the cooperation of the heart and lung teams. The heart is retracted toward the right and an inci-

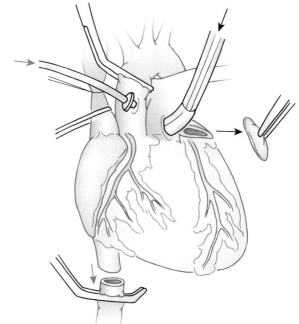

Figure 14–1 Drawing at time of cross-clamping showing placement of cannulas and venting of right and left side of the heart.
(Reprinted from Sundaresan S, Trachiotis GD, Aoe M, et al: Donor lung procurement: Assessment and operative technique. Ann Thorac Surg 56:1412, 1993, with permission from the Society of Thoracic Surgeons.)

sion is made with an 11-blade scalpel in the left atrium midway between the coronary sinus and the left pulmonary veins. Scissors are then used to extend the opening superiorly and inferiorly while visualizing the orifices of the left superior and inferior pulmonary veins. The remaining cuff of left atrium can be transected while internally visualizing the right pulmonary veins. The surgeon on the left side of the table can visualize the right vein orifices best and should divide the left atrial cuff over the right pulmonary veins. An appropriate residual atrial cuff should have a rim of left atrial muscle around each of the pulmonary vein orifices. An adequate cuff can be ensured if the interatrial groove is developed on the right (Figure 14-2). The superior vena cava is transected between ties, followed by both division of the aorta proximal to the cross-clamp and the PA at its bifurcation. The heart is then passed off the field.

Following extraction of the heart, we use a Foley catheter to deliver retrograde flush via the pulmonary vein orifices (approximately 300 ml of cold Perfadex in each orifice). During retrograde flushing residual blood and small clots are often flushed out of the opened pulmonary artery bifurcation. Alternatively this retrograde flush can be done on the back table prior to departure from the donor site. We incorporated this retrograde flushing into our donor procurements since experimental[27] and clinical[181] research found it to be superior to antegrade flush with less pulmonary edema, lower airway resistance, and better oxygenation during the first several hours after transplantation.

We then proceed with en-bloc removal of the contents of the thoracic cavity. Removal of the lungs by this technique

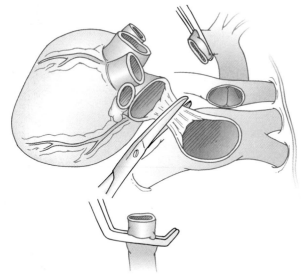

Figure 14–2 The heart is removed, leaving a cuff of left atrium. *(Reprinted from Sundaresan S, Trachiotis GD, Aoe M, et al: Donor lung procurement: Assessment and operative technique. Ann Thorac Surg 56:1412, 1993, with permission from the Society of Thoracic Surgeons.)*

prevents injury to the membranous trachea, pulmonary arteries, and pulmonary veins. The trachea is encircled two to three rings above the carina. The endotracheal tube is opened to atmosphere and the lungs are allowed to deflate to approximate end tidal volume while the endotracheal tube is backed into the proximal trachea. The trachea is sealed with a linear stapler and divided at least two rings above the carina (Figure 14-3). Immediately posterior, the

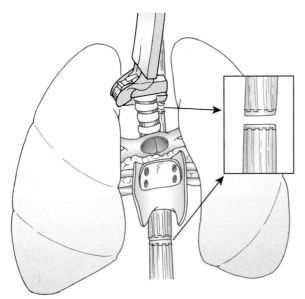

Figure 14–3 Drawing after removal of the heart, esophagectomy, and division of trachea prior to double-lung bloc extraction. *(Reprinted from Sundaresan S, Trachiotis GD, Aoe M, et al: Donor lung procurement: Assessment and operative technique. Ann Thorac Surg 56:1412, 1993, with permission from the Society of Thoracic Surgeons.)*

esophagus is encircled, stapled, and divided using a linear stapler. While retracting both lungs, heavy scissors are used to divide all the mediastinal tissue down to the spine. Staying directly on the spine the posterior mediastinal tissue is divided. At this point, the pericardium near the diaphragm is transected. The inferior pulmonary ligaments are sharply divided. The lower esophagus is encircled and divided with the linear stapler. Posterior mediastinal tissue is sharply divided to connect with the superior aspect of the dissection. The lungs are then removed en-bloc along with the thoracic esophagus and aorta.

If the lungs are returning to the same institution, they are tripled-bagged together, with cold preservation solution and transported on ice. Alternatively, if the lungs are to be used at separate institutions, they are divided on the back table. While the lung bloc is kept in an ice-slush bath, the donor esophagus and aorta are removed and the pericardium is excised. The lungs are separated by division of the posterior pericardium, left atrium between the pulmonary veins, division of the main pulmonary artery at the bifurcation, and division of the left bronchus above the take-off of the upper lobe bronchus. The left bronchus is divided between staples to maintain the inflation of each lung.

If the lungs have been transported en bloc they are separated as detailed above. The pulmonary artery and left atrial cuffs are freed from any pericardial attachments, which may cause kinking after the anastomosis is completed. The right and left pulmonary arteries are cleaned back to their first branches and inspected for any injuries or embolic material. The donor bronchus is divided two rings proximal to the upper lobe orifice. Care is taken to minimize dissection of the donor bronchus in order to preserve collateral flow through the peribronchial nodal tissue.

► RECIPIENT IMPLANTATION [96,117,119]

Prior to anesthetic induction, the majority of our patients have epidural catheters placed. If cardiopulmonary bypass (CPB) is planned we do not place an epidural because of the requirement for heparinization during CPB. Double lumen endotracheal intubation is routine. When the indication for transplantation is septic lung disease (cystic fibrosis, bronchiectasis), the patients are initially intubated with a large single lumen endotracheal tube to allow vigorous suctioning of purulent secretions through an adult fiberoptic bronchoscope. We believe that this step maximizes effective ventilation during independent lung ventilation and decreases the likelihood that cardiopulmonary bypass will be required.

Routine monitoring devices include a Swan–Ganz catheter, radial and femoral arterial lines, Foley catheter, and a transesophageal echocardiography probe. The patient is positioned supine with all extremities padded and arms tucked in at the sides. A heating blanket is placed just under the rib cage and the patient is securely strapped.

CPB is routinely used for children, for lobar transplants, in patients in whom a double lumen tube cannot be placed (small adults), during intracardiac procedures and in most patients with pulmonary hypertension. For the vast majority of our patients, however, we do not utilize CPB. We also do not routinely use the cell saver as the majority of our transplants are performed with less than 500 ml blood loss.

To reduce the need for CPB, the least functional lung, as determined by preoperative quantitative ventilation and perfusion imaging, is resected and replaced first. An attempt is made to detach all pleural adhesions and fully mobilize the hila of both lungs before the first lung is explanted. Great care is taken to avoid injuring the phrenic nerve as it passes just anterior to the hilum and the vagus nerve as it lies posterior to the hilum. This preliminary dissection shortens the time that the first implanted lung is exposed to the entire cardiac output, and thus lessens the likelihood of reperfusion edema in that lung. In this respect both donor lungs should be prepared for implantation prior to removing the recipient's lungs if possible.

The pulmonary arteries and pulmonary veins are dissected beyond their primary bifurcations to preserve the length of the main trunks. The right pulmonary artery is usually transected between firings of a vascular stapling device 1 cm beyond the ligated first branch to the right upper lobe. The left pulmonary artery is kept longer and transected between staple lines beyond the second branch to the left upper lobe. The vein branches are usually ligated with silk ties and divided at their secondary branch points to save length for the future recipient atrial cuff. The bronchus is transected between cartilaginous rings well into the mediastinum at a site suitable for anastomosis. The posterior bundle of lymphatics and bronchial arteries is exposed and divided with electrocautery or ligated and divided.

The lung is removed from the chest, and the operative field is prepared for implantation of the graft. The pulmonary artery stump is mobilized centrally, then grasped with a clamp and placed on traction anteriorly to afford better access to the bronchus. The pulmonary vein stumps are then grasped and retracted laterally to permit circumferential opening of the pericardium. With the pericardium freed, the vein stumps are retracted and temporarily fixed anteriorly. This assists in providing an excellent view of the bronchus. The left-sided double lumen endobronchial tube might impair the ability to trim the left bronchus to an appropriately short length, in which case the tube should be backed out a few millimeters. Meticulous hemostasis in the posterior mediastinum is achieved at this point, with the knowledge that reaching this portion of the operative field after implantation of the graft lung will be extremely difficult. Finally, a small-suction catheter is placed down the appropriate limb of the endotracheal tube to assist in aspiration of blood and iced saline during implantation.

The donor lung is placed within the recipient's chest cavity covered by a cold laparotomy pad. If space permits we place a layer of slush in the empty chest cavity first. We find it simplest to perform the anastomoses from posterior to anterior in the following sequence: bronchus, artery, and atrium. A silk traction suture is placed at the midpoint of the anterior bronchus of the recipient and used to retract the bronchus out of the mediastinum to help with visibility during the anastomosis. To begin the bronchial anastomosis, donor and recipient posterior peribronchial tissues are approximated. The membranous part of the bronchial anastomosis is then performed with a continuous suture (Figure 14-4). The cartilaginous airway is performed with interrupted figure-of-eight sutures (Figure 14-5A). Two sutures

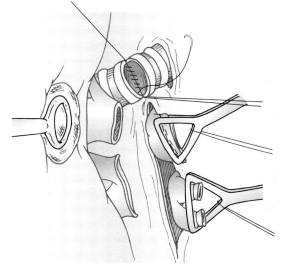

Figure 14–4 We prefer a running, continuous 4.0 PDS suture for the posterior membranous wall of the bronchial anastomosis. *(Reprinted with permission from Meyers BF, Patterson GA: Technical aspects of adult lung transplantation. Sem Thorac Cardiovasc Surg 10:213, 1998.)*

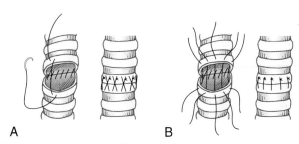

Figure 14–5 A, Normally we perform the anterior wall of the bronchial anastomosis with interrupted figure-of-eight 4.0 PDS suture. **B,** When the bronchus is small we prefer to perform the anterior wall of the bronchial anastomosis with interrupted 3.0 Vicryl sutures. *(Reprinted with permission from Meyers BF, Patterson GA: Technical aspects of adult lung transplantation. Sem Thoracic Cardiovasc Surg 10:213, 1998.)*

placed on each side of the previously placed silk suture usually suffice, although on occasion a single interrupted suture is necessary in the middle of the anterior wall. The silk suture marking the middle of the anterior wall is removed, and the airway is irrigated with cold saline. The anterior row sutures are then tied. If the bronchi are of small caliber, which is most commonly seen on the left side, we opt for reapproximating the anterior wall with simple interrupted 3.0 Vicryl sutures to prevent stricturing of the airway (Figure 14-5B). Once the bronchial anastomosis is completed, the suture used to reapproximate the posterior peribronchial tissues is continued around covering the anterior bronchial wall with peribronchial tissue as well. The entire bronchial anastomosis is constructed using 4-0 monofilament absorbable suture material.

Following this the pulmonary arteries of the donor and recipient are aligned in proper orientation. The recipient's

214 pulmonary artery is then clamped centrally with a small Satinsky clamp with care taken to avoid including the Swan–Ganz catheter in the jaws of the clamp. The vascular staple line is resected at a location that matches the size of the donor and recipient artery. Both donor and recipient pulmonary arteries are trimmed to prevent excessive length and possible kinking postoperatively. An end-to-end arterial anastomosis is performed with a running, continuous 5.0 polypropylene suture (Figure 14-6). This anastomosis must be made with precise, small suture bites to avoid any anastomotic stricture. Size discrepancies between recipient and donor pulmonary arteries can almost always be corrected during performance of the anastomosis by tiny corrections with each bite. Furthermore, to help with size discrepancies a larger recipient artery can be divided beyond the first ligated branch to match a smaller donor artery, while a smaller recipient artery is divided proximal to the first branch, or through it, to maximize circumference.

Both vein stumps are then retracted laterally and a Satinsky clamp is placed centrally on the recipient's left atrium. Once the clamp is placed, an umbilical tape is used to tie the clamp closed to minimize the likelihood of dislodgement during subsequent lateral retraction of the clamp. The ties are then cut off the recipient vein stumps and the bridge of atrium between vein stumps is divided to create the atrial cuff. Gentle lateral traction on the Satinsky clamp can bring this anastomosis to a more accessible location. Alternatively a retraction suture placed in the pericardium 2–3 cm above the inferior pulmonary vein with care taken to avoid injury to the phrenic nerve can be used to partially suspend the heart providing better exposure to the left atrial anastomosis. The anastomosis is performed with a continuous 4-0 polypropylene suture (Figure 14-7). Sutures are placed using a mattress technique, which achieves good intima-to-intima apposition and excludes all atrial muscle. This limits the thrombogenicity of this suture line. The last few sutures are left intentionally loose. The lung is partially inflated and the pulmonary artery clamp is

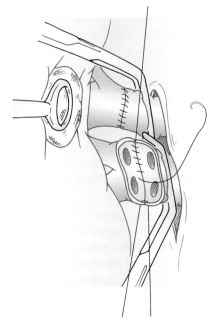

Figure 14–7 A running continuous suture of 4.0 Prolene is used to construct the left atrial anastomosis.
(*Reprinted with permission from Meyers BF, Patterson GA: Technical aspects of adult lung transplantation. Sem Thoracic Cardiovasc Surg 10:213, 1998.*)

loosened momentarily. The lung is flushed with the atrial clamp still in place so as to flush out residual pulmonary perfusate solution. The left atrial clamp is then opened momentarily to completely deair the atrium. The atrial suture line is then secured and clamps are removed completely. All suture lines as well as the cut edges of pericardium are then checked for hemostasis as ventilation and perfusion are restored.

The contralateral transplant is conducted in the same fashion. Traditionally we have drained the pleural space with two large-caliber chest tubes, one angled and one straight. More recently if hemostasis during the procedure was excellent we use two #19 Blake drains (Ethicon, Somerville, NJ) in each pleural space, one placed apically and one along the diaphragm. The ribs are reapproximated with interrupted figure-of-eight monofilament nonabsorbable suture. The pectoralis muscle and fascia are reapproximated with standard suture material, as is the subcutaneous layer. In women on occasion we drain the submammary space. Staples are used for the skin and then sterile dry dressings are applied. Prior to leaving the operating room, bronchoscopy is performed to inspect the bronchial anastomosis and clear any secretions.

▶ USE OF CARDIOPULMONARY BYPASS

When CPB is planned we prefer to do the majority of the dissection before administration of heparin and cannulation. A two-stage venous cannula is placed in the atrium and an aortic perfusion cannula is placed in the ascending aorta. We also routinely place a pulmonary artery vent. After cannulation, bypass is instituted at full flow and both lungs are

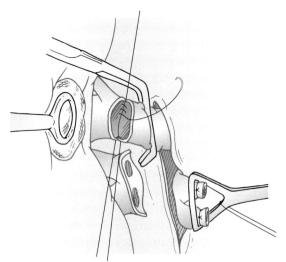

Figure 14–6 A running, continuous 5.0 Prolene suture is used for the pulmonary artery anastomosis.
(*Reprinted with permission from Meyers BF, Patterson GA: Technical aspects of adult lung transplantation. Sem Thoracic Cardiovasc Surg 10:213, 1998.*)

excised. After the first lung is implanted, the left atrium is deaired and the left atrial clamp is removed. The PA clamp is left in place. If the left atrial clamp is also left in place, there is often not enough atrium available for clamp placement on the opposite side. The lung is packed in iced saline and slush while the second lung is implanted.

▶ INCISION CONSIDERATIONS

Bilateral Anterolateral Thoracotomies

Our standard exposure is through bilateral anterolateral thoracotomies, which prevents the sternal healing complications seen with the "clamshell" incision (Figure 14-8).[115] The skin incision is performed along the inframammary crease at the level of the fourth intercostal space, and the skin over the sternum is not divided. The breast tissue and the lower edge of the pectoral muscle are elevated off the chest wall. The chest cavity is entered by dividing the intercostal muscle directly overlying the fifth rib. The internal mammary arteries are identified, isolated, ligated, and divided bilaterally. Alternatively the internal mammary arteries can be preserved if a 1-cm segment of costal cartilage of the fourth rib is resected at the sternal border allowing upward mobility of the fourth rib when retracted. More mobility is obtained by dividing intercostal muscle from within the pleural space to the paraspinal muscles. The serratus anterior muscle and the long thoracic nerve are not divided; rather they are pulled away from the chest wall to allow access to the posterolateral intercostal space. Optimal exposure is then obtained by appropriate placement of retractors at 90° angles from one another. For maximum exposure during hilar dissection, lung removal, and implantation, the table is tilted right or left as necessary. When an otherwise straightforward transplant requires CPB, we do not usually proceed with the clamshell incision since the **215** ascending aorta and right atrium can be easily cannulated through the medial aspect of the right anterolateral thoracotomy.

Transsternal Bilateral Thoracotomy (Thoracosternotomy) Incision

This incision provides excellent exposure to the hilar structures as well as the mediastinum and both pleural spaces (Figure 14-9). Bilateral retractors are used to elevate the chest wall upward. Currently we resort to the full clamshell incision under the following circumstances: (1) a concomitant heart operation is planned, (2) the patient has pulmonary hypertension with secondary cardiomegaly, and (3) the patient has restrictive lung disease and small chest cavities precluding adequate exposure via bilateral thoracotomies.

When a transverse sternotomy has been performed our preference is to reapproximate the sternum with a heavy gauge Steinmann pin and a single figure-of-eight #5 sternal wire. Other techniques to reapproximate the sternum have been developed.[18]

Posterolateral Thoracotomy and Anterolateral Thoracotomy

Patients with restrictive lung diseases and small chest cavities (Figure 14-10) and patients with secondary pulmonary hypertension and cardiomegaly may present with their

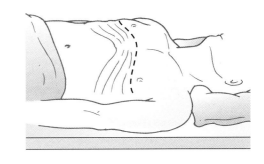

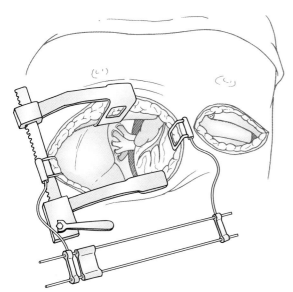

Figure 14–8 Our preferred incision for the majority of our bilateral lung transplants consists of bilateral anterolateral thoracotomies.
(Reprinted with permission from Meyers BF, Patterson GA: Technical aspects of adult lung transplantation. Sem Thoracic Cardiovasc Surg 10:213, 1998.)

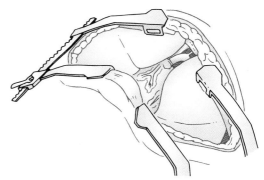

Figure 14–9 The transsternal bilateral thoracotomy incision provides excellent exposure to the hilar structures as well as the mediastinum and both pleural spaces and we continue to utilize this incision during certain circumstances (see text).
(Reprinted with permission from Shields TW, LoCicero J, Ponn RB: General Thoracic Surgery. Philadelphia: Lippincott Williams & Wilkins, 2000, p. 1193.)

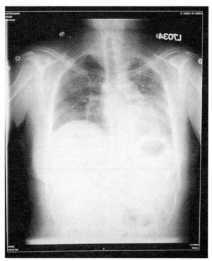

A

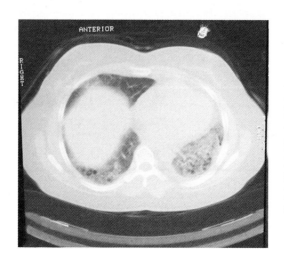

B

Figure 14–10 (A) Chest radiograph. **(B)** CT scan of patient with IPF showing the small size of the chest cavities, which almost entirely filled anteriorly on the left with the heart. In this patient we opted to perform a left posterolateral thoracotomy and a right anterolateral thoracotomy to obtain adequate exposure.

heart filling much of the left anterior hemithorax, making access to the left hilum via the anterior approach quite difficult. In these circumstances, CPB can be avoided by performing the left lung transplant first through a left posterolateral thoracotomy. The patient is then turned supine and the right lung transplant performed via a right anterolateral approach.

POSTOPERATIVE CARE

Immediately postoperatively, patients are transported intubated to the intensive care unit for constant monitoring. Once stabilized, a standard ventilator pressure support weaning protocol is initiated. All attempts are made to limit mean airway pressures to prevent barotrauma to the new anastomosis. Postoperatively a quantitative lung perfusion scan to assess for adequate patency and graft flow is usually performed. If a lobar or greater perfusion defect is appreciated further interrogation for the cause should be undertaken either by catheterization or operative exploration.

Careful fluid management is necessary to avoid substantial transplant lung edema, and usually negative fluid balance is attempted within the first 48 h. Adequate urine output is carefully maintained with combinations of blood, colloid, diuretics, and dopamine at 2–3 μg/kg/min. Prior to extubation, patients undergo bronchoscopy to ensure adequate clearance of secretions. Following extubation, the apical chest tubes are removed in the absence of an air leak, commonly within 48 h postoperatively. Because of the frequent occurrence and reoccurrence of pleural effusions postoperatively, especially in bilateral lung transplant candidates, the basal chest tubes remain for several days usually being removed on postoperative Day 5–7 (chest tube drainage <150 ml/24 h).

Vigorous chest physiotherapy, postural drainage, inhaled bronchodilators, and frequent clearance of pulmonary secretions are required in the postoperative care of these patients. Early and constant involvement of the physical therapy team ensures that transplant recipients are out of bed to chair, ambulatory with assistance, and utilizing the treadmill or exercise bikes as soon as possible even if they remain intubated. In patients with early allograft dysfunction requiring prolonged intubation, early tracheostomy allows easier mobility and better patient comfort, oral hygiene, and clearance of pulmonary secretions.

IMMUNOSUPPRESSION

The immunosuppression regimen utilized at Barnes-Jewish Hospital is shown in Table 14-1. Preoperatively we give azathioprine and at the time of graft reperfusion we give 500 mg intravenous (IV) methylprednisolone. Our postoperative regimen consists of triple therapy including cyclosporine A (Neoral, Novartis), azathioprine, and corticosteroids and perioperative use of an induction agent. We have chosen to use induction agents at our program because they have been shown to decrease the incidence of acute rejection.[62,130] Recently freedom from acute rejection has been shown to be the same whether using a cytolytic agent or interleukin (IL)-2R antagonists as induction strategy.[17] We have switched to using IL-2R antagonists because of their ease of administration (no premedication, central venous access not needed), fewer side effects, and potentially fewer secondary infections.

INFECTION PROPHYLAXIS

Our standard infectious prophylaxis regimen consists of IV cefepime and vancomycin except in patients with septic lung disease where our coverage is based on previously isolated bacterial organisms. Modifications are made based on intraoperative cultures. If *Candida albicans* is detected from airway cultures we treat with fluconazole, and if in the past the recipient was known to be colonized with *Aspergillus* species, we use itraconazole. In general we treat positive cultures for a total of 10–14 days, but if cultures are negative we discontinue antibiotics after 7 days. For the first year after transplantation we routinely give acyclovir (unless the patient is on ganciclovir or Valcyte) for herpes simplex

Table 14–1

Immunosuppressive Regimen at Barnes-Jewish Hospital

	Induction of anesthesia	*Time of reperfusion*	*Postoperative*[a]
Cyclosporine A (Neoral, Novartis)			Usually start 50–75 mg IV/PO POD 1 and increase for target trough 250–350 for first 6 months, then after 6 months 200–300
Azathioprine	2 mg/kg IV × 1		2 mg/kg IV/PO QD (round to nearest 25, maximum dose 150 mg QD)
Corticosteroids		500 mg IV methylprednisolone	Methylprednisolone or prednisone 0.5 mg/kg BID × 6 doses, then 0.5 mg/kg PO QD for first 3 months, taper to 15 mg QD between 3 and 6 months, then after 6 months decrease to 7.5 mg QD for diabetic patients or 15 mg QD for nondiabetics
Induction therapy (IL-2 receptor antagonist)	20 mg IV basiliximab (Simulect, Novartis) × 1		20 mg IV basiliximab POD #4

[a]If switch to tacrolimus adjust for target trough 10–14 first 6 months, then decrease 8–12 after 6 months. If switch to mycophenolate mofetil (CellCept) dose is 1–2 g/day given BID.

prophylaxis. To prevent *Candida albicans* we use nystatin (unless the patient is on fluconazole). In patients at high risk for cytomegalovirus (CMV) (donor+ / recipient− mismatch) our standard prophylaxis is 12 weeks of IV ganciclovir (5 mg/kg QD) usually starting 7–14 days posttransplantation. For transplants we use CMV-negative or leukocyte-reduced blood products.[54] We give lifelong prophylaxis for *Pneumocystis* with Bactrim DS or pentamidine starting approximately 3 weeks after transplantation.

In general after hospital discharge our patients continue with pulmonary rehabilitation at our center for the first 3 months and we see them weekly or biweekly in clinic during that time period. On each visit they receive blood work, chest radiograph, and pulmonary function tests. After 6 weeks we allow our patients to resume driving if they have stopped their pain medications. They may return home if they live far away at 3 months. We continue to follow the majority of our patients every 6–8 weeks for life. Currently we have over 300 surviving patients. If they do not live in the immediate area we see them biannually or annually assuming they have adequate follow-up at home. A large number of our transplant recipients return to work if they desire to do so.

We perform scheduled surveillance bronchoscopies with bronchoalveolar lavage (BAL) and transbronchial biopsies (TBBx) at 3, 6, and 12 weeks and 6 and 12 months postoperatively. In 25% of patients undergoing surveillance bronchoscopy with TBB and BAL, unsuspected infection or rejection requiring treatment is detected.[67] Considering

that some of these bronchoscopies are done as follow-up after treatment this number may actually be even higher. Our routine is to obtain at least 8–10 adequate size biopsy specimens. Debate continues about the necessity of surveillance bronchoscopy[*] and a few centers have elected to perform only diagnostic bronchoscopies based on clinical indications.[180] The time period that surveillance biopsies should be performed is also debated. Kesten and colleagues reported the yield of surveillance transbronchial biopsies beyond 4 years was very low.[92] Baz and colleagues reported patients free of acute rejection during the first 4 months following transplantation remained free and therefore surveillance bronchoscopy could be discontinued in this group after 4 months.[13] Since 10% of our patients who are free of acute rejection during the first 100 days still develop acute rejection during the remainder of the year, we perform surveillance bronchoscopy in all our recipients for the first year (Chakinala, unpublished data). After 1 year we perform bronchoscopy based on clinical or functional decline in the recipient lung function. Samples from the BAL are routinely sent for cytology, Gram's, KOH, and AFB stains, and immunostain for respiratory viruses, herpes simplex virus, and CMV. Additionally bacterial, mycobacterial, fungal, and viral cultures are performed. Open lung biopsies are performed on occasion when necessary and may be particularly useful at later time points.[25]

[*]References 13, 15, 67, 79, 151, 177, 196.

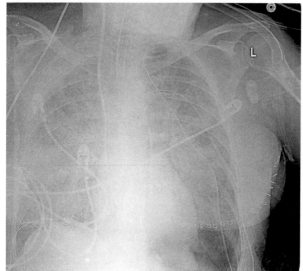

A

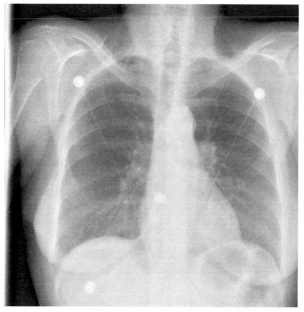

B

Figure 14–11 (**A**) Chest radiograph showing diffuse consolidation typical of ischemic reperfusion injury. The right lung was implanted first, which explains the increase injury appreciated on this side. (**B**) Radiograph of the same patient after complete recovery.

▶ POSTOPERATIVE COMPLICATIONS

Ischemia Reperfusion Injury

Ischemia reperfusion injury presents initially with pulmonary edema and pulmonary hypertension with the radiological findings of patchy infiltrates progressing to diffuse consolidation (Figure 14-11). Its etiology is complex but factors known to contribute clinically or in animal models include multiple cytokines, complement, and neutrophils. Primary graft failure (PGF) is believed to represent the extreme of severe reperfusion injury to the donor lung. Secondary causes of early allograft dysfunction such as a

technically inadequate vascular anastomosis need to be ruled out. The incidence of ischemia reperfusion varies depending on institutional definition between 13 and 35% of transplants.[30] Although it is the second most common cause of early mortality in lung transplant recipients, ischemia reperfusion injury plays a contributing role in the vast majority of early mortality. Mortality from primary graft failure is high with one series reporting 60% of patients dying prior to hospital discharge.[30] Fortunately severe reperfusion injury is not as commonly encountered in recent years.

Treatment of ischemia reperfusion is usually supportive with aggressive diuresis, continued mechanical ventilation, PEEP, and high levels of inspired oxygen. We use inhaled nitric oxide[41] or aerosolized prostacyclin[56] to improve oxygenation, which minimizes oxygen requirements and lowers pulmonary artery pressures in patients who have ischemia reperfusion injury. Paralytics and sedatives are used to minimize oxygen consumption. Extracorporeal membrane oxygenation (ECMO) may be required when refractory hypoxemia persists despite these therapies. We recently reviewed our experience with ECMO after lung transplantation.[120] Seven of the 12 patients requiring ECMO support were discharged from the hospital. All our survivors had ECMO instituted by postoperative Day 1, suggesting immediate lung dysfunction has the most potential for reversibility. A substantial risk is incurred with this therapy with high morbidity (bleeding, renal dysfunction, stroke) and mortality.

Because of the devastating results of severe ischemia reperfusion injury a significant amount of research has been focused on its prevention. Superior strategies of lung preservation have evolved.[111] It is clear from experimental[91,108] and clinical work[55] that low potassium dextran solution provides superior preservation over high potassium preservation solutions previously in use. In addition, experimental work suggests that nitric oxide added to the flush solution or inhaled at the time of harvest provides a preservation advantage.[60,195] Combination of an antegrade and retrograde[27,181] pulmonary vascular flush achieves more uniform distribution of flush solution and superior graft cooling. Lung hyperinflation is an excellent model of pulmonary edema. Therefore we are particularly careful to avoid lung hyperinflation during harvest and storage of the donor lungs. Each of these factors has contributed to a reduction in the frequency of reperfusion injury.

Recently the use of controlled reperfusion in combination with leukocyte depletion° has shown promise as a preventative strategy. Lick and colleagues[102] reported a nonrandomized small series in humans utilizing this technique and reported no reperfusion injury. At the time of reperfusion leukocyte filtered-modified perfusate is pumped at a controlled rate (200 ml/min) and pressure (less than 20 mm Hg) for 10 min through the transplanted lung. The lung was ventilated with 50% inspired oxygen concentration during the period.

Infectious Complications

Bacterial

Bacterial infections are most common in the early posttransplant period and remain the primary cause of mortality

---

°References 14, 31, 32, 57, 71–73.

in the early posttransplant period.[23] Most common organisms involved are those colonizing the donor or the recipient, or those known to populate individual institution's intensive care units. Gram-negative pathogens such as *Pseudomonas* ssp., *Klebsiella*, and *Haemophilus influenzae* are responsible for most early posttransplant bacterial pneumonias, but gram-positive organisms such as *Staphylococcus aureus* are also causes. Less commonly *Actinomyces* (Figure 14-12), *Mycobacterium tuberculosis*, and atypical *Mycobacterium* have been seen in lung transplant recipients.[11,23] Analysis of trends in individual hospital bacterial susceptibilities should guide selection of empiric therapy with adjustments as necessary when sensitivities are available.

Viral

CMV disease is the most commonly noted postoperative infectious complication. It occurs in 13–75% of transplant patients depending on definitions of CMV disease and use of CMV prophylaxis.[54,68] CMV induces heightened immunosuppression and patients therefore are at increased risk for other opportunistic infections and posttransplant lymphoproliferative disease.[155] Lung transplant recipients who are CMV negative and receive CMV-positive donor lungs are at the highest risk of developing severe life-threatening disease from primary infection, while it is not usually seen in donor-negative/recipient-negative transplants.[54] The diagnosis of CMV *infection* at our institution is based on a positive buffy coat or qualitative polymerase chain reaction from blood samples while the presence of "cytomegalic" cells (CMV inclusion bodies or positive immunoperoxidase stain) on tissue biopsies is indicative of CMV *disease* (Figure 14-13). Most CMV infections respond to 14–21 days of IV ganciclovir (5 mg/kg BID). The dose should be adjusted for leukopenia and renal dysfunction. When patients fail to respond to IV ganciclovir therapy, drug resistance is suspected and foscarnet or cidofovir therapy may be instituted.[199] For prevention of relapsing infection we have recently started using valganciclovir (Roche, Palo Alto, CA), an oral ganciclovir derivative with increased bioavailability.

The incidence and significance of noncytomegalovirus viral respiratory tract infections have been reported.[77,128] Most commonly isolated non-CMV viruses included herpes simplex virus (HSV), rhinovirus, and parainfluenza viruses. Less frequently isolated viruses are respiratory syncytial virus, influenza virus, adenovirus, and varicella zoster virus. HSV, parainfluenza, influenza, adenovirus, varicella zoster, and respiratory syncytial virus have been associated with a greater clinical severity of illness.[128,184] Treatment options are individualized and often limited; aerosolized ribavirin has been used for parainfluenza infections.[184]

Fungal

Fungal infections are a major problem after lung transplantation and occur early and late posttransplant. *Candida albicans* is commonly isolated posttransplant, but usually represents colonization,[23] although it may also be invasive.[89] *Aspergillus* spp. (Figure 14-14) can also represent colonization, but more often the presence of these organisms is more serious. In patients with a single lung transplant one potential reservoir of persistent *Aspergillus* is the native lung.[23] Aspergillomas found in the recipient explanted lungs have been associated with reduced posttransplant survival.[70] Invasive *Aspergillus* is often fatal.[20] Mortality directly related to *Aspergillus* infection has been reported in 4.3% of patients.[101] Other fungal infections such as *Histoplasma*, *Coccidioidomycosis*, *Mucormycosis*, *Nocardia*, *Zygomycetes*, and *Cryptococcus* are also reported.[23,83] *Scedosporium*

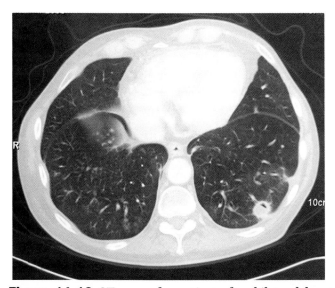

Figure 14–12 CT scan of a patient after bilateral lung transplantation who presented with fevers and chills and was found to have a lung abscess with actinomyces, resolved after treatment with ampicillin.

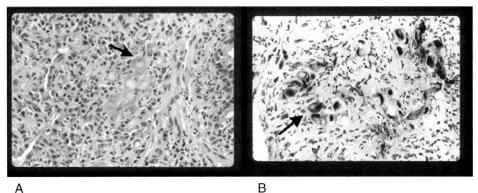

Figure 14–13 (**A**) Transbronchial lung biopsy showing CMV pneumonitis with demonstration of CMV inclusion bodies (see arrows) (hematoxylin and eosin). (**B**) Demonstration of CMV inclusion bodies by immunoperoxidase staining (see arrows).

A   B

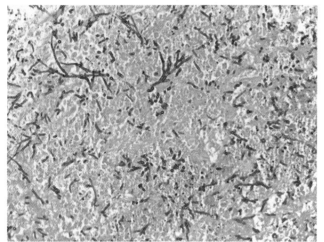

Figure 14–14 Histopathological examination of a patient with aspergillus (hematoxylin and eosin, × 20).

apiospermum is an uncommon cause of disseminated infection, but importantly it is inherently resistant to amphotericin B.[139]

Treatment is based on infection; amphotericin B is generally the drug of choice for *Aspergillus* and *Fusarium* while prolonged azole therapy may be used for *Scedosporium* (itraconazole, voriconazole). *Nocardia* infections are treated based on antimicrobial sensitivities, while pending imipenem and amikacin can be instituted.[83] Candidal infections can be treated with a combination of systemic and inhaled amphotericin B and fluconazole (some species are resistant). Single lung transplant should probably not be performed in patients with mycetomas as adequate removal of fungal organisms cannot be achieved.[70] Prolonged therapy is required for all fungal infections.

Acute Rejection

Acute rejection remains the "thorn in the side" of lung transplantation, being more prevalent in the lung than in any other solid organ transplant.[100,174] Although it is an uncommon cause of mortality, its danger lies in its proven association with the development of chronic rejection. The majority of episodes of acute rejection occur early in the postoperative period, and the incidence steadily declines after the first 3 months.[44,79,177] The clinical diagnosis of acute rejection remains imprecise. Normally symptomatic episodes present with dyspnea, hypoxemia, low-grade fever, and moderate leukocytosis, which can be difficult to differentiate from early infection. The chest radiograph findings of diffuse-perihilar interstitial infiltrates along with these clinical findings is consistent with rejection. Trulock[175] reported the frequent occurrence of radiographic abnormalities with early episodes of rejection, while episodes occurring after the first month frequently had a normal appearing chest radiograph. Monitoring of the allograft by spirometry is useful and a 10% or greater decline in baseline FEV_1 or forced vital capacity (FVC) indicates the need for further evaluation.

Suspicion of acute rejection should be evaluated by bronchoscopy with TBBx to confirm the diagnosis and rule out infection. A uniform grading system for classification of pulmonary transplant rejection (acute and chronic) was initially proposed in 1990[197] and subsequently revised in 1995 by the Lung Rejection Study Group (LRSG).[198] For acute rejection this grading system is based on histological criteria found on biopsy, with emphasis on perivascular and interstitial infiltration of mononuclear cells (Table 14-2 and Figure 14-15). Each grade should also note the coexistence of airway inflammation. The degree of perivascular inflammation is graded in the "A" category from 0 (no rejection) to 4 (severe rejection). The presence of small and large airway inflammation is listed as a "B" category and divided into five grades of increasing intensity or, alternatively, based on

Table 14–2
Grading of Acute Pulmonary Allograft Rejection[a]

Acute rejection	
Grade 0	None
Grade 1	Minimal
Grade 2	Mild
Grade 3	Moderate
Grade 4	Severe
Airway inflammation with or without lymphocytic bronchitis/bronchiolitis	
May grade	
Grade 0	None
Grade 1	Minimal
Grade 2	Mild
Grade 3	Moderate
Grade 4	Severe
Grade X	Ungradable

[a]Adapted from Yousem SA, Berry GJ, Cagle PT, et al: Revision of the 1990 working formulation for the classification of pulmonary allograft rejection: Lung rejection study group. J Heart Lung Transplant 15:1, 1996.

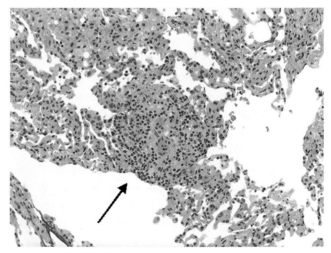

Figure 14–15 Histopathological examination of acute rejection, ISHLT grade 3 (see *arrow*) (hematoxylin and eosin, ×20).

institutional preference, simply noted as present or absent. Although perivascular infiltrates are the primary focus in this classification scheme, it was felt that the correlation of airway inflammation with the development of chronic rejection could not be ignored.[198]

Acute rejection is usually treated with IV methylprednisolone, 10–15 mg/kg/day for 3–5 days. Usually there is improvement in symptoms and radiographic findings within 8–12 h. Often this is followed with a steroid taper over 2–3 weeks. Another goal with therapy is to prevent future episodes; with this in mind the patient's maintenance therapy should be evaluated. New medications should be considered as they can decrease drug levels of calcineurin inhibitors by activating the cytochrome P-450 enzyme pathway and increasing their metabolism. The optimal initial maintenance immunosuppression regimen has not been clearly delineated. Two studies have shown a decrease in acute rejection episodes when tacrolimus (FK506; Prograf, Fujisawa) is chosen as the initial calcineurin inhibitor.[90,173] Other studies have shown a decreased recurrence in acute rejection after switching from cyclosporine to tacrolimus.[80,186] Based on these studies we often discontinue cyclosporine and start tacrolimus in patients with severe or recurrent acute rejection episodes. Mycophenolate mofetil (MMF) (Cellcept, Hoffmann-LaRoche) has not been shown to decrease acute rejection episodes compared to azathioprine in lung transplantation,[36,127] but based on its success in other organ transplants we often switch to this cell cycle inhibitor when patients have recurrent acute rejection episodes.[156] Novel immunosuppressive agents such as Sirolimus (rapamycin; Rapimmune, Wyeth and RAD rapamycin derivative, Novartis), a newer immunosuppressive agent that acts synergistically with CNIs plus has antiproliferative properties, and Leflunomide (Arava), a *de novo* pyrimidine nucleotide synthesis inhibitor, have shown promise in other organ transplants.[78,88,193] Their role in acute rejection in lung transplantation is being evaluated.[154] After treatment of acute rejection, we repeat bronchoscopy in 3–6 weeks to confirm an appropriate response to therapy. In approximately one third of cases persistence of acute rejection is detected on follow-up.[1,67,151,177] Treatment of acute rejection refractory to the above acute (steroids) and maintenance interventions is not uniform. A trial of cytolytic therapy is often initiated.[10,64,130,148] Other regimens have been attempted including aerosolized cyclosporine,[85] Alemtuzumab (Campath),[141] methotrexate,[21] extracorporeal photopheresis,[2,185] and total lymphoid irradiation.[179] No controlled trials have been performed comparing these therapies and reported studies are small with varying degrees of success reported.

Anastomotic Complications

The bronchial circulation to the donor lung is severed during extraction, and after implantation, the donor bronchus depends on retrograde flow from the pulmonary circulation until systemic collaterals develop. Anastomotic complications resulting from airway ischemia include infection, dehiscence, stenosis, and malacia. The reported incidence of these complications is 7–14%[29,65,146,149] of patients, although improvements in anastomotic techniques, pulmonary preservation, and care in preserving collateral circu-

lation during harvesting have lessened their occurrence. In our recent experience the incidence of airway complications was only 4%.[42]

Ischemia of the bronchial anastomosis can result in necrosis of tissue and a viable media for the growth of saprophytic fungus. These infections when they occur can be a significant source of morbidity. Nunley and colleagues[125] recently reviewed saprophytic fungal infections involving the bronchial anastomosis and found an occurrence of 25% in recipients surviving a minimum of 75 days posttransplantation. In 47% of those patients with fungal involvement of the anastomosis, airway complications occurred.

When a dehiscence occurs as a result of ischemia and necrosis at the suture line, it may present as the development of massive air leak or mediastinal emphysema in the early posttransplant period. If the dehiscence remains localized it usually will heal by granulation and reepithelialization as long as adequate drainage of the dehiscence is maintained.[135] Covered Wallstents (Schneider, Minneapolis, MN) have been utilized attempting to seal the anastomotic defect.[28] The location of the dehiscence is important in determining the long-term outcome. Membranous dehiscence generally heals without significant stricture formation, while dehiscence occurring in the anterior cartilaginous part of the anastomosis results in more frequent stricture formation. Complete dehiscence can result in mediastinal sepsis or uncontrolled air leaks requiring surgical intervention.[135]

A consequence of ischemia and necrosis at the bronchial anastomosis is the later development of a stricture. Bronchial anastomotic strictures can result from surgical stenosis, granulation tissue, infection, or bronchomalacia. Bronchoscopic assessment confirms the diagnosis and directs treatment. Management is based on etiology of the stricture. Bronchial stenosis can be treated by serial balloon dilation and if necessary stent placement and bronchomalacia by stent placement alone. Infections causing stenosis require debridement and appropriate antimicrobial therapy. Bronchial anastomotic strictures resulting from excessive granulation tissue are the most difficult to mange successfully because of the propensity to reoccur. Treatment of the granulation tissue consists of a combination of laser or forceps debridement, dilatation, and stenting.[29,168] Attempts to reduce the proliferation of granulation tissue with the use of topical antiproliferative agents like mitomycin C[52] and sirolimus (unpublished data) have shown promise. Complications from stent placement include restenosis, mucous plugging, migration, stent fracture, and creation of a false passage.[28,168]

Chronic Rejection

Chronic rejection of the lung allograft is the major limitation to long-term recipient survival. Five years after transplantation approximately 50% of recipients have developed chronic rejection.[75] Bronchiolitis obliterans (BO) is the histological finding of chronic rejection in the lung allograft (Figure 14-16). This entity, characterized by scarring and fibrosis of the small airways with or without an inflammatory component, was first described at Stanford in heart–lung recipients.[19] In the revised classification of pulmonary allograft rejection by the LRSG,[198] chronic rejection was categorized into "C" grade for chronic airway rejection

222

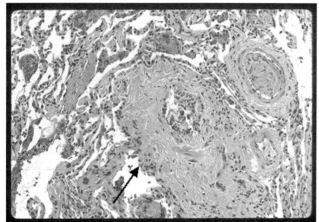

Figure 14–16 Transbronchial lung biopsy showing bronchiolitis obliterans with scarring and fibrosis of the small airways (see *arrow*) (hematoxylin and eosin).

Table 14–3		
Criteria for Bronchiolitis Obliterans Syndrome[a,b]		
BOS score	**Degree**	**Baseline FEV$_1$**
0	None	>90% and FEF$_{25-75}$ >75%
0-p	Potential	81–90% and/or FEF$_{25-75}$ $\leq$ 75%
1	Mild	66–80%
2	Moderate	51–65%
3	Severe	$\leq$50%

[a]Adapted from ISHLT, Cooper JD, Billingham M, et al: A working formulation for the standardization of nomenclature and for clinical staging of chronic dysfunction in lung allografts. J Heart Lung Transplant 12:713, 1993; and Estenne M, Maurer JR, Boehler A, et al: Bronchiolitis obliterans syndrome 2001: An update of the diagnostic criteria. J Heart Lung Transplant 21:297, 2002.
[b]Each BOS score or grade as a subcategory noting absence or presence of documented bronchiolitis obliterans histologically: "a"—without pathological evidence of bronchiolitis obliterans; "b"—with pathological evidence of bronchiolitis obliterans.

Box 14–3. Risk Factors for BOS/OB.[a]

Definitive role (accepted risk factors)
    Acute rejection
        Late rejection
    Lymphocytic bronchitis/bronchiolitis
        Late onset
Less clear role (potential risk factors)
    CMV
    Other infectious organisms
    HLA matching
Little or no role (hypothetic risk factors)
    Recipient and donor characteristics

[a]Adapted from Sharples LD, McNeil K, Stewart S, et al: Risk factors for bronchiolitis obliterans: A systematic review of recent publications. J Heart Lung Transplant 21:271, 2002.

(bronchiolitis obliterans) and "D" grade for chronic vascular rejection. In the "C" grade subcategories "a" and "b" were used to note the presence or absence of active airway inflammation (mononuclear cell infiltrates), respectively.

BO is a patchy heterogeneous process. Although transbronchial biopsy is useful for the diagnosis of infection and acute rejection, it is insensitive in the diagnosis of chronic rejection. Chamberlain and colleagues in a review of over 1000 transbronchial biopsies estimated the sensitivity to be only 17%.[22]

Because of the difficulties in documenting BO histologically, a classification system based on clinical parameters was proposed by the ISHLT, termed bronchiolitis obliterans syndrome (BOS).[86] In this classification scheme posttransplant FEV$_1$ is used to assess graft function. The best posttransplant FEV$_1$ is determined and defined as BOS 0. A decline from this baseline determines the stage of BOS, with stages 1–3 representing progressively worsening pulmonary function. Importantly other causes for a decrease in FEV$_1$ (i.e., infection, acute rejection) must be excluded. Patients cannot receive a diagnosis of BOS until at least 3 months after transplantation. BOS is a surrogate marker for chronic allograft rejection and does not require the presence of histologically documented BO. The absence or presence of BO is, however, noted by subcategories "a" and "b," respectively.

Revision, with the addition of a potential BOS stage (BOS-0-p), has recently been proposed based on limitations in the original staging system (Table 14-3).[53] BOS 0-p is defined by a drop in FEV$_1$ of 10–19% and/or a 25% or greater decline in baseline midexpiratory flow rate (FEF$_{25-75}$). The FEF$_{25-75}$ has been shown in several studies to be more sensitive than FEV$_1$ in the detection of early airflow obstruction in bilateral lung transplant recipients, but it has a wide variability with single lung transplants. The goal of introducing this potential stage of BOS is to raise clinical concern and increase surveillance.[53]

Numerous publications attempting to identify risk factors for BOS have been reported. Recently Sharples and colleagues[147] reviewed these studies and defined the reported risk factors as being accepted, potential, or hypothetical based on the available evidence (Box 14-3).

Treatment of patients with BOS/BO rarely reverses the lung dysfunction. Several therapies have been reported, but

in general the studies have been nonrandomized, small, and with short follow-up. Further complicating assessment of therapeutic benefit of a particular treatment has been the uncertain natural history of BOS. Although an almost certain decline in pulmonary function is seen after the onset of BOS, the rate of this decline can vary dramatically between individuals (Figure 14-17). Recently the acute and chronic onset BOS have been suggested to represent different entities.[87]

In general, therapy consists of the augmentation of standard immunosuppression regimens, addition of new immunosuppressive medicines, and immune modulating therapies.* Our standard therapy usually consists of modification of standard immunosuppression with a switch from

---

*References 40, 49, 51, 84, 93, 94, 126, 142–144, 152, 153, 157, 158, 182, 190.

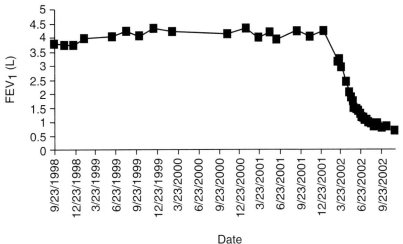

A

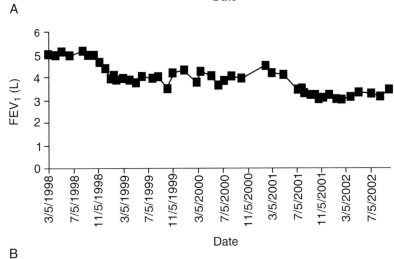

B

Figure 14–17 (**A**) Rapid decline in pulmonary function after development of BOS. This patient succumbed from respiratory failure despite multiple attempts to stabilize his lung function. (**B**) Slower, more chronic onset of decline in pulmonary function in a patient without clinical symptoms.

cyclosporine to tacrolimus, and possibly azathioprine to MMF. More recently we have added Rapamune, which has unique properties (antiproliferative, tolerogenic) that may make it particularly useful for treatment of BO/BOS. We have tried leflunomide on one occasion without success.

Cytolytic therapy is utilized if continued decline in pulmonary function is seen despite these changes. On occasion we have used total lymphoid irradiation. Other treatment options that have been tried include inhaled steroids,[157] aerosolized cyclosporine,[84] methotrexate,[51] cyclophosphamide,[182] and extracorporeal photopheresis[126,152]; a few have resulted in stabilization of the patient's pulmonary status but generally treatment is disappointing.

Recently a surgical treatment for BOS has been proposed by the Duke University Lung Transplant Group[43,98,129] for use in patients with BOS found to have gastroesophageal reflux. Gastroesophageal reflux disease (GERD) with resultant aspiration may contribute to BOS. GERD is prevalent in lung transplant recipients and for multiple reasons this group may be more likely to be affected even with silent aspiration of acid contents. Host defense mechanisms such as cough and mucociliary clearance of foreign bodies are markedly impaired after lung transplantation. Furthermore, vagal nerve injury during the transplant and the use of immunosuppressive agents after transplantation may result

in delayed gastric emptying and decreased gastrointestinal motility. The Duke University Lung Transplant Group has reported improvement in pulmonary function following a laparoscopic Nissen fundoplication for treatment of GERD.[43] Patients treated before they progressed to the later stages of BOS showed the most benefit. A survival advantage was also seen in the lung transplant group surgically treated for their GERD. Currently a prospective, randomized, multiinstitutional trial is being planned to further evaluate the role played by GERD in BOS.

Prevention of BOS through the promotion of immune tolerance of transplanted organs is being investigated. Long-term surviving transplant recipients have been found to have donor cells present in their tissues and blood (chimerism).[137,162] Based on these findings, the Pittsburgh Lung Transplant Group[137] attempted to increase chimerism in lung transplant recipients with concurrent infusion of donor BM cells at the time of transplantation. Overall these results were unimpressive but not surprising. Preconditioning (± BM infusion) of the host using different regimens may be required to achieve tolerance and chimerism in adults. Much ongoing research is now being directed toward achieving the state of tolerance in clinical transplantation.

Retransplantation may be an option in carefully selected patients with BOS. BOS does not appear to occur in an

224 accelerated manner after retransplantation. In the pulmonary retransplant registry 81 and 56% were free of BOS at 1 and 4 years after retransplantation, respectively.[124]

Posttransplant Lymphoproliferative Disease

Posttransplant lymphoproliferative disease (PTLD) is a well-recognized complication after solid-organ and bone marrow transplantation with an incidence between 4 and 10% after lung transplantation (Figure 14-18A).[4,7,99,131] We have previously reported a 6.1% incidence of PTLD after lung transplantation at our institution.[131] PTLD includes a spectrum of disease entities ranging from atypical lymphoid proliferation to malignant non-Hodgkin's lymphoma.[145,169] Most commonly the cells are of B cell origin, and although not absolute there is an association between PTLD and Epstein–Barr virus (EBV) (Figure 14-18B and C).[122] Cytotoxic T cells are involved in destroying cells presenting EBV in the context of MHC I. It has been proposed that an immunocompromised recipient undergoing a primary EBV

infection may not be capable of destroying the virus-infected B cells, resulting in EBV-driven B cell proliferation. In lung transplant recipients a strong correlation between negative EBV serology prior to transplantation and the development of PTLD has been reported. Studies have reported a 6.8 to 20-fold increased risk of development of PTLD in recipients who were EBV negative pretransplantation.[4,191] Some have proposed that EBV carried in the donor lymphocytes in the graft results in a primary infection in the recipient. However, reports have tended to show the recipient orgin of the lymphocytes in PTLD.[194] The use of induction therapy[170] and CMV infection[188] have been suggested as contributing factors to the development of PTLD.

PTLD, when it occurs in the first year after transplantation, shows a predilection for the thorax and commonly arises in the lung allograft.[4,7,99,131] Cases of PTLD that present after the first year in contrast usually are extrathoracic, commonly arising in the abdomen and pelvis.[131] In our series, of the 16 reported cases of PTLD that occurred after the first year 88% were extrathoracic. We recently reviewed

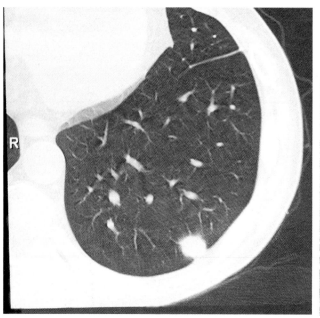

A

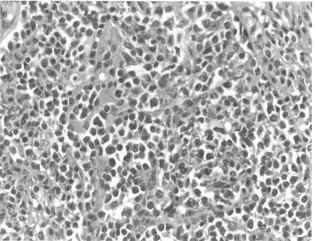

B

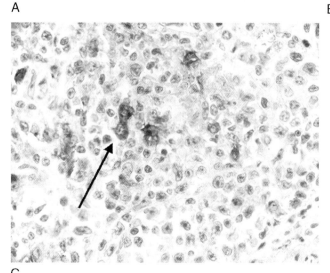

C

Figure 14–18 (**A**) CT scan of a patient with multiple pulmonary nodules developing several months after bilateral lung transplantation found to be PTLD. (**B**) Histopathological examination of a posttransplant lymphoproliferative nodule (hematoxylin and eosin). (**C**) Immunostaining of PTLD nodule positive for Epstein–Barr virus (see *arrow*).

our late cases of PTLD occurring in the abdomen and pelvis.[69] These cases occurred at a median time of 5.8 years after transplantation. Interestingly in all the late cases occurring in the abdomen and pelvis in our series, recipients were EBV positive pretransplant. Late-occurring abdominal and pelvic PTLD cases were most commonly malignant non-Hodgkin's lymphomas, and despite aggressive therapy, prognosis was poor. In contrast the patients who presented with early PTLD, unless disseminated at diagnosis, had a favorable prognosis often responding to simply decreasing immunosuppression.[69]

Treatment of PTLD is based on the stage and progression of disease. Initially a trial of reduction of immunosuppression is attempted, particularly with disease limited to the allograft. Many also have recommended the simultaneous of antiviral therapy.[191] Although chemotherapy (CHOP) has been used in patients with widespread disease or with progression of disease, treatment-related mortality is considerable. In one reported study 75% (3/4) of PTLD patients treated with chemotherapy died as a result of sepsis.[191] Recently Rituximab (Mabthera, Roche), a humanized anti-CD20 monoclonal antibody, has shown promise as a treatment option.[183] Only a few cases of its use in the lung transplant population have been reported. Verschuuren and colleagues[183] reported complete remission in three lung transplant patients treated with Rituximab. Complications, however, occurred in two, one relapsed with a partial CD20 negative PTLD, and the other developed hypogammaglobulinemia with subsequent sepsis and death.

Preventive strategies have been contemplated. In adult lung transplantation it does not appear prudent in matching recipient and donor EBV status, because greater then 90% of the population are EBV positive by the time they are 35; in children who would have a higher percentage of negative recipients this may have more value. Malouf and colleagues[110] reported that prophylactic use of antiviral therapy may reduce the incidence of PTLD.

Gastrointestinal Complications

Gastrointestinal (GI) complications are frequent in lung transplant recipients, occurring in as many as 50% of patients in some series.[107] Frequently reported nonsurgical GI complications include esophagitis, pancreatitis, gastric atony, adynamic colonic ileus, gastroesophageal reflux, peptic ulcer disease, gastritis, GI bleeding, CMV hepatitis, CMV colitis, diverticulitis, cholecystitis, and *Clostridium difficile* colitis/diarrhea. The majority of these nonsurgical GI complications occur in the first month postoperatively and most patients respond to conservative therapy.[107] Acute abdominal processes requiring surgical intervention have a reported incidence of 4–17% in lung transplant recipients and include, in decreasing occurrence, bowel perforation, appendicitis, cholecystitis, colitis, and pneumatosis intestinalis.[76] PTLD may present as an acute abdominal process, secondary to intussusception (see Figure 14-19) or bowel perforation. Surgical GI complications can occur at any time after transplantation and a high index of suspicion is needed because their severity may be masked initially by immunosuppression. Emergent operative exploration when required has significant morbidity and mortality associated

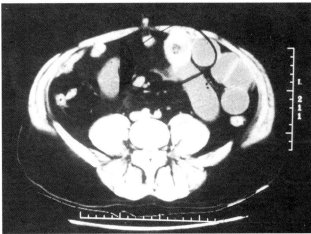

Figure 14–19 CT scan showing a patient with small bowel intussusception secondary to posttransplantation lymphoproliferative disease.

with it. Elective procedures, however, can be performed safely in this population with acceptable morbidity.[138]

▶ ## RESULTS

Over the past 20 years approximately 15,000 lung transplants including almost 8000 single lung and over 6400 double lung transplants have been performed.[75] However, the rapid early growth of the field has slowed because of the shortage of available donors. The major recipient indications for transplantation in the ISHLT registry include COPD (39.4%), IPF (16.9%), cystic fibrosis (16.1%), α_1-antitrypsin deficiency emphysema (9.3%), and PPH (4.6%). One-, three-, and five-year survival reported in this registry is 76, 57, and 43%, respectively. The most common causes of early deaths are graft failure and infections, with BOS being the primary cause of late death.[75] In the recipients undergoing lobar transplants for cystic fibrosis the 1-year survival is 73.8%, and in the recipients with other lung diseases the 1-year survival is 75%.[159]

We have performed 689 lung transplants since the inception of our program in 1988. Our most common indications for lung transplantation are COPD (42%), cystic fibrosis (16%), α_1-antitrypsin deficiency (14%), IPF (11%), PPH (6%), other (5%), bronchiectasis (3%), lymphangioleiomyomatosis (2%), and retransplant (1%). Actuarial survival rates for lung transplants at our program are 85, 72, and 55% at 1, 3, and 5 years, respectively.

Two hundred and thirty adult lung retransplants had been reported to the pulmonary retransplant registry at its last report,[124] with 1- and 3-year actuarial survivals of 47 and 33%, respectively. In this report 64% of the retransplants were for BO/BOS. Potential recipients who are nonambulatory and ventilator dependent are not considered good candidates for retransplantation. The best results after retransplantation occur in the more experienced centers, in nonventilated patients, and in recipients retransplanted more than 2 years following their initial transplant.

Hosenpud and colleagues[81] based on data from the joint United Network for Organ Sharing/International Society of

226 Heart and Lung Transplantation Thoracic Registry reported a survival benefit for patients undergoing lung transplantation for cystic fibrosis and IPF but not for patients transplanted for end-stage emphysema. Other studies have shown a survival benefit for emphysema in addition to IPF, CF, and pulmonary hypertension. The benefit of lung transplantation in patients with congenital heart disease has been questioned. Charman and colleagues[26] found no improvement in survival in patients transplanted for Eisenmenger's syndrome.

Multiple studies have addressed quality of life in lung transplant recipients.[33,66,105,140,171] Improvement in quality of life is seen posttransplant and usually becomes evident after 3–6 months. Mobility, energy, sleep, ADL dependency level, and dyspnea were reported to be improved following lung transplantation.[171] Pretransplant psychological status appears to affect posttransplant quality of life and adjustment.[33] Paris and colleagues evaluated return to work after lung transplantation and reported 22% were employed, 38% were unemployed but medically able to work, 29% were disabled, and 10% had retired.[132]

The economic impact of lung transplantation has recently been assessed in the United Kingdom. Anyanwu and colleagues[3] compared the costs of lung transplantation to the cost of remaining on the waiting list. They concluded that although lung transplantation is an expensive treatment, benefits in survival and quality of life gains are seen and bilateral lung transplantation appears to be more cost-effective than single lung transplantation.

▶ PEDIATRIC LUNG TRANSPLANTATION

According to the ISHLT registry approximately 60–70 pediatric lung transplants are performed each year with nearly 750 total having been reported.[16] The vast majority of these transplants are performed in children ages 11–17, but a number are also performed in patients <1 year of age. In contrast, the majority of pediatric donors are ≥18 years of age. In infants congenital heart disease, primary pulmonary hypertension, and pulmonary vascular disease are the main indications for lung transplantation. During childhood and adolescence cystic fibrosis accounts for the majority of lung transplants. Approximately 40% of pediatric lung transplant recipients survive 5 years. Bilateral lung transplant recipients show an improved survival compared to single lung transplant recipients, but this may be an effect of underlying disease and other recipient factors. The vast majority of pediatric lung transplants are bilateral (89%). As in adults, early mortality after pediatric lung transplantation is secondary to infections and graft failure and late mortality is attributed mostly to bronchiolitis obliterans with >50% developing BO by 5 years.[16]

Only 20–30 centers are currently performing pediatric lung transplants. Our center began its pediatric lung transplant program in July 1990 and performed its first infant lung transplant in 1993. Currently the largest pediatric lung transplant program worldwide, our center has performed 265 pediatric transplants since its inception. Of these 203 have been bilateral, 39 bilateral lobar (living donor), 14 heart–lung, and 9 single lung transplants (St Louis Children's Hospital Lung Transplant Registry; Huddleston,

personal communication). The indications for lung transplantation were in decreasing order cystic fibrosis (42%), pulmonary vascular disease (21%), bronchiolitis obliterans (10%), pulmonary alveolar proteinosis (6%), pulmonary fibrosis (7%), and other (12%). The average age of recipients at the time of transplantation was 9.5 ± 5.9 years.[82] Actuarial survival at our center was 77% at 1 year, 62% at 3 years, and 55% at 5 years. The most common cause of early mortality was graft failure. Late mortality was most commonly secondary to bronchiolitis obliterans (57%), infection (21%), and posttransplant malignancies (18%).[82]

REFERENCES

1. Aboyoun CL, Tamm M, Chhajed PN, et al: Diagnostic value of follow-up transbronchial lung biopsy after lung rejection. Am J Respir Crit Care Med 164:460, 2001.
2. Andreu G, Achkar A, Couetil JP, et al: Extracorporeal photochemotherapy treatment for acute lung rejection episode. J Heart Lung Transplant 14:793, 1995.
3. Anyanwu AC, McGuire A, Rogers CA, et al: An economic evaluation of lung transplantation. J Thorac Cardiovasc Surg 123:411, 2002.
4. Aris RM, Maia DM, Neuriner IP, et al: Post-transplantation lymphoproliferative disorder in the Epstein-Barr virus-naive lung transplant recipient. Am J Respir Crit Care Med 154:1712, 1996.
5. Aris RM, Neuringer IP, Weiner MA, et al: Severe osteoporosis before and after lung transplantation. Chest 109:1176, 1996.
6. Aris RM, Routh JC, LiPuma JJ, et al: Lung transplantation for cystic fibrosis patients with Burkholderia cepacia complex. Survival linked to genomovar type. Am J Respir Crit Care Med 164:2102, 2001.
7. Armitage JM, Kormos RL, Stuart RS, et al: Posttransplant lymphoproliferative disease in thoracic organ transplant patients: Ten years of cyclosporine-based immunosuppression. J Heart Lung Transplant 10:877, 1991.
8. Artemiou O, Birsan T, Taghavi S, et al: Bilateral lobar transplantation with the split lung technique. J Thorac Cardiovasc Surg 118:369, 1999.
9. Barbers RG: Cystic fibrosis: Bilateral living lobar versus cadaveric lung transplantation. Am J Med Sci 315:155, 1998.
10. Barlow CW, Moon MR, Green GR, et al: Rabbit antithymocyte globulin versus OKT3 induction therapy after heart-lung and lung transplantation: Effect on survival, rejection, infection, and obliterative bronchiolitis. Transplant Int 14:234, 2001.
11. Bassiri AG, Girgis RE, Theodore S: Actinomyces odontolyticus thoracopulmonary infections. Two cases in lung and heart-lung transplant recipients and review of the literature. Am J Respir Crit Care Med 152:374, 1995.
12. Battafarano RJ, Anderson RC, Meyers BF, et al: Perioperative complications after living donor lobectomy. J Thorac Cardiovasc Surg 120:909, 2000.
13. Baz MA, Layish DT, Govert JA, et al: Diagnostic yield of bronchoscopies after isolated lung transplantation. Chest 110:84, 1996.
14. Bhabra MS, Hopkinson DN, Shaw TE, et al: Controlled reperfusion protects lung grafts during a transient early increase in permeability. Ann Thorac Surg 65:187, 1998.
15. Boehler A, Vogt P, Zollinger A, et al: Prospective study of the value of transbronchial lung biopsy after lung transplantation. Eur Respir J 9:658, 1996.

16. Boucek MM, Edwards LB, Keck BM, et al: The registry of the international society for heart and lung transplantation: Fifth official pediatric report—2001 to 2002. J Heart Lung Transplant 21:827, 2002.

17. Brock MV, Borja MC, Ferber L, et al: Induction therapy in lung transplantation: A prospective, controlled clinical trial comparing OKT3, anti-thymocyte globulin, and daclizumab. J Heart Lung Transplant 20:1282, 2001.

18. Brown RP, Esmore DS, Lawson C: Improved sternal fixation in the transsternal bilateral thoracotomy incision. J Thorac Cardiovasc Surg 112:137, 1996.

19. Burke CM, Theodore J, Dawkins KD, et al: Post-transplant obliterative bronchiolitis and other late lung sequelae in human heart lung transplantation. Chest 86:824, 1984.

20. Cahill BC, Hibbs JR, Savik K, et al: Aspergillus airway colonization and invasive disease after lung transplantation. Chest 112:1160, 1997.

21. Cahill BC, O'Rourke MK, Strasburg KA, et al: Methotrexate for lung transplant recipients with steroid-resistant acute rejection. J Heart Lung Transplant 15:1130, 1996.

22. Chamberlain D, Maurer J, Chaparro C, et al: Evaluation of transbronchial lung biopsy specimens in the diagnosis of bronchiolitis obliterans after lung transplantation. J Heart Lung Transplant 13:963, 1994.

23. Chaparro C, Kesten S: Infections in lung transplant recipients. Clin Chest Med 18:339, 1997.

24. Chaparro C, Maurer J, Gutierrez C, et al: Infection with Burkholderia cepacia in cystic fibrosis: Outcome following lung transplantation. Am J Respir Crit Care Med 163:43, 2001.

25. Chaparro C, Maurer JR, Chamberlain DW, et al: Role of open lung biopsy for diagnosis in lung transplant recipients: Ten-year experience. Ann Thorac Surg 59:928, 1995.

26. Charman SC, Sharples LD, McNeil KD, et al: Assessment of survival benefit after lung transplantation by patient diagnosis. J Heart Lung Transplant 21:226, 2002.

27. Chen C, Gallagher RC, Ardery P, et al: Retrograde flush and cold storage for twenty-two to twent-five hours lung preservation with and without prostaglandin E1. J Heart Lung Transplant 16:658, 1997.

28. Chhajed PJ, Malouf MM, Tamm M, et al: Interventional bronchoscopy for the management of airway complications following lung transplantation. Chest 120:1894, 2001.

29. Chhajed PN, Malouf MA, Tamm M, et al: Interventional bronchoscopy for the management of airway complications following lung transplantation. Chest 120:1894, 2001.

30. Christie JD, Bavaria JE, Palevsky HI, et al: Primary graft failure following lung transplantation. Chest 114:51, 1998.

31. Clark SC, Sudarshan C, Khanna R, et al: Controlled reperfusion and pentoxifylline modulates reperfusion injury after single lung transplantation. J Thorac Cardiovasc Surg 115:1335, 1998.

32. Clark SC, Sudarshan CD, Dark JH: Controlled perfusion of the transplanted lung. Ann Thorac Surg 71:1755, 2001.

33. Cohen L, Littlefield C, Kelly P, et al: Predictors of quality of life and adjustment after lung transplantation. Chest 113:633, 1998.

34. Cohen RG, Barr ML, Schenkel FA, et al: Living-related donor lobectomy for bilateral lobar transplantation in patients with cystic fibrosis. Ann Thorac Surg 57:1423, 1994.

35. Cooper JD, Billingham M, Egan T: A working formulation for the standardization of nomenclature and for clinical staging of chronic dysfunction in lung allografts. J Heart Lung Transplant 12:713, 1993.

36. Corris PA, Glanville A, McNeil K, et al: One year analysis of an ongoing international randomized study of mycophenolate mofetil (MMF) versus azathioprine (AZA) in lung transplantation. J Heart Lung Transplant 20:149, 2001.

37. Couetil JA, Tolan MJ, Loulmet DF, et al: Pulmonary bipartitioning and lobar transplantation: A new approach to donor organ shortage. J Thorac Cardiovasc Surg 113:529, 1997.

38. Cummings J, Houck J, Lichtenfeld D: Positive effect of aggressive resuscitative efforts on cadaver lung procurement. J Transplant Coordi 5:103, 1995.

39. Dark JH, Patterson GA, Al-Jilaihawi AN, et al: Experimental en bloc double-lung transplantation. Ann Thorac Surg 42:394, 1986.

40. Date H, Lynch JP, Sundaresan S, et al: The impact of cytolytic therapy on bronchiolitis obliterans syndrome. J Heart Lung Transplant 17:869, 1998.

41. Date H, Triantafillou A, Trulock E, et al: Inhaled nitric oxide reduces human lung allograft dysfunction. J Thorac Cardiovasc Surg 111:913, 1996.

42. Date H, Trulock EP, Arcidi JM, et al: Improved airway healing after lung transplantation: An analysis of 348 bronchial anastomoses. J Thorac Cardiovasc Surg 110:1424, 1995.

43. Davis RD, Lau CL, Eubanks S, et al: Improved lung allograft function following fundoplication in lung transplant patients with GERD. J Thorac Cardiovasc Surg 125:533, 2003.

44. De Hoyos A, Chamberlain D, Schvartzman R, et al: Prospective assessment of a standardized pathologic grading system for acute rejection in lung transplantation. Chest 103:1813, 1993.

45. De Meester J, Smits JM, Persijn GG, et al: Listing for lung transplantation: Life expectancy and transplant effect, stratified by type of end-stage lung disease, the Eurotransplant experience. J Heart Lung Transplant 20:518, 2001.

46. Demikhov VP: Experimental Transplanation of Vital Organs (authorized translation from the Russian by Basil Haigh). New York: Consultants Bureau Enterprises, Inc., 1962.

47. Demikhov VP: Transplantation of Vital Organs in Experiments. Moscow: Medgiz, 1960.

48. Derom F, Barbier F, Ringoir S, et al: Ten-month survival after lung homotransplantation in man. J Thorac Cardiovasc Surg 61:835, 1971.

49. Diamond DA, Michalski JM, Lynch JP, et al: Efficacy of total lymphoid irradiation for chronic allograft rejection following bilateral lung transplantation. Int J Radiat Oncol 41:795, 1998.

50. Dodge JA, Morison S, Lewis PA, et al: Cystic Fibrosis in the United Kingdom, 1968–1988: Incidence, population, and survival. Paediatr Perinatal Epidemiol 7:157, 1993.

51. Dusmet M, Maurer J, Winston T, et al: Methotrexate can halt the progression of bronchiolitis obliterans syndrome in lung transplant recipients. J Heart Lung Transplant 15:948, 1996.

52. Erard AC, Monnier P, Spiliopoulos A, et al: Mitomycin C for control of recurrent bronchial stenosis: A case report. Chest 120:2103, 2001.

53. Estenne M, Maurer JR, Boehler A, et al: Bronchiolitis obliterans syndrome 2001: An update of the diagnostic criteria. J Heart Lung Transplant 21:297, 2002.

54. Ettinger NA, Bailey TC, Trulock EP, et al: Cytomegalovirus infection and pneumonitis. Impact after isolation lung transplantation. Am Rev Respir Dis 147:1017, 1993.

55. Fischer S, Matte-Martyn A, De Perrot M, et al: Low-potassium dextran preservation solution improves lung function after human lung transplantation. J Thorac Cardiovas Surg 121:594, 2001.

56. Fiser SM, Cope JT, Kron IL, et al: Aerosolized prostacyclin (epoprostenol) as an alternative to inhaled nitric oxide for patients with reperfusion injury after lung transplantation. J Thorac Cardiovasc Surg 121:981, 2001. [erratum appears in J Thorac Cardiovasc Surg 121(6):1136, 2001].

57. Fiser SM, Kron IL, Long SM, et al: Controlled perfusion decreases reperfusion injury after high-flow reperfusion. J Heart Lung Transplant 21:687, 2002.

228

58. Follette DM, Rudich SM, Babcock WD: Improved oxygenation and increased lung donor recovery with high-dose steroid administration after brain death. J Heart Lung Transplant 17:423, 1998.

59. Fremes SE, Patterson GA, Williams WG, et al: Single lung transplantation and closure of patent ductus arteriosus for Eisenmenger's syndrome. J Thorac Cardiovasc Surg 100:1, 1990.

60. Fujino S, Nagahiro I, Triantafillou AN, et al: Inhaled nitric oxide at the time of harvest improves early lung allograft function. Ann Thorac Surg 63:1383, 1997.

61. Gaca JG, Lesher A, Aksoy O, et al: Disseminated intravascular coagulation in association with pig-to-primate pulmonary xenotransplantation. Transplantation 73:1717, 2002.

62. Garrity ER Jr, Villanueva J, Bhorade SM, et al: Low rate of acute lung allograft rejection after the use of daclizumab, an interleukin 2 receptor antibody. Transplantation 71:773, 2001.

63. Gray-Donald K, Gibbons L, Shapiro SH, et al: Nutritional status and mortality in chronic obstructive pulmonary disease. Am J Respir Crit Care Med 153:961, 1996.

64. Griffith BP, Hardesty RL, Armitage JM, et al: Acute rejection of lung allografts with various immunosuppressive protocols. Ann Thorac Surg 54:846, 1992.

65. Griffith BP, Hardesty RL, Armitage JM, et al: A decade of lung transplantation. Ann Surg 218:310, 1993.

66. Gross CR, Raghu G: The cost of lung transplantation and the quality of life post-transplant. Clin Chest Med 18:391, 1997.

67. Guilinger RA, Paradis IL, Dauber JH, et al: The importance of bronchoscopy with transbronchial biopsy and bronchoalveolar lavage in the management of lung transplant recipients. Am J Respir Crit Care Med 152:2037, 1995.

68. Gutierrez CA, Chaparro C, Drajden M, et al: Cytomegalovirus viremia in lung transplant recipients receiving ganciclovir and immune globulin. Chest 113:924, 1998.

69. Hachem R, Patterson G-A, Trulock EP: Abdominal-pelvic lymphoproliferative disease after lung transplantation. J Heart Lung Transplant 22:S194, 2003.

70. Hadjiliadis D, Sporn TA, Perfect JR, et al: Outcome of lung transplantation in patients with mycetomas. Chest 121:128, 2002.

71. Halldorsson A, Kronon M, Allen BS, et al: Controlled reperfusion after lung ischemia: Implications for improved function after lung transplantation. J Thorac Cardiovasc Surg 115:415, 1998.

72. Halldorsson A, Kronon M, Allen BS, et al: Controlled reperfusion prevents pulmonary injury after 24-hours of lung preservation. Ann Thorac Surg 66, 1998.

73. Halldorsson AO, Kronon MT, Allen BS, et al: Lowering reperfusion pressure reduces the injury after pulmonary ischemia. Ann Thorac Surg 69:198, 2000.

74. Hardy JD, Webb WR, Dalton ML, et al: Lung homotransplantation in man. JAMA 186:1065, 1963.

75. Hertz MI, Taylor DO, Trulock EP, et al: The registry of the International Society for Heart and Lung Transplantation: Nineteenth official report—2002. J Heart Lung Transplant 21:950, 2002.

76. Hoekstra HJ, Hawkins K, de Boer WJ, et al: Gastrointestinal complications in lung transplant survivors that require surgical intervention. Br J Surg 88:433, 2001.

77. Holt ND, Gould FK, Taylor CE, et al: Incidence and significance of noncytomegalovirus viral respiratory infection after adult lung transplantation. J Heart Lung Transplant 16:416, 1997.

78. Hong JC, Kahan BD: Sirolimus rescue therapy for refractory rejection in renal transplantation. Transplantation 71:1579, 2001.

79. Hopkins PM, Aboyoun CL, Chhajed PN, et al: Prospective analysis of 1,235 transbronchial lung biopsies in lung transplant recipients. J Heart Lung Transplant 21:1062, 2002.

80. Horning NR, Lynch JP, Sundaresan SR, et al: Tacrolimus therapy for persistent or recurrent acute rejection after lung transplantation. J Heart Lung Transplant 17:761, 1998.

81. Hosenpud JD, Bennett LE, Keck BM, et al: Effect of diagnosis on survival benefit of lung transplantation for end-stage lung disease. Lancet 351:24, 1998.

82. Huddleston CB, Bloch JB, Sweet SC, et al: Lung transplantation in children. Ann Surg 236:270, 2002.

83. Husain S, McCurry K, Dauber J, et al: Nocardia infection in lung transplant recipients. J Heart Lung Transplant 21:354, 2002.

84. Iacono AT, Keenan R, Duncan SR, et al: Aerosolized cyclosporine in lung recipients with refractory chronic rejection. Am J Respir Crit Care Med 153:1451, 1996.

85. Iacono AT, Smaldone GC, Keenan RJ, et al: Dose-related reversal of acute lung rejection by aerosolized cyclosporine. Am J Respir Crit Care Med 155:1690, 1997.

86. ISHLT, Cooper JD, Billingham M, et al: A Working formulation for the standardization of nomenclature and for clinical staging of chronic dysfunction in lung allografts. J Heart Lung Transplant 12:713, 1993.

87. Jackson CH, Sharples LD, McNeil K, et al: Acute and chronic onset of bronchiolitis obliterans syndrome (BOS): Are they different entities? J Heart Lung Transplant 21:658, 2002.

88. Kahan BD: Efficacy of sirolimus compared with azathioprine for reduction of acute renal allograft rejection: A randomised multicentre study. The Rapamune US Study Group. Lancet 356:194, 2000.

89. Kanj SS, Welty-Wolf K, Madden J, et al: Fungal infections in lung and heart-lung transplant recipients. Medicine 75:142, 1996.

90. Keenan RJ, Konishi H, Kawai A, et al: Clinical trial of tacrolimus versus cyclosporine in lung transplantation. Ann Thorac Surg 60:580, 1995.

91. Keshavjee S, Yamazaki F, Cardoso PF, et al: A method for safe twelve-hour pulmonary preservation. J Thorac Cardiovasc Surg 98:529, 1989.

92. Kesten S, Chamberlain D, Maurer J: Yield of surveillance transbronchial biopsies performed beyond two years after lung transplantation. J Heart Lung Transplant 15:384, 1996.

93. Kesten S, Chaparro C, Scavuzzo M, et al: Tacrolimus as rescue therapy for bronchiolitis obliterans syndrome. J Heart Lung Transplant 16:905, 1997.

94. Kesten S, Rajagopalan N, Maurer J: Cytolytic therapy for the treatment of bronchiolitis obliterans syndrome following lung transplantation. Transplantation 61:427, 1996.

95. Konstantinov IE: A mystery of Vladimir P. Demikhov: The 50th anniversary of the first intrathoracic transplantation. Ann Thorac Surg 65:1171, 1998.

96. Lau C, Patterson GA: Technical considerations in lung transplantation. Chest Clin North Am 13(3):463, 2003.

97. Lau CL, Guthrie TJ, Scavuzzo M, et al: Lobectomy to downsize donor lungs for use in small recipients. J Heart Lung Transplant 22:S116, 2003.

98. Lau CL, Palmer SM, Howell DN, et al: Laparoscopic antireflux surgery in the lung transplant population. Surg Endosc 16:1674, 2002.

99. Levine SM, Angel L, Anzueto A, et al: A low incidence of posttransplant lymphoproliferative disorder in 109 lung transplant recipients. Chest 116:1273, 1999.

100. Levine SM, Bryan CL: Bronchiolitis obliterans in lung transplant recipients. The "thorn in the side" of lung transplantation. Chest 107:894, 1995.

101. Levine SM, Peters JI, Anzueto A, et al: Aspergillus infection in single lung transplant recipients. Am Rev Respir Dis 147:A599, 1993.

102. Lick SD, Brown PS, Jr., Kurusz M, et al: Technique of controlled reperfusion of the transplanted lung in humans. Ann Thorac Surg 69:910, 2000.

103. Lima O, Cooper JD, Peters WJ, et al: Effects of methylpred-nisolone and azathioprine on bronchial healing following lung autotransplantation. J Thorac Cardiovasc Surg 82:211, 1981.

104. Lima O, Goldberg M, Peters WJ, et al: Bronchial omen-topexy in canine lung transplantation. J Thorac Cardiovasc Surg 83:418, 1982.

105. Limbos MM, Chan CK, Kesten S: Quality of life in female lung transplant candidates and recipients. Chest 112:1165, 1997.

106. Liou TG, Adler FR, C. Cahill B, et al: Survival effect of lung transplantation among patients with cystic fibrosis. JAMA 286:2683, 2001.

107. Lubetkin EI, Lipson DA, Palevsky HI, et al: GI complica-tions after orthotopic lung transplantation. AJG 91:2382, 1996.

108. Maccherini M, Keshavjee SH, Slutsky AS, et al: The effect of low-potassium-dextran versus Euro-Collins solution for preservation of isolated type II pneumocytes. Transplantation 52:621, 1991.

109. Mal N, Andreassian B, Pamela F, et al: Unilateral lung trans-plantation in end-stage pulmonary emphysema. Am Rev Respir Dis 140:797, 1989.

110. Malouf MA, Chhajed PN, Hopkins P, et al: Anti-viral pro-phylaxis reduces the incidence of lymphoproliferative disease in lung transplant recipients. J Heart Lung Transplant 21:547, 2002.

111. Matsuzaki Y, Waddell TK, Puskas JD, et al: Amelioration of post-ischemic lung reperfusion injury by PGE1. Am Rev Respir Dis 148:882, 1993.

112. Maurer JR, Frost AE, Estenne M, et al: International guide-lines for selection of lung transplant candidates. J Heart Lung Transplant 17:703, 1998.

113. McLaughlin VV, Genthner DE, Panella MM, et al: Reduction in pulmonary vascular resistance with long-term epoprostenol (prostacyclin) therapy in primary pulmonary hypertension. N Engl J Med 338:273, 1998.

114. Meyer DM, Bennett LE, Novick RJ, et al: Single vs bilateral, sequential lung transplantation for end-stage emphysema: Influence of recipient age on survival and secondary end-points. J Heart Lung Transplant. 20:935, 2001.

115. Meyers BF, Lynch J, Trulock EP, et al: Lung transplantation: A decade of experience. Ann Surg 230:362, 1999.

116. Meyers BF, Lynch JP, Trulock EP, et al: Single versus bilat-eral lung transplantation for idiopathic pulmonary fibrosis: A ten-year institutional experience. J Thorac Cardiovasc Surg 120:99, 2000.

117. Meyers BF, Patterson GA: Bilateral lung transplantation. Oper Tech Thorac Cardiovasc Surg 4:162, 1999.

118. Meyers BF, Patterson GA: Lung transplantation versus lung volume reduction as surgical therapy for emphysema. World J Surg 25:238, 2001.

119. Meyers BF, Patterson GA: Technical aspects of adult lung transplantation. Sem Thorac Cardiovasc Surg 10:213, 1998.

120. Meyers BF, Sundt TM 3rd, Henry S, et al: Selective use of extracorporeal membrane oxygenation is warranted after lung transplantation. J Thorac Cardiovasc Surg. 120:20, 2000.

121. Meyers BF, Yusen RD, Guthrie TJ, et al: Outcome of bilat-eral lung volume reduction in patients with emphysema potentially eligible for lung transplantation. J Thorac Cardiovasc Surg 122:10, 2001.

122. Montone KT, Litzky LA, Wurster A, et al: Analysis of Epstein-Barr virus associated posttransplantation lympho-proliferative disorder after lung transplantation. Surgery 119:544, 1996.

123. Nelems W: Human lung transplantation. Chest 78:569, 1980.

124. Novick RJ, Stitt LW, Al-Kattan K, et al: Pulmonary retrans-plantation: Predictors of graft function and survival in 230 patients. Ann Thorac Surg 65:227, 1998.

125. Nunley DR, Gal AA, Vega JD, et al: Saprophytic fungal infections and complications involving the bronchial anasto-mosis following human lung transplantation. Chest 122:1185, 2002.

126. O'Hagan AR, Stillwell PC, Arroliga A, et al: Photopheresis in the treatment of refractory bronchiolitis obliterans compli-cating lung transplantation. Chest 115:1459, 1999.

127. Palmer SM, Baz MA, Sanders L, et al: Results of a random-ized, prospective, multicenter trial of mycophenolate mofetil versus azathioprine in the prevention of acute lung allograft rejection. Transplantation 71:1772, 2001.

128. Palmer SM, Jr., Henshaw NG, Howell DN, et al: Community respiratory viral infection in adult lung transplant recipients. Chest 113:944, 1998.

129. Palmer SM, Miralles AP, Howell DN, et al: Gastroesophageal reflux as a reversible cause of allograft dysfunction after lung transplantation. Chest 118:1214, 2000.

130. Palmer SM, Miralles AP, Lawrence CM, et al: Rabbit antithy-mocyte globulin decreases acute rejection after lung trans-plantation: Results of a randomized, prospective study. Chest 116:127, 1999.

131. Paranjothi S, Yusen RD, Kraus MD, et al: Lymphopro-liferative disease after lung transplantation: Comparison of presentation and outcome of early and late cases. J Heart Lung Transplant 20:1054, 2001.

132. Paris W, Diercks M, Bright J, et al: Return to work after lung transplantation. Journal of Heart and Lung Transplantation 17:430, 1998.

133. Pasque MK, Cooper JD, Kaiser LR, et al: An improved tech-nique for bilateral lung transplantation: Rationale and initial clinical experience. Ann Thorac Surg 49:785, 1990.

134. Pasque MK, Trulock EP, Kaiser LR, et al: Single-lung trans-plantation for pulmonary hypertension. Three month hemo-dynamic follow-up. Circulation 84:2275, 1991.

135. Patterson G: Airway complications. Chest Surg Clin North Am 3:157, 1993.

136. Patterson GA, Cooper JD, Goldman B, et al: Technique of successful clinical double-lung transplantation. Ann Thorac Surg 45:626, 1988.

137. Pham SM, Rao AS, Zeevi A, et al: Effects of donor bone mar-row infusion in clinical lung transplantation. Ann Thorac Surg 69:345, 2000.

138. Pollard TR, Schwesinger WH, Sako EY, et al: Abdominal operations after lung transplantation. Arch Surg 12:714, 1997.

139. Raj R, Frost AE: Scedosporium apiospermum fungemia in a lung transplant recipient. Chest 121:1714, 2002.

140. Ramsey SD, Patrick DL, Lewis S, et al: Improvement in quality of life after lung transplantation: A preliminary study. J Heart Lung Transplant 14:870, 1995.

141. Reams BD, Davis RD, Curl J, et al: Treatment of refractory acute rejection in a lung transplant recipient with campath 1H. Transplantation 74:903, 2002.

142. Revell MP, Lewis ME, Llewellyn-Jones CG, et al: Conservation of small-airway function by tacrolimus/ cyclosporine conversion in the management of bronchiolitis obliterans following lung transplantation. J Heart Lung Transplant 19:1219, 2000.

143. Ross DJ, Lweis MI, Kramer M, et al: FK 506 'rescue' immunosuppression for obliterative bronchiolitis after lung transplantation. Chest 112:1175, 1997.

144. Sarahrudi K, Carretta A, Wisser W, et al: The value of switch-ing from cyclosporine to tacrolimus in the treatment of refractory acute rejection and obliterative bronchiolitis after lung transplantation. Transplant Int 15:24, 2002.

145. Schaar CG, Van Der Pijl JW, Van Hoek B, et al: Successful outcome with a "quintuple approach" of posttransplant lym-phoproliferative disorder. Transplantation 71:47, 2001.

230

146. Schafers HJ, Haydock DA, Cooper JD: The prevalence and management of bronchial anastomotic complications in lung transplantation. J Thorac Cardiovasc Surg 101:1044, 1991.

147. Sharples LD, McNeil K, Stewart S, et al: Risk factors for bronchiolitis obliterans: A systematic review of recent publications. J Heart Lung Transplant 21:271, 2002.

148. Sheenib H, Massard G, Reynaud M, et al: Efficacy of OKT3 therapy for acute rejection in isolated lung transplantation. J Heart Lung Transplant 13:514, 1994.

149. Shennib H, Massard G: Airway complications in lung transplantation. Ann Thorac Surg 57:506, 1994.

150. Shields TW, LoCicero J, Ponn RB, editors: General Thoracic Surgery, Vol 1: Philadelphia: Lippincott Williams & Wilkins, 2000.

151. Sibley RK: The role of transbronchial biopsies in the management of lung transplant recipients. J Heart Lung Transplant 12:308, 1993.

152. Slovis BS, Loyd JE, L.E. King J: Photopheresis for chronic rejection of lung allografts. N Engl J Med 332:962, 1995.

153. Snell GI, Esmore DS, Williams TJ: Cytolytic therapy for the bronchiolitis obliterans syndrome complicating lung transplantation. Chest 109:874, 1996.

154. Snell GI, Levvey BJ, Chin W, et al: Rescue therapy: A role for sirolimus in lung and heart transplant recipients. Transplantation Proceedings 33:1084, 2001.

155. Snydman DR: Infections in solid organ transplantation. Transplant Infect Dis 1:21, 1999.

156. Sollinger HW, Group USRTMMS: Mycophenolate mofetil for the prevention of acute rejection in primary cadaveric renal allograft recipients. Transplantation 60:225, 1995.

157. Speich R, Boehler A, Russi EW, et al: A case report of a double-blind, randomized trial of inhaled steroids in a patient with lung transplant bronchiolitis obliterans. Respiration 64:375, 1997.

158. Speich R, Boehler A, Thurnheer R, et al: Salvage therapy with mycophenolate mofetil for lung transplantation bronchiolitis obliterans: Importance of dosage. Transplantation 64:533, 1997.

159. Starnes VA, Barr ML, Schenkel FA, et al: Experience with living-donor lobar transplantation for indications other than cystic fibrosis. Thorac Cardiovasc Surg 114:917, 1997.

160. Starnes VA, Lewiston NJ, Luikart H, et al: Current trends in lung transplantation: Lobar transplantation and expanded uses of single lungs. J Thorac Cardiovasc Surg 104:1060, 1992.

161. Starnes VA, Woo MS, MacLaughlin EF, et al: Comparison of outcomes between living donor and cadaveric lung transplantation in children. Ann Thorac Surg. 68:2279, 1999.

162. Starzl TE, Demetris AJ, M. T, et al: Systemic chimerism in human female recipients of male livers. Lancet 340:876, 1992.

163. Steen S, Sjoberg T, Pierre L, et al: Transplantation of lungs from a non-heart-beating donor. Lancet 357:825, 2001.

164. Straznicka M, Follette DM, Eisner MD, et al: Aggressive management of lung donors classified as unacceptable: Excellent recipient survival one year after transplantation. J Thorac Cardiovasc Surg 124:250, 2002.

165. Sundaresan S, Semenkovich J, Ochoa L, et al: Successful outcome of lung transplantation is not compromised by the use of marginal donor lungs. J Thorac Cardiovasc Surg 109:1075, 1995.

166. Sundaresan S, Shiraishi Y, Trulock EP, et al: Single or bilateral lung transplantation for emphysema? J Thorac Cardiovasc Surg 112:1485, 1996.

167. Sundaresan S, Trachiotis GD, Aoe M, et al: Donor lung procurement: Assessment and operative technique. Ann Thorac Surg 56:1409, 1993.

168. Susanto I, Peters JI, Levine SM, et al: Use of balloon-expandable metallic stents in the management of bronchial stenosis and bronchomalacia after lung transplantation. Chest 114:1330, 1998.

169. Swedlow SH: Classification of the posttransplant lymphoproliferative disorders: From the past to the present. Semin Diag Pathol 14:2, 1997.

170. Swinnen LJ, Costanzo-Nordin MR, Fisher SG, et al: Increased incidence of lymphoproliferative disorder after immunosuppression with the monoclonal antibody OKT3 in cardiac transplant recipients. N Engl J Med 323:1723, 1990.

171. TenVergert EM, Essink-Bot M-L, Geertsma A, et al: The effect of lung transplantation on health-related quality of life. Chest 113:358, 1998.

172. Toronto Lung Transplantation Group: Unilateral lung transplantation for pulmonary fibrosis. N Engl J Med 314:1140, 1986.

173. Treede H, Klepetko W, Reichenspurner H, et al: Tacrolimus versus cyclosporine after lung transplantation: A prospective, open, randomized two-center trial comparing two different immunosuppressive protocols. J Heart Lung Transplant 20:511, 2001.

174. Trulock EP: Lung transplantation. Am J Respir Crit Care Med 155:789, 1997.

175. Trulock EP: Management of lung transplant rejection. Chest 13:1566, 1993.

176. Trulock EP: Recipient selection. Chest Surg Clin North Am 3:1, 1993.

177. Trulock EP, Ettinger NA, Brunt EM, et al: The role of transbronchial lung biopsy in the treatment of lung transplant recipients: An analysis of 200 consecutive procedures. Chest 102:1049, 1992.

178. UNOS: UNOS policy 3.7.5.1. Allocation of thoracic organs, waiting time accrual for lung candidates with idiopathic pulmonary fibrosis (IPF). Richmond, VA: UNOS, 1997.

179. Valentine VG, Robbins RC, Wehner JH, et al: Total lymphoid irradiation for refractory acute rejection in heart-lung and lung allografts. Chest 109:1184, 1996.

180. Valentine VG, Taylor DE, Dhillon GS, et al: Success of lung transplantation without surveillance bronchoscopy. J Heart Lung Transplant 21:319, 2002.

181. Venuta F, Rendina EA, Bufi M, et al: Preimplantation retrograde pneumoplegia in clinical lung transplantation. J Thorac Cardiovasc Surg 118:107, 1999.

182. Verleden GM, Buyse B, Delcroix M, et al: Cyclophosphamide rescue therapy for chronic rejection after lung transplantation. J Heart Lung Transplant 18:1139, 1999.

183. Verschuuren EA, Stevens SJ, van Imhoff GW, et al: Treatment of posttransplant lymphoproliferative disease with rituximab: The remission, the relapse, and the complication. Transplantation 73:100, 2002.

184. Vilchez R, McCurry K, Dauber J, et al: Influenza and parainfluenza respiratory viral infection requiring admission in adult lung transplant recipients. Transplantation 73:1075, 2002.

185. Villanueva J, Bhorade SM, Robinson JA, et al: Extracorporeal photopheresis for the treatment of lung allograft rejection. Ann Transplant 5:44, 2000.

186. Vitulo P, Oggionni T, Cascina A, et al: Efficacy of tacrolimus rescue therapy in refractory acute rejection after lung transplantation. J Heart Lung Transplant 21:435, 2002.

187. Waddell TK, Bennett L, Kennedy R, et al: Heart-lung or lung transplantation for Eisenmenger syndrome. J Heart Lung Transplant 21:731, 2002.

188. Walker RC, Marshall WF, J.G. S, et al: Pretransplantation assessment of the risk of lymphoproliferative disorder. Clin Infect Dis 20:1346, 1995.

189. Weill D, Keshavjee S: Lung transplantation for emphysema: Two lungs or one. J Heart Lung Transplant 20:739, 2001.

190. Whyte RI, Rossi SJ, Mulligan MS, et al: Mycophenolate mofetil for obliterative bronchiolitis syndrome after lung transplantation. Ann Thorac Surg 64:945, 1997.

191. Wigle DA, Chaparro C, Humar A, et al: Epstein-Barr virus serology and posttransplant lymphoproliferative disease in lung transplantation. Transplantation 72:1783, 2001.

192. Wildevuur CRH, Benfield JR: A review of 23 human lung transplantations by 20 surgeons. Ann Thorac Surg 9:489, 1970.

193. Williams JW, Mital D, Chong A, et al: Experiences with leflunomide in solid organ transplantation. Transplantation 73:358, 2002.

194. Wood BL, Sabath D, Broudy VC, et al: The recipient origin of posttransplant lymphoproliferative disorders in pulmonary transplant patients. Cancer 78:2223, 1996.

195. Yamashita M, Schmid RA, Ando K, et al: Nitroprusside ameliorates lung allograft reperfusion injury. Ann Thorac Surg 62:791, 1996.

196. Yousem SA: Significance of clinically silent untreated mild acute cellular rejection in lung allograft recipients. Hum Pathol 27:269, 1996.

197. Yousem SA, Berry GJ, Brunt EM, et al: A working formulation for the standardization of nomenclature in the diagnosis of heart and lung rejection: Lung rejection study group. J Heart Lung Transplant 9:593, 1990.

198. Yousem SA, Berry GJ, Cagle PT, et al: Revision of the 1990 working formulation for the classification of pulmonary allograft rejection: Lung rejection study group. J Heart Lung Transplant 15:1, 1996.

199. Zamora MR: Controversies in lung transplantation: Management of cytomegalovirus infections. J Heart Lung Transplant 21:841, 2002.

Lung Cancer

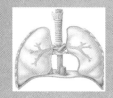

Screening for Lung Cancer

Robert J. Korst, Jeffrey L. Port, and Nasser Altorki

CHAPTER 15

INTRODUCTION

Lung cancer is the most common cause of cancer mortality in the United States, resulting in more deaths than breast, prostate, and colon cancer combined.[14] Although these latter three tumor types are associated with effective screening tests to detect early disease, no such examination exists for patients at risk for lung cancer. The current recommendations from the National Cancer Institute (NCI) as well as the American Cancer Society (ACS) are that no attempt at screening for lung cancer should be performed for patients thought to be at risk for this disease.[1,29,36] According to the ACS, "any test for the early detection of lung cancer" is not recommended, and "People with signs or symptoms of lung cancer should consult their physicians."[1] Given the high rates of lung cancer mortality (especially when signs or symptoms become apparent), combined with the lack of an effective screening tool, screening for lung cancer is the subject of active investigation, both at the clinical and laboratory levels.

The "ideal" screening tool should possess adequate sensitivity for detecting the disease in question, while simultaneously maintaining specificity, in order to reduce the number of false positive results. In addition, no harm should come to the patient as a result of screening. With regard to sensitivity, the "ideal" screening test should reduce mortality caused by the screened disease (disease-specific mortality). Conversely, the false positive rate should be as low as possible to ensure that patients without the disease do not undergo unnecessary testing, which may be associated with added morbidity. Finally, the "ideal" screening test should be painless, and not sequester an unreasonable amount of resources.

With this as a background, the goals of this chapter are to acquaint the reader with (1) the existing published data regarding lung cancer screening, (2) the nature of current clinical investigative efforts for the detection of early disease, and (3) the focus of studies involving "novel" screening techniques for this deadly disease.

HISTORY OF SCREENING FOR LUNG CANCER

Interest in screening high-risk patients for lung cancer was sparked when the association between cigarette smoking and lung cancer was first appreciated in the 1950s.[7] Plain chest radiograph (CXR) was the first modality used in a mass screening trial to detect lung cancer. The first mass screening project was conducted in London from 1960 to 1964, and although not a randomized trial, 55,034 men were assigned to undergo either CXR every 6 months for 3 years (the screened group) or a single CXR at the beginning of the study, followed by a repeat CXR at the end of the 3-year period (the "unscreened" group).[4] At the end of the 3-year period, more lung cancer was detected as a result of the screening protocol in the screened group compared to the "unscreened" group (132 versus 96 cases). In addition, resectability was enhanced in the screened group. Despite these findings, lung cancer-specific mortality was not different between the two groups, with 62 patients dying of lung cancer in the screened group compared to 59 patients in the "unscreened" group.[4]

In the 1970s, the National Cancer Institute funded three randomized trials that focused on the use of both CXR and sputum cytology to rigorously evaluate the value of screening for lung cancer.[12,27,44] At the time, refinements in the technology used for the cytological assessment of expectorated sputum encouraged the designers of two of these trials (the Johns Hopkins Lung Project and Memorial Sloan-Kettering Cancer Center [MSKCC] trial) to focus primarily on the effect of the addition of sputum cytology to interval CXRs (Table 15-1). In the MSKCC study, patients were randomized to either annual CXR alone or annual CXR plus the addition of sputum cytological assessment

Table 15-1

Study Design and Results of Two Randomized Controlled Trials Evaluating the Role of Sputum Cytological Examination for Lung Cancer Screening

Study institution/location	MSKCC[27]	Johns Hopkins[44]
Years of accrual	1974–1982	1973–1982
Screened arm		
Sample size	4968	5226
Protocol	Annual CXR; sputum cytology every 4 months	Annual CXR; sputum cytology every 4 months
Number of cancers (baseline)	30	39
Number of cancers (repeat screen)	114	194
Lung cancer mortality[a]	2.7	3.4
Unscreened arm		
Sample size	5072	5161
Protocol	Annual CXR	Annual CXR
Number of cancers (baseline)	23	40
Number of cancers (repeat screen)	121	202
Lung cancer mortality[a]	2.7	3.8

[a]Per 1000 person-years.

every 4 months.[27] Exactly the same number of cancers were detected in both groups. Patients who had sputum cytology in addition to CXR, however, tended to have their tumors detected at an earlier date than those undergoing CXR alone. Despite this, no difference was detected in resectability rates or lung cancer-specific mortality. This screening protocol was also utilized in the Johns Hopkins Lung Project randomized trial, with similar results (Table 15-1). No difference in the number of lung cancers or lung cancer-specific mortality was detected between the two groups.[44]

The Mayo Lung Project was designed differently than the MSKCC and Johns Hopkins trials, and focused on the combined impact of CXR and sputum cytology in screening for lung cancer (Table 15-2). Considered by many to be the most definitive of the four randomized trials, patients were randomized to undergo CXR as well as sputum cytological assessment every 4 months for 6 years (the screened group), or given the recommendation to undergo both of these examinations annually (the "unscreened" group).[12] Of significance in this trial, more than 50% of patients in the "unscreened" group underwent CXR during the study period, while an additional 25% of patients in the screened group were not compliant with the protocol. After a median follow-up period of 3 years, more lung cancers were detected in the screened group compared to the "unscreened" group. In addition, the resectability rate in the screened group was significantly higher; however, no reduction in lung cancer-specific mortality was found for the screened patients.[12]

Similar to the Mayo Lung Project, in the late 1970s, a screening trial was conducted in Czechoslovakia that also focused on the combined effects of CXR and sputum cytological examination for lung cancer screening (Table 15-2). In this trial, patients in the screened group underwent CXR

and evaluation of sputum cytology every 6 months for 3 years, while those in the "unscreened" group had an initial CXR and sputum cytological examination, both of which were repeated at the end of the 3-year period.[21,22] After the initial screening period, both groups underwent annual CXR and sputum assessment for an additional 3 years. Once again, more lung cancer was diagnosed in the screened group compared to the "unscreened" group (39 versus 27 cases). Despite this, no difference was appreciated in lung cancer-specific mortality.[21,22]

The interpretation of these four randomized trials continues to be a source of controversy. Opponents of lung cancer screening cite that although three of the four randomized trials described above demonstrated that screening may indeed lead to more effective diagnosis of early lung cancer, none was able to demonstrate a reduction in lung cancer-specific mortality.[2,8] Overdiagnosis bias has been cited as the most likely reason for this seemingly paradoxical result.[2] Overdiagnosis implies that a significant number of cancers detected by screening are indolent and would not lead to clinical disease in these patients. Indeed, if all screen-detected lung cancers were to grow, spread, and become clinically apparent, it would be expected that the lung cancer incidence rates would be unaffected by screening—if followed long enough, all tumors would become symptomatic, and be detected at equal rates in both screened and unscreened patients. In contrast, if screening led to the diagnosis of lung cancers that were clinically indolent (e.g., overdiagnosis), these tumors would be diagnosed in the screened population, but not in the unscreened group, resulting in higher rates of detection but no reduction in mortality in the screened group (as seen in the Mayo Lung Project and Czechoslovakia trials).

Table 15–2

Study Design and Results of Two Randomized Controlled Trials Evaluating the Role of CXR Combined with Sputum Cytological Examination for Lung Cancer Screening

Study institution/location	Mayo[12]	Czechoslovakia[21,22]
Years of accrual	1971–1983	1976–1980
Screened arm		
Sample size	4618	3172
Protocol	CXR and sputum cytology every 4 months for 6 years	CXR and sputum cytology every 6 months for 3 years[a]
Number of cancers (baseline)	Data not available	Data not available
Number of cancers (repeat screen)	206	39
Lung cancer mortality[b]	3.2	3.6
Unscreened arm		
Sample size	4593	3174
Protocol	Advised for annual CXR and sputum cytology	CXR and sputum cytology initially and after 3 years[a]
Number of cancers (baseline)	Data not available	Data not available
Number of cancers (repeat screen)	160	27
Lung cancer mortality[b]	3.0	2.6

[a]Followed by annual CXR and sputum cytology for an additional 3 years.
[b]Per 1000 person-years.

Proponents of lung cancer screening criticize the randomized trials using several arguments. First, none of the four randomized trials incorporated a completely unscreened control group, making any positive effects of screening more difficult to detect. Second, two of the trials (the MSKCC and Johns Hopkins trials) evaluated only the effect of sputum cytological evaluation, since both the experimental and control groups had annual CXRs.[27,44] Standard cytological examination of expectorated sputum is currently not thought to be a sensitive means to screen for lung cancer. Further, the patients diagnosed with lung cancer in both arms of these two trials had earlier stage disease and higher resectability and survival rates compared with historical controls of sporadically diagnosed lung cancer patients, implying that annual CXR may be beneficial for lung cancer screening. Third, there was a significant amount of crossover in the Mayo Lung Project, where more than half of the "unscreened" patients had CXRs and 25% of the screened patients were not compliant with the protocol.[12] Fourth, the Mayo Lung Project was designed to detect a 50% reduction in mortality and was underpowered to detect more subtle differences in mortality (19% chance of detecting a 10% decrease in mortality).[11]

In addition to these criticisms, advocates of screening argue that the concept of lung cancer overdiagnosis is erroneous, based on the following indirect evidence.[40,50] First, lung cancer is a virulent disease, with nearly 90% of patients diagnosed with lung cancer dying of their disease, making the overdiagnosis hypothesis contrary to the known biological behavior of this disease process.[14] Second, although the undiagnosed autopsy prevalence of some cancers (e.g.,

prostate) may be very high, this has not been found to be the case for lung cancer.[26] Finally, data from the surgical literature, both prospective and retrospective, suggest that suboptimal treatment or no treatment of early stage lung cancer is associated with an inferior prognosis when compared to optimally treated patients.[41] Taken together, this information calls the assumption of overdiagnosis into question.

▶ CURRENT LUNG CANCER SCREENING EFFORTS

PLCO Screening Trial

The Prostate, Lung, Colorectal and Ovarian (PLCO) cancer trial is a complex, multicenter trial sponsored by the NCI with a target accrual of 148,000 subjects.[13] Men and women, ages 55–74, were randomized to undergo an annual CXR [for 3 years (smokers) or 2 years (nonsmokers)] or routine medical care (unscreened group). Participants will be followed for at least 13 years after randomization to assess health status and cause of death. Accrual to the main phase began in 1994, and was completed in 2001. The PLCO trial has an 89% power to detect a 10% reduction in lung cancer-specific mortality. The results have yet to be reported.

Low-Dose Computed Tomography

Computed tomography (CT) of the chest was introduced into routine clinical practice in the early 1980s and has been demonstrated to be more sensitive than CXR for the detection of pulmonary nodules.* Furthermore, the sensitivity of CT for the detection of small pulmonary nodules is not compromised even with significant reductions in the radiation dose, with low-dose, helical scans now being performed during a single breath-hold.[25] Given these advancements, a new era of lung cancer screening using low-dose CT has begun.

In the 1990s, lung cancer screening projects using low-dose CT were initiated in North America, Europe, and Asia (Table 15-3), with five groups publishing prevalence data (baseline screening)[6,15,37,39,43] and four groups publishing incidence data (repeated screening).[16,37,38,42] Screening CXRs were also performed in three of these studies, allowing comparison of the sensitivity of CXR to low-dose CT in detecting lung cancer.[15,37,39] Four studies accrued only subjects with a significant history of smoking, while one accrued patients regardless of smoking history. The end points assessed in these large trials included the number, size, and radiographic character (including calcification) of nodules detected, as well as the number and stage of cancers detected. Nodule detection was followed by an algorithm for further workup, which was unique to each trial, but was consistently based on the size, number, radiographic characteristics, and growth rate of detected nodules.

As shown in Table 15-3, consistent results were obtained across all five studies. First, a large percentage of subjects were found to have noncalcified pulmonary nodules on low-dose CT, ranging from 11–51%. Second, far fewer lesions were suspicious for malignancy, with cancer detected in only 0.4–2.7% of the total patients screened. This wide variability in the incidence of malignancy is largely attributed to the selection of the study population. Third, although the number of cancers detected during repeat (incidence) screening was significantly less than that detected during baseline (prevalence) screening, nodules detected on repeat screening were more likely to be malignant. Fourth, the majority of cancers detected in all studies were stage 1. Finally, in the three programs where CXR was also performed, low-dose CT was far more sensitive than CXR in detecting lung cancer.

Similar to the randomized, controlled screening trials from the 1970s, the interpretation of these studies is once again the subject of intense controversy. Advocates of low-dose CT screening point to the high proportion of early, resectable lung cancers detected by this modality with an associated low proportion of unnecessary biopsy procedures. Critics, however, correctly indicate that these trials did not address perhaps the most important question—whether lung cancer-specific mortality is reduced in patients screened with low-dose CT.[2] If overdiagnosis bias truly exists, many patients may potentially be harmed by therapeutic interventions dictated by clinically irrelevant tumors. In addition, concern has been raised regarding the cost and potential harm to the large number of patients who are found to have noncalcified nodules on low-dose CT that require either follow-up scans or more invasive procedures, only to have a benign lesion (false positives).[2]

In summary, low-dose CT is clearly a more sensitive modality than CXR in the detection of pulmonary nodules and early lung cancer. Future direction for low-dose CT as a screening tool for early lung cancer detection will involve the conduction of large-scale randomized trials enrolling high-risk subjects with lung cancer-specific mortality as the primary end point. These trials will need to address the cost and potential harm that may come to patients as a result of false positive scans. Such large-scale trials are either in the final stages of planning or beginning accrual in several European countries as well as the United States. In addition, three-dimensional morphological analysis of pulmonary nodules on CT is currently being investigated with the goal of accurately detecting changes that may predict malignancy.[34]

*References 6, 15, 16, 37–39, 42, 43.

Table 15–3

Results of Five Low-Dose CT Lung Cancer Screening Studies

Study institution/organization	Mayo	Shinshu	ELCAP	ALCA	Munster
Reference number	42, 43	38, 39	15, 16	37	6
Prevalence					
Number of subjects	1520	5483	1000	1611	817
Abnormal CT result	51%	35%	23%	11.5%	43%
Number of cancers on CXR	NA	1	7	5	NA
Number of cancers on CT	26	19	27	14	11
Stage 1 NSCLC[a]	79%	84%	85%	71%	64%
Incidence					
Number of subjects	1438	4781	1184	1180	NP
Number of cancers on CT	10	37	7	19	NP
Stage 1 NSCLC[a]	67%	86%	82%	79%	NP
Interval cancers[b]	2	NA	2	3	NP

NA, not assessed; NP, not published; NSCLC, non-small-cell lung cancer.

[a]Percent of total non-small-cell lung cancers detected.

[b]Cancers not detected by screening CT.

► NOVEL TECHNOLOGIES WITH POTENTIAL SCREENING APPLICATION

Sputum Evaluation

The examination of expectorated sputum using standard cytological techniques is generally regarded as insensitive in screening for lung cancer based on the results of the MSKCC and Johns Hopkins Lung Projects, which randomized subjects to either annual CXR alone or CXR plus sputum cytological evaluation every 4 months (Table 15-1).[27,44] Both trials demonstrated that the examination of expectorated sputum did not enhance the ability to detect lung cancer.

To improve the sensitivity of sputum analysis as a screening tool, more sophisticated assays using sputum cells are being investigated. In a retrospective analysis of archived sputum specimens containing moderately atypical cells from the Johns Hopkins Lung Project, 64% of specimens possessing positive immunostaining for the nuclear ribonucleoprotein, hnRNP A2/B1, were from patients who eventually developed lung cancer, whereas 88% with negative staining did not develop cancer.[46] Further prospective investigations in a population of Chinese tin miners as well as North American patients with a history of resected, stage 1 non-small-cell lung cancer have echoed the retrospective data, with the sensitivity and specificity of hnRNP A2/B1 immunostaining reported as 77 and 82%, respectively, for the detection of second primary lung cancer and 82 and 65% for the detection of new primary lung cancer.[45,47] Whether these data will be reproducible and applicable to lung cancer screening remains to be determined.

Other sputum-based investigational approaches to early detection of lung cancer and potentially screening include the use of the polymerase chain reaction (PCR) to detect mutations in expectorated bronchial epithelial cells and the detection of malignancy-associated changes. Although PCR is a very sensitive assay (detects one mutated cell in an excess of 100,000 normal cells), and mutations in genes including K-*ras* and p53 have indeed been detected in the sputum of patients with lung cancer using PCR,[24] at the present time the utility of this technique remains unclear because these mutations are also found in the sputum of smokers without cancer, and many different mutations can exist for a particular gene (e.g., p53).[17,49]

The presence of malignant cells is thought to induce changes in the chromatin pattern in neighboring, nontransformed cells. These subtle, subvisual changes in DNA are termed malignancy-associated changes (MACs), and can be quantified using computer-assisted imaging technology.[18,19,28] In a retrospective analysis using archived sputum specimens from the Mayo Lung Project, MACs were present in 74% of the specimens from patients who went on to develop cancer.[32] One advantage of this technology is that a positive result is not dependent on the presence of malignant cells in the sputum, which may serve to offset some of the inefficiencies of the sputum induction process. The clinical application of image cytometry is the subject of ongoing investigation, including its combined role with low-dose CT in detecting early lung cancer.

It has become increasingly evident that abnormal methylation of the promoter region of a variety of specific genes may be responsible for the inhibition of gene expression seen in multiple tumor types (e.g., tumor suppressor genes).[33] Such "epigenetic" changes have also been shown to occur in lung cancers and can be demonstrated in the sputum of lung cancer patients.[31,33,48,51] Specifically, a recent study has demonstrated aberrant methylation of the p16 as well as O^6-methylguanine DNA methyltransferase (MGMT) genes in 100% of squamous cell cancers and their corresponding sputum specimens.[31] However, similar to the detection of mutations (genetic changes), false positives were relatively common, with aberrant methylation being demonstrable in nearly one out of four long-term smokers without cancer,[31] implying that this methodology may be most useful in identifying high-risk patients, as opposed to definite cancer cases.

Regardless of the technology used, when evaluating sputum for the presence of malignant cells, the quality of the sputum specimen remains a cause of some of the insensitivity associated with these techniques. As an example, in the study evaluating hnRNP A2/B1 immunostaining for the detection of second primary lung cancer by the Lung Cancer Early Detection Working Group, approximately 25% of sputum samples were unsatisfactory for analysis.[45] As a result of this problem, recent investigations have also focused on the development of technology that will enhance the quality of these specimens. Potential advances include the high-frequency chest wall oscillation vest,[10] as well as the use of inhaled uridine 5′-triphosphate (UTP), a compound that stimulates salt and water transport and cilia beat frequency in airway epithelium.[20]

Molecular Detection of Circulating Tumor Cells

In addition to the analysis of sputum, molecular diagnostic techniques are beginning to be evaluated for the detection of circulating tumor cells in the bloodstream in patients with lung cancer. In this regard, the use of methylation-specific PCR has revolutionized the detection of circulating, epigenetic alterations (aberrant promoter methylation).[33] Numerous genes have now been found to be abnormally methylated in both small-cell and non-small-cell lung cancer specimens, including p16, DAP-K, GSTP1, MGMT, adenomatous polyposis coli (APC), and the retinoic acid receptor-β.[3,9,30,33] Significantly, identical aberrant methylation is often found in the serum of patients from whom these tumor specimens are obtained, but not in the serum of patients whose tumors had unmethylated DNA, or serum from normal subjects.

Other detectable alterations in the blood of patients with lung cancer (mainly small cell) include microsatellite alterations as well as levels of prepro-gastrin-releasing peptide mRNA, the latter being detected using reverse transcriptase PCR.[5,35] Whether these findings as well as changes in promoter methylation will play a role in screening patients for lung cancer remains to be determined.

Fluorescence Bronchoscopy

Conventional, white-light bronchoscopy has an overall sensitivity of only approximately 40% for the detection of preinvasive lung cancer (carcinoma *in situ*).[23] Fluorescence bronchoscopy relies on the difference in autofluorescence

238 spectra between normal and malignant airway epithelia. Using the He-Cad laser (442 nm), normal epithelium fluoresces green, while malignant tissue fluoresces brown/red. In a recent review of the published literature regarding the use of fluorescence bronchoscopy for the detection of preinvasive lesions, Lam and colleagues found that the addition of fluorescence bronchoscopy to conventional white-light bronchoscopy improved the detection rate from 40 to 80%.[23] Future work regarding fluorescence bronchoscopy will entail the design and evaluation of thinner bronchoscopes, since the major limitation of this modality is related to the size of the instrument.

▶ SUMMARY

Lung cancer continues to be a deadly disease, curable only in its early stages. Over the past five decades, attempts have been made to screen high-risk patients for lung cancer, with the goal of detecting tumors in these earlier, curable stages, consequently reducing disease-specific mortality. Four reports of randomized, controlled trials of lung cancer screening currently exist, none of which has shown a reduction in lung cancer-specific mortality in the screened groups. As a result, it is currently not recommended that physicians perform screening for this disease. The interpretation of these four trials, however, has been the subject of several criticisms, with many clinicians questioning this conclusion in favor of screening.

Current clinical investigation has focused on the role of low-dose CT in screening for lung cancer, with multiple studies demonstrating that this modality is more sensitive than CXR for detecting early lung cancer. Despite this enhanced sensitivity, high numbers of false positive scans have raised issues including cost effectiveness and overdiagnosis of indolent disease, leading many to challenge the advocates of this strategy. This ensuing controversy underscores the need for large, randomized controlled trials of low-dose CT in this capacity.

Finally, novel technologies are currently being developed in the laboratory that may possess utility in the detection of preclinical lung cancer. These include assays for molecular alterations in sputum and peripheral blood, as well as novel imaging techniques including fluorescence bronchoscopy and computer-assisted imaging of expectorated sputum cells. Whether any of these new technologies will play a role in the future of lung cancer screening remains to be determined.

REFERENCES

1. American Cancer Society: Report on the cancer-related health checkup: Cancer of the lung. CA Cancer J Clin 30:199–207, 1980.
2. Bach PB, Kelley MJ, Tate RC, et al: Screening for lung cancer: A review of the current literature. Chest 123(1 Suppl): 72S–82S, 2003.
3. Bearzatto A, Conte D, Frattini M, et al: p16(INK4A) hypermethylation detected by fluorescent methylation-specific PCR in plasmas from non-small cell lung cancer. Clin Cancer Res 8:3782–3787, 2002.
4. Brett GZ: The value of lung cancer detection by six-monthly chest radiographs. Thorax 23:414–420, 1968.
5. Chen XQ, Stroun M, Magnenat JL, et al: Microsatellite alterations in plasma DNA of small cell lung cancer patients. Nat Med 2:1033–1035, 1996.
6. Diederich S, Wormanns D, Semik M, et al: Screening for early lung cancer with low-dose spiral CT: Prevalence in 817 asymptomatic smokers. Radiology 222:773–781, 2002.
7. Doll R, Hill AB: Smoking and carcinoma of the lung: Preliminary report. Br Med J 2:739–748, 1950.
8. Eddy DM: Screening for lung cancer. Ann Intern Med 111:232–237, 1989.
9. Esteller M, Sanchez-Cespedes M, Rosell R, et al: Detection of aberrant promoter hypermethylation of tumor suppressor genes in serum DNA from non-small cell lung cancer patients. Cancer Res 59:67–70, 1999.
10. Fink JB, Mahlmeister MJ: High-frequency oscillation of the airway and chest wall. Respir Care 47:797–807, 2002.
11. Fontana RS, Sanderson DR, Woolner LB, et al: Screening for lung cancer. A critique of the Mayo Lung Project. Cancer 67(4 Suppl):1155–1164, 1991.
12. Fontana RS, Sanderson DR, Taylor WF, et al: Early lung cancer detection: Results of the initial (prevalence) radiologic and cytologic screening in the Mayo Clinic study. Am Rev Respir Dis 130:561–565, 1984.
13. Gohagan JK, Prorok PC, Hayes RB, et al: The Prostate, Lung, Colorectal and Ovarian (PLCO) Cancer Screening Trial of the National Cancer Institute: History, organization, and status. Control Clin Trials 21(6 Suppl):251S–272S, 2000.
14. Greenlee RT, Murray T, Wingo PA: Cancer statistics. CA 50: 7–33, 2000.
15. Henschke CI, McCauley DI, Yankelevitz DF, et al: Early Lung Cancer Action Project: Overall design and findings from baseline screening. Lancet 354:99–105, 1999.
16. Henschke CI, Naidich D, Yankelevitz DF, et al: Early Lung Cancer Action Project: Initial findings on repeat screening. Cancer 92:153–159, 2001.
17. Hollstein M, Rice K, Greenblatt MS, et al: Database of p53 gene somatic mutations in human tumors and cell lines. Nucleic Acids Res 22:3551–3555, 1994.
18. Hu YC, Sidransky D, Ahrendt SA: Molecular detection approaches for smoking associated tumors. Oncogene 21:7289–7297, 2002.
19. Ikeda N, MacAulay C, Lam S, et al: Malignancy associated changes in bronchial epithelial cells and clinical application as a biomarker. Lung Cancer 19:161–166, 1998.
20. Johnson FL, Donohue JF, Shaffer CL: Improved sputum expectoration following a single dose of INS316 in patients with chronic bronchitis. Chest 122:2021–2029, 2002.
21. Kubik AK, Parkin DM, Zatloukal P: Czech Study on Lung Cancer Screening: Post-trial follow-up of lung cancer deaths up to year 15 since enrollment. Cancer 89(11 Suppl): 2363–2368, 2000.
22. Kubik A, Polak J: Lung cancer detection. Results of a randomized prospective study in Czechoslovakia. Cancer 57:2427–2437, 1986.
23. Lam S, MacAulay C, leRiche JC, et al: Detection and localization of early lung cancer by fluorescence bronchoscopy. Cancer 89: 2468–2473, 2000.
24. Mao L, Hruban RH, Boyle JO, et al: Detection of oncogene mutations in sputum precedes diagnosis of lung cancer. Cancer Res 54:1634–1637, 1994.
25. Mayo JR, Hartman TE, Lee KS, et al: Minimal tube current required for good image quality with the least radiation dose. Am J Roentgenol 164:603–607, 1995.
26. McFarlane MJ, Feinstein AR, Wells CK: Clinical features of lung cancers discovered as a postmortem "surprise." Chest 90:520–523, 1986.
27. Melamed MR, Flehinger BJ, Zaman MB, et al: Screening for early lung cancer. Results of the Memorial Sloan-Kettering study in New York. Chest 86:44–53, 1984.

28. McWilliams A, MacAulay C, Gazdar AF, et al: Innovative molecular and imaging approaches for the detection of lung cancer and its precurser lesions. Oncogene 21:6949–6959, 2002.

29. National Cancer Institute web site, Screening for lung cancer (PDQ): http://www.nci.nih.gov/cancerinfo/pdq/screening/lung/HealthProfessional#Section_15.

30. Oshita F, Sekiyama A, Suzuki R, et al: Detection of occult tumor cells in peripheral blood from patients with small cell lung cancer by promoter methylation and silencing of the retinoic acid receptor-beta. Oncol Rep 10:105–108, 2003.

31. Palmisano WA, Divine KK, Saccomanno G, et al: Predicting lung cancer by detecting aberrant promoter methylation in sputum. Cancer Res 60:5954–5958, 2000.

32. Payne PW, Sebo TJ, Doudkine A, et al: Sputum screening by quantitative microscopy: A reexamination of a portion of the National Cancer Institute Cooperative Early Lung Cancer Study. Mayo Clin Proc 72:697–704, 1997.

33. Plass C: Cancer epigenomics. Hum Mol Genet 11:2479–2488, 2002.

34. Ravenel JG, McAdams HP, Remy-Jardin M, et al: Multidimensional imaging of the thorax: Practical applications. J Thorac Imaging 16:269–281, 2001.

35. Saito T, Kobayashi M, Harada R, et al: Sensitive detection of small cell lung carcinoma cells by reverse transcriptase-polymerase chain reaction for prepro-gastrin-releasing peptide mRNA. Cancer 97:2504–2511, 2003.

36. Smith RA, von Eschenbach AC, Wender R, et al: American Cancer Society guidelines for the early detection of cancer: Update of early detection guidelines for prostate, colorectal, and endometrial cancers. Also: update 2001—testing for early lung cancer detection. CA Cancer J Clin 51:38–75, 2001.

37. Sobue T, Moriyama N, Kaneko M, et al: Screening for lung cancer with low-dose helical computed tomography: Anti-lung Cancer Association Project. J Clin Oncol 20:911–920, 2002.

38. Sone S, Li F, Yang Z-G, et al: Results of three-year mass screening programme for lung cancer using mobile low-dose spiral computed tomography scanner. Br J Cancer 84:25–32, 2001.

39. Sone S, Takashima S, Li F, et al: Mass screening for lung cancer with mobile spiral computed tomography scanner. Lancet 351:1242–1245, 1998.

40. Strauss GM, Gleason RE, Sugarbaker DJ: Screening for lung cancer. Another look; a different view. Chest 111:754–768, 1997.

41. Sugarbaker DJ, Strauss GM: Extent of surgery and survival in early lung carcinoma: Implications for overdiagnosis in stage IA nonsmall cell lung carcinoma. Cancer 89(11 Suppl): 2432–2437, 2000.

42. Swensen SJ, Jett JR, Hartman TE, et al: Lung cancer screening with CT: Mayo Clinic experience. Radiology 226:756–761, 2003.

43. Swensen SJ, Jett JR, Sloan JA, et al: Screening for lung cancer with low-dose spiral computed tomography. Am J Respir Crit Care Med 165:508–513, 2002.

44. Tockman M: Survival and mortality from lung cancer in a screened population: The Johns Hopkins study. Chest 89:325s–326s, 1986.

45. Tockman MS, Erozan YS, Gupta P, et al: The early detection of second primary lung cancers by sputum immunostaining. LCEWDG Investigators. Lung Cancer Early Detection Group. Chest 106(6 Suppl):385S–390S, 1994.

46. Tockman MS, Gupta PK, Myers JD, et al: Sensitive and specific monoclonal antibody recognition of human lung cancer antigen on preserved sputum cells: A new approach to early lung cancer detection. J Clin Oncol 6:1685–1693, 1988.

47. Tockman MS, Mulshine JL, Piantadosi S, et al: Prospective detection of preclinical lung cancer: Results from two studies of heterogeneous nuclear ribonucleoprotein A2/B1 overexpression. Clin Cancer Res 3(12 Pt 1):2237–2246, 1997.

48. Wang YC, Lu YP, Tseng RC, et al: Inactivation of hMLH1 and hMSH2 by promoter methylation in primary non-small cell lung tumors and matched sputum samples. J Clin Invest 111:887–895, 2003.

49. Wistuba II, Lam S, Behrens C, et al: Molecular damage in the bronchial epithelium of current and former smokers. J Natl Cancer Inst 89:1366–1373, 1997.

50. Yankelevitz DF, Kostis WJ, Henschke CI, et al: Overdiagnosis in chest radiographic screening for lung carcinoma: Frequency. Cancer 97:1271–1275, 2003.

51. Zochbauer-Muller S, Minna JD, Gazdar AF: Aberrant DNA methylation in lung cancer: Biological and clinical implications. Oncologist 7:451–457, 2002.

Lung Cancer Workup and Staging

Bernard J. Park and Valerie W. Rusch

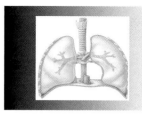

INTRODUCTION

It was estimated that by the year 2003 there would be approximately 171,900 new cases of lung cancer in the United States, with bronchogenic carcinoma remaining the leading cause of cancer-related deaths in both men and women.[25] Of these newly diagnosed cases, approximately 80% will be non–small cell lung cancer (NSCLC), and of these, 80% will present with disseminated or locally advanced disease. Unfortunately, only 20% will be potentially surgically curable patients with early stage disease where complete resection yields a 5-year survival rate approaching 70%.[48]

Thorough workup and staging of the lung cancer patient are critical for a number of reasons. First, determining a patient's clinical TNM (tumor, node, metastasis) stage allows appropriate therapeutic decisions to be made based on the specific stage of disease. This is particularly important in the setting of locally advanced disease where

multimodality approaches may be warranted, as well as in unresectable disease where unnecessary thoracotomy should be avoided. Second, accurate staging allows the clinician to give the patient valuable prognostic information. Third, staging allows evaluation of new therapeutic interventions and comparison of results of treatments between studies and institutions.

There are differences and controversies regarding the extent of workup and staging that should be performed, as well as the appropriate modalities employed. One modality that has had a significant impact on the evaluation and staging of lung cancer is positron emission tomography.

THE STAGING SYSTEM

Staging is a process through which the extent of lung cancer in a patient is measured by a combination of techniques that includes history, physical examination, radiographs, and invasive procedures. Prior to initiation of treatment, a clinical stage (cTNM) is generated. If surgical resection occurs, the operative findings and pathological features determine the final pathological stage (pTNM).

In 1974 the American Joint Committee for Cancer (AJCC) Staging developed a lung cancer staging system based on TNM descriptors.[41] Naruke and co-authors[45] devised the original lymph node mapping schema that placed nodes into stations based on clearly defined anatomical boundaries. Used to define the N nodal descriptors, it was modified for North America by the American Thoracic Society[1] and by Mountain and Dresler[43] into its current form (Figure 16-1). The AJCC system was used across North America through 1985, while the Union Internationale Contre de Cancer (UICC) has employed a separate, different system since 1978. Both systems functioned well for the most part, but each had several problems that became apparent when long-term survival statistics for the various subsets became available. In particular, it was noted that in stage I disease, patients in the subset with N1 disease had a much poorer prognosis; similarly, patients with stage III disease based on the local extent of tumor (T_3) seemed to have a better survival than stage III patients based on mediastinal nodal involvement (N_2 or N_3).

In 1986 the AJCC, UICC, and representatives from Japan and Germany proposed an International Staging System (ISS) for lung cancer that grouped patients with similar survival outcomes using anatomic and morphological criteria.[42] This system was originally applied to a database of over 3000 patients from the M.D. Anderson Cancer Center and the Lung Cancer Study Group (LCSG) and verified significant survival differences between stages. The

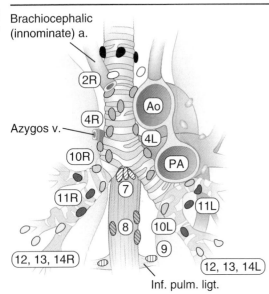

Brachiocephalic (innominate) a.

Azygos v.

Inf. pulm. ligt.

Ligamentum arteriosum

L. pulmonary a.

Phrenic n.

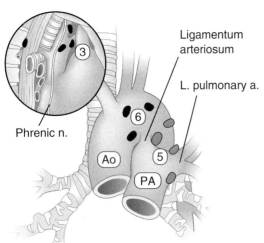

Superior Mediastinal Nodes

● 1 Highest mediastinal

○ 2 Upper paratracheal

● 3 Prevascular and retrotracheal

◐ 4 Lower paratracheal (including azygos nodes)

N2 = single digit, ipsilateral

N3 = single digit, contralateral or supraclavicular

Aortic Nodes

◐ 5 Subaortic (A-P window)

● 6 Para-aortic (ascending aorta or phrenic)

Inferior Mediastinal Nodes

⊘ 7 Subcarinal

⊘ 8 Paraesophageal (below carina)

⦀ 9 Pulmonary ligament

N₁ Nodes

◐ 10 Hilar

● 11 Interlobar

○ 12 Lobar

○ 13 Segmental

○ 14 Subsegmental

Figure 16–1 Regional lymph node stations for the staging of NSCLC.
(Adapted from Mountain CF, Dresler CM: Chest: Regional lymph node classification for lung cancer staging. Chest 111:1718–1723, 1997.)

applicability of the ISS was subsequently confirmed by studies from Naruke and colleagues[46] and Watanabe and co-workers.[71] The most recent version of the ISS, adopted in 1997, attempted to further minimize heterogeneity within stages and refine prognostic groupings after reviewing survival data on over 5000 patients[44] (Table 16-1). The significant changes included dividing stages I and II into A and B subsets, and incorporating $T_3 N_0 M_0$ tumors into stage IIB. In addition, the issue of satellite nodules was addressed. Those within the same lobe of the lung as the primary lesion indicate T_4 disease, whereas all other ipsilateral synchronous lesions are designated as M_1 (Table 16-2).

▶ DIAGNOSIS AND STAGING

Diagnosis and clinical staging take place concurrently, beginning with the initial history and physical examination. A variety of noninvasive and invasive tests are available to work up a patient suspected of having lung cancer, and often a single study serves the dual purpose of securing a diagnosis and further staging the patient. If a patient's treatment is nonsurgical or involves multimodality therapy, obtaining a tissue diagnosis prior to treatment is mandatory. If the patient's clinical stage appears most appropriately managed by surgical resection alone, tissue confirmation of malignancy can be secured either preoperatively or at the time of exploration, depending on the preference of the operating surgeon.

History and Physical Examination

Patients often present for evaluation with a number of studies already performed. However, the history and physical examination remain the most important initial steps in working up patients who are suspected of having lung cancer. This is the case for several reasons. A detailed history focusing on risk factors such as duration of cigarette smoking, exposure to asbestos and other industrial hazards, a prior history of lung cancer, and the presence of symptoms allows the clinician to assess the probability of the diagnosis of lung cancer. Bach and associates showed that the duration of tobacco smoking, more so than the amount of daily usage, increases an individual's risk of developing lung cancer.[3]

Table 16–1

TNM Classification and Revised International Staging of Lung Cancer[a]

Primary tumor (T)

T_x Tumor that cannot be assessed, or malignant cells in sputum or bronchial washings but not visualized by imaging or bronchoscopy

T_{is} Carcinoma *in situ*

T_0 No evidence of primary tumor

T_1 Tumor ≤3 cm, in a lobar bronchus or distal airways, and surrounded by lung or visceral pleura

T_2 Tumor that is either >3 cm, involving the main bronchus (≥2 cm of the carina), invading the visceral pleura, or with atelectasis or obstructive pneumonitis that extends to the hilar region but does not involve the entire lung

T_3 Tumor of any size that invades the chest wall (including superior sulcus tumors), diaphragm, mediastinal pleura, parietal pericardium; or tumor in the main bronchus <2 cm from, but not involving, the carina; or associated atelectasis or obstructive pneumonitis of the entire lung

T_4 Tumor of any size that invades the mediastinum, heart, great vessels, trachea, esophagus, vertebral body, carina; or presence of malignant/pericardial effusion; or satellite tumor nodule(s) within ipsilateral primary-tumor lobe of the lung

Lymph nodes (N)

N_x Regional lymph nodes cannot be assessed

N_0 No regional lymph node metastasis

N_1 Metastasis to ipsilateral peribronchial and/or ipsilateral hilar lymph nodes, and intrapulmonary nodes by direct extension

N_2 Metastasis to ipsilateral mediastinal and/or subcarinal lymph nodes

N_3 Metastasis to contralateral mediastinal, contralateral hilar, scalene, or supraclavicular lymph nodes

Distant metastasis (M)

M_x Distant metastasis cannot be assessed

M_0 No distant metastasis

M_1 Distant metastasis present

Stage	TNM subsets
0	$T_{is}\ N_0\ M_0$
IA	$T_1\ N_0\ M_0$
IB	$T_2\ N_0\ M_0$
IIA	$T_1\ N_1\ M_0$
IIB	$T_2\ N_1\ M_0$
	$T_3\ N_0\ M_0$
IIIA	$T_3\ N_1\ M_0$
	$T_{1-3}\ N_2\ M_0$
IIIB	$T_4\ N_{0-2}\ M_0$
	Any T $N_3\ M_0$
IV	Any T any N M_1

[a]Adapted from Mountain CF: Revisions in the international system for staging lung cancer. Chest 111:1710–1717, 1997.

Similarly, the risk associated with asbestos increases with the intensity and length of exposure, and together, tobacco use and asbestos exposure have a multiplicative effect. Certain symptoms, such as bone pain, hoarseness, weight loss, and neurological changes, can indicate the presence of metastatic disease and mandate further investigation.

A thorough physical examination is also critical for a number of reasons. It provides an estimate of a patient's overall health status, which has significant implications for the types of treatments available to that individual. Certain physical findings can support the suspicion of lung cancer, such as ptosis, miosis, and anhidrosis in Horner's syndrome, or the presence of clubbing. Furthermore, the physical examination can often demonstrate advanced disease even before any radiographic or other studies are performed. For

instance, palpation of the supraclavicular fossae can reveal lymph node metastases and auscultation of the lung fields can detect the presence of a malignant pleural effusion.

▶ NONINVASIVE MODALITIES

Chest Radiography

A standard posteroanterior and lateral chest radiograph remains the most common initial study in which a suspected lung cancer is identified. Lesions are detected on a chest X-ray performed for symptoms or for unrelated reasons, such as part of routine health assessment or preoperative clearance. Most lesions are not visible until they are at least

Table 16–2

Cumulative Survival by Stage[a]

Stage	TNM subset	5-year survival (%) clinical TNM	5-year survival (%) pathological TNM
IA	$T_1 N_0 M_0$	61	67
IB	$T_2 N_0 M_0$	38	57
IIA	$T_1 N_1 M_0$	34	55
IIB	$T_2 N_1 M_0$	24	39
	$T_3 N_0 M_0$	22	38
IIIA	$T_3 N_1 M_0$	9	25
	$T_{1-3} N_2 M_0$	13	23
IIIB	$T_4 N_{0-2} M_0$	7	
	Any T $N_3 M_0$	3	
IV	Any T	1	
	Any N M_1		

[a]Adapted from Mountain CF: Revisions in the international system for staging lung cancer. Chest 111:1710–1717, 1997.

7–10 mm in diameter,[58] at which time they contain roughly 1 billion cells, representing 30 doublings.[14] A high-quality chest radiograph can impart a large amount of information and should be reviewed carefully. It localizes the site of suspicious lesions (central or peripheral) and the local extent and effects of disease, showing areas of atelectasis, consolidation, or proximity to the pleural surface. The presence of a pleural effusion indicative of a T4 tumor can be seen, as well as elevation of the hemidiaphragm in the event of phrenic nerve involvement. Advanced disease may be identified in the case of rib destruction from bone metastases or synchronous lesions in the pulmonary parenchyma. Hilar and mediastinal lymph node metastasis is more difficult to identify, unless there is substantial enlargement.

Sputum Cytology

Cytological analysis of sputum for malignant cells is a simple diagnostic technique, although it is being employed less often than in the past because of the utilization of bronchoscopy and percutaneous needle biopsy. Samples obtained may be induced by saline nebulization or collected as a 3-day pool of sputum produced from spontaneous coughing in the morning. Induced specimens should be immediately fixed and stained. Pooled samples are pre-served in Saccomanno's solution (50% ethanol and 2% polyethylene glycol) or 70% ethanol until fixation and staining can be performed. Schreiber and McCrory[62] recently performed a meta-analysis of the published data on the diagnostic accuracy of sputum cytology in lung cancer. Most studies included a variety of indications for testing with only a few evaluating the sensitivity and specificity of sputum cytology in patients suspected of having lung cancer. Based on 16 published studies of at least 50 patients each, the overall sensitivity is 66% (range 42–97%) and the overall specificity is 99% (range of 68–100%). The false positive and false negative rates are 9 and 6%, respectively. When sputum cytology is utilized in patients suspected of having lung cancer on clinical grounds, the diagnostic yield is higher, with a sensitivity of 87% and specificity of 90%, as demonstrated by Jay and colleagues.[24]

A number of authors have shown that the sensitivity of sputum cytology for detecting lung cancer depends on the number of specimens collected per patient. Pilotti and co-workers,[54] Liang,[33] and Böcking[6] and co-workers confirmed that the optimal diagnostic sensitivity requires three specimens per patient. Several other factors influence the diagnostic sensitivity of sputum cytology including tumor location, size, and histological type. Schreiber and McCrory[62] reviewed 17 studies that compared the sensitivity of sputum cytology in central versus peripheral lung lesions. Meta-analysis showed that the overall sensitivity was 71% for central lesions and 49% for peripheral lesions. The likely explanation is that central tumors have a higher likelihood of shedding tumor cells into expectorated sputum because of their proximal bronchial location. Kato and associates[26] found that large tumors (greater than 3 cm), tumors associated with atelectasis or consolidation, and lower lobe location had higher diagnostic yields. In their study, the lowest sensitivity (20%) for sputum cytology occurred with peripheral tumors less than 3 cm in diameter. Histology of the tumor generally has less influence on the diagnostic accuracy of sputum cytology than the other factors mentioned. Squamous carcinomas are, however, more frequently diagnosed by sputum analysis than adenocarcinomas or large cell carcinomas. This is probably related to the fact that squamous tumors are more commonly central in location.

High-Resolution Computed Tomography (CT)

Once a suspicious lesion is detected on a chest X-ray (CXR) or low-dose CT, the standard next step in the evaluation is a high-resolution CT of the chest and upper abdomen. This will yield information about the features and local extent of a potential lung cancer, giving precise size measurements and demonstrating signs of malignancy within a given lesion (spiculation, ground glass opacification, lack of calcification). Evidence of invasion of contiguous structures, such as chest wall or mediastinal structures, can be assessed. This is especially critical when planning operative intervention, although unresectable involvement of surrounding structures may require surgical exploration for verification. CT also provides details about the remaining lung parenchyma and pleural spaces. Satellite or additional nodules, bullous or emphysematous changes, pleural thickening, masses, or effusion may be identified. Typically, the chest CT for a suspected lung cancer includes the upper abdomen, specifically the liver and adrenal glands. Although most asymptomatic, incidental lesions in the upper abdomen are benign (adrenal adenoma, hepatic cysts), unsuspected metastases are identified in a small percentage of patients.

In addition to providing information regarding the primary tumor and the possibility of distant metastases, the CT of the chest allows assessment of mediastinal lymph nodes. If not contraindicated, intravenous contrast is useful in distinguishing nodes from vascular structures. The most widely used criterion to define metastatic involvement is a short-axis diameter of ≥1 cm. Although it is the most effective radiographic method to measure lymph node enlargement, CT alone is inadequate to reliably predict metastatic nodal disease. In a prospective study of 143 patients with bronchogenic carcinoma in which CT findings were correlated with surgical pathological staging, McLoud and co-authors[35] reported the sensitivity of CT in predicting mediastinal nodal status was 64% with a specificity of 62%. Toloza and colleagues[67,68] reported results of a meta-analysis of 20 studies with 3438 evaluable patients that showed an overall sensitivity of 57% and specificity of 82%. Therefore staging of the mediastinum and subsequent therapeutic decisions should not be based solely on the results of the CT in most cases.

Positron Emission Tomography (PET)

Whole-body PET is a physiological imaging technique based on the detection of positrons emitted by low-atomic-weight isotopes (carbon, fluorine, oxygen, nitrogen).

[18F]Fluorodeoxyglucose (FDG) is a D-glucose analogue that is phosphorylated after cellular uptake and accumulates intracellularly, rather than being metabolized. Because lung cancer cells have an increased rate of glycolysis and overexpress the glucose transporter, there is preferential accumulation and visualization of FDG within the primary tumor and potential metastatic sites.[7] The criteria for an abnormal PET scan are either a standardized uptake value (SUV) of >2.5 or uptake in the lesion that is greater than the background activity of the mediastinum. Unlike CT, PET cannot assess local extent of tumor or its anatomic relationships to surrounding structures, and currently the lower limit of resolution of PET is approximately 1.0–1.2 cm. In addition, certain nonneoplastic processes (such as inflammatory conditions and infections) can produce "positive" PET findings. Despite its limitations, PET is becoming an increasingly valuable tool in staging (especially the mediastinum) and for detection of distant disease (Figure 16-2).

Several recent studies have shown that PET is superior to CT in staging the mediastinum in lung cancer patients. Pieterman and colleagues[53] prospectively compared standard staging approaches to PET for detection of mediastinal lymph node and distant metastases in 102 patients with resectable NSCLC who underwent histological staging of the mediastinum. The sensitivity and specificity of PET for detection of mediastinal nodal metastases were 91 and 86%, respectively, compared with a sensitivity of 75% and specificity of 66% for CT. Similarly, meta-analysis of 18 studies by Toloza and co-workers[67,68] demonstrated an overall sensitivity of 84% and specificity of 89%. Pieterman and associates[53]

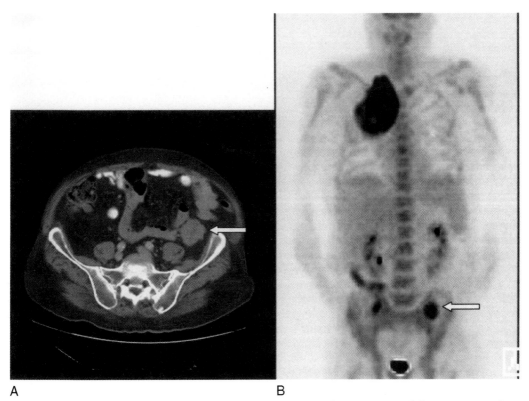

A   B

Figure 16–2 (A, B) PET-CT showing a right superior sulcus tumor and the presence of an asymptomatic retroperitoneal metastasis.

246 also showed that combining CT and PET resulted in the highest diagnostic accuracy with a sensitivity of 94% and specificity of 86%, supporting the utilization of both modalities for staging of the mediastinum.

Another significant result in the study by Pieterman and co-authors was the observation that PET resulted in a stage different from the one arrived at by the standard methods in 62 of 102 patients, correctly indicating a lower stage in 20 patients and identifying higher stage disease in 42 patients. More importantly, PET was effective in identifying occult metastatic disease. In 11 patients (11%) PET demonstrated distant metastatic disease that was not detected by the usual staging tests. The sites of metastasis included bone, liver, and adrenal gland.

Recently, integrated PET-CT scanners have been introduced into clinical practice to improve diagnostic accuracy and anatomic localization of disease.[5] Lardinois and colleagues[31] compared the diagnostic accuracy of integrated PET-CT with CT alone, PET alone, and visually correlated PET and CT in 50 patients with proven or suspected NSCLC. In 40 patients who underwent histological confirmation, tumor staging was significantly more accurate with integrated PET-CT than with CT alone ($p = .001$), PET alone ($p < .001$), or visual correlation of PET and CT ($p = .013$). In 37 patients with histological confirmation of nodal status, integrated PET-CT was more accurate in assessing the mediastinum than PET alone ($p = .013$). Moreover, unsuspected extrathoracic metastases were discovered in 16% (8 of 49 patients). PET is playing a larger role in the diagnosis and staging of lung cancer. Although its exact role is still evolving, PET clearly improves the noninvasive assessment of the mediastinum and may be extremely valuable in identification of occult distant metastatic disease.

Bone Scan

At present, metastatic bone involvement is typically assessed using technetium-99m methylene diphosphate (^{99m}Tc MDP) whole-body bone scan. When utilized as a result of a clinical assessment that suggests the possibility of bone metastases (i.e., bone pain or tenderness), radionuclide bone scanning is relatively sensitive, but not specific. In their meta-analysis of 7 studies and 633 patients, Toloza and colleagues[67,68] showed an overall sensitivity of 87% and specificity of 67%. False positive abnormalities are more common when scans are done in asymptomatic patients and can be the result of degenerative or traumatic skeletal injury. Follow-up imaging with magnetic resonance imaging may or may not aid in establishing a definitive diagnosis. False negative results, though uncommon, do occur, and in one series 6% of patients with an initially negative bone scan developed confirmed skeletal metastases within 1 year.[38]

Magnetic Resonance Imaging (MRI)

MRI of the chest for the evaluation and characterization of pulmonary lesions and mediastinum offers few advantages over CT in the diagnosis or staging of lung cancer. Heelan and co-workers[20] evaluated both CT and MRI in otherwise operable patients with NSCLC and found that MRI was no more accurate than CT in identifying hilar or mediastinal lymph node metastases and actually had a higher false posi-

tive rate. There are situations, however, in which MRI can be a useful investigation. When tumors are adjacent to the vertebral body or spinal canal, MRI provides superior visualization of the spinal canal and can more accurately detect subtle changes in the marrow suggestive of invasion. In addition, MRI can more accurately delineate a superior sulcus tumor's relationship to major vessels and the brachial plexus at the thoracic outlet.

▶ INVASIVE MODALITIES

Bronchoscopy

Rigid or flexible bronchoscopy with conventional white light allows visualization of the tracheobronchial tree and is a standard part of evaluating patients with a known or suspected lung cancer. It serves several critical purposes: diagnosis, staging, assessment of resectability, and visualization of the remaining bronchial tree. Flexible video-assisted bronchoscopy has become a widely employed technique, replacing rigid bronchoscopy for all but a few, special circumstances. Flexible bronchoscopy is generally performed as an outpatient procedure on a spontaneously breathing patient through the nasal or oral route, following topical anesthesia and sedation. The tracheobronchial tree up to the second or third subsegmental bronchi is easily visualized. The options available to secure a diagnosis include direct biopsy, brushing, saline lavage for cytology, or transbronchial needle aspiration (TBNA) with or without fluoroscopic guidance. Employing more than one technique (i.e., biopsy, brushing, and cytological lavage) generally improves the diagnostic yield.

When bronchoscopy reveals endobronchial tumor, biopsy is best accomplished with either a forceps or brush biopsy with sensitivities in the range of 80–100%.[13,63] Positive endobronchial findings are more common with squamous and small cell cancers because of their central location. In contrast, a normal bronchoscopic examination is usually seen with peripheral lesions, and the diagnostic sensitivity of bronchoscopy varies widely from 37 to 98% depending on the size and location of the target lesion. Increasing size and presence of a bronchus sign (bronchus leading to or contained within a lesion on CT) portend a higher diagnostic yield.[63] The use of fluoroscopy to guide a transbronchial biopsy or TBNA and lavage can improve diagnostic accuracy up to 80%.[61]

TBNA can also be used in cases in which there is bronchial distortion (thickening or blunting of the carina, extrinsic compression) secondary to the lesion or metastatic lymph nodes. Popularized by Wang and Terry, TBNA employs a 20- to 22-gauge, rigid needle through the channel of the fiberoptic bronchoscope to puncture the airway in the area of interest.[70] It is a safe and inexpensive procedure with an overall sensitivity of 50% and specificity of 96%.[13,63] As previously mentioned, diagnostic yield is enhanced by the use of fluoroscopy, as well as utilization of rapid, on-site cytopathology. A positive result, especially from a mediastinal lymph node station, can obviate further surgical staging, although a negative result should still be confirmed surgically. Limitations include a sensitivity of only 30% for small (<2 cm), peripheral lesions and inaccessibility of certain lymph node stations, including anterior, aortopulmonary, paraesophageal, and pulmonary ligament nodes.

Autofluorescence Bronchoscopy

Detection and treatment of subtle dysplastic or early invasive neoplastic lesions whose presence is suggested by positive sputum cytology remain a challenge. In one study, Woolner[74] reported that only 29% of the carcinoma *in situ* detected by sputum cytology could be localized by conventional bronchoscopy. Additional studies have shown that roughly one third of patients with positive sputum cytology, but radiographically occult lung cancers, require more than one bronchoscopy for localization.[4,11] In an effort to improve identification of superficial bronchial mucosal malignancy, Hung and associates[22] were able to demonstrate that normal and malignant bronchial mucosa have different autofluorescence intensities under blue light (wavelength 442 nm). This led to the development of the LIFE (Light Imaging Fluorescence Endoscope)-Lung System (Xillix Technologies, Richmond, British Columbia, Canada). Whereas normal bronchial mucosa appears green, premalignant and malignant tissue appears brown-red.[27] Subsequent prospective trials comparing white-light bronchoscopy alone to white-light bronchoscopy plus LIFE have shown enhanced sensitivity in detection of intraepithelial neoplasms and invasive carcinoma.[21,27–29] Lam and co-authors[29] reported the results of a multicenter North American trial of 173 patients that showed the relative sensitivity of white-light bronchoscopy plus LIFE versus white-light bronchoscopy alone to be 6.3 for intraepithelial lesions and 2.71 if invasive cancers were included. The role of LIFE currently is in preoperative screening for synchronous squamous carcinomas, follow-up of postoperative patients for recurrence or second primary tumors, and monitoring patients undergoing local, endobronchial treatments for early stage disease. LIFE may also be useful for obtaining tissue for molecular biological studies of carcinogenesis and monitoring areas of intraepithelial dysplasia in chemoprevention trials.

Percutaneous Transthoracic Needle Biopsy

Percutaneous transthoracic needle biopsy is a well-established procedure used in confirming a tissue diagnosis of lung cancer in patients who are not surgical candidates because of advanced disease or medical contraindications. However, with the identification of increasing numbers of noncalcified pulmonary nodules by low-dose CT, transthoracic needle biopsy is becoming a critical tool in the detection of early stage lung cancer. Although both fluoroscopic and CT guidance are employed, CT is the preferred modality for several reasons. CT allows planning precise trajectories that avoid aerated lung, blood vessels, bullae, and vital cardiovascular structures in the mediastinum. Smaller lesions can be biopsied, and CT can enable differentiation between necrotic and viable areas within a larger tumor, improving diagnostic yield.[55] The most common complications of the procedure are pneumothorax and mild hemoptysis. Although the reported incidence of pneumothorax varies greatly, the rate of postprocedure pneumothoraces requiring intervention ranges from 1.6 to 17%.[39,52] The most important risk factor

is underlying chronic obstructive pulmonary disease (COPD).[12] Hemoptysis occurs in 5–10% of cases and is usually self-limited. Massive hemoptysis is extremely rare with the use of 20-gauge or smaller needles.[40,73] Relative contraindications to transthoracic biopsy, therefore, are the presence of severe COPD, bleeding disorder, contralateral pneumonectomy, or severe pulmonary hypertension. When successful, the results of percutaneous transthoracic biopsy are positive in patients with lung cancer in roughly 90% of cases, with a low false positive rate of less than 2%.[10] However, false negative results can be frequent and should be considered indeterminate unless a specific benign diagnosis is made.

Cervical Mediastinoscopy

Because mediastinal lymph node involvement by metastatic carcinoma strongly influences treatment decisions, accurate assessment is paramount. Cervical mediastinoscopy is the most accurate prethoracotomy method of staging the mediastinum in bronchogenic carcinoma. Described by Carlens in 1959, mediastinoscopy employs a rigid, lighted scope placed in the avascular, pretracheal space to access the superior mediastinum.[9] Its efficacy is well established with a pooled procedural sensitivity of 81% and a specificity of 100% in a recent meta-analysis of 5687 patients.[68] Moreover, a negative mediastinoscopy predicts a high rate of complete resection at thoracotomy. Luke and colleagues[34] demonstrated that of 590 patients with a negative mediastinoscopy, 93% had complete tumor resection. Cervical mediastinoscopy is an outpatient procedure that is extremely safe. In a review of 2137 patients, Hammoud and co-workers[18] reported overall morbidity and mortality rates of 0.6 and 0.05%, respectively.

The indications for mediastinoscopy are often debated and routine mediastinoscopy is controversial. Most thoracic surgeons would agree that mediastinoscopy should be performed for the following: (1) lymph node enlargement greater than 1 cm in the short axis on CT, (2) hypermetabolic uptake on PET, and (3) possible enrollment into induction therapy protocols. Relative indications include the presence of T_2 or T_3 tumor, adenocarcinoma, or large cell carcinoma.[69] Those who support the practice of routine mediastinoscopy emphasize its low complication rate and accuracy, the high rate of complete resection following a negative mediastinoscopy, the relatively low sensitivity of CT, the prevalence of nodal disease even in T1 tumors (Table 16-3), and the ability to select patients who might benefit from induction therapy.

Left Anterior Mediastinotomy and Extended Cervical Mediastinoscopy

One limitation of mediastinoscopy can be in the setting of a left upper lobe cancer, in which aortopulmonary window and paraaortic lymph nodes (levels 5 and 6) may need to be sampled. In this situation there are two options for surgical staging. Most commonly, level 5 and 6 mediastinal lymph nodes can be accessed from a left anterior or parasternal approach, as described by McNeill and Chamberlain.[36] A transverse incision is placed over the second rib, and the costal cartilage is removed. The retrosternal extrapleural

Table 16–3

Prevalence of Nodal Metastases in cT1 NSCLC

Author (year)	n	Node + (%)	N1 (%)	N2 (%)	Skip N (%)
Ishida et al (1990)[23]	221	28	9	19	28
Naruke (1993)[47]	714	33	18	15	30
Asamura et al (1996)[2]	337	26	10	16	25
Oda et al (1998)[50]	524	22	8	14	51
Graham et al (1999)[16]	86	29	19	10	34

space is entered by blunt dissection and the paraaortic space is explored. Modifications of the procedure include preservation of the internal mammary vessels, use of the mediastinoscope for better visualization, and preservation of the cartilaginous rib. In three reported series totalling 194 patients with left upper lobe cancers who underwent a Chamberlain procedure, 38% (73 of 194) had positive biopsy results and resectability in those patients with a negative anterior mediastinotomy was 95%.[51] As with cervical mediastinoscopy, morbidity and mortality in previously reported series are low, 8 and 0%, respectively.

The second surgical approach to the anterior mediastinum in left upper lobe cancers is extended mediastinoscopy, as described by Ginsberg and associates.[15] Following a pathologically negative standard cervical mediastinoscopy, the mediastinoscope is withdrawn and blunt digital dissection is used to create a window between the innominate and left carotid arteries posterior to the innominate vein. The mediastinoscope is reinserted and advanced along the anterolateral surface of the aortic arch into the node-containing fat pad. Extended mediastinoscope should be avoided in patients with a dilated or calcified aortic arch or previous sternotomy.

Scalene Node Biopsy

Scalene node biopsy is used to assess suspicious nodes in the supraclavicular fossa, identified either by palpation or imaging (specifically PET). It has also been shown to be valuable to rule out N_3 disease in patients with proven N_2 disease. In the event that there are grossly palpable nodes in the supraclavicular fossa, a fine needle aspiration (FNA) in the office is often sufficient. Should an FNA be nondiagnostic or metastatic disease is suspected on imaging alone, a formal excision of the fat pad may be performed. A 3- to 4-cm incision is placed over the insertion of the sternocleidomastoid muscle parallel to the clavicle. Dissection is performed between the clavicular and sternal heads, exposing the scalene fat pad on top of the scalenus anterior muscle. Care must be taken to preserve the phrenic nerve lying posterior on the scalenus anterior muscle. Alternatively, Lee and

Ginsberg[32] reported a technique whereby scalene node biopsy can be done during a positive cervical mediastinoscopy employing a single incision. They showed that 15.4% (6/39) of patients with positive N_2 disease had positive scalene nodes as well, indicating N_3 disease.

Video-Assisted Thoracic Surgery (VATS)

VATS with the use of the thoracoscope and enhanced video optics and instrumentation provides another valuable tool for the diagnosis and staging of NSCLC. It requires general anesthesia and a patient that can tolerate single-lung ventilation. With the patient in a standard lateral decubitus position, the thoracoscope and endoscopic instruments are inserted through two or more operating ports placed via small incisions through the intercostal space. With this technique, the entire hemithorax can be explored, including the hilum, mediastinum, visceral and parietal pleural surfaces, and chest wall. The principal use of VATS has been to perform the excisional biopsy of peripheral lung nodules for diagnosis of primary lung cancer or to rule out synchronous or metastatic disease.[19,49] However, VATS is less effective for lesions located in the posterior paravertebral space or situated deep in the lung parenchyma. It is increasingly being used to evaluate mediastinal lymph nodes in patients with lung cancer. In particular, VATS can be used to sample nodes inaccessible by cervical mediastinoscopy (anterior, aortopulmonary, para-aortic) or anterior mediastinotomy (hilar, inferior pulmonary ligament).[30,57] Several studies have shown that the sensitivity and accuracy of VATS approach 100% for diagnosis and staging of lung cancer with minimal morbidity and mortality.

Thoracotomy

When other diagnostic and staging modalities have failed, thoracotomy is indicated for accurate diagnosis, staging, and subsequent curative treatment of potential lung cancers. With the myriad of accurate, less invasive diagnostic methods available, more than 95% of tumors can be characterized without thoracotomy. Exploratory thoracotomy, however, still allows the most thorough assessment of the primary lesion, the pleural space, and the ipsilateral mediastinal lymph nodes. The tumor is typically biopsied by Tru-Cut needle and the local extent and status of the mediastinal lymph nodes are assessed while the pathologists analyze the specimen by frozen section.

METASTATIC WORKUP

Approximately 40% of patients with newly diagnosed lung cancer are found to have extrathoracic metastases. Identifying these patients is critical to avoid unnecessary thoracotomy and delaying appropriate systemic therapy. Currently, the standard multiorgan imagings employed to rule out the most common metastases in patients with NSCLC (adrenal, liver, brain, bone) are CT of the chest and upper abdomen, a CT or MRI of the brain with contrast, and ^{99m}Tc MDP bone scan. Whole-body PET is showing promise in initial studies of its use for extrathoracic staging, disclosing non-CNS metastatic disease in up to 10–20% of cases missed by standard methods.[37,53,60,72] Although it is not yet a standard staging modality, with increasing data on its efficacy and new generation fusion PET-CT technology, PET is quickly becoming a ubiquitously employed staging technique.

Who should undergo evaluation for distant metastatic disease? There are precious few prospective randomized trials of extrathoracic imaging for NSCLC. It is well accepted that patients who have certain symptoms, abnormal physical findings, or laboratory abnormalities are at increased risk of having metastatic disease. Silvestri and coauthors showed in a large meta-analysis that a positive clinical evaluation was associated with a roughly 50% rate of abnormal scans.[65] These results underscore how critical the findings of the initial history, physical examination, and laboratory tests are in guiding subsequent workup. Patients with a positive clinical evaluation (Table 16-4) should undergo multiorgan scanning.

What about asymptomatic patients? Routine multiorgan imaging in patients without symptoms or signs is controversial. Several studies have shown that routine preoperative scanning in asymptomatic patients is associated with a low percentage (3–10%) of positive results with silent metastases in 2.7–15%.[56,59] In their meta-analysis, Silvestri and colleagues[65] calculated the probability that a scan will be negative if the clinical evaluation is negative (negative predictive value of the clinical evaluation). For CT of the abdomen, brain, and bone scan the negative predictive values were 94, 95 and 89%, respectively. The only prospective, randomized trial that compared routine multiorgan scanning with chest CT and mediastinoscopy in asymptomatic patients with clinically operable lung cancer showed no statistically significant difference in the rate of unnecessary thoracotomy, postoperative recurrence, or overall survival.[8] Based on this and the consequences of false positive results, most would not recommend routine preoperative multiorgan imaging in patients with clinical stage I or II disease and a negative clinical evaluation.

Which asymptomatic patients should be routinely scanned? Some authors have reported that more locally advanced lesions (T3 or N2) have a higher rate of asymptomatic distant metastases.[17,64] Others have shown that adenocarcinomas have a higher rate of asymptomatic cerebral metastases compared with squamous carcinomas.[59,66]

In summary, we feel that the following patients should undergo multiorgan scanning: (1) any patient with a positive clinical evaluation (symptoms, signs, bloodwork), (2) patients with locally advanced disease (stage IIIA) being considered for multimodality therapy, and (3) patients with early stage disease (stages I, II) who are marginal operative candidates.

SUMMARY

Lung cancer remains a challenging and deadly disease. Proper diagnosis and staging are critical in determining the best treatment strategy for each individual patient. The most important component of the workup is the initial history and physical examination. There are numerous noninvasive and invasive techniques that can be employed to establish an accurate and valid clinical estimate of tumor stage.

Table 16–4

Clinical Evaluation for Metastatic Disease

Clinical evaluation	Finding
Symptoms	Constitutional: weight loss >5% of body weight, malaise Musculoskeletal: focal skeletal pain Neurological: headache, seizure, mental status or personality changes
Physical signs	Focal neurological deficit Supraclavicular lymphadenopathy Hoarseness Superior vena cava syndrome Bony tenderness Skin or soft tissue mass Hepatomegaly
Laboratory tests	Anemia Elevated liver function tests (LFTs) Hypercalcemia

REFERENCES

1. American Thoracic Society: Medical section of the American Lung Association. Clinical staging of primary lung cancer. Am Rev Respir Dis 127:659–664, 1983.
2. Asamura H, Nakayama H, Kondo H, et al: Lymph node involvement, recurrence, and prognosis in resected small, peripheral, non-small-cell lung carcinomas: Are these carcinomas candidates for video-assisted lobectomy? J Thorac Cardiovasc Surg 111:1125–1134, 1996.
3. Bach PB, Kattan MW, Thornquist MD, et al: Variations in lung cancer risk among smokers. J Natl Cancer Inst 95:470–478, 2003.

250

4. Bechtel JJ, Kelly WR, Petty TL, et al: Outcome of 51 patients with roentgenographically occult lung cancer detected by sputum cytologic testing: A community hospital program. Arch Intern Med 154:975–980, 1994.

5. Beyer T, Townsend DW, Brun T, et al: A combined PET/CT scanner for clinical oncology. J Nucl Med 41:1369–1379, 2000.

6. Böcking A, Biesterfeld S, Chatelain R, et al: Diagnosis of bronchial carcinoma on sections of paraffin-embedded sputum: Sensitivity and specificity of an alternative to routine cytology. Acta Cytol 36:37–47, 1992.

7. Brown RS, Leung JY, Kison PV, et al: Glucose transporters and FDG uptake in untreated primary human non-small cell lung cancer. J Nucl Med 40:556–565, 1999.

8. The Canadian Lung Oncology Group: Investigating extra-thoracic metastatic disease in patients with apparently operable lung cancer. Ann Thorac Surg 71:425–434, 2001.

9. Carlens EJ: Mediastinoscopy: A method for inspection and tissue biopsy in the superior mediastinum. Dis Chest 36:343–352, 1959.

10. Charig MJ, Stutley JE, Padley SPG, et al: The value of negative needle biopsy in suspected operable lung cancer. Clin Radiol 44:147–149, 1991.

11. Cortese DA, Pairolero PC, Bergstralh EJ, et al: Roentgeno-graphically occult lung cancer: A 10-year experience. J Thorac Cardiovasc Surg 86:373–380, 1983.

12. Fish GD, Stanley JH, Miller KS, et al: Post-biopsy pneumo-thorax: Estimating the risk by chest radiography and pulmonary function tests. AJR Am J Roentgenol 150:71–74, 1988.

13. Gasparini S: Bronchoscopic biopsy techniques in the diagnosis and staging of lung cancer. Monaldi Arch Chest Dis 52:392–398, 1997.

14. Geddes DM: The natural history of lung cancer: A review board on rates of tumor growth. Br J Dis Chest 73:1–17, 1979.

15. Ginsberg RJ, Rice TW, Goldberg M, et al: Extended cervical mediastinoscopy. A single staging procedure for bronchogenic carcinoma of the left upper lobe. J Thorac Cardiovasc Surg 94:673–678, 1987.

16. Graham AN, Chan KJ, Pastorino U, et al: Systematic nodal dissection in the intrathoracic staging of patients with non-small cell lung cancer. J Thorac Cardiovasc Surg 117:246–251, 1999.

17. Grant D, Edwards K, Goldstraw P: Computed tomography of the brain, chest, and abdomen in the preoperative assessment of non-small cell lung cancer. Thorax 43:883–886, 1988.

18. Hammoud ZT, Anderson RC, Meyers BF, et al: The current role of mediastinoscopy in the evaluation of thoracic disease. J Thorac Cardiovasc Surg 118:894–899, 1999.

19. Hazelrigg SR, Nunchuck SK, LoCicero J III, et al: Video-assisted thoracic surgery study group data. Ann Thorac Surg 56:1039–1044, 1993.

20. Heelan RT, Martini N, Westcott JW, et al: Carcinomatous involvement of the hilum and mediastinum: Computed tomographic and magnetic resonance evaluation. Radiology 156:111–115, 1985.

21. Hirsch FR, Prindiville SA, Miller YE, et al: Fluorescence versus white-light bronchoscopy for detection of preneoplastic lesions: A randomized study. J Natl Cancer Inst 93:1385–1391, 2001.

22. Hung J, Lam S, LeRiche JC, et al: Autofluorescence of normal and malignant bronchial tissue. Laser Surg Med 11:99–105, 1991.

23. Ishida T, Yano T, Maeda K, et al: Strategy for lym-phadenectomy in lung cancer three centimeters or less in diameter. Ann Thorac Surg 50:708–713, 1990.

24. Jay SJ, Wehr K, Nicholson DP, et al: Diagnostic sensitivity and specificity of pulmonary cytology: Comparison of techniques used in conjunction with flexible fiberoptic bronchoscopy. Acta Cytol 24:304–312, 1980.

25. Jemal A, Murray T, Samuels A, et al: Cancer statistics, 2003. CA Cancer J Clin 53:5–26, 2003.

26. Kato H, Konako C, Ono J, et al: Cytology of the lung: Techniques and interpretation. Tokyo: Igaku-Shoin, 1983.

27. Kennedy TC, Lam S, Hirsch FR: Review of recent advances in fluorescence bronchoscopy in early localization of central airway lung cancer. Oncologist 6:257–262, 2001.

28. Lam S, Kennedy TC, Unger M, et al: Localization of bronchial intraepithelial neoplastic lesions by fluorescence bronchos-copy. Cancer 113:696–702, 1998.

29. Lam S, MacAulay C, LeRiche JC, et al: Detection and localization of early lung cancer by fluorescence bronchoscopy. Cancer 89:2468–2473, 2000.

30. Landreneau RJ, Hazelrigg SR, Mack MJ, et al: Thoracoscopic mediastinal lymph node sampling: Useful for mediastinal lymph node stations inaccessible by cervical mediastinoscopy. J Thorac Cardiovasc Surg 106:554–558, 1993.

31. Lardinois D, Weder W, Hany TF, et al: Staging of non-small-cell lung cancer with integrated positron-emission tomography and computed tomography. N Engl J Med 348:2500–2507, 2003.

32. Lee JD, Ginsberg RJ: Lung cancer staging: The value of ipsilateral scalene lymph node biopsy performed at mediastinoscopy. Ann Thorac Surg 62:338–341, 1996.

33. Liang XM: Accuracy of cytologic diagnosis and cytotyping of sputum in primary lung cancer: Analysis of 161 cases. J Surg Oncol 40:107–111, 1989.

34. Luke WP, Pearson FG, Todd TPU, et al: Prospective evaluation of mediastinoscopy for assessment of carcinoma of the lung. J Thorac Cardiovasc Surg 91:53–56, 1986.

35. McLoud TC, Bourgouin PM, Greenberg RW, et al: Bronchogenic carcinoma: Analysis of staging in the medi-astinum with CT by correlative lymph node mapping and sampling. Radiology 182:319–323, 1992.

36. McNeill T, Chamberlain J: Diagnostic anterior mediastino-tomy. Ann Thorac Surg 2:532–539, 1966.

37. MacManus MP, Hicks RJ, Matthews JP, et al: High rate of unsuspected distant metastases by PET in apparent stage III non-small-cell lung cancer: Implications for radical radiation therapy. Int J Radiat Oncol Biol Phys 50:287–293, 2001.

38. Michel F, Soler M, Imhof E, et al: Initial staging of non-small cell lung cancer: Value of routine radioisotope bone scanning. Thorax 46:469–473, 1991.

39. Moore EH, Shepard JO, McLoud TC, et al: Positional precautions in needle aspiration lung biopsy. Radiology 175:733–735, 1990.

40. Moore EH: Technical aspects of needle aspiration lung biopsy: A personal perspective. Radiology 208:303–318, 1998.

41. Mountain CF, Carr DT, Anderson WA: A system for the clinical staging of lung cancer. AJR Am J Roentgenol Radium Ther Nucl Med 120:130–138, 1974.

42. Mountain CF: A new international staging system for lung cancer. Chest 89:225–233, 1986.

43. Mountain CF, Dresler CM: Regional lymph node classification for lung cancer staging. Chest 111:1718–1723, 1997.

44. Mountain CF: Revisions in the international system for staging lung cancer. Chest 111:1710–1717, 1997.

45. Naruke T, Suemasu K, Ishikawa S: Lymph node mapping and curability at various levels of metastasis in resected lung cancer. J Thorac Cardiovasc Surg 76:832–839, 1978.

46. Naruke T, Goya T, Tsuchya R, et al: Prognosis and survival in resected lung cancer based on the new international staging system. J Thorac Cardiovasc Surg 96:440–447, 1988.

47. Naruke T: Significance of lymph node metastases in lung cancer. Semin Thorac Cardiovasc Surg 5:210–218, 1993.

48. Nesbitt JC, Putnam JB, Walsh GL, et al: Survival in early-stage non-small cell lung cancer. Ann Thorac Surg 60:466–472, 1995.

49. Nomori H, Horio H, Fuyuno G, et al: Lung adenocarcinomas diagnosed by open lung or thoracoscopic vs. bronchoscopic biopsy. Chest 114:40–44, 1998.

50. Oda M, Watanabe Y, Shimizu J, et al: Extent of mediastinal node metastasis in clinical stage I non-small-cell lung cancer: The role of systematic nodal dissection. Lung Cancer 22:23–30, 1998.

51. Olak J: Parasternal mediastinotomy (Chamberlain procedure). Chest Surg Clin North Am 6:31–39, 1993.

52. Permutt LM, Johnson WW, Dunnick NR: Percutaneous transthoracic needle aspiration: A review. AJR Am J Roentgenol 152:451–455, 1989.

53. Pieterman RM, van Putten JWG, Meuzelaar JJ, et al: Pre-operative staging of non-small-cell lung cancer with positron-emission tomography. N Engl J Med 343:254–261, 2000.

54. Pilotti S, Rilke F, Gribaudi G, et al: Sputum cytology for the diagnosis of carcinoma of the lung. Acta Cytol 26:649–654, 1982.

55. Pinstein ML, Scott RL, Salazar J: Avoidance of negative percutaneous lung biopsy using contrast-enhanced CT. AJR Am J Roentgenol 140:265–267, 1983.

56. Quinn DL, Ostrow LB, Porter DK, et al: Staging of non-small cell bronchogenic carcinoma: Relationship of the clinical evaluation to organ scans. Chest 89:270–275, 1986.

57. Rendina EA, Venura F, DeGiaconio T, et al: Comparative merits of thoracoscopy, mediastinoscopy, and mediastinotomy for mediastinal biopsy. Ann Thorac Surg 57:992–995, 1994.

58. Rigler LG: The earliest roentgenographic signs of carcinoma of the lung. JAMA 195:655–657, 1966.

59. Salvatierra A, Baamonde C, Llamas JM, et al: Extrathoracic staging of bronchogenic carcinoma. Chest 97:1052–1058, 1990.

60. Saunders CAB, Dussek JE, O'Doherty MJ, et al: Evaluation of fluorine-18-deoxyglucose whole body positron emission tomography imaging in the staging of lung cancer. Ann Thorac Surg 67:790–797, 1999.

61. Schenk DA, Bryan CL, Bower JH, et al: Transbronchial needle aspiration in the diagnosis of bronchogenic carcinoma. Chest 92:83–85, 1987.

62. Schreiber G, McCrory DC: Performance characteristics of different modalities for diagnosis of suspected lung cancer. Summary of published evidence. Chest 123:115S–128S, 2003.

63. Shure D: Fiberoptic bronchoscopy—diagnostic applications. Clin Chest Med 8:1–13, 1987.

64. Silvestri GA, Lenz JE, Harper SN, et al: The relationship of clinical findings to CT scan evidence of adrenal gland metastases in the staging of bronchogenic carcinoma. Chest 102:1748–1751, 1992.

65. Silvestri GA, Littenberg B, Colice GL: The clinical evaluation for detecting metastatic lung cancer: A meta-analysis. Am J Respir Crit Care Med 152:225–230, 1995.

66. Tarver RD, Richmond BD, Klatte EC: Cerebral metastases from lung carcinoma: Neurological and CT correlation work in progress. Radiology 153:689–692, 1984.

67. Toloza EM, Harpole L, McCrory DC: Noninvasive staging of non-small cell lung cancer. A review of the current evidence. Chest 123:137S–146S, 2003.

68. Toloza EM, Harpole L, Detterbeck F, et al: Invasive staging of non-small cell lung cancer. A review of the current evidence. Chest 123:157S–166S, 2003.

69. Vallieres E, Waters PF: Incidence of mediastinal node involvement in clinical T1 bronchogenic carcinomas. Can J Surg 30:341–342, 1987.

70. Wang KP, Terry PB: Transbronchial needle aspiration in the diagnosis and staging of bronchogenic carcinoma. Am Rev Respir Dis 127:344–347, 1983.

71. Watanabe Y, Shimizu, J, Oda M, et al: Proposals regarding some deficiencies in the new international staging system for non-small cell lung cancer. Jpn J Clin Oncol 21:160–168, 1991.

72. Weder W, Schmid RA, Bruchhaus H, et al: Detection of extrathoracic metastases by positron emission tomography in lung cancer. Ann Thorac Surg 66:886–893, 1998.

73. Wescott JL: Percutaneous transthoracic needle biopsy. Radiology 169:593–601, 1988.

74. Woolner LB: Pathology of cancer detected cytologically. In Atlas of Early Lung Cancer: National Cancer Institute, National Institutes of Health, U.S. Department of Health and Human Services. Tokyo: Igaku-Shoin, 1983, pp. 107–213.

Lung Cancer: Surgical Treatment

Dennis A. Wigle, Shaf Keshavjee, and Robert J. Ginsberg

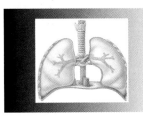

INTRODUCTION

The incidence of lung cancer remains at epidemic proportions, with the American Cancer Society projecting an incidence of 184,600 new cases for the year 2002.[4] Approximately 90% of these cases will occur in patients with histories of significant tobacco use. Unfortunately, roughly 90% of these patients are expected to ultimately die of their disease, despite the fact that 35% are surgical candidates.

Surgical resection for non-small-cell lung cancer is still regarded as the most effective method of controlling the primary tumor provided it is resectable for cure. Radiation therapy, used either alone or with chemotherapy, can be effective in palliation and has resulted in the occasional cure, but does not approach the success rate of surgery. Except for small-cell lung cancer, chemotherapy as a single modality is reserved for palliation of advanced tumors, as almost no cures have been reported unless combined with surgery or radiation therapy.

HISTORICAL NOTE

Surgery for lung cancer was first discussed in the literature around the turn of the last century. Pean reported in 1895[89] the successful removal of a lung cancer by partial excision;

254 the actual operation had been performed 30 years previously. Hugh Morriston Davies described the first dissection lobectomy for lung cancer in 1912,[22] with the patient unfortunately dying 8 days postoperatively with empyema. The modern era of surgical resection for lung cancer required the development of underwater drainage and advances in anesthetic techniques. The first one-stage lobectomy was reported by Brunn,[7] followed by Allan and Smith[2] who described a two-stage resection in 1930. Following Graham's historic pneumonectomy in 1932, surgical resection for lung cancer became prevalent, with pneumonectomy quickly becoming the procedure of choice.[14] The technique of segmentectomy was described by Churchill and Belsey.[15] More refined techniques were developed subsequent to this, including sleeve resection by Price-Thomas in 1947,[92] carinal resection by Mathey and associates[77] and Thompson,[119] and en bloc resection of the chest wall by Coleman[17] and for a superior sulcus tumor in 1956.[13] Although lesser resections had been performed by a variety of surgeons as compromise procedures in patients with poor pulmonary function, Jensik and colleagues[51] reported the first series of segmental resections as intentional curative procedures.

▶ SURGICAL PRINCIPLES IN THE MANAGEMENT OF LUNG CANCER

It is now standard practice to carefully stage all lung cancers at the time of initial presentation for diagnostic and prognostic purposes. Since 1986, the international tumor–node–metastasis (TNM) staging system has been employed by most oncologists. Briefly stated, tumors confined to the lung without any regional or distant metastases are classified as stage I. Tumors associated with only hilar or peribronchial lymph node involvement (N_1), or extension to the chest wall, mediastinum, or diaphragm, are classified as stage II. Locally advanced tumors with mediastinal or cervical lymph node metastases, or invasion into "unresectable" structures, are classified as stage III tumors, while tumors presenting with distant metastases are classified as stage IV.

The 5-year survival rate following complete resection of a lung cancer is stage dependent. Incomplete resection rarely, if ever, provides cure. Most recent series show that 60–70% of patients undergoing complete resection for T1N0 lung cancer survive for 5 years, and 80% never have recurrences. At the other extreme, less than 10% of patients undergoing resections for stage IIIB disease are cured.

It is not acceptable for a surgically curable lung cancer to be treated by resection without careful consideration of oncological principles. The following principles of oncological surgery must be employed:

1. Whenever possible, the tumor and all associated lymphatic drainage must be removed completely, most frequently by lobectomy or pneumonectomy.
2. Care must be taken not to transgress the tumor during resection to avoid tumor spillage.
3. En bloc resection of closely adjacent or invaded structures is preferable to discontinuous resection.
4. Resection margins should preferably be assessed by frozen section. Reexcision is preferred whenever possible if positive resection margins are encountered.

5. All accessible mediastinal lymph node stations should be sampled or removed for pathological evaluation. We prefer mediastinal lymph node dissection, with each node identified and properly labeled by the surgeon.

Surgical resection is the treatment of choice for stage I, II, and selected stage III non-small-cell lung cancers. It is generally offered to all patients with early stage disease, specific groups of patients with stage III disease, and those with solitary or limited pulmonary metastases and completely resectable primary disease.

▶ SURGICAL TECHNIQUES

Lobectomy

Lobectomy has been the preferred method of resection for early stage lung cancer since Churchill's report of long-term survival in the 1950s.[16] Entry into the pleural space via a posterolateral incision is the gold standard. For peripheral tumors, the fifth intercostal space is typically entered for upper or middle lobectomy, while the sixth space can be utilized for a lower lobectomy. In lower lobe tumors that are more centrally positioned, it can be advantageous to expose the hilum via the fifth intercostal space to facilitate safe dissection. Anterolateral muscle-sparing incisions typically require an approach one interspace higher than usual as the anterior aspect of the ribs is positioned more inferiorly. Anterior approaches through either a median sternotomy or anterior thoracotomy can provide excellent access to the superior pulmonary veins and main pulmonary arteries, but poorer access to the inferior pulmonary veins and bronchi.

Mobilization and Dissection

Adhesions encountered upon entering the pleural space are divided by either blunt or sharp dissection. The inferior pulmonary ligament is incised to the inferior pulmonary vein to mobilize the entire lung. The lung is then inspected and palpated to assess the extent of tumor involvement and determine if lobectomy is possible. The mediastinal pleura at the hilum is then completely excised to facilitate hilar and nodal dissection (Figures 17-1, 17-2, and 17-3).

The dissection of hilar structures for lobectomy is frequently more tedious and time consuming than that for a pneumonectomy (Figures 17-4 and 17-5). Any inflammatory process in the region can make the dissection difficult, and anatomical anomalies are much more frequent. Classically, one would first divide the artery, then the veins, and finally the bronchus. Some surgical oncologists have favored ligation of the veins first to prevent release of tumor cells into the circulation, but this has the disadvantage of creating significant venous congestion and retention of blood within the resected specimen. There is no evidence to suggest any survival advantage with the latter approach. In cases in which vessel dissection is difficult, the bronchus can be divided first to facilitate exposure. This approach was originally described for patients with associated lung abscesses to prevent spillage to the main bronchus and opposite lung. In patients with central tumors, it can be useful not to adhere to any predetermined sequence of ligation,

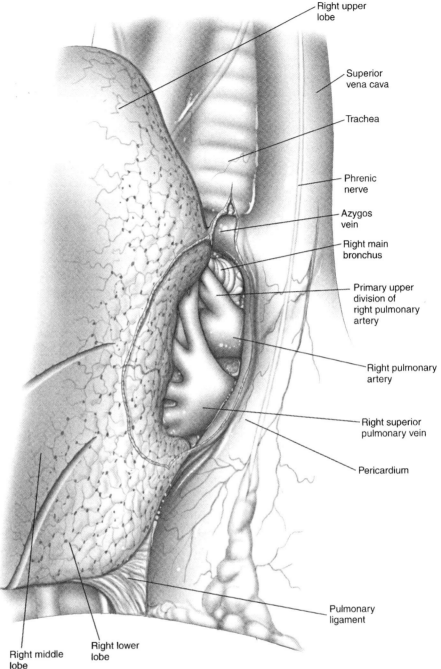

Figure 17-1 Anterior view of right hilum. The mediastinal pleura is open and the lung retracted posteriorly. *(From Martini N, Ginsberg RJ: Lobectomy. In Thoracic Surgery, 2nd ed. New York: Churchill Livingstone, 2002.)*

Labels (clockwise): Right upper lobe · Superior vena cava · Trachea · Phrenic nerve · Azygos vein · Right main bronchus · Primary upper division of right pulmonary artery · Right pulmonary artery · Right superior pulmonary vein · Pericardium · Pulmonary ligament · Right lower lobe · Right middle lobe

but rather remove that structure whose absence provides better exposure to the remaining structures. When encountering an extremely difficult dissection in which injury to the pulmonary arteries is possible, dissecting and encircling the main pulmonary artery can allow easy cross-clamping to prevent unnecessary blood loss should problems arise.

An incomplete fissure is frequently encountered in many lobectomies. Filmy, avascular adhesions can sometimes be bluntly dissected with a sponge stick, but frequently a fissure requires division with a linear stapler to access hilar structures.

Many approaches to the management of vessels have been described. Segmental pulmonary arteries are typically divided between ligatures. Pulmonary veins have a tendency to slip from a single ligature, and hence most surgeons prefer double ligation or ligation plus transfixation.

Bronchial closure is typically achieved with stapling. Excessive devascularization of the bronchial stump should be avoided. Frozen sections should be obtained from the margins of any questionable area. Many surgeons oversew the staple line with a running absorbable suture to avoid the occasional catastrophe of individual staples misfiring and coming loose at a later time. Some form of vascularized material such as pericardium, pleura, or intercostal muscle should be used to cover the bronchus where the risk of fistula formation is significant.

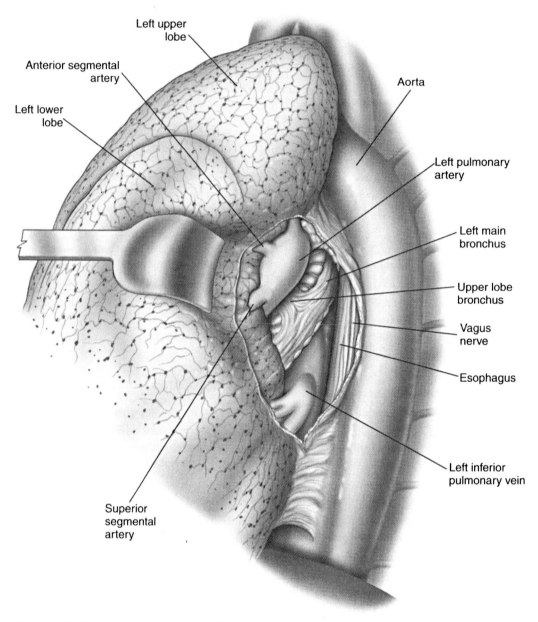

Figure 17-2 Posterior view of left hilum.
(From Martini N, Ginsberg RJ: Lobectomy. In Thoracic Surgery, 2nd ed. New York: Churchill Livingstone, 2002.)

Pneumonectomy

The first successful one-stage pneumonectomy for bronchogenic carcinoma was performed by Graham and Singer in 1933.[41] Pneumonectomy was long the procedure of choice for resectable lung cancer once these techniques became widespread in the 1940s. In the modern era, pneumonectomy is reserved for cancer operations where lobectomy or bronchial sleeve resection will not provide an R0 resection.

Entry into the pleural cavity for pneumonectomy is typically undertaken via posterolateral thoracotomy through the fifth intercostal space. Although many surgeons routinely remove a rib, this is not a strict requirement. Anterolateral thoracotomy unfortunately provides suboptimal access to

hilar structures and hence is rarely employed. Median sternotomy can provide excellent access to hilar structures for a right pneumonectomy, but the heart severely restricts access to the inferior veins for completion of a left pneumonectomy. Although some surgeons prefer this approach given the advantage of less postoperative pulmonary compromise, there is a theoretical increased risk of sternal infection in clean contaminated cases such as pulmonary resection.[18,114]

Although the division of the pulmonary veins should occur early in the procedure and before the division of the artery for oncological reasons, this may not always be possible. When not involved with tumor, their identification and dissection are usually straightforward. With tumor involvement, the veins should be manipulated gently to prevent

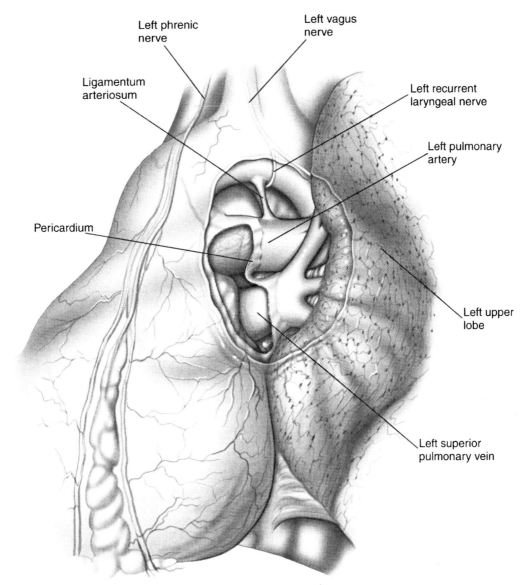

Figure 17–3 Intrapericardial exposure of left pulmonary hilum.
(From Waters PF: Pneumonectomy. In Thoracic Surgery, 2nd ed. New York: Churchill Livingstone, 2002.)

tumor emboli and a rapid decision made as to potential resectability. Although the vessels may be closed in a variety of ways, vascular staplers have become the most popular. Several millimeters of atria can also be taken with the resection if required, though we prefer to do this with an atrial clamp and oversewing of the resection margin.

The pulmonary artery is typically divided using a vascular stapler. A number of techniques are available when insufficient length is present to safely apply a stapler, including intrapericardial dissection, mobilization of the superior vena cava (SVC) on the right side, or division of the ligamentum arteriosum on the left. The division of the main bronchus is also a function of experience and preference. We prefer to use the bronchial stapler where possible. If a closure is sewn, absorbable sutures are preferable over nonabsorbable due to the incidence of suture granulomas and subsequent hemoptysis. The routine use of some form of patch to but-

tress the stump is a controversial issue, with options including omentum, intercostal muscle, or pericardial fat.

The management of a postpneumonectomy space attends to a potentially lethal problem. Steps are typically taken to normalize volume in the operated space to return the mediastinum to the midline. A tube is either left in place clamped to allow ongoing manipulation of space volume, or withdrawn early postoperatively after ensuring the mediastinum is midline. Failure to do so can result in significant impairment of venous return with occasional catastrophic consequences.

Segmentectomy

Anatomical segmental resection is the removal of one or more bronchopulmonary segments of an individual lobe through ligation and division of bronchovascular structures.

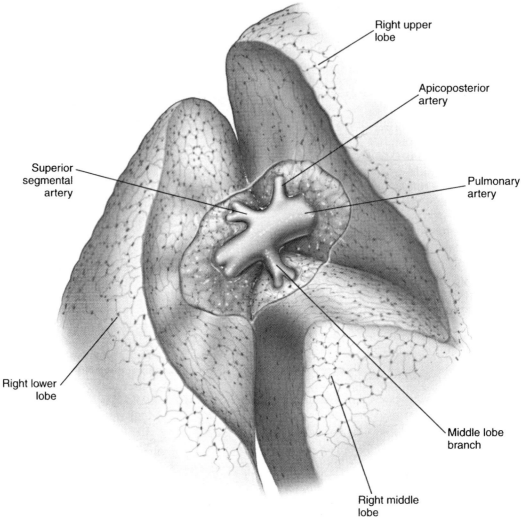

Figure 17–4 Anterior view of right major fissure. The fissure has been opened to expose the segmental arteries.
(From Martini N, Ginsberg RJ: Lobectomy. In Thoracic Surgery, 2nd ed. New York: Churchill Livingstone, 2002.)

This is to be differentiated from wedge resection, which involves the excision of portions of lobes via stapling devices, cautery, or laser ablation. Historically, segmental resection was first proposed by Churchill and Belsey in 1939,[15] who suggested that "the bronchopulmonary segment may replace the lobe as the surgical unit of the lung." The procedure was popularized as a means of removing irreversibly damaged lung, such as in bronchiectasis, with minimal loss of functioning lung parenchyma.

Segmental resection is technically more difficult than lobectomy and requires intimate knowledge of bronchovascular anatomy and possible arterial anomalies. The most reliable landmark of an individual segment is the bronchus. The segmental bronchus can usually be identified by repeated traction on a segment and finger palpation in the hilar area for the resultant tightening of the segmental bronchus. The order of division of segmental hilar structures may vary, but generally the arterial branches are divided first to allow identification of the segmental bronchus. As the venous drainage may not be readily apparent, ligation of veins is best performed last after the intersegmental plane has been developed. Establishment of the plane is performed by differential inflation. The excluded segment will remain airless after expansion of the lung with the segmental bronchus occluded. If collateral ventilation fills the diseased segment, the reverse procedure can be employed to demarcate the diseased segment by deflating the lung following occlusion of the segmental bronchus. Stapling devices can sometimes be difficult to employ at the tertiary hilum, and hence manual closure of the ligated segmental bronchus with silk sutures so as not to occlude other segmental orifices is sometimes required.

Limited Pulmonary Resection

A limited pulmonary resection is performed in a nonanatomical fashion without individual ligation of segmental bronchovascular structures (Figure 17-6). This approach is

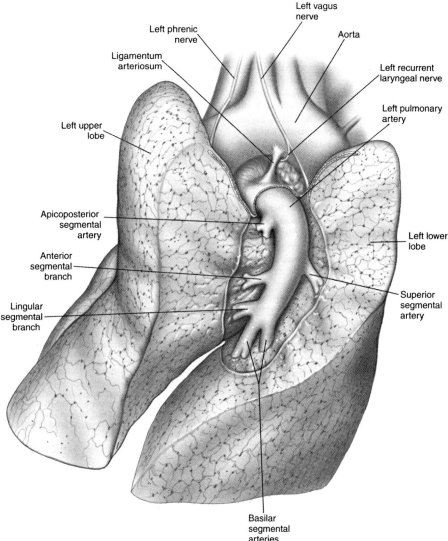

Figure 17–5 Interlobar view of left hilum. The segmental anterior supply to the upper and lower lobes is identified. *(From Martini N, Ginsberg RJ: Lobectomy. In Thoracic Surgery, 2nd ed. New York: Churchill Livingstone, 2002.)*

Labels on figure: Left vagus nerve; Left phrenic nerve; Aorta; Ligamentum arteriosum; Left recurrent laryngeal nerve; Left upper lobe; Left pulmonary artery; Apicoposterior segmental artery; Left lower lobe; Anterior segmental branch; Lingular segmental branch; Superior segmental artery; Basilar segmental arteries

typically used for excisional biopsy of lesions that if benign, require no further treatment. Limited resections for lung cancer should be reserved for patients with severely compromised pulmonary function where lobectomy or segmental resection would not be tolerated. The advent of mechanical stapling devices has made this the most popular approach for such limited resections.

Mediastinal Lymph Node Dissection

Intraoperative staging is an essential component of the surgical treatment of lung cancer, particularly in the assessment of nodal status. It is critical for the thoracic surgeon to accurately identify and properly label lymph node specimens submitted to the pathologist so that histological stage can be determined. Unfortunately determination of N status remains the most controversial aspect of the TNM staging system for lung cancer. Disagreement about the stage to which a specific lymph node level should be assigned (e.g., level 10), as well as competing definitions for a number of N levels (e.g., levels 2–4), accounts for much of the confusion. A graphic representation of current station definitions is shown in Figure 17-7.

In the right hemithorax, mediastinal lymphadenectomy can be accomplished through either a standard posterolateral thoracotomy or a muscle-sparing incision. The superior mediastinum, bordered by the azygous vein, the SVC, and the trachea, is exposed by retracting the lung inferiorly. The mediastinal fat pad is removed from the SVC posteriorly to the trachea, between the azygous vein inferiorly and the innominate artery superiorly. Right level 2 nodes are located within this tissue between the cephalic borders of the aortic arch and innominate vein, while right level 4 nodes sit distal to this point and proximal to the origin of the right upper lobe bronchus. Dissection between the esophagus and the membranous portion of the trachea will reveal retrotracheal level 3 nodes. Right level 10 nodes are found along the anterior border of the bronchus intermedius distal to the pleural reflection. Level 11 interlobar nodes can be exposed by retracting the lung anteriorly, while level 12 nodes are found adjacent to the distal lobar bronchus and are typically removed with the specimen.

Level 7 nodes are accessed by retracting the lung anteriorly and opening the mediastinal pleura to expose the subcarinal region. Tissue attachments to the right and left mainstem bronchi should be clipped prior to removal as

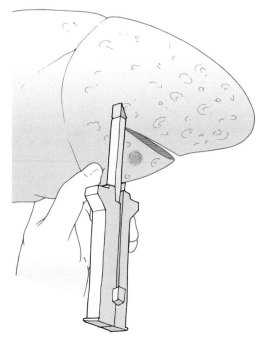

Figure 17–6 Stapled wedge resection.
(*Modified from Fell SC, Kirby TJ: Limited pulmonary resection. In Thoracic Surgery, 2nd ed. New York: Churchill Livingstone, 2002.*)

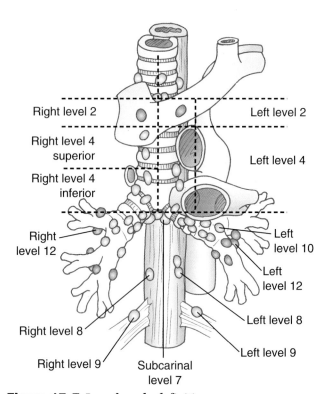

Right level 2
Left level 2
Right level 4 superior
Left level 4
Right level 4 inferior
Right level 12
Left level 10
Left level 12
Right level 8
Left level 8
Left level 9
Right level 9
Subcarinal level 7

Figure 17–7 Lymph node definitions.
(*Modified from Keller SM: Mediastinal lymph node dissection. In Thoracic Surgery, 2nd ed. New York: Churchill Livingstone, 2002.*)

there are often moderate sized vessels running to this region. Level 9 nodes are typically easily visualized along the inferior pulmonary ligament, though level 8 paraesophageal nodes are not always present.

On the left side, aortopulmonary (levels 5 and 6) and subcarinal nodes (level 7) can be exposed via a thoracotomy through the fifth interspace. Access to level 2 and 4 nodes typically requires mobilization of the aortic arch and is not done. Dissection within these regions is best done with blunt instruments and control of vessels accomplished with clips or ties to avoid electrical injury. The position of the phrenic nerve should be identified to avoid injury and subsequent diaphragmatic paralysis. Vocal cord paralysis is a rare but potential complication and hence the recurrent laryngeal nerve and proximal vagus must be protected. Level 7 nodes can be identified similar to the right side by retracting the lung anteriorly and following the left mainstem bronchus to the subcarinal region. Level 9 nodes are usually easily seen as they are on the right. Level 11 and 12 nodes are best seen with the lung retracted anteriorly, with level 12 nodes typically being removed with the specimen. Care should be taken here as the pulmonary artery is located immediately anterior and must be carefully avoided when clips or cautery are utilized.

► OCCULT LUNG CANCER

An occult lung cancer is defined as a tumor not evident on radiological imaging but discovered either incidentally at bronchoscopy or by sputum cytology. Fewer than 1% of lung cancers fall into this category. The majority of these patients either participate in early lung cancer detection programs or present with hemoptysis in the absence of any findings on routine chest radiographs.

Localization

Occult carcinomas require careful investigation for localization of the site of cancer. Flexible bronchoscopy makes inspection of the entire tracheobronchial tree down to segmental and subsegmental bronchi possible. A radiographically occult lung cancer can sometimes be located by this method alone. If a lesion is located centrally in a main or lobar bronchus it can be readily visualized and a biopsy obtained. In instances in which the tracheobronchial tree appears normal at bronchoscopy, a meticulous sampling of each segmental bronchus by selective, protected endoscopic brushing and cytological analysis becomes necessary. Only repeated positive brushings from an isolated segment is acceptable for such localization. A complete aerodigestive examination is also essential to rule out carcinoma in other sites. It has been reported that up to one third of patients with a normal chest radiograph and sputum positive for malignant squamous cells have a carcinoma in the head and neck region.[71] For this reason, a detailed head and neck examination should be performed in addition to a careful diagnostic quadroscopy, including bronchoscopy, laryngoscopy, nasopharyngoscopy, and esophagoscopy to complete the examination of the proximal aerodigestive tract.

More sophisticated techniques have been recently introduced to enhance the sensitivity and specificity of bronchoscopic localization. Specifically, the development of *in vivo* fluorescent staining of mucosal malignancies with hematoporphyrin derivatives and laser induced fluorescence excitation (LIFE) bronchoscopy has aided in the detection of mucosal abnormalities not apparent to the naked eye.[29,44,62,130]

Therapy

Following localization, the therapy of choice for a radiographically occult lung cancer remains surgical removal of the primary tumor by segmentectomy, lobectomy, or pneumonectomy, with or without a sleeve resection as necessary. Lesser resections are usually not possible due to the central localization of most occult primary tumors. The 5-year survival of patients treated surgically for radiographically occult lung carcinoma approaches 100%.

Although recurrences are rare, new lung primaries are observed in up to 45% of these patients, the majority of whom present with new endobronchial squamous cell cancers. Continued surveillance of these patients at regular intervals is therefore necessary.

Other therapeutic approaches to occult disease include the use of photodynamic therapy with transbronchoscopic laser-induced photoexcitation of hematoporphyrin derivatives. This has been reported by Hayata et al[44] and Cortese et al[19] to be effective in eradicating occult *in situ* endobronchial lung cancer, with recurrence rates around 20% in short-term follow-up of highly selected patients.

A new form of "chest radiograph-occult" lung cancer is being identified with routine computed tomography (CT) scanning or "low-dose" CT scanning used in early detection programs.[45] Many of these lesions are only a few millimeters in diameter and are difficult to diagnose as carcinoma. Wedge resection is often required to make a diagnosis. These lesions can be difficult to identify within a lobe, sometimes necessitating a lobectomy to ensure removal. The question as to whether a lesser resection is acceptable for such tumors is provocative but has not yet been completely addressed scientifically.

Given the adverse reports on lesser resection for stage I lung cancer,[39,127] many authors have attempted to address the role of limited resection in early peripheral disease. It has been found that even in tumors less than 1 cm in diameter, lymphatic permeation and lymph node metastases within the lung can occur. A lesser resection, particularly wedge resection, ignores this lymphatic permeation. If a wedge resection is required because of compromised pulmonary function, it appears that postoperative radiotherapy decreases the local-regional recurrence rate.[30,79] The role of postoperative radiotherapy following limited resection by video-assisted thoracoscopic surgery (VATS) has been studied recently by the CALGB Cooperative group in North America, with early reports suggesting less than satisfactory results. In Japan, where spiral CT scanning has been prevalent for almost 20 years, many centers have employed wedge resection and segmentectomy for early subcentimeter lesions. In these highly selected individuals, many with the ground-glass appearance typical of noninvasive bronchoalveolar carcinoma, limited resections have yielded up to 90% 5-year tumor-free survival[58,59,115,121] (Table 17-1).

STAGE I DISEASE (T_1N_0, T_2N_0)

This is the most common form of early lung cancer seen by most physicians. Many patients in this stage are detected on routine chest radiographs or CT scans of the chest and upper abdomen performed for unrelated medical conditions. Most are discrete peripheral lesions. Metastatic surveys by CT scanning are routinely done to assess the mediastinum, liver, and adrenal glands. Wider surveys have a low yield and thus have not been shown to be cost effective. Routine positron emission tomography (PET) scanning as a method of staging is still under investigation. The role of mediastinoscopy is still controversial in the case of a negative CT scan. Surgical therapy is the management of choice in a fit patient with no mediastinal involvement. At the time of surgery, systematic lymph node sampling or dissection is carried out to ensure that no hilar or mediastinal nodal metastases are present.

Lesser resections such as wedge excision or segmentectomy have been advocated by some for small peripheral tumors. Jensik[50] and Kulka and Forai[61] have reported on a large series of patients with stage I carcinoma treated in this conservative fashion. The Lung Cancer Study Group (LCSG) performed a multicenter randomized clinical trial of lobectomy versus a lesser resection by wedge or segmentectomy in stage I carcinomas presenting as small peripheral tumors.[39] This study suggests a 3-fold increase in the incidence of local recurrence in patients treated by resections smaller than lobectomy. This observation is

---

Table 17–1

Five-Year Survival Rates by Stage following Complete Resection for Lung Cancer[a]

Stage	Survival (%)
I (n = 539)	76
$\quad T_1N_0$	84
$\quad T_2N_0$	68
II (n=214)	47
IIIA	
$\quad T_3N_0$ (chest wall)	56
$\quad T_3N_0$ (carina)	36
$\quad T_3N_0$ (mediastinum)	29
$\quad N_2$ (surgery, n = 151)	30
$\quad N_2$ (chemotherapy + surgery) (n = 89)	26

[a]Adapted from Martini N, Bains MS, Burt ME, et al: Incidence of local recurrence and second primary tumors in resected stage I lung cancer. J Thorac Cardiovasc Surg 109:120, 1995.

262 corroborated by a report on segmental resections by Warren and Faber.[127] In the LCSG analysis, overall survival was decreased in the limited resection group. Although the apparent advantage of limited resection is in the conservation of lung tissue, this was not evident in the assessment of long-term pulmonary function following surgery. An important disadvantage is the 10–15% risk of local-regional recurrence. As a consequence, this form of therapy is usually reserved for patients with significantly limited lung reserve at the time of resection.

Isolated lesions located more centrally typically require a lobectomy or pneumonectomy for adequate resection. A Japanese study has demonstrated virtually no loss of pulmonary function 1 year following lobectomy and no significant differences in function following segmentectomy.[117] For tumors protruding from a lobar orifice into the main bronchus, a sleeve lobectomy should be considered whenever possible. This procedure conserves pulmonary parenchyma and offers lower morbidity and mortality than that associated with pneumonectomy, with comparable survival rates when a complete resection is accomplished.[35]

The role of ipsilateral mediastinal lymph node sampling vs. lymph node dissection in stage I disease remains unclear. Although it would seem intuitive that a formal lymph node dissection might provide the most accurate postsurgical staging, a randomized clinical trial comparing the two modalities has not demonstrated either survival or recurrence rate advantages to either therapeutic arm in stage I or II disease if mediastinoscopy was used in conjunction with intraoperative sampling. This question is currently being addressed in a large North American trial (American College of Surgeons Oncology Group, ACOSOG). This may provide the answer as to whether mediastinal lymph node dissection is of added value vs. lymph node sampling alone. Investigators are also currently assessing the value of intraoperative radioisotope and dye-based identification of sentinel lymph nodes based on experiences in breast cancer and melanoma. It remains to be determined whether this approach has value in deciding whether to perform a lymph node dissection.[65,112,120]

Survival

Patients with small tumors 3 cm or less in diameter that are confined to the lung parenchyma without evidence of regional lymphatic metastases or extension to chest wall, diaphragm, or pleura have a 5-year disease-free survival rate of 60–80% when treated by primary surgical resection.[76] Tumors greater than 3 cm in diameter that are still confined to the lung without metastases to lymph nodes or distant sites (stage IB) also have a favorable prognosis with a 5-year disease-free survival rate of ~70%. The modern-day overall 5-year survival rate in stage I carcinoma, whether T_1 or T_2, approaches 70% (Table 17-2). No adjuvant treatment is recommended for patients with stage I disease following complete resection, though this issue continues to be investigated in clinical trials. Of the 20–30% of patients who have recurrences following resection for stage I disease, the majority have relapses at distant sites, with more than 20% being solitary brain metastases. Close follow-up for the detection of solitary recurrences or second primaries is consequently advised.

► STAGE II DISEASE (T_1N_1, T_2N_1)

Tumors confined to the lung or bronchus with involvement of hilar or bronchopulmonary lymph nodes as the sole site of tumor spread (T_1N_1, T_2N_1 disease) account for less than 5% of the lung cancer population and less than 10% of all resected lung cancers.[75] Lobectomy is the surgical procedure of choice for this stage of disease. Recent series have suggested that the majority of T_1N_1 lesions can be removed with a lobectomy encompassing all disease. In the Memorial Sloan-Kettering Cancer Center series reported by Martini et al[75] on the surgical treatment of stage II lung cancer, a lobectomy was sufficient to encompass all disease in 34 of the 35 T_1N_1 lesions. Of interest was that ~50% of patients had only a single N_1 node involved, and 85% had nodal involvement at a single N_1 level. At this stage of disease, we believe it imperative that a complete lymph node dissection be performed given the high frequency of occult mediastinal metastases. This is particularly true if the nodal involvement is hilar.

The role of sleeve lobectomy and vascular sleeve resection for N_1 disease has been addressed.[48,63] Reports indicate that if a complete resection can be performed by sleeve lobectomy with or without vascular sleeve resection, the results of surgical treatment appear similar to those following pneumonectomy. This approach should be considered in patients with ipsilateral mediastinal disease for whom a sleeve resection will encompass all areas involved with tumor to preserve lung function.

Modern series suggest that the overall survival rate for stage II disease is approximately 40% at 5 years, with little difference in survival between T_1 and T_2 lesions.[75] The location of the primary tumor, the location of N_1 nodes, the extent of surgical resection, and the presence or absence of visceral pleural involvement also do not appear to influence survival. Factors positively influencing survival include the presence of a single positive lymph node vs. multiple nodes positive for tumor, with an associated 45% and 31% 5-year survival, respectively (Figure 17-8). Patterns of recurrence in stage II disease appear to be influenced by histology, with local or regional recurrences being more frequent in patients with squamous cell carcinoma, and patients with adenocarcinoma have a higher incidence of distant metastases. Data from the Lung Cancer Study Group[67] suggest that although postoperative radiotherapy in these patients may decrease the rate of local or regional recurrence, it does not appear to influence survival.

Despite the large number of patients developing distant metastases following complete (R0) resections for N_1 disease, the role of adjuvant and neoadjuvant treatment is still largely undefined. In practice, however, many patients are offered varying combinations of chemotherapy and irradiation despite the lack of clear evidence for adjuvant therapy. Many trials are ongoing in Europe and North America attempting to address this question. Previous trials of postoperative adjuvant chemotherapy, immunotherapy, or combinations of the two have shown little effect on survival rates in randomized studies.[46,67] Induction chemotherapy has been tested with some promise, as a French phase III trial has suggested a survival advantage in early stage disease.[23] Recent data from the International Adjuvant Lung Cancer Trial (IALT) investigators have also suggested a 5% differ-

Table 17–2

Five-Year Survival Rates in the Three Largest Series Reporting Stage-by-Stage Survival According to the 1997 Stage Classification[a]

Stage	Naruke[b]		Mountain[c]		Rami-Porta[d]	
	Number of patients	5-year survival (%)	Number of patients	5-year survival (%)	Number of patients	5-year survival (%)
I						
T_1N_0 (IA)	245	75	511	67	235	58
T_2N_0 (IB)	291	57	549	57	817	50
II						
T_1N_1 (IIA)	66	52	76	55	31	66
T_2N_1 (IIB)	153	38	288	39	290	42
T_3N_0 (IIB)	106	33	87	38		
IIIA						
T_3N_1 (IIIA)	85	39	55	38	389	25
T_1–$3N_2$ (IIIA)	368	15	344	23		
T_1–$3N_3$ (IIIB)	55	0	572	3	138	28
T_4 any N (IIIB)	104	0	458	6		
IV						
TN any M_1	293	7	1427	1	27	28

[a]Note that in the Naruke and Mountain series, the stage IV survival includes unresected patients, whereas the Rami-Porta series includes only resected patients. The Mountain series includes all IIIB patients whether resected or not.
[b]Naruke T, Goya T, Tsuchiya R, Suemasu K: Prognosis and survival in resected lung cancer based on the new international staging system. J Thorac Cardiovasc Surg 96:440, 1988.
[c]Mountain CF: Revisions in the International Staging System for Lung Cancer. Chest 111:1710, 1997.
[d]Rami-Porta R, for the Bronchogenic Carcinoma Cooperative Group of the Spanish Society of Pneumonology and Thoracic Surgery: Lung Cancer 29(Suppl 1):133, 2000.

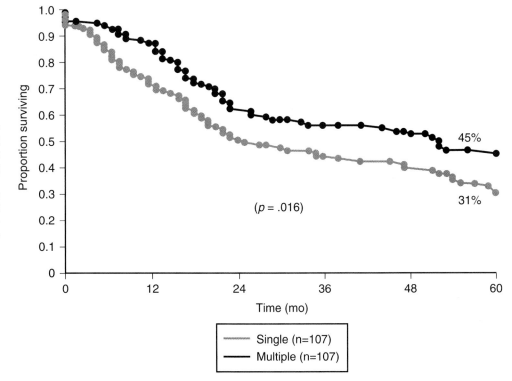

Figure 17–8 Survival by number of N_1 nodes involved following complete resection in stage II non-small-cell lung cancer.
(Adapted from Martini N, Bains MS, Burt ME, et al: Survival after resection in stage II non-small cell lung cancer. Ann Thorac Surg 54:460, 1992.)

ence in 5-year survival for patients receiving adjuvant chemotherapy in stages I, II, and III disease prior to surgery.[64]

▶ T_3N_0 DISEASE

Tumors invading adjacent structures that can be completely resected by en bloc resection are classified as T_3 lesions. These tumors have been recently recategorized as stage IIB disease given their favorable survival following surgical resection. With N_1 involvement, the overall survival following resection of T_3 tumors is decreased such that T_3N_{1-2} tumors are classed as stage IIIA disease.

Tumors Invading the Chest Wall

Cancers of the lung that invade the chest wall are usually peripheral in location and hilar or mediastinal lymph node metastases are generally less likely to occur in this group of patients. These tumors extend to invade the parietal pleura and may involve the muscles and ribs of the chest wall. Significant numbers of these patients are amenable to treatment by surgical resection even with chest wall invasion (reviewed in detail in Chapter 20). Factors that influence survival in this group of patients are (1) complete resectability of the tumor, (2) extent of invasion of the chest wall, and (3) the presence or absence of regional lymph node metastases. A recent review of 334 patients from Memorial Sloan-Kettering with carcinoma of the lung invading chest wall that were treated surgically showed an overall 5-year survival rate of 50% in those patients with a complete resection.[28] A recent Mayo Clinic report has also suggested a 35% 4-year survival for this stage of disease.[40] For those patients in whom resection was incomplete (macroscopic or microscopic disease) or not possible, the 5-year survival in both series was essentially zero. Postoperative radiation therapy in this group of patients did not impact their ultimate survival.

Superior Sulcus Tumors

Superior sulcus tumors or pancoast tumors represent a unique subset of carcinomas of the lung invading the chest wall (reviewed in detail in Chapter 21). By reason of their location in the pleural apex, they often invade adjoining tissues early with symptomatic consequences. Early invasion of the lower brachial plexus, particularly the T_1 nerve root, is common. Shoulder and arm pain radiating to the inner aspect of the upper arm (T_1) and the ulnar distribution in the fourth and fifth fingers of the hand (C8) is a common presenting symptom. Extension to the stellate ganglion with a consequent Horner's syndrome is seen in at least one third of patients. Extension to the ribs or vertebrae is also common.

Most superior sulcus tumors are initially diagnosed histologically or cytologically by a transcutaneous needle biopsy performed under CT guidance. Diagnostic bronchoscopy is less helpful in establishing a tissue diagnosis in this group of patients because of the peripheral position of the lesion, although transbronchoscopic biopsy using image intensification has been reported. Although the majority of superior

sulcus tumors are histologically squamous cell carcinomas or adenocarcinomas, up to 3–5% can be small-cell lung carcinomas (SCLC). Given the vastly different therapeutic implications of the presence of SCLC, an accurate tissue diagnosis prior to treatment is critical.

Modern series suggest a 5-year survival of ~40% for complete surgical resection of superior sulcus tumors. This decreases to less than 10% for incomplete (R1-microscopic or R2-grossly positive) resections. Both advanced stage and advanced nodal status precipitate poorer outcomes in pancoast tumors.[99] Although the role of preoperative treatment has been questioned by some, a recent North American Intergroup trial suggests that both T_3 and T_4 tumors benefit from preoperative chemoradiation with high complete pathological response rates (65%) and very high complete resection rates. The 2-year survival of 70% for patients who had a complete resection in this report is improved vs. historical controls.[100] A recent update of these data reported an impressive 53% 5-year survival after complete resection.[101]

Tumors in Proximity to the Carina

Another subset of stage IIB carcinomas that benefits from surgical management includes patients with central tumors extending to within 2 cm of the carina. In many instances the carina itself is not involved despite a T_3 presentation, and in many instances surgical removal of the tumor is possible. Nodal involvement severely affects prognosis, emphasizing the need for preoperative mediastinoscopy. Because most series report the results of either sleeve lobectomies or sleeve pneumonectomies, no definitive series exist reporting the results of surgical resection of T3 tumors due to their proximity to the carina. In patients in whom resection can be undertaken despite the proximity of the lesion to the carina but without its involvement, the 5-year anticipated survival rate following resection is currently reported to be ~35%.[74]

Although a pneumonectomy is the most common resection under these circumstances, the presence of tumor at a major lobar orifice and the need to conserve lung tissue are the main indications for sleeve resection. A pneumonectomy may still be required to encompass all of a tumor protruding from a lobar orifice into the main bronchus and to provide a clear margin of resection. In such situations a sleeve lobectomy can be a worthwhile alternative and has comparable morbidity and mortality rates to pneumonectomy. Faber et al[31] performed 101 sleeve lobectomies over a 21-year period, with only two postoperative deaths in the entire series. The survival rate in this group of patients was 30% at 5 years and 22% at 10 years. When the tumor involves not only the mainstem bronchus but also the proximal pulmonary artery, vascular sleeve resection can also be performed. Although early reports suggested a much higher mortality rate with very poor survival, recent reports with improved techniques suggest results equivalent to sleeve lobectomy alone or that of pneumonectomy.[94]

Tumors Invading the Mediastinum

Patients presenting with invasion of a primary tumor into the mediastinum generally do poorly if treated by surgery alone. Two thirds of these patients also have mediastinal lymph node metastases. Few centers have reported results in this subset of patients. A review of the Memorial Sloan-Kettering Cancer Center experience from 1974 to 1984 involving 225 patients undergoing thoracotomy for non-small-cell carcinoma invading only the mediastinum (T3) demonstrated that only 49 patients (22%) underwent complete resection of all intrathoracic disease.[9] The 5-year survival rate in this group was only 9%. Partial resection, implantation of isotopes to treat residual disease, plus external radiation therapy was carried out in 33 patients (15%) with a surprising 3- and 5-year survival rate of 22%. Partial resection without implantation was done in 42 patients (19%) and implantation without resection in 101 patients (45%). There were no 5-year survivors in the latter two groups. A more recent update of this experience analyzing only N0 patients showed a 19% 5-year survival from 102 patients resected. The only other large series in the literature[91] reported a 25% 5-year survival in 40 patients with disease invading the mediastinum. The adverse effect of N2 disease was apparent in that no survivors were reported in the nine patients with mediastinal invasion and concomitant N2 disease.

STAGE III DISEASE

In general, the majority of lung cancers at presentation are advanced tumors. When distant metastases are absent, but lymphatic metastases to the mediastinum are present, they are classified as stage III disease (N_2 or N_3 disease). Tumors invading "unresectable" adjacent organs (T_4) are also included in this stage. Many of these locally advanced tumors are amenable to surgical or combined modality therapy that includes surgery, particularly T_4 or N_2 disease. At this stage of disease, it is important to rule out distant metastases with preoperative organ scanning. Once again, mediastinoscopy is important in these patients with a high risk of having mediastinal lymph node metastases. It should be noted, however, that once a lesion is clinically staged as T_4 or N_2, the current accepted therapy in most cases is nonsurgical. Nonetheless, when induction therapy is used and no progression is noted, a number of randomized trials have suggested that surgical resection can lead to reasonable survival in responders.[64,96,97]

T_3N_{1-2}

The presence of hilar or mediastinal nodes adversely affects survival in this group of patients with T_3 tumors despite a complete resection. The survival rate following a complete resection in the presence of nodal disease is less than 20% at 5 years. When identified preoperatively, many of these patients are being offered neoadjuvant approaches with a strategy of reevaluation regarding resectability if a response occurs. No evidence exists to support preoperative radiation therapy alone for tumors invading the chest wall in the presence of N_1 or N_2 disease. Postoperative radiation therapy in patients who have evidence of mediastinal lymph node metastases or residual disease is usually advised in an attempt to decrease the incidence of local recurrence,[87] although the efficacy of this treatment is unknown. A randomized trial by the Lung Cancer Study Group to assess the value of postoperative radiotherapy in this group of patients was abandoned because of low accrual. Preoperative medi-

astinoscopy can identify patients unlikely to benefit from surgical resection alone when a tumor has been staged clinically as T_3. Hilar nodal involvement may also be revealed by preoperative PET scanning.

N_2 Disease

Metastasis to mediastinal lymph nodes (N_2 disease) is often the most frequent hurdle to cancer cure despite an otherwise localized presentation. Mediastinal metastases are present in nearly 50% of all limited disease patients at presentation with non-small-cell lung carcinoma. Given that the majority of these patients likely have occult micrometastatic disease already present elsewhere, many clinicians have traditionally viewed this large group of patients as having nonsurgical disease.[88,90]

Not Clinically Evident N_2 Disease: "Resectable"

This group of patients comprises those with ipsilateral N_2 disease identified at thoracotomy. Many can benefit from effective management by primary surgery. A series by Martini et al[72] describing 706 patients seen at Memorial Sloan-Kettering from 1974 to 1981 with mediastinal lymph node metastases found that only 151 (21%) were completely resectable. The overall 5-year survival rate of this group was 30%.[71] There was no difference in survival at 5 years between patients with adenocarcinoma (30%) and those with squamous cell carcinoma (32%). Mediastinoscopy at that time was not routinely performed as part of staging before thoracotomy, and clinical evidence of N_2 disease was based largely on radiographic and bronchoscopic findings. Patients with a normal-appearing mediastinum on routine chest radiographs and CT scan and a normal carina at bronchoscopy without compression or distortion of the trachea or main bronchi were classified as having N_0 or N_1 disease. Patients who had an abnormal mediastinum on chest radiographs, which was suggestive of N_2 disease ("bulky" nodal disease), and those with findings at bronchoscopy suggestive of carinal involvement, were considered to have clinically manifested N_2 disease. When nodal involvement was present, the number of nodes affected was significant. Patients with a single involved N_2 node did better than those with multiple nodes involved at one or more levels ($p = .005$) (Figure 17-9). A number of other reports have subsequently identified improved survival in patients with single-station N_2 nodal disease.

The role of primary surgery in the management of N_2 disease can be summarized as follows. Patients found at thoracotomy to have unsuspected N_2 disease (clinical N_1 disease) that can be completely resected should be offered that opportunity. If, at mediastinoscopy, a microscopic focus of N_2 disease is identified in one station only, primary surgery can be considered, although currently most centers offer patients combined modality therapy. Patients who do best are those in whom N_2 disease is discovered serendipitously at surgery following a negative mediastinoscopy. In these instances, ipsilateral mediastinal lymph node dissection (not just sampling) is strongly advised, and has been found in a recent analysis to improve survival.[57] In this interesting subset analysis of an intergroup study assessing postoperative radiation therapy, the authors identify the fact that an

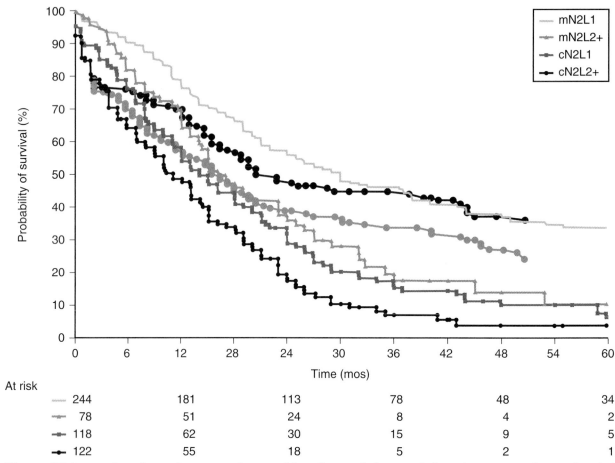

Figure 17–9 Lymph node involvement and survival based on pathologic and clinical staging. N_2 disease identified clinically (CN) has an extremely poor prognosis, as does more than one level of mediastinal lymph nodes (L2+) found at pathologic analysis.
(Adapted from Ginsberg RJ, Martini N: Non-small cell lung cancer—surgical management. In Thoracic Surgery, 2nd ed. New York: Churchill Livingstone, 2002.)

ipsilateral mediastinal lymph node dissection on the right side improved survival in patients with N_2 disease, but no such improvement was noted when left-sided mediastinal nodal dissection (levels 5, 6, and 7) was carried out. This suggests an important role of mediastinoscopy, particularly with suspected left hilar nodal involvement. Whether an extended lymph node dissection that includes superior mediastinal nodal stations when left-sided tumors are present is worthwhile awaits further study.

Adjuvant therapies in patients with surgically treated N_2 disease that has been completely or incompletely resected have unfortunately to date shown little benefit. Postoperative radiotherapy appears to decrease the incidence of local-regional recurrence but does not affect survival. Adjuvant chemotherapy and chemoradiotherapy have not been impressive in improving long-term and disease-free survival, and it is unlikely that major improvements will be demonstrated with the current spectrum of drugs available.

Clinically Evident N2 Disease: "Unresectable"

In contrast to patients with N2 disease identified at thoracotomy, patients presenting with radiological or endoscopic evidence of clinical N_2 disease have a poor survival rate. In the series reported by Martini et al,[72] only 18% of such patients had resectable disease, and only 9% of those treated by resection survived 5 years. None ultimately survived their cancer. These results have since been confirmed.[113,118,129] In all retrospective analyses, single-station mediastinal lymph node involvement yields a better prognosis than multistation involvement and shows the adverse effects of multiple levels of involved lymph nodes assessed at the time of surgery and assessed clinically. Only those patients with clinical N_1 disease had a survival greater than 10% following complete surgical resection. This result has been repeated multiple times in the literature. The importance of preoperative mediastinoscopy in any patient suspected to have clinical hilar or N_2 disease cannot be overstated. The identification of N_2 disease preoperatively suggests the need to consider a combined modality therapeutic approach since primary surgery yields such a poor survival outcome when clinically evident N_2 disease is present.

CT scanning is an integral part of staging and the presurgical evaluation of the mediastinum,[33,42,73] with the results correlating well with negative nodes less than 1 cm in transverse diameter (80–90% accuracy). Many centers accept this as evidence of mediastinal negativity and proceed with surgical resection based on this result. However, even patients with peripheral T1 tumors and no mediastinal lymphadenopathy according to CT may be found to have positive mediastinal lymph nodes in as many as 21% of cases.[105] Enlarged mediastinal lymph nodes (greater than 1 cm in shortest diameter) detected on CT scans should be confirmed to be positive by mediastinoscopy or other invasive staging before therapy is begun, since up to 30% of such cases do not contain tumors in the mediastinal nodes, and these patients can be offered primarily surgical therapy. The role of PET scanning in providing confirmatory evidence of N_2 disease without the need for invasive mediastinal staging has yet to be defined, although early reports look promising.[123] Unfortunately, positive PET scans in the mediastinum can reflect inflammatory changes, while negative PET scans can be falsely negative.

In summary then, patients with N_2 disease who benefit best from surgery as their primary therapy are those who present with peripheral tumors, an apparently normal mediastinum on plain chest radiographs and at bronchoscopy, and a normal mediastinum on CT scan and mediastinoscopy with a single, microscopic or encapsulated, discrete ipsilateral lymph node involvement that is discovered at surgery. The importance of CT scanning and mediastinoscopy is to identify significant mediastinal disease (i.e., involvement at multiple stations of N_2 nodes, invasion of mediastinal structures by nodal disease, or contralateral [N_3] nodal disease), thus avoiding primary surgery and a consequent poor outcome. Unfortunately, neither CT scan nor plain radiography correlates well with N_2 disease when the tumor in the lung is central or hilar in location or extends to the mediastinum, making it difficult to separate T_3 from N_2 disease. In these groups of patients, invasive mediastinal evaluation by mediastinoscopy can be helpful to make the distinction.

The role of preoperative radiation therapy alone for clinically evident N_2 disease has been extensively evaluated and does not appear to improve survival.[107,126] Most of these patients die because of distant metastases, and consequently radiation is not beneficial overall despite a reported increase in resectability, local-regional control, and apparent sterilization of some of the tumors in resected specimens. Several centers have assessed the benefit of preoperative chemotherapy or combined chemotherapy and radiation therapy in these locally advanced tumors that are usually considered incurable by primary surgery.[8,117] Phase II studies have suggested an improved survival compared with that in historical controls, and two randomized trials have confirmed the benefit of induction therapy compared with primary surgery.[8,60,96,97]

Numerous phase II trials over the past 20 years have investigated a variety of induction chemotherapy and chemoradiation regimens, most involving cisplatinum and mitomycin. More recently, attempts have been made to shorten the chemoradiation approaches with hyperfractionation techniques. The results of these phase II trials suggest that when used as induction therapy, chemotherapy and chemoradiation produce similar outcomes, similar morbidity, and similar long-term survival. The role of the surgeon in managing such patients should begin prior to any induction therapy, and must include preoperative assessment of the T (bronchoscopy) and N (mediastinoscopy) stages and a predetermination of the expected resection that might follow the induction therapy. After completion of such preoperative treatment, a careful reassessment is required to rule out the development of metastases, to determine whether the patient's disease is still potentially resectable, and whether the patient has sufficient cardiopulmonary capability to tolerate such a resection, keeping in mind the adverse cardiopulmonary toxicities of specific agents and radiotherapy. Following induction therapy, resection is possible in most responders, and survival following these regimens is contingent on attainment of a complete resection. Despite the preoperative regimens, surgical morbidity and mortality rates have not exceeded those expected following resection of locally advanced stage III lung cancer.

The two early phase III trials of induction chemotherapy have suggested a significant improvement in survival.[96,97] However, a recent trial[49] has failed to confirm these results. When one takes into account all of these trials, it is evident that persisting N_2 disease following induction therapy is an adverse prognostic factor, whereas a complete response or downstaging is a positive prognostic factor. In total, the sum of all reports on preoperative treatment to date can be viewed only as feasibility studies because of the small number of patients studied in each report. However, these studies demonstrate a high response to induction treatment with increased resectability in responders. The early survival data of these trials are sufficiently encouraging to support the initiation of large-scale randomized studies, which are currently in progress to assess fully the role of induction therapy and surgery vs. the current standard therapy, radiotherapy (with or without chemotherapy), in these "unresectable" N_2 patients. Recent reports suggest up to a 15% 5-year survival rate with chemoradiotherapy as the primary treatment,[27,104] results that are equivalent to those seen following induction therapy and surgery. Currently, a North American trial is being completed that compares these two approaches. As well, in North America and Europe, induction chemotherapy is now being tested in phase III trials that compare primary surgery with this combined modality approach in earlier stage disease.[64]

Stage IIIB Disease (T_4 or N_3)

Patients presenting with (1) supraclavicular or contralateral mediastinal lymph node metastases (N_3); (2) invasion of the spine, trachea, carina, esophagus, aorta, or heart (T_4), or satellite lesions within the same lobe; or (3) malignant pleural effusion (T_4) are currently grouped under stage IIIB disease and are considered inoperable. Most of these patients are treated by primary radiotherapy or chemoradiation. Few are considered for surgical therapy although a small group of T_4N_0 tumors can be completely resected. Currently, phase II clinical trials are assessing the potential role of combined modality therapy, including surgery, for this subset of patients. Occasionally, patients are found at thoracotomy to have completely resectable T_4 disease because they have been clinically overstaged. These comprise most of the reported long-term survivors. In a report by Stamatis and associates[111] in which the authors used induction chemoradiation followed by surgery for stage IIIB tumors, 9 of the 13 R0 resections for T_4 disease had complete pathological

268 responses, and 8 of the 14 R0 resections with N_3 disease had complete pathological responses at the time of the surgery. The 5-year survival rate of the various subgroups was identical to the number of patients who had complete responses, implying a negligible impact for surgical treatment.

Overstaging of IIIB patients is an area of particular concern. There should exist incontrovertible evidence before a patient is assigned to a T_4 or N_3 category on clinical grounds. Patients who are clinically staged as T_4 or N_3 can be of lower stage at the time of invasive staging or thoracotomy. If invasive approaches are not used for staging, inappropriate (nonsurgical) therapy may be prescribed for otherwise resectable tumors.

T_4 Disease

Carinal Involvement

Lesions that extend to and invade the carina have a much poorer prognosis than those in the mainstem bronchi. Pneumonectomy with tracheal sleeve resection and direct reanastomosis of the trachea to the contralateral mainstem bronchus has been offered to young patients who are good surgical risks with a 20% or greater 5-year survival rate, often in the face of 13–30% operative mortality rates.[24,52] In a recent update of the Massachusetts General experience, Mitchell and colleagues[80] reported on carinal resections or sleeve pneumonectomies from 58 primary bronchogenic carcinomas. The operative mortality for right carinal pneumonectomy was 15.9% (7 of 44) and for left carinal pneumonectomy was 30.8% (4 of 13). Dartevelle and colleagues[20] reported an impressive 42.3% 5-year survival rate for carinal pneumonectomy. Sleeve pneumonectomy should be reserved for young healthy patients with clinical N_0 or N_1 disease as determined by mediastinoscopy who have completely resectable disease. All other patients in general should be treated primarily with chemoradiation without resection. On occasion, small tumors around the carina but originating in the mainstem bronchus, usually squamous cell cancers, can be treated with carinal resection alone or carinal resection combined with lobectomy. If small tumors are involving the carina, nonsurgical approaches may be valuable.[19,55] Transbronchoscopic brachytherapy or photodynamic therapy may play an important adjuvant role in the future management of such localized tracheal invasion.

Satellite Nodules

Although ipsilobar satellite nodules are now considered T_4 tumors, the 5-year survival following resection of a tumor with an ipsilobar satellite lesion still warrants surgical resection. In many instances, the satellite lesion is discovered either at the time of pathological examination or by PET scanning. It is not possible to conclude that a satellite nodule seen on CT scan represents cancer as opposed to an inflammatory lesion. Given that the 5-year survival of this subset of T_4 disease is significant (>20%), the approach for these patients should be surgical unless there is evidence of disease elsewhere. Reports of survival in patients with ipsilobar satellite nodules vary. Although in most reports, the presence of satellite nodules is associated with a poor prognosis, it does not have the same prognosis as other T_4 lesions.[5]

Organ Involvement

T_4 lesions can be completely resected in selected instances for an occasional cure. This includes direct invasion of the vertebra, SVC, esophagus, or atrium. It is this group of patients for whom induction therapy, either chemotherapy or chemoradiotherapy, is currently being investigated. Early reports have suggested the down staging of such patients, allowing for less radical resections.[94] Others[21] approach such lesions without preoperative treatment, using imaging and invasive staging to assess operability and resectability of the involved adjacent structure.

With improved surgical techniques and the use of cardiopulmonary bypass where indicated, reports are emerging of patients having had main pulmonary arteries reconstructed, SVCs reconstructed, and total vertebrectomies being performed for this stage of disease. The rare, fortunate patient who has had an R0 resection can be cured of his or her tumor with this very aggressive approach.[110,131] If one highly selects such patients, up to a 25% 5-year survival can be expected in the presence of an R0 resection.

N_3 Disease

Contralateral mediastinal lymph node metastases are considered by most surgeons to be an absolute contraindication to surgery because long-term survival with surgery is rare and anecdotal. However, the Southwest Oncology Group has completed a phase II induction chemotherapy and radiotherapy program followed by surgery for this group of patients. The early results of this trial suggested a complete resection rate similar to that seen with induction therapy for N_2 disease.[98] Long-term results, including survival rates, in patients treated for N_3 disease by this aggressive fashion have been reported. None of the patients with N_3 disease due to contralateral mediastinal involvement survived 5 years. The only survivors were two patients with preoperatively proven scalene node involvement. At the time of surgery, no attempt was made to remove the cervical lymph nodes. It can be concluded that in this form of combined modality therapy the radiotherapy was responsible for curing the extrathoracic disease. Some centers in Japan use a median sternotomy to accomplish an extended lymph node dissection that includes contralateral mediastinal and ipsilateral or bilateral neck node dissection for patients with N_3 involvement. Occasional long-term survivors have been documented using this aggressive approach.[43,82,128] Although unlikely to provide substantial long-term benefit, these approaches are worthy of well-constructed clinical trials. At the present time, however, the standard of care for patients with proven N_3 involvement is chemotherapy and/or radiation without surgery.

In a recent update by Hata of 232 patients undergoing bilateral mediastinal lymph node dissection over a 20-year period, the overall survival of patients ultimately staged as having N_3 disease was 41% (47 patients). This was identical to that seen with those patients ultimately found to have N_2 disease. Of the 16 patients preoperatively identified as having N_3 disease, there was similar (46%) 5-year survival following bilateral lymphadenectomy. In patients identified as having supraclavicular nodal disease, Hata extended his resection to include not only bilateral mediastinal lymph nodes but also a bilateral neck dissection. In these 40 patients, a 20% 5-year survival was achieved. Spurred by this information, other surgeons in Japan are now exploring this very extended lymph node dissection. It is unknown what adjuvant therapies were used in the Hata series. As yet, surgeons in Europe and North America have not adopted this very aggressive approach, offering primary chemoradiation for those patients with preoperatively identified N3 disease. When bilateral mediastinal lymphadenectomy is used with or without cervical lymphadenectomy, the overall survival according to pathological stage exceeds that achieved by other surgical approaches regardless of combination with radiation or chemotherapy. Although the value of postoperative treatment in this group of aggressively treated patients is unknown, most surgeons advocate postoperative radiotherapy if an induction approach has not been used.

► SOLITARY METASTASES (M₁)

Brain

Patients occasionally present with resectable lung cancer and evidence of a solitary metastasis on complete organ scanning. These patients should be considered for resection of both the primary tumor and the solitary metastasis. PET scanning can be useful in ruling out other sites of disease. Brain metastases constitute nearly one third of all observed recurrences in patients with resected non-small-cell lung cancer,[12] and twice that incidence is found at autopsy of all patients dying of lung cancer. Most brain metastases occur in those patients with a histological diagnosis of adenocarcinoma as opposed to squamous or large-cell carcinoma. When local and regional control can be achieved but brain metastases develop as the sole site of metastasis, the therapy employed for the brain metastasis ultimately determines survival.

Untreated patients with brain metastases have a median survival of less than 3 months. When brain metastases are multiple or advanced systemic disease is also present, the therapy of choice is whole-brain irradiation. However, one third of patients presenting with brain metastases have solitary lesions. Therapy with surgery or radiation can be effective, with reports of 18% and 13% 3- and 5-year survival, respectively.[10] Those most likely to receive long-term benefit from surgical resection, or stereotactic radiosurgery, are patients with a single surgically accessible brain metastasis and no other evident systematic disease. Randomized trials suggest that surgery offers the best form of palliation despite other noncerebral metastases.[86] High-dose corticosteroid therapy should be the initial treatment prescribed for all patients, as it reduces edema and can cause regression of neurological symptoms that is sometimes complete. Surgery or radiation therapy is usually initiated after 3–4 days of steroid therapy.

Two studies now have demonstrated conclusively that surgical extirpation followed by whole-brain irradiation is superior to whole-brain irradiation alone in managing solitary cerebral metastases with regard to survival and quality of life. No study has compared the newer forms of stereotactic radiosurgery directed solely at the solitary metastatic focus, although the results of such nonsurgical therapies are encouraging.

When the brain lesion is detected first and the search for the primary tumor is negative, resection of the cranial metastasis is the therapy of choice.[10,68] When the brain metastasis presents subsequent to the resection of the lung carcinoma and no other site of recurrence is present or the patient has minimal disease elsewhere, resection of the intracranial lesion is again the therapy of choice. When both brain and lung lesions are detected simultaneously, if both lesions are resectable, craniotomy is done first and thoracotomy shortly thereafter, unless symptoms from the primary tumor (e.g., significant hemoptysis) dictate otherwise. If either the lung or brain lesion is suspected to be unresectable, surgical therapy is directed first to the site where resectability is questioned most; otherwise therapy by nonsurgical means is recommended. Postoperative whole-brain irradiation is usually prescribed for all patients who have had resected brain metastases because of its potential ability to sterilize the tumor bed, even in patients who have had an apparent complete surgical excision.

Patients undergoing resection for solitary brain metastases have a 1-year survival of 55% and a mean survival of just greater than 2 years.[10,68] The overall 5-year survival rate for such patients approaches 20%. Surgical therapy should be offered to patients with single surgically accessible brain metastases, no evident systemic disease elsewhere, and a primary cancer confined to the lung.

Lung

Despite the possibility of a second lesion being a metastatic deposit, most second lesions represent synchronous primary tumors and the patient should be considered for resection of both tumors whenever possible. The long-term results of those patients with true solitary lung metastases also suggest that many patients can be salvaged. Deslauriers et al[25] reviewed the solitary metastatic lesions identified in resected specimens and reported a 22% 5-year survival rate. Similarly, in patients with synchronous primary pulmonary metastases, about 25% achieve similar long-term survival when treated surgically.

Adrenal Gland

Solitary adrenal metastases are being detected with increasing frequency because of routine upper abdominal CT scanning in the preoperative workup.[3,11,84,102] Resection of the primary tumor and the solitary metastatic focus should be considered if both are completely resectable.[93,95,122] Although 5-year survivors have been reported, the long-term results of such aggressive therapy are unknown. This should be viewed in light of the fact that no 5-year survivors have been reported with nonsurgical therapy.

Bone and Other Sites

It is rare for true solitary metastases from a lung primary to occur in the bone, liver, and other common metastatic sites, such as the skin. However, if thorough preoperative staging procedures do not reveal any other sites of metastases and if both lesions (primary and solitary metastatic focus) are completely resectable, surgical therapy can be offered if the risks are low. This is preferably done in the setting of a clinical trial.

SMALL-CELL LUNG CANCER

Although surgery for small-cell lung cancer (SCLC) was the initial therapy of choice historically, this was abandoned following the results of a randomized trial by the Medical Research Council (MRC) in England that compared radiotherapy alone with surgery alone in patients with limited disease.[34,78] Despite the mean survival time for these patients being short (10 months), with only 5% survival at 5 years, the fact that all surviving patients were being treated in the radiation arm made this the standard form of therapy. Currently, chemotherapy is the standard therapy for limited stage SCLC.[66] For SCLC lesions presenting as a solitary pulmonary nodule, many groups around the world recommend pulmonary resection combined with multiple courses of combination chemotherapy with or without thoracic irradiation and prophylactic cranial irradiation.[36,37] The majority of these patients have peripheral stage T_1N_0 lesions determined to be SCLC at pathological review. Reports from the late 1970s and early 1980s demonstrate that surgery alone can provide curative therapy in up to 25% of such patients.[81,108]

It is difficult to compare the results of multimodal approaches that include surgery to chemoradiation alone for SCLC as most medical oncologists do not classify very limited peripheral tumors as a separate entity.[106] Retrospective analyses suggest mixed results; Osterlind and colleagues[85] reported no beneficial effect for surgical resection, whereas Shepherd and associates suggest a 2-fold improvement in survival when surgery was used as part of therapy.[103]

PALLIATIVE RESECTIONS

For surgery to be effective and potentially curative in controlling lung cancer, the resection must be complete. The role of surgery for the palliation of patients with unresectable tumors is debatable. There are specific situations, such as an unremitting lung abscess distal to an obstructing tumor, massive hemoptysis, or painful invasion of the chest wall (ribs or vertebrae) that have led surgeons to consider and perform palliative or incomplete resections in the hope of improving the patient's symptoms.

Lung Abscess

An unresolving lung abscess, caused by either a necrotizing tumor (usually a squamous cell carcinoma) or a lung abscess distal to an obstructing tumor, rarely requires surgical resection. Other options, such as endobronchial laser therapy to relieve the proximal obstruction followed by external radiotherapy or percutaneous drainage of the abscess, usually suffice to alleviate the symptoms. However, if complete resection is probable, a surgical approach should be considered. Otherwise the lesser measures described may relieve

symptoms and result in satisfactory palliation without the potential morbidity of noncurative surgery.

Massive Hemoptysis

Massive uncontrolled hemoptysis is a rare feature of untreated lung cancer. Most frequently it is the result of the development of a bronchovascular fistula following radiotherapy. The pulmonary artery, aorta, or eroded bronchial vessels are the common sources of bleeding. In most of these examples, exsanguination and/or suffocation lead to instantaneous death of the patient. Occasionally, persisting but significant hemoptysis can allow time to control the bleeding. Bronchoscopic treatment by cautery or laser coagulation or the placement of an endobronchial blocker or bronchial artery embolization by percutaneous angiography may relieve the problem. Rarely is thoracotomy indicated, irrespective of a tumor's resectability. In completely unresectable cases, hilar stripping of all vessels from the bronchi can relieve the problem. On occasion a palliative resection is required to control bleeding.

Chest Wall Invasion

When a patient with an otherwise unresectable tumor as a result of extensive nodal involvement or distant metastases presents with excruciating chest wall pain caused by invasion of the ribs or vertebrae, consideration is occasionally given to resection of the primary tumor for palliative purposes. This approach is typically combined with radiotherapy despite the usual prior failure of this modality. In most cases it is preferable to use other nonsurgical measures, such as external beam irradiation or narcotics and even a rhizotomy when necessary. However, on rare occasions, when thoracic vertebrae are invaded and destroyed and are causing extradural compression, attempts at resection of the primary tumor invading the vertebra together with vertebral body resection have been employed with reports of 5-year survival in selected cases.[32] This can be performed with or without the addition of brachytherapy in an attempt to protect the spine from high-dose external irradiation. Short-term pain relief can be obtained in this fashion. Unfortunately, in most instances, the tumor recurs within 3–6 months. The palliative benefit obtained by these surgical approaches has never been prospectively compared with that of less aggressive alternatives for pain control.

In summary, palliative resections should be avoided when less aggressive nonsurgical approaches are available that provide similar palliative results.

POSTOPERATIVE MORBIDITY AND MORTALITY RATES

Because most reported cures in carcinoma of the lung have occurred in patients treated surgically, it is natural to want to expand the role of surgery, either alone or combined with radiation, chemotherapy, or both. However, many nonsurgical physicians are justifiably concerned with the postoperative mortality figures of 5–20% quoted in the literature, along with morbidity rates as high as 40%.

Proper case selection and careful preoperative and perioperative management are essential to minimize postoperative complications. Major complications occur in nearly 10% of patients with stage I or II disease, and up to 20% of those requiring extended resections for the treatment of locally advanced stage III tumors.[26] In most series, the total morbidity following surgical resection for lung cancer approaches 40%, with approximately 20% of these events being major. Major complications would include the risk of intrathoracic hemorrhage, pneumonia, bronchopleural fistula, and empyema. Mortality rates, however, can vary significantly and are influenced by a number of factors. An analysis by Reed and colleagues[109] demonstrated that surgeons formally trained in cardiothoracic surgery perform oncological resections with lower morbidity and mortality rates. Other reports, however, suggest that the total volume of pulmonary resections performed does not influence these outcome measures.[6] It has been suggested that multimodality therapies may increase these rates of adverse outcome, particularly in the case of right pneumonectomy.[1]

The Lung Cancer Study Group analyzed 2000 consecutive resections for lung cancer and reported an overall postoperative mortality rate of 3.3%.[38] More recent retrospective analyses confirm that pneumonectomy carries an overall 6–7% mortality rate, whereas lobectomy and lesser resections should not exceed a 2% postoperative mortality figure. A Japanese review suggests an impressive 30-day mortality rate of 3.2% for pneumonectomy and 1.2% for lobectomy.[124] To minimize complications a lesser resection may be considered in elderly patients and in all physiologically compromised persons who present an increased risk for surgery.

▶ SPECIFIC CONSIDERATIONS

Intraoperative Tumor Spillage

Transgression of the tumor with spillage of cells intraoperatively theoretically can lead to pleural implants and local recurrence. If such tumor spillage occurs, the hemithorax should be copiously irrigated with large quantities of saline. Whether cell lysing agents (e.g., hypertonic saline, water, absolute alcohol, or chemotherapeutic agents) have any role to play in such irrigations is unknown.

Positive Resection Margins

Bronchial, vascular, and close-proximity margins should be always monitored by frozen-section analysis at the time of surgery. Reresection to negative margins is advised whenever a positive margin is identified. Although a 2-cm bronchial resection margin is ideal, we accept a negative margin, regardless of the distance from the tumor. *In situ* disease at the resection margin carries a much better prognosis than that caused by invasive disease or submucosal or adventitial lymphatic involvement.[54] Most surgeons advocate postoperative radiation in these circumstances because of the potential value of minimizing local-regional recurrence, although there is no evidence yet to suggest an improvement in long-term survival. Any remaining residual disease can potentially be approached with endoluminal

brachytherapy or photodynamic therapy using hematoporphyrin derivatives.

Perioperative Blood Transfusion

Retrospective data have not definitively confirmed an adverse prognostic effect of perioperative blood transfusion in the long-term survival of patients with resected lung cancers. Tartter et al[116] reported that perioperative blood transfusion adversely affects the prognosis after the resection of stage I non-small-cell lung cancer. In 165 patients with stage I disease, using disease-free survival rates as the end point, they found a significantly decreased disease-free survival rate in transfused patients. Hyman et al[47] also reported a significantly increased relative risk of dying in transfused patients among 105 patients with stage I or II resected lung cancer.

To determine the impact of perioperative transfusion on the recurrence-free interval, the status of 352 patients treated by resection for stages I and II non-small-cell lung cancer at Memorial Sloan-Kettering Cancer Center was investigated.[56] The recurrence rate was not significantly different in transfused patients compared with those who received no blood, even when stratified for stage. Furthermore the number of units transfused was not associated with the time to tumor recurrence. These results did not support the contention that perioperative blood transfusion is associated with a decreased recurrence-free interval. Despite this, unnecessary blood transfusions should be avoided whenever possible.

Lobectomy vs. Pneumonectomy

Intraoperatively, particularly with central lesions by virtue of the primary tumor or involved lymph nodes, a decision has to be made whether a lobectomy or pneumonectomy should be performed. Incomplete resections never cure. Before considering a lobectomy complete, all resection margins should be confirmed by frozen-section analysis. The "sump" lymph nodes lying on the pulmonary artery between the upper and lower lobes should be examined. If there is any question that these contain tumor, indicating that a larger resection (e.g., pneumonectomy) is required, frozen-section analysis of such lymph nodes should be performed. When performing an upper lobectomy, involvement of the sump lymph nodes between the upper and lower lobes necessitates a completion pneumonectomy. Following right lower lobectomy, involvement of the sump nodes around the middle lobe requires the addition of a middle lobectomy. Any lymph involvement proximal to the upper lobe takeoff along the mainstem bronchi necessitates pneumonectomy, as does involvement of the lymph nodes around the main pulmonary artery. In all instances the surgeon must remember that there is one good chance to cure the patient, and a complete resection is required for this to occur.

▶ LOCAL RECURRENCE FOLLOWING INITIAL PULMONARY RESECTION

The majority of patients undergoing pulmonary resection for lung cancer do experience recurrence particularly those

272 with greater than stage I disease. With all stages of disease, one third of recurrences are initially local, with two thirds occurring at distant sites. In highly selected patients, a local recurrence can be treated with resection with a hope of ultimate cure if there is no evidence of regional or distant metastases.

Local recurrences following limited pulmonary resections are frequently problematic given that the limited resection is usually performed initially due to concern that the patient cannot tolerate a larger resection. Nonetheless, serious consideration should be given to completion lobectomy. Most patients even with severe diminution of pulmonary function can tolerate a lobectomy.

Occasionally, endobronchial recurrences at the stump of a previous resection are limited to the mucosal and submucosal layers rather than occurring in peribronchial lymph nodes, which harbors a much poorer prognosis. In selected post-lobectomy patients, a sleeve resection or completion pneumonectomy may be indicated. Alternatively, endobronchial recurrences can be treated locally with brachytherapy or photodynamic therapy. In recent series, the postoperative mortality for completion pneumonectomy ranges from 0 to 15%, and 5-year survival averages approximately 25%. There appears to be no difference in outcome if the resection was performed for locally recurrent disease or for a second primary tumor (Table 17-3). In rare circumstances, reresection of the bronchial stump following pneumonectomy may be warranted, although it usually requires a carinal resection with postoperative mortality approaching 20%.

Mediastinal lymph nodes can harbor occult metastases following surgical resection, and recurrences can be isolated to these areas. Most instances of nodal recurrence in the mediastinum, however, present with extensive involvement, and patients typically have symptoms related to compression of the trachea, esophagus, or superior vena cava. If disease is limited to intraparenchymal or hilar lymph nodes, and this can be proven on staging investigations (mediastinoscopy or PET scanning), then completion pneumonectomy can be considered with a goal of cure. Adjuvant therapies may be beneficial in such circumstances but this is not known at present.

Recurrences within the chest wall or pleura unfortunately often represent more diffuse processes within the pleural space. The most common indication for surgical management of a pleural recurrence is the development of a malignant pleural effusion significant enough to cause symptoms. Pleural drainage and pleurodesis are often worthwhile if the residual lung is expandable. If the lung cannot be expanded following drainage, then ambulatory pleural catheters can be used to drain fluid and relieve symptoms.

In summary, most patients presenting with local recurrent disease will also be found to have concurrent metastatic disease. On occasion, local recurrences may be isolated and warrant reresection with curative intent.

▶ POSTRESECTION FOLLOW-UP FOR NON-SMALL-CELL LUNG CANCER

The overall survival figures for stage II disease remain at approximately 45% even with a curative R0 resection and pathologically negative margins. Although local and systemic interventions may improve survival after primary therapy in these patients, it is unclear if additional survival advantages exist from successful treatment of recurrent disease or second primaries if they develop. Given the substantial health care costs associated with regular routine postoperative follow-up by thoracic surgeons, the utility of this approach has been questioned.[125] After resection of an early stage lung cancer, new primaries develop at a rate of approximately 2–5% per year.[53] Although many protocols examining the question are currently underway, the optimal postresection follow-up strategy is yet to be defined. A balance of specialty care from the thoracic surgeon and general medical care from the patient's regular physician appears to be a reasonable approach. At the Toronto General Hospital, we routinely see patients at 1, 3, 6, 12, 18, and 24 months following resection, then yearly to 5 years. Patients would be discharged from routine thoracic surgical follow-up if they remain disease free beyond this point.

▶ MEDIASTINAL LYMPH NODE DISSECTION

It is widely acknowledged that routine mediastinal lymph node dissections provide the best surgical staging at the time of operation and may contribute to long-term survival in patients with occult N_2 disease. A current North American trial may ultimately resolve the role of mediastinal lymph node sampling vs. dissection in early stage tumors. In hilar N_1 and N_2 disease, mediastinal lymphadenectomy is advised and supported by a recent report of a North American intergroup trial.[57] The results of extending this lymph node

Table 17–3
Mortality and 5-Year Survival following Completion of Pneumonectomy for Recurrent or Second Primary Lung Cancer

Reference	Number of patients	Mortality (%)	5-Year survival (%)
McGovern (1988)	84	9.4	26.4
Gregoire (1993)	41	11.6	33
Terzi (1995)	32	3.6	28.7
Al-Katten (1995)	26	0	23
Verhagen (1996)	33	15.2	18.3
Muysoms (1998)	76	13.2	32.3
Regnard (1999)	62	5	35

dissection in patients with N_2 disease to include two-field lymphadenectomies has been explored in Japan.[43,82,128] Long-term survivors have been described using this approach even in the face of N_3 disease.

SUMMARY

Complete surgical resection continues to be the mainstay of potentially curative treatment in most patients with resectable lung cancers. Oncological principles dictate that incomplete resection is to be avoided. With advances in surgical technique, complex resections of advanced tumors for potential cure can be undertaken. Data from studies of lung volume reduction[83] suggest that curative lung resections can be achieved with acceptable morbidity and mortality even in patients with severely compromised lung function. In summary, careful and accurate staging with surgery plus or minus chemotherapy and/or radiotherapy in selected cases remains the optimal treatment of lung cancer today.

REFERENCES

1. Abolhoda A, Martin J, Ginsberg R, et al: Morbidity and mortality for pulmonary resections in lung cancer after induction treatment. 9th World Conference on Lung Cancer, Toyko, Japan, September, 2000.
2. Allan CI, Smith FJ: Primary carcinoma of the lung with report of case treated by operation. Surg Gynecol Obstet 55: 151, 1932.
3. Allard P, Yankaskas BC, Fletcher RH, et al: Sensitivity and specificity of computed tomography for the detection of adrenal metastatic lesions among 91 autopsied lung cancer patients. Cancer 66:457, 1990.
4. American Cancer Society: Cancer Facts and Figures 2001. American Cancer Society, 2002. http://www.cancer.org.
5. Battafarano RJ, Myers BF, Guthrie TJ, et al: Surgical resection of multifocal non-small cell lung cancer is associated with prolonged survival. Ann Thorac Surg 74:988–994, 2002.
6. Begg CB, Cramer LD, Hoskins WJ, Brennan MF: Impact of hospital volume on postoperative mortality for major cancer surgery. JAMA 280:1747, 1998.
7. Brunn HB: Surgical principles underlying one-stage lobectomy. Arch Surg 18:490, 1929.
8. Burkes RL, Ginsberg RJ, Shephard FA, et al: Induction chemotherapy with mitomycin, vindesine and cisplatin for stage III unresectable non-small-cell lung cancer: Results of the Toronto phase II trial. J Clin Oncol 10(4):580–586, 1992.
9. Burt ME, Pomerantz AH, Bains MS, et al: Results of surgical treatment of stage III lung cancer invading the mediastinum. Surg Clin North Am 67:987, 1987.
10. Burt M, Wronski M, Arbit E, et al: Resection of brain metastases from non-small cell lung carcinoma: Results of therapy. J Thorac Cardiovasc Surg 103:399, 1992.
11. Burt ME, Heelan R, Coit D, et al: Prospective evaluation of unilateral adrenal metastases in patients with operable non-small cell lung cancer: Impact of magnetic resonance imaging. J Thorac Cardiovasc Surg 107:584, 1994.
12. Ceresoli GL, Reni M, Chiesa G, et al: Brain metastases in locally advanced nonsmall cell lung carcinoma after multimodality treatment: Risk factors analysis. Cancer 95(3):605–612, 2002.
13. Chardak WM, MacCallun JD: Pancoast tumor (5 yr survival without recurrence or metastases following radical resection and postoperative irradiation). J Thorac Surg 31:535, 1956.
14. Churchill ED: The surgical treatment of carcinoma of the lung. J Thorac Surg 2:254, 1933.
15. Churchill E, Belsey HR: Segmental pneumonectomy in bronchiectasis. Ann Surg 109:481, 1939.
16. Churchill ED, Sweet RH, Sutter L, Scannel JG: The surgical management of carcinoma of the lung: A study of cases treated at the Massachusetts General Hospital from 1930–1950. J Thorac Cardiovasc Surg 20:349, 1950.
17. Coleman FP: Primary carcinoma of the lung with invasion of ribs: Pneumonectomy and simultaneous block resection of chest wall. Ann Surg 126:156, 1947.
18. Cooper JD, Nelems JM, Pearson FG: Extended indications for median sternotomy in patients requiring pulmonary resection. Ann Thorac Surg 26:413, 1978.
19. Cortese DA, Edell ES, Kinsey JH: Photodynamic therapy for early stage squamous cell carcinoma of the lung. Mayo Clin Proc 72:595, 1997.
20. Dartevelle PG: Extended operations for the treatment of lung cancer. Ann Thorac Surg 63:12, 1997.
21. Dartevelle PG, Macchiarini P: Surgical management of superior sulcus tumors. Oncologist 4:398, 1999.
22. Davies HM: Recent advances in the surgery of the lung and pleura. Br J Surg 1:228; 1913–1914.
23. Depierre A, Milleron B, Moro D, et al: Phase III trial of neoadjuvant therapy (NCT) in resectable stage I (except T1N0), II, IIIa non-small cell lung cancer (NSCLC): The French experience. Proc Am Soc Clin Oncol 18:465a, 1999.
24. Deslauriers J: Involvement of the main carina. In Delarue NC, Eschapasse H, editors: International Trends in General Thoracic Surgery. Philadelphia: W.B. Saunders, 1985, p. 139.
25. Deslauriers J, Brisson J, Cartier R, et al: Carcinoma of the lung: Evaluation of satellite nodules as a factor influencing prognosis after resection. J Thorac Cardiovasc Surg 97:504, 1989.
26. Deslauriers J, Ginsberg RJ, Dubois P, et al: Current operative morbidity associated with elective surgical resection for lung cancer. Can J Surg 32:335, 1989.
27. Dillman RO, Herndon J, Seagran SL, et al: Improved survival in stage III non-small cell lung cancer: Seven year follow up of cancer and leukemia group B (CALGB) trial 8433. J Natl Cancer Inst 88:1210, 1996.
28. Downey RJ, Martini N, Rusch VW, et al: Extent of chest wall invasion and survival in patients with lung cancer. Ann Thorac Surg 68:188, 1999.
29. Edell ES, Cortese DA: Bronchoscopic localization and treatment of occult lung cancer. Chest 96:919, 1989.
30. Errett LE, Wilson J, Chiu RC, Monroe DD: Wedge resection as an alternative procedure for peripheral bronchogenic carcinoma in poor-risk patients. J Thorac Cardiovasc Surg 90:656, 1985.
31. Faber LP, Jensik RJ, Kittle CF: Results of sleeve lobectomy for bronchogenic carcinoma in 101 patients. Ann Thorac Surg 37: 279, 1984.
32. Fadel E, Missenard G, Chapelier A, et al: En bloc resection of non-small cell lung cancer invading the thoracic inlet and intervertebral foramina. J Thorac Cardiovasc Surg 123(4):676–685, 2002.
33. Ferguson MK, MacMahon H, Little AG, et al: Regional accuracy of computed tomography of the mediastinum in staging of lung cancer. J Thorac Cardiovasc Surg 91:498, 1986.
34. Fox W, Scadding JG: Medical Research Council comparative trial of surgery and radiotherapy for primary treatment of small celled or oat called carcinoma of the bronchus: Ten year follow-up. Lancet 2:63, 1973.
35. Gaissert HA, Mathisen DJ, Moncure AC, et al: Survival and function after sleeve lobectomy for lung cancer. J Thorac Cardiovasc Surg 111(5):948–953, 1996.
36. Ginsberg RJ: Surgery and small cell lung cancer—an overview. Lung Cancer 5:232, 1989.

37. Ginsberg RJ, Karrer K: Surgery in small cell lung cancer—an overview. Lung Cancer 5:139, 1989.

38. Ginsberg RJ, Hill LD, Eagan RT, et al: Modern thirty-day operative mortality for surgical resections in lung cancer. J Thorac Cardiovasc Surg 86:498, 1983.

39. Ginsberg RJ, Rubinstein L, Lung Cancer Study Group: A randomized trial of lobectomy versus limited resection in patients with T1N0 non-small cell lung cancer. Ann Thorac Surg 60:615–622, 1995.

40. Gould PM, Bonner JA, Sawyer TE, et al: Patterns of failure and overall survival in patients with completely resected T3 N0 M0 non-small cell lung cancer. Int J Radiat Oncol Biol Phys 45:91, 1999.

41. Graham EA, Singer JJ: Successful removal of the entire lung for carcinoma of the bronchus. JAMA 101:1371, 1933.

42. Graves WG, Martinez MJ, Carter PL, et al: The value of computed tomography in staging bronchogenic carcinoma: A changing role for mediastinoscopy. Ann Thorac Surg 40:57, 1985.

43. Hata E, Hayakawa K, Miyamoto H, et al: The incidence and prognosis of the contralateral mediastinal node involvement of the let lung cancer patients who underwent bilateral mediastinal dissection and pulmonary resection through a median sternotomy (abstr). Lung Cancer 4:A87, 1988.

44. Hayata Y, Kato, Konaka C, et al: Photoradiation therapy with hematoporphyrin derivative in early and stage I lung cancer. Chest 86:169, 1984.

45. Henschke CI, McCauley DI, Yankelovitz DF, et al: Early lung cancer action project: Overall design and findings from baseline screening. Lancet 354:99, 1999.

46. Holmes EC, Gail M, Lung Cancer Study Group: Surgical adjuvant therapy for stage II and III adenocarcinoma and large cell undifferentiated carcinoma. J Clin Oncol 4:710, 1986.

47. Hyman NH, Foster RS Jr, DeMeules JE, Costanza MC: Blood transfusions and survival after lung cancer resection. Am J Surg 149:502, 1985.

48. Icard P, Regnard JF, Guibert L, et al: Survival and prognostic factors in patients undergoing parenchymal saving bronchoplastic operation for primary lung cancer: A series of 110 consecutive patients. Eur J Cardiothorac Surg 15: 426, 1999.

49. Ichinose Y, Tsuchiya R, Kato H: Randomized trial of chemotherapy versus surgery for stage IIIA non-small cell lung cancer. Lung Cancer 29(Suppl 2):173, 2000.

50. Jensik RJ: Miniresection of small peripheral carcinomas of the lung. Surg Clin North Am 67:951, 1987.

51. Jensik RJ, Faber LP, Milloy FJ, Monson DO: Segmental resection for lung cancer. A fifteen year experience. J Thorac Cardiovasc Surg 66:563, 1973.

52. Jensik RJ, Faber LP, Kittle CF, et al: Survival in patients undergoing tracheal sleeve pneumonectomy for bronchogenic carcinoma. J Thorac Cardiovasc Surg 84:489, 1982.

53. Johnson BE: Second lung cancers in patients after treatment for an initial lung cancer. J Natl Cancer Inst 90:1335, 1998.

54. Kaiser LR, Fleschner P, Keller S, Martini N: The significance of extramucosal residual tumor at the bronchial resection margin. Ann Thorac Surg 47:265, 1989.

55. Kato H, Okunaka T, Shimatani H: Photodynamic therapy for early stage bronchogenic carcinoma. J Clin Laser Med Surg 14:235, 1996.

56. Keller SM, Groshen S, Martini N, Kaiser LF: Blood transfusion and lung cancer recurrence. Cancer 62:606, 1988.

57. Keller SM, Adak S, Wagner H, et al: Complete mediastinal lymph node dissection improves survival in patients with resected stages I and IIIa non-small cell lung cancer. Ann Thorac Surg 70:358, 2000.

58. Kodama K, Doi O, Higashiyama M, Yokouchi H: Intentional limited resection for selected patients with T1N0M0 non-

59. Konaka C, Ikeda N, Hiyoshi T, et al: Peripheral non-small cell lung cancers 2.0 cm or less in diameter: Proposed criteria for limited pulmonary resection based upon clinicopathological presentation. Lung Cancer 27:185, 1988.

60. Kris MG, Gralla RJ, Martini N, et al: Preoperative and adjuvant chemotherapy in patients with locally advanced non-small cell lung cancer. Surg Clin North Am 67:1051, 1987.

61. Kulka F, Forai I: The segmental and apical resection of primary lung cancer. Proceedings of the IV World Conference on Lung Cancer, Toronto, Canada, 1985, p. 81.

62. Lam S, MacAulay C, Hung J, et al: Detection of dysplasia and carcinoma in situ with a lung imaging fluorescence endoscopic device. J Thorac Cardiovasc Surg 105:1035, 1993.

63. Lausberg HF, Graeter TP, Wendler O, et al: Bronchial and bronchovascular sleeve resection for treatment of central lung tumors. Ann Thorac Surg 70:367, 2000.

64. Le Chevalier T (for the IALT Investigators): Results of the randomized International Adjuvant Lung Cancer Trial (IALT): Cisplatin-based chemotherapy (CT) vs no CT in 1867 patients (pts) with resected non-small cell lung cancer (NSCLC). Proc Am Soc Clin Oncol 22:2, 2003.

65. Liptay MJ, Masters BA, Freed BH, Bakshey AG: Intraoperative radioisotope sentinel lymph node mapping in non-small cell lung cancer. Lung Cancer 29(Suppl 1):138, 2000.

66. Livingston RG: Current chemotherapy of small cell lung cancer. Chest 89:2585, 1986.

67. Lung Cancer Study Group: Effects of postoperative mediastinal radiation on completely resected stage II and stage III epidermoid cancer of the lung. N Engl J Med 315: 1377, 1986.

68. Magilligan DJ Jr, Duvernoy C, Malik G, et al: Surgical approach to lung cancer with solitary cerebral metastasis: Twenty-five years' experience. Ann Thorac Surg 42:360, 1986.

69. Martini N: Rationale for surgical treatment of brain metastasis in non-small cell lung cancer. Ann Thorac Surg 42:357, 1986.

70. Martini N, Flehinger BJ: The role of surgery in N2 lung cancer. Surg Clin North Am 67:1037, 1987.

71. Martini N, Melamed MR: Occult carcinomas of the lung. Ann Thorac Surg 30:215, 1980.

72. Martini N, Flehinger BJ, Zaman MB, Beattie EJ Jr: Results of resection in non-oat cell carcinoma of the lung with mediastinal lymph node metastases. Ann Surg 198:386, 1983.

73. Martini N, Heelan R, Westcott J: Comparative merits of conventional, computed tomographic and magnetic resonance imaging in assessing mediastinal involvement in surgically confirmed lung carcinoma. J Thorac Cardiovasc Surg 90:639, 1985.

74. Martini N, Bains MS, MacCormack PM, et al: Surgical treatment in non-small cell carcinoma of the lung: The Memorial Sloan-Kettering experience. In Hoogstraten B, Addis BJ, Hansen HH, et al, editors: (UICC) Current Treatment of Cancer, Lung Tumors. Heidelberg: Springer-Verlag, 1988, p. 111.

75. Martini N, Burt ME, Bains MS, et al: Survival after resection in stage II non-small cell lung cancer. Ann Thorac Surg 54: 460, 1992.

76. Martini N, Bains MS, Burt ME, et al: Incidence of local recurrence and second primary tumors in resected stage I lung cancer. J Thorac Cardiovasc Surg 109:120, 1995.

77. Mathey, J, Binet JP, Galey JJ, et al: Tracheal and tracheobronchial resections: Technique and results in 20 cases. J Thorac Cardiovasc Surg 51:1, 1966.

78. Miller AB, Fox W, Tall R: Five year follow-up of the Medical Research Council's comparative trial of surgery and radiother-

apy for primary treatment of small celled or oat celled carcinoma of the bronchus. Lancet 12:501, 1969.

79. Miller JI, Hatcher CR: Limited resection of bronchogenic carcinoma in the patient with marked impairment of pulmonary function. Ann Thorac Surg 44:340, 1987.

80. Mitchell JD, Mathisen DJ, Wright CD, et al: Clinical experience with carinal resection. J Thorac Cardiovasc Surg 117:39, 1999.

81. Mountain CF: Clinical biology of small cell lung cancer: Relationship to surgical therapy. Semin Oncol 5:272, 1978.

82. Naruke T, Goya T, Tsuchiya R, Suemasu K: Extended radical operation of N2 left lung cancer through median sternotome. Lung Cancer 4(Suppl):A87, 1988.

83. NETT Research Group: A randomized trial comparing lung volume reduction surgery with medical therapy for severe emphysema. N Engl J Med 348:2059, 2003.

84. Nielsen ME Jr, Heaston DK, Dunnick NR, Korobkin M: Preoperative CT evaluation of adrenal glands in non-small cell bronchogenic carcinoma. AJR Am J Roentgenol 139:317, 1982.

85. Osterlind K, Hansen M, Hansen HH, Dombernowsky P: Influence of surgical resection prior to chemotherapy on long-term results in small cell lung cancer. A study of 150 operable patients. Eur J Cancer 5:589, 1989.

86. Patchell RA, Tibbs PA, Walsh JW, et al: A randomized trial of surgery in the treatment of single metastases to brain. N Engl J Med 322:494, 1990.

87. Patterson GA, Ilves R, Ginsberg RJ, et al: The value of adjuvant radiotherapy in pulmonary and chest wall resection for bronchogenic carcinoma. Ann Thorac Surg 34:692, 1982.

88. Paulson DL, Urschel HC Jr: Selectivity in the surgical treatment of bronchogenic carcinoma. J Thorac Cardiovasc Surg 62:554, 1971.

89. Pean J: Chirurgie des poumons. Discussion Ranc Chir Proc Verh Paris 9:72, 1895.

90. Pearson FG: Mediastinal adenopathy—the N2 lesion. In Delarue NC, Eschapasse H, editors: International Trends in General Thoracic Surgery. Philadelphia: W.B. Saunders, 1985, p. 104.

91. Pitz CC, Brutel de la Riviere A, Elbers HR, et al: Results of resection of T3 non-small cell lung cancer invading the mediastinum or main bronchus. Ann Thorac Surg 62: 1016, 1996.

92. Price-Thomas C: Conservative resection of the bronchial tree. J R Coll Surg Edinb 1:169, 1956.

93. Raviv G, Klein E, Yellin A, et al: Surgical treatment of solitary adrenal metastases from lung cancer. J Surg Oncol 43:124, 1990.

94. Rendina EA, Venuta F, DeGiacomo T, et al: Induction chemotherapy for T4 centrally located non-small cell lung cancer. J Thorac Cardiovasc Surg 117:225, 1999.

95. Reyes L, Parvez Z, Nemoto T, et al: Adrenalectomy for adrenal metastasis from lung carcinoma. J Surg Oncol 44:32, 1990.

96. Rosell R, Gomez-Codina, J, Camps, C, et al: A randomized trial comparing preoperative chemotherapy plus surgery with surgery alone in patients with non-small cell lung cancer. N Engl J Med 330:153, 1994.

97. Roth JA, Fosella F, Komaki R, et al: A randomized trial comparing perioperative chemotherapy and surgery with surgery alone in resectable Stage IIIA non-small cell lung cancer. J Natl Cancer Inst 86:673, 1994.

98. Rusch VW, Albain KS, Crowley JJ, et al: Surgical resection of stage IIIA and stage IIIB non-small cell lung cancer after concurrent induction chemoradiotherapy: A Southwest Oncology Group trial. J Thorac Cardiovasc Surg 105:97, 1993.

99. Rusch VW, Parekh KR, Leon L, et al: Factors determining outcome after surgical resection of T3 and T4 lung cancers

of the superior sulcus. J Thorac Cardiovasc Surg 119:1147, 2000.

100. Rusch VW, Giroux DJ, Kranton J, et al: Induction chemoradiation and surgical resection for non-small cell lung carcinomas of the superior sulcus: Initial results of Southwest Oncology Group trial 9416 (intergroup trial 0160). J Thorac Cardiovasc Surg 121:472, 2001.

101. Rusch, VW, Giroux DJ, Kraut J, et al: Induction chemoradiotiotherapy and surgical resection for non-small cell lung carcinomas of the superior sulcus (pancoast tumors): Mature results of Southwest Oncology Group trial 9416 (intergroup trial 0160). American Society of Clinical Oncology, Chicago, 2003 (abstract).

102. Sandler MA, Paerlberg JL, Madrazo BL, et al: Computed tomographic evaluation of the adrenal gland in the preoperative assessment of bronchogenic carcinoma. Radiology 145:733, 1982.

103. Salzer GM, Muller LC, Huber H, et al: Operation for N2 small cell lung carcinoma. Ann Thorac Surg 49:759, 1990.

104. Schaake-Koning C, Van Den Bogaert W, Dalesio O, et al: Effects of concomitant cisplatin and radiotherapy on inoperable non-small cell lung cancer. N Engl J Med 326:524, 1992.

105. Seely JM, Mayo JR, Miller RR, Muller NL: T1 lung cancer: Prevalence of mediastinal nodal metastasis and diagnostic accuracy of CT. Radiology 186(1):129, 1993.

106. Shepherd FA, Ginsberg RJ, Evans WK, et al: Very limited small cell lung cancer (SCLC): Results of non-surgical treatment. Proc Annu Meet Am Soc Clin Oncol 3:223, 1984.

107. Shields TW, Higgins GA, Lawton R, et al: Preoperative x-ray therapy as an adjuvant in the treatment of bronchogenic carcinoma. J Thorac Cardiovasc Surg 59:49, 1970.

108. Shields TW, Higgins GA, Matthews NJ, et al: Surgical resection in the management of small cell carcinoma of the lung. J Thorac Cardiovasc Surg 84:481, 1982.

109. Silvestri GA, Handy J, Lackland D, et al: Specialists achieve better outcomes than generalists for lung cancer surgery. Chest 114:675, 1998.

110. Spaggiari L, Solli P, Leo F: Tracheal sleeve and superior vena cava resection for bronchogenic carcinoma. Lung Cancer 29 (Suppl 1):135, 2000.

111. Stamatis G, Eberhardt W, Stuben G, et al: Preoperative chemoradiotherapy and surgery for selected non-small cell lung cancer IIIB subgroups: Long term results. Ann Thorac Surg 68:1144, 1999.

112. Sugi K, Kaneda Y, Esato K: The identification of sentinel lymph node by staining in lung cancer patients. Lung Cancer 29(Suppl 1):139, 2000.

113. Suzuki K, Nagai K, Yoshida Y, et al: The prognosis of surgically resected N2 non-small cell lung cancer: The importance of clinical N status. J Thorac Cardiovasc Surg 118:145, 1999.

114. Takita H, Merrin C, Didolkar MS, et al: The surgical management of multiple lung metastases. Ann Thorac Surg 24:359, 1977.

115. Takizawa T, Terashima M, Koike T, et al: Pulmonary function after segmentectomy for small peripheral carcinoma of the lung. J Thorac Cardiovasc Surg 118:536, 1999.

116. Tartter PE, Burrows L, Kirschner P: Perioperative blood transfusion adversely affects prognosis after resection of stage I (subset N0) non-oat cell lung cancer. J Thorac Cardiovasc Surg 88:659, 1984.

117. Taylor SG IV, Trybula M, Bonomi PD, et al: Simultaneous cisplatin-fluorouracil infusion and radiation followed by surgical resection in regionally localized stage III, non-small cell lung cancer. Ann Thorac Surg 43:87, 1987.

118. Thomas PA, Piantadosi S, Mountain CF: Should subcarinal lymph nodes be routinely examined in patients with non-small cell lung cancer? J Thorac Cardiovasc Surg 95:883, 1988.

276

119. Thompson DT: Tracheal resection with left lung anastomosis following right pneumonectomy. Thorax 21:560, 1966.

120. Tiffet O, Davies T, Jenc O: Preoperative detection of the sentinel lymph node in non-small cell lung cancer with radioisotope and blue dye technique. Lung Cancer 29(Suppl 1):138, 2000.

121. Tsubota J, Ayabe K, Doi O, et al: Ongoing prospective study of segmentectomy for small lung tumors. Study group of extended segmentectomy for small lung tumor. Ann Thorac Surg 66:1787, 1998.

122. Twomey P, Montgomery C, Clark O: Successful treatment of adrenal metastases from large-cell carcinoma of the lung. JAMA 248:581, 1982.

123. Vesselle H, Pugsley JM, Vallieres E, et al: The impact of fluorodeoxyglucose F18 positron-emission tomography on the surgical staging on non-small cell lung cancer. J Thorac Cardiovasc Surg 124:511–517, 2002.

124. Wada H, Nakamura T, Nakamoto K: Thirty-day operative mortality for thoracotomy for lung cancer. J Thorac Cardiovasc Surg 115:70, 1998.

125. Walsh GL, O'Connor M, Willis KM, et al: Is follow-up of lung cancer patients after resection medically indicated and cost-effective? Ann Thorac Surg 60:1563, 1995.

126. Warram J (collaborative study): Preoperative irradiation of cancer of the lung: Final report of a therapeutic trial. Cancer 36:914, 1975.

127. Warren WH, Faber LP: Segmentectomy vs lobectomy in patients with stage I pulmonary carcinoma: Five year survival and patterns of intrathoracic recurrence. J Thorac Cardiovasc Surg 107:1087, 1994.

128. Watanabe Y, Ichihashi T, Iwa T: Median sternotomy as an approach for pulmonary surgery. J Thorac Cardiovasc Surg 36:227, 1988.

129. Watanabe Y, Shimizu J, Oda M, et al: Proposals regarding some deficiencies in the new international staging system for non-small cell lung cancer. Jpn J Clin Oncol 21:160, 1991.

130. Weigel TL, Kosco PJ, Dacic S, et al: Fluorescence bronchoscopic surveillance in patients with a history of non-small cell lung cancer. Diagn Ther Endosc 6:1, 1999.

131. York JE, Walsh GL, Lang FF, et al: Combined chest wall resection with vertebrectomy and spinal reconstruction for the treatment of Pancoast tumors. J Neurosurg. 91(1 Suppl):74, 1999.

Lung Cancer: Minimally Invasive Approaches

Mark Onaitis and Thomas A. D'Amico

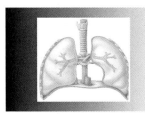

INTRODUCTION

The surgical approach in the management of patients with lung cancer is evolving. Conventional surgical approaches (including standard posterolateral thoracotomy, muscle-sparing thoracotomy, transsternal thoracotomy, and median sternotomy) remain the standard for the majority of patients with resectable lung cancer. Minimally invasive procedures, however, may be employed in selected patients with early-stage lung cancer to minimize operative morbidity without sacrificing oncological efficacy.

DEFINITION

Minimally invasive procedures, utilizing operative telescopes and video technology, are referred to synonymously as thoracoscopic procedures or video-assisted thoracic surgery (VATS). For clarity, the terms "VATS" or "thoracoscopic" refer to totally thoracoscopic approaches, where visualization is dependent on video monitors, and rib spreading is avoided. A hybrid procedure, which employs rib spreading and direct visualization in addition to thoracoscopy, may be referred to as video-assisted thoracotomy.

Thoracoscopy has been widely utilized diagnostically in the management of patients with lung cancer; thoracoscopic wedge resection to confirm malignancy prior to thoracotomy for anatomic resection is commonly performed. In addition, thoracoscopic therapeutic procedures, including pleurodesis for malignant pleural effusion and pericardial window for pericardial effusions, are also frequently performed. The application of thoracoscopic anatomic resections is comparatively new but increasing in utilization internationally.

Thoracoscopic lobectomy is defined as the anatomic resection of an entire lobe of the lung, using a videoscope and an access incision, without the use of a mechanical retractor and without rib spreading.[15,23,24,41] The anatomic resection includes individual dissection and stapling of the involved pulmonary vein, pulmonary artery, and bronchus and appropriate management of the mediastinal lymph nodes, as would be performed with thoracotomy. In selected patients, thoracoscopic anatomic segmentectomy may be formed, adhering to the same oncological principles that guide resection at thoracotomy.

Some surgeons have advocated simultaneous stapling of hilar structures with video assistance and the avoidance of rib spreading.[21,22] Such an approach has been termed video-assisted simultaneously stapled lobectomy. Although this technique has been utilized successfully in selected patients, the reference to "thoracoscopic lobectomy" is limited to anatomic resection with individual vessel ligation. VATS wedge resection describes nonanatomic thoracoscopic resection of a lesion, which is considered useful for diagnostic procedures.

To be considered a viable alternative to conventional lobectomy, thoracoscopic lobectomy must be applied with the same oncological principles: individual vessel ligation, complete anatomical resection with negative margins, complete hilar lymph node dissection, and appropriate management of the mediastinal lymph nodes. Theoretical advantages to minimally invasive resection include reduced surgical trauma, decreased postoperative pain, shorter chest tube duration, shorter length of stay, preserved pulmonary function, and superior cosmetic result when compared to lobectomy via open thoracotomy.[26,34,49]

HISTORY

The history of minimally invasive thoracic surgery began in 1910 when Jacobeus utilized a cystoscope to lyse adhesions in order to collapse the lung to treat tuberculosis.[12] This technique was widely applied in the early part of the century but was largely abandoned after streptomycin was introduced in 1945. However, with the emergence of laparoscopic cholecystectomy, minimally invasive approaches were applied more widely. The first descriptions of VATS to perform anatomic lobectomy were published in 1993 by Kirby and Rice[15] and Walker et al.[41] The first randomized trial of VATS lobectomy versus the conventional open approach was presented in 1994 and demonstrated no significant benefits for VATS.[16] With more widespread application of technology and refinements in technique, other groups have published series of VATS lobectomy* (Table 18-1).

INDICATIONS

In general, the indications for thoracoscopic lobectomy are similar to those for lobectomy using the open approach.[4,47] Thus, the procedure is applied to patients with known or suspected lung cancer (clinical stage I) that appears amenable to complete resection by lobectomy; preoperative staging and patient selection for thoracoscopic lobectomy should be con-

*References 3, 4, 10, 13, 21, 25, 32, 34, 38, 40, 47.

ducted as for conventional thoracotomy. Tumor size may preclude the option of thoracoscopic lobectomy in some patients, as some large specimens may not be amenable to removal without rib spreading; however, no absolute size criteria are used. Although controversial, some have also argued that the thoracoscopic approach may allow recruitment and resection of some patients considered "medically inoperable," who could not undergo conventional thoracotomy.[4,5,38] The minimal physiological requirements for resection have not been agreed upon; however, the selection of patients for thoracoscopic lobectomy must take into account that conversion to thoracotomy may be necessary.

CONTRAINDICATIONS

Absolute contraindications to thoracoscopic lobectomy include the inability to achieve complete resection with lobectomy, T_3 or T_4 tumors, N_2 or N_3 disease, and inability to achieve single-lung ventilation.[4,38] Relative contraindications include tumors that are visible at bronchoscopy, the presence of hilar lymphadenopathy that would complicate vascular

---

Table 18–1

Recent Series of Thoracoscopic Lobectomy[a]

Series	N	Conversion rate (%)	Method	LN dissection	Mortality (%)	Survival stage I (%)
Lewis and Caccavale[22]	200	0	SSL	Dissection	0	92 (3 years)
Hermansson et al[10]	30	6.7	SSL	Sampling	0	NA
Solaini et al[34]	125	10.4	IHD	Sampling	0	90 (3 years)
Brown[3]	105	7.6	IHD	Sampling	0	NA
Kaseda et al[13]	128	11.7	IHD	Dissection	0.8	94 (4 years)
McKenna et al[25]	212	7	IHD	Dissection	0.5	76 (4.5 years)
Roviaro et al[32]	171	19.9	IHD	Sampling	0	91 (1 year)
Walker[40]	150	11.8	IHD	Sampling	2	81 (5 years)
Yim et al[47]	214	0	IHD	Sampling	0.5	NA
Daniels et al[4]	110	1.8	IHD	Dissection	3.6	NA
Swanson et al[38]	97	8.5	IHD	Both	2.1	NA

[a]LN, Lymph node; IHD, individual hilar dissection; SSL, simultaneously stapled lobectomy; NA, not assessed.

dissection (benign or malignant), prior thoracic irradiation, and the use of induction therapy. Prior thoracic surgery, incomplete or absent fissures, and benign mediastinal adenopathy should not be considered contraindications.[4,5,38,48] Finally, chest wall involvement would obviate thoracoscopic resection for most patients, but successful en bloc resection via VATS has been reported.[43]

STRATEGY FOR THORACOSCOPIC LOBECTOMY

After bronchoscopy and mediastinoscopy (when indicated), single-lung anesthesia is established using a dual lumen endotracheal tube or bronchial blocker. The patient is positioned in a full lateral decubitus position with slight flexion of the table at the level of the hip, which provides splaying of the ribs to improve thoracoscopic access and exposure. Care must be taken to secure and pad the patient such that the risk of neurological injury is minimized. Once the patient is positioned, the anesthesiologist should reconfirm the desired position of the endotracheal tube. Prior to sterile preparation and draping, the chest is marked for the placement of thoracoscopic incisions.

Port placement is a matter of surgeon preference. Most surgeons use three or four incisions, although lobectomy can usually be accomplished using only two incisions.[4] The first incision, a 10-mm port access used predominantly for the thoracoscope, is placed in the seventh or eighth intercostal space in the midaxillary line. The location of this incision is chosen so that it does not compete with the anterior incision, yet still provides anterior and superior visualization of the hilum. A port is used for placement of the telescope, but ports are not used for the other incisions. Prior to making the second incision, evidence that the patient is unresectable should be sought, such as parietal pleural involvement.

The second incision, an anterior access incision (4.5–6.0 cm) for dissection and specimen retrieval, is placed in the fifth or sixth intercostal space, just inferior to the breast. The location of this incision, where the intercostal spaces are the widest, is chosen to provide access for hilar dissection and is usually not dependent on whether the planned procedure is an upper or lower lobectomy. Additional incisions may be employed, either in the axilla or posteriorly, to improve visualization or to provide retraction.

Instrumentation for thoracoscopic lobectomy is critical to successful completion of the procedure. The thoracoscope should be a 30° angled scope to optimize the ability to achieve panoramic visualization during dissection and to minimize competition with the operative instruments. A spectrum of surgical instruments may be employed for dissection, including conventional instruments and dedicated thoracoscopic or laparoscopic instruments. It is especially beneficial to use curved instruments for retraction during dissection, as it will minimize the tendency for instruments to compete or collide with each other. Thoracoscopic (linear) mechanical staplers, such as the EndoGIA (U.S. Surgical, Norwalk, CT), are employed for control of the vessels (2.0- or 2.5-mm staples), bronchus (3.5- or 4.8-mm staples), and fissure.

After the placement of the second incision, the surgeon performs thoracoscopic exploration, which includes confirmation of the location of the tumor, exclusion of the presence of pleural metastases, and division of the pulmonary ligament. If a malignant diagnosis has not been achieved preoperatively, thoracoscopic wedge resection is performed using an automatic stapling device, and the specimen is removed in a protective bag. After frozen section confirms a malignant diagnosis, thoracoscopic lobectomy may then be completed. Mediastinal lymph node dissection may be performed at this point or may be deferred until the lobectomy is completed.

The approach to the staging of mediastinal lymph nodes is controversial. Many advocate systematic sampling of mediastinal lymph nodes because of concerns about the adequacy and safety of formal dissection.[29] Others accomplish mediastinal lymph node dissection by complete resection of the mediastinal nodes thoracoscopically, including levels 2, 4, 7, 8, and 9 on the right and levels 5, 6, 7, 8, and 9 on the left.[4,13]

Hilar dissection is carried out through the access incision, to achieve visualization and mobilization of the hilar structures. For any anatomical thoracoscopic lobectomy, hilar dissection is begun with mobilization of the pulmonary vein. For upper lobectomy, the lung is reflected posteriorly and inferiorly to facilitate dissection. For lower lobectomy, the lung is retracted superiorly. Moving the thoracoscope to the anterior incision may improve visualization of the superior hilum and may facilitate placement of the linear stapler for upper lobectomy, if introduced through the midaxillary port.

The risk of intraoperative hemorrhage is minimized with careful hilar dissection, which is facilitated with the visual clarity and magnification available with the video thoracoscope. Unexpected bleeding from a major branch of the pulmonary artery or pulmonary vein may occur, however. In most cases, the source of the bleeding is easily identifiable and tamponade is possible, allowing conversion to thoracotomy. To minimize the risk of vascular injury, surgeons have employed a variety of techniques to isolate the pulmonary arterial and venous branches, including ligatures to retract the vessels and catheters to guide the stapling devices. These techniques may be helpful in difficult cases, but are not required for the majority of patients.

All lobectomy specimens are removed using a protective specimen bag, to prevent implantation of tumor cells in the incision. The lobectomy specimen and hilum are each inspected to ascertain that anatomic lobectomy has been performed. After retrieval, the hemithorax is irrigated with warm saline and the bronchial stump is inspected. If an air leak is encountered, repeat stapling or endoscopic suturing may be performed.[45]

SPECIFIC TECHNICAL CONSIDERATIONS

Left Upper Lobectomy

With the thoracoscope in the midaxillary incision, the horizontal and oblique fissures are inspected and the presence of the tumor in the left upper lobe is confirmed. The lung is retracted posteriorly, and the superior pulmonary vein is identified and mobilized. The left superior pulmonary vein is then encircled using a curved clamp; dissection behind the superior pulmonary vein allows identification of the

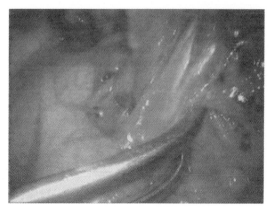

Figure 18–1 Left superior pulmonary vein, encircled with a curved clamp. (See color plate.)

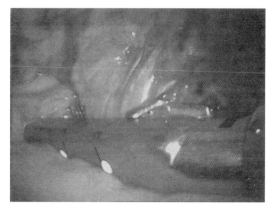

Figure 18–2 Left superior pulmonary vein, just prior to division with stapler. (See color plate.)

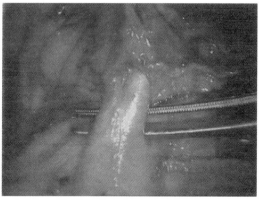

Figure 18–3 Apical anterior branches of left pulmonary artery. (See color plate.)

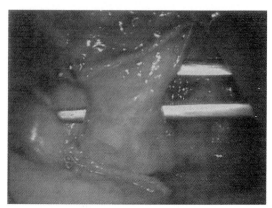

Figure 18–4 Left upper lobe bronchus, encircled with a curved clamp. (See color plate.)

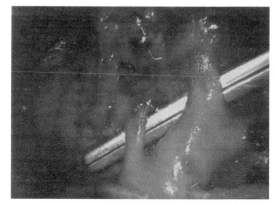

Figure 18–5 Posterior and lingular branches of left pulmonary artery. (See color plate.)

Right Upper Lobectomy

Right upper lobectomy is slightly more difficult than left upper lobectomy, because both the horizontal and oblique fissures must be managed. With the thoracoscope in the midaxillary incision, the horizontal and oblique fissures are inspected and the presence of the tumor in the right upper lobe is confirmed. The right lung is retracted posteriorly, and the superior pulmonary vein is identified and mobilized, to identify the division between the middle lobe and upper lobe venous branches. The upper lobe branches are encircled using a curved clamp; dissection behind the superior pulmonary vein allows identification of the pulmonary artery. The stapling device is then applied and the vein is divided, exposing the pulmonary artery. The pulmonary artery is mobilized, and the apical anterior trunk (truncus anterior) may then be stapled and divided. The right bronchus is now exposed, and the upper lobe bronchus may be stapled and divided. Subsequently, the posterior ascending arterial branch is stapled. Finally, the fissures are completed and the specimen retrieved.

Right Middle Lobectomy

With the thoracoscope in the midaxillary incision, the horizontal and oblique fissures are inspected and the presence of the tumor in the middle lobe is confirmed. The lung is retracted posteriorly, and the superior pulmonary vein is

pulmonary artery (Figure 18-1). The stapling device is then applied (Figure 18-2) and the superior pulmonary vein is divided, exposing the pulmonary artery. The pulmonary artery is mobilized, focusing on the apical and anterior branches (Figure 18-3), which may then be stapled and divided. The left upper lobe bronchus is now visualized and may be stapled and divided (Figure 18-4). Subsequently, the branches of the posterior and lingular arteries are stapled (Figure 18-5). Finally, the fissures are completed and the specimen retrieved.

identified and mobilized, to identify the division between the middle lobe and upper lobe venous branches. The middle lobe vein is encircled and stapled, exposing the middle lobe bronchus and artery. Retraction of the middle lobe laterally and posteriorly optimizes exposure of the bronchus. At this point, the bronchus is encircled and stapled, further exposing the middle lobe artery. The middle lobe artery is then stapled and divided as well, allowing completion of the fissures.

Lower Lobectomy (Right or Left)

The strategy for lower lobectomy is similar on the right and left sides. With the thoracoscope in the midaxillary incision, the presence of the tumor in the lower lobe is confirmed. The lung is retracted anteriorly, and the pleura incised between the lung and the esophagus. The lung is then retracted laterally and superiorly to incise the pleura overlying the inferior pulmonary vein, which may then be encircled and stapled, after ascertaining that the superior segment branch is included in the dissection. Further superior retraction of the lower lobe improves exposure of the bronchus, at the bifurcation of the lower lobe bronchus and the middle lobe bronchus (right lung) or lingular bronchus (left lung). The lower lobe bronchus is then encircled and stapled, exposing the lower lobe arterial trunk, which is then stapled and divided. Finally, the fissure is completed and the specimen retrieved.

Simultaneously Stapled Lobectomy

Although there are several ways to accomplish simultaneously stapled lobectomy, the goal is to optimize anatomical parenchymal resection and nodal staging, without individual vessel dissection. One strategy is to open the lobar fissure using a linear stapler, allowing the pulmonary artery, pulmonary vein, and the bronchus to be stapled simultaneously using a linear stapler. Alternatively, the pulmonary vein is easily mobilized in most patients, and independent division of the vein allows excellent hilar nodal staging. Subsequently, the lobectomy can be completed by simultaneously stapling the remaining hilar structures and the fissure to complete the resection.

Wedge Resection

Lobectomy is considered the procedure of choice in most patients with early stage lung cancer, as it is associated with a lower rate of local recurrence and higher overall survival, compared to wedge resection.[7] However, in patients with small peripheral tumors who will not tolerate anatomical resection, wedge resection followed by radiotherapy is an option.[1,33,37] VATS wedge resection of small (<3 cm) peripheral nodules is usually carried out using endoscopic stapling devices to transect lung parenchyma. Larger and more centrally located nodules are more challenging. Both a neodymium:yttrium–aluminum–garnet (Nd:YAG) laser[18] and monopolar floating ball device[45] are methods that have been reported to achieve precise tumor resection without unnecessary sacrifice of lung parenchyma.

RESULTS

The safety and efficacy of thoracoscopic lobectomy for patients with early-stage lung cancer have been established. Although there are no prospective, randomized series that compare thoracoscopic lobectomy to conventional approaches, a sufficient number of series have been published, both single-institution and multiinstitution experiences, to conclude that thoracoscopic lobectomy is a reasonable strategy for patients with clinical stage I lung cancer.°

Daniels and colleagues reported the results of thoracoscopic lobectomy in 110 consecutive patients.[4] The 30-day mortality was 3.6%, with no intraoperative deaths. The conversion rate was 1.8%, and none was emergent. The median chest tube duration was 3 days and median length of stay was 3 days. The Cancer and Leukemia Group B (CALGB) reported on the results of a multiinstitutional series of 97 patients who underwent thoracoscopic lobectomy.[38] In this series, the mortality was 2%, the operative time was 130 min, and the median length of stay was 3 days. Numerous other series have been published and are summarized in Table 18-1. In summary, thoracoscopic lobectomy has been demonstrated to be equivalent in terms of safety and oncological efficacy, as measured by complete resection rate, operative time, extent of lymph node dissection, operative mortality, and short-term survival, when compared to published results for thoracotomy and lobectomy.[2,7,9]

Morbidity and mortality associated with thoracoscopic resection are comparable or lower than expected for conventional thoracotomy and resection (Table 18-1). The mortality reported in several recent series ranges from 0 to 4%. Conversion rates range from 0 to 20% and appear to decrease over time with experience.

Persistent air leak, defined as lasting greater than 7 days, is the most common major complication but may be expected to decrease with experience and the use of endoscopic suturing.[45,46] Wound recurrence due to tumor implantation was first described in 1996,[6] but its risk may be minimized by use of specimen bags and copious irrigation. Perhaps the most feared major complication is hemorrhage into a closed chest, but careful hilar dissection has led to only rare cases.

POSTOPERATIVE PAIN

Postthoracotomy pain is related to rib spreading, which is obviated by the totally thoracoscopic approach. Many groups have analyzed acute pain after VATS. Although Kirby's randomized trial of VATS versus muscle-sparing lobectomy revealed no difference in postoperative pain, many of the VATS patients had undergone rib spreading during the operation.[15] This study also did not differentiate between acute and more chronic pain. Nomori and colleagues compared a group of age- and sex-matched patients who underwent thoracoscopic lobectomy (n = 33) or limited anterior thoracotomy (n = 33).[30] The patients who underwent thoracoscopic lobectomy experienced less pain between postoperative day (POD) 1 and POD 7 (p <.05–.001) and had lower analgesic requirements up to POD 7 (p <.001).

°References 4, 5, 13, 25, 32, 38, 40, 47.

282

Demmy and colleagues reported on their results in a series of patients who underwent either thoracoscopic lobectomy or conventional thoracotomy.[5] In this series, the percentage of patients reporting severe pain was 6% after thoracoscopic lobectomy and 65% after thoracotomy. Moreover, the percentage of patients reporting minimal or no pain was 63% after thoracoscopic lobectomy and 6% after thoracotomy. Other studies analyzing acute pain have concluded that VATS either causes less pain[8,17,26,39] or lower analgesia requirement[31,42] in the early postoperative period.

Chronic discomfort is also an important issue in postoperative recovery. Although more difficult to measure than acute pain, chronic pain and shoulder dysfunction have been studied. Stammberger and colleagues, in addressing long-term quality of life following VATS, reported that 53% of 173 patients undergoing VATS had insignificant pain 2 weeks following the operation. At 6 months, 75% had no complaints, and only 4% had mild or moderate discomfort at 2 years.[35] Landreneau's group questioned patients about shoulder dysfunction and concluded that although dysfunction is the same between VATS and conventional groups at 3 weeks, it lasted significantly longer in the conventional group.[17] This group's next examination of these issues revealed a significantly lower proportion of patients experiencing pain and shoulder dysfunction within the first year after operation.[19]

POSTOPERATIVE PULMONARY FUNCTION

Many have theorized that smaller incisions and absence of rib spreading may improve lung function in the postoperative period, and several studies have reported pulmonary function test (PFT) data following thoracoscopic resection. Two studies examined postoperative PaO_2 after both VATS and muscle-sparing thoracotomy and found that VATS patients had better oxygenation during the first postoperative week.[28,39] Others have revealed improvements in early postoperative forced expiratory volume in 1 s (FEV_1) and forced vital capacity (FVC) in the first weeks and months after VATS.[14,17,26] These differences likely disappear over time as Nakata et al revealed no PFT differences with longer than 1 year of follow-up.[28]

SYSTEMIC INFLAMMATORY EFFECTS

Minimally invasive procedures appear to produce less of a systemic insult than more conventional, invasive procedures.[20,26,36,49] Many have studied inflammatory mediators after VATS and open resection and have found lower levels of C-reactive protein and interleukins (IL) in those having undergone VATS.[20,26,49] Yim and colleagues analyzed the cytokine responses in a series of 36 matched patients who underwent thoracoscopic lobectomy or conventional thoracotomy and lobectomy. Analgesic requirement was significantly lower in the patients who underwent VATS lobectomy. In addition, the levels of IL-6 and IL-8 were lower in the VATS group, compared to the group that underwent thoracotomy. Leaver et al examined immunosuppression due to systemic effects of surgery and found

higher numbers of CD4 lymphocytes and natural killer cells and less suppression of lymphocyte oxidation in the VATS group.[20] Whether these trends toward more effective immune function after VATS resection will lead to faster recovery or toward better oncologic outcomes will be important end points of future studies.

ONCOLOGICAL EFFECTIVENESS

The ultimate acceptance of thoracoscopic lobectomy will be dependent upon its oncological effectiveness as compared with conventional lobectomy. Although there has been no prospective, randomized trial with sufficient power to assess differences between the operations, the studies performed are sufficient for limited analysis. First, no differences were seen in number of lymph nodes obtained either by dissection or sampling between conventional and VATS lobectomy.[5,11,31] Second, data from existing series reveal survival rates for stage I patients at least as good as those published in the literature for conventional thoracotomy (see Table 18-1). Some groups have documented improved survival when VATS was utilized.[13,22,45] Reasons for the possible differences are unclear, but it has been postulated that preservation of immune function and less systemic release of inflammatory cytokines may contribute.[44] Final resolution of these issues awaits a rigorously controlled prospective, randomized trial.

COST-EFFECTIVENESS

The assessment of cost effectiveness is controversial, because of the difficulty in identifying and including all costs. Clearly, VATS can be associated with high costs of consumables and with longer operative times in inexperienced hands. However, numerous disposable instruments that are essential to the performance of thoracoscopic lobectomy, such as linear endoscopic staplers, are also employed by many in performing either conventional thoracotomy or limited thoracotomy. Nakajima and colleagues recently published a study from Japan demonstrating that hospital charges were actually lower for the VATS approach.[27] One important variable in the assessment of cost effectiveness is length of stay. In a recent series of thoracoscopic lobectomy, the median length of stay was only 3 days.[4] As experience increases with thoracoscopic lobectomy, the operative time will become comparable to conventional approaches. In fact, the mean operative time in the CALGB multiinstitutional study was only 130 min.[38]

SUMMARY

Minimally invasive approaches to lung cancer treatment have been demonstrated to be safe and effective for patients with early-stage lung cancer. Thoracoscopic lobectomy is designed to achieve the same oncological result as conventional lobectomy: complete hilar dissection and individual vessel control. The recognized advantages of thoracoscopic anatomic resection include less short-term postoperative pain, shorter hospital stay, and preserved pulmonary function. Although there are no prospective randomized studies comparing the thoracoscopic approach to conventional thoracotomy, there are no data from published series to suggest any difference in oncological efficacy.

REFERENCES

1. Asamura H, Nakayama H, Kondo H, et al: Lymph node involvement, recurrence, and prognosis in resected small, peripheral non-small cell lung carcinomas: Are these carcinomas candidates for video-assisted lobectomy? J Thorac Cardiovasc Surg 111:1125–1134, 1996.
2. Battafarano RJ, Piccirillo JF, Meyers BF, et al: Impact of comorbidity on survival after surgical resection in patients with stage I non-small cell lung cancer. J Thorac Cardiovasc Surg 123:280–287, 2002.
3. Brown WT: Video-assisted thoracic surgery: The Miami experience. Semin Thorac Cardiovasc Surg 10(4):305–312, 1998.
4. Daniels LJ, Balderson SS, Onaitis MW, D'Amico TA: Thoracoscopic lobectomy: A safe and effective strategy for patients with stage I lung cancer. Ann Thorac Surg 74:860–864, 2002.
5. Demmy TL, Curtis JJ: Minimally invasive lobectomy directed toward frail and high-risk patients: A case control study. Ann Thorac Surg 68:194–200, 1999.
6. Downey RJ, McCormick P, LoCicero J, et al: Dissemination of malignant tumors after video-assisted thoracic surgery: A report of twenty-one cases. J Thorac Cardiovasc Surg 111:954, 1996.
7. Ginsberg RJ, Rubinstein LV: Lung Cancer Study Group randomized trial of lobectomy versus resection for T1 non-small cell lung cancer. Ann Thorac Surg 60:615, 1995.
8. Guidicelli R, Thomas P, Lonjon R, et al: Video-assisted minithoracotomy versus muscle-sparing thoracotomy for performing lobectomy. Ann Thorac Surg 58:712–718, 1994.
9. Harpole DH Jr, DeCamp MM, Dale J, et al: Prognostic models of 30-day mortality and morbidity after major pulmonary resection. J Thorac Cardiovasc Surg 117:969–979, 1999.
10. Hermansson U, Konstantinov IE, Aren C: Video-assisted thoracic surgery (VATS) lobectomy: The initial Swedish experience. Semin Thorac Cardiovasc Surg 10(4):285–290, 1998.
11. Iwasaki A, Shirakusa T, Kawahara K, et al: Is video-assisted thoracoscopic surgery suitable for resection of primary lung cancer? Thorac Cardiovasc Surg 45(1):13–15, 1997.
12. Jacobeus HC: Ueber die moglichkeit die zystoskopie bei untersuchung seroser hohlungen anzuwenden. Munchen Med Wochenschur 57:2090–2092, 1910.
13. Kaseda S, Aoki T, Hangai N: Video-assisted thoracic surgery (VATS) lobectomy: The Japanese experience. Semin Thorac Cardiovasc Surg 10(4):300–304, 1998.
14. Kaseda S, Aoki T, Hangai N, et al: Better pulmonary function and prognosis with video-assisted thoracic surgery than with thoracotomy. Ann Thorac Surg 70(5):1644–1646, 2000.
15. Kirby TJ, Rice TW: Thoracoscopic lobectomy. Ann Thorac Surg 56(3):784–786, 1993.
16. Kirby TJ, Mack MJ, Landreneau RJ, Rice TW: Lobectomy—video-assisted thoracic surgery versus muscle-sparing thoracotomy: A randomized trial. J Thorac Cardiovasc Surg 109:997, 1995.
17. Landreneau RJ, Hazelrigg SR, Mack MJ, et al: Postoperative pain-related morbidity: Video-assisted thoracic surgery versus thoracotomy. Ann Thorac Surg 56(6):1285–1289, 1993.
18. Landreneau RJ, Keenan RJ, Hazelrigg SR, et al: VATS wedge resection of the lung using the neodymium:yttrium-aluminum garnet laser. Ann Thorac Surg 56:758, 1993.
19. Landreneau RJ, Mack MJ, Hazelrigg SR, et al: Prevalence of chronic pain after pulmonary resection by thoracotomy or video-assisted thoracic surgery. J Thorac Cardiovasc Surg 107:1079–1086, 1994.
20. Leaver HA, Craig SR, Yap PL, et al: Lymphocyte responses following open and minimally invasive thoracic surgery. Eur J Clin Invest 30(3):320–328, 2000.
21. Lewis RJ, Caccavale RJ: Video-assisted thoracic surgical non-rib spreading simultaneously stapled lobectomy (VATS(n)SSL). Semin Thorac Cardiovasc Surg 10(4):332–339, 1998.
22. Lewis RJ, Caccavale RJ, Boncage JP, Widmann MD: Video-assisted thoracic surgical non-rib spreading simultaneously stapled lobectomy: A more patient-friendly oncologic resection. Chest 116:1119–1124, 1999.
23. Mason DP, Swanson SJ: Lung cancer: diagnosis and treatment. In Demmy TL, editor: Video-Assisted Thoracic Surgery (VATS). Georgetown: Landis Bioscience, 2001, pp. 71–98.
24. McKenna RJ: Thoracic lobectomy with mediastinal sampling in 80-year-old patients. Chest 106(6):1902–1904, 1994.
25. McKenna RJ, Fischel RJ, Wolf R, Wurnig P: Video-assisted thoracic surgery (VATS) lobectomy for bronchogenic carcinoma. Semin Thorac Cardiovasc Surg 10(4):321–325, 1998.
26. Nagahiro I, Andou A, Aoe M, et al: Pulmonary function, postoperative pain, and serum cytokine level after lobectomy: A comparison of VATS and conventional procedure. Ann Thorac Surg 72:362–365, 2001.
27. Nakajima J, Takamoto S, Kohno T, Ohtsuka T: Costs of video-assisted thoracoscopic surgery versus open resection for patients with lung carcinoma. Cancer 89:2497–2501, 2000.
28. Nakata M, Sakei H, Yokoyama N, et al: Pulmonary function after lobectomy: Video-assisted thoracic surgery versus thoracotomy. Ann Thorac Surg 70(3):938–941, 2000.
29. Naruke T, Tsuchiya R, Kando H, et al: Lymph node sampling in lung cancer: How should it be done? Eur J Cardiothorac Surg 16:S17–24, 1999.
30. Nomori H, Horio H, Naruke T, Suemasu K: What is the advantage of a thoracoscopic lobectomy over a limited anterior thoracotomy procedure for lung cancer surgery? Ann Thorac Surg 72:879–884, 2001.
31. Ohbuchi T, Morikawa T, Takeuchi E, et al: Lobectomy: Video-assisted thoracic surgery versus posterolateral thoracotomy. Jpn J Thorac Cardiovasc Surg 46(6):519–522, 1998.
32. Roviaro G, Varoli F, Vergani C, Maciocco M: Video-assisted thoracoscopic surgery (VATS) major pulmonary resections: The Italian experience. Semin Thorac Cardiovasc Surg 10(4):313–320, 1998.
33. Shennib H, Kohman L, Herndon JE, et al: CALGB 9335: A multicenter phase II prospective study of video-assisted wedge resection followed by radiotherapy for T1N0 NSCLC in high-risk patients: Preliminary analysis of technical outcome. American Association of Thoracic Surgery, Toronto, 2000.
34. Solaini L, Prusciano F, Bagioni P, et al: Video-assisted thoracic surgery major pulmonary resections. Present experience. Eur J Cardiothorac Surg 20:437–442, 2001.
35. Stammberger U, Steinacher C, Hillinger S, et al: Early and long-term complaints following video-assisted thoracoscopic surgery: Evaluation in 173 patients. Eur J Cardiothorac Surg 18(1):7–11, 2000.
36. Sugi K, Kaneda Y, Esato K: Video-assisted thoracoscopic lobectomy reduces cytokine production more than conventional open thoracotomy. Jpn J Thorac Cardiovasc Surg 48(3):161–165, 2000.
37. Swanson SJ, Bueno R, Jaklitsch MT, et al: Subcentimeter non-small cell lung cancer: Early detection and resection is warranted. 80th American Association of Thoracic Surgery, Toronto, 2000.
38. Swanson SJ, Herndon J, D'Amico TA, et al: Results of CALGB 39802: Feasibility of VATS lobectomy for lung cancer. Proc Am Soc Clin Oncol 21:290a, 2002.

284

39. Tschernko EM, Hofer S, Bieglmayer C, et al: Early postoperative stress: Video-assisted wedge resection/lobectomy vs conventional axillary thoracotomy. Chest 109(6): 1636–1642, 1996.

40. Walker WS: Video-assisted thoracic surgery: The Edinburgh experience. Semin Thorac Cardiovasc Surg 10(4):291–299, 1998.

41. Walker WS, Carnochan FM, Pugh GC: Thoracoscopic pulmonary lobectomy. Early operative experience and preliminary clinical results. J Thorac Cardiovasc Surg 106(6):1111–1117, 1993.

42. Walker WS, Pugh GC, Craig SR, et al: Continued experience with thoracoscopic major pulmonary resection. Int Surg 81(3):255–258, 1996.

43. Widmann MD, Caccavale RJ, Bocage JP, Lewis RJ: Video-assisted thoracic surgery resection of chest wall en bloc for lung carcinoma. Ann Thorac Surg 70:2138, 2000.

44. Yim APC: VATS major pulmonary resection revisited—controversies, techniques, and results. Ann Thorac Surg 74:615–623, 2002.

45. Yim APC: Video-assisted pulmonary resections. In Pearson FG, Cooper JD, Deslauriers J, et al, editors: Thoracic Surgery. Philadelphia: Churchill Livingstone, 2002, pp. 1073–1084.

46. Yim APC, Liu HP: Complications and failures from video-assisted thoracic surgery: Experience from two centers in Asia. Ann Thorac Surg 61:538, 1996.

47. Yim APC, Izzat MB, Liu H, Ma C: Thoracoscopic major lung resections: An Asian perspective. Semin Thorac Cardiovasc Surg 10(4):326–331, 1998.

48. Yim APC, Liu HP, Hazelrigg SR, et al: Thoracoscopic operations on reoperated chests. Ann Thorac Surg 65:328, 1998.

49. Yim APC, Wan S, Lee TW, et al: VATS lobectomy reduced cytokine responses compared with conventional surgery. Ann Thorac Surg 70(1):243–247, 2000.

Lung Cancer: Multimodal Therapy

Sudish C. Murthy, Thomas W. Rice, and Malcolm M. DeCamp

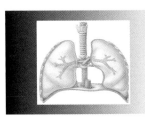

INTRODUCTION

Surgery alone, although long regarded as the best chance for a cure, has some serious shortcomings in the management of non–small cell lung cancer (NSCLC). Even in the most favorable of circumstances (i.e., resection of early-stage lung cancer), failure of therapy is expected in 20–40% of patients.[30,41,47] Moreover, because less than one third of patients initially have limited disease, surgical resection is only offered to a minority of patients with NSCLC.

To overcome these deficiencies, considerable effort has been directed toward developing preoperative (termed *induction* or *neoadjuvant*) and postoperative (termed *adjuvant*) strategies to both improve long-term outcomes after surgery and increase the number of eligible patients for surgical therapy. These strategies employ chemotherapy and radiation used singly, sequentially, or concurrently.

The ability to predict which patients fail surgical therapy alone allows for identification of patients most suitable for (and most likely to benefit from) multimodality therapy. Locoregional lymph node involvement[48] is a powerful predictor of outcome and should be thoroughly investigated during treatment planning. Tumor histology also impacts survival of resected patients; early-stage squamous cancers carry a more favorable prognosis than early-stage adenocarcinomas.[46] Finally, numerous genetic markers are being discovered that may aid outcome prognostication.[39] To this end, recent reports have proposed systems using histological and molecular criteria to stratify survival of resected patients.[13,37]

In developing strategies for combined therapies, the pattern of failure (recurrence) must be considered. Because locoregional recurrence after resection of stage I cancers is rare, additional therapy might include chemotherapy (to treat suspected systemic disease). Similarly, resected stage II cancers are twice as likely to fail systemically rather than locally,[27] suggesting that adjuvant systemic therapy (chemotherapy) might be more useful than adjuvant local therapy (radiotherapy).

ADJUVANT THERAPY

Despite enthusiasm for multimodality treatment of NSCLC, over 30 years of clinical trials have yet to demonstrate a consistent benefit of adjuvant therapy (chemotherapy or radiotherapy) for resected cancers. This may be due in part to the rapid evolution of chemotherapy and radiation protocols, which have fostered large numbers of difficult-to-compare studies. Few studies have been designed to critically examine treatment effects on specific NSCLC stages; most studies tend to group stages I–III in their treatment arms. This shortcoming has been compounded by lack of accurate pathological staging in most trials.

ADJUVANT CHEMOTHERAPY

Early randomized trials of adjuvant chemotherapy focused on the use of nitrogen mustard,[33,75] cyclophosphamide,[8,33] and combination lomustine (CCNU) and hydroxyurea.[73] Cumulatively, these trials demonstrated that treated patients had more postoperative complications without any survival benefit than did untreated patients. In fact, patients treated with postoperative cyclophosphamide experienced a poorer long-term survival than did untreated patients.[8] This was independently confirmed by meta-analysis.[73] Findings from these early studies have been largely discounted because histological type and pathological stage were not considered during trial design. Also, the chemotherapeutic agents used have since been demonstrated to be ineffective for NSCLC.

As several studies began documenting the efficacy of platinum regimens as primary therapy for advanced (stage IV) NSCLC, platinum-based combination chemotherapy became the preferred adjuvant choice. There was initial enthusiasm when one randomized trial, Lung Cancer Study Group trial 772,[34] suggested a disease-free and overall survival benefit in the treatment arm. Although the survival

286 advantage was not considered statistically significant, significant optimism was generated by the study. Subsequent trials, however, proved to be far less promising.

A randomized study of adjuvant CAP (cyclophosphamide, Adriamycin, cisplatin) therapy for resected stage I–II NSCLC[23] did not demonstrate treatment efficacy. This trial suffered from the inability to deliver the prescribed chemotherapeutic regimen (four cycles) over the prescribed time. Fewer than 30% of patients in the treatment arm actually received chemotherapy as intended. Other randomized studies have been similarly plagued by incomplete delivery of prescribed postoperative therapies,[52,56] which partly contributes to the negative findings of these trials. Additionally, the dose of cisplatin (40–60 mg/m²/cycle) is lower than that currently recommended (80–120 mg/m²/cycle).[59]

Although each of the early platinum trials was considered negative, subtle survival differences were noted between control and treated patients. Surprisingly, a meta-analysis of several randomized adjuvant platinum-based trials demonstrated a 13% reduction in the risk of death ($p = .08$) for treated patients.[10] This resulted in the institution of additional adjuvant chemotherapy trials.

The lessons learned from some of the earlier trials led to the design of three large, contemporary, randomized studies. Platinum dosing was adjusted so that patients were scheduled to receive 300–400 mg/m² (total dose). Adjuvant radiation therapy was at the discretion of participating centers. Two studies demonstrated trends for survival benefit in treated patients, although neither was considered to be a *positive* trial.[15,70] The most recently reported trial, the International Adjuvant Lung Cancer Trial (IALT),[6] however, demonstrated a survival benefit with adjuvant chemotherapy. This study included resected stage I–III patients and demonstrated a clear survival advantage (5% percent benefit after 5 years, $p = .003$) that favored the chemotherapy arm versus surgery alone. This survival advantage is similar in magnitude to that achieved by adjuvant chemotherapy for resected breast and colon cancers.[20,36] Given the results of these large trials, there is currently renewed enthusiasm for adjuvant chemotherapy for patients with resected stage I, II, or III NSCLC.

▶ ADJUVANT RADIOTHERAPY

Studies of the efficacy of adjuvant radiotherapy are confounded by many of the same factors that interfere with chemotherapy trials. Many randomized adjuvant radiotherapy studies are composed of patients from all stages of resected NSCLC. Consequently, the expected negligible (or deleterious) effects on patients with early-stage cancers may obscure small beneficial effects for patients with more advanced disease. Also, because the discipline of radiation oncology evolved so quickly, many of the early randomized studies became obsolete by the time the data matured. Moreover, most of the randomized trials were underpowered to demonstrate small but relevant differences in outcome. Consequently, it is not surprising that, although many feasibility and retrospective studies have yielded promising results of adjuvant radiotherapy to date, no randomized trial has documented a survival benefit of postoperative radiotherapy.

Currently there is no justification to include adjuvant radiotherapy in the management of resected stage I–II NSCLC. Three randomized trials,[7,38,80] as well as a meta-analysis of nine randomized trials (PORT study),[57] document a deleterious effect (survival disadvantage) of adjuvant radiotherapy for early-stage NSCLC. Reasons for this are poor radiotherapy planning,[80] larger fraction size,[7] greater total radiation dose,[7,38,80] outdated equipment, and poor quality control.[69]

Although there was optimism that hilar lymph node (N_1)–positive patients (stage II) would provide a good substrate for adjuvant radiotherapy, this appears not to be the case. From subgroup analysis of several randomized trials,[22,57,77] radiotherapy has no significant effect on either local control or overall survival for these patients.

There are insufficient randomized data to defend the use of adjuvant radiotherapy for resected stage III (N_2/N_3) disease. Even though improved local control has been reported,[22,49,77] it does not translate into a meaningful survival benefit for patients. The strongest argument to support adjuvant radiotherapy for resected stage III NSCLC comes from a nonrandomized, single-institution, retrospective study.[33,45] These investigators found that postoperative radiotherapy was the strongest independent predictor of survival for resected N_2-positive disease. This study, however, has been widely criticized.[69] The PORT meta-analysis did not demonstrate efficacy for radiotherapy after resection of stage III disease.[57]

▶ INDUCTION THERAPY

Induction therapy is any cytoreductive treatment (e.g., chemotherapy, radiotherapy, chemoradiotherapy) administered before definitive locoregional treatment (e.g., surgery). Although a tissue diagnosis is required before therapy begins, the pathological stage of the cancer may be less well defined before treatment commences. Aggressive surgical (mediastinoscopy or video-assisted thoracoscopic surgery [VATS]) or interventional (transbronchial needle aspiration or endoscopic ultrasound-guided fine-needle aspiration) staging is imperative to ensure that induction therapy protocols are applied to homogeneous patient populations. Some patients may be rendered inoperable because of serious induction therapy toxicity, and this must be considered during treatment planning. Recognizing this has led to more concerted efforts to develop induction strategies for more advanced cancers (i.e., less curable with surgery alone). Nonetheless, some recent data suggest a role of induction therapy for early-stage cancers.

Use of chemotherapy in the induction setting (preoperative/neoadjuvant) has several potential advantages. First, there is early treatment of micrometastases. Because distant recurrence is the most common mode of failure, early eradication of systemic disease might translate into a survival advantage. Second is the hypothesis that chemotherapy is most efficacious when tumor burden is small.[28] Third, drug delivery and toxic effects to the primary tumor may be enhanced as a result of preservation of tumor blood supply. This may increase both response and the probability of a complete resection. Perhaps most importantly, however, a higher percentage of patients likely will receive the intended dose of chemotherapy when drugs are delivered preoperatively.[55]

Radiotherapy has been used extensively in combination induction regimens with chemotherapy. Two large phase III trials comparing induction radiotherapy (40–50 Gy) followed by resection with primary resection alone were reported several decades ago. Both demonstrated inferior survival rates for radiated patients.[74,83] Since then, few data have emerged, suggesting a role for radiotherapy alone as an induction modality. Consequently, discussions of preoperative radiotherapy are in the context of chemoradiotherapy protocols.

Induction therapies are not without concerns. Subsequent resections generally are more technically challenging and may result in lung-sparing operations becoming less feasible. Morbidity and mortality rates for surgery after induction therapy may be greater,[15,61] and for an early-stage cancer with the potential for a relatively good survival, the risks may well exceed any benefits. Finally, serious preoperative complications (grade 4 toxicities or death) may preclude any attempt at curative resection.

► INDUCTION CHEMOTHERAPY FOR EARLY-STAGE NON–SMALL CELL LUNG CANCER

Interestingly, data support the use of induction chemotherapy for early-stage cancers. Such studies build on observations from other solid tumor treatment trials where chemotherapy response rates improve as similar drug regimens are applied to earlier stages of disease.[76] The feasibility of induction chemotherapy was recently demonstrated by the Bimodality Lung Oncology Team (BLOT) study.[55] This phase II trial examined the response, toxicity, resectability rate, surgical morbidity, and intermediate survival for patients treated preoperatively with carboplatinum and paclitaxel. Two preoperative cycles were administered and three postoperative cycles planned for patients undergoing complete resections. After induction therapy, 56% of patients had a major objective response; 86% of patients underwent complete resection. Impressively, 96% of patients received the intended preoperative chemotherapy, whereas 46% received the planned postoperative courses. Treated patients appeared to recover as well as patients who did not receive induction therapy.

A recent randomized trial suggests a benefit of induction chemotherapy for stages I and II NSCLC.[15] The induction regimen consisted of two cycles of mitomycin, ifosfamide, and cisplatin. Two additional cycles were given postoperatively for responding patients. The patient population was heterogeneous, with some stage IIIA patients included in the study. Nonetheless, despite a slightly higher mortality rate for chemotherapy-treated patients, disease-free survival was longer for treated patients than for untreated patients with stage I or II cancers.

► INDUCTION THERAPY FOR STAGE IIIA/B NON–SMALL CELL LUNG CANCER

Induction Chemotherapy

In 1982 Pearson and colleagues[54] reported on the dismal outcome of surgery for stage IIIA (N_2 lymph node–positive) patients. They noted a 9% 5-year survival rate for gross

mediastinal lymph node involvement and a 24% survival rate for patients with microscopically positive nodes. Even for occult, single-station N_2 disease, the best reported survival rate is less than 30% after 5 years.[42] Because the vast majority of these patients die of metastatic disease, the use of induction therapy as the systemic component of a multidisciplinary treatment approach for patients with locally advanced NSCLC has been investigated.

By the mid-1990s the recognized standard of care for resectable stage IIIA (N_2-positive) NSCLC was changed by the near-simultaneous reports of two small randomized trials designed to study the efficacy of induction chemotherapy followed by resection. Collectively, these studies represented data acquired from only 120 patients. Rosell and associates[63] compared surgery alone with three cycles of induction chemotherapy (platinum based) followed by surgery. All patients were scheduled to receive postoperative thoracic irradiation. A second trial from the M.D. Anderson Cancer Center was more chemotherapy intensive.[65] Three cycles of a cisplatin regimen were given as induction and an additional three cycles planned postoperatively for responding patients. In this trial radiotherapy was reserved for unresectable or incompletely resected patients. Entry into either trial required pathological confirmation of mediastinal lymph node involvement (N_2 disease) by mediastinoscopy or T_3 disease.

Both trials were stopped early because interim safety analyses demonstrated a significant advantage, favoring patients given induction chemotherapy. Mature, actual (not actuarial) survival updates have been published, with an average of 7 years of follow-up.[62,64] These reports document a durable and statistically significant survival benefit of induction chemotherapy and surgery versus surgery alone and translate into a 20% *better* 5-year survival rate.

The revised AJCC staging system for NSCLC has further homogenized stage IIIA disease.[48] Most patients within this designation have mediastinal (N_2) lymph node involvement. The shared survival estimates for these patients and the disappointing pattern of distant relapse after "curative" resection underscore the systemic nature of NSCLC once it is detectable in the lymphatic system. Contemporary treatment strategies with cure as their goal must provide solutions for both local and systemic disease in order to be viable.

Induction Chemoradiotherapy

The use of radiotherapy in sequence after chemotherapy (with or without surgery) has long been used to consolidate the local component of therapy for stage III NSCLC.[19,40,78] Concurrent chemoradiotherapy has several theoretic advantages over the sequential strategy. Many of the contemporary drugs active in NSCLC (e.g., cisplatin, paclitaxel) also are radiation sensitizers and allow for synergistic tumoricidal effect when given concurrently with ionizing radiation. Combined therapy clearly is more toxic[24]; however, several investigators have found the subsequent operative mortality and morbidity rates to be similar to induction chemotherapy alone if appropriate perioperative safeguards are in place.[14,61] Another hypothetical advantage of concurrent chemoradiation induction therapy is reduction in tumor bulk. This may allow inoperable lesions to be resected, or for lesser resections, to be performed (lobectomy versus pneumonectomy). Finally, delivery of ionizing radiation when tumor

288 vascularity has not been reduced by surgical dissection may enhance response.

Since 1990 the standard of care for patients with unresectable stage IIIA disease (bulky N_2 involvement) and most patients with stage IIIB NSCLC has been concurrent chemoradiotherapy.[71] Based on encouraging observations with regard to clinical response rates but a disappointing rate of local relapse, investigators began to explore the addition of surgery after this regimen to provide "definitive" local control.[4] The Southwest Oncology Group (SWOG) conducted the most widely reported, multiinstitutional, feasibility trial of this strategy, SWOG 8805. The treatment protocol consisted of two cycles of induction chemotherapy (cisplatin and etoposide) and 45 Gy of concurrent radiotherapy for patients with stage IIIA or IIIB NSCLC.[2] Of the 126 patients enrolled, 60% had stage IIIA disease and 40% were stage IIIB. Fifty-three percent of the stage IIIB patients had N_3 lymph node involvement. There was a 6% operative mortality rate even though nearly one third of the operations required pneumonectomy,[66] which compares favorably with contemporary surgical series without induction therapies.[25,32] This underscores the feasibility and safety of combined neoadjuvant therapy despite increased surgical complexity.[2]

Stage IIIB disease with N_3 lymph node involvement generally is considered inoperable because of the inability to obtain a complete resection and near-universal pattern of systemic failure after aggressive local therapy. Growing experience with surgery after induction chemoradiation has allowed certain centers to offer resection to selected stage IIIB patients. In SWOG 8805, stage IIIA and IIIB patients had equivalent clinical and pathological responses and, surprisingly, similar survival rates.[2] These investigators, as well as others,[5,11,21,31] noted that only patients who had sterilization of their mediastinal disease after induction treatment benefit from treatment. For patients experiencing complete pathological responses (i.e., no viable tumor found in the resected specimen), a 40–55% 5-year survival rate is expected.[14,31]

Our own experience using hyperfractionated radiotherapy with concurrent induction chemotherapy (cisplatin and paclitaxel) has identified an intermediate prognostic group.[79,84] Stage IIIA/B patients treated with this regimen were equally likely to benefit whether they had pretreatment N_2 or N_3 disease. Patients downstaged from N_3 to N_2, or those IIIA patients with residual N_2 disease at surgery, still had a median survival rate of 27 months and a 31% 5-year survival rate.[14]

Grunenwald and associates[31] advocate bilateral mediastinal lymph node dissection after chemoradiotherapy for N_3 disease. However, this treatment provides no obvious therapeutic benefit and appears useful only as a prognostic tool.

Concurrent chemoradiation used as induction therapy is evaluative only when followed by surgical resection. In SWOG 8805, 21% of resected patients had a complete pathological response with sterilization of primary and lymph node cancer (i.e., downstaged to stage 0). An additional 37% of patients had only microscopic residual cancer.[2] Such observations have led some investigators to question whether resection actually contributes to survival or merely provides prognostic information for these patients. To address the utility of surgery in stage III NSCLC, the National Cancer Institute sponsored a multiinstitutional phase III trial (INT 0139) in which 429 patients received two cycles of cisplatin and etoposide with concurrent thoracic radiotherapy (45 Gy), followed by either resection or additional chemoradiation therapy. Resected patients were scheduled for two postoperative cycles of chemotherapy, whereas patients randomized to the no-surgery arm were to receive uninterrupted radiation up to 61 Gy with two additional cycles of chemotherapy. Although there were more early deaths in the surgical arm (14 versus 3), disease-free survival rates were superior when resection was a component of treatment (log-rank, $p = .02$). The 3-year survival rate in the operated group was 29% compared with only 19% in the chemoradiation-alone cohort.[3]

Current investigative efforts to enhance survival in stage III disease are focused on novel induction chemotherapy drug combinations, different dose schedules and intensities, altered radiation fractionation schemes, and the use of biological response modifiers targeting inflammation, angiogenesis, tissue invasion, cellular proliferation, apoptosis, and metastasis.[12,35,85]

Surgery remains central in the accurate staging of these patients and enhances survival for some patients with either stage IIIA or IIIB NSCLC. Unfortunately, no patient or tumor characteristics can predict response to induction therapy. Moreover, clinical, noninvasive, and radiographic assessments of response have been disappointing.[78] Semiquantitative positron emission tomography (PET)[1] and some minimally invasive techniques (e.g., endoscopic ultrasound-guided fine needle aspiration,[82] VATS,[44] repeat mediastinoscopy[43,58,81]) may permit identification of patients most likely to benefit from resection after induction therapies. Nonresponders might be best served by alternative or experimental therapeutics. For these reasons, the optimal treatment of stage III NSCLC remains undefined. Induction therapy appears superior to an adjuvant strategy, with resection providing the only accurate assessment of response and superior survival, but only in downstaged patients. For successful advancement of this field, these multimodality regimens should only be offered to patients in the context of prospective clinical trials.

▶ SPECIAL CIRCUMSTANCES: SUPERIOR SULCUS TUMORS

Patients with superior sulcus (Pancoast) tumors represent a unique group who serve as attractive candidates for induction protocols. The biological behavior of some of these tumors seems different from that of other NSCLC in that extensive local disease can occur without the obligate systemic disease that accompanies other T_3 tumors.[17] Nonetheless, presence of regional lymph node involvement still remains a powerful negative predictor of survival after Pancoast tumor resection.

In approximately one third of Pancoast tumor resections, complete resection is not obtained.[16] This is significant because an incomplete resection is equivalent to no operation at all in terms of survival.[18,26,50,51] The common problem of local recurrence is peculiar to these tumors.

The first long-term survival after resection of a superior sulcus tumor occurred only after the addition of adjuvant radiation therapy.[9] Subsequently, an induction radiation therapy strategy was developed that gave treated patients vastly improved survival over historical controls.[53,72] Despite these advances, complete resection for node-negative T_3 tumors was possible in less than two thirds of patients. Locoregional disease was the most common form of recurrence.[68]

Recently a multiinstitutional phase II trial was completed that addressed the feasibility of induction chemoradiation therapy for patients with superior sulcus tumors.[67] The study population included N_2/N_3 node-negative patients with T_3 or T_4 tumors and adequate cardiopulmonary fitness to tolerate resection. Patients were given two cycles of cisplatin and etoposide concurrent with 45 Gy of radiation. The radiation field included the primary tumor and ipsilateral supraclavicular fossa, but excluded the hilum or mediastinum. Surgery was performed 3 to 5 weeks after the end of the induction therapy. Two cycles of "boost" (adjuvant) chemotherapy were scheduled after recovery from surgery (Figure 19-1).

Induction therapy was completed as planned in 92% of patients. The related mortality rate was 3%. Seventy-five percent of enrolled patients underwent surgery. Of these, 92% underwent complete resection. The 2-year survival for completely resected patients was a surprising 70%. We await mature results.

▶ RECOMMENDATIONS

The extent of NSCLC at initial diagnosis, as defined by AJCC staging, is currently the only reliable predictor of survival. It is therefore essential to exhaust all reasonable efforts to obtain accurate staging information before consideration of adjuvant or induction therapies. Multimodality therapy planning should then be used in a stage-dependent manner.

Staging protocols must include a thorough search for distant metastatic disease, as well as provide accurate information regarding locoregional lymph node involvement. We currently favor using PET as part of the metastatic survey and prefer mediastinoscopy for evaluation of mediastinal lymph nodes. Our institutional experience with PET to

Figure 19-1 CT scan images from a patient with an anterior Pancoast (T_4) tumor. Images **A** and **B** are before, and **C** and **D** are after, induction chemoradiation therapy. The treatment protocol is outlined in the text.[65] The patient went on to have a complete resection (which included the right innominate vein) and a complete pathological response (ypT_0N_0, stage 0).

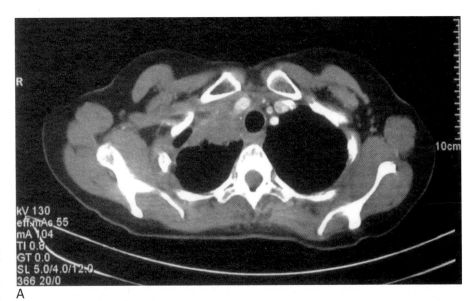

A

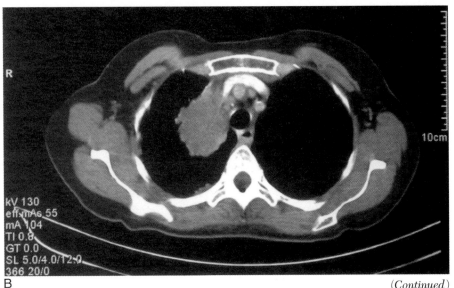

B

(Continued)

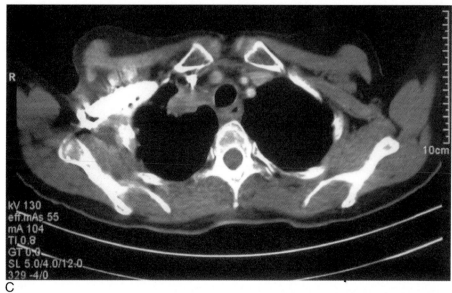

Figure 19–1 cont'd

stage the mediastinum has not measured up to that reported elsewhere[29,60] and has not replaced mediastinoscopy for this purpose in our practice.

Assuming that an accurate pretreatment stage can be obtained, there currently are no compelling data to include stage IA cancers into any multimodality protocol. We recommend, however, that lymphadenectomy (or extensive sampling) accompany any resection for early-stage cancer because complete resection is a hallmark of curative therapy, and also to more clearly identify patients with micrometastatic locoregional disease. With the recent publication of the IALT trial[6] and the BLOT study,[55] strong consideration for adjuvant or induction chemotherapy for stage IB, IIA, and IIB patients should be given. If possible, these patients should be entered into ongoing clinical trials to further clarify this area.

Patients with stage IIIA/B NSCLC do poorly with surgery alone. After numerous studies and much debate, the optimal use of induction chemoradiation therapy still remains largely unresolved. Clearly, pathological responders benefit, but pretherapy identification of these patients has proven elusive. Although we still consider induction therapy to be investigational for these patients, we do not offer resection without it.

REFERENCES

1. Akhurst T, Downey RJ, Ginsberg MS, et al: An initial experience with FDG-PET in the imaging of residual disease after induction therapy for lung cancer. Ann Thorac Surg 73(1):259–264; discussion 264–266, 2002.
2. Albain KS, Rusch VW, Crowley JJ, et al: Concurrent cisplatin/etoposide plus chest radiotherapy followed by surgery for stages IIIA (N2) and IIIB non-small-cell lung cancer: Mature results of Southwest Oncology Group phase II study 8805. J Clin Oncol 13(8):1880–1892, 1995.
3. Albain KS, Scott CB, Rusch VR, et al: Phase III comparison of concurrent chemotherapy plus radiotherapy (CT/RT) and CT/RT followed by surgical resection for stage IIIA (pN2) non-

small cell lung cancer (NSCLC): Initial results from intergroup trial 0139 (RTOG93-09). Proc Am Soc Clin Onc 22:621, 2003.

4. Albain KS: Induction therapy followed by definitive local control for stage III non-small-cell lung cancer. A review, with a focus on recent trimodality trials. Chest 103 (suppl 1):43S–50S, 1993.

5. Andre F, Grunewald D, Le Chevalier T: Persistence of viable tumor cells after radiation and chemotherapy for stage IIIB non-small cell lung cancer: An early marker of treatment failure. J Thorac Cardiovasc Surg 121(2):403, 2001.

6. Arriagada R, Bergman B, Dunant A, et al: Cisplatin-based adjuvant chemotherapy in patients with completely resected non-small-cell lung cancer. N Engl J Med 350(4):351–360, 2004.

7. Bonner JA: The role of postoperative radiotherapy for patients with completely resected non-small cell lung carcinoma: Seeking to optimize local control and survival while minimizing toxicity. Cancer 86(2):195–196, 1999.

8. Brunner KW, Marthaler T, Muller W: Effects of long-term adjuvant chemotherapy with cyclophosphamide (NSC-26271) for radically resected bronchogenic carcinoma. Cancer Chemother Rep 4(2):125–132, 1973.

9. Chardack WM, Maccallum JD: Pancoast tumor: Five-year survival without recurrence or metastases following radical resection and postoperative irradiation. J Thorac Surg 31(5):535–542, 1956.

10. Carbone DP, Minna JD: Chemotherapy in non-small cell lung cancer: A meta-analysis using updated data on individual patients from 52 randomised clinical trials. Non-small Cell Lung Cancer Collaborative Group. Br J Med 311(7010):889–890, 1995.

11. Choi NC, Carey RW, Daly W, et al: Potential impact on survival of improved tumor downstaging and resection rate by preoperative twice-daily radiation and concurrent chemotherapy in stage IIIA non-small-cell lung cancer. J Clin Oncol 15(2):712–722, 1997.

12. Ciardiello F, Caputo R, Bianco R, et al: Inhibition of growth factor production and angiogenesis in human cancer cells by ZD1839 (Iressa), a selective epidermal growth factor receptor tyrosine kinase inhibitor. Clin Cancer Res 7(5):1459–1465, 2001.

13. D'Amico TA, Massey M, Herndon JE 2nd, et al: A biologic risk model for stage I lung cancer: Immunohistochemical analysis of 408 patients with the use of ten molecular markers. J Thorac Cardiovasc Surg 117(4):736–743, 1999.

14. DeCamp MM, Rice TW, Adelstein DJ, et al: Value of accelerated multimodality therapy in stage IIIA and IIIB non-small cell lung cancer. J Thorac Cardiovasc Surg 126(1):17–27, 2003.

15. Depierre A, Milleron B, Moro-Sibilot D, et al: Preoperative chemotherapy followed by surgery compared with primary surgery in resectable stage I (except T1N0), II, and IIIa non-small-cell lung cancer. J Clin Oncol 20(1):247–253, 2002.

16. Detterbeck F: Diagnosis and Treatment of Lung Cancer: An Evidence-Based Guide for the Practicing Clinician, pp. 233–243. Philadelphia: W.B. Saunders, 2001.

17. Detterbeck FC: Changes in the treatment of Pancoast tumors. Ann Thorac Surg 75(6):1990–1997, 2003.

18. Detterbeck FC: Pancoast (superior sulcus) tumors. Ann Thorac Surg 63(6):1810–1818, 1997.

19. Dillman RO, Seagren SL, Propert KJ, et al: A randomized trial of induction chemotherapy plus high-dose radiation versus radiation alone in stage III non-small-cell lung cancer. N Engl J Med 323(14):940–945, 1990.

20. Early Breast Cancer Trialists Collaborative Group: Systemic treatment of early breast cancer by hormonal, cytotoxic, immune therapy: 133 randomised trials involving 31,000 recurrences and 24,000 deaths among 75,000 women. Lancet 339:1–15, 1992.

21. Eberhardt W, Wilke H, Stamatis G, et al: Preoperative chemotherapy followed by concurrent chemoradiation therapy based on hyperfractionated accelerated radiotherapy and definitive surgery in locally advanced non-small-cell lung cancer: Mature results of a phase II trial. J Clin Oncol 16(2):622–634, 1998.

22. Effects of postoperative mediastinal radiation on completely resected stage II and stage III epidermoid cancer of the lung. The Lung Cancer Study Group. N Engl J Med 315(22): 1377–1381, 1986.

23. Feld R, Rubinstein L, Thomas PA: Adjuvant chemotherapy with cyclophosphamide, doxorubicin, and cisplatin in patients with completely resected stage I non-small-cell lung cancer. The Lung Cancer Study Group. J Natl Cancer Inst 85(4):299–306, 1993.

24. Fowler WC, Langer CJ, Curran WJ Jr., et al: Postoperative complications after combined neoadjuvant treatment of lung cancer. Ann Thorac Surg 55(4):986–989, 1993.

25. Ginsberg RJ, Hill LD, Eagan RT, et al: Modern thirty-day operative mortality for surgical resections in lung cancer. J Thorac Cardiovasc Surg 86(5):654–658, 1983.

26. Ginsberg RJ, Martini N, Zaman M, et al: Influence of surgical resection and brachytherapy in the management of superior sulcus tumor. Ann Thorac Surg 57(6):1440–1455, 1994.

27. Ginsberg RJ, Vokes EE, Raben A: Non-small cell lung cancer. In Devita VTJ, Hellman S, Rosenberg SA, editors: Cancer Principles and Practice of Oncology, pp. 858–911. Philadelphia: Lippincott-Raven, 1997.

28. Goldie JH, Coldman AJ: A mathematic model for relating the drug sensitivity of tumors to their spontaneous mutation rate. Goldie Cancer Treat Rep 63(11–12):1727–1733, 1979.

29. Gonzalez-Stawinski GV, Lemaire A, Merchant F, et al: A comparative analysis of positron emission tomography and mediastinoscopy in staging non-small cell lung cancer. J Thorac Cardiovasc Surg 126(6):1900–1905, 2003.

30. Green FL, Page DL, Fleming ID: Cancer Staging Manual, pp. 167–177. New York: Springer-Verlag, 2002.

31. Grunenwald DH, Andre F, Le Pechoux C, et al: Benefit of surgery after chemoradiotherapy in stage IIIB (T4 and/or N3) non-small cell lung cancer. J Thorac Cardiovasc Surg 122(4):796–802, 2001.

32. Harpole DH Jr., DeCamp MM Jr., Daley J, et al: Prognostic models of thirty-day mortality and morbidity after major pulmonary resection. J Thorac Cardiovasc Surg 117(5): 969–979, 1999.

33. Higgins GA, Shields TW: Experience of the Veterans Administration Surgical Adjuvant Group. In Muggia F, Rozencwieg M, editors: Lung Cancer: Progress in Therapeutic Research, p. 433. New York: Raven Press, 1979.

34. Holmes EC, Gail M: Surgical adjuvant therapy for stage II and stage III adenocarcinoma and large-cell undifferentiated carcinoma. J Clin Oncol 4(5):710–715, 1986.

35. Huang SM, Harari PM: Epidermal growth factor receptor inhibition in cancer therapy: Biology, rationale and preliminary clinical results. Invest New Drugs 17(3):259–269, 1999.

36. International Multicentre Pooled Analysis of Colon Cancer Trials (IMPACT) Investigators: Efficacy of adjuvant fluorouracil and folinic acid in colon cancer. Lancet 345:939–944, 1995.

37. Kwiatkowski DJ, Harpole DH Jr., Godleski J, et al: Molecular pathologic substaging in 244 stage I non-small-cell lung cancer patients: Clinical implications. J Clin Oncol 16(7):2468–2477, 1998.

38. Lafitte JJ, Ribet ME, Prevost BM, et al: Postresection irradiation for T2 N0 M0 non-small cell carcinoma: A prospective, randomized study. Ann Thorac Surg 62(3):830–834, 1996.

39. Lau CL, D'Amico TA: Clinical and molecular prognostic factors and models for non-small cell lung cancer. In Pass HI, Mitchell JB, Johnson DH, editors: Lung Cancer: Principles and Practice, pp. 602–611. Philadelphia: Lippincott Williams & Wilkins, 2000.

40. Le Chevalier T, Arriagada R, Quoix E, et al: Radiotherapy alone versus combined chemotherapy and radiotherapy in nonresectable non-small-cell lung cancer: First analysis of a randomized trial in 353 patients. J Natl Cancer Inst 83(6):417–423, 1991.

41. Martini N, Bains MS, Burt ME, et al: Incidence of local recurrence and second primary tumors in resected stage I lung cancer. J Thorac Cardiovasc Surg 109(1):120–129, 1995.

42. Martini N, Flehinger BJ, Zaman MB, et al: Results of resection in non-oat cell carcinoma of the lung with mediastinal lymph node metastases. Ann Surg 198(3): 386–397, 1983.

43. Mateu-Navarro M, Rami-Porta R, Bastus-Piulats R, et al: Remediastinoscopy after induction chemotherapy in non-small cell lung cancer. Ann Thorac Surg 70(2):391–395, 2000.

44. Mentzer SJ, Swanson SJ, DeCamp MM, et al: Mediastinoscopy, thoracoscopy, and video-assisted thoracic surgery in the diagnosis and staging of lung cancer. Chest 112 (suppl 4):239S–241S, 1997.

45. Miller DL, McManus KG, Allen MS, et al: Results of surgical resection in patients with N2 non-small cell lung cancer. Ann Thorac Surg 57(5):1095–1000; discussion 1100–1101, 1994.

46. Mountain CF, Lukeman JM, Hammar SP, et al: Lung cancer classification: The relationship of disease extent and cell type to survival in a clinical trials population. J Surg Oncol 35(3):147–156, 1987.

47. Mountain CF: Prognostic implications of the International Staging System for Lung Cancer. Semin Oncol 15(3):236–245, 1988.

48. Mountain CF: Revisions in the International System for Staging Lung Cancer. Chest 111(6):1710–1717, 1997.

49. Muggia FM, Rozencweig M: Lung Cancer: Progressive Therapeutic Research, p. 443. New York: Raven Press, 1979.

50. Muscolino G, Valente M, Andreani S: Pancoast tumours: Clinical assessment and long-term results of combined radiosurgical treatment. Thorax 52(3):284–286, 1997.

51. Niwa H, Masaoka A, Yamakawa Y, et al: Surgical therapy for apical invasive lung cancer: Different approaches according to tumor location. Lung Cancer 10(1–2):63–71, 1993.

52. Ohta M, Tsuchiya R, Shimoyama M, et al: Adjuvant chemotherapy for completely resected stage III non-small-cell lung cancer. Results of a randomized prospective study. The Japan Clinical Oncology Group. J Thorac Cardiovasc Surg 106(4):703–708, 1993.

53. Paulson DL: Carcinomas in the superior pulmonary sulcus. J Thorac Cardiovasc Surg 70(6):1095–1104, 1975.

54. Pearson FG, DeLarue NC, Ilves R, et al: Significance of positive superior mediastinal nodes identified at mediastinoscopy in patients with resectable cancer of the lung. J Thorac Cardiovasc Surg 83(1):1–11, 1982.

55. Pisters KM, Ginsberg RJ, Giroux DJ, et al: Induction chemotherapy before surgery for early-stage lung cancer: A novel approach. Bimodality Lung Oncology Team. J Thorac Cardiovasc Surg 119(3):429–439, 2000.

56. Pisters KM, Kris MG, Gralla RJ, et al: Randomized trial comparing postoperative chemotherapy with vindesine and cisplatin plus thoracic irradiation with irradiation alone in stage III (N2) non-small cell lung cancer. J Surg Oncol 56(4): 236–241, 1994.

57. Postoperative radiotherapy in non-small-cell lung cancer: Systematic review and meta-analysis of individual patient data from nine randomised controlled trials. PORT Meta-analysis Trialists Group. Lancet 352(9124):257–263, 1998.

58. Rami-Porta R: Restaging after induction therapy for non-small cell lung cancer. Ann Thorac Cardiovasc Surg 8(6):325–327, 2002.

59. Rapp E, Pater JL, Willan A, et al: Chemotherapy can prolong survival in patients with advanced non-small-cell lung cancer: Report of a Canadian multicenter randomized trial. J Clin Oncol 6(4):633–641, 1988.

60. Reed CE, Harpole DH, Posther KE, et al: Results of the American College of Surgeons Oncology Group Z0050 trial: The utility of positron emission tomography in staging potentially operable non-small cell lung cancer. J Thorac Cardiovasc Surg 126(6):1943–1951, 2003.

61. Roberts JR, Eustis C, Devore R, et al: Induction chemotherapy increases perioperative complications in patients undergoing resection for non-small cell lung cancer. Ann Thorac Surg 72(3):885–888, 2001.

62. Rosell R, Gomez-Codina J, Camps C, et al: Preresectional chemotherapy in stage IIIA non-small-cell lung cancer: A 7-year assessment of a randomized controlled trial. Lung Cancer 26(1):7–14, 1999.

63. Rosell R, Gomez-Godina J, Camps C, et al: A randomized trial comparing preoperative chemotherapy plus surgery with surgery alone in patients with non-small cell lung cancer. N Engl J Med 330(3):153–158, 1994.

64. Roth JA, Atkinson EN, Fossella F, et al: Long-term follow-up of patients enrolled in a randomized trial comparing perioperative chemotherapy and surgery with surgery alone in resectable stage IIIA non-small-cell lung cancer. Lung Cancer 21(1):1–6, 1998.

65. Roth JA, Fossella F, Komaki R, et al: A randomized trial comparing perioperative chemotherapy and surgery with surgery alone in resectable stage IIIA non-small-cell lung cancer. J Natl Cancer Inst 86(9):673–680, 1994.

66. Rusch VW, Albain KS, Crowley JJ, et al: Surgical resection of stage IIIA and stage IIIB non-small-cell lung cancer after concurrent induction chemoradiotherapy. A Southwest Oncology Group trial. J Thorac Cardiovasc Surg 105(1):97–104; discussion 104–106, 1993.

67. Rusch VW, Giroux DJ, Kraut MJ, et al: Induction chemoradiation and surgical resection for non-small cell lung carcinomas of the superior sulcus: Initial results of Southwest Oncology Group Trial 9416 (Intergroup Trial 0160). J Thorac Cardiovasc Surg 121(3):472–483, 2001.

68. Rusch VW, Parekh KR, Leon L, et al: Factors determining outcome after surgical resection of T3 and T4 lung cancers of the superior sulcus. J Thorac Cardiovasc Surg 119(6):1147–1153, 2000.

69. Sawyer TE, Bonner JA: Postoperative irradiation in non-small cell lung cancer. In Pass HI, Mitchell JB, Johnson DH, editors: Lung Cancer: Principles and Practice, pp. 778–797. Philadelphia: Lippincott Williams & Wilkins, 2000.

70. Scagliotti GV, Fossati R, Torri V, et al: Randomized study of adjuvant chemotherapy for completely resected stage I, II, or IIIA non-small-cell lung cancer. J Natl Cancer Inst 95(19):1453–1461, 2003.

71. Schaake-Koning C, van den Bogaert W, Dalesio O, et al: Effects of concomitant cisplatin and radiotherapy on inoperable non-small-cell lung cancer. N Engl J Med 326(8):524–530, 1992.

72. Paulson DL: Carcinomas in the superior sulcus. J Thora Cardiovasc Surg 70(6):1095–1104, 1975.

73. Shields TW, Higgins GA Jr., Humphrey EW, et al: Prolonged intermittent adjuvant chemotherapy with CCNU and hydroxyurea after resection of carcinoma of the lung. Cancer 50(9):1713–1721, 1982.

74. Shields TW, Higgins GA Jr., Lawton R, et al: Preoperative x-ray therapy as an adjuvant in the treatment of bronchogenic carcinoma. J Thorac Cardiovasc Surg 59(1):49–61, 1970.

75. Slack NH: Bronchogenic carcinoma: Nitrogen mustard as a surgical adjuvant and factors influencing survival. University surgical adjuvant lung project. Cancer 25(5):987–1002, 1970.

76. Song S, Wientjes MG, Gan Y, et al: Fibroblast growth factors: An epigenetic mechanism of broad spectrum resistance to anticancer drugs. Proc Natl Acad Sci U S A 97(15):8658–8663, 2000.

77. Stephens RJ, Girling DJ, Bleehen NM, et al: The role of post-operative radiotherapy in non-small-cell lung cancer: A multicentre randomised trial in patients with pathologically staged T1-2, N1-2, M0 disease. Medical Research Council Lung Cancer Working Party. Br J Cancer 74(4):632–639, 1996.

78. Sugarbaker DJ, Herndon J, Kohman LJ, et al: Results of cancer and leukemia group B protocol 8935. A multiinstitutional phase II trimodality trial for stage IIIA (N2) non-small-cell lung cancer. Cancer and Leukemia Group B Thoracic Surgery Group. J Thorac Cardiovasc Surg 109(3):473–483; discussion 483–485, 1995.

79. Thames HD Jr., Peters LJ, Withers HR, et al: Accelerated fractionation vs hyperfractionation: Rationales for several treatments per day. Int J Radiat Oncol Biol Phys 9(2):127–138, 1983.

80. Van Houtte P, Rocmans P, Smets P, et al: Postoperative radiation therapy in lung cancer: A controlled trial after resection of curative design. Int J Radiat Oncol Biol Phys 6(8):983–986, 1980.

81. Van Schil P, van der Schoot J, Poniewierski J, et al: Remediastinoscopy after neoadjuvant therapy for non-small cell lung cancer. Lung Cancer 37(3):281–285, 2002.

82. Wallace MB, Silvestri GA, Sahai AV, et al: Endoscopic ultrasound-guided fine needle aspiration for staging patients with carcinoma of the lung. Ann Thorac Surg 72(6):1861–1867, 2001.

83. Warram J: Preoperative irradiation of cancer of the lung: Final report of a therapeutic trial. A collaborative study. Cancer 36(3):914–925, 1975.

84. Withers HR: Biologic basis for altered fractionation schemes. Cancer 55(suppl 9):2086–2095, 1985.

85. Woodburn JR: The epidermal growth factor receptor and its inhibition in cancer therapy. Pharmacol Ther 82(2–3):241–250, 1999.

Lung Cancer: Surgical Strategies for Tumors Invading the Chest Wall

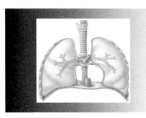

Michael Straznicka and Garrett L. Walsh

▶ INTRODUCTION AND HISTORY

Lung cancer continues to be the leading cause of cancer-related deaths in both men and women. Over 75% of non–small cell lung cancers (NSCLC) are in advanced stages at the time of presentation, with extensive locoregional disease or distant metastasis. The majority of resectable lung cancers are confined to the pulmonary parenchyma, but 5–8% extend beyond the lungs and invade the pleura, soft tissues, or osseous structures of the chest wall.[11,13] Chest wall invasion for surgical staging (T_3) is defined as any tumor involvement into or beyond the parietal pleura. Pathologists can further describe these tumors by their depth of chest wall invasion, but this is infrequently reported in this subset of T_3 patients.

Historically, chest wall invasion by a tumor of any histology was considered to be unresectable. Early surgical experience demonstrated that the surgical violation of the parietal pleura resulted in a sucking chest wound with immediate pulmonary collapse, often leading to the rapid demise of the patient. Dr. M. Michellau presented to the Institute of France in Paris in March of 1818 with a fungating mass protruding from his left chest wall. Dr. Richerand proposed a resection of the involved rib and pleura, an unprecedented operation at that time. On March 31, 1818, Dr. Richerand resected the left sixth and seventh ribs of Dr. Michellau with an unexpected occurrence of acute respiratory distress upon entrance into the chest cavity. The patient was saved by covering the aperture with a linen cloth plastered with cerate. Despite a rock postoperative course, Dr.

Michellau survived and returned home 27 days postoperatively. The pathology of the lesion is not known, but a primary rib malignancy is suspected.[46a]

In the summer of 1883 a brilliant young surgeon, H.M. Block, in what was then called Danzig, East Prussia, now Gdansk, Poland, carried out the first planned pulmonary resection. Dr. Block had performed successful open chest surgery on experimental animals and was eager to apply his experience to humans.[3] He chose a young female relative with a diagnosis of bilateral pulmonary tuberculosis and performed a thoracotomy to resect her diseased lung. Although the details of the operation are not known, we do know that the operation had a tragic end. A few days later, the short, brilliant career of Dr. Block ended with a self-inflicted gunshot wound to the head.[52]

Murphy[37] described his experiments and clinical experiences with open pneumothorax during his address to the American Medical Association in 1898. Parham,[44] in 1899, was the first in the United States to report resection of a bony chest wall tumor involving three ribs. A controlled pneumothorax with soft-tissue coverage was created. This patient survived, although many others who followed did not.

The difficulties of operating with an opened pleural space in a spontaneously breathing patient were all too apparent to the surgeons of those times. Working without adequate control of the airway and ventilator support was difficult, and the patient quickly deteriorated once the chest was open. Many ideas were investigated to overcome these deficiencies of the anesthetic techniques.

Major surgical and anesthesia advances were introduced in 1904 at the German Surgical Congress in Berlin. Two techniques, designed to surmount the open chest problem, were proposed. Ferdinand Sauerbruch,[47] from the surgical clinic of von Mickulykz at the University of Breslau, introduced his method of *"unterdruck"* (low pressure) ventilation. Lung expansion was maintained after thoracotomy by keeping an experimental animal's entire body inside a negative pressure chamber (at −15 cm H_2O) while the head remained outside the chamber with the anesthesiologist. Brauer[4] described the benefits of *"uberdruck"* (high pressure) anesthesia, in which the lung was kept expanded by placing the patient's head in a glass positive pressure chamber.

Surprisingly, the "unterdruck" method initially was the preferred technique. Sauerbruch and von Mickulykz built a negative-pressure operating room large enough to accommodate an entire surgical team, in which successful thoracic operations were carried out. These rooms continued to be built as late as 1918 in Munich by Sauerbruch, making this approach the favored method in Germany throughout the

296

1930s. Sauerbruch's ideas and methods so dominated his associates and contemporaries that little progress in other anesthetic techniques were issued from Germany during this era.

Major progress, however, had already begun and would continue in France, England, and the United States during roughly the same period. The use of positive pressure ventilation of the lungs was slowly being developed. Reliable delivery of positive pressure to the lungs was possible only by direct intubation of the trachea, and at that time, a tracheotomy was the only technique for tracheal intubation. Most surgeons were unwilling to perform a tracheotomy simply to deliver an anesthetic under positive pressure. The first systematic use of intubation through the mouth using bellows to inflate the lung was by the Frenchman DePaul, who intubated and resuscitated neonates in the mid-1800s. Other French surgeons, Tuffier, Quenu, and Doyen, and Milton in Egypt, also used positive pressure during thoracotomies in the last few years of the nineteenth century.

In the late 1800s two physicians from New York, Joseph O'Dwyer and George Fell, described intubation techniques and positive pressure ventilation. Dr. O'Dwyer developed a practical method of endotracheal intubation for the treatment of diphtheria, which was applied in thousands of cases and resulted in a gratifying decrease in the mortality rate of that dreaded disease.[40,42] Dr. Fell also used a crude device to maintain ventilation in patients suffering from drug overdoses.[14] In New Orleans Parham and Matas used the combined Fell–O'Dwyer apparatus in 1898 to administer positive pressure surgical anesthesia.[41]

The use of positive pressure ventilation identified the need for cuffed endotracheal tubes for the reliable delivery of anesthesia to the lungs. Eisenmenger first described a cuffed endotracheal tube in 1893. Placement of such tubes was facilitated by Kirstein,[28] who introduced direct laryngoscopy in 1895 for safe, reliable placement of endotracheal tubes in the trachea. In 1907 Chevalier Jackson improved the laryngoscope and produced the instrument that is still in use today and bears his name.[48] A practical endotracheal tube design for general use was introduced by Guedel in 1928,[22] and its use became widespread starting in the 1930s. In 1938 the first operative use of ventilators was made with the Freckner "Spiropulsator," developed in Sweden. In 1942 Griffith in Montreal, Canada, introduced curare to facilitate intraoperative controlled ventilation.[19]

With these international advances in intubation techniques and airway management, positive pressure anesthesia slowly became a clinical reality during the last few years of the nineteenth century and the first few decades of the twentieth century. As a direct result, surgeons were now willing to transgress the parietal pleura to address the complex pathologies of the thoracic cavity with increasing frequency. From 1904 to 1929, surgeons began to specialize and perform a series of pulmonary resections, and by 1929, thoracic surgery had become an established specialty. Most early lung resections and thoracoplasties were performed because of infections. Surgical morbidity and mortality rates were horrifying at first, and only the bravest patients and the most resilient surgeons chose to continue to work in the field. Sepsis was the predominant cause of death and was correlated mainly with an open pleural cavity.

In 1947 Coleman[9] reported long-term survival after en bloc excision of the chest wall with pulmonary resection.

Concurrently, significant strides in chest wall reconstructive techniques were occurring through the use of fascia lata grafts,

autogenous rib grafts, large cutaneous flaps, and latissimus dorsi muscle flaps, as described by Campbell in 1950[6a] and Grillo in 1966.[21] Over the past 40 years we have witnessed further refinements in surgical procedures, the use of prophylactic antibiotics, improved anesthesia delivery and monitoring, and the implementation and utilization of critical care units for postoperative ventilation. Today these advances permit the safe and effective resection of locally advanced lung cancer with extensive chest wall involvement on a routine basis.

Pancoast tumors comprise a distinct surgical entity and are discussed separately.

▶ DEMOGRAPHICS AND SYMPTOMS

Patients with lung cancer are usually 50–70 years old; lung cancer is rarely seen in patients younger than 30 years, although with the ongoing epidemic of children and young teenage smokers, advanced lung cancer can be seen even in these younger age groups (Figure 20-1). Lung cancer with chest wall invasion most typically presents in patients in their seventh decade, with a median age of 64–66 years (range, 38–93 years).[6,33,43] Overall, lung cancer incidence and mortality continue to be disproportionately higher in men than in women, although the gap is narrowing. Lung cancer with chest wall invasion has an overwhelming predominance in men; women represent only 10–30% of patients in several recent studies.[6,13,33,43] Current or previous smoking history is elicited in approximately two thirds of patients, with an average 50-pack-year history per patient.[6,13]

The lung parenchyma has no sensory nerve fibers, which accounts for the often late clinical presentation of most bronchogenic tumors. The majority of patients have presenting symptoms related to compression, invasion, or obstruction of the lung parenchyma or airways, or invasion of the chest wall or mediastinal structures. Metastasis to distant organs, including neurological symptoms and bone pain, unfortunately are common.

Patients whose lung cancer has invaded the chest wall have similar presenting symptoms, including chest pain (40–60%), cough (14%), recurrent lower respiratory tract infection (10–25%), dyspnea (11%), hemoptysis (12%), and weight loss (10–18%). However, as many as 25% of patients can be asymptomatic (Table 20-1).[6,13,33]

The right lung has a slight predominance in location of lung cancers, both in general and for those with chest wall invasion.[13] Okad described a marked predilection for the upper lobes in his series of lung cancers that invade the chest wall, although not all series confirm this finding.[43] Lung cancers in general have a slight predilection for upper lobes rather than lower lobes.

Squamous cell carcinoma is the classic smoking-related tumor, and for many years it was the most common histology. In recent years, however, adenocarcinoma has overtaken squamous cell carcinoma as the most common lung cancer worldwide. Several series of patients with lung cancer that invades the chest wall have demonstrated that the histological diagnosis of squamous cell carcinoma remains the most common, followed closely by adenocarcinoma; large cell carcinoma and adenosquamous carcinoma comprise fewer of these tumors.[13,33,43] Average tumor diameter in these patients, by computed tomography (CT) measurements, was 6.5 cm; tumors ranged from 2–18 cm in maximum diameter.[13]

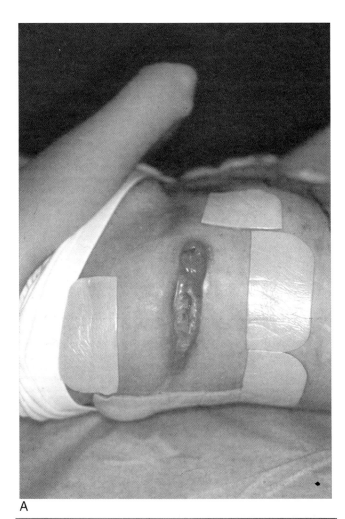

A

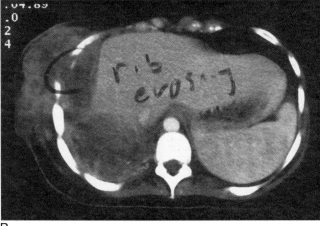

B

Figure 20–1 **A,** A 25-year-old woman presents to our institution with a nonhealing thoracotomy incision with a draining wound after an attempted decortication for what was initially felt to be a postpneumonic empyema. **B,** A CT scan demonstrates a large right lower lobe adenocarcinoma of the lung with direct invasion of the chest wall as the cause for the nonhealing wound.

Table 20–1

Presenting Symptoms in Lung Cancers with Chest Wall Invasion

Presenting symptom	Percent
Chest pain	40–60%
Recurrent lower respiratory tract infection	10–25%
Weight loss	10–18%
Cough	11%
Hemoptysis	12%
Dyspnea	11%
Asymptomatic	25%

is identified on routine chest X–rays in only a fraction of cases. Tissue diagnosis of malignancy in these T_3 lesions usually is obtained by transthoracic needle aspiration by our interventional radiologists.

Peripheral lung lesions with the suggestion of chest wall involvement may require additional radiographic testing to confirm invasion. These radiographic techniques include CT scans, nuclear medicine (scintigraphic) bone scans, magnetic resonance imaging (MRI), and positron emission tomography (PET) scans. Although gross tumor involvement of the chest wall is easily diagnosed with these radiographic modalities, confirmation of isolated parietal or mediastinal pleural invasion is more difficult and often unreliable.[17,18,29,45]

The use of CT scans has greatly increased the precision of tumor localization, allowed accurate evaluation of contiguous organ involvement, improved assessment of lymph nodes, and improved the identification of pulmonary metastasis. A CT scan is excellent for assessing rib destruction and intercostal muscle tumor extension, but is relatively inaccurate for invasion limited to the parietal or mediastinal pleura.[17,18,45] Helical three-dimensional reconstruction has been shown to be superior to standard two-dimensional images, but this technology is not in widespread use.[30] Shirakawa and associates[49] identified patients who had parietal pleural invasion by using inspiratory/expiratory CT scans. They demonstrated that a respiratory phase shift of greater than half of a vertebral body height in middle and lower lobe tumors reliably predicted the absence of parietal pleural invasion. The accuracy and negative predictive value were 90% and 86%, respectively, in tumors located in the lower and middle lobes. For upper lobe tumors, however, the respiratory phase shift did not correlate with operative findings regardless of whether invasion was present. This discrepancy is due to the minimal normal respiratory phase shift

▶ DIAGNOSIS

Chest roentgenography is useful for the identification of parenchymal lesions, although it has poor specificity and sensitivity for detecting chest wall involvement. Rib destruction is a reliable indicator of chest wall invasion, although it of these lung fields when the patients were studied in the supine position.

MRI has the advantages of multiplanar imaging and high differential signal intensity, which are invaluable for determining vascular invasion and spinal involvement. Conventional MRI, unfortunately, is just as limited as CT scans for evaluation of parietal and mediastinal pleural invasion. Kodalli and associates[29] used breath-hold inspiration and expiration MRI to assess parietal pleural invasion. Pleural invasion was excluded when tumor displacement exceeded 5 mm in reference to chest wall structures or relevant mediastinal structures (e.g., the aortic arch). This study identified 100% sensitivity and specificity for pleural invasion for tumors located in the middle lobe and basilar segments of the lower lobes. Studies of upper lobe tumors and those located in the apical segments of the lower lobes demonstrated a positive predictive value of only 40% but a negative predictive value of 100%. The superiority of MRI to CT scans lies in its ability to assess lung and diaphragm movement in a coronal plane. Insufficient respiratory motion is evident by less than 1-cm movement of the diaphragm on coronal images, and necessary scans could be repeated by asking the patient to take a deeper breath.

More invasive methods have been used for detection of parietal pleural invasion, including use of expiratory dynamic CT scans after the introduction of a diagnostic pneumothorax.[53,54] Lack of invasion was diagnosed on the basis of appearance of an air space between the mass and adjacent structures. Sensitivity was 100% in both studies for chest wall invasion, although sensitivity dropped to 76% in cases of mediastinal invasion. Specificity for tumor involvement was 80% in Watanabe's study.[53] Benign pleural adhesions caused false-positive results in both of these studies. Complications were reported as mild and included chest pain, shortness of breath, and subcutaneous emphysema.

Despite these results from a variety of imaging techniques, we do not feel that these tests are warranted because they potentially subject high-risk patients to the risks of a pneumothorax and ultimately are unlikely to alter the planned operative procedure.

▶ STAGING

Accurate staging of NSCLC is critical for effective clinical management. Standard staging includes a complete patient history and physical examination, laboratory tests (including complete blood cell counts, serum electrolytes, glucose, calcium, phosphorous, and liver function tests), electrocardiogram (ECG), chest X-ray, and CT scan of the chest and upper abdomen to include the adrenal glands. PET scans or combined CT–PET scans have become routine in our staging workup of lung cancer patients. MRIs of the brain are used whenever a patient has neurological symptoms or in whom the lesion is locally advanced or nodal disease is suspected.

Surgical–pathological staging is performed according to the new International Staging System for Lung Cancer, using information about the primary tumor (T), nodal status (N), and distant metastasis (M) (Table 20-2).[36] "T" status denotes characteristics of the primary tumor, including size and local aggressiveness. T_1 tumors are less than 3 cm in size and are surrounded by lung parenchyma. Primary tumors that

Table 20–2

Brief Description of the TNM Stage Groups for Lung Cancer

Stage 0	Carcinoma in situ		
Stage IA	T_1	N_0	M_0
Stage IB	T_2	N_0	M_0
Stage IIA	T_1	N_1	M_0
Stage IIB	T_2	N_1	M_0
	T_3	N_0	M_0
Stage IIIA	T_3	N_1	M_0
	T_1	N_2	M_0
	T_2	N_2	M_0
	T_3	N_2	M_0
Stage IIIB	T_4	N_0	M_0
	T_4	N_1	M_0
	T_4	N_2	M_0
	T_1	N_3	M_0
	T_2	N_3	M_0
	T_3	N_3	M_0
	T_4	N_3	M_0
Stage IV	Any T	Any N	M_1

involve only the visceral pleura are T_2. Chest wall involvement increases the T status to T_3. "Chest wall involvement," however, includes a wide pathological spectrum, from invasion of the parietal pleura only to full-thickness chest wall replacement by tumor. Other characteristics that denote a T_3 status include invasion of the diaphragm, involvement of the mediastinal pleura, involvement of the parietal pericardium, or a tumor within a main stem bronchus 2 cm or less from the carina, but not involving the carina. Full-thickness invasion into the mediastinum, including the heart, great vessels, trachea, and/or vertebral bodies denotes a T_4 classification. Satellite lesions located within the involved lobe also denote a T_4 classification. Most T_4 tumors are not considered suitable for surgical resection, although those patients in whom an R_0 (microscopically negative margins) resection is possible may be treated surgically.

Nodal status (N) comprises the second feature of the International Staging System. Clinical evidence of ipsilateral hilar node involvement is classified as N_1. N_1 disease is not considered a contraindication for surgical resection. Ipsilateral adenopathy of the mediastinum increases the nodal status to N_2. The most effective treatment modality for these patients is controversial and is discussed later. Spread of tumor to the contralateral mediastinal, contralateral hilar, or any scalene or supraclavicular nodal basins denotes an N_3 status; patients with N_3 disease generally are not considered surgical candidates.

Patients without evidence of distant metastatic disease are considered to have M_0 disease, and they may be candidates for surgical resection if T and N status are acceptable. Distant metastatic disease is noted as M_1; M_1 disease is almost always considered inoperable. Systemic treatment in the form of chemotherapy is currently the treatment of choice, often in combination with radiation therapy for local control.

In 1997 an important change was made to the TNM staging system. Before 1997 a NSCLC that was defined as $T_3 N_0 M_0$ was classified as stage IIIA. Survival data of patients with these tumors revealed that their clinical course with surgery alone was more favorable than those of other patients with stage IIIA disease (i.e., those with hilar or mediastinal lymph node involvement; T_3N_1, T_3N_2, T_1N_2, or T_2N_2). Subsequently, these tumors have been downstaged to stage IIB.

Because the survival rate of lung cancer patients with chest wall involvement and nodal disease is significantly worse than that of patients with chest involvement alone, the clinical challenge for surgeons is to identify nodal involvement by noninvasive imaging or minimally invasive biopsy techniques before subjecting patients to extensive chest wall resections.

The importance of correct pretreatment staging cannot be overemphasized. Hilar and mediastinal lymph nodes can be assessed before surgery by using CT scans, MRI, and PET scans. The utility of conventional CT scans has been surpassed by that of helical CT scans and MRI scans. More sophisticated tests such as PET scan measure biological characteristics of tissues and can detect disease in otherwise normal-appearing nodal tissue.

Despite advances in nuclear imaging techniques, mediastinoscopy remains the most sensitive and specific test for evaluating the mediastinal nodes and should be considered before undertaking a major chest wall resection in these patients. Because of its anatomical location, the preoperative assessment of N_1 disease is more problematic. Patients with T_3N_1 disease still should be considered for en bloc resections and have a better survival rate than those with N_2 disease.

Flexible bronchoscopy is performed for transbronchial biopsies, brushings, and washings. Although it is unlikely that peripheral chest wall tumors extend into the airway, it is the authors' practice to perform bronchoscopy immediately before resection to identify any unsuspected endobronchial disease and to assess the airway anatomy.

Extrathoracic metastases are found in up to 50% of patients with newly diagnosed lung cancer.[27] Patients with symptoms suggestive of central nervous system involvements are evaluated with an MRI scan of the brain. Symptoms or laboratory findings suggestive of disseminated malignancy, such as weight loss, bone pain, or elevated alkaline phosphatase, are evaluated with bone scintigraphy scans. CT scans of the chest are performed with intravenous (IV) contrast and include imaging of the liver and adrenal glands. Any abnormality suggestive of metastatic disease to the liver or adrenal glands is further investigated with dedicated abdominal CT scans, MRI, or liver ultrasound. Appropriate biopsies of suspicious lesions need to be performed before thoracic surgery.

Bone scintigraphy scans are used to detect occult bony metastases and confirm bony lesions in symptomatic patients. The vertebral column is the most commonly affected region for bone metastases. MRI is accepted as the most accurate imaging modality in detecting bone metastases within the vertebral column, and focal imaging can be guided by bone scan abnormalities or symptoms.[15,24,50] Suspicious uptake in bones other than the vertebral column also requires further investigation, although MRI scans become less useful. False positives are seen within the bony thorax when a history of rib fractures or trauma is noted. False negatives can be appreciated when bone scans are correlated with PET scans. Positive lesions on PET scans, which are not seen on bone scans, may represent soft tissue metastasis.[12] Durski and associates[12] recommend that all patients be staged with a PET scan, and bone scans should be performed only if symptomatically indicated when PET scans are negative. In their series, the use of bone scans in addition to PET scans did not change the clinical stage of any of their patients, although it allowed more precise localization of skeletal abnormalities.

PET scans using F18-fluorodeoxyglucose (FDG) are routinely used in addition to CT scans for both initial diagnosis and staging of NSCLC. One study suggests that performing both a PET and CT scan is more cost-effective than performing a CT scan alone for staging.[16] The reported sensitivity and specificity of PET for thoracic lymph node involvement are 70–100% and 81–100%, respectively. CT has a sensitivity and specificity of 25–81% and 56–94%, respectively.[2,8,23,35,51] Adrenal adenomas can be effectively diagnosed and biopsy avoided in cases where adrenal gland enlargement of 1 cm or more does not correlate with high FDG uptake on PET.

▸ TREATMENT

Patients with confirmed N_2 disease who are devoid of distant metastatic disease are offered treatment on protocol with neoadjuvant chemotherapy. Surgery is offered to those patients whose tumors show an objective response to chemotherapy and whose disease can be completely resected.[33] Progression of disease while on chemotherapy is generally regarded as a contraindication to surgery, as is evidence of N_3 disease. Preoperative radiation therapy has not been shown to increase survival in several studies, but has demonstrated an increased operative mortality.[1,11,33] Preoperative radiation therapy therefore is not widely used and is not recommended at our institution.

Patients with evidence of metastatic spread should not be considered surgical candidates except in extraordinary circumstances. These circumstances may include isolated brain metastases that can be resected before lung resection.

▸ PREOPERATIVE ASSESSMENT

The most important risk factors for perioperative complications for patients who are undergoing resection of lung tumors are cardiovascular and pulmonary disease, metabolic disorders (e.g., diabetes), and malnutrition. A complete preoperative assessment therefore includes physiological testing for cardiac and pulmonary reserve, optimal management of diabetes, and nutritional support when needed. Spirometry, arterial blood gases, alveolocapillary diffusion (DLCO), and xenon ventilation scans determine pulmonary reserve and predict postoperative function. Cardiac

300

evaluation, including ECG, echocardiography, stress testing, and even cardiac catheterization, may be required to identify correctable disease in high-risk patients. Nutritional assessment includes aggressive diabetic control, optimization of protein stores, and possible enteral or parenteral feeds for severely malnourished patients. Serial measurements of prealbumin levels may be used as a guide to nutritional improvement.

Most surgeons try to leave a patient with at least 33% of predicted forced expiratory volume in one second (FEV_1) postoperatively. The use of spirometry, xenon scanning, and exercise oxygen testing are helpful in identifying patients who are truly medically inoperable based on these pulmonary function criteria. There are no studies, however, that can accurately predict the increased postoperative pulmonary compromise of patients with T_3 lesions who require chest wall resections. It is often difficult to predict preoperatively the extent of required rib resections and the requirement for chest wall stabilization and reconstruction. Often a surgeon may end up removing more chest wall than anticipated. The overall effect on chest wall mechanics must be taken into account when evaluating the medical condition of the patient and the extent of pulmonary resection. Occasionally in patients with marginal lung function, a nonanatomical or subsegmental resection of the lung may be required if the chest wall component of the operation is extensive.

OPERATIVE TECHNIQUES

Good communication and cooperation with our anesthesia colleagues is crucial to the success of these operations. Several anesthetic techniques have dramatically improved our intraoperative course and our patients' postoperative recovery. The placement of an epidural catheter before the institution of general anesthesia is encouraged in all of our patients. A double-lumen endotracheal tube is useful for these cases and greatly facilitates visualization during the surgery.

In the great majority of patients, the tumor can be approached via a posterolateral thoracotomy. In tumors that involve the chest wall and the apex of the chest (either superior sulcus tumors proper or large upper lobe tumors with chest wall and neck extensions), an initial anterior neck approach to dissect the subclavian vessels and the brachial plexus may be beneficial before addressing the posterior chest wall component (Figure 20-2). Depending on the tumor location, the incision may be tailored more posteriorly

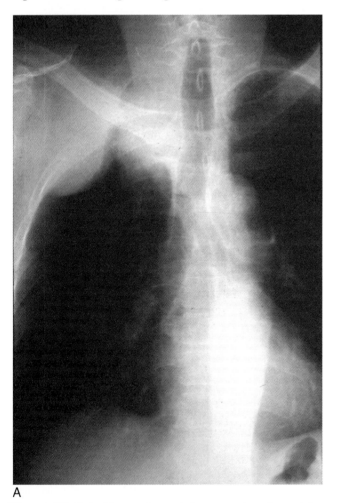

A

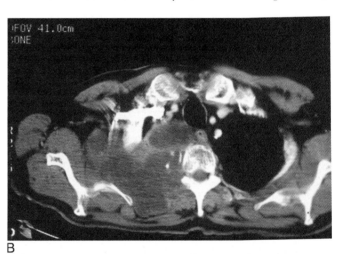

B

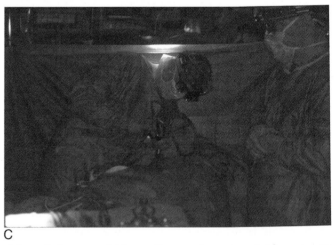

C

Figure 20–2 A, Chest radiograph demonstrating a large right upper lobe apical tumor, which was diagnosed a sarcomatoid carcinoma by transthoracic needle biopsy. **B,** A CT scan demonstrates the full thickness chest wall involvement with tumor extension into the posterior chest wall musculature. **C,** A mediastinoscopy is performed routinely to rule out N_2 or N_3 nodal involvement before proceeding with the extensive lung and chest wall resection. (See color plate for part **C.**)

and extended superiorly between the scapula and spinous processes. Review of the radiographic studies and palpation of the interspaces should identify an intercostal space at least one rib space below the inferior margin of the tumor for entry into the chest cavity. Upon entry into the hemithorax, careful digital examination of the lung and chest wall is performed to determine tumor attachment and assess chest wall fixation. The chest cavity is examined closely for pleural dissemination or metastatic deposits at other sites. Great care should be taken to prevent disruption of thin adhesions of the tumor to the parietal pleura that may be involved with tumor.

When tumor invasion into the chest wall is radiographically evident before surgery, an en bloc chest wall resection should be carried out with at least one uninvolved rib and intercostal muscle above and below the mass.[46] An en bloc resection is defined as removal of lung parenchyma in continuity with a portion of the adjacent parietal pleura and chest wall soft tissues. The overlying integument generally is

left intact, although complete extension of tumors through the skin can be seen (Figure 20-3).

On rare occasions when the tumor is large, its bulk can impede the exposure of the hilar structures. In this situation, several firings of a stapler through normal, uninvolved pulmonary parenchyma can permit the initial removal of the tumor and chest wall, with safer dissection of the delicate hilar vessels without the risk of torsion and traction created by the weight of the tumor and attached chest wall. An en bloc resection is preferred whenever it is feasible.

It is more difficult to determine the extent of malignant pleural involvement when the adhesions are thin and filmy between the tumor and the chest wall. The tumor may be somewhat mobile on palpation. A surgeon must resist the temptation to simply lyse these adhesions. An extrapleural dissection must be initiated. If the plane is not easily identified at any time during the extrapleural dissection, then the extrapleural dissection must be immediately halted and a

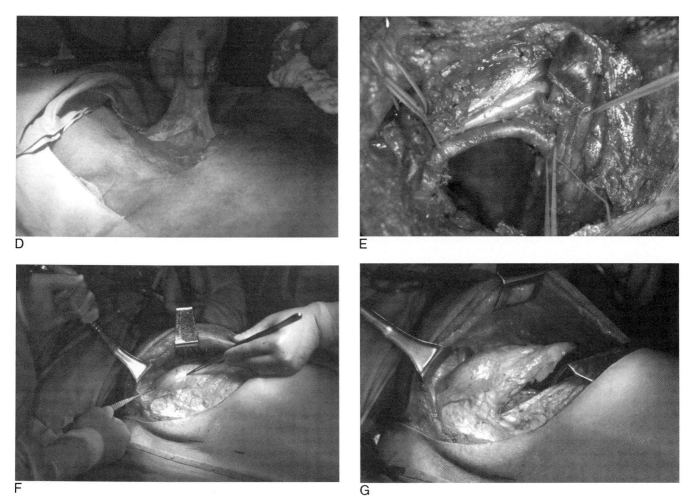

Figure 20–2 cont'd D, An initial supraclavicular neck dissection is performed to dissect the subclavian vessels and brachial plexus. This is the initial hockey-stick skin incision along the anterior border of the sternocleidomastoid muscle and along the clavicle. **E,** A close-up of the resection of the first and second ribs from the anterior approach with resection of the subclavian vein and preservation of the subclavian artery and brachial plexus as shown. **F,** The patient is repositioned. The initial dissection is through a posterolateral thoracotomy with elevation of the scapula after division of the latissimus dorsi muscle and reflection of the serratus anterior muscle. The tumor bulge into the interspaces of the chest wall can be appreciated. There is no gross tumor involvement of the external surface of the chest wall, however. **G,** An interspace is entered caudal to the inferior extent of the tumor involvement. (See color plate for parts **D** and **F**.)

(Continued)

302

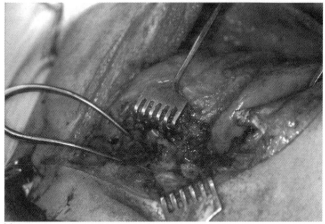

H

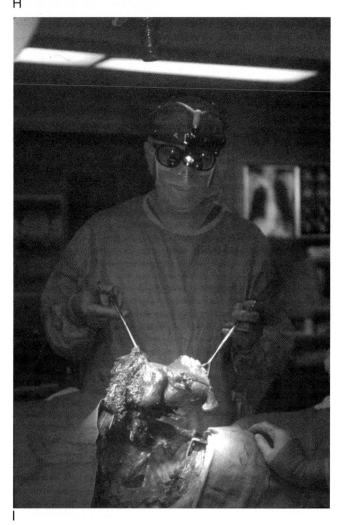

I

Figure 20–2 cont'd H, The posterior elevation of the paraspinous muscles and disarticulation of the posterior ribs from the transverse processes and vertebral bodies. **I,** Complete en bloc removal of the chest wall (ribs one to five) and the right upper lobe (See color plate.)

full-thickness chest wall resection performed. If the extrapleural dissection appears to proceed easily, frozen section analysis of the parietal pleura is recommended.[13] If the tumor transgresses the parietal pleura on frozen section, then an additional resection of the chest wall is required.

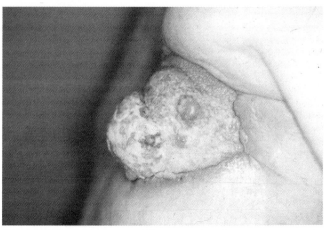

Figure 20–3 A 75-year-old man with a fungating tumor in the left anterior chest wall originating from a bronchogenic carcinoma of the lingula with transmural invasion of the chest wall and skin.

Circumferential margins of 2 cm generally are regarded as adequate, although some surgeons advocate a larger margin of 4 cm on the rib resection.[6,20] In these studies the mean number of ribs resected was three, with a range of one to five.[6,13] The oncological resection should never be compromised by less than a complete resection.

Several circumstances deserve additional mention. Special attention needs to be paid to tumors extending into the intervertebral foramen without intraspinal extension. Disarticulation of the ribs is performed through the costotransverse joints with ligation of the nerve roots as they exit the spinal column.[55] Tumors that extend into the vertebral column may require a laminectomy to expose the epidural tumor and involved nerve root. The tumor is dissected free from the dura, and the nerve roots are identified and transected. In cases where the tumor invades the vertebral bodies themselves, a partial resection of the vertebral body may be performed without the need for instrumentation. Resection should be carried out to grossly uninvolved bone and can include complete vertebrectomy with spinal reconstruction (Figure 20-4). Further discussion regarding vertebral resection and reconstruction is beyond the scope of this chapter.

Anterior tumors that invade into the sternum are resected en bloc with the involved portion of the sternum and attached ribs. A complete resection is mandatory and may necessitate a complete sternectomy. Reconstruction with a rigid prosthesis to prevent flail usually is required after a complete sternectomy. If the resection is limited to either the manubrium or less than one third of the sternum, reconstruction is often unnecessary.[38]

The resected portion of the chest wall remains attached to the lung and is allowed to drop into the hemithorax, where pulmonary resection is then carried out in the usual manner. The extent of pulmonary resection is determined by the amount of parenchymal involvement, as well as the pulmonary reserve of the patient. A crucial determinant for long-term survival is the ability to achieve a complete (R_0) resection.[11] The survival rate of patients who undergo incomplete resection (R_1) is comparable to that of patients who have not had a resection at all.[11] Most frequently, lobectomy is sufficient to achieve an R_0 resection.

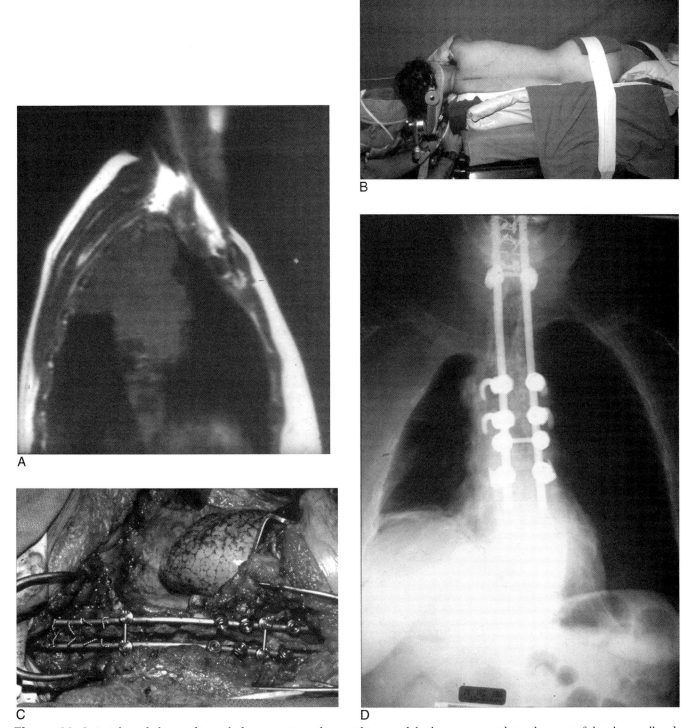

Figure 20–4 **A,** A lateral chest radiograph demonstrating a large right upper lobe lung cancer with involvement of the chest wall and T_1 through T_3 vertebral bodies. **B,** Operative positioning of the patient with the head in cervical tongs to immobilize it and to maintain the alignment of the cervical and thoracic spines. The patient is additionally secured on a beanbag and taped with the appropriate padding of the anterior superior iliac spine. **C,** Intraoperative photograph showing the resected chest wall, right upper lobe, and multilevel vertebral body resection with reconstruction with posterior rods and anterior stabilization. **D,** Chest radiograph posteroanterior (PA) demonstrating postoperative instrumentation. (See color plate for part **B.**)

304

Burkhart and associates,[6] in 95 operations for bronchogenic carcinoma with chest wall involvement, performed a lobectomy in 80% of patients in their series, pneumonectomy in 13%, bilobectomy in 4%, and sublobar resection in 3%. Okada,[43] in his series of 132 patients, favored a more lung-preserving approach, with 49% undergoing lobectomy, 15% segmentectomy, 13% sleeve lobectomy, 10% pneumonectomy, 8% lobectomy with partial resection, and 5% sleeve bilobectomy or sleeve pneumonectomy. In both series a complete mediastinal and hilar lymph node dissection was performed in each patient. In all cases the operating surgeon confirmed the clinical impression of an R_0 resection. In our practice we would agree with the general recommendation to perform a complete mediastinal and hilar nodal dissection in these patients.

▶ RECONSTRUCTION

Reconstruction of the chest wall defect is controversial. Some surgeons do not routinely reconstruct chest wall defects in any patients, and they report minimal morbidity. Facciolo and associates[13] performed 104 thoracotomies with full-thickness chest wall resection without prosthetic reconstruction of the costal elements in any patient. Chest wall defects were closed with scapula repositioning or chest wall muscle transfers. Exact details regarding location and complexity of the defects were not described, although the results were excellent.

In general, all full-thickness skeletal defects that have the potential for paradox should be considered for reconstruction. Both the size and location of the chest wall resection should guide the decision for reconstruction. When the defect is small, approximately 5 cm or less, the skeletal component can be ignored and the defect closed with overlying soft issues only. Posterior defects up to 10 cm in diameter may not require reconstruction because the overlying scapula provides support. Exceptions include midthoracic posterior defects that allow the scapular tip to become entrapped in the bony thorax during full range of motion of the ipsilateral arm. In these cases either the chest wall can be reconstructed or the scapular tip can be amputated.

Many complex chest wall chest defects require not only skeletal stabilization, but also skin and soft-tissue coverage to protect the reconstruction. Indications for reconstruction include the need for structural stability, cosmesis for anterior and lateral chest wall defects, obliteration of dead space, and recruitment of healthy soft tissue from nonanatomical areas to restore the chest wall integrity.

Reconstruction can be performed using autogenous tissues, such as fascia lata grafts or muscle transpositions, or various prosthetic materials, including mesh, metals, or soft-tissue patches. The use of autogenous tissue is favored when the wound to be closed is contaminated. Grossly contaminated wounds may need to remain open for a period of time for aggressive local wound care before attempted closure, sometimes at the expense of prolonged mechanical ventilation.

The most commonly used autogenous grafts are locally advanced muscle flaps. Although transposition of the latissimus dorsi muscle for chest wall coverage was described in 1896 by Tansini, it was Jurkiewicz and associates who reintroduced the musculocutaneous concept in 1977 and created a surge of interest in muscle and musculocutaneous flap reconstruction of the thoracic cavity.[5] The use of muscle flaps should be anticipated before surgery, and the operation conducted to protect the muscle of choice and its vascular pedicle at all times (Figure 20-5).

The most widely used local muscle flaps are the latissimus dorsi, pectoralis major, rectus abdominis, trapezius, and deltoid muscles. The latissimus dorsi muscle has excellent versatility because of its large size and wide arc of motion, allowing it to reach both the anterior and posterior thorax. The pectoralis major muscle also displays great versatility, with significant limitations only seen when posterior thoracic coverage is needed. In those cases it can be used as a free flap. Less frequently, the transverse rectus abdominis musculocutaneous (TRAM) flap is used. It is used almost exclusively for anterior defects and is rotated about its vascular pedicle.

When muscle flaps are not available or cannot be used, a variety of prosthetic materials are available. In fact, because of the availability and easy handling of synthetic materials, many surgeons prefer to use synthetic grafts for reconstruction even if muscle flaps are available. The choice of prosthetic material can vary, but the type of material used often depends upon the surgeon's preference. LeRoux and Shama have set forth the ideal characteristics of a prosthetic material: rigidity to abolish paradoxical chest motion, inertness to permit ingrowth of fibrous tissues and decrease the likelihood of infection, malleability so that it can be fashioned to the appropriate shape at the time of the operation, and radiolucency to allow for follow-up of the underlying problem.[34]

Additional desirable features include hypoallergenicity, lack of proven carcinogenicity, the ability to withstand sterilization, the ability to not be modified by bodily fluids, and adequate strength. Although no substance to date perfectly fulfills all of these criteria, various synthetic and alloplastic materials can be used with satisfactory results.

Polypropylene mesh (PM) (Marlex, Cranston RI) with or without methylmethacrylate sandwich, polytetrafluoroethylene (PTFE) mesh, and Vicryl mesh are examples of materials that have been used in different situations. PTFE is made in a variety of thickness sizes; 2-mm thickness is required for chest wall reconstruction to tolerate the tension generated during closure. Some surgeons consider PTFE to be easier to handle than PM because it lends itself to a slight stretch, can be sutured with less wrinkles and surface irregularities, and may create a watertight seal of the pleural space.[38] However, Deschamps and associates[10] compared PM mesh to PTFE and observed no significant differences in outcomes or complications.

Polypropylene mesh with methylmethacrylate (PPMM) sandwich provides the most rigidity and perhaps the best cosmetic result, at the price of greater difficulty of implantation. In cases where the chest wall resection is extensive and the possibility of paradoxical movement of the reconstruction is suspected, this level of rigidity is desired. A few key points need to be kept in mind when working with this unyielding material. After the specimen in removed, the patient is returned to a neutral position by unflexing the operating table if initially flexed on positioning. An imprint of the defect is made to determine the size of the reconstruction, and the mesh is tailored to leave approximately 2–3 cm of extra material circumferentially with which to secure the patch to the remaining chest wall. A thin layer of methylmethacrylate is applied directly to the mesh, leaving 2–3 cm of mesh circumferentially free of cement. A second layer of mesh, of identical size, is quickly applied to the cement, thereby creating the "sandwich." The cement generates a significant amount of heat as it hardens, so care must be taken to avoid contact with unprotected tissue. When the reconstruction is of the lateral chest wall, it is important to recreate the curvature of the thorax. This may be accomplished by allowing the sandwich to harden on a malleable retractor that has been shaped appropriately, or by allowing the sandwich to harden on the patient's (protected) iliac crest.

Regardless of the material used, the patch is secured taut with heavy interrupted nonabsorbable sutures either through or around the remaining ribs. If the spine constitutes the posterior border of the defect, the sutures may be placed through the transverse processes. The patch is then covered with adequate healthy soft tissue. Intrathoracic chest tubes are tunneled a distance from the reconstruction and positioned to avoid direct contact with the synthetic material. Subcutaneous closed suction drains should be used when extensive flaps have been raised and a large potential dead space has been created.

The simplest and most practical method of coverage is local tissue advancement. There are occasional cases in which the local muscle flaps may be unavailable because the muscles have been extirpated or the vascular pedicle has been destroyed by surgical ablation or irradiation. In those cases free tissue transfer of flaps utilizing microvascular reconstruction can be used with excellent results.[39] Often these complex cases require the close interaction of the thoracic surgical team with our plastic surgeon colleagues. Available grafts can include contralateral latissimus dorsi and serratus anterior muscles, as well as both ipsilateral and contralateral TRAM flaps.[39] The omentum is an excellent salvage flap that can be used in cases where the pedicled muscle flap fails. Suction drains frequently are used to eliminate dead space, or in cases of large raw surfaces over the prosthetic reconstruction. Drains usually are removed when the daily drainage is less than 25 ml/day in each drain.

Lung tumors that involve the chest wall are exceedingly rare in children, but children present a unique challenge to the thoracic surgeon when reconstruction is necessary. Depending on the age of the child, growth of the chest wall continues, thereby limiting the ability to use prosthetic materials for reconstruction. As the child outgrows the

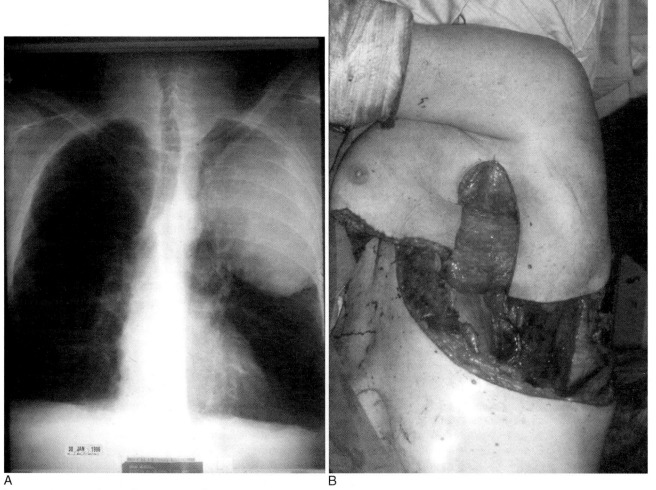

A   B

Figure 20–5 A, Chest radiograph (PA) demonstrating a large squamous cell carcinoma of the left upper lobe involving ribs one through seven. Mediastinoscopy was negative. **B,** Lateral operative positioning with the entail skin incision raised for muscle flaps.

(Continued)

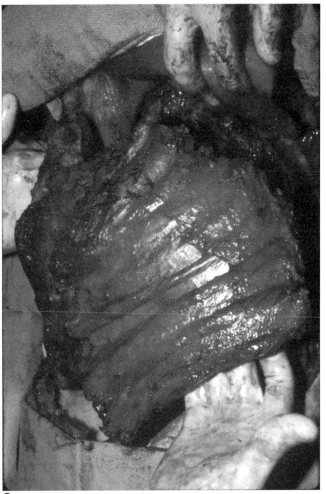

C

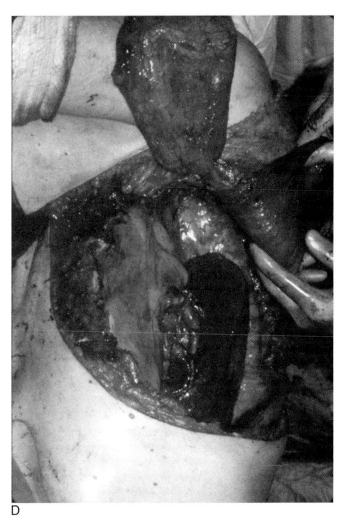

D

Figure 20–5 cont'd C, Operative photo demonstrating extensive chest wall resection of seven ribs with en bloc left upper lobe attached. **D,** Resulting surgical chest wall defect with previously mobilized muscle flaps (latissimus, serratus, and pectoralis) that are used to cover the prosthetic chest wall reconstruction. (See color plate.)

reconstruction, the mesh may cut through its anchors and recreate the defect. If a more solid reconstruction is used, it can act as a tether, eventually leading to contracture and deformity. Ideally reconstruction should be performed with rotational muscle flaps whose nerve supplies are carefully preserved, to allow for growth and a dynamic contribution to chest wall development.[25]

POSTOPERATIVE CARE

Postoperative care should be tailored to each individual patient. A patient with good preoperative pulmonary function who had a limited resection and reconstruction should be extubated in the operating room at the conclusion of the case and convalesced on a telemetry ward. A frailer patient with an extensive resection and reconstruction may require intubation for 24–48 hours in the intensive care unit, with meticulous respiratory hygiene. For all patients the authors prefer to continue epidural analgesia until the chest tubes are removed or up to 7 days after surgery (whichever comes first). Aggressive pulmonary hygiene, including early ambulation, incentive spirometry, and bronchodilators, is essen-

tial and is attended by a full-time respiratory therapy staff on the wards. All patients remain on telemetry monitors throughout their hospital stay. The use of antibiotics postoperatively usually is limited to three doses of a broad-spectrum cephalosporin, but some physicians advocate the use of antibiotics until the chest tubes and drains have been removed. Chest tubes are removed when air leaks have been sealed and when drainage is less than 100 ml per 8-hour shift. Additional postoperative care is similar to that of thoracotomy patients.

COMPLICATIONS

Complications specific to chest wall resection and reconstruction include wound seroma formation, wound infection involving the prosthesis, and respiratory mechanical changes subsequent to prosthetic placement.[10,32] Small seromas are best managed with observation because the majority resolve with time. Large or symptomatic seromas can be repeatedly aspirated under strict sterile conditions with little risk of contamination. Surgical obliteration is infrequently necessary and is reserved for recalcitrant seromas.[10]

Wound infections that occur with synthetic grafts usually require removal of the prosthesis and replacement with either autogenous reconstruction or open wound care with delayed closure. Prolonged air leaks from violated visceral pleural surfaces or fissures can allow respiratory bacteria to infect the overlying prosthesis. Every attempt must be made to seal or oversew any raw lung surfaces and decrease the remaining free space within the hemithorax before placement of the prosthetic material. In all pulmonary resections, including the upper lobes, the inferior pulmonary ligament should be divided to permit sufficient mobility of the remaining lung in the hemithorax. Chest tubes should be placed in the hemithorax, minimizing their direct contact with the mesh. Polypropylene mesh is preferable to PTFE when significant air leaks are present. The smooth surface of PTFE often makes it more difficult for a lung prosthesis apposition to occur and can result in a localized bronchopleural fistula that declares itself months later. Polypropylene mesh permits more vigorous adhesions and rapid ingrowth of the lung and is better suited for a "contaminated" environment of an air leak.

The development of a bronchopleural fistula after pneumonectomy is an extremely morbid complication to treat, and in cases with chest wall resection and synthetic reconstruction, the treatment options are limited and complex. The majority of cases require removal of the prosthesis and prolonged open wound care. Patients who survive the initial sepsis and demonstrate signs of wound healing may be considered for complex reconstructions, which may include muscle flaps, omental flaps, and even thoracoplasty. Frequently these complicated cases are best handled using a multispecialty approach, with the aid of talented plastic surgeons familiar in reconstructive techniques.

Delayed wound infections can occur as a result of seroma aspiration or hematogenous seeding from distant infection. In these cases careful inspection of the prosthesis in the operating room is required. The majority of early prosthesis infections require removal of the prosthesis, followed by local wound care. In infections that present months after the primary surgery, removal of the prosthesis without replacement is often well tolerated without pulmonary compromise. After several months, sufficient fibrous tissue has developed to support the chest wall mechanics. Delayed wound infections may have had adequate time for incorporation of the prosthesis by granulation tissue, especially polypropylene, making prosthesis removal difficult and even unnecessary. Deschamps and associates[10] allowed those prostheses that were well incorporated by granulation tissue to remain in situ, using aggressive wound débridement and frequent dressing changes. They were able to salvage about one half of these infected reconstructions without removal of their prosthesis, and without development of delayed wound infections or draining sinus tracts.

Postoperative respiratory mechanical changes often are difficult to measure, but do vary based upon the type of prosthesis used. The loss of viscoelasticity and inhomogeneity is due to the replacement of a dynamic chest wall with a rigid structure that prevents chest wall mobility. Animal studies suggest that PTFE is favorable to PPMM because it allows the chest wall to remain dynamic during the respiratory cycle.[32] Human studies are limited, but demonstrate good pulmonary function 6 months postoperatively. Lardinois and associates[31] studied patients preoperatively and 6 months postoperatively and found no significant deterioration of FEV_1, and they noted concordant chest wall to prosthesis movements in the majority of patients.

Cerebrospinal fluid (CSF) leaks can occur when the dura is violated during dissection within the intervertebral foramina or during partial or complete vertebrectomies. The nerve roots should be ligated distal to the emergence of the external sheath covering the cord. Potential spinal fluid leaks should be carefully evaluated during the initial operation. If a small dural tear has occurred during the resection, it needs to be repaired with fine monofilament sutures and covered with an autogenous tissue transfer using intercostal muscle, diaphragm, or pleura. Negative intrathoracic pressure coupled with positive pressure created in the CSF can lead to a chronic CSF leak. Initial treatment includes a lumbar drain and patient immobility in a supine position to minimize the CSF pressure. Supine bed rest of a postthoracotomy patient can be associated with significant pulmonary complications.

Patients who have required these extensive, combined lung and chest wall resections, which extend to the region of the vertebral bodies and dural sac, can have fascinating delayed complications. One example is shown (Figure 20-6). A patient in whom a small dural rent was identified and repaired during the resection of a tumor involving the vertebrae required a chest tube for 10 days for a prolonged air leak that occurred during the dissection of the interlobar fissure. The patient had no problems after the removal of the chest tubes and discharge from the hospital. Several months later, he had mental status changes and a seizure that was felt, on clinical grounds, to likely represent metastatic disease to the

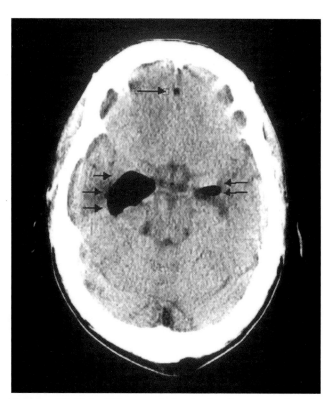

Figure 20–6 A CT scan of the brain demonstrating the pathognomic finding of air within the ventricular system of the brain secondary to a bronchopleural-subarachnoid fistula from a combined chest wall, lung, and vertebral body resection.

308 brain. A CT scan was done and demonstrated a significant amount of air within the brain, which originated from a small bronchopleural subarachnoid fistula. This required an additional thoracotomy with interposition of a pedicled omental flap between the lung and the dural sac to close the small communication. Within 48 hours, the patient's neurological status normalized.

▶ PATHOLOGY

A complete resection (R_0) is defined as pathological evidence of disease-free (negative) tissue margins on final pathology and an assessment by the surgeon that all grossly detectable disease, including nodal disease, has been removed. Patients who had complete gross resection at thoracotomy but were found to have positive margins on final microscopic pathological review are classified as having undergone an incomplete (R1) resection. Gross residual disease after an attempted resection is classified as an R_2 resection, including residual nodal disease that could not be removed.

Depth of chest wall invasion can be grouped into three levels on the basis of the final pathological examination: parietal pleura only; parietal pleura and soft tissues; and parietal pleura, soft tissues, and bone. Complete pathological stage (TNM) is based on microscopic examination of the primary mass, all surrounding margins, and nodes.

The evaluation of the world literature pertaining to chest wall resections in patients with lung cancer often is complicated, based on varied surgical practices. Some surgeons proceed directly to en bloc full-thickness chest wall resections rather than attempting to strip the parietal pleura by extrapleural maneuvers. In Facciolo and associates' series of 104 patients who underwent full-thickness, en bloc resections of lung with attached chest wall, the pathological depth of invasion was limited to parietal pleura in only 27%, parietal pleura and soft tissues in 35%, and parietal pleura, soft tissue, and bone in 38%.[13] All margins were microscopically negative on final pathological review. All lymph nodes were negative in 80% (N_0), 5% had positive hilar or lobar nodes (N_1), and 15% had positive mediastinal (N_2) nodes.

Chapelier and associates[7] also exclusively performed full-thickness resection of any tumors found by the naked eye to be invading at least the parietal pleura. A total of 100 patients were treated by this method. Pathological evaluation revealed parietal pleural invasion in 29% of cases, parietal pleura and intercostal muscle invasion in 47% of cases, and osseous invasion in 24% of cases. Microscopically negative margins were attained in all but one patient. Nodal status was 65% N_0, 28% N_1, and 7% N_2.

Burkhart and associates[6] reviewed their experience with 95 resections with bronchogenic carcinoma with invasion of the chest wall, all treated with full-thickness chest wall resection. Depth of invasion extended into the parietal pleura only in 31% of patients, into the parietal pleura and soft tissues in 45% of patients, and into the osseous structures in 24% of patients. Seventeen percent of patients had pathologically involved N_1 nodes, and 15% had pathologically involved N_2 nodes. A presumed R_0 resection was obtained in all cases.

Downey and associates[11] reported on 334 patients who underwent thoracic exploration for T_3 tumors involving the chest wall at Memorial Sloan-Kettering Hospital. Intra-

operative results included 175 patients who achieved an R_0 resection, 94 who achieved an R_1 or R_2 resection, and 65 who underwent exploration only. Of the 175 patients who did attain an R_0 resection, 80 (46%) underwent an extrapleural resection based on intraoperative surgeon judgment of the level of invasion. All 80 had evidence of parietal invasion only. The remaining 95 patients underwent full-thickness chest wall resection, of which 19% had parietal pleural invasion, 25% had parietal pleural and soft tissue invasion, and 56% had invasion involving the osseous structures.

Magdeleinat and associates[33] attempted an extrapleural resection in all patients whose parietal pleura could be easily removed. Intraoperative frozen sections were obtained when any doubt existed about negative margins. Tumors fixed to the deeper structures were removed with the associated full-thickness chest wall. A total of 201 patients were studied, of which 89 (44%) had tumor invasion limited to the parietal pleura. Ten of these patients underwent a full-thickness chest wall resection because the surgeon suspected deeper invasion intraoperatively. Only one patient who underwent an extrapleural resection had an underestimation of invasion, with microscopic residual identified at final pathology. Thirty-four patients (17%) did not achieve an R_0 resection, most often because of residual tumor at the lateral edges of the resection. Nodal disease was absent in 58% (N_0), hilar nodal disease was seen in 26% (N_1), and mediastinal nodal disease was seen in 13% (N_2). Three percent of patients had T_4 disease.

Okada and associates[43] reported on 132 patients with preoperative assessment of T_3 tumors who were surgically treated with R_0 resection. All criteria for T_3 inclusion were studied, including chest wall invasion, tumors <2 cm from the carina, and mediastinal pleural invasion. Pathological examination demonstrated that 37% had parietal pleural invasion only, 34% had invasion involving the soft tissues and/or bone, 14% had extension through the intralobar pleura, 9% were within 2 cm of the carina, and 5% had invasion of the mediastinal pleura. All involved adjacent structures were removed en bloc to attain an R_0 resection. Complete nodal resection was accomplished to complete an R_0 resection.

▶ RESULTS

Operative mortality is defined as mortality within 30 days of surgery or within the same hospitalization. Improvements in preoperative screening, anesthetic techniques, and postoperative care have decreased the incidence of postoperative mortality in many studies. Long-term results are affected most importantly by complete resection to microscopically negative margins and by absence of N_2 nodal involvement.[26] The extent (number of ribs) of chest wall resection is not a determinant for 5-year survival as long as an R_0 resection is accomplished. These results are validated by several studies.

Facciolo and associates[13] reported no operative mortality and a major complication rate of 20%, which included atrial fibrillation, bleeding, prolonged air leak, and empyema. Forty percent of patients received postoperative radiation therapy, and all patients with N_2 disease received postoperative chemotherapy. The overall 5-year survival rate was 61%, with a median survival period of 74 months. Statistically worse 5-year survival rates were noted in patients with N_2

disease when compared with patients with N_0 disease (18% vs 67%). Depth of invasion also affected survival rates, with a 79% survival rate at 5 years for pleural involvement only compared with a 56% survival rate for pleural, soft-tissue, and bone involvement. An impressive 90% 5-year survival rate was noted in the subset of patients with N_0 disease whose tumors were limited to the parietal pleural invasion only. The addition of postoperative radiation therapy dramatically increased 5-year estimated survival rates from 47% to 74%, although the criteria for administering postoperative radiation are not clearly defined.

Chapelier and associates[7] had different results. The operative mortality rate was 4%, and postoperative complications were noted in 16% of patients. The median survival period was 18 months, the 2-year survival rate was 41%, and the 5-year survival rate was 18%. Significantly worse 5-year survival rates were noted with N_2 disease when compared with N_0 or N_1 disease (0% vs 22% vs 9%, respectively). Patients with more than 2 ribs resected had better survival rates when compared with patients with less than 2 ribs resected ($p = .03$). Invasion limited to the pleura only was an independent factor favoring long-term survival when compared with deeper invasion ($p = .02$). The long-term survival rate for patients with well-differentiated tumors was significantly better than that for those with poorly differentiated or undifferentiated ones ($p = .005$). Postoperative radiation therapy or adjuvant chemotherapy did not improve survival in this study.

Burkhart and associates[6] summarized the Mayo Clinic experience, with somewhat higher mortality and morbidity rates. The operative mortality rate was 6.3%, and the complication rate was 45%. The overall 5-year actuarial survival rate was 39%, with best survival rates noted in Stage IIB (T_3 N_0 M_0) patients (44%), and worse rates for stage IIIA patients (26%). Interestingly, women in their study had a significantly improved 5-year survival rate than men (53% vs 39%, respectively), and women without evidence of nodal disease had the best survival rate (61% 5-year survival). Survival rates in all groups were affected by depth of invasion; tumors that invaded the parietal pleura only resulted in a 5-year survival rate of 50%, compared with 35% in patients with tumor invasion into the soft tissues, and 31% in patients with osseous involvement. Although these results did not reach statistical significance, the trend is suggestive of results seen at other institutions. Of their patients, 10% received neoadjuvant chemotherapy and/or radiation therapy, with a disappointing increase in operative mortality rates noted in those patients who had received radiation. No improvement in survival rates was seen in pretreated patients.

The Memorial Sloan-Kettering experience, as summarized by Downey and associates,[11] is comparable with other reports. The operative mortality rate, including all patients who underwent surgery, was 3%. Patients who left the operating room with either R_1 or R_2 disease had a dismal 5-year survival rate of 4%, which was comparable to those patients who underwent exploration without resection (0%). Patients who received R_0 resection had a 6% postoperative mortality rate and an overall 5-year survival rate of 32%. Further analysis in the R_0 group demonstrated survival advantage in node-free patients; 5-year survival rate in T_3 N_0 M_0 = 49%, T_3 N_1 M_0 = 27%, and T_3 N_2 M_0 = 15% ($p < .0003$). After either complete extrapleural or en bloc resection, there was no significant difference in survival rates between histological groups, nor was there any difference in survival rates by univariate analysis of pathological demonstration of extension of tumor into the pleura, into the pleura and soft tissues, or into the pleura, soft tissues, and ribs. Overall there was no observed significant difference in survival rates after a complete extrapleural resection compared with a complete en bloc resection. However, further subgroup analysis demonstrated that patients with N_0 disease had a prolonged survival period when receiving an extrapleural resection versus an en bloc resection (65 months vs 21 months, respectively, $p < .01$). This result could not be explained further. They also noted no survival advantage to radiation therapy given preoperatively, intraoperatively, or postoperatively.

Magdeleinat and associates[33] documented a 7% operative mortality rate and a 36% complication rate. Predictably, perioperative complications were more frequent in older patients and in patients with limited pulmonary reserve. Actuarial 5-year and 10-year survival rates for the entire population were 21% and 13%, respectively. After complete and incomplete resection, 5-year survival rates were 24% and 13%, respectively. The highest survival rate was noted again in the subgroup of patients without nodal involvement. The authors noted an increased 5-year survival rate in patients whose tumor did not extend beyond the parietal pleura (37%) as compared with those whose tumor did extend past the parietal pleura into the chest wall proper (15%). Of note, in patients with disease limited to the pleura, the type of resection (extrapleural or chest wall) did not affect survival rates (37% and 31%, respectively).

The focus of Okada and associates' study[43] was slightly different than that of the other reports, with emphasis on the significance of T_3 classification in its various definitions. The 132 patients reviewed were divided by definitions of T_3 based on chest wall invasion, interlobar invasion, main bronchus involvement, mediastinal pleural invasion, and diaphragm invasion. The operative mortality rate was 1.5%, but hospital complication rates were not reported. The authors confirmed improved 5-year survival rates in patients with N_0 disease (48%) as compared with N_1 disease (32%) or N_2 disease (19%) ($p < .005$). There was no statistically significant difference in survival between patients whose tumors involved the parietal pleura only, the parietal pleura and chest wall, or the interlobar pleura. However, patients with tumors localized to the main stem bronchus <2 cm from the carina had an impressive 5-year survival rate of 88%. Complete resection was again stressed as a prerequisite to long-term survival (Table 20-3).

▶ SUMMARY

In summary, bronchogenic lung cancer with invasion into the chest wall is seen in less than 10% of patients with resectable disease. Although chest wall invasion denotes a T_3 tumor classification, it does not preclude resectability. Extensive preoperative staging is required because metastatic disease is a contraindication for surgical treatment. Patients diagnosed with N_2 disease should not be considered candidates for primary surgical treatment. When available, these patients should be considered for protocol

Table 20-3

Results of Surgical Resection of Lung Cancer with Chest Wall Invasion

Author	Mortality (%)	Major morbidity (%)	5-year survival (%)	Median survival	5-year survival with N_0 (%)	5-year survival with N_2 (%)	5-year survival with pleural invasion only (%)	5-year survival with invasion beyond pleura (%)	5-year survival with R_1 or R_2 resection (%)
Facciolo et al	0°	19°	61°	74 months°	67°	18°	79°	54°	N/A (all R_0)
Chapelier et al	4°	16°	18°	18 months°	22°	0°			N/A (all R_0)
Burkhart et al	6.3°	45°	39°	N/A	44°	26°	50°	31°	N/A (all R_0)
Downey et al	6	N/A	32°	23 months	49	15	33°	34°	4
Magdeleinat et al	7	36	24°	N/A	25°	21°	37	15	13

N/A, Not applicable.
° In patients who achieved R_0 resection.

treatments that may include neoadjuvant chemotherapy or radiation therapy followed by surgery if an appropriate response is seen.

The operative approach may include an extrapleural resection only when tumor invasion is limited to the parietal pleura, or it may include a more extensive en bloc resection when deeper soft-tissue and bony chest wall invasion are demonstrated. The most important predictor of long-term patient survival is the achievement of an R_0 resection. Reconstruction generally is required for anterior and lateral defects when a flail segment is created, and for large posterior defects that may cause a trapped scapula. Reconstruction options are numerous, including autogenous tissue flaps, rotational muscle flaps, and a variety of prosthetic materials. The choice of reconstruction is based upon each individual patient and his or her clinical situation, surgeon preference, and the availability of specialized plastic surgical assistance.

Long-term results are encouraging in those patients who, after final pathological review, are found to have N_0 disease (stage IIB). The role of postoperative adjuvant treatment in patients with incidental N_1 or N_2 (IIIA) disease is not defined.

REFERENCES

1. Albertucci M, DeMeester TR, Rothberg M, et al: Surgery and the management of peripheral lung tumors adherent to the parietal pleura. J Thorac Cardiovasc Surg 103:8–13, 1992.
2. Albes JM, Lietzenmayer R, Schott U, et al: Improvement of non-small-cell lung cancer staging by means of positron emission tomography. J Thorac Cardiovasc Surg 47:42–47, 1999.
3. Block HM: Experimentelles zur Lungenresection. Deutche Med Wochenschrift 7:634–636, 1881.
4. Brauer L: Die ausschaltung der pneumothoraxfolgen met hilfe des uberdruckverfahrens. Mitteilungen aus den grenzebieten der medizin und chirurgie, 398–486, 1904.
5. Brown R, Fleming W, Jurkiewicz M: An island flap of the pectoralis major muscle. Br J Plast Surg 30:161–165, 1977.
6. Burkhart HM, Allen MS, Nichols FC III, et al: Results of en bloc resection for bronchogenic carcinoma with chest wall invasion. J Thorac Cardiovasc Surg 123:670–675, 2002.
6a. Campbell DA: Reconstruction of anterior thoracic wall. J Thorac Cardiovasc Surg 19:456–461, 1950.
7. Chapelier A, Fadel E, Macchiarini P, et al: Factors affecting long-term survival after en-bloc resection of lung cancer invading the chest wall. Eur J Cardiothorac Surg 18:513–518, 2000.
8. Chin R, Ward R, Keyes JW, et al: Mediastinal staging of non-small-cell lung cancer with positron emission tomography. Am J Respir Crit Care Med 152:2090–2096, 1995.
9. Coleman FP: Primary carcinoma of the lung, with invasion of the ribs: pneumonectomy and simultaneous black resection of chest wall. Ann Surg 126:168, 1947.
10. Deschamps C, Tirnaksiz BM, Darbandi R, et al: Early and long-term results of prosthetic chest wall reconstruction. J Thorac Cardiovasc Surg 117:588–591, 1999.
11. Downey RJ, Martini N, Rusch VW, et al: Extent of chest wall invasion and survival in patients with lung cancer. Ann Thorac Surg 68:188–193, 1999.
12. Durski JM, Srinivas S, Segall G: Comparison of FDG-PET and bone scans for detecting skeletal metastases in patients with non-small cell lung cancer. Clinical Positron Imaging 3:97–105, 2000.
13. Facciolo F, Cardillo G, Lopergolo M, et al: Chest wall invasion in non-small cell lung carcinoma: A rationale for en bloc resection. J Thorac Cardiovasc Surg 121:649–656, 2001.

14. Fell GW: Forced respiration. JAMA 16:325, 1891.
15. Frank JA, Ling A, Patronas NJ, et al: Detection of malignant bone tumors: MR imaging vs.scintigraphy. Am J Roentgenol 155:1043–1048, 1990.
16. Gambhir SS, Hoh CK, Phelps ME, et al: Decision tree sensitivity analysis for cost-effectiveness of FDG-PET in the staging and management of non-small-cell lung carcinoma. J Nucl Med 37:1428–1436, 1996.
17. Glazer HS, Duncanmeyer J, Aronberg DJ, et al: Pleural and chest wall invasion in bronchogenic-carcinoma: CT evaluation. Radiology 157:191–194, 1985.
18. Glazer HS, Kaiser LR, Anderson DJ, et al: Indeterminate mediastinal invasion in bronchogenic-carcinoma: CT evaluation. Radiology 173:37–42, 1989.
19. Griffith HR, Johnson GE: The use of curare in general anesthesia. Anesthesiology 3:418–420, 1942.
20. Grillo HC: Technical considerations in stage III disease: Pleural and chest wall involvement. In Delarue NC, Eschapasse H, editors: International Trends in General Thoracic Surgery, 1st ed, pp. 134–138. Philadelphia: W.B. Saunders, 1985.
21. Grillo HC, Greenberg JJ, Wilkins EW Jr.: Resection of bronchogenic carcinoma involving thoracic wall. J Thorac Cardiovasc Surg 51:417–421, 1966.
22. Guedel AE: A new intratracheal catheter. Curr Res Anes Anal 7:238–239, 1928.
23. Gupta NC, Graeber GM, Rogers JS, et al: Comparative efficacy of positron emission tomography with FDG and computed tomographic scanning in preoperative staging of non-small cell lung cancer. Ann Surg 229:286–291, 1999.
24. Hauboldreuter BG, Duewell S, Schilcher BR, et al: The value of bone scintigraphy, bone marrow scintigraphy and fast spin-echo magnetic resonance imaging in staging of patients with malignant solid tumors: A prospective study. Eur J Nucl Med 20:1063–1069, 1993.
25. Hosalkar H, Thatte MR, Yagnik MG: Chest-wall reconstruction in spondylocostal dysostosis: Rare use of a latissimus dorsi flap. Plast Reconstr Surg 110:537–540, 2002.
26. Incarbone M, Pastorino U: Surgical treatment of chest wall tumors. World J Surg 25:218–230, 2001.
27. Jemal A, Thomas A, Murray T, et al: Cancer statistics, 2002. Cancer J Clin 52:23–47, 2002.
28. Kirstein A: Autoskopie des larynx und der trachea (laryngoscopia directa, euthyskopie, besichtigung ohne spiegel. Arch Laryngol Rhinol 3:156–164, 1895.
29. Kodalli N, Erzen C, Yuksel M: Evaluation of parietal pleural invasion of lung cancers with breathhold inspiration and expiration MRI. Clin Imaging 23:227–235, 1999.
30. Kuriyama K, Tateishi R, Kumatani T, et al: Pleural invasion by peripheral bronchogenic-carcinoma: Assessment with 3-dimensional helical Ct. Radiology 191:365–369, 1994.
31. Lardinois D, Müller M, Furrer M, et al: Functional assessment of chest wall integrity after methylmethacrylate reconstruction. Ann Thorac Surg 69:919–923, 2000.
32. Macedo-Neto AV, Santos LV, Menezes SL, et al: Respiratory mechanics after prosthetic reconstruction of the chest wall in normal rats. Chest 113:1667–1672, 1998.
33. Magdeleinat P, Alifano M, Benbrahem C, et al: Surgical treatment of lung cancer invading the chest wall: Results and prognostic factors. Ann Thorac Surg 71:1094–1099, 2001.
34. Mansour KA, Thourani VH, Losken A, et al: Chest wall resections and reconstruction: A 25-year experience. Ann. Thorac Surg 73:1720–1725, 2002.
35. Marom EM, McAdams HP, Erasmus JJ, et al: Staging non-small cell lung cancer with whole-body PET. Radiology 212:803–809, 1999.
36. Mountain CF: Revisions in the international system for staging lung cancer. Chest 111:1710–1717, 1997.
37. Murphy JB: Surgery of the lung. JAMA 31:165, 1898.
38. Nesbitt JC, Wind GG: Thoracic Surgical Oncology Exposures and Techniques. Philadelphia: Lippincott Williams & Wilkins, 2003.
39. Netscher DT, Valkov PL: Reconstruction of oncologic torso defects: Emphasis on microvascular reconstruction. Semin Surg Oncol 19:255–263, 2000.
40. Northrop WP, O'Dwyer J: His methods of work on intubation: The measure of his success; the interest of both to young graduates. Med Rec 65:561, 1904.
41. O'Dwyer J: Chronic stenosis of the larynx treated by a new method with report of a case. Med Rec 29:641, 1886.
42. O'Dwyer J: Fifty cases of croup in private practice treated by intubation of the larynx, with a description of the method and of the dangers incident thereto. Med Rec 32:557, 1887.
43. Okada M, Tsubota N, Yoshimura M, et al: How should interlobar pleural invasion be classified? Prognosis of resected T3 non-small cell lung cancer. Ann Thorac Surg 68: 2049–2052, 1999.
44. Parham FW: Thoracic resection for tumors growing from the bony wall of the chest. Trans South Surg Gynecol Assoc 11:223–363, 1898.
45. Pennes DR, Glazer GM, Wimbish KJ, et al: Chest wall invasion by lung-cancer: Limitations of CT evaluation. Am J Roentgenol 144:507–511, 1985.
46. Ravitch MM, Steichen FM: Pulmonary resections. In Ravitch MM, Steichen FM, editors: Atlas of General Thoracic Surgery, pp. 189–292. Philadelphia: W.B. Saunders, 1988.
46a. Richerand A, Deschamps JFP, Percy P-F, et al. Account of a resection of the ribs and the pleura. Read before the Royal Academy of Sciences of the Institute of France, April 27, 1818. Translated by Thomas Wilson. Philadelphia, printer for the translator by Thomas Town, 1818.
47. Sauerbruch F: Uber die auschaltung der schadlichen wirkung des pneumothorax bei intrathorakelen operationen. Zentralbl Chir 31:146–149, 1904.
48. Scott J: Oral endotracheal intubation. In Dailey RH, Simon B, Young GP, editors: The Airway: Emergency Management, pp. 73–91. St Louis: Mosby, 1993.
49. Shirakawa T, Fukuda K, Miyamoto Y, et al: Parietal pleural invasion of lung masses: Evaluation with CT performed during deep inspiration and expiration. Radiology 192:809–11, 1994.
50. Smoker WRK, Godersky JC, Knutzon RK, et al: The role of MR imaging in evaluating metastatic spinal disease. Am J Roentgenol 149:1241–1248, 1987.
51. Steinert HC, Hauser M, Allemann F, et al: Non-small cell lung cancer: Nodal staging with FDG PET versus CT with correlative lymph node mapping and sampling. Radiology 202:441–446, 1997.
52. Walton GL: Letter from Berlin. Resection of the lung as proposed by Dr. Block. Boston Med Surg J 108:262, 1883.
53. Watanabe A, Shimokata K, Saka H, et al: Chest CT combined with artificial pneumothorax: value in determining origin and extent of tumor. Am J Roentgenol 156:707–710, 1991.
54. Yokoi K, Mori K, Miyazawa N, et al: Tumor invasion of the chest wall and mediastinum in lung-cancer: Evaluation with pneumothorax CT. Radiology 181:147–152, 1991.
55. York JE, Walsh GL, Lang FF, et al: Combined chest wall resection with vertebrectomy and spinal reconstruction for the treatment of Pancoast tumors. J Neurosurg 91:74–80, 1999.

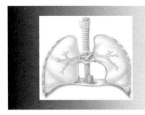
Anterior Approach to Pancoast Tumors

Philippe G. Dartevelle and Sacha Mussot

Presentation
Preoperative Studies
Treatment
Anterior Transcervical Technique
Surgical Morbidity and Mortality
Results and Prognosis

▶ PRESENTATION

Superior sulcus lesions of non-small-cell histology account for less than 5% of all bronchial carcinomas, as reported by Ginsberg and associates.[7] They cause steady, severe, and unrelenting shoulder and arm pain along the distribution of the eighth cervical nerve trunk and first and second thoracic nerve trunks. They also cause Horner's syndrome (i.e., ptosis, miosis, and anhidrosis) and weakness and atrophy of the intrinsic muscles of the hand, a clinical entity known as Pancoast's syndrome.[10] These tumors may arise from either upper lobe and tend to invade the parietal pleura, endothoracic fascia, subclavian vessels, brachial plexus, vertebral bodies, and first ribs. However, their clinical features are influenced by their location. Tumors located anterior to the anterior scalene muscle may invade the platysma and sternocleidomastoid muscles, external and anterior jugular veins, inferior belly of the omohyoid muscle, subclavian and internal jugular veins and their major branches, and the scalene fat pad (Figure 21-1). They invade the first intercostal nerve and first rib more frequently than the phrenic nerve or superior vena cava, and patients usually complain of pain distributed to the upper anterior chest wall.

Tumors located between the anterior and middle scalene muscles may invade the anterior scalene muscle with the phrenic nerve lying on its anterior aspect; the subclavian artery with its primary branches, except the posterior scapular artery; and the trunks of the brachial plexus and middle scalene muscle (Figure 21-2). These tumors present with signs and symptoms related to the compression or infiltration of the middle and lower trunks of the brachial plexus (e.g., pain and paresthesia radiating to the shoulder and upper limb).

Tumors lying posterior to the middle scalene muscles are usually located in the costovertebral groove and invade the nerve roots of T1, the posterior aspect of the subclavian and vertebral arteries, paravertebral sympathetic chain, inferior cervical (stellate) ganglion, and prevertebral muscles. Some of these posterior tumors can invade transverse processes (Figure 21-3), and even the vertebral bodies (only those abutting the costovertebral angle or extending into the intraspinal foramen without intraspinal extension may yet be resected). Because of the peripheral location of these lesions, pulmonary symptoms, such as cough, hemoptysis, and dyspnea, are uncommon in the initial stages of the disease. Abnormal sensation and pain in the axilla and medial aspect of the upper arm in the distribution of the intercostobrachial (T_2) nerve are more frequently observed in the early stage of the disease process. With further tumor growth, patients may present with full-blown Pancoast's syndrome.

▶ PREOPERATIVE STUDIES

Any patient presenting with signs and symptoms that suggest the involvement of the thoracic inlet should undergo a careful and detailed preoperative evaluation to establish the diagnosis of bronchial carcinoma and assess operability. These patients usually present with small apical tumors that are hidden behind the clavicle and the first rib on routine chest radiographs. The diagnosis is established by history and physical examination, biochemical profile, chest radiographs, bronchoscopy and sputum cytology, fine-needle transthoracic or transcutaneous biopsy and aspiration, and computed tomography of the chest. A video-assisted thoracoscopy occasionally might be indicated to obtain tissue proof when the other investigations are negative and to eliminate the possibility of pleural metastatic disease. If there is evidence of mediastinal adenopathy on chest radiographs or computed tomographic scanning, histological proof is mandatory because patients with clinical N_2 disease are not suitable for operation. Neurological examination, magnetic resonance imaging, and electromyography delineate the tumor's extension to the brachial plexus, phrenic nerve, and epidural space. Vascular invasion is evaluated by venous angiography, subclavian arteriography, Doppler ultrasonography (cerebrovascular disorders may contraindicate sacrifice of the vertebral artery), and magnetic resonance imaging (Figure 21-4). Magnetic resonance imaging has to be performed routinely when tumors approach the intervertebral foramina to rule out invasion of the extradural space (Figure 21-5).

The initial evaluation also includes all preoperative cardiopulmonary functional tests routinely performed before any major lung resection and investigative procedures to identify the presence of any metastatic disease.

▶ TREATMENT

Despite their small size and general lack of extrathoracic metastasis at presentation, one of the most perplexing

314

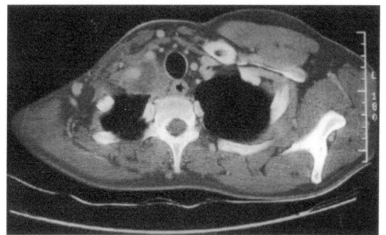

Figure 21–1 Computed tomography showing a right superior sulcus bronchial carcinoma invading the anterior thoracic inlet, including the subclavian artery.
(From Fadel E, Chapelier A, Bacha E, et al: Subclavian artery resection and reconstruction for thoracic inlet cancers. J Vasc Surg 29:584, 1999.)

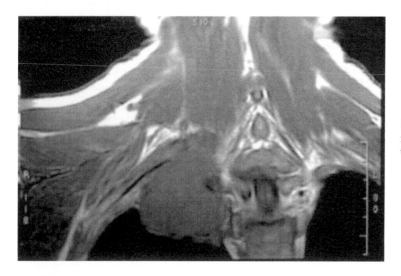

Figure 21–2 Magnetic resonance image showing a right superior sulcus bronchial carcinoma invading the middle thoracic inlet.

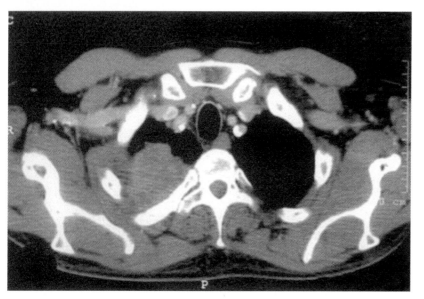

Figure 21–3 Computed tomography showing a right superior sulcus bronchial carcinoma invading the posterior arch and the transverse process of the first rib and abutting the costovertebral angle.

characteristics of superior sulcus tumors has been almost universal and rapid mortality. For many years, it was believed that these tumors were not amenable to surgery until Chardack and MacCallum[2] successfully performed a lobectomy and chest wall excision followed by radiation therapy. Five years later, Shaw and colleagues[11] approached superior sulcus tumors with preoperative radiation therapy (30–45 Gy in 4 weeks, including the primary tumor, mediastinum, and supraclavicular region) followed by surgical resection. This radiosurgical approach shortly became the

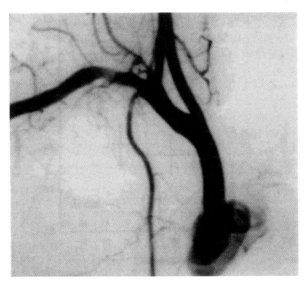

Figure 21–4 Angiography illustrating a massive tumoral invasion of the intrascalenic right subclavian artery beyond origin of vertebral artery.
(From Fadel E, Chapelier A, Bacha E, et al: Subclavian artery resection and reconstruction for thoracic inlet cancers. J Vasc Surg 29:585, 1999.)

Macchiarini and Dartevelle[9] reviewed surgical approaches for the treatment of superior sulcus lesions. All of them must be known because the ultimate hope for cure depends on whether a complete resection is performed. As a general rule, superior sulcus tumors not invading the thoracic inlet are completely resectable through the classic posterior approach of Shaw and associates[11] alone. Because the posterior approach does not allow direct and safe visualization, manipulation, and complete oncological clearance of all anatomical structures that compose the thoracic inlet, superior sulcus lesions extending to the thoracic inlet should be resected by the anterior transcervical approach as described by Dartevelle and colleagues.[4] In addition this operative procedure is increasingly accepted as a standard approach for all benign and malignant lesions of the thoracic inlet structures, including nonbronchial cancers[8] (e.g., osteosarcomas of the first rib and tumors of the brachial plexus), and for exposing the anterolateral aspects of the upper thoracic vertebrae.

Contraindications to this approach include extrathoracic metastasis, invasion of the brachial plexus above the T1 nerve root, invasion of the vertebral canal and sheath of the medulla, massive invasion of the scalene muscles and extrathoracic muscles, mediastinal lymph node metastasis, and significant cardiopulmonary disease.

standard treatment, yielding better disease control and survival than other treatments. More recently, Ginsberg and colleagues[7] provided evidence that en bloc resection of the chest wall and the involved adjacent structures as well as lobectomy must be considered the standard surgical approach for superior sulcus tumors combined with external radiation (preoperative, postoperative, or both). The goal of the operation is the complete and en bloc resection of the upper lobe in continuity with the invaded ribs, transverse processes, subclavian vessels, T1 nerve root, upper dorsal sympathetic chain, and prevertebral muscles.

▶ ANTERIOR TRANSCERVICAL TECHNIQUE

One-lung anesthesia with measurements of urine output and body temperature are necessary, as is an arterial line opposite the primary lesion and at least two venous lines for volume expansion as necessary. The patient is supine with the neck hyperextended and the head turned away from the involved side. A bolster behind the shoulder elevates the operative field. The skin preparation extends from the mastoid downward to the xiphoid process and from the midaxillary line laterally to the contralateral midclavicular line medially.

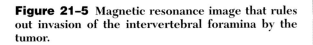
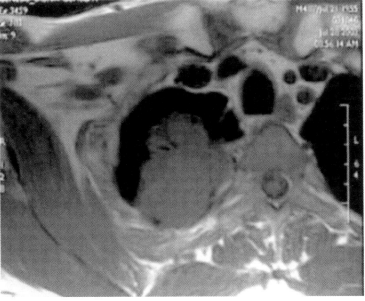

Figure 21–5 Magnetic resonance image that rules out invasion of the intervertebral foramina by the tumor.

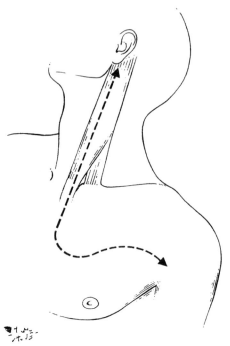

Figure 21–6 Anterior transcervical approach: L-shaped skin incision.
(From Dartevelle P, Macchiarini P: Anterior approach to apical lesions. In Pearson FG, et al, editors: Thoracic Surgery, 2nd ed. New York: Churchill Livingstone, 2002, p. 1039.)

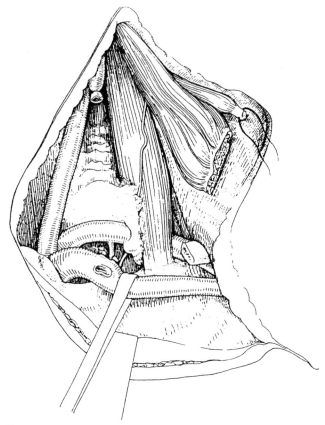

Figure 21–7 Illustrative view after having divided the sternal head of the sternocleidomastoid and the inferior belly of the omohyoid muscles, resected the scalene fat pad and the internal half of the clavicle. Thereafter, the exposure, dissection, and division of the external and internal jugular vein greatly facilitate the exposure of the subclavian vein and permit assessment of tumor resectability.
(From Dartevelle P, Macchiarini P: Anterior approach to apical lesions. In Pearson FG, et al, editors: Thoracic Surgery, 2nd ed. New York, Churchill Livingstone, 2002, p. 1039.)

An L-shaped cervicotomy incision is made, including a vertical presternocleidomastoid incision carried horizontally below the clavicle up to the deltopectoral groove (Figure 21-6). The incision is then deepened with cautery. The sternal attachment of the sternocleidomastoid muscle is divided. The cleidomastoid muscle, along with the upper digitations of the ipsilateral pectoralis major muscle, is scraped from the clavicle. A myocutaneous flap is then folded back, providing full exposure of the neck and cervicothoracic junction.

Once the inferior belly of the omohyoid muscle is divided, the scalene fat pad is dissected and pathologically examined to exclude scalene lymph node metastasis. Inspection of the ipsilateral superior mediastinum after division of the sternothyroid and sternohyoid muscles is then made by the operator's finger along the tracheoesophageal groove. The tumor's extension to the thoracic inlet is then carefully assessed. We recommend resection of the medial half of the clavicle only if the tumor is deemed resectable.

The jugular veins are dissected first, so that branches to the subclavian vein can eventually be divided. On the left side, ligation of the thoracic duct is usually required. Division of the distal part of the internal, external, and anterior jugular veins facilitates visualization of the venous confluence at the origin of the innominate vein; do not hesitate to suture-ligate the internal jugular vein to increase exposure of the subclavian vein (Figure 21-7). If the subclavian vein is involved, it can be easily resected after proximal and distal control has been achieved. Direct extension of the tumor to the innominate vein does not preclude resection.

Next, the anterior scalene muscle is divided with cautery either at its insertion on the scalene tubercle of the first rib or in a tumor-free margin (Figure 21-8). If the tumor has invaded the upper part of this muscle, it needs to be divided at its insertions on the anterior tubercles of the transverse processes of C3–C6. Before dealing with the anterior scalene muscle, the status of the phrenic nerve is carefully assessed because its unnecessary division has a deleterious influence on the postoperative course. It should be preserved whenever possible.

The subclavian artery is then dissected (Figure 21-9). To improve its mobilization, its branches are divided; the vertebral artery is resected only if invaded and if no significant extracranial occlusive disease was detected on preoperative Doppler ultrasound. If the tumor rests against the wall of the subclavian artery, the artery can be freed following a subadventitial plane. If there is invasion of the arterial wall, resection of the artery to obtain tumor-free margins is necessary. After proximal and distal control is obtained, the artery is divided on either side of the tumor (Figure 21-10). Revascularization is performed at the end of the procedure either with a polytetrafluoroethylene graft (6 or 8 mm) or, more often, with an end-to-end anastomosis after freeing

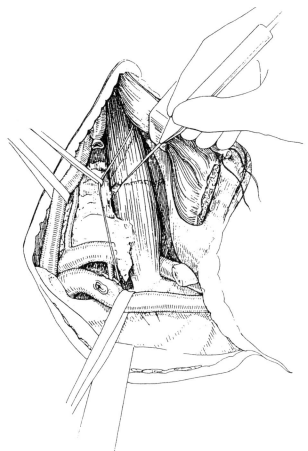

Figure 21–8 The subclavian artery is exposed after division of the insertion of the anterior scalenus muscle on the first rib; the phrenic nerve is protected and preserved.
(From Dartevelle P, Macchiarini P: Anterior approach to apical lesions. In Pearson FG, et al, editors: Thoracic Surgery, 2nd ed. New York, Churchill Livingstone, 2002, p. 1040.)

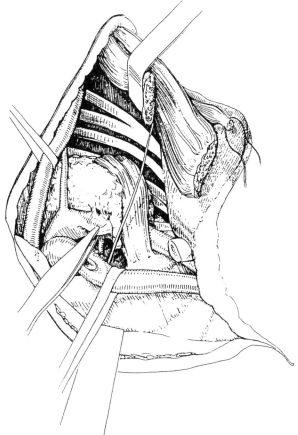

Figure 21–9 The retraction of the anterior scalenus muscles allows the identification of the interscalenic trunks of the brachial plexus; the subclavian artery might be gently freed from the tumor by dividing all collateral branches (the vertebral artery is generally preserved if not invaded).
(From Dartevelle P, Macchiarini P: Anterior approach to apical lesions. In Pearson FG, et al, editors: Thoracic Surgery, 2nd ed. New York, Churchill Livingstone, 2002, p. 1040.)

the carotid and subclavian arteries. During these maneuvers, the pleural space is usually opened by dividing Sibson's fascia.

The middle scalene muscle is divided above its insertion on the first rib or higher, as indicated by the extension of the tumor. This might require division of its insertions on the posterior tubercles of the transverse processes of vertebrae C2–C7, especially for apical tumors invading the middle compartment of the thoracic inlet. The nerve roots of C8 and T1 are then easily identified and dissected free from outside to inside up to where they join to form the lower trunk of the brachial plexus. Thereafter, the ipsilateral prevertebral muscles are resected, along with the paravertebral sympathetic chain and stellate ganglion, from the anterior surface of the vertebral bodies of C7 and T1 (Figure 21-11). This permits oncological clearance of the major lymphatic vessel draining the thoracic inlet and the visualization of the intervertebral foramina as well. The T1 nerve root is usually divided proximally beyond visible tumor, just lateral to the T1 intervertebral foramen. Although the tumor's spread to the brachial plexus may be high, neurolysis is usually achieved without division of the nerve roots above T1

(Figure 21-12). Injury of the lateral and long thoracic nerves should be avoided because it may result in a winged scapula.

Before the upper lobectomy, the chest wall resection is completed (Figure 21-13). The anterolateral arch of the first rib is divided at the costochondral junction. The second rib is divided at the level of its middle arch, and the third rib is scraped on the superior border toward the costovertebral angle. The specimen is then progressively freed. The divided ribs are disarticulated from the transverse processes of the first two or three thoracic vertebrae. It is through this cavity that an upper lobectomy can be performed to complete the operation, although it is technically demanding. In effect, unlike the original description by Dartevelle and colleagues,[4] it has become evident that an additional posterior thoracotomy is usually not required. The upper lobectomy and chest wall resection of the first four ribs can be performed through the transcervical approach only, without resorting to a posterolateral thoracotomy. The cervical incision is closed in two layers after the sternal insertion of the sternocleidomastoid muscle is sutured, and conventional postlobectomy drainage of the ipsilateral chest cavity is carried out.

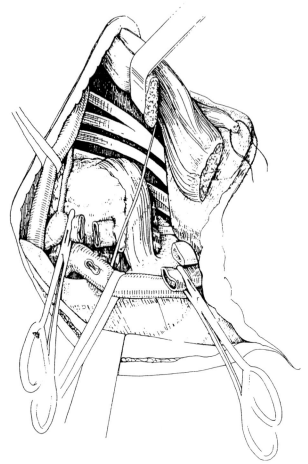

Figure 21-10 If involved by the tumor, the subclavian artery might be divided after its proximal and distal control.
(*From Dartevelle P, Macchiarini P: Anterior approach to apical lesions. In Pearson FG, et al, editors: Thoracic Surgery, 2nd ed. New York, Churchill Livingstone, 2002, p. 1041.*)

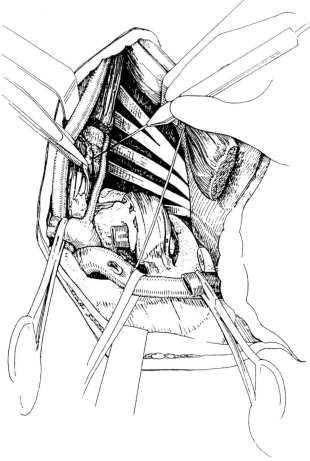

Figure 21-11 The prevertebral muscles are extensively detached from the vertebral bodies and both the stellate ganglion and dorsal sympathetic chain are isolated and finally released, using raspatories, from all surrounding attachments.
(*From Dartevelle P, Macchiarini P: Anterior approach to apical lesions. In Pearson FG, et al, editors: Thoracic Surgery, 2nd ed. New York, Churchill Livingstone, 2002, p. 1041.*)

There is increasing concern about the functional and esthetic benefit of preserving the clavicle. We believe that the indications for preserving and reconstructing the clavicle are limited to the combined resection of the serratus anterior muscle and the long thoracic nerve because this causes the scapula to rotate and draw forward. This entity (scapula alata), combined with the resection of the internal half of the clavicle, pushes the shoulder anteriorly and medially and leads to severe cosmetic and functional discomfort. If this circumstance is anticipated, we recommend an oblique section of the manubrium that fully preserves the sternoclavicular articulation, its intraarticular disc, and the costoclavicular ligaments rather than the simple sternoclavicular disarticulation. Clavicular osteosynthesis can then be accomplished by placing metallic wires across the lateral clavicular edges and across the divided manubrium.

Dartevelle[3] developed a technique for resecting posteriorly located superior sulcus tumors extending into the intervertebral foramen without intraspinal extension (Figure 21-14). The underlying principle is that a radical procedure can be performed by resecting the intervertebral foramen and dividing the nerve roots inside the spinal canal by a combined anterior transcervical and posterior midline approach. The first step of the operation includes the transcervical approach, during which resectability is assessed and all tumor-bearing areas are freed in tumor–free margins, as described. On completion, the patient is placed in a ventral position, and a median vertical incision is extended from spinal processes C7–T4. After a unilateral laminectomy on three levels, the nerve roots are divided inside the spinal canal at their emergence from the external sheath covering the spinal cord. After division of the ipsilateral hemivertebral bodies, the specimen is resected en bloc with the lung, ribs, and vessels through the posterior incision (Figure 21-15). On the side of the tumor, spinal fixation is performed from the pedicle above to the pedicle below the resected hemivertebrae; on the contralateral side, a screw is placed in each pedicle (Figure 21-16). However, the presence of an anterior spinal artery penetrating the spinal canal through an invaded intervertebral foramen contraindicates surgery. Tumors involving transverse processes should be resected with the anterior approach. The maneuver is similar to what

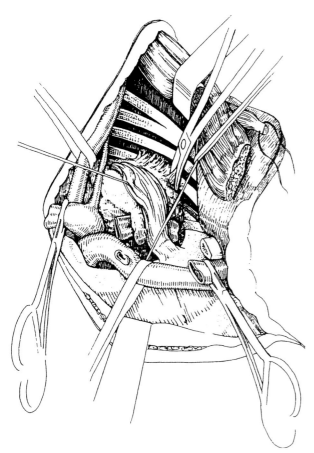

Figure 21–12 The tumor's involvement of the brachial plexus requires an out-inside neurolysis if the upper trunks are involved or a resection of T1 if the lower trunk or nerve roots are involved. *(From Dartevelle P, Macchiarini P: Anterior approach to apical lesions. Pearson FG, et al, editors: Thoracic Surgery, 2nd ed. New York, Churchill Livingstone, 2002, p. 1042.)*

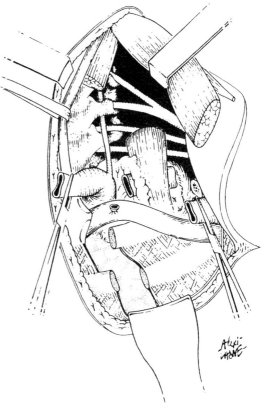

Figure 21–13 Once structures above the thoracic inlet are freed from the tumor, the first two ribs might be separated anteriorly at its chondrocostal junction and resected posteriorly in tumor-free margins. The third rib is scraped on its superior border toward the costovertebral angle and retracted inferiorly. *(From Dartevelle P, Macchiarini P: Anterior approach to apical lesions. Pearson FG, et al, editors: Thoracic Surgery, 2nd ed. New York, Churchill Livingstone, 2002, p. 1042.)*

Figure 21–14 Magnetic resonance image of a left superior sulcus bronchial carcinoma extending into the intervertebral foramen without intraspinal extension (*arrow*).

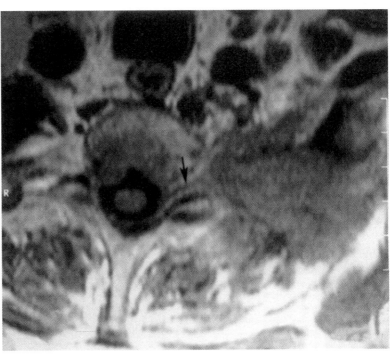

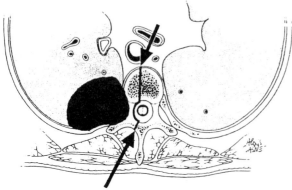

Figure 21–15 **Right-sided apical tumor involving the costotransverse space and intervertebral foramen and part of the ipsilateral vertebral body.** This tumor is first approached anteriorly as described in the text and then the operation is completed through a hemivertebrectomy performed through the posterior midline approach.
(From Dartevelle P, Macchiarini P: Anterior approach to apical lesions. Pearson FG, et al, editors: Thoracic Surgery, 2nd ed. New York, Churchill Livingstone, 2002, p. 1044.)

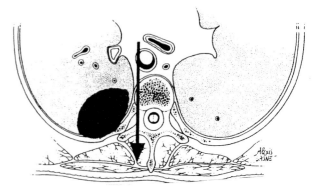

Figure 21–17 **Right-sided apical tumor involving the posterior arch of the rib only and resected from the anterior cervical approach by a vertical en bloc resection of part of the lateral vertebral body, the costotransverse space, and transverse process.**
(From Dartevelle P, Macchiarini P: Anterior approach to apical lesions. In Pearson FG, et al, editors: Thoracic Surgery, 2nd ed. New York, Churchill Livingstone, 2002, p. 1044.)

2. *Horner's syndrome and nerve deficits.* Although division of the T1 nerve root does not induce significant muscular palsy in the nerve's distribution, resection of the lower trunk of the brachial plexus may result in atrophic paralysis of the forearm and small muscles of the hand, with paralysis of the cervical sympathetic system (Klumpke–Déjérine syndrome). This should be discussed with the patient preoperatively. Relief of the preoperative pain and cure are worth the nerve sacrifice, however, and adaptation is usually reasonable.
3. *Hemothorax* may result from extensive pleural adhesion, chest wall resection, or blood spillage from veins around the intervertebral foramina.
4. *Chylothorax* should be prevented intraoperatively by detailed and extensive ligation of the cervical and intrathoracic lymphatic vessels. Whenever this occurs, continued chest tube drainage, lung expansion, or reoperation may be necessary.
5. *Prolonged ventilatory support.* Because of chest wall dyskinesia and phrenic nerve resection—or even temporary paresis from the dissection—patients having a combined transcervical and midline approach are more likely than others to develop postoperative atelectasis and perfusion–ventilation mismatch. Thus, they are unable to breathe spontaneously in the early postoperative course.

The postoperative course is usually characterized by atelectasis because of the extended chest wall resection, with or without phrenic nerve sacrifice. Treatment involves measures to achieve complete lung expansion by ensuring the following:

- Adequate ventilation, using mechanical support if necessary.
- Satisfactory chest tube function.
- Prevention of retained secretions by mobilization; coughing; chest physiotherapy; nasotracheal, orotracheal, or bronchoscopic suctioning; or a temporary tracheostomy.
- Adequate analgesia.
- Increase of the transpulmonary pressure with incentive spirometry or continuous positive airway pressure mask.

Fluid overload should be avoided and diuretics used judiciously to avoid adult respiratory distress syndrome. Chest

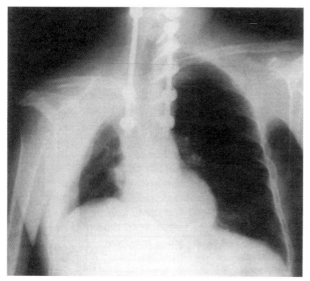

Figure 21–16 **Chest radiograph showing bilateral spinal fixation with metal rods interposed.**
(From Dartevelle P: Extended operations for lung cancer. Ann Thorac Surg 63:12, 1997.)

is used with the posterior approach but from the front to the back, with a finger placed behind the transverse process of T1 and T2 to give the correct direction of the chisel (Figure 21-17).

▶ SURGICAL MORBIDITY AND MORTALITY

There are many surgical complications.

1. *Spinal fluid leakage.* The risks of air embolism into the subarachnoid space, ventricles, and central canal of the brain and spinal cord justify reoperation, for which a cerebral ventricular-venous shunt may be required.

Table 21–1

Results of Patients Treated Surgically for Superior Sulcus Tumors[a]

Author (year)	Number of cases	5-year survival (%)	Mortality (%)
Paulson D. L. (1985)	79	35	3
Anderson et al (1986)	28	34	7
Devine et al (1986)	40	10	8
Miller et al (1987)	36	31	NS[b]
Wright et al (1987)	21	27	—
Shahian et al (1987)	18	56	—
McKneally et al (1987)	25	51	NS
Komaki et al (1990)	25	40	NS
Sartori et al (1992)	42	25	2.3
Maggi et al (1994)	60	17.4	5
Ginsberg et al (1994)	100	26	4
Okubo et al (1995)	18	38.5	5.6
Dartevelle P. (1998)	70	34	—
Total	562	33±12[c]	3.5±3[c]

[a]Adapted from Dartevelle P, Macchiarini P: Optimal management of tumors in the superior sulcus. In Franco KL, Putman J Jr, editors: Advanced Therapy in Thoracic Surgery. Hamilton, Ontario: B.C. Decker, 1998.
[b]NS, not stated.
[c]Values are number ± standard deviation.

Box 21–1. Factors Influencing Survival and Disease-Free Survival.[a,b]

Adverse prognostic factors
    Female gender
    Positive bronchoscopy
    Abnormal serum carcinoembryonic antigen (CEA)
    Full-blown Pancoast–Tobias syndrome
    Positive lymph nodes (N1–3)
Factors without prognostic influence
    Side and site of the tumor
    Type of surgery (wedge versus lobectomy)
    Subclavian vessel invasion (absent versus present)
    Invasion of the intervertebral foramen

[a]In completely resected patients whose superior sulcus tumors invaded the thoracic inlet and were surgically resected through the anterior approach. By multivariate analysis, only the nodal status adversely affected disease-free survival.
[b]Adapted from Macchiarini P, Dartevelle P: Extended resections for lung cancer. In Roth JA, Hong WK, Cox JD, editors: Lung Cancer, 2nd ed. Cambridge, MA: Blackwell Scientific Publications, 1998.

within 1–2 months. The radial pulse should be closely followed to control the patency of the revascularized subclavian artery; after a preoperative loading dose of intravenous heparin, anticoagulant treatment should be switched to oral doses for a 6-month postoperative period only.

RESULTS AND PROGNOSIS

The overall 5-year survival rates after combined radiosurgical (posterior approach) treatment of superior sulcus tumors due to bronchial carcinoma range from 18–56% (Table 21-1). The best prognosis is found in patients without nodal involvement who have had a complete resection, as noted by Arcasoy and Jett[1] and Ginsberg and colleagues.[7] Dartevelle and Macchiarini[5,9] reported a complete resection rate of 100% with no postoperative mortality or major complications. The 5-year and median survival rates were approximately 35% and 18 months, respectively. The local recurrence rate was less than 1.8% using our approach. Fadel and colleagues[6] reported 17 en bloc resections of non-small-cell lung cancers invading the thoracic inlet and intervertebral formina with a 5-year and median survival rates of 20% and 27 months, respectively. Among the adverse prognostic factors, the nodal status is the only predictor of disease-free survival (Box 21-1).

REFERENCES

1. Arcasoy SM, Jett JR: Superior pulmonary sulcus tumors and Pancoast's syndrome. N Engl J Med 337:1370, 1997.
2. Chardack WM, MacCallum JD: Pancoast syndrome due to bronchogenic carcinoma: Successful surgical removal and postoperative irradiation: A case report. J Thorac Surg 54:831, 1953.
3. Dartevelle P: Extended operations for lung cancer. Ann Thorac Surg 63:12, 1997.
4. Dartevelle P, Chapelier A, Macchiarini P, et al: Anterior transcervical-thoracical approach for radical resection of lung

tubes remain in place until all air leaks have stopped and there is complete lung expansion and almost no fluid drainage. Incomplete lung expansion with persistent intrapleural air space should be ignored because ultimately it will be filled with serous fluid.

Resection of the subclavian vein should be accompanied by elevation of the ipsilateral forearm to facilitate venous drainage and generation of a collateral venous pathway

322

tumors invading the thoracic inlet. J Thorac Cardiovasc Surg 105:1025, 1993.

5. Dartevelle P, Macchiarini P: Optimal management of tumors in the superior sulcus. In Franco KL, Putman J Jr, editors: Advanced Therapy in Thoracic Surgery. Hamilton, Ontario: B.C. Decker, 1998.

6. Fadel E, Missenard G, Chapelier A et al: En bloc resection of non-small cell lung cancer invading the thoracic inlet and intervertebral foramina. J Thorac Cardiovasc Surg 123:676, 2002.

7. Ginsberg RJ, Martini N, Zaman M, et al: Influence of surgical resection and brachytherapy in the management of superior sulcus tumor. Ann Thorac Surg 57:1440, 1994.

8. Macchiarini P, Dartevelle P, Chapelier A, et al: Technique for resecting primary or metastatic non-bronchial carcinomas of the thoracic outlet. Ann Thorac Surg 55:6, 1993.

9. Macchiarini P, Dartevelle P: Extended resections for lung cancer. In Roth JA, Hong WK, Cox JD, editors: Lung Cancer, 2nd ed. Cambridge, UK: Blackwell Scientific Publications, 1998.

10. Pancoast HK: Importance of careful roentgen-ray investigations of apical chest tumors. JAMA 83:1407, 1924.

11. Shaw RR, Paulson DL, Kee JLJ: Treatment of the superior sulcus tumor by irradiation followed by resection. Ann Surg 154:29, 1961.

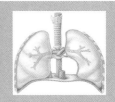

Other Primary Tumors of the Lung

John R. Roberts

▶ CARCINOID TUMORS

Carcinoid tumors are the most common "other" tumors of the lung, accounting for about 1% of lung neoplasms.[122] These lesions were originally described in 1888 in the ileum, and, until recently, they were often called "bronchial adenomas" because of their generally benign course (Box 22-1).[62] More recently, their occasional malignancy has prompted other designations (e.g., typical vs. atypical; Kulchitsky tumors; neuroendocrine carcinoma). The term *carcinoid tumor* has remained in common usage, however, and will be used here.

Box 22–1. Changing Names of Unusual Tumors.

Rare tumors' names may change during the history of the tumor. Thus "bronchial adenoma" becomes "carcinoid." Similarly, "intravascular bronchioalveolar tumor" becomes "epithelioid hemangioendothelioma." Sometimes this happens because something basic about the lesion is learned that was not understood before. Bronchial adenomas were considered to always be benign lesions; when some were found to metastasize, a new name was needed. The table below lists some of the tumors that have changed their names.

Old name	New name
Bronchial adenoma	Carcinoid tumor
No name given	Large-cell neuroendocrine tumor
Intravascular bronchioalveolar tumor	Epithelioid hemangioendothelioma
Embryoma	Pulmonary blastoma
Oat-cell carcinoma	Small-cell carcinoma

Carcinoid tumors are perplexing neoplasms. Together, neuroendocrine lesions can include lesions that never metastasize (carcinoid tumors), lesions that occasionally metastasize (atypical carcinoid), lesions that quite often recur after resection (large cell neuroendocrine carcinoma), and lesions that so commonly metastasize that they are never treated with surgery alone and are considered the prototypical cancer (small-cell carcinoma). Although carcinoids are rarely mistaken for small-cell carcinoma, they can be mistaken for atypical carcinoids and large-cell neuroendocrine lesions.

▶ CLINICAL FEATURES OF CARCINOID TUMORS

Signs and Symptoms of Carcinoid Tumors

Carcinoid tumors may present either as peripheral lesions (rarely) or as central lesions (more commonly). Peripheral lesions rarely cause symptoms or signs but rather present radiologically. Central lesions may present with all of the sequelae of endobronchial obstruction (e.g., hemoptysis, persistent pneumonia, bronchitis, wheezing, chest pain) that other lung malignancies do. Most patients are symptomatic, and many will have been treated for asthma for some time before the diagnosis is made.

Because these lesions are slow growing, symptom onset may be unusually insidious. The most common presentation is asymptomatic, although some patients present with asthma, wheezing, stridor, bronchiectasis, lung abscesses, and empyema.

Endocrinopathies

Pulmonary carcinoid tumors seldom present with the carcinoid syndrome, although Harpole and others[45] reported an unusually high incidence of 12% (Box 22-2). Carcinoid tumors may cause Cushing's syndrome (increased adrenal cortical tropic hormone [ACTH] production), excessive pigmentation (melanocyte-stimulating hormone), hypo-

glycemia (insulin production), polyuria (inappropriate anti-diuretic syndrome), and acromegaly (high levels of growth hormone and insulin-like growth factor-1).[73]

Cushing's syndrome is the second most common endocrinopathy found in carcinoid tumors (1–2%). Conversely, bronchial carcinoid (25%) is the most frequent cause of ectopic production of ACTH, followed by small-cell lung cancer (11%) and disseminated neuroendocrine tumors (7%).[2] Any patient with Cushing's disease who has no evidence of pituitary or adrenal lesions should then be evaluated for thoracic masses. The most common causes of thoracic Cushing's disease are carcinoid tumors, small-cell carcinoma of the lung, and carcinoid tumor of the thymus.

▶ DIAGNOSIS OF CARCINOID TUMORS

Like most lesions in the lung, no single diagnostic maneuver is always successful. Chest radiographs and chest computed tomography (CT) scans may be suspicious, but they are not diagnostic. Peripheral lesions can undergo fine-needle aspiration, and bronchoscopy can be used in the biopsy of proximal lesions. In both cases, these small biopsies may be confused for either benign lesions or small-cell carcinoma.

Radiology of Carcinoid Tumors

Peripheral lesions may not be seen well on regular chest radiographs, but they can be seen on chest CT scans. Central or hilar lesions can also be seen on CT scan, and

Box 22–2. Neuroendocrine Tumor.

Pulmonary carcinoid tumors (typical and atypical), along with small-cell carcinoma and large-cell neuroendocrine carcinomas, make up the spectrum of neuroendocrine tumors. These lesions are also called *Kulchitsky tumors*. Therapy for these tumors ranges widely, however, from resection alone to resection and occasional chemoradiation to chemoradiation alone. These differences in treatment are due to the great differences in the ability of these lesions to metastasize. Although carcinoid tumors rarely metastasize, atypical carcinoids occasionally metastasize, large-cell neuroendocrine tumors often metastasize, and small-cell carcinoma always metastasizes. Small-cell carcinoma is only rarely treated surgically.

Carcinoid → Atypical carcinoid → Large-cell neuroendocrine → Small-cell carcinoma
Kulchitsky cell I tumor → Kulchitsky II tumor → Kulchitsky III tumor
Surgery alone →_____ → Chemoradiation alone

When pulmonary carcinoids do recur or metastasize, they are difficult to treat, because they are resistant to most chemotherapeutic agents and radiation. Systemic octreotide is the chemotherapy that is most commonly used for metastatic carcinoid. By contrast, cisplatin and etoposide are the agents that are most commonly used for small-cell carcinoma. For carcinoid tumors that act more aggressively than they are expected to, treatment with the chemotherapy regimen typically used for small-cell disease can be effective.

these may narrow or obstruct bronchi. Diffuse or punctate calcifications can be seen in approximately 30% of lesions and support a diagnosis of carcinoid.[64] Typical carcinoids demonstrate homogeneous contrast enhancement, whereas atypical carcinoids generally show little or no contrast enhancement and have more irregular contours. None of these differences, however, reliably separate carcinoid lesions from other pulmonary lesions.

Pulmonary carcinoids are generally hypometabolic on positron emission tomography (PET) scan,[116] although some studies have found lesions smaller than 3 cm to be hypermetabolic and thus positive on PET scan.[65]

Carcinoid tumors overexpress somatostatin receptors.[54] Immunoscintigraphy using somatostatin analogues (e.g., octreotide, lanreotide, and pentetreotide) has some use in the diagnostic evaluation of neuroendocrine lung tumors. Scintigraphic visualization of carcinoid tumors with octreotide has a sensitivity of 86% but a low specificity; it is also positive in many other tumors, granulomata, and autoimmune diseases.[57] The combination of iodine-131–metaiodobenzylguanidine and indium-111–pentetreotide gives a higher sensitivity (95%), but it still has a low specificity.[116] Because of this poor specificity, the technique cannot be used to exclude a carcinoid tumor. For the time being, immunoscintigraphy is a confirmatory diagnostic tool only.

Bronchoscopic Evaluation

More carcinoid tumors (75%) can be accessed at bronchoscopy than can other lung malignancies. However, the risk of significant bleeding is also greater than for other lung malignancies, and it can occasionally be massive.[28,127] The overlying mucosa is often intact, so brushings or washings are nondiagnostic. Small biopsies can be safely done, especially if dilute epinephrine is used to control bleeding; however, biopsies of lesions suspected to be carcinoid should generally be done with rigid bronchoscopy so that massive bleeding can be controlled.

Fine-needle aspiration biopsies of carcinoid tumors—whether of peripheral lesions or of endobronchial lesions through the bronchoscope—can be mistakenly diagnosed as small-cell carcinoma. This is most likely to occur when there is a biopsy atypical carcinoid or frozen sections are obtained.

Greater accuracy is possible when frozen sections and needle biopsies are avoided.

STAGING OF CARCINOIDS

Prognosis depends only on histology (typical vs. atypical), presence or absence of nodal metastases, and presence or absence of distant metastases. Although application of the TNM staging system used for non–small-cell lung cancer is often used, it does not accurately predict prognosis. Most "typical" carcinoids present as solitary masses with no nodal metastases, whereas most "atypical" carcinoids present with nodal metastases (Table 22-1).

PATHOLOGY

The derivation of carcinoid tumors has been controversial. Initially, these tumors were believed to arise from amine precursor uptake of amino acid decarboxylase; more recent analysis suggests that carcinoids arise from bronchial epithelial cells.[17] Further, the tumor markers (ACTH, antidiuretic hormone, calcitonin, bombesin), enzymes (neuron-specific enolase and synaptophysin), and amino acids (serotonin) found in carcinoids are also found in small-cell carcinoma. These data suggest a relationship among carcinoid, atypical carcinoid, large-cell neuroendocrine carcinoma, and small-cell carcinoma that has become generally accepted (Box 22-3).

TYPES OF CARCINOID

Typical Carcinoid

The majority of these lesions (80%) can be seen with a bronchoscope; the remainder (20%) is peripheral. The lesions are glossy, highly vascularized lesions, and they are usually sessile. They generally spread beyond the bronchial wall and cannot be completely resected endoscopically.

Microscopically, typical carcinoids differ from atypical carcinoids by the presence of well-differentiated clusters of

---

Table 22–1

Differentiating Typical Carcinoids, Atypical Carcinoids, and Small-Cell Carcinoma

	Nodal metastases	Location	Mitoses	Smoking history	5-year survival[44]
Carcinoids	Rare (10–15%)	Central (80%)	Rare	Common	87–100%
Atypical	Frequent (~60%)	Peripheral (60%)	Frequent	Very common	37–71%
Large cell	Frequent (~60%)	Variable	Common	Very common	15–45%
Small cell	Common (80%)	Central	Common	90–100%	0–20%

interlacing cells and the absence of mitoses and nodal metastases.

Atypical Carcinoid

These tumors were first described 60 years ago, almost simultaneously by several investigators.[3,29] As opposed to typical carcinoid tumors, a slight majority of these lesions are located peripherally, and a majority (50–70%) present with nodal or distant metastases.[120] Several studies evaluating smoking history have found that approximately a third of patients with typical carcinoid smoke, and 60–80% of patients with atypical carcinoid have smoking histories.[8,31,48]

These tumors reveal striking pleomorphism and high mitotic activity. The histological appearance of these tumors is usually very different from typical carcinoid, but it may be quite similar to that of small-cell carcinoma (Table 22-1). Atypical carcinoids demonstrate high degrees of pleomorphism, high mitotic rates, nuclear abnormalities, and cellular necrosis. As we will discuss later, the treatments for all three of these lesions are strikingly different.

Unusual Carcinoids

Tumorlets

Tumorlets are isolated foci of atypical hyperplastic bronchial epithelium that are histologically similar to neuroendocrine tissue.[126] They are usually incidental findings in lung that has been resected for other reasons, or they may be found at autopsy. Patients with any type of lung disease may have these lesions, but they are especially common in those with emphysema or restrictive lung disease.[75]

Tumorlets have a different immunohistochemical profile than carcinoids, which suggests that they are not tumors but rather proliferations of neuroendocrine cells.[22]

Melanocytic Carcinoid

This rare tumor was initially reported in the 1980s.[14,41] The presentation and treatment are generally similar to those of atypical carcinoids.

Oncocytic Carcinoid

This rare lesion is a variable mixture of eosinophilic oncocytes and cells that are more typical of carcinoid tumor.[38]

▶ MANAGEMENT AND TREATMENT

Except for patients with distant metastases, resection is the therapy of choice for carcinoid disease.

Endobronchial Resection or Laser Therapy

Endobronchial resection, with or without laser ablation, is appropriate when large lesions in frail patients make a safe complete resection unlikely. Before the development of modern techniques of resection and postoperative care, endoluminal resection was commonly done. In this case, the hope is that these indolent lesions would not progress rapidly as they recurred. In general, this is an alternative therapy for those patients who are too ill (e.g., patients with pneumonia) or too frail (e.g., older patients or those with poor pulmonary function) to undergo resection.

In selected patients, some authors recommend bronchoscopic removal and then close follow-up.[18,56,114,123] At our center, we advocate the use of either high-resolution CT scanning or endobronchial ultrasound to evaluate the wall thickness of the bronchus and to thus assess the early recurrence. This is a minority opinion, however; anatomical resection is necessary for cure for the majority of patients, and less-invasive therapies should be reserved only for those who are unable to undergo resection. However, these techniques can be helpful to prepare patients for definitive resection by clearing the airway of tumor obstruction and allowing for antibiotic therapy and clearing of pneumonia before surgical resection.

Resection

Complete removal of the tumor with preservation of as much lung as possible is the treatment goal. Surgery offers the only chance of cure and thus is the treatment of choice. Typical carcinoids, in which nodal metastases are rare, can be resected with less than a lobectomy (wedge or segmentectomy) if negative margins can be obtained with the lesser resection. Atypical carcinoids, however, are more likely to have nodal metastases and thus to have lymphatic spread within a lobe. Lobectomy should be planned when atypical carcinoids are suspected (Table 22-2).

Surgical staging with complete lymphadenectomy is necessary in any lung resection but perhaps even more so when the diagnosis is carcinoid tumor. Many tumors will appear to be typical carcinoid until nodal metastases are discovered; this diagnosis would not be possible without lymphadenectomy.

Bronchotomy

Tumors isolated to specific areas of the airway (e.g., the trachea, the left main stem bronchus, or the bronchus intermedius) can be removed with resections of the airway only and preservation of the parenchyma.[37] Unlike endoscopic removal, this allows for resection of the bronchial wall as

Table 22–2

Carcinoid: Frequency of Surgical Resections[12,35,36,68,70,104]

Procedure	Frequency
Lobectomy (including bronchoplastic procedures)	51–58%
Bilobectomy	9–15%
Segmentectomy or wedge resections	2–15%
Bronchoplastic procedures	5–18%
Pneumonectomy	6–16%

well as lymphadenectomy. Occasionally this technique can be applied to the carina, again with preservation of all or most of the pulmonary parenchyma.[113]

Wedge and Segmental Resections

These procedures are appropriate for limited lesions either in the parenchyma or in the tertiary bronchi; only typical carcinoids are likely to be completely resected with these approaches. Neither of these limited resections is appropriate without frozen section evaluation of the regional lymph nodes to ensure the absence of metastases. If nodal metastases are found, lobectomy should be done.

Lobectomy, With or Without Sleeve Resection

Because most carcinoids develop at the orifice of lobar bronchi, lobectomy (occasionally with sleeve resection) is the most common procedure performed for carcinoid tumor. Complete lymphadenectomy should be done at resection, and margins should be checked to ensure complete resection. Sleeve resections allow for the preservation of distal parenchyma, and they are preferred over pneumonectomy for this reason. Endoscopic resection of obstructing lesions allows for the evaluation of distal lung tissue and the treatment of ongoing infection caused by the obstruction, and it can facilitate parenchyma-sparing resections.

Pneumonectomy

With the increasing experience with bronchoplastic or sleeve resections, pneumonectomy should be rarely needed for the surgical therapy of carcinoid tumors.

Radiation

Radiotherapy should not be the primary modality used for the treatment of carcinoids, because these tumors are gen-

erally resistant to radiotherapy. Of course, some reports have identified cases of inoperable tumors that responded to radiotherapy.[6]

Treating tumors with mediastinal nodal involvement is controversial; Martini and colleagues[67] reported only one local recurrence in patients with mediastinal nodal involvement who were treated with radiotherapy at Memorial Sloan-Kettering Cancer Center. However, a large epidemiological study from the Netherlands did not demonstrate any benefit from postoperative radiotherapy in those patients with nodal involvement.[98]

Chemotherapy

Effective drug therapy for metastatic carcinoid is limited. These treatments are not curative, even when they are combined with radiotherapy, and they are used to treat symptoms of carcinoid syndrome.

It is accurate to say that there is no standard chemotherapy for carcinoid syndrome. Chronic infusions of octreotide are often used for the treatment of symptoms, and these have response rates of 60%.[88] Octreotide can also be combined with interferon-alfa[40] or with metaiodobenzylguanidine to control severe symptoms.[116] The most common second-line therapy is probably the combination of fluorouracil and streptozotocin, whereas third-line therapy consists of cisplatin and etoposide.

Response can be followed by clinical improvement, radiological regression, or biochemical marker improvement. Chromogranin A is a glycoprotein that is important in the storage and secretion of neuroendocrine substances that can be secreted into the plasma, and it is the most sensitive biochemical marker for carcinoid disease. Those patients with carcinoid syndrome can be monitored by examining the urinary excretion of 5-hydroxyindolacetic acid; elevated levels are found in approximately two thirds of patients.[40]

► PROGNOSIS OF CARCINOIDS

Mucous Gland and Salivary Gland Type Tumors

The submucosal serous and mucous glands of the trachea and bronchi are similar to the salivary glands and can give rise to similar tumors. Adenoid cystic carcinoma, mucoepidermoid carcinoma, and mixed tumors of salivary gland type are rare malignant lesions that can develop in the airway. Together they make up slightly less than 1% of all of the tumors that develop in the lung and the respiratory tree.[93,118] The most common of the three is adenoid cystic carcinoma, followed by epidermoid carcinoma and then salivary gland carcinoma.[92] Significant characteristics of these three tumors are summarized in Table 22-3.

Adenoid Cystic Carcinoma

Adenoid cystic carcinoma, which is also called cylindroma, is most common in the salivary glands. However, it can also develop in the lung, breast, prostate, esophagus, cervix, and skin. Although it is uncommon in respiratory tree overall, adenoid cystic carcinoma is the most common lesion in the trachea, accounting for more than 30% of all malignant

Table 22–3

Comparison of Adenoid Cystic, Mucoepidermoid, and Mixed Tumor of Salivary Glands in the Tracheobronchial Tree[a]

	Location	Sputum cytology	Nodal disease	Diagnosis	Treatment	5-year survival
Adenoid cystic	Trachea, bronchi, lung	Negative	Common	Bronchial	Surgery, radiation therapy	~85%
Mucoepidermoid	Bronchi	Negative	Rare	Bronchial	Surgery	Variable
Mixed tumor of salivary glands	Trachea, bronchi	Negative	Very rare	Bronchial	Surgery	~85%

[a]Comparison with respect to location of tumor, identification with sputum cytology, likelihood of nodal disease, best means of diagnosis, best means of treatment, and 5-year survival. All three tumors are best treated with surgery, if possible.

lesions in this area.[39] These lesions can also present peripherally in the lung parenchyma, but they will usually be the result of metastases from an undiscovered primary in the head and neck or the trachea.[25,48]

Pathological Features

Grossly, adenoid cystic carcinomas of the airway are often firm and rubbery and white or pale pink in color. The overlying mucosa is usually intact, although it may be ulcerated, and the tumor *always* extends superiorly and inferiorly into the submucosa and along the nerves. Because of this tendency, getting a complete resection (i.e., "negative margins") is not straightforward.

Histologically, three specific patterns are recognized: cribriform, tubular, and solid. Although all are dangerous, tumors with solid elements metastasize more commonly than the other patterns; however, a single tumor can show more than one type.[86] The tumors contain mature ductal cells and immature myoepithelial cells.[7] A high proportion of immature cells correlates with an increased invasiveness. These tumors typically stain with antibodies against S-100 proteins, various keratins, vimentins, and muscle-specific actin.[4]

Clinical Features

Unlike their effect on lung cancer and carcinoids, smoking and other environmental factors do not cause adenoid cystic carcinoma. The tumors may occur in patients of any adult age, and they are detected only after they cause symptoms as a result of obstruction of the airway.

Patients may present with cough, fever, hemoptysis, purulent sputum, wheezing, pneumonia or recurrent pneumonias, or chest pain. Because these tumors grow slowly and extraluminally, the development of symptoms can be particularly insidious. The physical examination may be normal, or it may demonstrate only diminished breath sounds, a unilateral wheeze, or stridor.

Radiological Features

Unless the tumor obstructs the trachea, mainstem bronchus, or lobar bronchus and causes atelectasis, the lung fields on a chest radiograph will appear normal. Occasionally some narrowing of the trachea in the chest or low in the neck can be seen to suggest a tracheal mass. Mediastinal or hilar masses can occasionally be seen, again along with some narrowing of the trachea. Tumor masses in the cervical trachea are easily seen on neck radiographs.

CT scans give much more detail about both the intraluminal and extraluminal extent of adenoid cystic carcinomas.[111] However, because of volume averaging (and the tumor's tendency to submucosal spread), CT radiography does not accurately predict the longitudinal extent of tumor.[60a] CT scanning will also accurately demonstrate enlarged lymph nodes, but it is no more accurate for the identification of nodal involvement than it is for lung cancer.

Shanley and others[106] found magnetic resonance imaging to be superior to CT scanning for the determination of longitudinal extent, partly because of the multiple views that if offers.

Diagnosis

These lesions may present as polypoid lesions that obstruct the airway or as diffuse multinodular infiltrative lesions. Cytology of the airway (sputum analysis, bronchial washings, and even bronchial brushings) seldom yields a diagnosis of adenoid cystic carcinoma, because the tumors are often covered with normal bronchial epithelium. Transbronchial biopsies identify the majority of these lesions, and severe bleeding is rarely a problem.

Therapy

Surgical Therapy

Surgical resection is the treatment of choice, and it is the only modality likely to result in cure. Because of the likelihood of submucosal and perineural spread, intraoperative frozen sections must be used to confirm negative margins.[94] Intraoperative transmucosal bronchoscopic biopsies can direct operative planning.[95] Unfortunately, a surgeon must occasionally accept a microscopically positive margin rather than extend the longitudinal extent of resection and risk the dehiscence of a tense anastomosis.[19] With complete resection and lymphadenectomy, even patients with mediastinal nodal metastases can have long-term survival.[42]

Radiation Therapy

Adenoid cystic carcinomas are relatively radiosensitive, so radiotherapy can be used for those patients who are too frail for surgery or for those who have incomplete resections. The rate of complete response correlates significantly with a dose of 6000 cGy or more.[34] Most authors have used either preoperative or postoperative radiotherapy and found a low recurrence rate.[42,94,95]

Because these tumors can be extremely indolent, frail patients can be managed with laser debulking and radiation therapy. Most of these patients will have few if any symptoms after 6 months,[11] and they have a significant chance of long-term survival.[26] Laser therapy should precede radiation therapy, especially in those patients with significant endobronchial obstruction, because edema from radiation therapy may temporarily exacerbate the airway obstruction.[83,96] Finally, endobronchial brachytherapy can be used to extend the palliative treatment of adenoid cystic carcinoma, although there is not extensive reported experience.[15,103]

Chemotherapy

Prognosis

Complete resection yields the best long-term survival. Perelman and Koroleva[95] reported that 66% of their patients were alive at 5 years and that 56% were alive at 15 years. Pearson and others[94] found that 75% of their completely resected patients were alive at 8 years; the remainder had died of unrelated causes. Grillo and Mathisen[42] found that only 12% (7 out of 60) resected patients died from their tumors during a 26-year follow-up period.

Because these lesions grow slowly, even patients with incompletely resected lesions can survive for long periods. Carter and Eggleston[13] summarized several studies involving patients treated both definitively and palliatively and found 5-year, 10-year, and 20-year survival rates of 85%, 55%, and 20%, respectively.

Mucoepidermoid Carcinoma

Mucoepidermoid carcinoma is an uncommon tumor of the airway that accounts for about 1% of all primary malignant bronchial gland tumors and 0.2% of all lung neoplasms. This tumor is histologically similar to tumors of the same name of the salivary glands.[109]

Bronchial mucoepidermoid carcinomas are classified as either high-grade or low-grade on the basis of their histological appearance. Low-grade tumors can have both cystic and solid histological characteristics, although the cystic component usually predominates. By contrast, high-grade tumors are more likely to show solid characteristics, which may be the dominant type. High-grade mucoepidermoid carcinoma can be difficult to differentiate from adenosquamous carcinoma of the lung.[52]

Clinical Features

In general, men and women are affected with equal frequency.[121] Low-grade lesions are more likely in patients who are less than 30 years old, and high-grade lesions more likely in patients who are more than 30 years old, although both tumors have been found in very young and very old patients.[129] Tobacco use or other environmental exposure is not believed to be important, a characteristic that is also found for adenoid cystic carcinoma. The typical symptoms are those of airway obstruction; however, as discussed above, tracheal tumors and obstructions are uncommon as compared with adenoid cystic carcinoma.

The radiographic appearance of mucoepidermoid carcinoma is similar to adenoid cystic carcinoma. Parenchymal lesions are rare, and the scans typically demonstrate endobronchial tumors. CT scans may demonstrate the enlarged nodes that are common in high-grade lesions.

Again, as is found with adenoid cystic carcinoma, the mucosa overlying the tumor is usually intact, so sputum cytology, bronchial washings, and bronchial brushings are nondiagnostic. Transbronchial biopsies are necessary to make the diagnosis. Significant hemorrhage is uncommon.[19]

Treatment

Surgical resection is the primary treatment of mucoepidermoid carcinomas of the airway. Bronchoplastic techniques should be used to preserve as much lung as possible. Hilar and mediastinal lymph node resection is also recommended. Patients with high-grade and low-grade lesions are approached similarly, although the high-grade lesions are often unresectable. The role of radiation therapy is controversial; at least two authors found adjuvant radiotherapy to be ineffective for high-grade lesions,[46,121] although others have found significant response.[58] The prognosis for low-grade lesions is very good, with high cure rates, whereas 2-year survival in patients with high-grade lesions is rare. Surveillance with both bronchoscopy and CT scans is indicated. The differences between low-grade and high-grade mucoepidermoid carcinoma of the airway are summarized in Table 22-4.

Mixed Tumor of Salivary Gland Type

Otherwise known as pleomorphic adenomas, these tumors are exceedingly rare, with some summaries reporting a total of only eight cases in the literature.[81] The histological features are similar to those of the mixed tumors that arise in salivary glands in the head and neck: epithelial cells in a chondroid stroma.

The tumors usually grow slowly, and they rarely metastasize to either nodes or distant sites. The therapeutic goal is complete resection, and cure can be expected.

330

Table 22–4

Characteristics of High- and Low-Grade Mucoepidermoid Carcinoma

	Bronchial wall involvement	Cystic or solid histology	Nodal metastases	Common age	2-year survival
Low grade	Uncommon	Mostly cystic	Never	<30 years	~75%
High grade	Common	Mixed	Common	>30 years	~0%

Uncommon Primary Malignant Tumors of the Lung

Most of the uncommon histologies that develop elsewhere in the body also occur in the lungs. Most of these lesions are sarcomas, but others include blastomas, pulmonary lymphomas, pulmonary melanomas, and malignant teratomas (Box 22-4). Most of these lesions are initially asymptomatic and peripheral.[85] Resection is the therapy of choice, and adjuvant chemotherapy should be used when appropriate for the histology.

Sarcomas

Mesenchymal tumors may arise from either stromal cells of the bronchus, blood vessels, or parenchyma (Box 22-5). Because these lesions do not arise from the epithelium or endothelium, they usually do not cause an ulcer, and they can rarely be diagnosed with sputum cytological evaluations. A Mayo Clinic review found that sarcomas made up 18% of the rare pulmonary tumors.[74]

Most patients are asymptomatic and present with a well-circumscribed mass that is seen in the lung parenchyma on chest radiographs that are done for unrelated reasons.[32] Those patients with symptoms have nonspecific ones such as chest pain, cough, and hemoptysis. The lesions may invade the pleura and chest wall, and they rarely cavitate; they are equally common on both sides.[115] The lesions are often large, and, in one series, averaged 7 cm in diameter.[66]

Like other sarcomas, pulmonary sarcomas rarely metastasize to lymphatics but rather to distant organs via the bloodstream. Distant metastases are often late manifestations of advanced disease.[125] The therapy of choice for all of these tumors is resection, but the results vary, with relatively high cure rates for chondrosarcoma and lower rates for osteosarcoma.[50] The largest reported series identified 43 patients; 29 underwent resection, 6 received radiation therapy, 2 received radiation and chemotherapy, and 6 were not treated.[71] The overall 1-year, 3-year, and 5-year survival rates were 55%, 31%, and 25%, respectively. Smaller tumors (<5 cm) correlated with longer survival, as did resection as compared with other therapies.

Fibrosarcoma and Leiomyosarcoma

These tumors may develop either in the pulmonary hilum (endobronchially) or the periphery of the lung. Most patients have cough or hemoptysis and are young. Resection is usually curative, although mitotic rate, size of the tumor, and involvement of adjacent structures predict poorer outcomes.[43,85]

Pulmonary Rhabdomyosarcoma

These rare lesions often replace 1 or more pulmonary lobes and invade adjacent structures.[63] Most reported cases occurred in children.[107]

Malignant Fibrous Histiocytoma of the Lung

These lesions are rarer than fibrosarcomas or leiomyosarcomas of the lung. The average patients with this condition are 55 years old, with a broad range.[130] They presented with

---

Box 22–4.   Uncommon Primary Malignant Tumors of the Lungs.

Soft-tissue sarcoma
   Parenchymal and bronchial sarcomas
   Sarcomas of blood vessels
Carcinosarcoma
Pulmonary blastoma
Lymphoma
Melanoma
Malignant teratoma

Box 22–5.   Primary Soft-Tissue Sarcomas of the Lung.

Leiomyosarcoma
Fibrosarcoma
Spindle-cell sarcoma
Rhabdomyosarcoma
Malignant fibrous histiocytoma
Angiosarcoma
Malignant hemangiopericytoma
Neurogenic sarcoma
Synovial sarcoma
Kaposi's sarcoma
Liposarcoma
Chondrosarcoma
Osteosarcoma

cough, chest pain, weight loss, or hemoptysis, and a mass was present on chest radiograph. The primary therapy has been resection, with increased size, extension into other organs, and incomplete resection being predictors of poor outcome.[72]

Pulmonary Chondrosarcoma

Most chondrosarcomas in the lung result from hematogenous metastases or direct extension into the chest wall. Chondrosarcoma may develop in the lung but from the cartilaginous portions of the airway. Several authors have described 1 or 2 cases[47,79,82]; Morgan and Salama[78] described the largest series (8 cases). Patients ranged in age from 23–72 years (average age, 46 years). The most common clinical symptoms were cough, chest pain, and dyspnea. Radiologically and macroscopically, these lesions often demonstrate calcification. All patients underwent surgery; 3 out of 6 patients with follow-up were free of disease 3 or more years after resection; the others died of recurrent disease.

Pulmonary Osteosarcoma

Primary pulmonary osteosarcoma is also rare, with most such tumors presenting in the lungs as metastases. Loose[61] reported 2 cases and reviewed 8 others. In that report, 3 criteria were chosen as being necessary to confirm that a pulmonary osteosarcoma was a primary tumor rather than a metastasis: (1) the tumor was a uniform sarcomatous tumor that excluded malignant mixed mesenchymal tumor; (2) osteoid or bone was found in the tumor; and (3) no primary osseous tumor was found elsewhere. Most of the patients in that study presented with chest pain. Resection was recommended for these tumors, although long-term survival was rare.

Others have been able to demonstrate the presence of primary pulmonary osteogenic sarcoma before resection by a combination of CT and pleural biopsies[20] or nuclear medicine scans (bone scans).[97]

Sarcomas of Large-Vessel Origin

In contrast with the lesions described above, which are exceedingly rare, sarcomas of large-vessel origin are only rare. The most common types are undifferentiated sarcoma,[124] leiomyosarcoma,[5] and fibrosarcoma.[87] These lesions may present in patients of any age, and they are slightly more likely to occur in women. Patients most commonly present with dyspnea or chest pain, and they may have a murmur.

The lesions present as mediastinal or hilar masses.[10,76] In some cases, patients have presented with symptoms consistent with pulmonary embolus.[69] These tumors are usually active on PET scan.[117]

Prolonged survival is unusual; one large study found that no patients survived for more than 3.5 years.[90] Kruger[55] found that adjuvant therapy increased survival, but the chance for cure is small.

Sarcomas of Small-Vessel Origin

Angiosarcoma, epithelioid hemangioendothelioma, hemangiopericytoma, and hemangioendothelioma are malignant vascular tumors that present as lung masses.

Angiosarcoma

This rare tumor can present as a solitary lesion or as multiple lesions. A review of the literature in 1983 identified only 10 cases.[112] When multiple, the lesions may actually be metastases from tumors in the right ventricle, pulmonary artery, or a distant site.[128] Patel and Ryu[91] reported 15 cases from the Mayo Clinic, but these were not clearly primary disease. In one series, 3 out of 7 patients with diffuse disease underwent autopsy; in all 3, a distant primary site was identified.[1]

The presentation of these lesions can vary. Some may present as a bilateral infiltrate and masquerade as pulmonary hemorrhage.[108] The most common presenting symptom is hemoptysis; others include weight loss, cough, and chest pain.

Naka and others[84] described the largest series, in which 99 patients were identified; most had primary sites elsewhere (29% in the head and face; 17% in the liver; 13% in the trunk; 12% in the heart; 7% in the extremities). Predisposing factors were chronic pyothorax, use of Thorotrast, and radiotherapy. The 5-year survival rate in this study was only 17%.

Epithelioid Hemangioendothelioma

This is a vascular tumor that was first described by Dail and Liebow[23] and subsequently further reviewed by Dail and others.[24] In the 1970s and 1980s, the lesion was called "intravascular bronchioalveolar tumor," but it subsequently came to be considered epithelioid hemangioendothelioma.

The tumor is 4 times more common in women than it is in men. Most patients have no symptoms, although clubbing is relatively common. Chest radiographs and CT scans typically reveal many small nodules.[100] Those patients with pleural effusions or spindle tumor cells had shorter survival times.[51] In fact, some of the patients with the best histology demonstrated spontaneous regression.

Hemangiopericytomas

These tumors develop from capillary pericytic cells and are thus found throughout the body, and in the chest and mediastinum. They may present as Pancoast tumors,[16] mediastinal tumors,[77,80] esophageal tumors,[110] or cardiac tumors,[89] and they are prone to cause hemoptysis or thromboembolic disease.[101] Approximately a third of patients have no symptoms, whereas the remainder report hemoptysis, chest pain, and cough.[131]

Magnetic resonance imaging may be useful when planning the extent of resection.[102] The only known therapy is surgical resection. The indicators of poor prognosis are as follows: (1) chest symptoms, (2) tumor size greater than 8 cm, (3) pleural and bronchial wall invasion, (4) tumor necrosis, and (5) more than 3 mitoses per 10 high-power fields. Chemotherapy and radiation therapy have not been effective against these lesions.[30,33]

Pulmonary Blastoma

Pulmonary blastomas are composed of both malignant mesenchymal and epithelial components that resemble the lung at

332 3 months' gestation. It is not surprising, then, that this tumor can present in infants and children.[105] Koss and others[53] reviewed 52 cases of pulmonary blastoma and divided the tumors into 2 classes based on their histological features: well-differentiated fetal adenocarcinomas and biphasic blastomas.

The average age of patients in this particular study was 35 years (range, 1–72 years). Forty-one percent of the patients were free of symptoms, with the others complaining of cough, hemoptysis, or dyspnea. The majority of patients had a normal physical examination.

Chest radiographs revealed a unilateral pulmonary mass located in either the hilum or the periphery. Bronchoscopy and fine-needle aspiration were only occasionally helpful for making the diagnosis.

The fetal lesions were more likely to be well-differentiated fetal adenocarcinomas and to present as pleural lesions.[9] Adjuvant chemotherapy may be of benefit, but surgical resection is the primary therapy.

Pulmonary Lymphoma

Lymphomas of the lung, as in other parts of the body, are classified as Hodgkin's or non-Hodgkin's. Primary lymphomas are rare; most are secondary, resulting from spread from the mediastinum. The incidence ranges from 0.33–0.50% of all lung tumors.[60,75] Secondary involvement of the lung as a result of spread from mediastinal disease is common.

Discussion of the intricacies of diagnosis and treatment of lymphoma is beyond the scope of this text. Thoracic surgeons are most often involved in the care of patients with lymphoma either to diagnose mediastinal adenopathy or to resect lung lesions. The diagnosis of lymphoma is difficult for the pathologist; when lymphoma is suspected, the surgeon has several additional responsibilities (Box 22-6). Tissue submitted in formalin will decrease some of the nuclear detail, and it will also not allow for cytogenetic or flow cytometric studies. Therefore, the surgeon is responsible for notifying the pathologist in advance and for ensuring that adequate tissue is obtained for these additional studies (and, thus, not all put in formalin).

The most common scenario is that of a patient undergoing mediastinoscopy for suspected mediastinal nodal involvement by either small-cell or non–small-cell carcinoma. If the tissue is sent in formalin, then the opportunity to evaluate the lymphoma is lost.

Primary Pulmonary Lymphoma

Eighteen percent of patients have lymph nodes or nodal tissue within the lungs.[119] These tissues have had multiple names (e.g., bronchial-associated lymphoid tissue, mucosa-associated lymphoid tissue). The classifications of lymphomas are many and confusing, but one that has been reasonably well accepted and that is relatively simple was proposed by Costa and Martin (Box 22-7).[21] Those lesions that are resected completely will often require only postoperative chemotherapy rather than chemoradiation.

Secondary Pulmonary Lymphomas

Approximately three quarters of patients with Hodgkin's disease will have some thoracic involvement, most commonly in the anterior mediastinum or paratracheal regions.[27] Spread occurs by contiguity, from mediastinal to hilar nodes to the lungs. Only with bulk disease in the mediastinum is involvement in the lungs, pleura, or pericardium common; exceptions to this pattern suggest some disease other than Hodgkin's lymphoma. By contrast, non-Hodgkin's disease is much less predictable. Risdall and others[99] found pulmonary involvement in 54% of patients undergoing autopsy.

Recurrent lymphoma after treatment is much less predictable. Recurrent disease, from either Hodgkin's disease or non-Hodgkin's disease, may present with pulmonary

---

Box 22–6. Pathologic Preparation of Tissue Suspected to be Lymphoma.

1. Touch preparations
2. Fresh tissue for cytogenetic studies
3. Tissue fixed in B-5 solution to preserve nuclear detail
4. Fresh tissue for flow cytometric studies

Box 22–7. Pulmonary Lymphoreticular Disorders.

Benign primary pulmonary lymphoreticular disorders

Pseudolymphoma
Lymphocytic interstitial pneumonia

Primary non-Hodgkin's lymphoma of the lung

Rappaport Classification	Working Formulation
Low grade	
Well-differentiated lymphocytic	Small lymphocytic
Nodular, poorly differentiated lymphocytic	Follicular, small cleaved cells
Intermediate grade	
Nodular histiocytic	Follicular, large cells
Diffuse, poorly differentiated lymphocytic	Diffuse, small cleaved cells
Diffuse, mixed lymphocytic and histiocytic	Diffuse, mixed small and large
High grade	
Diffuse histiocytic	Large cell, immunoblastic
Lymphoblastic	Lymphoblastic, convoluted
Angiocentric	
Immunoproliferative lesions	
Lymphocytic vasculitis	
Lymphomatoid granulomatosis	
Angiocentric large cell lymphoma	
Plasma cell disorders	
Waldenström's macroglobulinemia	
Plasmacytoma	
Multiple myeloma	

Hodgkin's disease

Modified from Costa J, Martins S: Pulmonary lymphoreticular disorders. In Jaffe ES (editor): Surgical Pathology of the Lymph Nodes and Related Organs. Philadelphia: WB Saunders, 1985, p. 282.

nodules, pulmonary masses, pulmonary consolidation, infiltrates, pleural masses, or hilar/mediastinal adenopathy.[59]

SUMMARY

All of the lesions described in this chapter are rare, and thus the appropriate management difficult to summarize or to recall. Surgeons must review appropriate literature every time they manage an unusual tumor to ensure appropriate care for their patients.

REFERENCES

1. Adem C, Aubry MC, Tazelaar HD, Myers JL: Metastatic angiosarcoma masquerading as diffuse pulmonary hemorrhage: clinicopathologic analysis of 7 new patients. Arch Pathol Lab Med 125:1562–1565, 2001.
2. Aniszewski JP, Young WF Jr, Thompson GB, et al: Cushing syndrome due to ectopic adrenocorticotropic hormone secretion. World J Surg 25:934–940, 2001.
3. Arrigoni MG, Woolner LB, Bernatz TE: Atypical carcinoid tumours of the lung. J Thorac Cardiovasc Surg 64:413–421, 1972.
4. Azumi N, Battifora H: The cellular composition of adenoid cystic carcinoma: an immunohistochemical study. Cancer 60:1589–1598, 1987.
5. Baker PB, Goodwin RA: Pulmonary artery sarcomas. A review and report of a case. Arch Pathol Lab Med 109:35–39, 1985.
6. Baldwin JN, Grimes OF: Bronchial adenomas. Surg Gynecol Obstet 124:813–818, 1967
7. Balazs M: Adenoid cystic (cylindromatous) carcinoma of the trachea: an ultrastructural study. Histopathology 10:425–435, 1986.
8. Beasley MB, Thunnissen FBJM, Brambilla E, et al: Pulmonary atypical carcinoid: predictors of survival in 106 cases. Hum Pathol 31:1255–1265, 2000.
9. Bekassy AN, Garwicz S, Wiebe T, Hagerstrand I: Uncertain role of high dose chemotherapy with autologous stem cell support in pediatric pleuro-pulmonary blastoma (PPB). Med Pediatr Oncol 28:75–76, 1997.
10. Britton PD: Primary pulmonary artery sarcoma—a report of two cases, with special emphasis on the diagnostic problems. Clin Radiol 41:92–94, 1990.
11. Brutinel WM, Cortese DA, McDougall JC, et al: A two-year experience with the neodymium-YAG laser in endobronchial obstruction. Chest 91:159–165, 1987.
12. Carretta A, Ceresoli GL, Arrigoni G, et al: Diagnostic and therapeutic management of neuroendocrine lung tumors: a clinical study of 44 cases. Lung Cancer 29:217–225, 2000.
13. Carter D, Eggleston J: Fascicle 17. Tumors of the Lower Respiratory Tract. Washington, DC: Armed Forces Institute of Pathology, 1979.
14. Cebelin MS: Melanocytic bronchial carcinoid tumor. Cancer 46:1843–1848, 1980.
15. Chin HW, Demeester T, Chin RY, et al: Endobronchial adenoid cystic carcinoma. Chest 100:1464–1465, 1991.
16. Chong KM, Hennox SC, Sheppard MN: Primary hemangiopericytoma presenting as a Pancoast tumor. Ann Thorac Surg 55:9, 1993.
17. Churg A: Tumors of the lungs. In Thurlbeck WM (editor): Pathology of the Lung. Stuttgart: Thieme Medical Publishers, 1988.
18. Codrington H, Sutedja T, Golding R, et al: Unusual pulmonary lesions: case 2. Endobronchial carcinoid of the lung. J Clin Oncol 20:2747–2748, 2002.
19. Conlan AA, Payne WS, Woolner LB, et al: Adenoid cystic carcinoma (cylindroma) and mucoepidermoid carcinoma of the bronchus. Factors affecting survival. J Thorac Cardiovasc Surg 76:369–377, 1978.
20. Connolly JP, McGuyer CA, Sageman WS, Bailey H: Intrathoracic osteosarcoma diagnosed by CT scan and pleural biopsy. Chest 100:265–267, 1991.
21. Costa J, Martin S: Pulmonary lymphoreticular disorders. In Jaffee E (editor): Surgical Pathology of the Lymph Nodes and Related Organs. Philadelphia: WB Saunders, 1985, p. 289.
22. Cutz E, et al: Immunoperoxidase staining for serotonin, bombesin, calcitonin, and leuenkephalin in pulmonary tumorlets, bronchial carcinoids, and oat cell carcinomas. Lab Invest 46:16A, 1982.
23. Dail D, Liebow AA: Intravascular bronchioalveolar tumor [abstract]. Am J Pathol 78:6, 1975.
24. Dail DH, Liebow AA, Gmelich JT, et al: Intravascular, bronchiolar, and alveolar tumor of the lung (IVBAT): an analysis of twenty cases of a peculiar sclerosing endothelial tumor. Cancer 51:452–464, 1983.
25. Dalton L, Garling RR: Peripheral adenoid cystic carcinoma of the lung. South Med J 83:577, 1990.
26. Diaz-Jiminez JP, Canela-Cardona M, Maestre-Alcacer J: Nd:YAG laser photoresection of low-grade malignant tumors of the tracheobronchial tree. Chest 97:920, 1990.
27. Diehl LF, Hopper KD, Giguere J, et al: The pattern of intrathoracic Hodgkin's disease assessed by computed tomography. J Clin Oncol 9:438–443, 1991.
28. Donahue JK, Weichert RR, Ochsner JL: Bronchial adenoma. Ann Surg 167:873–885, 1968.
29. Englebreth-Holm J: Benign bronchial adenomas. Acta Chir Scand 90:383, 1944.
30. Enzinger FM, Smith BH: Hemangiopericytoma. An analysis of 106 cases. Hum Pathol 7:61–82, 1976.
31. Erasmus JJ, McAdams HP, Patz ER Jr, et al: Evaluation of primary pulmonary carcinoid tumors using FDG PET. AJR Am J Roentgenol 170:1369–1373, 1998.
32. Fadhli HA, Harrison AW, Shaddock SH: Primary pulmonary leiomyosarcoma. Dis Chest 48:431–, 1965.
33. Feldman F, Seaman WB: Primary thoracic hemangiopericytoma. Radiology 82:998–1009, 1964.
34. Fields JN, Rigaud G, Emani BN: Primary tumors of the trachea. Results of radiation therapy. Cancer 63:2429–2433, 1989.
35. Filosso PL, Rena O, Donati G, et al: Bronchial carcinoid tumors: surgical management and long-term outcome. J Thorac Cardiovasc Surg 123:303–309, 2002.
36. Fink G, Krelbaum T, Yellin A, et al: Pulmonary carcinoid: presentation, diagnosis, and outcome in 142 cases in Israel and review of 640 cases from the literature. Chest 119:1647–1651, 2001.
37. Frist WH, Mathisen DJ, Hilgenberg AD, et al: Bronchial sleeve resection with and without pulmonary resection. J Thorac Cardiovasc Surg 93:350–357, 1987.
38. Ghadially FN, Block HJ: Oncocytic carcinoma of the lung. J Submicrosc Cytol Pathol 17:435–442, 1985.
39. Goldstraw P, Lamb D, McCormack RJ, et al: The malignancy of bronchial adenoma. J Thorac Cardiovasc Surg 72:309–314, 1976.
40. Granberg D, Eriksson B, Wilander E, et al: Experience in treatment of metastatic pulmonary carcinoid tumors. Ann Oncol 12:1383–1391, 2001.
41. Grazer R, Cohen SM, Jacobs JB, et al: Melanin-containing peripheral carcinoid of the lung. Am J Surg Pathol 6:73–78, 1982.

42. Grillo HC, Mathisen DJ: Primary tracheal tumors: treatment and results. Ann Thorac Surg 49:69–77, 1990.

43. Guccion JG, Rosen SH: Bronchopulmonary leiomyosarcoma and fibrosarcoma: a study of 32 cases and review of the literature. Cancer 30:836–847, 1972.

44. Hage R, Brutel de la Riviere A, Seldenrijk CA, et al: Update in pulmonary carcinoid tumors: a review article. Ann Surg Oncol 10:697–704, 2003.

45. Harpole Jr DH, Feldman JM, Buchanan S, et al: Bronchial carcinoid tumors: a retrospective analysis of 126 patients. Ann Thorac Surg 54:50–54, 1992.

46. Heitmiller RF, et al: Mucoepidermoid lung tumors. Ann Thorac Surg 49:394–399, 1990.

47. Huang HY, Hsieh MJ, Chen WJ, et al: Primary mesenchymal chondrosarcoma of the lung. Ann Thorac Surg 2002 73:1960–1962, 2002.

48. Inoue H, Iwashita A, Kanegae H, et al: Peripheral pulmonary adenoid cystic carcinoma with substantial submucosal extension to the proximal bronchus. Thorax 46:147–148, 1991.

49. Kayser K, Kayser C, Rahn W, et al: Carcinoid tumors of the lung: immuno- and ligandohistochemistry, analysis of integrated optical density, syntactic structure analysis, clinical data, and prognosis of patients treated surgically. J Surg Oncol 63:99–106, 1996.

50. Keller SM, Katariya K. Primary lung tumors other than bronchogenic carcinoma: benign and malignant. In Fishman AP (editor): Fishman's Pulmonary Diseases and Disorders. McGraw-Hill, 1998.

51. Kitaichi M, Nagai S, Nishimura K, et al: Pulmonary epithelioid haemangioendothelioma in 21 patients, including three with partial spontaneous regression. Eur Respir J 12:89–96, 1998.

52. Klacsmann PG, Olson JL, Eggleston JC: Mucoepidermoid carcinoma of the bronchus. Cancer 43:1720–1733, 1979.

53. Koss MN, Hochholzer L, O'Leary T: Pulmonary blastomas. Cancer 67:2368–2381, 1991.

54. Kristofferson A, Olsson T, Bjornebrink J, et al: Diagnosis of ectopic ACTH production from a bronchial carcinoid by imaging with octreotide scintigraphy. Eur J Surg 162:515–518, 1996.

55. Kruger I: Symptoms, diagnosis, and therapy of primary sarcomas of the pulmonary artery. Thorac Cardiovasc Surg 38:91–95, 1990.

56. Kurimoto N, Murayama M, Yoshioka S, et al: Assessment of usefulness of endobronchial ultrasonography in determination of depth of tracheobronchial tumor invasion. Chest 115:1500–1506, 1999.

57. Kwekkeboom DJ, Krenning EP, Bakker WH, et al: Somatostatin analogue scintigraphy in carcinoid tumors. Eur J Nucl Med 20:283–292, 1993.

58. Leonardi HK, Jung-Legg Y, Legg MA, et al: Tracheobronchial mucoepidermoid carcinoma: clinicopathological features and results of treatment. J Thorac Cardiovasc Surg 76:431–438, 1978.

59. Lewis ER, Caskey CI, Fishman EK: Lymphoma of the lung: CT findings in 31 patients. AJR Am J Roentgenol 156:711–714, 1991.

60. L'Hoste Jr RJ, Lieberman PH, Filippa DA, et al: Primary pulmonary lymphomas. Cancer 54:1397–1406, 1984.

60a. Li L, Ellerbroek NA, Libshitz HI: Primary malignant tumors of the trachea: a radiologic and clinical study. Cancer 66:894–899, 1990.

61. Loose JH: Primary osteosarcoma of the lung. Report of two cases and review of the literature. J Thorac Cardiovasc Surg 100:867–873, 1990.

62. Lubarch O: Ueber den primaren krebs des ileum, nebst bemerkungen uber das gleichzeitige vorkommen von krebs und tuberkolose. Virchows Arch 111:280–317, 1888.

63. Luck SR, Reynolds M, Raffensperger JG: Congenital bronchopulmonary malformations. Curr Probl Surg 23:251–314, 1986.

64. Magid D, Siegelman SS, Eggleston JC, et al: Pulmonary carcinoid tumors. CT assessment. J Comput Assist Tomogr 13:244–247, 1989.

65. Marom EM, Sarvis S, Herndon JE II, Patz EF Jr: T1 lung cancers: sensitivity of diagnosis with fluorodeoxyglucose PET. Radiology 223:453–459, 2002.

66. Martini N, Hajdu SI, Beattie Jr EJ: Primary sarcoma of lung. J Thorac Cardiovasc Surg 61:33–38, 1971.

67. Martini N, Zaman MB, Bains MS, et al: Treatment and prognosis in bronchial carcinoid involving regional lymph nodes. J Thorac Cardiovasc Surg 107:1–6, 1994.

68. Marty-Ane CH, Costes V, Pujol JL, et al: Carcinoid tumors of the lung: do atypical features require aggressive management? Ann Thorac Surg 59:78–83, 1995.

69. Mattoo A, Fedullo PF, Kapelanski D, Ilowite JS: Pulmonary artery sarcoma: a case report of surgical cure and 5-year follow-up. Chest 122:745–747, 2002.

70. McCaughan BC, Martini N, Bains MS: Bronchial carcinoids. Review of 124 cases. J Thorac Cardiovasc Surg 89:8–17, 1985.

71. McCormack PM, Martini N: Primary sarcomas and lymphomas of the lung. In Martini N, Vogt-Moykopf I (editors): Thoracic Surgery: Frontiers and Uncommon Neoplasms, Part 3, Uncommon Pulmonary Neoplasms, vol 5. St. Louis, Mosby, 1989, pp. 260–274.

72. McDonnell T, Kyriakos M, Roper C, et al: Malignant fibrous histiocytoma of the lung. Cancer 61:137–145, 1988.

73. Melmed S, Ziel FH, Braunstein GD, et al: Medical management of acromegaly due to ectopic production of growth hormone-releasing hormone by a carcinoid tumor. J Clin Endocrinol Metab 67:395–399, 1988.

74. Miller DL, Allen MS: Rare pulmonary neoplasms. Mayo Clin Proc 68:492–498, 1993.

75. Miller M, Mark G, Kanarek D: Multiple peripheral pulmonary carcinoid and tumorlets of carcinoid type with restrictive and obstructive lung disease. Am J Med 65:373–378, 1978.

76. Moffat RE, Chang CHJ, Slaven JE: Roentgen considerations in primary pulmonary artery sarcoma. Radiology 104:283–288, 1972.

77. Morandi U, Stefani A, De Santis M, et al: Preoperative embolization in surgical treatment of mediastinal hemangiopericytoma. Ann Thorac Surg 69:937–939, 2000.

78. Morgan AD, Salama FD: Primary chondrosarcoma of the lung: case reports and reviews of the literature. J Thorac Cardiovasc Surg 64:460–466, 1972.

79. Morgenroth A, Pfeuffer HP, Viereck HJ, et al: Primary chondrosarcoma of the left inferior lobar bronchus. Respiration 56:241–244, 1989.

80. Mori M, Nakanishi N, Furuya K: Hemangiopericytoma of the mediastinum causing spontaneous hemothorax. Ann Thorac Surg 58:1525–1527, 1994.

81. Mori M, Furuya K, Kimura T, et al: Mixed tumor of salivary gland type arising in the bronchus. Ann Thorac Surg 52:1322–1324, 1991.

82. Mukhopadhyay S, Khurana KK, Dexter E, et al: Pathologic quiz case: chest wall mass in a 74-year-old man. Extraskeletal myxoid chondrosarcoma. Arch Pathol Lab Med 127:e413–e414, 2003.

83. Munsch C, Westaby S, Sturridge M: Urgent treatment for a nonresectable, asphyxiating tracheal cylindroma. Ann Thorac Surg 43:663–664, 1987.

84. Naka N, Ohsawa M, Tomita Y, et al: Angiosarcoma in Japan. A review of 99 cases. Cancer 75:989–996, 1995.

85. Nascimento AG, Unni KK, Bernatz PE: Sarcomas of the lung. Mayo Clin Proc 57:355–359, 1982.

86. Nomori H, Kaseda S, Kobayashi K, et al: Adenoid cystic carcinoma of the trachea and mainstem bronchus. J Thorac Cardiovasc Surg 96:271–277, 1988.

87. Nonomura A, Kurumaya, H, Kono, N, et al: Primary pulmonary artery sarcoma: report of two autopsy cases studied by immunohistochemistry and electron microscopy, and review of 110 cases reported in the literature. Acta Pathol Jpn 38:883–896, 1988.

88. Oberg K: Chemotherapy and biotherapy in the treatment of neuroendocrine tumours. Ann Oncol 12:S111–S1114, 2001.

89. Ohtani M, Ohnishi K, Imagawa H, et al: Cardiac hemangiopericytoma growing in the left atrium. Ann Thorac Surg 58:1544–1546, 1994.

90. Parish JM, Rosenow EC, Swensen SJ, Crotty TB: Pulmonary artery sarcoma. Clinical features. Chest 110:1480–1488, 1996.

91. Patel AM, Ryu JH: Angiosarcoma in the lung. Chest 103:1531–1535, 1993.

92. Paulson DL, Ginsberg RJ: Bronchial adenoma. In Shields TW (editor): General Thoracic Surgery, ed 3. Philadelphia: Lea & Febiger, 1989.

93. Payne WS, Schier J, Woolner LB: Mixed tumors of the bronchus (salivary gland type). J Thorac Cardiovasc Surg 49:663–668, 1965.

94. Pearson FG, Todd TRJ, Cooper JD: Experience with primary neoplasms of the trachea and carina. J Thorac Cardiovasc Surg 88:511–518, 1984.

95. Perelman MI, Koroleva NS: Primary tumors of the trachea. In Grillo H, Eschapasse H (editors): International Trends in General Thoracic Surgery, vol 2. Philadelphia: WB Saunders, 1987.

96. Personne C, Colchen A, Leroy M, et al: Indications and technique for endoscopic laser resections in bronchology: a critical analysis based upon 2284 resections. J Thorac Cardiovasc Surg 91:710–715, 1987.

97. Petersen M: Radionuclide detection of primary pulmonary osteogenic sarcoma: a case report and review of the literature. J Nucl Med 31: 1110–1114, 1990.

98. Quaedvlieg PFHJ, Visser O, Lamers CBHW, et al: Epidemiology and survival in patients with carcinoid disease in the Netherlands. An epidemiological study with 2391 patients. Ann Oncol 12:1295–1300, 2001.

99. Risdall R, Hoppe TR, Warnke R: Non-Hodgkin's lymphoma: a study of the evolution of the disease based upon 92 autopsied cases. Cancer 44:529–542, 1979.

100. Ross GJ, Viola L, Friedman AC, et al: Intravascular bronchioloalveolar tumor: CT and pathologic correlation. J Comput Assist Tomogr 13:240–243, 1989.

101. Rothe TB, Karrer W, Gebbers JO. Recurrent haemoptysis in a young woman: a case of a malignant haemangiopericytoma of the lung. Thorax 49:188–189, 1994.

102. Rusch VW, Shuman WP, Schmidt R, et al: Massive pulmonary hemangiopericytoma: an innovative approach to evaluation and treatment. Cancer 64:1928–1936, 1989.

103. Ryan KL, Lowy J, Harrell JH: Management of adenoid cystic carcinoma. Chest 89(Suppl):503, 1986.

104. Schreurs AJM, Westermann CJJ, Van den Bosch JMM, et al: A twenty-five year follow-up of ninety-three resected typical carcinoid tumors of the lung. J Thorac Cardiovasc Surg 104:1470–1475, 1992.

105. Seballos RM; Klein RL: Pulmonary blastoma in children: report of two cases and review of the literature. J Pediatr Surg 29:1553–1556, 1994.

106. Shanley DJ, Daum-Kowalski R, Embry RL: Adenoid cystica carcinoma of the airway: MR findings. AJR Am J Roentgenol 156:1321–1322, 1991.

107. Shariff S, Thomas JA, Shetty N, et al: Primary pulmonary rhabdomyosarcoma in a child, with review of the literature. J Surg Oncol 38:261–264, 1988.

108. Sheppard MN, Hansell DM, Du Bois RM, et al: Primary epithelioid angiosarcoma of the lung presenting as pulmonary hemorrhage. Hum Pathol 28:383–385, 1997.

109. Smetana HF, Iverson L, Swan LL: Bronchogenic carcinoma, an analysis of 100 autopsy cases. Milit Surg 111:335–351, 1952.

110. Smith RT, Small WC, Mansour K: Case report: haemangiopericytoma of the oesophagus. Br J Radiol 68:1031–1033, 1995.

111. Spizarny DL, Shepard JA, Mcloud TC, et al: CT of adenoid cystic carcinoma of the trachea. AJR Am J Roentgenol 146:1129–1132, 1986.

112. Spragg RG, Wolf PL, Haghighi P, et al: Angiosarcoma of the lung with fatal pulmonary hemorrhage. Am J Med 74:1072–1076, 1983.

113. Stamatis G, Freitag L, Greschuchna D: Limited and radical resection for tracheal and bronchopulmonary carcinoid tumors: report on 227 cases. Eur J Cardiothorac Surg 4:527–532, 1990.

114. Suredja G, Golding RP, Postmus PE: High resolution computed tomography in patients referred for intraluminal bronchoscopic therapy with curative intent. Eur Respir J 9:1020–1023, 1996.

115. Suster S: Primary sarcomas of the lung. Semin Diagn Pathol 12:140–157, 1995.

116. Taal BG, Hoefnagel CA, Valdes Olmos RA, et al: Palliative effect of metaiodobenzylguanidine in metastatic carcinoid tumors. J Clin Oncol 14:1829–1838, 1996.

117. Thurer RL, Thorsen A, Parker JA, et al: FDG imaging of a pulmonary artery sarcoma. Ann Thorac Surg 70:1414–1415, 2000.

118. Toole A, Stern H: Carcinoid and adenoid cystic carcinoma of the bronchus. Ann Thorac Surg 13:63–81, 1972.

119. Trapnell DH: Recognition and incidence of intrapulmonary lymph nodes. Thorax 19:44–50, 1964.

120. Travis WD, Colby TV, Corrin B: Histological Typing of Lung and Pleural Tumors, ed 3. Berlin: Springer, 1999.

121. Turnbull AD, Huvos AG, Goadner JT, et al: Mucoepidermoid tumors of bronchial glands. Cancer 28:539–544, 1971.

122. Vadasz P, Palffy G, Egervary M, et al: Diagnosis and treatment of bronchial carcinoid tumors: clinical and pathological review of 120 operated patients. Eur J Cardiothorac Surg 7:8–11, 1993.

123. Van Boxen TJ, Golding RP, Venmans BJ, et al: High-resolution CT in patients with intraluminal typical bronchial carcinoid tumors treated with bronchoscopic therapy. Chest 117:125–128, 2000.

124. Wackers FJ, Van Der Schoot JB, Hampe JR: Sarcoma of the pulmonary trunk associated with hemorrhagic tendency: a case report and review of the literature. Cancer 23:339–351, 1969.

125. Watson WL, Anlyan AJ: Primary leiomyosarcoma: a clinical evaluation of six cases. Cancer 7:250–258, 1954.

126. Whitwell F: Tumourlets of the lung. J Pathol 70:529–541, 1955.

127. Wilkins, Jr, EW, Grillo, HC, Moncure, AC et al: Changing times and surgical management of bronchopulmonary carcinoid tumor. Ann Thorac Surg 38:339–344, 1984.

128. Yousem SA: Angiosarcoma presenting in the lung. Arch Pathol Lab Med 110:112–115, 1986.

129. Yousem SA, Hochholzer L: Malignant fibrous histiocytoma of the lung. Cancer 60:2532–2541, 1987.

130. Yousem SA, Hochholzer L: Mucoepidermoid tumors of the lung. Cancer 60:1346–1352, 1987.

131. Yousem SA, Hochholzer L: Primary pulmonary hemangiopericytoma. Cancer 59:549–555, 1987.

Secondary Lung Tumors

Evelio Rodriguez, Herbert E. Cohn, and Joseph S. Friedberg

CHAPTER 23

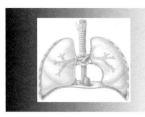

INTRODUCTION

After the liver, the lung is the second most common site for metastatic involvement in neoplastic disease when all histologies are considered. Consequently, 20–54% of patients with cancer will have pulmonary metastases at some point in the natural history of their disease. In the absence of extrathoracic metastases (~25% of patients with disseminated disease), complete resection is associated with increased survival, regardless of histology. With appropriate patient selection, life expectancy will often be improved with pulmonary metastasectomy. Cures are reported, either with resection alone or in combination with chemotherapy.[11,22] Even in the context of unresectability, surgical forms of palliation may serve to improve quality of life. For other patients (e.g., nonseminomatous germ cell tumors) surgery may have a more diagnostic role such as defining residual disease potentially amenable to salvage forms of therapy.

HISTORY

The first, and perhaps most famous, planned pulmonary metastasectomy in the United States was performed in 1933 by Barney and Churchill.[12] Soon after resection of a renal cell carcinoma they noted that the patient's pulmonary nodule, seen on chest X-ray (CXR) preoperatively and presumed to be tuberculosis, had doubled in size. The lesion, thought to represent metastatic disease, was treated with radiation therapy. They noted a poor response and elected to resect the nodule. The patient went on to live 23 years, eventually dying of coronary artery disease with no evidence of tumor recurrence on autopsy.[57]

During the nineteenth century there were sporadic reports of lung resections for metastatic tumors reported in the European literature. The first one of these reports was in 1855, by the French surgeon Sédillot, who removed a chest wall tumor and excised disease extending into the lung.[193] Almost 30 years later, in 1882, Weinlechner was credited for the first resection of a true pulmonary metastases. He excised pulmonary metastases from a rib sarcoma at the same time as the resection of the primary tumor.[199] The following year, Kronlein reported the first long-term survivor following a pulmonary metastasectomy. In this report, he described removal of a small metastatic nodule in the lung of a patient with a recurrent chest wall sarcoma. The patient went on to survive 7 years, eventually succumbing to recurrent pulmonary disease.[6,90,127] Despite the early discovery that survival could be improved by resection of

338 metastatic disease, it was not for another 40 years that metastasectomy was performed as a separate procedure by Divis in Europe.[42] This was followed soon after by similar reports in the American literature by Torek and Tudor Edwards in the early twentieth century.[44,186]

These early reports, and others like them, paved the way toward general acceptance of pulmonary metastasectomy. Although initial indications for surgery were reserved for those with a solitary metastasis, with time and experience more aggressive metastasectomies were performed. In 1947 Alexander and Haight reported the first series of pulmonary metastasectomies.[2] In their description of 24 cases of pulmonary metastasectomies they described a woman, in her twenties, with a spindle cell neurogenic sarcoma. She initially underwent a right lower lobectomy for metastatic disease in 1939. She subsequently had a recurrence in 1940 for which she underwent a left upper lobectomy. By the 1950s there were numerous case series with similar accounts. Today the indications for resection of secondary pulmonary malignancies have been broadened to include patients not only with recurrent disease, but those with multiple metastases, bilateral lesions, and essentially all histologies.[108]

PATHOPHYSIOLOGY OF METASTASIS TO LUNG

The generation of a metastasis involves a complex series of events known as the *metastatic cascade*. The initial tumor growth is supported by nutrients supplied by the organ's microenvironment mainly by diffusion. For the primary tumor to exceed 1–2 mm in size, *neovascularization or angiogenesis* must occur. This process is stimulated by both host and tumor-derived factors such as fibroblast growth factor (FGF), basic fibroblast growth factor (bFGF), and vascular endothelial growth factor (VEGF).[100] The next step in the metastatic cascade is tumor *invasion*. This phase is characterized by production of proteolytic enzymes (matrix metalloproteinases, collagenases; serine proteinases and cysteine proteinases) derived from the host and the tumor. This serves to facilitate spread by extracellular matrix breakdown, reduced tumor cell adhesiveness, stimulation of cell migration, and chemotaxis. In addition, during the invasion stage, tumor cells down-regulate the expression of adhesive proteins.[49] The balance between these angiogenic, proteinase, and adhesive molecules stimulating and inhibiting different cell factors helps to determine the metastatic potential of a given tumor.

Once the tumor cells have detached from adjacent cells, they migrate through the degraded basement membrane and gain access into lymphatics and blood vessels in a process called *intravasation*. The tumor cells that have gained access to the circulatory system are then able to *arrest* in capillary beds of different organs and/or lymph nodes. Only 0.1% of tumors cells in circulation will go on to generate metastases.[101] These cells must overcome destruction by the host's immune system such as natural killer cells and macrophages. In additions, they must withstand the physical forces of transport, such as shear forces and deformation, before they can *arrest* and seed a capillary network.

Hematogenous dissemination through the pulmonary arteries, and much less commonly through the bronchial arteries or lymphatics, is the most common form of spread for secondary pulmonary malignancies. This is thought to be the result of the lung's role as the primary capillary filter for the drainage of most organs.[133] Lymphatic spread in pulmonary metastases is unusual and more commonly represents hematogenous dissemination with extension to the lymphatics. Direct tracheobronchial dissemination is also rare and accounts for only 2–5% of pulmonary metastases, most commonly associated with renal cell and breast carcinomas.[168] Mediastinal involvement is also unusual and is frequently associated with concomitant parenchymal spread. Pleural effusions, when they occur, are typically manifestations of visceral or parietal pleural involvement, commonly seen with breast carcinoma.

Once arrest has occurred, tumor cells must then invade the interstitium in a process known as *extravasation*. Disruption of endothelial cells and their basement membrane occurs in a manner similar to intravasation. Once deposited in their new metastatic site cytokines, such as epidermal growth factor (EGF), transforming growth factor-α (TGF-α), platelet-derived growth factor (PDGF), and human growth factor (HGF), act as chemical messengers between the host and tumor to foster growth. Conversely, the host organ produces inhibitors, such as TGF-β, mammastatin, and amphiregulin, to prevent metastatic implantations.[49] These compounds are under investigation to assess their ability to control metastatic disease.

Do Metastases Metastasize?

In 1975, Hoover and Ketcham demonstrated, experimentally, that metastases do have the ability to metastasize.[73] In their experiment, mice had their primary tumor amputated after pulmonary metastasis developed. These mice were then placed into parabiosis with normal syngeneic partners. Metastases were demonstrated in the non-tumor-bearing partners. In addition, both autopsy and other experimental data have defined the concept of metastases from metastatic disease.[134] It is still poorly understood, however, when and how metastases are able to metastasize and more importantly how this process can be prevented from happening. It is thought that metastases need to follow the same steps as the primary tumor to metastasize: angiogenesis, intravasation, arrest, and extravasation.

Does Lung Cancer Metastasize to Lung?

Lung cancer is able to metastasize via lymphatic channels to the ipsilateral lung and, as suggested by some autopsy series, less commonly to the contralateral lung. These are patients with one primary lung cancer and intrapulmonary metastases. According to the 1997 lung cancer staging revision of the American Joint Commission of Cancer and the Union Internationale Contre Cancer, these patients are considered to have M1 disease.[130] It is difficult, however, to determine if these patients have synchronous lesions or a primary lung cancer with intrapulmonary metastases. Ichinose et al have used DNA flow cytometry to evaluate these lesions.[76,77] With this technique, lesions are determined to be synchronous if they demonstrate completely different DNA ploidy. If both tumors show diploidy or when at least one DNA index of abnormal clones between two aneuploidy tumors was the same or almost identical, then the tumors are considered metastatic. In addition, loss of heterozygosity and p53 mutational status have been used to distinguish multicentric lung cancers from intrapulmonary metastases.[83,110,170] With these criteria, it appears that lung cancer can metastasize to lung. These new molecular genetic techniques will continue to assist us in determining whether two lung lesions are synchronous primary lung tumors or a single primary lung tumor with lung metastasis.

SYMPTOMS AND PRESENTATION

Approximately 75–90% of patients with secondary pulmonary malignancies are asymptomatic and, therefore, their disease is most commonly discovered incidentally on routine or follow-up radiological examinations.[135,185] The usual lack of symptoms may, in part, be secondary to the common, nonobstructing peripheral location of pulmonary metastases. The asymptomatic nature of pulmonary metastases emphasizes the importance of obtaining lung imaging studies in the follow-up of cancer patients.

Symptoms, when they do occur, typically result from a delayed diagnosis with endobronchial or pleural involvement, large bulky disease, or central tumors. Patients may present with cough and hemoptysis suggesting an endobronchial lesion and thus warranting bronchoscopic examination. Endobronchial metastatic lesions are extremely rare, less than 2%, in patients who die of solid tumors with breast, kidney, pancreas, colon, and melanoma as the most common sources.[175] Another presenting symptom may be dyspnea, which is usually secondary to airway obstruction, a pleural effusion, parenchymal replacement by multiple metastatic lesions, or lymphatic spread. Finally, chest pain, wheezing, or pneumothorax may occur, but these are unusual presenting symptoms.

During physical examination one may appreciate wheezing, a sign of airway obstruction. Occasionally, a pericardial rub is heard representing pericardial involvement. Pleural and pericardial involvement are usually due to ovarian, breast, or lung adenocarcinomas. Also, thymomas are notorious for their pleural involvement when they metastasize.[63] In addition, decreased breath sounds and egophony may be appreciated when an obstructing lesion is present with associated lobar or segmental atelectasis that could be seen on CXR as postobstructive pneumonias.

RADIOGRAPHIC APPEARANCE

Every patient with a history of cancer should be routinely followed up and depending on the primary tumor with a plain CXR and/or a computerized assisted tomography (CT) of the chest. The presence of a new solitary pulmonary nodule in a patient with a prior malignancy essentially confirms the diagnosis of cancer. In one study in which 800 extrathoracic cancer patients presented with a new solitary pulmonary nodule, 87% were found to have a malignancy (63% primary lung cancer, 24% metastatic disease).[24] The likelihood that a nodule is malignant is less if found in a patient with no known cancer. In another study of 955 patients, 73% had no known history of previous

extrathoracic malignancy and only 49% of their nodules were malignant. Of note, 19% of these malignant lesions (9% total) represented metastatic disease.[187] The likelihood of finding metastases in a cohort of patients, all with no known cancer, therefore, is even lower. In one such study only 3% of solitary pulmonary lesions in 887 such patients were metastatic (see Box 23-1).[178]

Once a nodule has been found on a CXR, in a patient with a history of previous extrathoracic cancer, a diagnostic dilemma exists in determining whether the lesion represents metastatic or primary disease. This distinction has significant implications with respect to treatment and prognosis. The likelihood that a given pulmonary nodule is metastatic is dependent on the histology of the primary tumor (Table 23-1).[24,133]

Metastatic lung nodules themselves are most commonly described as being well circumscribed with smooth margins and spherical shape as well as located in the periphery of the lung[35] (Figure 23-1). In addition, there is a predilection for a more basilar distribution consistent with this region's increased blood flow in the upright position.[133] Of interest, patients with choriocarcinoma have an increased tendency for metastases in the posterior portions of the upper lobes of their lungs. This curious variation is thought to result from hematogenous dissemination to this region during supine resections of the uterine primary cancers.[69] Irregular borders and associated linear densities are more frequently associated with primary bronchogenic lung cancer.[35]

Metastatic nodules are frequently small in size, usually less then 1 cm. However, in the setting of multiple nodules, the probability that a nodule represents a metastasis increases with increasing nodule size.[175] Gross et al found

---

Box 23–1. Likelihood That a Pulmonary Nodule Is Metastatic.[24,178]

Solitary lung nodule in a patient who has a known extrathoracic primary	24% metastatic
Solitary lung nodule in a patient with no known primary	3% metastatic

---

Table 23–1

Likelihood of Metastatic versus Primary Lung Cancer[24]

Type of primary	Solitary nodule found on CXR
Sarcoma, melanoma	More commonly metastatic cancer
Carcinoma (e.g., breast, squamous cell)	More commonly primary lung cancer
Adenocarcinoma (e.g., colorectal)	Equally likely to be metastatic as primary

340

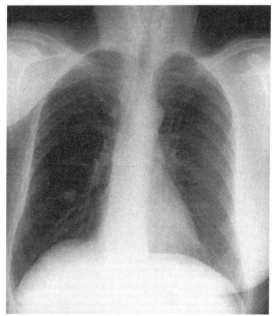

A

B

Figure 23–1 Radiography (A) and CT scan (B) demonstrating the usual characteristics of pulmonary metastasis (i.e., peripheral well-circumscribed lesions).
(Reproduced with permission from Greelish JP, Friedberg J: Secondary pulmonary malignancy. Surg Clin North Am 80: 633–657, 2000.)

that 87% of lesions greater than 2.5 cm in size were metastatic.[65] Also of significance, 75% of secondary malignancies of the lung will present with multiple lesions. Consequently, multiple lesions in the lung predict metastatic involvement 73% of the time.[65] Less commonly, multiple pulmonary nodules represent granulomatous disease, multifocal primary lung cancer, intraparenchymal lymph nodes, or pneumoconiosis.

Calcifications and nodule cavitation are frequently seen during the evaluation of pulmonary nodules and may help differentiate between benign, primary malignancies, and metastatic lung lesions. Calcifications, classically associated

with benign lesions of the lung such as granulomas and hamartomas, are rarely seen in metastatic pulmonary disease. When present, however, they are most commonly associated with osteosarcomas, chondrosarcomas, and breast and ovarian primaries. Cavitation, a characteristic of some benign lesions such as abscesses, aspergillosis, and tuberculosis, may be a sign of central tumor necrosis (5% of metastases).[97] This is most commonly seen with squamous cell carcinomas, sarcomas, and testicular tumors. Cavitation may also occur in a metastasis following chemotherapy and radiation therapy.[135]

One should pay attention in evaluating the mediastinum since metastatic disease involves the mediastinum 2–3% of the time.[65,175] Head and neck tumors, testicular tumors, breast carcinomas, melanomas, and especially renal cell carcinomas have been known to present as mediastinal disease.

► RADIOLOGICAL WORKUP

Secondary pulmonary malignancies are found most frequently by CXR obtained either incidentally or as part of a metastatic workup. In this context, CXR serves as a screening test and provides a baseline for future studies.[133] The sensitivity of plain radiographs is low, however, and in some series may only be 48% when compared to CT. Once a nodule is found or suspected on plain film, a CT of the chest should be obtained. Furthermore, in the metastatic workup of pneumotrophic primary malignancies (see Boxes 23-2 and 23-3), chest CT should be obtained as a primary study.

CT is the imaging modality of choice in the evaluation of pulmonary nodules because of its increased sensitivity, resolution, and three-dimensional nature.[136] Whereas the resolution of a routine CXR is approximately 9 mm, that of high-resolution (thin-section) CT scan is 1–2 mm.[85,183]

Box 23–2. Primary Malignancies Most Commonly Metastatic to the Lung.[64, a]

Breast
Colon
Kidney
Uterus
Prostate
Oropharyngeal
Carcinoma

ªMost common because of greater prevalence.

Box 23–3. Tumors with the Highest Predilection for Pulmonary Metastases.[64]

Choriocarcinoma
Osteosarcoma
Testicular tumors
Melanoma
Ewing's sarcoma
Kaposi's sarcoma

Approximately, 70–80% of tumor nodules less than 6 mm will be detectable by CT of the chest.[40,165] In addition, CT scan may further define the number and location of the nodules, aiding in assessment of resectability. For example, CT scans may help to distinguish an endobronchial lesion from a parenchymal lesion invading the bronchus. They may also demonstrate pericardial or pleural involvement and assist in visualizing any associated effusions. In so characterizing a lesion, a better estimate of the likelihood of malignancy and its resectability may be made. Earlier studies have demonstrated that CT scan of the chest may still underestimate the number of nodules when compared to those palpated at thoracotomy.[29,159,165] However, modern high-resolution CT scan techniques are able to detect lesions in the 2–3 mm range that are often difficult to be palpated during thoracotomy.

In addition to CXR and CT scan, other imaging modalities such as magnetic resonance imaging (MRI) may also be of use when assessing resectability and attempting to visualize potential involvement of the spine or surrounding structures.[48] The resolution of this study, however, is still inferior to CT. Positron emission tomography (PET) scans may have a role in characterizing metastatic pulmonary nodules, for breast carcinoma,[43] colorectal tumors,[75] and cholangiocarcinomas.[87] This modality, based on the differential metabolism of glucose, is currently under investigation as a tool in distinguishing metastatic lesions from primary pulmonary neoplastic disease.[68,180] Spiral CT has been shown to be superior to PET scans in diagnosing metastases from primary bone tumors (i.e., osteosarcomas and Ewing sarcomas).[53]

Occasionally, nuclear radiological techniques are useful in determining lung metastases from thyroid tumors as well as other neuroendocrine tumors.

TISSUE DIAGNOSIS

Obtaining tissue diagnosis prior to thoracotomy may be advantageous during the workup of a patient with a pulmonary nodule. When presented with a solitary pulmonary nodule in a patient with a history of cancer, the lesion may be benign or malignant. If malignant, the lesion may represent a primary lung cancer or metastatic disease. Under normal circumstances, the standard of care for a primary lung cancer is a formal anatomical resection while metastatic disease may be removed by simple wedge resection. Consequently, this diagnosis has significant implications regarding the therapeutic options for the patient. Furthermore, some patients may not be surgical candidates but still require a tissue diagnosis for appropriate nonsurgical management.

Sputum cytology is often nondiagnostic since most of the pulmonary metastases are peripherally located and is generally not indicated.[194] Bronchoscopic examination and diagnosis of pulmonary metastases are useful in the case of endobronchial and/or centrally located lesions. In a recent study a total of 113 patients with proven pulmonary metastases were analyzed. An endobronchial lesion was identified in 50.4% of the patients.[39] This value is higher than most series, but does point out the potential utility of bronchoscopy.

Fine needle aspiration (FNA) is another option for obtaining a tissue diagnosis. It is associated with a risk of pneumothorax, in some series as high as 27%.[34] In addition, the sensitivity of this procedure may be relatively low (80%). Equivocal or "negative" results do not establish a diagnosis of benign disease. Generally this procedure is thought to yield useful information only when it establishes a diagnosis of cancer.[113] When a nonsurgical therapy is indicated for a suspected histological diagnosis, or when a patient is not a surgical candidate, FNA represents an excellent diagnostic option. Success of this procedure depends not only on the skill of the operator, but also upon the diagnostic prowess of the interpreting cytologist.

Video-assisted thoracoscopy (VATS) for excisional biopsy has a sensitivity and specificity approaching 100%.[38,105,122] It is a procedure of significantly greater magnitude than FNA and requires general anesthesia with selective lung ventilation. It is indicated when FNA has failed, or is unlikely, to establish a diagnosis or when more information or tissue is required for treatment purposes. Also, under appropriate circumstances, it may be therapeutic as well as diagnostic in that the nodules can be completely excised.

Occasionally, we will perform a thoracoscopic FNA in cases of multiple lesions not amenable for complete surgical resection when a transthoracic FNA has been nondiagnostic.[179] In these cases, a diagnosis can be established in the operating room without excision of lung parenchyma and proper treatment may be initiated.

INDICATIONS FOR SURGERY

Indications for surgery, in the context of secondary pulmonary malignancy, are determined by the desire for curative resection, tissue diagnosis, or evaluation of residual disease after chemotherapy (see nonseminomatous germ cell tumors). Prior to proceeding with resection, a number of questions should be considered in the preoperative assessment of the patient.

Does the Pulmonary Nodule Represent One Site of Multiorgan Spread, Likely Precluding Resection with Curative Intent?

Pulmonary metastases are common in the advanced stages of cancer, with as many as one third of patients presenting with secondary nodules. Of these patients, however, the majority of pulmonary nodules (75–85%) are a manifestation of widespread disease. Consequently, only 15–25% of patients will have lesions confined to the lung and, as such, are appropriate candidates for curative resection (see Table 23-2). Preoperative evaluation, in general, should exclude extrathoracic disease. Occasional cases of isolated liver and lung metastases in good-risk patients might be considered for surgical resection.

When pleural or pericardial effusions are present, thoracentesis or pericardiocentesis should be performed to rule out malignancy. Positive cytology, if returned, contraindicates resection. Cytology, however, may be falsely negative in up to 40–60% of cases.[46,146] Consequently, a negative cytology returned in the context of a high index of suspicion for malignancy warrants pericardial and/or pleural

Table 23–2

Most Common Site of Metastasis and Percentage with Isolated Disease

Histology	Most common site of metastasis	Second most common site of metastasis	Percentage of those with isolated pulmonary metastases (all patients)
Breast carcinoma	Lung (59–65%)[196]		22%[177]
Colorectal	Liver[31]	Lung[31]	2–4%[22]
Germ cell tumors	Lung[95]		
Head and neck squamous cell carcinoma	Lung (75%)[36]		
Melanoma	Lung[a] (18–36%)[10,b]		5%[66]
Osteosarcoma	Lung (85%)[91]		
Renal cell carcinoma	Lung[99]		4%[99]
Soft tissue sarcoma	Lung (80–90%)[136]		20%[56]
All histologies	Liver	Lung[203]	15–20%[47,58]

[a]Secondary to skin, subcutaneous, lymph nodes.
[b]In clinical series, 70–87% in autopsy series.

biopsy. Bronchoscopy should always be performed prior to thoracoscopy or thoracotomy to rule out endobronchial lesions.

Is There a Nonsurgical Therapeutic Option?

Although a significant survival advantage may result for patients undergoing surgical resection of secondary pulmonary malignancies, nonsurgical management may be more appropriate for certain histologies. For example, in the context of nonseminomatous germ cell tumors, great success has been obtained with chemotherapy alone with cure rates approaching 90% (see germ cell tumors). In addition, high-dose multidrug chemotherapy and bone marrow rescue are the primary form of treatment offered to patients for disseminated pulmonary involvement secondary to breast carcinoma, although this is an area of controversy (see breast carcinoma).

Will the Patient Tolerate the Procedure?

Risk factors associated with metastatic disease, such as smoking and advanced age, require that patients being considered for surgical resection receive a thorough medical assessment with particular attention to their pulmonary and cardiac status. Stress testing, echocardiograms, arterial blood gases, pulmonary function testing, and ventilation perfusion scans may be necessary to assess a patient's tolerance for a proposed resection or their ability to undergo single lung ventilation. In addition, previously administered chemotherapeutic agents such as bleomycin or mitomycin may result in additional compromise of pulmonary function. Likewise, doxorubicin may be associated with cardiac impairment. The thoracic surgeon expecting to perform a metastasectomy must always be prepared to perform a formal anatomical resection should the pathology reveal a primary lung cancer or should wedge resection result in incomplete resection. For this reason, preoperative assessment with an eye toward a potential segmentectomy, lobectomy, or even pneumonectomy is prudent.

Are the Lesions Resectable?

Unresectability is defined as noncontiguous involvement beyond the visceral pleural envelope.[135] This is best determined at operation. Consequently, resectability may only be estimated preoperatively with the aforementioned imaging modalities. In addition, thoracoscopy can sometimes be useful to assess for disseminated disease and bulky tumors involving major structures precluding complete resection, or to access a pleural or pericardial effusion that cannot be reached percutaneously. If the pericardium or pleura is involved with neoplastic disease from direct extension of an underlying parenchymal lesion, but with no associated effusion, they should be resected en bloc with the specimen. Direct metastases to the pleura or pericardium in a discontinuous manner, disseminated spread, and malignant pleural or pericardial effusions are generally a contraindication for resection.

Is the Primary Tumor Controlled?

Efficacy of pulmonary metastasectomy is dependent upon, among other factors, the ability to control the primary neoplasm. The primary neoplasm, therefore, should generally be addressed prior to resection of the pulmonary metastases. A thorough preoperative testing should be performed to rule out other possible metastatic sites, or local recurrence of the primary tumor, prior to pulmonary metastasectomy.

Alexander and Haight,[2] in the 1940s, were the first to describe specific selection criteria in the consideration of pulmonary metastasectomy. They realized that the benefits of surgical resection depended on primary tumor control, absence of extrathoracic spread, and adequate patient selection. Of note, approximately one third of patients will meet these selection criteria. In so doing, they may appropriately undergo metastatic resection (Box 23-4).

▶ SURGICAL APPROACH

The goal of metastasectomy is complete resection of the lesions with maximal preservation of normal parenchyma. By fulfilling this goal the surgeon facilitates patient recovery and quality of life. Parenchymal sparing surgery also provides the potential for repeat resection, should it be necessary at some future date. Operative mortality should not exceed 1%.

A number of approaches to the thorax may be applied for metastasectomy. The choice of incision should reflect the extent of disease, the goal of complete resection, and the patient's ability to undergo the procedure. Median sternotomy is a good approach if bilateral disease is present that can be resected with that exposure.[160,190] In addition, median sternotomy has been, by some surgeons, the preferred approach for pulmonary metastasectomy in children.[37] This approach, while providing excellent exposure to

---

Box 23–4. Selection Criteria for Metastasectomy.[30,a]

- ✓ Local control of the primary tumor or ability to completely resect the primary with synchronous presentations
- ✓ Radiological findings consistent with metastatic disease
- ✓ Absence of extrathoracic metastases, that is, confined to the lung
- ✓ Ability to perform a complete resection of the metastases
- No significant comorbidity that would preclude surgery
- No alternative therapy that is superior to surgery

[a]Approximately one third of patients with metastatic disease will meet these criteria.

---

most of the chest, is limited for large posterior central lesions and left lower lobe lesions. Relative contraindications to median sternotomy include a history of radiation therapy, diabetes, obesity, chronic obstructive pulmonary disease (COPD), previous median sternotomy, and the use of steroids.[117] Under these conditions alternative approaches should be given consideration.

Lateral thoracotomy is commonly used for unilateral disease, but it precludes assessment of the contralateral lung. The morbidity associated with thoracotomy should also be considered in patients with marginal pulmonary status. Liberal use of epidural anesthesia should be considered for all thoracotomy patients for postoperative pain control. Modifications of standard thoracotomies, such as muscle-sparing incisions, are another option.[59,143] Bilateral staged thoracotomies, frequently 6 weeks apart, and a bilateral thoracosternotomy (clamshell incision) are alternatives for those patients with bilateral disease. The clamshell approach entails bilateral anterior thoracotomies with a transverse sternotomy and thus allows excellent access to both hemithoraces. A study of 90 patients at Memorial Sloan-Kettering Cancer Center noted no perioperative deaths or significant morbidity after clamshell thoracotomy.[8] A hemiclamshell incision, consisting of a unilateral anterior thoracotomy with a limited or complete median sternotomy, may also be used. Once thoracotomy is performed, thorough inspection and palpation of the pulmonary tissue are necessary to ensure that complete resection is possible and to exclude disseminated disease. Some surgeons have advocated marking each nodule during assessment.[192]

The next question is the following: Is VATS comparable to thoracotomy in the management of unilateral pulmonary metastases? Although VATS has a number of advantages and may be useful in the tissue diagnosis of lung nodules, its role for therapeutic metastatic resection is controversial.[195] VATS is generally limited to resection of lesions in the outer third of the lung and lesions smaller than 3 cm in size. One study claimed that intraoperative palpation of the lung often revealed additional nodules that eluded preoperative imaging studies. There is also concern that the VATS approach offers only a limited opportunity to palpate the lung.[114,160] It should be noted, however, that these studies were performed with earlier generation imaging devices. Other studies have shown that VATS is a reasonable approach in the management of pulmonary metastases, especially when less than three lesions are present; they are peripherally located, less than 3 cm in size; and a preoperative chest CT confirmed unilateral disease.[98,126,128] VATS results have been compared to thoracotomy results for colorectal metastases with similar 3-year survival rates.[197] More studies are needed to definitively decide whether VATS should be the procedure of choice for pulmonary metastasectomy. With enhanced imaging techniques, however, VATS may prove to be an equal or superior approach.

When a unilateral procedure is performed for the treatment of presumed unilateral pulmonary metastases, based on preoperative imaging, the question is whether this approach will miss undiagnosed contralateral disease and whether this would be detrimental to the patient. A few studies have tried to answer this question. One study looked at sternotomy versus unilateral thoracotomy in patients with metastases that appeared unilateral in preoperative imaging studies.[161] Utilizing the latter approach (unilateral thoracotomy) the contralateral lung was not assessed. One would expect there to be residual disease in the unevaluated thorax, thus resulting in a worse prognosis for this group. In fact, no such difference in long-term survival was found. Furthermore, repeat resection of recurrences has been shown to improve survival and, consequently, any missed subclinical disease could subsequently be resected.[161,164] These results have been corroborated by a more recent study by Younes et al.[208] In this study, patients undergoing unilateral thoracotomy for unilateral disease ($n = 179$) and patients undergoing bilateral thoracotomies for bilateral disease ($n = 88$) were investigated. The two groups of patients with confirmed bilateral metastases (synchronous or metachronous) were compared. Patients who experienced recurrence in the contralateral lung within 3, 6, or 12 months had an overall 5-year survival rate of 24, 30, and 37%, respectively. When patients with recurrence in the contralateral lung were compared to patients with bilateral metastases on admission, there was no significant difference in overall survival. The only two predictors of contralateral recurrence were histology and the number of pathologically proven metastases. The authors concluded that bilateral exploration of presumed unilateral lung metastases is not warranted in all cases.[208] In light of these studies, most thoracic surgeons feel comfortable treating unilateral disease, based on a good preoperative chest CT, without exploring the contralateral chest.

The metastasectomy itself most commonly consists of a wedge resection. This is facilitated by the tendency of metastatic disease to be found at the periphery of the lung and is easily performed utilizing lung clamps and a pulmonary stapling device. Excision with electrocautery or laser may also be performed under select circumstances.[3,19,88] The posterior areas of the lung may be better assessed from an anterior approach by filling the hemithorax with saline to allow the lung to float anteriorly. Alternatively, posterior packs may be used. Only rarely are metastases found in regional lymph nodes, thus formal nodal dissection is generally not indicated.[135] In distinction to primary lung cancer where lobectomy has been shown to improve survival in comparison to wedge resections, no such difference has been found with metastasectomy.[60] Resection with a 1–2 cm margin of uninvolved tissue has proven to be adequate in this setting. Lobectomy is indicated if a lesser procedure would result in an incomplete resection, or is not technically possible. This is most commonly the case with large centrally located lesions. Chest wall resection of contiguous lesions not associated with other disease, and even pneumonectomy, has been shown to improve survival when utilized in the appropriate setting.[70,89,176]

RESULTS OF PULMONARY METASTASECTOMY

Pulmonary metastasectomy in appropriately selected patients has been shown to improve survival. When all histologies are considered, the 5-year survival rates for patients undergoing resection of secondary pulmonary malignancy

are 25–35% (see Table 23-3). In an attempt to more clearly define those patients most likely to benefit from metastasectomy, many series have evaluated potential prognostic indicators. For example, short *tumor doubling time* is frequently a sign of an aggressive lesion. It has been proposed that patients with such tumors, therefore, might not derive a survival benefit from resection. Reports of such studies, however, are equivocal.[28,36,82,148] Moreover, the practical application of such a measurement is difficult. *Disease-free interval* has also been studied in an attempt to predict outcomes. Longer disease-free intervals, however, have not been consistently associated with a better prognosis.[14,119,148,149] An increased *number of nodules* seen on preoperative testing might intuitively be associated with a poor prognosis. In general, patients with multiple nodules do more poorly then those with a solitary nodule. Again, however, there is great variability.[137,138,148,149] The number of

Table 23–3

Five-Year Survival Rates of Various Histological Metastatic Resections

Histology	5-year survival without metastasectomy	5-year survival with metastasectomy
All histologies		25–40%[115,149]
Breast cancer	11%[177]	35–50%[54,93,118]
Colorectal cancer	<5%[144]	40–45%[116,152]
Germ cell tumors		68%[149]
Head and neck squamous cell carcinoma		29–60%[149]
Melanoma	3–4%[66,181]	21–36%[66,149,181,204]
Osteosarcoma	0–17%[32,91]	20–40%[13,41,122,149]
Renal cell carcinoma		13–54%[141]
Soft tissue sarcomas		20–40%[109,149]
Urinary tract cancer		25–43%[141]

nodules above which resection is unwarranted is also unclear. As many as 20–30 metastasectomies can be performed at one operation with good results.[108] In addition, the number of nodules estimated with preoperative testing is often inaccurate. As such, multiplicity may be more appropriately used to assist in the assessment of tumor resectability. None of these criteria for predicting positive outcome from metastasectomy has been universally established. Most studies have proposed that *complete resectability* is the only universal determinant of prognosis across all histologies (see Box 23-5).[138]

Many of the aforementioned studies attempting to evaluate prognostic determinants in pulmonary metastasectomy have been faulted for insufficient statistical power. One group, however, reported 5206 cases of pulmonary metastases from various sites from the 18 medical centers of the International Registry of Lung Metastases. In this retrospective review, three parameters were shown to have prognostic significance regardless of primary histology: resectability, a disease-free interval of over 36 months, and solitary versus multiple metastasis.[137] As a result, they have proposed a four-group staging system based on the number of poor prognostic indicators present in a given patient (see Table 23-4). Although staging systems such as this one may better define those patients most likely to benefit from metastasectomy, survival in patients following surgery, even with poor prognostic indicators, is superior to any other treatment. Consequently, some feel that metastasectomy should be offered to appropriate patients regardless of these factors, with the possible exception of inability to perform complete resection.[137]

In addition to the aforementioned factors equivocally associated with prognosis, other factors have been clearly shown not to affect outcome. These factors include unilateral versus bilateral disease, age, gender, and wedge resection versus formal lobectomy (see Box 23-6).

Recurrence is the most common cause of death following complete pulmonary resection of metastatic disease. Despite this, repeat resections have contributed to prolonged survival for a number of histologies.[149,157,159,164] The most studied of these is soft tissue sarcomas. In a study by the National Cancer Institute in which patients underwent reresection for soft tissue sarcomas, no difference in the actuarial 5-year survival was found in those undergoing one, two, and even three resections for recurrence.[157] Preoperative selection criteria similar to those utilized with the initial resection are important in appropriately choosing patients for repeat resection. This ensures the absence of disseminated disease and the ability of a given patient to tolerate the proposed procedure. Once screened, therefore,

resection of recurrent disease will be offered to the majority of patients (approximately 70%) should no extrathoracic dissemination be present and should the lesion be amenable to resection.

► METASTASES TO THE LUNG

Osteosarcoma

Like soft tissue sarcomas, osteosarcoma has a strong predilection for metastasis to the lung. In addition, the lesions themselves are frequently multiple and often recur despite resection. Consequently pulmonary involvement is responsible for the majority of deaths in patients with this disease. Approximately 10–20% of patients will have distant metastases on initial evaluation, and, as with other histologies, CT of the chest is the imaging modality of choice for detection.

Prior to the introduction of chemotherapy, the overall survival from osteogenic sarcoma was only 10–20%.[13,91] In the early 1970s, however, the use of chemotherapy, especially high-dose methotrexate, substantially improved outcomes.[158] Later, with the introduction of multimodality therapy, chemotherapy (doxorubicin, high-dose cyclophosphamide, and cisplatin) combined with resection, improved 5-year survival rates to 32–40%.[122,138,173] In some cases treatment resulted in cure. As a consequence of these improved results early in the history of metastasectomy,

Table 23–4

Prognostic Staging System[138]

Prognostic stage	Number of prognostic indicators[a]	5-year survival
I	None	61%
II	One	34%
III	Two	24%
IV	Unresectable	14%

[a]Resectability, disease-free interval over 36 months, and solitary versus multiple metastasis.

Box 23–5. Prognostic Factors in Metastasectomy.[137]

Absolute	Equivocal
Complete resectability	Tumor doubling time
	Disease-free survival
	Number of nodules
	Histology
	Nodal status

Box 23–6. Factors Not Affecting Prognosis in Metastasectomy.[135,148]

Age
Gender
Unilateral versus bilateral disease
Wedge resection versus formal lobectomy

346 a more aggressive approach toward resection of pulmonary metastases developed. Furthermore, simultaneous resection of the primary osteosarcoma and lung metastasectomy after neoadjuvant chemotherapy has been associated with improved outcomes.[7]

Despite the survival advantage imparted by surgical resection in osteogenic carcinoma, 50% of patients will have a recurrence within 1 year. Eventually, 85% of these patients relapse with recurrent pulmonary disease, this occurring despite lack of earlier evidence of gross secondary disease and adequate removal of the primary tumor. Resection of these recurrences is indicated as numerous studies have demonstrated improved survival.[5,84] If the patient is not a surgical candidate, radiotherapy maybe an option.[169] Brachytherapy has been used successfully in patients with metastatic endobronchial lesions.[123]

No prognostic factors, except for complete resection, have consistently been associated with improved survival following metastasectomy.[138] A number of studies have looked at the aforementioned characteristics (age, sex, location, doubling time, disease-free survival, number of nodules, resectability). Few consistent conclusions can be drawn.* Most studies do correlate a worse outcome with increased number of nodules.[16,137] In addition, every study concludes that complete surgical resection is associated with increased survival.[62,120,137,138] In addition, the location of the primary lesion has been associated with worse prognosis in the case of pelvic and vertebral tumors.[155]

Recently, Her-2/*neu* expression has also been associated with increased risk for pulmonary metastases.[209] These findings suggest that these patients may benefit from additional biological therapy. Finally, Phase I/II gene therapy trials using an adenovirus vector containing a murine osteocalcin promoter for the treatment of refractory osteosarcomas metastatic to the lung are in development.[17]

Soft Tissue Sarcoma

Soft tissue sarcomas are a group of nonossifying malignant neoplasms derived from mesenchymal connective tissue. Most soft tissue sarcomas metastasize within the first 2 years of diagnosis, with the lungs being the most common site (80–90% of the time).[145] Consequently, secondary pulmonary disease is the primary cause of death in these patients. The predilection for dissemination to the lungs also emphasizes the importance of pulmonary surveillance in following up sarcoma patients. One follow-up recommendation is to obtain a CXR every 1–2 months for the first year, then every 3–6 months thereafter with a CT of the chest should metastases be suspected. It is our practice to obtain routine surveillance CT scans, starting out every 3 months and gradually extending to once a year as a durable remission is demonstrated.

Unfortunately, the improved survival and response rates following chemotherapy in patients with osteosarcoma have not been paralleled in soft tissue sarcomas.[94] Of those with soft tissue sarcomas, however, 20% will have isolated disease and are candidates for resection. Unlike pulmonary metastases from melanoma and carcinoma that are commonly solitary, sarcomatous involvement of the lung tends

to be multiple. Five-year survival rates following resection of secondary pulmonary disease are 20–30%, a significant improvement over those patients who are not resected.[28,137,157,182]

As with osteosarcoma, a number of prognostic indicators have been studied in an attempt to select those patients with soft tissue sarcomas most likely to benefit from resection. With the exception of resectability, however, no consistent criteria arise.[174] Histologically, malignant fibrous histiocytomas do tend to have a better prognosis.[28] In addition, as with osteosarcoma, most studies demonstrate a decreased survival associated with an increased number of nodules.[148,159] A large retrospective study from Memorial Sloan-Kettering reviewed 3149 patients with soft tissue sarcomas. Of these patients, 719 developed pulmonary metastases, and 248 underwent at least one pulmonary resection. Three independent negative prognostic factors were identified: three or more lesions, largest metastases' diameter more than 2 cm, and high-grade primary tumor histology.[200] A much smaller study, including 23 patients, found similar prognostic factors associated with poor outcomes. These included three or more lesions and disease-free interval of less than 6 months.[15] Similar to osteogenic sarcoma, the majority of patients undergoing pulmonary resection do go on to develop recurrent disease. In these patients, reoperation is warranted if extrathoracic involvement is absent.[15,141,157,191]

Colorectal Carcinoma

The incidence of colorectal carcinoma in the United States is high, with approximately 100,000 new cases occurring each year. Approximately, 10–30% of these patients will go on to have metastases. Because of this high incidence of recurrence it is important to follow up these patients very closely. Routine physical examinations and radiographic imaging, as well as carcinoembryonic antigen (CEA) levels are useful. Higher levels of CEA are more likely to be seen when resulting from metastatic involvement (of the liver and/or lung) compared to locoregional recurrence and should prompt the physician to a metastatic workup.[150] The most common extraabdominal location of secondary disease is metastasis to the lung. Unfortunately, such pulmonary involvement is also frequently associated with disseminated disease, usually involving the liver. Ten percent of colorectal cancer patients with metastatic involvement of the lung, or 1–3% of those with colorectal cancer, will have isolated pulmonary disease.[116,166] These patients benefit from resection.[61,116] Five-year survival rates following resection of colorectal metastases to the lung are 20–40% and 10-year survival is 20%.[61,78,111,116]

The preoperative selection criteria for resection of colorectal metastases of the lung are similar to those previously mentioned. Because liver resections for metastatic colorectal carcinoma have resulted in 25–35% 5-year survival rates,[150] there is rationale to consider resection for a patient with synchronous involvement of the liver and the lung. In several series examining this issue, the 5-year survival rates following dual metastasectomy have been reported to range from 21 to 52%.[129,153,174] In addition, patients who develop a pulmonary recurrence after a hepatic resection for colorectal metastases appear to benefit from pulmonary metastasectomy.[92,207] Even in the face of the presence of

---

*References 16, 26, 62, 137, 138, 158, 173.

extrapulmonary metastases, as long as they are resectable, patients have increased survival when the pulmonary metastases are removed.[78]

Those colorectal cancer patients found to have a solitary pulmonary nodule on follow-up have an equal likelihood that their lesion will be a primary lung cancer as metastatic disease. For this reason, video-assisted thoracoscopy and tissue diagnosis by wedge resection may be indicated. Reoperation for recurrent metastatic disease is also warranted. As with other histologies, no consistent conclusions can be made regarding prognostic indicators in tailoring patient selection for resection.[61,116,129] The only positive prognostic factors that are consistent among four recent series of patients after pulmonary metastasectomy for colorectal metastases are complete resection and a normal CEA level prior to thoracotomy.[154,156,162,163]

Breast Carcinoma

Breast cancer accounts for 30,000 deaths each year and is currently the second most common cause of cancer deaths in females in the United States, behind lung cancer. Pulmonary involvement in breast cancer is most commonly associated with widespread disease, thereby contraindicating resection in the majority of patients. A thorough preoperative workup, specifically searching for extrapulmonary disease, is necessary in considering patients for pulmonary resection. When properly screened, up to 20% of patients will be found to have isolated pulmonary disease and may potentially benefit from metastasectomy.

Considering that a pulmonary nodule in a patient with known breast carcinoma is more likely to be primary lung cancer,[27] histological diagnosis is needed to proceed with appropriate management. A diagnosis of adenocarcinoma on biopsy obtained by FNA or wedge resection, however, requires the use of further assays (e.g., ER/PR receptor status and cytokeratin stains) to establish a diagnosis of breast cancer.[3,151]

Five-year survival rates after metastatic resection range from 35% to 62%.[54,93,118,172,177] Despite these results, high-dose multidrug chemotherapy and bone marrow rescue are the primary forms of treatment currently offered to patients with disseminated pulmonary involvement. Consequently, few patients are referred for complete resection. As is the case with nonseminomatous germ cell disease, surgery may also have a role in the evaluation of residual disease found after chemotherapy and thus help in assessing any component of active disease. Patients with ER-receptor-positive metastases and/or complete resection appear to have a more favorable prognosis.[54,93]

Germ Cell Tumors

Germ cell tumors account for only 1% of all cancers, but are the most common malignancy in males between 15 and 35 years of age. The vast majority of these tumors arise from the testicle. Approximately half of germ cell tumors are seminomas while the remainder are nonseminomatous (embryonal, teratocarcinoma, choriocarcinoma, and yolk sac tumors).[21] The majority (70%) of this latter group may be diagnosed by an elevation of human chorionic gonadotropin-β (hCG-β), α-fetoprotein (AFP), or both. The

most common site of distant metastasis for these tumors is the lung.[95]

Germ cell tumors are unusual in their response to chemotherapy, even in the context of disseminated disease.[9] Overall, greater then 90% of germ cell tumors will be cured with cisplatin-based chemotherapy and, therefore, the primary treatment is nonsurgical.[79] Of those patients with non-seminomatous germ cell tumors with pulmonary metastases, 70% will have normalization of tumor markers and radiographic clearance of disease, a complete response, following chemotherapy. Patients with residual radiographic evidence of pulmonary involvement, despite normal serum markers (AFP, hCG-β) after chemotherapy, are frequently referred for resection to determine if viable tumor exists in these partial responders and nonresponders.[9,20,79] Of those who do not respond to initial chemotherapy, 25% will respond to salvage forms of treatment.[103] In addition, patients with radiological evidence of disease and abnormal serum markers may also be candidates for surgical salvage if their disease is considered resectable.[125]

In performing resections, for residual disease, approximately 15–20% of specimens will contain viable germ cell tumor. Forty percent of such patients will have necrotic or fibrotic tissue. Another 40% will have undergone maturation of their malignancy into a mature (nonmalignant) teratoma.[25,107] Because no reliable method of preoperative diagnosis exists, and the potential for malignant and chemoresistant degeneration of benign teratomas may occur, resection of any residual disease is indicated.[1] Approximately 90% of those resections revealing fibrotic tissue or teratomas will be cured with resection alone. "Sterilized" lesions, i.e., those composed of fibrotic and necrotic tissue with no viable tumor cells, require no further therapy. Viable tumor in resected residual masses serves as an indication for salvage chemotherapy. In these patients 60–70% will be cured.[205]

Controversy exists surrounding the appropriate management of residual pulmonary masses found in seminoma patients following chemotherapy. Less then 25% of such residual disease will represent viable tumor and less than 5% will reveal teratoma. For this reason, and the morbidity associated with resection, expectant management is advocated by some.[52,104] However, a recent report of 15 patients who underwent resection for residual disease after cisplatin-based chemotherapy revealed complete response in only 37% of the patients after cisplatin treatment. After surgical resection of the residual disease, complete response was seen in 80% of the patients.[74] In addition, the size of the residual mass determines whether there is residual viable tumor since it has been reported that 27% of residual masses greater than 3 cm in diameter, compared to 3% of those less than 3 cm, contain viable seminomatous tumor.[147] For patients with larger masses, radiation therapy, as the only treatment or preceded by resection, may be indicated.[205]

Melanoma

Melanoma is responsible for 1–2% of cancer deaths. The lung is involved in secondary disease 15% of the time.[54,181] Although the lungs are one of the most common sites of distant spread, only 5% of patients with such involvement have

348 an absence of extrathoracic involvement. More commonly, lesions found on CXR are a manifestation of widespread disease at the time of diagnosis and such patients are traditionally treated with chemotherapy. A thorough search for dissemination is indicated in melanoma patients being considered for resection. Although melanoma does have the lowest 5-year survival rate following metastasectomy,[66,142] long-term survival benefits have been reported in many cases.[33,124,184,204] Thus, the surgeon may wish to apply more rigorous criteria in selecting patients with melanoma for pulmonary metastasectomy.[131]

In an effort to elucidate prognostic factors associated with improved survival after pulmonary metastasectomy for melanoma, Leo et al reviewed 328 patients identified in the international registry of lung metastases who underwent resection of melanotic pulmonary metastases.[96] Of these patients, 282 underwent complete resection. Independent unfavorable prognostic factors included multiple metastases and time to pulmonary metastases of less than 36 months. Patients without risk factors experienced the best survival (29% at 5 years), followed by those with one risk factor only (20% at 5 years). On the other hand, those with two risk factors or incomplete resection showed a significantly poorer survival (7 and 0% at 5 years).[96]

We have performed resections of metastatic melanoma, in patients who cannot be completely resected, to harvest tumor for a human vaccine protocol available at our institution. Preliminary results of this study are encouraging.[18] Only in very rare circumstances should an incomplete resection be planned outside of an experimental protocol.

Head and Neck Squamous Cell Carcinoma

Forty percent of patients with head and neck squamous cell carcinoma will go on to develop distant disease. In these patients the lung is the most commonly affected organ.[188] Some of the same risk factors that predispose patients to head and neck cancer also put patients at risk for primary cancer of the lung. As a result, a solitary nodule found in follow-up is more likely to be primary lung cancer. For this reason, these lesions should be treated as such until proven otherwise. Five-year survival rates following metastatic resection range from 29 to 60%.[50,102,198] Positive prognostic factors include single lesion, disease-free interval of more than 2 years, locoregional control, and complete resection.[50,102,200]

Urological Tumors

Of approximately 30,000 patients diagnosed with renal cell carcinoma each year, 60–70% will go on to develop metastases. The most common metastatic site is the lung.[106,141,189] Unresected, less than 5% of patients will survive 5 years. In contrast, after complete pulmonary metastasectomy 5-year survivals range between 37 and 54%.[55,139,140] Positive prognostic factors include complete resection, disease-free interval of more than 2 years, and fewer than seven lesions. In view of these results, and the fact that renal cell carcinomas are chemoresistant and radioresistant, surgical resection of pulmonary metastases is indicated for most cases.[55]

Of patients with transitional cell carcinoma 50% will also develop pulmonary metastases. Although reports in the literature are sparse, isolated disease, when completely resected, may result in 5-year survival rates of approximately 25%.[22]

Endocrine Tumors

Pulmonary metastases from these tumors are rare. Occasionally resection may be indicated to alleviate symptoms of hormone production.[51,80] A review of 25 patients who underwent pulmonary metastasectomy for different types of endocrine tumors showed a 61% 5-year survival. Independent predictors of poor survival included positive mediastinal lymph nodes, incomplete resection, and short disease-free interval.[86]

Gynecological Tumors

Uterine and cervical cancers have also been shown to respond to metastasectomy in appropriate candidates. A 24–52% 5-year survival following pulmonary metastasectomy has been reported.[4,167,171] For choriocarcinoma multidrug chemotherapy is the primary form of treatment. Resistant lesions should be considered for resection. Five-year survival rates approaching 50% have been reported.[81,206]

ALTERNATIVE FORMS OF THERAPY IN SECONDARY PULMONARY DISEASE

Isolated Lung Perfusion

Systemic toxicity of chemotherapeutic agents frequently limits the dose that would otherwise eradicate micrometastatic disease in the lung. Isolated regional lung perfusion therapy is a novel form of delivery that has shown some promise. This technique is analogous to isolated limb perfusion, a therapy used in the treatment of advanced sarcoma and melanoma.[45] With isolation of the circulation to a region, a 25-fold higher tissue concentration of chemotherapeutic agent may be achieved and, in general, less systemic toxicity will occur.[132,203,204] The nearly closed nature of the pulmonary circulation, with only 5% being perfused by the bronchial circulation, makes the lung an ideal organ for isolated perfusion. Isolated lung perfusion has been applied to a number of histological types including colorectal carcinomas, sarcomas, melanoma, and renal cell carcinoma.[132] Eight patients with unresectable pulmonary metastases from soft tissue sarcomas were enrolled in a Phase I trial that demonstrated that the technique was safe and feasible but none of the patients responded to the therapy.[23] All human studies involving isolated lung perfusion have, to date, provided some evidence that the technique is feasible and safe. Further studies are needed to assess its efficacy in terms of response.[23,45,71,132]

Radiofrequency Ablation

Radiofrequency ablation (RFA) delivers thermal energy through a catheter delivery system resulting in coagulation necrosis. It has been extensively used in hepatic tumors. Initial studies in rabbits demonstrated the feasibility of this technique in eradicating pulmonary tumors.[121] A recent study reported 18 patients with malignant pulmonary tumors treated with RFA.[72] The authors concluded that RFA is a viable option for small peripheral lesions. In the future, this technique may be used in the management of metastatic disease to the lungs. Further studies investigating the role of this technique are needed.

Palliative Therapy

Palliative therapy should be considered for symptomatic patients whose disseminated disease or unresectability precludes curative forms of therapy. Endobronchial lesions are frequently symptomatic. Commonly they are associated with unresectable disease and frequently require palliative therapy.[67,112,187] Those patients with endobronchial lesions who present with hemoptysis may respond well to a short course of external beam radiation.

Obstructive lesions may be treated bronchoscopically with mechanical debridement, laser ablation, brachytherapy, or stenting. Nd:YAG laser provides the best penetration, coagulation, and thermal necrosis and may be administered through a flexible fiberoptic system.

Photodynamic therapy (PDT) is a technique for killing cells that employs nontoxic compounds, photosensitizers, that tends to concentrate in tumor cells and can subsequently be activated with visible light. When the photosensitizer is exposed to the correct wavelength of light, it has the ability to transfer energy to oxygen. It is the excited species of oxygen that eventually cause cell death. PDT is thought to work by both direct tumor cell kill as well as destruction of the tumor's neovascularization. The advantage of PDT in this setting is that the palliation is generally more durable than with other bronchoscopic treatments, but the therapy also causes a transient cutaneous photosensitivity that some patients may feel is unacceptable. PDT is currently approved for obstructing as well as early stage endobronchial lesions and, in select cases, may be a good option.

Malignant effusions secondary to neoplastic disease may be voluminous and consequently symptomatic. When they occur, they may be treated by VATS or bedside drainage followed by talc pleurodesis. Internal shunting or external drainage of a pleural effusion is an option for a failed pleurodesis or, occasionally, as the primary palliative procedure. We are currently underway with a Phase II trial of VATS-delivered PDT for select cases of malignant effusions without evidence of extrapleural disease.

Pericardial effusions occurring in the setting of disseminated disease may become symptomatic. Percutaneous drainage, subxiphoid window, or VATS window procedures are the options for this condition.

▶ SUMMARY

Patients with pulmonary metastases were previously relegated to palliative medical management. Since the first metastasectomies in the nineteenth century general acceptance of this technique has occurred. Although initial indications for resection of pulmonary metastases were limited to patients with solitary nodules, over time indications have broadened to include multiple lesions, recurrent disease,

and nearly all histologies. With appropriate patient selection, and the absence of extrathoracic disease, complete resection is associated with an increase in patient survival for the majority of cancers.

REFERENCES

1. Ahmed T, Bosl GJ, Hajdu SI: Teratoma with malignant transformation in germ cell tumors in men. Cancer 56:860, 1985.
2. Alexander J, Haigh C: Pulmonary resection for solitary metastatic sarcomas and carcinomas. Surg Gynecol Obstet 85:129–146, 1947.
3. Alsabeh R, Wilson CS, Ahn CW, et al: Expression of bcl-2 by breast cancer: A possible diagnostic application. Mod Pathol 9, 439–444, 1996.
4. Anderson TM, McMahon JJ, Nwogu CE, et al: Pulmonary resection in metastatic uterine and cervical malignancies. Gynecol Oncol 83(3):472–476, 2001.
5. Antunes M, Bernardo J, Salete M, et al: Excision of pulmonary metastases of osteogenic sarcoma of the limbs. Eur J Cardio-Thorac Surg 15(5):592–596, 1999.
6. Attinger B, Jaggi F, Haag M, et al: The first successful lung resection. Schweiz Rundsch Med Prax 82:435–440, 1993.
7. Bacci G, Mercur M, Briccoli A, et al: Osteogenic sarcoma of the extremity with detectable lung metastases at presentation. Results of treatment of 23 patients with chemotherapy followed by simultaneous resection of primary and metastatic lesions. Cancer 79(2):245–254, 1997.
8. Bains MS, Ginsberg RJ, Jones WG II, et al: The clamshell incision: An improved approach to bilateral pulmonary and mediastinal tumors. Abstract. The Society of Thoracic Surgeons, 1994.
9. Bajorin D, Herr H, Motzer R, et al: Current perspectives on the role of adjunctive surgery in combined modality treatment for patients with germ cell tumors. Sem Oncol 19:148–158, 1992.
10. Balch C, Houghton AN, Peters LJ: In Devita VT, Hellman S, Rosenberg SA, editors: Cancer: Principles and Practice of Oncology. Philadelphia, J. B. Lippincott Co., 1993, pp. 1612–1661.
11. Barney JD, Churchill EJ: Adenocarcinoma of the kidney with metastasis to the lung: Cured by nephrectomy and lobectomy. J Urol 42:269, 1961.
12. Barney JD: Twelve-year cure following nephrectomy for adenocarcinoma and lobectomy for solitary metastasis. J Urol 52:406–407, 1944.
13. Beattie EJ Jr, Matini N, Rosen G: The management of pulmonary metastases in children with osteogenic sarcoma with surgical resection combined with chemotherapy. Cancer 35:618–621, 1975.
14. Beattie EJ, Harvey JC, Marcove R, Martini N: Results of multiple pulmonary resections for metastatic osteogenic sarcoma after two decades. J Surg Oncol 46:154–155, 1991.
15. Belal A, Salah, Haijar W, et al: Pulmonary metastatectomy for soft tissue sarcomas: Is it valuable? J Cardiovasc Surg 42(6):835–840, 2001.
16. Belli L, Scholl S, Livartowski A, et al: Resection of pulmonary metastases in osteosarcoma. A retrospective analysis of 44 patients. Cancer 63:2546–2550, 1989.
17. Benjamin R, Helman, Meyers P, et al: A phase I/II dose escalation and activity study of intravenous injections of OCaP1 for subjects with refractory osteosarcoma metastatic to lung. Human Gene Ther 12(12):1591–1593, 2001.
18. Berd D, Sato T, Cohn H, et al: Treatment of metastatic melanoma with autologous, hapten-modified melanoma

350

vaccine: Regression of pulmonary metastases. Int J Cancer. 94(4):531–539, 2001.

19. Branscheid D, Krysa S, Wollkopf G, et al: Does Nd-YAG laser extend the indications for resection of pulmonary metastases? Eur J Cardiothorac Surg 6:590–597, 1992.

20. Brenner PC, Herr HW, Morse MJ, et al: Simultaneous retroperitoneal, thoracic, and cervical resection of post-chemotherapy residual masses in patients with metastatic nonseminomatous germ cell tumors of the testis. J Clin Oncol 14:1765, 1996.

21. Brown LM, Pottern LM, Hoover RN, et al: Testicular cancer in US. Trends in incidence and mortality. Int J Epidemiol 15: 164, 1986.

22. Burt M: In Fishman AP, editor: Pulmonary Disease. Philadelphia: J. B. Lippincott Co., 1998, pp. 1851–1860.

23. Burt ME, Liu D, Abolhoda A, et al: Isolated lung perfusion for patients with unresectable metastases from sarcoma: A phase I trial. Ann Thorac Surg 69(5):1542–1549, 2000.

24. Cahan W, Castro E, et al: Benign solitary lesions in patients with cancer. Ann Surg 187:241–249, 1978.

25. Carsky S, Ondrus D, Schnorrer M, et al: Germ cell testicular tumours with lung metastases: Chemotherapy and surgical treatment. Int Urol Nephrol 24:305, 1992.

26. Carter SR, Grimer RJ, Sneath RS, et al: Results of thoracotomy in osteogenic sarcoma with pulmonary metastases. Thorax 46:727–731, 1991.

27. Casey JJ, Stempel BG, Scanlon EF, Fry WA: The solitary pulmonary nodule in the patient with breast cancer. Surgery 96: 801–805, 1984.

28. Casson AG, Putnam JB, Natarajan G, et al: Five-year survival after pulmonary metastasectomy for soft tissue sarcoma. Cancer 69:662–668, 1992.

29. Cerfolio RJ, Allen MS, Deschamps C, et al: Pulmonary resection of metastatic renal cell carcinoma. Ann Thorac Surg 57:339–344, 1994.

30. Chen PW, Pass HI: Indication for resection of pulmonary metastases. In Baue AE, Geha AS, Laks H, et al editors: Glenn's Thoracic and Cardiovascular Surgery. Stamford, CT: Appleton & Lange, 1996, pp. 499–510.

31. Cohen AL, Minsky BD, Schilsky RL: In DeVita V T, Hellman S, Rosenberg SA, editors: Cancer: Principles and Practice of Oncology. Philadelphia: J. B. Lippincott Co., 1993, pp. 929–977.

32. Coley BL: Neoplasms of Bone and Related Conditions: Etiology, Pathogenesis, Diagnosis and Treatment. New York: Hoeber, 1960.

33. Creech O: Metastatic melanoma of the lung treated by pulmonary resection: A report of a case. Med Rec Ann 45:4426–4427, 1951.

34. Crosby JH, Kager B, Hoeg K: Transthoracic fine needle aspiration. Cancer 56:2504–2507, 1985.

35. Crow J, Slavin G, Kreel L: Pulmonary metastasis: A pathologic and radiologic study. Cancer 47:2595–2601, 1981.

36. D'Amico TA, Sabiston DC: Surgical management of pulmonary metastases. In Sabiston DC, Spencer FC, editors: Surgery of the Chest. Philadelphia: W. B. Saunders Co., 1995, pp. 669–675.

37. De Oliveira-Filho AG, Neto LS, Epelman S: Median sternotomy for the resection of bilateral pulmonary metastases in children. Pediatr Surg Int 13(8):560–563, 1998.

38. DeCamp MM Jr, Jaklitsch MT, Mentzer SJ, et al: The safety and versatility of video-thoracoscopy: A prospective analysis of 895 consecutive cases. J Am Coll Surg 181:165–167, 1995.

39. Diaz G, Jimenez D, Dominguez-Reboiras S, et al: Yield of bronchoscopy in the diagnosis of neoplasm metastatic to lung. Respir Med 97(1):27–29, 2003.

40. Diederich S, et al: Helical CT of pulmonary nodules in patients with extrathoracic malignancy: CT-surgical correlation. Am J Radiol 172:353–360, 1999.

41. Di Lorenzo M, Collin PP: Pulmonary metastases in children: Results of surgical treatment. J Pediatr Surg 23: 762–765, 1988.

42. Divis G: Ein Beitrag Zur Operativen Behandlung der Lungeschwulste. Acta Chir Scand 62:329–341, 1927.

43. Dose J, Bleckmann C, Bachmann S, et al: Comparison of fluorodeoxyglucose positron emission tomography and "conventional diagnostic procedures" for the detection of distant metastases in breast cancer patients. Nucl Med Commun 23(9):857–864, 2002.

44. Edwards AT: Malignant disease of the lung. J Thorac Surg 4, 107–124, 1934.

45. Eggermont AM, Schraffordt J, Koops H, et al: Isolated limb perfusion with tumor necrosis factor and melphalan for limb salvage in 186 patients with locally advanced soft tissue extremity sarcomas. The cumulative multicenter European experience. Ann Surg 224:756–764, 1996.

46. Emad A, Rezaian GR: Closed percutaneous pleural brushing: A new method for diagnosis of malignant pleural effusions. Respir Med 92:659–663, 1998.

47. Farrell JJ: Pulmonary metastasis: A pathologic, clinical, roentgenologic study based on 78 cases seen at necropsy. Radiology 24:444, 1935.

48. Feuerstein IM, Jicha DL, Pass HI, et al: Pulmonary metastases: MRI imaging with surgical correlation—A prospective study. Radiology 182:123–129, 1992.

49. Fidler IJ: Molecular biology of cancer: Invasion and metastasis. In De Vita V, Hellman S, Rosenberg SA, editors: Principles and Practice of Oncology. Philadelphia: J. B. Lippincott Co., 1997, pp. 135–152.

50. Finley RK 3rd, Verazin GT, Driscoll DL, et al: Results of surgical resection of pulmonary metastases of squamous cell carcinoma of the head and neck. Am J Surg 164(6):594–598, 1992.

51. Flye MW, Brennan MR: Surgical resection of metastatic parathyroid carcinoma. Ann Surg 193:425–435, 1981.

52. Fossa SD, Borge L, Gass N, et al: The treatment of advanced metastatic seminoma: Experience in 55 cases. J Clin Oncol 5:1071, 1987.

53. Franzius Z, Daldrup-Link HE, Sciuk J, et al: FDG-PET for detection of pulmonary metastases from malignant primary bone tumors: Comparison with spiral CT. Ann Oncol 12(4): 479–486, 2001.

54. Friedel G, Linder A, Toomes, H: The significance of prognostic factors for the resection of pulmonary metastases of breast cancer. Thorac Cardiovasc Surg 42:71–75, 1994.

55. Friedel G, Hurtgen M, Penzenstadler M, et al: Resection of pulmonary metastases from renal cell carcinoma. Anticancer Res 19(2C):1593–1596, 1999.

56. Gadd M, Casper E, Woodruff J, et al: Development and treatment of pulmonary metastases in adult patients with extremity soft tissue sarcoma. Ann Surg 218:705–712, 1993.

57. Gerulanos ML: Eine Studie uber den operativen Pneumothorax im Anschluss an einem Fall von Lungenrecsectino wegen Brustwandsarcom. Deutsche Ztschr Chir 49:497–536, 1898.

58. Gilbert HA, Kagan AR: In Weiss L, editor: Fundamental Aspects of Metastasis. Amsterdam: North Holland Publishing Co. Inc., 1976, p. 315.

59. Ginsberg RJ: Alternative (muscle-sparing) incisions in thoracic surgery. Ann Thorac Surg 56:752–754, 1993.

60. Ginsberg RJ, Rubinstein LV: Randomized trial of lobectomy versus limited resection for T1N0 non-small cell lung cancer. Ann Thorac 60:615–622, 1995.

61. Girard P, Ducreux M, Baldeyrou P, et al: Surgery for lung metastases from colorectal cancer: Analysis of prognostic factors. J Clin Oncol 14:2047–2053, 1996.

62. Goorin AM, Delorey MJ, Lack EE, et al: Prognostic significance of complete surgical resection of pulmonary metastases

in patients with osteogenic sarcoma: Analysis of 32 patients. J Clin Oncol 2:425–431, 1984.

63. Graeber GM, Tamim W: Current status of the diagnosis and treatment of thymoma. Sem Thorac Cardiovasc Surg 12(4): 268–1277, 2000.

64. Greelish JP, Friedberg JS: Secondary pulmonary malignancy. Surg Clin North Am 80:633–657, 2000.

65. Gross BH, Glazer GM, Brookstein FL: Multiple pulmonary nodules detected by computed tomograph, diagnostic implications. J Comput Assist Tomogr 9:880–885, 1985.

66. Harpole DH, Johnson CM, Wolfe WG, et al: Analysis of 945 cases of pulmonary metastatic melanoma. J Thorac Cardiovasc Surg 103:743–750, 1995.

67. Harvey JC, Lee K, Beattie, EJ: Surgical management of pulmonary metastases. Chest Surg Clin North Am 4:55–66, 1994.

68. Hawkins RA, Hon C, Choi Y, et al: The role of positron emission tomography in oncology and other whole-body applications. Sem Nucl Med 4:268–284, 1992.

69. Hendin AS: Gestational trophoblastic tumors metastatic to the lung. Cancer 53:58–61, 1984.

70. Hendriks JM, van Putte B, Romijn S: Pneumonectomy for lung metastases: Report of ten cases. Thorac Cardiovasc Surg 51(1):38–41, 2003.

71. Hendriks JM, et al: Isolated lung perfusion with melphalan and tumor necrosis factor for metastatic pulmonary adenocarcinoma. Ann Thorac Surg 66:1719–1725, 1998.

72. Herrera LJ, Fernando HC, Perry Y, et al: Radiofrequency ablation of pulmonary malignant tumors in nonsurgical candidates. J Thorac Cardiovasc Surg 125(4):929–937, 2003.

73. Hoover HC Jr, Ketcham AS: Metastasis of metastases. Am J Surg 130(4):405–411, 1975.

74. Horvath LG, McCaughan BC, Stockle M, Boyer MJ: Resection of residual pulmonary masses after chemotherapy in patients with metastatic non-seminomatous germ cell tumours. Int Med J 32(3):79–83, 2002.

75. Hung GU, Shiau YC, Tsai SC, et al: Value of 18F-fluoro-2-deoxyglucose positron emission tomography in the evaluation of recurrent colorectal cancer. Anticancer Res 21(2B): 1375–1378, 2001.

76. Ichinose Y, Hara N, Ohta M, et al: DNA ploidy patterns of tumors diagnosed as metachronous or recurrent lung cancers. Ann Thorac Surg 52(3):469–473, 1991.

77. Ichinose Y, Hara N, Ohta M: Synchronous lung cancers defined by deoxyribonucleic acid flow cytometry. J Thorac Cardiovasc Surg 102(3):418–424, 1991.

78. Irshad K, Ahmad F, Morin JE, et al: Pulmonary metastases from colorectal cancer: 25 years of experience. Can J Surg 44(3):217–221, 2001.

79. Israel A, Bosl G, Golbey R, et al: the results of chemotherapy for extragonadal germ-cell tumors in the cisplatin era: The Memorial Sloan-Kettering Cancer Center experience (1975–1982). J Clin Oncol 3:1073–1079, 1985.

80. Jensen JC, Pass HI, Sindelar WF, et al: Recurrent or metastatic disease in select patients with adrenocortical carcinoma. Arch Surg 126:457–461, 1991.

81. Jones WB, Romain K, Erlandson RA, et al: Thoracotomy in the management of gestational choriocarcinoma. A clinicopathologic study. Cancer 72(7):2175–2181, 1993.

82. Joseph WL, Morton DL, Adkins PC: Prognostic significance of tumor doubling time in evaluating operability in pulmonary metastatic disease. J Thorac Cardiovasc Surg 61: 23–32, 1971.

83. Kandioler D, Dekan G, End A, et al: Molecular genetic differentiation between primary lung cancers and lung metastases of other tumors. J thorac Cardiovasc Surg 111:827–831, 1996.

84. Kandioler D, Kromer E, Tuchler H, et al: Long-term results after repeated surgical removal of pulmonary metastases. Ann Thorac Surg 65(4):909–912, 1998.

85. Khahn A, et al: Solitary pulmonary nodules: Comparison of classification with standard, thin-section, and reference phantom CT. Radiology 179:477–481, 1991.

86. Khan JH, McElhinney DB, Rahman SB, et al: Pulmonary metastases of endocrine origin: The role of surgery. Chest 114(2):526–534, 1998.

87. Kluge R, Schmidt F, Caca K, et al: Positron emission tomography with [(18)F]fluoro-2-deoxy-D-glucose for diagnosis and staging of bile duct cancer. Hepatology 33(5):1029–1035, 2001.

88. Kodama K, Doi O, Higashiyama M, et al: Surgical management of lung metastases. Usefulness of resection with the neodymium:yttrium-aluminum-garnet laser with median sternotomy. J Thorac Cardiovasc Surg 101:901–908, 1991.

89. Koong HN, Pastorino U, Ginsberg RJ: Is there a role for pneumonectomy in pulmonary metastases? International registry of lung metastases. Ann Thorac Surg 68(6): 2039–2043, 1999.

90. Kronlein RU: Ueber Lungenchirurgie. Berl Klin Wchnschr 21:129–132, 1884.

91. La Quaglia MP: Osteosarcoma: Specific tumor management and results. Chest Surg Clin North Am 8:77–95, 1998.

92. Labow DM, Buell JE, Yoshida A, et al: Isolated pulmonary recurrence after resection of colorectal hepatic metastases—is resection indicated? Cancer J 8(4):342–347, 2002.

93. Lanza LA, Natarajan G, Roth JA, et al: Long-term survival after resection of pulmonary metastases from carcinoma of the breast. Ann Thorac Surg 54:244–248, 1992.

94. Lanza LA, Putnam JB, Benjamin RS, et al: Response to chemotherapy does not predict survival after resection of sarcomatous pulmonary metastases. Ann Thorac Surg 51:219–224, 1991.

95. Lee M, Hendrickson FR: Analysis of pattern of recurrence in nonseminomatous testicular tumor. Radiology 127:775, 1978.

96. Leo F, Cagini L, Rocmans P, et al: Lung metastases from melanoma: When is surgical treatment warranted?. Br J Cancer 83(5):569–572, 2000.

97. Libshitz HI, North LB: Pulmonary metastases. Radiol Clin North Am 20:437, 1982.

98. Lin JC, Wiechmann RJ, Szwerc MF: Diagnostic and therapeutic video-assisted thoracic surgery resection of pulmonary metastases. Surgery 126(4):636–642, 1999.

99. Linehan WM, Shipley WU, Parkinson DR: Cancer of Kidneys and ureter. In DeVita VT, Hellman S, Rosenberg SA, editors: Cancer: Principles and Practice of Oncology. Philadelphia: J. B. Lippincott Co., 1993, pp. 1023–1051.

100. Liotta LA: Cancer metastasis and angiogenesis: An imbalance of positive and negative regulation. Cell 64:327–336, 1991.

101. Liotta LA, et al: The significance of hematogenous tumor cell clumps in the metastatic process. Cancer Res 36:889–894, 1976.

102. Liu D, Labow DM, Dang N, et al: Pulmonary metastasectomy for head and neck cancers. Ann Surg Oncol 6(6): 572–578, 1999.

103. Loehrer PJ, Lauer R, Roth BJ, et al: Salvage therapy in recurrent germ cell cancer: Ifosfamide and cisplatin plus either vinblastine or etoposide. Ann Intern Med 109:540, 1988.

104. Loehrer PJS, Birch R, Williams SD, et al: Chemotherapy of metastatic seminoma: The Southeastern Cancer Study Group experience. J Clin Oncol 5:1212, 1987.

105. Mack MJ, Hazelrigg SR, Landreneau RJ, Acuff TE: Thoracoscopy for the diagnosis of the indeterminate solitary pulmonary nodule. Ann Thorac Surg 56:830–832, 1993.

106. Maldazys JD, deKernion JB: Prognostic factors in metastatic renal carcinoma. J Urol 136:376–379, 1986.

107. Mandelgaum I, Yaw P, Einhorn L, et al: The importance of one-stage median sternotomy and retroperitoneal node dissection in disseminated testicular cancer. Ann Thorac Surg 5:524, 1983.

352

108. Martini N, McCormack PM: Evolution of the surgical management of pulmonary metastases. Chest Surg Clin North Am 8:13–27, 1998.

109. Martini N, McCormack PM, Bains MS, et al: Surgery for solitary and multiple pulmonary metastases. NY State J Med 78: 1711–1713, 1978.

110. Matsuzoe D, Hideshima T, Ohshima K, et al: Discrimination of double primary lung cancer from intrapulmonary metastasis by p53 gene mutation. 79(9–10):1549–1552, 1999.

111. McAfee MK, et al: Colorectal lung metastases: Results of surgical excision. Ann Thorac Surg 53:780–785; discussion 785–786, 1992.

112. McCormack PM, Ginsberg RJ: Current management of colorectal metastases to lung. Chest Surg Clin North Am 8: 119–126, 1998.

113. McCormack PM: Surgical resection of pulmonary metastases. Semi Surg Oncol 6:297, 1990.

114. McCormack P, Bains MS, Begg CB, et al: Role of video-assisted thoracic surgery in the treatment of pulmonary metastases: Results of a prospective trial. Ann Thorac Surg 62:213–217, 1996.

115. McCormack PM, Bains MS, Beatti JR, et al: Pulmonary resection for metastatic disease. Chest 73:163–166, 1978.

116. McCormack PM, Burt ME, Bains MS, et al: Lung resection for colorectal metastases. 10 years results. Arch Surg 127: 1403–1406, 1992.

117. McDonald WS, Brame M, Sharp C, Eggerstedt J: Risk factors for median sternotomy dehiscence in cardiac surgery. S Med J 82:1361–1364, 1989.

118. McDonald ML, Deschamps C, Ilstrup DM, et al: Pulmonary resection for metastatic breast cancer. Ann Thorac Surg 58: 1599–1602, 1994.

119. Meyer WH, Schell MJ, Kumar AP, et al: Thoracotomy for pulmonary metastatic osteosarcoma. An analysis of prognostic indicators of survival. Cancer 59:374–379, 1987.

120. Meyers PA, Heller G, Healey JH, et al: Osteogenic sarcoma with clinically detectable metastasis at initial presentation. J Clin Oncol 11:449–453, 1993.

121. Miao Y, Ni Y, Bosmans H, et al: Radiofrequency ablation for eradication of renal tumor in a rabbit model by using a cooled-tip electrode technique. Ann Surg Oncol 8(8): 651–657, 2001.

122. Mitruka S, et al: Diagnosing the indeterminate pulmonary nodule: Percutaneous biopsy versus thoracoscopy. Surgery 118:676–684, 1995.

123. Mogulkoc N, Goker E, Atasever A, et al: Endobronchial metastasis from osteosarcoma of bone: Treatment with intraluminal radiotherapy. Chest 116(6):1811–1814, 1999.

124. Morton DL, Joseph WL, Ketcham AS, et al: Surgical resection and adjunctive immunotherapy for selected patients with multiple pulmonary metastases. Ann Surg 178:361–366, 1973.

125. Murphy BR, Breeden ES, Donohue JP, et al: Surgical salvage of chemorefractory germ cell tumors. J Clin Oncol 11:324, 1993.

126. Mutsaerts EL, Zoetmulder FA, Meijer S: Outcome of thoracoscopic pulmonary metastasectomy evaluated by confirmatory thoracotomy. Ann Thorac Surg 72(1):230–233, 2001.

127. Naef AP: The Story of Thoracic Surgery: Milestones and Pioneers. Toronto: Hogrefe and Huber, 1990.

128. Nakajima J, Takamoto S, Tanaka M, et al: Thoracoscopic surgery and conventional open thoracotomy in metastatic lung cancer. Surg Endosc 15(8):849–853, 2001.

129. Okimura S, Kondo H, Tsubai M, et al: Pulmonary resection for metastatic colorectal cancer: Experience with 159 patients. J Thorac Cardiovasc Surg 112:867–874, 1996.

130. Olak J, Ferguson MK: Surgical management of second primary and metastatic lung cancer. In Pass HI, Mitchell JB, Johnson DH, et al, editors: Lung Cancer Principles and Practice. Philadelphia: J. B. Lippincott Co., 2000, pp. 730–741.

131. Ollila DW, Morton DL: Surgical resection as the treatment of choice for melanoma metastatic to the lung. Chest Surg Clin North Am 8:183–196, 1998.

132. Pass HI, Mew DJ, Kranda KC: Isolated lung perfusion with tumor necrosis factor for pulmonary metastases. Ann Thorac Surg 61:1609–1617, 1996.

133. Pass HI: Treatment of metastatic lung cancer. In De Vita V, Hellman S, Rosenberg SA, editors: Principles and Practice of Oncology. Philadelphia: J. B. Lippincott, Co. 1993, pp. 2186–2200.

134. Pass HI, Temeck BA: Biology of metastatic disease. Chest Surg Clin North Am 8:1–11, 1998.

135. Pass HI, Donington JS: Metastatic cancer of the lung. In De Vita V, Hellman S, Rosenberg SA, editors: Principles and Practice of Oncology. Philadelphia: J.B. Lippincott, 1997, pp. 2536–2551.

136. Pass HI, Dwyer, A, Makuch R et al: Detection of pulmonary metastases in patients with osteogenic and soft-tissue sarcomas: The superiority of CT scan compared to conventional linear tomograms using dynamic analysis. J Clin Oncol 3: 1261–1265, 1985.

137. Pastorino U, Buyse M, Friedel G, et al: Long-term results of lung metastasectomy: Prognostic analyses based on 5206 cases. J Thorac Cardiovasc Surg 113:37–49, 1997.

138. Pastorino U, McCormack PM, Ginsberg RJ: A new staging proposal for pulmonary metastases: The results of analysis of 5206 cases of resected pulmonary metastases. Chest Surg Clin North Am 8:197–202, 1998.

139. Pfannschmidt J, Hoffmann H, Muley T, et al: Prognostic factors for survival after pulmonary resection of metastatic renal cell carcinoma. Ann Thorac Surg 74(5):1653–1657, 2002.

140. Piltz S, Meimarakis G, Wichmann MW, et al: Long-term results after pulmonary resection of renal cell carcinoma metastases. Ann Thorac Surg 73(4):1082–1087, 2002.

141. Pogrebniak HW, Haas G, Linehan M, et al: Renal cell carcinoma: Resection of solitary and multiple metastases. Ann Thorac Surg 54:33–38, 1992.

142. Pogrebniak H, Stovroff M, Roth J, Pass H: Resection of pulmonary metastases form malignant melanoma: Results of a 16-year experience. Ann Surg 52:197–203, 1988.

143. Poon MA, O'Connel MJ, Moertel CG, et al: Biochemical modulation of fluorouracil: Evidence of significant improvement of survival and quality of life in patients with advanced colorectal carcinoma. J Clin Oncol 7:1407–1414, 1989.

144. Ponn RB, Ferneini A, D'Agostino RS, et al: Comparison of late pulmonary function after posterolateral and muscle-sparing thoracotomy. Ann Thorac Surg 53:675–679, 1992.

145. Potter DA, Glenn J, Kinsella T, et al: Patterns of recurrence in patients with high-grade soft-tissue sarcomas. J Clin Oncol 3:353–366, 1985.

146. Prakash UB, Reiman HM: Comparison of needle biopsy with cytologic analysis for the evaluation of pleural effusion: Analysis of 414 cases. Mayo Clinic Proc 60:158–164, 1985.

147. Puc H, Hellan R, Mazumdar M, et al: Management of residual mass in advanced seminoma: Results and recommendations from the Memorial Sloan-Kettering Cancer Center. J Clin Oncol 14:454, 1996.

148. Putnam JB Jr, Roth JA, Wesley MN, et al: Analysis of prognostic factors in patients undergoing resection of pulmonary metastases from soft tissue sarcomas. J Thorac Cardiovasc Surg 87:260–267, 1984.

149. Putnam JB Jr, Roth JA, Wesley MN, et al: Survival following aggressive resection of pulmonary metastases from osteogenic sarcoma: Analysis of prognostic factors. Ann Thorac Surg 36:516–523, 1983.

150. Quentmeier A, Archlag P, Herfarth C: Key role of the CEA test in the diagnosis and surgical therapy of recurrent colorectal cancer. Chirug 57:83–87, 1986.

151. Raab SS, Berg LC, Swanson PE, et al: Adenocarcinoma in the lung in patients with breast cancer: A prospective analysis of the discriminatory value of immunohistology. Am J Clin Pathol 100:27–35, 1993.

152. Regnard JF, Grunenwald D, Spaggiari L, et al: Surgical treatment of hepatic and pulmonary metastases from colorectal cancers. Ann Thorac Surg 66:214–219, 1998.

153. Regnard JF, Nicolosi M, Coggia M, et al: Results of surgical treatment of lung metastases from colorectal cancer. Gastroenterol Clin Biol 19:378–384, 1995.

154. Rena O, Casadio C, Viano F, et al: Pulmonary resection for metastases from colorectal cancer: Factors influencing prognosis. Twenty-year experience. Eur J Cardio-Thorac Surg 21(5):906–912, 2002.

155. Renard AJ, Veth RP, Schreuder HW, et al: Osteosarcoma: Oncologic and functional results. A single institutional report covering 22 years. J Surg Oncol 72(3):124–129, 1999.

156. Rizk NP, Downey RJ: Resection of pulmonary metastases from colorectal cancer. Sem Thorac Cardiovasc Surg 14(1):29–34, 2002.

157. Rizzoni WE, Pass HI, Wesley MN, et al: Resection of recurrent pulmonary metastases in patients with soft-tissue sarcomas. Arch Surg 121:1248–1252, 1986.

158. Rosen G, Suwansirikul S, Kwon C, et al: High-dose methotrexate with citrovorum factor rescue and adreamycin in childhood osteogenic sarcoma. Cancer 33:1151–1163, 1974.

159. Roth JA, Pass HI, Wesley MN, et al: Differing determinants of prognosis following resection of pulmonary metastases from osteogenic and soft tissue sarcoma patients. Cancer 1361–1366, 1985.

160. Roth J, Pass H, Wesley M, et al: Comparison of median sternotomy and thoracotomy for resection of pulmonary metastases in patients with adult soft tissue sarcoma. Ann Thorac Surg 42:134–138, 1986.

161. Roth JA: Resection of pulmonary metastases. In Roth, J, Ruckdeschel J, Weiseberger T, editors: Thoracic Oncology. Philadelphia: W.B. Saunders Co., 1989, pp. 619–630.

162. Saito Y, Omiya H, Kohno K, et al: Pulmonary metastasectomy for 165 patients with colorectal carcinoma: A prognostic assessment. J Thorac Cardiovasc Surg 124(5):1007–1013, 2002.

163. Sakamoto T, Tsubota N, Iwanaga K, et al: Pulmonary resection for metastases from colorectal cancer. Chest 119(4):1069–1072, 2001.

164. Saltzman DA, Snyder CL, Ferrell KL, et al: Aggressive metastasectomy for pulmonic sarcomatous metastases: A follow-up study. Am J Surg 17:543–547, 1993.

165. Schaner EG, Chang E, Doppman JL, et al: Comparison of computed and conventional whole lung tomography in detecting pulmonary nodules: A prospective radiologic pathologic stugy. Am J Roentgenol 131:51–54, 1978.

166. Schulten MF, Heiskell CA, Shields TW: The incidence of solitary pulmonary metastasis from carcinoma of the large intestine. Surg Gynecol Obstet 143:727–729, 1976.

167. Seki M, et al: Surgical treatment of pulmonary metastases from uterine cervical cancer. Operation method by lung tumor size. J Thorac Cardiovasc Surg 104:876–881, 1992.

168. Shapshay SM, Strom MS: Tracheobronchial obstruction form metastatic distant malignancies. Ann Otol Rhinol Laryngol 91:648–651, 1982.

169. Shibamoto Y, Horii N, Takahashi M: Long-term control of multiple lung metastases from osteosarcoma obtained by conventional radiotherapy: A case report. Oncol Rep 6(5):1085–1087, 1999.

170. Shimizu S, Yatabe Y, Koshikawa T, et al: High frequency of clonally related tumors in cases of multiple synchronous lung cancers as revealed by molecular diagnosis. Clin Cancer Res 6(10):3994–3999, 2000.

171. Shiromizu K, Kasamatsu T, Takahashi M, et al: A clinicopathological study of postoperative pulmonary metastasis of uterine cervical carcinomas. J Obstet Gynaecol Res 25(4):245–249, 1999.

172. Simpson R, Kennedy C, Carmalt H, et al: Pulmonary resection for metastatic breast cancer. Austr New Zeal J Surg 67(10):717–719, 1997.

173. Skinner K, Eilber F, Holmes E, et al: Surgical treatment and chemotherapy for pulmonary metastases from osteosarcoma. Arch Surg 127:1065–1071, 1992.

174. Smith JW, Fortner JG, Burt ME: Resection of hepatic and pulmonary metastases from colorectal cancer. Surg Oncol 1:399–404, 1992.

175. Snyder BJ, Pugatch RD: Imaging characteristicc of metastatic disease to the chest. Chest Surg Clin North Am 8(1):29–48, 1998.

176. Spaggiari L, Grunenwald DH, Girard P, et al: Pneumonectomy for lung metastases: Indications, risks, and outcome. Ann Thorac Surg 66(6):1930–1933, 1998.

177. Staren ED, Salerno C, Rongione A, et al: Pulmonary resection for metastatic breast cancer. Arch Surg 127:1282–1284, 1992.

178. Steele JD: The solitary pulmonary nodule. J Thorac Cardiovasc Surg 46:21–36, 1963.

179. Sterman DH, Sztejman E, Rodriguez E, Friedberg J: Diagnosis and staging of "other bronchial tumors." Chest Surg Clin North Am 13(1):79–94, 2003.

180. Strauss LG, Conti PS: The applications of PET in clinical oncology. J Nucl Med 32:633–648, 1991.

181. Tafra L, Dale PS, Wanek LA, et al: Resection and adjuvant immunotherapy for melanoma metastatic to the lung and thorax. J Thorac Cardiovasc Surg 110:119–124, 1995.

182. Temple LK, Brennan MF: The role of pulmonary metastasectomy in soft tissue sarcoma. Sem Thorac Cardiovasc Surg 14(1):35–44, 2002.

183. Templeton PA, Zerhouni EA: High-resolution computed tomography of focal lung disease. Sem Roentgenol XXVI:143–150, 1991.

184. Todd TR: Pulmonary metastectomy. Current indication for removing lung metastases. Chest 103:401S, 1993.

185. Toomes H, Delphendahl A, Manke H, et al: The coin lesion of the lung. Cancer 51:534–539, 1983.

186. Torek F: Removal of metastatic carcinoma of the lung and mediastinum. Arch Surg 21:1416–1424, 1930.

187. Udelsman R, Roth JA, Lees D, et al: Endobronchial metastases from soft tissue sarcoma. J Surg Oncol 32:145–149, 1986.

188. Vaidya AM, Petruzzelli GJ, Clark J, Emami B: Patterns of spread in recurrent head and neck squamous cell carcinoma. Otolaryngol Head Neck Surg 125(4):393–396, 2001.

189. van der Poel HG, Roukema JA, Horenblas S, et al: Metastasectomy in renal cell carcinoma: A multicenter retrospective analysis. Eur Urol 35(3):197–203, 1999.

190. Van der Veen AH, van Geel AN, Hop WC, et al: Median sternotomy: The preferred incision for resection of lung metastases. Eur J Surg 164(7):507–512, 1998.

191. van Geel AN, Pasterino U, Jauch KW, et al: Repeat resection of recurrent pulmonary metastatic soft tissue sarcoma. Eur J Surg Oncol 20:436–440, 1994.

192. Vandoni RE, Cuttat JF, Wicky S, Suter ML: CT-guided methylene-blue labelling before thoracoscopic resection of pulmonary nodules. Eur J Cardio-Thorac Surg 14:265–270, 1998.

193. Viadana E, Bross IDJ, Pickern JW: Cascade spread of bloodborne metastases in solid and non solid cancer of humans. In Weiss L, Gilbert HA, editors: Pulmonary Metastasis. Boston: G.K. Hall, 1978, pp. 143–167.

194. Vincent RG, Choksi LB, Takita H: Surgical resection of solitary pulmonary metastasis. In Weiss L, Gilbert HA, editors: Pulmonary Metastasis. Boston: G.K. Hall, 1978, 232–242.

354

195. Walsh GL, Nesbitt JC: Tumor implants after thoracoscopic resection of a metastatic sarcoma. Ann Thorac Surg 59: 215–216, 1995.

196. Warren S, Witman E: Studies on tumor metastases: The distribution of metastases in cancer of the breast. Surg Gynecol Obstet 57:1018, 1937.

197. Watanabe M, Deguchi H, Sato M, et al: Midterm results of thoracoscopic surgery for pulmonary metastases especially from colorectal cancers. J Laparoendosc Adv Surg Tech, Part A 8(4):195–200, 1998.

198. Wedman J, Balm AJ, Hart AA, et al: Value of resection of pulmonary metastases in head and neck cancer patients. Head Neck 18(4):311–316, 1996.

199. Weinlechner JW: Zur Kasuistik der Tumoren an der Brustwand und deren Behandlung (Resektion der Rippen, Eroffnung der Brusthohle, partielle Entfernung der Lunge). Wein Med Wochenschr 32:589–591, 624–628, 1882.

200. Weiser MR, Downey RJ, Leung DH, et al: Repeat resection of pulmonary metastases in patients with soft-tissue sarcoma. J Am Coll Surg 191(2):184–190, 2000.

201. Weksler B, Schneider A, Ng B, et al: Isolated single lung perfusion in the rat. J Appl Physiol 74:2736–2739, 1993.

202. Weksler B, Lenert J, Ng B, et al: Isolated single lung perfusion with doxorubicin is effective in eradicating soft tissue

203. Willis RA: Secondary tumors of the lungs. In The Spread of Tumors in the Human Body. London: Butterworths, 1973, pp. 167–174.

204. Wong JH, Euhus DM, Morton DL: Surgical resection for metastatic melanoma to the lung. Arch Surg 23:1091–1095, 1988.

205. Xiao H, Liu D, Bajorin D, et al: Medical and surgical management of pulmonary metastases from germ cell tumors. Chest Surg Clin North Am 8:131–143, 1998.

206. Xu LT, Sun CF, Wang, YE, et al: Resection of pulmonary metastatic choriocarcinoma in 43 drug-resistant patients. Ann Thorac Surg 39:257–259, 1985.

207. Yamada H, Katoh H, Kondo S, et al: Surgical treatment of pulmonary recurrence after hepatectomy for colorectal liver metastases. Hepato-Gastroenterology 49(46):976–979, 2002.

208. Younes RN, Gross JL, Deheinzelin D: Surgical resection of unilateral lung metastases: Is bilateral thoracotomy necessary? World J Surg 26(9):1112–1116, 2002.

209. Zhou H, Randall RL, Brothman AR, et al: Her-2/neu expression in osteosarcoma increases risk of lung metastasis and can be associated with gene amplification. J Pediatr Hematol/Oncol 25(1):27–32, 2003.

sarcoma lung metastases in a rat model. J Thorac Cardiovasc Surg 107:50–54, 1994.

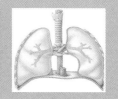

Congenital Chest Wall Deformities

CHAPTER 24

Robert C. Shamberger

▶ INTRODUCTION

A great variety of congenital abnormalities of the chest wall occur. Their physiological implications are also quite varied and span the spectrum from the rare entities of ectopia cordis and asphyxiating thoracic dystrophy, which are often lethal, to the much more common pectus excavatum and pectus carinatum with their limited physiological impact. In this chapter anterior thoracic deformities are considered in five categories: pectus excavatum, pectus carinatum, Poland's syndrome, sternal defects including ectopia cordis, and miscellaneous conditions including asphyxiating thoracic dystrophy (Jeune's syndrome).

▶ PECTUS EXCAVATUM

Pectus excavatum is the most frequent anterior chest wall deformity. The central depression of the chest is produced by posterior angulation of the sternum and the costal cartilages. The first and second costal cartilages and the manubrium are usually in a normal position (Figure 24-1), but the lower costal cartilages, which insert into the sternum and the body of the sternum, are depressed. The most anterior segment of the ossified portion of the ribs may also be curved posteriorly in older adolescents and adults. The extent of sternal and cartilaginous deformity is quite variable. Numerous methods of grading these deformities have been proposed by Hümmer and Willital,[60] von der Oelsnitz,[132] Welch,[140] Haller and associates,[48] and others, but none has been universally accepted. Asymmetry of the depression is often present. The right side is frequently more depressed than the left, and the sternum may be rotated as well. Many children with pectus excavatum have a characteristic physique with a broad thin chest, dorsal lordosis, "hook shoulder" deformity, costal flaring, and poor posture.

Pectus excavatum is present at birth or within the first year of life in the majority of affected children (86%), as shown in Figure 24-2. The deformity rarely resolves with increasing age, and it may worsen during the period of rapid growth in adolescence. Waters and associates identified scoliosis in 26% of 508 patients with pectus excavatum. Hence, it is important that all patients with pectus deformities are evaluated clinically for scoliosis. Asymmetrical pectus excavatum with a deep right gutter and sternal rotation often is

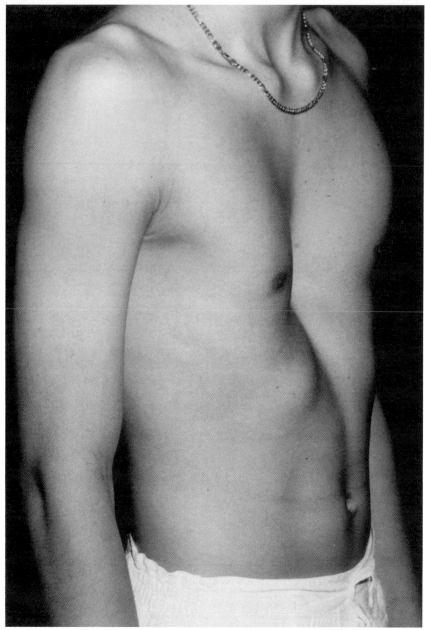

Figure 24–1 A 16½-year-old boy with a symmetrical pectus excavatum deformity. Note that the depression extends to the sternal notch.

Pectus Excavatum

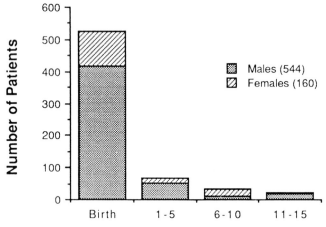

Figure 24–2 Age at appearance of pectus excavatum deformity in 704 infants and children. Note the large proportion identified at birth or within the first year of life and the predominance of males with this deformity.
(*From Shamberger RC, Welch, KJ: Surgical repair of pectus excavatum. J Pediatr Surg 23:615, 1988, with permission.*)

accompanied by scoliosis.[135] Congenital heart disease was identified in 1.5% of infants and children undergoing chest wall correction at the Children's Hospital in Boston (Table 24-1).[119] The frequency of chest wall deformities among all patients with congenital heart disease evaluated at this institution was only 0.17%.

Table 24–1

Congenital Heart Disease Associated with Pectus Excavatum and Carinatum

Congenital heart disease	Number of cases
Aortic ring	1
Aortic regurgitation	1
Atrial septal defect primum	2
Atrial septal defect secundum	3
Complete atrioventricular canal	3
Dextrocardia	3
Ebstein's malformation	1
Idiopathic hypertrophic subaortic stenosis	2
Patent ductus arteriosus	1
Pulmonic stenosis	1
Total anomalous pulmonary venous return	1
Transposition of great arteries	6
Tetralogy of Fallot	3
Tricuspid atresia	1
Truncus arteriosus	1
Ventricular septal defect	6

From Shamberger RC, Welch KJ, Castaneda AR, Keane JF, Fyler DC: Anterior chest wall deformities and congenital heart disease. J Thorac Cardiovasc Surg 96:427, 1988, with permission.

Asthma may be identified in association with pectus excavatum and carinatum. In a review of 694 consecutive cases, 35 patients with asthma were identified (5.2%), a frequency comparable to that of asthma in the general pediatric population.[119]

Etiology and Incidence

Ravitch reported that pectus excavatum may occur as frequently as 1 in 300 to 400 live births and that it is rare in blacks. It occurs move frequently in boys than girls, by almost a 4:1 ratio.[101] Although the sternal depression appears to be caused by overgrowth of costal cartilages, the etiology of pectus deformities is unknown. Lester attributed its development to an abnormality of the diaphragm, which tethered the sternum posteriorly.[75] This theory was supported by the occurrence of pectus excavatum in children after repair of agenesis of the diaphragm and the frequent association of pectus excavatum and congenital diaphragmatic hernia.[44,131] Histopathological changes in the costal cartilages similar to those seen in scoliosis, aseptic osteonecrosis, and inflammatory processes are reported, but the etiology of these findings and their significance are unknown.[53]

A family history of chest wall deformity in 37% of 704 patients suggests a genetic predisposition to pectus excavatum.[120] Three of four siblings were affected in one family. A high incidence of chest wall deformities occurs in children with Marfan's syndrome, and these deformities are often severe and usually accompanied by scoliosis.[114] Pectus excavatum is also commonly seen in individuals with the abdominal musculature deficiency syndrome (prune-belly syndrome).[141] Pectus excavatum also occurs in association with other myopathies and chromosomal defects such as Turner's syndrome. A summary of the associated musculoskeletal abnormalities is shown in Table 24-2.

Symptoms

Pectus excavatum is well tolerated in infancy and childhood. The anterior depression in an infant with a flexible chest may be accentuated by upper airway obstruction as from tonsillar and adenoidal hypertrophy, but this obstruction does not produce the pectus deformity. Older children may complain of pain in the area of the deformed cartilages or of precordial pain after sustained exercise. Symptomatic limitations to sustained exercise may also appear in these children and teenagers and limit their participation in athletic activities. Palpitations, presumably due to transient atrial arrhythmias, are occasionally reported. These patients may have mitral valve prolapse.

Pathophysiology

The cardiopulmonary implications of the pectus excavatum deformity have been debated for many decades. Although some believe this deformity has a limited physiological effect, many patients report increased stamina after surgical repair. These findings date back to the first surgical repair performed by Sauerbruch in 1913.[110] The patient was an 18-year-old boy who developed dyspnea and palpitations with very limited exercise. Three years after his operation, he could work 12–14 hours a day without tiring and without palpitations. Anecdotal reports during the next three decades

Table 24–2

Musculoskeletal Abnormalities Identified in 130 of 704 Cases of Pectus Excavatum

Musculoskeletal abnormality	Number of cases
Scoliosis	107
Kyphosis	4
Myopathy	3
Marfan's syndrome	2
Pierre Robin syndrome	2
Prune-belly syndrome	2
Neurofibromatosis	3
Cerebral palsy	4
Tuberous sclerosis	1
Congenital diaphragmatic hernia	2

From Shamberger RC, Welch KJ: Surgical repair of pectus excavatum. J Pediatr Surg 23:615, 1988, with permission.

repeated this observation. Investigators have sought to identify the physiological abnormality or combination of abnormalities that could explain this symptomatic improvement after surgery. Early physiological measurements of cardiac and pulmonary function were crude and did not yield convincing evidence of a cardiopulmonary deficit. In many early studies the results fell within the broad range of normal values, if often at the lower limits.[121]

A systolic ejection murmur is frequently present in individuals with pectus excavatum, and it is magnified by a short interval of exercise. This murmur is attributed to the close proximity between the sternum and the pulmonary artery, which results in transmission of a flow murmur.

Electrocardiographic abnormalities are common and result from the abnormal configuration of the chest wall producing displacement of the heart into the left thoracic cavity.[113] Patients with a history of palpitations should have a 24-h electrocardiogram as well as an echocardiogram to evaluate for mitral valve prolapse. Resolution of these supraventricular arrhythmias has been anecdotally reported after correction of a pectus excavatum deformity.

Many authors attribute the symptomatic improvement after surgery to improvement in pulmonary function. This has been difficult to prove, however, with the wide range of pulmonary function that exists from individual to individual

and its dependence on physical training and body habitus. Several of the key studies will be reviewed.

Pulmonary Function Studies

As early as 1951, Brown and Cook performed pulmonary evaluations on patients before and after surgical repair.[17] They demonstrated that although vital capacity (VC) was normal, the maximum breathing capacity was diminished (50% or more) in 9 of 11 cases and increased an average of 31% after surgical repair. Weg and associates in 1967 evaluated 25 Air Force recruits with pectus excavatum and compared them with 50 unselected basic trainees.[138] Although the lung compartments of both groups were equal, as were the vital capacities, the maximum voluntary ventilation was significantly lower in those with pectus excavatum than in the control population. Castile and co-workers in 1982 evaluated seven patients with pectus excavatum, five of whom were symptomatic with exercise.[21] The mean total lung capacity of the group was 79% of predicted. Flow volume configurations were normal, excluding airway obstruction as a cause of the symptoms. Workload tests demonstrated normal response to exercise in the dead space to tidal volume ratio and alveolar–arterial oxygen difference. The measured oxygen uptake, however, increasingly exceeded predicted values as workload approached maximum in the four "symptomatic" subjects with pectus excavatum. This pattern of oxygen consumption was different from that in normal subjects and in the three asymptomatic subjects with pectus excavatum in whom a linear response was seen. The mean oxygen uptake in the symptomatic subjects at maximal effort exceeded the predicted values by 25.4%. The three asymptomatic subjects, on the other hand, demonstrated normal linear oxygen uptake during exercise. Increased oxygen uptake suggests increased work of breathing in these symptomatic individuals despite the normal or mildly reduced vital capacities. Increases in tidal volume with exercise were uniformly depressed in those with pectus excavatum.

Cahill and co-workers in 1984 performed preoperative and postoperative studies in five children and adolescents with pectus carinatum and in 14 with pectus excavatum.[19] No abnormalities were demonstrated in the pectus carinatum group. The low normal vital capacities in excavatum patients were unchanged by operation, but a small improvement in the total lung capacity and a significant improvement in the maximal voluntary ventilation were seen. Exercise tolerance improved in those with pectus excavatum after operation, as determined both by total exercise time and maximal oxygen consumption. In addition, at any given workload, those with pectus excavatum demonstrated a lower heart rate, stable oxygen consumption, and higher minute ventilation after repair. Mead and associates in 1985 studied rib cage mobility by assessing intraabdominal pressure.[80] Normal abdominal pressure tracings in pectus excavatum suggested normal rib cage mobility.

Blickman and colleagues in 1985 assessed pulmonary function in 17 children with pectus excavatum by xenon perfusion and ventilation scintigraphy before and after surgery.[9] Ventilation studies were abnormal in 12 children before surgery and improved in 7 children after repair. Perfusion scans were abnormal in 10 children before surgery and improved after operation in 6 children. The ventilation–perfusion ratios were abnormal in 10 of the 17 children preoperatively and normalized after repair in 6 children.

Derveaux and associates in 1989 evaluated 88 patients with pectus excavatum and carinatum by pulmonary function tests before and 1 to 20 years after repair (mean was 8 years).[31] The surgical technique used a fairly extensive chest wall dissection. Preoperative studies were within the normal range (>80% of predicted) except in subjects who had both scoliosis and pectus excavatum. The postoperative values for forced expiratory volume in 1 s (FEV_1) and VC expressed as percentage of expected were decreased in all groups, although the absolute values at follow-up may have been greater than at preoperative evaluation. Improved chest wall configuration was confirmed by radiological evaluation, so the relative deterioration in pulmonary function was not the result of recurrence of the pectus deformity. An inverse relationship was found between preoperative and postoperative function. Those with less than 75% of predicted function had improved function after surgery, but function was worse after repair if the preoperative values were greater than 75% of predicted. Almost identical results were found in a study by Morshuis and co-workers in 1994.[86] They evaluated 152 subjects before and a mean of 8 years after surgery for pectus excavatum. These results of pulmonary evaluation were in contrast to the subjective symptomatic improvement reported by the patients and their improved chest wall configuration. The decline in pulmonary function in the postoperative studies was attributed to the operation because the preoperative pulmonary defect appeared to be stable regardless of the age at initial repair. Both studies were marred by the obvious lack of an age- and severity-matched control group without surgery.

Derveaux and colleagues in 1988 evaluated transpulmonary and transdiaphragmatic pressures at total lung capacity in 17 individuals with pectus excavatum.[32] Preoperative and long-term follow-up evaluations were performed a mean of 12 years apart. Reduced transpulmonary and transdiaphragmatic pressures demonstrated that the increased restrictive defect was produced by extrapulmonary rather than pulmonary factors, suggesting that surgery produced increased rigidity of the chest wall.

Wynn and others in 1990 assessed 12 children with pectus excavatum by pulmonary function tests and exercise testing.[147] Eight children had repair and were evaluated preoperatively and postoperatively. Four children had two sets of evaluations, but no operation. A decline in total lung capacity was identified in the repaired children compared with stable values in the control group. Cardiac output and stroke volume increased appropriately with exercise before and after operation in both groups, and the operation was believed to have produced no physiologically significant effect on the response to exercise.

Kaguraoka and associates in 1992 evaluated pulmonary function in 138 individuals before and after repair of pectus excavatum.[66] A decrease in VC occurred during the first 2 months after surgery, with recovery to preoperative levels by 1 year after operation. At 42 months, the values were maintained at baseline, despite a significant improvement in the chest wall configuration. Tanaka and co-workers in 1993 found similar results in individuals who had the more extensive sternal turnover technique; in fact, they demonstrated a more significant and long-term decrease in VC.[129] Morshuis

and co-workers in 1994 evaluated 35 subjects who had had pectus excavatum repaired as teenagers or young adults; the ages were 17.9 ± 5.6 years.[87] Preoperative evaluations were performed and repeated 1 year after surgery. Preoperative total lung capacity (86.0 ± 14.4% of predicted) and VC (79.7 ± 16.2%) were significantly decreased from predicted values and decreased further after surgery (−9.2 ± 9.2% and −6.6 ± 10.7%, respectively). The efficiency of breathing at maximal exercise improved significantly after operation. Exercise was limited by ventilation in 43% of the subjects before repair. A tendency toward improvement occurred after operation. However, the group with no ventilatory limitation initially demonstrated one after operation with a significant increase in oxygen consumption.

Quigley and colleagues in 1996 evaluated 36 adolescents with pectus excavatum and 10 age-matched healthy controls at baseline and then an average of 8 months after surgery in 15 subjects and 9 months in controls.[96] Adolescents with pectus excavatum had a decrease in VC compared with controls, although the mean values remained in the normal range. The mean total lung capacity was also normal. There was no difference in workload performance between subjects with pectus excavatum and the controls, with both groups achieving a similar duration and level of exercise. No significant change in pulmonary function tests was seen in follow-up in either group. The duration of exercise as well as the level of work increased significantly in those who had surgery, but not in the controls. The absence of adverse effects on pulmonary function after surgery was attributed to a less extensive surgical procedure than was used in the studies reported by Derveaux et al[32] and Morshuis et al.[86,87] Two series report the effects on pulmonary function of the new minimally invasive repair of pectus excavatum—MIRPE described by Nuss.[12,124] In these series there were limited or no preoperative abnormalities and mild or no significant change after repair.

In composite, these studies of pulmonary function over the last four decades have failed to document consistent improvement in pulmonary function resulting from surgical repair. In fact, some studies have demonstrated deterioration in pulmonary function at long-term evaluation that was attributed to increased chest wall rigidity after repair. Despite this finding, workload studies have shown improvement in exercise tolerance after repair.

Cardiovascular Studies

Posterior displacement of the sternum can produce a deformity of the heart, particularly indentation of the right ventricle. Displacement of the heart to the left, often with a sternal "imprint" on the anterior wall of the right ventricle, was demonstrated angiographically by Garusi and D'Ettorre in 1964[42] and Howard[59] demonstrated its resolution after surgical repair. Elevated right heart pressures have been reported by some authors, as have pressure curves similar to those seen in constrictive pericarditis. In 1962, Bevegård studied 16 individuals with pectus excavatum by right heart catheterization and exercise testing.[8] The physical work capacity in pectus excavatum at a given heart rate was significantly lower in the sitting than the supine position. Those with 20% or greater decline in physical work capacity from the supine to the sitting position had shorter sternovertebral distances

360 than did those with less decrease in their physical work capacity. The measured stroke volume at rest decreased from supine to sitting positions a mean of 40.3%, similar to normal subjects. In the supine position, stroke volume increased with exercise 13.2%. In the sitting position, the increase in stroke volume from rest to exercise was 18.5% for the pectus excavatum group, significantly lower ($p <0.001$) than the 51% increase seen in normal subjects. Thus, in the pectus excavatum group, an increased cardiac output could be achieved primarily by increased heart rate because only limited enhancement of the stroke volume could occur. Intracardiac pressures measured at rest and with exercise were normal in all subjects despite this apparent limitation of ventricular volume. Gattiker and Bühlmann in 1967 confirmed this limitation of the stroke volume in a study of 19 subjects.[43] In the upright position at a heart rate of 170 beats per minute, the physical work capacity was lower than in the supine position (mean 18% decrease) because of the decrease in stroke volume. Beiser and associates in 1972 performed cardiac catheterization in six adolescents and young adults with moderate degrees of pectus excavatum.[7] Normal pressure and cardiac index were obtained at rest in the supine position. The cardiac index during moderate exercise was normal, but the response to upright exercise was below that predicted in two patients and at the lower limit of normal in three patients. The cardiac index was 6.8 ± 0.8 liters/min/m² compared with 8.9 ± 0.3 liters/min/m² in a group of 16 normal controls ($p <0.01$). The difference in cardiac performance again appeared to be produced primarily by a smaller stroke volume in the group with pectus excavatum in an upright position. Stroke volume was 31% lower and cardiac output 28% lower during upright as compared with supine exercise. Postoperative studies were performed in three individuals: two of them achieved a higher level of exercise tolerance after surgery. The cardiac index increased an average of 38%. Because heart rate at maximal exercise was not higher after repair, an enhanced stroke volume response was responsible for this increase.

Peterson and associates in 1985 performed radionuclide angiography and exercise studies in 13 children with pectus excavatum.[94] Ten of 13 were able to reach the target heart rate before surgical repair, four without symptoms. After operation, all but one child reached the target heart rate during the exercise protocol, and 9 of 13 reached the target without becoming symptomatic. The left and right ventricular end-diastolic volumes were consistently increased after repair at rest, and the mean stroke volume was increased 19% after repair. These findings substantiated the ventricular volume changes previously demonstrated by cardiac catheterization, although an increase in the cardiac index was not demonstrated. Recent echocardiographic studies by Kowalewski and associates of 42 patients before and 6 months after surgery revealed statistically significant changes in the right ventricular volume indices after surgery.[69] There was no correlation seen, however, between the pectus index and the changes in the right ventricular volume indices. Similar echocardiographic results have been demonstrated after the minimally invasive repair of pectus excavatum, with a significant improvement in the stroke volume.[124]

Additional studies are needed to further define the relationship between pectus excavatum and cardiopulmonary function. Recent dynamic or exercise studies have been most promising in this area. Methods to more effectively evaluate preoperative cardiopulmonary function are needed to identify which children may achieve symptomatic and physiological improvement from surgical repair.

Echocardiographic Studies

Bon Tempo, Salomon, and Schutte and their associates reported mitral valve prolapse in patients with narrow anterior-posterior chest diameters, anterior chest wall deformities, and scoliosis.[11,108,115] Prospective echocardiographic studies of adults with pectus excavatum demonstrated mitral valve prolapse in 6 of 33 (18%) subjects studied by Udoshi and associates and in 11 of 17 subjects (65%) of Saint-Mezard and colleagues.[107,130] Anterior compression of the heart by the depressed sternum may deform the mitral annulus or the ventricular chamber and produce mitral valve prolapse in these patients. Preoperative evaluation by echocardiogram of children and adolescents with pectus excavatum by the author and associates identified 23 with mitral valve prolapse.[122] Postoperative studies did not demonstrate mitral valve prolapse in 10 (43%) of these children, suggesting its resolution after correction of the chest wall deformity.

Surgical Repair

The first surgical corrections of pectus excavatum were reported by Meyer in 1911 and Sauerbruch in 1920 and Ochsner and DeBakey summarized the early experience with various techniques.[83,89,110] In 1949, Ravitch reported a technique that included excision of all deformed costal cartilages with the perichondrium, division of the xiphoid from the sternum, division of the intercostal bundles from the sternum, and a transverse sternal osteotomy securing the sternum anteriorly in an overcorrected position.[97] Kirschner wire fixation was utilized in the first two patients and silk suture fixation in later patients.

Baronofsky (1957) and Welch (1958) subsequently reported a technique for the correction of pectus excavatum that emphasized total preservation of the perichondrial sheaths as well as the attachment of the upper sheaths and intercostal bundles to the sternum.[6,139] Anterior fixation of the sternum was achieved with silk sutures. Haller and associates later developed a technique that they labeled *tripod fixation*.[49] Subperichondrial resection of the abnormal cartilages is performed followed by a posterior sternal osteotomy. The most cephalad normal cartilages are then divided obliquely in a posterolateral direction. When the sternum is elevated, the sternal ends of the cartilage rest on the costal ends, providing further anterior support of the sternum. Support of the sternum by metallic struts after mobilization of the costal cartilages has been promoted by several authors. Rehbein developed struts that could be placed into the marrow cavity of the ribs at the costochondral junction.[102] An arch was then formed by the struts anterior to the sternum, and the sternum was secured to this arch. Paltia and associates placed a transverse strut through the caudal end of the sternum, firmly fixing its location.[92] The two ends of the strut are supported by the ribs laterally. Adkins and Blades and Jensen and associates used retrosternal elevation by a metallic strut.[1,145] Willital employed a similar retrosternal strut after creating multiple chondrotomies in the costal cartilages to provide flexibility.[145]

Recent innovations in these methods include bioabsorbable struts, or use of Marlex mesh or a Dacron vascular graft as a strut, but there is no evidence these methods are preferable to traditional methods with metallic struts.[72] Robicsek described a large series of chest wall deformities.[105] For those patients with pectus excavatum the sternum is mobilized more extensively with this technique than in others, except for the sternal turnover. The sternum is divided from the intercostal muscles and perichondrial sheaths from its tip to the upper extent of the deformity. It is then supported in an anterior position by a "hammock" of Marlex mesh that is sewn to the ends of the ribs to each side. The advantages of this extensive mobilization and permanent implantation of the mesh are not clear. No randomized studies have compared the recurrence or complication rates between suture or strut fixation techniques. von der Oelsnitz and Hecker and co-workers, using suture fixation, reported satisfactory repairs in their large series in 90–95%.[53,132]

The *sternal turnover* was first proposed by Judet and Judet in 1954 and Jung in 1956 in the French literature.[64,65] The sternum is mobilized and the costal cartilages are divided, allowing the sternum to be rotated 180°. Wada and colleagues in 1970[133] reported a very large series from Japan using this technique, which is essentially a free graft of sternum. It is a radical approach and has been associated with major complications if infection occurs. Modifications of this technique by Taguchi and associates in 1975 have involved either preservation of the internal mammary vessels by wide dissection or reimplantation of the internal mammary artery.[128] These modifications were developed because of the reported incidence of osteonecrosis and fistula formation, which occurred in up to 46% of patients older than 15 years.

Allen and Douglas implanted Silastic molds into the subcutaneous space to fill the depression in pectus excavatum.[2] Although this approach may improve the external contour of the chest, extrusion of the molds has occurred, and this method does nothing to increase the volume of the thoracic cavity or relieve compression on the heart. Recently other authors have reported favorable cosmetic results in adults with no pulmonary restrictions, but with a significant frequency of seroma and hematoma formation.[137]

A method of elevation of the sternum with a retrosternal bar without resection or division of the costal cartilages was first reported by Nuss in 1998.[88] He repaired 42 patients under 15 years of age (median age 5 years) by placing a convex steel bar under the sternum and anterior to the heart through small bilateral thoracic incisions. A long clamp was passed blindly behind the sternum and out an opening in the contralateral chest (Figure 24-3A and B). A tape was then drawn across the chest in the clamp and used to pull the bar through the chest. The bar was initially placed with the concave side anteriorly and was then rotated once it was in position (Figure 24-3C, E, and F). The bar was left in position for 2 years before removal when presumed permanent remodeling of the cartilages had occurred. Although Nuss in his initial report warned that the "upper limits of age for this procedure require further evaluation," the technique has been widely used in older patients, and long-term results from this population have not yet been reported. In 2002 the results by Nuss and his associates using this technique in 303 patients was reported by Croitoru et al.[25] This included a group of children older than in the initial report (range 21 months to 29 years;

median age 12.4 years). Two bars were required in 12.5% of the patients. Routine use of thoracoscopy to avoid cardiac injury was instituted in 1998. Lateral stabilizers were placed in 69.4% of the cases and were routinely used after 1998 and were wired to the bar in 65.4% of cases (Figure 24-3D). Epidural analgesic was employed for 2–4 days and the median length of stay was 5 days with a range of 3–10 days. The frequency of early complications was low. It included pneumothorax requiring aspiration 1.0%, pericarditis 2.3%, with only 0.3% requiring drainage, pneumonia 0.7%, hemothorax 0.3%, transient extremity paralysis 0.3%, superficial wound infection 2.3%, and bar infection requiring eventual removal of the bar 0.7%.

Late complications in this series included bar displacement requiring repositioning in 8.6%, which included a high proportion (over 50%) of patients in whom a stabilizer was not utilized or in whom the stabilizer was not wired to the bar. When both modifications were employed displacement occurred in only 5% of the patients. An unexpected occurrence of allergies to the metal bar was encountered in 1% of the patients who presented with rashes in the area of the bars. This required revision to bars composed of other alloys. Late hemothorax occurred in two patients, one secondary to undefined trauma. The occurrence of a mild overcorrection in the deformity was seen in 3.6% and a pectus carinatum deformity developed in 1.3%, all of whom had either Marfan's syndrome or Ehlers–Danlos syndrome. The reported outcome of children in this large series was excellent appearance in 84.5%, good in 14.8%, and failed in only one patient, however, the bars had been removed at the time of the report in only 23.4% of the patients.

Hebra and associates reported the results of a survey of members of the American Pediatric Surgery Association who had employed the minimally invasive (Nuss) technique.[52] Thirty institutions contributed 251 cases, although it should be noted that 42% were performed by one surgeon. The complications reported were similar to those of Nuss and his associates, but the frequency was higher, presumably because the procedures were performed by more individuals less familiar with the operation. Displacement of the bar occurred in 9.2% of cases and pneumothorax requiring tube thoracostomy in 4.8%. Less frequently encountered complications included thoracic outlet syndrome, pericarditis, blood loss requiring a transfusion, cardiac injury, persistent cardiac arrhythmias, and erosion of the sternum by the bar. Many of the surgeons had adopted the use of thoracoscopy to improve the safety of passing the clamp anterior to the heart. Other surgeons elevate the sternum with a bone hook during passage of the clamp to open the retrosternal space anterior to the heart.

Engum and co-authors reported their series of 21 patients with a mean age of 8.2 years.[36] Their patients had an average hospital stay of 4.9 days, which was comparable with the open repair. Complications encountered in their series were similar to the experience of others and included rotation of the bar, production of a marked pectus carinatum deformity, progressive chest wall asymmetry, and chronic persistent pain requiring removal of the bar in one case.

Molik and colleagues later enlarged this single institution review and in a retrospective analysis compared 68 patients with standard surgical repair with 35 patients with a Nuss repair.[85] The Nuss procedure required less time (3.3 h)

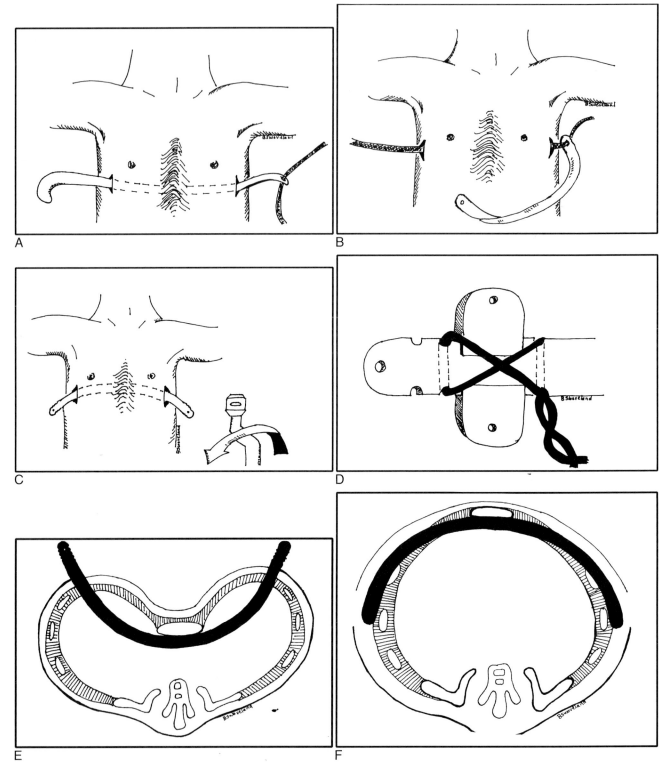

Figure 24–3 A, A long Lorenz tunneler is passed across the chest behind the sternum and anterior to the heart. (Walter Lorenz Surgical, Inc. Jacksonville, FL). **B,** Two umbilical tapes are then drawn back across the chest with the device and to one is secured the convex steel Lorenz bar that is guided into the substernal tunnel using the umbilical tape to keep it on track. **C,** The Lorenz bar is shown with its convex aspect directed posteriorly. It is then rotated 180 degrees with a special device, the Lorenz flipper, compressing the sternum anteriorly. **D,** A stainless steel cross-piece is then secured to one end of the bar (or both ends in some patients needing extra support) with heavy #3 wire. Once it is wired together the whole apparatus is then sutured to the soft tissues of the chest with multiple absorbable sutures to achieve secure fixation to the chest wall to prevent rotation of the bar and loss of correction of the deformity or side-to-side movement of the bar. The entrance of the bar under the rib is at the inner aspect of the pectus ridge. **E,** Schematic depiction of the Lorenz bar after placement and then **(F)** after rotation 180 degrees producing anterior displacement of the sternum and costal cartilages.
(Reproduced with permission from Donald Nuss, M.D. Children's Hospital of The King's Daughters, Norfolk, VA.)

compared with the open technique (4.7 h), but had a higher complication rate (43%) than the open method (20%). Four patients with the standard operation (6%) and eight with the Nuss technique (29%) required reoperation. Length of stay was comparable between the open (4.8 days) and Nuss (4.0 days) techniques. The Nuss patients had a higher frequency of epidural analgesics postoperatively and an increased duration of patient-controlled analgesia after surgery.

Fonkalsrud and associates reported a similar retrospective comparison of the two techniques each utilized at one institution.[38] During a 5-year interval, 68 patients had the minimally invasive procedure and 139 had the open technique. There was a higher incidence of reoperations and hospitalizations in the Nuss group, but it was noted that 90% of the complications of this method occurred in the first 25 cases, again clearly demonstrating the role of experience in determining the frequency of surgical complications. It was difficult to determine in this study whether the differences noted in the use of epidural catheters and intravenous narcotics were attributable to truly different patient requirements or were a manifestation of institutional bias for analgesic techniques. There was a shorter mean hospitalization noted for the open procedure (2.9 days) compared with the minimal access procedure (6.5 days), and a similar difference between mean time before return to work or school (12 versus 18 days). These authors concluded that "long-term follow-up also will be required to assure both health professionals and the public that this is the procedure of choice for patients with pectus excavatum."

The occurrence of "overcorrection" of the deformity or production of a true carinate deformity was first reported by Croitoru and associates and was associated with underlying connective tissue disorders (Marfan's syndrome and Ehlers–Danlos syndromes).[25] It was reported, however, by Hebra to have occurred in an otherwise healthy 13-year-old boy 1 year after Nuss repair.[51] What factors predispose some patients to this complication is not understood.

A prospective multiinstitutional study of patients undergoing repair of pectus excavatum is in progress. It is hoped that this study will better define the role as well as the risks and benefits of the open and minimally invasive surgical procedures in the repair of pectus excavatum.

Children should be followed up long-term after repair by any technique until they reach full stature. Only by so doing can each surgeon assess the ultimate results of his or her surgical technique. Regrettably, recurrence can occur until full stature is achieved.

Surgical Technique

The open surgical technique for correction of pectus excavatum is depicted in Figure 24-4. In girls, particular attention is taken to place the incision within the projected inframammary crease, thus avoiding the complications of breast deformity and development described by Hougaard and Arendrup.[57] Skin flaps are mobilized by electrocautery to the angle of Louis superiorly and a shorter distance to the xiphoid inferiorly. Pectoral muscle flaps are elevated off the sternum and costal cartilages, preserving the entire pectoralis major and portions of the pectoralis minor and serratus anterior muscles in the flap (see Figure 24-4A). Ellis and associates described elevating the skin and muscle together

in a single flap, which is a reasonable, but not widely adopted alternative method.[35]

Perioperative antibiotics are used, giving one dose of cefazolin immediately before operation and three postoperative doses. The Hemovac drain is removed when the drainage is less than 15 ml for an 8-h period. All patients are warned to avoid ibuprofen or aspirin-containing compounds for 2 weeks before surgery.

I currently use the retrosternal bar (Baxter Healthcare Co., Deerfield, IL) for internal fixation to secure the sternum firmly in an anterior position and to avoid the need to skeletonize the sternum to achieve adequate mobility for suture fixation. Although correction of pectus excavatum is technically most easily performed in a young child, I have become increasingly concerned about long-term recurrence in these children as well as impairment in growth of the chest wall. I currently delay surgery until the children are well into their pubertal growth. At this age, the chest has less remaining growth and opportunity for recurrence of the pectus excavatum (Figure 24-5). Fonkalsrud also recommends delay until at least 10 years of age because of recurrence most frequently occurring during pubertal growth.[38] In contrast, Backer and associates have found no correlation between the age at repair and frequency of recurrence.[5,61]

The closed technique developed by Donald Nuss is depicted in Figure 24-3. Various modifications have been developed to minimize the risk of cardiac injury during passage of the clamp behind the sternum. Some surgeons place a small incision along the lower margin of the sternum through which a bone hook is placed to elevate the sternum and increase the retrosternal space. Others create a small additional opening into the chest through which a small thoroscope is placed to observe passage of the clamp behind the sternum and anterior to the pericardium.

Complications

Complications are few and relatively unimportant, except for major recurrence which occurred in 17 of 704 patients in one reported series (Table 24-3).[119] Pneumothorax occurred in 2% of the patients and required only observation or aspiration. Tube thoracostomy was required in only four patients in the entire series and in no patients during the last two decades of the report. Wound infection is rare with use of perioperative antibiotic coverage.

The most distressing complication after surgical correction of pectus excavatum is major recurrence of the deformity. It is difficult to predict which patients will have a major recurrence, but it appears to occur with increased frequency in children with poor muscular development and an asthenic or "marfanoid" habitus. All children with Marfan's syndrome should be repaired with strut fixation because of the high risk of recurrence reported without strut fixation. Scherer and associates reported a low recurrence rate (one of eight cases) using a retrosternal strut.[114]

Although recurrences appear symmetrical, many are in fact right sided, with a deep right parasternal gutter and sternal obliquity. The third, fourth, and fifth rib ends migrate medially, with apparent "foreshortening" of the costal cartilages. Correction of recurrent pectus excavatum is generally a

Text continued on pg. 368

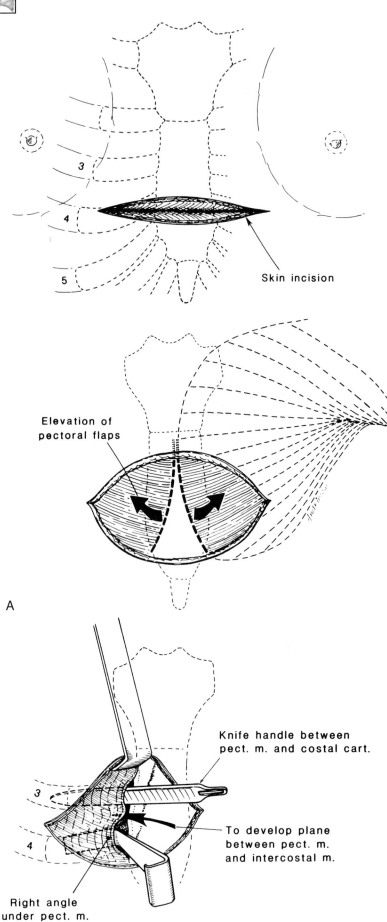

Skin incision

Elevation of
pectoral flaps

A

Knife handle between
pect. m. and costal cart.

To develop plane
between pect. m.
and intercostal m.

Right angle
under pect. m.

B

Figure 24–4 Open surgical technique for repair of pectus excavatum. **A,** A transverse incision is placed below and well within the nipple lines and, in females, at the site of the future inframammary crease. The pectoralis major muscle is elevated from the sternum along with portions of the pectoralis minor and serratus anterior bundles. **B,** The correct plane of dissection of the pectoral muscle flap is defined by passing an empty knife handle directly anterior to a costal cartilage after the medial aspect of the muscle is elevated with electrocautery. The knife handle is then replaced with a right-angle retractor, which is pulled anteriorly. The process is then repeated anterior to an adjoining costal cartilage. Anterior distraction of the muscles during the dissection facilitates identification of the avascular areolar plane and avoids entry into the intercostal muscle bundles. Muscle elevation is extended bilaterally to the costochondral junctions of the third to fifth ribs and a comparable distance for ribs 6 and 7.

Figure 24–4 cont'd
C, Subperichondrial resection of the costal cartilages is achieved by incising the perichondrium anteriorly. It is then dissected away from the costal cartilages in the bloodless plane between perichondrium and costal cartilage. Cutting back the perichondrium 90 degrees in each direction at its junction with the sternum (inset) facilitates visualization of the back wall of the costal cartilage. **D,** The cartilages are divided at their junction with the sternum with a knife having a Welch perichondrial elevator held posteriorly to elevate the cartilage and protect the mediastinum (inset). The divided cartilage can then be held with an Allis clamp and elevated. The costochondral junction is preserved with a segment of costal cartilage on the osseous ribs by incising the cartilage with a scalpel. Costal cartilages three through seven are generally resected, but occasionally the second costal cartilages must be removed if posterior displacement or funneling of the sternum extends to this level, as may be seen in older patients (see Figure 24-1). Segments of the sixth and seventh costal cartilages are resected to the point where they flatten to join the costal arch. Familiarity with the cross-sectional shape of the medial ends of the costal cartilages facilitates their dissection. The second and third cartilages are broad and flat, the fourth and fifth are circular, and the sixth and seventh are narrow and deep.

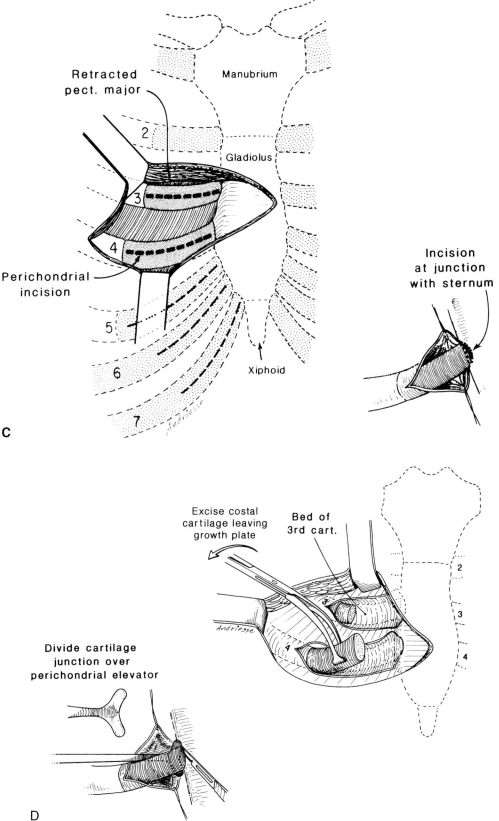

(Continued)

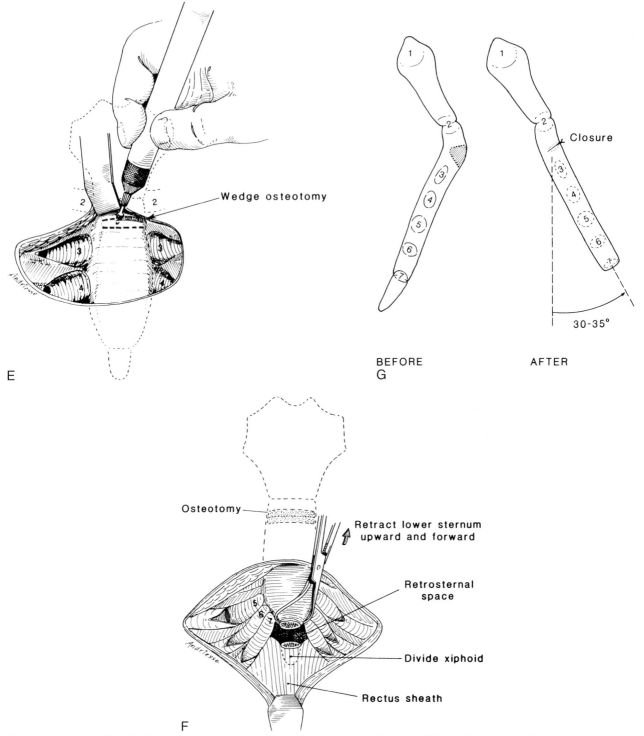

Wedge osteotomy

BEFORE
G

1

2

3

4

5

6

7

Closure

30-35°

AFTER

E

Osteotomy

Retract lower sternum
upward and forward

Retrosternal
space

Divide xiphoid

Rectus sheath

F

Figure 24–4 cont'd E, The sternal osteotomy is created above the level of the last deformed cartilage and the posterior angulation of the sternum, generally the third cartilage but occasionally the second. Two transverse sternal osteotomies are created through the anterior cortex with a Hall air drill (Zimmer USA, Inc., Warsaw, IN) 3–5 mm apart. **F,** The base of the sternum and the rectus muscle flap are elevated with two towel clips, and the posterior plate of the sternum is fractured. The xiphoid can be divided from the sternum with electrocautery, allowing entry into the retrosternal space. This step is not necessary with the use of a retrosternal strut unless the xiphoid is protruding anteriorly when the sternum is in its corrected position. Preservation of the attachment of the perichondrial sheaths and xiphoid avoids an unsightly depression that can occur below the sternum. **G,** Correction of the abnormal position of the sternum is achieved by creation of a wedge-shaped osteotomy, which is then closed with elevation by the strut, bringing the sternum anteriorly into a slightly overcorrected position.

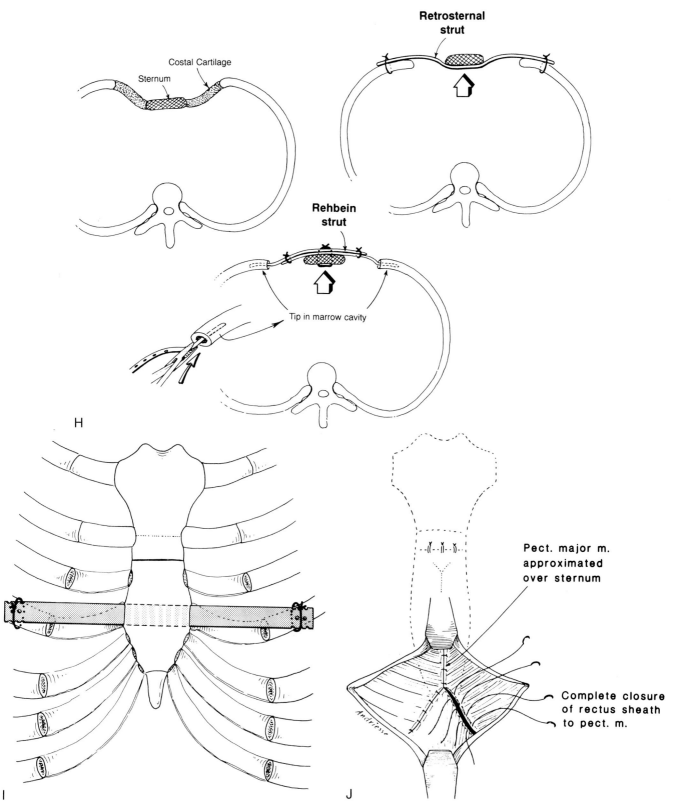

Figure 24–4 cont'd **H,** This figure demonstrates the use of both retrosternal struts and Rehbein struts. Rehbein struts are inserted into the marrow cavity (inset) of the third or fourth rib, and the struts are then joined medially to create an arch anterior to the sternum. The sternum is sewn to the arch to secure it in its new anterior position. The retrosternal strut is placed behind the sternum and is secured to the rib ends laterally to prevent migration. **I,** Anterior depiction of the retrosternal strut. The perichondrial sheath to either the third or fourth rib is divided from its junction with the sternum, and the retrosternal space is bluntly dissected to allow passage of the strut behind the sternum. It is secured with two pericostal sutures laterally to prevent migration. The wound is then flooded with warm saline and cefazolin solution to remove clots and inspect for a pleural entry. A single-limb medium Hemovac drain (Snyder Laboratories, Inc., New Philadelphia, OH) is brought through the inferior skin flap to the left of the sternum and placed in a parasternal position to the level of the highest resected costal cartilage. **J,** The pectoral muscle flaps are secured to the midline of the sternum, advancing the flaps inferiorly to obtain coverage of the entire sternum. The rectus muscle is then joined to the pectoral muscle flaps, closing the mediastinum.

*(**A–G** and **J** from Shamberger RC, Welch KJ: Surgical repair of pectus excavatum J. Pediatr Surg 23:615, 1988, with permission. **D** and **F** adapted from original figures. **H** and **I** from Shamberger RC: Chest Wall Deformities in General Thoracic Surgery, 5th ed. by Thomas W. Shields with permission.)*

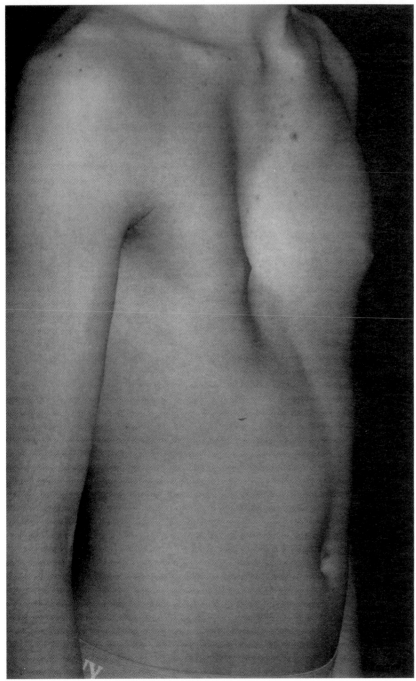

Figure 24–5 (**A**) Preoperative photographs of a 14-year-old boy with pectus excavatum.

A

formidable task. Sanger and associates reported their experience in secondary correction.[109] They resected the regenerated fibrocartilage plate, repeated the osteotomy, and closed the pectoral muscles behind the sternum. Ten patients had an early good result. In the Boston Children's Hospital experience, 12 children and adolescents underwent secondary repair. Resection of the segments of the third to fifth costal cartilages was necessary to correct the deformity. After clearing the tip of the sternum, resection of the left fibrocartilage plate to the level of the third or second perichondrial sheath allowed the sternum to be brought forward and rotated into an acceptable position. Ten of 12 repeat operations were accomplished without pleural entry. Follow-up of patients with secondary correction ranged from 10 to 17 years. Eight

have acceptable thoracic contour, two have a broad shallow depression, and two have frank recurrence. I recommend use of strut fixation on all patients with secondary repair because cartilage regeneration will be slower and less adequate than that after primary operation.

In 1990, Martinez and associates first described a deficiency in thoracic growth in children after repair of pectus excavatum during the preschool years.[78] Subsequently in 1996, Haller reported three boys who presented in their teens with apparent limited growth of the ribs after resection of the costal cartilages at an early age.[46] This produced a bandlike narrowing of the mid chest, which was labeled acquired Jeune's disease by the authors (Figure 24-6). In some cases, the first and second ribs in which the costal cartilages had not

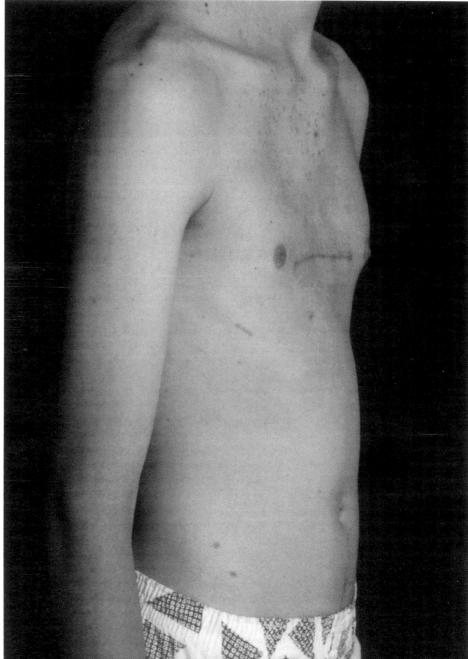

B

Figure 24–5 cont'd (B) Postoperative photograph 7 months after repair using a retrosternal strut.

been resected had relative overgrowth, producing anterior protrusion of the upper sternum (Figure 24-6C). Haller et al attributed this to injury of the costochondral junctions during surgical repair.[46] As these junctions are the longitudinal growth centers for the ribs, early operation resulted in decreased growth of the ribs and of the sternum resulting from injury to its growth centers or vascular supply.

Martinez and associates demonstrated experimentally in 6-week-old rabbits that resection of the costal cartilages produced a marked impairment in chest growth, particularly the anterior-posterior diameter, during a 5.5-month period of observation.[78] Less severe impairment occurred if only the medial three fourths of the costal cartilage was resected, preserving the growth centers at the costochondral junction.

This impairment was attributed to fibrosis and scarring within the perichondrial sheaths. Perichondrial sheaths, bone, or other prosthetic tissues that cannot grow also should not be joined posterior to the sternum because they will form a bandlike stricture across the chest. This complication of delayed thoracic growth was described primarily in children repaired in early childhood and can be avoided by delaying surgery until the children are older. Preservation of the costochondral junction by leaving a segment of the cartilage on the osseous portion of the rib may partially minimize growth impairment. Weber and Kurkchubasche described a method of improving the severe pulmonary impairment encountered in one patient with the "acquired Jeune's syndrome."[136] A sternotomy was performed and

Table 24–3

Complications of Pectus Excavatum Repair: 70 Cases in 704 Patients

Complication	Number of cases
Pneumothorax[a]	11
Wound infection	5
Wound hematoma	3
Wound dehiscence	5
Pneumonia	3
Seroma	1
Hemoptysis	1
Hemopericardium	1
Major recurrence	17
Mild recurrence	23

From Shamberger RC, Welch KJ: Surgical repair of pectus excavatum. J Pediatr Surg 23:615, 1988, with permission.

[a]Four patients required chest tube placement.

wedged open permanently with rib struts. The pleura was opened bilaterally along with subperichondrial resection of six ribs. Pulmonary function was improved after the procedure in this patient.

Patients are followed after surgery to full growth: age 16 for girls and 19 for boys. Use of clinical and Moiré photography for initial evaluation and follow-up studies leads to improved clinical assessment of results and obviates the need for multiple radiographic examinations.[123]

► PECTUS CARINATUM

Pectus carinatum, an anterior protrusion of the sternum or chest wall, is much less frequent than pectus excavatum; 16.7% of all chest wall deformities in the Boston Children's Hospital experience. The anterior protrusion occurs in a spectrum of configurations often divided into four categories (Table 24-4).[118] The most frequent form, termed *chondrogladiolar* by Brodkin, consists of anterior protrusion of the body of the sternum with protrusion of the lower costal cartilages.[15] It is described as appearing as if a giant hand had pinched the chest from the front, forcing the ster-

num and medial portion of the costal cartilages forward and the lateral costal cartilages and ribs inward (Figure 24-7).[58] Asymmetric deformities with anterior displacement of the costal cartilages on one side and normal cartilages on the contralateral side are less common (Figure 24-8). Mixed lesions have a carinate deformity on one side and a depression or excavatum deformity on the contralateral side, often with sternal rotation. Some authors classify these as a variant of the excavatum deformities. The least frequent deformity is the chondromanubrial or "pouter pigeon" deformity with protrusion of the upper chest involving the manubrium and second and third costal cartilages and relative depression of the body of the sternum (Figure 24-9).

Etiology

The etiology of pectus carinatum is no better understood than that of pectus excavatum. It appears as an overgrowth of the costal cartilages with forward buckling of the cartilages and anterior displacement of the sternum. Again, there is a clear-cut increased family incidence, which suggests a genetic basis. In a review by the author and colleagues of 152 patients, 26% had a family history of chest wall deformity and 12% of scoliosis.[118] It is much more frequent in boys than in girls by a three to one ratio. Scoliosis and other deformities of the spine are the most common associated musculoskeletal anomalies (Table 24-5).[118]

Pectus carinatum is rarely present at birth, and in almost one half of the patients, the deformity was not identified until after the eleventh birthday (Figure 24-10). The deformity often progresses during early childhood, particularly in the period of rapid growth at puberty. The chondromanubrial deformity, in contrast with the chondrogladiolar form, is often noted at birth and is associated with a truncated, comma-shaped sternum with absent sternal segmentation or premature obliteration of the sternal sutures (Figure 24-11). Currarino and Silverman described its association with an increased risk of congenital heart disease.[27] Lees and Caldicott reviewed 1915 thoracic radiographs and identified 135 children with sternal fusion anomalies.[73] Eighteen percent of these children had documented congenital heart disease.

Surgical Repair

Correction of carinate deformities has had a colorful history, beginning with the first repair by Ravitch in 1952 of an upper chondromanubrial deformity.[98] He resected multiple costal cartilages and performed a double sternal osteotomy. In 1953, Lester reported two methods of repair for a lower chondrogladiolar deformity.[74] The first approach, resection of the anterior portion of the sternum, was abandoned because of excessive blood loss and unsatisfactory results. The second method, subperiosteal resection of the entire sternum, was a no less radical technique. Chin and later Brodkin (1958),[16] in a technique called the xiphosternopexy, advanced the transected xiphoid and the attached rectus muscles to a higher site on the sternum.[16,22] This produced posterior displacement of the sternum in younger patients with a flexible chest wall. Howard combined this method with subperichondrial resection of the costal cartilages and a sternal osteotomy.[58] Ravitch reported

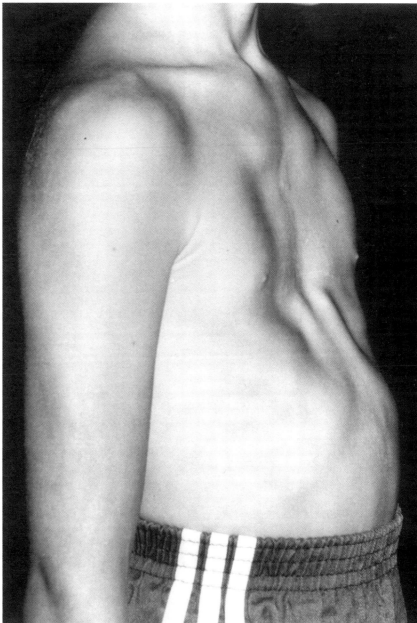

Figure 24–6 Sequence of photographs demonstrating deterioration in the quality of a repair that can occur with time. This boy had an initial excellent result from a Welch repair with suture fixation of the sternum at age 4 years 3 months. The follow-up photographs at 7 years 6 months (**A**),

A

repair of the chondrogladiolar deformity by resection of costal cartilage in a one- or two-stage procedure, with placement of "reefing" sutures to shorten and posteriorly displace the perichondrium.[99] A sternal osteotomy was used in one of three cases. Robicsek and associates described repair by subperichondrial resection of costal cartilages, transverse sternal osteotomy, and resection of the protruding lower portion of the sternum.[104] The xiphoid and rectus muscles were reattached to the new lower margin of the sternum, pulling it posteriorly. In 1973, Welch and Vos reported an approach to these deformities that I continue to use today.[142] Recent attempts at treating children with pectus carinatum by orthotic bracing have been reported, and success has been achieved in younger children, but compliance is limited in older patients because of the pain associated with the bracing.[34,45,84]

Surgical Technique

The placement of the skin incision, mobilization of the pectoral muscle flaps, and subperichondrial resection of the involved costal cartilage are identical to the method described for pectus excavatum. Management of the sternum is shown in Figure 24-12 for the various deformities. In the chondromanubrial deformity, the costal cartilages must be resected from the second cartilage inferiorly.[121] A single-limb medium Hemovac drain (Snyder Laboratories, Inc., New Philadelphia, OH) is brought through the inferior skin flap, as for excavatum patients, with the suction ports in a parasternal position to the level of the highest resected costal cartilage. The pectoralis muscle flaps and skin flaps are closed. Perioperative antibiotics are used as in pectus excavatum.

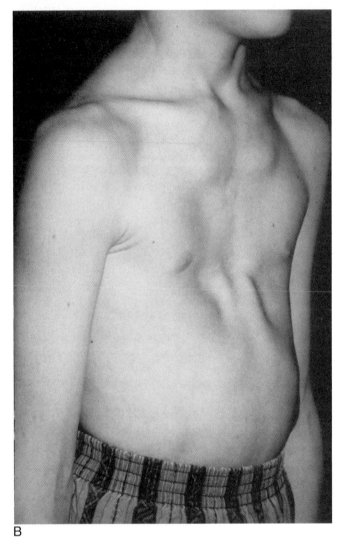

B

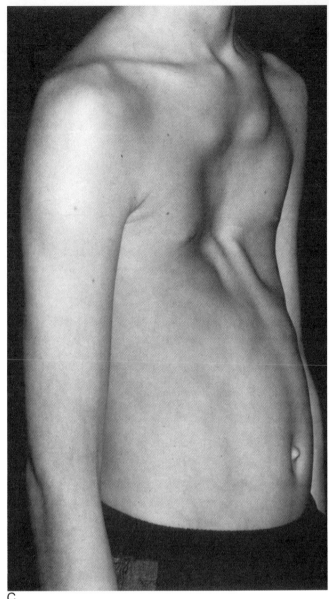

C

Figure 24–6 cont'd 9 years 3 months (**B**), and 12 years 9 months (**C**) demonstrate progressive depression of the sternum and costal cartilages and relative "overgrowth" of the upper chest.

Table 24–4	
Frequency of Pectus Carinatum Deformities	
Deformity	*Number of cases*
Chondrogladiolar	
Symmetrical	89
Asymmetrical	49
Mixed carinatum and excavatum	14
Chondromanubrial	3
Total	155

From Shamberger RC, Welch KJ: Surgical correction of pectus carinatum. J Pediatr Surg 22:48, 1987.

Operative Results

Results are overwhelmingly successful in these patients. In a review of 152 cases, postoperative recovery was generally uneventful.[118] Blood transfusions are rarely required, and none has been given in the last 10 years of the report. There is a 3.9% complication rate (Table 24-6). Only three patients have required revision, each having additional lower costal cartilages resected for persistent unilateral malformation of the costal arch.

▶ POLAND'S SYNDROME

In 1841, Poland, while a medical student, described congenital absence of the pectoralis major and minor muscles associated with syndactyly.[95] Despite a prior report of this entity by Froriep in 1839, the eponym Poland's syndrome has been used since 1962, when Clarkson first applied it to a group of similar patients.[23,41] Subsequent reports have described other components of the syndrome, including

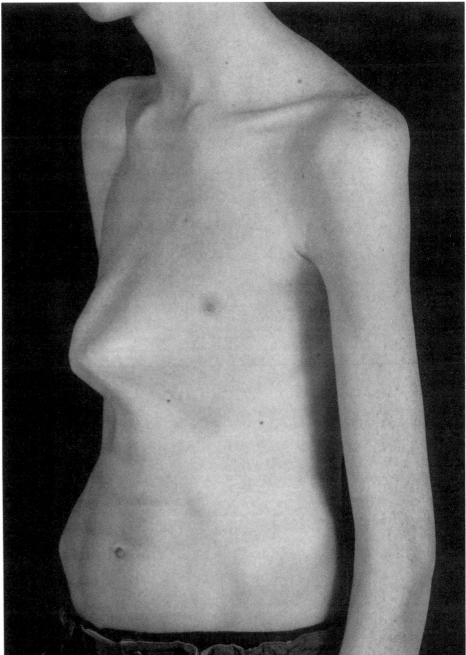

Figure 24–7 Symmetrical chondrogladiolar pectus carinatum in an 11½-year-old boy.

absence of ribs, chest wall depression, and abnormalities of the breasts. Each component of the syndrome occurs with variable severity. The extent of thoracic involvement may range from hypoplasia of the sternal head of the pectoralis major and minor muscles with normal underlying ribs to complete absence of the anterior portions of the second to fifth ribs and costal cartilages (Figures 24-13 and 24-14). Breast involvement is frequent, ranging from mild hypoplasia to complete absence of the breast (amastia) and nipple (athelia) (Figure 24-13C). Minimal subcutaneous fat and an absence of axillary hair are additional components of the syndrome. Hand deformities may include hypoplasia of the fingers (brachydactyly) and fused fingers (syndactyly), primarily involving the central three digits. The most severe expression of the anomaly, mitten or claw deformity

(ectromelia), is rare.[23,134] Poland's syndrome may also occur in combination with Sprengel's deformity, in which there is decreased size, elevation, and winging of the scapula.

Poland's syndrome is present at birth and has an estimated incidence of 1 in 30,000 to 1 in 32,000 births.[40,79] Abnormalities of the breast can be defined at birth by absence of the underlying breast bud and the hypoplastic nipple, which is often superiorly displaced. The etiology of Poland's syndrome is unknown. Bouvet and associates proposed hypoplasia of the ipsilateral subclavian artery as the origin of this malformation, but, as noted by David, decreased blood flow to the extremity may be the result of decreased muscle mass of the hypoplastic limb rather than its cause.[13,30] Although some forms of syndactyly are autosomal dominant traits, a similar pattern has not been

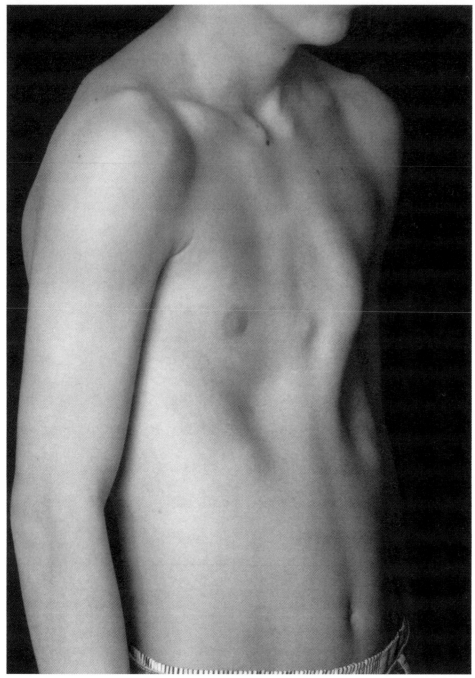

Figure 24–8 A 15-year-old boy with marked asymmetrical pectus carinatum demonstrates protrusion of the costal cartilages limited to the left side of his chest.

demonstrated in patients with Poland's syndrome, which is generally sporadic. Multiple cases within a family are rare.[24,29,127] Poland's syndrome is associated with a second rare syndrome, the Möbius syndrome; bilateral or unilateral facial palsy and abducens oculi palsy. Nineteen such cases have been identified, but a unifying etiology is lacking. An unusual association between Poland's syndrome and childhood leukemia has also been reported.[10,39]

The Boston Children's Hospital's experience with Poland's syndrome from 1970 to 1987 included 41 children and adolescents, of whom 21 were males.[116] The lesion was right sided in 23 patients, left sided in 17 patients, and bilateral in 1 patient. Hand anomalies were noted in 23 (56%) and breast anomalies in 25 (61%). In 10 children the underlying thoracic

abnormality required reconstruction, and in three children, rib or cartilage grafts were needed for complete repair.

Surgical Repair

Assessment of the extent of involvement of the various musculoskeletal components is critical for optimal thoracic reconstruction. If the deformity is limited to the sternal component of the pectoralis major and minor muscles without underlying chest wall deformity, there is little functional deficit and repair is unnecessary, except to facilitate breast augmentation in females (see Figure 24-14). If the underlying costal cartilages are depressed or absent, repair must be considered to minimize the concavity, to eliminate the

Text continued on pg. 378

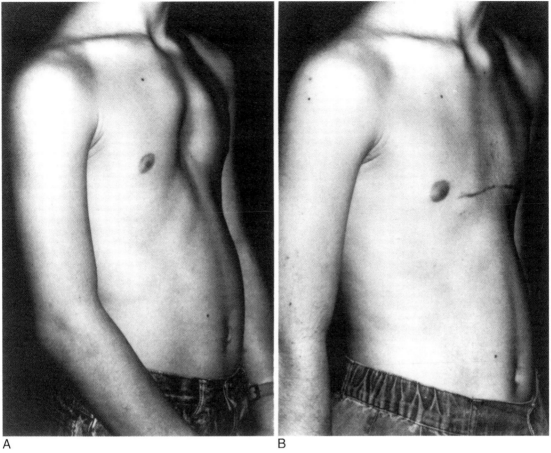

A B

Figure 24–9 A, A 15-year-old boy with the chondromanubrial deformity. Note the posterior depression of the lower sternum, accentuated by the anterior bowing of the second and third costal cartilages. **B,** After repair, the sternal contour is improved and costal cartilages are reformed in a more appropriate fashion.

Table 24–5

Musculoskeletal Abnormalities Identified in 30 of 152 Cases of Pectus Carinatum

Musculoskeletal abnormality	Number of cases
Scoliosis	23
Neurofibromatosis	2
Morquio's disease	2
Vertebral anomalies	1
Hyperlordosis	1
Kyphosis	1

From Shamberger RC, Welch KJ: Surgical correction of pectus carinatum. J Pediatr Surg 22:48, 1987, with permission.

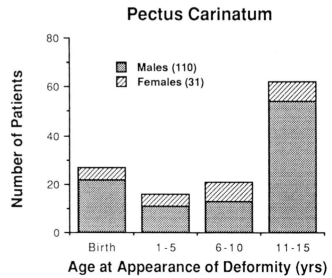

Figure 24–10 Age at appearance of pectus carinatum deformity in 141 infants and children. Note the appearance of protrusion in almost one half of the children at puberty. *(From Shamberger RC, Welch KJ: Surgical correction of pectus carinatum. J Pediatr Surg 22:48–53, 1987, with permission.)*

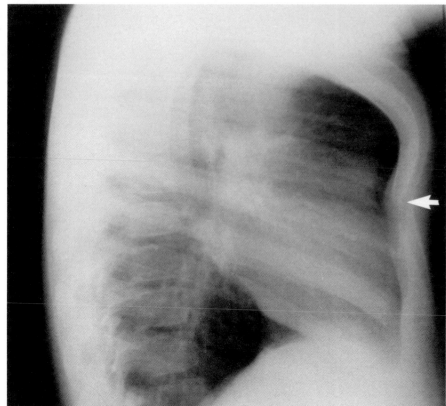

Figure 24–11 Lateral chest radiograph of a boy with chondromanubrial pectus carinatum. The short, comma-shaped sternum lacking segmentation is apparent. Arrow is at the tip of the truncated sternum.
(From Shamberger RC, Welch KJ: Surgical correction of chondromanubrial deformity [Currarino Silverman syndrome]. J Pediatr Surg 23:319, 1988, with permission.)

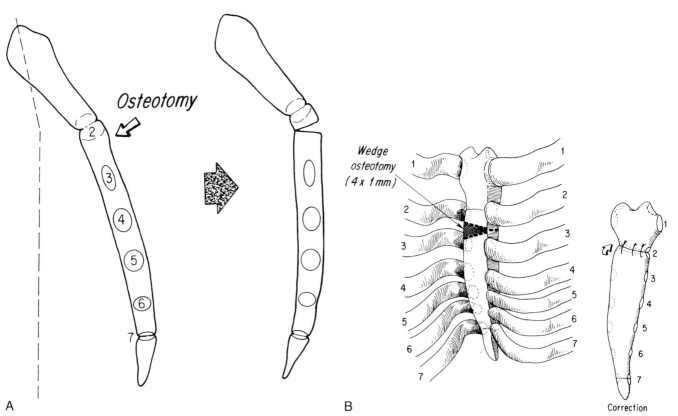

Figure 24–12 A, A single or double osteotomy after resection of the costal cartilages allows posterior displacement of the sternum to an orthotopic position. **B,** The mixed pectus deformity is corrected by full and symmetrical resection of the third to seventh costal cartilages, followed by transverse offset (0–10 degrees wedge-shaped sternal osteotomy). Closure of this defect achieves both anterior displacement and rotation of the sternum.
(From Shamberger RC, Welch KJ: Surgical correction of pectus carinatum. J Pediatr Surg 22:48, 1987, with permission.)

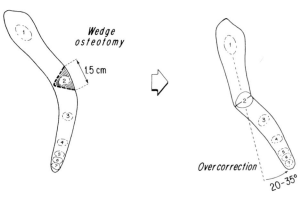

Wedge osteotomy

1.5 cm

Overcorrection

20-35°

Chondromanubrial (very rare)

C

Figure 24–12 cont'd C, The chondromanubrial type of deformity is depicted with a broad, wedge-shaped sternal osteotomy placed through the anterior cortex of the obliterated sternomanubrial junction. Closure of the osteotomy after fracture of the posterior cortex achieves a posterior displacement of the superior portion of the sternum, which is secured only by its attachment to the first rib. The lower portion of the sternum is overcorrected 20–35° and is secured in position by strut or suture fixation. (*From Shamberger RC, Welch KJ: Surgical correction of chondromanubrial deformity. J Pediatr Surg 23:319, 1988, with permission.*)

Table 24–6

Complications of Pectus Carinatum Repair: 7 Cases in 152 Patients

Complication	Number of cases
Pneumothorax[a]	4
Atelectasis	1
Wound infection	1
Local tissue necrosis	1

[a]Two patients required chest tube placement.

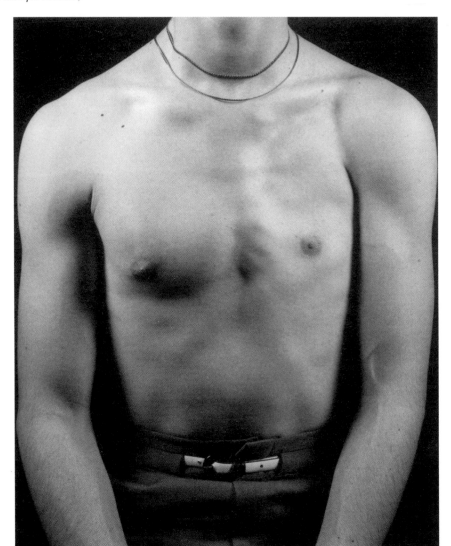

Figure 24–13 **A,** Muscular 15-year-old boy with Poland's syndrome with loss of the left axillary fold owing to absence of the pectoralis major muscle. He has an orthotopic sternum and normal cartilages. He compensates adequately for loss of the pectoralis major and minor muscles. Surgery is not indicated in males with these findings.

A

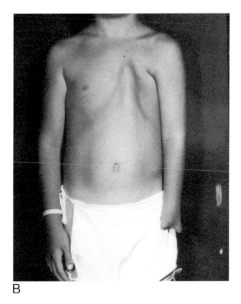

B

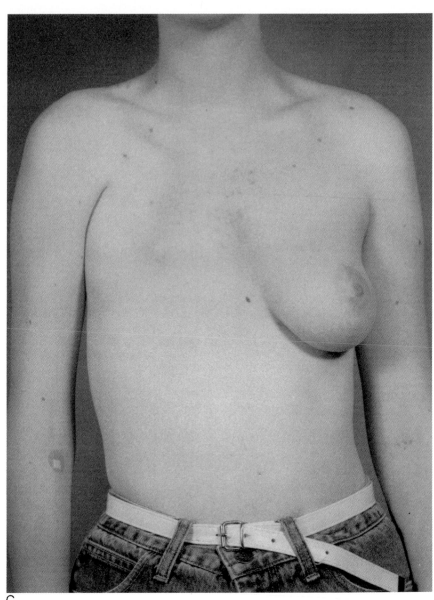

C

Figure 24–13 cont'd B, Eight-year-old boy with Poland's syndrome and more extensive thoracic involvement. The pectoralis major and minor muscles and the serratus to the level of the fifth rib are absent. There is sternal obliquity, and the third to fifth ribs are aplastic, ending at the level of the nipple. The corresponding costal cartilages are absent. The endothoracic fascia lies beneath a thin layer of subcutaneous tissue. Note the hypoplastic nipple and ectromelia of the ipsilateral hand, the most severe malformation of the hand associated with Poland's syndrome. **C,** Fourteen-year-old girl with Poland's syndrome. Note the high position of the right nipple, amastia, sternal rotation, and depressed right chest. The anterior second to fourth ribs and cartilages were missing. Breast augmentation will be required after the ipsilateral breast achieves full growth.

paradoxic motion of the chest wall if ribs are absent, and in girls to provide an optimal base for breast reconstruction. Ravitch reported correction of posteriorly displaced costal cartilages by unilateral resection of the cartilages, a wedge osteotomy of the sternum allowing rotation of the sternum, and fixation with Rehbein struts and Steinmann pins.[100] I have achieved suitable repair in most cases with bilateral costal cartilage resection and an oblique osteotomy, which corrects both the sternal rotation and posterior displacement, as in the patients with mixed pectus carinatum and excavatum deformity (Figure 24-15). The sternum is then displaced anteriorly and is supported with a retrosternal strut, which allows correction of the posteriorly displaced costal cartilages. An unappreciated carinate deformity is often present on the contralateral side, which accentuates the ipsilateral concavity (see Figure 24-14B).

Absence of the medial portion of the ribs can be managed with split rib grafts taken from the contralateral side. These must be secured to the sternum medially and to the "dagger point" ends of the hypoplastic ribs laterally. The grafts can be covered with a prosthetic mesh if needed for further support. In these cases, it must be remembered that there is little tissue present between the endothoracic fascia and the fascial remnants of the pectoral muscles.

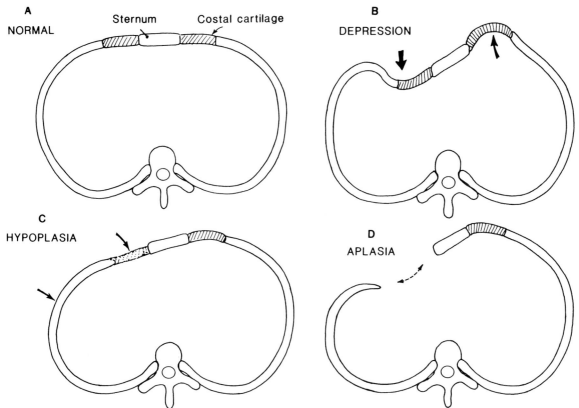

Figure 24–14 These figures depict the spectrum of thoracic abnormality seen in Poland's syndrome. **A,** Most frequently, an entirely normal thorax is present, and only pectoral muscles are absent. **B,** Depression of the involved side of the chest wall, with rotation and often depression of the sternum. A carinate protrusion of the contralateral side is frequently present. **C,** Hypoplasia of ribs on the involved side but without significant depression may be seen. It usually does not require surgical correction. **D,** Aplasia of one or more ribs is usually associated with depression of adjacent ribs on the involved side and rotation of the sternum.
(From Shamberger RC, Welch KJ, Upton J III: Surgical treatment of thoracic deformity in Poland's syndrome. J Pediatr Surg 24:760, 1989, with permission).

Soft tissue coverage of the area can be augmented with transfer of a latissimus dorsi muscle flap. This is particularly helpful in girls who will require breast augmentation.[47,90] Flap rotation is seldom, if ever, required in boys and has the disadvantage of adding a second posterior thoracic scar and decreasing the strength of the latissimus dorsi muscle.

► STERNAL DEFECTS

Sternal defects are rare compared with pectus excavatum and carinatum, yet they have received a great deal of attention in the medical literature because of their dramatic presentation and often fatal outcome. Deformities resulting from failure of ventral fusion of the sternum can be divided into four groups: (1) cleft sternum, (2) thoracic ectopia cordis, (3) thoracoabdominal ectopia cordis, and (4) cervical ectopia cordis. The heart is in a normal position in cleft sternum, but is displaced in the other three entities. In thoracic ectopia cordis, the heart protrudes anteriorly and there are no tissues covering the heart. In cervical ectopia cordis, the protrusion is even more pronounced and the heart is often fused with the head. In thoracoabdominal ectopia cordis,

the heart is covered, but often displaced into the abdomen through a defect in the diaphragm.

► CLEFT STERNUM

An infant with cleft sternum has a complete or partial separation of the sternum, but a normally positioned intrathoracic heart. This deformity results from failure of fusion of the sternal bars, which should occur about the eighth week of gestation. In all such cases, despite the sternal separation, normal skin coverage is present, with an intact pericardium and a normal diaphragm. Abdominal wall defects such as omphalocele do not occur in these children. The condition causes few functional problems. A dramatic increase in the protrusion of the deformity occurs with crying or Valsalva's maneuver. The sternal defects described in 109 cases are summarized in Table 24-7.[117] The cleft involves primarily the upper sternum, whereas patients with thoracic or thoracoabdominal ectopia cordis have clefts primarily of the lower sternum.

The second distinction between cleft sternum and the other sternal defects is that children with cleft sternum rarely have intrinsic congenital heart disease. An unexplained

Text continued on pg. 382

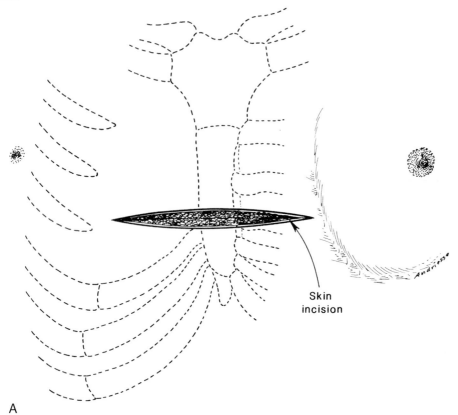

Skin
incision

A

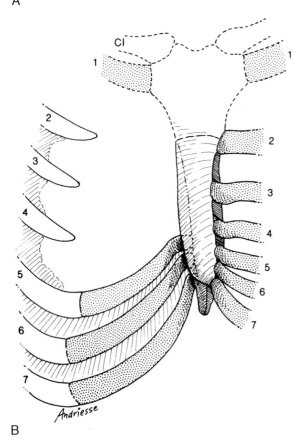

B

Figure 24–15 A, A transverse incision is placed below the nipple lines and, in females, in the inframammary crease. **B,** Schematic depiction of the deformity, with rotation of the sternum, depression of the cartilages of the involved side, and carinate protrusion of the contralateral side.

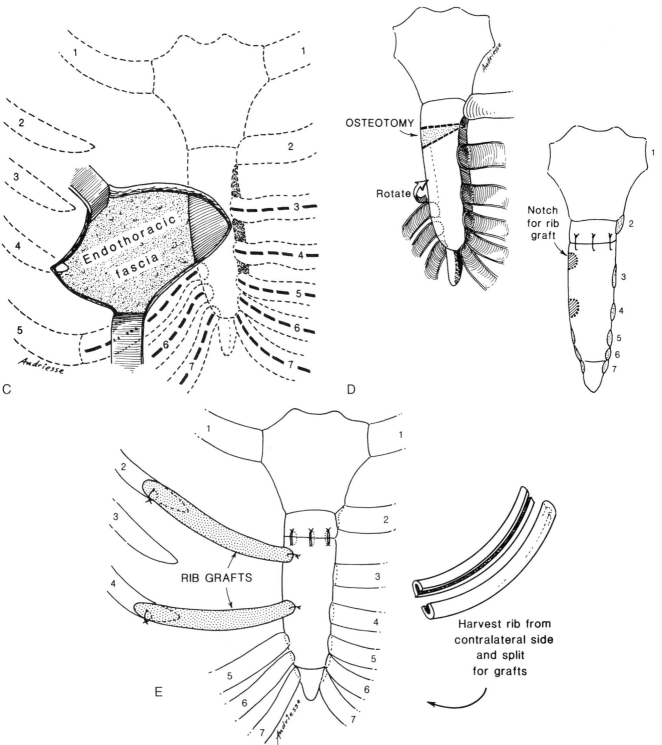

Figure 24–15 cont'd C, In patients with aplasia of the ribs, the endothoracic fascia is encountered directly below the attenuated subcutaneous tissue and pectoral fascia. The pectoral muscle flap is elevated on the contralateral side and the pectoral fascia, if present, on the involved side. Subperichondrial resection of the costal cartilages is then carried out, as shown by the bold dashed lines. Rarely, this must be carried to the level of the second costal cartilages. **D,** A transverse, offset, wedge-shaped sternal osteotomy is created below the second costal cartilage. Elevation of the sternum with a retrosternal strut corrects both the posterior displacement and the rotation of the sternum. **E,** In patients with rib aplasia, split rib grafts are harvested from the contralateral fifth or sixth rib and then secured medially with wire sutures into previously created sternal notches and with wire to the native ribs laterally. Ribs are split as shown along their short axis to maintain maximum mechanical strength.

(From Shamberger RC, Welch KJ, Upton J III: Surgical treatment of thoracic deformity in Poland's syndrome. J Pediatr Surg 24:760, 1989, with permission.)

Table 24–7

Sternal Defects Reported in 109 Cases of Cleft Sternum

Sternal defect	Number of cases
Upper cleft	46
Upper cleft to xiphoid	33
Complete cleft	23
Lower defect with manubrium or midsegment intact	5
Central (skin ulceration noted in only three cases) defect with manubrium and xiphoid intact	2

From Shamberger RC, Welch KJ: Sternal defects. Pediatr Surg Int 5:156, 1990, with permission.

association does exist, however, between cleft sternum and cervicofacial hemangiomas, which were reported in 14 cases since the first description of this association by Fischer in 1879.[37]

Surgical Repair

Maier and Bortone accomplished the first primary repair of cleft sternum in 1949 in a 6-week-old infant.[76] The flexibility of the newborn chest allows approximation of the sternal bars without producing cardiac compression (Figure 24-16). A summary of the reported repairs for cleft sternum in 69 cases is shown in Table 24-8.

Sabiston reported reconstruction of cleft sternum using multiple oblique chondrotomies.[106] The chondrotomies increase the chest wall dimensions and flexibility. The technique is useful in older infants and children with a less flexible chest and a wide defect. Meissner described a variation of repair in which the cartilages are divided laterally and swung medially to cover the defect.[81] Autologous grafts of costal cartilage, split ribs, and segments of the costal arch have been used since Burton first repaired this defect with a portion of the costal arch.[18] Repairs with prosthetic material are far less satisfactory because of the risks of infection and the inability of these tissues to grow with the child. Most

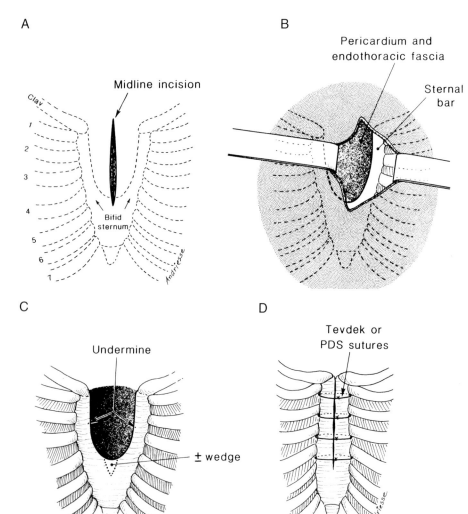

Figure 24–16 A, Repair of bifid sternum is best performed through a longitudinal incision extending the length of the defect. **B,** Directly beneath the subcutaneous tissues the sternal bars are encountered, with pectoral muscles present lateral to the bars. **C,** The endothoracic fascia is mobilized off the sternal bars posteriorly with blunt dissection to allow safe placement of the sutures. Approximation of the sternal bars may be facilitated by excising a wedge of cartilage inferiorly. **D,** Closure of the defect is achieved with 2-0 Tevdek or PDS (Ethicon, Inc., Sommerville, NJ) sutures.
(From Shamberger RC, Welch KJ: Sternal defects. Pediatr Surg Int 5:156, 1990, with permission.)

authors now recommend treatment of cleft sternum in the newborn period, when simple direct closure is possible without the use of prosthetic materials or grafts.

Ectopia Cordis

Although treatment of isolated cleft sternum is routinely successful, surgical repair of ectopia cordis has a high mortality, particularly thoracic ectopia cordis. The lethal factor in thoracic ectopia cordis and cervical ectopia cordis is the extrathoracic location of the heart, which makes tissue coverage difficult. In thoracoabdominal ectopia cordis (the Cantrell pentalogy), the major impediment to survival is the high incidence of intrinsic congenital heart disease.[20]

Etiology

The etiology of thoracic ectopia cordis and thoracoabdominal ectopia cordis is much debated. Some consider these anomalies to be the result of disruption of the amnion and possibly disruption of the chorionic layer or yolk sac as well.[55,56,67,91] This disruption occurs during the third or fourth week of gestation at a time when cardiac chamber formation is occurring rapidly. This timing may account for the high incidence of abnormal cardiac development. VonPraagh (personal communication, 1987) has the intriguing notion, based on embryology studies by Patten and Bremer, that acute hyperflexion of the craniocervical segment of the embryo pins the heart down in the extrathoracic position with the submental cardiac apex.[14,93] The abnormal fetal configuration produced by oligohydramnios may persist to delivery and oppose traction by the gubernaculum cordis, which normally pulls the cardiac apex into caudal alignment. Chromosome abnormalities have been reported.[68,112,126]

Thoracic Ectopia Cordis

Thoracic ectopia cordis is one of the most dramatic occurrences in the delivery room (Figure 24-17). The naked beating heart is external to the thorax. Clearly visible are the atrial appendages, coronary vasculature, and cephalic orientation of the cardiac apex. The gubernaculum cordis initially extends to the supraumbilical raphe. Thoracic ectopia cordis was first reported by Stensen in 1671.[125] Stensen's report was later translated by Willius.[146] Stensen identified the four components of the tetralogy of Fallot in this patient with thoracic ectopia cordis (such is the fate of eponyms). Cardiac anomalies are unusually frequent in thoracic ectopia cordis. Table 24-9 lists the associated cardiac anomalies reported up to 1990. Only four of 75 cases had no intrinsic cardiac anomalies.

Infants with thoracic ectopia cordis are severely deficient in the midline somatic tissues that normally cover the heart. Many attempts at primary closure fail because of the inability to mobilize adequate tissues for coverage. An abdominal defect is often present as well. Recent computed tomogram evaluation by Haynor and associates also shows reduced intrathoracic volume in these infants.[50] Most allegedly successful repairs have been not of true thoracic ectopia cordis but, rather, of thoracoabdominal ectopia cordis. Cutler and Wilens first attempted repair in 1925 by skin flap coverage, but failed because of cessation of cardiac function, presumably from compression of the heart.[28] Only three survivors of more than 29 attempts have been recorded (Table 24-10).

The first successful repair of ectopia cordis was achieved by Koop in 1975 and was reported by Saxena.[111] An infant with a normal heart had skin flap coverage at 5 h of age, with inferior mobilization of the anterior attachments of the diaphragm. The sternal bars were 2 inches apart and could not be approximated primarily without cardiac compression and compromise. At 7 months of age, an acrylic resin of Dacron and Marlex mesh was inserted to close the sternal cleft, followed by primary skin closure. Necrosis of the skin flaps complicated the postoperative course with infection of the prosthetic material, which was later removed. This child is alive at age 20 years and is reported to be entirely well.

Successful closure in two other infants is reported. Dobell and associates also achieved closure in two stages.[33] Skin flap coverage was provided for the newborn. Rib strut grafts were placed over the sternal defect at 19 months of age and covered with pectoral muscle flaps. The pericardium was divided from its anterior attachments to the chest wall, allowing the heart to fall back partially into the thoracic cavity. Only Amato and colleagues achieved complete coverage of the heart in one stage.[3] The unifying theme of successfully managed cases is mobilization of adequate soft tissue to cover the heart in its extrathoracic location and avoiding attempts to return the

Table 24–8	
Methods of Repair of Cleft Sternum in 69 Cases	

Method of repair	*Number of cases*
Primary approximation and repair	25
Primary repair with sliding chondrotomies (Sabiston)	19
Primary repair with rotating chondrotomies (Meissner)	3
Primary repair with other chondrotomy	4
Bone or cartilage graft	8
Prosthetic mesh graft	4
Sternocleidomastoid muscle transposition	3
Transposition of local soft tissues	2
Skin closure with excision of ulcer	1

From Shamberger RC, Welch KJ: Sternal defects. Pediatr Surg Int 5:156, 1990, with permission.

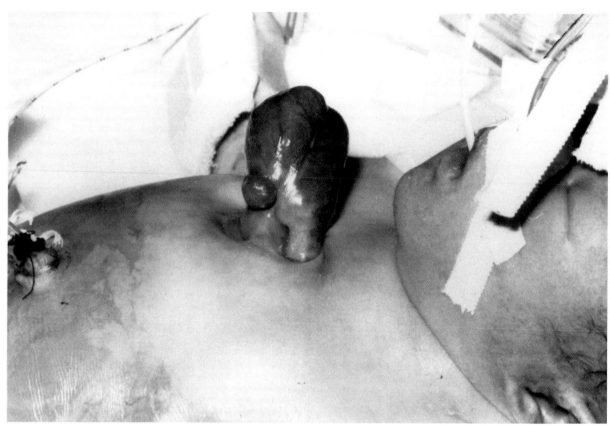

Figure 24–17 An infant with thoracic ectopia cordis with no abdominal wall defect. The cardiac apex is cephalad. Any movement of the heart results in bradycardia and arrest. The patient had complex tetralogy of Fallot.

heart to an orthotopic location. Of note, in the successful cases, intrinsic cardiac lesions and associated abdominal defects were absent. These are the characteristics that most distinguish the successes from the failures, rather than any differences in surgical techniques. Coverage of the heart with autologous tissues, whether by flap rotation or bipedicle flaps, generally produces excessive compression on the heart, which limits cardiac output either by kinking outflow vessels or impeding cardiac filling. In most instances, attempts are abandoned in the operating room because of severe impairment of cardiac function. In patients who are repaired with autologous tissue grafts (bone or cartilage) or synthetic materials, infection and extrusion of the graft invariably occur. Ultimate success with this lesion will be achieved only by accomplishing tissue coverage of the heart that avoids posterior displacement into an already limited thoracic space. This will require use of tissues from sites distant from the chest wall or tissue engineered materials. Severe intracardiac defects associated with thoracic ectopia cordis in most cases also limit survival. The only recent advancement in management of this lesion has been early ultrasonographic diagnosis including definition of the intracardiac lesion and termination of the pregnancy, if acceptable to the parents.[71,82]

Abdominal wall defects are also frequent in these patients, including an upper abdominal omphalocele or diastasis recti and, rarely, eventration of the abdominal viscera (Figure 24-18). Associated abdominal wall defects are summarized in Table 24-11. The presence of abdominal defects should not, however, lead to classification of these lesions as thoracoab-

dominal ectopia cordis. This term should be reserved for those infants in whom the heart is covered at birth.

Thoracoabdominal Ectopia Cordis (Cantrell's Pentalogy)

In thoracoabdominal ectopia cordis, the heart is covered by an omphalocele-like membrane or thin skin, which is often pigmented. The sternum is generally cleft inferiorly, and the heart lacks the severe anterior rotation present in thoracic ectopia cordis. An early report of this lesion by Wilson in 1798 clearly defined the associated somatic defects of the abdominal wall, diaphragm, and pericardium (Figure 24-19) as well as the intrinsic cardiac anomalies. This entity was subsequently reviewed by Major in 1953 and Cantrell and associates in 1958.[20,77] It is now frequently called Cantrell's pentalogy, although it was described long before Cantrell's relatively recent review. The five essential features of thoracoabdominal ectopia cordis are a cleft lower sternum; a half moon-shaped anterior diaphragmatic defect resulting from lack of development of the septum transversum; absence of the parietal pericardium at the diaphragmatic defect; omphalocele (Table 24-12); and, in most patients, an intrinsic cardiac anomaly (Table 24-13 and Figure 24-19). A left ventricular diverticulum occurs with surprising frequency in this anomaly. In many cases, the diverticulum protrudes through the diaphragmatic and pericardial defects into the abdominal cavity.

Successful repair and long-term survival are more frequent in thoracoabdominal ectopia cordis than in thoracic

Table 24–9

Intrinsic Cardiac Lesions Reported: 75 Cases of Thoracic Ectopia Cordis

Cardiac lesion	Number of cases
Tetralogy of Fallot	16
Pulmonary artery stenosis	6
Transposition of great arteries and pulmonary artery stenosis or atresia	8
Patent ductus arteriosus (PDA)	2
Tricuspid and pulmonary atresia	3
Ventricular septal defect (VSD) and atrial septal defect (ASD)	6
VSD	5
ASD and PDA	4
ASD	1
Truncus arteriosus	3
Coarctation, ASD, and PDA	1
Coarctation	1
Aortic hypoplasia	1
Double-outlet left ventricle	2
Double-outlet right ventricle	2
Aortic stenosis, ASD, and PDA	1
Single atrium, single ventricle	3
Double atrium, single ventricle	3
Cor triatriatum	1

Table 24–9

Intrinsic Cardiac Lesions Reported: 75 Cases of Thoracic Ectopia Cordis—cont'd

Cardiac lesion	Number of cases
Aberrant right subclavian artery	1
Bilateral superior vena cava[a]	1
Normal	4

From Shamberger RC, Welch KJ: Sternal defects. Pediatr Surg Int 5:156, 1990, with permission.

[a]Also present in association with many of the listed anomalies.

Table 24–10

Reported Survivors of Thoracic Ectopia Cordis and Their Repair

Cardiac author	Year	Lesion	Method of sternal closure
Koop and Saxena[111]	1975	None	Skin flap closure at 5 h; acrylic resin applied to sternal cleft at 7 months
Dobell et al[33]	1982	None	Perinatal skin closure in one stage; second stage repair with skin grafts
Amato, Cotroneo, and Gladieri[3]	1988	None	Skin flaps mobilized, diaphragm moved inferiorly, Gore-Tex[a] membrane used to close defect with skin flaps over it; child survived, but died of aspiration at 11 months of age

From Shamberger RC, Welch KJ: Sternal defects. Pediatr Surg Int 5:156, 1990, with permission.

[a]Gore-Tex: WL Gore & Associates, Inc., Flagstaff, AZ.

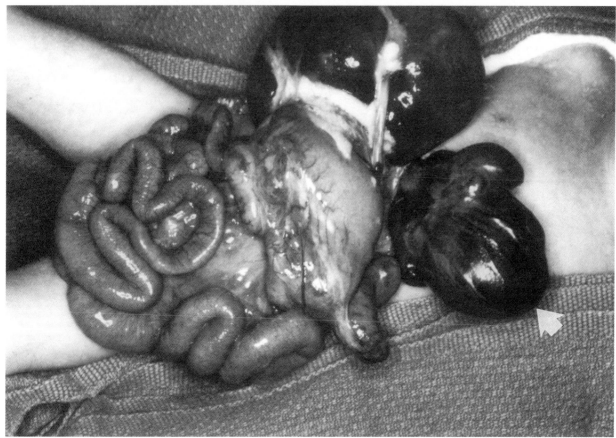

Figure 24–18 Infant with thoracic ectopia cordis *(arrow)* and eventration of the abdominal viscera. *(From Shamberger RC: Sternal defects. Pediatr Surg Int 5:156, 1990, with permission.)*

ectopia cordis. Arndt attempted the first repair in 1896, but return of the heart to the thoracic cavity resulted in death.[4] Wieting performed the first successful surgical repair in 1912.[143] He achieved primary closure of the diaphragm and abdominal wall fascia, but ignored the ventricular diverticulum. Initial surgical intervention must address the skin

defects overlying the heart and abdominal cavity. Primary excision of the omphalocele with skin closure avoids infection and mediastinitis, although several cases have been successfully managed by local application of topical astringents, thus allowing secondary epithelialization to occur. Several early cases, as in that of Cullerier in 1806, document the long-term viability of individuals with thoracoabdominal ectopia cordis with intact skin coverage despite the abnormal location and coverage of the heart.[26]

Advances in cardiac surgery now allow correction of the intrinsic cardiac lesions, which were previously fatal. An aggressive approach to repair in infants with thoracoabdominal ectopia cordis is appropriate. Repair of the abdominal wall defect or diastasis has been achieved by primary closure or prosthetic mesh (Table 24-14). Primary closure of the thoracoabdominal defect may be difficult to achieve because of the wide separation of the rectus muscles and their superior attachment to the costal arches. Complete repair of the intracardiac defect is best performed before placement of prosthetic mesh overlying the heart. Repair of the abdomen and chest wall is important primarily for mechanical protection of the heart and abdominal viscera. Early diagnosis by prenatal ultrasound has not altered the surgical approach or overall mortality of this lesion. Three patients in the Boston Children's Hospital series had severe pulmonary hypoplasia, which was lethal in two, a previously unreported association.[117]

Table 24–11

Abdominal Wall Defects Reported in 75 Cases of Thoracic Ectopia Cordis

Abdominal wall defect	Number of cases
Omphalocele	36
Diastasis recti (or ventral hernia)[a]	6
Eventration	4

From Shamberger RC, Welch KJ: Sternal defects. Pediatr Surg Int 5:156, 1990, with permission.
[a]Often covered by thin, pigmented dermis.

Text continued on pg. 389

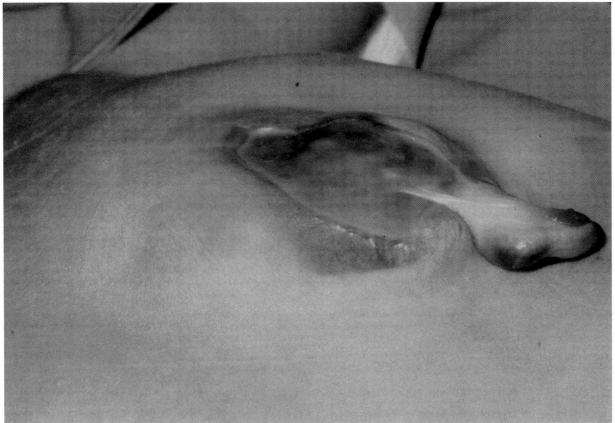

Figure 24–19 **Newborn male with thoracoabdominal ectopia cordis**. The head is to the left. Note the epigastric omphalocele extending superior to the umbilicus. The cardiac apex was visible below the costal arch just at the superior aspect of the omphalocele.

Table 24–12

Abdominal Wall Defects Reported in Patients with Thoracoabdominal Ectopia Cordis

Abdominal wall defect	Number of cases
Omphalocele	64
Diastasis recti (or ventral hernia)	40
Diaphragmatic defect	71
Pericardial defect	46

From Shamberger RC, Welch KJ: Sternal defects. Pediatr Surg Int 5:156, 1990, with permission.

Table 24–13

Intrinsic Cardiac Lesions Reported in Patients with Thoracoabdominal Ectopia Cordis

Cardiac lesion	Number of cases
Tetralogy of Fallot	13
Tetralogy of Fallot and diverticulum of left ventricle	1
Diverticulum of left ventricle	16
Diverticulum of left ventricle and ventricular septal defect (VSD)	9
Diverticulum of left ventricle, pulmonary stenosis, and VSD	1
Diverticulum of left ventricle and atrial septal defect (ASD)	1
Diverticulum of left ventricle, ASD, and VSD	1

(Continued)

Table 24–13

Intrinsic Cardiac Lesions Reported in Patients with Thoracoabdominal Ectopia Cordis—cont'd

Cardiac lesion	Number of cases
Diverticulum of left ventricle, VSD, and mitral stenosis	1
Diverticulum of left ventricle, hypoplastic left ventricle, and VSD	1
VSD	8
VSD and ASD	2
VSD and single atrium	1
ASD	3
ASD, VSD, and total anomalous pulmonary venous connection	1
Truncus arteriosus	5
Single atrium and single ventricle	5
Pulmonary atresia and single ventricle	2
Pulmonary atresia, VSD, and patent ductus arteriosus	1
Pulmonary stenosis and VSD	3
Tricuspid atresia	4
Double-outlet left ventricle	2
Double-outlet right ventricle	2
Transposition of the great arteries, mitral atresia, and pulmonary artery hypoplasia	1
Transposition of the great arteries and pulmonary artery stenosis	2
Transposition great arteries and VSD	1

Table 24–13

Intrinsic Cardiac Lesions Reported in Patients with Thoracoabdominal Ectopia Cordis—cont'd

Cardiac lesion	Number of cases
Aortic stenosis, ASD, and VSD	1
Bilateral superior vena cava[a]	1
Normal	5

From Shamberger RC, Welch KJ: Sternal defects. Pediatr Surg Int 5:156, 1990, with permission.
[a]Also present in association with many of the listed anomalies.

Table 24–14

Reported Methods of Repair of Thoracoabdominal Ectopia Cordis

Method of repair	Number of cases
Primary closure of diaphragm and abdominal wall defect	8
Primary closure of skin only and excision of omphalocele	7
Primary closure of diaphragm	4
Primary closure of abdominal wall defect	2
Coverage of abdominal defect with Silastic pouch and secondary epithelialization	3
Resection of lower ribs and sternum to increase room in chest with inferior attachment of diaphragm and primary skin coverage	1
Staged repair with initial skin closure with secondary prosthetic mesh closure of the abdominal and thoracic defect	1
Staged repair with initial skin closure with secondary closure of the abdominal wall and diaphragm	1

From Shamberger RC, Welch KJ: Sternal defects. Pediatr Surg Int 5:156, 1990, with permission.

THORACIC DEFORMITIES IN DIFFUSE SKELETAL DISORDERS

Asphyxiating Thoracic Dystrophy (Jeune's Disease)

In 1954, Jeune and colleagues described a newborn with a narrow rigid chest and multiple cartilage anomalies.[63] The patient died of respiratory insufficiency early in the perinatal period. Subsequent authors have further characterized this form of osteochondrodystrophy, which has variable degrees of skeletal involvement. It is inherited in an autosomal recessive pattern and is not associated with chromosomal abnormalities. Its most prominent feature is a narrow, bell-shaped thorax and protuberant abdomen. The thorax is narrow in both the transverse and sagittal axis and has little respiratory motion due to the horizontal direction of the ribs (Figure 24-20). The ribs are short and wide, and the splayed costochondral junctions barely reach the anterior axillary line. The costal cartilage is abundant and irregular, like a rachitic rosary. Microscopic examination of the costochondral junction demonstrates disordered and poorly progressing endochondral ossification, resulting in decreased rib length.

Skeletal abnormalities associated with this syndrome include short stubby extremities with relatively short and wide bones. The clavicles are in a fixed and elevated

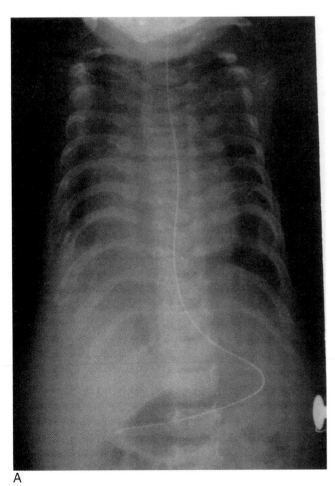

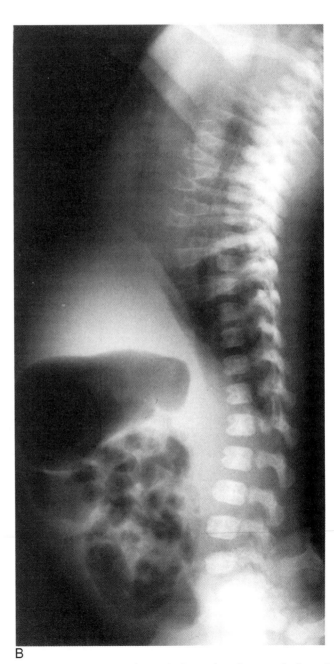

Figure 24–20 Jeune's disease (asphyxiating thoracic dystrophy). **A,** Anteroposterior radiograph shows short horizontal ribs and narrow chest. **B,** Lateral radiograph demonstrates that the short ribs end at the midaxillary line. Abnormal flaring at the costochondral junctions is also present. The patient died of progressive respiratory insufficiency at 1 month of age. There was no surgical intervention. Postmortem examination revealed alveolar hypoplasia.

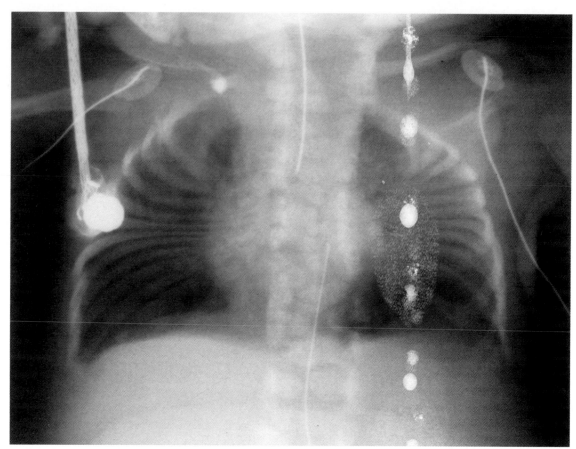

Figure 24–21 **Chest radiograph of an infant with spondylothoracic dysplasia.** Severe abnormality of the spine is apparent, with multiple alternating hemivertebrae producing a "crablike" configuration to the ribs.

position, and the pelvis is small and hypoplastic, with square iliac bones.

The syndrome has a variable extent of pulmonary impairment. Although the initial cases reported resulted in neonatal deaths, subsequent reports by Kozlowski and Masel and others have documented that infants can survive for longer intervals of time with this syndrome.[70] The pathological findings in autopsy cases reveal a range of abnormal pulmonary development. In most cases, the bronchial development is normal and there are fewer alveolar divisions, as described by Williams and associates.[144]

Spondylothoracic Dysplasia (Jarcho–Levin Syndrome)

Spondylothoracic dysplasia is an autosomal recessive deformity with multiple vertebral and rib malformations, described by Jarcho and Levin in 1938.[62] Infants and children with this syndrome have multiple alternating hemivertebrae in most, if not all, of the thoracic and lumbar spine. The vertebral ossification centers rarely cross the midline, although bone formation is normal. Multiple posterior fusions of the ribs and remarkable shortening of the thoracic spine result in a "crab-like" appearance of the ribs on the chest radiograph (Figure 24-21).

The thoracic deformity is secondary to the spine anomaly, which results in close posterior approximation of the origin of the ribs. Although most infants with the entity succumb before 15 months of age, as reviewed by Roberts and colleagues, no surgical efforts have been proposed or attempted.[103] One third of patients with this syndrome have associated malformations, including congenital heart disease and renal anomalies. Heilbronner and Renshaw have reported its occurrence primarily in Puerto Rican families (15 of 18 cases).[54]

REFERENCES

1. Adkins PC, Blades B: A stainless steel strut for correction of pectus excavatum. Surg Gynecol Obstet 113:111–113, 1961.
2. Allen RG, Douglas M: Cosmetic improvement of thoracic wall defects using a rapid setting silastic mold: A special technique. J Pediatr Surg 14:745–749, 1979.
3. Amato JT, Krauss AH, Gladiere R: Repair of complete ectopia cordis. Presented at American College of Surgeons Clinical Congress, Chicago, October 23–28, 1988.
4. Arndt C: Nabelschnurbruch mit Herzhernie: Operation durch Laparotomie mit todlichem Ausgang. Centralbl Gynakol 20:632–633, 1896.
5. Backer OG, Brunner S, Larsen V: The surgical treatment of funnel chest. Initial and follow-up results. Acta Chir Scand 121:253–261, 1961.
6. Baronofsky ID: Technique for the correction of pectus excavatum. Surgery 42:884–890, 1957.

7. Beiser GD, Epstein SE, Stampfer M, et al: Impairment of cardiac function in patients with pectus excavatum, with improvement after operative correction. N Engl J Med 287:67–272, 1972.

8. Bevegård S: Postural circulatory changes at rest and during exercise in patients with pectus excavatum. Acta Med Scand 171:695–713, 1962.

9. Blickman J: Pectus excavatum in children. Radiology 156:781–782, 1985.

10. Boaz D, Mace JW, Gotlin RW: Poland's syndrome and leukemia. Lancet 1:349–350, 1971.

11. Bon Tempo CP, Ronan JA Jr, de Leon AC Jr, et al: Radiographic appearance of the thorax in systolic click-late systolic murmur syndrome. Am J Cardiol 36:27–31, 1975.

12. Borowitz D, Cerny F, Zallen G, et al: Pulmonary function and exercise response in patients with pectus excavatum after Nuss repair. J Pediatr Surg 38:544–547, 2003.

13. Bouvet JP, Lerque D, Bermetieres F, Gros JJ: Vascular origin of Poland syndrome? A comparative rheographic study of the vascularization of the arms in eight patients. Eur J Pediatr 128:17–26, 1978.

14. Bremer L: Textbook of Embryology. Philadelphia: W.B. Saunders, 1936.

15. Brodkin H: Congenital chondrosternal prominence (Pigeon breast) a new interpretation. Pediatrics 3:286–295, 1949.

16. Brodkin H: Pigeon breast—Congenital chondrosternal prominence. Arch Surg 77:261–270, 1958.

17. Brown AL, Cook O: Cardio-respiratory studies in pre and postoperative funnel chest. Dis Chest 20:378–391, 1951.

18. Burton JF: Method of correction of ectopia cordis. Arch Surg 54:79–84, 1947.

19. Cahill JL, Lees GM, Robertson HT: A summary of preoperative and postoperative cardiorespiratory performance in patients undergoing pectus excavatum and carinatum repair. J Pediatr Surg 19:430–433, 1984.

20. Cantrell JR, Haller JA, Ravitch MM: A syndrome of congenital defects involving the abdominal wall, sternum, diaphragm, pericardium, and heart. Surg Gynecol Obstet 107:602–614, 1958.

21. Castile RG, Staats BA, Westbrook PR: Symptomatic pectus deformities of the chest. Am Rev Respir Dis 126:564–568, 1982.

22. Chin EF: Surgery of funnel chest and congenital sternal prominence. Br J Surg 44, 360–376,1957.

23. Clarkson P: Poland's syndactyly. Guy's Hosp Rep 111:335–346, 1962.

24. Cobben J: Poland anomaly in mother and daughter. Am J Med Genet 33:519–521, 1989.

25. Croitoru DP, Kelly RE Jr, Goretsky MJ, et al: Experience and modification update for the minimally invasive Nuss technique for pectus excavatum repair in 303 patients. J Pediatr Surg 37:437–445, 2002.

26. Cullerier M: Observation sur un deplacement remarquable du coeur; par M. Deschamps, medecin a Laval. J General Med Chir Pharm 26:275, 1806.

27. Currarino G, Silverman, FN: Premature obliteration of the sternal sutures and pigeon-breast deformity. Radiology 70:532–540, 1958.

28. Cutler GD, Wilens G: Ectopia cordis: Report of a case. Am J Dis Child 30:76–81, 1925.

29. David TJ: Familial Poland anomaly. J Med Genet 19:293–296, 1982.

30. David TJ: Vascular origin of Poland syndrome? Eur J Pediatr 130:299–301, 1979.

31. Derveaux L, Clarysse I, Ivanoff I, et al: Preoperative and postoperative abnormalities in chest x-ray indices and in lung function in pectus deformities. Chest 95:850–856, 1989.

32. Derveaux L, Ivanoff I, Rochette F, et al: Mechanism of pulmonary function changes after surgical correction for funnel chest. Eur Respir J 1:823–825, 1988.

33. Dobell AR, Williams HB, Long RW: Staged repair of ectopia cordis. J Pediatr Surg 17:353–358, 1982.

34. Egan JC, DuBois JJ, Morphy M, et al: Compressive orthotics in the treatment of asymmetric pectus carinatum: A preliminary report with an objective radiographic marker. J Pediatr Surg 35:1183–1186, 2000.

35. Ellis DG, Snyder CL, Mann CM: The 're-do' chest wall deformity correction. J Pediatr Surg 32:1267–1271, 1997.

36. Engum S, Rescorla F, West K, et al: Is the grass greener? Early results of the Nuss procedure. J Pediatr Surg 35:246–251; discussion 257–248, 2000.

37. Fischer H: Fissura sterno congenita mit partieller Bauchspalte. Dtsch Z Chir 12:367, 1879.

38. Fonkalsrud EW, Beanes S, Hebra A, et al: Comparison of minimally invasive and modified Ravitch pectus excavatum repair. J Pediatr Surg 37:413–417, 2002.

39. Fontaine G, Ovlaque S: Le syndrome de Poland-Mobius. Arch Fr Pediatr 41:351–352, 1984.

40. Freire-Maia N, Chautard EA, Opitz JM, et al: The Poland syndrome—Clinical and geneaological data, dermatoglyphic analysis, and incidence. Hum Hered 23:97–104, 1973.

41. Froriep R: Beobachtung eines Falles von Mangel der Brustdruse. Notizen aus dem Gebiete der Naturund Heilkunde 10:9–14, 1839.

42. Garusi GF, D'Ettorre A: Angiocardiographic patterns in funnel chest. Cardiologia 45:312–330, 1964.

43. Gattiker H, Bühlmann A: Cardiopulmonary function and exercise tolerance in supine and sitting position in patients with pectus excavatum. Helv Med Acta 33:122–138, 1966.

44. Greig JD, Azmy AF: Thoracic cage deformity: A late complication following repair of an agenesis of diaphragm. J Pediatr Surg 25:1234–1235, 1990.

45. Haje SA, Bowen JR: Preliminary results of orthotic treatment of pectus deformities in children and adolescents. J Pediatr Orthop 12:795–800, 1992.

46. Haller JA Jr, Colombani PM, Humphries CT, et al: Chest wall constriction after too extensive and too early operations for pectus excavatum. Ann Thorac Surg 61:1618–1624; discussion 1625, 1996.

47. Haller JA Jr, Colombani PM, Miller D, et al: Early reconstruction of Poland's syndrome using autologous rib grafts combined with a latissimus muscle flap. J Pediatr Surg 19:423–429, 1984.

48. Haller JA Jr, Kramer SS, Lietman SA: Use of CT scans in selection of patients for pectus excavatum surgery: A preliminary report. J Pediatr Surg 22:904–906, 1987.

49. Haller JA Jr, Peters GN, Mazur D, et al: Pectus excavatum. A 20 year surgical experience. J Thorac Cardiovasc Surg 60:375–383, 1970.

50. Haynor DR, Shuman WP, Brewer DK, et al: Imaging of fetal ectopia cordis: Roles of sonography and computed tomography. J Ultrasound Med 3:25–27, 1984.

51. Hebra A: Pectus carinatum as a sequela of minimally invasive pectus excavatum repair. Pediatr Endosurg Innovative Tech 6:41–44, 2002.

52. Hebra A, Swoveland B, Egbert M, et al: Outcome analysis of minimally invasive repair of pectus excavatum: Review of 251 cases. J Pediatr Surg 35:252–257; discussion 257–258, 2000.

53. Hecker WC, Procher G, Dietz HG: [Results of operative correction of pigeon and funnel chest following a modified procedure of Ravitch and Haller (author's transl)]. Z Kinderchir 34:220–227, 1981.

54. Heilbronner DM, Renshaw TS: Spondylothoracic dysplasia. J Bone Joint Surg 66A:302–303, 1984.

55. Hersh JH, Wadterfill D, Rutledge J, et al: Sternal malformation/vascular dysplasia association. Am J Med Genet 21:177–186, 1985.

56. Higginbottom MC, Jones KL, Hall VD, et al: The amniotic band disruption complex: Timing of amniotic rupture and variable spectra of consequent defects. J Pediatr 95:544–549, 1979.

57. Hügaard K, Arendrup H: Deformities of the female breasts after surgery for funnel chest. Scand J Thorac Cardiovasc Surg 17:171–174, 1983.

58. Hüward R: Pigeon chest (protrusion deformity of the sternum). Med J Aust 45:664–666, 1958.

59. Howard R: Funnel Chest: Its effect on cardiac function. Arch Dis Child 32:5–7, 1959.

60. Hümmer HP, Willital GH: Morphologic findings of chest deformities in children corresponding to the Willital-Hümmer classification. J Pediatr Surg 19:562–566, 1984.

61. Humphreys GH 2nd, Jaretzki A 3rd: Pectus excavatum. Late results with and without operation. J Thorac Cardiovasc Surg 80:686–695, 1980.

62. Jarcho S, Levin PM: Hereditary malformation of the vertebral bodies. Bull Johns Hopkins Hosp 62:216–262, 1938.

63. Jeune M, Caroon R, Beraud C, et al: Polychondrodystrophie avec blocage thoracique d'evolution fatale. Pediatrie 9:390–392, 1954.

64. Judet J, Judet R: Thorax en entonnoir. Un Procede operatoire. Rev Orthop 40:248–257, 1954.

65. Jung A: Le traitement du thorax en entoinnoir par le "retournement pedicule" de la cuvette sterno-chondrale. Mem Acad Chir 82:242–249, 1956.

66. Kaguraoka H, Ohnuki T, Itaoka T, et al: Degree of severity of pectus excavatum and pulmonary function in preoperative and postoperative periods. J Thorac Cardiovasc Surg 104:1483–1488, 1992.

67. Kaplan LC, Matsuoka R, Gilbert EF, et al: Ectopia cordis and cleft sternum: Evidence for mechanical teratogenesis following rupture of the chorion or yolk sac. Am J Med Genet 21:187–199,1985.

68. King CR: Ectopia cordis and chromosomal errors. Pediatrics 66:328, 1980.

69. Kowalewski J, Brocki M, Dryjanski T, et al: Pectus excavatum: Increase of right ventricular systolic, diastolic, and stroke volumes after surgical repair. J Thorac Cardiovasc Surg 118:87–92; discussion 92–83, 1999.

70. Kozlowski K, Masel J: Asphyxiating thoracic dystrophy without respiratory disease: Report of two cases of the latent form. Pediatr Radiol 5:30–33, 1976.

71. Kragt H, Aarnoudse JG, Meyboom EJ, et al: Case report: Prenatal ultrasonic diagnosis and management of ectopia cordis. Eur J Obstet Gynecol Reprod Biol 20:177–180, 1985.

72. Lansman S, Serlo W, Linna O, et al: Treatment of pectus excavatum with bioabsorbable polylactide plates: Preliminary results. J Pediatr Surg 37:1281–1286, 2002.

73. Lees RF, Caldicott JH: Sternal anomalies and congenital heart disease. Am J Roentgenol Radium Ther Nucl Med 124:423–427, 1975.

74. Lester CW: Pigeon breast (pectus carinatum) and other protrusion deformities of the chest of developmental origin. Ann Surg 137:482–489, 1953.

75. Lester CW: The etiology and pathogenesis of funnel chest, pigeon breast, and related deformities of the anterior chest wall. J Thorac Surg 34:1–10, 1957.

76. Maier HC, Bortone F: Complete failure of sternal fusion with herniation of pericardium. J Thorac Surg 18:851–859, 1949.

77. Major JW: Thoracoabdominal ectopia cordis. J Thorac Surg 26:309–317, 1953.

78. Martinez D, Juame J, Stein T: The effect of costal cartilage resection on chest wall development. Pediatr Surg Int 5:170–173, 1990.

79. McGillivray BC, Lowry RB: Poland syndrome in British Columbia: Incidence and reproductive experience of affected persons. Am J Med Genet 1:65–74, 1977.

80. Mead J, Sly P, Le Souef P, et al: Rib cage mobility in pectus excavatum. Am Rev Respir Dis 132:1223–1228, 1985.

81. Meissner F: Fissura sterni congenita. Zentralbl Chir 89:1832–1839, 1964.

82. Mercer LJ, Petres RE, Smeltzer JS: Ultrasound diagnosis of ectopia cordis. Obstet Gynecol 61:523–525, 1983.

83. Meyer L: Zur chirurgischen behandlung der angeborenen trichterbrust. Verh Berliner Med Gesellschaft 42:364–373, 1911.

84. Mielke CH, Winter RB: Pectus carinatum successfully treated with bracing. A case report. Int Orthop 17:350–352, 1993.

85. Molik KA, Engum SA, Rescorla FJ, et al: Pectus excavatum repair: Experience with standard and minimal invasive techniques. J Pediatr Surg 36:324–328, 2001.

86. Morshuis W, Folgering H, Barentsz J, et al: Pulmonary function before surgery for pectus excavatum and at long-term follow-up. Chest 105:1646–1652, 1994.

87. Morshuis WJ, Folgering HT, Barentsz JO, et al: Exercise cardiorespiratory function before and one year after operation for pectus excavatum. J Thorac Cardiovasc Surg 107:1403–1409, 1994.

88. Nuss D, Kelly RE Jr, Croitoru DP, et al: A 10-year review of a minimally invasive technique for the correction of pectus excavatum. J Pediatr Surg 33:545–552, 1998.

89. Ochsner A, DeBakey M: Chone-chondrosternon: Report of a case and review of the literature. J Thorac Surg 8:469–511, 1939.

90. Ohmori K, Takada H: Correction of Poland's pectoralis major muscle anomaly with latissimus dorsi musculocutaneous flaps. Okast Reconstr Surg 65:400, 1980.

91. Opitz JM: Editorial comment following paper by Hersh et al and Kaplan et al on sternal cleft. Am J Med Genet 21:201–202, 1985.

92. Paltia V: Operative technique in funnel chest: Experience in 81 cases. Acta Chir Scand 116:90–98, 1958.

93. Patten BM: Human Embryology. Philadelphia: Blakiston, 1946.

94. Peterson RJ, Young WG Jr, Godwin JD, et al: Noninvasive assessment of exercise cardiac function before and after pectus excavatum repair. J Thorac Cardiovasc Surg 90:251–260, 1985.

95. Poland A: Deficiency of the pectoralis muscles. Guy's Hosp. 6:191–193, 1841.

96. Quigley PM, Haller JA Jr, Jelus KL, et al: Cardiorespiratory function before and after corrective surgery in pectus excavatum. J Pediatr 128:638–643, 1996.

97. Ravitch MM: The operative treatment of pectus excavatum. Ann Surg 129:429–444, 1949.

98. Ravitch MM: Unusual sternal deformity with cardiac symptoms—operative correction. J Thorac Surg 23:138–144, 1952.

99. Ravitch MM: The operative correction of pectus carinatum (pigeon breast). Ann Surg 151:705–714, 1960.

100. Ravitch MM: Atypical deformities of the chest wall—Absence and deformities of the ribs and costal cartilage. Surgery 59:438–449, 1966.

101. Ravitch MM: Congenital Deformities of the Chest Wall and Their Operative Correction. Philadelphia: W.B. Saunders, 1977.

102. Rehbein F: The operative treatment of the funnel chest. Arch Dis Child 32:5–8, 1957.

103. Roberts AP, Conner AN, Tolmie JL, et al: Spondylothoracic and spondylocostal dysostosis: Hereditary forms of spinal deformity. J Bone Joint Surg 70B:123–126, 1988.

104. Robicsek F, Sargar PW, Taylor FH, et al: The surgical treatment of chondrosternal prominence (pectus carinatum). J Thorac Cardiovasc Surg 45:691–701, 1963.

105. Robicsek F, Fokin A: Surgical correction of pectus excavatum and carinatum. J Cardiovasc Surg (Torino) 40:725–731, 1999.

106. Sabiston DC Jr: The surgical management of congenital bifid sternum with partial ectopia cordis. J Thorac Surg 35:118–122, 1958.

107. Saint-Mezard G, Duret JC, Chanudet X, et al: Mitral valve prolapse and pectus excavatum. Fortuitous association or syndrome? Presse Med 15:439, 1986.

108. Salomon J, Shah PM, Heinle RA: Thoracic skeletal abnormalities in idiopathic mitral valve prolapse. Am J Cardiol 36:32–36, 1975.

109. Sanger PW, Robicsek F, Daugherty HK: The repair of recurrent pectus excavatum. J Thorac Cardiovasc Surg 56:141–143, 1968.

110. Sauerbruch F: Die Chirurgie der Brustorgane. Berlin: Springer, 1920.

111. Saxena NC: Ectopia cordis child surviving: Prosthesis fails. Pediatr News 10:3, 1976.

112. Say B, Wilsey CE: Chromosome aberration in ectopia cordis. Am Heart J 95:274–275, 1978.

113. Schaub VF, Wegmann T: Elektrokardiographische veranderungen bei trichterbrust. Cardiologia 24:39–46, 1954.

114. Scherer LR, Arn PH, Dressel DA, et al: Surgical management of children and young adults with Marfan syndrome and pectus excavatum. J Pediatr Surg 23:1169–1172, 1988.

115. Schutte J, Gaffney FA, Blend L, et al: Distinctive anthropometric characteristics of women with mitral valve prolapse. Am J Med 71:533–538, 1981.

116. Shamberger R, Welch KJ, Upton J III: Surgical treatment of thoracic deformity in Poland's syndrome. J Pediatr Surg 24:760–765, 1989.

117. Shamberger R, Welch KJ: Sternal defects. Pediatr Surg Int 5:156–164, 1990.

118. Shamberger RC, Welch KJ: Surgical correction of pectus carinatum. J Pediatr Surg 22:48–53, 1987.

119. Shamberger RC, Welch KJ: Cardiopulmonary function in pectus excavatum. Surg Gynecol Obstet 166:383–391, 1988.

120. Shamberger RC, Welch KJ: Surgical correction of chondromanubrial deformity (Currarino Silverman syndrome). J Pediatr Surg 23:319–322, 1988.

121. Shamberger RC, Welch KJ: Surgical repair of pectus excavatum. J Pediatr Surg 23:615–622, 1988.

122. Shamberger RC, Welch KJ, Sanders SP: Mitral valve prolapse associated with pectus excavatum. J Pediatr 111:404–407, 1987.

123. Shochat SJ, Csongradi JJ, Hartman GE, et al: Moire phototopography in the evaluation of anterior chest wall deformities. J Pediatr Surg 16:353–357, 1981.

124. Sigalet DL, Montgomery M, Harder J: Cardiopulmonary effects of closed repair of pectus excavatum. J Pediatr Surg 38:380–385, 2003.

125. Stensen N: An unusually early description of the so-called tetralogy of Fallot. Acta Med Phil Hafnienca 1:202, edited by T. Bartholin, 1671–1672.

126. Stoll SC, Vivier M, Renaud R: A supraumbilical midline raphe with sternal cleft in a 47,XXX woman. Am J Med Genet 27:229–231, 1987.

127. Sujansky E, Riccardi VM, Matthew AL: The familial occurrence of Poland syndrome. Birth Defects 13:117–132, 1977.

128. Taguchi K, Mochizuki T, Nakagaki N, Kato K: A new plastic operation for pectus excavatum: Sternal turnover surgical procedure with preserved internal mammary vessels. Chest 67:606–608, 1975.

129. Tanaka F, Kitano M, Shindo T, et al: [Postoperative lung function in patients with funnel chest]. Nippon Kyobu Geka Gakkai Zasshi 41:2161–2165, 1993.

130. Udoshi MB, Shah A, Fisher VJ, et al: Incidence of mitral valve prolapse in subjects with thoracic skeletal abnormalities—a prospective study. Am Heart J 97:303–311, 1979.

131. Vanamo K, Peltonen J, Rintala R, et al: Chest wall and spinal deformities in adults with congenital diaphragmatic defects. J Pediatr Surg 31:851–854, 1996.

132. von der Oelsnitz G: [Anomalies of the chest (author's transl)]. Z Kinderchir 33:229–236, 1981.

133. Wada J, Ikeda K, Ishida T, et al: Results of 271 funnel chest operations. Ann Thorac Surg 10:526–532, 1970.

134. Walker JC, Meijer R, Aranda D: Syndactylism with deformity of the pectoralis muscle—Poland's syndrome. J Pediatr Surg 4:569–572, 1969.

135. Waters P, Welch K, Micheli LJ, et al: Scoliosis in children with pectus excavatum and pectus carinatum. J Pediatr Orthop 9:551–556, 1989.

136. Weber TR, Kurkchubasche AG: Operative management of asphyxiating thoracic dystrophy after pectus repair. J Pediatr Surg 33:262–265, 1998.

137. Wechselberger G, Ohlbauer M, Haslinger J, Schoeller T: Silicone implant correction of pectus excavatum. Ann Plast Surg 47:489–493, 2001.

138. Weg JG, Krumholz RA, Harkleroad LE: Pulmonary dysfunction in pectus excavatum. Am Rev Respir Dis 96:936–945, 1967.

139. Welch K: Satisfactory surgical correction of pectus excavatum deformity in childhood: A limited opportunity. J Thorac Surg 36:697–713, 1958.

140. Welch K: Chest Wall Deformities: Philadelphia: W.B. Saunders, 1980.

141. Welch KJ, Kraney GP: Abdominal musculature deficiency syndrome prune belly. J Urol 111:693–700, 1974.

142. Welch KJ, Vos A: Surgical correction of pectus carinatum (pigeon breast). J Pediatr Surg 8:659–667, 1973.

143. Wieting: Eine operative behandelte Herzmissbildung. Dtsch Z Chir 114:293–295, 1912.

144. Williams AJ, Vauterg G, Reid LM: Lung structure in asphyxiating thoracic dystrophy. Arch Pathol Lab Med 108:658–661, 1984.

145. Willital GH: [Indication and operative technique in chest deformities (author's transl)]. Z Kinderchir 33:244–252, 1981.

146. Willius FA: An unusually early description of the so-called tetralogy of Fallot. Proc Staff Meet Mayo Clin 23:316–320, 1948.

147. Wynn SR, Driscoll DJ, Ostrom NK, et al: Exercise cardiorespiratory function in adolescents with pectus excavatum. Observations before and after operation. J Thorac Cardiovasc Surg 99:41–47, 1990.

Chest Wall Tumors

Peter C. Pairolero

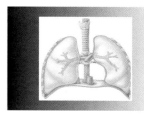

CHAPTER **25**

INTRODUCTION

Tumors of the chest wall encompass a variety of bone and soft tissue disorders.[3,5,22] Primary and metastatic neoplasms of both the bony skeleton and soft tissues are included as well as primary neoplasms that invade the thorax from adjacent structures such as the breast, lung, pleura, and mediastinum. Also included are benign, nonmalignant conditions of the chest wall such as infections, cysts, and fibromatosis. Almost all of these tumors have been irradiated as the treatment of choice or have been irradiated in combination with chest wall resection.[4] It is also not uncommon to have patients present with a postradiation necrotic chest wall neoplasm. The thoracic surgeon is frequently asked to establish a diagnosis for most of these patients; to treat some for cure; and to manage a few for necrotic, foul-smelling chest wall ulcers. All of these entities represent a diagnostic and therapeutic challenge. In many patients, surgical extirpation is often the only remaining method of treatment, and this may be compromised by an incorrect diagnosis or an inability to reconstruct large chest wall defects. From a practical standpoint, however, chest wall resection is most frequently used to treat primary chest wall neoplasms.[3,5,21,22]

Because primary chest wall neoplasms are uncommon, relatively few series historically have been reported. Moreover, most early reports included only patients with bone tumors.[12,24,27] When bone tumors are combined with primary soft tissue tumors, however, the soft tissues become a major source of chest wall neoplasms and today account for nearly half of all tumors.*

---

*References 3, 5, 7–9, 11, 15, 17, 21–23.

The incidence of malignancy in primary chest wall neoplasms varies and ranges from 50 to 80%. The higher malignancy rates occur in soft tissue tumors. Consequently, when bone and soft tissue tumors are combined, malignant fibrous histiocytomas (fibrosarcomas), chondrosarcomas, and rhabdomyosarcomas are the most common primary malignant neoplasms and cartilaginous tumors (osteochondroma and chondroma) and desmoid tumors are the most common primary benign tumors[5,21] (Box 25-1).

CLINICAL PRESENTATION

Chest wall tumors generally present as slowly enlarging, asymptomatic masses. With continued growth, pain invariably occurs. Initially, the pain is often generalized and the patient is frequently treated for a neuritis or a musculoskeletal complaint. Nearly all malignant neoplasms eventually become painful as compared to only two thirds of benign tumors. In some patients with rib tumors, a mass may not be apparent on physical examination but is detected on conventional chest X-ray.

Evaluation of patients with suspected chest wall tumors should include a careful history, physical examination, and laboratory examination followed by conventional X-rays of the involved area. Previous chest X-rays are important to determine the rate of growth. In general, magnetic resonance imaging (MRI) is the preferred method of imaging chest wall tumors. Not only does MRI distinguish the tumor from nerves and blood vessels, but it also allows visualization in different planes, such as coronal or sagittal planes. MRI, however, does not accurately assess pulmonary nodules or the extent of calcification within the lung. Thus, if the lung parenchyma needs evaluation for metastatic disease, computed tomography is preferable.

SURGICAL MANAGEMENT

Chest wall neoplasms that are clinically suspected of being primary tumors require tissue diagnosis. Those tumors suspected of being a metastasis from a known primary neoplasm elsewhere can be accurately diagnosed by incisional or needle biopsy. However, if a primary chest wall neoplasm (either benign or malignant) is suspected, an excisional biopsy rather than incisional or needle biopsy should be done because the latter two limited biopsies tend to underdiagnose certain low-grade malignancies, (e.g., chondrosarcoma, as being benign). Consequently, wide resection is invariably not done and the opportunity for cure is denied. Also, the location of the excisional biopsy should not interfere with subsequent treatment. An improperly placed biopsy site, extensive soft

396

Box 25–1. Primary Chest Wall Neoplasm.

Malignant

Malignant fibrous histiocytoma
Chondrosarcoma
Rhabdomyosarcoma
Myeloma
Ewing's sarcoma
Liposarcoma
Neurofibrosarcoma
Osteogenic sarcoma
Hemangiosarcoma
Leiomyosarcoma
Lymphoma

Benign

Osteochondroma
Chondroma
Desmoid
Lipoma
Fibroma
Neurilemoma

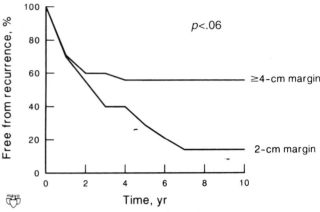

Figure 25–1 Percentage of patients with malignant chest wall tumors free from recurrent tumor by extent of resection margin. Zero time on abscissa represents day of chest wall resection.
(Reprinted from King RM, Pairolero PC, Trastek VF, et al: Primary chest wall tumors: Factors affecting survival. Ann Thorac Surg 41:597–601, 1986, with permission from The Society of Thoracic Surgeons.)

tissue dissection, and wound infection can all complicate subsequent treatment by delaying definitive resection, radiation, or chemotherapy. If frozen tissue diagnosis of a primary chest wall malignancy cannot be established at the time of excisional biopsy, the chest wound should be closed, most often without skeletal reconstruction, since the chest wall defect is usually small. If the neoplasm is later determined to be benign, no further surgical therapy is required. If, however, malignancy is diagnosed, wide resection is then required, which must also include en bloc resection of the entire biopsy site (skin, subcutaneous tissue, and muscle) because of potential tumor contamination of the overlying muscle, subcutaneous tissue, and skin.

Wide resection of a primary malignant chest wall neoplasm is now recognized as being essential to successful management. However, the extent of resection should not be compromised because of an inability to close large chest wall defects.[3,5,21,22] Opinions differ with regard to what constitutes wide resection. In a report from the Mayo Clinic that analyzed the effect of the extent of resection on long-term survival in patients with primary malignant chest wall neoplasm,[17] 56% of patients with a 4-cm or greater margin of resection remained free from cancer at 5 years compared with only 29% for patients with a 2-cm margin (Figure 25-1). For many surgeons, a resection margin of 2 cm is considered to be adequate. Although this margin may be adequate for chest wall metastases and benign tumors, a 2-cm margin for resection is *inadequate* for malignant neoplasms. Moreover, more aggressive malignant tumors, such as osteogenic sarcoma and malignant fibrous histiocytoma, have the potential to spread within the marrow cavity or along tissue plains such as the periosteum or parietal pleura. Consequently, all primary malignant neoplasms that are initially diagnosed by excisional biopsy should be resected further to include at least a 4-cm margin of normal tissue on all sides. High-grade malignancies should also have the entire involved bone resected. For neoplasms of the rib, this includes removal of the entire involved rib, the corresponding anterior costal arch if the tumor is located anteriorly, and partial resecection of several ribs above and below the neoplasm. For tumors of the sternum and manubrium, resection of the entire involved bone and corresponding costal arches bilaterally is indicated. Any attached structures such as lung, thymus, pericardium, or chest wall muscles should also be excised.

The role of resection for chest wall metastases and recurrent breast cancer is controversial. Nonetheless, most thoracic surgeons would agree that tumor ulceration is an indication for excision. For these patients, wound hygiene is crucial, and surgical excision is frequently the only treatment option available. The goal in treating patients with necrotic tumors should be a healed wound following local excision. Although the length of survival is not increased after resection, the quality of life is certainly improved.

The ability to close large chest wall defects is of prime importance in the surgical treatment of chest wall neoplasms. The critical questions of whether the reconstructed thorax will support respiration and protect the underlying organs must be answered when considering both the extent of resection and the method of reconstruction. Adequate resection and dependable reconstruction are the mandatory ingredients for successful treatment. These two important items are accomplished most safely by the joint efforts of a thoracic and a plastic surgeon.

Reconstruction of chest wall defects involves consideration of many factors.[3,5,22] The location and size are of utmost importance, but the medical history and local conditions of the wound may drastically alter a reconstructive choice. Primary closure remains the best option available if possible. If full-thickness reconstruction is required, which is usually the situation in most primary neoplasms that have not been previously treated, consideration must be given to both structural stability of the thorax and soft tissue coverage.

Skeletal Reconstruction

Reconstruction of the bony thorax is controversial. Differences of opinion exist both as to who should be reconstructed and as to what type of reconstruction should be done. In general, all full-thickness skeletal defects that have the potential for pneumothorax should be reconstructed. The decision not to reconstruct the skeleton depends on the size and location of the defect. Defects less than 5 cm in greatest diameter anywhere on the thorax are usually not reconstructed. Likewise, high posterior defects less than 10 cm do not require reconstruction because the overlying scapula provides support. However, if the defect is located near the tip of the scapula, the defect should be closed to avoid impingement of the tip of the scapula into the chest with movement of the arm. Alternatively, the lower half of the scapula could be resected. Finally, all larger defects located anywhere on the chest should be reconstructed and either autogenous tissue, such as fascia lata or ribs, or prosthetic material, such as the various meshes, polytetrafluoroethylene soft tissue patch, metals, or a combination of mesh impregnated with methylmethacrylate, may be used. All work equally well and the final selection is the surgeon's choice.

All large, full-thickness skeletal defects resulting from resection of neoplasm in both the sternum and lateral chest wall should be reconstructed if the wound is not contaminated. If the wound is contaminated from previous radiation necrosis or necrotic neoplasm, reconstruction with prosthetic material is not advised as the prosthesis may subsequently become infected resulting in obligatory removal. In this situation, reconstruction with a musculocutaneous flap is preferred. Similarly, resection of full-thickness bony thorax in a patient who has been previously irradiated may not require skeletal reconstruction since the lung is frequently adherent to the underlying parietal pleura and pneumothorax may not occur with chest wall resection.

Soft Tissue Reconstruction

Both muscle and omentum can be utilized to reconstruct soft tissue chest wall defects. Muscle can be transposed as muscle alone or as a musculocutaneous flap and is the tissue of choice for closure of most full-thickness soft tissue defects. All of the major chest wall and abdominal muscles can be mobilized on a single axis of rotation and transposed to another location on the chest wall.[2,6,15,19] The omentum should be reserved for partial thickness reconstruction or as a back-up procedure when muscle either is not available or has failed in a previous full-thickness repair.[16]

BENIGN CHEST WALL TUMORS

Osteochondroma

This is the most common benign bone neoplasm, constituting nearly 50% of all benign rib tumors. The incidence, however, may actually be higher since most patients are asymptomatic and the tumors are often not removed. Men are affected three times more frequently than women. The neoplasm begins in childhood and continues to grow until skeletal maturity is reached. The onset of pain in a previously asymptomatic tumor may indicate malignant degeneration.

Osteochondromas arise from the metaphyseal region of the rib and present as a stalked bony protuberance with a cartilaginous cap. A rim of calcification may be present at the periphery of the tumor, and stippled calcification is often found within the tumor. Microscopically, bony proliferation occurs to varying degrees, and the thickness of the cartilaginous cap also varies.

All osteochondromas occurring in children after puberty or in adults should be resected. Asymptomatic osteochondromas may occur before puberty, but if pain or increase in size occurs, the tumor should be resected.

Chondroma

Chondromas constitute 15% of all benign neoplasms of the rib cage. Most occur anteriorly at the costochondral junction. Both sexes are affected equally, and the tumor can occur at any age. These neoplasms usually present as a slowly enlarging mass that may be nontender or slightly painful. Radiographically, chondroma is an expansile lesion causing thinning of the cortex. The differentiation between a chondroma and a chondrosarcoma is impossible on clinical and radiographic examination. Grossly, chondroma presents as a lobulated mass. Microscopically, the tumor is characterized by lobules of hyaline cartilage. The microscopic differentiation between a chondroma and a low-grade chondrosarcoma can be extremely difficult. All chondromas must be considered malignant and should be treated by wide excision. Although this extent of resection may seem extensive for what may turn out to be a benign tumor, modern reconstructive techniques make the risk negligible, and long-term results are excellent.

Desmoid

Desmoid tumor deserves special consideration. Forty percent of all desmoids occur in the shoulder and chest wall. Encapsulation of the brachial plexus and the vessels of the arm and neck is common. The tumor often extends into the pleural cavity, markedly displacing mediastinal structures. Initially, the tumor presents as a poorly circumscribed mass with little or no pain. Paresthesias, hyperesthesia, and motor weakness occur later, following neural encasement. Veins or arteries are rarely occluded. Desmoid occurs most commonly between puberty and 40 years of age and is rarely observed in infants or the very old. Men and women are affected equally.

Grossly, the tumor originates in muscle and fascia and frequently extends along tissue planes. Microscopically, a monotonous pattern of elongated spindle-shaped cells infiltrating the surrounding tissue is invariably seen. Most pathologists consider desmoid to be a form of benign fibromatosis.[10,14] Because these tumors can invade adjacent structures and have been reported to have malignant degeneration, other pathologists consider desmoid to be a low-grade fibrosarcoma.[13,26] Whatever the cause, the tumor tends to be recurrent if inadequately excised and should be treated with wide resection. Encapsulation of thoracic outlet structures presents a special problem in management.

398 Enucleation of the tumor from these structures followed by radiation therapy is the current practice.

MALIGNANT CHEST WALL TUMORS

Malignant Fibrous Histiocytoma

Malignant fibrous histiocytoma is the most common primary chest wall neoplasm the thoracic surgeon is asked to evaluate.[17,21] The tumor characteristically occurs in late adult life, with the majority of cases occurring between the ages of 50 and 70. These neoplasms are rare in childhood, and approximately two thirds occur in men. Malignant fibrous histiocytoma often presents as a painless, slowly enlarging mass. Pregnancy, however, may accelerate the growth rate, resulting in pain. Fever and leukocytosis with neutropenia or eosinophilia are occasionally present.[28] Excellent circumstantial evidence suggests that some chest wall malignant fibrous histiocytomas are radiation induced.[28]

Grossly malignant fibrous histiocytoma tends to be lobulated and to spread for considerable distances along fascial planes or between muscle fibers, which accounts for its high recurrence rate following resection. The neoplasm is unresponsive to both irradiation and chemotherapy and should be treated by wide resection. Five-year survival is approximately 38%.

Chondrosarcoma

Chondrosarcoma accounts for 30% of all primary malignant bone tumors. It occurs most frequently in the anterior chest wall, with 75% arising in either the costochondral arches or the sternum. The tumor most commonly occurs in the third and fourth decades of life and is relatively uncommon in persons under the age of 20. Chondrosarcoma is more frequent in men. Nearly all patients present with a slowly enlarging mass, which has usually been painful for many months. Differentiation from chondroma may be extremely difficult. From a practical standpoint, all tumors arising in the costal cartilages should be considered to be malignant and should be treated by wide resection.

The cause of chondrosarcoma is unknown. Although malignant degeneration of benign cartilaginous tumors—secondary chondrosarcoma—has been reported, most chondrosarcomas arise *de nova*. An association has been suggested between trauma and chondrosarcoma.[14] In the Mayo Clinic series, 12.5% of patients had sustained severe crushing injury to the ipsilateral chest wall.[18]

Definitive diagnosis of chondrosarcoma can only be made pathologically. Histological confirmation, however, may be difficult since most tumors are well differentiated. This well-differentiated tendency frequently results in a misdiagnosis of chondroma and subsequent undertreatment, leading to local recurrences. For this reason, excisional biopsy rather than incisional or needle biopsy of all chest wall masses suspected of being chondrosarcoma is indicated.

Chest wall chondrosarcoma typically grows slowly and recurs locally. If it is left untreated, metastases occur late. Prompt, complete control of the primary neoplasm is the main determinant of survival; the objective of the first operation should be resection wide enough to prevent local recurrence. This involves resection of a 4-cm margin of normal tissue on all sides. Wide resection results in cure in nearly all patients.[1,18]

Rhabdomyosarcoma

This is the second most common chest wall soft tissue malignant neoplasm and occurs most frequently in children and young adults. These tumors are rare after the age of 45, and men are affected only slightly more often than women. Rhabdomyosarcomas present as a rapidly enlarging mass that is usually deep-seated and is intimately associated with striated muscle tissue. Generally, the tumor is neither painful nor tender, despite evidence of rapid growth. Both grossly and microscopically, it has few neoplastic characteristics. As with most rapidly growing tumors, the overall appearance reflects the degree of cellularity and the extent of secondary changes such as hemorrhage and necrosis.

Modern therapy has profoundly altered the clinical course of this disease. Wide resection followed by irradiation and multidrug chemotherapy has resulted in 5-year survivals of 70%. Inadequately treated, the tumor rapidly recurs both locally and metastatically.

CLINICAL EXPERIENCE

Since the early 1980s over 500 chest wall resections for primary neoplasms were performed at the Mayo Clinic by one team of surgeons.[3,5,21,22] Nearly two thirds of these neoplasms were malignant. Malignant fibrous histiocytoma and chondrosarcoma were the most common malignant neoplasms, and desmoid tumor was the most common benign tumor. Patients' ages ranged from 11 to 85 years with a median of 45.2 years. An average of 3.9 ribs were resected. Total or partial sternectomies were performed in 23 patients. Skeletal defects were closed with prosthetic material in 67 patients and with autogenous ribs in 5. Eighty-eight patients underwent 126 muscle transpositions including 48 pectoralis major, 35 latissimus dorsi, 16 serratus anterior, 3 external oblique, 2 rectus abdominis, 2 trapezius, and 20 other. The omentum was transposed in 14 patients. Median hospitalization was 8.5 days. There were no 30-day operative deaths. Patients were generally extubated during the evening of the operation or on the following morning. Three patients required tracheostomy. Most other patients had only minor changes in pulmonary function.[20]

Long-term survival of patients with primary chest wall malignant neoplasm is dependent on cell type and the extent of chest wall resection. In the Mayo Clinic series overall 5-year survival was 57%.[17] Wide resection for chondrosarcoma resulted in a 5-year survival of 96% as compared to only 70% for patients who had local excision[20] (Figure 25-2). Five-year overall survival for patients with either chondrosarcoma or rhabdomyosarcoma was 70% in contrast to only 38% for patients with malignant fibrous histiocytoma[17] (Figure 25-3). Recurrent neoplasm, however, was an ominous sign as only 17% of patients in whom recurrence developed survived 5 years.

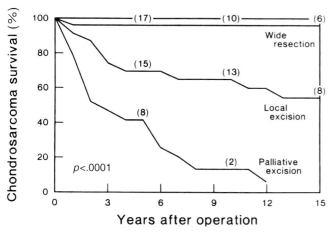

Figure 25–2 Survival of patients with chest wall chondrosarcoma by extent of operation. Zero time on abscissa represents day of chest wall resection.
(Reprinted from McAfee MK, Pairolero PC, Bergstralh EJ, et al: Chondrosarcoma of the chest wall: Factors affecting survival. Ann Thorac Surg 40:535–541, 1985, with permission from The Society of Thoracic Surgeons.)

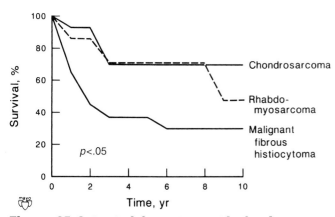

Figure 25–3 Survival for patients with chondrosarcoma and rhabdomyosarcoma compared with malignant fibrous histiocytoma. Zero time on abscissa represents day of chest wall resection.
(Reprinted from King RM, Pairolero PC, Trastek VF; et al: Primary chest wall tumors: Factors affecting survival. Ann Thorac Surg 41:597–601, 1986, with permission from The Society of Thoracic Surgeons.)

SUMMARY

The key to successful treatment of primary chest wall neoplasms remains early diagnosis and aggressive surgical resection. This procedure can generally be performed in one operation with minimal respiratory insufficiency and with low operative mortality. When combined with current methods of reconstruction, potential cure is likely for most patients with primary chest wall neoplasm.

REFERENCES

1. Arnold PG, Pairolero PC: Chondrosarcoma of the manubrium. Resection and reconstruction with pectoralis major muscle. Mayo Clin Proc 53:54–57, 1978.
2. Arnold PG, Pairolero PC: Use of pectoralis major muscle flaps to repair defects of anterior chest wall. Plast Reconstr Surg 63:205–213, 1979.
3. Arnold PG, Pairolero PC: Chest wall reconstruction: Experience with 100 consecutive patients. Ann Surg 199:725, 1984.
4. Arnold PG, Pairolero PC: Surgical management of the radiated chest wall. Plast Reconstr Surg 77:605–612, 1986.
5. Arnold PG, Pairolero PC: Chest wall reconstruction: An account of 500 consecutive patients. Plast Reconstr Surg 98(5):804, 1996.
6. Arnold PG, Pairolero PC, Waldorf JC: The serratus anterior muscle: Intrathoracic and extrathoracic utilization. Plast Reconstr Surg 73:240–248, 1984.
7. Eng J, Sabanathan S, Pradhan GN, Mearns AJ: Primary bony chest wall tumours. J R Coll Surg Edinb 5:44–47, 1990.
8. Evans KG, Miller RR, Muller NL, Nelems B: Chest wall tumours. Can J Surg 33:229–232, 1990.
9. Farley JH, Seyfer AE: Chest wall tumors: Experience with 58 patients. Military Med 156:413–415, 1991.
10. Goellner JR, Soule EH: Desmoid tumors: An ultrastructural study of eight cases. Hum Pathol 11:43, 1980.
11. Graeber GM, Snyder RJ, Fleming AW, et al: Initial and long-term results in the management of primary chest wall neoplasms. Ann Thorac Surg 34:664, 1982.
12. Groff DB, Adkins PC: Chest wall tumors. Ann Thorac Surg 4:260, 1967.
13. Hajdu SI: Pathology of Soft Tissue Tumors. Philadelphia: Lea & Febiger, 1979, p 122.
13a. Hodgkinson DJ, Arnold PG: Chest wall reconstruction using the external oblique muscle. Br J Plast Surg 33:216–220, 1980.
14. Hayry P, Reitamo JJ, Totterman S, et al: The desmoid tumor. II. Analysis of factors possibly contributing to the etiology and growth behavior. Am J Clin Pathol 77:674, 1982.
15. Hodgkinson DJ, Arnold PG: Chest wall reconstruction using the external oblique muscle. Br J Plast Surg 33:216–220, 1980.
16. Jurkiewicz MJ, Arnold PG: The omentum: An account of its use in the reconstruction of the chest wall. Ann Surg 185:548–554, 1977.
17. King RM, Pairolero PC, Trastek VF, et al: Primary chest wall tumors: Factors affecting survival. Ann Thorac Surg 41:597–601, 1986.
18. McAfee MK, Pairolero PC, Bergstralh EJ, et al: Chondrosarcoma of the chest wall: Factors affecting survival. Ann Thorac Surg 40:535, 1985.
19. McCraw JB, Arnold PG: McCraw and Arnold's Atlas of Muscle and Musculocutaneous Flaps. Norfolk: Hampton Press Publishing Company, 1986.
20. Meadows JA III, Staats BA, Pairolero PC, et al: Effect of resection of the sternum and manubrium in conjunction with muscle transposition on pulmonary function. Mayo Clin Proc 60:604–609, 1985.
21. Pairolero PC, Arnold PG: Chest wall tumors: Experience with 100 consecutive patients. J Thoracic Cardiovasc Surg 90:367–372, 1985.
22. Pairolero PC, Arnold PG: Thoracic wall defects: Surgical management of 205 consecutive patients. Mayo Clin Proc 61:557–563, 1986.
23. Pairolero PC, Arnold PG: Primary tumors of the anterior chest wall. Surg Rounds 19–24, 1986.

400

24. Pascuzzi CA, Dahlin DC, Clagett OT: Primary tumors of the ribs and sternum. Surg Gynecol Obstet 104:390, 1957.

25. Ryan MB, McMurtrey MJ, Roth JA: Current managment of chest wall tumors. Surg Clin North Am 69(5):1061–1080, 1989.

26. Soule EG, Scanlon PW: Fibrosarcoma arising in an extraabdominal desmoid tumor: Report of a case. Mayo Clin Proc 37:443, 1962.

27. Stelzer P, Gay WA Jr: Tumors of the chest wall. Surg Clin North Am 60:779, 1980.

28. Weiss SW, Enzinger FM: Malignant fibrous histiocytoma: An analysis of 200 cases. Cancer 41:2250, 1978.

Chest Wall Reconstruction

Mark S. Allen

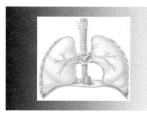

INTRODUCTION

Indications for chest wall resection include primary or metastatic chest wall neoplasms, tumors contiguous from breast or lung, radiation necrosis, congenital defects, and trauma or infectious processes from osteomyelitis or median sternotomy or lateral thoracotomy wounds.[12] Improvements in preoperative imaging, intraoperative anesthetic management, techniques available for reconstruction, and postoperative care allow almost any pathological process to be successfully managed by chest wall resection and reconstruction. The tenets of chest wall resection and reconstruction are (1) remove all devitalized tissue, (2) restore rigidity to the chest wall if the defect is large to prevent a flail chest, and (3) cover with healthy soft tissue to seal the pleural space, protect underling organs, and prevent infection. Since successful management of chest wall lesions often requires input from multiple different specialties, these types of problems are best cared for by a team of physicians including plastic surgeons, pulmonologists, anesthesiologists, as well as the thoracic surgeon. This chapter will review the history, indications, methods, and outcomes of chest wall resection and reconstruction.

HISTORY

Holden reported the first successful partial sternectomy in 1878, and in 1898 Parham reported resection of the chest wall in continuity with a pulmonary tumor.[17] Reconstruction was particularly difficult in these early efforts because of the problems involved in sealing the pleural cavity. With the advent of endotracheal intubation, the difficulties of pneumothorax during chest wall resection were mitigated. Closed-chest drainage, positive-pressure ventilation, and antibiotics further enhanced the success rate of chest wall resection and reconstruction. The 1940s and the war injuries seen in World War II advanced the management of an infected pleural space and ventilation mechanics, and brought advances in soft tissue coverage. Watson and James described the use of fascia lata grafts to close chest wall

defects.[19] The use of rib grafts to reinforce the anterior chest wall after sternectomy was discussed by Bisgard and Swenson.[3] The advent of musculocutaneous flaps to cover defects in the chest wall is a major advance in the reconstruction of chest wall defects. The latissimus dorsi musculocutaneous flap was initially described by Tansini in 1906 for coverage of the chest wall after a radical mastectomy.[18] The musculocutaneous flap was again described in the late 1930s and by Campbell in 1950, but, for unknown reasons, was not noticed until 20 years later. The idea of a musculocutaneous flap was then repopularized by Blades and Paul, Converse et al, and Myre and Kirklin.[5,7,16] In the field of thoracic surgery, Jurkiewicz expanded the idea of using muscle flaps to reconstruct the chest wall. Through him and the residents he trained, these techniques are now commonly in use.

Recently there have been numerous reports using the chest wall musculature to reconstruct the chest wall. Muscles used now include almost all the thoracic muscles, including the latissimus dorsi, pectoralis major and minor, serratus anterior, rectus abdominus, and external obliques. Tissue expanders have been added to facilitate transfer of the muscle, and free microvascular transfer has been described to cover chest wall defects. Currently, aggressive resections are almost always possible to cover with autologous tissue using modern techniques.

For stabilization of the resected bony chest wall, either autologous tissue or synthetic materials have been described. The use of transposed ribs or diced cartilage is of historic interest only and is rarely used today. Fascia lata for reconstruction of chest wall deformities was first described in 1947 by Watson and James.[19] Synthetic materials are the most commonly used objects today. Marlex, as a material to reconstruct the chest wall, was first described in 1960 by Graham et al.[11] Similar meshes were developed using prolene and vicryl. More recently, Gore-Tex patches have been constructed for this purpose.

INDICATIONS

Malignancies, primary, metastatic, or those with contiguous invasion of the chest wall, are the primary indication for a chest wall resection. It has been shown that lung cancer that invades the chest wall is best treated by resection of the bony chest wall in continuity with pulmonary resection. Similar, although much less common, is breast cancer that invades the chest wall directly from the breast tissue. This is uncommon today since most breast cancer is found when small. Primary tumors of the chest wall also dictate a full-thickness resection and often require reconstruction of the bony and soft tissues. Infection necessitates a chest wall resection usu-

402

Box 26–1. Etiology of Chest Wall Defects.[17]

Neoplasm
  Primary chest wall
    Chondrosarcoma
    Osteosarcoma
    Solitary plasmacytoma
    Ewing's tumor
    Desmoid tumor
  Contiguous lung cancer
  Contiguous breast cancer
  Metastatic chest wall
    Breast
    Kidney
    Colon
    Thyroid
    Sarcoma
Infection
  Median sternotomy wound
  Lateral thoracotomy wound
  Osteomyelitis
Radiation necrosis
Trauma

ally after an infected median sternotomy has not healed properly after an initial attempt to close it. Resection of all devitalized tissue with open packing and serial debridement is often necessary to obtain a closed healed wound. Radiation therapy can cause serious problems in the chest wall. Although hopefully less common today because of more accurate portals and improved knowledge of the dangers of radiation therapy, this problem is still seen all too commonly. A fungating, painful, infected, or bleeding mass on the chest wall that results from radiation therapy can be resected with a great improvement of quality. Traumatic lesions are another reason to resect and reconstruct the chest wall but are not as common. Finally, congenital defects exist that require chest wall reconstruction.

Reasons for resection of the chest wall vary among different series. The four main reasons are shown in Box 26-1. In a large series by Arnold and Pairolero, chest wall tumor was

the indication in 275 patients, infected median sternotomy in 142, radiation necrosis in 119, and a combination of reasons in the remaining 121 patients[2] (see Table 26-1). In Cohen's series of 113 patients, the indications for resection were infection in 76 patients, mostly infected median sternotomies, radiation necrosis in 23, tumor in 12, and trauma in 2 patients.[6] Finally in another large series by Mansour et al the indications were malignancy in 171 patients, infection in 31, radiation necrosis in 29, and other reasons in 29 patients.[12] The actual distribution is largely determined by the practice patterns of each reporting physician.

When a portion of the bony chest wall is removed, reconstruction is not always necessary. Restoration of chest wall stability minimizes paradoxical movement and ensures adequate ventilatory mechanics. If the defect is less than 5 cm in diameter, it is unlikely it will cause much physiological impairment of ventilation. Thus, whether to reconstruct becomes a question of cosmetic outcome. If the defect is located anteriorly and the patient is thin or is going to lose a great deal of weight, most defects should be reconstructed to avoid a noticeable deformity of the chest wall. Conversely, if the defect is small and located posteriorly or if it will be covered by the scapula, reconstruction is not necessary. However, when the defect is at or near the tip of the scapula it should be reconstructed to prevent the tip of the scapula from catching on the edge of the chest wall and causing an uncomfortable sensation for the patient. Resection of the upper thoracic ribs, as occurs when resecting a Pancoast tumor, does not require reconstruction of the bony chest wall, since the scapula will cover the defect.

In general, it is not necessary to replace the sternum with prosthetic material after removal. It has been shown that reconstruction of the sternum with rigid material does not improve the mechanics of breathing or pulmonary function.[13,14] However, the defect should be covered with muscle and skin to obtain a closed wound.

▶ METHODS OF RECONSTRUCTION

Once the resection of all devitalized or malignant tissue has been accomplished, the chest wall must be closed to provide for adequate respiratory mechanics, to protect the underly-

Table 26–1
Indications for Chest Wall Resection: Selected Series

Series	Malignancy	Infection	Radiation necrosis	Other	Total
Arnold and Pairolero[2]	275	142	119		536
Mansour et al[12]	171	31	29	29	260
Cohen and Ramasastry[6]	12	76	23	2	113
Total (%)	458 (50.4%)	249 (27.4%)	171 (18.8%)	31 (3.4%)	909

ing organs and vessels, and to obtain an acceptable cosmetic outcome. If the defect is small, as mentioned previously, the bony chest wall does not need reconstruction, and the soft tissue can be closed primarily. With larger resections, the bony chest wall and the soft tissues will need some more creative techniques to obtain a closed wound.

To reconstruct the bony chest wall, some type of firm tissue needs to be placed. Usually this means synthetic material; however, Murakawa et al described using fascia lata in eight patients who had a chest wall resection.[15] All had a good outcome, and they claimed harvesting the graft was easy since it did not require repositioning and was markedly cheaper than using synthetic material. They did acknowledge the disadvantage of having to make another incision to harvest the graft.

The specific type of synthetic tissue to use is a confusing choice and is usually based on surgeon preference. A 2-mm-thick expanded polytetrafluoroethylene (PTFE) or Gore-Tex (W.L. Gore & Associates, Inc, Flagstaff, AZ) patch is the preferred material despite its high cost. Advantages include its impermeability to water and air, strength, and ease of use. It is sutured into place by large (#0) polypropylene sutures. Use of the thinner 1-mm patch is not recommended in chest wall reconstruction since it does not hold sutures as well as the thicker patch. Since the patch is fairly rigid in all directions it is easier to place tightly into the chest wall defect than other synthetic materials that are knitted. The PTFE has a characteristic appearance on follow-up computed chest tomography (Figure 26-1).

Synthetic mesh made of polypropylene either single knitted (Marlex by Davol and Bard, Cranston, RI) or double-stitch knitted (Prolene by Ethicon, Inc, Somerville, NJ) is an excellent material for reconstruction. The material is not impermeable to water and air, which is of some concern for chest wall reconstructions. It is less expensive than PTFE and has been shown to yield just as good results as PTFE.[8]

These meshes can also be combined with methylmethacrylate to form a rigid prosthesis for the chest wall. This is rarely necessary as shown by Arnold and Pairolero.[2] They used this rigid material only once in 500 reconstructions and it had to be removed 2 months later for infection. The material must be used with care because when mixed, the reaction is exothermic and the heat given off may damage lung or surrounding tissues. It can be useful for reconstructing a huge defect where a curved prosthesis is needed. With a piece of lead plate formed to the correct shape, a marlex methylmethacrylate sandwich can be formed over the lead template. Once this mixture has cooled, it can be sutured into the defect in the chest wall by passing large sutures through the marlex that is at the perimeter of the prosthesis. Infection of a rigid prosthesis remains a problem. The constant motion of the chest wall tends to loosen the material unless it is secured very carefully. In one series, three of the nine prostheses had to be removed for infection even though all were placed in clean incisions.[9] It was felt that methylmethacrylate led to more chest wall pain and respiratory problems than other synthetic materials.

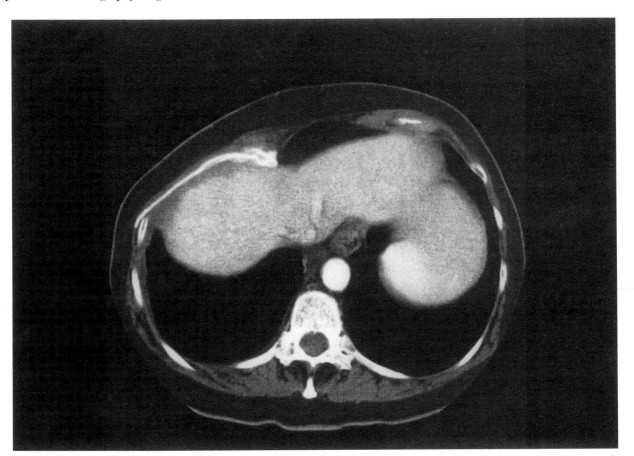

Figure 26–1 Postoperative chest computed tomography on a patient who has had a 2-mm Gore-Tex patch placed in the right lower anterior chest wall.

404

Whatever prosthetic material is chosen, it should be securely attached to the chest wall. The suture material should be nonabsorbable polypropylene, usually #0 or #1. The sutures can be passed around the rib for a secure closure and should be placed interrupted so that if one fails, the patch does not fail. The patch should be placed on the outside edge of the bony chest wall for the best cosmetic result. If the diaphragm is involved in the resection, it can be attached to the patch in a similar manner. The patch should be under tension after it is sewn in place; therefore, if a patient is in a flexed lateral decubitus position, the flex in the operation room should be removed before placing the patch.

Seromas will often occur after a synthetic material is used to reconstruct the chest wall. It is unclear whether placing a drain at the time of surgery to prevent the formation of a seroma is a good idea. The drain will certainly decrease the incidence of seromas but may increase the incidence of infection, a far more serious problem. Postoperative seromas can be managed by observation with a gentle pressure dressing or, if the seroma is large, aspiration under strict aseptic conditions. Aspiration may have to be performed several times until the problem resolves. Infection of a prosthetic patch is a grave problem and usually means the patch must be removed. Usually a fibrin layer has formed under the patch so the risk of creating an open pneumothorax is low if the patch has been in place for sufficient time, usually a week or two. If the patch is made of Gore-Tex, it is rela-

tively easy to slip the patch out, place drains in the space, and allow the incision to heal by secondary intention. Marlex is much more difficult to remove because of the ingrowth of fibrous tissue.

▶ SOFT TISSUE COVERAGE

Once the bony chest wall has been stabilized, the incision is closed. This is best accomplished by primary closure with local tissue. Unfortunately, this is often not possible because much of the overlying skin and muscle required resection. In this situation, myocutaneous flaps have become an invaluable resource to cover the prosthetic material and provide closure. A variety of different myocutaneous flaps are available; the choice of which one to use depends on the location of the defect and what is available.

For anterior central chest wall defects, the pectoralis major is an excellent choice. In Arnold's series, this muscle was used in 355 patients.[2] It is mobilized preserving the thoracromial neurovascular leash and can easily reach the midline (Figure 26-2). Mobilization in this fashion permits another median sternotomy to be done in the future without dividing the blood supply of the flaps.

Another extremely versatile myocutaneous flap is based on the latissimus dorsi muscle (Figure 26-2). This flap covers anterior or anterior lateral defects quite well. It is

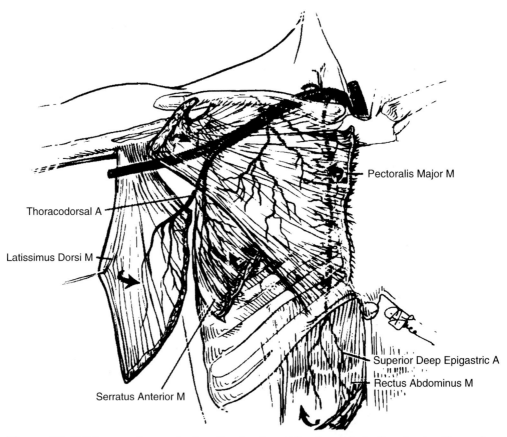

Pectoralis Major M

Thoracodorsal A

Latissimus Dorsi M

Superior Deep Epigastric A

Rectus Abdominus M

Serratus Anterior M

Figure 26–2 Diagram demonstrating the dominant blood supply to the chest wall muscles. *(From Black SB, Mendez-Eastman SK: Repair and care of chest wall defects. Plast Surg Nurs 21:13–21, 2001. Originally from Shaw, Aston, Zide, 1990.)*

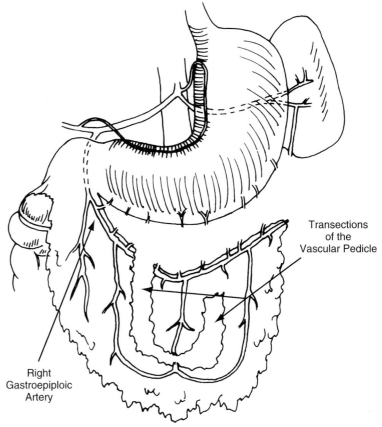

Figure 26–3 Diagram demonstrating the blood supply of the omentum and the divisions necessary to harvest the omentum based on the right gastroepiploic artery and the omental arcade. *(From Graeber GM: Chest wall resection and reconstruction. Sem Thorac Cardiovasc Surg 11:251–263, 1999.)*

Transections of the Vascular Pedicle

Right Gastroepiploic Artery

transposed on the dominant thoracodorsal neurovascular leash and can retain its function when the nerve is left intact. It is an extremely reliable source of tissue coverage.

The serratus anterior muscle is rarely used for chest wall defects but can be rotated into the chest cavity to cover defects in the airway (Figure 26-2).

For lower anterior chest wall defects, the rectus abdominus can be used for coverage. The muscle can be harvested with its overlying skin as a transverse rectus abdominus myocutaneous flap, known as the TRAM flap. This will provide excellent coverage for the lower chest wall. The muscle depends on the blood supply from the superior epigastric artery so if the ipsilateral mammary artery has been taken, this flap is not the first choice.

The external oblique can also be used to cover lower anterior chest wall defects. It is not commonly used. It can reliably cover up only to the inferior mammary crease.

The omentum can also be used to provide viable tissue on a damaged chest wall. It is not thick enough to cover prosthetic material, but it can be used when the bony chest is intact and the skin and subcutaneous tissue have been lost due to radiation damage or infection. It requires a laparotomy for harvest. Laparoscopic harvesting has been described, but most patients with a chest wall defect do not tolerate the pneumoperitoneum required for a laparoscopic approach. It is usually based on the right gastroepiploic arcade and if the omental arc is divided, the tissue can reach almost anywhere on the chest wall (Figure 26-3). The omentum is most useful for coverage of the chest wall after radiation damage. In the large series by Arnold, omentum was

of little use for treatment of an infected median sternotomy.[2]

► **SUMMARY**

In summary, resection and reconstruction of chest wall lesions can be a challenging endeavor. However, by approaching the problems of each patient with a careful, well-thought plan, the results should be excellent in the majority of patients. Use of expertise of a variety of other specialties, including plastic surgeons, anesthesiologists, and pulmonary medicine will greatly facilitate successful results.

REFERENCES

1. Akiba T, et al: Reconstruction of thoracic wall defects after tumor resection using a polytetrafluoroethylene soft tissue (Gore-Tex) patch. Jpn J Cardiovasc Surg 46:526–529, 1998.
2. Arnold PG, Pairolero PC: Chest-wall reconstruction: An account of 500 consecutive patients. Plast Reconstr Surg 98:804–810, 1996.
3. Bisgard JD, Swenson SA Jr: Tumors of the sternum: Report of a case with special operative technique. Arch Surg 56:570, 1948.
4. Black SB, Mendez-Eastman SK: Repair and care of chest wall defects. Plast Surg Nurs 21:13–21, 2001.
5. Blades B, Paul JS: Chest wall tumors. Ann Surg 131:976, 1950.

406

6. Cohen M, Ramasastry SS: Reconstruction of complex chest wall defects. Am J Surg 172:35–40, 1996.

7. Converse JM, Campbell RM, Watson WL: Repair of large radiation ulcers situated over the heart and the brain. Ann Surg 133:95, 1951.

8. Deschamps C, et al: Early and long-term results of prosthetic chest wall reconstruction. J Thorac Cardiovasc Surg 117:588–592; 1999.

9. Gayer G, Yellin A, Rozenman Y: Reconstruction of the sternum and chest wall with methyl methacrylate: CT and MRI appearance. Eur Radiol 8:239–243, 1998.

10. Graeber GM: Chest wall resection and reconstruction. Sem Thorac Cardiovasc Surg 11:251–263, 1999.

11. Graham J, Usher FC, Perry JL, Barkley HT: Marlex mesh as a prosthesis in the repair of thoracic wall defects. Ann Surg 151:469–479, 1960.

12. Mansour KA, et al: Chest wall resections and reconstruction: A 25-year experience. Ann Thorac Surg 73:1720–1726, 2002.

13. McCormack PM: Use of prosthetic materials in chest-wall reconstruction: Assets and liabilities. Surg Clin North Am 69:965–976, 1989.

14. Meadows JA III, Statts BA, Pairolero PC: Effect of resection of the sternum and manubrium in conjunction with muscle transposition on pulmonary function. Mayo Clin Proc 60:604, 1985.

15. Murakawa T, et al: Reappraisal of fascia lata grafts for the reconstruction of chest wall defects. Asia Cardiovasc Thorac Ann 10:285–286, 2002.

16. Myre TT, Kirklin JW: Resection of tumors of the sternum. Ann Surg 144:1023, 1956.

17. Sabanathan S, et al: Chest wall resection and reconstruction. Br J Hosp Med 57:255–259, 1997.

18. Tansini I: Sopra il mio nuovo processo di amputazione della mammella. Gazz Med Ital Torino 57:141, 1906.

19. Watson WL, James AG: Fascia lata grafts for chest wall defects. J Thorac Surg 16:399–406, 1947.

Thoracic Outlet Syndrome and Dorsal Sympathectomy

Harold C. Urschel, Jr. and Amit N. Patel

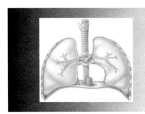

▶ INTRODUCTION

Thoracic outlet syndrome, a term coined by Rob and Standover,[57] refers to compression of the subclavian vessels and brachial plexus at the superior aperture of the chest. It was previously designated according to presumed etiologies as scalenus anticus, costoclavicular, hyperabduction, cervical rib, and first thoracic rib syndromes. The various syndromes are similar, and the compression mechanism is often difficult to identify. Most compressive factors operate against the first rib[16,76] (Figure 27-1).

▶ HISTORICAL ASPECTS

Until 1927, the cervical rib was commonly thought to be the cause of symptoms of this syndrome. Galen and Vesalius first described the presence of a cervical rib.[8] Hunauld, who published an article in 1742, is credited by Keen[36] as being the first to describe the importance of the cervical rib in causing symptoms. In 1818, Cooper treated symptoms of cervical rib with some success,[3] and in 1861, Coote[19] did the first cervical rib removal. Halsted[29] stimulated interest in dilatation of the subclavian artery distal to cervical ribs, and Law[40] reported the role of adventitious ligaments in the cervical rib syndrome. In 1927, Adson and Coffey[3] suggested the role of the scalenus anticus muscle in cervical rib syndrome. Naffziger and Grant[48] and Ochsner and associates[49] popularized section of the scalenus anticus muscle. Falconer and Weddell[26] and Brintnall and colleagues[12] incriminated the costoclavicular membrane in the production of neurovascular compression. In 1945, Wright[91] described the hyperabduction syndrome with compression in the costoclavicular area by the tendon of the pectoralis minor. Rosati and Lord[61] added claviculectomy to anterior exploration, scalenotomy, cervical rib resection, when one was present, and section of the pectoralis minor and subclavian muscles, as well as the costoclavicular membrane. The

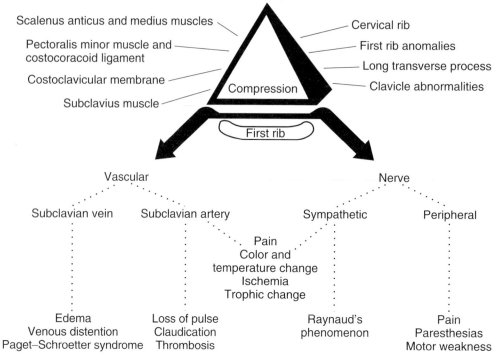

Figure 27–1 Schematic diagram showing the relation of muscle, ligament, and bone abnormalities in the thoracic outlet that may compress neurovascular structures against the first rib.

role of the first rib in causing symptoms of neurovascular compression was recognized by Bramwell[9] in 1903. Murphy[47] is credited with the first resection of the first rib. Brickner,[10] Brickner and Milch,[11] and Telford and co-workers[70,71] suggested that the first rib was the culprit. Clagett[16] emphasized the first rib and its resection through the posterior thoracoplasty approach to relieve neurovascular compression. In 1962, Falconer and Li[25] reported the anterior approach for first rib resection, whereas Roos[58] introduced the transaxillary route for first rib resection and extirpation. Krusen and Caldwell[13] introduced the method of measuring motor conduction velocities across the thoracic outlet in diagnosing thoracic outlet syndrome. Urschel and associates[85] popularized reoperation for recurrent thoracic outlet syndrome.

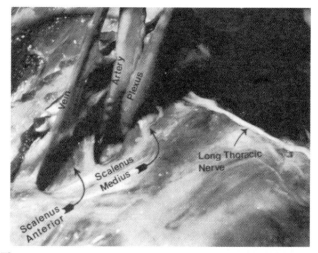

Figure 27–2 Anatomical dissection from the transaxillary approach, showing the relation of the neurovascular bundle, the scalenus anterior muscle, and the long thoracic nerve along the posterior border of the scalenus medius muscle.

SURGICAL ANATOMY

At the superior aperture of the thorax, the subclavian vessels and the brachial plexus traverse the cervicoaxillary canal to reach the upper extremity. The cervicoaxillary canal is divided by the first rib into two sections: the proximal one, composed of the scalene triangle and the costoclavicular space, and the distal one, composed of the axilla. The proximal division is the more critical for neurovascular compression. It is bounded superiorly by the clavicle, inferiorly by the first rib, anteromedially by the costoclavicular ligament, and posterolaterally by the scalenus medius muscle and the long thoracic nerve. The scalenus anticus muscle, which inserts on the scalene tubercle of the first rib, divides the costoclavicular space into two compartments: the anteromedial one containing the subclavian vein and the posterolateral one containing the subclavian artery and the brachial plexus (Figure 27-2). The latter compartment, which is bounded by

the scalenus anticus anteriorly, the scalenus medius posteriorly, and the first rib inferiorly, is called the scalene triangle.

FUNCTIONAL ANATOMY

The cervicoaxillary canal, particularly its proximal segment, the costoclavicular area, normally has ample space for passage of the neurovascular bundle without compression. Narrowing of this space occurs during functional maneuvers. It narrows during abduction of the arm because the clavicle rotates backward toward the first rib and the insertion of the scalenus anticus muscle. In hyperabduction, the neurovascular bundle is pulled around the pectoralis minor tendon, the coracoid process, and the head of the humerus. During this maneuver, the coracoid process tilts downward and thus exaggerates the tension on the bundle. The sternoclavicular joint, which ordinarily forms an angle of 15–20°, forms a smaller angle when the outer end of the clavicle descends (as in drooping of the shoulders in poor posture), and narrowing of the costoclavicular space may occur.[61] Normally, during inspiration, the scalenus anticus muscle raises the first rib and thus narrows the costoclavicular space. This muscle may cause an abnormal lift of the first rib, as in cases of severe emphysema or excessive muscular development, which is seen in young adults.

The scalene triangle, which normally occurs between the scalenus anticus anteriorly, the scalenus medius posteriorly, and the first rib inferiorly, permits the passage of the subclavian artery and the brachial plexus, which are in direct contact with the first rib. The space of the triangle is 1.2 cm at its base and approximately 6.7 cm in height (Figure 27-3). There is a close-fitting relationship between the neurovascular bundle and this triangular space. Anatomical variations may narrow the superior angle of the triangle, cause impingement on the upper components of the brachial plexus, and produce the upper type of scalenus anticus syndrome that involves the trunk containing elements of C5 and C6. If the base of the triangle is raised, compression of the subclavian artery and the trunk containing components of C7, C8, and T1 results in the lower type of scalenus anticus syndrome. Both types have been described by Swank and Simeone.[68]

COMPRESSION FACTORS

Many factors may cause compression of the neurovascular bundle at the thoracic outlet, but the basic factor is deranged anatomy, to which congenital, traumatic, and, occasionally, atherosclerotic factors may contribute[61] (Box 27-1). Bony abnormalities are present in approximately 30% of patients, either as cervical rib, bifid first rib, and fusion of first and second ribs, clavicular deformities, or previous thoracoplasties.[76] These abnormalities can be visualized on the plain posteroanterior chest film, but special X-ray views of the lower cervical spine may be required in some cases of cervical ribs.

SYMPTOMS AND SIGNS

The symptoms of thoracic outlet syndrome depend on whether the nerves or blood vessels, or both, are compressed in the cervicoaxillary canal. Neurogenic manifestations are observed more frequently than vascular ones. Symptoms consist of pain and paresthesias, which are present in approximately 95% of cases, and motor weakness and occasionally atrophy of hypothenar and interosseous muscles, which is the ulnar type of atrophy, in approximately 10%. The symptoms occur most commonly in areas supplied by the ulnar nerve, which include the medial aspects

> **Box 27–1. Etiological Factors of Neurovascular Compression Syndromes.**
>
> **Anatomical**
>
>   Potential sites of neurovascular compression
>   Interscalene triangle
>   Costoclavicular space
>   Subcoracoid area
>
> **Congenital**
>
>   Cervical rib and its fascial remnants
>   Rudimentary first thoracic rib
>   Scalene muscles
>   Anterior
>   Middle
>   Minimus
>   Adventitious fibrous bands
>   Bifid clavicle
>   Exostosis of first thoracic rib
>   Enlarged transverse process of C7
>   Omohyoid muscle
>   Anomalous course of transverse cervical artery
>   Brachial plexus postfixed
>   Flat clavicle
>
> **Traumatic**
>
>   Fracture of clavicle
>   Dislocation of head of humerus
>   Crushing injury to upper thorax
>   Sudden, unaccustomed muscular efforts involving shoulder
>   girdle muscles
>   Cervical spondylosis and injuries to cervical.spine
>
> **Atherosclerosis**

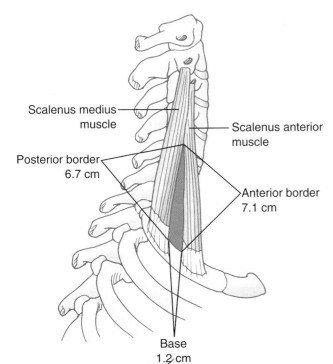

Scalenus medius muscle

Scalenus anterior muscle

Posterior border
6.7 cm

Anterior border
7.1 cm

Base
1.2 cm

Figure 27–3 Schematic drawing of the scalene (anterior) triangle showing its measurements and the narrow interval through which the neurovascular bundle passes.
(From Rosati LM, Lord JV: Neurovascular compression syndromes of the shoulder girdle. New York: Grune & Stratton, 1961.)

410 of the arm and hand, the fifth finger, and the lateral aspects of the fourth finger. The onset of pain is usually insidious and commonly involves the neck, shoulder, arm, and hand. The pain and paresthesias may be precipitated by strenuous physical exercise or sustained physical effort with the arm in abduction and the neck in hyperextension. Symptoms may be initiated by sleeping with the arms abducted and the hands clasped behind the neck. In other cases, trauma to the upper extremities or the cervical spine is a precipitating factor. Physical examination may be noncontributory. When present, objective physical findings usually consist of hypesthesia along the medial aspects of the forearm and hand. Atrophy, when evident, is usually described in the hypothenar and interosseous muscles with clawing of the fourth and fifth fingers. In the upper type of thoracic outlet syndrome in which components of C5 and C6 are involved in compression, pain is usually in the deltoid area and the lateral aspects of the arm. The presence of this pain should

induce action to exclude a herniated cervical disk.[61] Entrapment of C7 and C8 components that contribute to the median nerve produces symptoms in the index and sometimes the middle fingers. Components of C5, C6, C7, C8, and T1 can occur at the thoracic outlet by a cervical rib and produce symptoms of various degrees in the distribution of these nerves (Figure 27-4).

In some patients, the pain is atypical, involving the anterior chest wall or parascapular area, and is termed pseudoangina because it simulates angina pectoris. These patients may have normal coronary arteriograms and ulnar nerve conduction velocities decreased to values of 48 m/s and less, which strongly suggests the diagnosis of thoracic outlet syndrome. The shoulder, arm, and hand symptoms that usually provide the clue for the diagnosis of thoracic outlet syndrome may initially be absent or minimal compared with the severity of the chest pain. The diagnosis of thoracic outlet syndrome is frequently overlooked; many of these

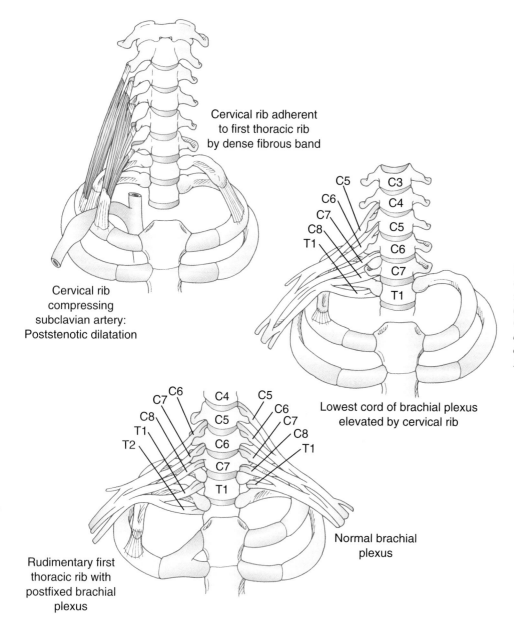

Figure 27–4 Compression caused by congenital rib abnormalities.
(Copyright 1971. CIBA-GEIGY Corporation. Modified and reproduced with permission from Clinical Symposia by Frank H. Netter, MD. All rights reserved.)

patients are committed to becoming "cardiac cripples" without an appropriate diagnosis or develop severe psychological depression when told that their coronary arteries are normal and that they have no significant cause for their pain.[86]

Symptoms of arterial compression include coldness, weakness, easy fatigability of the arm and hand, and pain that is usually diffuse.[76,77] Raynaud's phenomenon is noted in approximately 7.5% of patients with thoracic outlet syndrome.[76] Unlike Raynaud's disease, which is usually bilateral and symmetrical and elicited by cold or emotion, Raynaud's phenomenon in neurovascular compression is usually unilateral and is more likely to be precipitated by hyperabduction of the involved arm, turning of the head, or carrying of heavy objects. Sensitivity to cold may also be present. Symptoms include sudden onset of cold and blanching of one or more fingers, followed slowly by cyanosis and persistent rubor. Vascular symptoms in neurovascular compression may be precursors of permanent arterial thrombosis.[61] Arterial occlusion, usually of the subclavian artery, when present, is manifested by persistent coldness, cyanosis or pallor of the fingers, and in some instances, ulceration or gangrene. Palpation in the parascapular area may reveal prominent pulsation, which indicates poststenotic dilatation or aneurysm of the subclavian artery[62] (Figure 27-5).

Less frequently, the symptoms are those of venous obstruction or occlusion, commonly recognized as effort thrombosis, or Paget–Schroetter syndrome. The condition characteristically results in edema, discoloration of the arm, distention of the superficial veins of the limb and shoulder, and some degree of aches and pains. In some patients, the condition is observed on waking; in others, it follows sustained efforts with the arm in abduction. Sudden backward and downward bracing of the shoulders or heavy lifting or strenuous physical activity involving the arm may constrict the vein and initiate venospasm, with or without subsequent thrombosis. On examination, in cases of definite venous thrombosis, there is usually moderate tenderness over the axillary vein and a cord-like structure may be felt that corresponds to the course of the vein. The acute symptoms may subside in a few weeks or days as the collateral circulation develops. Recurrence follows with inadequacy of the collateral circulation.[42]

Objective physical findings are more common in patients with primarily vascular rather than neural compression. Loss or diminution of radial pulse and reproduction of symptoms can be elicited by the three classic clinical maneuvers: the Adson or scalene test,[2] the costoclavicular test, and the hyperabduction test.[78]

DIAGNOSIS

The diagnosis of thoracic outlet syndrome includes history, physical and neurological examinations, films of the chest and cervical spine, electromyogram, and ulnar nerve conduction velocity (UNCV). In some cases with atypical manifestations, other diagnostic procedures such as cervical myelography, peripheral[62] or coronary arteriography, or phlebography[1] should be considered. A detailed history and physical and neurological examinations can often result in a tentative diagnosis of neurovascular compression. This diagnosis is strengthened when one or more of the classic clinical maneuvers is positive and is confirmed by the finding of decreased UNCV.[77]

Clinical Maneuvers

The clinical evaluation is best based on the physical findings of loss or decrease of radial pulses and reproduction of symptoms that can be elicited by the following three classic maneuvers:

1. Adson or scalene test[2] (Figure 27-6). This maneuver tightens the anterior and middle scalene muscles and thus decreases the interspace and magnifies any preexisting compression of the subclavian artery and brachial plexus. The patient is instructed to take and hold a deep breath, extend the neck fully, and turn the head toward the side. Obliteration or decrease of the radial pulse suggests compression.[61,78]
2. Costoclavicular test (military position) (Figure 27-7). The shoulders are drawn downward and backward. This maneuver narrows the costoclavicular space by approximating the clavicle to the first rib and thus tends to compress the neurovascular bundle. Changes in the radial pulse with production of symptoms indicate compression.[61,78]
3. Hyperabduction test (Figure 27-8). When the arm is hyperabducted to 180 degrees, the components of the neurovascular bundle are pulled around the pectoralis minor tendon, the coracoid process, and the head of the humerus. If the radial pulse is decreased, compression should be suspected.[61,78]

Radiographic Findings

Films of the chest and cervical spine are helpful in revealing bony abnormalities, particularly cervical ribs (Figure 27-9) and bony degenerative changes. If osteophytic changes and intervertebral space narrowing are present on plain cervical films, a cervical computed tomography (CT) scan should be performed to rule out bony encroachment and narrowing of the spinal canal and the intervertebral foramina.

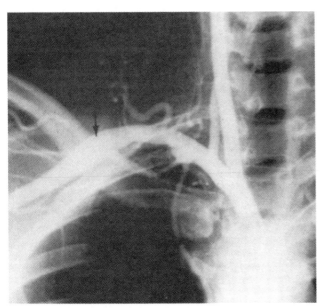

Figure 27–5 Arteriogram showing poststenotic dilatation (*arrow*) of the right subclavian artery secondary to thoracic outlet compression.

412

Adson maneuver
for diagnosis of
scalenus anticus syndrome

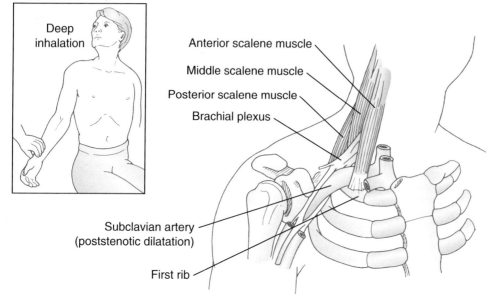

Deep
inhalation

Anterior scalene muscle

Middle scalene muscle

Posterior scalene muscle

Brachial plexus

Subclavian artery
(poststenotic dilatation)

First rib

Figure 27–6 Adson's maneuver. Relation of the scalene triangle to the neurovascular bundle. *(Copyright 1971. CIBA-GEIGY Corporation. Modified and reproduced with permission from Clinical Symposia by Frank H. Netter, MD. All rights reserved.)*

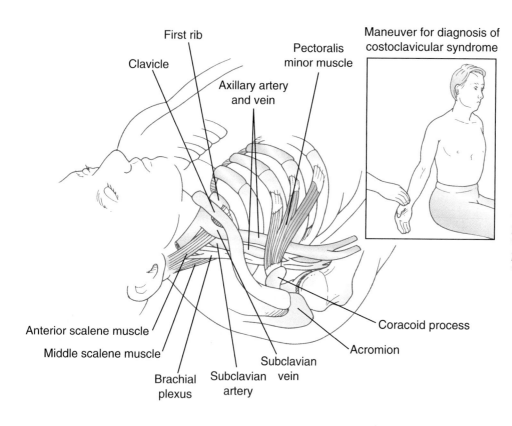

First rib

Clavicle

Pectoralis
minor muscle

Maneuver for diagnosis of
costoclavicular syndrome

Axillary artery
and vein

Anterior scalene muscle

Middle scalene muscle

Brachial
plexus

Subclavian
artery

Subclavian
vein

Coracoid process

Acromion

Figure 27–7 Costoclavicular maneuver (military position). Relation of the costoclavicular space to the neurovascular bundle. *(Copyright 1971. CIBA-GEIGY Corporation. Modified and reproduced with permission from Clinical Symposia by Frank H. Netter, MD. All rights reserved.)*

Nerve Conduction Velocity and Electromyography

This test is widely used in differential diagnosis of the causes of arm pain, tingling, and numbness with or without motor weakness of the hand. Such symptoms may result from compression at various sites: in the spine; at the thoracic outlet; around the elbow, where it causes tardy ulnar nerve palsy; or on the flexor aspects of the wrist, where it produces carpal tunnel syndrome. For diagnosis and localization of the site of compression, cathodal stimulation is applied at various points along the course of the nerve. Motor conduction velocities of the ulnar, median, radial, and musculocutaneous nerves can be measured reliably.[34] Caldwell and colleagues[13] have improved the technique of measuring UNCV for evaluation of patients with thoracic outlet compression. Conduction velocities over proximal and distal

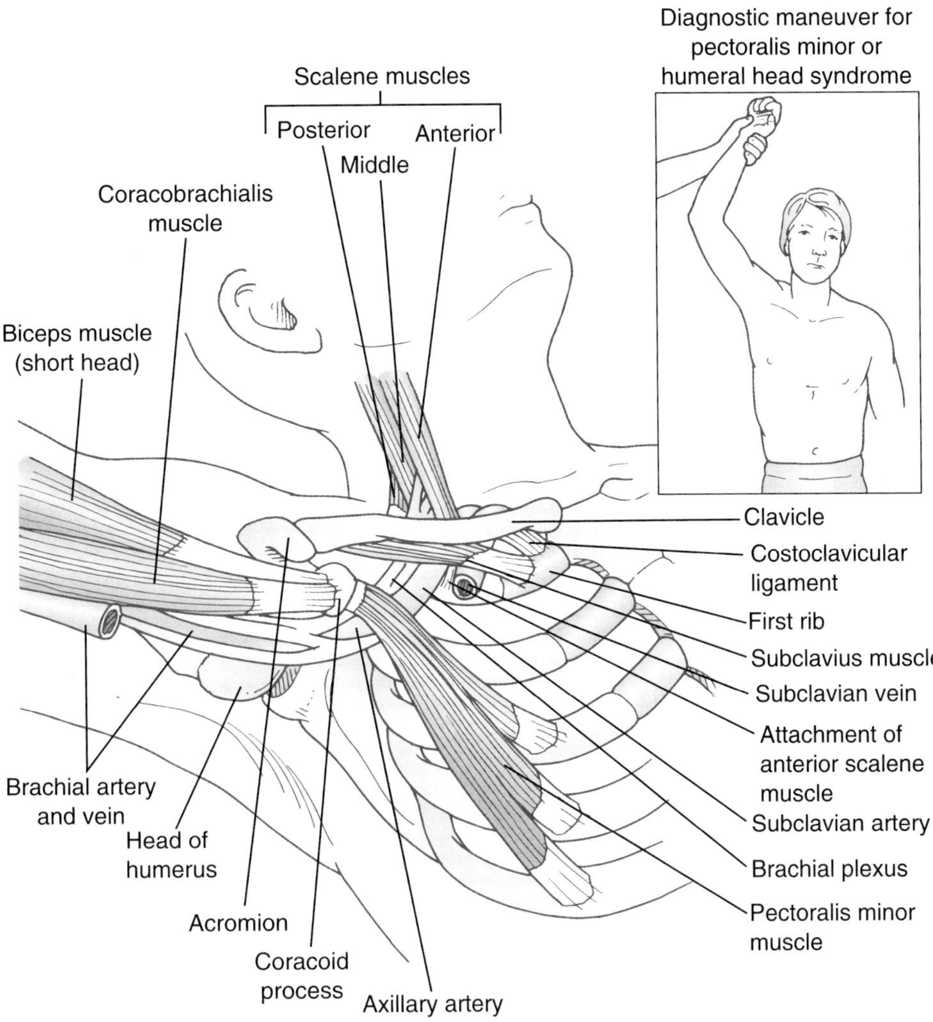

Diagnostic maneuver for
pectoralis minor or
humeral head syndrome

Scalene muscles

Posterior   Anterior

Middle

Coracobrachialis
muscle

Biceps muscle
(short head)

**Figure 27–8 Hyperabduction
maneuver.** Relation of the neurovascular bundle to the pectoralis
minor tendon, the coracoid process,
and the humeral head (pulley
effect).
*(Copyright 1971. CIBA-GEIGY
Corporation. Modified and reproduced with permission from Clinical
Symposia by Frank H. Netter, MD.
All rights reserved.)*

Clavicle

Costoclavicular
ligament

First rib

Subclavius muscle

Subclavian vein

Attachment of
anterior scalene
muscle

Subclavian artery

Brachial plexus

Pectoralis minor
muscle

Brachial artery
and vein

Head of
humerus

Acromion

Coracoid
process   Axillary artery

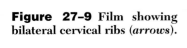

Figure 27–9 Film showing
bilateral cervical ribs (*arrows*).

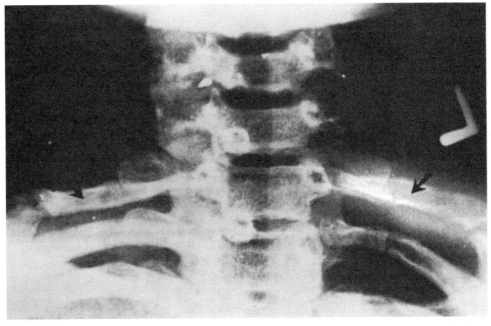

414 segments of the ulnar nerve are determined by recording the action potentials generated in the hypothenar or first dorsal interosseous muscles. The points of stimulation are the supraclavicular fossa, middle upper arm, below the elbow, and at the wrist[77] (Figure 27-10).

Method of Measuring Conduction Velocities

Equipment

Electromyographic examination of each upper extremity and determination of the conduction velocities are done with the Meditron 201 AD or 312 or the TECA-3 electromyograph; coaxial cable with three needles or surface electrodes are used to record muscle potentials, which appear on the fluorescent screen (Figure 27-11).

Technique

The conduction velocity is determined by the Krusen–Caldwell technique.[13] The patient is placed on the examination table with the arm fully extended at the elbow and in

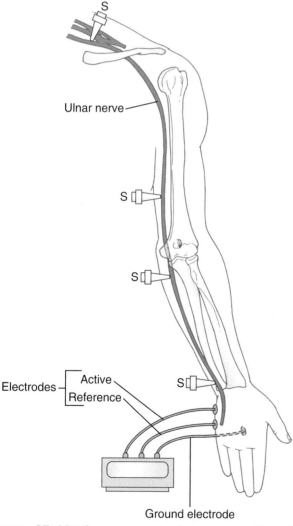

Figure 27–10 Ulnar nerve stimulation points (5) in the supraclavicular fossa (over the trunks of the plexus), above the elbow, below the elbow, and at the wrist.

about 20° of abduction at the shoulder to facilitate stimulation over the course of the ulnar nerve. The ulnar nerve is stimulated at the four points by a special stimulation unit (Figure 27-12) that imparts an electrical stimulus with strength of 350 V with the patient's load, which is approximately equal to 300 V with the patient's load with a skin resistance of 5000 Ω. Supramaximal stimulation is used at all points to obtain maximal response. The duration of the stimulation is 0.2 ms, except for muscular individuals, for whom it is 0.5 ms. Time of stimulation, conduction delay, and muscle response appear on the TECA screen; time markers occur each millisecond on the sweep.

The latency period to stimulation from the four points of stimulation to the recording electrode is obtained from the TECA digital recorder or calculated from the tracing on the screen.

Calculation of Velocities

After the latencies, which are expressed in milliseconds, are obtained, the distance in millimeters between two adjacent sites of stimulation is measured with steel tape. The velocities, which are expressed in meters per second, are calculated by subtracting the distal latency from the proximal latency and dividing the distance between two points of stimulation by the latency difference (Figure 27-13) according to the following formula:

$$\text{Velocity (m/s)} = \frac{\text{distance between two adjacent stimulation points (mm)}}{\text{difference in latency (ms)}}$$

Normal UNCVs

The normal values of the UNCVs according to the Krusen–Caldwell technique[13] are 72 m/s or above across the outlet, 55 m/s or above around the elbow, and 59 m/s or above in the forearm. Wrist delay is 2.5–3.5 ms. Decreased velocity in a segment or increased delay at the wrist indicates compression, injury, neuropathy, or neurological disorders. Decreased velocity across the outlet is consistent with thoracic outlet syndrome. Decreased velocity around the elbow signifies ulnar nerve entrapment or neuropathy. Increased delay at the wrist is encountered in carpal tunnel syndrome.

Grading of Compression

The clinical picture of thoracic outlet syndrome correlates fairly well with the conduction velocity across the outlet. Any value less than 70 m/s indicates neurovascular compression. The severity is graded according to decrease of velocity across the thoracic outlet: compression is called slight when the velocity is 66 to 69 m/s, mild when the velocity is 60 to 65 m/s, moderate when the velocity is 55 to 59 m/s, and severe when the velocity is 54 m/s and below.

Angiography

Simple clinical observations usually suffice to determine the degree of vascular impairment in the upper extremity. Peripheral angiography[39,62] is indicated in some cases, as in

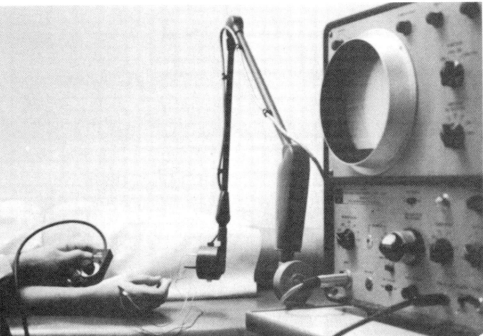

Figure 27–11 TECA-3 electromyograph using a coaxial cable and three needles to record generated action potentials.

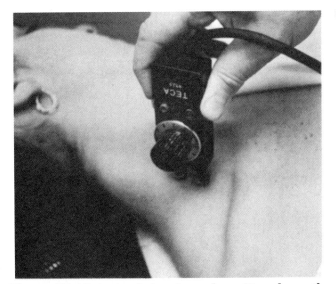

Figure 27–12 A stimulating electrode positioned over the cords of the brachial plexus at Erb's point in the supraclavicular fossa posterior to the sternocleidomastoid muscle, which is the stimulation site of the brachial plexus across the outlet.

the presence of a paraclavicular pulsating mass, the absence of radial pulse, or the presence of supraclavicular or infraclavicular bruits. Retrograde or antegrade arteriograms of the subclavian and brachial arteries to demonstrate or localize the pathology should be obtained. In cases of venous stenosis or obstruction, as in Paget–Schroetter syndrome, phlebograms are used to determine the extent of thrombosis and the status of the collateral circulation (Figure 27-14).

▶ DIFFERENTIAL DIAGNOSIS

The thoracic outlet syndrome should be differentiated from various neurological, vascular, cardiac, pulmonary, and esophageal conditions[61,76,77,86] (Box 27-2).

Neurological causes of pain in the shoulder and arm are more difficult to recognize and may arise from involvement of the nervous system in the spine, the brachial plexus, or the peripheral nerves. A common neurological cause of pain in the upper extremities is a herniated cervical intervertebral disk. The herniation almost invariably occurs at the interspace between the fifth and the sixth or the sixth and the seventh cervical vertebrae and produces characteristic symptoms. Onset of pain and stiffness of the neck is manifested with varying frequency. The pain radiates along the medial border of the scapula into the shoulder, occasionally into the anterior chest wall, and down the lateral aspect of the arm, at times into the fingers. Numbness and paresthesias in the fingers may be present. The segmental distribution of pain is a prominent feature. A herniated disk between the C5 and the C6 vertebrae, which compresses the C6 nerve root, causes pain or numbness primarily in the thumb and to a lesser extent in the index finger. The biceps muscle and the radial wrist extensor are weak, and the reflex of the biceps muscle is reduced or abolished. A herniated disk between the C6 and the C7 vertebrae, which compresses the C7 nerve root, produces pain or numbness in the index finger and weakness of index finger flexion and ulnar wrist extension; the triceps muscle is weak and its reflex is reduced or abolished. Any of these herniated disks may cause numbness along the ulnar border of the arm and hand due to spasm of the scalenus anticus muscle. Rarely, pain and paresthesias in the ulnar distribution may be related to herniation between the C7 and the Tl vertebrae, which causes compression of the C8 nerve root. Compression of the latter

Calculation of UNCV

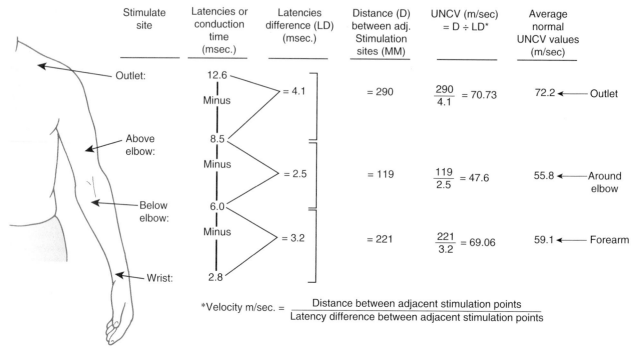

Stimulate site	Latencies or conduction time (msec.)	Latencies difference (LD) (msec.)	Distance (D) between adj. Stimulation sites (MM)	UNCV (m/sec) = D ÷ LD*	Average normal UNCV values (m/sec)
Outlet:	12.6	= 4.1	= 290	$\frac{290}{4.1}$ = 70.73	72.2 ◄── Outlet
	Minus				
Above elbow:	8.5	= 2.5	= 119	$\frac{119}{2.5}$ = 47.6	55.8 ◄── Around elbow
	Minus				
Below elbow:	6.0	= 3.2	= 221	$\frac{221}{3.2}$ = 69.06	59.1 ◄── Forearm
	Minus				
Wrist:	2.8				

*Velocity m/sec. = $\dfrac{\text{Distance between adjacent stimulation points}}{\text{Latency difference between adjacent stimulation points}}$

Figure 27–13 The sites of stimulation and the formula for calculating velocities.

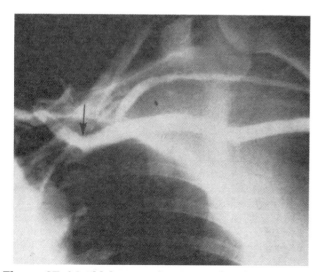

Figure 27–14 Phlebogram showing total occlusion *(arrow)* with minimal collateral circulation of the left subclavian vein due to thoracic outlet compression. At operation, no thrombus was present in the vein, and obstruction was relieved by removing the first rib.

nerve root produces weakness of intrinsic hand muscles.[37,61] Although rupture of the fifth and sixth disks produces hypesthesia in this area, only rupture of the seventh disk produces pain down the medial aspect of the arm.[61]

The diagnosis of a ruptured cervical disk is based primarily on the history and physical findings; lateral films of the cervical spine reveal loss or reversal of cervical curvature with the apex of the reversal of curvature at the level of the disk involved. Electromyography can localize the site and extent of the nerve root irritation. When a herniated disk is

Box 27–2. Differential Diagnosis of Thoracic Outlet Syndrome Nerve Compression.

Cervical spine ruptured intervertebral disk
Degenerative disease
Osteoarthritis
Spinal cord tumors
Brachial plexus superior sulcus tumors
Trauma-postural palsy
Peripheral nerves entrapment neuropathy
Carpal tunnel-median nerve
Ulnar nerve-elbow
Radial nerve
Suprascapular nerve
Medical neuropathies
Trauma
Tumor
Vascular phenomena
Arterial arteriosclerosis-aneurysm occlusive
Thromboangiitis obliterans
Embolism
Functional
Raynaud's disease
Reflex vasomotor dystrophy
Causalgia
Vasculitis, collagen disease, panniculitis
Venous thrombophlebitis
Mediastinal venous obstruction
Malignant
Benign
Other diseases
Angina pectoris
Esophageal
Pulmonary

suspected, cervical myelography should be done to confirm the diagnosis.[37,61]

Another condition that causes upper extremity pain is cervical spondylosis, a degenerative disease of the intervertebral disk and the adjacent vertebral margin that causes spur formation and the production of ridges into the spinal canal or intervertebral foramina. Films and a CT scan of the cervical spine and electromyography help in making the diagnosis of this condition (Figure 27-15).

Several arterial and venous conditions can be confused with thoracic outlet syndrome (see Box 27-2); the differentiation can often be made clinically.[61]

In atypical patients who present with chest pain alone, it is important to suspect the thoracic outlet syndrome in addition to angina pectoris. Exercise stress testing and coronary angiography may exclude coronary artery disease when there is a high index of suspicion of angina pectoris.[78,86]

THERAPY

Patients with thoracic outlet syndrome should be given physiotherapy when the diagnosis is made.

Proper physiotherapy includes heat massages, active neck exercises, stretching of the scalenus muscles, strengthening of the upper trapezius muscle, and posture instruction. Because sagging of the shoulder girdle, which is common among the middle-aged, is a major cause in this syndrome, many patients with less severe cases are improved by strengthening the shoulder girdle and by improving posture.[37]

Most patients with thoracic outlet syndrome who have UNCVs of more than 60 m/s improve with conservative management. If the conduction velocity is below that level,

most patients, despite physiotherapy, may remain symptomatic, and surgical resection of the first rib and correction of other bony abnormalities may be needed to provide relief of symptoms.[76,77,87]

If symptoms of neurovascular compression continue after physiotherapy, and the conduction velocity shows slight or no improvement or regression, surgical resection of the first rib and cervical rib, when present, should be considered.[76,77,87] Clagett[16] popularized the high posterior thoracoplasty approach for first rib resection, Falconer and Li[25] emphasized the anterior approach, and Roos[58] introduced the transaxillary route.

The transaxillary route is an expedient approach for complete removal of the first rib with decompression of the seventh and eighth cervical and first thoracic nerve roots and the lower trunks of the brachial plexus. First rib resection can be performed without the need for major muscle division, as in the posterior approach;[16] the need for retraction of the brachial plexus, as in the anterior supraclavicular approach;[25] and the difficulty of removing the posterior segment of the rib, as in the infraclavicular approach. In addition, first rib resection shortens the postoperative disability and provides better cosmetic results than the anterior and posterior approaches, particularly because 80% of patients are female.[76,77,87]

Technique of Transaxillary Resection of the First Rib

The patient is placed in the lateral position with the involved extremity abducted to 90° by traction straps wrapped around the forearm and attached to an overhead pulley. An appropriate weight, usually 2 lb, is used to maintain this position without undue traction[78] (Figure 27-16).

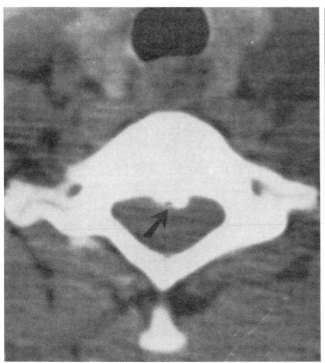

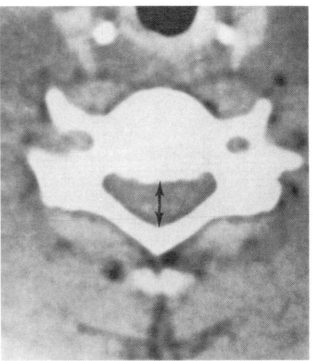

A   B

Figure 27-15 Computed tomography scan showing osteophytic ingrowth in the spinal canal (A) and narrowing of the anteroposterior diameter of the spinal canal (B) in a patient with the typical clinical picture of thoracic outlet syndrome.

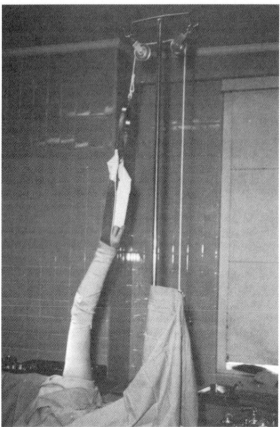

Figure 27–16 The arm is abducted to 90° by traction straps on the forearm and is attached to an overhead pulley.

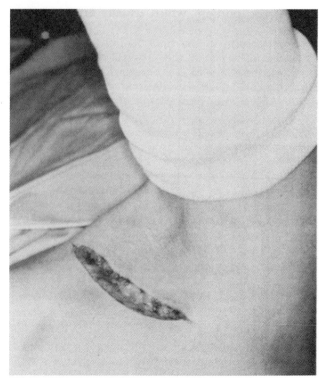

Figure 27–17 A transverse incision is made in the axilla below the hairline between the pectoralis major and the latissimus dorsi muscles and is extended to the chest wall.

A transverse incision is made in the axilla below the hairline between the pectoralis major and the latissimus dorsi muscles and deepened to the external thoracic fascia (Figure 27-17). Care should be taken to prevent injury to the intercostobrachial cutaneous nerve, which passes from the chest wall to the subcutaneous tissue in the center of the operative field.

The dissection is extended cephalad along the external thoracic fascia up to the first rib. With gentle dissection, the neurovascular bundle and its relation to the first rib and both scalenus muscles are clearly outlined to avoid injury to its components (Figure 27-18). The insertion of the scalenus anticus muscle is identified, skeletized, and divided (Figure 27-19). The first rib is dissected subperiosteally with a periosteal elevator and separated carefully from the underlying pleura to avoid pneumothorax. A segment of the middle portion of the rib is resected, followed by subperiosteal dissection and resection of the anterior portion of the rib at the costochondral junction. After the costoclavicular ligament is cut, the posterior segment of the rib is similarly dissected subperiosteally and resected in fragments, including the articulation with the transverse process, the neck, and the head. The scalenus medius muscle should not be cut from its insertion on the second rib but rather stripped with a periosteal elevator to avoid injury to the long thoracic nerve that lies on its posterior margin. The neck and head of the first rib are removed completely with a long, special Urschel double-action pituitary and Urschel Lexel rongeurs. The

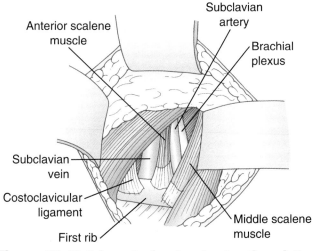

Figure 27–18 Schematic drawing showing the relationship of the neurovascular bundle to the scalene muscles, first rib, costoclavicular ligament, and subclavius muscle.

Anterior scalene muscle

Subclavian artery

Brachial plexus

Subclavian vein

Costoclavicular ligament

First rib

Middle scalene muscle

eighth cervical and first thoracic nerve roots may be visualized at this point. If a cervical rib is present, its anterior portion, which usually articulates with the first rib, should be resected at a point when the middle portion of the first rib is removed. The remaining segment of the cervical rib should be removed after removal of the posterior segments of the first rib. The wound is drained, and only the subcutaneous tissues and skin require closure, because no large muscles have been divided. The patient is encouraged to use the arm for self-care but to avoid heavy lifting until at least 3 months after operation. Cervical muscle stretching should be started

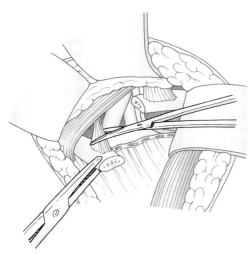

Figure 27–19 Schematic drawing showing division of the insertion of the scalenus anterior muscle on the first rib and removal of a segment of the midportion of the first rib.

at the end of the first week, and gentle exercising of the arm can be started at the end of the third week after operation.

It is preferable to remove the first rib entirely, including the head and neck, to avoid future irritation of the plexus, because a residual portion, particularly if long, will cause recurrence of symptoms.

EFFORT THROMBOSIS: PAGET–SCHROETTER SYNDROME

"Effort" thrombosis of the axillary-subclavian vein (Paget–Schroetter syndrome) is generally secondary to unusual or excessive use of the arm in addition to the presence of one or more compressive elements in the thoracic outlet.[1,35]

Historically, Paget[50] in 1875 in London and Von Schroetter[58] in 1884 in Vienna described this syndrome of thrombosis of the axillary-subclavian vein, which bears their names. The word effort[6] was added to thrombosis because of the frequent association with exertion producing either direct or indirect compression of the vein. The thrombosis is caused by trauma[15] or is associated with unusual occupations requiring repetitive muscular activity, as has been observed in professional athletes, Linotype operators, painters, and beauticians. Cold and traumatic factors, such as carrying skis over the shoulder, tend to increase the proclivity for thrombosis.[20] Elements of increased thrombogenicity also increase the incidence of the problem and exacerbate its symptoms on a long-term basis.

Adams and colleagues[1,21] reported long-term results in patients treated conservatively with elevation and warfarin sodium (Coumadin). There was a 12% incidence of pulmonary embolism. Development of occasional venous distention occurred in 18%, and late residual arm symptoms of swelling, pain, and superficial thrombophlebitis were noted in 68% of patients (deep venous thrombosis with postphlebitic syndrome). Phlegmasia cerulea dolens was present in one patient.

For many years, therapy included elevation of the arm and use of anticoagulants, with subsequent return to work. If symptoms recurred, the patient was considered for a first

rib resection, with or without thrombectomy,[21] as well as resection of the scalenus anterior muscle and removal of any other compressive element in the thoracic outlet, such as the cervical rib or abnormal bands.[32,54,59]

Increased availability of thrombolytic agents[63,67,92] combined with prompt surgical decompression of the neurovascular compressive elements in the thoracic outlet[69] reduced morbidity and the necessity for thrombectomy and substantially improved clinical results, including the ability to return to work.[82]

One advantage of urokinase over streptokinase is the direct action of urokinase on the thrombosis distal to the catheter, producing a local thrombolytic effect.[7,23,24] Streptokinase produces a systemic effect involving potential complications. Heparin is given postoperatively until the catheter is removed. Another advantage is that the need for thrombectomy decreases after use of the thrombolytic agent followed by aggressive surgical intervention because some of the long-term disability is related to morbidity from thrombectomy as well as recurrent thrombosis.[14,22,51]

The natural history of Paget–Schroetter syndrome suggests moderate morbidity[18,28,72] with conservative treatment alone. Bypass with vein or other conduits[30,31,33] has limited application. Causes other than thoracic outlet syndrome must be treated individually[43,66] using the basic principles mentioned. Intermittent obstruction of the subclavian vein[46] can lead to thrombosis, and decompression should be employed prophylactically.[31,33] Over 600 patients with Paget–Schroetter syndrome have now undergone operations. By far the best results are to lyse the clot, less than 6 weeks following the occlusion, the axillary-subclavian vien, and then promptly remove the first rib and provide neurovascular decompression. This gives uniformly good results. If the time of treatment is greater than 6 weeks from the time of the initial thrombosis, the results are less good, but again the same procedure should be performed to obtain optimal results.[83]

After successful thrombolysis, there often appears to be a stenosis in the vein on venography. Because of this, interventional radiologists or cardiologists tend to dilate this thinking it is an "internal" problem rather than the result of external compression. Because the stenosis immediately closes down after balloon dilatation they may insert intravascular stents. These have all failed in our experience[75] and in the experiences of others.[64]

DORSAL SYMPATHECTOMY AND THORACIC OUTLET SYNDROME MANAGEMENT WITH VIDEO-ASSISTED THORACIC SURGERY

Dorsal sympathectomy and the management of thoracic outlet syndrome are significantly improved with video assistance through magnification and an improved light system. Video-assisted thoracic surgery (VATS) offers better visualization of anatomical structures in a "deep hole," with an additional bonus of excellent visualization for other members of the team, particularly surgical residents. In addition, for sympathectomy alone, it offers less pain to the patient and a shorter hospitalization.

Video assistance is employed in two techniques. One involves the sympathectomy through three ports, with the

420 standard VATS. The second technique involves a transaxillary incision with removal of the first rib using video-assistance magnification and light; the surgeon operates either directly or secondarily while visualizing the image through the television set. This last technique was popularized by Martinez.[45]

Major indications for dorsal sympathectomy include hyperhidrosis, Raynaud's phenomenon and Raynaud's disease, causalgia, reflex sympathetic dystrophy (RSD), and vascular insufficiency of the upper extremity. Except for hyperhidrosis, all of the other indications require the usual diagnostic techniques, including cervical sympathetic block to assess whether the symptoms are relieved by temporary blockade of the sympathetic ganglia. When Raynaud's phenomenon of a minor to moderate degree is associated with thoracic outlet syndrome, the simple removal of the first rib with any cervical rib, in addition to stripping the axillary-subclavian artery (neurectomy), will relieve most symptoms following the initial operation.[76]

It is rarely necessary to perform a sympathectomy unless Raynaud's is a very severe type, in which case a dorsal sympathectomy is carried out with first rib resection. In contrast, with recurrent thoracic outlet syndrome and causalgia, it has been found that the dorsal sympathectomy should be performed with the initial reoperation procedure.[80,85]

Pathophysiology

The principal physiological effect expected of sympathectomy is the release of vasomotor control and hyperactive tone of the arterioles and smaller arteries that have a muscular element in the vessel wall. Circulation to the skin, peripheral extremity, and bone receives major improvement, but the effect on skeletal muscle of the arm is minimal. The other known function is the control over cutaneous weating, which is profuse and undesirable. Sympathectomy eliminates perspiration in that quadrant of the body but increases perspiration elsewhere. RSD is associated with pain, neuroesthenia, and cutaneous atrophy (Sudeck–Leriche) and posttraumatic limb. These patients also benefit from a sympathectomy if a diagnostic block is effective. Sympathectomy is not recommended in diabetic neuropathy. Nor should it be performed in any of the vascular vasospastic syndromes until after conservative management, including cessation of tobacco products and institution of β-blockers, peripheral vasodilators, and calcium channel blockers, has been tried.[17]

Preganglionic sympathetic nerves derived from the spinal cord do not follow a corresponding relationship to the accompanying somatic nerves. The cervical ganglia of C1 to C4 are fused into a superior cervical ganglion, C5 and C6 into the middle cervical ganglion, and C7 and C8 into the inferior ganglion, which combines with the ganglion from T1 to the larger stellate ganglion. Cervical ganglionectomy is not used for denervation of the upper extremity, since the preganglionic sympathetic outflow from the spinal cord to the arm is usually from T2 through T9, mostly from T2 through T4. In about 10% of cases, T1 preganglionic fibers also supply the upper extremity. For removal of preganglionic fibers to the upper extremity in most patients, removal of paravertebral ganglia T2 and T3 with the interconnecting chain is sufficient. Postganglionic fibers from these two segments

often join and branches then follow the nerves of the brachial plexus. The joined T2 and T3 fibers that bypass the stellate ganglion are known as the nerve of Kuntz.[38] For all of the remaining patients who have a T1 connection through the stellate ganglion to obtain adequate sympathetic denervation, the lower third of the stellate ganglion should also be removed, as recommended by Palumbo.[52,53]

Patients with RSD or sympathetic maintained pain syndrome (SMPS) must complain of pain outside a peripheral nerve distribution.[44] Although the injury itself may have been minor, the pain appears out of proportion to the injury. We have seen two types of RSD or SMPS; one involves the hand or even a greater majority of the upper extremity and a second is localized to one or more digits. In no instance can the patient's pain be completely accounted for by an injury to a specific nerve, although injury to a specific nerve may cause the more diffuse symptoms. The patient also demonstrates diminished hand function. Several patients have been referred with a diagnosis of SMPS, and, on examination, it is quite apparent that although they may complain of diffuse pain, the hand functions normally with a full range of movement and motor power is demonstrated. These patients, of course, do not have SMPS. The patient must also demonstrate some joint stiffness. The skin and soft tissue trophic changes demonstrate varying amounts of vasomotor instability, depending on the stage of SMPS.

According to Mackinnon and Dellon[44] there are early, intermediate, and late stages of SMPS. In the early stages, vasomotor instability is noted, with very dramatic sympathetic overactivity apparent in the hand or digit involved. Instability, with symptoms varying between redness and warmth and cyanosis and sweating, is noted in this early stage. Edema is also a classic finding in the early stage. In the intermediate stage of SMPS, pain is a less dramatic component and is usually elicited by attempts to move the joints. At rest, the patient may be quite comfortable. The edema and vasomotor changes have settled by this time, and the hand has the appearance of a "burned out" dystrophic hand, with marked stiffness and atrophy of the soft tissue noted. The normal wrinkles on the dorsum of the hand are no longer apparent. The fingertips may have a tapered appearance. The nail growth is usually more exaggerated than in the normal hand, and the hand is often cool and pale. The intermediate stage will extend over a number of months. During the late stage, all the superimposed problems of disuse atrophy may take effect. During this stage, problems with the elbow and shoulder are very common, even though the initial SMPS involved only the hand or one or more digits. The degree of pain experienced during the late phase is variable and is often the result of disuse and stiffness. SMPS can affect other areas of the body and has been observed in the foot, face, and penis.

Complications

Horner's Syndrome

If the fibers of C7 and C8 (the upper part of the stellate ganglion) are removed, Horner's syndrome results. This involves miosis, enophthalmos, drooping of the eyelid (ptosis), and flushing of that side of the face, with loss of sweating in that area.[27]

Postsympathetic Neuralgia

The complication of postsympathectomy neuralgia is less common in the upper extremities than in the lower extremities. The pain usually occurs in the shoulder and upper arm on the lateral aspect. Clinical history usually substantiates this diagnosis if the symptoms occur within the first 3 months. The confirmation may be obtained by a test involving skin resistance of pseudomotor activity detection. Tests reveal increased sympathetic activity and suggest a rebound phenomenon from the nonsympathectomized adjacent dermatomes. Rebound may be a regeneration of nerve fibers or an increased response of peripheral nerves to catecholamines. Symptoms are usually resolved in 3–6 weeks with conservative management. Phenytoin sodium (Dilantin), carbamazepine (Tegretol), and calcium channel blockers are all used in the medical management of these symptoms.[41]

Recurrent Symptoms

Occasionally following an excellent sympathectomy, with a warm hand and good circulation, recurrent symptoms may present as early as 3 months. These may be secondary to the regeneration or sprouting and rehooking of nerves or failure to strip the sympathetic nerves from the artery itself and the transfer of sympathetic tone through these nerves. Therefore, stripping of the axillary-subclavian artery of its local sympathetic nerves is performed in each case at the initial operation.[73] Also, during the initial procedure cauterization of the bed of the sympathectomy area produces sympathetic effects that usually last at least 3 years or longer.

Surgical Approaches for Dorsal Sympathectomy

Historically, the anterior cervical approach has been used, with the division of the scalenus-anticus muscle as the approach to the cervical sympathetic chain.[89] The stellate ganglion lies on the transverse process of C6, and this approach is used primarily by both neurosurgeons and vascular surgeons. For hypertension, Smithwick[65] and Urschel and Razzuk[79] popularized the posterior approach using a longitudinal parasternal incision with the patient in the prone position. A small piece of the first and second ribs is removed and the sympathetic chain is identified in the usual position. This approach has the advantage of allowing bilateral procedures at the same time without changing the patient's surgical position.

The most common approach is the transaxillary transthoracic approach, which is performed through the second or third interspace with the transverse subhairline incision.[4,5,52,53] This is more painful than the other approaches, but with video-assisted thoracoscopy, it can be performed with minimal discomfort. The approach most frequently employed when combined with thoracic outlet syndrome is the transaxillary approach with resection of the first rib, retraction of the pleura caudad, and a dorsal sympathectomy.[76,87] This combined procedure causes minimal pain and low morbidity. Video assistance is used frequently for this approach as well.

Variations of Dorsal Sympathectomy

Standard sympathectomy involves removal of the sympathetic chain with thoracic ganglia 1, 2, and 3. This involves removing the lower third of the stellate ganglion[80] with the second and third ganglia and the interconnecting sympathetic chain. This is the standard approach for hyperhidrosis, Raynaud's phenomena, causalgia, and RSD. It is advantageous that Horner's syndrome does not occur following removal of C8 or the upper two thirds of the stellate ganglia. Complete dorsal sympathectomy includes the removal of C8 with the total stellate ganglion including 1, 2, and 3 and the cervical chain in between. This procedure is primarily for patients with Raynaud's disease and actual ulceration of the fingers, as well as recurrent problems from the other indications. Newer evidence suggests that removal of only T2 and T3 ganglia, avoiding the stellate ganglia altogether, offers adequate sympathectomy for the standard indications of hyperhidrosis, Raynaud's phenomena, causalgia, and RSD. This is yet to be proved in the authors' experience, since careful attention to anatomy virtually eliminates the possibility of Horner's syndrome; thus, there is no advantage in leaving T1 if it presents potential problems.

Technique

Two approaches are employed. The first is the transaxillary approach with a transthoracic sympathectomy.[56] This involves leaving the first rib, collapsing the lung, and performing the sympathectomy with video-assisted techniques.[74] The second is a transaxillary removal of the first rib and the retraction of the pleura with a dorsal sympathectomy, which was used in most patients.

Transaxillary Approach with a Transthoracic Sympathectomy

The patient is placed in the lateral thoracotomy position with an axillary roll under the downside arm. The upper arm is suspended at 90 degree from the chest wall over a pulley system with a 1-pound weight.[5] An arm holder is employed to ensure that no hyperabduction or hyperextension of the shoulder occurs and that relaxation occurs every 3 min. Three ports are used between the second and the fourth interspaces. The camera should be placed either anteriorly or in the midaxillary port. A double-lumen endobracheal tube is employed, and the upside lung is collapsed, ventilating only the downside lung.[90] This shunts blood through the downside lung selectively, and excellent oxygenation usually results.

The lung is retracted and the sympathectomy performed. The mediastinal pleura are cut open and the sympathetic chain identified on the vertebral body near the neck of the ribs. Nerve hooks are employed to elevate the dorsal sympathetic chain, and the nerve connections, including the gray and white remi, are clipped before cutting or cauterization. The stellate ganglion is divided at the junction of the lower third, where it looks like a "cat's claw." The lower third is cut, but it is not photoablated or cauterized because Horner's syndrome may result from either heat or light injury in the adjacent C8 ganglion. The lower ganglia can be cauterized, photoablated with the laser, or cut. Hemostasis

422 is achieved with the cautery. The pleura are left open and the chest tube placed through one of the ports for purposes of drainage. There is a curvature of the sympathetic chain so that in many cases the stellate ganglion lies transversely, rather than vertically, on the transverse process of the vertebral body. Special knowledge of the anatomy is important, especially the location of the thoracic duct, which can simulate the sympathetic chain and be injured if not appropriately identified.

Transaxillary First Rib Resection for Thoracic Outlet Syndrome with Retraction of the Pleura and Sympathectomy

This technique differs slightly from the usual video-assisted thoracoscopy in that an actual incision is made transversely below the axillary hairline and the technique for rib resection is carried out.

A right-angle breast retractor with a light is employed, and a Dever retractor is placed on the other side of the incision. The video camera is a standard thoracoscope, a Wolf scope, or an Olympus flexible operating esophogastroscope.

The pleura are retracted inferiorly using a sponge stick, and the sympathetic chain is identified on the transverse process of the vertebral bodies. It is vertical between T2 and T3 ganglia. However, T1, the lower part of the stellate ganglion, angles anteriorly and lies in almost a transverse position. Clips are placed on all the communicating rami of the sympathetic chain. T2 and T3 ganglia are resected. The stellate ganglion is divided at the junction of its lower third and T1 is removed. This division is carried out with a sharp knife. Cauterization or laser photoablation is not employed in the stellate ganglion. Cautery is used after the removal of the sympathetic chain to prevent sprouting. Hemostasis is secured. A large, round Jackson-Pratt drain is placed and methylprednisolone acetate (Depo-Medrol) is injected over the nerve roots and plexus that have undergone neurolysis. The camera is removed and the wound closed in the usual manner.

Results

In 926 patients, sympathectomy alone or in conjunction with first rib removal for thoracic outlet syndrome has been successful (Urschel, 1999). In only six patients has sympathetic activity recurred in less than 6 months. All of these were treated conservatively initially. Three of the six required repeat sympathectomy. Postsympathectomy neuralgia occurred in only two of 926 patients. Both of these were managed successfully in a conservative manner. In the patients in whom Horner's syndrome was not created deliberately, four patients developed the syndrome. All resolved spontaneously in several months. Forty-two cases of Raynaud's phenomena were successfully treated with first rib resection alone or with periarterial neurectomy without initial sympathectomy.[73,74]

▶ REOPERATION FOR RECURRENT THORACIC OUTLET SYNDROME

Extirpation of the first rib relieves symptoms in patients with thoracic outlet syndrome not relieved by physiotherapy. Of the surgically treated patients, 10% develop various degrees of shoulder, arm, and hand pain and paresthesias that are usually mild and short-lasting and that respond well to a brief course of physiotherapy and muscle relaxants. In a few patients (1.6%), symptoms persist, become progressively more severe, and often involve a wider area of distribution because of entrapment of the immediate trunk in addition to the lower trunk and C8 and T1 nerve roots. Symptoms may recur 1 month to 7 years after rib resection; in most patients, they recur within the first 3 months. Symptoms consist of an aching or burning type of pain, often associated with paresthesias, involving the neck, shoulder, parascapular area, anterior chest wall, arm, and hand. Vascular lesions are uncommon and consist of causalgia minor and an occasional injury of the subclavian artery with subsequent false aneurysm formation caused by the sharp edge of a remaining posterior stump of an incompletely resected first rib (Figure 27-20). Recurrence is diagnosed on the basis of history, physical examination, and decreased nerve conduction velocity across the outlet. Diagnostic evaluation should also include thorough neurological evaluation, chest and cervical spine films (Figure 27-21), cervical myelography, subclavian artery angiography, and magnetic resonance imaging of cervical spine and brachial plexus,[55] when indicated.

Two groups of patients who require reoperation can be identified. Pseudorecurrence occurred in patients who did not have relief of symptoms after the initial operation. These patients can be separated etiologically as those in whom the second rib was mistakenly resected instead of the first; the first rib was resected, leaving a cervical rib; a cervical rib was resected, leaving an abnormal first rib; or a second rib was resected, leaving a rudimentary first rib. True recurrence occurred in patients whose symptoms were relieved after

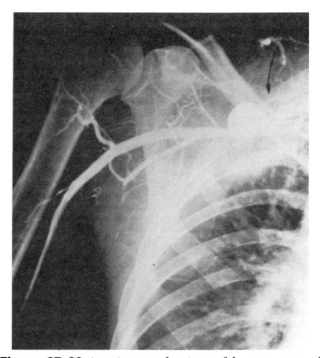

Figure 27–20 Arteriogram showing a false aneurysm of the right subclavian artery caused by the pointed end of a posterior stump (*arrow*) of an incompletely resected first rib.

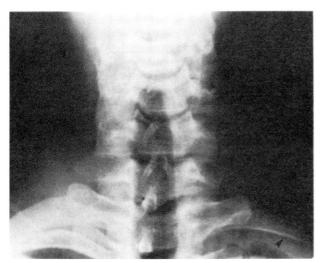

Figure 27–21 Cervical film showing a posterior remnant (arrow) of an incompletely resected first rib in a patient who developed recurrent thoracic outlet syndrome.

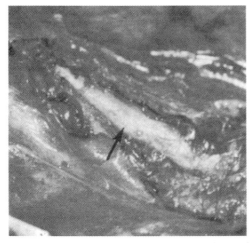

Figure 27–22 A long posterior remnant (*arrow*) of an incompletely resected first rib in a patient with recurrent thoracic outlet syndrome.

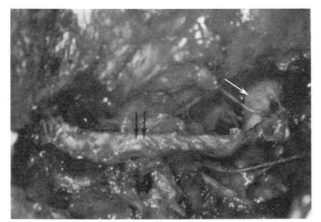

Figure 27–23 Fibrocalcific band (*double arrows*) of regenerated periosteum in continuity with a posterior remnant (*single arrow*) of the first rib in a patient with recurrent thoracic outlet syndrome.

the first operation but who retained a significant segment of the first rib or who had complete resection of the first rib but showed excessive scar formation around the brachial plexus.

Physiotherapy should be given to all patients with symptoms of neurovascular compression after first rib resection. If the symptoms persist and the conduction velocity remains below normal, reoperation is indicated.

Reoperation for thoracic outlet syndrome is performed with the posterior thoracoplasty approach to provide better exposure of the nerve roots and brachial plexus, which reduces the danger of injury to these structures and provides adequate exposure of the subclavian artery and vein. This incision also provides a wider field for resection of any bony abnormalities or fibrous bands and allows extensive neurolysis of the nerve roots and brachial plexus, which is not always possible with the limited exposure of the transaxillary approach. The anterior or supraclavicular approach is inadequate for reoperation.

The basic elements of reoperation include resection of persistent or recurrent bony remnants of a cervical first rib, neurolysis of the brachial plexus and nerve roots, and dorsal sympathectomy. Sympathectomy removes TI, T2, and T3 thoracic ganglia. Care is taken to avoid damage to the C8 ganglion (upper aspect of the stellate ganglion), which produces Horner's syndrome. The reoperation provides relief of major and minor causalgia and alleviates the paresthesias in the supraclavicular and infraclavicular areas. The incidence of "postsympathetic" syndrome has been negligible in this group of patients. A nerve stimulator is used to differentiate scar from nerve root to avoid damage with reoperations in these patients.

The technique of the operation includes a high thoracoplasty incision that extends from 3 cm above the angle of the scapula, halfway between the angle of the scapula and the spinous processes, and caudad 5 cm from the angle of the scapula. The trapezius and rhomboid muscles are split the length of the incision. The scapula is retracted from the chest wall by making a subperiosteal incision over the fourth rib. The posterior superior serratus muscle is divided and the sacrospinalis muscle retracted medially. The first rib remnant and cervical rib remnant, if present, are located and removed subperiosteally. After the rib remnants (Figure 27-22) have been resected, the regenerated periostium is removed (Figure 27-23). In the authors' experience, most regenerated ribs occur from the end of an unresected rib segment rather than from periosteum, although the latter is possible. For a reduction in the incidence of bony regeneration, it is important in the initial operation to remove the first rib totally in all patients with primarily nerve compression and pain.

After removal of a bony rib remnant, if there is excessive scar it may be prudent to do the sympathectomy initially. A 1-inch segment of the second rib is resected posteriorly to locate the sympathetic ganglion. In that way, the first thoracic nerve may be easier to locate below rather than through the scar.

Neurolysis of the nerve root and brachial plexus is done with a nerve stimulator and is carried down to but not into the nerve sheath. Neurolysis is extended peripherally over the brachial plexus as far as any scarring persists. Excessive neurolysis is not indicated, and opening of the nerve sheath

424 produces more scarring than it relieves. For scarring to be minimized the initial operation for thoracic outlet syndrome should include complete extirpation of the first rib, avoidance of hematomas with adequate drainage either by catheter or by opening the pleura, and avoidance of infection.

The subclavian artery and vein are released if symptoms mediate. The scalenus medius muscle is debrided. The dorsal sympathectomy is completed by extrapleural dissection. Meticulous hemostasis is effected, and a large, round Jackson-Pratt catheter drain is placed in the area of, but not touching, the brachial plexus and is brought out through the subscapular space via a stab wound into the axilla. Sepraseal (hyaluronidase) and methylprednisolone acetate (Depo-Medrol; 80 mg) are left in the area of the brachial plexus, but the patient is not given systemic steroids unless keloid formation has occurred. The wound is closed in layers with interrupted heavy Vicryl and Neurolon sutures to provide adequate strength. Range-of-motion exercises are performed to prevent shoulder limitation, but overactivity is avoided to minimize excessive scar formation.

When the problem is vascular and involves false or mycotic aneurysms, special techniques are used for reoperation. A bypass graft is interposed from the innominate or carotid artery proximally, through a separate tunnel distally, to the brachial artery. The graft is usually performed with the saphenous vein, although other conduits may be used. The arteries supplying and leaving the infected aneurysm are ligated. Subsequently, the aneurysm is resected by a transaxillary approach with no fear of bleeding or ischemia of the arm.

Special instruments have been devised to provide adequate resection through the transaxillary or posterior route and include a modified strengthened pituitary rongeur and a modified Leksell double-action rongeur for removal of the first rib without danger to the nerve root.

The sympathectomy relieves chest wall pain that resembles angina pectoris, esophageal disease, or even a tumor in the lung by denervating the deep fibers that accompany the arteries and bone.

The results of reoperation are good if an accurate diagnosis is made and the proper procedure is used.[80] More than 1200 patients have been followed up for 6 months to 15 years. All patients improved initially after reoperation, and in 79%, the improvement was maintained for more than 5 years. In 14% of the patients, symptoms were managed with physiotherapy; 7% required a second reoperation, in every case because of rescarring. There were no deaths, and only two patients had infections that required drainage.[84]

▶ SUMMARY

Thoracic outlet syndrome is recognized in approximately 8% of the population. Its manifestations may be neurological or vascular, or both, depending on the component of the neurovascular bundle predominantly compressed. The diagnosis is suspected from the clinical picture and is usually substantiated by determination of the UNCV. Treatment is initially conservative, but persistence of significant symptoms is an indication for first rib resection and occurs in approximately 5% of patients with diagnosed thoracic outlet

syndromes. Primary resection is performed preferably through the transaxillary approach. Symptoms of various degrees may recur after first rib resection in approximately 10% of patients. Most of the patients improve with physiotherapy, and only 1.6% require reoperation. Reoperation for recurrent symptoms is performed through a high posterior thoracoplasty incision.[80,84]

REFERENCES

1. Adams JT, DeWeese JA: Effort thrombosis of the axillary and subclavian veins. J Trauma 11:923, 1971. Adams JT, DeWeese JA, Mahoney EB, Rob CG: Intermittent subclavian vein obstruction without thrombosis. Surgery 63:147, 1968.
2. Adson AW: Cervical ribs: Symptoms and differential diagnosis for section of the scalenus anticus muscle. J Int Coll Surg 16:546, 1951.
3. Adson AW, Coffey JR: Cervical rib: A method of anterior approach for relief of symptoms by division of the scalenus anticus. Ann Surg 85:839, 1927.
4. Atkins HJB: Peraxillary approach to the stellate and upper thoracic sympathetic ganglia. Lancet 2:1152, 1949.
5. Atkins HJB: Sympathectomy by the axillary approach. Lancet 1:538, 1954.
6. Aziz R, Straenley CJ, Whelan TJ: Effort-related axillasubclavian vein thrombosis. Am J Surg 152:57, 1986.
7. Becker GJ, Holden RW, Robe FE, et al: Local thrombolytic therapy for subclavian and axillary vein thrombosis. Radiology 149:419, 1983.
8. Borchardt M: Symptomatologie und therapie der Halsrippen. Berl Klin Wochenschr 38:1265, 1901.
9. Bramwell E: Lesion of the first dorsal nerve root. Rev Neurol Psychiatr 1:236, 1903.
10. Brickner WM: Brachial plexus pressure by the normal first rib. Ann Surg 85:858,1927.
11. Brickner WM, Milch H: First dorsal vertebra simulating cervical rib by maldevelopment or by pressure symptoms. Surg Gynecol Obstet 40:38,1925.
12. Brintnall ES, Hyndman OR, VanAllen WM: Costoclavicular compression associated with cervical rib. Ann Surg 144:921, 1956.
13. Caldwell JW, Crane CR, Krusen EM: Nerve conduction studies in the diagnosis of the thoracic outlet syndrome. South Med J 64:210, 1971.
14. Campbell CB, Chandler JG, Tegtmeyer CJ: Axillary, subclavian and brachiocephalic vein obstruction. Surgery 82:816, 1977.
15. Cikrit DF, Dalsing MC, Bryant BJ et al: An experience with upper-extremity vascular trauma. Am J Surg 160:229, 1990.
16. Clagett OT: Presidential address: Research and prosearch. J Thorac Cardiovasc Surg 44:153, 1962.
17. Cooley DA, Wukasch DC: Techniques in Vascular Surgery. Philadelphia: W. B. Saunders, 1979, pp. 211–212.
18. Coon WW, Willis PW: Thrombosis of axillary subclavian veins. Arch Surg 94:657, 1966.
19. Coote H: Pressure on the axillary vessels and nerve by an exostosis from a cervical rib; Interference with the circulation of the arm; removal of the rib and exostosis; recovery. Med Times Gaz 2:108, 1861.
20. Daskalakis E, Bouhoutsos J: Subclavian and axillary vein compression of musculoskeletal origin. Br J Surg 67:573, 1980.
21. DeWeese JA, Adams JT, Gaiser DI: Subclavian venous thrombectomy. Circulation 16(Suppl. 2J):158, 1970.
22. Drapanas T, Curran WL: Thrombectomy in the treatment of "effort" thrombosis of the axillary and subclavian veins. J Trauma 6:107, 1966.

23. Drury EM, Trout HH, Giordono JM et al: Lytic therapy in the treatment of axillary and subclavian vein thrombosis. J Vasc Surg 2:821, 1984.

24. Eisenbud DE, Brener BJ, Shoenfeld R, et al: Treatment of acute vascular occlusions with intra-arterial urokinase. Am J Surg 160:160, 1990.

25. Falconer MA, Li FWP: Resection of the first rib in costoclavicular compression of the brachial plexus. Lancet, 11:59, 1962.

26. Falconer MA, Weddell G: Costoclavicular compression of the subclavian artery and vein: Relation to scalenus syndrome. Lancet 2:539, 1943.

27. Galbraith NF, Urschel HC Jr, Wood RE, et al: Fracture of first rib associated with laceration of subclavian artery: Report of a case and review of literature. J Thorac Cardiovasc Surg 65:649, 1973.

28. Gloviczki P, Razmier RJ, Hollier LH: Axillary-subclavian venous occlusion: The morbidity of a nonlethal disease. J Vasc Surg 4:333,1986.

29. Halsted WS: An experimental study of circumscribed dilation of an artery immediately distal to a partially occluding band, and its bearing on the dilation of the subclavian artery observed in certain cases of cervical rib. J Exp Med 24:271, 1916.

30. Hansen B, Feins RS, Detmar DE: Simple extra-anatomic jugular vein bypass for subclavian vein thrombosis. J Vasc Surg 2:291, 1985.

31. Hashmonai M, Schramek A, Farbstein J: Cephalic vein cross-over bypass for subclavian vein thrombosis: A case report. Surgery 80:563, 1976.

32. Inahara T: Surgical treatment of "effort" thrombosis of the axillary and subclavian veins. Am Surg 34:479, 1968.

33. Jacobson JH, Haimov M: Venous revascularization of the arm: Report of three cases. Surgery 81:599, 1977.

34. Jebsen RH: Motor conduction velocities in the median and ulnar nerves. Arch Phys Med 48:185,1967.

35. Johnston RW: Neurovascular conditions involving the upper extremity. In Rutherford RB, editor: Vascular Surgery, 3rd ed. Philadelphia: W. B. Saunders, 1989, pp. 801–898.

36. Keen WW: The symptomatology, diagnosis and surgical treatment of cervical ribs. Am J Sci 133:173, 1907.

37. Krusen EM: Cervical pain syndromes. Arch Phys Med 49:376, 1968.

38. Kuntz A: Distribution of the sympathetic rami to the brachial plexus. Arch Surg 15:871, 1927.

39. Lang ER: Roentgenographic diagnosis of the neurovascular compression syndromes. Radiology 79:58, 1962.

40. Law AA: Adventitious ligaments simulating cervical ribs. Ann Surg 72:497, 1920.

41. Litwin MS: Postsympathectomy neuralgia. Arch Surg 84:591,1962.

42. Lord JW, Urschel HC: Total claviculectomy. Surg Rounds 11:17, 1988.

43. Loring WE: Venous thrombosis in the upper extremities as a complication of myocardial failure. Am J Med 12:397, 1952.

44. Mackinnon SE, Dellon AL: Surgery of the Peripheral Nerve. New York: Thieme Medical, 1988, pp. 210–214.

45. Martinez NS: Posterior first rib resection for total thoracic outlet sundrome decompression. Contemp Surg 15: 13, 1979.

46. McLaughlin CW, Popma AM: lntermittent obstruction of the subclavian vein. JAMA 113:1960, 1939.

47. Murphy T: Brachial neuritis caused by pressure of first rib. Aust Med J 15:582, 1910.

48. Naffziger HC, Grant WT: Neuritis of the brachial plexus—Mechanical in origin: The scalenus syndrome. Surg Gynecol Obstet 67:722, 1938.

49. Ochsner A, Gage M, DeBakey M: Scalenous anticus (Naffziger) syndrome. Am J Surg 28:699, 1935.

50. Paget J: Clinical Lectures and Essays. London: Longmans Green, 1875.

51. Painter TD, Rarpf M: Deep venous thrombosis of the upper extremity: 5 years' experience at a university hospital. Angiology 35:743, 1984.

52. Palumbo LT: Upper dorsal sympathectomy without Homer's syndrome. Arch Surg 71:743, 1955.

53. Palumbo LT: Anterior transthoracic approach for upper extremity thoracic sympathectomy. Arch Surg 72:659, 1956.

54. Prescott SM, TIkoff G: Deep venous thrombosis of the upper extremity: A reappraisal. Circulation 59:350, 1979.

55. Rapoport S, Blair DN, McCarthy SM, et al: Brachial plexus: Correlation of MR imaging and CT pathologic findings. Radiology 167:161, 1988.

56. Ravitch MM, Steichen FM: Atlas of General Thoracic Surgery. Philadelphia: W. B. Saunders, 1988, pp. 101–109.

57. Rob CG, Standover A: Arterial occlusion complicating thoracic outlet compression syndrome. Br Med J 2:709, 1958.

58. Roos DB: Transaxillary approach for first rib resection to relieve thoracic outlet syndrome. Ann Surg 163:354, 1966.

59. Roos DB: Thoracic outlet nerve compression. In Rutherford RB, editor: Vascular Surgery, 3rd ed. Philadelphia: W. B. Saunders, 1989, pp. 858–875.

60. Roos DB, Owens JC: Thoracic outlet syndrome. Arch Surg 93:71, 1966.

61. Rosati LM, Lord JW: Neurovascular compression syndromes of the shoulder girdle. Modem Surgical Monographs. New York: Grune & Stratton, 1961.

62. Rosenberg JC: Arteriography demonstrations of compression syndromes of the thoracic outlet. South Med J 59:400, 1966.

63. Rubenstein N, Greger WP: Successful streptokinase therapy for catheter-induced subclavian vein thrombosis. Arch Intern Med 140:1370, 1980.

64. Sharafuddin MD, Melhem J: Endovascular management of venous thrombotic diseases of the upper torso and extremities. J Vasc Radiol 13:975, 2002.

65. Smithwick RH: Modified dorsal sympathectomy for vascular spasm (Raynaud's disease) of the upper extremity. Ann Surg 104:339, 1936.

66. Stoney WS, Addlestone RB, Alford WC Jr, et al: The incidence of venous thrombosis following long-term transvenous pacing. Ann Thorac Surg 22:166, 1976.

67. Sundqvist SB, Hedner U, Rullenberg RHE, et al: Deep venous thrombosis of the arm: A study of coagulation and fibrinolysis. Br Med J 283:265, 1981.

68. Swank WL, Simeone FA: The scalenous anticus syndrome. Arch Neurol Psychiatr 51:432, 1944.

69. Taylor LN, McAllister WR, Dennis DL, et al: Thrombolytic therapy followed by first rib resection for spontaneous subclavian vein thrombosis. Am J Surg 149:644, 1985.

70. Telford ED, Mottershead S: Pressure of the cervicobrachial junction. J Bone Joint Surg Am 30:249,1948.

71. Telford ED, Stopford JSB: The vascular complications of the cervical rib. Br J Surg 18:559, 1937.

72. TiIney NL, Griffiths HFG, Edwards EA: Natural history of major venous thrombosis of the upper extremity. Arch Surg 101:792, 1970.

73. Urschel HC Jr: Dorsal sympathectomy and management of thoracic outlet syndrome with VATS. Ann Thorac Surg 56: 717, 1993.

74. Urschel HC Jr: Video-assisted sympathectomy and thoracic outlet syndrome. Chest Surg Clin North Am 3:299, 1993.

75. Urschel HC Jr, Patel AN: Paget-Schroetter syndrome therapy: Failure of intravenous stents. Ann Thorac Surg 75:1693–1696, 2003. (Presented at STSA Meeting, Miami, FL; Nov. 8, 2002.)

76. Urschel HC Jr, Paulson DL, McNamara JJ: Thoracic outlet syndrome. Ann Thorac Surg 6:1, 1968.

426

77. Urschel HC Jr, Razzuk MA: Current concepts: Management of the thoracic outlet syndrome. N Engl J Med 286:1140, 1972.

78. Urschel HC Jr, Razzuk MA: Thoracic outlet syndrome. Surg Ann 5:229, 1973.

79. Urschel HC Jr, Razzuk MA: Posterior thoracic sympathectomy. In Malt RA, editor: Surgical Techniques Illustrated: A Comparative Atlas. Philadelphia: W. B. Saunders, 1985, pp. 612–615.

80. Urschel HC Jr, Razzuk MA: The failed operation for thoracic outlet syndrome: The difficulty of diagnosis and management. Ann Thorac Surg 42:523, 1986.

81. Urschel HC Jr, Razzuk MA: Thoracic outlet syndrome. In Grillo HC, editor: International Trends in General Thoracic Surgery, Vol. 2. St. Louis: C. V. Mosby, 1986, pp. 130–134.

82. Urschel HC Jr, Razzuk MA: Improved management of the Paget-Schroetter syndrome secondary to thoracic outlet compression. Ann Thorac Surg 52:1217, 1991.

83. Urschel HC Jr, Razzuk MA: Paget–Schroetter syndrome: What is the best management? Ann Thorac Surg 69:2; 1693, 2000.

84. Urschel HC Jr, Razzuk MA: Neurovascular decompression in the thoracic outlet: Changing management over 50 years. Ann Thorac Surg 228:609, 1998.

85. Urschel HC Jr, Razzuk MA, Albers JE, Paulson DL: Reoperation for recurrent thoracic outlet syndrome. Ann Thorac Surg 21:19, 1976.

86. Urschel HC Jr, Razzuk MA, Hyland JW, et al: Thoracic outlet syndrome masquerading as coronary artery disease. Ann Thorac Surg 16:239, 1973.

87. Urschel HC Jr, Razzuk MA, Wood RE, Paulson DL: Objective diagnosis (ulnar nerve conduction velocity) and current therapy of the thoracic outlet syndrome. Ann Thorac Surg 12:608, 1971.

88. Von Schroetter L: Erkrankungen der Gefossl. In Nathnogel AK, editor: Handbuch der Pathologie und Therapie. Wein: Holder, 1884.

89. White JC, Smithwick RH, Simeone FA: The Autonomic Nervous System: Anatomy, Physiology and Surgical Application, 3rd ed. New York: Macmillan, 1952, pp. 104–108.

90. Wood RE, Campbell DC, Razzuk MA, et al: Surgical advantages of selective unilateral ventilation. Ann Thorac Surg 14:2, 1972.

91. Wright IS: The neurovascular syndrome produced by hyperabduction of the arm. Am Heart J 29:1, 1945.

92. Zimmerman R, Marl H, Harenberg J, et al: Urokinase therapy of subclavian axillary vein thrombosis. Klin Wochenschr, 59:851, 1981.

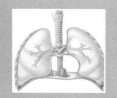

Benign Pleural Disease

Spontaneous Pneumothorax

Sean C. Grondin and Willard A. Fry

Etiology
Diagnosis
Initial Treatment
    Clinically Stable Patient
        Observation
        Tube Thoracostomy
        Needle Aspiration
    Clinically Unstable Patient
Persistent Air Leaks
Operation
Secondary Pneumothoraces

Etard first introduced the term *pneumothorax* in 1803. It was not until 1819, however, that Laennec described the signs and symptoms associated with this entity. Pneumothorax is an accumulation of air in the pleural space leading to lung collapse. Pneumothoraces are classified based on their etiology or clinical presentation. Although most pneumothoraces can be managed successfully with tube thoracostomy, patients with recurring pneumothoraces should be considered for operative intervention.

ETIOLOGY

Primary pneumothoraces occur because of the rupture of the visceral pleura (subpleural blebs) in a patient with no known pulmonary disease. Secondary pneumothoraces occur because of an existing lung condition, trauma, or an iatrogenic injury (Table 28A-1). Primary pneumothoraces are more common than secondary pneumothoraces. A male preponderance of 3:1 is reported, with tall, thin males between the ages of 15 (post-puberty) and 30 most commonly affected. Cigarette smoking increases the risk of primary pneumothorax by a factor of 20.

DIAGNOSIS

Most cases of spontaneous pneumothorax present with sudden-onset ipsilateral pleuritic chest pain with some short-ness of breath and occur when the patient has been at rest. Physical examination can be deceivingly normal, particularly for a small pneumothorax (<15% of the hemithorax). Patients presenting with larger pneumothoraces may have dyspnea and tachycardia. Findings on respiratory examination may include diminished or absent breath sounds, hyper-resonant percussion note, decreased movement of the chest wall, and diminished fremitus on the affected side. A chest radiograph assists in confirming the diagnosis by document-ing the presence of a thin visceral pleural line displaced from the chest wall on the upright posterior-anterior chest radi-ograph. Although a chest radiograph performed during expi-ration may assist in identifying a small pneumothorax, it is rarely needed. A variety of methods have been devised to estimate the extent of collapse observed in a pneumothorax. Often it is simplest to describe the degree of pneumothorax in terms of the number of centimeters that the lung is down from the apex of the chest cavity, how far down along the lat-eral wall the lung is retracted, and how far away it is from the lateral border of the chest wall in the midthorax. Occasionally a computed tomography (CT) scan of the chest is helpful in planning surgical intervention.

▶ INITIAL TREATMENT

Clinically Stable Patient

Observation

Historically, spontaneous pneumothoraces were treated with observation. Today, observation is reserved for asymp-tomatic patients who present with a pneumothorax of less than 20%. In such a case, the patient should be observed in the emergency department for 4–6 hours and discharged home if a repeat chest radiograph excludes progression of the pneumothorax. On discharge, the patient should be pro-vided with careful instructions for follow-up within 12–48 hours, depending on circumstances. A repeat chest radi-ograph is obtained at the follow-up visit to document reso-lution of the pneumothorax. If the patient lives a distance away from emergency services or is considered unreliable, it is safest to admit this patient to the hospital for observation and follow-up chest radiographs.

Table 28A–1

Classification of Pneumothorax

Spontaneous

Primary
    Subpleural bleb rupture
Secondary
    Bullous disease, including chronic obstructive lung disease
    Cystic fibrosis
    Asthma
    Connective tissue diseases, especially Marfan's syndrome
    Interstitial lung diseases, especially eosinophilic granuloma
    Pneumocystis carinii pneumonia
    Pneumonia with lung abscess
    Catamenial
    Metastatic cancer, especially sarcomas
    Lung cancer
    Esophageal perforation
Neonatal

Acquired

Iatrogenic
    Central line placement
    Pacemaker insertion
    Transthoracic needle biopsy
    Transbronchial needle biopsy
    Thoracocentesis
    Chest tube malfunction
    After laparoscopic surgery
Barotrauma
Traumatic
    Blunt trauma
        Motor vehicle accident
        Falls
        Sports related
    Penetrating trauma
        Gunshot wounds
        Stab wounds

Tube Thoracostomy

Larger pneumothoraces (>20%) usually are treated with prompt reexpansion of the lung by tube thoracostomy. In patients with emphysema or with significant symptoms, a lesser degree of pneumothorax often is treated to reexpand the lung. The size of the chest tube for insertion varies depending on the patient's habitus and the surgeon's preference. Today, chest tubes usually are made of plastic (Argyle tube) with a number scale marking the distance to the first hole on the tube. A tube larger than 20 Fr rarely is required. In many instances, a small 8 Fr pigtail catheter is effective, although care must be taken to ensure the tube does not kink or obstruct. An intravenous or intramuscular narcotic often is given before insertion to relax the patient and assist with analgesia. Normally the tube is placed under generous local anesthesia (1% or 2% lidocaine) in the fourth or fifth intercostal space in the anterior or midaxillary line and is directed toward the apex of the affected hemithorax. The tube is tunneled over the rib to form a subcutaneous tract

that can be compressed on removal of the tube. This technique is effective in preventing a hole that may lead to an air leak when a tube must remain in place for more than a few days. Insertion of the tube through the chest wall into the pleural space can be accomplished using a clamp, a finger technique, or trocar technique. The Advanced Trauma Life Support course sponsored by the American College of Surgeons recommends the clamp and finger technique. Trocar insertion or pigtail catheter insertion using the Seldinger technique is reserved for experienced surgeons familiar with chest wall anatomy. These latter techniques are usually quicker and more comfortable for the patient.

Catheters or chest tubes can be attached to a variety of chest drainage systems. Typically a Heimlich valve is used for outpatient management, and the water seal device is used for inpatient care. The tube is left in place until the air leak resolves and the lung is fully expanded. If the lung fails to reexpand, the position of the chest tube is reassessed radiographically (chest X-ray or occasionally CT scan), and suction is applied to a water seal device. Reliable patients who are unwilling to be hospitalized may be discharged home from the emergency department with a small-bore catheter attached to a Heimlich valve if the lung has reexpanded after the removal of pleural air. If a Heimlich valve is used, some provision for fluid drainage is required, such as a bronchoscopic mucus trap with some absorbent gauze or a vented urinary drainage bag. These patients usually are seen in follow-up within 48 hours.

In most instances, a primary spontaneous pneumothorax responds to tube thoracostomy. Generally the air leak from the lung seals after 1 to 2 days, and the chest tube can be removed. Patients also are counseled to avoid underwater diving, to avoid isolated travel experiences (e.g., camping trip), and to stop smoking if applicable. Air travel is discouraged for at least 1 week. Patients are informed that there is approximately a 30% chance of recurrence. The risk of recurrence increases to 60% to 70% if a second pneumothorax develops. Given these rates, surgery is recommended for patients with recurrent pneumothoraces.

In some instances, operative intervention is indicated after the first episode of spontaneous pneumothorax as would be the case for a patient with a prior pneumonectomy, a patient with a history of untreated bilateral pneumothoraces, or a patient with occupational hazards such as an airplane pilot or diver. The U.S. Air Force does not allow a pilot to fly until he or she has undergone surgical therapy after a spontaneous pneumothorax.

Needle Aspiration

The role of simple aspiration of a pneumothorax without chest tube placement is controversial. In most cases, simple aspiration is not appropriate for the treatment of spontaneous pneumothoraces because there is commonly an air leak for a short time after tube thoracostomy. Occasionally, surgeons are called to evaluate a patient who has had a pneumothorax for several days (the presence of a small hydrothorax with pneumothorax is a clue that the pneumothorax is a few days old) or a patient whose lung has not reexpanded with observational therapy. In these instances, needle aspiration using the disposable thoracentesis kit can be effective. The kits supply a small-diameter plastic catheter that can be passed over an aspirating needle to minimize the risk of lung injury and a large syringe with a one-way valve.

To perform the aspiration, local anesthetic is injected into the skin and the interspace in the second intercostal space in the midclavicular line. The needle/catheter is inserted gently into the affected hemithorax (above the third rib) until air is aspirated. The catheter is passed over the needle, and the needle is withdrawn. The syringe and one-way valve are attached, and the pleural cavity is aspirated until no further air can be removed.

At this time, the catheter is removed, and a postaspiration chest radiograph is obtained. Some surgeons favor leaving the catheter in place until the chest radiograph is completed. The advantage of this technique is that it allows further aspiration to be performed if the lung is not reexpanded or the option to attach the tube to a Heimlich valve.

Although needle aspiration has gained popularity in the United Kingdom, most surgeons suggest that this technique has limited applicability with success rates of less than 50% reported. Reasons for the failure of this technique include the inability to evacuate the pneumothorax completely, resulting in failure to approximate the visceral and parietal pleurae, and the lack of pleural scarring that can occur after placement of a foreign body, such as a chest tube in the thoracic cavity. In addition, this method does not treat the underlying etiology of the pneumothorax, pleural blebs.

Clinically Unstable Patient

In rare instances, a patient presents with a history consistent with spontaneous pneumothorax and a physical examination showing anxiety, absent breath sounds, tachycardia, cyanosis, hypotension, and deviation of the trachea to the uninvolved side. In this case, a clinical diagnosis of tension pneumothorax should be made without a confirming chest radiograph. Tension pneumothorax occurs when alveolar air enters continuously into the pleural space without evacuation resulting in increased pressure and shift of the mediastinum to the uninvolved side. Prompt decompression of the pleural space by insertion of a needle or chest tube is required to prevent circulatory collapse.

In a trauma patient with multiple injuries, the safest and most conservative treatment of a traumatic pneumothorax is to place a chest tube. This maneuver prevents the possibility of progression of the pneumothorax, eliminating this variable as a cause of respiratory or hemodynamic instability in a trauma patient. Rarely a patient presents with a significant hemothorax associated with the pneumothorax (i.e., hemopneumothorax). If the bleeding persists after chest tube placement (>100 ml/hr), immediate operative intervention is indicated to secure a torn vascular pleural adhesion.

PERSISTENT AIR LEAKS

Occasionally the air leak persists for several days after tube thoracostomy. For patients with air leaks that persist for more than 3 days, surgical intervention is recommended to attempt air leak closure, and a pleurodesis is performed to prevent recurrence. In special circumstances in which surgery is contraindicated or the patient refuses surgery, chemical pleurodesis by instillation of a sclerosing agent (e.g.,

doxycycline or talc slurry) through the chest tube can be used to promote pleural symphysis.

Rarely, there is a massive persistent air leak from the lung after chest tube placement with or without complete reexpansion of the lung. In this setting, immediate operative intervention is indicated to seal a large torn bulla.

▶ OPERATION

Indications for surgery after spontaneous pneumothorax include (1) recurrent pneumothorax, (2) persistent air leak or incomplete reexpansion of the lung, (3) massive air leak with incomplete reexpansion of the lung, (4) history of bilateral pneumothoraces either simultaneously or on separate occasions, (5) occupational hazard or possible lack of access to medical care, (6) history of tension pneumothorax or prior pneumonectomy, and (7) hemopneumothorax with persistent bleeding. Historically, operative approaches to treat spontaneous pneumothorax have included thoracotomy (anterior, lateral, or transaxillary) and median sternotomy. In the 1980s, results from muscle-sparing incisions, such as transaxillary thoracotomy, were good. In the 1990s, technological advances led to the development of video-assisted thoracic surgery (VATS) approaches for pneumothorax. Regardless of the technique selected, the ability of the surgeon to remove the offending bullae and obtain pleural symphysis is key to the success of the procedure.

VATS is performed by a thoracic surgeon in the operating room using double-lumen endotracheal general anesthesia. Patients are positioned in the lateral decubitus position and draped to allow open thoracotomy if necessary. The first thoracoscopic port (5 or 10 mm) is placed through the seventh interspace in the midaxillary line using a direct cutdown technique. The 30-degree thoracoscope is inserted into the hemithorax, and a careful visual inspection of the entire pleural space is performed. Two further ports are placed in the fourth or fifth interspace in the anterior axillary line or in the space between the spine and the medial border of the scapula (i.e., auscultatory triangle). Using lung graspers, the offending bleb is located and removed. Staple bullectomy is the most common approach for eliminating bullae. Other options for bullectomy may include electrocoagulation, laser ablation, or hand sewing depending on institutional experience and expertise using these techniques. If the bleb cannot be located, gentle insufflation of the lung with instillation of sterile saline solution into the thoracic cavity may help to locate the leaking bleb. If no bleb or leak is noted, the apex of the lung is removed using the stapler. The entire lung surface should be inspected to determine whether bullae are present elsewhere in the lung (other than the apex), such as the superior segment of the lower lobe.

For most patients undergoing surgery, intraoperative pleurodesis should be performed using parietal pleural abrasion or resection. Abrasion can be performed using a gauze plug, such as a Kittner dissector, or with the "the scouring pad" from the Bovie electrocautery unit. Apical parietal pleurectomy from the fifth rib superiorly also can be used as an effective technique to obtain pleural symphysis. Generally the intraoperative instillation of a chemical sclerosing agent such as talc is not recommended for young patients with benign disease. One or two chest tubes can be inserted through the VATS port sites and positioned accurately at the

430 chest apex. Postoperatively the chest tubes are kept to suction for at least 24 hours (preferably 48 hours) to promote complete lung reexpansion and pleural symphysis.

Overall the success rate for VATS and transaxillary approaches in the operative management of spontaneous pneumothorax is excellent. The VATS technique is thought to be associated with decreased perioperative pain, shorter hospital stay, and more rapid return to work. Formal cost-effective analyses have not been performed, however. The recurrence rate after the VATS approach is approximately 2–5% compared with 1–2% for the limited thoracotomy approach. It is hypothesized that the slightly higher recurrence rate associated with the VATS technique is secondary to inadequate exposure of bullae in the chest cavity or to less effective pleural abrasion than may be seen with thoracotomy. In most reported series, the intraoperative conversion rate from VATS to open thoracotomy due to technical difficulties is less than 5% for primary pneumothoraces and 29% for secondary pneumothoraces.

SECONDARY PNEUMOTHORACES

Patients with secondary pneumothoraces generally have significant comorbid diseases and are debilitated from a respiratory standpoint and require that treatment be individualized. Treatment should include chemical or surgical pleurodesis in combination with complete lung reexpansion to seal air leaks. Tube thoracostomy alone is associated with a high recurrence rate. Two subgroups of secondary pneumothoraces are worthy of further discussion—patients with acquired immunodeficiency syndrome (AIDS) and patients with pneumothoraces complicating chronic obstructive pulmonary disease.

Since the 1980s, there have been an increasing number of reports describing the association between spontaneous pneumothorax and AIDS. There seems to be a predilection for bilateral pneumothoraces arising from disease at the apex of both lungs. Most commonly, the pneumothorax is secondary to *Pneumocystis carinii* pneumonia; however, pneumothorax also can occur in patients with Kaposi's sarcoma, pneumonia caused by mycobacteria or cytomegalovirus, and necrotizing bacterial pneumonias. Whenever possible, initial management should be conservative with observation alone; however, tube thoracostomy frequently is required to treat large air leaks. CT scan of the chest is useful to evaluate the extent of disease and in planning surgery. Operative intervention with resection of the diseased area and pleurectomy is usually well tolerated.

Pneumothorax secondary to chronic obstructive pulmonary disease is the most common variety of secondary pneumothorax. Typically, this pneumothorax occurs in patients older than age 50 and may be difficult to confirm clinically and radiologically. Chest CT is often necessary to localize the pneumothorax and to distinguish between large bullae and the pneumothorax. Treatment consists of tube thoracostomy, which may need to be continued for a prolonged time compared with that for a primary spontaneous pneumothorax. If the air leak persists more than 14 days, operative intervention or chemical pleurodesis should be considered. Surgical management varies based on the location and extent of disease. Stapling of the bullae and subtotal parietal pleurectomy is our favored approach.

REFERENCES

1. Baumann MH, Strange C, Heftner JE, et al: Management of spontaneous pneumothorax—an American College of Chest Physicians Delphi Consensus Statement. Chest 119:590–602, 2001.
2. Beauchamp G: Spontaneous pneumothorax and pneumomediastinum. In Pearson FG, DesLauriers J, Ginsberg RJ, et al (eds): Thoracic Surgery, New York: Churchill Livingstone, 1995, p. 1037.
3. Harvey J, Prescott RJ: Simple aspiration versus intercostal tube drainage for spontaneous pneumothorax in patients with normal lungs. British Thoracic Society Research Committee BMJ 309:1338–1339, 1994.
4. Hatz RA, Kaps MF, Meimarakis G, et al: Long-term results after video-assisted thoracoscopic surgery for first-time and recurrent spontaneous pneumothorax. Ann Thorac Surg 70:253–257, 2000.
5. Sahn SA, Heffner JE: Spontaneous pneumothorax. N Engl J Med 342:868–874, 2000.

Benign Pleural Disease

Empyema Thoracis

Robert B. Lee

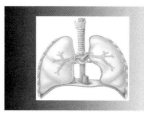

HISTORY

"When empyemata are opened by cautery or by knife; and the pus flows pure and white, the patient survives, but if it is mixed with blood; muddy and foul smelling, he will die."
Hippocrates 460-377 B.C.

Thoracic surgery in its infancy evolved as techniques were developed to treat complications of intrathoracic infections, particularly empyema thoracis. Hippocrates further described his observations of the clinical and physical findings of empyema thoracis:

Empyema may be recognized by the following symptoms: the fever is constant, less during the day and greater at night, and copious sweats supervene. There is a desire to cough, and the patient expectorates nothing worth mentioning.

Hippocrates' observations regarding the natural history of empyema were uncanny and remain true today: "In pleuritic afflictions when the disease is not purged off in fourteen days it usually results in empyema." Regarding treatment, he pronounced adequate drainage by intercostal incision or rib resection, followed by packing as the only means for cure. Treatment was virtually unchanged 2000 years later, when Dieffenbach condemned the American surgeon Antony who, on March 3, 1821, resected portions of the fifth and sixth ribs and "all disorganized parenchyma of the lung, [for] an extensive abscess about this carious bone." Little changed between that time and 1989, when Lawrence described drainage, rib resection, and thoracoplasty as management techniques for empyema.

The current therapy for management of empyema has progressed and evolved over the past 15 years to include computed tomography (CT)–guided catheter drainage, use of fibrinolytics, diagnostic and therapeutic thoracoscopy, and extrathoracic muscle flap interposition. These advanced techniques as well as thoracotomy with decortication, Eloesser flaps, and other well-established surgical approaches are described.

DEFINITIONS AND DETERMINATIONS

Empyema, from the Greek, is defined simply as "pus in the pleural cavity." The precursor of empyema is bacterial pneumonia and subsequent parapneumonic effusion. Other causes of empyema include ruptured lung abscess, bronchogenic carcinoma, esophageal rupture (Boerhaave's syndrome), penetrating or blunt chest trauma, mediastinitis with pleural extension, extension of a subphrenic abscess, infected congenital abnormalities, cervical and thoracic spine infection, and postresection bronchopleural fistula. A common cause of empyema, bronchopleural fistulas, is discussed elsewhere.

The general thoracic surgeon often is involved in the diagnosis and treatment of patients with persistent parapneumonic effusions and subsequent empyema. When the surgeon's involvement is delayed during repeated attempts at "medical management," the sequelae of empyema occur. parapneumonic effusions occur in 20–60% of patients hospitalized for bacterial pneumonia; 5–10% of these parapneumonic effusions progress to empyema (approximately 32,000 patients per year in the United States). The mortality rate of empyema is significant: 25–75% in the elderly and debilitated.

Pleural fluid first must be determined as exudative or transudative, which is accomplished by examination of pleural fluid obtained by thoracentesis. In the 1970s, Light established differential criteria based on levels of lactate dehydrogenase (LDH) and protein concentrations found in pleural fluid compared with the patient's serum. Light's criteria establish an exudate as having any one of the following characteristics: (1) pleural fluid protein divided by serum protein concentration greater than 0.5, (2) pleural fluid LDH concentration divided by serum LDH concentration greater than 0.6, (3) pleural fluid LDH concentration greater than two thirds of the upper limit of normal serum LDH concentration, and (4) a pH less than 7.0. Parapneumonic effusions are exudative and progress through three stages to an empyema; knowing the stage guides therapy.

The *first* or *exudative stage*, characterized by relatively low LDH, normal glucose, and normal pH, may be treated successfully by antibiotics. Untreated or inappropriately treated, the *second* or *fibropurulent stage* evolves with invasion of pleural fluid by bacteria, increased fibrin deposition, cellular debris, and white blood cells with the ultimate formation of limiting fibrin membranes producing loculations. The *third* or *organization stage* occurs as fibroblasts grow into the exudative fibrin sheet coating the visceral and

432 parietal pleura with an inelastic membrane or pleural "peel" encasing the lung and rendering it functionless. Empyema is established by pus obtained on thoracentesis, glucose concentration less than 60 mg/dl, LDH greater than three times the upper limit of normal, and pH less than 7.0. A meta-analysis was performed of multiple smaller studies evaluating criteria of defining pleural infection and empyema. This study defined pH as the most accurate and sensitive criteria for empyema and need for drainage. This analysis identified a slightly higher pH of 7.21–7.29 as the best indicator for drainage as opposed to a pH of 7.0 established by Light in the 1970s. Empyema is determined by analysis of the pleural fluid, and treatment is guided by radiological assessment.

RADIOLOGICAL ASSESSMENT AND INTERVENTION

The initial radiographical assessment should include the standard posterior-anterior and lateral projections of a chest radiograph. Pleural fluid is subject to the laws of gravity, collecting in the most dependent area of the involved hemithorax: initially the costophrenic angle, then laterally anteriorly, and finally superiorly. As much as 75–100 ml of pleural fluid may go undetected. As much as 175–500 ml is needed to blunt the lateral costophrenic angle. Free-flowing fluid or pus follows the coercion of gravity, making the right and left decubitus film the next essential study. The well-performed, overpenetrated decubitus film can detect 5 ml of fluid, reveal subpulmonic collections, reveal pseudotumors, and identify loculations. The ubiquitous posterior-anterior and lateral chest X-ray can separate the broad air-fluid level of an empyema from the more spherical fluid collection surrounded by lung parenchyma characteristic of lung abscess.

Ultrasonography is widely available in most institutions and frequently employed after the initial chest X-ray. Ultrasound is rapid, portable, and less expensive than CT. This technique can localize small amounts of fluid and loculations; identify and quantify pleural peels; and define solid lesions such as pleural or parenchymal tumors. Using a 3.5- or 5.0-mHz transducer and an intercostal acoustic window, an empyema is characterized as having acoustic homogeneity. Complex or advanced empyemas have debris and floating fronds. An organized empyema has an echogenic pleural peel, and the lung appears immobile or entrapped. Diagnostic thoracentesis, catheter drainage, or tube thoracostomy can be guided by ultrasound.

CT of the chest became clinically applicable in 1975 and widely available by the early 1980s. During the subsequent 20 years, CT has become the radiographic technique most frequently relied on for characterization of an empyema and for treatment. Present helical CT scanners have scan rates of 1 second, reliably reproducing cross-sectional images of the thorax, readily showing the anatomical separation between lung parenchyma, pleural space, and chest wall. Intravenous contrast material is necessary to define pulmonary blood vessels and enhance the parietal pleura. Exudative effusions (empyema) have abnormally high Hounsfield units (−20 HU) compared with transudative effusions (−100 HU). Differentiating empyema, lung abscess, transudative pleural fluid, and subdiaphragmatic fluid (ascites) is often difficult without CT. Lung abscesses generally are seen as air-fluid spherical lesions forming

acute angles with the lung parenchyma. The lung appears destroyed rather than compressed. There is an abrupt cut-off of vessels and bronchi. Empyemas appear laterally, pushing or compressing lung parenchyma, vessels, and bronchi. The shape is not uniform, and angles with the pleura are acute. Lateral lung abscesses or abscesses in the basilar segments of the lung near the diaphragm may be difficult to distinguish from the pleural location of an empyema.

Magnetic resonance imaging has been used to image the pleural space and offers the advantage of coronal, sagittal, and axial planes. This modality is more expensive and cumbersome, adds little information beyond CT, and rarely is used.

MEDICAL MANAGEMENT

Medical management of empyema is a misnomer. Medical management or conservative noninterventional therapy is rarely effective and often contraindicated for management of empyema. Thoracentesis and culture sensitivity–based antibiotic therapy are appropriate and generally successful for stage I parapneumonic effusions but not stage II effusions or stage III empyema. Drainage of the pleural space by radiologically guided catheters or surgical drainage must be employed for successful management of empyema.

Thoracentesis not only may be diagnostic as previously discussed, but also occasionally therapeutic. When the amount of pleural fluid is small to moderate, free flowing (not loculated), and fluent, the initial "diagnostic" thoracentesis using a vacuum bottle may clear the pleural space completely and become a therapeutic drainage procedure. If the fluid does not reaccumulate, no further intervention is required. If the fluid reaccumulates and the initial analysis of the fluid has defined an empyema, however, a drainage procedure should be initiated.

Historically, tube thoracostomy using a large-bore chest tube (32–38 Fr) was the initial intervention when empyema was established. These chest tubes were converted to an "empyema tube" at 14 to 21 days when pleural symphysis had occurred. The tube was withdrawn slowly over several weeks. Patients often were discharged with the tube connected to a drainage bag. When the initial drainage by chest tube was unsuccessful or the empyema loculated, open surgical drainage was performed. An empyema tube rarely is used today and has infrequent indications.

Image-guided catheter placement should be the initial method of drainage unless lung entrapment has been proved. This is effectively accomplished by placement of one or more flexible polyethylene pigtail catheters (8 Fr to 14 Fr) using CT guidance. After catheter placement, fibrinolytics are administered until the pleural space is cleared radiographically and the patient's clinical condition is improved. Streptokinase initially was used by Tillet and Sherry in 1949. Subsequently, urokinase was used and found to be more efficacious (90–92%) compared with streptokinase (66%) and less likely to cause a febrile or allergic reaction. Most authors report using 250,000 U of streptokinase on 3 consecutive days. We have used 100,000 U of urokinase in 100 ml of normal saline in similar fashion. The U.S. Food and Drug Administration (FDA) recalled urokinase from most institutions in 1999 for apparent quality control issues, making it no longer available. I am currently using tissue plasminogen activator (Activase) for fibrinolysis. Tissue plasminogen activator, 10 mg, is diluted in 50 ml of normal saline and injected into the catheter on 3 consecutive days. Results have been similar to urokinase. This is not an FDA-approved use for this drug, so it cannot be recommended. No prospective randomized trials have been done to evaluate fibrinolytic therapy with tissue plasminogen activator.

Urokinase first was used by transcatheter delivery for management of loculated intrathoracic effusion in 1989. Clinical trials comparing streptokinase with placebo, comparing different doses of streptokinase, and comparing different amounts of saline for diluting the streptokinase have been performed using tube thoracostomy as the standard for drainage. Most studies show increased drainage and clearance of chest X-ray findings using fibrinolytics but lack sophistication to make statistically based conclusions. Only one study by Bouros et al was conducted in a prospective, randomized, double-blinded fashion. The study compared 250,000 U of streptokinase with 100,000 U of urokinase, delivered in similar fashion in matched patient populations. Drainage amounts were similar, urokinase was more expensive, and length of stay was similar. Fever was more common in the streptokinase group (28%). No study has compared streptokinase, urokinase, and tissue plasminogen activator.

SURGICAL MANAGEMENT

Success rates with image-guided catheter placement and fibrinolytics approach 70–80% for early stage III parapneumonic effusion (empyema) when the appropriate dosage of drug is given repeatedly until the chest X-ray clears or the clinical condition improves. Of these patients, 20–30% require a surgical drainage procedure. These patients often can be identified early in their course by findings on chest CT, such as multiple loculations and contrast enhancement of the parietal pleura suggesting a "peel or rind."

Thoracoscopy should be the next therapeutic maneuver after attempted fibrinolysis. Some authors argue that thoracoscopy early in the management of the fibrinopurulent stage of empyema is more effective. Initially performed in 1910 for lysis of pleural adhesions in a tuberculous empyema by Jacobaeus, this technique has become remarkably safe and effective since the introduction of charged coupled device ("chip") cameras for video assistance. Video-assisted thoracic surgery (VATS) has become an extension of the thoracic surgeon's physical examination. VATS affords the advantage of being able to visualize the infected pleural space and determine if complete drainage of all empyema fluid and disruption of all adhesions and loculations can be accomplished. If not, decortication is indicated to free the entrapped lung. Performed early before collagen deposition on the visceral pleura and entrapment of the lung, VATS can be used to disrupt fibrinous adhesions, completely drain all infected fluid, débride the parietal and visceral pleura, and accurately place large-bore chest tubes under direct vision. VATS must accomplish two therapeutic goals to be successful: (1) establish a unified pleural space and (2) ensure total reexpansion of the lung parenchyma with obliteration of the pleural cavity. Wait et al at Parkland Memorial Hospital, Dallas, Texas, performed a randomized trial on 20 patients

comparing VATS and standard tube thoracostomy with streptokinase fibrinolysis (250,000 U streptokinase in 100 ml of normal saline repeated over 3 days). The VATS group had significantly less chest tube drainage, fever, and intensive care unit and hospital days and a higher success rate. Although this is a small group of patients, it supports the concept of early intervention using VATS.

I perform VATS within 48–72 hours (three treatments) after fibrinolytic therapy if fibrinolysis has failed to clear the pleural space effectively and reexpand the lung. VATS has been described using various techniques, under local anesthesia, in the awake patient, using flexible or rigid scopes, and with and without single-lung ventilation. A 0-degree or 30-degree lens and Chip camera using port access and single-lung ventilation of the contralateral side is the technique most widely accepted and used. When a double-lumen endotracheal tube is positioned correctly, the patient is placed in the lateral decubitus position with affected side up. I use the tube thoracostomy site for my camera port when present. When a chest tube is not present, a site in the midaxillary line along the fifth or sixth intercostal space may be used, in line with the thoracotomy incision should this be necessary.

On examination of the pleural space, a determination is made as to (1) whether all fluid can be drained and (2) the extent of lung entrapment. When the lung is not entrapped, débridement, irrigation, and disruption of all adhesions and loculations can be accomplished through a second appropriately placed port using a sponge forceps and suction-irrigating device. Two 32-Fr chest tubes are placed using video assistance and left to suction drainage for 3 to 5 days. Success depends on whether the lung is entrapped by a thick visceral peel (chronic organized phase of empyema). Only the fibrinopurulent, multiloculated stage of empyema is amenable to thorascopic management. If the lung is found to be entrapped, conversion to thoracotomy for decortication is advised. Decortication using VATS is frequently frustrating and often results in parenchymal lung injury and bleeding.

Decortication via a thoracotomy should be performed when the third or fibrotic stage of empyema is suggested by CT scan that reveals visceral pleural enhancement without fibrin septation in multiple areas of loculation. Entrapment should be suspected when this has occurred and when the pleural process is known to have been ongoing for greater than 10 to 14 days. I almost always attempt to use the videoscope to perform an initial evaluation, then convert to a 10- to 15-cm vertical incision in the midaxillary line for a muscle-sparing thoracotomy and decortication when lung entrapment is found. Using this incision, a complete pleurectomy-decortication can be performed quickly and effectively. The videoscope can be used through the incision to access the hard-to-reach areas better, such as the diaphragmatic sulcus; place chest tubes; and ensure full reexpansion of the lung parenchyma. The first objective of this operation is to remove all purulent fluid, fibrinous debris, and thickened parietal pleura from the pleural space. When partial or complete pleurectomy is required to accomplish this, complete hemostasis must occur, or a resulting hemithorax may occur, defeating the initial purpose. The second, more difficult, but most critical task is to resect the visceral pleural peel. A plane of separation

434 between the peel and visceral pleura must be established; this is accomplished with knife, scissors, sharppointed clamp, or even bluntly with a Kittner dissector. When the proper plane is established, the peel is stripped completely from the entire lung surface. The lung must be freed entirely from the rib cage, mediastinum, and diaphragm. All of the fibrotic visceral peel must be removed, even within the lung fissures. The costophrenic angle should be reestablished. Complete and total reexpansion of all lung parenchyma must be accomplished to ensure success. Decortication is achieved most easily through the sixth intercostal space, which allows better access to the diaphragm and costophrenic angle. This is a major operation and physiologically challenging to a compromised or debilitated patient. When the operative morbidity or mortality seems prohibitive, a lesser open drainage procedure may be considered.

The Eloesser flap or procedure originally was described by Eloesser in 1935 as a drainage procedure for tuberculous empyema. He described forming a U-shaped flap of skin and subcutaneous tissue and sewing it into the most dependent portion of the empyema cavity after resecting a portion of the underlying two or three ribs and attached intercostal muscles. With the flap acting as a tubeless, one-way valve, air is allowed to egress against less resistance than air entering. The lung is allowed to reexpand and obliterate the cavity. This procedure is most effective when a unilocular empyema is present and located inferiorly or laterally. The procedure can be accomplished under local anesthesia with intravenous sedation in a high-risk surgical patient with an empyema. Miller and others at Emory University reported a 90% success rate in 84 patients (1974-1998) using the inverted-U modified Eloesser flap.

▶ SUMMARY

The heterogeneity of empyema thoracis, the underlying primary disease process, and the patient's physiological status make no single therapy a universal first intervention. The diagnosis of pus in the pleural space must be made and the pace and progression of the disease process recognized to avoid sequelae. Optimal therapy and cost containment require selection of the most appropriate initial intervention. Thourani, Miller, and I reviewed our experience with 77

empyema thoracis patients at Emory University and Crawford Long Hospitals in Atlanta, Georgia (1990-1997). The treatment modalities previously discussed were employed. Of the effusions, 65% were parapneumonic, and 68% were multiloculated. There were 35% of effusions that failed primary intervention (image-directed catheter or tube thoracostomy [CT] and antibiotics), subsequently requiring surgical intervention. We found that 94% of cases requiring decortication as a primary or delayed intervention had a multiloculated effusion. Seventy-eight percent of the image-directed catheter failures were in patients with multiloculations. Early surgical decortication in patients with multiple loculations was more effective and resulted in decreased length of stay (5 days) and decreased cost (approximately $20,000 per patient).

Findings of this study have led me to adopt and recommend the following: (1) thoracic surgeons should be involved early in the treatment planning of a patient with empyema thoracis, the goal being complete drainage of the pleural space and reexpansion of the lung parenchyma; (2) early stage empyema (before the fibrinopurulent stage) that is unilocular is treated most effectively by image-directed catheters and fibrinolytic therapy; and (3) a multiloculated empyema, an empyema in the fibrinopurulent stage with an established visceral peel, and an empyema that has not cleared within 48 to 72 hours of treatment with an image-directed catheter and fibrinolytics should be treated by surgical intervention. The physiologically sound patient with empyema thoracis should be considered for early decortication.

REFERENCES

1. Bouros D, Schiza S, Siafakas N: Fibrinolytics in the treatment of a parapneumonic effusions. Monaldi Arch Chest Dis 54:258–263, 1999.
2. Lee RB: Radiologic evaluation and intervention for empyema thoracis. Chest Clin North Am 6:439, 1996.
3. Light RW, Rodriguez RM: Management of parapneumonic effusions. Clin Chest Med 19:373–382, 1998.
4. Thourani VH, Brady KM, Mansour KA, et al: Evaluation of treatment modalities for thoracic empyema: A cost-effectiveness analysis. Ann Thorac Surg 66:1121–1127, 1998.
5. Wait MA, Sharma S, Hohn J, et al: A randomized trial of empyema therapy. Chest 111:1548–1551, 1997.

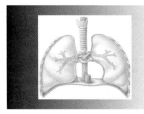

Benign Pleural Disease

Fibrothorax and Decortication of the Lung

CHAPTER 28C

Thomas J. Watson

Pathogenesis
Diagnosis and Evaluation
Indications and Contraindications
Operative Techniques
Outcomes
Summary

The pleural space is normally a potential cavity bordered by the visceral and parietal pleurae. A variety of pathological conditions may cause fibrous thickening of these pleural membranes, leading to their fusion or entrapment of the underlying pulmonary parenchyma. *Decortication* refers to the process of peeling this restrictive fibrous layer from the pleura, promoting lung reexpansion and improving thoracic excursion. As opposed to thoracoplasty, which collapses the rigid thorax to obliterate pleural space disease, decortication allows for the disentrapment of lung parenchyma, even when chronically involved, to bring about resolution of pleural pathology, improve pulmonary function, and increase chest wall dynamics.

PATHOGENESIS

Any pleural fluid left undrained, regardless of cause, has the potential to initiate an inflammatory response with fibrin deposition on the visceral and parietal pleural surfaces (Table 28C-1).

The severity of such a reaction depends on the initiating cause. Chronic transudative effusion may lead to a thin, translucent membrane, whereas empyema thoracis and hemothorax tend to cause a thick, irregular, fibrous peel. The parietal reaction is typically thicker than the visceral one. The fibrous layer develops over the lung, chest wall, diaphragm, and mediastinal surfaces.

The pulmonary parenchyma generally is unaffected by the pleural reaction per se, unless the pleural disease was initiated by an underlying lung infection, inflammatory process, or trauma. The peel that forms over the lung is discrete from the underlying visceral pleura and generally can be separated from it in the process of decortication. The goal of surgical therapy is removal of the encasing fibrotic membrane without damaging the normal pleura or, more importantly, the underlying pulmonary parenchyma.

DIAGNOSIS AND EVALUATION

The clinical presentation of a fibrothorax depends on the underlying cause, its severity and extent, and whether appropriate therapy was initiated. Because most fibrothoraces are secondary to parapneumonic empyema or traumatic hemothorax, associated parenchymal damage is common and may contribute substantially to the symptom complex. No inciting cause may be elicited in 50% of cases.

The most common presenting symptom of fibrothorax is dyspnea on exertion. Other common complaints include chest pain, pressure or tightness fever malaise and cough. The onset of these symptoms may be insidious without an obvious antecedent respiratory infection or acute traumatic event. Physical examination may reveal diminished breath sounds on the affected side with dullness to percussion. Deep inspiration shows decreased chest wall excursion with relative fixation of the hemidiaphragm.

Chest radiography is the mainstay of diagnostic testing for chronic empyema and fibrothorax. Milder cases show pleural-based radiodensities involving the lower hemithorax and diaphragmatic surface with obliteration of the costophrenic angle. Discrete loculations may occur more superiorly as well. In more severe cases, most of the pleural space can be involved with encasement of the entire lung. Closer inspection of the structures surrounding the lung may reveal narrowing of the intercostal spaces, elevation of the ipsilateral hemidiaphragm, and shift of the mediastinum toward the fibrothorax. Pleural calcification can occur in more chronic cases and provides an accurate assessment of the thickness of the pleural rind.

Computed tomography (CT) scans provide a more detailed evaluation of the extent of pleural disease and associated parenchymal pathology, which can be difficult to differentiate on plain chest radiographs. Specifically, densities seen on chest X-ray in large part may represent parenchymal consolidation, especially in the earlier stages of disease, with a relatively small pleural component. Similarly the CT scan may show an underlying carcinoma, fibrosis, atelectasis, or bronchiectasis that was missed on conventional chest x-ray and may affect the outcome of decortication. Finally, CT may help determine the chronicity of the pleural pathology, the degree of fluid component to the process, the extent of loculations, and the thickness of the visceral pleural membrane.

When a patient is considered for surgery, physiological testing can provide an assessment of the degree of respiratory compromise and a baseline against which to compare the

436

Table 28C-1
Common Causes of Fibrothorax
Empyema thoracis
Retained hemothorax
Tuberculosis
Chronic pneumothorax

Pleural effusions
   Transudative
   Exudative
   Chylous
   Pancreatic

outcome of intervention. Conventional pulmonary function testing with spirometry, lung volumes, and diffusion capacity for carbon monoxide show a restrictive ventilatory defect with diminished lung volumes (total lung capacity and vital capacity) and expiratory flows (forced expiratory volume in 1 second). If the lung parenchyma is not diseased, the diffusion capacity of the lungs corrected for the reduced volumes is normal, indicative of extrapulmonary chest wall restriction. Fibrothorax may cause a more severe impairment in respiratory function than might be anticipated from radiographical findings. Similarly, pleural restriction may compromise lung function more than parenchymal consolidation.

▶ INDICATIONS AND CONTRAINDICATIONS

The timing of intervention for pleural effusion, infection, or hemothorax is crucial to the outcome and determines the appropriate therapy. When effusions are thin, simple aspiration may suffice. Purulent collections and acute hemothoraces generally mandate closed tube thoracostomy with underwater seal drainage. Fibrinopurulent, loculated empyema and clotted hemothorax may be managed successfully with thoracoscopic irrigation, débridement, and evacuation. If these processes are not resolved at this stage, however, fibrin deposition ensues with resultant fibrothorax.

Decortication of the lung is indicated for patients with symptomatic extrapulmonary restriction due to fibrothorax. Decortication becomes necessary if malignant pleural disease is excluded, and less invasive measures have failed to drain the pleural space, reexpand the lung, or control pleural infection. In tuberculosis, decortication is indicated if long-term antituberculous therapy has failed to bring about resolution of pleural disease and thoracentesis does not eliminate an associated pleural effusion. Because decortication generally requires a thoracotomy, the degree of symptoms and respiratory compromise must be weighed carefully against the patient's comorbidities and the inherent risks of surgical intervention. Many patients being evaluated for surgical therapy have significant acute or chronic pulmonary disease that can affect their candidacy for decortication and the timing of operation.

In general, the longer surgical intervention is delayed, the more mature the pleural peel becomes. For this reason, traditional teaching has been to wait a period of approximately 4 to 6 weeks before operating on patients with fibrosing empyema thoracis or organizing hemothorax. This time allows for an easier plane of dissection between the fibrous rind and the underlying visceral pleura. A delay also allows any underlying parenchymal infectious consolidation to resolve, as otherwise lung reexpansion does not always follow successful decortication.

In practice, the recommendation to postpone surgical therapy is not always feasible. The onset of disease may be difficult to ascertain from historical information, and the pleural rind may be mature at the time of presentation to the surgeon. The patient may be hospitalized with acute symptoms and may be unwilling to delay definitive therapy. Unresolved pleural infection may need to be addressed in an urgent fashion. The costs of a prolonged hospitalization must be considered, and the treating physicians may feel pressure to discharge the patient as expeditiously as possible. Finally, excessive delays may lead to more extensive fibrosis with obliteration of the plane between the fibrous peel and visceral pleura, making decortication difficult and hazardous. It has been our practice to recommend decortication when CT shows the absence of any serious parenchymal consolidation or fibrosis, such that pulmonary reexpansion can be anticipated when the restrictive fibrous membrane is removed. Decortication is contraindicated in the setting of serious comorbidities, such that the patient is not a candidate for thoracotomy; chronic debility; and ongoing parenchymal disease, especially when secondary to associated bronchial obstruction.

▶ OPERATIVE TECHNIQUES

Bronchoscopy always is indicated at the time of surgery to rule out an associated endobronchial obstruction from tumor, foreign body, or broncholith that might impede expansion of entrapped lung. Single-lung ventilation is established with the use of a double-lumen endotracheal tube or single-lumen tube with or without a bronchial blocker. This ventilation strategy allows a variety of intraoperative manipulations to aid in the process of decortication, such as intermittent positive-pressure ventilation of the involved side alternating with lung collapse.

The patient is placed in the lateral decubitus position, providing access to the preferred operative approach, the posterolateral thoracotomy. We generally divide the latissimus dorsi and spare the serratus anterior muscle. The pleural cavity is entered through the fifth, sixth, or seventh intercostal space, depending on the location of the pleural pathology. Generally the fibrotic process is most dense within the inferior aspect of the hemithorax and along the hemidiaphragmatic surface, making the sixth or seventh interspace preferable. A portion or the entirety of one or two ribs may be resected to allow access because the chest wall typically is rigid and contracted, making exposure difficult. Often, by freeing the thickened parietal pleura from the chest wall before placing a rib retractor, however, rib resection can be avoided.

The thickened parietal membrane is incised, and the pleural cavity is entered. Although violating the empyema cavity has the potential to contaminate the thoracotomy wound, it is generally unavoidable. Clinically significant postoperative wound infections are uncommon, however, if perioperative antibiotics are administered and complete lung expansion is achieved with obliteration of the pleural space. If the lung is densely fused to the chest wall by the fibrotic process, entry may be gained into the pleural space closer to the mediastinum, where the adhesions typically are less dense. The intrapleural fluid and fibrinopurulent debris are evacuated with suction and forceps. Cultures are taken for microbiologic analysis, including acid-fast and fungal smears and cultures, when indicated.

Pulmonary decortication starts by incising the fibrous peel that encases the lung. Depending on the inciting cause and the severity of disease, several layers may be penetrated before the thin visceral pleura is reached. Ideally, dissection continues just superficial to the pleura, stripping the rind in continuous sheets. A variety of techniques can be used to separate the peel from the pleura, including sharp dissection with a knife or scissors, blunt dissection with a suction tip or Kittner dissector, and stripping using DeBakey or Russian forceps. The lung may be intermittently ventilated to show the correct tissue plane, the extent of any ongoing restriction, and the adequacy of the decortication at bringing about complete lung expansion. Most of the dissection is performed best with the lung collapsed, to minimize damage to the visceral pleura and underlying lung parenchyma. The difficulty of stripping the different lung surfaces may be variable and unpredictable. In regions where a tissue plane is difficult to detect, patches of the fibrotic rind may be left on the lung. Areas of lung parenchyma that are superficially denuded of pleura generally can be left alone because air leaks resolve with spontaneous ventilation, especially if the lung is fully expanded, and the parenchyma apposes the chest wall. More extensive parenchymal injury leading to bleeding and large air leaks must be controlled with cautery or suture.

The extent of parietal pleurectomy has been the subject of considerable controversy. The advantage of freeing the chest wall, diaphragm, and mediastinum of the restrictive peel is the improvement of chest ventilatory dynamics that can be expected. The counterargument has been the potential for increased blood loss, operative time, and damage to neighboring structures. Likewise, complete pulmonary expansion may facilitate subsequent resolution of thick parietal membranes. Our practice has been to add at least a partial, if not complete, parietal pleurectomy if it can be done expeditiously, safely, and conservatively. The plane of dissection along the chest wall is generally between the parietal pleura and endothoracic fascia. Bleeding is managed with manual pressure and electrocautery. Care must be taken in regions that are difficult to visualize because the control of bleeding may be a challenge. A dental mirror can aid in viewing areas not seen under direct vision. As the mediastinum is approached, the surgeon must be continually vigilant as to the location of the esophagus, major vascular structures, pericardium, nerves (phrenic, vagus, brachial plexus, and sympathetic chain) and diaphragm. Damage to any of these structures can have devastating consequences.

If there is associated parenchymal pathology to be addressed, lung resection may be necessary at the time of decortication. Depending on the extent of resection, complete filling of the residual pleural space may be an issue. If adequate lung expansion is not provided by decortication, a small tailoring thoracoplasty or parietal wall collapse without rib resection ("pleural tent") can be added. A variety of muscle flaps also may be used to obliterate pleural space and obviate the need for thoracoplasty.

The involved lung is inflated fully under positive pressure on completion of the procedure. The pleural space is drained with at least two chest tubes, given the likelihood of some postoperative air leak, the possibility of ongoing bleeding, and the potential for areas of incomplete lung expansion. Positioning of the tubes depends on the particular outcome of decortication, although at least one tube generally should be placed inferiorly to drain the costophrenic sulcus. The double-lumen endotracheal tube may be changed back to a single-lumen tube at the termination of the procedure if bronchoscopy is necessary to suction excessive airway secretions or purulence. The chest tubes are left to suction via an underwater seal drainage system.

▶ OUTCOMES

Operative mortality reported in most series is low (<5%), which reflects careful patient selection. Common postoperative complications include hemorrhage, prolonged air leaks, and residual empyema. With appropriate attention to operative technique, however, including control of bleeding and lung parenchymal damage and achieving adequate lung expansion, the incidence of these adverse outcomes should be minimized. Proper patient selection is crucial to ascertain that underlying lung pathology is managed adequately preoperatively or intraoperatively, allowing for maximum return of lung volume and function. Several authors have noted that the absence of underlying lung disease is the best predictor of improved pulmonary function after decortication. Although patients with diseases of a shorter duration might be expected to achieve a better operative result, even chronically entrapped lungs of many years' duration can expand fully after decortication, attesting to the relative sparing of the visceral pleura and parenchyma by the fibrotic process. Operative injury to the phrenic nerve, esophagus, or diaphragm can bring about postoperative complications with suboptimal, or even catastrophic, outcomes. Decortication, with the associated thoracotomy, is a major surgical undertaking with the potential for postthoracotomy pain and the loss of some degree of chest wall and upper extremity function.

▶ SUMMARY

Despite improvements in imaging techniques and the ability of physicians to intervene early in the course of pleural space diseases, patients still present to thoracic surgeons with the sequelae of chronic empyema, retained hemothorax, and eventually fibrothorax. The disease processes leading to fibrothorax may present insidiously, such that the patient does not seek medical attention until the sequelae of fibrothorax are already firmly established or may go unrecognized by the treating physician. Despite the desire to avoid a major surgical undertaking, less invasive medical or surgical therapies are doomed to fail in the setting of a lung

438 that is chronically entrapped by a restrictive pleural rind. Symptomatic improvement can be anticipated only after surgical intervention designed to remove this encasing membrane from the lung parenchyma, chest wall, and diaphragm. In properly selected patients, surgical decortication can be performed with low mortality; acceptable morbidity; and resultant improvements in pleural sepsis, respiratory dynamics, and symptoms. With appropriate attention to operative technique, even lungs that have been chronically entrapped can be decorticated successfully and restored to premorbid level of function, assuming underlying pulmonary parenchymal pathology has been managed.

REFERENCES

1. Deslauriers J, Perrault LP: Fibrothorax and decortication. In Pearson FG, et al., editors: Thoracic Surgery, New York, 1995, Churchill-Livingstone, p. 1107.
2. Rice TW: Fibrothorax and decortication of the lung. In Shields TW, et al, editors: General thoracic surgery, Philadelphia, 2000, Lippincott Williams & Wilkins, p. 729.
3. Samson PC, Burford TH: Total pulmonary decortication: its evolution and present concepts of indications and operative technique. J Thorac Surg 16:127, 1947.
4. Wright GW, et al: Physiologic observations concerning decortication of the lung. J Thorac Surg 18:372, 1949.

Benign Pleural Disease

Postpneumonectomy Empyema and Bronchopleural Fistula

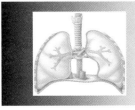

Jean Deslauriers and Philippe Demers

| Etiology
| Treatment
| Summary

Postpneumonectomy bronchopleural fistulas (BPF) are uncommon but life-threatening events. As a result of improvements in surgical techniques, the prevalence of BPF has declined markedly since the 1970s to a current level of less than 5%. When it occurs, however, BPF remains associated with reported mortalities of 30% to 50%. Empyemas without BPF are seldom seen, and although patients may have a prolonged course of management with multiple interventions, this complication rarely in itself is associated with death.

▶ ETIOLOGY

Several risk factors have been associated with the development of postpneumonectomy BPF (Table 28D-1). Because the most important aspect in the management of postpneumonectomy BPF is their prevention, every effort should be made to identify clearly all predisposing factors, especially factors relating to preoperative management and technical conduct of the operation. It is well known that there is a higher risk of BPF in older patients and in patients with diabetes mellitus, hypoalbuminemia, and prolonged steroid therapy. If these conditions cannot be controlled adequately preoperatively, the bronchus is at risk of dehiscence. Prophylactic reinforcement of the bronchial stump with pericardium, pericardial fat, or intercostal muscle has been shown to reduce the risk of BPF in such cases.

The influence of induction therapies is controversial, although several reports have shown increased incidence of BPF in patients who have received more than 45 gy of radiation therapy preoperatively. Because these bronchi are at much higher risk of dehiscence, coverage of the stump with large transposed intrathoracic muscles or omentum is recommended. In one report, the operative mortality rate associated with right pneumonectomy was close to 25% when the operation was done in the context of induction chemotherapy.

In patients who have obstructive pneumonia secondary to lung cancer, the infection ideally should be controlled before surgery. The same principle applies to patients undergoing pneumonectomy for tuberculosis; the incidence of BPF can be 20% in such cases. Patients with bronchiectasis are not at risk for BPF because they already have an increased vascular supply to the bronchus due to bronchial artery hyperplasia associated with this pathology.

The development of postpneumonectomy BPF is associated with several intraoperative factors, one of which is the inexperience of the operator who may not be familiar with the local anatomy or surgical principles involved in healthy bronchial closure. Most authors have reported a higher incidence of BPF after right pneumonectomy; this is not surprising because the right main bronchus vascular supply usually is provided by only one bronchial artery (versus two for the left main bronchus), making it more susceptible to devascularization during extensive nodal dissection. In addition, the left main bronchus retracts underneath the aortic arch after pneumonectomy and is protected better by mediastinal tissues. Whether there is a higher incidence of BPF in manually sutured bronchi than in stapled bronchi is unclear from the literature. The technique of bronchial closure is probably not important so long as the bronchus has not been devitalized, there is no tension at the sutured or stapled line, and there is good mucosal approximation.

In all cases, the bronchus must be closed near the carina to avoid excessively long stumps and pooling of secretions. Although residual malignancy in the bronchial resection margin impairs healing and increases the incidence of BPF, it is sometimes advisable to accept a positive resection line rather than increase the operative mortality by extending the resection to the lower end of the trachea.

Other intraoperative factors that have been shown to increase the potential risks for BPF development include surgery for higher stage tumors with more extensive mediastinal node dissections, pneumonectomy through an already infected pleural space, and contamination of the space during the operation. This last-mentioned factor is always a high possibility when pneumonectomy is done for benign disease, and sometimes contamination can be avoided by extrapleural dissection. It is important that these intraoperative risk factors be recognized and that bronchi at risk be covered with vascularized tissues. The benefits of routine coverage of low-risk bronchi are not clear, however, despite the fact that most surgeons tend to cover all right main bronchi with local tissues, such as pleura, pericardium, or mediastinal fat.

Perhaps the most significant risk factor for bronchial dehiscence is the need for postoperative mechanical ventilation.

440

Predisposing Risk Factors for Postpneumonectomy Bronchopleural Fistula and Empyema

Preoperative Factors

Age (>70 years)
Chronic obstructive pulmonary disease (predicted FEV_1 <0.8 liter)
Comorbidities (diabetes mellitus, collagen vascular disease)
Malnutrition (low serum albumin)
Prolonged steroid therapy
Induction therapies (chemotherapy, radiation therapy)
Pulmonary infection
Pneumonectomy through an empyema cavity

Intraoperative Factors

Right pneumonectomy (versus left)
Extended pneumonectomy or completion pneumonectomy
Higher stage tumors
Extensive nodal dissection (devascularization and devitalization of bronchial stump)
Unhealthy bronchus (ossification of bronchial cartilage, endobronchial mucosal disease)
Inadequate bronchial closure (with tension or poor mucosal approximation)
Residual cancer in bronchial margin
Inexperienced operator
Long bronchial stump
Contamination of pleural space during pneumonectomy

Postoperative Factors

Need for mechanical ventilation
Hemothorax or empyema

FEV_1, forced expiratory volume in 1 second.

In several multivariate analyses, this factor was an independent predictor of BPF development. Postoperative mechanical ventilation is sometimes unavoidable. If mechanical ventilation is necessary, the tip of the intratracheal tube must be as far as possible from the sutured bronchus, and suctioning must be gentle. High peak pressures and positive end-expiratory pressure levels must be avoided. Although the use of high-frequency ventilation has been recommended for this purpose, this mode of ventilation can be applied successfully only to a few individuals. In most cases of BPF occurring in patients being mechanically ventilated, it is a terminal event for which nothing much can be done.

▶ TREATMENT

In patients with suspected BPF, early diagnosis is paramount because the sooner it is made, the better the prognosis. Early dehiscence (within 2 weeks) usually is associated with increased dyspnea, expectoration of serosanguineous fluid, increased subcutaneous emphysema, and bulging of the thoracotomy incision. Serial x-rays often show a decreasing air-fluid level and mediastinal shift toward the remaining lung. In those cases, bronchoscopy is a crucial part of the evaluation because it usually documents the dehiscence and its exact site and size. It also documents the quality of the endobronchial mucosa and the length of the involved main bronchus. If the BPF is not seen, indirect signs, such as the presence of fibrin or bubbling within the bronchus, can be helpful. Occasionally, water-sealed drainage of the pleural space reveals an air leak.

Late-occurring BPF or empyemas without fistulas (up to 3 months postoperatively) may be difficult to diagnose. Bronchoscopy and thoracentesis in cases of empyema are important parts of the evaluation when these diagnoses are suspected.

Although the management of an acute postpneumonectomy BPF remains a major problem, immediate drainage of the pleural space is often lifesaving because it may prevent flooding of the contralateral lung by what already has accumulated within the pneumonectomy space. The size of the BPF does not correlate with the importance of aspiration. When the patient's clinical condition has been stabilized, the next step in management is to attempt closure of the BPF. If the fistula is small (i.e., <2–3 mm), several authors have reported successful endobronchial closure through local bronchoscopic application of fibrin sealants. If this can be accomplished, videothoracoscopy may be used to evacuate the space completely, remove all necrotic tissue, and insert two thoracostomy tubes that later will be used for continuous irrigation of the hemithorax.

If the BPF is large (>3 mm), direct reclosure of the bronchial stump through repeat thoracotomy should be performed as soon as possible. In instances in which gross disruption of the bronchus has occurred, the reclosed stump should be reinforced with intercostal or pectoralis major muscles. Occasionally, one also can use a flap of diaphragm or the omentum to cover the stump. The omentum, which is brought through the diaphragm, is particularly useful because of its extendibility, good adherence to inflammatory surfaces, ability for neovascularization, and immunologic properties. When this is accomplished, two chest tubes are left to irrigate further and attempt to sterilize the space, or an open thoracic window is created. When the bronchial stump is too short for reclosure, the transposed muscle flap or omentum is sutured circumferentially around the defect to obtain an airtight closure. When the chest cavity is cleaned, the tubes are removed, or the patient is taken back to the operating room for chest wall reclosure if he or she has an open thoracic window.

Early empyemas without BPF are uncommon, and they are managed best by videothoracoscopic débridement of the space, tube irrigation, and systemic antibiotics. With this regimen, most infected spaces can be sterilized, avoiding the need for an open thoracic window or thoracoplasty. When the space has been sterilized, as documented by two or three negative cultures, it is filled with the débridement antibiotic solution, and the tubes are removed. In all of these patients, special emphasis must be placed on maintaining adequate nutrition during the recovery period.

Treatment strategies for late occurring BPF (>4 weeks postoperatively) are different because the risks of aspiration in the remaining lung are low. Initial tube drainage is important, and occasionally, small BPF close spontaneously, especially in cases in which the fistula is secondary to an empyema. Drainage also can be accomplished by fenestration when the space and fistula site can be inspected and débrided on a daily basis. Large BPF usually require surgical reclosure, which is accomplished best by a transpericardial approach via a median sternotomy (Figure 28D-1). The main advantages of this approach are the uninfected operative field and the well-defined anatomy. When doing this procedure, the bronchus must be fully redivided, rather than stapled in continuity, and the closure must be reinforced with vascularized pericardium, mobilized thymus, or omentum, which is obtained easily through an extension of the sternotomy. Occasionally the BPF can be closed via a cervical approach using a videomediastinoscope (Figure 28D-2). Ultimately the residual empyema cavity can be sterilized by tube irrigation or open fenestration.

An alternative method is to drain the hemithorax initially by way of an open thoracic window. When the cavity appears healthy, the patient is returned to the operating room for muscle or omental transposition to achieve fistula closure and space obliteration.

Controversy remains regarding the role of thoracoplasty with or without added myoplasty to achieve space obliteration and fistula closure. In our experience, these procedures are well tolerated, and for most patients, they achieve the desired goals.

► SUMMARY

In all patients with postpneumonectomy BPF, definitive surgery should be considered only when the medical and nutritional status of the patient have been optimized; when the cavity is cleaned and healthy; when the BPF has been

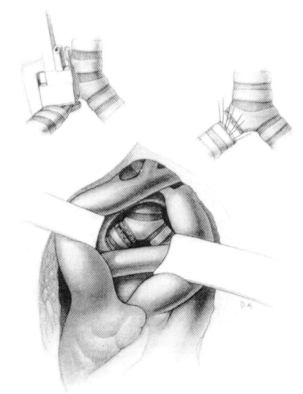

Figure 28D–1 Chronic right main bronchus fistula treated by division and reclosure of the proximal and distal stumps. *(From Ginsberg RJ, Person FG, Cooper JD, et al: Closure of chronic pseudopneumonectomy bronchopleural fistula using the transsternal transpericardical approach. Ann Thorac Surg 47:232–235, 1989.)*

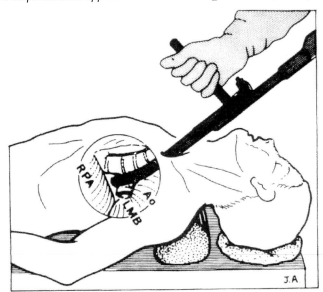

Figure 28D–2 Closure of BPF through cervicotomy. *(From Azorin JF, Francisci MP, Tremblay R, et al: Closure of bronchopleural fistula by video-assisted mediastinal pneumonectomy. Presse Med 25:805–806, 1996.)*

carefully categorized (site, size, quality of mucosa, length of stump) by bronchoscopy and CT scan; when the patient no longer requires or is unlikely to require mechanical ventilation; and when the patient has no evidence of recurring carcinoma. Although mortality and morbidity remain

442 high in these patients, careful understanding of the complication and systematic and aggressive management can be successful in some cases. Prevention is the most important consideration.

REFERENCES

1. Deschamps C, Bernard A, Nichols FC 3rd, et al: Empyema and bronchopleural fistula after pneumonectomy: factors affecting incidence. Ann Thorac Surg 72:243–247, 2001.

2. Ginsberg RJ, Pearson FG, Cooper JD, et al: Closure of chronic postpneumonectomy fistula using the trans-sternal transpericardial approach. Ann Thorac Surg 47:231–235, 1989.

3. Grégoire R, Deslauriers J, Beaulieu M, et al: Thoracoplasty: its forgotten role in the management of non tuberculous postpneumonectomy empyema. Can J Surg 30:343–345, 1987.

4. Hollaus PH, Lax F, Wurnig PN, et al: Video-thoracoscopic debridement of the postpneumonectomy space in empyema. Eur J Cardiothorac Surg 16:283–286, 1999.

5. Regnard JF, Alifano M, Puys P, et al: Open window thoracostomy followed by intrathoracic flap transposition in the treatment of empyema complicating pulmonary resection. J Thorac Cardiovasc Surg 120:270–275, 2000.

Benign Pleural Disease

Chylothorax

Robert M. Cortina and David W. Johnstone

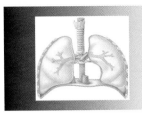

- **Definition and Diagnosis**
- **Medical Management**
- **Surgical Management**
- **Summary**

DEFINITION AND DIAGNOSIS

Chylothorax is the presence of lymph in the pleural space. Chylothorax may be caused by congenital or primary lymphatic disease but usually is due to intrathoracic malignancies with intrinsic or extrinsic obstruction, iatrogenic injury, and blunt or penetrating trauma. Postoperative chylothorax may complicate surgical procedures anywhere along the path of the thoracic duct between the diaphragm and the neck.

The initial symptom of intrathoracic chyle accumulation is dyspnea resulting from compressive atelectasis of the lung. Prolonged drainage leads to dehydration, malnutrition, and immunological compromise due to loss of fluid, fats, protein, and T lymphocytes. Before the advent of thoracic duct ligation, the mortality of postoperative and traumatic chylothorax was nearly 50%.

Although chyle can be clear in the fasting state, it becomes milky after oral intake that includes fats. Biochemical and microscopic examination of the effusion confirm the diagnosis. The concentration of triglycerides is higher than that of plasma; fluid with a triglyceride level of more than 110 mg/dl has a 99% chance of being chylous compared with a 5% chance when less than 50 mg/dl. The presence of chylomicrons in the fluid is specific for the diagnosis of chylothorax. Prompt diagnosis is essential to effective therapy because of the severity of complications from prolonged chylous drainage.

MEDICAL MANAGEMENT

Conservative (nonsurgical) management of chylothorax may be appropriate as an initial strategy, particularly in the first few days after surgery or trauma or in cases of malignant chylothoraces that may respond to treatment of the underlying neoplasm (particularly lymphoma). The components of initial management are drainage of the pleural space, reduction of chyle flow, maintenance of hydration, and provision of adequate nutrition.

Evacuation of the pleural space is achieved most commonly by tube thoracostomy. This provides lung reexpan-

sion, continuous drainage, and accurate measurement of chyle flow. Close attention must be paid to tube patency, position, and changes in drainage because prolonged drainage can lead to tube obstruction or loculation away from other portions of the pleural space. Chyle is bacteriostatic, and infection from the indwelling tube is unlikely.

In 1934, Hepner stated that chylous fistulas close by obliteration of the adjacent pleural space rather than healing of the lymphatic vessels themselves. To accelerate pleural symphysis, various chemical sclerosants have been applied to the pleural space, including antibiotics (tetracycline, doxycycline), antineoplastic agents (bleomycin), biologic modifiers (OK-432, interferon, and interleukins), and talc. Chemical pleurodesis may be most appropriate for patients with malignant chylothoraces, in whom direct closure of the leak is impossible, but we have had a low success rate in this setting.

Maintenance of nutrition, prevention of dehydration, and reduction of chyle flow are closely related. Large losses of fluid, electrolytes, protein, fat, fat-soluble vitamins, and lymphocytes may result in severe metabolic and immunological derangement. A reduction in enteral intake and specifically in the dietary intake of long-chain fatty acids is associated with a significant reduction in lymphatic flow. The substitution of dietary fat with medium-chain triglycerides is practiced widely, predicated on the preferential uptake of medium-chain triglycerides by the portal circulation. These diets have had variable degrees of success. The reason may be that intestinal triglycerides derive from endogenous and exogenous sources and that any oral intake increases chyle production. When a fat-free, nonelemental diet was compared with total parenteral nutrition (TPN), the closure rate of chylous fistulas favored TPN. Many authors prefer complete bowel rest and TPN as the optimal means of nutritional support to reduce chyle production.

Traumatic chylothoraces that close with conservative management do so within 2 weeks in most cases. When the chest drainage is low, the pleural space is evacuated, and the lung is expanded, oral intake can be resumed. When the patient is eating a normal diet with no evidence of persistent chyle leak, the chest tube can be removed.

When chylothorax is secondary to lymphatic obstruction by tumor, treatment of the primary condition with radiotherapy and/or chemotherapy may control the chyle fistulas either by producing local fibrosis or by relieving lymphatic obstruction. Pleuroperitoneal shunting may be appropriate in these patients because nutritional losses are minimized while dyspnea is relieved. Success has been reported to be 75–90% in

444 treating pediatric chylothoraces and 80% in adults. The procedure is associated with minimal discomfort, but the subcutaneous chamber must be compressed several hundred times per day to shunt an adequate volume. In debilitated cancer patients, this is not a useful solution. Intermittent external drainage with either thoracentesis or a semipermanent catheter may be a reasonable palliative alternative.

Other methods of conservative management include positive-pressure ventilation, inhaled nitric oxide at 20 ppm, and percutaneous embolization of the thoracic duct. The institution of positive-pressure ventilation and/or nitric oxide reportedly has resulted in a marked reduction in chest tube drainage and has stopped the chyle leak. It is believed that systemic venous hypertension may be a significant contributing factor to a persistent chyle leak. Nitric oxide, a predominately pulmonary arterial vasodilator, may decrease systemic venous pressures by augmenting forward flow through the right side of the heart.

Percutaneous transabdominal duct catheterization and embolization can be a safe and effective alternative treatment for persistent chylothorax and may be warranted in patients too frail to undergo duct ligation. Patients with previous major abdominal surgery involving retroperitoneal organs may not be suitable for this intervention because they may have occlusion of the major retroperitoneal lymphatic ducts and cisterna chyli.

▶ SURGICAL MANAGEMENT

Before Lampson's report of transpleural thoracic duct ligation in 1948, repeated thoracentesis and oral nutritional support commonly were employed. Mortality from traumatic chylothorax was greater than 50%, and nontraumatic chylothorax was usually fatal. After the introduction of thoracic duct ligation, the mortality rate improved to 10%.

There is general consensus that failed conservative management warrants surgical intervention. There is less agreement on clinical parameters necessitating surgical intervention. In 1971, Selle et al proposed the following parameters for surgical intervention. Idiopathic chylothorax in neonates and nontraumatic chylothorax should be managed nonoperatively. Indications for thoracic duct ligation in traumatic chylothorax are an average daily loss of greater than 1500 ml/day in adults or greater than 100 ml/year of age in children over 5 days persistent leak for more than 2 weeks despite conservative management, and nutritional or metabolic complications. In 1981, Strausser et al recommended operative therapy for nontraumatic chylothorax as well. In their report, only 3 of 13 patients responded to non-operative therapy, whereas 3 of 4 patients who had transthoracic duct ligation had permanent relief of their chylothorax.

Lymphangiography provides useful information regarding the lymphatic anatomy and fistula site, but it is laborious. We generally have reserved lymphangiography for refractory chylothoraces that have failed initial surgical closure. Other methods used to locate the leak include preoperative subcutaneous injection of 1% Evans blue dye in the thigh or enteral administration of a fat source, such as cream or olive oil. Methylene blue may be added to the fat source to highlight the site of the fistula.

The surgical options for control of chylothorax are direct ligation of the thoracic duct, mass ligation of the thoracic duct with and without thoracotomy, thoracoscopic ligation of the thoracic duct, pleurectomy, application of fibrin glue, and placement of a pleuroperitoneal shunt. If the chyle leak can be identified, direct ligation with nonabsorbable ligatures should be performed on either side of the leak. If the leak cannot be identified, extensive dissection should be avoided. Mass ligation of all tissue between the aorta, spine, esophagus, and pericardium is performed most easily above the diaphragmatic hiatus via the right pleural space. This ligation traditionally has been performed via a right thoracotomy through the sixth or seventh interspace. Parietal pleurectomy may promote pleural symphysis and should be considered when control of the duct is uncertain. Pulmonary decortication may be necessary if the lung is entrapped in a benign peel.

Since its introduction in the early 1990s, thoracoscopic ligation of the thoracic duct has become a therapeutic option. There are few reported series but multiple successful case reports. Enteral administration of 50 ml of heavy cream is given shortly before surgery. Thoracoscopy is performed with the patient under general anesthesia using single-lung ventilation. A trocar is placed in the right sixth or seventh intercostal space in the midaxillary line. A 30-degree scope is inserted, and the pleural space is evaluated. A second port in the right eight posterior intercostal space is used for dissection and division of the inferior pulmonary ligament. A third port is placed in the anterior axillary line superiorly for retraction of the lung. The pleura is incised above the diaphragm. If the duct can be identified easily, it is dissected free. A small segment usually is taken for pathological confirmation, then both ends are doubly clipped. If the thoracic duct cannot be identified easily, mass ligation of all tissue in the position previously described is performed using clips. Chest drainage is established. The chest drain is removed when chyle drainage has ceased with the patient on a normal diet.

Chylothorax complicates esophagectomy in 2–4% of transthoracic approaches and 10% of transhiatal resections. A recognized intraoperative thoracic duct injury should be closed immediately. Most postoperative chylothoraces in this setting do not heal with conservative management. Early surgical closure of the duct is optimal. Thoracoscopic closure of the duct has been reported, but the gastric conduit can make exposure difficult, and a low thoracotomy is often the best approach.

Chylothorax after pulmonary resection is unusual. An initial course of conservative management is prudent after lobectomy if the lung is fully expanded. If a large residual pleural space remains after bilobectomy or pneumonectomy, we recommend early surgical closure of the duct. Pleuroperitoneal shunts may be appropriate in some patients with obligatory pleural spaces.

▶ SUMMARY

Chylothorax may be iatrogenic, traumatic, or spontaneous because of congenital or acquired disorders. Early recognition is crucial to preventing serious complications of chronic lymphatic loss. Initial drainage, combined with measures to reduce chyle flow and maintain nutrition, may resolve the condition. For cases that do not show prompt response, particularly in the postoperative or trauma setting, early surgical ligation of the thoracic duct should be performed with the expectation of prompt resolution. Thoracoscopy offers a minimally invasive approach and warrants consideration by experienced surgeons. Other alternatives require consideration of the underlying etiology, consideration of the patient's medical condition and prognosis, and an understanding of the limitations of these approaches.

REFERENCES

1. Bessone LN, Ferguson TB, Burford TH: Chylothorax: collective review. Ann Thorac Surg 12:527–550, 1971.
2. Johnstone DW, Feins RH: Chylothorax. Chest Surg Clin N Am 4:617–628, 1994.
3. Kent RB 3rd, Pinson TW: Thoracoscopic ligation of the thoracic duct. Surg Endosc 7:52–53, 1993.
4. Lampson RS: Traumatic chylothorax: a review of the literature and report of a case treated by mediastinal ligation of the thoracic duct. J Thorac Surg 17:778, 1948.

Malignant Pleural and Pericardial Effusions

Todd L. Demmy and Chukwumere Nwogu

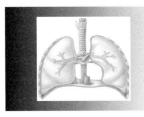

INTRODUCTION

Pleural effusions are common clinical problems occurring in over one million patients each year.[110,125] In some settings, up to 22% of these effusions are caused by malignant disease and over 100,000 malignant effusions require treatment annually.[120] Affected patients with advanced neoplastic diseases experience considerable morbidity as a result of these pleural fluid collections.

ETIOLOGY

Physiology

Pleural effusion results from a derangement in the normal physiology such that there is increased production of pleural fluid or a change of its composition with or without a reduction in the absorption of the fluid. This may be due to primary or secondary tumors of the pleura with seeding of the intrapleural space and lymphatic obstruction. Free floating tumor cells block absorption of fluid and produce vasoactive substances that in turn increase the production and block the absorption of intrapleural protein and fluid.[109]

Demographics

Of pleural neoplasms 95% arise from a metastatic source, with lung and breast carcinoma accounting for 75% of all cases.[58] Other common causes are lymphoma, gastric cancer, and ovarian cancer. Adenocarcinomas of unknown primary constitute a distinct entity in patients in whom the source of the pleural malignancy is never found. They are associated with exposure to environmental tobacco smoke.[7]

About half of patients with breast cancer develop a pleural effusion within their lifetime, as compared with one fourth of patients with lung cancer and one third of patients with lymphoma.[13,53] Breast cancer, lymphoreticular neoplasms, and melanoma take on average 30 months longer than other malignancies to manifest malignant effusions.[199]

Most pediatric effusions, on the other hand, are benign. If malignant, lymphomas or leukemias account for half with the remainder a mix of tumors such as neuroblastoma, Wilms' tumor, and germ cell neoplasms.[73]

EVALUATION

Historical and Physical Findings

Patients with malignant pleural effusions are typically symptomatic and complain of dyspnea, cough, or chest pain. The discomfort often is independent of respiration and but is aggravated by activity. With invasive pleural metastases, the affected nerve roots may radiate pain.[34] Like pericardial effusions, rapid fluid accumulation amplifies the symptoms.[13] For at least 10% of patients, the dyspnea is multifactorial and does not improve after drainage.[27] Physical findings indicating pleural effusion are decreased tactile fremitus and dullness to percussion on examination of the posterior chest. As the effusion increases in size, there may be hyperresonance on percussion immediately

448 above the fluid level because of compression and overdistention of the lung.[43] Bronchial airway signs may be prominent. As effusions become massive, tracheal deviations from mediastinal shifts are detectable. Malignant pleural effusions rarely cause hemodynamic compromise from tension hydrothorax.[149]

Imaging

Early evidence of pleural effusion by chest radiograph is costodiaphragmatic sulcus blunting caused by as little as 125 ml of fluid depending on the quality of the film (Figure 29-1). Occasionally, a spur-like shadow projects into the fissure.[34] Massive effusions are uncommon; however, when they occur they are more likely malignant. In patients in whom the finding is uncertain, a decubitus film might show shifting of the fluid. Effusions wider than 10 mm by decubitus film often are tapped successfully.[108]

There are specific computed tomography (CT) criteria for pleural effusions. In general, loculation, pleural thickening, pleural nodules, and extrapleural fat of increased density are present only in exudative effusions.[8] Multiple pleural nodules and nodular pleural thickening are generally limited to effusions of malignant etiology (Figure 29-2). Pleural thickening greater than 1 cm also is a reliable criterion.[210] Magnetic resonance imaging (MRI) has limited use, but it may be slightly more useful for certain pleural tumors such as lipoma, and it also can be helpful in determining the extent of invasion for mesothelioma.[137] Thoracic ultrasound shows the optimal site for diagnostic thoracentesis of a small pleural effusion. It also helps select ideal entry points for thoracoscopes or pleural biopsy instruments by avoiding adhesions.[121]

Nuclear medicine scans may detect early pleural metastases before other imaging tests. The mechanism by which this occurs is not clear, but in the case of bone scans may represent passive transudation of the technetium colloid.[100,195] If nuclear imaging reveals pleural activity and pleural fluid is scant, diagnostic thoracoscopy is necessary to exclude pleural disease provided this staging is relevant. Although the data are preliminary, activity in the pleural cavity, as demonstrated by fluorodeoxyglucose-positron emission tomography, also indicates pleural metastases.[51,72]

Diagnostic Procedures

The diagnosis of pleural effusion is confirmed by thoracentesis. Withdrawing only a small portion of pleural fluid is indicated occasionally when full lung reexpansion is unlikely or as a prelude to a definitive drainage procedure. It is usually preferable to attempt drainage of as much pleural fluid as possible (Figure 29-3).

Several commercial kits facilitate drainage by allowing insertion of soft catheters with side holes to completely evacuate the fluid. The catheters can be readjusted during

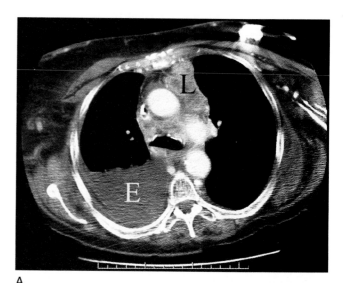

A

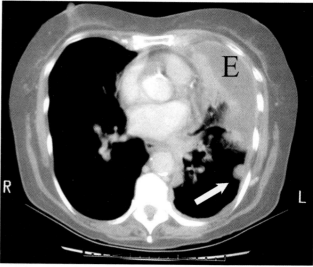

B

Figure 29–2 (**A**) CT images of a malignant pleural effusion. E, effusion; L, prevascular lymphadenopathy. (**B**) Chest CT of a breast carcinoma patient with recurrent basilar left pleural effusion after partially successful chemical sclerosis. The image shows partial pleurodesis, pleural thickening, and a pleural nodule (arrow) at level of mid thorax. E, effusion.

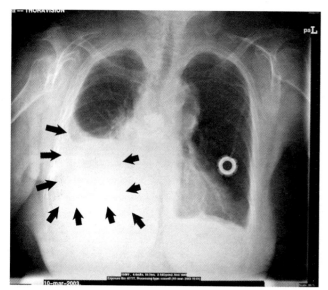

Figure 29–1 Chest roentgenogram showing large right pleural effusion outlined by arrows.

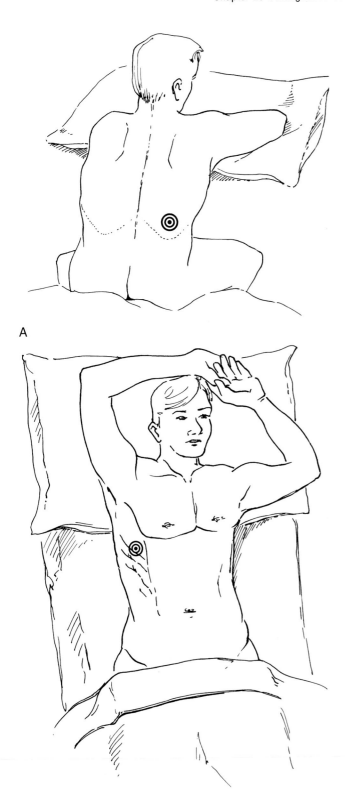

drainage in case the lung temporarily occludes the holes. Needles with retractable blunt obturators (e.g., Turkel needle) also prevent lung injury during pleural entry. Ultrasound or other imaging guides optimal needle or chest tube placement for effusion drainage (Figure 29-4). This is particularly useful for a small effusion or pleural disease of long duration complicated by lung consolidation or pleural loculation. While marking of the area of "deepest" fluid is useful, it is important to perform the thoracentesis with the patient in the same position as during the imaging. Attempts to completely aspirate chronic effusions should be undertaken carefully. High vacuum applied to the pleural space, by either syringe aspiration or vacuum bottle, is sufficient to rupture alveoli and cause a complicated hydropneumothorax.

Standard Chemistry and Cell Counts

Practically all malignant pleural effusions are exudates. Laboratory criteria to establish exudative effusions are based on absolute values or ratios to systemic parameters. One of the most useful criteria sets to classify effusions as exudative was described by Light: pleural fluid/serum total protein ratio greater than 0.5, pleural fluid/serum lactate dehydrogenase (LDH) ratio greater than 0.6, and pleural fluid LDH greater than 200 U/liter (>two thirds of the laboratories' upper limit of normal for serum).[110,186]

Low glucose (<60 mg/dl) and low pH (<7.20) levels are common in malignant pleural effusions.[182] This is attributed to glucose usage and acid production by the malignant cells, leukocytes within the pleural fluid, and also increased pleural membrane metabolism. Investigators have alternatively implicated abnormal pleural membrane transport of glucose, carbon dioxide, and hydrogen ion.[70] Cholesterol levels greater than 60 mg/dl suggest exudative etiology.[74] Pleural fluid amylase is elevated in about 10% patients with malignant pleural effusions even without pancreas gland disease.[109] In fact, the most common cause of an amylase-rich pleural effusion is neoplasm.[219] The cell count can also indicate malignancy. For some investigators, bloody fluid is the strongest positive predictor of malignant effusion.

Figure 29–3 (**A**) Common patient position for insertion of a thoracentesis needle or catheter. Posterior approach allows access to the most dependent (posterior pleural) sulcus to allow maximal drainage of nonloculated fluid. (**B**) Lateral patient positioning for thoracentesis or chest tube placement is also useful for effusions with large lateral collections of fluid. The patient's arm is abducted and flexed over his head to facilitate access to the lateral chest.

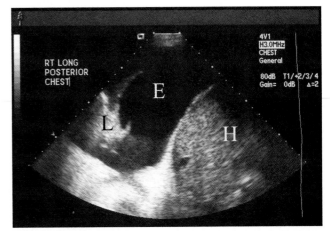

Figure 29–4 Ultrasound of right lateral chest to facilitate safe pleural access. E, effusion; H, hepatic lobe; L, lung.

450

Immunocytochemistry and Special Chemistry

Many investigators focused their explorations on staining patterns of cells obtained from pleural fluid to confirm malignancy, and, if present, correctly classify its origin. Unfortunately, markers are not yet sufficiently sensitive and specific, but they generally show twice the positivity of cytology alone (80% vs. 40%).[25] These tests usually are used after standard cytological screening and also are combined with cytogenetic and other miscellaneous tests to establish a diagnosis. A more complete list is displayed in Table 29-1.

Some of these markers, such as p53, predict a worse prognosis for malignant effusions that are p53-negative.[102] Another marker, Ki-67, is associated with a worse prognosis when its labeling index is low.[200]

Vascular endothelial growth factor (VEGF) has been found to be a useful discriminator for malignant effusions.[142] Other special chemistry values displayed in Table 29-2 are occasionally useful to categorize malignancy. The sensitivities and specificities vary by specific cell types.

Cytogenetics

DNA testing by flow cytometry or chromosome analysis predicts the likelihood of malignancy. The evidence of a marker chromosome, aneuploidy, or a hyperdiploid state suggests malignancy. Aneuploid samples (by flow cytometry) yield predictive values as high as 96%.[54,145] No aneuploidy was found in benign reactive effusions in one series.[42,146] A hyperdiploid chromosome 8 may be another useful marker.[150] Telomerase activity occurs in 92% of malignant effusions and in only 6% of benign effusions (with a specificity of 94.2%).[209,230]

Pleural Cytology and Biopsy

Cytological evaluations with standard staining (Papanicolaou's smears) generally confirm malignant pleural effusions. In very unusual cases (0.5%), the results are falsely positive.[89] In cytological specimen reviews, lung adenocarcinoma is the most frequent diagnosis. Breast cancer effusion specimens have a higher cytology diagnostic yield (about 78%) than lung or other tissue primaries.[47,83,89,199] The sensitivity of pleural fluid cytology frequently is greater than undirected pleural biopsy.

When standard pleural effusion cytology is nondiagnostic, pleural needle biopsy occasionally provides some additional useful diagnostic information (48% in one series).[220] However, whether pleural biopsy adds much over fluid cytological evaluation in cases of suspected malignancy is controversial. In another series, only 7% of the cases had a diagnosis made by use of pleural biopsy when the cytology result was negative.[173] For difficult cases, cytology combined with needle biopsy results are inferior to those obtained by video-assisted thoracic surgery (VATS) (41% vs. 97%).[20] In several series, a typical yield of undirected pleural needle biopsy of 50–60% was far inferior to biopsies obtained by VATS. Use of a directed VATS approach in these cases achieves greater than 90% success.[35,75,135,140,162] Yet, pleural needle biopsy may be useful with a known diagnosis such as breast carcinoma, in that it can provide additional tissue for hormone receptor determination.[106]

With idiopathic effusions (20% in some series), uncertainty is reduced to 4% using thoracoscopy.[19] The complication rate from thoracoscopic biopsy is low, with a mortality rates less than 1% and complication rates less than 10%.[5,41] Figure 29-5 shows thoracoscopy images that confirmed pleural malignancy.

A technique variation that might shift results of "blind" biopsy toward those by directed means is the use of a pleural brush to increase the cytological yield. In one series, this technique was positive in 90% of the cases, as opposed to 67% with the routine cytological aspirate and 58% with biopsy.[50] Thoracotomy to perform pleural biopsy is unusual given successful directed methods such as VATS.

When patients remain without a definitive diagnosis following VATS or thoracotomy, about one third will demonstrate a cause (typically lymphoma or mesothelioma) months to years later.[189] For patients with massive malignant effusions of uncertain etiology, fiberoptic bronchoscopy may establish lung cancer. When effusions are mild to moderate and without associated symptoms, the chance of finding a neoplasm is not great enough to warrant bronchoscopy.[171]

In summary, clinical information, conventional cytology results, immunocytochemistry, flow cytometry, and special chemistry test results all must be integrated to yield the most accurate diagnosis.[26]

▶ TREATMENT

The optimal treatment for malignant pleural effusion is controversial. Multiple technologies exist that control malignant pleural effusions successfully. The best selection for a patient is guided by factors including the individual's frailty and the prognosis of the primary malignancy. The need for additional pleural tissue or directed biopsy as well as concomitant diagnostic or therapeutic procedures requiring general anesthesia also guides the choice and timing of pleural interventions.

The anatomical state of the affected thorax is important. For instance, a pleural effusion of relatively rapid onset typically yields full expansion of the lung and pleural coaptation after the effusion is evacuated. On the other hand, malignant disease of long duration can prevent full lung expansion because of visceral pleural restriction, endobronchial obstruction, parenchymal fibrosis, or replacement by tumor. To help with planning, good diagnostic imaging is important.

Treatment options can be classified into those that rely on drainage alone or those that also obliterate the pleural space. Since there is an inflammatory response associated with most pleural effusions, persistent and complete pleural drainage may also achieve pleural fusion. Recent evidence shows cytokine activation from repetitive pleural draining that supports this view.[30] While pleural malignancy traditionally means surgical incurability, there are some investigational multidisciplinary methods that include operations for selected cases designed to improve the chance for cure.

A chest radiograph after pleurodesis commonly shows multiloculated fluid collections suggestive of empyema.[138] This finding probably represents regions of rapid pleural adhesion formation with intervening accumulations of

Table 29–1

Immunocytochemistry Markers

Reference	Test	Benign mesothelial	MM	General CA	Adeno CA	Other CA	Other Type
25	AFP					+ +	Hepatocellular
130	Alcian blue	0		+			
17	B 72.3		0	+ +	+ + +		
25	B-19					+ +	Prostate
118	BCA-225	0		+ +			
10,44,145,146,203	BER-EP4	0	0	+ +/+ + +	+ + +		
25	CA 15.3					+ + +	Breast
25	CA 19.9					+ + +	Gastric
29,39,97,98	Calretinin	+ + +	+ + +	0	0		
15	CD44 s	+ + +		–			
153	CD44 v 3-10	0		+			
10,25,31,130,201 98	CEA	0		+ + +	+ +	+ + +	Colorectal
39,66	Desmin	+ +/+ + +	0	0			
97,197	E-cadherin	0		+ + +	+ +		
130,201,203	EMA	–		+ + +	+ + +		
23	GLUT1	–		+ + +			
31,130	Keratin	0		+ + +	+	+ + +	
193	Ki67	0		+ +			
10	Leu MI				+ +		
25	MCA					+ +	Breast

(Continued)

Table 29–1

Immunocytochemistry Markers—cont'd

Reference	Test	Benign mesothelial	MM	General CA	Adeno CA	Other CA	Other Type
203	MCA-b-12	–		+ + +			
144	MOC31	0			+ + +		
98	Mucicarmine				+		
31	Mucin	0			+		
39	N-cadherin	+ +	+ + +	+			
133,147	p53	–/0		+			
184	UEA	0		+			

MM, malignant mesothelioma; General CA, nonspecific diagnosis of cancer; Adeno CA, specific diagnosis of adenocarcinoma; Other CA, specific diagnosis of certain, histological type; CEA, carcinoembryonic antigen; GLUT1, glucose transport protein; UEA, *Ulex eurapeaus* agglutinin.
Scale: + + +, >90%; + +, 60–90%; +, 30–59%; –, 10–29%; 0, <10%.

Table 29–2

Sensitivity and Specificity of Various Pleural Fluid Assays in the Detection of Malignancy

Reference	Assay	Sensitivity	Specificity
4	Ca 19-9	36	83
4,93,237	Ca 15.3	80–95	93
4,64	CEA	52	77
4	CYFRA 21-1	91	90
235	Ferritin ratio	94	96
156	MUC-1 >0.126	64	95.7
156	MUC-5AC >0.028	72	98
88	Sialic acid >0.075	68	77
105	Sialyl EA	64	95
153	TNF ratio	84	90
4	TSA	80	67

CEA, carcinoembryonic antigen; EA, embryonic; TNF, tumor necrosis factor; TSA, tumor-specific antigen.

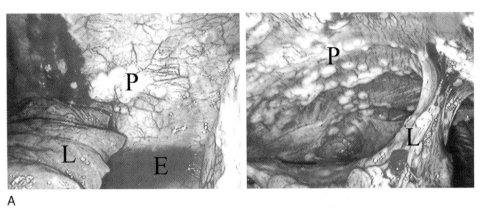

A

Figure 29–5 (**A**) Carcinoma parietal and visceral pleural implants with residual effusion are displayed. E, residual effusion; L, lung; P, parietal pleura. (**B**) Malignant mesothelioma—a characteristic "Grape clustering" pattern of pleural tumors. L, lung; P, parietal pleura.

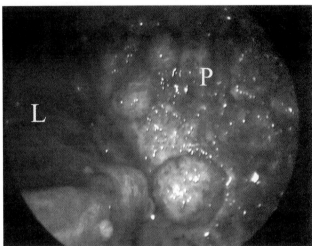

B

inflammatory fluid. This is probably an acceptable variation rather than a nonuniform distribution of sclerosing agent.

This imaging appearance generally resolves by 1–3 weeks; however, to avoid this phenomenon, some physicians wait for effusion drainage rates to decrease before instilling pleurodesis agents. It is not clear whether this practice is necessary. Long delays before pleurodesis may simply reduce the thoracic cavity area to which the instilled agent is exposed when significant pleural adhesions have already occurred in regions remote to the drainage catheter. Occasionally, significant pleural thickening or even fibrothoraxes occur as a long-term sequelae of pleurodesis. The use of thoracic ultrasound (Figure 29-4) can guide the optimal drainage site for small pleural effusions or the optimal point of entry of a thoracoscope to avoid adhesions.[121]

Drainage-Based Methods of Malignant Effusion Control

Serial thoracenteses appropriately control malignant pleural effusions for some patients. This option is not effective for durable effusion control but provides temporary symptomatic relief in cases with extremely poor prognoses. Thoracentesis is also ideal when alternate therapy should cause a major reduction in the patient's effusion. For example, a lymphoma-related effusion may resolve with chemotherapy.

Occasionally thoracentesis creates a hydropneumothorax because of poor compliance or entrapment of the ipsilateral lung. If the pneumothorax and dyspnea symptoms remain stable and noncompelling, tube thoracostomy should be avoided since pleural coaptation and effective ventilation from that lung are unlikely. Fluid will replace the air space over time.

Small Catheter Drainage

Implantation of a long-term pleural catheter or percutaneous medium-durability pleural catheter placement for continuous or intermittent drainage is better than serial percutaneous aspirations.[154] These methods have the advantage of obtaining near complete removal of the pleural fluid in the same way that a tube thoracostomy evacuates the pleural space. Needle aspiration rarely evacuates the fluid completely and rarely maintains the lung expansion long enough for a spontaneous pleurodesis to occur. Even without introduction of any pleural sclerosing agents, pleurodesis occurs simply by maintaining pleural apposition in a select group of patients probably from the underlying inflammation and invasive effects of the neoplasms.[176]

Using a small silicone catheter (Figure 29-6) with a valve that allows drainage only when connected to a closed system, about 50% success at 30 days has been achieved in prospective randomized clinical trials compared to traditional pleurodesis methods.[176]

This research was replicated with the Tenckoff, the pigtail catheter, and the Pleuracan device.[27,172,180,191] All controlled dyspnea in greater than 90% of the cases. Intermittent pleural drainage is an attractive option for patients in whom pleurodesis is less likely to occur because

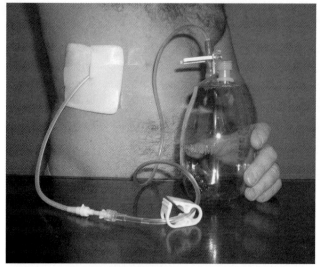

A

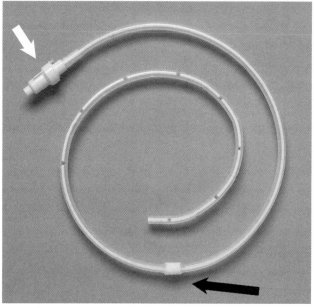

B

Figure 29–6 (**A**) Pleurx catheter. Patient connecting Pleurx catheter to bottle for self-drainage. (**B**) Close-up of Pleurx catheter. White arrow shows a one-way valve mechanism and black arrow shows Velcro cuff to provide tissue ingrowth.

of the inability of the visceral pleura to touch the parietal pleura. As a consequence, this type of methodology is often used in a complimentary fashion to sclerosis options at various centers.

Pleuroperitoneal Shunting

Another way to drain pleural fluid is to pump it into the peritoneal cavity using a device similar to that crafted to drain ascites into the venous system. This generally requires the patient to pump the shunt chamber (Figure 29-7) at least 20 times four times a day and perhaps more because of the need to overcome the negative intrapleural pressure.[32]

Over 80% of patients reported excellent results with this method, and it avoided the need for an appliance to traverse the skin.[114] Unfortunately with this technology, at least 10–20% of the patients will occlude their shunt possibly requiring revision; furthermore, determination of shunt obstruction may be difficult.[170,211] Otherwise, this shunt appears to have survival rates similar to talc pleurodesis.[170] Also, there is generally no evidence of peritoneal deposits resulting from this pleuroperitoneal shunting technology.[65] The decision to use the shunt can be made during thoracoscopy when pleural coaptation seems unlikely and it is also relatively easy to place the shunt while the patient is under general anesthesia.[198]

Sclerosis-Based Pleural Effusion Management

Generally, accelerating the process of pleurodesis (which might not occur by prolonged drainage alone) is done by accessing the pleural space, draining the majority of fluid, and then inserting a substance that increases the inflammatory response and, thus, causes intense adhesions within the pleural envelope. There is controversy regarding how pleural fluid characteristics affect the success of pleurodesis or the prognosis of the patient. For instance, investigators have shown that a low pleural fluid glucose (<60 mg), low pH (<7.2), low performance status (Karnofsky <70), massive effusion, and high pleural LDH levels (>600 U/l) are associated with a higher rate of failure with pleurodesis efforts. These values also predict positive pleural fluid cytology and a poor overall prognosis.[82,127,192,194] However, other investigators have contradicted this finding particularly with respect to pleural effusion pH.[2,22,77,78] Experimental evidence supports the concept that the inflammatory effect needed by some sclerosant agents is inhibited by steroid use, thereby decreasing the effectiveness of the pleurodesis.[67]

Rolling the patient into different positions after instilling the desired sclerosant is another common practice. This is unnecessary in patients with normal pleural spaces in whom aqueous sclerosing agents were used. Rapid intrapleural dispersion occurs in just one position as demonstrated by radiopharmaceutical labeling and nuclear medicine imaging.[116] However, when the pleural space is loculated or there is lack of full lung expansion, rolling may be useful. Sclerosing agents that are particulate, like talc slurry, might have more uniform distribution by rolling, but this has been disproved in one small prospective trial.[123] There also appears to be variations in the practice of pleurodesis with surgeons more likely to use an agent such as talc and other physicians using bleomycin or cycline-based drugs.[134]

Another practice that is controversial is the need for the pleural effusion drainage rate to taper off before instilling a sclerosing agent. This may be unnecessary. Investigators have shown that the daily amount of pleural fluid drainage is much less useful than having full pleural fluid evacuation and lung reexpansion on chest roentgenogram.[218]

A surrogate measurement of pleural coaptation (besides routine chest imaging) may better predict successful pleurodesis. This has been attempted by using elastance measurements of the pleural space.[103] High elastance indicates trapped lung and therefore a less likely favorable result. Pleurodesis appears to have only a minor adverse effect on respiratory function, although the studies on this are limited.[212]

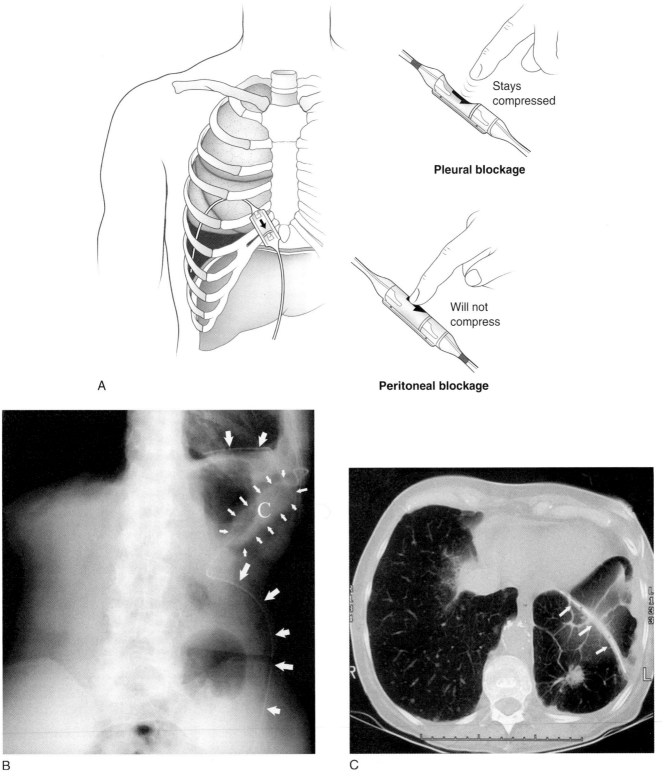

Figure 29–7 (**A**) Pleuroperitoneal shunt. Diagram showing shunt position and signs of proximal and distal obstruction. (Modified and reprinted with permission from the Ann Thorac Surg 51:605–609, 1991.) (**B**) Lower chest/upper abdomen roentgenogram showing left pleuroperitoneal shunt (*arrows*) with the chamber placed at the costal margin for patient self-pumping. C, Chamber. (**C**) CT image that shows the catheter in the left lower pleural space. This is a CT image 3 months after shunt placement in the same patient whose left lower lung loculated pleural breast carcinoma effusion is depicted in Figure 29-2B.

Finally, whereas sclerosis of the pleural cavity is generally practiced on inpatients, there have been successful outpatient pleurodesis programs.[167,190]

When pleurodesis is performed as an inpatient, a chest tube is generally inserted. There can be quite a significant variation in chest tube size ranging from 20 to 36 French depending on local institution or operator preference. Also, there appears to be considerable variation in sedation practices with occasional episodes of high discomfort and anxiety during the insertion of chest tubes.[119] Generally, patients with dyspnea from malignant effusions are not decompensated enough to require emergent placement without analgesic preparation. It is appropriate to establish a protocol to standardize intravenous sedative and analgesic use to supplement the generous use of local anesthetics during placement of a chest catheter.

There has been a trend toward the use of smaller catheters both for drainage and for the pleurodesis of malignant pleural effusions. In a prospective randomized study, a 12 French catheter was comparable to a standard large bore tube.[165] This has been reproduced in other studies using both inpatient and outpatient pleurodeses with the pigtail, Cystofix, Elecath, and PleuRx catheters and talc, doxycycline, or similar traditional sclerosing agents.[33,83,164,176,190]

Techniques of Sclerosis

Chemical Sclerosis—Talc

Talc was first used to create pleural adhesions in 1935 for tuberculosis management, and about 25 years later it started to become popular for controlling malignant effusions.[16] Generally, there are two ways to administer talc into the pleural space. One is in an insufflated powder (talc poudrage) and the other is instillation of particulate slurry with talc in a liquid vehicle. The dose of talc needed depends somewhat on the route of delivery and its preparation method. A fine powder from an aerosol gives a broader distribution with less mass (Figure 29-8). Nevertheless, reported successful talc pleurodeses generally used between 2 and 8 g with a dose of 5 g being the most common used in multicenter trials.*

Talc is often prepared preferentially in the hospital pharmacy rather than purchasing it from expensive vendors. In fact, the cost compares favorably to most other agents ($12.36 compared to bleomycin, $955.83, for example).[236] The use of purified but not sterilized talc may be acceptable

---

*References 1, 37, 174, 181, 207, 224.

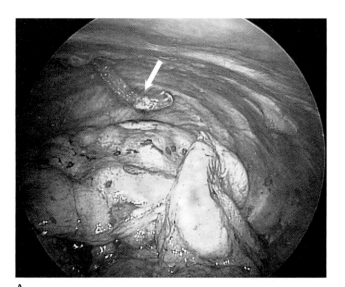

A

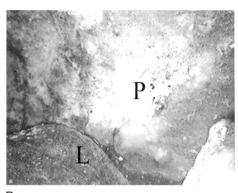

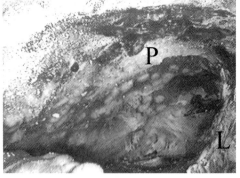

B

Figure 29–8 (**A**) Thoracoscopic image of left chest before insufflation of talc. Angled tip on insufflation catheter facilitates directing talc to desired areas. (**B**) Thoracoscopic image of left chest (from Figure 29-5A) after insufflation of talc. L, lung; P, Parietal pleura.

because a tremendous inflammatory response kills contaminating bacteria.[225] Nevertheless, the standard, preferred practice is to use talc sterilized by prolonged baking at 132° C, ethylene oxide sterilization (talc in cellophane pouches), or gamma radiation.[96]

Although the use of talc for malignant pleural effusions has become widespread and is considered a safe clinical practice, some patients sustain an inflammatory response severe enough to cause respiratory insufficiency. Such responses have prompted experts to question its use.[111] Clinical outcomes and laboratory testing show that talc administered intrapleurally is distributed systemically. The extent that this might adversely affect somewhat frail patients who receive it is unclear. Some investigators have suggested that the patient should be observed as inpatient for up to 72 h after its use.[178] Talc causes mesothelial denuding and an exudative neutrophilic pleural effusion similar to what occurs with the tetracycline class of sclerosis agents. In these studies, talc was found outside the pleural space in 20–40% of the animals studied.[95] For some tumors, such as mesothelioma, talc may also induce apoptosis.[148] On the other hand, if there is evidence of increased fibrinolytic activity then talc sclerosis may be less effective.[183]

Table 29-3 lists good to excellent results of talc and other sclerosant agents in noncomparative studies. Hospital stays ranged from 3.3 to 4.4 days.[1,2,37] Associated mortality ranges from 0 to 16% and morbidity ranges between 4 and 14% with respiratory complications being most frequent.°

When talc is tested in comparison trials (Table 29-4), the results are not as favorable but still are equal or superior to other common pleurodesis methods. Most of these investigations had good risk profiles with complications rates less than 20% and mortality attributed to the talc less than 5%. Yet there are unusual but disturbing reports with complication rates exceeding 50% of the procedures.[21]

Are the differences in results dependent on the patient population or, perhaps, the method or composition of the talcum powder used? Particle size might affect dissemination.[57] At least 20% of the patients who receive talc pleurodesis will have a transient interstitial haziness occur on the chest roentgenogram possibly from endothelial damage and capillary leak syndrome.[196] Talc slurry was thought to be a more risky delivery route because there seemed to be more anecdotal reports of respiratory distress associated with this method. Some investigators feel that intraoperative talc leads to shorter hospital stays.[52] A recently completed prospective study has not shown a significant difference between talc poudrage administered in the operating room compared to bedside talc slurry based on 30-day prevention of an effusion.[48]

Chemical Sclerosis—Cycline Drugs and Bleomycin

Multiple doses of chemical sclerosants have been studied, but a single dose is probably sufficient. A dose of tetracycline at 20 mg/kg was found to be effective as a single dose regimen.[104] Now doxycycline is available for clinical use rather than tetracycline. A dose of doxycycline is typically 500 mg in 100–200 ml of 0.9% saline.[179] Although there has been interest in using cycline-based drugs intraoperatively,

Table 29–3

Nonrandomized Trials of Common Sclerosant Agents

Agent/reference	N	Success[a] (%)
Talc poudrage		
38	40	90
1	42	82
155[b]	44	96
37[b]	24	88
194	125	87
233	69	94
11	213	93
2	25	88
183	52	81
216	360	90
227	360	85
123	20	85
Talc slurry		
207	15	81
95	58	81
174	31	82
225	34	100
Bleomycin		
163	38	63
18	20	85
159	200	62
68	21	71
167	19	79
Cyclines		
71	25	59
179	21	88
79	31	65
175	31	100
Others		
Iodopovidone[157]	52	96
Vincristine[217]	15	80

[a]Percent success was defined by most investigators as complete or near complete control of pleural effusion at 30 days after pleurodesis based on both symptom control and repeat chest imaging.

[b]Two of the studies used 30-day symptomatic control without repeat imaging as primary end points. While 1 month was a uniform interval for assessing this end point, some investigators used longer follow-up and studies also differed on whether early deaths were considered failures.

there is no advantage to this over bedside use.[53] Results of noncomparison studies with tetracycline and bleomycin are presented in Table 29-3.

Bleomycin, in general, shows results that are equivalent or just less than that of talc pleurodesis. A dose of 1 U/kg has been reported while a maximum dose of 60 U has been suggested.[159] Pleural effusions from breast tumors may respond better than that of other tumors to this drug. Many times these drugs may work better in the pleural cavity than in other spaces such as the peritoneal cavity.

458

Table 29–4

Randomized Trials of Common Sclerosant Agents: Percent Success[a]

Reference	N	Talc slurry	Talc poudrage	Bleomycin	Tetracycline	Other	Other compound name
48	469[b]	70	79				
151	26	79		75			
158	18	89		70			
236	35	90		79			
56	33	92			48		
76	134		97	64	33		
45	36		87	59			
126	62			64	52		
187	115[b]			64	33		
49	60			25	35	70	Bleomycin and tetracycline
166	106			72		79	Doxycycline
160	38			74		43	*Corynebacterium parvum*
81	32			13		65	*Corynebacterium parvum*
99	40			50		80	Mepacrine
117	40				80	60	Methenamine
12	18				83	90	Quinacrine
235	22				69	11	Nothing

[a]Percent success was defined typically as complete or near complete control of pleural effusion at 30 days after pleurodesis based on symptom control and repeat chest imaging.

[b]Multicenter trial.

Pain and transient fever occurred in 5% of patients after intrapleural instillation in a multicenter trial.[159] In other studies the fever can occur in as high as 60% of patients. It is unclear why there is so much variation in the reporting of these side effects.

Reports of pleural sclerosis need to be compared based on how long the treatment effects are followed. One investigation found 70% long-term success with combined bleomycin and tetracycline. Although a favorable early result was found with either agent, after 4 months the single sclerosant success fell to 25–35%.[49]

Other Sclerosing Compounds

Other compounds have been used including three doses of *Corynebacterium parvum* (7 mg in 20 ml saline). Good results (76–100% success) were obtained, but this drug is no longer available.* Intrapleural interferon-β 5–20 million units (maximum of three administrations) can be used alone but there is only a 30% remission rate.[185] Yet, when it is cycled with immunotherapy such as interleukin-2 and interferon-α and -β, a 56–70% response rate occurs.[69,113] Tumor necrosis factor therapy yielded an 87% recurrence-free rate at 4 weeks with a dose of 0.15–1.01 mg/patient. These patients have flu-like symptoms including fevers, chills, and fatigue.[177]

Radiopharmaceutical Interventions

Radioactive compounds were employed in the 1960s to control malignant pleural effusions but have seen renewed interest. The most commonly used is an intracavitary colloidal suspension of chromic phosphate (^{32}P) because of its safer emission and faster decay than elements like gold. Results of these therapies in uncontrolled trials have 75% success rates.[90] Generally, a dose of 6–12 mCi of ^{32}P is used and has a half-life of 14 days.[91] A therapeutic thoracentesis (maximal drainage) is performed using a temporary thoracentesis catheter. The catheter remains in place until the ^{32}P is instilled. It is then flushed and withdrawn. The patient may then be discharged provided that there are no complications.

Mechanical Abrasion or Laser

Limited data exist regarding the use of mechanical pleural abrasion that is effective for other types of pleural disease such as pneumothorax. Experimental data suggest that the mechanical abrasions are no better than the addition of sclerosing agents such as talc.[36,92] Similarly, laser treatments that cause superficial pleural destruction are probably not as effective in controlling effusions. Both are inhibited by their erratic effects in poorly healing neoplastic tissue.

Pleurectomy

The poor prognoses of patients with malignant pleural effusions limit enthusiasm for aggressive surgical options given the anticipated recovery times for such operations.[14] However, the less invasive therapies noted above are employed when thoracoscopy is needed to achieve a directed diagnosis of the pleural pathology. The use of thoracotomy and pleurectomy is accepted more for patients with malignant mesothelioma in whom early mortality from distant metastases is less certain.[202] The mortality rate for pleurectomy of malignant effusions is at least 12%.[61] Patients were considered for pleurectomy if they failed traditional drainage and sclerosing agents, had trapped lung, or were diagnosed as having malignant pleural effusion or pleural carcinomatosis at the time of thoracotomy. Nevertheless, these indications are now unusual outside a clinical trial.[128] To reduce the concern regarding thoracotomy morbidity, there is interest in VATS pleurectomy (Figure 29-9), which results in a shorter hospital stay and good effusion control.[221] In a series of VATS pleurectomy patients, there was 0% mortality with a mean hospital stay of 5 days. Six of 19 patients died within 12 months and of the remaining 13 patients, 2 developed recurrent effusions.[221]

▶ PROGNOSIS AND FUTURE TRENDS

The prognoses of patients with malignant effusions vary between clinical settings because of population variations in primary cell types and regional preferences in therapies used to control effusions. A survival less than 50% at 6 months and 6% at 2 years after malignant pleural effusion diagnosis is typical.[75,89,214,224,233] Also in these series, patients treated only by serial thoracenteses rather than more aggressive therapies had a particularly short survival (13.9 weeks). Alternatively, a longer interval between the initial diagnosis of cancer and the malignant effusion favors survival.

Breast cancer effusions are associated with a more favorable survival, particularly when estrogen receptor positive and the cells show a morula clustering pattern on cytology.[46,227] The presence of large clusters of malignant cells on smears also has a favorable prognosis in other cancers.[229] Unfavorable tumor surface receptors adversely affects prognosis (see the section on immunocytochemistry).

Like other treatment modalities, patient performance status is an important factor in determining optimal therapy. A Karnovsky score ≥70 is preferred prior to more aggressive

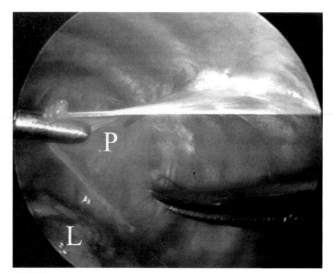

Figure 29–9 A VATS image of parietal pleurectomy is displayed. L, lung; P, parietal pleural peel.

---

*References 24, 55, 59, 136, 139, 160.

surgical approaches like thoracoscopy that require general anesthesia. This yields a survival, which makes the morbidity risk tenable.[22]

Occasionally, trivial malignant effusions are discovered with minimal nearby carcinomatous pleuritis at the time of thoracotomy. If there is only a small primary tumor with little other regional disease, it may be reasonable to perform a formal resection if the patient has good pulmonary function.[63,84] Although controversial, the logic for this follows from the finding that occult pleural metastases by pleural washings may have prolonged survival or cure.[50] Accordingly, for patients with minimal pleural carcinomatosis and N0 tumors, there is interest in performing ablative therapy of the pleura to improve cancer control and possibly affect cure. One of these treatments has been the use of pleurectomy and intracavitary photodynamic therapy, which has been used for mesothelioma but may also be useful for primary lung cancer.[60,206]

Hyperthermic chemotherapy and hypotonic chemotherapy are other investigational methods of effusion control.[85,132] Thrombolytic agents may disrupt loculations for more effective pleurodesis or pleural ablation therapy.[40] Transfer of lymphokine-activated killer cells improved tumor lysis in the pleural space while intrapleural interleukin-2 induced a 37% complete response in a multiinstitutional study possibly by restoring the immunocompetence of effusion-associated lymphocytes.[28,107,208,232] Cytokine therapy, particularly the use of vascular endothelial growth factor receptor blocker, can control some pleural effusions.[215,231] In related research, indomethacin blocks prostanoid-related endothelial cell permeability associated with adenocarcinomas.[168] Intrapleural steroids, however, do not slow effusion reaccumulation.[152]

Finally, intrapleural chemotherapy can control effusions without pleurodesis, per se. Mixed results have occurred with agents such as cisplatin and cytarabine, and doxorubicin.[131,143,188] One of the trials by the Lung Cancer Study Group showed a combined complete and partial response at 3 weeks of 49%.[188] Vincristine and paclitaxel as intrapleural therapy yielded an overall response rate of 80% and 93%, respectively.[169,217] More commonly, systemic chemotherapy is administered and recent drugs used for this include gemcitabine and vinorelbine or combinations with cisplatin, ifosfamide, and irinotecan.[62,112]

Fusing of a sclerosing agent with a chemotherapy agent is another novel approach. A bioadhesion compound linked to adriamycin achieved a 100% response rate in 14 patients in a preliminary report.[205] Similarly, microspheres can deliver chemotherapy intrapleurally at high local concentrations with low systemic exposures.[86]

Diverse managements are offered for patients with malignant pleural effusions. Optimally, the treatment selected conforms to the patient's anticipated survival based on histological diagnosis, molecular markers, extent of metastatic disease, and other comorbidities. There is some promising research but the overall prognoses of these patients are limited and therapy should focus on improving quality of life. Accordingly, less invasive outpatient small catheter-based methods are replacing impatient therapies such as the traditional chest tube with talc slurry. A multicenter trial (CALGB 30102) has been designed to test chest tube talc slurry with intermittent small catheter drainage.

Because malignant pleural effusions are a common problem with considerable morbidity, future multicenter studies will help determine the optimal therapy for those patients so afflicted.

MALIGNANT PERICARDIAL EFFUSIONS

Pericardial effusion is the most common cardiac problem in malignant disease and is reported in 1.5 to 21% of cancer cases.[101] Moreover, nonmalignant conditions also cause pericardial effusions in cancer patients. Examples of these conditions are infection, uremia, congestive heart failure, hypothyroidism and autoimmune disorders. Radiation, drug-induced pericarditis and idiopathic pericarditis are also known etiologies.

The most common malignancies to involve the pericardium are metastatic lung cancer, breast cancer, leukemia, lymphoma and melanoma. Less commonly, secondary involvement by esophageal, gastric, colonic, oral, nasopharyngeal, prostrate and ovarian carcinoma may be seen. Primary tumors of the pericardium are rare and include mesothelioma, fibrosarcoma, angiosarcoma and malignant teratoma.

MECHANISM

Tumors spread to the pericardium by direct extension or by hematogenous or lymphatic spread. Mediastinal lymph node metastases subsequently spread to the pericardium by retrograde movement through lymphatic vessels draining that space. Increased visceral pericardial fluid production may result from direct involvement of the serosal surface by tumor.[124] Flow obstructions by tumor increases lymphatic and venous hydrostatic pressure also driving pericardial fluid accumulation. The hemodynamic consequences of a pericardial effusion depend on its rate of accumulation and the pericardial compliance. Thus, large effusions may cause no symptoms if they accumulate slowly within compliant pericardia.

EVALUATION

Frequent pericardial effusion symptoms are dyspnea, cough, and chest pain. Physical examination findings are tachycardia, pulsus paradoxus, diminished heart sounds, elevated jugular venous pressure, hypotension, and pulsus alternans. Pericardial tamponade is more likely after rapid accumulations of fluid and may be the initial clinical presentation of malignant pericardial disease.

The chest radiograph often shows an enlarged cardiac silhouette, mediastinal widening, or hilar densities. Alternatively, a normal plain radiograph does not exclude pericardial effusion. Electrocardiographic effusion criteria are sinus tachycardia, nonspecific ST segment or T wave changes, low voltage tracings, and electrical alternans.

Echocardiography is very sensitive in detecting the presence of fluid and has become the most useful diagnostic tool for pericardial effusions (Figure 29-10). Right atrial or right ventricular compression with decreased left ventricular dimension and failure of the inferior vena cava to collapse

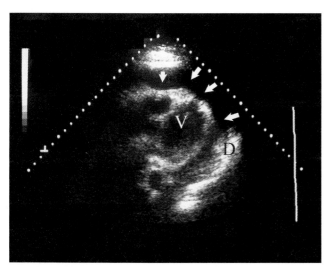

Figure 29–10 Echocardiogram showing a large pericardial effusion (*arrows*). D, diaphragmatic pericardium; V, ventricle.

on deep inspiration suggests hemodynamic compromise.[58] The echocardiogram also guides pericardiocentesis and/or drainage catheter placement safely. Cytological examination of the pericardial fluid may then be performed. The rate of positive cytological results reported in published series ranges from 57% to 100% among patients with malignancy.[124] Both CT and MRI provide excellent anatomical detail of the pericardial space but do not yield physiological or functional information (Figure 29-11).

TREATMENT

Various therapeutic interventions are used alone or in combination for patients with malignant pericardial effusions. One of the main objectives is obliteration of any potential pericardial space by fusion of the epicardium and pericardium.[204] Patient performance status, medical comorbidities, malignant disease stage, prognosis, and response to other cancer treatments influence selections of these options.

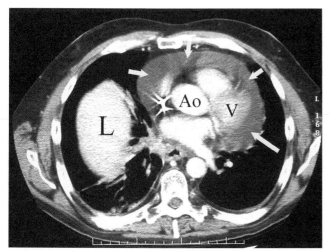

Figure 29–11 CT scan showing moderately large pericardial effusion (*arrows*). Ao, aortic root; L, liver dome (right); V, atrioventricular junction with adjacent pulmonary outflow tract.

Pericardiocentesis provides immediate decompression of the pericardial space and is usually performed with echocardiographic guidance. Hemodynamic impairment is thereby relieved but can recur quickly. Recurrence rates as high as 25% have been reported.[213] Thus, this procedure is seldom durable enough except for terminal patients with brief anticipated survival.

A pericardial catheter left in place at the time of pericardiocentesis allows drainage of additional fluid with or without administration of a sclerosing agent. Numerous investigators induced pericardial sclerosis to avoid pericardial effusion recurrences and described their small series.* Some of the agents administered were thiotepa, tetracyclines, OK-432 (an immunomodulator), bleomycin, aclarubicin, 5-fluorouracil, and radiocolloids such as ^{32}P and ^{154}Au. Doxycycline may produce intense pain and, as with bleomycin, may produce a febrile response in a significant number of patients.[67] Thiotepa does not cause pain and rarely evokes a fever. It is inexpensive and is the sclerosant of choice at some centers because of these advantages. Intrapericardial sclerosis has an overall success rate over 80%.[213] A few centers use intrapericardial radiocolloids but their popularity is limited in part because of logistic problems related to their administration. Intrapericardial interferon has also been used.[228] It reportedly enhances cell-mediated cytotoxicity and has an antiproliferative effect. Colchicine has also been described to have an inhibitory effect on leukocyte chemotaxis and decreases the production of interleukin-1 by monocytes.[9] These effects have been exploited in the use of colchicine in the treatment of refractory malignant pericardial effusion. The minimally invasive nature of these catheter-based interventions is attractive and reduces the recurrence rate after simple pericardiocentesis to an acceptable level. When less invasive options fail, surgical treatment can still be offered to appropriate candidates.

Of the surgical options, subxiphoid pericardial "window" creation has been utilized most extensively (Figure 29-12). It can be performed using local or general anesthesia with low complication rates and does not require single lung ventilation like some thoracoscopic methods. Success rates over 90% have been reported.[213] Much of the pericardial fluid drainage occurs in the space posterior to the ascending aorta through abundant carinal lymphatic systems. A relatively small tumor burden in that space (which is not visible to surgeons performing subxiphoid pericardial windows) may create an effusion. This accounts for some pericardial window specimens that do not show malignancy by pathological review.

Thoracotomy may be used to either create a pleuropericardial window or perform pericardiectomy. The latter has been claimed to have the greatest durability of all the surgical procedures. However, it does require general anesthesia and optimal single lung ventilation, and has relatively high morbidity and mortality rates.

Thoracoscopic approaches aim to provide the same quality of pericardial drainage without the morbidity of a thoracotomy.[115,122] This has been well tolerated in very ill patients but still requires single lung ventilation and general anesthesia. When both pleural and pericardial effusions are present, a thoracoscopic approach should be favored (Figure 29-13). This permits treatment of both spaces. Also,

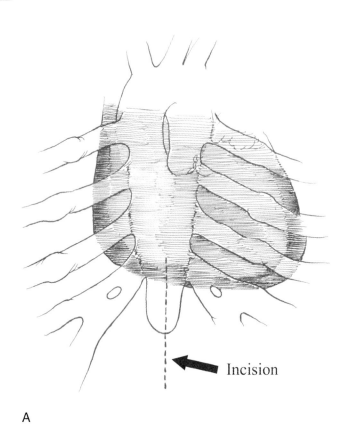

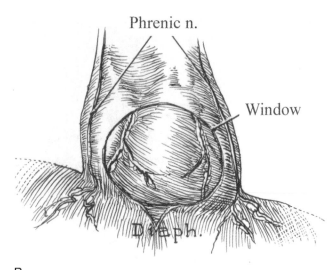

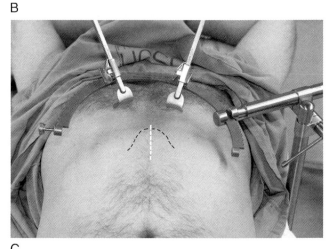

Figure 29–12 (**A**) Relation of pericardial effusion to planned subxiphoid incision. (**B**) *Large* pericardial window has been resected. Exposure for this can be facilitated by partial excision of the subxiphoid cartilage. Drainage may be facilitated by placement of a drainage tube, opening of the pleural spaces, or preperitoneal space depending on surgeons preference. (**C**) Exposure can also be facilitated by a self-retaining retractor system that lifts the costal margin and sternum anteriorly to expose the superior pericardium. The model is positioned under a partial ring of Bookwalter retractor system with small blades that provide this traction. Black lines show the costal margin and the white line overlies the xiphoid process denoting the planned incision.
(**A, B:** *Reprinted with permission from Ravitch M, Steichen F: Atlas of General Thoracic Surgery, p. 175.*)

excellent visualization of the thoracic cavity permits directed biopsies in undiagnosed cases.

Percutaneous balloon pericardial window creation has been reported.[161,222,238] Complications included pleural effusions requiring drainage, transient fever, and small pneumothoraces. This was performed with patients under local anesthesia and usually permitted prompt hospital discharge.

The Denver pleuroperitoneal shunt has also been used to drain pericardial effusions into the peritoneal space.[223] This requires only local anesthesia and a short hospital stay. The patients need to compress the pumping chamber of the device several times daily. Possible shortcomings of this drainage method include lack of patient cooperation and shunt thrombosis.

Passive pericardioperitoneal shunting can be accomplished using a video-assisted technique.[141] This essentially involves a laparoscopic approach to creating a generous transdiaphragmatic pericardial window without an external drain.

Chemotherapy and radiation therapy can be quite effective in patients with neoplasms that are sensitive to these modalities. They can be used in conjunction with direct pericardial interventions.

The choice of procedure is patient dependent and must be individualized. No modality is clearly superior to others, but the degree of invasiveness, morbidity, and cost vary widely. The clinical focus should be placed on providing rapid and durable relief from the effusion with the least possible morbidity.

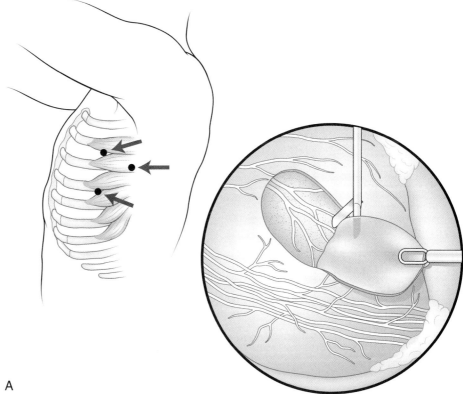

Figure 29–13 (**A**) Trocar positions for patient in preparation for thoracoscopic pericardial window. The patient is in a decubitus position. The camera trocar site lies most posteriorly. The remaining two sites are used for manipulating instruments. (**B**) Thoracoscopic image of left thoracoscopic pericardial window (left chest). H, heart; L, lung; P, pericardium. (*A Modified from Inderbitzi R, Furrer M, Leupi F: Pericardial biopsy and fenestration. Eur Heart J 14:135–137, 1993.*)

A

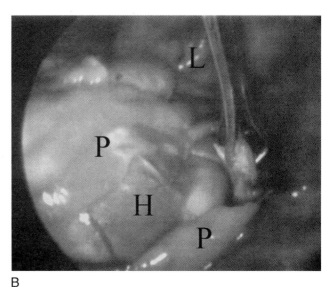

B

REFERENCES

1. Aelony Y, King R, Boutin C: Thoracoscopic talc poudrage pleurodesis for chronic recurrent pleural effusions. Ann Intern Med 115:778–782, 1991.
2. Aelony Y, King RR, Boutin C: Thoracoscopic talc poudrage in malignant pleural effusions: Effective pleurodesis despite low pleural pH. Chest 113:1007–1012, 1998.
3. Ahn MJ, Noh YH, Yoon HJ, et al: Detection of malignant cells in pleural fluid or ascites by CD44v8–10/CD44v10 competitive RT-PCR. Korean J Intern Med 16:30–35, 2001.
4. Alatas F, Alatas O, Metintas M, et al: Diagnostic value of CEA, CA 15-3, CA 19-9, CYFRA 21-1, NSE and TSA assay in pleural effusions. Lung Cancer 31:9–16, 2001.
5. Allen MS, Deschamps C, Jones DM, et al: Video-assisted thoracic surgical procedures: The Mayo experience. Mayo Clin Proc 71:351–359, 1996.
6. Anderson TM, Ray CW, Nwogu CE, et al: Pericardial catheter sclerosis versus surgical procedures for pericardial effusions in cancer patients. J Cardiovasc Surg (Torino) 42:415–419, 2001.
7. Ang P, Tan EH, Leong SS, et al: Primary intrathoracic malignant effusion: A descriptive study. Chest 120:50–54, 2001.
8. Arenas-Jimenez J, Alonso-Charterina S, Sanchez-Paya J, et al: Evaluation of CT findings for diagnosis of pleural effusions. Eur Radiol 10:681–690, 2000.
9. Austin EH, Flye MW: The treatment of recurrent malignant pleural effusion. Ann Thorac Surg 28:190–203, 1979.

10. Bailey ME, Brown RW, Mody DR, et al: Ber-EP4 for differentiating adenocarcinoma from reactive and neoplastic mesothelial cells in serous effusions. Comparison with carcinoembryonic antigen, B72.3 and Leu-M1. Acta Cytol 40:1212–1216, 1996.

11. Bal S, Hasan SS: Thoracoscopic management of malignant pleural effusion. Int Surg 78:324–327, 1993.

12. Bayly TC, Kisner DL, Sybert A, et al: Tetracycline and quinacrine in the control of malignant pleural effusions. A randomized trial. Cancer 41:1188–1192, 1978.

13. Belani CP, Ziskind AA, Dhawan M et al: Management of malignant pleural and pericardial effusions. In Aisner J, et al, editors: Comprehensive Textbook of Thoracic Oncology. Baltimore: Williams & Wilkins, 1996, pp. 880–905.

14. Bernard A, de Dompsure RB, Hagry O, et al: Early and late mortality after pleurodesis for malignant pleural effusion. Ann Thorac Surg 74:213–217, 2002.

15. Berner HS, Davidson B, Berner A, et al: Differential expression of CD44s and CD44v3-10 in adenocarcinoma cells and reactive mesothelial cells in effusions. Virchows Arch 436:330–335, 2000.

16. Bethune N: Pleural poudrage: A new technique for deliberate production of pleural adhesions as preliminary to lobectomy. J Thorac Cardiovasc Surg 4:251–261, 1935.

17. Betta PG, Pavesi M, Pastormerlo M, et al: Use of monoclonal antibody B72.3 as a marker of metastatic carcinoma cells in neoplastic effusions. Pathologica 83:99–104, 1991.

18. Bitran JD, Brown C, Desser RK, et al: Intracavitary bleomycin for the control of malignant effusions. J Surg Oncol 16:273–277, 1981.

19. Boutin C, Astoul P, Seitz B: The role of thoracoscopy in the evaluation and management of pleural effusions. Lung 168(Suppl): 1113–1121, 1990.

20. Boutin C, Viallat JR, Cargnino P, et al: Thoracoscopy in malignant pleural effusions. Am Rev Respir Dis 124: 588–592, 1981.

21. Brant A, Eaton T: Serious complications with talc slurry pleurodesis. Respirology 6:181–185, 2001.

22. Burrows CM, Mathews WC, Colt HG: Predicting survival in patients with recurrent symptomatic malignant pleural effusions: An assessment of the prognostic values of physiologic, morphologic, and quality of life measures of extent of disease. Chest 117:73–78, 2000.

23. Burstein DE, Reder I, Weiser K, et al: GLUT1 glucose transporter: A highly sensitive marker of malignancy in body cavity effusions. Mod Pathol 11:392–396, 1998.

24. Casali A, Gionfra T, Rinaldi M, et al: Treatment of malignant pleural effusions with intracavitary Corynebacterium parvum. Cancer 62:806–811, 1988.

25. Cascinu S, Del Ferro E, Barbanti I, et al: Tumor markers in the diagnosis of malignant serous effusions. Am J Clin Oncol 20:247–250, 1997.

26. Chen LM, Lazcano O, Katzmann JA, et al: The role of conventional cytology, immunocytochemistry, and flow cytometric DNA ploidy in the evaluation of body cavity fluids: A prospective study of 52 patients. Am J Clin Pathol 109:712–721, 1998.

27. Chen YM, Shih JF, Yang KY, et al: Usefulness of pig-tail catheter for palliative drainage of malignant pleural effusions in cancer patients. Support Care Cancer 8:423–426, 2000.

28. Chen YM, Yang WK, Ting CC, et al: Cross regulation by IL-10 and IL-2/IL-12 of the helper T cells and the cytolytic activity of lymphocytes from malignant effusions of lung cancer patients. Chest 112:960–966, 1997.

29. Chhieng DC, Yee H, Schaefer D, et al: Calretinin staining pattern aids in the differentiation of mesothelioma from adenocarcinoma in serous effusions. Cancer 90:194–200, 2000.

30. Chung CL, Chen YC, Chang SC: Effect of repeated thoracenteses on fluid characteristics, cytokines, and fibrinolytic activity in malignant pleural effusion. Chest 123:1188–1195, 2003.

31. Cibas ES, Corson JM, Pinkus GS: The distinction of adenocarcinoma from malignant mesothelioma in cell blocks of effusions: The role of routine mucin histochemistry and immunohistochemical assessment of carcinoembryonic antigen, keratin proteins, epithelial membrane antigen, and milk fat globule-derived antigen. Hum Pathol 18:67–74, 1987.

32. Cimochowski GE, Joyner LR, Fardin R, et al: Pleuroperitoneal shunting for recalcitrant pleural effusions. J Thorac Cardiovasc Surg 92:866–870, 1986.

33. Clementsen P, Evald T, Grode G, et al: Treatment of malignant pleural effusion: Pleurodesis using a small percutaneous catheter. A prospective randomized study. Respir Med 92:593–596, 1998.

34. Cohen RG, DeMeester TR, Lafontaine E: The pleura. In Sabiston DC, Spencer FC, editors: Surgery of the Chest. Philadelphia: W.B. Saunders, 1995, pp. 523–575.

35. Colt HG: Thoracoscopy. A prospective study of safety and outcome. Chest 108:324–329, 1995.

36. Colt HG, Russack V, Chiu Y, et al: A comparison of thoracoscopic talc insufflation, slurry, and mechanical abrasion pleurodesis. Chest 111:442–448, 1997.

37. Danby CA, Adebonojo SA, Moritz DM: Video-assisted talc pleurodesis for malignant pleural effusions utilizing local anesthesia and I.V. sedation. Chest 113:739–742, 1998.

38. Daniel TM, Tribble CG, Rodgers BM: Thoracoscopy and talc poudrage for pneumothoraces and effusions. Ann Thorac Surg 50:186–189, 1990.

39. Davidson B, Nielsen S, Christensen J, et al: The role of desmin and N-cadherin in effusion cytology: A comparative study using established markers of mesothelial and epithelial cells. Am J Surg Pathol 25:1405–1412, 2001.

40. Davies CW, Traill ZC, Gleeson FV, et al: Intrapleural streptokinase in the management of malignant multiloculated pleural effusions. Chest 115:729–733, 1999.

41. DeCamp MM Jr, Jaklitsch MT, Mentzer SJ, et al: The safety and versatility of video-thoracoscopy: A prospective analysis of 895 consecutive cases. J Am Coll Surg 181:113–120, 1995.

42. Decker D, Stratmann H, Springer W, et al: Benign and malignant cells in effusions: Diagnostic value of image DNA cytometry in comparison to cytological analysis. Pathol Res Pract 194:791–795, 1998.

43. DeGowin EL, DeGowin RL: The thorax and cardiovascular system. In DeGowin EL, DeGowin RL, editors: Bedside Diagnostic Examination. New York: Macmillan, 1981, pp. 229–471.

44. Delahaye M, van der HF, van der Kwast TH: Complementary value of five carcinoma markers for the diagnosis of malignant mesothelioma, adenocarcinoma metastasis, and reactive mesothelium in serous effusions. Diagn Cytopathol 17:115–120, 1997.

45. Diacon AH, Wyser C, Bolliger CT, et al: Prospective randomized comparison of thoracoscopic talc poudrage under local anesthesia versus bleomycin instillation for pleurodesis in malignant pleural effusions. Am J Respir Crit Care Med 162:1445–1449, 2000.

46. Dieterich M, Goodman SN, Rojas-Corona RR, et al: Multivariate analysis of prognostic features in malignant pleural effusions from breast cancer patients. Acta Cytol 38:945–952, 1994.

47. Dines DE, Pierre RV, Franzen SJ: The value of cells in the pleural fluid in the differential diagnosis. Mayo Clin Proc 50:571–572, 1975.

48. Dresler CM, Herndon J, Daniel TM, et al: Cancer and Leukemia Group B (CALGB) 9334: A phase III, intergroup

study of sclerosis of malignant pleural effusion by talc. Proceeding of ASCO, 2000, p. 2455 (abstract).

49. Emad A, Rezaian GR: Treatment of malignant pleural effusions with a combination of bleomycin and tetracycline. A comparison of bleomycin or tetracycline alone versus a combination of bleomycin and tetracycline. Cancer 78:2498–2501, 1996.

50. Emad A, Rezaian GR: Closed percutaneous pleural brushing: A new method for diagnosis of malignant pleural effusions. Respir Med 92:659–663, 1998.

51. Erasmus JJ, McAdams HP, Rossi SE, et al: FDG PET of pleural effusions in patients with non-small cell lung cancer. AJR Am J Roentgenol 175:245–249, 2000.

52. Erickson KV, Yost M, Bynoe R, et al: Primary treatment of malignant pleural effusions: Video-assisted thoracoscopic surgery poudrage versus tube thoracostomy. Am Surg 68:955–959, 2002.

53. Evans TR, Stein RC, Pepper JR, et al: A randomised prospective trial of surgical against medical tetracycline pleurodesis in the management of malignant pleural effusions secondary to breast cancer. Eur J Cancer 29A:316–319, 1993.

54. Falor WH, Ward RM, Brezler MR: Diagnosis of pleural effusions by chromosome analysis. Chest 81:193–197, 1982.

55. Felletti R, Ravazzoni C: Intrapleural Corynebacterium parvum for malignant pleural effusions. Thorax 38:22–24, 1983.

56. Fentiman IS, Rubens RD, Hayward JL: A comparison of intracavitary talc and tetracycline for the control of pleural effusions secondary to breast cancer. Eur J Cancer Clin Oncol 22:1079–1081, 1986.

57. Ferrer J, Montes JF, Villarino MA, et al: Influence of particle size on extrapleural talc dissemination after talc slurry pleurodesis. Chest 122:1018–1027, 2002.

58. Fiocco M, Krasna MJ: The management of malignant pleural and pericardial effusions. Hematol Oncol Clin North Am 11:253–265, 1997.

59. Foresti V: Intrapleural Corynebacterium parvum for recurrent malignant pleural effusions. Respiration 62:21–26, 1995.

60. Friedberg JS, Metz J, Mick R, et al: Multimodality treatment including pleural photodynamic therapy (PDT) for non-small cell lung cancer (NSCLC) patients with pleural carcinomatosis. Proceeding of ASCO, 2001.

61. Fry WA, Khandekar JD: Parietal pleurectomy for malignant pleural effusion. Ann Surg Oncol 2:160–164, 1995.

62. Fujita A, Takabatake H, Tagaki S, et al: Combination chemotherapy in patients with malignant pleural effusions from non-small cell lung cancer: Cisplatin, ifosfamide, and irinotecan with recombinant human granulocyte colony-stimulating factor support. Chest 119:340–343, 2001.

63. Fukuse T, Hirata T, Tanaka F, et al: The prognostic significance of malignant pleural effusion at the time of thoracotomy in patients with non-small cell lung cancer. Lung Cancer 34:75–81, 2001.

64. Garcia-Pachon E, Padilla-Navas I, Dosda MD, et al: Elevated level of carcinoembryonic antigen in nonmalignant pleural effusions. Chest 111:643–647, 1997.

65. Genc O, Petrou M, Ladas G, et al: The long-term morbidity of pleuroperitoneal shunts in the management of recurrent malignant effusions. Eur J Cardiothorac Surg 18:143–146, 2000.

66. Gill SA, Meier PA, Kendall BS: Use of desmin immunohistochemistry to distinguish between mesothelial cells and carcinoma in serous fluid cell block preparations. Acta Cytol 44:976–980, 2000.

67. Girardi LN, Ginsberg RJ, Burt ME: Pericardiocentesis and intrapericardial sclerosis: Effective therapy for malignant pericardial effusions. Ann Thorac Surg 64:1422–1427, 1997.

68. Goff BA, Mueller PR, Muntz HG, et al: Small chest-tube drainage followed by bleomycin sclerosis for malignant pleural effusions. Obstet Gynecol 81:993–996, 1993.

69. Goldman CA, Skinnider LF, Maksymiuk AW: Interferon instillation for malignant pleural effusions. Ann Oncol 4:141–145, 1993.

70. Good JT Jr, Taryle DA, Sahn SA: The pathogenesis of low glucose, low pH malignant effusions. Am Rev Respir Dis 131:737–741, 1985.

71. Gravelyn TR, Michelson MK, Gross BH, et al: Tetracycline pleurodesis for malignant pleural effusions. A 10-year retrospective study. Cancer 59:1973–1977, 1987.

72. Gupta NC, Rogers JS, Graeber GM, et al: Clinical role of F-18 fluorodeoxyglucose positron emission tomography imaging in patients with lung cancer and suspected malignant pleural effusion. Chest 122:1918–1924, 2002.

73. Hallman JR, Geisinger KR: Cytology of fluids from pleural, peritoneal and pericardial cavities in children. A comprehensive survey. Acta Cytol 38:209–217, 1994.

74. Hamm H, Brohan U, Bohmer R, et al: Cholesterol in pleural effusions. A diagnostic aid. Chest 92:296–302, 1987.

75. Harris RJ, Kavuru MS, Mehta AC, et al: The impact of thoracoscopy on the management of pleural disease. Chest 107:845–852, 1995.

76. Hartman DL, Gaither JM, Kesler KA, et al: Comparison of insufflated talc under thoracoscopic guidance with standard tetracycline and bleomycin pleurodesis for control of malignant pleural effusions. J Thorac Cardiovasc Surg 105:743–747, 1993.

77. Heffner JE, Nietert PJ, Barbieri C: Pleural fluid pH as a predictor of pleurodesis failure: Analysis of primary data. Chest 117:87–95, 2000.

78. Heffner JE, Nietert PJ, Barbieri C: Pleural fluid pH as a predictor of survival for patients with malignant pleural effusions. Chest 117:79–86, 2000.

79. Heffner JE, Standerfer RJ, Torstveit J, et al: Clinical efficacy of doxycycline for pleurodesis. Chest 105:1743–1747, 1994.

80. Hillerdal G, Dernevik L, Almgren SO, et al: Prognostic value of malignant cells in pleural lavage at thoracotomy for bronchial carcinoma. Lung Cancer 21:47–52, 1998.

81. Hillerdal G, Kiviloog J, Nou E, et al: Corynebacterium parvum in malignant pleural effusion. A randomized prospective study. Eur J Respir Dis 69:204–206, 1986.

82. Houston MC: Pleural fluid pH: Diagnostic, therapeutic, and prognostic value. Am J Surg 154:333–337, 1987.

83. Hsu WH, Chiang CD, Chen CY, et al: Ultrasound-guided small-bore elecath tube insertion for the rapid sclerotherapy of malignant pleural effusion. Jpn J Clin Oncol 28:187–191, 1998.

84. Ichinose Y, Tsuchiya R, Koike T, et al: Prognosis of resected non-small cell lung cancer patients with carcinomatous pleuritis of minimal disease. Lung Cancer 32:55–60, 2001.

85. Ichinose Y, Yano T, Asoh H, et al: Intraoperative intrapleural hypotonic cisplatin treatment for carcinomatous pleuritis. J Surg Oncol 66:196–200, 1997.

86. Ike O, Shimizu Y, Hitomi S, et al: Treatment of malignant pleural effusions with doxorubicin hydrochloride-containing poly(L-lactic acid) microspheres. Chest 99:911–915, 1991.

87. Imamura T, Tamura K, Takenaga M, et al: Intrapericardial OK-432 instillation for the management of malignant pericardial effusion. Cancer 68:259–263, 1991.

88. Imecik O, Ozer F: Diagnostic value of sialic acid in malignant pleural effusions. Chest 102:1819–1822, 1992.

89. Irani DR, Underwood RD, Johnson EH, et al: Malignant pleural effusions. A clinical cytopathologic study. Arch Intern Med 147:1133–1136, 1987.

90. Izbicki R, Weyhing BT, III, Baker L, et al: Pleural effusion in cancer patients. A prospective randomized study of pleural drainage with the addition of radioactive phsophorous to the pleural space vs. pleural drainage alone. Cancer 36:1511–1518, 1975.

91. Jackson GL, Blosser NM: Intracavitary chromic phosphate (32P) colloidal suspension therapy. Cancer 48:2596–2598, 1981.

92. Jensen MO, Matthees DJ, Antonenko D: Laser thoracoscopy for pleural effusion. Am Surg 58:667–669, 1992.

93. Kandylis K, Vassilomanolakis M, Baziotis N, et al: Diagnostic significance of the tumour markers CEA, CA 15-3 and CA 125 in malignant effusions in breast cancer. Ann Oncol 1:435–438, 1990.

94. Kawashima O, Kurihara T, Kamiyoshihara M, et al: Management of malignant pericardial effusion resulting from recurrent cancer with local instillation of aclarubicin hydrochloride. Am J Clin Oncol 22:396–398, 1999.

95. Kennedy L, Rusch VW, Strange C, et al: Pleurodesis using talc slurry. Chest 106:342–346, 1994.

96. Kennedy L, Vaughan LM, Steed LL, et al: Sterilization of talc for pleurodesis. Available techniques, efficacy, and cost analysis. Chest 107:1032–1034, 1995.

97. Kitazume H, Kitamura K, Mukai K, et al: Cytologic differential diagnosis among reactive mesothelial cells, malignant mesothelioma, and adenocarcinoma: Utility of combined E-cadherin and calretinin immunostaining. Cancer 90:55–60, 2000.

98. Ko EC, Jhala NC, Shultz JJ, et al: Use of a panel of markers in the differential diagnosis of adenocarcinoma and reactive mesothelial cells in fluid cytology. Am J Clin Pathol 116:709–715, 2001.

99. Koldsland S, Svennevig JL, Lehne G, et al: Chemical pleurodesis in malignant pleural effusions: A randomised prospective study of mepacrine versus bleomycin. Thorax 48:790–793, 1993.

100. Kosuda S, Yokoyama K, Nishiguchi I, et al: Bone scanning in patients with pleural effusion—experience in 76 cases. Ann Nucl Med 4:55–58, 1990.

101. Kralstein J, Frishman WH: Malignant pericardial diseases: Diagnosis and treatment. Cardiol Clin 5:583–589, 1987.

102. Lai CL, Tsai CM, Tsai TT, et al: Presence of serum anti-P53 antibodies is associated with pleural effusion and poor prognosis in lung cancer patients. Clin Cancer Res 4:3025–3030, 1998.

103. Lan RS, Lo SK, Chuang ML, et al: Elastance of the pleural space: A predictor for the outcome of pleurodesis in patients with malignant pleural effusion. Ann Intern Med 126:768–774, 1997.

104. Landvater L, Hix WR, Mills M, et al: Malignant pleural effusion treated by tetracycline sclerotherapy. A comparison of single vs repeated instillation. Chest 93:1196–1198, 1988.

105. Lee YC, Chern JH, Lai SL, et al: Sialyl stage-specific embryonic antigen-1: A useful marker for differentiating the etiology of pleural effusion. Chest 114:1542–1545, 1998.

106. Levine MN, Young JE, Ryan ED, et al: Pleural effusion in breast cancer. Thoracoscopy for hormone receptor determination. Cancer 57:324–327, 1986.

107. Li DJ, Wang YR, Tan XY, et al: A new approach to the treatment of malignant effusion. Chin Med J (Engl) 103:998–1002, 1990.

108. Light RW: Pleural effusions. Med Clin North Am 61:1339–1352, 1977.

109. Light RW: Tumors of the pleura. In Murray JF, Nadel JA, editors: Textbook of Respiratory Medicine. Philadelphia: W.B. Saunders, 1988, pp. 1770–1780.

110. Light RW: Pleural diseases. Dis Mon 38:261–331, 1992.

111. Light RW: Talc should not be used for pleurodesis. Am J Respir Crit Care Med 162:2024–2026, 2000.

112. Lilenbaum R, Cano R, Schwartz M, et al: Gemcitabine and vinorelbine in advanced nonsmall cell lung carcinoma: A phase II study. Cancer 88:557–562, 2000.

113. Lissoni P, Barni S, Tancini G, et al: Intracavitary therapy of neoplastic effusions with cytokines: Comparison among interferon alpha, beta and interleukin-2. Support Care Cancer 3:78–80, 1995.

114. Little AG, Kadowaki MH, Ferguson MK, et al: Pleuro-peritoneal shunting. Alternative therapy for pleural effusions. Ann Surg 208:443–450, 1988.

115. Liu HP, Chang CH, Lin PJ, et al: Thoracoscopic management of effusive pericardial disease: Indications and technique. Ann Thorac Surg 58:1695–1697, 1994.

116. Lorch DG, Gordon L, Wooten S, et al: Effect of patient positioning on distribution of tetracycline in the pleural space during pleurodesis. Chest 93:527–529, 1988.

117. Loutsidis A, Bellenis I, Argiriou M, et al: Tetracycline compared with mechlorethamine in the treatment of malignant pleural effusions. A randomized trial. Respir Med 88:523–526, 1994.

118. Loy TS, Diaz-Arias AA, Bickel JT: Value of BCA-225 in the cytologic diagnosis of malignant effusions: An immunocytochemical study of 197 cases. Mod Pathol 3:294–297, 1990.

119. Luketich JD, Kiss M, Hershey J, et al: Chest tube insertion: A prospective evaluation of pain management. Clin J Pain 14:152–154, 1998.

120. Lynch TJ Jr: Management of malignant pleural effusions. Chest 103:385S–389S, 1993.

121. Macha HN, Reichle G, von Zwehl D, et al: The role of ultrasound assisted thoracoscopy in the diagnosis of pleural disease. Clinical experience in 687 Cases. Eur J Cardiothorac Surg 7:19–22, 1993.

122. Mack M, Acuff T, Hazelrigg S, et al: Thoracoscopic approach for the pericardium. Endosc Surg Allied Technol 1:271–274, 1993.

123. Mager HJ, Maesen B, Verzijlbergen F, et al: Distribution of talc suspension during treatment of malignant pleural effusion with talc pleurodesis. Lung Cancer 36:77–81, 2002.

124. Maher EA, Shepherd FA, Todd TJ: Pericardial sclerosis as the primary management of malignant pericardial effusion and cardiac tamponade. J Thorac Cardiovasc Surg 112:637–643, 1996.

125. Marel M, Zrustova M, Stasny B, et al: The incidence of pleural effusion in a well-defined region. Epidemiologic study in central Bohemia. Chest 104:1486–1489, 1993.

126. Martinez-Moragon E, Aparicio J, Rogado MC, et al: Pleurodesis in malignant pleural effusions: A randomized study of tetracycline versus bleomycin. Eur Respir J 10:2380–2383, 1997.

127. Martinez-Moragon E, Aparicio J, Sanchis J, et al: Malignant pleural effusion: Prognostic factors for survival and response to chemical pleurodesis in a series of 120 cases. Respiration 65:108–113, 1998.

128. Martini N, Bains MS, Beattie EJ Jr: Indications for pleurectomy in malignant effusion. Cancer 35:734–738, 1975.

129. Martinoni A, Cipolla CM, Civelli M, et al: Intrapericardial treatment of neoplastic pericardial effusions. Herz 25:787–793, 2000.

130. Mason MR, Bedrossian CW, Fahey CA: Value of immunocytochemistry in the study of malignant effusions. Diagn Cytopathol 3:215–221, 1987.

131. Masuno T, Kishimoto S, Ogura T, et al: A comparative trial of LC9018 plus doxorubicin and doxorubicin alone for the treatment of malignant pleural effusion secondary to lung cancer. Cancer 68:1495–1500, 1991.

132. Matsuzaki Y, Shibata K, Yoshioka M, et al: Intrapleural perfusion hyperthermo-chemotherapy for malignant pleural dissemination and effusion. Ann Thorac Surg 59:127–131, 1995.

133. Mayall F, Heryet A, Manga D, et al: P53 immunostaining is a highly specific and moderately sensitive marker of malignancy in serous fluid cytology. Cytopathology 8:9–12, 1997.

134. McAlpine LG, Hulks G, Thomson NC: Management of recurrent malignant pleural effusion in the United Kingdom: Survey of clinical practice. Thorax 45:699–701, 1990.

135. McLean AN, Bicknell SR, McAlpine LG, et al: Investigation of pleural effusion: An evaluation of the new olympus LTF

135. semiflexible thoracofiberscope and comparison with Abram's needle biopsy. Chest 114:150–153, 1998.

136. McLeod DT, Calverley PM, Millar JW, et al: Further experience of Corynebacterium parvum in malignant pleural effusion. Thorax 40:515–518, 1985.

137. McLoud TC: CT and MR in pleural disease. Clin Chest Med 19:261–276, 1998.

138. McLoud TC, Isler R, Head J: The radiologic appearance of chemical pleurodesis. Radiology 135:313–317, 1980.

139. Millar JW, Hunter AM, Horne NW: Intrapleural immunotherapy with Corynebacterium parvum in recurrent malignant pleural effusions. Thorax 35:856–858, 1980.

140. Mohamed KH, Mobasher AA, Yousef AI, et al: Pleural lavage: A novel diagnostic approach for diagnosing exudative pleural effusion. Lung 178:371–379, 2000.

141. Molnar TF, Biki B, Horvath OP: Pericardioperitoneal shunt: Further development of the procedure using VATS technique. Ann Thorac Surg 74:593–595, 2002.

142. Momi H, Matsuyama W, Inoue K, et al: Vascular endothelial growth factor and proinflammatory cytokines in pleural effusions. Respir Med 96:817–822, 2002.

143. Monjanel-Mouterde S, Frenay C, Catalin J, et al: Pharmacokinetics of intrapleural cisplatin for the treatment of malignant pleural effusions. Oncol Rep 7:171–175, 2000.

144. Morgan RL, De Young BR, McGaughy VR, et al: MOC-31 aids in the differentiation between adenocarcinoma and reactive mesothelial cells. Cancer 87:390–394, 1999.

145. Motherby H, Friedrichs N, Kube M, et al: Immunocytochemistry and DNA-image cytometry in diagnostic effusion cytology. II. Diagnostic accuracy in equivocal smears. Anal Cell Pathol 19:59–66, 1999.

146. Motherby H, Kube M, Friedrichs N, et al: Immunocytochemistry and DNA-image cytometry in diagnostic effusion cytology I. Prevalence of markers in tumour cell positive and negative smears. Anal Cell Pathol 19:7–20, 1999.

147. Mullick SS, Green LK, Ramzy I, et al: P53 gene product in pleural effusions. Practical use in distinguishing benign from malignant cells. Acta Cytol 40:855–860, 1996.

148. Nasreen N, Mohammed KA, Dowling PA, et al: Talc induces apoptosis in human malignant mesothelioma cells in vitro. Am J Respir Crit Care Med 161:595–600, 2000.

149. Negus RA, Chachkes JS, Wrenn K: Tension hydrothorax and shock in a patient with a malignant pleural effusion. Am J Emerg Med 8:205–207, 1990.

150. Ning J, Liu S, Cheng S: [Numerical alteration of chromosome 8 in pleural effusions]. Zhonghua Zhong Liu Za Zhi 22:8–10, 2000.

151. Noppen M, Degreve J, Mignolet M, et al: A prospective, randomised study comparing the efficacy of talc slurry and bleomycin in the treatment of malignant pleural effusions. Acta Clin Belg 52:258–262, 1997.

152. North SA, Au HJ, Halls SB, et al: A randomized, phase III, double-blind, placebo-controlled trial of intrapleural instillation of methylprednisolone acetate in the management of malignant pleural effusion. Chest 123:822–827, 2003.

153. Odeh M, Sabo E, Srugo I, et al: Tumour necrosis factor alpha in the diagnostic assessment of pleural effusion. QJM 93:819–824, 2000.

154. Ohm C, Park D, Vogen M, et al: Use of an indwelling pleural catheter compared with thoracoscopic talc pleurodesis in the management of malignant pleural effusions. Am Surg 69:198–202, 2003.

155. Ohri SK, Oswal SK, Townsend ER, et al: Early and late outcome after diagnostic thoracoscopy and talc pleurodesis. Ann Thorac Surg 53:1038–1041, 1992.

156. Okamoto I, Morisaki T, Sasaki J, et al: Molecular detection of cancer cells by competitive reverse transcription-polymerase chain reaction analysis of specific CD44 variant RNAs. J Natl Cancer Inst 90:307–315, 1998.

157. Olivares-Torres CA, Laniado-Laborin R, Chavez-Garcia C, et al: Iodopovidone pleurodesis for recurrent pleural effusions. Chest 122:581–583, 2002.

158. Ong KC, Indumathi V, Raghuram J, et al: A comparative study of pleurodesis using talc slurry and bleomycin in the management of malignant pleural effusions. Respirology 5:99–103, 2000.

159. Ostrowski MJ, Halsall GM: Intracavitary bleomycin in the management of malignant effusions: A multicenter study. Cancer Treat Rep 66:1903–1907, 1982.

160. Ostrowski MJ, Priestman TJ, Houston RF, et al: A randomized trial of intracavitary bleomycin and Corynebacterium parvum in the control of malignant pleural effusions. Radiother Oncol 14:19–26, 1989.

161. Ovunc K, Aytemir K, Ozer N, et al: Percutaneous balloon pericardiotomy for patients with malignant pericardial effusion including three malignant pleural mesotheliomas. Angiology 52:323–329, 2001.

162. Page RD, Jeffrey RR, Donnelly RJ: Thoracoscopy: A review of 121 consecutive surgical procedures. Ann Thorac Surg 48:66–68, 1989.

163. Paladine W, Cunningham TJ, Sponzo R, et al: Intracavitary bleomycin in the management of malignant effusions. Cancer 38:1903–1908, 1976.

164. Parker LA, Charnock GC, Delany DJ: Small bore catheter drainage and sclerotherapy for malignant pleural effusions. Cancer 64:1218–1221, 1989.

165. Parulekar W, Di Primio G, Matzinger F, et al: Use of small-bore vs large-bore chest tubes for treatment of malignant pleural effusions. Chest 120:19–25, 2001.

166. Patz EF Jr, McAdams HP, Erasmus JJ, et al: Sclerotherapy for malignant pleural effusions: A prospective randomized trial of bleomycin vs doxycycline with small-bore catheter drainage. Chest 113:1305–1311, 1998.

167. Patz EF Jr, McAdams HP, Goodman PC, et al: Ambulatory sclerotherapy for malignant pleural effusions. Radiology 199:133–135, 1996.

168. Payne DK, Fuseler JW, Owens MW: Modulation of endothelial cell permeability by lung carcinoma cells: A potential mechanism of malignant pleural effusion formation. Inflammation 18:407–417, 1994.

169. Perng RP, Chen YM, Wu MF, et al: Phase II trial of intrapleural paclitaxel injection for non-small-cell lung cancer patients with malignant pleural effusions. Respir Med 92:473–479, 1998.

170. Petrou M, Kaplan D, Goldstraw P: Management of recurrent malignant pleural effusions. The complementary role talc pleurodesis and pleuroperitoneal shunting. Cancer 75:801–805, 1995.

171. Poe RH, Levy PC, Israel RH, et al: Use of fiberoptic bronchoscopy in the diagnosis of bronchogenic carcinoma. A study in patients with idiopathic pleural effusions. Chest 105:1663–1667, 1994.

172. Pollak JS, Burdge CM, Rosenblatt M, et al: Treatment of malignant pleural effusions with tunneled long-term drainage catheters. J Vasc Interv Radiol 12:201–208, 2001.

173. Prakash UB, Reiman HM: Comparison of needle biopsy with cytologic analysis for the evaluation of pleural effusion: Analysis of 414 cases. Mayo Clin Proc 60:158–164, 1985.

174. Prevost A, Costa B, Elamarti R, et al: Long-term effect and tolerance of talc slurry for control of malignant pleural effusions. Oncol Rep 8:1327–1331, 2001.

175. Pulsiripunya C, Youngchaiyud P, Pushpakom R, et al: The efficacy of doxycycline as a pleural sclerosing agent in malignant pleural effusion: A prospective study. Respirology 1:69–72, 1996.

176. Putnam JB Jr, Light RW, Rodriguez RM, et al: A randomized comparison of indwelling pleural catheter and doxycycline

468

pleurodesis in the management of malignant pleural effusions. Cancer 86:1992–1999, 1999.

177. Rauthe G, Sistermanns J: Recombinant tumour necrosis factor in the local therapy of malignant pleural effusion. Eur J Cancer 33:226–231, 1997.

178. Rinaldo JE, Owens GR, Rogers RM: Adult respiratory distress syndrome following intrapleural instillation of talc. J Thorac Cardiovasc Surg 85:523–526, 1983.

179. Robinson LA, Fleming WH, Galbraith TA: Intrapleural doxycycline control of malignant pleural effusions. Ann Thorac Surg 55:1115–1121, 1993.

180. Robinson RD, Fullerton DA, Albert JD, et al: Use of pleural Tenckhoff catheter to palliate malignant pleural effusion. Ann Thorac Surg 57:286–288, 1994.

181. Rodriguez-Panadero F: Talc pleurodesis for treating malignant pleural effusions. Chest 108:1178–1179, 1995.

182. Rodriguez-Panadero F, Lopez MJ: Low glucose and pH levels in malignant pleural effusions. Diagnostic significance and prognostic value in respect to pleurodesis. Am Rev Respir Dis 139:663–667, 1989.

183. Rodriguez-Panadero F, Segado A, Martin JJ, et al: Failure of talc pleurodesis is associated with increased pleural fibrinolysis. Am J Respir Crit Care Med 151:785–790, 1995.

184. Rosen-Levin E, Patil JR, Watson CW, et al: Distinguishing benign from malignant pleural effusions by lectin immunocytochemistry. Acta Cytol 33:499–504, 1989.

185. Rosso R, Rimoldi R, Salvati F, et al: Intrapleural natural beta interferon in the treatment of malignant pleural effusions. Oncology 45:253–256, 1988.

186. Roth BJ, O'Meara TF, Cragun WH: The serum-effusion albumin gradient in the evaluation of pleural effusions. Chest 98:546–549, 1990.

187. Ruckdeschel JC, Moores D, Lee JY, et al: Intrapleural therapy for malignant pleural effusions. A randomized comparison of bleomycin and tetracycline. Chest 100:1528–1535, 1991.

188. Rusch VW, Figlin R, Godwin D, et al: Intrapleural cisplatin and cytarabine in the management of malignant pleural effusions: A lung cancer study group trial. J Clin Oncol 9:313–319, 1991.

189. Ryan CJ, Rodgers RF, Unni KK, et al: The outcome of patients with pleural effusion of indeterminate cause at thoractomy. Mayo Clin Proc 56:145–149, 1981.

190. Saffran L, Ost DE, Fein AM, et al: Outpatient pleurodesis of malignant pleural effusions using a small-bore pigtail catheter. Chest 118:417–421, 2000.

191. Sahin U, Unlu M, Akkaya A, et al: The value of small-bore catheter thoracostomy in the treatment of malignant pleural effusions. Respiration 68:501–505, 2001.

192. Sahn SA, Good JT Jr: Pleural fluid pH in malignant effusions. Diagnostic, prognostic, and therapeutic implications. Ann Intern Med 108:345–349, 1988.

193. Saleh H, Bober P, Tabaczka P: Value of Ki67 immunostain in identification of malignancy in serous effusions. Diagn Cytopathol 20:24–28, 1999.

194. Sanchez-Armengol A, Rodriguez-Panadero F: Survival and talc pleurodesis in metastatic pleural carcinoma, revisited. Report of 125 cases. Chest 104:1482–1485, 1993.

195. Sandler ED, Hattner RS, Parisi MT, et al: Clinical utility of bone scan features of pleural effusion: Sensitivity and specificity for malignancy based on pleural fluid cytopathology. J Nucl Med 35:429–431, 1994.

196. Scalzetti EM: Unilateral pulmonary edema after talc pleurodesis. J Thorac Imaging 16:99–102, 2001.

197. Schofield K, D'Aquila T, Rimm DL: The cell adhesion molecule, E-cadherin, distinguishes mesothelial cells from carcinoma cells in fluids. Cancer 81:293–298, 1997.

198. Schulze M, Boehle AS, Kurdow R, et al: Effective treatment of malignant pleural effusion by minimal invasive thoracic surgery: Thoracoscopic talc pleurodesis and pleuroperitoneal shunts in 101 patients. Ann Thorac Surg 71:1809–1812, 2001.

199. Sears D, Hajdu SI: The cytologic diagnosis of malignant neoplasms in pleural and peritoneal effusions. Acta Cytol 31:85–97, 1987.

200. Shiba M, Kakizawa K, Kohno H, et al: Prognostic implication of Ki-67 immunostaining in treating subclinical pleural cancer found at thoracotomy in lung cancer patients. Ann Thorac Surg 71:1765–1771, 2001.

201. Shield PW, Callan JJ, Devine PL: Markers for metastatic adenocarcinoma in serous effusion specimens. Diagn Cytopathol 11:237–245, 1994.

202. Soysal O, Karaoglanoglu N, Demiracan S, et al: Pleurectomy/decortication for palliation in malignant pleural mesothelioma: Results of surgery. Eur J Cardiothorac Surg 11:210–213, 1997.

203. Stoop JA, Hendriks JG, Berends D: Identification of malignant cells in serous effusions using a panel of monoclonal antibodies Ber-EP4, MCA-b-12 and EMA. Cytopathology 3:297–302, 1992.

204. Sugimoto JT, Little AG, Ferguson MK, et al: Pericardial window: Mechanisms of efficacy. Ann Thorac Surg 50:442–445, 1990.

205. Sugitachi A, Takatsuka Y, Kido T, et al: Bio-adhesio-chemo (BAC) therapy for patients with malignant pleural effusion. Am J Clin Oncol 12:156–161, 1989.

206. Takita H, Mang TS, Loewen GM, et al: Operation and intracavitary photodynamic therapy for malignant pleural mesothelioma: A phase II study. Ann Thorac Surg 58:995–998, 1994.

207. Thompson RL, Yau JC, Donnelly RF, et al: Pleurodesis with iodized talc for malignant effusions using pigtail catheters. Ann Pharmacother 32:739–742, 1998.

208. Topalian SL, Solomon D, Avis FP, et al: Immunotherapy of patients with advanced cancer using tumor-infiltrating lymphocytes and recombinant interleukin-2: A pilot study. J Clin Oncol 6:839–853, 1988.

209. Toshima S, Arai T, Yasuda Y, et al: Cytological diagnosis and telomerase activity of cells in effusions of body cavities. Oncol Rep 6:199–203, 1999.

210. Traill ZC, Davies RJ, Gleeson FV: Thoracic computed tomography in patients with suspected malignant pleural effusions. Clin Radiol 56:193–196, 2001.

211. Tzeng E, Ferguson MK: Predicting failure following shunting of pleural effusions. Chest 98:890–893, 1990.

212. Ukale V, Bone D, Hillerdal G, et al: The impact of pleurodesis in malignant effusion on respiratory function. Respir Med 93:898–902, 1999.

213. Vaitkus PT, Herrmann HC, LeWinter MM: Treatment of malignant pericardial effusion. JAMA 272:59–64, 1994.

214. van de Molengraft FJ, Vooijs GP: Survival of patients with malignancy-associated effusions. Acta Cytol 33:911–916, 1989.

215. Verheul HM, Hoekman K, Jorna AS, et al: Targeting vascular endothelial growth factor blockade: Ascites and pleural effusion formation. Oncologist 5(Suppl 1):45–50, 2000.

216. Viallat JR, Rey F, Astoul P, et al: Thoracoscopic talc poudrage pleurodesis for malignant effusions. A review of 360 cases. Chest 110:1387–1393, 1996.

217. Vidyasagar MS, Ramanujam AS, Fernandes DJ, et al: Vincristine (Vinca-Alkaloid) as a sclerosing agent for malignant pleural effusions. Acta Oncol 38:1017–1020, 1999.

218. Villanueva AG, Gray AW Jr, Shahian DM, et al: Efficacy of short term versus long term tube thoracostomy drainage

before tetracycline pleurodesis in the treatment of malignant pleural effusions. Thorax 49:23–25, 1994.

219. Villena V, Perez V, Pozo F, et al: Amylase levels in pleural effusions: A consecutive unselected series of 841 patients. Chest 121:470–474, 2002.

220. Von Hoff DD, LiVolsi V: Diagnostic reliability of needle biopsy of the parietal pleura. A review of 272 biopsies. Am J Clin Pathol 64:200–203, 1975.

221. Waller DA, Morritt GN, Forty J: Video-assisted thoracoscopic pleurectomy in the management of malignant pleural effusion. Chest 107:1454–1456, 1995.

222. Wang HJ, Hsu KL, Chiang FT, et al: Technical and prognostic outcomes of double-balloon pericardiotomy for large malignancy-related pericardial effusions. Chest 122:893–899, 2002.

223. Wang N, Feikes JR, Mogensen T, et al: Pericardioperitoneal shunt: An alternative treatment for malignant pericardial effusion. Ann Thorac Surg 57:289–292, 1994.

224. Webb WR, Ozmen V, Moulder PV, et al: Iodized talc pleurodesis for the treatment of pleural effusions. J Thorac Cardiovasc Surg 103:881–885, 1992.

225. Weissberg D: Talc pleurodesis: A controversial issue. Poumon Coeur 37:291–294, 1981.

226. Weissberg D, Ben Zeev I: Talc pleurodesis. Experience with 360 patients. J Thorac Cardiovasc Surg 106:689–695, 1993.

227. Wiley EL, Von Roenn J: Metastatic breast carcinoma in pleural fluid. Correlation of morphology with estrogen receptor activity and morphology of the primary carcinoma. Acta Cytol 34:169–174, 1990.

228. Wilkins HE III, Cacioppo J, Connolly MM, et al: Intrapericardial interferon in the management of malignant pericardial effusion. Chest 114:330–331, 1998.

229. Yamada S, Takeda T, Matsumoto K: Prognostic analysis of malignant pleural and peritoneal effusions. Cancer 51:136–140, 1983.

230. Yang CT, Lee MH, Lan RS, et al: Telomerase activity in pleural effusions: Diagnostic significance. J Clin Oncol 16:567–573, 1998.

231. Yano S, Herbst RS, Shinohara H, et al: Treatment for malignant pleural effusion of human lung adenocarcinoma by inhibition of vascular endothelial growth factor receptor tyrosine kinase phosphorylation. Clin Cancer Res 6:957–965, 2000.

232. Yasumoto K, Ogura T: Intrapleural application of recombinant interleukin-2 in patients with malignant pleurisy due to lung cancer. A multi-institutional cooperative study. Biotherapy 3:345–349, 1991.

233. Yim AP, Chung SS, Lee TW, et al: Thoracoscopic management of malignant pleural effusions. Chest 109:1234–1238, 1996.

234. Yinnon A, Konijn AM, Link G, et al: Diagnostic value of ferritin in malignant pleural and peritoneal effusions. Cancer 62:2564–2568, 1988.

235. Zaloznik AJ, Oswald SG, Langin M: Intrapleural tetracycline in malignant pleural effusions. A randomized study. Cancer 51:752–755, 1983.

236. Zimmer PW, Hill M, Casey K, et al: Prospective randomized trial of talc slurry vs bleomycin in pleurodesis for symptomatic malignant pleural effusions. Chest 112:430–434, 1997.

237. Zimmerman RL, Fogt F, Goonewardene S: Diagnostic value of a second generation CA 15-3 antibody to detect adenocarcinoma in body cavity effusions. Cancer 90:230–234, 2000.

238. Ziskind AA, Pearce AC, Lemmon CC, et al: Percutaneous balloon pericardiotomy for the treatment of cardiac tamponade and large pericardial effusions: Description of technique and report of the first 50 cases. J Am Coll Cardiol 21:1–5, 1993.

Pleural Tumors

Siyamek Neragi-Miandoab, David J. Sugarbaker,
and Philip A. Linden

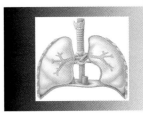

► ANATOMY AND HISTOLOGY OF THE PLEURA

The pleura is a thin contiguous membrane that lines the chest wall and covers the lungs, creating two distinct pleural spaces in the right and left chest. The internal aspect of the pleural membrane, which adheres to the lung parenchyma, is called the visceral pleura; the external aspect is called the parietal pleura. The visceral and parietal layers of the pleura meet at the hilum. The parietal pleura can be subdivided into four parts: cervical, costal, mediastinal, and diaphragmatic. Blood is supplied to the parietal pleura via branches from the intercostal, internal mammary, superior phrenic, and anterior mediastinal arteries. The visceral pleura derives blood from the lung parenchyma. Venous blood from the visceral pleura drains into the pulmonary vein, and lymphatic drainage is directed toward the mediastinal lymph nodes. Lymphatic drainage from the parietal pleura follows the arterial blood supply. The cervical parietal pleura drains into the axillary lymph nodes, the costal component into the intercostal and sternal nodes, the diaphragmatic into the phrenic nodes, and the mediastinal parietal pleura into mediastinal lymph nodes. Each pleura is moistened by small amounts of fluid produced by mesothelial cells, which facilitates movement of the lungs in the chest cavity.

From an embryological perspective, the pleura is composed of two lamellae originating from the mesoderm. The parietal pleura fuses with the ectoderm forming the somatopleure, and the visceral pleura fuses with endoderm giving rise to the splanchnopleure. Thus, all three germ layers are present in the pleura, and a mesothelioma can be composed of both epithelial and mesenchymal elements.

472

A layer of mesothelial cells covers the pleura, mesentery, and pericardium. In the chest, both visceral and parietal pleural layers are covered with mesothelial cells, a basement membrane, and a layer of well-vascularized connective tissue.[141,181] The normal mesothelial cells have a flat or low cuboidal shape and contain apical tight junctions, desmosomes, surface microvilli, and bundles of cytoplasmic tonofilaments. This layer is cytokeratin positive. The submesothelial layer, which is formed from connective tissue, contains collagen fibers, elastic fibers, blood cells, lymphatics, nerves, and submesothelial spindle cells.[16] The submesothelial spindle cells display fibroblastic features, expressing vimentin but not cytokeratin. These spindle cells lack cellular junctions and are more similar to fibroblasts, showing extended rough endoplasmic reticulum. When the surface mesothelial cells are injured, there is a proliferation of submesothelial cells that begins to exhibit myofibroblastoid features and is cytokeratin positive.[22] It is believed that these cells are capable of differentiating into surface mesothelial cells.

▶ BENIGN PLEURAL MASSES

Solitary or Localized Fibrous Tumor

Solitary fibrous tumors (formerly called benign mesothelioma) are connective tissue tumors, originating from the submesothelial connective tissue of the pleura. Although the tumors consist mostly of connective tissue and fibroblasts, they may contain nests or papillae of entrapped cuboidal mesothelial or bronchoalveolar cells. Most tumors are pedunculated, arise from the visceral pleura, and extend into the pleural space. Growth into the parenchyma and/or fissure can occasionally be seen. Grossly, they are lobulated, firm, and gray-white to yellow-white in color. In distinction to malignant mesothelioma, these tumors are well circumscribed, rarely show atypia, have no necrosis, exhibit a low mitotic rate, and do not invade adjacent tissues. Lack of invasion into adjacent tissues is the key microscopic feature that distinguishes these tumors from those labeled malignant.[44] Under the microscope they appear as whorls of fibroblasts with abundant collagen and elastin but without any identifiable architecture. Hence, the term "patternless pattern" is applied. These benign tumors stain positive for vimentin; negative for carcinoembryonic antigen (CEA) and S-100; and, in contrast to malignant mesothelioma, are negative for cytokeratin.[36] CD34 positivity has been noted.[171] These tumors are not associated with asbestos exposure. They are found with equal frequency in men and women, with a peak incidence after the fifth decade of life. Most fibrous tumors are asymptomatic and are discovered incidentally on a radiological study. Larger tumors are more likely to present with symptoms of cough, chest pain, and dyspnea. A small percentage of patients, usually with larger tumors, may display systemic syndromes resulting from the benign tumors. These include hypoglycemia, hypertrophic pulmonary osteoarthropathy, and clubbing. Occasionally, the hypoglycemia may be severe, resulting in seizures and coma. Overall, only 3–4% of these tumors present with hypoglycemia, and commonly they are greater than 10 cm in diameter. Several theories have been proposed to explain

hypoglycemia, including increased glucose utilization by the tumor and increased production of insulin-like substances, such as somatomedin. More recently, the production of insulin-like growth factor has been demonstrated in these tumors.[48] Prompt relief of the hypoglycemia accompanies excision of the tumor. The mechanism for hypertrophic pulmonary osteoarthropathy and clubbing is less clear. Nonetheless, relief of symptoms of hypertrophic pulmonary osteoarthropathy is common after complete removal of the tumor.

The treatment of localized fibrous tumor consists of localized resection including a margin of normal lung. Usually, this can be performed thoracoscopically. Lesions within the lung may require anatomical resections. Recurrences are rare following adequate resection (2%).[60] Patients should be followed up with computed tomography (CT) scans: reresection is usually possible for recurrences.

Calcifying Fibrous Pseudotumors

Calcifying fibrous pseudotumors (CFPT) are rare, benign tumors that can arise from either the parietal or visceral pleura. These usually are seen in the first three decades of life and exhibit slow growth. They demonstrate histological similarities to other inflammatory pseudotumors, such as pulmonary granulomas and plasma cell granulomas. Common characteristics include dense hyalinization, fibrous proliferation, and a lymphocytic cell infiltrate.[13] Calcifications may be apparent in certain radiographic studies.[61] Many have psammomatous features. These tumors do not have any potential for malignancy and are cured by excision.[147] A previous empyema or hemothorax can lead to a calcified fibrous pleuritis that can usually be distinguished from CFPT. Calcification from an old empyema or hemothorax is generally more diffuse, contains a calcified rim, is often associated with a residual effusion, and shows widening of the extrapleural fat.

Pleural Cysts

Pleural cysts arise mainly from the parietal pleura, generally at the pleuropericardial reflection. On radiographs, they appear as round masses on the right side of the heart. CT and CT-guided biopsy aid in the diagnosis. Chest radiographs are sufficient for follow-up. These cysts can be drained or resected.

Pleural Plaques

Pleural plaques arise from the parietal pleura and appear most commonly on the diaphragmatic surface or inferior areas of the chest. The thickness of the plaques is usually no greater than 5 mm, and the diameter is usually several centimeters, although, on occasion, plaques wider than 10 cm are noted. Characteristically, they are multiple, bilateral, and spare the costophrenic angles and apices.[112] They are considered to be a manifestation of very low asbestos exposure and occur in 1–10% of the population. Most commonly, they are associated with remote exposure to amosite and crocidolite asbestos fibers. These plaques are asymptomatic and have no malignant potential. Intraoperatively, asbestos plaques are dense, hard, white flat or nodular lesions and are almost always free of adhesions to adjacent structures.

Histological examination of these plaques reveals collagenous scarring and intersecting bands of collagen.

MALIGNANT TUMORS OF THE PLEURA

Primary malignant tumors of the pleural space, other than diffuse malignant mesothelioma, are extremely rare. The most common tumor of the pleural space is metastatic carcinoma, arising from lung and other remote organs. Occasionally, a small lung primary with extensive pleural spread may mimic diffuse malignant mesothelioma; this condition is termed pseudomesotheliomatous carcinoma of the lung. The differentiation of this condition from mesothelioma can be difficult and is discussed below. Thymomas not uncommonly metastasize to the pleural space, and diffuse spread of these tumors can also mimic mesothelioma. All other primary tumors of the pleural space including sarcomas, primary thymoma, and nerve sheath tumors have been described in case reports only.

Sarcoma

Liposarcoma, although one of the more common subtypes of soft tissue sarcoma, is rarely found in the chest. Of the 1067 cases of liposarcoma recorded by the Armed Forces Institute of Pathology, 29 were located in the chest, with a majority in the mediastinum. Only 9 cases have ever been described as arising in the pleural space.[186] These tumors tend to be very large upon presentation. The smallest pleural liposarcoma reported was 1 kg in size. Its CT characteristics are that of an inhomogeneous tumor with vague margins, fat infiltration, and, occasionally, calcification. Wide resection, including all involved soft tissue, with adequate margins is required. Because of the generally poor prognosis of liposarcomas of the trunk, adjuvant radiation should be considered.

Synovial sarcoma typically involves joints of the extremity, but can arise in the trunk. Gaertner et al, from the Armed Forces Institute of Pathology, reported five biphasic synovial sarcomas arising in the pleural cavity.[63] These sarcomas are termed biphasic because they are composed of both epithelial and spindled areas. The patients in this series were younger on average, ranging in age from 9 to 50 years. All patients died of their disease or suffered recurrence within 1–2 years of resection. Whereas the gross appearance of this sarcoma is different from mesothelioma, the immunohistochemistry can be similar.

Moran et al[108] described five smooth muscle tumors of the pleural space reviewed at the Armed Forces Institute of Pathology, including three leiomyosarcomas and two smooth muscle tumors of undetermined malignant potential. All but one of these patients were younger than 50 years and most presented with tumors larger than 10 cm. All tumors stained positive for smooth muscle actin, and only one stained positive for keratin.

Vascular tumors involving the pleural space have also been described. Weiss and Enzinger described 14 cases of hemangioendothelioma and angiosarcoma of the pleural space.[183] Epithelioid hemangioendothelioma occurs by proliferation of epithelioid endothelial cells most commonly originating in superficial or deep soft tissue in extremities. In rare cases, this tumor involves the peritoneal or pleural cavity and mimics diffuse mesothelioma.[189] The presence of abortive vessel formation and strong expression of vimentin and the absence of cytokeratin suggest endothelial tumors rather than mesotheliomas.[92]

Thymoma

Thymomas almost always originate in the anterior mediastinum. It is not uncommon for aggressive malignant thymomas to spread to the pleural space diffusely. Rarely, thymomas have also been seen to occur in the neck, thyroid, pulmonary hilum, and pulmonary parenchyma without a mediastinal component. Several cases of ectopic pleural thymoma without evidence of a mediastinal component have also been described.[108] In these cases, patients presented with shortness of breath and/or weight loss with radiographic findings of pleural thickening and encasement of the lung but no prominent mediastinal component. The diagnosis was established, microscopically, with the finding of a biphasic population of both lymphoid and epithelial cells.

Stage IVa malignant thymoma or diffuse thymic carcinoma originating in the mediastinum with extensive spread to the pleural space is a much more common phenomenon than extensive spread from a primary pleural thymoma.[114a] The diagnosis can be established via thoracoscopy.

Pseudomesotheliomatous adenocarcinoma is a term used to describe metastatic adenocarcinoma (usually from lung) with extensive involvement of the pleura, first described by Harwood et al.[72] In these lung adenocarcinomas, the majority of the growth occurs into and along the pleural space, with relatively little tumor burden found in the lung. Some ultrastructural and immunohistochemical features suggest that this variety of adenocarcinoma is derived from type II pneumocytes, known as Clara cells.[55] The radiographic and gross appearance and pattern of spread of these tumors may mimic diffuse malignant pleural mesothelioma Microscopically, the tubulopapillary growth seen in association with a desmoplastic reaction also mimics mesothelioma and may lead to misdiagnosis as a mesothelioma. Curiously, the average length of survival from time of diagnosis is not dissimilar from medically managed diffuse malignant pleural mesothelioma.[55] The differentiation between the two tumors must be made by immunohistochemical techniques, as will be detailed later in the section on diagnosis of malignant pleural mesothelioma.

Malignant Pleural Mesothelioma

Malignant pleural mesothelioma (MPM) is a diffuse tumor arising from mesothelial cells. It can occur in any body cavity covered by mesothelial cells, i.e., the peritoneum, pleura, pericardial sac, tunica vaginalis, and testis. The pleura, however, is the most common site. Mesothelial cells are derived from coelomic epithelium, which is developed from the mesodermal layer.[121] Malignant mesothelioma can demonstrate a wide variety of mesenchymal differentiation, ranging from fibrosarcomatous, malignant fibrous histiocytoma-like, chondroid, osteoblastic, and liposarcomatous forms, which can occur alone or in concordance with epithelial differentiation.[65] There is often diffuse pleural thickening involving both parietal and visceral layers of the pleura.[65] The tumor grows preferentially over serosal surfaces, penetrating the

474 interlobar fissures resulting in a lung completely encased with overlying tumor.[16]

The most common presentation consists of multiple gray or white nodules in a diffusely thickened pleura. Rarely, mesothelioma presents as a local pleural mass.[51] Microscopically, it may build papillae or pseudoacini or grow as solid nests. The cytoplasm looks abundant and acidophilic. In early stages it may be confused with mesothelial hyperplasia.[163] Features consisting of invasion of the deep tissue, prominent atypical cell colonies, and necrosis favor the diagnosis of malignancy.[100]

Epidemiology of Mesothelioma

It has been more than 40 years since Wagner et al[178] studied the increased risk of mesothelioma in miners of crocidolite asbestos in South Africa. It is estimated that 1.3 million employees in construction and general industry are exposed to significant amounts of asbestos each year. The heaviest exposure occurs in the construction industry. There are around 3000 new cases per year in the United States, and considering the 30- to 40-year latency period between exposure and expression of the disease, there will be an estimated 300,000 cases before the year 2030. Epidemiological studies predict that approximately 250,000 Europeans will develop mesothelioma in the next few decades, while the incidence of this disease has increased in the United States by 90% in the past 20 years.[32] The exact number of mesothelioma cases, however, is unknown, because the numbers are only projections of the Surveillance, Epidemiology and End Results (SEER) program. The SEER program provides population-based, tumor-specific data on all histologically proven cancers occurring in selected geographic sites in the United States, including about 12% of the U.S. population.[36] Asbestos exposure is not recorded in the SEER database. The mortality of mesothelioma continues to increase worldwide (5–10% a year). This increase is likely to continue in Europe and the United States until year 2020. Unregulated use of asbestos in less industrialized countries will most likely lead to an increased incidence of mesothelioma in these countries as well.[31]

Asbestos Exposure and Malignant Pleural Mesothelioma

Asbestos is the generic name for a group of highly fibrous asbestiform minerals with thin fibers. The combined used of light microscopy, electron microscopy, and X-ray analysis offers the most accurate approach to evaluating and estimating the concentration of asbestos in air or bulk samples. In the 1970s, Langer and Pooly[87] introduced the use of electron microscopy to identify and quantitate asbestos in lung tissue.

Asbestos fibers are heat resistant, which makes them a suitable material for insulation purposes. Because of their highly regarded resistant qualities, however, once these fibers invade the lung, they remain there for very long periods of time.

The increased incidence of mesothelioma has been closely linked to the rise of the asbestos industry and the use of asbestos in fireproofing and insulation. In the early 1930s several publications in major medical journals began revealing the deleterious effect of asbestos exposure, linking it to cancer. In the following years, materials such as fiberglass were developed to replace asbestos. Manufacturer awareness about product liability in the 1970s led to the rapid replacement of asbestos with alternative materials as well as the initiation of new organizational and educational efforts among worker groups regarding environmental health and expansion of occupational medicine clinics.[52] In young adults mesothelioma is primarily linked to occupations such as carpenters, plumbers, electricians, and insulation installers, where workers are exposed to amphibole fibers.[102]

Different Types of Asbestos Fibers

There are two general types of asbestos, amphibole and serpentine. Chrysotile asbestos is the only serpentine type, whereas crocidolite, amosite, tremolite, anthophyllite, and actinolite all belong to the amphibole group. Crocidolite asbestos is mined mainly in South Africa and Western Australia, and in fact, the first reports linking asbestos exposure to mesothelioma were from cohort studies of miners in these countries. Chrysotile asbestos accounts for the majority of worldwide asbestos production (in excess of 95%), and for some time it was believed to be noncarcinogenic or significantly less carcinogenic than amphibole types. Inhalational exposure to asbestos requires the material to be released into the air. This occurs during construction and also during asbestos removal; only very low levels of airborne asbestos are present in buildings maintained in good condition.

The normal host response involves removal of asbestos fibers via macrophage-mediated phagocystosis. The long amphibole fibers cannot be phagocytosed. They persist in the lung, a characteristic termed "biopersistence." The asbestos fibers can reach the pleura through the lymphatics or by direct penetration from the lung, where they can cause fibrosis, pleural plaques, or mesothelioma. Mesothelioma is believed to originate on the parietal and diaphragmatic pleurae as opposed to the visceral pleura.[24]

Certain individuals have proposed that amphibole fibers (crocidolite, amosite, and tremolite) cause cancer, and that serpentine (chrysotile) fibers do not. This assumption is based on observations in the 1970s that serpentine fibers were cleared from the body much more quickly than amphibole fibers, and that exposure to chrysotile, a serpentine fiber, did not seem to increase the incidence of mesothelioma. It is known that chrysotile fibers break down (as seen under electron microscopy),[113] allowing macrophages to clear the fibers, while amphibole fibers remain in the lungs for many years after exposure. This biopersistence of fibers in the lung directly correlates to the increased risk of malignancy in animals.[105,106] There is evidence that these "biopersistent" fibers cause malignancy in humans as well.[102] Stanton et al[151] demonstrated in a rat model that the carcinogenicity of mineral particles is primarily a function of their dimension (diameter and length of fiber), rather than their physicochemical properties. It is impossible, however, to view the diameter and length of a fiber separate from its physicochemical properties, as these factors all affect biopersistence and surface area available for free radical production.[83] Wagner et al,[179] Stanton and Wrench,[151] and Davis[54a] all believe that long (>8 μm) and thin fibers are important determinants of carcinogenicity.

Recently, evidence has emerged that chrysotile may be a major cause of malignant pleural mesothelioma.[149] Chrysotile fibers are less persistent in tissue than amphibole fibers and are not seen as easily as amphibole fibers under the microscope, thus explaining their apparent absence in mesothelioma specimens. Several recent articles present cogent arguments for the carcinogenicity of chrysotile fibers.[113,149] All this is confounded by the fact that most forms of chrysotile are contaminated with small amounts of amphibole asbestos.[97] Recently, The Commission of the European Union passed guidelines obligating member states to prohibit the use and marketing of chrysotile asbestos, which had applied previously only to amphibole asbestos.[188]

Contribution of Asbestos to the Development of Mesothelioma

The development of malignant mesothelioma after asbestos exposure is a multifactorial, multistep process. Different kinds of asbestos fibers may have different carcinogenic mechanisms or may act with other environmental or genetic factors. Sanden published a series of articles on shipyard workers in a prospective cohort study[142] that suggested that asbestos fibers may function as initiating agents in the development of mesothelioma and as promoters or cocarcinogens in lung cancer.

Two theories attempt to explain the long latency between exposure and expression of mesothelioma. The first suggests that transformation to the carcinogenic state occurs early in the course of exposure, but the tumor takes a very long time to grow. This seems unlikely, since unlike other tumors, there is no evidence for the existence of a premalignant noninvasive phase with mesothelioma. Moreover, if such a phase exists, it would have to be very short-lived and not detectable with current diagnostic techniques.[36] The second theory suggests that the genetic changes brought about by asbestos exposure accumulate over time, finally reaching a threshold of malignant transformation. This theory implies that cells pass on their chromosomal damage over many years. Opponents of this theory argue that given the high toxicity of asbestos, the damaged cell or daughter cell could not survive so many years carrying damaged genetic material.[36]

Human mesothelial cells are very sensitive to asbestos, and they often die after phagocytosis of asbestos fibers.[21] The phagocytosis of asbestos by macrophages produces oxygen radicals and lymphokines, which damage the DNA as well as suppress the immune system. The immunosuppressive effect of asbestos occurs in a local and systemic fashion.[131,167] Asbestos fibers can produce superoxide (O^{2-}), hydroxyl radical ($\cdot OH$), and hydrogen peroxide. The production of oxygen radicals can be catalyzed by iron or surface reactions on the fiber surface[70] or after mobilization of iron from fibers.[94] Moreover, the unsuccessful phagocytosis of asbestos fibers may generate oxygen radicals and increase oxidative stress.[71] Mossman et al[110] reported that there was increased nitrite oxide found in macrophages of asbestos-exposed lung. Macrophages release chemokines, which attract leukocytes and cytokines and cause proliferation and altered differentiation in mesothelial cells.[184] Inflammatory cells are commonly found in the bronchoalveolar lavage of asbestos workers.[130] Attracted neutrophils induce cell damage by induction of inflammation via oxidative stress.[84] The asbestos-induced inflammation may cause damage to cell replication and the genetic material of cells, which may play a role in the initiation and promotion as well as progression of the tumor.

Growth factor release, induced in part by asbestos exposure, results in the proliferation of mesothelial cells, making them more susceptible to DNA damage and genetic susceptibility.[109] It has been reported that direct exposure to amphibole fibers increases DNA synthesis in mesothelial cells, possibly via increased production of hepatocyte growth factor (HGF).[5] Eagles et al[58] observed increased levels of HGF in the pleural effusions of patients with malignant mesothelioma. Epidermal growth factor (EGF) is required for growth of normal mesothelial cells,[64,88] and mesothelial cells demonstrate EGF receptors.[20] Mesothelial cells exposed to asbestos produce transforming growth factor-α (TGF-α), which binds to EGF receptors with high affinity, increasing the proliferation rate. This effect can be antagonized by TGF-α antibody.[180]

Asbestos-Like Fibers

Exposure to erionite, a naturally occurring fiber with a length-to-diameter ratio similar to asbestos, has also been linked to the development of mesothelioma. Erionite is present in large quantities in volcanic rock in certain regions of Eastern Europe. Several areas in Turkey, including South Anatolia, and the villages of Tuzkoy, Karain, and Sarihidir, have an increased incidence of mesothelioma.[49,96] A high concentration of erionite fibers has been found in the lung tissue of many patients in these villages,[145] and in some of these villages, mesothelioma is the most common cause of death. Fibrous erionite is widespread; some cases of mesothelioma in the Rocky Mountains may be linked to erionite.[85] Erionite fibers are hypothesized to cause a mobilization of Mg, K, and Ca cations, inducing a catalytic reaction producing free oxygen radicals.[57] The combination of the biopersistence of the fibers and large surface area (200 m²/g surface area for erionite vs. 10 m²/g for crocidolite)[47,117] available for catalytic activity may explain their carcinogenicity.

Non-Asbestos-Related Mesothelioma

In a review of the mesothelioma literature Peterson et al[122] reported that asbestos exposure in mesothelioma patients varied from 13%[30] to 100%,[46] implying that there are many non-asbestos-related mesotheliomas. The increased incidence in women and children with no asbestos exposure suggests that other environmental or genetic factors may contribute to induction of malignant mesothelioma.[81] Other authors support this view.[45] A portion of these non-asbestos-related mesothelioma cases have been linked to unrecognized exposure in some patients.[103] Factors that may contribute to induction of mesothelioma include radiation,[91] nonasbestos mineral fibers, organic chemicals, viruses, genetic predisposition, pleural scarring,[76] and chronic inflammation.[53] Based on the best available data, only about 80% of mesotheliomas are associated with asbestos exposure. In fact, a history of asbestos exposure is lacking in 400–600 mesothelioma patients a year in the United States, suggesting that many other factors may play a role in the pathogenesis of mesothelioma.

Mesothelioma in Children

Our knowledge about pediatric mesothelioma is very limited. Grundy and Miller[69] identified 31 cases of mesothelioma in children. The histological analysis demonstrated the majority

476

of those tumors to be sarcomatous. None of the tumors was exclusively epithelial. The longest survival was only 24 months after the onset of symptoms. No specific environmental exposure was identified. Brenner et al[30] reported seven cases of pediatric mesothelioma, in which parental, occupational, or nonoccupational asbestos exposure was absent. Fraire et al[62] reported on a series of 80 children (only 10 cases were pathologically documented) with a survival time ranging from 8 to 59 months. Only one of the children was found to have asbestos exposure. Given the known long latency of asbestos-related mesothelioma in adults, it is unlikely that mesothelioma in children is due to asbestos exposure.[79]

The Role of Radiation

Ionizing radiation has been suspected of contributing to the development of mesothelioma since the 1970s. Sanders and Jackson[143] showed that 27% of rats given intraabdominal injections of radioactive material developed mesothelioma. Maurer and Egloff[99] published a case report of peritoneal mesothelioma after administration of Thorotrast, widely used as an X-ray contrast agent in the 1930s and 1940s.[133] Stock et al reported a case of peritoneal mesothelioma in a patient 16 years after 32 Gy radiation to the abdomen and pelvis for seminoma.[155] Gilks et al reported a separate case of peritoneal mesothelioma after radiation therapy (38 Gy to the pelvis and 36 Gy to the upper abdomen) for a seminoma.[66] Recently, there have been reports about the development of mesothelioma after radiation therapy for breast cancer,[146] Hodgkin's disease,[86a] cervical cancer,[18a] and Wilm's tumor.[81] Weissman et al reported four cases of pleural mesothelioma in Hodgkin's patients treated with radiation. None of the patients had asbestos exposure and the mean interval was 15 years. Shannon et al[146] described two cases of pleural mesothelioma following radiation therapy for breast cancer. Austin et al[11] reported mesothelioma in a patient who had been irradiated for Wilm's tumor. Other studies also suggest an increased risk of mesothelioma in children with Wilm's tumor[9] following chemoradiation. Radiation-induced malignant mesothelioma appears to have the same prognosis as asbestos-related mesothelioma.[41] The incidence of radiation-induced mesothelioma seems to be increasing, as the numbers of long-term survivors of radiation-treated malignancies increase. Further investigation is needed to identify the relationship between second malignancies, including malignant mesothelioma, and therapeutic modalities in relation to their effect on environmental factors and underlying predisposition.

The Role of Genetics and Tumor Suppressor Genes

The absence of asbestos exposure in a significant percentage of mesothelioma patients is used by some to argue for a genetic predisposition.[47] In addition, the fact that only a small proportion (5%) of South African asbestos mine workers developed mesothelioma indicates that other environmental or genetic factors are involved.

The epidemiological studies of mesothelioma in Central Anatolia, Turkey, have contributed valuable knowledge about the genetic components of mesothelioma. About 50% of people in this region die of this cancer. The stones used to construct houses in this region are mined from volcanic caves and contain a high level of erionite. Yet mesothelioma is often clustered in certain families in these regions of Turkey, and not just in houses with high levels of erionite. Roushdy-Hammady spent 2.5 years in Central Anatolia, Turkey, examining the pedigree of six generations in 526 individuals and creating an epidemiological map.[132] The results of her analysis suggest that the predisposition for developing malignant mesothelioma in this population is transmitted in an autosomal dominant fashion. Erionite is an environmental factor that may contribute to or accelerate the induction of malignant mesothelioma in this population. Attempts have been made to isolate the affected or mutated gene, which might be the target for erionite fibers.[36]

Karyotypic studies have shown some chromosomal loss in most human mesotheliomas, including deletion of some regions in the short arms (p) of chromosomes 1, 3, 9, and the long arm (q) of 6, 13, and 15. Monosomy 4 and 14 as well as defects in chromosome 22 have been reported.[36,169] Loss and/or inactivation of tumor suppressor genes may play a role in the pathogenesis of mesothelioma. Tumor suppressor gene loss has been identified by analyzing the loss of heterogenicity (LOH) with polymorphic DNA markers.[36] Crocidolite asbestos has the capability of stimulating protooncogens c-*fos* and c-*jun*. These two genomes encode transcription factors, which activate genes responsible for the initiation of DNA synthesis.[129] A continuous stimulation of these transcription factors by asbestos may result in enhanced cell division. Mesothelioma may commence with increased proliferation in stem cells and progressive accumulation of genetic mistakes or mutations over decades. These mutations may occur spontaneously or as a result of alterations in tumor suppressor genes and/or asbestos-related misaggregation of chromosomes.

The Role of SV40

Simian virus 40 (SV40) has the capacity to induce tumors via the large T antigen (Tag) protein. This 90-kDa protein has been shown to bind and inactivate a variety of tumor suppressor genes including p53, pRb, and p130. Subsequent uncontrolled cell division leads to cellular immortalization. Inhibition of p53 also leads to interruption of cellular DNA repair mechanisms.

SV40 was introduced in large scale to the population of the United States and Europe in the 1950s and 1960s during Salk poliovirus (IPV) vaccinations. An estimated 90 million U.S. citizens were vaccinated with contaminated polio vaccine. Thirty percent of the vaccine may have been contaminated with SV40.[86,169] SV40 was first linked to mesothelioma in animal experiments when SV40 was injected into the pleural cavity and found to induce pleural mesothelioma in a high percentage of hamsters.[38] Carbone et al[37] examined human malignant mesothelioma samples and found SV40-like DNA in 29 of 48 patients.

Mesothelioma specimens from countries such as Turkey and Finland, where the polio vaccine was not contaminated with SV40, do not show evidence of SV40. Hirvonen et al examined tumor tissue in 49 Finnish patients (born between 1912 and 1953) with malignant mesothelioma after asbestos exposure. Using polymerase chain reaction (PCR) and Southern blotting technique, they found no evidence of SV40 DNA in mesothelioma samples.[77] Similar studies in Turkey showed no evidence of SV40-like DNA in mesothelioma samples.[59]

A variety of studies have linked the presence of SV40 to angiogenesis. SV40 enhances the production of vascular endothelial cell growth factor (VEGF) by mesothelial cells.[55] Likewise, SV40 T antigen-positive mesothelial cells demonstrate an increased VEGF level. Increased VEGF or fibroblast growth factor-β levels correlate with poor prognosis.[156] While VEGF is a fairly specific angiogenic factor, it has also been shown to be a growth factor for mesothelioma cells *in vitro*.[156] SV40 inactivation of p53 leads to decreased expression of thrombospondin-1, an angiogenesis inhibitor.[127] Increased hepatocyte growth factor (HGF; also termed scatter factor) production and receptor (Met) activation in SV40-infected mesothelial cells lead to increased mesothelial VEGF production.[55,185] Among its many properties, HGF is an angiogenic factor.

Thus, although it is clear that many cases of mesothelioma (especially in Europe) occur without SV40 infection, there is a high incidence (approaching 50%) of SV40 in malignant mesothelioma in the United States. Thus, SV40-induced transformation may act in synergy with DNA damage induced through asbestos exposure to foster the development of malignant mesothelioma. There is also considerable evidence that SV40 infection is associated with an increase in the angiogenic state, that is, a reduction in endogenous angiogenesis inhibitors and an increase in angiogenic stimulators.

Clinical Presentation

In the early stages of the disease, symptoms are subtle. In an asymptomatic patient, a small pleural effusion with associated pleural thickening may be present. Cough and dyspnea are the most frequent early complaints. At presentation, most will have dyspnea (80%) and cough (69%), and some (40%) will have weight loss.[95] Fatigue, weakness, and weight loss typically occur later. Pain is also common later in the disease, as the tumor invades the chest wall and/or mediastinum. Worsening dyspnea and a sense of chest tightness occur as the tumor encases the lung and invades adjacent structures. Shortness of breath is worsened by tumor encasement of the lung, resulting in shunting of blood and $\dot{V}/\dot{Q}$ mismatch.[6] Late in the course of the disease cachexia, severe fatigue, and invasion of the adjacent structures such as chest wall, esophagus, and vertebrae are common findings.[152] Occasionally, a bulky tumor can be palpated between the ribs indicating chest wall invasion. Invasion through the diaphragm may result in abdominal ascites. Bowel obstruction can be observed in advanced disease.[162] Invasion near or into the esophagus may result in dysphagia. Invasion into the pericardium and heart may result in a pericardial effusion, tamponade, arrhythmia, and myocardial dysfunction.

Radiological Evaluation

Radiological studies including chest X-ray (Figure 30–1), CT (Figure 30–2), and magnetic resonance imaging (MRI) (Figure 30–3) are all useful in the workup of malignant mesothelioma. Pleural thickening usually can be diagnosed on plain chest radiograph. In the presence of pleural thick-

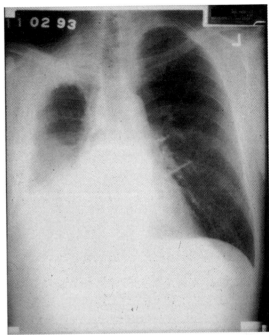

Figure 30–1 **Chest X-ray of mesothelioma.** Plain chest radiograph of a patient with mesothelioma showing a large pleural effusion and pleural rind.

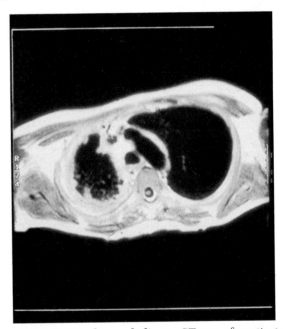

Figure 30–2 **CT of mesothelioma.** CT scan of a patient with mesothelioma displaying circumferential pleural thickening.

ening and effusion, the diagnosis of malignant mesothelioma should be considered, especially with a known history of asbestos exposure.[162] After tapping the pleural effusion, irregular and nodular pleural thickening can often be seen in malignant mesothelioma.[175] A pleural tumor, exudative effusion, and mediastinal pleural involvement are suggestive of malignant disease.[168] In advanced cases, mediastinal shift and narrowing of the intercostal spaces can be seen on plain film. Rib erosion and periosteal reaction are indications of chest wall invasion. Contralateral effusion, pleural

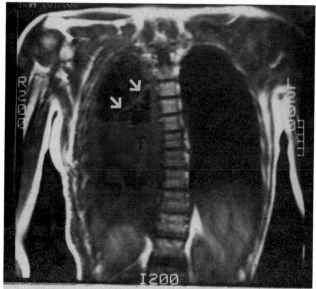

A

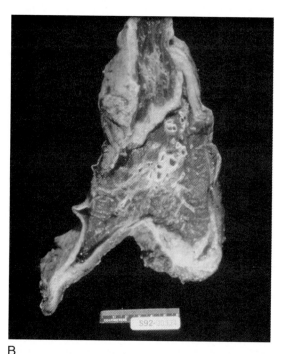

B

Figure 30–3 MRI of mesothelioma (A) and photo of gross specimen (B). A, Sagittal MRI of a patient with mesothelioma showing pleural tumor with extension into the major fissure. B, Photo of the gross specimen shows growth of disease into the major fissure.

thickening, or pulmonary nodules may be an indication of metastatic disease.

CT aids in defining the exact anatomical extent of tumor. A pleural effusion with nodular pleural thickening is common, and in more advanced cases, circumferential encasement of the lung may be visible. Several findings on CT may be suggestive of tumor invasion of adjacent structures. Infiltration of extrapleural fat and intercostal muscle and displacement and/or destruction of ribs can be seen with CT. Infiltration of mediastinal fat planes is suggestive of

medisatinal invasion. Invasion of great vessels, trachea, or esophagus is often accompanied by evidence of the tumor surrounding greater than 50% of the structure.[120] Invasion of the diaphragm can be difficult to detect by CT, but preservation of the fat planes below the diaphragm and a smooth diaphragmatic contour are reassuring for the absence of invasion through the diaphragm.[98]

MRI is generally superior to CT in evaluating diaphragmatic or mediastinal invasion.[120] A study comparing CT and MRI from 1992 showed the diagnostic accuracy in overall staging to be nearly equivalent between the modalities at 50–65%.[120] Differences have also been seen in the ability to determine diaphragmatic invasion (CT accuracy 55% vs. MRI accuracy 82%) and the ability to determine invasion of endothoracic fascia (CT accuracy 46% vs. MRI accuracy 69%).[74] It is clear from these numbers that neither modality approaches 100% accuracy, and when resectability is in question, operative exploration is mandated. Overall, MRI and CT findings that suggest resectability include preserved extrapleural fat planes, normal CT and MRI attenuation values in structures neighboring the tumor, absence of extrapleural soft tissue masses, and a smooth diaphragmatic surface on sagittal and coronal images.[120]

Fluorodeoxyglucose positron emission tomography (FDG-PET) scan is useful in assessing the overall extent of intrathoracic disease and the presence of extrathoracic metastasis. In a highly selected group of 28 patients, FDG-PET diagnosed 22 of 24 pleural malignancies (two of these positive scans were later found to be diffuse pleural adenocarcinomatosis). Two cases of mesothelioma were PET negative. In addition, one out of four benign pleural processes was read as PET positive.[19] Another study showed a sensitivity of 91% and a specificity of 100% in differentiating benign from malignant pleural disease.[82] Thus, although PET is about 90% sensitive for differentiating malignant from benign pleural disease, it cannot distinguish mesothelioma from adenocarcinoma, and false positives are possible with benign inflammatory pleural disease.

Tissue Diagnosis

The pleural fluid associated with MPM is exudative. A frankly bloody effusion is more suggestive of adenocarcinoma than mesothelioma. Cytological examination will often reveal mesothelial cells, inflammatory cells, and red blood cells; however, a definitive cytological diagnosis of mesotheliomia is rare. The sensitivity of pleural effusion cytology has been reported to be 16–26%.[134] Similar difficulties are encountered when attempts are made to diagnose MPM using transthoracic fine-needle aspiration with cytology. It is usually not possible to distinguish reactive mesothelial cells from malignant pleural cells. Core-needle pleural biopsy may allow for the diagnosis of MPM. Pleural biopsy using a reverse bevel needle, such as Abrams or Cope needles, without imaging guidance has a sensitivity range of 21–43% for detecting malignant mesothelioma. CT-guided needle biopsy (with 14- and 18-gauge core needles) in one report of 21 patients had a significantly higher sensitivity (86%) and a specificity of 100%.[3] Local radiation therapy after CT-guided needle biopsy was employed in this study and was shown to reduce the chance of tumor seeding on the biopsy or thoracoscopy track.[25] Pleural biopsy can be associated with complications such as pneumothorax, vaso-vagal syncope, hemothorax, biopsy site hematoma, and ipsi-lateral shoulder pain.[123] Thoracoscopic biopsy has a sensitivity of 91–98% for the diagnosis of pleural disease.[23] Because of the risk of seeding and the low sensitivity of cyto-logical examination,[125] we recommend proceeding directly to VATS, if malignant mesothelioma is suspected. The inci-sion should be placed in the line of the proposed thoraco-tomy incision. Seeding of the thoracoscopy incision is not uncommon with mesothelioma, and the thoracoscopy inci-sion should routinely be excised during thoracotomy. A VATS biopsy can provide sufficient tissue for histopathology, immunohistochemistry, and electron microscopy.[28] The VATS technique is nearly 100% effective in obtaining suffi-cient tissue and establishing a diagnosis with no mortality. If the patient is not a candidate for future thoracotomy (either pleurectomy or extrapleural pneumonectomy), then drainage of effusion and talc pleurodesis may be performed at the time of initial diagnostic thoracoscopy.

Pathology

Histopathology

The diagnosis of MPM can be difficult. First, differentiation must be made between benign proliferative mesothelial processes and malignant mesothelioma. Patients at risk for these two disease processes have nearly identical risk factors (i.e., asbestos exposure). Patient history and even clinical presentation are often similar in benign and malignant pleu-ral processes. Second, differentiating between epithelial mesothelioma and pleural carcinomatosis and between sar-comatoid mesothelioma and sarcoma can be difficult. The differentiation is most critical between metastatic carcino-matosis of the pleural space and malignant mesothelioma, as surgical debulking is of no benefit and must be avoided in carcinomatosis. Fortunately, there has been significant progress in the microscopic and immunohistochemical dif-ferentiation of these processes.

It may often be difficult to differentiate between a benign and a malignant proliferation of the pleura. Definite stromal invasion is the most reliable indicator of malignancy for both epithelial and spindle cell mesotheliomas. If the biopsy sample is small, assessment of stromal invasion may not be possible. Invasion of fat or the chest wall by thick-ened and fibrotic pleura is indicative of malignancy.

Atypical mesothelial cells may be seen with either benign or malignant pleural processes and their presence is not use-ful in distinguishing between the two. A superficial entrap-ment of mesothelial cells in an area of inflammatory fibrin deposition is common in benign processes and is not syn-onymous with true invasion. Likewise, invasion of stroma and fat by inflammatory cells can be found with benign or malignant proliferation. Densely packed mesothelial cells in the pleural space are consistent with benign disease, but if they are found within the stroma, they are more suggestive of mesothelioma.[44] The presence of branching glands and papillae is suggestive of malignancy. Necrosis occurs more commonly with a malignant process, but can be seen in benign processes, especially after talc poudrage. Keratin staining is useful for assessing penetration of mesothelial cells into the stroma or adjacent structures, but cannot be

used for the differentiation of malignant mesothelioma from benign proliferations, since both are keratin positive.

The three histological subtypes of malignant mesothe-lioma are classified according to the relative proportion of epithelial and spindle cells. These are the epithelial, spindle (sarcomatoid), and mixed (epithelial and sarcomatoid) sub-types. The epithelial type (Figure 30-4) accounts for more than 50% of all cases of mesothelioma; its subtypes include tubular, papillary, solid, large/giant cell, small cell, clear cell, signet cell, glandular, microcystic, myxoid, and adenoid cys-tic.[4,50] About 15–20% of all mesotheliomas are sarcoma-toid,[17] which should be differentiated from primary and secondary pleural-based sarcomas and spindle cell carcino-mas.[74a] The sarcomatoid type (Figure 30-5) is characterized by ovoid-to-spindle-shaped cells similar to cells seen in fibrosarcomas.

In a recent study, Suzuki reviewed the pathological spec-imens in 1517 mesothelioma patients. The data included 436 insulation workers, 20 UNARCO workers, 225 Cancer and Leukemia Group B (CALGB) cases, some mesothe-lioma panel cases, and 836 random cases. The cell type was documented in 1511 of the 1517 cases, with the majority

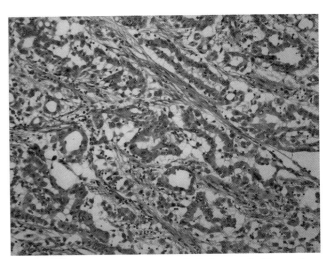

Figure 30–4 Photograph of epithelial mesothelioma. Low-power magnification of epithelial type mesothelioma, with apparent glandular formation mimicking adenocarcinoma.

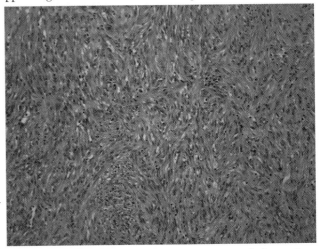

Figure 30–5 Photograph of sarcomatoid mesothelioma. Low-power magnification of sarcomatoid mesothelioma.

480 representing the epithelial cell type (930; 61.5%), followed by biphasic (334; 22.1%) and fibrosarcomatous (247; 16.4%). The latency period in Suzuki's series was longer than 20 years in 98.1% of the 800 documented cases.[164]

Mesothelioma cells derived from the mesothelium consist of glands and tubules that imitate adenocarcinoma, whereas malignant cells originating from the deep connective tissue of the mesothelial surface resemble fibrosarcoma. If only the epithelial components are apparent, differentiation from adenocarcinoma may be very difficult.[170] Microscopically, malignant mesothelioma displays large spherical cells arranged in solid masses and columns mostly within lymphatics. As with adenocarcinoma, there may be glandular formation. The cells are more regular and uniform than those of adenocarcinoma. The dominance of cuboidal cells favors the diagnosis of mesothelioma, whereas columnar-shaped cells, as well as cellular crowding and nuclear molding, are suggestive of adenocarcinoma.[16] In malignant mesothelioma, the cells are more frequently binucleated or multinucleated and arranged in clumps, and the nuclear and nucleolar sizes are proportionally larger.[16]

Electron microscopy may aid in the differentiation of mesothelioma from adenocarcinoma. Mesothelial cells possess long microvilli (Figure 30-6), possibly in contact with extracellular collagen as the basement membranes are incomplete. They often contain cytoplasmic glycogen, lipid, and bundles of intermediate filaments. Adenocarcinoma cells possess short microvilli and a cytoplasm with secretory vesicles. The basement membrane underlying adenocarcinoma cells has a more complete structure than that underlying mesothelioma cells.[56] MPM demonstrates large numbers of desmosomes, tonofilaments, and long slender branching microvilli, whereas adenocarcinomas have fewer desmosomes and tonofilaments, and short, stubby unbranched microvilli.[116] The length-to-diameter ratio (LDR) of microvilli can be used to make this differentiation. Whereas LDR ≥15 is suggestive of mesothelioma, LDR ≤10 is more suggestive of adenocarcinoma.[182]

Histochemistry is useful in distinguishing mesothelioma from adenocarcinoma. Periodic acid–Schiff (PAS) stains neutral mucopolysaccharides found in secretory vacuoles in adenocarcinomas, whereas these are usually absent in mesothelioma specimens. Mayer's mucicarmine stain (also a mucopolysaccharide stain) is likewise usually strongly positive in adenocarcinoma and negative in mesothelioma. The presence of hyaluronic acid strongly supports the diagnosis of mesothelioma. The reliability of these stains depends upon appropriate fixation and other technical details, which may vary from laboratory to laboratory.

Immunohistochemistry

There is no single immunohistochemical marker that has sufficient specificity and sensitivity to differentiate among mesothelioma, adenocarcinoma, sarcoma, and reactive mesothelial hyperplasia. A panel of immunohistochemical markers is currently employed to aid in the differentiation.[128] The immunohistochemical profile, after evaluation with light and electron microscopy, is usually required to establish a diagnosis. Antibodies such as carcinoembryonic antigen (CEA), calretinin, and cytokeratin have gained widespread use. CEA is highly specific in differentiating adenocarcinoma from mesothelioma; 2% of mesothelioma specimens do show some positive staining for CEA. Low-molecular-weight cytokeratins can be found in all histological subtypes of mesothelioma, whereas the high-molecular-weight cytokeratins are present only in the epithelial type.[18] Cytokeratin subtypes 5 and 6 are moderately specific for MPM.[115] LeuM1 (CD15) is not found in mesothelioma, and positivity strongly argues against the diagnosis. Calretinin has also demonstrated good specificity for mesothelial cells.[90] Immunostaining for BerEP4 was initially believed to be highly specific for non-mesothelial pleural tumors. More recently, deficiencies of this stain have become apparent. Ordonez found reactivity in 84–100% of pulmonary and nonpulmonary adenocarcinomas, but also in 26% of mesothelioma specimens.[115]

Recently, two additional stains have been employed to distinguish adenocarcinoma from mesothelioma: TTF-1 (thyroid transcription factor-1) and E-cadherin. In a study of 41 malignant mesotheliomas and 35 lung adenocarcinomas, all mesothelioma specimens were negative for TTF-1 and all adenocarcinoma specimens were positive for E-cadherin.[1] The authors of this study recommend starting with staining for TTF-1 and E-cadherin, and proceeding, if necessary, to a secondary panel of antibodies, including BerEP4, LeuM1 (CD15), calretinin, cytokeratin 5/6, and N-cadherin. A summary of conventional and new immunohistochemical staining patterns for mesothelioma is given in Tables 30-1 and 30-2.

Bueno et al recently employed the novel technique of microarray RNA profiling in an attempt to distinguish mesothelioma from adenocarcinoma.[67] A large number of gene products can be evaluated, and comparisons of the relative levels of these products can be used to estimate the likelihood of diagnosis of either mesothelioma or adenocarcinoma. They report about 95–99% accuracy in diagnosing MPM and adenocarcinoma. This technique represents an exciting and potentially powerful tool in the diagnosis of malignant pleural mesothelioma.

Staging

Accurate staging is important in selecting appropriate therapy, in determining a prognosis, and in accurately evaluating the effectiveness of new therapies. A variety of staging

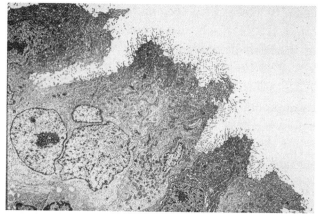

Figure 30–6 **Electron micrograph of mesothelioma.** Electron microscopy of mesothelioma showing characteristic long microvilli.

Table 30–1

Comparison of Conventional Antibodies with New Antibodies in Mesothelioma[a]

Antibody/antigen[b]	Positive (%)	Negative (%)
CEA	2	98
BerEP4	7	93
HBME-1	63	37
LeuM1 (CD15)	0	100
Calretinen	80	20
Cytokeratin 5/6	63	37
E-cadherin	22	78
N-cadherin	78	22
SP-A	98	2
SP-A	98	2
Thrombomodulin	53	47
TTF-1	0	100

[a]Reproduced with permission from: Abutaily AS, Addis BJ, Roche WR: Immunohistochemistry in the distinction between malignant mesothelioma and pulmonary adenocarcinoma: A critical evaluation of new antibodies. J Clin Pathol 55:662–668, 2002.

[b]CEA, carcinoembryonic antigen; SP-A, surfactant apoprotein A; TTF-1, thyroid transcription factor 1.

systems have evolved. These include the Butchart staging system (Table 30-3),[33] the TNM staging system proposed by the Union Internationale Contre le Cancer (UICC) (Table 30-4),[136] the International Mesothelioma Interest Group (IMIG) staging system based on TNM status (Table 30-5),[139] and the Brigham and Women's Hospital/Dana Farber Cancer Institute Modified Staging System (Table 30-6).[157]

Butchart's staging system was first proposed in 1976, and was evaluated in a relatively small cohort of patients (Table 30-3).[33] Many clinicians continue to use it for its simplicity. Stage I disease in Butchart's system describes a tumor involving the pleural envelope, lung, pericardium, and diaphragm. Stage II disease extends to the chest wall, esophagus, heart, and contralateral pleura, with or without thoracic lymph node involvement. Stage III tumors invade through the diaphragm into the peritoneum or have extrathoracic lymph node involve-

ment. Stage IV disease is associated with the presence of distant metastases. Unfortunately, Butchart's system fails to provide any information predictive for survival and prognosis. It also fails to take into account the intricacies of patterns of spread, since anything beyond stage I is unresectable.

The UICC also proposed a TNM-based staging system (Table 30-4), which provides a more detailed description of tumor size (T) than prior systems. However, mesothelioma can invade beyond the boundaries proposed by this system, making the T variable inapplicable in some cases. The nodal status follows the same guidelines used for non-small-cell lung cancer, described by the same group (UICC). Considering the locally aggressive nature of malignant pleural mesothelioma, with its tendency to completely fill the pleural space, nodal status can be difficult to evaluate. The M status is rarely encountered, owing to the very short survival time of patients with malignant mesothelioma. Thus, the UICC system fails to correlate with patient survival and prognosis of the disease, and thus most clinicians have abandoned this staging system.

The IMIG, at a meeting in June 1994, proposed another staging system utilizing TNM status (Table 30-5).[139] This system attempts to reconcile the unique characteristics of MPM with the universally accepted TNM system. T_{1a} refers to the involvement of ipsilateral parietal pleura with or without diaphragmatic involvement; T_{1b} tumor involves the visceral pleura. T_2 is tumor that invades the lung parenchyma to the extent that the tumor cannot be fully removed without resecting the underlying lung. There may also be involvement of diaphragmatic muscle, fissure, pulmonary parenchyma, or pleural effusion. T_3 tumors are more advanced, but are still amenable to surgical resection. There is invasion of the endothoracic fascia, mediastinal fat, localized chest wall, or pericardium. T_4 tumors are unresectable and consist of diffuse invasion of tumor into the chest wall through the diaphragm and into underlying peritoneum, or direct extension to the contralateral side, mediastinal organs, the spine, internal surface of the pericardium, or myocardium. N_1 tumors involve the ipsilateral bronchopulmonary and hilar lymph nodes, and N_2 describes the involvement of the subcarinal and ipsilateral mediastinal as well as ipsilateral mammary nodes. N_3 tumors metastasize to the contralateral side or ipsilateral/contralateral supraclavicular lymph nodes.[139] The IMIG staging system presumes that thoracoscopy, thoracotomy, and mediastinoscopy will be used for staging whenever possible.

The Brigham and Women's Hospital/Dana Farber Cancer Institute staging system proposed by Sugarbaker et al[157] (Table 30-6) is based on prognostic factor analysis in 52 patients treated with comprehensive trimodality therapy. It is thus directed at the unique pattern of spread, prognosis, and treatment of mesothelioma. This system stratifies patients according to survival and accounts for the following variables: resectability, tumor histology, and nodal status. It is comprised of four stages:

Stage I: resectable tumors without lymph node involvement.
Stage II: resectable tumors with lymph node involvement.
Stage III: tumors that have been rendered unresectable as a result of tumor invading the mediastinum or through the diaphragm.
Stage IV: tumors associated with extrathoracic metastasis.

Subsequent analysis in a series of 120 patients at our institution has confirmed the validity of this system.[158]

Table 30–2

Percentages of Tumors Labeling with New Antibodies and Staining Patterns[a]

Antibody/ antigen[b]	Adenocarcinoma			Mesothelioma		
	Positive (%)	Negative (%)	Staining pattern	Positive	Negative (%)	Staining pattern (%)
Calretinin	6	94	Cytoplasm and nuclei	80	20	Cytoplasm and nuclei
Cytokeratin 5/6	6	94	Pericellular and cytoplasm	63	37	72% pericellular and cytoplasmic 28% cytoplasm only
E-cadherin	100	0	Cell membrane	22	78	Cell membrane
N-cadherin	26	74	22% cell membrane	78	22	22% membrane 78% cytoplasm 31% cytoplasm 47% both
SP-A	100	0	26% cell membrane	98	2	82% membrane 74% cytoplasm 18% cytoplasm
Thrombomodulin	6	94	Cell membrane	53	47	Cell membrane
TTF-1	69	31	Nuclear	0	100	

[a]Reproduced with permission from Abutaily AS, Addis BJ, Roche WR: Immunohistochemistry in the distinction between malignant mesothelioma and pulmonary adenocarcinoma: A critical evaluation of new antibodies. J Clin Pathol 55:662–668, 2002.
SP-A, surfactant apoprotein A; TTF-1, thyroid transcription factor 1.

Prognosis

Although there is no universally accepted staging system, all of the current staging systems recognize the prognostic importance of T status, N status, and M status. Aside from stage, several independent prognostic variables are important: age, performance status, and histological type. Less important negative prognostic variables include chest pain, dyspnea, presence of pleural effusion, asbestos exposure, weight loss, low hemoglobin level, high white blood cell count, platelet count >400, and lactate dehydrogenase level >500 IU/liter.[75]

The median survival without treatment ranges between 4 and 12 months.[42,89,134] The most common mode of death is respiratory failure or pneumonia. Other causes of death include small bowel obstruction from direct invasion, as well as myocardial invasion.[9] The most recent study on the natural history of mesothelioma treated with palliative intent shows the median survival to be only 7 months. In this Canadian study some patients received talc pleurodesis, some radiation, and some chemotherapy. None underwent pleurectomy or extrapleural pneumonectomy. Epithelial histology was an independent predictor of improved survival in this group.[104] In the absence of randomized trials, the 7-month survival represents a benchmark of best medical therapy against which surgical and multimodality therapies can be measured.

Table 30–3

Butchart Staging System[a]

Stage	Definition
I	Within the capsule of the parietal pleura: ipsilateral pleura, lung, pericardium, diaphragm
II	Invading the chest wall or mediastinum: esophagus, heart, opposite pleura, positive lymph node within the chest
III	Through the diaphragm to peritoneum; opposite pleura, positive lymph node outside the chest
IV	Distant blood-borne metastases

[a]Reproduced with permission from Butchart EG, Ashcroft T, Barnsley WC, et al: Pleuropneumonectomy in the management of diffuse malignant mesothelioma of the pleura. Experience with 29 patients. Thorax 31:15–24, 1976.

Table 30–4

UICC Staging System Proposed by Union Internationale Contre le Cancer[a]

T: Primary tumor and extent

T_x: Primary tumor cannot be assessed

T_0: No evidence of primary tumor

T_1: Primary tumor limited to ipsilateral parietal or visceral pleura

T_2: Tumor invades to any of the following organs: ipsilateral lung, endothoracic fascia, diaphragm, pericardium

T_3: Tumor invades any of the following: ipsilateral chest wall muscle, ribs, mediastinal organs or tissue

T_4: Tumor extends any of the following: contralateral pleura or lung by direct extension, peritoneum or intraabdominal organs by direct extension, cervical tissue

N: Lymph nodes

N_x: Regional lymph node cannot be assessed

N_0: No regional lymph node metastases

N_1: Metastases in ipsilateral bronchopulmonary or hilar lymph nodes

N_2: Metastases in ipsilateral mediastinal lymph nodes

N_3: Metastases in contralateral mediastinal, internal mammary, supraclavicular, or scalene lymph nodes

M: Metastases

M_x: Presence of distant metastases cannot be assessed

M_0: No (known) distant metastases

M_1: Distant metastases present

Table 30–4

UICC Staging System Proposed by Union Internationale Contre le Cancer[a]—cont'd

Staging
Stage I: T_1, N_0, M_0
           T_2, N_0, M_0
Stage II: T_1, N_1, M_0
           T_2, N_1, M_0
Stage III: T_3, N_0, M_0
           T_3, N_1, M_0
           T_1, N_2, M_0
           T_2, N_2, M_0
           T_3, N_2, M_0
Stage IV: Any T, N_3, M_0
           T_4, any N, M_0
           Any T, any N, M_1

[a] Reproduced with permission from Rusch VW, Ginsberg RJ: New concepts in the staging of mesothelioma. Invited comment to Chapter 26. In Deslauriers J, Lacquet LK, editors: Thoracic Surgery: Surgical Management of Pleural Diseases, International Trends in Thoracic Surgery, Vol. 6. St. Louis: C. V. Mosby, 1990, pp. 336–343.

Table 30–5

New International Staging System for Diffuse Malignant Pleural Mesothelioma (International Mesothelioma Interest Group)[a]

T_1
T_{1a}: Tumor limited to the ipsilateral parietal pleura, including mediastinal and diaphragmatic pleura; no involvement of visceral pleura
T_{1b}: Tumor involving the ipsilateral parietal pleura, including mediastinal and diaphragmatic pleura; scattered foci of tumor also involving the visceral pleura

T_2: Tumor involving each of the ipsilateral pleura surfaces (parietal, mediastinal, diaphragmatic, and visceral pleura) associated with one of the following aspects:
  Involvement of diaphragmatic muscle
  Confluent visceral pleural tumor (including the fissures) or extension of the tumor from the visceral pleura into the underlying pulmonary parenchyma

T_3: Describes locally advanced but potentially resectable tumor
  Tumor involving all of the ipsilateral pleural surfaces (parietal, mediastinal, diaphragmatic, and visceral pleura) with one or more of the following features:
    Involvement of the endothoracic fascia
    Extension into the mediastinal fat
    Solitary, completely resectable focus of tumor extending into the soft tissue of the chest wall
    Nontransmural involvement of the pericardium

484

Table 30-5

New International Staging System for Diffuse Malignant Pleural Mesothelioma (International Mesothelioma Interest Group)[a]—cont'd

T_4:   Locally advanced and technically unresectable tumor
    Tumor involving all of the ipsilateral pleural surfaces (parietal, mediastinal, diaphragmatic, and visceral) with one or more of the following aspects:
    Diffuse extension or multifocal masses of the tumor in the chest wall, with or without rib destruction
    Direct transdiaphragmatic extension of the tumor to the peritoneum
    Direct extension of the tumor to the contralateral pleura
    Direct extension of the tumor to one or more mediastinal organs
    Direct extension of the tumor into the spine
    Tumor extending through to the internal surface of the pericardium with or without a pericardial effusion, or tumor involving the myocardium

N: Lymph nodes
    N_x: Regional lymph node cannot be assessed
    N_0: No regional lymph node metastases
    N_1: Metastases in the ipsilateral bronchopulmonary or hilar lymph nodes
    N_2: Metastases in the subcarinal or ipsilateral mediastinal lymph nodes, including the ipsilateral internal mammary nodes
    N_3: Metastases in the contralateral mediastinal, contralateral mammary, ipsilateral, or contralateral supraclavicular lymph nodes

M: Metastases
    M_x: Distance metastases cannot be assessed
    M_0: No distant metastases
    M_1: Distant metastases present

Stage I: Ia: $T_{1a}N_0M_0$
             Ib: $T_{1b}N_0M_0$
Stage II: $T_2N_0M_0$
Stage III: Any T_3M_0
             Any N_1M_0
             Any N_2M_0
Stage IV: Any T_4
             Any N_3
             Any M_1

[a]Reproduced with permission from Rusch VW: A proposed new international TNM staging system for malignant pleural mesothelioma. From the International Mesothelioma Interest Group. Chest 108:1122–1128, 1995.

Table 30-6

Brigham and Women's Hospital/DFCI Staging System

Stage	Definition
I	Disease confined to capsule of the parietal pleura: ipsilateral pleura, lung, pericardium, diaphragm, or chest wall disease limited to prior biopsy site
II	All of Stage I with positive intrathoracic (N_1 or N_2) lymph nodes
III	Local extension of disease into chest wall or mediastinum; heart, or through diaphragm, peritoneum; with or without extrathoracic or contralateral (N_3) lymph node involvement
IV	Distant metastatic disease

Treatment

Radiation Therapy

The radiosensitivity of mesothelioma cells is modest. It is more radiosensitive than non-small-cell lung cancer, but less sensitive than small-cell cancer.[39] The effectiveness of radiation therapy in the treatment of MPM, however, is limited by the diffuse nature of the tumor and by the radiosensitivity of adjacent vital structures. Radiation limits of adjacent vital structures include lung (20 Gy), liver (30 Gy), spinal cord (45 Gy), heart (45 Gy), and esophagus (50 Gy). Radiation pneumonitis and esophagitis are not infrequent complications. Myelitis and hepatitis are less common.[78]

No large studies have compared radiation to no treatment, and thus it is difficult to assess the solitary value of radiation therapy in altering the course of the disease.

Successful palliation has been seen in small groups of patients, and generally requires the application of greater than 40 Gy to the hemithorax. In a study of 23 patients by Ball and Cruickshank, those patients receiving less than 40 Gy did not have effective palliation, while the majority treated with higher doses were palliated.[15] A study by the Joint Center for Radiation Therapy in Boston reviewing radiation treatments in 29 patients confirmed that a dose of 40 Gy seemed necessary for palliation.[68]

Radiation is effective in the prevention of local recurrence after thoracentesis or thoracoscopic biopsy. A prospective, randomized trial of radiation delivered to needle biopsy and thoracoscopy port sites showed that 0 of 20 patients developed site metastases after directed radiation, whereas 8 of 20 control patients developed site metastases. Treatment within 15 days of the procedure was required.[27] Radiation is usually ineffective in controlling disease after partial surgical resections. Dosages must be limited to 20 Gy because of toxicity to the remaining lung. Only one of eight patients received adequate local control when treated in this manner following failed surgical excision.[27]

Two thirds of all recurrences following extrapleural pneumonectomy occur in the ipsilateral hemithorax. In a nonrandomized trial, 31% of patients treated with radiation had a local recurrence, whereas 45% of patients not treated had such recurrence (the difference was not statistically significant). Postoperative radiation was found to possibly benefit patients with positive resection margins; those with negative margins did not show any decrease in local recurrence after postoperative radiation.[14] Radiation therapy is employed following extrapleural pneumonectomy as part of multimodality therapy at the Brigham and Women's Hospital. A dose of 30 Gy is delivered to the postpneumonectomy hemithorax, and 40 Gy is delivered to the mediastinum. Larger doses to the hemithorax are avoided as they have been associated with significant neutropenia from marrow suppression of the entire hemithorax. A boost dose of 5 Gy may be given for positive margins or nodes. Higher doses have been recommended by Yajnik et al, from the Memorial Sloan-Kettering Cancer Center. Hemithoracic radiation (median dose: 54 Gy, range: 45–54 Gy) after extrapleural pneumonectomy (EPP) in 35 patients demonstrated excellent local control. The radiation therapy targeted the entire hemithorax, including the pleural folds as well as the thoracotomy and chest tube incision sites. The total dose of 5400 cGy was delivered in 30 fractions of 180 cGy. There were no major complications. The authors concluded that high-dose hemithoracic radiation therapy following EPP was effective and well tolerated. The dose distributions were adequate, using a combined photon and electron technique with blocking of critical normal structures.[187]

Chemotherapy

Mesothelioma is relatively chemoresistant. Most chemotherapeutic agents have demonstrated response rates less than 20%. No single agent has been shown to have an effect on overall survival. As single agents, only the antimetabolites, anthracyclines, and platinum compounds appear to be active. Anthracyclines, including doxorubicin, mitomycin, epirubicin, pirarubicin, and detorubicin, have shown response rates between 11% and 26% as solitary agents. Epirubicin at a dose of 110 mg/m² every 3 weeks had a response rate of 15%, with side effects of myelosupression and gastrointestinal toxicity. A study of detorubicin in 35 patients yielded a 26% response rate, higher than that for doxorubicin.[12] The antimetabolite methotrexate given at a dose of 3000 mg every 10 days with leucovorin rescue showed a 37% response rate in a phase II trial of 63 patients. Toxicity was seen in 58% of patients.[150]

The platinum analogs, cisplatin and carboplatin, have response rates of 14% and 11% respectively. One third of patients receiving cisplatin at a dose of 100 mg/m² every 23 weeks discontinued treatment owing to side effects. Carboplatin at a dose of 400 mg/m² every 4 weeks was somewhat better tolerated without any improvement in response rate.[12] The effectiveness of individual chemotherapeutic regimens is summarized in Table 30-7. Combination chemotherapy is generally not much more effective than single agent therapy. A trial combining three of the more active chemotherapeutic agents (cisplatin, doxorubicin, and mitomycin C) resulted in a response rate of 21%, which is not better than any of the single agents alone. In a CALGB randomized trial of cisplatin and doxorubicin vs. cisplatin and mitomycin each arm had a response rate of only 13%.[43]

Table 30–7

Single-Agent Response Rates in Malignant Mesothelioma with More Than Five Patients[a]

Agent	Evaluable	Responding	Response rate (%)
Anthracyclines and related compounds			
Doxorubicin	164	29	18
Pirarubicin	85	11	12
Epirubicin	69	8	43
Detorubicin	21	9	10
Actinomycin D	10	1	5
Menogaril	22	1	3
Mitoxantrone	34	1	
Alkylating agents			
Cyclophosphamide	14	4	28
Ifosfamide	82	8	10
Mechlorethamine	6	2	
Thiotepa	7	1	
Melphalan	3	2	
Procarbazine	6	2	
Mitomycin C	12	2	17
Cisplatin	56	8	14
Cisplatin (weekly)	9	4	44
Carboplatin	97	11 (2 CRs)	11
Carboplatin	7	0	
Vincas and related compounds			
Vincristine	23	0	
Etoposide	51	3	6
Vindesine	37	1	3
Antimetabolites			
5-Fluorouracil	28	4	14
Methotrexate, high dose	69	26	38
	60	22	
Didezazfolic acid (CB3717)	18	1	6
5-Azacytidine	7	0	
Dihydro-5-azacytidine	55	4 (1 CR)	7
Bleomycin	6	1	
Trimetrexate	52	6	12
Miscellaneous			
AMSA	19	1	5
Cyclolencine	7	2	
AZQ	20	0	0
Biologicals			
BCG (after surgery)	30	Inevaluable	
RNA (intrapleural)	10	8	80

Table 30-7

Single-Agent Response Rates in Malignant Mesothelioma with More Than Five Patients[a]—cont'd

Agent	Evaluable	Responding	Response rate (%)
Interferon			
α	38	4	11
β	14	0	
γ (intrapleural)	99	24 (7 CRS)	24
γ (intrapleural)	89	17	20
Interleukin-2			
(intrapleural)	24	10	42
Doxorubicin-containing combinations with			
5-Azacytidine	36	8	27
Ifosfamide	49	12	24
Cisplatin	60	17	28
Cisplatin, bleomycin, mitomycin	25	(1 CR)11	44
Cyclophosphamide +/− DTIC[b]	81	6	7
Cyclophosphamide, DTIC, vincristine	30	8	21
Interferon	25	4	16
Radiotherapy	24	4	16
Non-doxorubicin-containing combinations			
Epirubicin, ifosfamide	17	1	6
Cisplatin, etoposide	26	3	12
Cisplatin, pirarubicin	39	6	15
Cisplatin, vinblastine	20	5	25
Cisplatin, mitomycin C	32	10	31
Cisplatin, mitomycin C, interferon-α	19	2	11
Rubidizone, DTIC	23	0	0

[a]Reproduced with permission from Antman KH, Pass HI, Schiff PB: Benign and malignant mesothelioma. In De Vita D, Hellman S, Rosenberg S, editors: Principles and Practice of Oncology. Philadelphia: Lippincott-Raven, 1997, pp. 1853–1978.

[b]DTIC, dacarbazine.

Gemcitabine, a pyrimidine antimetabolite, is ineffective when used as a single agent. In combination with cisplatin, however, there is increased activity. A regimen of cisplatin 100 mg/m² followed by gemcitabine at 1000 mg/m² for a total of six cycles resulted in an initially promising response rate of 48%. Toxicity included nausea and vomiting in 21% and leucopenia in 36%.[34] A subsequent multicenter trial led by the same group with 53 patients, however, showed a response rate of only 26%.

Intrapleural drug delivery can achieve a high local drug concentration with less systemic toxicity. In theory, this should result in more effective delivery of medication with fewer side effects. Studies investigating the effect of combined intrapleural and systemic chemotherapy, however, have shown no improvement in the locoregional recurrence rate over systemic chemotherapy alone.[126,135]

Recently, pemetrexed (Alimta) has been introduced for the treatment of malignant mesothelioma. It is an antifolate that inhibits the enzymes thymidylate synthase, dihydrofolate reductase, and glycinamide ribonucleotide formyltransferase.[144] A phase I study of pemetrexed in combination with cisplatin showed a remarkable response rate of approximately 50% in patients with the epithelial subtype of MPM.[173] Hughes et al[80] conducted a phase II study with 27 patients to determine the maximum tolerated dose (MTD) of combined pemetrexed and carboplatin, as well as their efficacy. The recommended dose of the combination is for pemetrexed 500 mg/m² and for carboplatin AUC 5 mg/ml•min. The combination seemed to be active and well tolerated in MPM. The main toxicity was short-term neutropenia.[80] A phase III trial[176] compared the efficacy of the pemetrexed and cisplatin combination with cisplatin alone. A total of 456 patients with no prior therapy were recruited for the study. Of this total, 226 received pemetrexed and cisplatin and 222 received cisplatin alone. The patients who did not get therapy served as the controls. These patients were not eligible for surgery. Median survival varied from 12.1 months after pemetrexed/cisplatin therapy versus 9.3 months in the control group. The response rate of 51.3% in the pemetrexed/cisplatin group was significantly higher than the control group, which had a 16.7% response rate. Folic acid and vitamin B$_{12}$ supplementation was found to significantly reduce toxicity. Moreover, the combination of pemetrexed, cisplatin, and vitamin supplementation was shown to improve mean survival.[176]

Surgery

Achieving a cure for malignant pleural mesothelioma is difficult, even with maximal therapy including aggressive surgery, radiation, and chemotherapy. Palliation and improved survival, however, are common with appropriately aggressive treatment. Pleurodesis is typically less effective for MPM than for other malignant effusions because the effusions are typically loculated, and tumor encasement of the lung prevents lung expansion. Pleurodesis often requires pleurectomy in order to free up the entrapped lung so that it can expand and fuse with the chest wall. Even complete pleurectomy will leave some disease in the fissures, and thus it is a palliative, rather than curative operation. The same can be said for extrapleural pneumonectomy in diffuse MPM, though extrapleural pneumonectomy is a more effective cytoreductive procedure than pleurectomy. Even when the tumor appears to be contained within the pleural envelope, however, there are often microscopic areas left in the chest wall, around the great vessels, esophagus, or at the diaphragmatic insertions. Thus extrapleural pneumonectomy, although having the capacity for cure, is, more often than not, a palliative procedure. Postresection topical therapy, including intraoperative heated chemotherapy, is an attempt to treat residual disease. Pleurectomy and extrapleural pneumonectomy are effective in palliation and in improving survival over best supportive care.

Preoperative Evaluation

The preoperative evaluation should include chest CT, MRI, echocardiography, pulmonary function testing including DL_{CO}, and differential $\dot{V}/\dot{Q}$ scan. CT and MRI are used to define the anatomical extent of the tumor. Echocardiography may show invasion into heart, will reveal any significant valvular disease, and can estimate pulmonary artery pressures. Great care must be used in performing pneumonectomy in patients with systolic pulmonary artery pressures greater than 40–45. Patients are candidates for resectional therapy if the tumor has not spread outside the hemithorax, if there is no or minimal invasion into the chest wall, and if there is no invasion into vital structures such as great vessels, myocardium, or esophagus. Patients are considered for EPP provided their Karnofsky performance status is greater than 70, their creatinine is <1.5, left ventricular ejection fraction >45%, the predicted FEV_1 >1 liter, Pco_2 <45, and Po_2 >65 mm Hg.[159] The eligibility criteria for EPP are summarized in Table 30-8. Patients who do not meet the above criteria are often candidates for pleurectomy. The most common reason for exclusion from extrapleural pneumonectomy is disease not amenable to complete gross resection, followed by poor pulmonary function, and, less often, comorbid disease.

Technical Aspects of Extrapleural Pneumonectomy

Right Side After induction of anesthesia, a double-lumen tube is introduced. The patient is positioned in a left lateral decubitus position. Placement of a nasogastric tube facilitates palpation of the esophagus and empties the stomach to prevent aspiration. Routine monitoring includes an arterial line, pulse oximeter, and central venous pressure line. An epidural catheter is used for postoperative pain management. If there is a suspicion of transdiaphragmatic invasion into the peritoneal space, laparoscopy or a small limited laparotomy should be performed prior to thoracotomy.

The incision has to provide access to the apex of the chest, as well as the diaphragm. An extended right posterolateral thoracotomy is created. The incision extends from midway between the posterior scapula and the spine, under the tip of the scapula, along the course of the sixth rib to the costochondral junction. The latissimus and serratus muscles are divided (Figure 30-7). Any prior thoracoscopy port site incisions are excised. The pleura is dissected bluntly from the chest wall, with the aid of sharp dissection as needed. The fused pleural surface is dissected away from the chest wall until there is adequate room for placement of a chest retractor. Dissection should be performed in a systematic manner, and after leaving an area of dissection, packing should be placed to limit blood loss. Sharp dissection or blunt dissection with a sponge stick can be used to extend the pleural dissection toward the apex. Superiorly, caution should be paid to the brachial triangle to avoid injury to the subclavian artery or vein. The dissection is extrapleural and the pleura should be pushed away from the azygos vein and esophagus until the right mainstem bronchus and the upper lobe appear. During the pleural dissection the surgeon needs to reorient continuously to avoid injuries to the esophagus, heart, and other mediastinal structures. Medially, attention has to be paid to mammary vessels, which should be left on the chest wall. The superior vena cava and azygos vein can be dissected free from adjacent tissue. Posteriorly,

Table 30–8	
Eligibility Criteria for Extrapulmonary Pneumonectomy	
I	Histological verification of mesothelioma via immunohistochemistry
II	Tumor contained to the ipsilateral hemithorax
III	No invasion of heart, great vessels, esophagus, or chest wall by CT and MRI
IV	Predicted postoperative FEV_1 and DL_{CO} >40%
V	Estimated pulmonary artery pressure <45 systolic; ejection fraction >45%
VI	RA ABG not required, but if done, Pco_2 <45 and Po_2 >65
VII	Absence of severe hepatic or renal dysfunction (creatinine <1.5)
VIII	Absence of ongoing angina or significant coronary artery disease

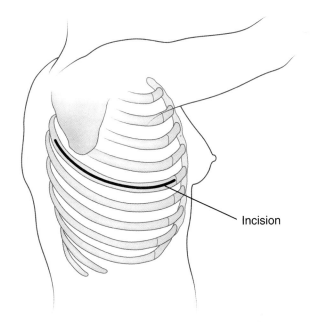

Figure 30–7 Incision for EPP. The incision extends from halfway up the height of the scapula, posteriorly, to the costal cartilage of the sixth rib, anteriorly. The latissimus and serratus are divided, and the sixth rib is removed.

488 dissection is continued with care not to avulse the intercostal vessels and to leave the esophagus unharmed (Figure 30-8).

Palpation of the stiff nasogastric tube aids in identifying the esophagus. At this point, dissection down to the hilum has been completed with the exception that the anterior dissection has stopped at the pericardium and the diaphragm has not yet been resected. If the tumor is deemed resectable,

then dissection of the diaphragm begins at the anterior border of the pericardium, and the diaphragm dissected from the chest wall is divided circumferentially. Sharp dissection of the diaphragm around the esophagus and inferior vena cava is preferred; dissection from the peritoneum can be done bluntly with a sponge stick pushing away the peritoneum (Figure 30-9). The pericardium is opened caudally and the

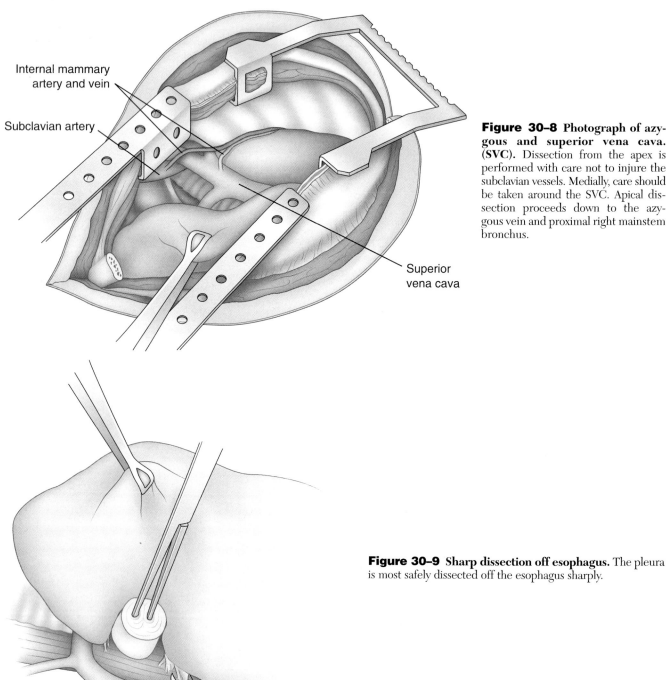

Internal mammary artery and vein

Subclavian artery

Superior vena cava

Figure 30–8 Photograph of azygous and superior vena cava. (SVC). Dissection from the apex is performed with care not to injure the subclavian vessels. Medially, care should be taken around the SVC. Apical dissection proceeds down to the azygous vein and proximal right mainstem bronchus.

Figure 30–9 Sharp dissection off esophagus. The pleura is most safely dissected off the esophagus sharply.

incision is extended to the cranial side toward the superior vena cava (Figure 30-10). The lung with pleura and diaphragm can then be pulled anteriorly, so that the posterior attachment to the pericardium can be dissected. The pericardial incision should be completed with anteromedial dissection toward the phrenic nerve and hilar vessels. The main pulmonary artery and pulmonary veins can be separated and isolated intrapericardially using a soft-flanged catheter passed around the pulmonary artery to guide the vascular stapler, avoiding traction injury (Figure 30-11) as described by Sugarbaker et al.[160] The pericardial dissection is completed by dividing the pericardium posterior to the hilum. The specimen, including the lung and pleura, can be pulled anteriorly and the dissection is then continued posterolaterally to the pericardium and esophagus. After subcarinal lymph node dissection, the bronchus is dissected and divided using a heavy

489

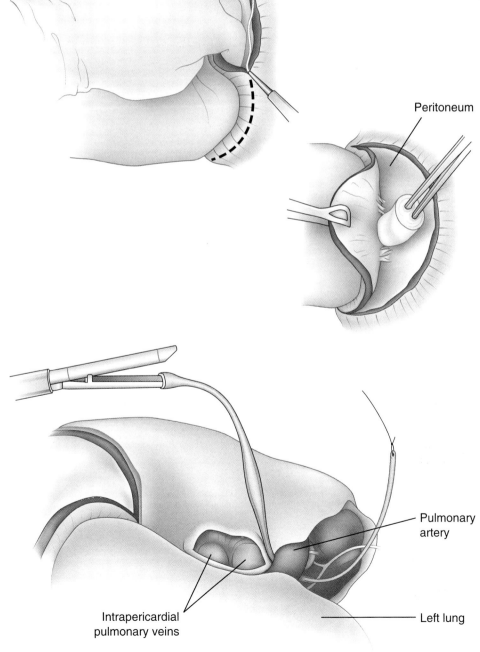

Figure 30–10 Dissection off diaphragm. Removal of the diaphragm begins anteriorly and is done bluntly, tearing the insertions off the chest wall. Attempts are made to preserve the integrity of the underlying peritoneum. Great care must be taken around the inferior vena cava hiatus.

Diaphragmatic incision

Peritoneum

Figure 30–11 Endoleader. The pulmonary vessels are taken intrapericardially, using a red rubber endoleader to aid in passing the stiff staplers around the delicate vessels.

Pulmonary artery

Intrapericardial pulmonary veins

Left lung

gauge wire bronchial stapler (Figure 30-12) (TA-30, Ethicon Endo-Surgery, Johnson & Johnson). The specimen is sent to pathology, where the status of the resection margins will be evaluated. Many sections are taken to assess the microscopic margins along the chest wall, diaphragm, mediastinal structures, and lymph nodes. The bronchial stump is covered with a piece of pericardial fat pad, which can be sewed around the stump. The diaphragm is reconstructed with a 2-mm impermeable patch (Gore-Tex, WL Gore and Associates INC, Flagstaff, AZ). The 2-0 sutures are placed circumferentially 1 cm from the edge of the patch; the awl is used to thread the sutures through the chest wall 2–3 cm away from the rib

edge. Buttons and a small piece of impermeable patch (Gore-Tex) are used to secure the patch to the chest wall and prevent the sutures from pulling through. The sutures are threaded using an intravenous angiocatheter. Excess tension should be avoided when tying the sutures. A recent advancement has been the construction of the diaphragmatic patch from two separate pieces of Gore-Tex. These two patches are sewn together peripherally, but centrally they are not sewn, leaving room for expansion and minimizing tension on the neodiaphragm. This is believed to lessen the incidence of diaphragmatic patch rupture with bowel herniation into the chest (Figure 30-13). The pericardium on the right side is

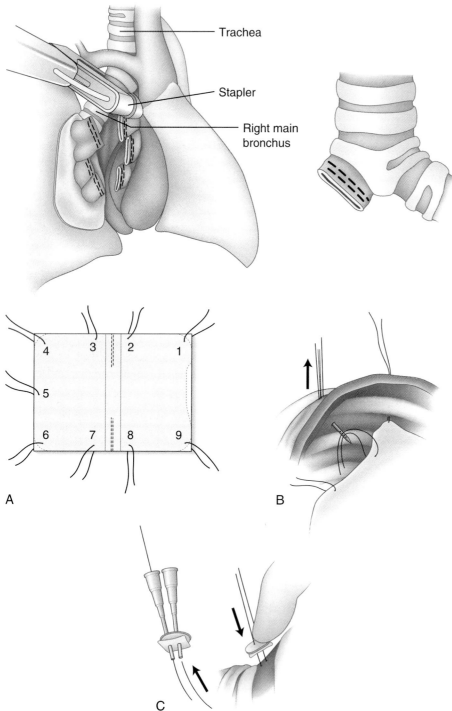

Figure 30–12 TIA 30 of bronchus. The bronchus is stapled close to the carina. After clamping down, but prior to firing the stapler, ease in ventilation of the contralateral lung must be ensured.

Figure 30–13 Diaphragm patch. Two separate 2-mm-thick Gore-Tex patches are attached (**A**) with two firings from a TA45 stapler. Securing 0 silk sutures are placed (**B**) through the patch, through the chest wall, and then tied down (**C**) over a button. The hinge creates a dynamic patch that absorbs sudden increases in abdominal pressures, lessening the risk of patch rupture.

always reconstructed with a prosthetic patch to prevent cardiac displacement and herniation. A 0.1-mm synthetic membrane (Gore-Tex, WL Gore and Associates INC, Flagstaff, AZ) is secured to posterior, inferior, and anterior pericardial margins; inferiorly it is sutured to the diaphragmatic patch. The patch must be generous, as the right heart may dilate following pneumonectomy. The pericardial patch should be fenestrated to prevent a cardiac tamponade by postoperative pericardial effusion after pericardiotomy (Figure 30-14).

Use of permeable patches in this situation can result in peritoneal fluid filling the right pneumonectomy space, leading to severe mediastinal shift or cardiac tamponade. It is also important to leave the pericardial patch loose, as a tight patch can result in constriction of the filling of heart, diastolic dysfunction, and development of an iatrogenic tamponade. Thorough hemostasis with an argon laser coagulator is necessary to decrease postoperative bleeding. The chest is closed in the usual watertight fashion. A 12-French red rubber catheter is inserted at the anterior edge of the wound to permit mediastinal positioning. After turning the patient to the supine position and before extubation, the pneumonectomy space is reduced in size by aspiration (750 cm^3 of air in women and 1000 cm^3 in men) using a 50-cm^3 syringe attached to a red rubber catheter. The mediastinum can be evaluated by follow-up chest radiographs and air may be removed or introduced as needed. The rubber catheter is removed on postoperative Day 1.

Left Side An endobronchial blocker or a right double-lumen tube is used to isolate the left lung. Anatomical differences when approaching from the left include the position of the esophagus, the presence of the aorta, and the absence of the inferior vena cava. During resection of the posterior and posteromedial plane of the aorta, attention should be paid to prevent avulsion of the intercostal vessels and dissection of the aorta, which can easily occur. The intercostal vessel should be clipped. Injury of intercostal vessels can occur during dissection of the aortodiaphragmatic hiatus, which can be prevented if care is taken to enter the correct plane during cautious dissection. The assessment of the aorta is important, as it can be the determining factor in gauging the resectability of the tumor. The esophagus should be located to prevent its injury while resecting the diaphragm. Pulmonary veins can be divided

intrapericardially. The left main pulmonary artery is usually divided extrapericardially to prevent encroachment of the main pulmonary artery. The left main bronchus must be divided and buttressed close to the carina. A short bronchial stump is favored.

The pericardium on the left side is not routinely reconstructed. The heart cannot rotate around the axis of the superior and inferior vena cava as it can on the right. Provided the amount of pericardium resected is not too small, the heart will not become entrapped in the orifice of the pericardium. The diaphragm is reconstructed in a manner similar to that for the right side. Given the smaller size of the left hemithorax, less air has to be aspirated from it at the end of the operation (500 cm^3 in women, 750 cm^3 in men).

The average blood loss is estimated to be between 500 and 750 ml. During resection of the specimen, hemostasis can be accomplished by electrocautery. After removal of lung and pleura, the argon beam coagulator can be used to coagulate the small vessels. Hemostasis is critical as postoperative bleeding is associated with high morbidity.[165]

Pleurectomy

Pleurectomy is a palliative debulking procedure used to reduce the size of the tumor. It is effective palliative therapy for patients in whom pneumonectomy is contraindicated. An identical posterolateral thoracotomy is performed. Anterior, posterior, and apical dissection of pleura from the chest wall is identical to that for extrapleural pneumonectomy. After dissection is completed down to the hilum, the thickened pleura is then separated off the lung parenchyma using a combination of blunt stripping and sharp dissection. Bleeding from the lung is controlled with high cautery and argon beam coagulation. The parietal pleura can be removed widely, whereas the mediastinal pleura cannot be entirely resected. The pleura and any disease that extends into the fissures should be removed as completely as possible, if necessary, down to the pulmonary artery in the fissure. The diaphragmatic pleura can be completely resected only if the diaphragm is resected. Reconstruction of the diaphragm is not always needed if the lung is not removed, as the inflated lung should prevent herniation of contents into the chest. Major complications of this procedure include bronchopleural fistulae,

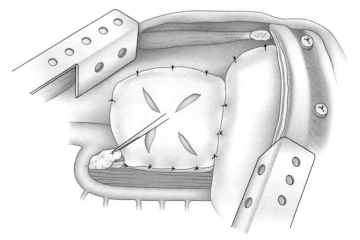

Figure 30–14 Completed pericardial and diaphragmatic patch. The pericardial patch is constructed loosely and fenestrated to prevent tamponade. A pericardial or thymic fat pad is harvested and placed over the bronchial stump.

492

hemorrhage, pneumonia, subcutaneous emphysema, empyema, and in rare cases vocal cord paralysis.[29,119]

Postoperative Management

The postoperative management includes pain management, meticulous attention to fluid status, and early diagnosis with aggressive treatment of deep venous thrombosis, pulmonary embolus, vocal cord paralysis, chylothorax, empyema, bronchopulmonary fistula, and excessive mediastinal shift.[165] Adequate pain control can minimize postoperative atelectasis. Patients are monitored in a thoracic care unit with arterial and central venous lines, oximetry, and monitoring of the ECG and respiratory rate. Anticoagulation with subcutaneous heparin and pneumatic boots is necessary to prevent the risk of deep venous thrombosis and pulmonary emboli. Forty-eight hours after extrapleural pneumonectomy, chest physical therapy and ambulation are initiated.[165]

Pulmonary edema is one of the most feared complications following pneumonectomy, and every effort is made to avoid fluid overload. Patients are given a strict fluid restriction of 1000 ml/day for the first 5 days. Active diuresis is performed until end points of either hypotension or a prerenal state are achieved. Daily chest X-rays have to be performed to evaluate the mediastinum and any lung edema or excessive shifting. The nasogastric tube is left in overnight and removed the following day provided the output is not high. Oral intake should be delayed until full gastric function is ensured, and the diet should be advanced slowly. Injury to one of the vagus nerves is not uncommon as a result of dissection near the esophagus. Aspiration can have devastating consequences in this patient population.

Operative Results

Pleurectomy and extrapleural pneumonectomy are major operations associated with significant morbidity. Several large series of pleurectomy for MPM have been reported. Allen et al reported a series of 56 patients and described a perioperative mortality rate of 5.4%, morbidity of 26.8%, and 1-year survival of 30%.[7] Achatzy et al reviewed 245 pleurectomy patients treated in Germany undergoing partial and complete pleurectomy and showed an 8.5% 30-day mortality rate and a median survival of 9.2 months.[2] At Memorial Sloan Kettering, McCormack and others looked at 64 patients and quoted a mortality rate of 1.8%, a complication rate of 25%, and 1-year survival of 49%.[101] Finally, Brancatisano et al[29] reported their series of 45 pleurectomy patients. They had a perioperative mortality rate of 2.2%, a morbidity rate of 16%, and a median survival of 16 months. They stated that 98% of pleural effusions were controlled by pleurectomy. Overall, these studies show that perioperative mortality at large U.S. centers should be less than 5%, with effective palliation and improved survival over patients treated nonsurgically.

Extrapleural pneumonectomy carries a higher perioperative mortality in most series, although the low mortality rate of 3.8% at the Brigham and Women's Hospital approaches that of pleurectomy. In the initial series published by Butchart in 1978 the perioperative mortality rate was 30%.[33] Other studies in the 1970s had similar results. Since then, several series at large academic centers have established that the operation can be done with mortality rates of less than 10%. DaValle et al recorded a mortality rate of 9%[54] and Rusch et al reported a perioperative mortality rate of 6%.[137] In the largest reported trial of EPP employing multimodality therapy, involving 183 patients, Sugarbaker et al reported a perioperative mortality rate of 3.8%.[157] Major morbidity occurred in 25% of the patients and included cardiovascular morbidity in 7 patients, pulmonary complications in 15 patients, bleeding and/or cardiac tamponade in 9, vocal cord paralysis in 10, and diaphragmatic patch rupture in 2.

Multimodality Treatment

The failure of single modality treatments to increase the survival of patients with MPM has resulted in a multimodality approach. No large randomized studies have been performed comparing either pleurectomy/decortication (P/D) with EPP or comparing surgery (P/D or EPP) to chemotherapy. Although significant discomfort (pain and shortness of breath) is caused by the inability to control local disease, a significant number of patients are found at autopsy to have metastatic disease as well. Thus, both local and systemic treatments are necessary. Treatment plans involving two modalities—chemotherapy and surgery, radiation and surgery, and chemotherapy and radiation—have shown some improvement over single modality treatment in nonrandomized studies. Radiation and chemotherapy without surgery has had very limited success.[93,148] Trials involving surgery (P/D or EPP) with radiation or chemotherapy have shown some improvement in survival vs. historical controls. Notably, between 1976 and 1988, Memorial Sloan Kettering treated 105 MPM patients with P/D combined with intraoperative brachytherapy and 42 Gy of postoperative external beam radiation. The median survival was 12.5 months. Radiation pneumonitis occurred in 18% of patients. Local relapse was the most common site of treatment failure.[135] In a later study from the same institution, Rusch et al looked at 28 patients who underwent P/D followed by intrapleural cisplatin at 100 mg/m^2 and mitomycin at 8 mg/m^2. Three to five weeks later, systemic cisplatin and mitomycin were administered. Overall survival was 68% at 1 year and 40% at 2 years. Locoregional disease was the most common site of relapse.[138] The trimodality multidisciplinary approach includes either EPP or P/D with combination radiation, systemic chemotherapy, and, most recently, intrapleural treatments. The largest series of patients undergoing trimodality therapy has been compiled at the Brigham and Women's Hospital.[157] Between 1980 and 1997, 183 patients underwent EPP followed by chemotherapy and radiation. Chemotherapy was begun 6 weeks following pneumonectomy, if the patient's condition permitted. Patients were treated with cisplatin 70 mg/m^2, doxorubicin 50–60 mg/m^2, and cyclophosphamide 600 mg/m^2. After 1995, patients received carboplatin 6 mg/m^2 and paclitaxel 200 mg/m^2. Two cycles of chemotherapy were administered 3 weeks apart, followed by radiation therapy. Three to four weeks after completion of the radiation therapy, two additional cycles of chemotherapy were given.

Radiation treatment consisted of 30 Gy delivered to the hemithorax in 1.5 Gy fractions and 40 Gy delivered to the mediastinum. Boost doses were given to areas of gross residual disease, areas of positive margins, and to regions where lymph nodes returned positive.

Perioperative (30 day) mortality was 3.8%; three of the seven deaths resulted from pulmonary embolus. The median survival of the remainder of the patients was 19 months; the 2 and 5 year survival was 38% and 15%. Five-year survival was 21% for those patients with epithelial histology; no patients with either sarcomatoid or mixed type mesothelioma lived 5 years. Epithelial type histology, clean resection margins, and negative extrapleural nodes all favored 5-year survival. Patients with all three of these variables had an impressive 5-year survival of 46%. Although the study was retrospective and did not include a control, the overall median survival of 19 months is almost three times as long as the median survival of patients treated with palliative intent only.[104]

Failure after this form of trimodality therapy was evaluated by Baldini et al.[14] Forty-nine patients undergoing EPP (35 with adjuvant chemoradiation, 14 with adjuvant chemotherapy) were followed for a median of 23 months. Twenty-five (54%) had a recurrence; the median time to first recurrence was 19 months. The ipsilateral hemithorax was the first site of recurrence in 35% of the patients, the abdomen in 26%, contralateral thorax in 17%, and distant sites in 8%. Disease in the abdomen most likely represented local spread from the chest, and thus the percent of patients suffering from failure of local control was in excess of 50%. The inability of conventional systemic chemotherapy or external beam radiation therapy led to the development of an intraoperative, intrapleural heated chemotherapy protocol at the Brigham and Women's Hospital.

Emerging Treatments

EPP and Intraoperative Hyperthermic Cisplatin Lavage (Heated Chemotherapy)

Prior attempts to control local recurrence, such as administering intrapleural chemotherapy, have neglected the abdomen as a common site of relapse. Rusch et al[137,140] and Sugarbaker et al[14,162] showed that multimodality treatments may prolong the survival of patients diagnosed at an early stage. One of the novel approaches in treatment of malignant mesothelioma is the use of intraoperative intracavitary hyperthermic chemotherapy. Hyperthermia, itself, is capable of inducing cell death. Possible mechanisms include acceleration of apoptosis, rapid cell necrosis without cycle progression, and alteration of the cell cycle.[111] The combination of hyperthermia and chemotherapy has synergistic tumoricidal effects.[172] Hyperthermia may antagonize certain drugs such as cytosine arabinoside and amsacrine,[111] but it has a synergistic effect with others such as cisplatin and mitomycin C.

The cytotoxic activity of hyperthermia has been reported by Stehlin.[153] He pioneered the use of hyperthermia for the treatment of melanoma, where its synergistic effect increases the efficacy of chemotherapy.[153] The hyperthermic effect can be confined to target areas, which makes it a suitable combination with chemotherapy following cytoreduction. Ratto et al[124] demonstrated a higher tissue concentration with hyperthermic cisplatin lavage than with normothermic perfusion. We have used a new approach, administering hyperthermic cisplatin lavage intraoperatively following EPP. After pleural pneumonectomy including diaphragm resection, cisplatin lavage is performed into both the pleural and peritoneal cavities. Sodium thiosulfate is administered intravenously at the same time in an effort to minimize nephrotoxicity. Under the nephroprotective effect of sodium thiosulfate, the cisplatin dose could be escalated without serious toxic effects (unpublished data from Brigham and Women's Hospital). Complications associated with the use of intracavitary heated cisplatin include an increased incidence of deep vein thrombosis (DVT) and diaphragmatic patch dehiscence.[161] The increased incidence of DVT may be due to the increased temperature of the pelvis and pelvic veins. The increased incidence of diaphragmatic patch dehiscence may be caused by intraabadominal swelling after local hyperthermic treatment. There was no increase in gastrointestinal complications overall. The mortality of hyperthermic bicavitary chemotherapy is comparable to EPP alone.

Antiangiogenic Therapy Three angiogenesis inhibitors are currently undergoing trials in the treatment of mesothelioma: thalidomide, SU5416, and bevacizumab. SU5416, an inhibitor of the VEGF-1 (vascular endothelial growth factor) receptor flk-1, is being studied in a National Cancer Institute (NCI) phase II trial with the end point being time to progression and objective response rate; results are pending. Thalidomide, one of the very few available oral antiangiogenic agents, is being evaluated in phase II trials at the University of Maryland and in the Netherlands. Bevacizumab is a recombinant anti-VEGF monoclonal antibody. It is being evaluated with gemcitabine and cisplatin in a randomized double blind phase II trial at M.D. Anderson, University of Chicago, and the University of Pennsylvania with the end points being time to progression and response rate.[114]

Photodynamic Therapy

Photodynamic therapy (PDT) involves the administration of a compound (photofrin) that is selectively concentrated in malignant cells. Upon exposure to light of a certain wavelength, the compound is activated, forming free radicals, resulting in cell death. Because of the limited depth of absorption of light in tissues, treatment via PDT is limited to superficial areas and may be ideally suited to the treatment of mesothelioma following debulking. Several centers have studied PDT in MPM. Takita and Dougherty reported on a phase II trial of either P/D or EPP followed by PDT. Photofrin was injected 48 h prior to the procedure, and after tumor excision, 25 J/cm² of 630-nm light was administered to the pleural space. Median survival for patients in stage I or II was 21 months.[166]

At the NCI, Pass et al performed a phase III prospective randomized trial of PDT after either P/D or EPP. Provided debulking could be performed down to 5 mm of residual tumor, the patient was randomized to receive PDT or not. Out of a total of 63 patients, 48 were randomized. Median survival was 14 months; there was no advantage in either survival or time to recurrence in the PDT group.[118]

494

Recent studies[174] have focused on optimization of such factors as drug dose, drug-light interval, fluence rate, and total light dose (or fluence) to improve the effectiveness of PTD. Tumor response correlates strongly with the drug-light interval. Oxygen consumption by photochemical reaction during PDT can cause oxygen deficit more rapidly than it can be replenished, which could limit the efficacy of PDT. A new photosensitizer, *meta*-tetrahydroxyphenylchlorin (mTHPC), has recently been introduced. Nicotinamide injection and carbogen breathing can influence tumor oxygenation and increase the tumor response for PDT after photosensitizer injection.[174]

Immunotherapy

Various immunomodulators, including interleukin-2 (IL-2), interferon (IFN)-α, IFN-β, IFN-γ, and granulocyte-macrophage colony-stimulating factor (GM-CSF), have been examined in mesothelioma patients.[177] IFN-γ and IL-2 have shown some effectiveness in small study populations. IFN-γ has been shown to have a direct cytotoxic effect on mesothelioma cells *in vitro*; it facilitates cellular differentiation and activates T lymphocytes and natural killer cells. Boutin et al administered intrapleurally 40 million units of recombinant IFN-γ in patients with Butchart's stage I and II mesothelioma. There were eight complete responders, documented by surgical biopsy, and nine additional patients had at least a 50% reduction in tumor mass. The overall response rate was 20%.[26] The same group performed a phase II trial involving intrapleural infusion of activated macrophages and IFN-γ in the treatment of MPM with limited success.[107]

IL-2, a cytokine known to stimulate T cell proliferation, has been tried in small numbers of mesothelioma patients. Astoul et al infused IL-2 intrapleurally in 22 patients over 5 days with a 50% partial response rate. Responders survived an average of 28 months, whereas nonresponders lived only an average of 8 months.[10] Their results have not been duplicated. In a different study, repeated intrapleural instillation of 9,000,000 IU IL-2 twice weekly for 4 weeks following needle thoracentesis was able to palliate pleural fluid collection in 28 of 31 (90%) patients. Pleurisy recurred only in 1 of 28 patients after 19 months. Median survival was 15 months (range 5–39) in all patients.[40]

Introducing activated macrophages and IFN-γ into the pleural space in a small series of patients with stage IA, IB, IIA disease was tolerated without major complications. The antitumor activity was modest, and the regression of tumor was far below expectation (14%). After completion of the immunotherapy, 10 patients underwent chemotherapy as their disease progressed. The median survival of patients, including those who received chemotherapy, was 29.2 months.[107] A combined immunotherapeutic and chemotherapeutic approach has been evaluated in phase I and phase II trials in mesothelioma patients, but has failed to demonstrate any convincing effect on survival or relapse rate.[73,107]

Gene Therapy

An early trial involving injection of adenoviral vectors carrying the herpes simplex virus thymidine kinase gene (HSV-tk) was performed on MPM patients. The agent was instilled into the pleural space via a chest tube. Tumor cells incorporating the gene were then susceptible to eradication via treatment by ganciclovir, which was administered in a dose of 5 mg/kg twice daily on days 6 to 20. Gene expression was verified in most patients in this study. There was a partial response rate of 4% and complete response rate of 4% in this initial group of 25 patients. Although the response rate was poor, this was an early trial and it did show successful transfection of the desired vector.[154]

REFERENCES

1. Abutaily AS, Addis BJ, Roche WR: Immunohistochemistry in the distinction between malignant mesothelioma and pulmonary adenocarcinoma: A critical evaluation of new antibodies. J Clin Pathol 55:662–668, 2002.
2. Achatzy R, Beba W, Ritschler R, et al: The diagnosis, therapy and prognosis of diffuse malignant mesothelioma. Eur J Cardiothorac Surg 3:445–447; discussion 448, 1989.
3. Adams RF, Gleeson FV: Percutaneous image-guided cutting-needle biopsy of the pleura in the presence of a suspected malignant effusion. Radiology 219:510–514, 2001.
4. Adams VI, Unni KK: Diffuse malignant mesothelioma of pleura: Diagnostic criteria based on an autopsy study. Am J Clin Pathol 82:15–23, 1984.
5. Adamson IY, Bakowska J: KGF and HGF are growth factors for mesothelial cells in pleural lavage fluid after intratracheal asbestos. Exp Lung Res 27:605–616, 2001.
6. Aisner J: Current approach to malignant mesothelioma of the pleura. Chest 107:332S–344S, 1995.
7. Allen KB, Faber LP, Warren WH: Malignant pleural mesothelioma. Extrapleural pneumonectomy and pleurectomy. Chest Surg Clin North Am 4:113–126, 1994.
8. Antman KH, Blum RH, Greenberger JS, et al: Multimodality therapy for malignant mesothelioma based on a study of natural history. Am J Med 68:356–362, 1980.
9. Antman KH, Pass HI, Schiff PB: Benign and malignant mesothelioma. In De Vita D, Hellman S, Rosenberg S, editors: Principles and Practice of Oncology. Philadelphia: Lippincott-Raven, 1997, pp. 1853–1978.
10. Astoul P, Picat-Joossen D, Viallat JR, et al: Intrapleural administration of interleukin-2 for the treatment of patients with malignant pleural mesothelioma: A Phase II study. Cancer 83:2099–2104, 1998.
11. Austin MB, Fechner RE, Roggli VL: Pleural malignant mesothelioma following Wilms' tumor. Am J Clin Pathol 86:227–230, 1986.
12. Baas P: Chemotherapy for malignant mesothelioma: From doxorubicin to vinorelbine. Semin Oncol 29:62–69, 2002.
13. Bahadori M, Liebow AA: Plasma cell granulomas of the lung. Cancer 31:191–208, 1973.
14. Baldini EH, Recht A, Strauss GM, et al: Patterns of failure after trimodality therapy for malignant pleural mesothelioma. Ann Thorac Surg 63:334–338, 1997.
15. Ball DL, Cruickshank DG: The treatment of malignant mesothelioma of the pleura: Review of a 5-year experience, with special reference to radiotherapy. Am J Clin Oncol 13:4–9, 1990.
16. Barker F, Krausz T: The pleura. In McGee JOD, editor: Oxford Textbook of Pathology, Vol. 2A. Oxford: Oxford University Press, 1992, pp. 1042–1050.
17. Battifora H, McCaughey WTE: Tumour and pseudotumor of the serosal membrane. In Atlas of Tumour Pathology, 3rd Series Fascicle 15. Washington D.C.: Armed Forces Institute of Pathology. 1995, pp. 37–47.

18. Battifora H: The pleura. In Sternberg SS, editor: Diagnostic Surgical Pathology. 1989, pp. 828–855.

18a. Beier KM, Gallup DG, Burgess R, Stock RJ: Occurrence of malignant peritoneal mesothelioma after surgery and radiation for cervical cancer. Gynecol Oncol 17:375–380, 1984.

19. Benard F, Sterman D, Smith RJ, et al: Metabolic imaging of malignant pleural mesothelioma with fluorodeoxyglucose positron emission tomography. Chest 114:713–722, 1998.

20. Bermudez E, Everitt J, Walker C: Expression of growth factor and growth factor receptor RNA in rat pleural mesothelial cells in culture. Exp Cell Res 190:91–98, 1990.

21. Bocchetta M, Di Resta I, Powers A, et al: Human mesothelial cells are unusually susceptible to simian virus 40-mediated transformation and asbestos cocarcinogenicity. Proc Natl Acad Sci USA 97:10214–10219, 2000.

22. Bolen JW, Hammar SP, McNutt MA: Reactive and neoplastic serosal tissue. A light-microscopic, ultrastructural, and immunocytochemical study. Am J Surg Pathol 10:34–47, 1986.

23. Boutin C, Astoul P, Seitz B: The role of thoracoscopy in the evaluation and management of pleural effusions. Lung 168(Suppl): 1113–1121, 1990.

24. Boutin C, Dumortier P, Rey F, et al: Black spots concentrate oncogenic asbestos fibers in the parietal pleura. Thoracoscopic and mineralogic study. Am J Respir Crit Care Med 153:444–449, 1996.

25. Boutin C, Frenay C, Astoul P: [Endoscopic diagnosis of mesothelioma]. Rev Mal Respir 16:1257–1262, 1999.

26. Boutin C, Nussbaum E, Monnet I, et al: Intrapleural treatment with recombinant gamma-interferon in early stage malignant pleural mesothelioma. Cancer 74:2460–2467, 1994.

27. Boutin C, Rey F, Viallat JR: Prevention of malignant seeding after invasive diagnostic procedures in patients with pleural mesothelioma. A randomized trial of local radiotherapy. Chest 108:754–758, 1995.

28. Boutin C, Rey F: Thoracoscopy in pleural malignant mesothelioma: A prospective study of 188 consecutive patients. Part 1: Diagnosis. Cancer 72:389–393, 1993.

29. Brancatisano RP, Joseph MG, McCaughan BC: Pleurectomy for mesothelioma. Med J Aust 154:455–457, 460, 1991.

30. Brenner J, Sordillo PP, Magill GB, et al: Malignant mesothelioma of the pleura: Review of 123 patients. Cancer 49:2431–2435, 1982.

31. Britton M: The epidemiology of mesothelioma. Semin Oncol 29:18–25, 2002.

32. Bussolino F, Di Renzo MF, Ziche M, et al: Hepatocyte growth factor is a potent angiogenic factor which stimulates endothelial cell motility and growth. J Cell Biol 119:629–641, 1992.

33. Butchart EG, Ashcroft T, Barnsley WC, et al: Pleuropneumonectomy in the management of diffuse malignant mesothelioma of the pleura. Experience with 29 patients. Thorax 31:15–24, 1976.

34. Byrne MJ, Davidson JA, Musk AW, et al: Cisplatin and gemcitabine treatment for malignant mesothelioma: A phase II study. J Clin Oncol 17:25–30, 1999.

35. Cacciotti P, Strizzi L, Vianale G, et al: The presence of simian-virus 40 sequences in mesothelioma and mesothelial cells is associated with high levels of vascular endothelial growth factor. Am J Respir Cell Mol Biol 26:189–193, 2002.

36. Carbone M, Kratzke RA, Testa JR: The pathogenesis of mesothelioma. Semin Oncol 29:2–17, 2002.

37. Carbone M, Pass HI, Rizzo P, et al: Simian virus 40-like DNA sequences in human pleural mesothelioma. Oncogene 9:1781–1790, 1994.

38. Carbone M, Rizzo P, Grimley PM, et al: Simian virus-40 large-T antigen binds p53 in human mesotheliomas. Nat Med 3:908–912, 1997.

39. Carmichael J, Degraff WG, Gamson J, et al: Radiation sensitivity of human lung cancer cell lines. Eur J Cancer Clin Oncol 25:527–534, 1989.

40. Castagneto B, Zai S, Mutti L, et al: Palliative and therapeutic activity of IL-2 immunotherapy in unresectable malignant pleural mesothelioma with pleural effusion. Results of a phase II study on 31 consecutive patients. Lung Cancer 31: 303–310, 2001.

41. Cavazza A, Travis LB, Travis WD, et al: Post-irradiation malignant mesothelioma. Cancer 77:1379–1385, 1996.

42. Chahinian AP, Ambinder RM, Mandel EM, et al: Evaluation of 63 patients with diffuse malignant mesothelioma [abstract]. Proc Am Soc Clin Oncol 21:360, 1980.

43. Chahinian AP, Antman K, Goutsou M, et al: Randomized phase II trial of cisplatin with mitomycin or doxorubicin for malignant mesothelioma by the Cancer and Leukemia Group B. J Clin Oncol 11:1559, 1993.

44. Churg A, Colby TV, Cagle P, et al: The separation of benign and malignant mesothelial proliferations. Am J Surg Pathol 24:1183–1200, 2000.

45. Churg AM: Pathology of the Lung. In Thurlbeck WM, Churg AM, editor: Disease of the Pleura, 2nd ed. New York: Thieme, 1995, pp. 1067–1110.

46. Cochrane JC, Webster I: Mesothelioma in relation to asbestos fibre exposure. A review of 70 serial cases. S Afr Med J 54:279–281, 1978.

47. Coffin D, Peters S, Palekar L, et al: A study of the biological activity of erionite in relation to its chemical and structural characteristics. In Wehner A, Felton DL, editors: Biological Interaction of Inhaled Mineral Fibers and Cigarette Smoke. Columbus, OH: Battelle Press, 1989, pp. 313–323.

48. Cole FHJ, Ellis RA, Goodman RC, et al: Benign fibrous pleural tumor with elevation of insulin-like growth factor and hypoglycemia. South Med J 83:690–694, 1990.

49. Constantopoulos SH, Goudevenos JA, Saratzis N, et al: Metsovo lung: Pleural calcification and restrictive lung function in northwestern Greece. Environmental exposure to mineral fiber as etiology. Environ Res 38:319–331, 1985.

50. Corson JM: Pathology of diffuse malignant pleural mesothelioma. Semin Thorac Cardiovasc Surg 9:347–355, 1997.

51. Crotty TB, Myers JL, Katzenstein AL, et al: Localized malignant mesothelioma. A clinicopathologic and flow cytometric study. Am J Surg Pathol 18:357–363, 1994.

52. Cullen MR: The amphibole hypothesis of asbestos-related cancer—gone but not forgotten. Am J Public Health 86:158–159, 1996.

53. Das PB, Fletcher AG, Deodhare SG: Mesothelioma in an agricultural community of India: A clinicopathological study. Aust NZ J Surg 46:218–226, 1976.

54. DaValle MJ, Faber LP, Kittle CF, et al: Extrapleural pneumonectomy for diffuse, malignant mesothelioma. Ann Thorac Surg 42:612–618, 1986.

54a. Davis JM, Addison J, Bolton RE, et al: The pathogenicity of long versus short fibre samples of amosite asbestos administered to rats by inhalation and intraperitoneal injection. Br J Exp Pathol 67:415–430, 1986.

55. Dessy E, Pietra GG: Pseudomesotheliomatous carcinoma of the lung. An immunohistochemical and ultrastructural study of three cases. Cancer 68:1747–1753, 1991.

56. Dewar A, Valente M, Ring NP, et al: Pleural mesothelioma of epithelial type and pulmonary adenocarcinoma: An ultrastructural and cytochemical comparison. J Pathol 152: 309–316, 1987.

57. Dumortier P, Coplu L, Broucke I, et al: Erionite bodies and fibres in bronchoalveolar lavage fluid (BALF) of residents from Tuzkoy, Cappadocia, Turkey. Occup Environ Med 58:261–266, 2001.

58. Eagles G, Warn A, Ball RY, et al: Hepatocyte growth factor/scatter factor is present in most pleural effusion fluids from cancer patients. Br J Cancer 73:377–381, 1996.

59. Emri S, Kocagoz T, Olut A, et al: Simian virus 40 is not a cofactor in the pathogenesis of environmentally induced malignant pleural mesothelioma in Turkey. Anticancer Res 20:891–894, 2000.

60. England DM, Hochholzer L, McCarthy MM: Localized benign and malignant fibrous tumors of the pleura. A clinicopathologic review of 223 cases. Am J Surg Pathol 15:640–658, 1989.

61. Erasmus JJ, McAdams HP, Patz EF Jr, et al: Calcifying fibrous pseudotumor of pleura: Radiologic features in three cases. J Compt Assist Tomogr 20:763–765, 1996.

62. Fraire AE, Cooper S, Greenberg SD, et al: Mesothelioma of childhood. Cancer 62:838–847, 1988.

63. Gaertner E, Zeren EH, Fleming MV, et al: Biphasic synovial sarcomas arising in the pleural cavity. A clinicopathologic study of five cases. Am J Surg Pathol 20:36–45, 1996.

64. Gerwin BI, Lechner JF, Reddel RR, et al: Comparison of production of transforming growth factor-beta and platelet-derived growth factor by normal human mesothelial cells and mesothelioma cell lines. Cancer Res 47:6180–6184, 1987.

65. Gibbs AR, Whimster WF: Tumors of lung and pleura. In Fletcher CD, editor: Diagnostic Histopathology of Tumours, Vol. 1. London: Churchill Livingstone, 1995.

66. Gilks B, Hegedus C, Freeman H, et al: Malignant peritoneal mesothelioma after remote abdominal radiation. Cancer 61:2019–2021, 1988.

67. Gordon GJ, Jensen RV, Hsiao LL, et al: Translation of microarray data into clinically relevant cancer diagnostic tests using gene expression ratios in lung cancer and mesothelioma. Cancer Res 62:4963–4967, 2002.

68. Gordon W Jr, Antman KH, Greenberger JS, et al: Radiation therapy in the management of patients with mesothelioma. Int J Radiat Oncol Biol Phys 8:19–25, 1982.

69. Grundy GW, Miller RW: Malignant mesothelioma in childhood. Report of 13 cases. Cancer 30:1216–1218, 1972.

70. Gulumian M, van Wyk JA: Hydroxyl radical production in the presence of fibres by a Fenton-type reaction. Chem Biol Interact 62:89–97, 1987.

71. Hansen K, Mossman BT: Generation of superoxide ($O2^-$) from alveolar macrophages exposed to asbestiform and nonfibrous particles. Cancer Res 47:1681–1686, 1987.

72. Harwood TR, Gracey DR, Yokoo H: Pseudomesotheliomatous carcinoma of the lung. A variant of peripheral lung cancer. Am J Clin Pathol 65:159–167, 1976.

73. Hasturk S, Tastepe I, Unlu M, et al: Combined chemotherapy in pleurectomized malignant pleural mesothelioma patients. J Chemother 8:159–164, 1996.

74. Heelan RT, Rusch VW, Begg CB, et al: Staging of malignant pleural mesothelioma: Comparison of CT and MR imaging. AJR Am J Roentgenol 172:1039–1047, 1999.

74a. Henderson DW: Pathology and diagnosis of mesothelioma. In Henderson DW, Shilkin KB, Whitaker D, et al: Malignant mesothelioma. New York: Hemisphere Publishing, 1982, pp. 183–222.

75. Herndon JE, Green MR, Chahinian AP, et al: Factors predictive of survival among 337 patients with mesothelioma treated between 1984 and 1994 by the Cancer and Leukemia Group B. Chest 113:723–731, 1998.

76. Hillerdal G, Berg J: Malignant mesothelioma secondary to chronic inflammation and old scars. Two new cases and review of the literature. Cancer 55:1968–1972, 1985.

77. Hirvonen A, Mattson K, Karjalainen A, et al: Simian virus 40 (SV40)-like DNA sequences not detectable in Finnish mesothelioma patients not exposed to SV40-contaminated polio vaccines. Mol Carcinog 26:93–99, 1999.

78. Ho L, Sugarbaker DJ, Skarin AT: Malignant pleural mesothelioma. Cancer Treat Res 105:327–373, 2001.

79. Hubbard R: The aetiology of mesothelioma: Are risk factors other than asbestos exposure important? Thorax 52:496–497, 1997.

80. Hughes A, Calbert P, Azzabi A, et al: Phase I clinical and pharmacokinetic study of pemetrexed and carboplatin in patients with malignant pleural mesotheliomia. J Clin Oncol 20:3533–3544, 2002.

81. Huncharek M: Non-asbestos related diffuse malignant mesothelioma. Tumori 88:1–9, 2002.

82. Jaklitsch MT, Grondin SC, Sugarbaker DJ: Treatment of malignant mesothelioma. World J Surg 25:210–217, 2001.

83. Janssen YM, Marsh JP, Absher MP, et al: Oxidant stress responses in human pleural mesothelial cells exposed to asbestos. Am J Respir Crit Care Med 149:795–802, 1994.

84. Kamp DW, Dunn MM, Sbalchiero JS, et al: Contrasting effects of alveolar macrophages and neutrophils on asbestos-induced pulmonary epithelial cell injury. Am J Physiol 266:184–191, 1994.

85. Kelsey KT, Yano E, Liber HL, et al: The in vitro genetic effects of fibrous erionite and crocidolite asbestos. Br J Cancer 54:107–114, 1986.

86. Kops SP: Oral polio vaccine and human cancer: A reassessment of SV40 as a contaminant based upon legal documents. Anticancer Res 20:4745–4750, 2000.

86a. Kramer G, Gans S, Rijnders A, Leer J: Long-term survival of a patient with malignant pleural mesothelioma as a late complication of radiotherapy for Hodgkin's disease treated with 90yttrium-silicate. Lung Cancer 27:205–208, 2000.

87. Langer AM, Pooly FD: Identification of single asbestos fiber in human tissue. In Bogovski P, Gilson JC, Timbrell V, editors: Biologic Effects of Asbestos. Lyon: IARC, 1973, pp. 119–125.

88. Laveck MA, Somers AN, Moore LL, et al: Dissimilar peptide growth factors can induce normal human mesothelial cell multiplication. In Vitro Cell Dev Biol 24:1077–1084, 1988.

89. Law MR, Hodson ME, Turner-Warwick M: Malignant mesothelioma of the pleura: Clinical aspects and symptomatic treatment. Eur J Respir Dis 65:162–168, 1984.

90. Leers MP, Aarts MM, Theunissen PH: E-cadherin and calretinin: A useful combination of immunochemical markers for differentiation between mesothelioma and metastatic adenocarcinoma. Histopathology 32:209–216, 1998.

91. Lerman Y, Learman Y, Schachter P, et al: Radiation associated malignant pleural mesothelioma. Thorax 46:463–464, 1991.

92. Lin BT, Colby T, Gown AM, et al: Malignant vascular tumors of the serous membranes mimicking mesothelioma. A report of 14 cases. Am J Surg Pathol 20:1431–1439, 1996.

93. Linden CJ, Mercke C, Albrechtsson U, et al: Effect of hemithorax irradiation alone or combined with doxorubicin and cyclophosphamide in 47 pleural mesotheliomas: A nonrandomized phase II study. Eur Respir J 9:2565–2572, 1996.

94. Lund LG, Aust AE: Mobilization of iron from crocidolite asbestos by certain chelators results in enhanced crocidolite-dependent oxygen consumption. Arch Biochem Biophys 287: 91–96, 1991.

95. Maggi G, Casadio C, Cianci R, et al: Trimodality management of malignant pleural mesothelioma. Eur J Cardiothorac Surg 19:346–350, 2001.

96. Magnani C, Leporati M: Mortality from lung cancer and population risk attributable to asbestos in an asbestos cement manufacturing town in Italy. Occup Environ Med 55: 111–114, 1998.

97. Mancuso TF: Relative risk of mesothelioma among railroad machinists exposed to chrysotile. Am J Ind Med 13:639–657, 1988.

98. Marom EM, Erasmus JJ, Pass HI, et al: The role of imaging in malignant pleural mesothelioma. Semin Oncol 29:26–35, 2002.

99. Maurer R, Egloff B: Malignant peritoneal mesothelioma after cholangiography with thorotrast. Cancer 36:1381–1385, 1975.

100. McCaughey WT, Al-Jabi M: Differentiation of serosal hyperplasia and neoplasia in biopsies. Pathol Annu 21(Pt 1): 271–293, 1986.

101. McCormack PM, Nagasaki F, Hilaris BS, et al: Surgical treatment of pleural mesothelioma. J Thorac Cardiovasc Surg 84: 834–842, 1982.

102. McDonald JC, Armstrong BG, Edwards CW, et al: Case-referent survey of young adults with mesothelioma: I. Lung fibre analyses. Ann Occup Hyg 45:513–518, 2001.

103. McDonald JC, McDonald AD: Epidemiology of mesothelioma from estimated incidence. Prev Med 6:426–442, 1977.

104. Merritt N, Blewett CJ, Miller JD, et al: Survival after conservative (palliative) management of pleural malignant mesothelioma. J Surg Oncol. 78:171–174, 2001.

105. Miller BG, Jones AD, Searl A, et al: Influence of characteristics of inhaled fibres on development of tumours in the rat lung. Ann Occup Hyg 43:167–179, 1999.

106. Miller BG, Searl A, Davis JM, et al: Influence of fibre length, dissolution and biopersistence on the production of mesothelioma in the rat peritoneal cavity. Ann Occup Hyg 43:155–166, 1999.

107. Monnet I, Breau JL, Moro D, et al: Intrapleural infusion of activated macrophages and gamma-interferon in malignant pleural mesothelioma: A phase II study. Chest 121:1921–1927, 2002.

108. Moran CA, Suster S, Koss MN: Smooth muscle tumours presenting as pleural neoplasms. Histopathology 27:227–234, 1995.

109. Mossman BT, Gruenert DC: SV40, growth factors, and mesothelioma: Another piece of the puzzle. Am J Respir Cell Mol Biol 26:167–170, 2002.

110. Mossman BT, Kamp DW, Weitzman SA: Mechanisms of carcinogenesis and clinical features of asbestos-associated cancers. Cancer Invest 14:466–480, 1996.

111. Myerson RJ, Moros E, Roti JL: Hyperthermia. In Perez CA, Brady LW, editors: Principles and Practice of Radiation Oncology, 3rd ed. Philadelphia: Lippincott-Raven, Inc., 1997, pp. 637–683.

112. Naidich DP, Zerhouni EA, Siegelmann SS: Computed Tomography and Magnetic Resonance of the Thorax, 2nd ed. New York: Raven Press, 1991.

113. Nicholson WJ: The carcinogenicity of chrysotile asbestos— a review. Ind Health 39:57–64, 2001.

114. Nowack AK, Lake RA, Kindler HL, et al: New approaches for mesothelioma: Biologies, vaccines, gene therapy, and other novel agents. Semin Oncol 29:82–96, 2002.

114a. Okumura M, Ohta M, Tateyama H, et al: The WHO histologic classification system reflects the oncologic behavior of thymoma: A clinical study of 273 patients. Cancer 94:624–632, 2002.

115. Ordonez NG: Value of cytokeratin 5/6 immunostaining in distinguishing epithelial mesothelioma of the pleura from lung adenocarcinoma. Am J Surg Pathol 22:1215–1221, 1998.

116. Oury TD, Hammar SP, Roggli VL: Ultrastructural features of diffuse malignant mesotheliomas. Hum Pathol 29: 1382–1392, 1998.

117. Palekar LD, Eyre JF, Coffin DL: Transplantation and chromosomal analysis of cell lines derived from mesotheliomas induced in rats with erionite and UICC chrysotile asbestos. IARC Sci Publ 167–172, 1989.

118. Pass HI, Temeck BK, Kranda K, et al: Phase III randomized trial of surgery with or without intraoperative photodynamic therapy and postoperative immunochemotherapy for malig-

119. Pass HI, Temeck BK, Kranda K, et al: Preoperative tumor volume is associated with outcome in malignant pleural mesothelioma. J Thorac Cardiovasc Surg 115:310–317; discussion 317–318, 1998.

120. Patz EF Jr, Shaffer K, Piwnica-Worms DR, et al: Malignant pleural mesothelioma: Value of CT and MR imaging in predicting resectability. AJR Am J Roentgenol 159:961–966, 1992.

121. Pepper C, Jasani B, Navabi H, et al: Simian virus 40 large T antigen (SV40LTAg) primer specific DNA amplication in human pleural mesothelioma tissue. Thorax 51:1074–1076, 1996.

122. Peterson JT Jr, Greenberg SD, Buffler PA: Non-asbestos-related malignant mesothelioma. A review. Cancer 54: 951–960, 1984.

123. Prakash UB, Reiman HM: Comparison of needle biopsy with cytologic analysis for the evaluation of pleural effusion: Analysis of 414 cases. Mayo Clin Proc 60:158–164, 1985.

124. Ratto GB, Civalleri D, Esposito M, et al: Pleural space perfusion with cisplatin in the multimodality treatment of malignant mesothelioma: A feasibility and pharmacokinetic study. J Thorac Cardiovasc Surg 117:759–765, 1999.

125. Renshaw AA, Dean BR, Antman KH, et al: The role of cytologic evaluation of pleural fluid in the diagnosis of malignant mesothelioma. Chest 111:106–109, 1997.

126. Rice TW, Adelstein DJ, Kirby TJ, et al: Aggressive multimodality therapy for malignant pleural mesothelioma. Ann Thorac Surg 58:24–29, 1994.

127. Roberts DD: Regulation of tumor growth and metastasis by thrombospondin-1. FASEB J 10:1183–1191, 1996.

128. Roberts F, McCall AE, Burnett RA: Malignant mesothelioma: A comparison of biopsy and postmortem material by light microscopy and immunohistochemistry. J Clin Pathol 54:766–770, 2001.

129. Robledo R, Mossmann B: Cellular and molecular mechanisms of asbestos induced fibrosis. J Cell Physiol 180:158–166, 1999.

130. Rom WN, Bitterman PB, Rennard SI, et al: Characterization of the lower respiratory tract inflammation of nonsmoking individuals with interstitial lung disease associated with chronic inhalation of inorganic dusts. Am Rev Respir Dis 136:1429–1434, 1987.

131. Rosenthal GJ, Simeonova P, Corsini E: Asbestos toxicity: An immunologic perspective. Rev Environ Health 14:11–20, 1999.

132. Roushdy-Hammady I, Siegel J, Emri S, et al: Genetic-susceptibility factor and malignant mesothelioma in the Cappadocian region of Turkey. Lancet 357:444–445, 2001.

133. Roussy G. OC, Guerin M.: Ueber sarkomerzeugung durch kolloidales thoriumdioxd bei der weissen Ratte. Strahlentherapy 56:160–167, 1936.

134. Ruffie P, Feld R, Minkin S, et al: Diffuse malignant mesothelioma of the pleura in Ontario and Quebec: A retrospective study of 332 patients. J Clin Oncol 7:1157–1168, 1989.

135. Rusch V, Saltz L, Venkatraman E, et al: A phase II trial of pleurectomy/decortication followed by intrapleural and systemic chemotherapy for malignant pleural mesothelioma. J Clin Oncol 12:1156–1163, 1994.

136. Rusch VW, Ginsberg RJ: New concepts in the staging of mesothelioma. Invited comment to Chapter 26. In Deslauriers J, Lacquet LK, editors: Thoracic Surgery: Surgical Management of Pleural Diseases, International Trends in Thoracic Surgery, Vol. 6. St. Louis: C. V. Mosby, 1990, pp. 336–343.

137. Rusch VW, Piantadosi S, Holmes EC: The role of extrapleural pneumonectomy in malignant pleural mesothelioma.

A lung cancer study group trial. J Thorac Cardiovasc Surg 102:1–9, 1991.

138. Rusch VW, Rosenzweig K, Venkatraman E, et al: A phase II trial of surgical resection and adjuvant high-dose hemithoracic radiation of malignant pleural mesothelioma. J Thorac Cardiovasc Surg 117:54–63; discussion 63–65, 2001.

139. Rusch VW: A proposed new international TNM staging system for malignant pleural mesothelioma. From the International Mesothelioma Interest Group. Chest 108:1122–1128, 1995.

140. Rusch VW: Pleurectomy/decortication in the setting of multimodality treatment for diffuse malignant pleural mesothelioma. Semin Thorac Cardiovasc Surg 9:367–372, 1997.

141. Sahn SA: State of the art. The pleura. Am Rev Respir Dis 138:184–234, 1988.

142. Sanden A, Jarvholm B, Larsson S, et al: The risk of lung cancer and mesothelioma after cessation of asbestos exposure: A prospective cohort study of shipyard workers. Eur Respir J 5:281–285, 1992.

143. Sanders CL, Jackson TA: Induction of mesotheliomas and sarcomas from "hot spots" of 239 PuO 2 activity. Health Phys 22:755–759, 1972.

144. Scagliotti GV, Shin DM, Kindler HL, et al: Phase II study of pemetrexed with and without folic acid and vitamin B12 as a front-line therapy in malignant pleural mesothelioma. J Clin Oncol 21:1556–1561, 2003.

145. Sebastien P, Gaudichet A, Bignon J, et al: Zeolite bodies in human lungs from Turkey. Lab Invest 44:420–425, 1981.

146. Shannon VR, Nesbitt JC, Libshitz HI: Malignant pleural mesothelioma after radiation therapy for breast cancer. A report of two additional patients. Cancer 76:437–441, 1995.

147. Shields TW, Yeldandi AV: Uncommon tumors of the pleura. In Shields TW, LoCicero JI, Ponn RB, editors: General Thoracic Surgery, Vol. 1, 5th ed. Philadelphia: Lippincott, Williams & Wilkins, 2000, pp. 791–794.

148. Sinoff C, Falkson G, Sandison AG, et al: Combined doxorubicin and radiation therapy in malignant pleural mesothelioma. Cancer Treat Rep 66:1605–1607, 1982.

149. Smith AH, Wright CC: Chrysotile asbestos is the main cause of pleural mesothelioma. Am J Ind Med 30:252–266, 1996.

150. Solheim OP, Saeter G, Finnanger AM, et al: High-dose methotrexate in the tretment of malignant mesothelioma of the pleura: A phase II study. Br J Cancer 65:956, 1992.

151. Stanton MF, Wrench C: Mechanisms of mesothelioma induction with asbestos and fibrous glass. J Natl Cancer Inst 48: 797–821, 1972.

152. Steel TR, Allibone J, Revesz T, et al: Intradural neurotropic spread of malignant mesothelioma. Case report and review of the literature. J Neurosurg 88:122–125, 1998.

153. Stehlin JS Jr: Hyperthermic perfusion for melanoma of the extremities: Experience with 165 patients, 1967 to 1979. Ann NY Acad Sci 335:352–355, 1980.

154. Sterman DH, Kaiser LR, Albelda SM: Advances in the treatment of malignant pleural mesothelioma. Chest 116: 504–520, 1999.

155. Stock RJ, Fu YS, Carter JR: Malignant peritoneal mesothelioma following radiotherapy for seminoma of the testis. Cancer 44:914–919, 1979.

156. Strizzi L, Catalano A, Vianale G, et al: Vascular endothelial growth factor is an autocrine growth factor in human malignant mesothelioma. J Pathol 193:468–475, 2001.

157. Sugarbaker DJ, Flores RM, Jaklitsch MT, et al: Resection margins, extrapleural nodal status, and cell type determine postoperative long-term survival in trimodality therapy of malignant pleural mesothelioma: Results in 183 patients. J Thorac Cardiovasc Surg 117:54–63; discussion 63–55, 1999.

158. Sugarbaker DJ, Garcia JP, Richards WG, et al: Extrapleural pneumonectomy in the multimodality therapy of malignant pleural mesothelioma. Results in 120 consecutive patients. Ann Surg 224:288–294; discussion 294–296, 1996.

159. Sugarbaker DJ, Norberto JJ, Swanson SJ: Extrapleural pneumonectomy in the setting of multimodality therapy for diffuse malignant pleural mesothelioma. Semin Thorac Cardiovasc Surg 9:373–382, 1997.

160. Sugarbaker DJ, Norberto JJ: Multimodality management of malignant pleural mesothelioma. Chest 113:61S–65S, 1998.

161. Sugarbaker DJ, Zellos L, Bueno RB: Feasibility of pleurectomy and intraoperative bicavitary hyperthermic cisplatin lavage for mesothelioma: A phase I-II study. (abstract) ASCO Annual Meeting, 2003.

162. Sugarbaker DJ, Norberto JJ, Swanson SJ: Surgical staging and work-up of patients with diffuse malignant pleural mesothelioma. Semin Thorac Cardiovasc Surg 9:356–360, 1997.

163. Suzuki Y: Diagnostic criteria for human diffuse malignant mesothelioma. Acta Pathol Jpn 42:767–786, 1992.

164. Suzuki Y: Pathology of human malignant mesothelioma—preliminary analysis of 1,517 mesothelioma cases. Ind Health 39:183–185, 2001.

165. Swanson SJ, Grondin SC, Sugarbaker DJ: Technique of pleural pneumonectomy in diffuse mesothelioma. In Shields TW, LoCicero JI, Ponn RB, editors: General Thoracic Surgery, Vol. 1, 5th ed. Philadelphia: Lippincott Williams & Wilkins, 2000, pp. 783–790.

166. Takita H, Dougherty TJ: Intracavitary photodynamic therapy for malignant pleural mesothelioma. Semin Surg Oncol 11:368–371, 1995.

167. Tanaka S, Choe N, Hemenway DR, et al: Asbestos inhalation induces reactive nitrogen species and nytrosine formation in the lung and pleura of the rat. J Clin Invest 102:445–454, 1998.

168. Teirstein AS: Diagnosing malignant pleural mesothelioma. Chest 114:713–722, 1998.

169. Testa JR, Pass HI, MC: Molecular biology of mesothelioma. In De Vita V, Hellman S, Rosenberg S, editors: Principles and Practice of Oncology, 6 ed. Philadelphia: Lippincott Williams & Wilkins, 2001, pp. 1937–1943.

170. Thurlbeck W, Miller RR: The respiratory system, disease of the pleura. In Rubin E FJ, editor: Pathology, Vol 1. Philadelphia: Lippincott, 1988, pp. 615–619.

171. van de Rijn M, Lombard CM, Rouse RV: Expression of CD34 by solitary fibrous tumors of the pleura, mediastinum, lung. Am J Surg Pathol 18:814–820, 1994.

172. van de Vaart PJ, van der Vange N, Zoetmulder FA, et al: Intraperitoneal cisplatin with regional hyperthermia in advanced ovarian cancer: Pharmacokinetics and cisplatin-DNA adduct formation in patients and ovarian cancer cell lines. Eur J Cancer 34:148–154, 1998.

173. van Meerbeeck JP, Baas P, Debruyne C, et al: A phase II EORTC study of temozolomide in patients with malignant pleural mesothelioma. Eur J Cancer 20:3533–3544, 2002.

174. van Veen P, Scouwink JH, Star WM, et al: Wedge-shaped applicator for additional light delivery and dosimetry in the diaphragmatic sinus during photodynamic therapy for malignant pleural mesothelioma. Phys Med Biol 46:1873–1883, 2001.

175. Viallat JR, Boutin C: [Malignant pleural effusions: Recourse to early use of talc]. Rev Med Interne 19:811–818, 1998.

176. Vogelzang N, Rusthoven JJ, Symanowski J, et al: Multimodality management of malignant pleural mesothelioma. J Clin Oncol 21:2636–2644, 2003.

177. Von Hoff DD, Metch B, Lucas JG, et al: Phase II evaluation of recombinant interferon-beta (IFN-beta ser) in patients with diffuse mesothelioma: A Southwest Oncology Group study. J Interferon Res 10:531–534, 1990.

178. Wagner IC, Sleggs CA, Marchand P: Diffuse pleural mesothelioma and asbestos exposure in the Northwestern Cape Province. Br Ind Med 17:260–271, 1960.
179. Wagner JC, Griffiths DM, Hill RJ: The effect of fibre size on the in vivo activity of UICC crocidolite. Br J Cancer 49:453–458, 1984.
180. Walker C, Everitt J, Ferriola PC, et al: Autocrine growth stimulation by transforming growth factor alpha in asbestos-transformed rat mesothelial cells. Cancer Res 55:530–536, 1995.
181. Wang NS: Anatomy and physiology of the pleural space. Clin Chest Med 6:3–16, 1985.
182. Warhol MJ, Hickey WF, Corson JM: Malignant mesothelioma: Ultrastructural distinction from adenocarcinoma. Am J Surg Pathol 6:307–314, 1982.
183. Weiss SW, Enzinger FM: Epithelioid hemangioendothelioma, a vascular tumor often mistaken for carcinoma. Cancer 50: 970–981, 1982.
184. Weitzman SA, Weitberg AB, Clark EP, et al: Phagocytes as carcinogens: Malignant transformation produced by human neutrophils. Science 227:1231–1233, 1985.
185. Wojta J, Kaun C, Breuss JM, et al: Hepatocyte growth factor increases expression of vascular endothelial growth factor and plasminogen activator inhibitor-1 in human keratinocytes and the vascular endothelial growth factor receptor flk-1 in human endothelial cells. Lab Invest 79:427–438, 1999.
186. Wong WW, Pluth JR, Gordo GL, et al: Liposarcoma of the pleura. Mayo Clinic Proc 69:882–885, 1994.
187. Yajnik S, Rosenzweig KE, Mychalczak B, et al: Intensity-modulated radiotherapy following extrapleural pneumonectomy for the treatment of malignant mesothelioma: Clinical implementation. Int J Radiat Oncol Biol Phys 55:606–616, 2003.
188. Yano E, Wang ZM, Wang XR, et al: Cancer mortality among workers exposed to amphibole-free chrysotile asbestos. Am J Epidemiol 154:538–543, 2001.
189. Yousem SA, Hochholzer L: Unusual thoracic manifestations of epithelioid hemangioendothelioma. Arch Pathol Lab Med 111:459–463, 1987

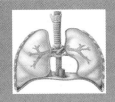

Surgery of the Diaphragm: A Deductive Approach

Daniel C. Wiener and Michael T. Jaklitsch

And on a day we meet to walk the line
And set the wall between us once again.
We keep the wall between us as we go...
He only says, 'Good fences make good neighbors.'
                        —Robert Frost, "Mending Wall"

▶ INTRODUCTION

The muscular diaphragm acts as a boundary between the positive pressure abdominal cavity and the negative pressure thoracic cavity. Perhaps because it is a boundary structure, or perhaps because the horizontal diaphragm is poorly visualized by a plain chest radiograph and computed tomography (CT) scan, discussion of the surgical approach to the diaphragm is neglected in many surgical textbooks.

In our opinion there is some misinformation regarding the surgical treatment of the diaphragm in the current literature. This misinformation seems to reflect a lack of understanding of the basic anatomy and physiology of the diaphragm. Although diaphragmatic disease is infrequent,

exposure to the diaphragm is commonplace, because it is visualized during every thoracic surgical procedure and most intraabdominal operations. Therefore the basic principles advocated by this chapter can be verified or denied by the curious reader in the operating room.

Two fundamental principles can be applied to all surgical approaches to the diaphragm: (1) The muscles contract in a radial manner like the spokes of a wheel, and (2) the balance of positive pressure pushing up from the abdomen and negative pressure within the thorax created by the elastic recoil of the lung during quiet expiration displaces the central tendon into the chest, whereas contraction of the diaphragmatic muscle pulls the tendon back toward the costal margin and elevates the lower ribs, enlarging the volume of the thorax. We hope to apply these two fundamental principles in an understanding of the physiology and pathophysiology of the diaphragm. Furthermore, we believe that these two principles will allow the reader to use new technologies and develop better operations to treat diaphragmatic disease.

▶ EMBRYOLOGY

In utero the diaphragm forms from the septum transversum and pleuroperitoneal folds.[28] The septum transversum is an unpaired ventral membrane that separates the pericardium from the remainder of the thorax and creates the central trileaflet of the diaphragmatic tendon (Figure 31-1).[17] One of the trileaflet tendons lies within the right hemithorax, one within the left hemithorax, and the third beneath the pericardium. The dorsolateral portions of the diaphragm start with the formation of pleuroperitoneal folds. The mesothelium of the pleura binds to the mesothelium of the peritoneum in a membrane only two cell layers deep. Myotomes from C3, C4, and C5 then migrate from the lateral border toward the center of each hemithorax within the interspace between these two mesothelial layers in the seventh week of life. The outer rim of muscle of the diaphragm is from myotomes, which carry nerve innervation from T7 through T12.[17] The intestines return to the abdomen from the yolk sac in the tenth week of life and will displace into the chest if the diaphragm has not successfully formed (a congenital diaphragmatic hernia).

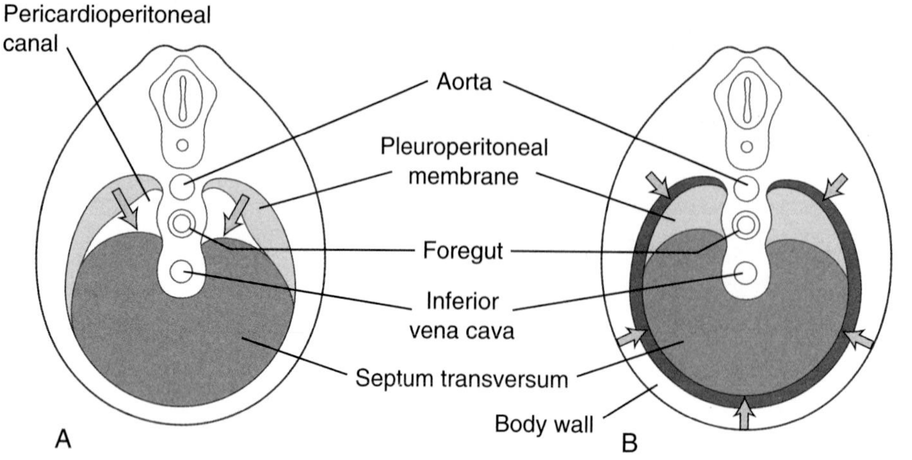

Pericardioperitoneal
canal

Aorta

Pleuroperitoneal
membrane

Foregut

Inferior
vena cava

Septum transversum

Body wall

A   B

**Figure 31–1 (A, B) Transverse
schematic of developing embryo during
weeks 5–7.** Bilateral pleuroperitoneal folds extend anteriorly to reach
the posterior edge of the septum transversum, thus forming the posterior
portions of the diaphragm. Septum transversum develops into the majority of the
central tendon.
*(From Larsen W: Human embryology.
2nd Ed. New York: Churchill Livingston,
1997.)*

▶ STRUCTURE AND FUNCTION

This simplified embryological description provides several fundamental concepts of diaphragm function and pathology. Muscle contraction is in a radial manner along the lines of migration of the myotomes. Thus fiber shortening is along the lines of a wheel spoke, between the central tendon and the circumferential ribcage. Furthermore, any congenital loss of muscle or tendon may present as a hernia within the diaphragm.

In the adult each hemidiaphragm resembles the surface of an upside-down fairway wooden golf club. The fan-shaped tendon is like the flat metal sole plate, and the circumferential muscle curves away into the sulcus like the curved wooden club head. The muscle fascicles of the crus coalesce and attach to the lumbar spine, just as the wooden club curves down to attach to the metal shaft.

There are three natural openings within the diaphragm (Figures 31-2 and 31-2B). The aortic opening is the most posterior of the three and is formed from fibers comprising the right and left diaphragmatic crura.[10] This tunnel is actually behind the diaphragm, and not within it, and contains the aorta, azygos vein, and thoracic duct. The esophageal hiatus is slightly more ventral from the aortic hiatus and consists of fibers passing between the aorta and the esophagus toward the right crus, and fibers converging on the pericardial tendon. The opening of the inferior vena cava lies within the confluence of the tendons of the right hemithorax and the tendon beneath the pericardium.

The fan-shaped muscle of the diaphragm arises from the internal circumference of the thorax, with attachments to the sternum, the lower six or seven ribs, and the vertebral bodies of the lumbar vertebrae. Posteriorly the muscle fibers originate from the aponeurotic arch of the ligamentum arcuatum externum, which overrides the psoas and quadratus lomborum muscle. Laterally the fibers of the diaphragm interdigitate with slips from the transversalis muscle of the abdomen as they originate from the ribs.[10] The right crus is larger and longer than the left and arises from the bodies of the upper three or four lumbar vertebrae. The left crus arises from the upper two lumbar vertebral bodies.

During inspiration the first rib is elevated and fixed by the scalene muscles of the neck. The external intercostal muscles raise, in turn, each of the lower ribs. Raising these ribs, like a bucket handle that is attached to the sternum and vertebral column, enlarges the thorax and creates the negative pressure that ventilates the lung.[10]

The diaphragm is the major muscle of inspiration.[5] In the resting state the central tendon is displaced cephalad into the thorax by the positive intraabdominal pressure. During contraction the radial muscle fibers pull the tendon down toward the abdominal cavity like a drumhead. This further augments the negative intrathoracic pressure and further increases the positive pressure in the abdomen. The diaphragmatic crura contribute to the magnitude of displacement of the central tendon. In fact, if there were only circumferential attachments to the ribcage, the diaphragm would be limited in its ability to displace the lower ribs and enlarge the thoracic cavity. The thicker fascicles of the crura, which lie at a 45–90° angle to the plane of the fan, pull on the anchoring lumbar spine like a lever and thus fix the central tendon in place. In descending, the fan of the diaphragm displaces the intraabdominal viscera, which do not yield completely because they are bolstered by the anterior abdominal wall. The central tendon becomes a fixed point from which the radial muscles of the fan contract and are thus able to elevate the lower ribs. Even though the points of muscle attachment to the lumbar spine are more caudal than the attachments to the ribcage, the domed tendon acts as fulcrum cephalad to the attachments to the ribcage. In fact, contraction of the diaphragm can only raise the lower ribs if the intraabdominal viscera are in situ, and not if the organs have been removed.[10] Injuries to the crura have a more disproportionate effect on the respiratory function of the ipsilateral diaphragm than a similar injury to the peripheral muscle.

A forced inspiration descends the central tendon from one to two rib interspaces. Under normal respiration, each hemidiaphragm provides between 15 and 25% of respiratory muscle function, with each side of the combined intercostals providing the remaining percentage.[3,39] Under strained respiration, however, the diaphragm can increase its workload to provide up to 80% of the work of breathing.

▶ PLEURAL AND PERITONEAL ATTACHMENTS

The pleura is tightly adherent to the top surface of the diaphragmatic central tendon and most of the musculature. It is impossible to separate the pleura from the central

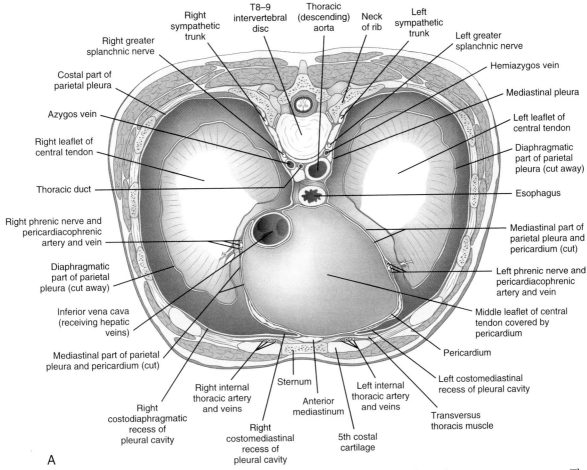

Figure 31-2 Superior (A) and inferior (B) view of the diaphragm, including phrenic nerve anatomy. The intradiaphragmatic course of the phrenic nerves is often difficult to visualize at the time of surgery. Familiarity with the nerve's path as it traverses the muscle is helpful when deciding where to make diaphragmatic incisions.

tendon of each hemidiaphragm. As the pleura curves off the chest wall and folds back upon itself on the surface of the diaphragm, there is a circumferential diaphragmatic recess of approximately 1 cm that does not contain pleura.[38] This recess of uncovered diaphragm is used to good advantage during an extrapleural dissection when the surgeon wraps his or her fingers into this recess and pulls downward, thus exposing the diaphragmatic musculature for division (Figure 31-3).

The peritoneum is less adherent to the undersurface of the diaphragm and can be bluntly mobilized off the diaphragm during extraperitoneal approaches to the abdominal aorta. The plane of dissection lies between the inferior phrenic artery and vein on the muscle side and the peritoneal membrane. The peritoneum separates from the central tendon of the right diaphragm to form the falciform ligament and produces an area directly under the central tendon, which does not have peritoneal covering. This is known as the bare area.

ARTERIAL AND VENOUS ANATOMY

The superior phrenic arteries are located on the thoracic surface of the diaphragm. They are small branches from the lower thoracic aorta and traverse the posterior diaphragm over the top portion of each crus close to the mediastinum.[10] They terminate in small anastamoses with the musculophrenic and pericardiophrenic arteries, which are both branches from the internal mammary artery. These latter two arteries also supply blood to the phrenic nerve and the pericardial fat pad.[1]

The inferior phrenic arteries lie on the undersurface of the crus and the dome of the diaphragm (Figure 31-4). They are small paired vessels with frequent anatomical variations. They can originate separately or as a common trunk from the aorta above the celiac artery or from the celiac artery itself. Alternatively, a common trunk arising from either the aorta or celiac artery gives rise to these two arteries. Occasionally one vessel originates from the aorta, whereas the other emerges from one of the renal arteries. Diverging near the crura, the inferior phrenic arteries then course obliquely superior and lateral along the inferior surface of the diaphragm. The left inferior phrenic artery passes posterior to the esophagus, and then runs anteriorly along the lateral side of the esophageal hiatus. The right inferior phrenic artery passes behind the inferior vena cava.[10]

Close to the posterior aspect of the central tendon, both the left and right inferior phrenic arteries divide into a

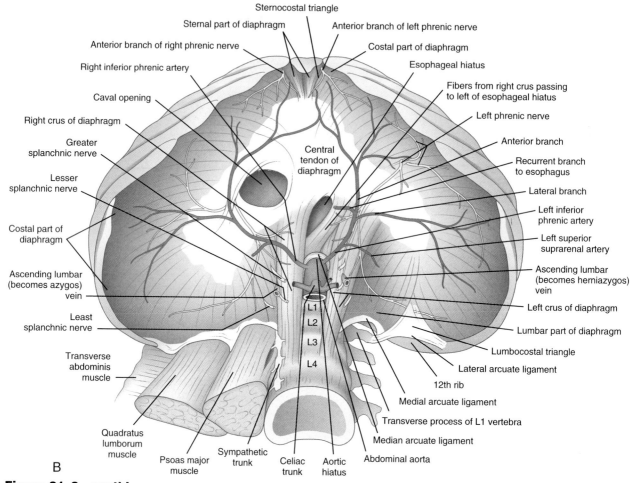

Sternocostal triangle
Sternal part of diaphragm
Anterior branch of left phrenic nerve
Anterior branch of right phrenic nerve
Costal part of diaphragm
Right inferior phrenic artery
Esophageal hiatus
Caval opening
Fibers from right crus passing to left of esophageal hiatus
Right crus of diaphragm
Left phrenic nerve
Greater splanchnic nerve
Central tendon of diaphragm
Anterior branch
Recurrent branch to esophagus
Lesser splanchnic nerve
Lateral branch
Left inferior phrenic artery
Costal part of diaphragm
Left superior suprarenal artery
Ascending lumbar (becomes azygos) vein
Ascending lumbar (becomes herniazygos) vein
Left crus of diaphragm
Least splanchnic nerve
Lumbar part of diaphragm
Lumbocostal triangle
Transverse abdominis muscle
Lateral arcuate ligament
12th rib
Medial arcuate ligament
Quadratus lumborum muscle
Transverse process of L1 vertebra
Median arcuate ligament
Psoas major muscle
Sympathetic trunk
Celiac trunk
Aortic hiatus
Abdominal aorta

L1
L2
L3
L4

B

Figure 31–2, cont'd

medial and a lateral branch. The medial branch extends anteriorly, close to the mediastinum. Branches of this vessel traverse the muscular portion of the diaphragm to anastamose with the musculophrenic and pericardiophrenic arteries. The lateral branch of the inferior phrenic artery courses laterally and forms anastamoses with the lower intercostal arteries. The left inferior phrenic artery provides a minor contribution to the blood supply of the lower esophagus. Both the right and left inferior phrenic arteries have branches to the ipsilateral suprarenal gland. These branches are called the right and left superior suprarenal arteries.[10]

In general the venous anatomy in this region parallels that of the arteries. The superior phrenic veins are small and drain anteriorly to the internal mammary vein. The much larger inferior phrenic veins parallel the course of the inferior phrenic arteries. The right vein empties directly into the inferior vena cava. The left vein usually has two branches, one of which drains into the left renal or suprarenal vein and the other passes anterior to the esophageal hiatus and empties into the inferior vena cava.[10]

LYMPHATICS

The lymphatics of the diaphragm drain toward the internal mammary chain anteriorly and the thoracic duct posteriorly. Smaller lateral lymphatic branches follow the course of the intercostal vessels along the lateral and posterior margins of the chest wall.[10] Although these vessels are rarely seen in the nonpathological state, engorged vessels are frequently seen on both the upper and lower surfaces of the diaphragm in patients who have congenital heart disease with elevated central venous pressures, and in primary pathological conditions of the lymphatics, such as cavernous lymphangioma.

DIAPHRAGMATIC INNERVATION

The phrenic nerve originates from the C3, C4, and C5 nerve roots and then enters the chest anterior to the subclavian artery. On the left side the nerve lies medial to the internal mammary artery (IMA) 64% of the time, and on the right side it lies medial to the IMA only 46% of the time.[24] Thus

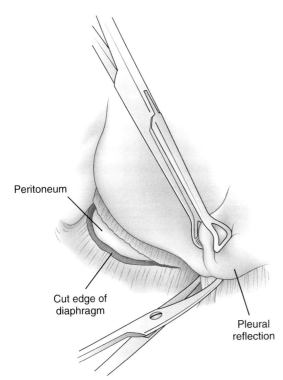

Figure 31–3 The parietal pleura folds off the ribcage and onto the diaphragm but does not extend into the deep recess of the diaphragmatic sulcus. A bare area of diaphragmatic muscle can be exposed with traction on the parietal pleura.

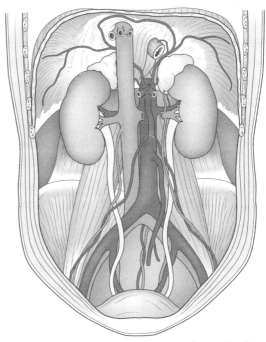

Figure 31–4 Arterial anatomy of the inferior diaphragmatic surface.

the left nerve is more prone to injury during mobilization of the left internal mammary artery through a median sternotomy incision.

As mentioned earlier, the majority of diaphragmatic muscle originates from cervical myotomes innervated by fibers from the spinal nerve roots at cervical levels C3, C4, and C5. These fibers join and form the phrenic nerve, which elongates as the septum transversum migrates caudally. There is, however, an outer rim of diaphragmatic muscle that originates from migrating mesenchymal cells of the nearby body wall innervated by spinal nerves from thoracic levels T7–T12. Additionally, there is a contribution from mesenchyme associated with the foregut at levels L1–L3 that coalesces to form the right and left crura.[10,17]

Despite the contributions from the thoracic and spinal nerve roots, the majority of the diaphragm is innervated by the phrenic nerve. Although the origin of the phrenic nerve and its proximal course through the mediastinum are well known, the distal extent of the nerve as it branches into the diaphragm proper is less well described. In 1956 Merendino and colleagues[20] published the most descriptive and often-cited reference regarding this intradiaphragmatic portion of the phrenic nerve. Their anatomical findings and frequently adapted schematized drawings are based on electrical stimulation studies and gross dissection in dogs, as well as intraoperative dissection of approximately 40 human diaphragms.

The phrenic nerve usually divides at the level of the diaphragm or just above it. The right phrenic nerve enters the diaphragm just lateral to the inferior vena cava within

the central tendon. The left phrenic nerve enters lateral to the left border of the heart just anterior to the central tendon within the muscle itself. The intradiaphragmatic course of the phrenic nerve can be predicted, even when not directly seen, by knowing the distribution of the four main motor divisions. The phrenic nerve first splits into an anterior and a posterior trunk (see Figure 31-2B). The anterior trunk subsequently divides into a sternal and an anterolateral branch near the anteromedial border of the central tendon. The posterior trunk likewise divides into a crural and a posterolateral branch along the posteromedial border of the central tendon. The sternal and crural branches are short and continue to run in an anteromedial and posteromedial direction, respectively. The anterolateral and posterolateral branches are much longer and run close to the muscular fiber insertions into the central tendon. These two branches innervate the majority of the diaphragm. Their anatomical relation to one another is often described as a pair of handcuffs or manacles. Often these branches are within the muscle layers and are not readily visible.

DIAPHRAGMATIC INCISIONS

There are a variety of suitable locations for diaphragmatic incisions that one can deduce from knowledge of diaphragmatic anatomy and function. Certain areas of the diaphragm can be incised safely without causing significant damage or loss of function. Other regions are apt to result in bleeding, structural weakness, and/or diaphragmatic hemiparesis if incised or cauterized inappropriately.

Diaphragmatic incisions can be divided into three groups: circumferential, central tendon, or radial. Circumferential incisions in the periphery result in little loss of function.

These circumferential incisions, however, must be at least 5 cm lateral to the edge of the central tendon to avoid the posterolateral and anterolateral branches of the phrenic nerve. These incisions can be difficult to correctly realign after a long operation. Placing surgical clips on each side of the muscular incision can greatly facilitate the correct spatial orientation on closing (Figure 31-5).

Incisions in the central tendon, as far centrally as within 2 cm of the entrance of the phrenic nerve, do not interrupt any major branch of the nerve itself. This type of incision can provide excellent visualization of the abdomen from the thorax, and vice versa. These incisions are easy to open and close.

A transverse radial incision made from the midaxillary line centrally is relatively safe because it courses between the distal aspects of the anterolateral and posterolateral branches of the phrenic nerve (i.e., through the opening of the handcuffs). Radial incisions from the costal margin extending all the way to the esophageal hiatus, however, may result in segmental diaphragmatic paralysis if the incision transects the crural or posterolateral branches of the phrenic nerve.

▶ TRAUMATIC DIAPHRAGMATIC INJURY

Both blunt and penetrating trauma can injure the diaphragm. Penetrating injuries to the lower thorax and upper abdomen place the diaphragm at risk of injury. The nipples, marking the most cephalad displacement of the

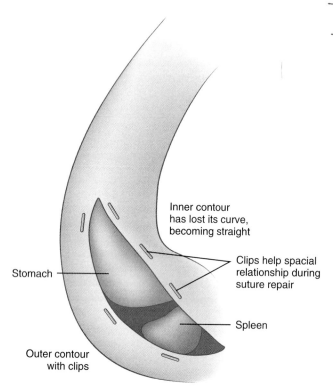

Inner contour has lost its curve, becoming straight

Clips help spacial relationship during suture repair

Stomach

Spleen

Outer contour with clips

Figure 31–5 Curvilinear diaphragmatic incision between strategically placed surgical clips. Diaphragmatic incisions disrupt the radial tension and distort the muscular anatomy. Placement of surgical clips before incision facilitates closure with proper realignment of the diaphragmatic musculature.

central tendon, and the base of the twelfth rib, marking the most caudal attachment of the muscle, are important landmarks that identify a potential diaphragmatic injury from penetrating trauma. Any missile traversing this area or knife wound within this zone may create a diaphragmatic laceration.

Blunt trauma that dramatically increases the intraabdominal pressure may cause a central tendon rupture of the diaphragm. Diaphragmatic rupture occurs in 0.8–1.6% of patients arriving at the emergency room with blunt trauma.[27] Because the liver protects the right hemidiaphragm from this latter mechanism of injury, most diaphragmatic ruptures from blunt trauma are recognized on the left side.

An abnormal diaphragm contour on plain chest X-ray (CXR) or CT scan after a traumatic injury should raise the possibility of diaphragmatic injury. These findings may be easier to appreciate if a radiopaque nasogastric tube is in place at the time of imaging. Nonetheless, radiographic findings may still be as subtle as blurring of the costophrenic angle. Because of this subtlety, delayed diagnoses are not uncommon. Review of the literature suggests that the diagnosis is missed in as many as 66% in some series.[31]

Diaphragmatic injuries that are diagnosed promptly should be explored from the abdomen with either a laparotomy or laparoscopy because of the frequent association of other abdominal organ injury (liver, spleen, stomach, kidney). In those cases with a significant delay in diagnosis, injuries generally should be explored from the thorax, with either thoracotomy or thoracoscopy, because the herniated abdominal structure is frequently adhesed to the ipsilateral lung.

Diaphragmatic injuries need to be repaired when they are recognized. Repair corrects and/or prevents complications, such as respiratory compromise or herniation of abdominal viscera with the associated risk of incarceration and strangulation. If no other indication for surgical exploration is present and the diagnosis of diaphragmatic rupture remains in question, exploratory thoracoscopy is a simple and effective diagnostic procedure. Small tears can be sutured with thoracoscopic techniques after reduction of abdominal contents displaced across the defect. Thoracoscopic exploration and repair require general anesthesia with single lung ventilation. Timing therefore depends on underlying pulmonary and neurological function.

▶ DIAPHRAGMATIC ELEVATION

The two most common causes of diaphragmatic elevation are congenital eventration of the diaphragm and phrenic nerve palsy.

Congenital eventration of the diaphragm is a spectrum of disorders that share the underlying cause of impaired fetal myotome migration.[2] Mild cases may only lack the central tendon, whereas severe cases may lack the central tendon and the entire muscular diaphragm. The area of congenitally missing muscle tissue is usually closed with a fused single membrane of pleura and peritoneum. This membrane generally is displaced within the ipsilateral hemithorax because of the absence of muscle.

Phrenic nerve paralysis in children can be due to a viral palsy, iatrogenic injury (typically after pediatric thoracic surgery), or a traction injury to the phrenic nerve at the base of the neck after a forceps delivery. In addition, there can be congenital absence of the phrenic nerve.

Diaphragmatic elevation is poorly tolerated in neonates. The flaccid diaphragm itself compresses the lower lobe of the ipsilateral lung. In addition, if there is a large displacement of abdominal components into the negative pressure thorax, this bulk mechanically shifts the mediastinum with compression of the contralateral lung. Thus there is atelectasis of the ipsilateral lower lobe, compression of the left atrium and impediment to pulmonary venous blood flow, and contralateral lung compression with additional atelectasis.[19] The end result may be complete pulmonary failure requiring intubation. Mechanical ventilation reinflates the atelectatic lungs and balances the mobile mediastinum. The ipsilateral diaphragm is shifted into the abdomen.

A variety of techniques have been described in the literature for plication of the diaphragm. Severe forms of congenital eventration of the diaphragm with only a pleuroperitoneal membrane requires patching.[2] A rim of rudimentary diaphragmatic tissue generally can be found around the lateral contour of the chest with enough substance to hold sutures to anchor the patch. Along the medial side, the patch can be stitched to the pericardium and the anterior thoracic spinal ligaments.

The easiest technique of plication is to place imbricating stitches within the central tendon of the diaphragm.[6,29] These stitches can be easily placed both thoracoscopically as well as through a minithoracotomy.[21] If the sutures extend far enough from the edge of the diaphragmatic tendon, they can produce substantial caudal displacement of the tendon toward the abdominal cavity and allow expansion of the ipsilateral lower lobe, as well as balancing the mediastinum (Figure 31-6).[33] The drawback of this technique, however, is that the majority of the pleats will fold the noncompliant central tendon. The compliant muscular remnant can be expected to stretch with time. It has been our experience that the central tendon pleating technique is associated with reelevation of the diaphragm to the level of the hilum within several years. Long-term follow-up of this technique has included reports of recurrent diaphragmatic elevation requiring additional intervention in as many as 19% of treated patients.[34] Furthermore, the phrenic vessels and branches of the nerve travel near the insertion of the muscle into the edge of the tendon and cannot be visualized from the thoracic surface of the diaphragm. Yet, to adequately displace the central tendon, these stitches need to extend into the muscle area, and this places the branches of the nerve at risk of injury.

Figure 31-2 shows the top view of the diaphragm and illustrates the radial spokes of the muscle fibers from their origin along the costal margin toward the central tendon. The phrenic nerve can be seen along the mediastinal pleura, but then pierces the diaphragmatic muscle close to the inferior vena cava on the right and the tip of the acute angle of the heart on the left. The phrenic vessels and phrenic nerve cannot be visualized from the thoracic surface of the diaphragm beyond these areas.

Dr. David State[36] described a subcostal radial plication technique for congenital eventration of the diaphragm in 1949. The original description of this technique included a generous incision across the right upper quadrant of the

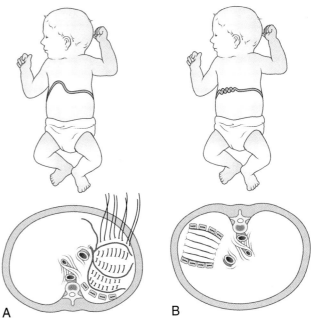

Figure 31–6 Diaphragmatic plication by pleating the central tendon. Sutures extend beyond the junction of the central tendon with the muscle and should not directly strike the branches of the phrenic nerve. Unfortunately, the phrenic branches lie within the muscle and frequently cannot be visualized.

abdomen and placement of radial sutures along the muscular portion of the diaphragm, pulling it toward the lateral chest wall (Figure 31-7). A transthoracic radial plication also has been described.[30,33]

Dr. John Foker at the University of Minnesota has used a transthoracic radial plication technique since 1976 to treat 35 children with elevation of the diaphragm.[13] The repairs were performed with interrupted horizontal mattress-pledgeted sutures imbricating the muscular portion of the diaphragm in a radial manner toward the chest wall via a posterolateral thoracotomy (Figure 31-8). The plication sutures extended in an unbroken band from the xyphoid area to the vertebral body. No sutures were placed along the mediastinal pleura. The goal was to produce a taut diaphragm that appeared as a straight-angled line from mediastinum to chest wall on anteroposterior (AP) view of the chest roentgenogram. We believe that this produces a plication that mimics the contraction of the fan-shaped muscle while minimizing injury to the branches of the nerve or vessels.

In this series, 31 of the 36 operations (86%) led to extubation within 3 days, even though 15 patients had been ventilator dependent before plication.[13] There were no deaths within 30 days, and no morbidity directly attributed to plication. Only one (3%) patient suffered a recurrence requiring repeat plication. Twenty-six of these patients survived long term (median 12 years at time of analysis), and 18 of these patients were reevaluated with diaphragmatic ultrasound in 1996. Some degree of function had returned to 14 (78%) of the diaphragms.

We have extended this technique to a thoracoscopic approach in adults with elevated hemidiaphragms with some success. Currently we use a three-port technique, with an anterior and posterior port at the sixth and eighth intercostal

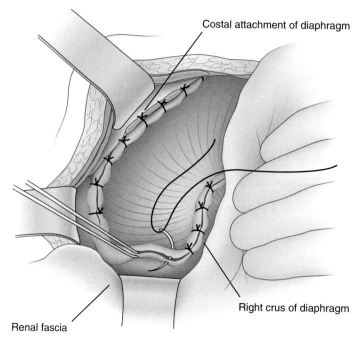

Costal attachment of diaphragm

Right crus of diaphragm

Renal fascia

Figure 31–7 Original description of a radial plication technique by Dr. David State in 1949. A generous subcostal incision was used, and the muscle was sewn circumferentially to the lateral chest wall and crus to make the tendon taught.

space, respectively. The third port is subcostal and is used to pass an 0-ring clamp through the abdominal cavity to grasp the undersurface of the central tendon of the diaphragm. This allows the vigorous caudal displacement of the muscle to see the muscular imbrications for plication. The posterior thoracic port is then used to plicate the anterior and lateral borders of the muscle, whereas the anterior thoracic port is used to plicate the lateral and posterior borders.

▶ DIAPHRAGMATIC HERNIAS

There are several types of hernias involving the diaphragm, including hernias of the foramen of Morgagni, the foramen of Bochdalek, as well as central tendon and paraesophageal hernias.

The foramen of Morgagni is a potential space that lies in the parasternal area, where the internal mammary vessels pass from the thoracic cavity into the upper abdominal cavity. Slips of diaphragmatic muscle insert medially onto the back of the xiphisternum, and laterally to the costal margin (see Figure 31-2B). This produces a small triangular gap of muscle tissue around the mammary vessels.

In the presence of increased intraabdominal pressure, omentum, small intestine, or colon can pass through this defect into the anterior mediastinum. Dull pain along the right subcostal area is the most common presenting symptom. Others are found incidentally on radiographic imaging for unrelated reasons. Foramen of Morgagni hernias are more common in women, obese individuals, and on the right side because the left side is partially occluded by the

presence of the pericardial sac. These hernias appear as a density in the parasternal area. CT scans of the chest are helpful in distinguishing these hernias from the pericardial fat pad or a pericardial cyst.[23]

Foramen of Morgagni hernias are frequently repaired from an abdominal approach. Both laparoscopic and thoracoscopic repairs have been described.[11,12] A small rim of the internal transthoracic muscle is frequently found behind the sternum and is sutured to the diaphragm to close the hernia. We perform this closure with interrupted mattress sutures using a heavy nonabsorbable suture. Alternatively, the posterior rectus sheath or a rib can be used to help close the hernia. Rarely the hernia cannot be closed without tension, and a patch is used.

Foramen of Bochdalek hernias can occur in adults. These are rare disorders, which are either found incidentally on radiographs for other reasons or are recognized after organ incarceration or volvulus.[15] Most of these hernias are small and are repaired primarily. This can be performed with minimally invasive techniques. Larger defects may require a patch.

A congenital hernia can occur in each of the three central tendons of the trileaflet diaphragm. Radiographically these can be confused with tumors lying over the dome of the diaphragm. When the hernia occurs in the central trileaflet, it is frequently associated with a congenital absence of the inferior pericardial sac. This can lead to the phenomenon of abdominal contents within the pericardial sac. Repair of these hernias is straightforward because of the laxity of the central tendon. Primary repair is frequently possible. Very large defects may require patching.

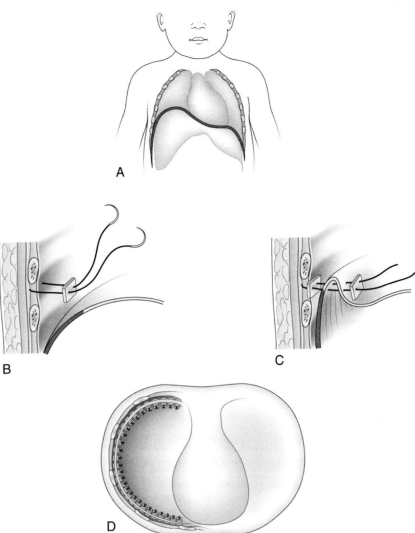

Figure 31–8 Radial plication of the diaphragm with interrupted double-pledgeted sutures extending from the xyphoid to the vertebral spine. Each suture pleats the flaccid muscle to the lateral chest wall.

The most frequent diaphragmatic hernia is the paraesophageal hernia. The most commonly used descriptive classification system defines four types of hiatal hernias. A sliding, or type I hiatal hernia, accounts for as many as 95% of paraesophageal hernias and involves the circumferential weakening of the phrenoesophageal ligament with symmetrical displacement of the proximal stomach into the thoracic cavity. This is frequently associated with a shortened esophagus. Most type I hernias are asymptomatic, discovered incidentally on radiographic studies or endoscopy. When symptoms occur, they are primarily related to the associated loss of lower esophageal sphincter tone and gastroesophageal reflux. The likelihood of these symptoms increases in proportion to the size of the hernia.[25]

A paraesophageal, or type II hiatal hernia, involves a focal weakening of the phrenoesophageal ligament. These hernias tend to occur either anterior or lateral to the esophagus. The gastric cardia remains within the abdomen, and the lower esophageal sphincter remains at the level of the diaphragm. A portion of the gastric fundus, however, rolls through the defect into the chest and produces extrinsic compression of the lower esophagus.

A mixed, or type III hiatal hernia, has both a sliding and a rolling component. The lower esophageal sphincter has been displaced up into the thorax because of a shortened esophagus. A portion of the gastric fundus then rolls through the enlarged hiatal hernia, producing extrinsic compression of the distal esophagus as well. We agree with Pearson and colleagues[26] that a type II hernia with the gastroesophageal junction below the diaphragm is rarely seen, and types I and III with the gastroesophageal junction displaced into the thorax are far more common.

Type IV hernias are associated with a large enough defect in the phrenoesophageal membrane to allow other organs, such as the colon, spleen, and small intestine, to enter the hernia sac and the chest cavity. Unrepaired type I, II, or III hiatal hernias can progress, resulting in a large defect between the crura of the diaphragm. As the hernia enlarges, the stomach has a tendency to migrate into the thoracic cavity. The positive pressure in the abdomen and the negative thoracic pressure can lead to the herniation of the greater curvature of the stomach into the right side of the chest and twisting the stomach upon itself. This gastric volvulus produces a gastric outlet obstruction. If air or gastric juices

510 distend the proximal stomach above the gastric outlet, the intraluminal pressure can exceed the perfusion pressure of the organ. This leads to ulceration, bleeding, and the potential for gastric rupture. Recognition of a gastric volvulus or displacement of intraabdominal organs into the chest is an indication for urgent surgical repair. Because of this potential life-threatening complication, most surgeons recommend repair of these hernias even in the asymptomatic patient.

The initial step in operative repair of a hiatal hernia is to clearly delineate the muscular limits of the hiatal defect. Some experienced surgeons advocate a transthoracic approach for long-standing hernias to facilitate lysis of inflammatory adhesions under direct vision, but at the cost of more postoperative pain. More recently, laparoscopic approaches have proven somewhat superior in this goal of identifying the limits of hiatal hernia. This is due to the cephalad displacement of the diaphragmatic muscle during insufflation of carbon dioxide into the abdomen, making the two crura of the diaphragm taut. This tautness and extra space between the stomach and the diaphragmatic muscle greatly facilitates the dissection.

The fat between the proximal stomach and the diaphragmatic muscle needs to be removed. Dividing the muscular fibers of the left diaphragmatic crus in a straight lateral manner can enlarge tight hiatal rings. This will not divide the branches of the phrenic nerve that lie far anteriorly, nor the phrenic vein, which lies medially. The left inferior phrenic artery may be divided without causing ischemia because anastamosing vessels continue to perfuse the area. The enlargement of the tight hiatal ring can greatly facilitate the reduction of a large bulky hernia. Alternatively, a red rubber catheter can be passed across the neck of the hiatal hernia and air insufflated within the sac to facilitate reduction of the hernia contents. This breaks the natural vacuum that occurs when trying to reduce the abdominal contents through the hiatal neck.

The diaphragmatic defect needs to be closed as part of the surgical repair of the hiatal hernia. In fact, it is the pathology of the diaphragm that has contributed to the disease of gastroesophageal reflux by disrupting the lower esophageal sphincter. Closure of the dilated esophageal diaphragmatic hiatus is frequently performed by placement of sutures reapproximating the right and left crura of the diaphragm. In large hiatal hernias this defect can be sizable. If the fibers of the diaphragmatic crura have been thinned, we frequently use pledgeted nonabsorbable sutures to reapproximate the right and left muscle bundles. Rarely a synthetic patch may need to be used to close a large defect that has been present for a long time, because the diaphragmatic muscles will not hold approximating sutures.

The postoperative complication rate after laparoscopic antireflux surgery is approximately 8%. Between 3 and 6% of all patients undergoing antireflux surgery require reoperation for recurrent, persistent, or new symptoms secondary to complications of the initial repair.[37] In one published series of 627 patients, 7% of the entire group had demonstrable anatomical failure, the majority of which were due to intrathoracic migration of the wrap with or without disruption of the fundoplication.[35] A number of factors have been attributed to this problem, including inadequate closure of the crura, lack of appreciation of a shortened esophagus, and physiological factors that increase intraabdominal pressure such as valsalva, coughing, or retching in the postoperative period.

We believe that one of the most common errors in the surgical repair of hiatal hernias is not recognizing that an esophagus has shortened. If the esophagus is not of adequate length to allow the fundoplication to reside within the abdomen without undue pressure, the fundoplication will likely herniate into the thorax within a few years. We have a low threshold for extending the length of the esophagus with a Collis gastroplasty to ensure that the fundoplication will lie beneath the diaphragmatic hiatus without tension.

A rare but devastating complication of fundoplication herniation into the chest from an unrecognized shortened esophagus is a gastropericardial fistula (Figure 31-9).[22] This rare condition has an associated mortality rate of more than 50% and is most often seen in patients with prior gastroesophageal surgery. Most likely these fistulas originate at the site of gastric ulcerations. Approximately 3–5% of open Nissen fundoplication procedures are complicated by gastric ulceration. In most cases the ulcerations occur high on the lesser curvature of the stomach, in proximity to the fundoplication, and are seen most often in patients with recurrent hiatal hernias. Fistulas from the stomach to the aorta, diaphragm, pericardium, right ventricle, and bronchus have been reported as late complications from open Nissen fundoplication.[22]

Repair of a gastropericardial fistula involves the removal of a circle of pericardium (Figure 31-9, *B*) and the fistulous entry into the stomach. The muscle of the diaphragm can then be used as a pedicled muscle flap to lie between the exposed heart and the staple line along the lesser curve of the stomach. In our experience, we have used pledgeted sutures to close the muscles of the crura and secure the wrap beneath the diaphragm.[22]

DIAPHRAGMATIC PACING

Diaphragmatic pacing may have a role to play for patients with compromised pulmonary function and diaphragmatic paralysis. The technology was first used clinically in 1967, and over 700 patients with chronic hypoventilation have been treated in this manner, some for as much as 18 years.[7] Expertise in this technique, however, is limited to a few centers. Technical details of long-term continuous pacing were mostly worked out by William Glenn of Yale. He and his colleagues rapidly moved from a successful animal model in 1964[9] to treatment of a patient with central hypoventilation in 1967.[14] Excellent detailed reviews of this subject have recently been published by Glenn and Koda[7] and Elefteriades and Quin, also from Yale.[4]

Diaphragmatic pacing largely has been supplanted by noninvasive methods of ventilatory support, including bilevel positive airway pressure (BiPAP) and continuous positive airway pressure (CPAP), particularly in the setting of temporary respiratory compromise or comorbid disease, such as chronic obstructive pulmonary disease (COPD). A select subset of patients, however, may be helped by this diaphragmatic pacing. The ideal patient for this technique

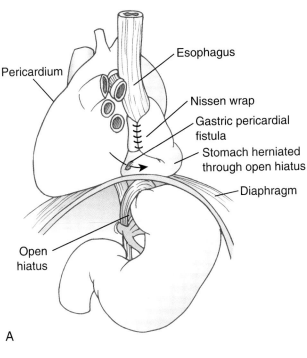

A

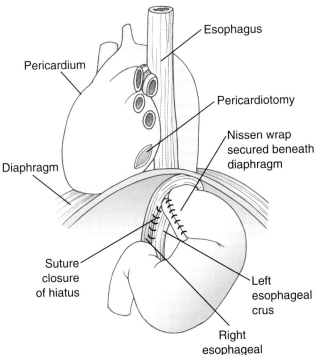

B

Figure 31–9 **A,** Gastropericardial fistula is a devastating complication of a fundoplication herniating into the chest from failure to close the diaphragmatic crura. The fistula is typically along the lesser curve of the stomach distal to the fundoplication. **B,** We repaired this fistula by using the diaphragm as a muscle flap to place between the heart and the stomach.

has central nervous system or upper motor neuron disease, and an intact phrenic nerve and diaphragm.[4] The major experience with phrenic nerve pacing has come from quadriplegic patients and central alveolar hypoventilation patients. Patients with spinal cord injury above C3 are espe-

cially good candidates, because the whole phrenic nerve is denervated from upper motor neurons but intact within the chest. Because pacing will not produce normal excursion of an atrophied diaphragmatic muscle, it is recommended that the pacemaker be placed soon after the neurological insult.

The major therapeutic objective of diaphragmatic pacing is oxygenation, rather than the elimination CO_2. Expiratory flow must be adequate, thus limiting the use of pacing in severe COPD or other conditions that have significantly altered the shape of the chest wall or diaphragm.[4] Sufficient diaphragmatic strength, near normal function of the distal phrenic nerve, and satisfactory excursion of the thoracic skeleton must be demonstrated.

The topic of phrenic nerve pacing is frequently discussed in the setting of phrenic nerve palsy. It is important to realize that the inherent lack of electrical conductivity of skeletal muscle, unlike the heart, does now allow uniform contraction of the muscle by multiple surface electrodes. An intact lower motor neuron (i.e., phrenic nerves) is thus required to deliver the electric impulse via neurotransmitters throughout the muscle for coordinated contraction. Because axonal damage precludes conduction of electrical impulses to the neuromuscular junction, direct phrenic nerve injury is not amenable to pacing. These patients may be better treated with direct intervention (i.e., primary phrenic nerve repair or nerve transplant with an intercostal or recurrent laryngeal nerve) or supportive measures (i.e., diaphragmatic placation, nocturnal BiPAP, or tracheostomy).[4]

The best placement of the phrenic nerve pacemaker, with current technology, is within the upper thorax via an anterolateral thoracotomy through the third intercostal space. This allows placement of the electrode around the main phrenic trunk below the entry of the accessory nerve from the C5 nerve root, which frequently joins the phrenic nerve within the upper thorax.[8] Although the nerve trunk is easily found in the neck, in 76% of patients the phrenic nerve is missing the C5 accessory nerve at this level.[16] Furthermore, placement of the electrode over the superior vena cava avoids direct conduction of the electrical signal to the atrium, which can occur lower in the thorax. Electrodes can now be placed thoracoscopically.[4] Implantation via the cervical approach has largely been abandoned because of its inability to bring the pacing electrode in proximity to the C5 branch of the phrenic nerve.

The phrenic nerve should be tested transcutaneously for patients with a central nervous system cause of hypoventilation to verify intact nerve and muscle function. This test was described by Shaw and Glenn in 1975.[32] An indifferent electrode is placed on the skin of the neck, and a pacing electrode delivering 5–10 mA for 1 ms is placed at the lateral border of the sternocleidomastoid muscle. A forceful contraction of the diaphragm signifies normal or near-normal diaphragmatic function. Forceful diaphragmatic movement can be observed by physical examination. Quantification of diaphragmatic excursion can be made by fluoroscopy or ultrasound. An excursion of at least 5 cm should be seen to consider pacing intervention.[4]

The initial diaphragmatic pacemaker consisted of a monopolar electrode attached to an antenna and a radiofrequency generator. A bipolar electrode would be used if the patient also has a cardiac pacemaker. To overcome the lack

512 of natural electric conductivity of the skeletal muscle of the diaphragm, a train of pulse currents with increasing amplitude is delivered by the pacemaker to stimulate all axons within the nerve.[4] One consequence of the pulse train to induce uniform muscle contraction is that every fascicle is stimulated to contract. Because 24% of the fascicles are fast-twitch, fatigue-prone, type IIB fibers,[18] full-time pacing can occur only after a period of muscle conditioning. Part-time pacing in quadriplegic patients does not start for 14 days to avoid pleural effusion.[4] Pacing starts at 15 minutes per hour and changes every 7–14 days. Conditioning thus takes 3–6 months. A permanent tracheostomy is recommended for all patients on full-time, continuous phrenic nerve pacing.[4]

Three pacing systems are currently available: the Avery model (Avery Labs, Glen Cove, NY), the Arotech OY (Tampere, Finland), and MedImplant (Vienna, Austria). All models have a two-part system with an extracorporeal radiofrequency generator and implantable receiver/nerve electrode. Further technological improvements may make diaphragmatic pacing a more generalizable technique for patients with long-term but ultimately reversible dysfunction, such as viral palsies and iatrogenic injuries.

In summary, diaphragmatic pacing is useful for carefully selected patients with intact phrenic nerve and diaphragmatic muscle function, but impaired upper motor neurons. The potential exists for a large group of patients with lower motor neuron disease (i.e., temporary or permanent phrenic nerve injury) to benefit once further advances in technology can produce smooth coordinated muscular contraction of the diaphragm with direct muscular stimulation

► DIAPHRAGMATIC RESECTION AND REPAIR WITH PROSTHETIC PATCH

Partial diaphragmatic resections are necessary to remove tumors that have invaded a portion of the diaphragm. The redundancy of the muscle frequently allows primary repair for small to modest resections. Larger defects are easily repaired with the use of a mesh or impermeable graft sutured to the remnant of muscle. We use mesh for patients with lung tissue remaining in the ipsilateral hemithorax, and impermeable grafts for patients who have had a pneumonectomy, to prevent fluid shifts between the thorax and abdomen.

Complete diaphragmatic resection may be required for large tumors invading the diaphragm, such as lung cancer of the lower lobe or sarcomas of the chest. We have gained our extensive experience with complete diaphragmatic resection as part of an extrapleural pneumonectomy for mesothelioma.[38]

An extrapleural pneumonectomy is the complete removal of the pleural envelope and all its contents, including the ipsilateral lung, lateral pericardium, and underlying diaphragm. Because the pleura cannot be separated from the central tendon of the diaphragm, the diaphragm must be resected if the pleural envelope is to be kept intact during removal.

Diaphragmatic resection begins with the traction of the pleura away from the chest wall deep into the diaphragmatic sulcus. This exposes the bare area of the lateral diaphragm where the pleura folds off the ribcage and back onto the upper surface of the diaphragm (Figure 31-10).[38] The division of these lateral radial bands of the fan-shaped portion of the diaphragm is started at the most anterior portion of the chest close to the pericardium. The fingers of the surgeon bluntly dissect the peritoneum from beneath the muscle, then pull the fibers taut to facilitate visualization to divide the muscle with cautery. It is not unusual for the posterolateral portion of the diaphragm to be beyond the direct vision of the surgeon. Fibers in this area can be bluntly avulsed with minimal risk of bleeding. Once the ligamentum arcuatum externum (external arcuate ligament) is reached in the paravertebral sulcus, the perinephric fat of Gerota's fossa, and not the peritoneum, is directly beneath the fan-shaped muscle. This part of the dissection quickly progresses to the lateral margin of the crus. The diaphragm can then be separated from the peritoneum up toward the lateral border of the pericardium. Defects in the peritoneum are closed as they are recognized.

An extrapleural pneumonectomy requires the removal of the lateral portion of the pericardium because the mediastinal pleura cannot be removed from that structure. The pericardium is opened anteriorly. The phrenic nerve is divided cephalad to the pulmonary artery. The trileaflet of the diaphragmatic tendon is divided along the line demarcating the central tendon of the ipsilateral muscle from the tendon lying beneath the pericardium. This cut is made medial to the insertion of the phrenic nerve into the anterior muscle. This medial cut is extended along the fused portion of diaphragmatic tendon and pericardium to the inferior vena cava on the right, or the esophageal hiatus on the left.

At this point the only attachment of the diaphragm remaining is the crus. Blunt dissection of the pleura of the deep diaphragmatic sulcus needs to be completed before division of the crus to prevent buttonholing the inferior extent of the posterolateral pleura. The superior phrenic

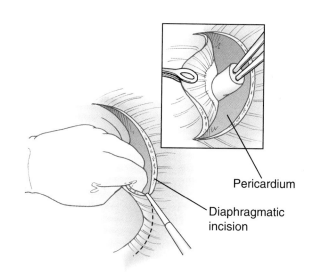

Pericardium

Diaphragmatic incision

Figure 31–10 Circumferential incision of the right hemidiaphragm exposing the underlying peritoneum. Pericardial and crural attachments remain after division of the fan-shaped muscle.

arteries are surgically inconsequential and rarely identified. The inferior phrenic vessels, however, lie on the deep surface of the crus and are easily seen and ligated. These vessels may bifurcate low over the crus, and a second branch may therefore be found after ligation of a branch thought to be the main trunk. The left inferior phrenic vein usually has two branches, one of which drains into the left renal or suprarenal vein and another that passes anterior to the esophageal hiatus and empties into the inferior vena cava. The right inferior phrenic vein empties directly into the inferior vena cava and therefore requires careful dissection and ligation. Vigorous lateral traction can avulse this vessel from the inferior vena cava, close to the insertion of the hepatic veins. Once these vessels have been divided, the crus is easily divided. This completes the diaphragmatic resection.

The postpneumonectomy space fills with fluid. To prevent fluid shifts between the thorax and abdomen, we use a 2-mm impermeable Gore-Tex prosthetic patch to reconstruct the resected diaphragm. This patch prevents herniation of abdominal contents into the chest, holds the abdominal viscera out of the thoracic radiation field, and also bolsters the contralateral diaphragm by fixing the medial edge of the fan into place. This then facilitates the function of the opposite diaphragm by allowing its central tendon to become the anchor point for the lateral fan fascicles. Without patching the ipsilateral diaphragmatic defect, the contralateral muscle function is compromised.

After the patch has been cut to the shape of the removed diaphragm, the medial edge is sewn to the pericardial tendon with a soft nonabsorbable stitch. We prefer 0-Ethibond for this suture. This suture line runs from the free edge of the divided anterior fan muscles, along the pericardial edge, to either the inferior vena cava or esophageal hiatus. A reliable lateral anchorage system has been devised, requiring a sterilized leatherworking awl (Figure 31-11). Loops of suture material that have been passed through the lateral edge of the patch are then brought through the chest wall with the awl. The sutures are then passed through a small postage stamp–sized patch of the same material, as well as a sterile plastic button, with the assistance of two angiocaths. The loop of suture is then tied down to itself onto the button, resulting in excellent lateral displacement of the patch.

The posterior mediastinum between the thoracic spine and the inferior vena cava or esophagus is the area where patch ruptures occur, with abdominal contents herniating into the chest. This is due to a lack of strong mediastinal tissue available to anchor the patch. Our group of surgeons have developed the following three potential solutions: (1) a suture anchoring the patch to the anterior spinal ligament, (2) a tongue of extra patch material folded inferiorly along the lumbar spine in simulation of the diaphragmatic crus, and (3) a composite of two patches of 2 mm Gore-Tex stapled together in the middle with a thoracoabdominal (TA) stapler to create a dynamic patch at the center with less tension at the lateral suture lines. The first technique uses the dense spinous ligament to anchor the posterior mediastinal portion of the patch and decreases the free defect between the anterior suture line at the inferior vena cava and the thoracic spine to a few centimeters. The second technique allows the medial portion of the patch to partially displace

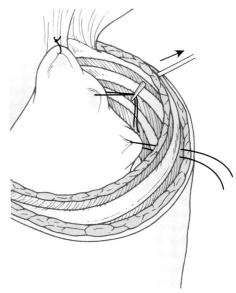

Figure 31–11 Diaphragmatic resection for extrapleural pneumonectomy necessitates patch closure. A sterile leatherworking awl is used to pass anchoring sutures through the chest wall to recreate radial lines of tension. These sutures are secured along the outside of the ribcage using angiocaths through the holes of sterile buttons.

into the chest, but prevents visceral herniation unless the entire tongue becomes displaced into the chest. The last technique allows the prosthetic patch to "give" without rupture if the patient experiences abdominal distention.

▶ CONCLUSION

The diaphragm serves several functions as a result of its unique anatomical location. It is the major muscle of respiration, by creating the intrathoracic vacuum and moving the lower ribs. It is a barrier between the positive pressure abdomen and the negative pressure thorax. It is important in the function of the lower esophageal sphincter.

Surgical approaches to the diaphragm are easily learned and depend on an understanding of the anatomy and physiology of the muscle, nerve, and blood vessels. A variety of incisions are possible once the location of the nerve and vessel branches have been learned. These structures frequently lie within the muscle itself and are not seen on the surface of the structure. Therefore the concept of a handcuff around the junction of the central tendon to the muscle is helpful.

Diaphragmatic repair and patching is helpful in traumatic injuries, congenital absence of a part of the diaphragm, and diaphragmatic hernias. Diaphragmatic pacing is not useful in phrenic nerve palsies, because an intact lower motor neuron is required for the current level of technology to function. Plication of the diaphragm for these cases is useful. We prefer a radial plication technique that mimics the radial contraction of the fan-shaped muscle to that of a central tendon pleat.

514

Repair of gastroesophageal reflux depends on the creation of a new lower esophageal sphincter. A major contributor of the pathology, however, is a diaphragmatic hernia between the crura: a hiatal hernia. Therefore we believe that tightening of the crus around the repair and lengthening of a shortened esophagus are important steps to keep the repair within the abdomen, and prevent complications such as gastropericardial fistula.

The entire hemidiaphragm can be resected. Small resections can be repaired primarily, but large resections should be patched to assist the function of the contralateral muscle. The choice between permeable or impermeable patches depends on the remaining presence of ipsilateral lung. The principles of the patch repair include a tight apposition to the medial remnant of the diaphragm, and then radial lateral displacement of anchoring sutures.

Although the diaphragm acts as a boundary between the thorax and abdomen, it should not serve as a boundary between the realm of thoracic surgeons and gastrointestinal surgeons. The diaphragm makes a good fence, but neighbors on both sides of that fence should know its anatomy, physiology, and surgical principles of resection and repair.

REFERENCES

1. Anderson T, Miller J: Surgical technique and application of pericardial fat pad and pericardiophrenic grafts. Ann Thorac Surg 59:1590–1591, 1995.
2. Beck W, Motsay D: Eventration of the diaphragm. Arch Surg 65:557–563, 1952.
3. Bergofsky E: Relative contributions of the rib cage and the diaphragm to ventilation in man. J Appl Physiol 19:698–706, 1964.
4. Elefteriades J, Quin J: Diaphragm pacing. Chest Surg Clin N Am 8(2):331–357, 1998.
5. Epstein S: An overview of respiratory muscle function. Clin Chest Med 15:619–639, 1994.
6. Garbaccio C, Gyepes M, Fonkalsrud E: Malfunction of the intact diaphragm in infants and children. Arch Surg 105:57–61, 1972.
7. Glenn W, Koda H: Pacing the diaphragm in chronic ventilatory insufficiency. In Shields TW, editor: Thoracic Surgery, pp. 595–610. Philadelphia: Lea & Febiger, 1989.
8. Glenn W, Sairenji H: Diaphragm pacing in the treatment of chronic ventilatory insufficiency. In Roussos C, Macklem P, editors: The Thorax, pp. 1407–1449. New York: Marcel Dekker, 1985.
9. Glenn WW, Hageman JH, Mauro A, et al: Electrical stimulation of excitable tissue by radio-frequency transmission. Ann Surg 160:338–350, 1964.
10. Gray H: Anatomy, Descriptive and Surgical. Pick T, Howden R, editors. Revised American, from the 15th English ed., p.1257. New York: Bounty Books, 1977.
11. Huntington T: Laparoscopic transabdominal preperitoneal repair of a hernia of foramen of Morgagni. J Laparoendosc Surg 6:131–133, 1996.
12. Hussong R, Landrenau R, Cole F: Diagnosis and repair of a Morgagni hernia with video-assisted thoracic surgery. Ann Thorac Surg 63:1474–1475, 1997.
13. Jaklitsch M, et al: Twenty year experience with peripheral radial plication of the diaphragm. In 33rd Annual Meeting of the Society of Thoracic Surgeons, San Diego, 1997.
14. Judson J, Glenn W: Radiofrequency electrophrenic respiration: Long-term application to a patient with primary hypoventilation. JAMA 203:1033–1037, 1968.
15. Karanikas ID, Dendrinos SS, Liakakos TD, et al: Complications of congenital posterolateral diaphragmatic hernia in adults. J Cardiovasc Surg (Torino) 35:555–558, 1994.
16. Kelley W: Phrenic nerve paralysis: Special consideration of the accessory phrenic nerve. J Thorac Cardiovasc Surg 19:923–928, 1950.
17. Larsen W: Human Embryology, 2nd ed., pp. 136–137. New York: Churchill Livingstone, 1997.
18. Lieberman D, Faulkner JA, Craig AB Jr, et al: Performance and histochemical composition of guinea pig and human diaphragm. J Appl Physiol 34:233–237, 1973.
19. Marcos J, Grover F, Trinkle J: Paralyzed diaphragm—Effect of plication on respiratory mechanics. J Surg Res 16:523–526, 1974.
20. Merendino KA, Johnson RA, Skinner HH, et al: The intradiaphragmatic distribution of the phrenic nerve with particular reference to the placement of diaphragmatic incisions and controlled segmental paralysis. Surgery 39:189–198, 1956.
21. Mouroux J, Padovani B, Poirier NC, et al: Technique for the repair of diaphragmatic eventration. Ann Thorac Surg 62:905–907, 1996.
22. Murthy S, Looney J, Jaklitsch M: Brief report: Gastropericardial fistula after laparoscopic surgery for reflux disease. N Engl J Med 346:328–332, 2002.
23. Naunheim K: Adult presentation of unusual diaphragmatic hernias. Chest Surg Clin N Am 8(2):359–369, 1998.
24. Owens W, Gladstone D, Heylings D: Surgical anatomy of the phrenic nerve and internal mammary artery. Ann Thorac Surg 58:843–844, 1994.
25. Patti MG, Goldberg HI, Arcerito M, et al: Hiatal hernia size affects lower esophageal sphincter function, esophageal acid exposure, and the degree of mucosal injury. Am J Surg 171:182–186, 1996.
26. Pearson FG, Cooper JD, Ilves R, et al: Massive hiatal hernia with incarceration: A report of 53 cases. Ann Thorac Surg 35(1):45–51, 1983.
27. Reber PU, Schmied B, Seiler CA, et al: Missed diaphragmatic injuries and their long term sequelae. J Trauma 44(1):183–188, 1998.
28. Schumpelick V, Steinau G, Schluper I, et al: Surgical embryology and anatomy of the diaphragm with surgical applications. Surg Clin North Am 80(1):213–239, xi, 2000.
29. Schwartz M, Filler R: Plication of the diaphragm for symptomatic phrenic nerve paralysis. J Pediatr Surg 13(3):259–263, 1978.
30. Sethi G, Reed W: Diaphragmatic malfunction in neonates and infants: Diagnosis and treatment. J Thorac Cardiovasc Surg 62(1):138–143, 1971.
31. Shah R, Sabanthan S, Mearns AJ, et al: Traumatic rupture of diaphragm. Ann Thorac Surg 60:1444–1449, 1995.
32. Shaw R, Glenn W, Holcomb W: Phrenic nerve conduction studies in patients with diaphragm pacing. Surg Forum 26:195–197, 1975.
33. Shoemaker R, Palmer G, Brown JW, et al: Aggressive treatment of acquired phrenic nerve paralysis in infants and small children. Ann Thorac Surg 32(3):251–259, 1981.
34. Smith C, Sade RM, Crawford FA, et al: Diaphragmatic paralysis and eventration in infants. J Thorac Cardiovasc Surg 91:490–497, 1986.

35. Soper N, Dunnegan D: Anatomic fundoplication failure after laparoscopic antireflux surgery. Ann Surg 229(5):669–676, 1999.
36. State D: The surgical correction of congenital eventration of the diaphragm in infancy. Surgery 25:461–468, 1949.
37. Stein H, Feussner H, Siewert J: Failure of antireflux surgery: Causes and management strategies. Am J Surg 171(1):36–39, 1996.
38. Sugarbaker D, Mentzer S, Strauss G: Extrapleural pneumonectomy in the treatment of malignant pleural mesothelioma. Ann Thorac Surg 54:941–946, 1992.
39. Wade O: Movements of the thoracic cage and diaphragm in respiration. J Physiol 124:193–212, 1954.

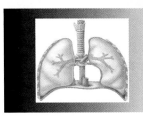

Congenital Diaphragmatic Hernia

Dario O. Fauza, Nikki Allmendinger, and Jay M. Wilson

CHAPTER **32**

DEFINITION

Many congenital diaphragmatic anomalies include some sort of defect that allows for herniation of abdominal contents into the chest. Yet the term congenital diaphragmatic hernia (CDH), or Bochdalek's hernia, refers specifically to congenital defects located on the posterolateral aspect of the diaphragm. Despite the name diaphragmatic "hernia," only in approximately 15% of the cases is there a true hernia sac.

HISTORY

The first known written description of a diaphragmatic herniation was made by Ambroise Paré in 1579.[221] However, the two cases described by Paré were caused by trauma. In his *Sepulchretum,* published in 1679, Teophile Bonet attributed the first description of a congenital case to Lazare Rivere at the beginning of the seventeenth century, even if it was from the necropsy of an adult.[39] The first report of a CDH in a newborn was made by George Macaulay in 1754, also as a necropsy finding, in an infant who died from respiratory failure a little more than 1 hour after birth.[184]

In 1761 Giambattista Morgagni, then a pupil of Valsalva, wrote a review of diaphragmatic herniations and credited Stehenius with the first observation that CDH was associated with pulmonary hypoplasia.[195] In the review Morgagni described the first case of a parasternal hernia in an elderly man, henceforth termed Morgagni's hernia. In 1848 Vincent Alexander Bochdalek reported two cases in which he described the location of the diaphragmatic defect as being in the posterolateral aspect of the muscle, hence the origins of the terms Bochdalek's hernia and Bochdalek's foramen.[33] Although widely employed, these terms actually are incorrect, given that the mechanisms and exact location proposed by Bochdalek, namely, "rupture of the lumbocostal triangle," are inaccurate.[44,286,290]

The link between CDH and deviations of the embryonic development of the pleuroperitoneal membrane only started to be established from the studies by Broman in 1902 and 1905.[46,47] Nevertheless, although this anatomical location for the diaphragmatic defect is universally accepted, it is not yet known where the primary disorder that leads to CDH takes place.

The first successful repair of a CDH was performed by Aue in a 9-year-old boy in 1901, but was published only in 1920.[16] The first publication of a successful CDH repair was by Hedenhain in 1905, where he reported a procedure, also in a 9-year-old boy, that took place in 1902.[135] In 1940 the first survival of a neonate, who underwent CDH repair on the second day of life, was reported by Ladd and Gross.[168]

518 In 1946 Gross was also the first to report on a good outcome after repair before the first 24 hours of life.[117]

In 1977 German et al[111] reported the first child with CDH to survive after being placed on extracorporeal membrane oxygenation (ECMO). Ever since the mid-1980s it has become clear that ECMO plays a major role in maximizing the survival rates of neonates with CDH.[63,201,304]

In 1989 Harrison and associates[128] presented the first series of CDH treated by open prenatal repair of the diaphragmatic defect in humans, leading to live births, but no midterm survival. Survival after this procedure was reported by this same group in 1992, but only in 28.6% of the operated fetuses.[122]

In the early 1990s, from the work of Wung et al,[308,309] the concept of avoiding hyperventilation and minimizing barotrauma was introduced. These principles have since led to marked reduction in iatrogenic insult to the lungs, which was very common in the old, aggressive ventilation strategies, and consequent significant improvement in survival.[38,153,201,304]

The first successful lung transplantation for the treatment of CDH was performed in a newborn in 1992, by the groups of Shochat and Starnes.[247,277] Also in 1992 Wilson and associates[300] first showed, in an ovine model of CDH, that fetal lung growth could be significantly accelerated after occlusion of the fetal trachea, leading to reversal of the pulmonary hypoplasia associated with experimental CDH. In 1994 Harrison's group first applied this maneuver successfully in a human fetus with CDH.[2] Nonetheless, the results of fetal tracheal occlusion, whether performed openly or videofetoscopically, remain worse than those of postnatal care at the most advanced centers.[100,123,127]

In 1994 the Congenital Diaphragmatic Hernia Registry was created as a meta-institutional organization dedicated to the exchange and analysis of data related to this disease, as well as to the design and implementation of multicentric prospective trials. This initiative was molded after the pediatric oncology groups established in the 1980s and, as such, has begun to have a major beneficial impact on CDH survival and management guidelines.

In 1995 we demonstrated experimentally that lung growth could also be accelerated after birth, through continuous intrapulmonary distension with a perfluorocarbon.[92] The first series of patients that received this treatment, under ECMO support, was presented in 2000,[93] and a multicentric prospective trial is being organized. Also in 2000 the use of a tissue-engineered construct for the repair of the diaphragmatic defect was first proposed in an animal model.[94] Current development efforts are aimed at defining the patients that would benefit from lung growth acceleration, enhancing diaphragmatic repair through tissue engineering, and minimizing morbidity of the increasingly more common long-term survivors.

▶ EPIDEMIOLOGY

The prevalence of CDH has been reported as being anywhere between 1:1200 and 1:12,000 births.* Likely the main reason for such disparities is the so-called hidden mortality of CDH, which relates to the fact that many babies die before making it to a referral center and thus are not included in the statistics.[253] The better-controlled studies show CDH as occurring in 1:2107 to 1:3163 births.* The largest series ever studied, by Torfs et al,[268] involving more than 718,000 births and stillbirths in part of California, revealed that CDH occurred in 1:3163 births and in 1:3340 live births. Among the major congenital anomalies, CDH is one of the most common, accounting for approximately 8% of the cases.[206]

There are no clear racial differences in the prevalence of CDH.[239,268] The study by Torfs et al[268] showed a higher prevalence in rural rather than in urban areas, but this has not yet been confirmed by other series. The prevalence of prematurity and weight deviations in neonates with CDH is no different from that of the general population.[268] Although isolated CDH is a little more common in boys than in girls (1.5:1), sex distribution is normal in CDH associated with other congenital anomalies and in the whole CDH population.[43,268]

There is limited controversy as to the risk of CDH recurrence within families. In the vast majority of cases CDH is sporadic, with no genetic component described to date and with the risk for further offspring being practically equal to that of the general population.[51,73] At the same time, many families with more than one case of CDH, usually siblings, have been identified.† Less frequently, relatives other than siblings also can display this anomaly.[178,214,271] The epidemiological profile of familial cases of CDH differs little from that of the total of cases: It is slightly more common in male patients (approximately 2:1)[186,190,271,285] and there are conflicting data regarding the other variables.[214,307] The occurrence of familial CDH follows a pattern suggestive of multifactorial inheritance as the most likely mode of transmission, with recurrence estimated between 1.3% and 2%.[105,206,268,307] The possibility that a genomic imprinting phenomenon takes place also has been proposed recently.[17]

▶ EMBRYOLOGY OF THE DIAPHRAGM

The diaphragm comes from the mesoderm. Its development is complex and not yet fully understood. It results from the fusion of four embryonic components: two odd ones, namely, the transverse septum and the mediastinum (also known as the dorsal mesentery of the esophagus), and two paired structures, namely, both sides of the body wall musculature and both pleuroperitoneal membranes (Figure 32-1).[46]

The diaphragm begins to develop during the third and fourth weeks of gestation, with the appearance of the first component of the diaphragm, the transverse septum (see Figure 32-1). At this point the transverse septum is an incomplete mesenchymal divider, related cranially to the pericardial cavity and caudally to the midgut. Dorsally the transverse septum blends with the mediastinum. On each side of the mediastinum there are the pleural canals, which connect the pericardial and peritoneal cavities. The subsequent development of the diaphragm depends on the closure of these dorsal pleural canals, which gives rise to the pleural cavities.

---

*References 51, 70, 73, 89, 125, 172, 226, 230, 239, 268, 270, 287.

*References 51, 70, 73, 172, 239, 268.
†References 17, 55, 70, 105, 178, 190, 206, 268, 285, 307.

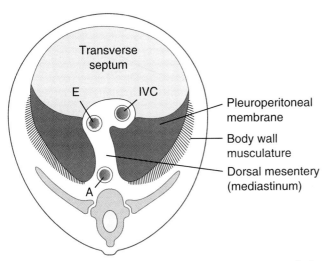

Figure 32–1 The four embryonic components of the diaphragm. A, Aorta; E, esophagus; IVC, inferior vena cava.

During the fourth week of gestation, the pulmonary buds, which are developing inside the mediastinum, begin to protrude into the pleural canals. At this stage the pleural canals are very small and the pericardial cavity is very large. Crests formed on both extremities of the pleural canals separate the future pleural cavities from the pericardial cavity cranially, and from the peritoneal cavity caudally. The cranial crest gives rise to the pleuropericardial membrane, and the caudal crest forms the pleuroperitoneal membrane (see Figure 32-1).

The enlargement of what are now the pleural cavities leads to a progressive narrowing of the opening between them and the pericardial cavity, as well as to the development of the pleuropericardial membrane. In like manner, there is progressive narrowing of the pleuroperitoneal canals and the development of the pleuroperitoneal membranes.[44,286] The definitive closure of the pleuroperitoneal canals, now small, occurs during the eighth week of gestation.[44]

After closure of the pleuroperitoneal canals, the pleural cavities continue to expand in parallel to lung growth. Cranially they spread out beyond the limits of the pericardial space.

Caudally they extend into the body wall.[44] During this process, which takes place from the ninth to the twelfth week, the mesoderm in the posterior thoracic wall is carved by the caudal borders of the expanding pleural cavities, so that its inner portion becomes part of the diaphragm. At the same time a similar process happens at another more lateral and anterior portion of both the thoracic and the abdominal walls. As a consequence, part of the diaphragmatic muscle originates from the musculature of the thoracic and the abdominal walls.[44,194]

Despite the almost universal acceptance of this explanation for the development of the diaphragmatic muscle, there is some controversy related to the role of the phrenic nerve in that process. In accordance with the principle that muscles in general retain their original segmental innervation, certain authors believe that myoblasts derived from the caudal portion of the infrahyoid mesoderm migrate, together with the phrenic nerve, from the third and fourth cervical somites toward the diaphragm, so that this would be the origin of the diaphragmatic muscle.[86,176] However, the phenomenon of myoblast migration, together with the phrenic nerve, has not yet been proven; it is but a partially accepted theory. The fact that the tendinous center of the diaphragm is a fibrous structure completely devoid of muscle fibers speaks against this theory.[286] In any event, even if myoblasts from the superior cervical myotomes do follow the phrenic nerve, at least part of the diaphragmatic innervation should be later transferred to muscular portions derived from the thoracic and abdominal walls.

Deviations from the normal development of each one of the various components of the diaphragm bring about different variants of diaphragmatic anomalies. Table 32-1 shows the diverse embryonic origins of the diaphragm and their relation to different diaphragmatic defects.

▶ PATHOLOGY

Etiology

The etiology of CDH is unknown. Only in a few rare syndromes in which a diaphragmatic defect is present is there a well-defined genetic cause, such as in trisomies of the

Table 32–1

Embryonic Origins of the Diaphragm and Corresponding Diaphragmatic Defects

Embryonic structure	Time (weeks)	Portion formed	Diaphragmatic defect
Transverse septum	3 and 4	Central tendon	Pericardial hernia (ventral defect)
Pleuroperitoneal membranes	7 and 8	Primitive diaphragm	Bochdalek's hernia (posterolateral defect)
Mediastinum (dorsal mesentery)	—	Median portion and crura	—
Body wall	9–12	Muscle periphery (ventrolateral and dorsal)	Morgagni's hernia (parasternal defect) and eventration

520 chromosomes 13 and 18. Experimental CDH can be produced in diverse animal species through different manipulations, including exposure to diet deficient in either vitamin A,[10,282] zinc,[142] or cadmium[19] and administration of thalidomide,[83] anti-rat rabbit serum,[45] 2,4-dichlorophenyl-p-nitrophenyl ether (nitrofen, an herbicide),[8,144,162] or polybromate biphenyls.[24,264] However, to date there has been no clear relationship between these experimental models and clinical or epidemiological data in humans.

Pathogenesis

The pathogenesis of CDH also is unknown. Normally, before the return of the bowel from the umbilical cord to the abdominal cavity, which occurs during the tenth week of gestation, it is necessary for the pleuroperitoneal canal and the lumbocostal triangle to firmly close, which happens between the eighth and tenth weeks. In case such closure does not take place, the bowel passes through the pleuroperitoneal canal, sometimes also through the lumbocostal triangle, and invades the chest, resulting in a "herniation" without a hernia sac. In case there is only a membranous closure, the same phenomenon happens, albeit with a hernia sac that may or not rupture some time later. In any case, although it is well established that the diaphragmatic defect is at the level of the pleuroperitoneal canal,[44,46,47,286] the sequence of events that culminates in disturbances of its closure remains to be determined.

The prevailing theory regarding CDH development has been that the incomplete closure of the pleuroperitoneal canal was a primarily diaphragmatic defect and that the abdominal viscera herniated to the thorax impeded normal lung development and resulted in the pulmonary hypoplasia and hypertension observed almost universally in association with CDH. This perception was widely confirmed by animal models in which a diaphragmatic defect was surgically produced in fetuses of different species,[74,95,156] or in which the diphragmatic herniation was mimicked by an inflatable prosthesis placed in the pleural cavity.[126] All of these models resulted in lung hypoplasia and pulmonary hypertension at birth.

Nonetheless, the foremost notion today is that the primary defect is not in the diaphragm, but in the lung buds, and that the diaphragmatic defect is actually secondary to a primary pulmonary hypoplasia. Such pulmonary hypoplasia, in turn, could be intensified even more by the presence of abdominal viscera herniated into the chest. Starting at the fourth week of gestation, the growth of the pulmonary buds and pleural cavities results in a progressive narrowing of the pleuroperitoneal canals and in the formation of the pleuroperitoneal membranes.[44,286] The development of the diaphragm, more specifically of the pleuroperitoneal membranes, is intimately related to lung development itself. Researchers who have worked with the experimental model of CDH induced by nitrofen have shown that, at least in that model, the pulmonary hypoplasia precedes the diaphragmatic defect.[144,162,193,203] These findings are in accordance with the fact that nitrofen exposure can lead to pulmonary hypoplasia independently of the existence of CDH.[113,157,272] Iritani[144] has concluded that the lung buds, which are primarily hypoplastic because of the exposure to nitrofen,

cause hypoplasia of the posthepatic mesenchymal plate, which in turn develops in intimate association with the lung buds. The hypoplasia of this mesenchymal plate, which is one of the precursor portions of the primitive diaphragm, would then give rise to the diaphragmatic defect and, consequently, the CDH. Moreover, it is thought that the morphogenesis and differentiation of the pulmonary respiratory epithelium is intimately dependent on the kind of extracellular matrix synthesized by the mesenchyme.[161,162,265] Kluth et al[161] have shown that lungs of embryos exposed to nitrofen display an abnormal expression of factors normally found in the extracellular mesenchymal matrix, with a delayed pattern of epithelial differentiation. Iritani[144] and others[48,250] speculate further that CDH is more common on the left side in humans because lung bud development tends to be slower on the left side than on the right and, also, the fusion of the pleuroperitoneal membranes happens later on the left side than on the right.[74] Independently of the possibility of a primary pulmonary hypoplasia in the nitrofen model, Alles et al[7] have shown that there is also cell death in the mesoderm of some cervical somites, which are precursors of the diaphragm, suggesting a concomitant primary disorder of diaphragmatic development. Consequently, the mechanism behind the emergence of CDH in this model still needs to be clarified.

There are still a number of other, less accepted theories for the pathogenesis of CDH.[86,108,136,141] Whatever the location and nature of the primary defect may be, the presence of a diaphragmatic defect per se usually leads to herniation of abdominal viscera to the chest, which in turn at least contributes to worsen the pulmonary hypoplasia.[74,95,156] The sooner the herniation occurs in gestation and/or the larger the herniation content, the more intense is the pulmonary hypoplasia.

Pathological Anatomy

Gross Findings

The diaphragmatic defect, or Bochdalek's foramen, is located in the posterolateral aspect of the diaphragm, involving at least the area that originates from the pleuroperitoneal membrane and, many times, also the area immediately posterior to it, namely, the lumbocostal triangle (Figure 32-2). The size of the defect is highly variable, from less than 1 cm in diameter, to an almost complete absence of the hemidiaphragm, extending beyond the dome practically to the midline, preserving merely a small anterolateral band of muscle. There is no fibrosis or any evidence of inflammation at the level of the diaphragmatic opening. The left side is affected in approximately 80–90% of the cases, the right side is affected in 10–20%, and bilateral cases are rare, occurring in approximately 1% of patients.[63,312]

In most cases the pleura and the peritoneum are in continuity over the borders of the diaphragmatic defect, which may render the identification of the residual posterior muscle band difficult. A hernia sac is present in only approximately 15% of patients. There is no relationship between the size of the diaphragmatic opening and the volume of the herniation.

Because of the herniation to the chest, the mediastinum is usually deviated to the contralateral side of the hernia (Figure 32-3). Both lungs, but particularly the one ipsilateral to the

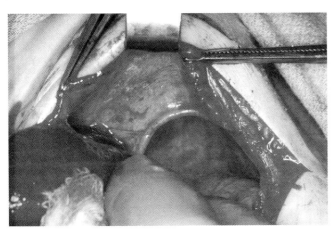

Figure 32–2 Typical intraoperative finding, through a left subcostal laparotomy, in a neonate with congenital diaphragmatic hernia (CDH). Note the defect on the posterolateral aspect of the left diaphragm.

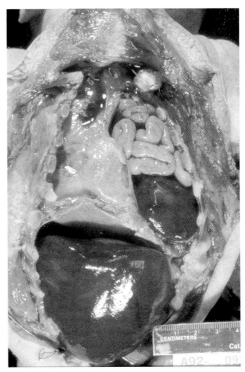

Figure 32–3 Typical gross necropsy finding in a neonate with congenital diaphragmatic hernia (CDH). Note the abdominal organs herniated to the left hemithorax through the posterolateral defect on the ipsilateral diaphragm and the mediastinum deviation to the right. There is no hernia sac.

defect, are smaller than normal in both volume and weight (Figure 32-4).[23,36,159] Pulmonary lobulation ordinarily is normal, but may be compromised in a few cases.[13,159] On the other hand, the shape of the pulmonary lobes is commonly distorted.[13,159] The pulmonary ligament is almost always absent on the side of the hernia.[159] The number of airway generations and their dimensions are reduced, especially in the ipsilateral side of the defect.[13,159] The pulmonary arteries, as well as the number and dimensions of their branches, are smaller than normal, in proportion to the reduced size of the lungs, also particularly on the side of the hernia.[159]

The herniation of abdominal contents to both the thorax and the pulmonary hypoplasia may lead to the appearance of many other abnormalities. Because of that, such abnormalities are not exactly considered to be other anomalies associated with CDH, but actually are integral components of the so-called CDH syndrome.[96] The most frequent of such abnormalities are persistent ductus arteriosus, persistent foramen ovale, and intestinal malrotation.[96] Less frequently, the following abnormalities also can be a direct consequence of CDH: gastric volvulus, abnormally sized chest cavity, accessory spleen and/or congenital splenic fibrosis in left CDH, abnormal hepatic lobulation in right CDH, and hypoplasia and/or fibrosis of the lobe of the liver ipsilateral to the hernia.[96,166] Also, the volume of the abdominal cavity is frequently reduced.

Microscopy

Except for the defect itself, the diaphragm does not exhibit any other deformity. A local decrease of the density of branches of the phrenic and intercostal nerves has been described by some[86] but is not yet confirmed by others and is considered of limited value.[7]

The impact of CDH on the lungs vary within an ample spectrum. The lung ipsilateral to the hernia is impaired the most, but both lungs are affected. In a given patient the effects of the hernia are not uniform on the different portions of each lung.

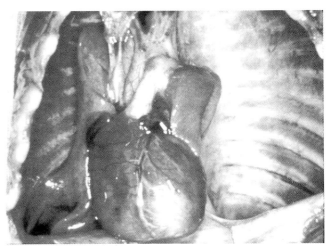

Figure 32–4 Thoracic cavity in the same neonate shown in Figure 32-3, after removal of the abdominal organs herniated to the left hemithorax. Notice the reduced size of the lungs, especially on the left side.

The airway branching order is abnormal, with a reduced number of generations of lower bronchi and bronchioli, often with complete absence of the latter, so that bronchi may end directly in alveoli.[13,23,159] Given that normal airway branching is complete by the sixteenth week of gestation,[48,233] the reduction in airway generations observed both

522

grossly and microscopically is further evidence of the fact that CDH and/or pulmonary hypoplasia start before this time, more specifically between the tenth and twelfth weeks of gestation. On the other hand, the development of airway cartilage itself does not seem to be affected, so that the proportion of cartilage-bearing airways to the total number of airways is normal.[13,159] However, the number of bronchi containing mucous glands is diminished.[13]

The total alveolar number is reduced, both in absolute terms and in relation to total lung volume.[13,23,159] However, the number of alveoli per acinus may be either reduced or normal, suggesting that the reduction in total alveolar number is mostly a consequence of the lower number of terminal bronchioli.[23,159] The alveoli also are smaller than normal.[159] The fate of type II pneumocytes is not yet completely clear. Many studies uncover evidence that the surfactant system is depressed, but it is not absolutely clear whether or not this has to do with a reduction in the density of type II pneumocytes.[°]

In parallel to the lower number of airway generations, the absolute number of arterial branches is reduced,[159] yet the density of intraacinar arteries may be normal.[23] The arterial diameters are reduced.[23,159] There is hypertrophy of the arterial muscle layer at all levels, as well as extension of such muscle layers into more distal branches, which normally would not bear any muscle.[23,109,159,202] There seems to be a direct relationship between pulmonary hypoplasia and arterial muscularization, so that the more hypoplastic the lung, the more intense is the abnormally augmented muscularization.[202]

Pathophysiology

The cardinal aspects of CDH pathophysiology are pulmonary hypertension with persistence of a fetal circulatory pattern, along with a reduction in both pulmonary tidal volume and compliance. The intensity of such manifestations vary a great deal, from almost nonexistent to incompatible with life, depending mostly on the severity of the anatomical abnormalities of a given patient. According to many authors, a deficiency of the surfactant system also is part of CDH pathophysiology[15,31,139,293]; however, this notion has not yet been universally accepted.[160,201,263]

In children, total peripheral airway cross-sectional area is proportionally larger than in adults; hence the reduction in airway generation present in CDH usually does not lead to significant increases in airway resistance.[306] The difficulty in ventilating children with CDH stems mostly from the lower pulmonary compliance and lower tidal volumes. The pressure–volume curves of these hypoplastic lungs are abnormal, so that at a given pressure, lung volume is lower than normal.[252] Microscopic analyses under insufflation show that although certain airspaces may open at 15–20 cm H_2O, many are still closed at 30–35 cm H_2O.[76] Thus higher inspiratory pressures are transferred only to the alveoli that are open, leading to alveolar rupture and a tendency to develop pneumothorax.[77] It is not yet clear whether the decreased pulmonary compliance is a result of a quantitative and/or qualitative depression of the surfactant system, or a relative increase in the total amount of collagen in the

lungs.[31,133,139,293] The lower tidal volumes are a direct consequence of the reductions in both lung volume and total alveolar number.[13,23,36,159] All of these ventilatory abnormalities are the main reasons for the tendency of infants with CDH to retain CO_2.[77]

Contrary to what happens with the airways, the peripheral vessels (lower arteries, arterioles, and capillaries) account for most of the pulmonary vascular resistance (PVR). Therefore as a result of the reduction in the total number of arterial branches and their lower-than-normal diameters, the total arterial cross-sectional area is diminished and the PVR is usually significantly increased in CDH.[174,213] Further contributing factors to the increased PVR are the hypermuscularization of the arteries and amplified arterial reactivity. Because of the latter, certain physiological stimuli such as alveolar hypoxia, hypoxemia, hypercapnia, acidosis, cyanosis, hypothermia, and any "disturbances," such as certain inflammatory mediators and simple manipulations of the patient, may trigger intense pulmonary vasoconstriction and marked increase in PVR.[246,283] Other than the possibility of a role played by the muscular hypertrophy present in pulmonary arteries and arterioles, the reason why these vessels tend to overreact to stimuli is not yet known. Apparently the pulmonary vasculature's ability to synthesize nitric oxide is preserved and thus is not part of the mechanism.[151] The possibility of an imbalance involving prostanoids, which are vasoactive agents that include prostaglandins, playing a role has been proposed, but is not yet confirmed.[102,213,259] Nonetheless, there is evidence that disturbances in the homeostasis of other endogenous vasoactive agents, namely, the peptides endothelins, contribute to the increase in PVR.[163,213]

This increase in PVR leads to pulmonary hypertension, which is almost universally observed in neonates with CDH.[76,119,213] Pulmonary hypertension leads to a decrease in total blood flow to the lungs, an increase in end-diastolic pressure in the right ventricle, and a tendency for persistence of a fetal circulatory pattern, with right-to-left shunt through the ductus arteriosus and foramen ovale.[76,283] The decrease in total pulmonary blood flow and the right-to-left shunt lead to hypoxemia, hypercapnia, and acidosis, which in turn are stimuli to pulmonary vasoconstriction, which worsens the pulmonary hypertension, with consequent intensification of the fetal circulatory pattern and so forth, establishing a vicious cycle that is difficult to break. Not infrequently, patients may be satisfactorily oxygenated and fairly stable, until a random stimulus triggers the vicious cycle of fetal circulation. Such a period of temporary stability that precedes the emergence or worsening of pulmonary hypertension has been coined the "honeymoon" period. It was described for the first time by Collins et al in the mid-1970s and remains a frequent observation in neonates with CDH.[67,213] Patients who display symptoms of persistent hypoxemia soon after birth without ever going through a "honeymoon" period usually have severe pulmonary hypoplasia and serious abnormalities of the pulmonary vasculature.[109]

In the fetus the oxygenated blood that comes from the placenta returns to the right side of the heart through the umbilical vein and crosses either the foramen ovale or the ductus arteriosus toward the aorta, so that only approximately 7% of the cardiac output goes through the

---

°References 15, 31, 107, 139, 201, 263, 293.

lungs.[104] Therefore the hemodynamic disturbances associated with pulmonary hypertension almost never manifest in utero. After birth, however, the hemodynamic status tends to deteriorate, often with overload and potential failure of the right side of the heart. Thus cardiac failure is typically part of the pathophysiology of CDH,[75,137] and survival depends to a great extent on the ability of the myocardium to withstand the overload imposed by the pulmonary vasculature.[75,76] The deviation of the mediastinum by the herniated content may lead to a decrease in the venous return to the heart, possibly contributing to further worsening of the patient's hemodynamic status.

Recently it has been suggested that neonates with CDH may have adrenal insufficiency, with an inadequate response to stress.[223] At the same time there is preliminary experimental evidence pointing to the possibility that lower-than-normal glucocorticoid levels may contribute to the abnormal lung development and maturation found in CDH.[198] The true meaning of these findings in CDH pathophysiology remains to be better defined.

Among the different aspects of the pathophysiology of CDH, it is the pulmonary hypertension that is most responsible for mortality in the neonatal period. Because otherwise healthy neonates who undergo total pneumonectomy are often able to maintain good oxygenation and ventilation without clinically relevant pulmonary hypertension, the lack of pulmonary parenchyma alone cannot explain all the manifestations commonly observed in infants with CDH.[249] Rarely in CDH is the bilateral lung impairment intense enough to cause a neonate to have less than half of the normal total alveolar surface area. Consequently, it appears that, more often than not, the pulmonary vasculature abnormalities are clinically much more relevant than the lack of alveoli (pulmonary hypoplasia).

CLINICAL MANIFESTATIONS

Ninety percent of the patients with CDH are symptomatic within the first 24 hours of life.[273] However, this disease may first manifest at any age and, more rarely, go unnoticed until very late in life, or even never be diagnosed.[9,101,218]

When a child is symptomatic within the first 24 hours of life, the main clinical manifestation is respiratory distress. The earlier the onset of signs and symptoms, the more severe is the pulmonary disease. Newborns that are symptomatic in the first 6 hours after birth are considered high risk and account for 88% of the cases.[273] Tachypnea associated with sternal, subcostal, and supraclavicular retraction is common. Cyanosis and/or pallor also are frequent. Apgar scores tend to be low. If untreated, the dyspnea tends to worsen with time, for the following three reasons: (1) the progressive distension of the intrathoracic bowel by gas, which is accelerated by aerophagy, common in children in respiratory distress; (2) the gradual increase of the volume herniated to the chest, which is a result of the negative pressure exerted during respiration; and (3) the escalating hypoxemia, hypercapnia, and acidosis caused by the vicious cycle generated by persistent pulmonary hypertension. The abdomen is often scaphoid because of the migration of abdominal viscera to the chest. However, because of possible bowel distension inside the abdominal cavity, the abdomen may assume a normal appearance with time. The chest may be asymmetrical, larger on the side of the hernia, especially after the bowel fills with gas. The heart sounds are commonly dislocated to the contralateral side of the hernia. Sometimes the same thing happens with the trachea. In the ipsilateral hemithorax the respiratory sounds may be diminished or absent altogether, whereas bowel sounds may be present. There may be hemodynamic instability, with a tendency to arterial hypotension, because of a decreased venous return to the heart as a result of the mediastinal deviation and/or because of right ventricular failure caused by pulmonary hypertension. Occasionally, mediastinal deviation also can lead to superior vena cava syndrome.[112] If untreated, a symptomatic newborn usually expires in a few minutes or hours.

Rarely in the neonatal period there may be manifestations stemming from perforations and/or strangulation of a hollow viscus, gastric or midgut volvulus, and/or rupture of a herniated spleen, such as gastrointestinal obstructions, empyema, hemothorax, fever, arterial hypotension, coagulopathy, anemia, and/or hypovolemic shock. An association between CDH and septicemia with group B streptococcus in premature babies also has been described.[90]

When CDH first manifests after the neonatal period, partial or complete gastrointestinal (GI) obstructions are more common than respiratory distress, which, if at all present, tends to be mild. Unlike in the neonates, the spectrum of manifestations of late presentation CDH is broad, including, in addition to GI obstruction and respiratory distress, sudden death, growth retardation, perforations and/or strangulations of intrathoracic hollow viscus (which may lead to sepsis, empyema, pneumothorax, and/or hemothorax), rupture of a herniated spleen (with hemothorax, anemia, and possibly hypovolemic shock), airway infections and/or recurrent pneumonias, urinary tract obstruction caused by herniation of the ureter, chest pain, abdominal pain, vomiting, diarrhea, anorexia, acute condition in the abdomen, intrathoracic appendicitis, and other rare presentations.[9,218]

In bilateral CDH, both sides do not always manifest at the same time, since staggered presentation has been described.[18]

DIAGNOSIS

The majority of cases are diagnosed before birth, during routine prenatal ultrasound.[301] The relative proportion of cases diagnosed in utero is constantly climbing because of both the increasing application of prenatal ultrasound screening and improvements in ultrasound technology and resolution. Fetal ultrasonography should always be performed whenever there is polyhydramnios, given that CDH is one of its causes, apparently because of a reduction in the volume of amniotic fluid swallowed by the fetus, probably as consequence of the GI obstruction caused by the hernia. A few authors also recommend careful ultrasonographic examination whenever an amniocentesis shows abnormally low levels of lecithin and sphingomyelin because of the possibility of an association between CDH and a deficiency in the surfactant system.[15,139] Such an association, however, is not always present.[263] CDH can be diagnosed by prenatal ultrasound from the eleventh week of gestation until term;

524 previously negative examinations may become positive at any time during pregnancy.[149,301] False-negative and false-positive examinations may occur; fetal ultrasonography is precise in approximately 90% of the cases.[244,283] Not infrequently, the herniated content identified by prenatal ultrasound may move in and out of the chest, as if the hernia were a dynamic process.[3] A case of CDH diagnosed in the second trimester of pregnancy that seemed to have resolved spontaneously during the third trimester, with delivery of a normal infant, has been reported.[245] There may be inaccuracies regarding the side of the hernia, when it is unilateral, and sometimes a bilateral CDH may be diagnosed as unilateral.[3] The differential diagnosis of CDH identified by prenatal ultrasound include congenital cystic adenomatoid malformation of the lung (CCAM), diaphragmatic eventration, Morgagni's hernia, hiatal hernia, pentalogy of Cantrell, primary diaphragmatic agenesis, pericardial hernia, pulmonary sequestration, lung cysts, diaphragmatic duplication, leiomyosarcoma of the lung, mediastinal teratoma, esophageal atresia with tracheoesophageal fistula, primary pulmonary agenesis, primary pulmonary hypoplasia, and intrathoracic duplications of the GI tract.[155,283] Color Doppler, three-dimensional ultrasonography, and magnetic resonance imaging (MRI) may all facilitate the prenatal diagnosis of CDH.[84,182] In extremely rare, select cases, if in doubt, more invasive examinations may be considered, such as amniography, computed tomography (CT), or ultrasonography with concomitant intrathoracic or intraabdominal injection of saline as a "contrast."[3,118] However, as MRI becomes more accessible, these more invasive examinations will soon be of historical interest only. At most referral centers the prenatal diagnosis of CDH automatically leads to an amniocentesis, a chorionic villus sampling, or an umbilical cord sampling, so that the fetal karyotype can be determined. If a chromosomal abnormality is detected, pregnancy termination may be considered.

After birth, a plain chest radiograph is almost always enough to confirm the diagnosis. The typical image is that of bowel loops seen within the lung field(s), with deviation of the mediastinum to the contralateral side of the hernia, and decrease or absence of gas in the abdomen (Figure 32-5). When the radiograph is obtained before the GI tract could be filled with gas, or if the intestines are not herniated (which is more common in right-sided hernias), there may be confusion in the diagnosis. The introduction of a radiopaque gastric tube often helps, in case the stomach is herniated (Figure 32-5). Should any uncertainty persist, which is highly uncommon, the diagnosis can be confirmed through a radiograph performed after infusion of contrast through the gastric tube. Even less frequently, an ultrasound may be helpful. More rarely, a CT, MRI, or contrast enema may have a role. The differential diagnosis of CDH after birth includes diaphragmatic eventration, pneumonia, CCAM, lung cysts, pneumothorax, pleural collections, Morgagni's hernia, hiatal hernia, primary agenesis of the diaphragm, primary pulmonary agenesis, primary pulmonary hypoplasia, pericardial hernia, pulmonary sequestration, cardiac tumors, and duplication of the diaphragm. Despite all of these possibilities, the diagnosis of CDH after birth tends to be relatively simple.

With late presentation CDH the diagnosis is usually made through a simple chest radiograph as well. Also in these cases, a gastric tube may be helpful during the inter-

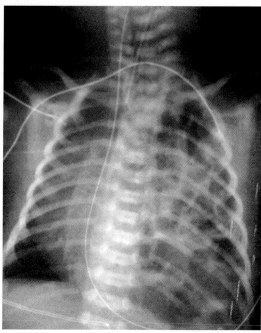

Figure 32–5 Typical aspect of plain radiograph from a neonate with a left congenital diaphragmatic hernia (CDH). Notice the presence of bowel loops in the left hemithorax, the mediastinal deviation to the right, and the gastric tube in the chest.

pretation of the radiograph. Many times there is previous history of a normal chest X-ray.[27] The possibility of late presentation CDH should always be considered; otherwise the diagnosis will likely be delayed and confused with pneumonia, pneumatoceles, CCAM, pneumothorax, pleural collections, diaphragmatic eventration, lung cysts, lung nodules, or pulmonary sequestrations. Because late presentation CDH is relatively rare, the need for other examinations in addition to the chest radiograph is somewhat more common. Such examinations may include an upper GI (often with the patient in the Trendelenburg position), ultrasound, CT, MRI, fluoroscopy, and, more rarely, a contrast enema. CDH may be diagnosed as an incidental imaging finding in an asymptomatic patient.[197]

ASSOCIATED ANOMALIES

Children bearing any major congenital anomaly are known to carry a much higher risk of having another anomaly than the general population. Neonates with CDH are no exception to that rule. The incidence of other anomalies associated to CDH in the literature varies from "rare" to 56%.[96,125,226,239,268] There are several different explanations for this disparity: the inclusion, or not, of the other anomalies directly linked to CDH and considered integral components of the so-called CDH syndrome, as described earlier; the inclusion, or not, of stillbirths and/or patients who die before reaching a referral center; variable diagnostic routines; variable autopsy rates; variable patient populations in terms of the proportion of high-risk neonates included in the analysis; and variable regional prevalences of certain congenital anomalies. These studies have identified

Table 32–2

Associated Anomalies Identified in 166 High-Risk Patients with Congenital Diaphragmatic Hernia[a]

Anomaly	Number of patients
Cardiac	
Heart hypoplasia	13
Atrial septal defect	10
Ventricular septal defect	9
Hypoplasia of aortic isthmus	3
Aortic coarctation	3
Persistent left superior vena cava	3
Ebstein's anomaly	2
Parachute mitral valve	2
"Abnormal" mitral valve	1
"Abnormal" tricuspid valve	1
Absent left pericardium	1
Absent right pulmonary artery	1
Bicommisural aortic valve	1
Bifid apex of the heart	1
Common atrioventricular canal	1
Cor triatriatum	1
Double outlet of right ventricle	1
Double coronary ostea	1
Scimitar syndrome	1
Single coronary artery	1
Gastrointestinal	
Meckel's diverticulum	6
Absent gallbladder	1
Absent vermiform appendix	1
Accessory pancreas	1
Annular pancreas	1
Duodenal atresia	1
Ectopic liver	1
Ectopic pancreas	1
Esophageal atresia with TEF	1
Imperforate anus	1
Neuroenteric cyst	1
Phyrigian cap deformity of gallbladder	1
Chromosomal	
Trisomy 18	2
"Abnormal" chromosome 14 centromere	1
Balanced 12/15 translocation	1
Chromosome 7Q deletion	1
Chromosome 12P	1
Mosaic trisomy	1
Tetraploidy 21	1
Trisomy 13	1
Genitourinary	
Undescended testes	6
Bicornuate uterus	2
Hydronephrosis	2
Horseshoe kidneys	1
Hypospadias	1
Renal dysplasia	1

Table 32–2

Associated Anomalies Identified in 166 High-Risk Patients with Congenital Diaphragmatic Hernia[a]—cont'd

Anomaly	Number of patients
Genitourinary—cont'd	
Single kidney	1
UPJ obstruction	1
Vaginal/uterine atresia	1
Central Nervous System	
Hydrocephalus	4
Rachyschesis	2
Circle of Willis anomaly	1
Microcephaly	1
Myelomeningocele	1
Open spine	1
Vascular malformation of spinal cord	1
Musculoskeletal	
Hemivertebrae	2
Absent rib	1
"Abnormal" rib	1
Accessory rib	1
Hip dislocation	1
"Limb dystrophy"	1
Polydactyly	1
Sacral dysgenesis	1
Scoliosis	1
Pulmonary	
Pulmonary sequestration	2
Pulmonary lymphangiectasia	1
Trifurcated trachea	1
Other	
Inguinal hernia	2
Omphalocele	2
Cleft lip/palate	1
Conotruncal facies	1
Torticollis	1

TEF, Tracheoesophageal fistula; UPJ, ureteropelvic junction.

From Fauza DO, Wilson JM: Congenital diaphragmatic hernia and associated anomalies: Their incidence, identification, and impact on prognosis. J Pediatr Surg 29:1113–1117, 1994.

[a]Excluding pulmonary hypoplasia, persistent ductus arteriosus, persistent of the foramen ovale, intestinal malrotation, gastric volvulus, size abnormalities of the chest wall, accessory spleen and/or congenital splenic fibrosis in left congenital diaphragmatic hernia (CDH), abnormalities of liver lobulation in right CDH, and hypoplasia and/or fibrosis of the liver lobe ipsilateral to the hernia.

526

many different associated anomalies, in all body systems, usually with a predominance of cardiac malformations.

In a detailed review of 166 high-risk neonates (i.e., symptomatic within the first 6 hours of life), we noticed that approximately 40% of the children had one or more congenital anomaly associated with CDH.[96] This index was obtained even after exclusion of all the other anomalies that are part of the CDH syndrome. Cardiac anomalies were by far the most common, found in 63% of the patients who had an associated anomaly, followed by anomalies in the genitourinary tract (23%), GI tract (17%), central nervous system (CNS) (14%), muscles and skeleton (10%), chromosomes (10%), lungs (5%), and others (5%); in many children there were more than one associated anomaly (Table 32-2).[96] Our results were comparable to those from another study involving 237 children in whom CDH was diagnosed at up to 1 year of age.[268] In our series it was interesting to notice that the prenatal diagnosis of CDH, especially if made before 25 weeks of gestation, was a risk factor for the presence of other anomalies that were also life threatening, namely, cardiac anomalies of the CNS, chromosomes, and omphalocele.[96]

The high proportion of cardiac anomalies associated with CDH in many series deserves special attention. In our review, for example, they were more frequent than all the other anomalies put together (see Table 32-2).[96] Among cardiac anomalies, heart hypoplasia was the most common.[96] This finding is in accordance with many observations pointing to the fact that the cardiac hypoplasia associated with CDH, especially that of the cardiac chambers ipsilateral to the hernia, occurs, like the pulmonary hypoplasia itself, at least in part because of compression of the heart by the the herniated content, and perhaps should also be considered as part of the CDH syndrome, because it likely plays a role in the cardiac failure often manifested clinically.[96,116,152,237] The presence of an associated cardiac anomaly leads to significant further reduction of the postductal oxygen pressure (PO_2) when compared with isolated CDH.[96] In fact, in neonates with an excessively low postductal PO_2, particular care should be taken in searching for a potential associated cardiac anomaly.

Patients with late presentation CDH also seem to have a higher prevalence of other anomalies than the general population. However, the related series published thus far are too small for definitive conclusions. For example, in a review of 26 patients spanning 20 years, Berman et al[28] found one or more associated anomalies in 31%.

▶ PROGNOSTIC FACTORS

The search for reliable prognostic markers has been an essential aspect of the study of CDH for many years. Given the broad pathology spectrum related to CDH, such markers are critical for any meaningful comparisons among different therapeutic strategies, as well as for the identification of cases that are incompatible with life, in which further efforts would not be justified.

Certain clinical variables are known to be associated with different survival rates. Ever since the study by Young in 1969, there is a well-established reverse relationship between age at the beginning of symptoms and mortality rates.[89,311] Neonates who are symptomatic within the first 6 hours of life are considered high risk, because the lowest survival rates are

found in this group of patients.[89] There is no difference in mortality between the sexes in isolated CDH; however, higher mortality rates have been reported in female patients than in male patients when CDH is associated with other anomalies.[268] Some studies have shown that the lower the gestational age at birth, or the lower the birth weight, the lower is the survival rate.[89,280] Lower Apgar scores, particularly in the fifth minute, also are linked to higher mortality.[89] Contrary to what a few studies have suggested, the side of the hernia has not had any prognostic impact in the larger series.[89] At the same time, children who have to receive a prosthesis for closure of the defect seem to be have lower survival than those in whom a primary repair is feasible.[89] It is not yet known whether the presence of a hernia sac is of any prognostic significance. The variable with the highest impact on CDH survival rates is the possible presence of other associated congenital anomalies. The prognosis of neonates with associated anomalies, especially cardiac anomalies, is much worse than that of infants with isolated CDH.[89,96,255]

Since the beginning of the 1970s until today, countless studies have tried to correlate mortality to blood gas values and/or ventilation parameters, either independently or mutually integrated in often intricate equations. Examples include pH values; "best" PCO_2 or "best" PO_2, either postductal or preductal; alveolar–arterial O_2 gradient; mean airway pressure; respiratory rate; pulmonary compliance; dead space; and tidal volume, to name a few.* In the relatively recent past, perhaps the most popular of these markers was the "best" postductal PO_2 obtained during "maximal" mechanical ventilation, either before surgical repair of the hernia or before placing the patient on ECMO. Children with values higher than 100 mm Hg were labeled "responsive" and had a better prognosis, and vice versa.[217,302] Other parameters also used until recently were the so-called Bohn criteria, which related PCO_2 with the ventilation index (VI = respiratory rate multiplied by mean airway pressure); among the many different combinations, for example, PCO_2 >40 mm Hg with VI ≥1000 suggests high mortality.[34,217,302] Some authors have proposed that preductal blood gases are more predictive of the degree of pulmonary hypoplasia than postductal blood gases, given that the latter are more influenced by the intensity of pulmonary hypertension and right-to-left shunt, a preductal PO_2 <100 mm Hg and a preductal PCO_2 >60 mm Hg are related to very high mortality.[38,256] As a result of the now almost universal acceptance of the principle of gentle ventilation, permissive hypercapnia, and minimization of iatrogenic injury related to mechanical ventilation, even preductal blood gases have had increasingly limited prognostic value, at the same time that postductal gases such as "best" PO_2 during maximal ventilation have been practically abandoned.

Imaging criteria as severity predictors also have been extensively studied. One example is the value of prenatal ultrasonography. Until the early 1990s, a positive prenatal ultrasound was considered a marker of bad prognosis, particularly if the hernia was diagnosed before the twenty-fifth week of gestation.[4,204] Lately, probably as a result of the widespread use of fetal ultrasound during routine prenatal care, the improvements in ultrasound technology, and the novel therapeutic strategies for CDH, it is clear that the prenatal

---

*References 14, 34, 37, 217, 256, 302.

diagnosis of an isolated CDH is, by itself, of no prognostic value, regardless of the gestational age in which it is made.[255,301] In the event that other associated anomalies, especially cardiac anomalies, are diagnosed prenatally in addition to the diaphragmatic hernia, the prognosis is still comparable to that if the diagnosis is made after birth.[96] Several specific findings on fetal ultrasound have been proposed as bad prognostic markers, such as polyhydramnios, herniation of the liver and/or the stomach into the chest, "underdevelopment" of the left side of the heart, disproportionate cardiac ventricles, high ratio of the herniated area to the cardiac area, low ratio of the lung area to the total thoracic area, depression or absence of fetal breathing movements, severe mediastinal deviation, reduction of liquid flow through the nose and oropharynx during fetal breathing movements, and disturbances of blood flow modulation through the ductus arteriosus.[4,103,131,149,204] The merit of all these markers, however, is highly controversial and has limited acceptance. Recently the value of liver herniation, as well as of the so-called lung-to-head ratio (LHR), which measures the relative proportion between the areas of the lung and the head at predetermined locations, has been emphasized by a few groups.[120,129] For example, fetuses with the liver in the chest and an LHR <1 have a particularly poor prognosis. The possible presence of the liver in the chest does seem to be valuable prognostic information; however, the same cannot be said of the LHR, which has been shown to be inconsistent, especially across different institutions.[273] Measurements of fetal lung volume through MRI are now being refined and may be helpful in the near future.[84]

In like manner, some studies suggest that certain postnatal imaging findings, either independently or in combination, also can be linked to poor outcome. On plain chest radiograph, examples of such findings include presence of the stomach in the chest, ipsilateral or contralateral pneumothorax presence of interstitial emphysema, and a low ratio of aerated ipsilateral lung area to that of the contralateral lung.[49,251,270] On echocardiogram, examples include decreased left ventricular mass, disproportionate dimensions between both pulmonary arteries, and a disproportionately large pulmonary artery trunk in relation to the aorta.[52,130] Finally, on pulmonary arteriogram, examples include reduced dimensions of both pulmonary arteries, reduced size of the ipsilateral lung, and severe peripheral compromise.[217] Yet, analogous to what happens with prenatal imaging, the predictive value of these proposed postnatal findings is questionable, to say the least, and very few institutions adopt any of them at this time.

To date, only the following variables have been clearly validated by well-controlled, extensive multicentric data as being of predictive value in CDH: age at the onset of symptoms, birth weight, 5-minute Apgar score, and the presence of an associated cardiac anomaly.[89] The meaning of all other suggested prognostic markers is debatable and of limited acceptance.[216] One of the most common shortcomings of the studies involving prognostic markers is that most of them are reviews from a single institution. Hence the data are unavoidably linked to the unique patient population and peculiar therapeutic strategies of each service, which are aspects known to still be highly variable from one center to another in CDH. On the other hand, even if well-controlled multicentric trials were accomplished, the fact that the treatment of CDH is a constantly evolving moving target could lessen the significance of their results. The introduction of ECMO and of the principle of gentle ventilation are clear examples of the vulnerability of this kind of data, because these therapies rendered the conclusions obtained before their availability nearly useless, even within a given institution.

TREATMENT

Except for the rare cases in which there may be strangulation of the herniated content, CDH is not a surgical emergency. CDH is a physiological emergency. In fact, not infrequently, mechanical aspects of respiration tend to deteriorate after the repair of the hernia.[57,205] Indeed, emergency surgery is not only unnecessary and often deleterious, but a period of preoperative stabilization is known to improve outcome.[288,309] The child should not go to the operating room while unstable. The time needed for stabilization may vary anywhere from less than 12 hours to several days. A few authors even suggest that waiting until well after stabilization has been reached is beneficial.[309] In certain premature neonates at higher surgical risk, the surgeon may wait weeks, or even more than a month, before proceeding to make the repair.[273]

The therapeutic strategy in children with CDH and other associated anomalies must be individualized for each patient. More often than not, the hernia is repaired before the other anomaly(ies). However, when CDH is associated with cardiac anomalies, such strategy may lead to unacceptably high mortality.[96,273] Unless the cardiac defect is very mild, the current tendency is to repair the heart before the diaphragm, or, occasionally, to repair both during the same intervention. However, the best guidelines for the different scenarios are still being defined.

One of the benefits of the prenatal diagnosis of CDH is that delivery can be planned at a tertiary referral center. Although no study has yet shown significant differences in survival between inborn and outborn children at referral centers, the initial results of postnatal resuscitation are known to be maximized when the presence of CDH is detected before birth.[301] Unless there is any obstetrical contraindication, vaginal delivery is preferred over cesarean section.

Preoperative Care

The neonate should be intubated in the delivery room. Ventilation by mask before intubation should be avoided because of the risk for distension of hollow viscera inside the chest. A gastric tube should be introduced and kept under mild continuous suction to minimize such distension and to drain air that may have been swallowed. Central venous access is established, usually through the umbilical vein (occasionally, however, particularly in right-sided CDH, there may be significant distortions of the liver anatomy because of the herniation, which may impede the use of this vein). One of the umbilical arteries is catheterized for blood pressure and postductal blood gas monitoring. Preductal blood gases are obtained through access to the right radial artery, or to one of the superficial temporal arteries. Transcutaneous pulse oximetry monitors and, if available, transcutaneous PO_2 and PCO_2 monitors are placed on both preductal and postductal

528

territories. Monitors for body temperature and respiratory rate also should be positioned. A Foley catheter is introduced, at least in the high-risk cases. The volumes of intravenous infusions should be carefully controlled to minimize the chances of a pulmonary edema developing. Prophylactic antibiotics covering both gram-positive and gram-negative bacteria are commonly administered. Whenever possible, inotropic agents should be avoided, given that these drugs usually not only increase cardiac output, but also increase peripheral vascular resistance, both of which may, together with the ever-present pulmonary hypertension, lead to excessive cardiac overload not always tolerated, especially when there is some degree of cardiac hypoplasia.[96,152] When the use of these drugs is inescapable, many prefer dobutamine, amrinone, or epinephrine to dopamine or norepinephrine, because the former drugs may produce pulmonary vasodilatation at low doses.[283] Any manipulation or interaction with the infant should be kept to a minimum because of the great volatility of the pulmonary vasculature.

Every neonate with CDH should undergo an echocardiogram with Doppler, given the relatively common occurrence and prognostic impact of associated cardiac anomalies. Should any cardiac disease be identified, depending on the specific diagnosis, its treatment must either be coordinated with that of the hernia, or, in those cases in which the association of anomalies is deemed incompatible with life, bold therapeutic efforts such as ECMO or even surgery itself should not be undertaken.[96] Certain variables, namely, prenatal diagnosis before the twenty-fifth week of gestation, low Apgar scores, and "excessively low" postductal Po_2, have been shown to be risk factors for the presence of other associated anomalies.[96] If these variables are present, further examinations such as genitourinary tract and head ultrasounds, as well as a karyotype (if this was not already done during pregnancy) should be strongly considered in addition to the echocardiogram.[96]

Up until recently, neonates were sedated, paralyzed, hyperventilated, and also received systemic alkalinization with sodium bicarbonate or thrometamine to minimize pulmonary hypertension. Ventilation parameters used to be controlled by postductal blood gases. This strategy, which unfortunately is still practiced by many centers today, is clearly associated with unacceptably high risks for iatrogenic lung injury. Pulmonary hypoplasia and, in particular, pulmonary hypertension are both expected to lead to low Po_2 and high Pco_2, especially in postductal gases. Attempts to normalize postductal blood gas values often lead to marked increases in ventilator parameters, namely, respiratory rate (RR), inspired O_2 fraction (FIo_2), peak inspiratory pressure (PIP), positive end-expiratory pressure (PEEP), and mean airway pressure (MAP), which in turn commonly lead to hyperdistension of the lungs and severe barotrauma, not to mention the toxicity of high FIO2 levels. A recent survey involving clinical and autopsy data of 68 children with CDH treated in this fashion showed a tremendously high frequency and severity of iatrogenic insult to the pulmonary parenchyma.[237] In that study 91% of the patients had evidence of diffuse alveolar damage with development of hyaline membrane, which was more obvious in the ipsilateral lung. Moreover, 65% of the children developed pneumothorax, 51% had pulmonary hemorrhage, and 6% already had variable degrees of interstitial fibrosis.[237] Other studies also

showed alveolar ruptures, damage to the alveolar basal membrane, alveolar hemorrhage, and edema, all of which contributed to atelectasis, a decline in lung compliance, and even further deterioration of gas exchange.[201,304] In addition to barotrauma, to which neonates with CDH are particularly vulnerable,[76] pulmonary hyperdistension leads to even further increases of the already elevated pulmonary vascular resistance, thus worsening the effects associated with pulmonary hypertension.[175,187] Systemic alkalinization with sodium bicarbonate may lead to increases in Pco_2 and to both volume and sodium overloads. Thrometamine may be useful at times in the short term, but relatively large volumes of this drug are usually necessary, which tends to result in both generalized and pulmonary edema.

For a number of years it has been clear that a completely different strategy, first proposed by Wung et al,[308,309] should be offered to high-risk neonates with CDH. It is based on the following guidelines: minimal sedation; no muscle paralysis; respiration merely assisted by the mechanical ventilator, if possible, through pressure support under flow synchronization, or, if this is not available, then through simple or synchronized intermittent mandatory volume; permissive hypercapnia with no hyperventilation; and no systemic alkalinization. Patient monitoring is mostly through preductal gases. Ventilator parameters are left at a minimum necessary to maintain preductal O_2 saturation (Sao_2) ≥90%, whatever the postductal values may be, with tolerance of high Pco_2 levels. In general, the ventilator parameters are left at base RR ≤40 breaths per minute (bpm), PIP and PEEP no higher than 30 and 5 cm H_2O, respectively, and the FIo_2 should be the lowest possible to prevent severe preductal hypoxemia. In other words, unless there is metabolic acidosis, suggesting excessively low O_2 delivery, low postductal Po_2 and Sao_2 should be tolerated as long as there is an adequate amount of oxygen in the preductal blood that is going to the brain and heart. As long as the pH is at "acceptable" levels, hypercapnia should be tolerated. The main goal of this therapeutic strategy is the prevention of barotrauma, probably the most common cause of death whenever the old "conventional" hyperventilation strategy is employed.[38,304,309] Despite the known benefits of sedation in CDH, which raises the excitability threshold of the pulmonary vasculature[274], in this "new" strategy sedation must be used with great caution so that the child may be able to effectively activate the mechanical ventilator, preferably in pressure support under flow synchronization. When the child is able to control both the RR and the air flow from the respirator, he or she can contribute more to the minute volume without compromising the functional residual capacity. This therapeutic strategy also avoids the side effects of systemic alkalinization.

As discussed earlier, the lungs of newborns with CDH are particularly vulnerable to barotrauma, so the occurrence of pneumothorax is relatively common. Other than in very rare, select occasions, one should not drain a pneumothorax ipsilateral to the hernia before surgical repair, given the risk of iatrogenic injury to the herniated content.

Pulmonary Vasodilators

Regardless of the ventilation strategy, many vasodilators administered systemically have been used in an attempt to control the pulmonary hypertension. Examples of these agents include tolazoline, nitroglycerin, nitroprusside, acetylcholine, prostaglandin E_1, prostaglandin D_2, prostacyclin, isoprenaline, and nifedipine. Despite the theoretical appeal of these drugs, they are not selective enough to the pulmonary vasculature and usually lead to a drop in both total peripheral vascular resistance and systemic arterial pressure. Therefore their effects on the pressure gradient through the ductus arteriosus is either minimal or inexistent, so that the tendency to right-to-left shunt is unchanged. Furthermore, they may lead to vasodilation of poorly ventilated areas of the lungs, which may even worsen the intrapulmonary right-to-left shunt. The drop in systemic arterial pressure, on the other hand, may lead to the administration of volume and/or inotropics, both of which should be avoided. Bos et al[41] reported a reduction of both the alveolar–arterial O_2 gradient and the oxygenation index (OI = MAP × FIo_2/Po_2) after administration of prostacyclin in high-risk patients with CDH, but this had no impact on survival. The use of prostacyclin also is associated with an increase of the bleeding time, which is obviously undesirable in surgical patients.[32,41] Inhalatory prostacyclin has been investigated experimentally, but has found no clinical applicability as yet.[30,281] The response to prostaglandin D_2 is variable, and systemic hypotension is a common side effect.[30,41,213] The most popular of these vasodilators was perhaps tolazoline, an adrenergic α-receptor blocking agent with a mild inotropic and chronotropic effect on the myocardium. This drug also lowers the levels of thromboxane B_2, which is possibly a mediator of pulmonary hypertension in CDH and which also has histamine-like effects.[54,283] Children who respond to tolazoline usually do so within 4 hours after an initial bolus of 1–2 mg/kg, which may be noticed through an increase in the postductal Po_2. This bolus is commonly followed by a continuous infusion of 1 mg/kg/hr. The infusion of vasodilators directly into the pulmonary artery has been shown not to have any advantage over their systemic or peripheral administration.[291] Side effects of tolazoline may be severe and include systemic arterial hypotension, upper GI hemorrhage, thrombocytopenia, hyponatremia, and skin rubor.[54,283] In case of upper GI hemorrhage, priority should be given to antacids and gastric lavage, given that tolazoline may inhibit the effects of cimetidine.[5] Tolazoline, as well as these other vasodilators, may occasionally contribute to the stabilization of the patient, sometimes lengthening the "honeymoon" period. However, this is often not the case and, even when there is some improvement in oxygenation, no beneficial impact on survival has been demonstrated.[41,288,309] Indeed, most referral centers no longer use systemically administered pulmonary vasodilators.

Nitric Oxide

The most potent selective pulmonary vasodilator known is nitric oxide (NO) administered by the endotracheal route. NO is a natural mediator of smooth muscle relaxation in general, but acts only locally because of its extremely short half-life. It is responsible for the biological activity of the so-called endothelial-derived relaxing factor.[219] When given as part of the inspired air, NO crosses the alveolar–capillary membrane by diffusion and stimulates the cyclic guanosine 3′,5′-monophosphate (cyclic GMP) in the smooth muscle of the pulmonary arterioles, inducing vasodilatation. Its effects are limited to the pulmonary vasculature because it quickly combines with hemoglobin and is deactivated.

At first there was great enthusiasm in relation to the use of NO for the treatment of CDH. Nonetheless, clinical experience has been disappointing. Occasionally NO does help in stabilizing the patient; however, even when there is an initially satisfactory response, there may be tachyphylaxis and, to date, improvements in outcome related to its use remain to be demonstrated.[173,243,273] In fact, studies involving term neonates with respiratory failure of different causes have shown that inhalatory NO improves oxygenation and lowers the need for ECMO in all diagnosis, except in CDH.[97] The underlying reason why CDH neonates are unresponsive to NO remains unknown. There has been some evidence that, if combined with the administration of surfactant or with liquid ventilation, NO may improve oxygenation and lower the PVR of children with CDH.[150,201] However, the role of NO in CDH, if any, remains to be clearly outlined.

Surfactant

Given the possibility of a deficiency in the surfactant system in children with CDH, endotracheal instillation of exogenous surfactant has been studied as a therapeutic adjunct for more than a decade. The results obtained thus far, however, do not justify its widespread application (i.e., other than when prematurity itself is the indication for its use).[181,240,294]

Prenatal administration of corticosteroids is known to induce, or at least increase, the production of endogenous surfactant.[98] Although the precise mechanisms behind this phenomenon have yet to be elucidated, studies exploring this response in the treatment of CDH have been proposed.[98]

Alternative Forms of Mechanical Ventilation

Alternative forms of mechanical ventilation also have been employed in CDH. One example is high-frequency oscillatory ventilation (HiFi), which mobilizes volumes smaller than the anatomical dead space at frequencies of up to 40 Hz. Gas exchange seems to occur not from the delivery of gas under positive pressure, as in conventional mechanical ventilation, but through a diffusion process. Compared with conventional ventilation, it is thought that HiFi minimizes barotrauma and facilitates gas exchange, especially CO_2 elimination, in select circumstances. This form of ventilation, either isolated or combined with NO, has been tested in many institutions for the support of patients with CDH, usually with less-than-satisfactory results.[158,273] Like NO, HiFi seems to be an option only in select cases, yet to be better defined. When analyzed as a whole, the experience with HiFi in CDH has been disappointing.[201] However, Bohn[35] has recently proposed that, as long as HiFi is not used for lung recruitment, but with MAPs no higher than 14–16 cm H_2O and peak-to-peak airway pressures limited to 35–45 cm H_2O, it can lead to improved survival, especially if employed early, rather than in a rescue mode.

Intratracheal pulmonary ventilation (ITPV), a form of ventilation that promotes active expiration, drastically

530 lowering dead space, thus enhancing CO_2 elimination and minimizing barotrauma, has been employed in a handful of CDH cases, with very promising preliminary results.[305] Regrettably, broader, definitive studies have been stalled by regulatory constraints and conflicting patents.

Liquid ventilation with a perfluorocarbon (PFC) also has been examined for some time. PFCs are bioinert, nonabsorbable by the alveolar–capillary membrane, and may carry large amounts of both O_2 (in particular) and CO_2. Also, they display low surface tension levels, thus acting as truly artificial surfactants. Hybrid liquid ventilation (i.e., with a PFC and a gas) is known to increase pulmonary compliance and improve gas exchange, especially oxygenation.[295] The improved oxygenation, in turn, optimizes redistribution of pulmonary blood flow, hence alleviating the pulmonary hypertension.[295] Liquid ventilation, either isolated or in combination with NO, has been applied in a few CDH cases, with encouraging results.[225,295] However, its impact on outcome and role in the treatment of CDH, if any, has yet to be established.[115,201]

Extracorporeal Membrane Oxygenation

Since the mid-1980s extracorporeal life support has left the realm of experimental therapy and has become part of the standard therapeutic options in CDH. Several early studies showed that the introduction of ECMO resulted in a significant increase in survival of these patients.[20,254,261,288,304] The significance of these studies, however, was limited by the relatively small number of patients and by the fact that each involved a single institution. Recently a multicentric review by the Congenital Diaphragmatic Hernia Registry, involving 632 patients from 65 centers, showed that ECMO improved survival from 53–77% in children with high mortality markers and comparable prognosis.[201] That same study also showed a direct relationship between the severity of the cases and the beneficial impact of ECMO on outcome.

During extracorporeal support there is not enough time for the lungs to grow to the point of reversing the pulmonary hypoplasia. However, ECMO acts as a bridge, lessening, if not eliminating, the component of pulmonary vascular hyperreactivity and allowing for maximum pulmonary remodeling, with an increase in compliance of the pulmonary arteries and arterioles, which normally takes place after birth,[23,109] as well as reducing barotrauma to a minimum. There is still some debate regarding the best moment to place the patient on ECMO in relation to the time of surgical repair of the hernia.[63] There were no differences in survival when preoperative versus postoperative commencement of ECMO was compared.[228,303] The current trend at most referral centers, however, is to use ECMO during preoperative stabilization, with repair of the hernia performed either after ECMO decannulation or while the patient is still under bypass.[170,299,304] Despite the need for anticoagulation during ECMO, it has been shown that certain pharmacological precautions and technical principles allow for safe surgical intervention during bypass, with a minimum risk of hemorrhagic complications.[80,298,299,304] Occasionally a patient may be stable without the need for ECMO in the preoperative period, deteriorating either during or soon after the operation and then needing to undergo bypass.

A few authors have proposed criteria for the contraindication of both ECMO and surgical repair, which are supposedly linked to pulmonary disease incompatible with life.[36,38,256,288,309] Given the many reports by other groups showing survival of patients who had met such criteria,[64,261,303,304] not to mention the controversies related to the prognostic markers of CDH in general,[216] we offer ECMO and surgery to every patient, unless the presence of other associated anomalies is deemed incompatible with life.[96]

The specific criteria for placing a patient on ECMO are equally debatable. Given the many controversies surrounding prognostic markers in CDH, it is no surprise that the many proposed indications for ECMO in this disease have not been widely accepted. Usually the indications for ECMO in other diseases do not apply to CDH, mainly because the mechanical ventilation parameters used in other diagnoses before ECMO is considered would be unacceptably toxic to the lungs of children with CDH, which are particularly vulnerable to iatrogenic injury.[275] In most centers ECMO is considered when the CDH patient cannot be adequately maintained without the use of "toxic" ventilator parameters. The definition of such "toxic" parameters varies from one institution to another. As mentioned earlier, in general we do not allow the PIP and PEEP to be higher than 30 and 5 cm H_2O, respectively; it should be possible to gradually lower the FIo_2 to 60% or less in no more than 72 hours, and the base RR on the ventilator should not exceed 40 bpm, although a much higher RR from the child is tolerated when he or she is under flow synchronization on the ventilator. The ventilation parameters are controlled mostly by preductal blood gases. In case the patient cannot be maintained under these guidelines, the use of HiFi and/or NO may be considered in select cases. However, most of the time, extracorporeal bypass is indicated right away. Whenever possible, venovenous ECMO is preferred to the venoarterial model.[228,304] In case ECMO is initiated preoperatively, we perform the repair during bypass.

Surgery

If the patient is placed on ECMO, we begin a continuous infusion of aminocaproic acid (AMICAR), an inhibitor of fibrinolysis, approximately 2 hours before the operation, concomitantly with reductions of the activated clotting time (ACT).[80,299] If the patient is placed on HiFi and/or NO administration, these methods do not need to be discontinued during the procedure; instead, they can be useful in select cases. If neither ECMO, HiFi, nor NO are being used, the best form of intraoperative ventilation is one at low pressures and high respiratory rates, with a dedicated infant/pediatric ventilator. Conventional anesthesia ventilators are excessively compliant and have too much dead space; hence they are are not suitable for these children.

In addition to general inhalatory anesthesia, we recommend the routine introduction of a catheter for continuous epidural anesthesia, which allows for early withdrawal of curare in the postoperative period, as well as for maintenance of abdominal wall relaxation.[304] All of these effects, in turn, facilitate early postoperative resumption of flow synchronization, as well as minimize volume retention, commonly associated with the continued use of curare. Nitrous oxide (N_2O) should not be used because it tends to cause bowel distension, which may hinder hernia reduction and abdominal closure.

The patient is positioned supine and slightly tilted to the side contralateral to the hernia by a small support placed under the ipsilateral thoracoabdominal transition. An abdominal access is preferred over a thoracic one, usually through a subcostal laparotomy.[63] After careful reduction of the herniated content, the ipsilateral lung should always be inspected. If it is not visible, the presence of a hernia sac, which is not always easily identifiable, must be investigated. If present, the hernia sac should be separated from the diaphragm and at least partially resected. Very often the posterior aspect of the residual diaphragm must be detached from the posterior abdominal wall after opening the peritoneum and the pleura, which usually cover that area.

Whenever possible, a primary repair of the hernia is performed, with nonabsorbable sutures (Figure 32-6). Yet a primary repair should not be forced under tension because of the following potentially harmful consequences: the diaphragm becomes flat and tense, minimizing, if not eliminating, its functionality; there is an excessive enlargement of the thoracic cavity, which may lead to alveolar hyperextension in the ipsilateral lung and consequent worsening of the pulmonary hypertension and barotrauma; the tension exerted on the diaphragm may be transmitted to the rib cage, resulting in chest wall deformities; and, finally, there is further decrease of the abdominal cavity volume, hampering closure of the laparotomy.[21] In a review by the Congenital Diaphragmatic Hernia Registry, 51% of the patients had to receive a "patch" of some kind to have the diaphragm closed.[63] In case a tension-free primary repair is not possible, several alternative techniques have been proposed, including abdominal or thoracic muscle flaps, free fascia lata grafts, and a myriad of prostheses, such as lyophilized dura mater, silicone, Dacron, polypropylene (Marlex), polytetrafluoroethylene (PTFE, or Teflon), and others.° Regardless of the technique used, care should be taken not to leave the diaphragm too flat, but with a slight to moderately sized dome, so that the same problems associated with primary closure under tension may be avoided.[21] The dome should not be too pronounced; otherwise local paradoxical respiration may ensue. We do not favor muscle flaps because of the residual defects left in the abdominal or thoracic walls, as well as the increased risk for local hemorrhage, particularly if ECMO is or may be employed. At most U.S. centers, pediatric surgeons prefer the use of a prosthesis made of expanded Teflon (Figure 32-7). The reasons for such a preference derive at least partly from a study showing improved Teflon incorporation by the host and a better motility pattern of this prosthesis in the short term when compared with silicone prosthesis and muscle flaps.[208] A number of acellular biological prostheses, including acellular human dermis and small intestinal submucosa (SIS), also have been studied experimentally, with conflicting results.[72,165,169,229] Among these, SIS has already been used clinically, with disappointing results (unpublished data). When the posterior residual diaphragm is not large enough for proper suturing, one option is to pass the suture around the subadjacent rib after gentle anterior traction of the rib with a clamp to avoid injury to its neurovascular bundle.

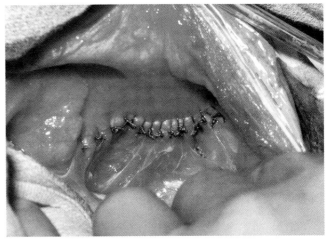

Figure 32–6 Primary repair of a diaphragmatic defect in a newborn with congenital diaphragmatic hernia (CDH).

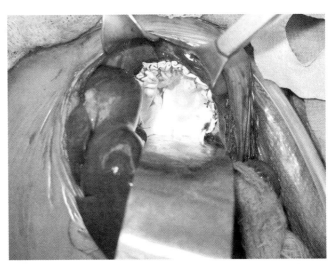

Figure 32–7 Prosthetic repair of a diaphragmatic defect with expanded Teflon, in a newborn with congenital diaphragmatic hernia (CDH).

Soon before completion of the diaphragmatic closure, a multiperforated tube is placed into the pleural cavity, exteriorized through the chest, and typically placed just under the water seal. Continuous suction through the chest is usually avoided because of the possibility of pulmonary overdistension, which is highly detrimental in CDH. Many authors even recommend that a chest tube not be placed at all.[309,310] In the review by the Congenital Diaphragmatic Hernia Registry, 24% of the patients did not receive a chest tube.[63]

We prefer to correct the intestinal malrotation, which is almost always present. However, most centers do not perform this maneuver.[63] In most institutions, including ours, an appendectomy is not routinely done, to minimize morbidity.[63] Given the reduced abdominal volume, difficulty in closing the abdominal wall is not uncommon. If there is excessive intraabdominal tension after abdominal wall

---

°References 26, 29, 43, 63, 164, 180, 248, 288.

532 closure, a syndrome of compression of the inferior vena cava may develop, along with a decrease in thoracic expansibility and tidal volume. To prevent this, repeated digital distension of the abdominal wall and evacuation of intestinal gas may be helpful. Some have suggested a routine gastrostomy as an additional means to decompress the stomach, facilitate abdominal closure, and minimize postoperative respiratory complications, but there has been no evidence-based support for this idea.[170,191] When tension-free closure of the abdominal wall is not possible, the use of an abdominal silo should be considered, followed by postoperative serial reductions and definitive primary closure.[241,288,309] Another option is simply to close the skin, leaving the proper, definitive closure for a later date.[299] The need for either of these maneuvers, however, should be extremely rare.

In children placed on ECMO, a few technical precautions should be taken to prevent excessive bleeding: The skin should be open with needle-tip electrocautery; when primary diaphragmatic closure is unlikely, the posterior residual diaphragm should not be dissected if it is adhered to the posterior abdominal wall, but the stitches should be passed around the subadjacent rib, as described in the preceding; finally, fibrin glue should be applied to the diaphragmatic suture line and other raw surfaces.[299] We do not leave a drain in the abdomen. If the abdominal wall cannot be closed primarily and a silo is implanted, serial reductions should commence only after the child comes off bypass.

More recently, thoracoscopic and laparoscopic repairs of CDH have been employed in select, very stable cases.[177,276] During thoracoscopy, reduction of the hernia can even be facilitated by the mild positive intrathoracic pressure often applied intraoperatively. The precise indications, pros, and cons of the so-called minimally invasive repair of CDH are yet to be clarified.

Postoperative Care

If the patient was not placed on ECMO during surgery, mild ventilatory support under flow synchronization, as described in the preceding, should resume as soon as possible, if necessary, with pharmacological reversal of the muscle paralysis in case it needed to be used. This transition can be facilitated tremendously if the child was placed under continuous epidural anesthesia intraoperatively.[304] The principles guiding mechanical ventilation described for the preoperative period also apply to the postoperative period. The same is true for the criteria to place the patient on ECMO.

Although some children improve after repair of the hernia, frequently there is (at least temporary) deterioration of the respiratory mechanics in the immediate postoperative period.[205,236] This phenomenon is thought to be due to anatomical distortions on the diaphragm and thoracic cavity, hyperinflation of both lungs, and an increase of the intraabdominal pressure.[236] Under these circumstances, the ventilator parameters may need to be temporarily "increased," sometimes to the point that alternative modes of ventilation and even ECMO may have to be used. Occasionally, children who had been on bypass preoperatively and were decannulated before the operation may need to go back on ECMO (this also is one of the reasons why we prefer to perform the repair during bypass).

Another potential complicating factor is the administration of intravenous fluids, which must be controlled very carefully. Concomitantly to the common risk of hypovolemia, related to surgical trauma and bleeding, neonates with CDH, more so than newborns with other surgical diseases, initially behave as if with inappropriate secretions of antidiuretic hormone and may tend to retain excessive amounts of water.[241] The explanation for this phenomenon is not yet clear. This predisposition must be recognized early; otherwise patients can be easily overloaded with fluids, with harmful consequences to their respiratory and cardiac status.

Sometimes intraabdominal pressure may rise significantly in the immediate postoperative period. The surgeon should be attentive to signs of inferior vena cava syndrome, which may lead to a decrease in the venous return to the heart, impairment of renal blood flow, and/or a reduction in tidal volume. If there is any evidence of renal insufficiency and/or major worsening of respiratory and cardiac status, muscle paralysis must be considered, which may lower the intraabdominal pressure. In the more severe cases it may be necessary to take the child back to the operating room for placement of an abdominal silo.

Whenever used, the chest tube is not continuously aspirated, but only placed under a passive water seal to avoid pulmonary hyperdistension, which may occur in both lungs because of the large empty residual space within the ipsilateral pleural cavity.[236,309] The chest tube should be removed only after the patient is extubated, usually after liquid drainage ceases. Not infrequently, liquid drainage lasts for a long time, until the lung can occupy the whole pleural space. In these circumstances the surgeon may consider removing the chest tube while it is still draining fluid and tolerate a temporary pleural collection.

Children placed on ECMO should continue to receive AMICAR, in parallel to the maintenance of ACT levels lower than usual for bypass.[299] When AMICAR is not used, or when the technical precautions described in the preceding are not duly followed, the incidence and severity of hemorrhagic complications tend to be high.[279,288] If bleeding occurs, surgical dressings must be regularly weighted and the losses through the chest tube and abdominal drain (if present) must be quantified. In our service, either blood losses equal or greater than 20% of a patient's total blood content in 8 hours or less, or progressive abdominal distension, are criteria for surgical reexploration. Frequently, specific areas of bleeding cannot be found during reoperation, only a diffuse oozing throughout the operative field. In these cases more aggressive pharmacological management related to AMICAR and ACT levels must be pondered. In addition to these potential surgical complications related to ECMO, the common risks associated with extracorporeal bypass itself are obviously a possibility.

More rarely, GI obstruction caused by adhesions, gastric volvulus, or midgut volvulus may occur even in the immediate postoperative period.[284] Other rare complications are chylothorax and/or chylous ascites.[183,267,292] In the few cases reported to date, the causes for these chylous collections have not been clearly determined. Their treatment should be based on parenteral nutrition, feedings with middle-chain triglycerides, and, if necessary, occasional needle drainages.[183,267,292]

Late Presentation Congenital Diaphragmatic Hernia

Regardless of its initial clinical presentation, including cases of purely incidental findings, late presentation CDH should be repaired as soon as possible because of the risks of incarceration and strangulation of the herniated content, and even sudden death.[62,215,222] In these cases a laparotomy is still the preferred method of access; however, a thoracotomy may be considered much more frequently than in neonates whenever the presence of firm adhesions within the herniated content into the chest is suspected. Often it cannot be determined preoperatively whether a laparotomy or a thoracotomy is the best method of access, and personal, somewhat subjective preferences may play a role in the decision process.

RESULTS

Even among referral centers with all known therapeutic options for treatment of CDH available, there may be a sizable variability of the survival rates associated with this disease. There are several reasons for these differences. On one hand, patient population profiles may vary with regard to the proportion of high-risk neonates from one institution to another. Also, patients may die before reaching a center and thus not be included in the final numbers; it is the so-called hidden mortality, originally described by Harrison.[124] At the same time, a few authors deliberately exclude children considered to have pulmonary hypoplasia incompatible with life, often based on arguable criteria, which artificially improve survival rates.[38,256] The same is true for the possible inclusion of children bearing other congenital anomalies associated with CDH.[96,255] In addition, there are still major differences among institutions related to therapeutic protocols or strategies. Such heterogeneities, combined with the different sizes of the review series and the constant evolution of the treatment options for CDH, may limit the interpretation of the results.

Bearing in mind the limitations described in the preceding, the latest meaningful reviews have shown that overall survival for isolated CDH at many referral centers has been close to 90%, a sharp increase from the depressing figures of less than 20 years ago, when ECMO was not widely available and aggressive hyperventilation was still the norm.[38,153,201,309] At our institution over 80% of the patients are diagnosed prenatally. As a consequence, their delivery can be planned, usually at one of two sister institutions linked to our hospital. The few cases diagnosed only after birth within our referral base are rapidly transferred to us; consequently, our "hidden mortality" is practically zero and our patient population is large and illustrative. In accordance with the data from other referral centers, our survival rates for high-risk neonates (about 90% of our cases) had varied between approximately 85–90% for isolated CDH and had been approximately 70% when all cases, including those with other associated anomalies, were considered.[201,212,304] These numbers were intimately related to the application of the principle of gentle ventilation and permissive hypercapnia, as well to the liberal and early indication for ECMO. In the past 3 years, our overall survival rate has surpassed 90% by adding careful attention to the right side of the heart to the management principles outlined earlier.[81]

In non–high-risk patients (i.e., when an isolated CDH becomes symptomatic after 6 hours of life) the survival rate is close to 100%.[38,201]

LONG-TERM FOLLOW-UP

At the same time that CDH survival rates have almost skyrocketed lately, perhaps predictably so, morbidity rates have worsened. High-risk children who otherwise would have died not long ago now survive, often with multiple problems, in various systems, and need to be followed by a dedicated, multidisciplinary team.* Although this seems to be somewhat more evident in patients who had to be placed on ECMO, it is currently a universal trend, which also applies to those who did not need bypass.[183,199,200,212] In many series, including ours, there is a direct relationship between the need for prosthetic diaphragmatic repair and the incidence and severity of late complications.[71,199,200,212]

One of the most common problems in CDH survivors is gastroesophageal reflux disease (GERD).† In our experience, virtually every child has some manifestation of GER, but only about 20% need to undergo a fundoplication.[200] It has been suggested that, in addition to GER, esophageal motility is often abnormal, not infrequently with concurrent esophageal dilatation, hindering management of the GER itself.[260,266] In our series, over half of the children stayed below the 25th percentile for weight during the first year of life, despite a higher-than-normal caloric intake.[200] Up to two thirds of the children may need a gastric tube or gastrostomy to be adequately fed, usually because of oral feeding difficulties.[71,183,260] Prolonged endotracheal intubation is predictive for severe oral aversion, which was found in one fourth of our patients during the first year of life.[200] Most of these GI and nutritional complications tend to improve with age.[200]

Bronchopulmonary dysplasia, or "chronic lung disease" is present in one to two thirds of patients.[40,71] The need for continuous oxygen delivery through a nasal catheter for more than 2 years after hospital discharge is not uncommon (16% of the cases, in our experience) in some patients.[71,199,212,273] Volume restrictions, usually through diet based on hyperosmolar formula, may help minimize pulmonary complications.[183] Diuretics, sometimes in association with broncodilators and/or steroids, also may be useful.[71,199] In our patients, prophylaxis against respiratory syncytial virus has been proposed as a means to decrease both the incidence and severity of acute respiratory failure related to this disease.[199]

Although the alveoli continue to multiply during the first 8 years of life,[85,233] their total numbers do not reach normal values in CDH.[13,23,140,159] Emphysematous changes occasionally may be seen on plain chest radiographs, especially in the more caudal portions of the lungs.[146] Radioisotopic pulmonary scans usually show reductions on both ventilation and perfusion, which also are typically disproportionate to each other.[146,199] Interestingly, despite all of these initial

---

*References 71, 183, 199, 200, 212, 257.
†References 71, 170, 183, 200, 212, 257, 260, 288.

534 disturbances, pulmonary function seems to normalize in the long term.[50,232,306] Pulmonary artery pressure, estimated by Doppler echocardiogram, tends to normalize with time in most children. However, deaths from right-sided cardiac failure have been reported as late as 18 months of age.[288]

Different factors, including hypoxemia, ventilation strategy, and ECMO, may affect neurodevelopmental outcome. In general, the overall incidence of neurological complications in patients who received ECMO for CDH is comparable to that found in infants who underwent bypass because of other diseases.[258,278] However, there is some controversy regarding purely cognitive development. Although a few authors have found cognition problems to be more frequent in children with CDH than in those who were placed on ECMO for other reasons, others have not confirmed such findings.[212,258,278] In most cases such impairment is mild or moderate.[71,183,212,258,278] Children with continued need for oxygen therapy and/or with failure to thrive are more susceptible to neurodevelopmental complications. Otherwise, neurodevelopmental delays tend to disappear, or at least improve, with age.[183,212]

Hearing deficits and need for hearing aids have been noticed in up to one fifth of the children, for reasons yet to be completely clarified.[71,183,212,257] Putative causes include prolonged alkalosis, the use of aminoglycoside antibiotics, and the administration of high doses of furosemide.[183] ECMO is also a risk factor.[88] Every child with CDH, particularly those with speech delays, must undergo screening audiometry and brainstem auditory evoked response testing periodically, given that hearing deficits may have a delayed onset.[183,212]

Chest wall development may be affected by both the disease itself and its treatment. The volume of the ispsilateral thoracic cavity may be reduced, apparently as a consequence of the reduced size of the lungs.[192] Overall, up to one third of the children have some degree of chest wall deformity, more commonly pectus excavatum and thoracic scoliosis (the latter is a risk factor for hernia recurrence in children who receive a diaphragmatic prosthesis).[183,212] In general, chest wall deformities associated with CDH are mild and rarely need surgical repair.[183,212]

Several other complications have been reported in different systems. Intestinal obstruction is the most frequent reason for reoperation in our experience, occurring in just under 20% of cases.[183] Its most common causes are adhesions, followed by midgut volvulus and gastric volvulus.[71,183,212] A number of other ailments also have been reported in association with CDH, albeit much less frequently, including vesicoureteral reflux, cholelithiasis, asymptomatic renal calculi, chylothorax, hypertrophic pyloric stenosis, retinal vasculopathy without functional visual deficit, and chronic superior vena cava syndrome (the latter two complications were likely related to ECMO).[71,183,212]

Diaphragmatic Hernia Recurrence

Overall postoperative recurrence rates have been reported to be between 6 and 80%.[170,183,196,278,288] Hernia recurrence is more common within the first 18 months of age, but can happen at any age.[196] The vast majority of the cases occur in children in whom a prosthetic patch was used for repair of the hernia, with a little over half of them progressing with a recurrence in the larger or longer series.[170,183,196,278]

Diaphragmatic repair with a prosthesis also has been associated with higher rates of infection, adhesions, and both thoracic and spinal column deformities when compared with primary repair.[69,71,114] The main mechanism behind hernia recurrence is believed to be related to normal growth, which is supposed to lead to traction and eventual detachment of the prosthesis, usually at its posteromedial aspect.[170] The most common clinical manifestations of hernia recurrence are intestinal obstruction and respiratory distress, in that order.[196,212] Asymptomatic recurrences are not uncommon,[183,196] nor are patients with multiple recurrences.[196] Diagnosis is usually made through a plain chest radiograph. However, sometimes a contrast GI radiograph is necessary. Occasionally, depending on the herniated content, ultrasound, CT, or, more rarely, a contrast enema may be helpful. Hernia recurrence should be surgically repaired because of the risk for incarceration or strangulation. In select cases of short-term "small" and stable recurrences, reoperation may be postponed, depending on the patient's overall condition.[66] Given that hernia recurrence is frequently asymptomatic at first, a plain chest radiograph should be performed at least once a year postoperatively in every patient who underwent prosthetic repair.[183]

▶ FUTURE PERSPECTIVES

Since the mid-1990s, much progress has been made regarding the treatment of CDH. Survival rates consistently hovering around 90% are now commonplace at major referral centers. At the same time it could be said that a formerly fatal illness has been turned into a chronic disease, because morbidity rates have increased in parallel to survival. The challenges ahead relate to both minimizing morbidity and rescuing the cases with extreme pulmonary hypoplasia, which remains the leading cause of death in this disease. These challenges have been the stimuli for some of the most fertile research efforts in pediatric surgery lately. Summarized accounts of some of these efforts follow, along with a few brief historical notes.

Despite a few anecdotal successes, the results of the actual repair of the hernia in the fetus were disappointing.[122,128] One of the reasons for the bad results was that the reduction of the hernia increased intraabdominal pressure, hampering umbilical blood flow, and also frequently led to kinking of the umbilical vein and the ductus venosus.[122,185] Just over 10 years ago, Wilson and others showed that a complete occlusion of the fetal trachea drastically accelerated fetal lung growth, reversing both the pulmonary hypoplasia and its associated pulmonary vascular abnormalities in experimental CDH, resulting in marked improvements of lung function at birth (Figure 32-8).[78,79,300] This led almost immediately to clinical trials, in which fetal tracheal occlusion was accomplished first through open surgery, then videofetoscopically.[22,121,123,127,220] The tracheal occlusion device is removed at birth before occluding the umbilical cord, during a so-called ex-utero, intrapartum (EXIT) procedure. Once again, despite a few, mostly isolated successes, results have been significantly worse than that of postnatal care, mostly because of postoperative preterm labor, dislodgment of the tracheal occlusion device, erratic secretion of the pulmonary liquid by the fetus, and pulmonary dysfunction in a few patients in whom there was reversal of the lung hypoplasia (the cause of which remains to be determined).[100,121,123,127] Even so, recent experimental developments may contribute to refine and optimize fetal tracheal occlusion in the future.[59,60,87,91]

The acceleration of pulmonary growth observed after fetal tracheal occlusion depends on sustained intrapulmonary distension by retained lung liquid, which is actively secreted by the alveolar–capillary membrane.[78,79,300] One development of this finding was our demonstration that lung growth also can be accelerated after birth by continuous intrapulmonary distension with a liquid medium, namely, PFC, which is bioinert and nonabsorbable by the alveolar–capillary membrane.[92] This phenomenon cannot be reproduced in the lungs of adult individuals.[210] Thus apparently, liquid-based pulmonary distention simply accelerates normal growth and cannot induce hyperplasia in mature, developed lungs. Long-term studies in animal models have revealed no deleterious effects of PFC-based lung distension.[211] The first series of neonates who underwent pulmonary distention with PFC under extracorporeal support was presented in 2000, with encouraging results (Figure 32-9).[93] A larger, multicentric study with longer distention times than those allowed by the U.S. Food and Drug Administration (FDA) in the first series are now being organized.

The concept of lung transplantation in CDH involves the notion that the transplanted lung (or lobe) should maintain the patient only until the native lung contralateral to the hernia develops enough to allow for resection of the graft, so that immunosuppression is no longer necessary. Successful conventional lung transplantations have been performed in CDH in very few cases.[247,277] Survival after living donor,

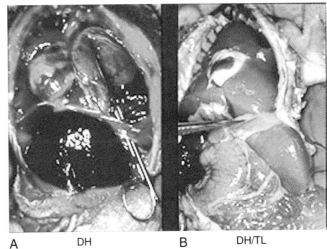

Figure 32–8 (**A**) Gross necropsy finding in a newborn lamb with experimental congenital diaphragmatic hernia (CDH). The scissors are placed through a defect on the left diaphragm. Abdominal viscera are present in the left hemithorax. The lungs are small and not visible. (**B**) Gross necropsy finding in a newborn lamb with experimental CDH and complete tracheal occlusion. The forceps are holding the left diaphragm. Both lungs are markedly enlarged. The left lung has completely reduced the herniated abdominal viscera and has grown into the abdomen, through the diaphragmatic defect.
(*From DiFiore JW, Fauza DO, Slavin R, et al: Experimental fetal tracheal ligation reverses the structural and physiological effects of pulmonary hypoplasia in congenital diaphragmatic hernia. J Pediatr Surg 29:248–257, 1994.*)

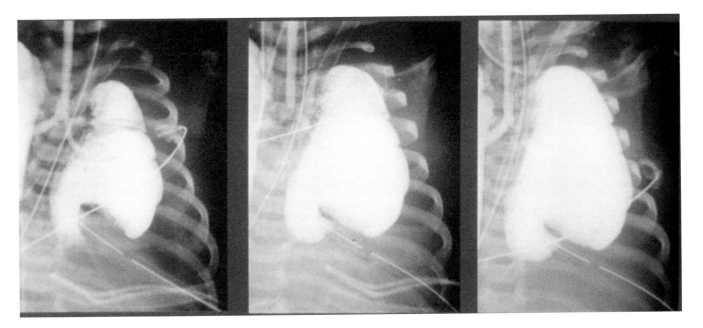

Day 1   Day 3   Day 7

Figure 32–9 Plain chest radiographs from a neonate with congenital diaphragmatic hernia (CDH) showing the progress of the ipsilateral lungs during intrapulmonary distension with a perfluorocarbon (radiopaque) for 7 days. Notice their obvious increase in size, which did not happen in the contralateral lungs.
(*From Fauza DO, Hirschl R, Wilson JM: Continuous intrapulmonary distension with a perfluorocarbon accelerates lung growth in infants with congenital diaphragmatic hernia: Initial experience. J Pediatr Surg 36:1237–1240, 2001.*)

536 reduced lung transplantations has been achieved as well, albeit only experimentally.[68] Chronic donor shortage and the many difficulties yet to be overcome in reduced lung transplantation to newborns render these options of limited, if any, value, at least for the foreseeable future.

Diaphragmatic reconstruction with an autologous engineered construct was first proposed in 2000 and has since continued to develop experimentally as a viable and potentially improved alternative for diaphragmatic replacement in the neonatal period.[94,106] Recent data showed that diaphragmatic repair with an autologous tendon engineered from mesenchymal cells isolated from the amniotic fluid leads to improved mechanical and functional outcomes when compared with an equivalent acellular bioprosthetic repair, given a suitable scaffold environment.[106] We hope to translate these findings into clinical practice in the not-too-distant future.

Fundamental knowledge and basic aspects of the management of CDH also should continue to improve. A better understanding of the pathogenesis and pathophysiology of this disease are expected. A large, detailed, multicentric sudy sponsored by the National Institutes of Health aimed at uncovering genetic aspects of CDH is underway. The search for prognostic markers will continue, for example, through ever-improving imaging methods such as three-dimensional anatomical measurements via MRI.[84] The role of so-called adjunct therapies, such as surfactant, NO, and alternative ventilation methods, should be better defined.

The role of the Congenital Diaphragmatic Hernia Registry is as important as any of the previously mentioned initiatives. Like its pediatric oncology counterparts, this organization, now embracing 65 centers, has had a major impact on both the understanding and treatment of this disease, and its influence should only continue to flourish.

▶ OTHER DIAPHRAGMATIC ANOMALIES

In addition to "classical" CDH, many other congenital diaphragmatic anomalies have been described. An overview of their location and frequency at different ages can be seen in Figure 32-10.[249] Classical CDH is by far the most common diaphragmatic anomaly of the neonatal period. Hiatal hernia rarely manifests before adulthood. In this section only general aspects of these other diaphragmatic anomalies are briefly discussed.

Diaphragmatic Eventration

Eventration is a term used to describe an abnormal elevation of the diaphragm. It can be congenital or acquired. Acquired cases, also known as diaphragmatic paralysis or paresis, usually result from damage to the phrenic nerve, which in turn may be due to traumatic delivery, thoracic surgery, tumors, inflammation, or CNS conditions such as poliomyelitis and Werdnig–Hoffmann disease.[1,61,189] In congenital cases the phrenic nerve is almost always normal. Often it is difficult to differentiate a congenital case from one caused by obstetric trauma. Acquired eventration should be suspected whenever there is a history of complications at delivery and/or concomitant signs of injury to the brachial plexus.

In congenital eventration, either the whole diaphragm may be affected, or only part of it—usually its dome, which is not a meeting point of embryonic components. Indeed it is thought that diaphragmatic eventration represents a failure of muscularization of the diaphragm, not a failed fusion of all its embryonic components. Its cause is unknown. It can be present on either side, but is more frequent on the left. Bilateral cases have been reported.[188] Diaphragmatic

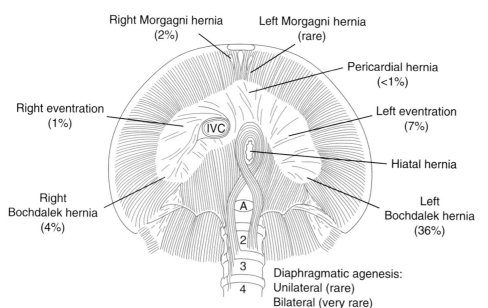

Figure 32–10 Overall relative incidence and location of different diaphragmatic anomalies at all ages, including children and adults. Bochdalek's hernia is by far the most common in infants. Hiatal hernia rarely manifests before adulthood. A, Aorta; IVC, inferior vena cava.

Right Morgagni hernia (2%)
Left Morgagni hernia (rare)
Pericardial hernia (<1%)
Right eventration (1%)
Left eventration (7%)
IVC
Hiatal hernia
Right Bochdalek hernia (4%)
Left Bochdalek hernia (36%)
A
2
3
4
Diaphragmatic agenesis:
Unilateral (rare)
Bilateral (very rare)
Diaphragmatic duplication (very rare)

thickness and its muscle fiber density vary within a broad spectrum in the eventrated area, ranging from normal, with practically all fibers present, to very thin, without any fibers. The eventrated portion of the diaphragm does not function. In certain cases the differentiation with CDH containing a hernia sac is purely arbitrary. As in CDH, there may be associated pulmonary hypoplasia, intestinal malrotation, and other anomalies in various systems.[145,171,231]

Clinical manifestations also vary within an ample spectrum, which, to a certain extent, is analogous to that of CDH. However, presentation after the neonatal period is much more common and symptoms are usually much less exuberant than in CDH. In older children (often recurrent), pneumonia may be the first manifestation. GI symptoms, usually obstructive in nature, and/or failure to thrive are not uncommon. In cases linked to Werdnig–Hoffmann disease, respiratory distress caused by the eventration may the initial manifestation of disease.[189] The patient also may be completely asymptomatic. The diagnosis is typically made through a plain chest radiograph, although sometimes it may have to be confirmed through an ultrasonography or fluoroscopy examination, both of which also may be helpful in an eventual differential with CDH. In the latter two examinations, paradoxical respiration on the affected area should be noticeable, as long as the patient is not being artificially ventilated.

Symptomatic patients should undergo surgical repair. In asymptomatic patients, surgery is recommended when there is a large eventration and/or pulmonary function tests are abnormal, given that lung growth may be compromised if the eventration is not treated. In a few patients with an asymptomatic acquired eventration, there may be variable degrees of recovery of the diaphragmatic function with time and spontaneous reversal of the eventration, so that a so-called conservative treatment may be justified initially, but not for long.

During surgery, plication of the diaphragm with nonabsorbable sutures is usually preferred, but, in select patients, partial resection followed by overlapped reconstruction of the residual diaphragm may be the best option (simple end-to-end suturing commonly leads to recurrence). In right eventrations, most authors prefer to perform the repair through a thoracotomy. In left eventrations, there is some controversy regarding whether a thoracotomy or a laparotomy would be the most suitable method of access. We favor the thoracic method of access, mostly because it allows for visualization of the branches of the phrenic nerve, which thus can be preserved during diaphragmatic plication. This is particularly relevant in view of the fact that, after plication, there may be at least partial recovery of diaphragmatic function.[11] When a thoracotomy is used, regardless of the side, usually the seventh intercostal space is the one to be opened. An abdominal method of access may be preferred in certain bilateral cases. Over the last few years, thoracoscopic repair in the less severe cases increasingly has been favored by many centers.[138] The minimally invasive approach may well become the method of choice for many patients.

Morgagni's Hernia

Also known as retrosternal or parasternal hernia, this type of diaphragmatic hernia occurs through the parasternal spaces, also called Morgagni's foramina, or Larrey's clefts, which are small, triangular portions of the diaphragm on each side of the inferior limit of the sternum that form as a result of the union between the transverse septum and the thoracic wall. This hernia can occur on both sides, but is more common on the right. Bilateral cases have been reported.[99,207] If a hernia sac is present, the superior epigastric artery normally stays lateral to it. This type of hernia is more frequent in adults and in older children. In childhood this type of hernia occurs in a proportion of approximately 1:20 in relation to classical CDH.[56,207,224] Predisposing factors include obesity and a history of trauma. It is usually asymptomatic. Only occasionally does it lead to mild symptoms such as respiratory discomfort, vague GI manifestations, and/or epigastric tenderness. It tends to be symptomatic more often in children than in adults.[207] Most of the time this type of hernia is diagnosed as an incidental finding on a chest roentgenogram. A lateral radiograph is usually more helpful than an anteroposterior image, sometimes after a barium swallow or, more rarely, after a contrast enema. Occasionally, ultrasound or CT also can be valuable to confirm the diagnosis.[207]

Incarceration of the herniated content is rare. Open repair is frequently performed through a supraumbilical, usually subcostal laparotomy. After hernia reduction and resection of the hernia sac (if present), the diaphragm is sutured to the posterior sheath of the rectus abdominis muscle. A prosthesis is rarely necessary for diaphragmatic repair. Also, the laparoscopic approach increasingly has been used in select patients.[25,110,179]

Various other anomalies can be associated with Morgagni's hernia, more frequently cardiac anomalies.[207,224] Intestinal malrotation is somewhat common.[207] Morgagni's hernia may be part of the pentalogy of Cantrell, if associated with defects of the inferior aspect of the sternum, the supraumbilical abdominal wall, and the pericardium (all of which lead to cardiac ectopia), in addition to a cardiac anomaly.[53] In these cases the surgeon usually tries to suture the diaphragm to the sternum and may need to use a prosthesis more frequently than in isolated hernias.

Hiatal Hernia

Hernias that occur through the esophageal hiatus can be divided into the following four main types: (1) sliding esophageal hernia, the most common, in which the esophagus moves freely through the hiatus so that the esophagogastric junction may be located either in the chest or in the abdomen at different times; (2) paraesophageal hernia, in which the esophagogastric junction remains below the diaphragm and the stomach rolls up into the chest parallel to the esophagus; (3) combined hernia, in which the two previous types coexist; and (4) the controversial congenital short esophagus. Hiatal hernia may manifest as early as the neonatal period; however, most cases first present in adulthood. Vomiting is the most common manifestation; yet patients often may be asymptomatic. The diagnosis is usually made through a contrast upper GI. An upper GI endoscopy is frequently part of the diagnostic evaluation as well. Surgical treatment is the norm, particularly because of the risks of incarceration and strangulation. Through either a laparoscopy or a laparotomy, the hernia is reduced, the diameter of the esophageal hiatus is normalized, and a gastroesophageal fundoplication is performed. The treatment

538 of choice for certain cases of short esophagus remains a subject of much debate. Hiatal hernia is discussed in more detail in Chapter 35.

Pericardial Hernia

This anomaly, also known as hernia of the central diaphragmatic tendon, is the rarest and least understood of the diaphragmatic defects that may lead to a hernia. In this defect there is a communication between the peritoneal and pericardial cavities, with or without herniation.[58] In general, there is no hernia sac.[58,154,297] It has been identified from soon after birth up to late adulthood, with most of the cases diagnosed in neonates.[234,289,297] It is thought that the primary defect affects the transverse septum directly.[249] There are not enough data for typical clinical manifestations to be described; pericardial hernia can be asymptomatic and only incidentally suspected on a plain chest radiograph.[234,289] Surgical repair through laparotomy is recommended.[234]

Diaphragmatic Agenesis

This entity is customarily confused with CDH in which the diaphragmatic defect is particularly large, especially if the residual posterior diaphragm is not dissected from the abdominal wall. True diaphragmatic agenesis is rare. It is usually unilateral, is more common on the left side, and rarely is bilateral.[65,134,235] It is generally identified in the neonatal period, but cases uncovered only in adulthood have been described.[147,242] It can be associated with multiple other anomalies, especially if bilateral.[65,148] Clinical manifestations, diagnosis, and treatment are analogous to those of CDH, with the exception that a prosthesis is always necessary for diaphragmatic closure.[242] Survival data are unreliable, because in many studies the differentiation with classical CDH is not clear. In general, it is thought that its prognosis is worse than that for classical CDH, given the dimensions of the diaphragmatic defect.

Diaphragmatic Duplication

Diaphragmatic duplication, whether partial or complete, is exceedingly rare.[167,296] It consists of a fibromuscular membrane that separates the affected hemithorax in two cavities and represents a duplication of the pleuroperitoneal membrane. In most cases the accessory diaphragm is not innervated by the phrenic nerve. The accessory diaphragm may be eminently muscular, whereas the orthopic diaphragm is fibrous, and vice versa.[132,238] The accessory diaphragm may be in such a location within the chest that the ipsilateral lung is divided in two compartments; it also may be associated with anomalous airways or pulmonary vessels, as well as with partial pulmonary agenesis.[6,82,132,262] Clinically it may cause respiratory distress in the neonatal period, recurrent airway infections during childhood, and "chronic pulmonary inflammation" in adulthood, occasionally with bronchiectasis.[82,296] Apparently it also can be asymptomatic.[6,209] Given that, when present, symptoms are nonspecific, the diagnosis is commonly confirmed only intraoperatively. In the rare cases in which a diaphragmatic duplication was resected, this resulted in improvement of respiratory symptoms. At least one case of association between (right-sided) CDH and diaphragmatic duplication in a neonate has been reported.[143]

Cribriform Diaphragm

A case of incidental intraoperative finding of a cribriform aspect of the right diaphragm, with several portions of the liver protruding to the chest through the many diaphragmatic defects, has been described in an elderly patient.[12] It is not yet possible to know whether this is another diaphragmatic anomaly, with a distinct embryonic pathogenesis, or an extremely rare variant of CDH, or even simply an acquired diaphragmatic defect.

REFERENCES

1. Abad P, Lloret J, Martinez Ibanez V, et al: [Diaphragmatic paralysis: pathology at the reach of the pediatric surgeon]. Cir Pediatr 14:21–24, 2001.
2. Adzick NS: Personal communication, 1994.
3. Adzick NS, Harrison MR, Glick PL, et al: Diaphragmatic hernia in the fetus: Prenatal diagnosis and outcome in 94 cases. J Pediatr Surg 20:357–361, 1985.
4. Adzick NS, Vacanti JP, Lillehei CW, et al: Fetal diaphragmatic hernia: Ultrasound diagnosis and clinical outcome in 38 cases. J Pediatr Surg 24:654–657; discussion 657–658, 1989.
5. Ahlquist RP, Huggins RA, Woodbury RA: The pharmacology of benzyl-imidazoline (Priscoline). J Pharmacol Exp Ther 89:271–274, 1947.
6. Allen L: Transpleural muscles. J Thorac Surg 19:290–291, 1950.
7. Alles AJ, Losty PD, Donahoe PK, et al: Embryonic cell death patterns associated with nitrofen-induced congenital diaphragmatic hernia. J Pediatr Surg 30:353–358; discussion 359–360, 1995.
8. Ambrose AM, Larson PS, Borzelleca JF, et al: Toxicologic studies on 2,4-dichlorophenyl-p-nitrophenyl ether. Toxicol Appl Pharmacol 19:263–275, 1971.
9. Amirav I, Kramer SS, Schramm CM: Radiological cases of the month. Delayed presentation of congenital diaphragmatic hernia. Arch Pediatr Adolesc Med 148:203–204, 1994.
10. Andersen DH: Incidence of congenital diaphragmatic hernia in the young of rats bred on a diet deficient in vitamin A. Am J Dis Child 62:888, 1941.
11. Anderson KD: Congenital diaphragmatic hernia. In Welch KJ, Randolph JG, Ravitch MM, et al, editors: Pediatric Surgery, p. 599. Chicago: Year Book Medical Publishers, 1986.
12. Appelquist E, Hoier-Madsen K: Cribriform diaphragm: A variant of congenital diaphragmatic herniation. A case report. Scand J Thorac Cardiovasc Surg 20:185–187, 1986.
13. Areechon W, Reid L: Hypoplasia of the lung with congenital diaphragmatic hernia. Br Med J 1:230–233, 1963.
14. Arnold JH, Bower LK, Thompson JE: Respiratory deadspace measurements in neonates with congenital diaphragmatic hernia. Crit Care Med 23:371–375, 1995.
15. Asabe K, Tsuji K, Handa N, et al: Immunohistochemical distribution of surfactant apoprotein-A in congenital diaphragmatic hernia. J Pediatr Surg 32:667–672, 1997.
16. Aue O: Uber angeborene Zwerchfellhernien. Deutsch Z Chir 160:14, 1920.
17. Austin-Ward ED, Taucher SC: Familial congenital diaphragmatic hernia: Is an imprinting mechanism involved? J Med Genet 36:578–579, 1999.

18. Barker DP, Hussain S, Frank JD, et al: Bilateral congenital diaphragmatic hernia—delayed presentation of the contralateral defect. Arch Dis Child 69:543–544, 1993 (letter).

19. Barr M Jr: The teratogenicity of cadmium chloride in two stocks of Wistar rats. Teratology 7:237–242, 1973.

20. Bartlett RH, Gazzaniga AB, Toomasian J, et al: Extracorporeal membrane oxygenation (ECMO) in neonatal respiratory failure. 100 cases [published erratum appears in Ann Surg 205(1):11A, 1987]. Ann Surg 204:236–245, 1986.

21. Bax NM, Collins DL: The advantages of reconstruction of the dome of the diaphragm in congenital posterolateral diaphragmatic defects. J Pediatr Surg 19:484–487, 1984.

22. Bealer JF, Skarsgard ED, Hedrick MH, et al: The 'PLUG' odyssey: Adventures in experimental fetal tracheal occlusion. J Pediatr Surg 30:361–364; discussion 364–365, 1995.

23. Beals DA, Schloo BL, Vacanti JP, et al: Pulmonary growth and remodeling in infants with high-risk congenital diaphragmatic hernia. J Pediatr Surg 27:997–1001; discussion 1001–1002, 1992.

24. Beaudoin AR: Teratogenicity of polybrominated biphenyls in rats. Environ Res 14:81–86, 1977.

25. Becmeur F, Chevalier-Kauffmann I, Frey G, et al: [Laparoscopic treatment of a diaphragmatic hernia through the foramen of Morgagni in children. A case report and review of eleven cases reported in the adult literature]. Ann Chir 52:1060–1063, 1998.

26. Benjamin HB: Agenesis of the left diaphragm. J Thorac Cardiovasc Surg 46:265–270, 1963.

27. Berman L, Stringer D, Ein SH, et al: The late-presenting pediatric Bochdalek hernia: A 20-year review. J Pediatr Surg 23:735–739, 1988.

28. Berman L, Stringer DA, Ein S, et al: Childhood diaphragmatic hernias presenting after the neonatal period. Clin Radiol 39:237–244, 1988.

29. Bianchi A, Doig CM, Cohen SJ: The reverse latissimus dorsi flap for congenital diaphragmatic hernia repair. J Pediatr Surg 18:560–563, 1983.

30. Bindl L, Fahnenstich H, Peukert U: Aerosolised prostacyclin for pulmonary hypertension in neonates. Arch Dis Child Fetal Neonatal Ed 71:F214–F216, 1994.

31. Blackburn WR, Logsdon P, Alexander JA: Congenital diaphragmatic hernia: Studies of lung composition and structure. Am Rev Respir Dis 115S:275, 1977.

32. Bloss RS, Aranda JV, Beardmore HE: Congenital diaphragmatic hernia: Pathophysiology and pharmacologic support. Surgery 89:518–524, 1981.

33. Bochdalek VA: Einige Betrachtungen uber die Entstehung des angelborenen Zwerchfellbruches. Als Bietrag zur pathologischen. Anatomie der Hernien. Vjsch Prakt Heik 19:89–97, 1848.

34. Bohn D: Ventilatory and blood gas parameters in predicting survival in congenital diaphragmatic hernia. Pediatr Surg Int 2:336–340, 1987.

35. Bohn D: Congenital diaphragmatic hernia. Am J Respir Crit Care Med 166:911–915, 2002.

36. Bohn D, Tamura M, Perrin D, et al: Ventilatory predictors of pulmonary hypoplasia in congenital diaphragmatic hernia, confirmed by morphological assessment. J Pediatr 111:423–431, 1987.

37. Boix-Ochoa J, Peguero G, Seijo G, et al: Acid-base balance and blood gases in prognosis and therapy of congenital diaphragmatic hernia. J Pediatr Surg 9:49–57, 1974.

38. Boloker J, Bateman DA, Wung JT, et al: Congenital diaphragmatic hernia in 120 infants treated consecutively with permissive hypercapnea/spontaneous respiration/elective repair. J Pediatr Surg 37:357–366, 2002.

39. Bonetus T: De Suffocatione. Observatio XLI. Suffocatio excitata a tenuium intestorum vulnus diaphramatis, in thoracem ingrestu. Sepulchretum sive anatomia practica et cadareribus morbo denatus: Geneva, 1679.

40. Bos AP, Hussain SM, Hazebroek FW, et al: Radiographic evidence of bronchopulmonary dysplasia in high-risk congenital diaphragmatic hernia survivors. Pediatr Pulmonol 15:231–234, 1993.

41. Bos AP, Tibboel D, Koot VC, et al: Persistent pulmonary hypertension in high-risk congenital diaphragmatic hernia patients: incidence and vasodilator therapy. J Pediatr Surg 28:1463–1465, 1993.

42. Boychuk RB, Nelson JC, Yates KA: Congenital diaphragmatic hernia (an 8-year experience in Hawaii). Hawaii Med J 42:400–402, 1983.

43. Bray RJ: Congenital diaphragmatic hernia. Anaesthesia 34:567–577, 1979.

44. Bremer JL: The diaphragm and diaphragmatic hernia. Arch Pathol 36:539–549, 1943.

45. Brent RL: Antibodies and malformations. In Tuchmann-Duplessis H, editor: Malformations Congénitales des Mammiféres, pp. 187–222. Paris: Masson City, 1971.

46. Broman I: Uber die Entwicklung des Zwerchfells beim Menschen. Verh Anat Ges 16:9–17, 1902.

47. Broman I: Ueber die Entwicklung und Bedeutung der Mesenterien und der Körperhöhlen bei den Wirbeltieren. Ergeb Anat Entw 15:332–409, 1905.

48. Bucher U, Reid L: Development of the intrasegmental bronchial tree: The pattern of branching and development of cartilage at various stages of intrauterine life. Thorax 16:207–218, 1961.

49. Burge DM, Atwell JD, Freeman NV: Could the stomach site help predict outcome in babies with left sided congenital diaphragmatic hernia diagnosed antenatally? J Pediatr Surg 24:567–569, 1989.

50. Butler MW, Stolar CJ, Altman RP: Contemporary management of congenital diaphragmatic hernia. World J Surg 17:350–355, 1993.

51. Butler N, Claireaux AE: Congenital diaphragmatic hernia as a cause of perinatal mortality. Lancet 1:659–663, 1962.

52. Callahan PF, Short BL, Rais-Bahrami K, et al: Pulmonary artery size is larger in nonsurvivors with congenital diaphragmatic hernia. In 10th Annual Children's National Medical Center ECMO Symposium. Keystone, Colo: EUA, 1994.

53. Cantrell JR, Haller JA, Ravitch MM: A syndrome of congenital defects involving the abdominal wall, sternum, diaphragm, pericardium and heart. Surg Gynecol Obstet 107:602–614, 1958.

54. Caplan MS, MacGregor SN: Perinatal management of congenital diaphragmatic hernia and anterior abdominal wall defects. Clin Perinatol 16:917–938, 1989.

55. Carmi R, Meizner I, Katz M: Familial congenital diaphragmatic defect and associated midline anomalies: Further evidence for an X-linked midline gene? Am J Med Genet 36:313–315, 1990.

56. Carter REB, Waterston DJ, Aberdeen E: Hernia and eventration of the diaphragm in childhood. Lancet 1:656–659, 1962.

57. Cartlidge PH, Mann NP, Kapila L: Preoperative stabilisation in congenital diaphragmatic hernia. Arch Dis Child 61:1226–1228, 1986.

58. Casey AE, Hidden EH: Nondevelopment of septum transversum, with congenital absence of anterocentral portion of the diaphragm and the suspensory ligament of the liver and presence of an elongated ductus venosus and a pericardioperitoneal foramen. Arch Pathol 38:370–374, 1944.

59. Chang R, Komura M, Andreoli S, et al: Hyperoncotic enhancement of pulmonary lung growth after fetal tracheal occlusion: A comparison between dextran and albumin. J Pediatr Surg 39:324–328; discussion 324–328, 2004.

540

60. Chang R, Komura M, Andreoli S, et al: Rapidly polymerizing hydrogel prevents balloon dislodgment in a model of fetal tracheal occlusion. J Pediatr Surg:39:557–560, 2004.

61. Christensen P: Eventration of the diaphragm. Thorax 14:311–319, 1959.

62. Chui PP, Tan CT: Sudden death due to incarcerated Bochdalek hernia in an adult. Ann Acad Med Singapore 22:57–60, 1993.

63. Clark RH, Hardin WD Jr, Hirschl RB, et al: Current surgical management of congenital diaphragmatic hernia: A report from the Congenital Diaphragmatic Hernia Study Group. J Pediatr Surg 33:1004–1009, 1998.

64. Clark RH, Yoder BA, Sell MS: Prospective, randomized comparison of high-frequency oscillation and conventional ventilation in candidates for extracorporeal membrane oxygenation [see comments]. J Pediatr 124:447–454, 1994.

65. Coca MA, Landin F: Malformations congénitales multiples avec absence presque complète de diaphragme. Semin Hop Paris 33:3839, 1957.

66. Cohen D, Reid IS: Recurrent diaphragmatic hernia. J Pediatr Surg 16:42–44, 1981.

67. Collins DL, Pomerance JJ, Travis KW, et al: A new approach to congenital posterolateral diaphragmatic hernia. J Pediatr Surg 12:149–156, 1977.

68. Crombleholme TM, Adzick NS, Hardy K, et al: Pulmonary lobar transplantation in neonatal swine: A model for treatment of congenital diaphragmatic hernia. J Pediatr Surg 25:11–18, 1990.

69. Cullen ML: Congenital diaphragmatic hernia: Operative considerations. Semin Pediatr Surg 5:243–248, 1996.

70. Czeizel A, Kovacs M: A family study of congenital diaphragmatic defects. Am J Med Genet 21:105–117, 1985.

71. D'Agostino JA, Bernbaum JC, Gerdes M, et al: Outcome for infants with congenital diaphragmatic hernia requiring extracorporeal membrane oxygenation: The first year. J Pediatr Surg 30:10–15, 1995.

72. Dalla Vecchia L, Engum S, Kogon B, et al: Evaluation of small intestine submucosa and acellular dermis as diaphragmatic prostheses. J Pediatr Surg 34:167–171, 1999.

73. David TJ, Illingworth CA: Diaphragmatic hernia in the south-west of England. J Med Genet 13:253–262, 1976.

74. deLorimier AA, Tierney OF, Parker HR: Hypoplastic lungs in fetal lambs with surgically produced congenital diaphragmatic hernia. Surgery 62:12–17, 1967.

75. Dibbins AW: Neonatal diaphragmatic hernia: A physiologic challenge. Am J Surg 131:408–410, 1976.

76. Dibbins AW: Congenital diaphragmatic hernia: Hypoplastic lung and pulmonary vasoconstriction. Clin Perinatol 5:93–104, 1978.

77. Dibbins AW, Wiener ES: Mortality from neonatal diaphragmatic hernia. J Pediatr Surg 9:653–662, 1974.

78. DiFiore JW, Fauza DO, Slavin R, et al: Experimental fetal tracheal ligation reverses the structural and physiological effects of pulmonary hypoplasia in congenital diaphragmatic hernia. J Pediatr Surg 29:248–256; discussion 256–257, 1994.

79. DiFiore JW, Fauza DO, Slavin R, et al: Experimental fetal tracheal ligation and congenital diaphragmatic hernia: A pulmonary vascular morphometric analysis [see comments]. J Pediatr Surg 30:917–923; discussion 923–924, 1995.

80. Downard CD, Betit P, Chang RW, et al: Impact of AMICAR on hemorrhagic complications of ECMO: A ten-year review. J Pediatr Surg 38:1212–1216, 2003.

81. Downard CD, Jaksic T, Garza JJ, et al: Analysis of an improved survival rate for congenital diaphragmatic hernia. J Pediatr Surg 38:729–732, 2003.

82. Drake EH, Lynch JP: Bronchiectasis associated with anomaly of the right pulmonary vein and right diaphragm: Report of a case. J Thorac Surg 19:433, 1950.

83. Drobeck HP, Coulston F, Cornelius D: Effects of thalidomide on fetal development in rabbits and on establishment of pregnancy in monkeys. Toxicol Appl Pharmacol 7:165–178, 1965.

84. Duncan KR: Fetal and placental volumetric and functional analysis using echo-planar imaging. Top Magn Reson Imaging 12:52–66, 2001.

85. Dunnill MS: Postnatal growth of the lung. Thorax 17:329–333, 1962.

86. Dussault J, Godlewski G, Pignodel C: Pathogenesis of congenital diaphragmatic hernia of the newborn infant: Apropos of 2 cases. Bull Assoc Anat (Nancy) 65:77–81, 1981.

87. Dzakovic A, Kaviani A, Jennings RW, et al: Positive intrapulmonary oncotic pressure enhances short-term lung growth acceleration after fetal tracheal occlusion. J Pediatr Surg 37:1007–1010; discussion 1007–1010, 2002.

88. ECMO Registry Report, Ann Arbor, MI: Extracorporeal Life Support Organization, 2004.

89. Estimating disease severity of congenital diaphragmatic hernia in the first 5 minutes of life. The Congenital Diaphragmatic Hernia Study Group. J Pediatr Surg 36:141–145, 2001.

90. Falcao MC, Carvalho MF, Tannuri U, et al: [Early-onset neonatal sepsis and late-appearing diaphragmatic hernia]. Rev Hosp Clin Fac Med Sao Paulo 53:152–155, 1998.

91. Fauza DO, Barnewolt C, Brown SD, et al: Ultrasound-guided fetal tracheal occlusion. J Pediatr Surg 37:300–302, 2001.

92. Fauza DO, DiFiore JW, Hines MH, et al: Continuous intrapulmonary distention with perfluorocarbon accelerates postnatal lung growth: Possible application for congenital diaphragmatic hernia. Surg Forum 46:666–669, 1995.

93. Fauza DO, Hirschl RB, Wilson JM: Continuous intrapulmonary distention with perfluorocarbon accelerates lung growth in infants with congenital diaphragmatic hernia: initial experience. J Pediatr Surg 36:1237–1240, 2001.

94. Fauza DO, Marler JJ, Koka R, et al: Fetal tissue engineering: Diaphragmatic replacement. J Pediatr Surg 36:146–151, 2001.

95. Fauza DO, Tannuri U, Ayoub AA, et al: Surgically produced congenital diaphragmatic hernia in fetal rabbits. J Pediatr Surg 29:882–886, 1994.

96. Fauza DO, Wilson JM: Congenital diaphragmatic hernia and associated anomalies: Their incidence, identification, and impact on prognosis. J Pediatr Surg 29:1113–1117, 1994.

97. Finer NN, Barrington KJ: Nitric oxide therapy for the newborn infant. Semin Perinatol 24:59–65, 2000.

98. Finer NN, Tierney A, Etches PC, et al: Congenital diaphragmatic hernia: Developing a protocolized approach. J Pediatr Surg 33:1331–1337, 1998.

99. Fitchett CW, Tavarez V: Bilateral congenital diaphragmatic herniation: Case report. Surgery 57:305–308, 1965.

100. Flake AW, Crombleholme TM, Johnson MP, et al: Treatment of severe congenital diaphragmatic hernia by fetal tracheal occlusion: Clinical experience with fifteen cases. Am J Obstet Gynecol 183:1059–1066, 2000.

101. Folkman J: Personal communication, 1995.

102. Ford WD, James MJ, Walsh JA: Congenital diaphragmatic hernia: Association between pulmonary vascular resistance and plasma thromboxane concentrations. Arch Dis Child 59:143–146, 1984.

103. Fox HE, Badalian SS: Ultrasound prediction of fetal pulmonary hypoplasia in pregnancies complicated by oligohydramnios and in cases of congenital diaphragmatic hernia: A review. Am J Perinatol 11:104–108, 1994.

104. Fox WW, Duara S: Persistent pulmonary hypertension in the neonate: Diagnosis and management. J Pediatr 103:505–514, 1983.

105. Frey P, Glanzmann R, Nars P, et al: Familial congenital diaphragmatic defect: Transmission from father to daughter. J Pediatr Surg 26:1396–1398, 1991.

106. Fuchs JR, Kaviani A, Oh JT, et al: Diaphragmatic reconstruction with autologous tendon engineered from mesenchymal amniocytes. J Pediatr Surg 39:834–838, 2004.

107. Gandy G, Bradbrooke JG, Naidoo BT, et al: Comparison of methods for evaluating surface properties of lung in perinatal period. Arch Dis Child 43:8–16, 1968.

108. Gattone VHD, Morse DE: A scanning electron microscopic study on the pathogenesis of the posterolateral diaphragmatic hernia. J Submicrosc Cytol 14:483–490, 1982.

109. Geggel RL, Murphy JD, Langleben D, et al: Congenital diaphragmatic hernia: Arterial structural changes and persistent pulmonary hypertension after surgical repair. J Pediatr 107:457–464, 1985.

110. Georgacopulo P, Franchella A, Mandrioli G, et al: Morgagni-Larrey hernia correction by laparoscopic surgery. Eur J Pediatr Surg 7:241–242, 1997.

111. German JC, Gazzaniga AB, Amlie R, et al: Management of pulmonary insufficiency in diaphragmatic hernia using extracorporeal circulation with a membrane oxygenator (ECMO). J Pediatr Surg 12:905–912, 1977.

112. Giacoia GP: Right-sided diaphragmatic hernia associated with superior vena cava syndrome. Am J Perinatol 11:129–131, 1994.

113. Gray LE Jr, Kavlock RJ, Chernoff N, et al: Prenatal exposure to the herbicide 2,4-dichlorophenyl-p-nitrophenyl ether destroys the rodent Harderian gland. Science 215:293–294, 1982.

114. Greenholz SK: Congenital diaphragmatic hernia: An overview. Semin Pediatr Surg 5:216–223, 1996.

115. Greenspan JS, Fox WW, Rubenstein SD, et al: Partial liquid ventilation in critically ill infants receiving extracorporeal life support. Philadelphia Liquid Ventilation Consortium. Pediatrics 99:E2, 1997.

116. Greenwood RD, Rosenthal A, Nadas AS: Cardiovascular abnormalities associated with congenital diaphragmatic hernia. Pediatrics 57:92–97, 1976.

117. Gross RE: Congenital hernia of the diaphragm. Am J Dis Child 71:579–592, 1946.

118. Haeusler MC, Ryan G, Robson SC, et al: The use of saline solution as a contrast medium in suspected diaphragmatic hernia and renal agenesis. Am J Obstet Gynecol 168:1486–1492, 1993.

119. Haller JA Jr, Signer RD, Golladay ES, et al: Pulmonary and ductal hemodynamics in studies of simulated diaphragmatic hernia of fetal and newborn lambs. J Pediatr Surg 11:675–680, 1976.

120. Harrison MR, Adzick NS, Bullard KM, et al: Correction of congenital diaphragmatic hernia in utero. VII: A prospective trial. J Pediatr Surg 32:1637–1642, 1997.

121. Harrison MR, Adzick NS, Flake AW, et al: Correction of congenital diaphragmatic hernia in utero. VI: Hard-earned lessons. J Pediatr Surg 28:1411–1417; discussion 1417–1418, 1993.

122. Harrison MR, Adzick NS, Flake AW, et al: Correction of congenital diaphragmatic hernia in utero. VIII: Response of the hypoplastic lung to tracheal occlusion. J Pediatr Surg 31:1339–1348, 1996.

123. Harrison MR, Albanese CT, Hawgood SB, et al: Fetoscopic temporary tracheal occlusion by detachable balloon for congenital diaphragmatic hernia. Am J Obstet Gynecol 185:730–733, 2001.

124. Harrison MR, Bjordal RI, Langmark F, et al: Congenital diaphragmatic hernia: The hidden mortality. J Pediatr Surg 13:227–230, 1978.

125. Harrison MR, de Lorimier AA: Congenital diaphragmatic hernia. Surg Clin North Am 61:1023–1035, 1981.

126. Harrison MR, Jester JA, Ross NA: Correction of congenital diaphragmatic hernia in utero. I. The model: Intrathoracic balloon produces fatal pulmonary hypoplasia. Surgery 88:174–182, 1980.

127. Harrison MR, Keller RL, Hawgood SB, et al: A randomized trial of fetal endoscopic tracheal occlusion for severe fetal congenital diaphragmatic hernia. N Engl J Med 349:1916–1924, 2003.

128. Harrison MR, Langer JC, Adzick NS, et al: Correction of congenital diaphragmatic hernia in utero. V: Initial clinical experience. J Pediatr Surg 25:47–55; discussion 56–57, 1990.

129. Harrison MR, Mychaliska GB, Albanese CT, et al: Correction of congenital diaphragmatic hernia in utero. IX: Fetuses with poor prognosis (liver herniation and low lung-to-head ratio) can be saved by fetoscopic temporary tracheal occlusion. J Pediatr Surg 33:1017–1022; discussion 1022–1023, 1998.

130. Hasegawa S, Kohno S, Sugiyama T, et al: Usefulness of echocardiographic measurement of bilateral pulmonary artery dimensions in congenital diaphragmatic hernia. J Pediatr Surg 29:622–624, 1994.

131. Hasegawa T, Kamata S, Imura K, et al: Use of lung-thorax transverse area ratio in the antenatal evaluation of lung hypoplasia in congenital diaphragmatic hernia. J Clin Ultrasound 18:705–709, 1990.

132. Hashida Y, Sherman FE: Accessory diaphragm associated with neonatal respiratory distress. J Pediatr 59:529–532, 1961.

133. Hassett MJ, Glick PL, Karamanoukian HL, et al: Pathophysiology of congenital diaphragmatic hernia. XVI: Elevated pulmonary collagen in the lamb model of congenital diaphragmatic hernia. J Pediatr Surg 30:1191–1194, 1995.

134. Hatzitheofilou C, Conlan AA, Nicolaou N: Agenesis of the diaphragm. A case report. S Afr Med J 62:999–1001, 1982.

135. Heidenhain L: Gesichte eines Falles von chronisher Incarceration des Mageus in einer angehorenen Zwerchfellhernie welcher durcher Laparotomie geheilt wurde, mitansheissenden Bermerkungen uber die Moglichkeit, das Kardiacarcinom der Speiserihre zu reseciren. Deutsch Z Chir 76:394–407, 1905.

136. Heine H: Zur Entwicklungsgeschichte angeborener Zwerchfellhernien bei Saugetieren. Anat Anaz 133:382–393, 1973.

137. Hill AC, Adzick NS, Stevens MB, et al: Fetal lamb pulmonary hypoplasia: pulmonary vascular and myocardial abnormalities. Ann Thorac Surg 57:946–951, 1994.

138. Hines MH: Video-assisted diaphragm plication in children. Ann Thorac Surg 76:234–236, 2003.

139. Hisanaga S, Shimokawa H, Kashiwabara Y, et al: Unexpectedly low lecithin/sphingomyelin ratio associated with fetal diaphragmatic hernia. Am J Obstet Gynecol 149:905–906, 1984.

140. Hislop A, Reid L: Persistent hypoplasia of the lung after repair of congenital diaphragmatic hernia. Thorax 31:450–455, 1976.

141. Holder RM, Ashcraft KW: Congenital diaphragmatic hernia. In Ravitch MM, Welch KJ, Benson CD, et al, editors: Pediatric Surgery, pp. 432–445. Chicago: Year Book Medical Publishers, 1979.

142. Hurley LS: Teratogenic aspects of manganese, zinc, and copper nutrition. Physiol Rev 61:249–295, 1981.

143. Ildstad ST, Stevenson RJ, Tollerud DJ, et al: High apical insertion of the right diaphragm in an infant with right-sided Bochdalek diaphragmatic hernia. J Pediatr Surg 25:553–555, 1990.

144. Iritani I: Experimental study on embryogenesis of congenital diaphragmatic hernia. Anat Embryol (Berl) 169:133–139, 1984.

145. Irving IM, Booker PD: Congenital diaphragmatic hernia and eventration of the diaphragm. In Lister J, Irving IM: editors:

Neonatal Surgery, 3rd ed., pp. 199–200. London: Butterworth, 1990.

146. Jeandot R, Lambert B, Brendel AJ, et al: Lung ventilation and perfusion scintigraphy in the follow up of repaired congenital diaphragmatic hernia. Eur J Nucl Med 15:591–596, 1989.

147. Jenkinson EL: Absence of half of the diaphragm (thoracic stomach; diaphragmatic hernia). AJR 26:899–903, 1931.

148. Kajii T, Oikawa K, Itakura K, et al: A probable 17-18 trisomy syndrome with phocomelia, exomphalos, and agenesis of hemidiaphragm. Arch Dis Child 39:519–522, 1964.

149. Kamata S, Hasegawa T, Ishikawa S, et al: Prenatal diagnosis of congenital diaphragmatic hernia and perinatal care: Assessment of lung hypoplasia. Early Hum Dev 29:375–379, 1992.

150. Karamanoukian HL, Glick PL, Wilcox DT, et al: Pathophysiology of congenital diaphragmatic hernia. VIII: Inhaled nitric oxide requires exogenous surfactant therapy in the lamb model of congenital diaphragmatic hernia. J Pediatr Surg 30:1–4, 1995.

151. Karamanoukian HL, Glick PL, Wilcox DT, et al: Pathophysiology of congenital diaphragmatic hernia. X: Localization of nitric oxide synthase in the intima of pulmonary artery trunks of lambs with surgically created congenital diaphragmatic hernia. J Pediatr Surg 30:5–9, 1995.

152. Karamanoukian HL, Glick PL, Wilcox DT, et al: Pathophysiology of congenital diaphragmatic hernia. XI: Anatomic and biochemical characterization of the heart in the fetal lamb CDH model. J Pediatr Surg 30:925–928; discussion 929, 1995.

153. Kays DW, Langham MR, Jr., Ledbetter DJ, et al: Detrimental effects of standard medical therapy in congenital diaphragmatic hernia. Ann Surg 230:340–348; discussion 348–351, 1999.

154. Keith A: Diaphragmatic herniae. Br Med J 2:1297, 1910.

155. Kelly DR, Grant EG, Zeman RK, et al: In utero diagnosis of congenital diaphragmatic hernia by CT amniography. J Comput Assist Tomogr 10:500–502, 1986.

156. Kent GM, Olley PM, Creighton RE, et al: Hemodynamic and pulmonary changes following surgical creation of a diaphragmatic hernia in fetal lambs. Surgery 72:427–433, 1972.

157. Kimbrough RD, Gaines TB, Linder RE: 2,4-Dichlorophenyl-p-nitrophenyl ether (TOK): Effects on the lung maturation of rat fetus. Arch Environ Health 28:316–320, 1974.

158. Kinsella JP, Truog WE, Walsh WF, et al: Randomized, multicenter trial of inhaled nitric oxide and high-frequency oscillatory ventilation in severe, persistent pulmonary hypertension of the newborn. J Pediatr 131:55–62, 1997.

159. Kitagawa M, Hislop A, Boyden EA, et al: Lung hypoplasia in congenital diaphragmatic hernia. A quantitative study of airway, artery, and alveolar development. Br J Surg 58:342–346, 1971.

160. Kitterman JA: Fetal lambs with surgically produced congenital diaphragmatic hernia (CDH) are deficient in pulmonary surfactant. J Pediatr Surg 28:1218–1219, 1993 (letter; comment).

161. Kluth D, Keijzer R, Hertl M, et al: Embryology of congenital diaphragmatic hernia. Semin Pediatr Surg 5:224–233, 1996.

162. Kluth D, Tenbrinck R, von Ekesparre M, et al: The natural history of congenital diaphragmatic hernia and pulmonary hypoplasia in the embryo. J Pediatr Surg 28:456–462; discussion 462–463, 1993.

163. Kobayashi H, Puri P: Plasma endothelin levels in congenital diaphragmatic hernia. J Pediatr Surg 29:1258–1261, 1994.

164. Koot VC, Bergmeijer JH, Bos AP, et al: Incidence and management of gastroesophageal reflux after repair of congenital diaphragmatic hernia. J Pediatr Surg 28:48–52, 1993.

165. Koot VC, Bergmeijer JH, Molenaar JC: Lyophylized dura patch repair of congenital diaphragmatic hernia: Occurrence of relapses. J Pediatr Surg 28:667–668, 1993.

166. Kovarik JL, Jensen NK: Congenital aplasia of the right hepatic lobe with right-sided diaphragmatic hernia and intestinal malrotation. Int Surg 51:499–503, 1969.

167. Krzyzaniak R, Gray SW: Accessory septum transversum. The first case report. Am Surg 52:278–281, 1986.

168. Ladd WE, Gross RE: Congenital diaphragmatic hernia. N Engl J Med 233:917–925, 1940.

169. Lally KP, Cheu HW, Vazquez WD: Prosthetic diaphragm reconstruction in the growing animal. J Pediatr Surg 28:45–47, 1993.

170. Lally KP, Paranka MS, Roden J, et al: Congenital diaphragmatic hernia. Stabilization and repair on ECMO. Ann Surg 216:569–573, 1992.

171. Laxdal OE, McDougal H, Mellin GW: Congenital eventration of the diaphragm. N Engl J Med 205:401–408, 1954.

172. Leck I, Record RG, McKeown T, et al: The incidence of malformations in Birmingham, England, 1950–1959. Teratology 1:263–280, 1968.

173. Leveque C, Hamza J, Berg AE, et al: Successful repair of a severe left congenital diaphragmatic hernia during continuous inhalation of nitric oxide. Anesthesiology 80:1171–1175, 1994.

174. Levin DL: Congenital diaphragmatic hernia: A persistent problem. J Pediatr 111:390–392, 1987.

175. Levine G, Goetzman B, Milstein J, et al: Influence of airway state on hemodynamics of the pulmonary circulation in newborn lambs. Pediatr Res 31:314A, 1992.

176. Lewis WH: The development of the muscular system. In Keibel F, Mall FP, editors: Manual of Human Embryology. Philadelphia: J.B. Lippincott, 1910.

177. Liem NT: Thoracoscopic surgery for congenital diaphragmatic hernia: A report of nine cases. Asian J Surg 26:210–212, 2003.

178. Lilly JR, Paul M, Rosser SB: Anterior diaphragmatic hernia: Familial presentation. Birth Defects Orig Artic Ser 10:257–258, 1974.

179. Lima M, Domini M, Libri M, et al: Laparoscopic repair of Morgagni-Larrey hernia in a child. J Pediatr Surg 35:1266–1268, 2000.

180. Lister J: Recent advances in the surgery of the diaphragm in the newborn. Prog Pediatr Surg 2:29–39, 1971.

181. Lotze A, Knight GR, Anderson KD, et al: Surfactant (beractant) therapy for infants with congenital diaphragmatic hernia on ECMO: Evidence of persistent surfactant deficiency [see comments]. J Pediatr Surg 29:407–412, 1994.

182. Luks FI, Carr SR, Ponte B, et al: Preoperative planning with magnetic resonance imaging and computerized volume rendering in twin-to-twin transfusion syndrome. Am J Obstet Gynecol 185:216–219, 2001.

183. Lund DP, Mitchell J, Kharasch V, et al: Congenital diaphragmatic hernia: The hidden morbidity. J Pediatr Surg 29:258–262; discussion 262–264, 1994.

184. Macaulay G: An account of viscera herniation. Phil Trans Roy Coll Phys 6:25–35, 1754.

185. MacGillivray TE, Jennings RW, Rudolph AM, et al: Vascular changes with in utero correction of diaphragmatic hernia. J Pediatr Surg 29:992–996, 1994.

186. Mäkelä V: Hernia diaphragmatica congenita spuria. Finska Läk Sällsk Handl 58:1107–1127, 1916.

187. Mansell AL, McAteer AL, Pipkin AC: Maturation of interdependence between extra-alveolar arteries and lung parenchyma in piglets. Circ Res 71:701–710, 1992.

188. McNamara JJ, Eraklis AJ, Gross RE: Congenital posterolateral diaphragmatic hernia in the newborn. J Thorac Cardiovasc Surg 55:55–59, 1968.

189. Mellins RB, Hays AP, Gold AP, et al: Respiratory distress as the initial manifestation of Werdnig-Hoffmann disease. Pediatrics 53:33–40, 1974.

190. Mishalany H, Gordo J: Congenital diaphragmatic hernia in monozygotic twins. J Pediatr Surg 21:372–374, 1986.

191. Mishalany HG, Nakada K, Woolley MM: Congenital diaphragmatic hernias: Eleven years' experience. Arch Surg 114:1118–1123, 1979.

192. Moessinger AC, Harding R, Adamson TM, et al: Role of lung fluid volume in growth and maturation of the fetal sheep lung. J Clin Invest 86:1270–1277, 1990.

193. Molenaar JC, Bos AP, Hazebroek FW, et al: Congenital diaphragmatic hernia, what defect? J Pediatr Surg 26:248–254, 1991.

194. Moore KL: The Developing Human, 4th ed. Philadelphia: W.B. Saunders, 1988.

195. Morgagni GB: The seats and causes of disease investigated by anatomy. Alexander BT, translator: pp. 205–206. London: Miller & Caldwell, 1769.

196. Moss RL, Chen CM, Harrison MR: Prosthetic patch durability in congenital diaphragmatic hernia: A long-term follow-up study. J Pediatr Surg 36:152–154, 2001.

197. Movsowitz HD, Jacobs LE, Movsowitz C, et al: Transesophageal echocardiographic evaluation of a transthoracic echocardiographic pitfall: A diaphragmatic hernia mimicking a left atrial mass. J Am Soc Echocardiogr 6:104–106, 1993.

198. Muglia LJ, Bae DS, Brown TT, et al: Proliferation and differentiation defects during lung development in corticotropin-releasing hormone-deficient mice. Am J Respir Cell Mol Biol 20:181–188, 1999.

199. Muratore CS, Kharasch V, Lund DP, et al: Pulmonary morbidity in 100 survivors of congenital diaphragmatic hernia monitored in a multidisciplinary clinic. J Pediatr Surg 36:133–140, 2001.

200. Muratore CS, Utter S, Jaksic T, et al: Nutritional morbidity in survivors of congenital diaphragmatic hernia. J Pediatr Surg 36:1171–1176, 2001.

201. Muratore CS, Wilson JM: Congenital diaphragmatic hernia: Where are we and where do we go from here? Semin Perinatol 24:418–428, 2000.

202. Naeye RL, Shochat SJ, Whitman V, et al: Unsuspected pulmonary vascular abnormalities associated with diaphragmatic hernia. Pediatrics 58:902–906, 1976.

203. Nakao Y, Iritani I, Kishimoto H: Experimental model of congenital diaphragmatic hernia induced chemically. Teratology 24:11A, 1981.

204. Nakayama DK, Harrison MR, Chinn DH, et al: Prenatal diagnosis and natural history of the fetus with a congenital diaphragmatic hernia: Initial clinical experience. J Pediatr Surg 20:118–124, 1985.

205. Nakayama DK, Motoyama EK, Tagge EM: Effect of preoperative stabilization on respiratory system compliance and outcome in newborn infants with congenital diaphragmatic hernia. J Pediatr 118:793–799, 1991.

206. Narayan H, De Chazal R, Barrow M, et al: Familial congenital diaphragmatic hernia: Prenatal diagnosis, management, and outcome. Prenat Diagn 13:893–901, 1993.

207. Nawaz A, Matta H, Jacobsz A, et al: Congenital Morgagni's hernia in infants and children. Int Surg 85:158–162, 2000.

208. Newman BM, Jewett TC, Lewis A, et al: Prosthetic materials and muscle flaps in the repair of extensive diaphragmatic defects: An experimental study. J Pediatr Surg 20:362–367, 1985.

209. Nigogosyan G, Ozarda H: Accessory diaphragm: A case report. AJR 83:309–311, 1961.

210. Nobuhara KK, Fauza DO, DiFiore JW, et al: Continuous intrapulmonary distension with perfluorocarbon accelerates neonatal (but not adult) lung growth. J Pediatr Surg 33:292–298, 1998.

211. Nobuhara KK, Ferretti ML, Siddiqui AM, et al: Long-term effect of perfluorocarbon distension on the lung. J Pediatr Surg 33:1024–1028; discussion 1028–1029, 1998.

212. Nobuhara KK, Lund DP, Mitchell J, et al: Long-term outlook for survivors of congenital diaphragmatic hernia. Clin Perinatol 23:873–887, 1996.

213. Nobuhara KK, Wilson JM: Pathophysiology of congenital diaphragmatic hernia. Semin Pediatr Surg 5:234–242, 1996.

214. Norio R, Kaariainen H, Rapola J, et al: Familial congenital diaphragmatic defects: Aspects of etiology, prenatal diagnosis, and treatment. Am J Med Genet 17:471–483, 1984.

215. Nunez R, Rubio JL, Pimentel J, et al: Congenital diaphragmatic hernia and intrathoracic intestinal volvulus. Eur J Pediatr Surg 3:293–295, 1993.

216. O'Rourke PP: Congenital diaphragmatic hernia: Are there reliable clinical predictors? Crit Care Med 21:S380–S381, 1993.

217. O'Rourke PP, Vacanti JP, Crone RK, et al: Use of the postductal PaO_2 as a predictor of pulmonary vascular hypoplasia in infants with congenital diaphragmatic hernia. J Pediatr Surg 23:904–907, 1988.

218. Osebold WR, Soper RT: Congenital posterolateral diaphragmatic hernia past infancy. Am J Surg 131:748–754, 1976.

219. Palmer RM, Ferrige AG, Moncada S: Nitric oxide release accounts for the biological activity of endothelium-derived relaxing factor. Nature 327:524–526, 1987.

220. Papadakis K, Luks FI, Deprest JA, et al: Single-port tracheoscopic surgery in the fetal lamb. J Pediatr Surg 33:918–920, 1998.

221. Paræo A: Opera Chirurgica, p. 230. Frankfurt, Germany: 1610.

222. Phillpott JW, Cumming WA: Torsion of the spleen: An unusual presentation of congenital diaphragmatic hernia. Pediatr Radiol 24:150–151, 1994.

223. Pittinger TP, Sawin RS: Adrenocortical insufficiency in infants with congenital diaphragmatic hernia: A pilot study. J Pediatr Surg 35:223–225; discussion 225–226, 2000.

224. Pokorny WJ, McGill CW, Harberg FJ: Morgagni hernias during infancy: Presentation and associated anomalies. J Pediatr Surg 19:394–397, 1984.

225. Pranikoff T, Gauger PG, Hirschl RB: Partial liquid ventilation in newborn patients with congenital diaphragmatic hernia. J Pediatr Surg 31:613–618, 1996.

226. Puri P, Gorman F: Lethal nonpulmonary anomalies associated with congenital diaphragmatic hernia: Implications for early intrauterine surgery. J Pediatr Surg 19:29–32, 1984.

227. Puri P, Gorman WA: Natural history of congenital diaphragmatic hernia: Implications for management. Pediatr Surg Int 2:327–330, 1987.

228. Rais-Bahrami K, Short BL: The current status of neonatal extracorporeal membrane oxygenation. Semin Perinatol 24:406–417, 2000.

229. Ramadwar RH, Carachi R, Young DG: Collagen-coated Vicryl mesh is not a suitable material for repair of diaphragmatic defects. J Pediatr Surg 32:1708–1710, 1997.

230. Ravitch MM, Barton BA: The need for pediatric surgeons as determined by the volume of work and the mode of delivery of surgical care. Surgery 76:754–763, 1974.

231. Reed JA, Borden DL: Eventration of the diaphragm. Arch Surg 31:30–64, 1935.

232. Reid IS, Hutcherson RJ: Long-term follow-up of patients with congenital diaphragmatic hernia. J Pediatr Surg 11:939–942, 1976.

233. Reid LM: Lung growth in health and disease. Br J Dis Chest 78:113–134, 1984.

234. Rogers JF, Lane WZ, Gibbs R: Herniation through the diaphragm into the pericardium. Conn Med J 22:653–656, 1958.

235. Sagal Z: Absence of left diaphragm associated with inverted thoracic stomach. AJR 30:206–214, 1933.

236. Sakai H, Tamura M, Hosokawa Y, et al: Effect of surgical repair on respiratory mechanics in congenital diaphragmatic hernia. J Pediatr 111:432–438, 1987.

544

237. Sakurai Y, Azarow K, Cutz E, et al: Pulmonary barotrauma in congenital diaphragmatic hernia: A clinicopathological correlation. J Pediatr Surg 34:1813–1817, 1999.

238. Sappington TB Jr, Daniel RA Jr: Accessory diaphragm: A case report. Am Surg 21:212–216, 1951.

239. Sarda P, Devaux P, Lefort G, et al: Epidemiology of diaphragmatic hernia in Languedoc-Roussillon. Genet Couns 2:77–81, 1991.

240. Scheffers EC, H IJ, Tenbrinck R, et al: Evaluation of lung function changes before and after surfactant application during artificial ventilation in newborn rats with congenital diaphragmatic hernia. J Pediatr Surg 29:820–824, 1994.

241. Schnitzer JJ, Kikiros CS, Short BL, et al: Experience with abdominal wall closure for patients with congenital diaphragmatic hernia repaired on ECMO. J Pediatr Surg 30:19–22, 1995.

242. Shaffer JO: Prosthesis for agenesis of the diaphragm. JAMA 188:1000–1002, 1964.

243. Shah N, Jacob T, Exler R, et al: Inhaled nitric oxide in congenital diaphragmatic hernia. J Pediatr Surg 29:1010–1014; discussion 1014–1015, 1994.

244. Sherer DM, Abramowicz JS, D'Angio C, et al: Hepatic interlobar fissure sonographically mimicking the diaphragm in a fetus with right congenital diaphragmatic hernia. Am J Perinatol 10:319–322, 1993.

245. Sherer DM, Woods JR Jr: Second trimester sonographic diagnosis of fetal congenital diaphragmatic hernia, with spontaneous resolution during the third trimester, resulting in a normal infant at delivery. J Clin Ultrasound 19:298–302, 1991.

246. Shochat SJ: Pulmonary vascular pathology in congenital diaphragmatic hernias. Pediatr Surg Int 2:331–335, 1987.

247. Shochat SJ: Personal communication, 1995.

248. Simpson JS, Gossage JD: Use of abdominal wall muscle flap in repair of large congenital diaphragmatic hernia. J Pediatr Surg 6:42–44, 1971.

249. Skandalakis JE, Gray SW, Ricketts RR: The diaphragm. In Skandalakis JE, Gray SW, editors: Embryology for Surgeons, p. 502. Baltimore: Williams & Wilkins, 1994.

250. Skandalakis JE, Gray SW, Symbas P: The trachea and the lungs. In Skandalakis JE, Gray SW, editors: Embryology for Surgeons, p. 415. Baltimore: Williams & Wilkins, 1994.

251. Srouji MN, Buck B, Downes JJ: Congenital diaphragmatic hernia: Deleterious effects of pulmonary interstitial emphysema and tension extrapulmonary air. J Pediatr Surg 16:45–54, 1981.

252. Starrett RW, de Lorimier AA: Congenital diaphragmatic hernia in lambs: Hemodynamic and ventilatory changes with breathing. J Pediatr Surg 10:575–582, 1975.

253. Stauffer UG, Rickham PP: Congenital diaphragmatic hernia and eventration of the diaphragm. In Rickham PP, Lister J, Irvings JM, editors: Neonatal Surgery, p. 163. London: Butterworth, 1978.

254. Steimle CN, Meric F, Hirschl RB, et al: Effect of extracorporeal life support on survival when applied to all patients with congenital diaphragmatic hernia. J Pediatr Surg 29:997–1001, 1994.

255. Steinhorn RH, Kriesmer PJ, Green TP, et al: Congenital diaphragmatic hernia in Minnesota. Impact of antenatal diagnosis on survival. Arch Pediatr Adolesc Med 148:626–631, 1994.

256. Stolar C, Dillon P, Reyes C: Selective use of extracorporeal membrane oxygenation in the management of congenital diaphragmatic hernia. J Pediatr Surg 23:207–211, 1988.

257. Stolar CJ: What do survivors of congenital diaphragmatic hernia look like when they grow up? Semin Pediatr Surg 5:275–279, 1996.

258. Stolar CJ, Crisafi MA, Driscoll YT: Neurocognitive outcome for neonates treated with extracorporeal membrane oxygenation: Are infants with congenital diaphragmatic hernia different? J Pediatr Surg 30:366–371; discussion 371–372, 1995.

259. Stolar CJ, Dillon PW, Stalcup SA: Extracorporeal membrane oxygenation and congenital diaphragmatic hernia: Modification of the pulmonary vasoactive profile. J Pediatr Surg 20:681–683, 1985.

260. Stolar CJ, Levy JP, Dillon PW, et al: Anatomic and functional abnormalities of the esophagus in infants surviving congenital diaphragmatic hernia. Am J Surg 159:204–207, 1990.

261. Stolar CJ, Snedecor SM, Bartlett RH: Extracorporeal membrane oxygenation and neonatal respiratory failure: Experience from the extracorporeal life support organization. J Pediatr Surg 26:563–571, 1991.

262. Sullivan HJ: Supernumerary diaphragm with agenesis of upper lobe. J Thorac Surg 34:544–547, 1957.

263. Sullivan KM, Hawgood S, Flake AW, et al: Amniotic fluid phospholipid analysis in the fetus with congenital diaphragmatic hernia. J Pediatr Surg 29:1020–1023; discussion 1023–1024, 1994.

264. Sutherland MF, Parkinson MM, Hallett P: Teratogenicity of three substituted 4-biphenyls in the rat as a result of the chemical breakdown and possible metabolism of a thromboxane A2-receptor blocker. Teratology 39:537–545, 1989.

265. Taderera JV: Control of lung differentiation in vitro. Dev Biol 16:489–512, 1967.

266. Taylor GA, Short BL: Esophageal dilatation and reflux in neonates on extracorporeal membrane oxygenation after diaphragmatic hernia repair. AJR Am J Roentgenol 151:1055, 1988 (letter).

267. Tilmont P, Alessandri JL, Duthoit G, et al: Epanchement chyleaux apres cure chirurgicale d'une hernie diaphragmatique chez 2 nouveau-nes. Arch Fr Pediatr 50:783–786, 1993.

268. Torfs CP, Curry CJ, Bateson TF, et al: A population-based study of congenital diaphragmatic hernia. Teratology 46:555–565, 1992.

269. Touloukian RJ, Cole D: A state-wide survey of index pediatric surgical conditions. J Pediatr Surg 10:725–732, 1975.

270. Touloukian RJ, Markowitz RI: A preoperative x-ray scoring system for risk assessment of newborns with congenital diaphragmatic hernia. J Pediatr Surg 19:252–257, 1984.

271. Turpin R, Petit P, Chigot P, et al: Hernie diaphragmatique congénitale de type embryonnaire (fente pleuro-péritonéale gauche). Coincidence chez deux cousins germains de cette malformation isolée. Ann Pédiatr 35:272–279, 1959.

272. Ueki R, Nakao Y, Nishida T, et al: Lung hypoplasia in developing mice and rats induced by maternal exposure to nitrofen. Cong Anom 30:133–143, 1990.

273. Unpublished data from the Department of Surgery, Children's Hospital, Boston: Boston, 2001.

274. Vacanti JP, Crone RK, Murphy JD, et al: The pulmonary hemodynamic response to perioperative anesthesia in the treatment of high-risk infants with congenital diaphragmatic hernia. J Pediatr Surg 19:672–679, 1984.

275. van der Staak FH, Thiesbrummel A, de Haan AF, et al: Do we use the right entry criteria for extracorporeal membrane oxygenation in congenital diaphragmatic hernia? J Pediatr Surg 28:1003–1005, 1993.

276. van der Zee DC, Bax NM: Laparoscopic repair of congenital diaphragmatic hernia in a 6-month-old child. Surg Endosc 9:1001–1003, 1995.

277. Van Meurs KP, Rhine WD, Benitz WE, et al: Lobar lung transplantation as a treatment for congenital diaphragmatic hernia. J Pediatr Surg 29:1557–1560, 1994.

278. Van Meurs KP, Robbins ST, Reed VL, et al: Congenital diaphragmatic hernia: Long-term outcome in neonates

treated with extracorporeal membrane oxygenation. J Pediatr 122:893–899, 1993.

279. Vazquez WD, Cheu HW: Hemorrhagic complications and repair of congenital diaphragmatic hernias: Does timing of the repair make a difference? Data from the Extracorporeal Life Support Organization. J Pediatr Surg 29:1002–1005; discussion 1005–1006, 1994.

280. Walker LK: Use of extracorporeal membrane oxygenation for preoperative stabilization of congenital diaphragmatic hernia. Crit Care Med 21:S379–S380, 1993.

281. Walmrath D, Schneider T, Pilch J, et al: Aerosolised prostacyclin in adult respiratory distress syndrome. Lancet 342:961–962, 1993.

282. Warkany J, Roth CB: Congenital malformations induced in rats by maternal vitamin A deficiency. II. Effect of varying the preparatory diet upon the yield of abnormal young. J Nutr 35:1–12, 1948.

283. Weinstein S, Stolar CJ: Newborn surgical emergencies. Congenital diaphragmatic hernia and extracorporeal membrane oxygenation. Pediatr Clin North Am 40:1315–1333, 1993.

284. Welch KJ: The thoracic parietes. In Welch KJ, editor: Complications of Pediatric Surgery, pp. 170–181. Philadelphia: W.B. Saunders, 1982.

285. Welch RG, Cooke RT: Congenital diaphragmatic hernia. Lancet 1:975, 1962.

286. Wells LJ: Development of the human diaphragm and pleural sacs. Contrib Embryol Carnegie Inst Wash 35:109, 1954.

287. Wenstrom KD, Weiner CP, Hanson JW: A five-year statewide experience with congenital diaphragmatic hernia. Am J Obstet Gynecol 165:838–842, 1991.

288. West KW, Bengston K, Rescorla FJ, et al: Delayed surgical repair and ECMO improves survival in congenital diaphragmatic hernia. Ann Surg 216:454–460; discussion 460–462, 1992.

289. Wetzel H: Parasternale Zwerchfellhernie mit Verlagerung des Colon in den Herzbeutel. Fortschr Rontgenstr 98:501–503, 1963.

290. White JJ, Suzuki H: Hernia through the foramen of Bochdalek: A misnomer. J Pediatr Surg 7:60–61, 1972.

291. Wiener ES: Congenital posterolateral diaphragmatic hernia: New dimensions in management. Surgery 92:670–681, 1982.

292. Wiener ES, Owens L, Salzberg AM: Chylothorax after Bochadalek herniorrhaphy in a neonate. Treatment with intravenous hyperalimentation. J Thorac Cardiovasc Surg 65:200–206, 1973.

293. Wigglesworth JS, Desai R, Guerrini P: Fetal lung hypoplasia: Biochemical and structural variations and their possible significance. Arch Dis Child 56:606–615, 1981.

294. Wilcox DT, Glick PL, Karamanoukian H, et al: Pathophysiology of congenital diaphragmatic hernia. V. Effect of exogenous surfactant therapy on gas exchange and lung mechanics in the lamb congenital diaphragmatic hernia model. J Pediatr 124:289–293, 1994.

295. Wilcox DT, Glick PL, Karamanoukian HL, et al: Partial liquid ventilation and nitric oxide in congenital diaphragmatic hernia. J Pediatr Surg 32:1211–1215, 1997.

296. Wille L, Holthusen W, Willich E: Accessory diaphragm. Report of 6 cases and a review of the literature. Pediatr Radiol 4:14–20, 1975.

297. Wilson AK, Rumel WR, Ross OL: Peritoniopericardial diaphragmatic hernia: Report of a case in a newborn infant, successfully corrected by surgical operation with recovery of patient. AJR 57:42–49, 1947.

298. Wilson JM, Bower LK, Fackler JC, et al: Aminocaproic acid decreases the incidence of intracranial hemorrhage and other hemorrhagic complications of ECMO. J Pediatr Surg 28:536–540; discussion 540–541, 1993.

299. Wilson JM, Bower LK, Lund DP: Evolution of the technique of congenital diaphragmatic hernia repair on ECMO. J Pediatr Surg 29:1109–1112, 1994.

300. Wilson JM, DiFiore JW, Peters CA: Experimental fetal tracheal ligation prevents the pulmonary hypoplasia associated with fetal nephrectomy: possible application for congenital diaphragmatic hernia. J Pediatr Surg 28:1433–1439; discussion 1439–1440, 1993.

301. Wilson JM, Fauza DO, Lund DP, et al: Antenatal diagnosis of isolated congenital diaphragmatic hernia is not an indicator of outcome. J Pediatr Surg 29:815–819, 1994.

302. Wilson JM, Lund DP, Lillehei CW, et al: Congenital diaphragmatic hernia: Predictors of severity in the ECMO era. J Pediatr Surg 26:1028–1033; discussion 1033–1034, 1991.

303. Wilson JM, Lund DP, Lillehei CW, et al: Delayed repair and preoperative ECMO does not improve survival in high-risk congenital diaphragmatic hernia. J Pediatr Surg 27:368–372; discussion 373–375, 1992.

304. Wilson JM, Lund DP, Lillehei CW, et al: Congenital diaphragmatic hernia—a tale of two cities: The Boston experience. J Pediatr Surg 32:401–405, 1997.

305. Wilson JM, Thompson JR, Schnitzer JJ, et al: Intratracheal pulmonary ventilation and congenital diaphragmatic hernia: A report of two cases. J Pediatr Surg 28:484–487, 1993.

306. Wohl ME, Griscom NT, Strieder DJ, et al: The lung following repair of congenital diaphragmatic hernia. J Pediatr 90:405–414, 1977.

307. Wolff G: Familial congenital diaphragmatic defect: Review and conclusions. Hum Genet 54:1–5, 1980.

308. Wung JT, James LS, Kilchevsky E, et al: Management of infants with severe respiratory failure and persistence of the fetal circulation, without hyperventilation. Pediatrics 76:488–494, 1985.

309. Wung JT, Sahni R, Moffitt ST, et al: Congenital diaphragmatic hernia: Survival treated with very delayed surgery, spontaneous respiration, and no chest tube. J Pediatr Surg 30:406–409, 1995.

310. Yazbeck S, Cloutier R, Laberge JM: La hernie diaphragmatique congénitale: Les résultas changent-ils vraiment? Chir Pediatr 27:37–40, 1986.

311. Young D: Diaphragmatic hernia in infancy. In Wilkinson AW, editor: Recent Advances in Paediatric Surgery, pp. 142–151. London: Churchill Livingstone, 1969.

312. Zamir O, Eyal F, Lernau OZ, et al: Bilateral congenital posterolateral diaphragmatic hernia. Am J Perinatol 3:56–57, 1986.

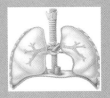

Esophageal Anatomy and Function

CHAPTER **33**

John C. Lipham and Tom R. DeMeester

▶ INTRODUCTION

The esophagus is a muscular tube that starts as the continuation of the pharynx and ends as the cardia of the stomach. Knowledge of the anatomy of the esophagus and its relationship with other organs and structures is essential for the surgeon to evaluate the location of lesions seen by endoscopy, barium swallow, or computed tomography; to interpret esophageal function studies; and to safely expose the esophagus during surgery (Figure 33-1). Similarly, a knowledge of foregut embryology is key to the understanding of the pathogenesis of congenital malformations of the esophagus.

▶ EMBRYOLOGY AND ANATOMY

The embryonic esophagus forms when paired longitudinal grooves appear on each side of the laryngotracheal diverticulum. These grooves subsequently grow medially and fuse to form the tracheoesophageal septum. This septum divides the foregut into the ventral laryngotracheal tube and the dorsal esophagus. Incomplete fusion of the two lateral grooves was formerly thought to be the major factor in the pathogenesis of congenital tracheoesophageal fistula, but the anomaly is now attributed to abnormal growth and differentiation of the lung buds. Initially the esophagus is short, but it rapidly elongates, with the relative final length attained by the seventh week of gestation.[27] This is followed by endodermal proliferation, which nearly obliterates the esophageal lumen. Subsequent recanalization occurs by the development of large vacuoles that coalesce. The adult position of the vagal nerves on the lower third of the esophagus results from the unequal growth of the greater and lesser curvature of the stomach, so the left vagus rotates anteriorly and the right vagus posteriorly.

The cricopharyngeal sphincter and the most proximal 1–2 cm of the cervical esophagus are primarily striated muscle. The striated muscle is derived from the caudal branchial arches and innervated by the vagus nerve and its recurrent laryngeal branches. The cricopharyngeal sphincter is made up primarily of the cricopharyngeus muscle, but it is also aided by the inferior pharyngeal constrictors and the circular muscles of the upper esophagus. Recent studies have indicated that the transition from predominately striated to predominately smooth muscle occurs in the proximal 4–5 cm of the esophagus and that only 1 cm of the proximal esophagus below the cricopharyngeal sphincter is entirely striated muscle.[33] In contrast with the proximal portion of the cervical esophagus, the thoracic and abdominal esophagus and the lower esophageal sphincter (LES) consist entirely of smooth muscle and are composed of an inner circular and outer longitudinal layer. Throughout the length of the esophagus, there is no serosa overlying the muscle layers. The smooth muscle of the lower esophagus arises from the splanchnic mesenchyme and is supplied by nerves of the esophageal plexus derived from neural crest cells.[27]

Cervical Esophagus

The cervical portion of the esophagus is about 5 cm long. It starts below the cricopharyngeus muscle, and it appears as a continuation of the inferior constrictor muscle of the pharynx. A space between the right and left inferior constrictor

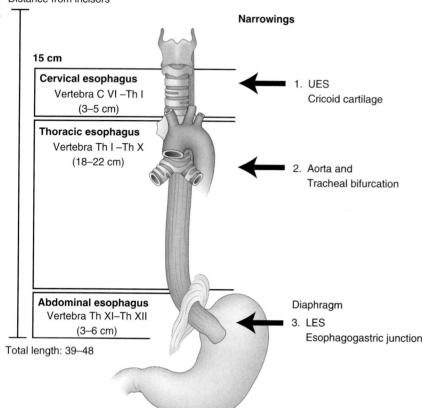

Distance from incisors

Narrowings

15 cm

Cervical esophagus
Vertebra C VI – Th I
(3–5 cm)

Thoracic esophagus
Vertebra Th I –Th X
(18–22 cm)

Abdominal esophagus
Vertebra Th XI–Th XII
(3–6 cm)

Total length: 39–48

1. UES
   Cricoid cartilage

2. Aorta and
   Tracheal bifurcation

Diaphragm
3. LES
   Esophagogastric junction

Figure 33–1 Classical division of the esophagus and relationships to the cervical and thoracic vertebrae as radiological landmarks. The approximate lengths and narrowings (*arrows*) of the esophagus are shown. UES, upper esophageal sphincter; LES, lower esophageal sphincter.

muscles posteriorly just above the cricopharyngeus muscle is the site where a Zenker's diverticulum develops (Figure 33-2). The beginning of the cervical esophagus is marked by the level of C6, and the end by the lower border of T1 curves slightly to the left in its descent. Anteriorly, it abuts the trachea and larynx and can be dissected off both organs. Posteriorly the cervical esophagus lies on the vertebral bodies in a prevertebral or retroesophageal space. This space continues with a retropharyngeal space superiorly and is continuous with the posterior mediastinum. Laterally the omohyoid muscle crosses the cervical esophagus obliquely, and it is usually divided to expose this portion of the esophagus. The carotid sheaths lie laterally, and the lobes of the thyroid and the strap muscles lie anteriorly. The recurrent laryngeal nerves lie in the grooves between the esophagus and the trachea. The right recurrent nerve runs a more lateral and oblique course to read the groove and is more prone to anatomical variation. The surgical approach to the cervical esophagus may be from either side of the neck through an incision along the medial border of the sternocleidomastoid muscle. The left-sided approach is preferred to avoid injury to the right recurrent nerve.

Thoracic Esophagus

The thoracic portion of the esophagus is approximately 20 cm long (see Figure 33-1) and starts at the thoracic inlet.

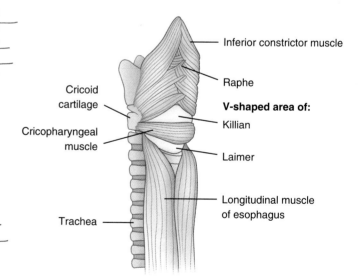

Figure 33–2 Muscular architecture of the pharyngoesophageal junction, which is the region of the upper esophageal sphincter. The triangular areas of the sparse muscle cover are shown in the scheme. Zenker's diverticulum arises from Killian's triangle.
(*Modified from Liebermann-Meffert D: Anatomy, embryology, and histology. In Pearson FG, Deslauriers J, Ginsberg RJ, et al [editors]: Esophageal Surgery. New York: Churchill Livingstone, 1995, pp. 1–25.*)

Inferior constrictor muscle

Raphe

V-shaped area of:

Killian

Laimer

Longitudinal muscle of esophagus

Cricoid cartilage

Cricopharyngeal muscle

Trachea

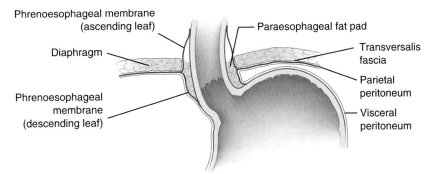

Figure 33–3 Attachments of the phreno-esophageal membrane.

In the upper portion of the thorax, it is closely related to the posterior wall of the trachea. This close relationship is responsible for the early spread of cancer of the upper esophagus into the trachea, and it may limit the surgeon's ability to resect such a tumor. Above the level of the tracheal bifurcation, the esophagus courses to the right of the descending aorta and then moves to the left, passing behind the tracheal bifurcation and the left main bronchus.

In the lower portion of the thorax, the esophagus again deviates to the left and anteriorly to pass through the diaphragmatic hiatus. The lower thoracic esophagus is buttressed only by mediastinal pleura on the left, making this portion the weakest and the most common the site of perforation in Boerhaave's syndrome. The azygos vein is closely related to the esophagus as it arches from its paraspinal position over the right main bronchus to enter the superior vena cava. The thoracic duct ascends behind and to the right of the distal thoracic esophagus, but at the level of T5 it passes posterior to the aorta and ascends on the left side of the esophagus, which is posterior and medial to the left subclavian artery.

Abdominal Esophagus

The abdominal portion of the esophagus is approximately 2 cm long and includes a part of the LES. It begins as the esophagus passes through the diaphragmatic hiatus and is surrounded by the phrenoesophageal membrane, a fibroelastic ligament that arises from the subdiaphragmatic fascia as a continuation of the transversalis fascia lining the abdomen (Figure 33-3). The upper leaf of the membrane attaches in a circumferential fashion around the esophagus about 1–2 cm above the level of the hiatus. The lower limit of the phrenoesophageal membrane blends with the serosa of the stomach, and its end is marked anteriorly by a prominent fat pad, which corresponds approximately with the gastroesophageal junction. The lower esophageal sphincter is a zone of high pressure 3–4 cm long at the lower end of the esophagus[17] and does not correspond with any macroscopic anatomical change except for a slight thickening of the esophageal muscular wall. Its function is derived from the microscopic architecture of the muscle fibers. The esophageal hiatus is surrounded by the right and left crura, which together form a sling of skeletal muscle around the esophagus that originates from tendinous bands attached to the anterolateral surface of the first lumbar vertebrae (Figure 33-4). The relative contribution of the right and left crura to this sling is variable. Posterior to the esophagus, the crura are united by a tendinous arch—the median arcuate ligament—that lies just anterior to the aorta.

Blood Supply, Lymphatics, and Innervation

The cervical portion of the esophagus receives its main blood supply from the inferior thyroid artery. The thoracic portion receives blood from the bronchial and esophageal arteries. Seventy-five percent of individuals have one right-sided and two left-sided bronchial arteries, and usually two esophageal branches arise directly from the aorta. The blood supply of the abdominal portion of the esophagus comes from the ascending branch of the left gastric artery and from the right and left inferior phrenic arteries (Figure 33-5). After the vessels have entered the muscular wall of the esophagus, branching occurs at right angles to provide an extensive longitudinal vascular plexus. The rich blood supply provided by this vascular plexus allows for mobilization of the esophagus from the stomach to the aortic arch without causing ischemic injury.[28]

The capillaries of the esophagus drain into a submucosal and periesophageal venous plexus, from which the esophageal veins originate. In the cervical region, the esophageal veins empty into the inferior thyroid vein; in the thoracic region, they empty into the bronchial, azygos, or hemiazygos veins; and in the abdominal region, they empty into the coronary vein (Figure 33-6).

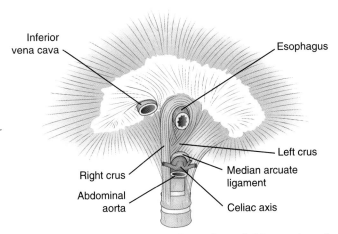

Figure 33–4 Diaphragm and esophageal hiatus viewed from the abdomen.

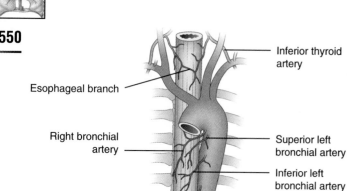

The lymphatics channels are located almost exclusively below the muscularis mucosa in the submucosa of the esophagus. They are so dense and interconnected that they constitute a plexus (Figure 33-7) with more lymph vessels than blood capillaries. Lymph flow in the submucosal plexus runs in a longitudinal direction, and, after the injection of a contrast medium, the longitudinal spread is six times that of the transverse spread. In the upper two thirds of the esophagus, the lymphatic flow is mostly cephalad; in the lower third, it is mostly caudad. In the thoracic portion of the esophagus, the submucosal lymph plexus extends over a long distance in a longitudinal direction before penetrating the muscle layer to enter lymph vessels in the adventitia. As a consequence of this nonsegmental lymph drainage, the lymphatic spread of tumor cells can extend for a considerable distance superiorly and inferiorly within the submucosal lymphatics before the cells pass through lymphatic channels in the muscularis and on into the regional lymph nodes. By contrast, the cervical esophagus has a more segmental lymph drainage into the regional lymph nodes, and, as a result, tumors in this portion of the esophagus have less submucosal extension.

Lymph from the cervical esophagus drains into the paratracheal and deep cervical lymph nodes, whereas lymph from

Figure 33-5 Arterial blood supply of the esophagus.
(Modified from Rothberg M, DeMeester TR: Surgical anatomy of the esophagus. In Shields TW [editor]: General Thoracic Surgery, ed 3. Philadelphia: Lea & Febiger, 1989, p. 84.)

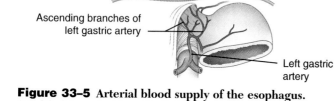

Figure 33-6 Venous drainage of the esophagus.
(Modified from Rothberg M, DeMeester TR: Surgical anatomy of the esophagus. In Shields TW [editor]: General Thoracic Surgery, ed 3. Philadelphia: Lea & Febiger, 1989, p. 85.)

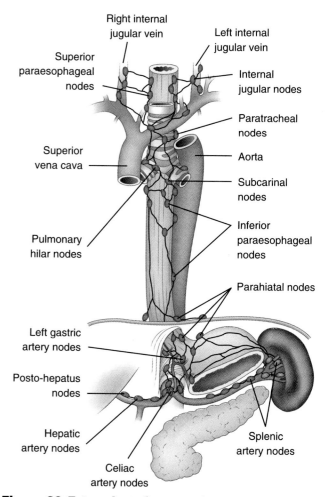

Figure 33-7 Lymphatic drainage of the esophagus.
(From DeMeester TR, Barlow AP: Surgery and current management for cancer of the esophagus and cardia: Part 1. Curr Probl Surg 25:498, 1988.)

the upper thoracic esophagus flows mainly into the paratracheal lymph nodes. The lymph from the lower thoracic esophagus drains into the subcarinal and inferior pulmonary nodes. Lymph from the distal thoracic and abdominal portion of the esophagus drains into the parahiatal and left gastric nodes.[27]

The parasympathetic innervation of the pharynx and esophagus is provided mainly by the Xth cranial or vagal nerve. The constrictor muscles of the pharynx receive branches from the pharyngeal plexus, which is located on the posterior lateral surface of the middle constrictor muscle and is formed by pharyngeal branches of the vagus nerve, with a small contribution from the IXth and XIth cranial nerves. The cricopharyngeal sphincter and the cervical portion of the esophagus receive branches from both the right and left recurrent laryngeal nerves (Figure 33-8). Damage to these recurrent nerves interferes not only with the movement of the vocal cords but also with the function of the cricopharyngeal sphincter and the motility of the cervical esophagus and predisposes the patient to pulmonary aspiration on swallowing. The upper thoracic esophagus receives innervation from the left recurrent laryngeal nerve and both vagal nerves. The esophageal plexus, which is formed by the branches of the right and left vagal nerves and thoracic sympathetic chain, lies on the anterior and posterior walls of the esophagus and innervates the lower thoracic portion.[29] The branches of the plexus coalesce into the left (anterior) and right (posterior) vagal trunks.

Afferent visceral sensory fibers from the esophagus end without synapse in the first four segments of the thoracic spinal cord using a combination of sympathetic and vagal pathways. These pathways are also occupied by afferent visceral sensory fibers from the heart, which explains the similarity of symptoms in esophageal and cardiac diseases.

PHYSIOLOGY

To comprehend the mechanics of alimentation, it is useful to visualize the gullet as a series of pumps and valves. In the pharyngeal segment, the tongue and pharyngeal muscle function as pumps, whereas the soft pallet, the epiglottis, and the cricopharyngeus serve as the valves that regulate flow. In the esophageal segment, the esophageal body functions as the pump to propel the food bolus, whereas the lower esophageal sphincter serves as a one-way valve to allow transport into the stomach and to prevent the flow of gastric contents back into the esophagus.

The Swallowing Mechanism

Swallowing can be started at will, or it can be reflexively elicited by the stimulation of the anterior and posterior tonsillar pillars or the posterior lateral walls of the hypopharynx. The afferent sensory nerves of the pharynx are the glossopharyngeal nerves and the superior laryngeal branches of the vagal nerves. Once aroused by stimuli entering via these nerves, the swallowing center in the medulla coordinates the complete act of swallowing by discharging impulses through the Vth, VIIth, Xth, XIth, and XIIth cranial nerves and the motor neurons of C1 through C3. Discharges through these nerves always occur in a specific pattern and last for approximately 0.5 seconds. Little is known about the

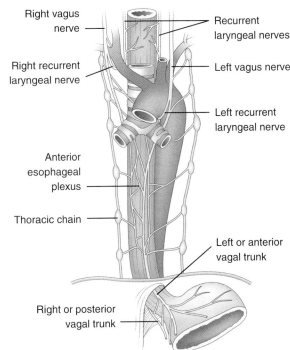

Figure 33–8 Innervation of the esophagus.
(*Modified from Rothberg M, DeMeester TR: Surgical anatomy of the esophagus. In Shields TW [editor]: General Thoracic Surgery, ed 3. Philadelphia: Lea & Febiger, 1989, p. 85.*)

swallowing center except that it can trigger swallowing after a variety of different inputs. Once triggered, the swallow response is always a rigidly ordered pattern of outflow neurogenic impulses.

The act of alimentation requires the passage of food and drink from the mouth into the stomach. Food is taken into the mouth in a variety of bite sizes, after which it is broken up by the teeth, mixed with saliva, and lubricated. When food is ready for swallowing, the tongue, acting as a pump, moves the bolus into the posterior oropharynx and forces it into the hypopharynx (Figure 33-9). Concomitantly with the posterior movement of the tongue, the soft palate is elevated, thereby closing the passage between the oropharynx and nasopharynx. With the initiation of the swallow, the hyoid moves superiorly and anteriorly, thereby elevating the larynx and enlarging the retropharyngeal space. At the same time, the epiglottis covers the laryngeal inlet to prevent aspiration.

During swallowing, the pressure in the hypopharynx rises abruptly to 60 mm Hg as a result of the backward movement of the tongue and contraction of the posterior pharyngeal constrictors. A sizable pressure difference develops between the hypopharyngeal pressure and the subatmospheric midesophageal or intrathoracic pressure (Figure 33-10). This pressure gradient speeds the movement of food from the hypopharynx into the esophagus when the cricopharyngeus or upper esophageal sphincter (UES) relaxes. The bolus is both propelled by the peristaltic contraction of the posterior pharyngeal constrictors and sucked into the thoracic esophagus by this pressure gradient.

Critical to receiving the bolus is the compliance of the cervical esophageal muscle and the timing and degree of relaxation of the UES. Abnormalities of compliance and

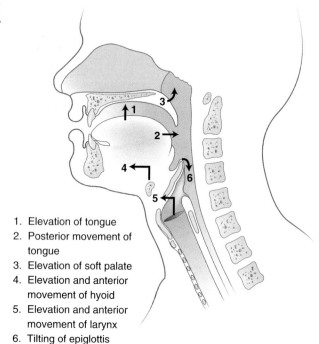

1. Elevation of tongue
2. Posterior movement of tongue
3. Elevation of soft palate
4. Elevation and anterior movement of hyoid
5. Elevation and anterior movement of larynx
6. Tilting of epiglottis

Figure 33–9 **Sequence of events during the oropharyngeal phase of swallowing.**
(From DeMeester TR, Stein HJ, Fuchs KH: Physiologic diagnostic studies. In Zuidema GD, Orringer MB [editors]: Shackelford's Surgery of the Alimentary Tract, ed 3, vol 1. Philadelphia: W.B. Saunders, 1991, p. 95.)

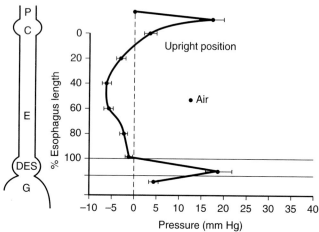

Figure 33–10 **Resting pressure profile of the foregut showing the pressure differential between the atmospheric pharyngeal pressure (P) and the less-than-atmospheric midesophageal pressure (E) and the greater-than-atmospheric intragastric pressure (G), with the interposed high-pressure zones of the cricopharyngeus (C) and the distal esophageal sphincter (DES).** The necessity for relaxation of the cricopharyngeus and DES pressure to move a bolus into the stomach is apparent. Esophageal work occurs when a bolus is pushed from the midesophageal area with a pressure that is less than atmospheric (E) and into the stomach, which has a pressure that is greater than atmospheric (G).
(From Waters PF, DeMeester TR: Foregut motor disorders and their surgical management. Med Clin North Am 65:1237, 1981.)

UES opening result in pharyngeal dysphagia. During the transfer of the bolus from the mouth into the esophagus, the UES is mechanically pulled open. Elevation of the larynx by muscles attached to the hyoid bone pulls the UES open at the time muscle relaxation of the UES occurs. This is an active relaxation caused by a reduction in the tone of the tonic cricopharyngeus muscle, and it is dependent on a neurologically mediated reflex. This is an all-or-nothing event; partial relaxation does not normally occur. The upper esophageal sphincter closes within 0.5 seconds of the initiation of the swallow, with a postrelaxation contraction pressure that is approximately twice the resting pressure of 30 mm Hg. The postrelaxation contraction continues down the esophagus as a peristaltic wave (Figure 33-11). The high closing pressure and the initiation of the peristaltic wave prevent reflux of the bolus from the esophagus back into the pharynx. After completion of the swallow, the pressure of the UES returns to its normal resting pressure.

The pharyngeal activity in swallowing initiates the esophageal phase of swallowing. Because of the helical arrangement of its circular muscles, the body of the esophagus functions as a worm-drive propulsive pump, and it is responsible for transmitting a bolus of food into the stomach. With the act of swallowing, the longitudinal muscle of the esophageal body shortens, thus enlarging the lumen to accept the bolus (this is called the "on response"), after which the circular smooth muscle contraction forms the peristaltic wave (the "off response"). During the esophageal phase of swallowing, the bolus is moved into the stomach over a gradient of 12 mm Hg (i.e., from a negative intrathoracic pressure environment of –6 mm Hg to a positive intraabdominal pressure environment of +6 mm Hg). Effective and coordinated smooth-muscle function in the lower two thirds of the esophageal body is important to allow this movement to occur.

The peristaltic wave generates an occlusive pressure that varies from 30–120 mm Hg. The wave rises to a peak in 1 second, remains at the peak for about 0.5 second, and then subsides in about 1.5 seconds. The whole course of the rise and fall of an occlusive contraction may occupy one point in the esophagus for 3–5 seconds.[40,41] The peak of the primary peristaltic contraction moves down the esophagus at a rate of 2–4 cm per second and reaches the distal esophagus about 9 seconds after swallowing starts. A consecutive swallow in 20 seconds produces a similar primary peristaltic wave; however, if the swallow occurs sooner, the esophagus is inhibited and unresponsive.

To be effective, peristaltic contractions must be of sufficient amplitude to occlude the esophageal lumen and sufficiently organized in a peristaltic waveform to propel a bolus aborally. Low-amplitude contractions that do not occlude the lumen merely indent a semisolid bolus rather than propel it, and simultaneous contractions throughout the body of the esophagus result in splitting the bolus or even propelling it orally. Clinically, defects in peristalsis occur in three broad categories, depending on which major feature is the most impaired. First, there is a neural abnormality that results in the defective organization of the peristaltic wave; this is recognized by the presence of simultaneous contractions with a loss of the peristaltic sequence and results in typical primary motility disorders (e.g., diffuse esophageal spasm). The second category of defects is evident when there is a reduction of the amplitude of the contraction but the

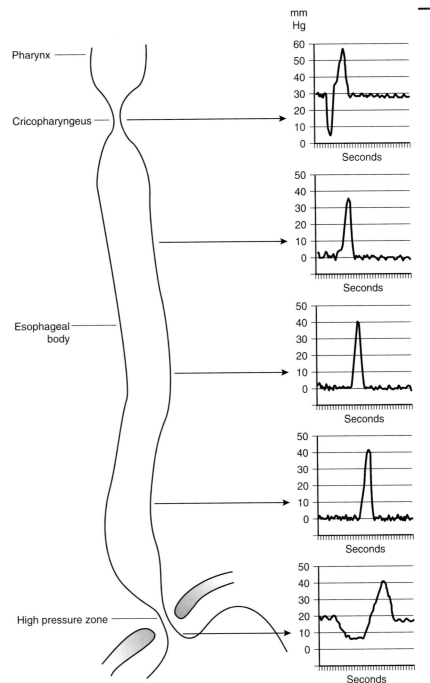

Figure 33-11 Intraluminal esophageal pressures in response to swallowing.
(From Waters PF, DeMeester TR: Foregut motor disorders and their surgical management. Med Clin North Am 65:1237, 1981.)

peristaltic sequence remains; this is usually due to the result of muscle damage and the formation of fibrous tissue within the muscle. Examples include end-stage gastroesophageal reflux disease and connective tissue disorders such as scleroderma. The third type of defect involves the altered anatomy of the esophageal body. A loss in the efficiency of the peristaltic sequence can result when the esophagus is not anchored distally, as occurs with a large sliding hiatal hernia; this will look like an accordion esophagus on barium swallow, with ineffective clearance of barium from the esophagus.

Lower Esophageal Sphincter

The LES represents the barrier that confines the gastric juice to the stomach and protects the acid-sensitive squamous esophageal mucosa from injury by refluxed gastric juice. As is true for any valve, failure of the LES can occur in two completely opposite ways, which lead to two distinct clinical disease entities. Regardless of the type of LES failure, the secondary effects are produced proximally in the esophagus. Failure of the LES to relax or to open appropriately leads to

554 the inability of the esophagus to propel food into the stomach, esophageal distention, and the condition known as *achalasia*. On the other hand, failure of the LES to remain closed leads to an increased exposure of the squamous epithelium to gastric juice and the condition known as *gastroesophageal reflux disease* (GERD).

The LES has no anatomical landmarks, but its presence can be identified by a rise in pressure over gastric baseline pressure when a pressure transducer is pulled from the stomach into the esophagus. This high-pressure zone is normally present, except in two situations: (1) after a swallow, when it is momentarily dissipated or relaxes to allow passage of food into the stomach, and (2) during a belch, when it allows gas to be vented from a distended fundus. The common denominator for virtually all episodes of gastroesophageal reflux is the loss of this normal high-pressure zone or barrier. When the barrier is absent, resistance to the flow of gastric juice from an environment of higher pressure (the stomach) to an environment of lower pressure (the esophagus) is lost. In early GERD, this is usually caused by a transient loss of the barrier. In advanced GERD, there is usually a permanent loss of the barrier.[9]

There are three characteristics of the LES or high-pressure zone that maintain its function as a barrier to intragastric and intraabdominal pressure challenges. Two of these characteristics—the overall length and pressure of LES—work together and depend on each other to provide resistance to the flow of gastric juice from the stomach into the esophagus.[3] The shorter the overall length, the higher the pressure must be for the LES to maintain sufficient resistance to remain competent (Figure 33-12). Consequently, the effect of a normal LES pressure can be nullified by a short overall LES length, and the effect of a normal overall LES length can be nullified by a low LES pressure. For practical purposes, the pressure of the LES is measured at a single point, but, in actuality, pressure is applied over the entire length of the LES; this allows for the computer formation of a three-dimensional image of the LES or barrier (Figure 33-13). The volume of this image reflects the LES's resistance to the flow of fluid through it, which is called the "sphincter pressure vector volume." A calculated volume below that of the fifth percentile of normal resting subjects indicates a permanently defective LES.[48] A fundamental principle for surgeons to understand is that the length of the barrier or LES is critical to its function. Shortening of LES length occurs naturally with gastric filling as the terminal esophagus is "taken up" by the expanding fundus (Figure 33-14)[31]; this is similar to the shortening of the neck of a balloon as it is inflated. With excessive gastric distention (e.g., with overeating), the length of the LES shortens to a critical point at which it gives way, the pressure drops precipitously, and reflux occurs (Figure 33-15).[39] If the length of the LES is permanently shortened, then further shortening caused by the normal gastric distention with normal-volume meals results in postprandial reflux. In this situation, competency of the barrier is an ever-constant clinical problem. The observation that gastric distention results in the shortening of the LES down to a critical length so that the pressure dissipates, the lumen opens, and reflux occurs provides a mechanical explanation for transient LES relaxations (tLESRs) without invoking a neuromuscular reflex. If only the LES pressure and not its length is measured (e.g., with

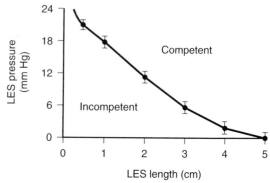

Figure 33–12 The relationship of the lower esophageal sphincter pressure (measured at the respiratory inversion point) and overall lower esophageal sphincter length with the resistance to the flow of fluid through the barrier. Note that the shorter the overall length of the high-pressure zone, the higher the pressures must be to maintain sufficient resistance to remain competent. Competent, no flow; incompetent, flow of varied volumes.

a Dent sleeve), the event appears as a spontaneous relaxation of LES pressure.[12] In reality, it is the progressive shortening of the LES rather than the tLESRs that results in the loss of LES pressure.

Variations in the anatomy of the cardia, from a normal acute angle of His to an abnormal dome architecture of a sliding hiatal hernia, influence the ease with which the sphincter is shortened by gastric distention. A hernia can result from the pulsion force of abdominal pressure on the esophageal hiatus or from the traction produced by inflammatory fibrosis of the esophageal body. The resulting alteration in the geometry of the cardia places the sphincter at a mechanical disadvantage in maintaining its length with progressive degrees of gastric distention. Greater gastric distention is necessary to open the barrier in patients with an intact angle of His than in those with a hiatal hernia.[20] The reason is that the dome or funnel shape of a hiatal hernia allows the wall tension forces that pull open the barrier with gastric distention to be more effectively applied to the gastroesophageal junction,[30] and it accounts for the common association of a hiatal hernia with GERD. Kahrilas and colleagues[25] demonstrated this mechanical disadvantage by studying the effect of intragastric air infusion on the number of tLESRs or "shortenings" per hour. Patients with hiatal hernias had significantly more tLESRs per hour than did control subjects without hernias. The reduction in length became significant 20–30 minutes after the beginning of air infusion and occurred in a distal-to-cephalad direction before a loss of LES pressure was observed.

The third characteristic of the LES high-pressure zone is its position. A portion of the overall length of the high-pressure zone is normally exposed to the positive intraabdominal pressure environment and is commonly referred to as the abdominal length of the LES.[11] During periods of increased intraabdominal pressure, the resistance of the LES would easily be overcome if its position were such that abdominal pressure were unable to be applied equally to the LES and the stomach.[24,36,37] Think of sucking on a soft soda straw immersed in a bottle of liquid; the positive hydrostatic

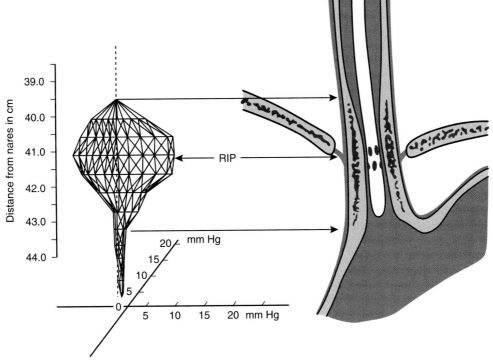

Figure 33–13 A graphic illustration of how a three-dimensional computerized image of the lower esophageal sphincter can be constructed by measuring the pressure of the high-pressure zone in 4 quadrants at 0.5-cm intervals over the entire length of the zone. RIP, respiratory inversion point.
(From Stein HJ, DeMeester TR, Naspetti R, et al: Three-dimensional imaging of the lower esophageal sphincter in gastroesophageal reflux disease. Ann Surg 215:374–384, 1991.)

pressure of the fluid and the negative pressure inside the straw from sucking causes the straw to collapse instead of allowing the liquid to flow up the straw in the direction of the negative pressure. If the LES is positioned so that the abdominal length is inadequate, it cannot collapse in response to applied positive intraabdominal pressure. On the other hand, intragastric pressure would be augmented by the applied positive intraabdominal pressure, and the sphincter pressure would be easily overcome; the negative intrathoracic pressure will encourage reflux to occur. More than 1 cm of the LES needs to be exposed to the abdominal pressure environment for it to respond effectively to changes in intraabdominal pressure.[12]

If, in the fasting state, the LES has an abnormally low pressure, a short overall length, or a minimal length exposure to the abdominal pressure environment, the result is a permanent loss of resistance with unhampered reflux of gastric contents into the esophagus; this is known as a *permanently defective* barrier or LES. The most common consequence of a permanently defective LES is increased esophageal exposure to gastric juice, which results in inflammatory injury to the mucosa and the muscularis propria of the esophageal body, thereby causing a reduced contraction amplitude of the esophageal body and interrupted or dropped sequences. If the reflux is not brought under control, the progressive loss of effective esophageal clearance results in an ever-increasing esophageal exposure to gastric juice with further organ injury (Figure 33-16).[47,50]

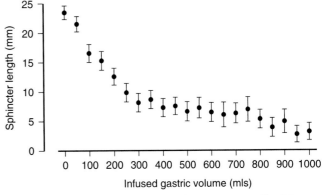

Figure 33–14 The relationship between overall sphincter length to gastric distention with increasing volumes of water.
(From Mason RJ, Lund RJ, DeMeester TR, et al: Nissen fundoplication prevents shortening of the sphincter during gastric distention. Arch Surg 132:719–726, 1997.)

Causes and Consequences of the Failure of the Gastroesophageal Barrier

Early GERD is initiated by increased transient losses of the barrier as a result of gastric overdistention from excessive air and food ingestion.[1,9] The tension vectors produced by gastric wall distention pull on the gastroesophageal junc-

556

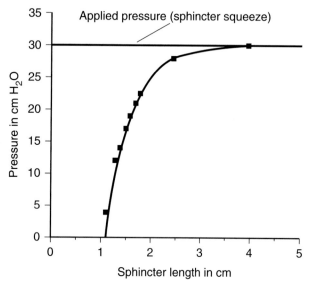

Figure 33–15 **The relationship between resting lower esophageal sphincter (LES) pressure measured by manometry and LES length when applied pressure or "sphincter squeeze" is kept constant.** Analysis was made with a model of the LES high-pressure zone. Note that, as the LES length decreases, the pressure recorded within the LES decreases only slightly until a length of 2 cm is reached, when LES pressure drops precipitously and its competency is lost. *(From Pettersson GB, Bombeck CT, Nyhus LM: The lower esophageal sphincter: mechanisms of opening and closure. Surgery 88:307–314, 1980.)*

tion, which results in the terminal esophagus being "taken up" into the stretched fundus, thereby reducing the length of the LES. With overeating, a critical length is reached (usually about 1–2 cm) at which the sphincter gives way; its pressure drops precipitously, and reflux occurs (see Figure 33-14). If the swallowed air is vented, gastric distention is reduced, the length of the LES is restored, and compe-

tency returns until subsequent distention again shortens it and further reflux occurs. Aerophagia is common in patients with GERD, because they swallow their saliva more frequently to neutralize the acidic gastric juice that is refluxed into the esophagus.[4] Together, the actions of overeating and air swallowing result in the common complaint of postprandial bloating, repetitive belching, and heartburn in patients with early GERD. The high prevalence of the disease in the Western world is thought to be a result of the eating habits of Western society.[21] Gastric distention from overeating, along with delayed gastric emptying resulting from the increased ingestion of fatty foods, lead to prolonged periods of postprandial gastric distention with shortening of the LES and repetitive transient loss of the barrier. A Nissen fundoplication prevents the shortening of the barrier with progressive degrees of gastric distention by diverting the forces produced by gastric wall tension that pull on the gastroesophageal junction.[39]

In advanced GERD, permanent loss of sphincter length occurs from inflammatory injury that extends from the mucosa into the muscular layers of the LES. Fletcheer and colleagues[16] showed that, in the fasting state, there is a persistent region of high acidity in the area of the gastroesophageal junction and that this region of acidity migrates 2 cm proximally after meals. This migration occurs from distention of the stomach with eating and pulling apart of the distal high-pressure zone or LES, thus allowing the area of high acidity to move proximal to the squamocolumnar junction. This proximal movement exposes the distal esophageal squamous mucosa to acid and results in the formation of cardiac mucosa. Cardiac mucosa is an acquired mucosa and results from inflammatory injury to the squamous mucosa in the terminal esophagus.[35] The inflammatory process extends into the muscular layer of the LES, thereby resulting in muscle cell injury with permanent shortening of the high-pressure zone or LES and a concomitant reduction in the amplitude of the high-pressure zone or barrier pressure.[10,35,49] A defective barrier is recognized when the length

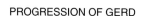

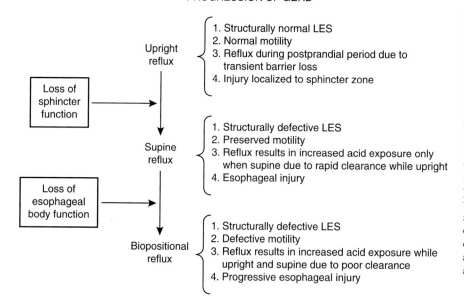

Figure 33–16 **Schema of the progression of gastroesophageal reflux disease.** Initially esophageal acid exposure occurs only after meals and when the patient is in the upright, awake position, as a result of the transient losses of the barrier. With inflammatory injury to the lower esophageal sphincter, the barrier becomes permanently defective, and an increase in the esophageal acid exposure occurs with the patient in the supine position, whereas gravity and the esophageal body effectively clear the refluxed acid during the day when the patient is upright. Inflammatory injury to the esophageal body from supine acid exposure results in the loss of esophageal body clearance function and increased esophageal acid exposure during the day and night; this is known as *bipositional reflux.*

or pressure of the LES measured during the fasting state is below the 2.5 percentile of normal.[8] For clinicians, the finding of a permanently defective LES has several implications. First, patients with a defective LES can be difficult to control symptomatically, and mucosal damage may be difficult to control with medical therapy.[26] Surgery is usually required to achieve consistent long-term symptom relief in these patients and to interrupt the natural history of the disease. It has been shown repeatedly that a laparoscopic Nissen fundoplication can restore the length and pressure of the LES to normal.[38] Second, a permanently defective LES is commonly associated with reduced contractility and abnormal wave progression of the esophageal body[46]; this makes the clearance of reflux acid difficult and leads to excessive esophageal exposure to acid. Third, a permanently defective LES and the loss of effective esophageal clearance leads to increased esophageal exposure to gastric juice with mucosal injury and the potential for Barrett's metaplasia, repetitive regurgitation, aspiration, and pulmonary fibrosis.

EVALUATION OF ESOPHAGEAL FUNCTION

A thorough understanding of the patient's underlying anatomical and functional deficits is fundamental to the successful treatment of esophageal disease. The diagnostic tests that are employed to evaluate the esophagus are those used to visualize structural abnormalities, detect functional abnormalities, and measure esophageal exposure to gastric juice.

Radiographical Evaluation

Radiographical assessment of the anatomy and function of the esophagus and stomach is one of the more important aspects of the esophageal evaluation, provided that the surgeon has a working knowledge of esophageal physiology. The first diagnostic test in patients with suspected esophageal disease should be a barium swallow that includes a full assessment of the stomach and the duodenum.[13] Videotaping the study greatly aids in the evaluation by providing the surgeon with a real-time visualization of bolus transport and the size and reducibility of the hiatal hernia. The study also provides anatomical information, such as the presence of obstructing lesions and structural abnormalities of the foregut.

The pharynx and the upper esophageal sphincter are evaluated in the upright position, with the performance of an assessment of the relative timing and coordination of the events of pharyngeal transit.[15] This includes oropharyngeal bolus transport, pharyngeal contraction, opening of the pharyngoesophageal segment, and the degree of airway protection during swallowing. It readily identifies a diverticulum, stasis of the contrast medium in the valleculae, a cricopharyngeal bar, and/or narrowing of the pharyngoesophageal segment.[45] These are anatomical manifestations of neuromuscular disease and result from the loss of muscle compliance from the deinnervation of the skeletal muscle of the pharynx and the cervical esophagus.[14]

The assessment of peristalsis on a video esophagram often adds to or complements the information obtained by esophageal manometry. Esophageal motility is optimally assessed by observing several individual swallows of barium with the patient in both the upright and supine positions;

the study can be performed with both liquid and solid bolus material. During normal swallowing, a primary peristaltic wave is generated that completely strips the bolus out of the esophagus and into the stomach. Residual material rarely stimulates a secondary peristaltic wave, rather an additional pharyngeal swallow is usually required.

Normal subjects in the prone position can clear at least 3 out of 5 10-cc liquid barium boluses with 1 swallow and have only 1 episode of proximal escape or distal retention of a barium bolus with the 5 swallows. Normal subjects can clear a solid barium bolus with 4 or more swallows in the upright position. Motility disorders with disorganized or simultaneous esophageal contraction give a segmented appearance to the barium column. This can often give a beading or corkscrew appearance to the barium within the esophagus. In patients with dysphagia, the use of a barium-impregnated marshmallow, piece of bread, or hamburger can identify an esophageal transport disturbance that is not evident on the liquid barium study.

A hiatal hernia is present in a high percentage of patients with gastroesophageal reflux.[44] These hernias are best demonstrated with the patient in the prone position; the increased intraabdominal pressure produced in this position promotes displacement of the hernia above the diaphragm. The presence of a hiatal hernia is an important component of the underlying pathophysiology of reflux. A large (>5 cm) or irreducible hiatal hernia suggests a shortening of the esophagus, and a paraesophageal hernia can explain the complaint of dysphagia. Reflux is not easily seen on video esophagram, and only rarely in patients with classic symptoms of GERD does the radiologist observe spontaneous reflux (i.e., unprovoked retrograde flow of barium from the stomach into the esophagus). When spontaneous reflux is seen by the radiologist, it is a very dependable sign of GERD; however, failure to observe reflux does not indicate the absence of disease.

A full-column technique with distention of the esophageal wall can discern extrinsic compression of the esophagus, and a fully distended esophagogastric region is necessary to identify narrowing from a ring, stricture, or obstructing lesion. Mucosal relief or double-contrast films can be obtained to enhance the detection of small neoplasms, esophagitis, and varices. Assessment of the stomach and duodenum during the barium study is helpful for the evaluation of the patient with esophageal symptoms. A gastric or duodenal ulcer, a neoplasm, or poor gastroduodenal transit can mimic many of the symptoms that are suggestive of an esophageal disorder.

Endoscopic Examination

Endoscopic evaluation of the esophagus in practice is the physical examination of the foregut and is a critical part of the assessment of a patient with esophageal disease and is indicated even if the video esophagram is normal. A barium study obtained before esophagoscopy is helpful to the endoscopist by directing attention to locations of subtle change and alerting the examiner to such potential danger spots as a cervical vertebral osteophyte, an esophageal diverticulum, a deeply penetrating ulcer, or a carcinoma. Regardless of the radiologist's interpretation of an abnormal finding, each structural abnormality of the esophagus should be examined visually with an endoscope.

During every examination, the locations of the diaphragmatic crura, gastroesophageal junction, and squamocolumnar junction are measured. The crura are usually evident, and their location can be confirmed by having the patient sniff. The squamocolumnar junction is the location at which the velvet and darker-rose–colored columnar epithelium changes to the lighter squamous epithelium. The anatomical gastroesophageal junction is the location at which the gastric rugal folds meet the tubular esophagus; it is often at or just below the squamocolumnar junction. Particular effort should be exerted to detect esophagitis and Barrett's columnar-lined esophagus when gastroesophageal reflux disease is suspected. Barrett's esophagus is a condition in which the tubular esophagus is lined with columnar epithelium as opposed to the normal squamous epithelium. Histologically, it appears as columnar mucosa with globlet cells and is called *intestinal metaplasia*.[6,42,43] It is suspected at endoscopy when there is difficulty with visualizing the squamocolumnar junction at its normal location and by the appearance of a redder, more luxuriant mucosa than is normally seen in the lower esophagus; its presence is confirmed by biopsy. Multiple biopsies should be taken in a cephalad direction to determine the length of the metaplastic mucosa. Barrett's esophagus is susceptible to ulceration, bleeding, stricture formation, and malignant degeneration.[18] The earliest histological sign of the latter is severe dysplasia or intramucosal adenocarcinoma.[52] These dysplastic changes have a patchy distribution, so a minimum of 4 biopsies every 2 cm should be taken from the Barrett's-lined portion of the esophagus.

Abnormalities of the cardia or gastroesophageal junction can be visualized by retroflexion of the endoscope. Hill and others[19] have graded the appearance of the gastroesophageal valve from I to IV according to the degree of unfolding or deterioration of the normal architecture (Figure 33-17).

A hiatal hernia is confirmed by finding a pouch lined with gastric rugal folds lying 2 cm or more above the margins of the diaphragmatic crura. A prominent sliding hiatal hernia is frequently associated with GERD. When a hernia is observed, particular attention is taken to exclude a gastric ulcer or gastritis within the herniated stomach.

As the endoscope is removed, the esophagus is again examined, and biopsy samples are taken. The location of the cricopharyngeus is identified, and the larynx and vocal cords are visualized. Acid reflux may result in inflammation of the larynx. Vocal cord movement should also be recorded, both as a reference for subsequent surgery and as an assessment of the patient's ability to protect the airway.

Esophageal Manometry

Fundamental to the evaluation of a patient with benign esophageal disease is the assessment of esophageal contractility and sphincter function. Stationary esophageal manometry is performed by passing a catheter containing pressure

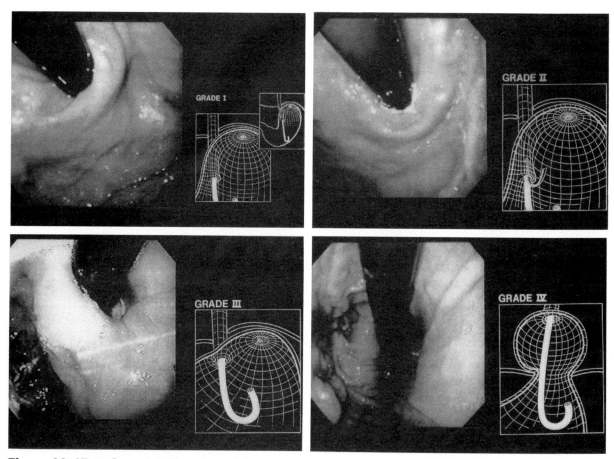

Figure 33–17 Endoscopic Hill grading of the gastroesophageal valve.

sensor ports (usually spaced 5 cm apart) into the esophagus to measure contraction pressures and waveform in the esophageal body and the resting pressure and response to swallowing of the sphincters. Manometry is indicated whenever a motor abnormality of the esophagus is suspected by the symptoms of dysphagia, odynophagia, chest pain, heartburn, and regurgitation.[5] It is particularly necessary to confirm the diagnosis of specific primary esophageal motility disorders such as achalasia, diffuse esophageal spasm, nutcracker esophagus, and hypertensive LES.[2] It can also identify ineffective esophageal motility (IEM) abnormalities that result from GERD and systemic disease such as scleroderma, dermatomyositis, polymyositis, or mixed connective tissue disease. In patients with symptomatic GERD, esophageal manometry can identify a mechanically defective LES and evaluate the adequacy of the esophageal body contraction amplitudes and waveform.

Esophageal manometry is performed by inserting a lubricated manometric catheter through the nostril and into the esophagus (Figure 33-18). The catheter is advanced until all recording ports are in the stomach. A complete manometric study assesses the characteristics of the LES, the degree of LES relaxation, the esophageal body contraction amplitude and waveform, and the measurement of the UES function.

Lower Esophageal Sphincter

As the catheter is slowly withdrawn in 1-cm increments, the high-pressure zone of the LES is reached by the uppermost

pressure port. The lower (distal) border of the LES is the point at which the resting pressure rises above the gastric baseline; the upper border is the point at which sphincter pressure reaches the esophageal baseline. The respiratory inversion point (RIP) is identified when the positive excursions that occur with breathing in the abdominal environment change to negative deflections in the thoracic environment. The RIP is the functional division between the abdomen and thorax. The *resting pressure* of the LES is the pressure above gastric baseline measured during midrespiration at the RIP. The *overall length* of the sphincter is the distance from the distal border to the proximal border. The *abdominal length* is the distance from the distal border to the RIP and represents the portion of the LES that is subject to fluctuations in intraabdominal pressure (Figure 33-19). The measurements for each of these components from each transducer are expressed as an average. A mechanically defective sphincter is identified by the presence of 1 or more of the following characteristics: (1) an average LES pressure of less than 6 mm Hg, (2) an average abdominal length of less than 1 cm, and (3) an average overall length of less than 2 cm. As compared with normal volunteers, these values are below the 2.5 percentile. A defect in 1 or even 2 components of the LES may be compensated by good esophageal body function, but when all 3 components are defective, excessive esophageal acid exposure is inevitable.[51]

Lower Esophageal Sphincter Relaxation

The catheter is positioned with 4 pressure ports at the same level in the LES, 1 port in the stomach, and at least 1 in the esophageal body. A series of swallows are obtained by giving the patient 5-mL boluses of water. The LES pressure normally drops to gastric baseline immediately after the swallow, before the oncoming peristaltic wave reaches the lower esophagus.

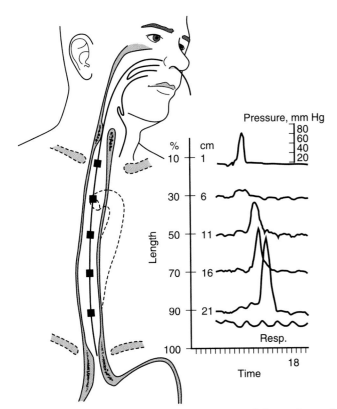

Figure 33-18 Illustration of the position of the 5-channel esophageal motility catheter during the esophageal body portion of the study.

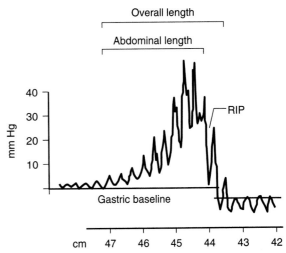

Figure 33-19 Manometric tracing as a transducer is pulled across the lower esophageal sphincter, showing pressure, overall length, and abdominal length. RIP, respiratory inversion point.

560

Esophageal Body Motility

To evaluate the esophageal body, the catheter is positioned so that the pressure-sensing ports span the length of the esophagus, and the peristaltic response to 10 swallows of 5 mL of water is measured. The features of individual contractions are the amplitude, duration, slope, and morphology (i.e., whether single-, double-, or triple-peaked) (Figure 33-20). Transmission of waves from one level to the next is assessed by the speed of wave propagation and by noting any interruption. Most commercially available manometric systems automatically measure these features and compare the results with those of normal subjects (Figures 33-21 and 33-22).

Upper Esophageal Sphincter

The position, length, and resting pressure of the UES and its relaxation with swallowing are assessed with a technique similar to that used for the LES. The key features to be assessed are the adequacy of pharyngeal contraction and the timing and extent of UES relaxation. An indirect measure of UES stiffness or loss of compliance is the intrabolus pressure, which appears as a pressure rise or shoulder on the upstroke of the pharyngeal contraction (Figures 33-23 and 33-24).

Ambulatory 24-Hour pH Monitoring

The development of 24-hour pH monitoring was a major advance in the unraveling of the pathophysiology of GERD. All previous tests had relied on the identification of reflux by a provocative maneuver, which had little relevance to the patient's daily activities. Twenty-four–hour pH monitoring made it possible to determine if the time of esophageal exposure to gastric juice in a patient over a 24-hour period was greater than what was found in normal subjects.

Twenty-four–hour pH monitoring is considered by many to be the gold standard for the diagnosis of GERD, because it has the highest sensitivity and specificity of all tests currently available. It is indicated in any patient with symptoms suggestive of GERD, unless the symptoms are trivial or permanently abolished by a short course of acid-suppression therapy. The need for continued acid suppression should stimulate objective study. A 24-hour pH monitoring study is especially important in patients who are being considered for antireflux surgery. Atypical presentations of GERD are also a common indication; they include such symptoms as noncardiac chest pain (i.e., pain despite a normal cardiac evaluation) and respiratory symptoms such as shortness of breath, cough, nocturnal wheezing, and chronic hoarseness. Twenty-four–hour pH monitoring in such patients allows for confirmation of the diagnosis of GERD and can relate the occurrence of the symptoms to an episode of reflux.[34]

To perform the test, a small pH electrode is passed transnasally into the esophagus and placed 5 cm above the upper border of the LES, a position that has been previously determined by manometry. Different probes are available, but bipolar glass electrodes are preferred for their greater reliability[22] and their elimination of the need for an external reference electrode. The electrode is connected to an external portable digital storage device that is strapped to the patient's side, and pH values are continuously recorded at 6-second intervals for 24 hours (i.e., a complete circadian cycle). Precalibration and postcalibration of the system to pH levels of 1 and 7 is important to exclude electrode drift. The patient is instructed to carry out normal daily activities but to avoid strenuous exertion. He or she is asked to remain in the upright position while awake during the day, lying down supine only at night while sleeping, and to ingest 2 meals at the usual time. The diet is standardized only by its absence of food and beverages with a pH value of less than 5.0 and greater than 6.0. The patient notes in a diary the

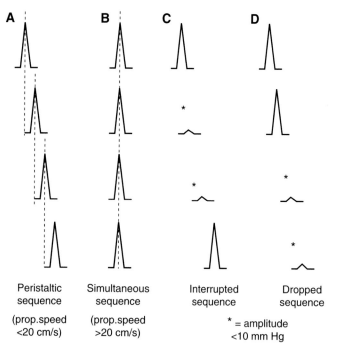

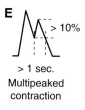

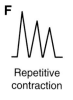

Figure 33–20 Classification of esophageal contraction waves on stationary manometry. **A,** A complete peristaltic sequence is a series of detectable contractions at each esophageal level, with a progression speed of less than 20 cm per second. **B,** A simultaneous sequence is a series of detectable contractions at each esophageal level, with a progression speed of more than 20 cm per second. **C,** An interrupted sequence is a series of detectable contractions in which an initial contraction is followed by no detectable contractions (<10 mm Hg), with a normal contraction subsequently reappearing. **D,** A dropped sequence is a series of detectable contractions in which an initial contraction is followed by no detectable contractions (<10 mm Hg). The morphology of the contractions is classified as normal, multi-peaked, or repetitive. The difference between multi-peaked (**E**) and repetitive (**F**) contractions is that, in the latter, the pressure between 2 consecutive peaks returns to baseline.

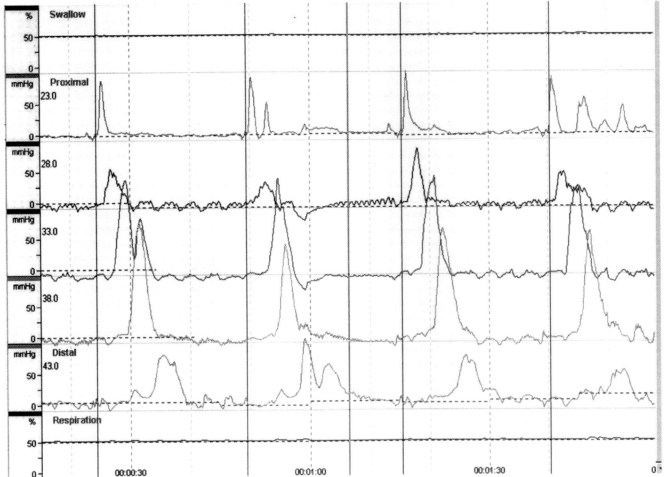

Figure 33–21 Illustration of progressive peristaltic contraction sequences in response to wet swallows.

times of meals, retiring for sleep, and rising the following morning as well as the presence and duration of any symptoms. Figure 33-25 shows typical 24-hour pH tracings from a healthy subject and from a patient with GERD. Medications such as H_2 blockers and prokinetics should be discontinued for 48 hours before the testing begins. Proton-pump inhibitors (e.g., omeprazole) should be stopped for 2 weeks before pH monitoring because of their long-lasting action.

It is important to emphasize that 24-hour esophageal pH monitoring should not be considered a test for reflux but rather a measurement of the esophageal exposure to gastric juice. The measurement is expressed as the percentage of time that the esophageal pH was below 4 during the 24-hour period. Just measuring the percentage of time that the pH is less than 4, although concise, does not reflect how the exposure has occurred; for example, it may have occurred in a few long or several short reflux episodes. Consequently, two other assessments are necessary: (1) the frequency of the reflux episodes and (2) their duration. For this reason, esophageal exposure to gastric juice is best assessed by the following measurements[10]:

1.–3. The cumulative time that the esophageal pH is below 4 expressed as the percentage of the total, upright, and supine monitored times;
2. The frequency of reflux episode is when the pH drops below 4, expressed as the number of episodes per 24 hours;
3. The number of episodes during which the pH remained below 4 for longer than 5 minutes per 24 hours; and
4. The time in minutes of the longest recorded reflux episode is the longest time the pH consistently remained below 4.

Normal values for these six components of the 24-hour record were derived from 50 asymptomatic control subjects. The upper limits of normal were established at the 95th percentile.[32] If the values of symptomatic patients are outside of the 95th percentile of normal subjects, they are considered to be abnormal for the component measured. There is a uniformity of normal values for these six components as reported by centers throughout the world. The normal values for the six components obtained from 50 healthy volunteers are shown in Table 33-1. A composite scoring system has been derived that integrates the different components of the pH record into a single measurement of esophageal acid exposure.

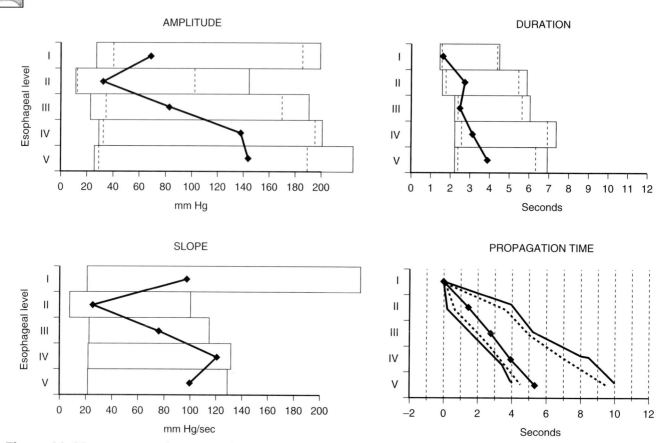

Figure 33–22 Computerized printout of an esophageal body motility study. Median patient values are related to the normal range obtained from healthy volunteers. The 2.5th and 97.5th percentiles are shown by solid lines; the 5th and 95th percentiles are shown by dotted lines.

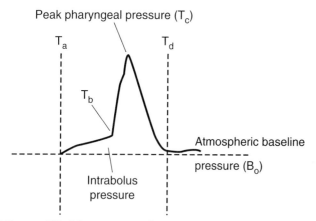

Figure 33–23 Diagram of a typical pharyngeal pressure tracing. T_a, arrival of the bolus head; T_b, the bolus tail; T_c, peak pressure of the pharyngeal-stripping wave; T_d, completion of the pharyngeal pressure wave; B_0, baseline atmospheric pressure.

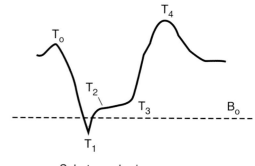

Subatmospheric pressure

Figure 33–24 Diagram of a typical upper esophageal sphincter pressure and its relaxation on swallowing. T_0, pressure at beginning of the swallow; T_1, complete opening of the sphincter (with complete opening, pressure is subatmospheric); T_2, transition from subatmospheric to a supra-atmospheric pressure as the head of the bolus flows into the sphincter; T_3, pressure at the bolus tail ahead of the pharyngeal stripping wave; T_4, peak pressure after luminal closure by the pharyngeal stripping wave; B_0, baseline atmospheric pressure.

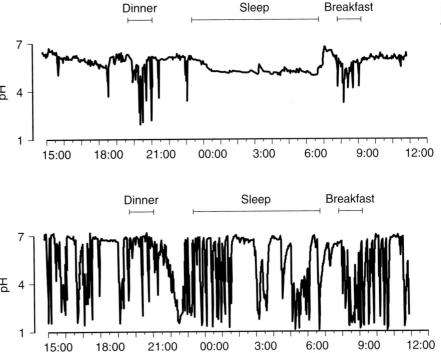

Figure 33–25 Twenty-four hour pH monitoring of the distal esophagus in a healthy subject *(top)* and in a patient with gastroesophageal reflux disease *(bottom)*. Physiological reflux occurs in the normal subject, mainly when in the upright position after meals. The patient's record shows the presence of an increased number of reflux episodes, both in the upright and supine positions, some of them with prolonged clearing time.

This composite score is calculated from the 6 parameters using their standards deviation as weighing factors.[23]

In patients with symptoms of chronic cough, hoarseness, or pulmonary aspiration, placement of an additional pH electrode in the proximal part of the esophagus or pharynx can be helpful.[7] If the accumulated reflux episodes are greater than 1% in the proximal esophagus or the number of reflux episodes is greater than 7 (particularly if there is a temporal relationship between the reflux episodes and the onset of the symptoms), reflux can be documented and

Table 33–1

Normal Values for Ambulatory Esophageal pH Monitoring in 50 Healthy Volunteers

	Mean	Standard deviation	Median	Minimum	Maximum	95th percentile
Percentage of total time with pH <4	1.5	1.4	1.2	0	6.0	4.5
Percentage of upright time with pH <4	2.2	2.3	1.6	0	9.3	8.4
Percentage of supine time with pH <4	0.6	1.0	0.1	0	4.0	3.5
Number of episodes of pH <4	19.0	12.8	16.0	2.0	56.0	46.9
Number of episodes of pH <4 with a duration of >5 minutes	0.8	1.2	0	0	5.0	3.5
Longest episode (minutes)	6.7	7.9	4.0	0	46.0	19.8
Composite score	6.0	4.4	5.0	0.4	18.0	14.7

564 assumed to be the cause of the patient's respiratory symptoms.

Additional testing may be necessary if the standard methods of assessing esophageal function fail to yield conclusive results. The 24-hour esophageal bile probe can be useful for detecting the presence of bilirubin during a 24-hour period in those patients that reflux a preponderance of duodenal contents. Ambulatory 24-hour esophageal manometry can give a much more comprehensive picture of esophageal function during a patient's normal daily activity, especially during meals. In normal subjects, the esophagus becomes progressively more organized from the supine position to the upright position to the meal period; this feature is reflected in the higher prevalence of effective peristaltic waves during meals. Loss of this improved organization of esophageal activity during meals is a subtle sign of a motility disorder. Lastly, the assessment of gastric function can be important in many patients with esophageal symptoms. Disorders of gastric emptying frequently can contribute to or be confused with esophageal disease, especially GERD.

Advances in technology have made pH testing more comfortable for the patient. The recent development of a catheter-free miniaturized pH electrode has revolutionized the way that standard 24-hour pH testing is performed. The Bravo System (Medtronics, Minneapolis, MN) allows for the transnasal or transoral deployment of a small capsule attached to the esophageal mucosa that is capable of transmitting pH data via radiotelemetry to a pager-sized receiver, thus eliminating the need for an unpleasant catheter. It may also provide a more accurate physiologic picture by allowing patients to perform their normal daily activities without the social restrictions imposed by the catheter. Further potential promise is seen in the development of multichannel intraluminal esophageal impedance (MII) measurement. This type of measurement determines the resistance to the flow of current through a given medium (impedance). The impedance to current changes as the composition of the medium in which the current is traveling changes (i.e., air, liquids, or solids). The application of this technology provides a better insight into esophageal bolus transport, and, when coupled with a pH probe, differentiates acid reflux from nonacid reflux. These technological advances—and others yet to come—will undoubtedly provide a better understanding of esophageal physiology and function and ultimately lead to the improved treatment of esophageal disorders.

REFERENCES

1. Barham CP, Gotley DC, Mills A, Alderson D: Precipitating causes of acid reflux episodes in ambulant patients with gastro-oesophageal reflux disease. Gut 36:505–10, 1995.
2. Benjamin SM, Richter JE, et al: Prospective manometric evaluation with pharmacologic provocation of patients with suspected esophageal motility dysfunction. Gastroenterology 84:893–901, 1983.
3. Bonavina L, Evander A, DeMeester TR, et al: Length of the distal esophageal sphincter and competency of the cardia. Am J Surg 151:24–34, 1986.
4. Bremner RM, Hoeft SF, Costantini M, et al: Pharyngeal swallowing: the major factor in clearance of esophageal reflux episodes. Ann Surg 218:364–370, 1993.
5. Castell DO, Richter JE, Dalton CB (editors): Esophageal Motility Testing. New York: Elsevier, 1987.
6. Chandrasoma P: Norman Barrett: so close, yet 50 years away from the truth. J Gastrointest Surg 3:7–14, 1999.
7. DeMeester TR: Prolonged oesophageal pH monitoring. In Read NW (editor): Gastrointestinal Motility: Which Test? Petersfield, England: Wrightson Biomedical, 1989, p. 41.
8. DeMeester TR, Ireland AP: Gastric pathology as an initiator and potentiator of gastroesophageal reflux disease. Dis Esophagus 10:1–8, 1997.
9. DeMeester TR, Peters JH, Bremner CG, Chandrasoma P: Biology of gastroesophageal reflux disease: pathophysiology relating to medical and surgical treatment. Annu Rev Med 50:469–506, 1999.
10. DeMeester TR, Wang CI, Wernly JA, et al: Technique, indications and clinical use of 24-hour esophageal pH monitoring. J Thorac Cardiovasc Surg 79:656–670, 1980.
11. DeMeester TR, Wernly JA, Bryant GH, et al: Clinical and in vitro analysis of gastroesophageal competence: a study of the principles of antireflux surgery. Am J Surg 137:39–46, 1979.
12. Dent J: A new technique for continuous sphincter pressure measurement. Gastroenterology 71:263–267, 1976.
13. Dodds WJ: Current concepts of esophageal motor function: clinical implications for radiology. AJR Am J Roentgenol 128:549–561, 1977.
14. Donner MW: Swallowing mechanism and neuromuscular disorders. Semin Roentgenol 9:273–282, 1974.
15. Ekberg, Walgreen L: Dysfunction of pharyngeal swallowing: a cineradiographic investigation in 854 dysphagial patients. Acta Radiol Diagn 26:389–395, 1985.
16. Fletcheer J, Wirz A, Young J, et al: Unbuffered highly acidic gastric juice exists at the gastroesophageal junction after a meal. Gastroenterology 121:775–783, 2001.
17. Gray SW, Rowe JS Jr, Skandalakis JE: Surgical anatomy of the gastroesophageal junction. Am Surg 45:575–587, 1979.
18. Hameeteman W, Tytgat GNJ, Houthoff HJ, et al: Barrett's esophagus: development of dysplasia and adenocarcinoma. Gastroenterology 96:1249–1256, 1989.
19. Hill LD, Kozarek RA, Kraemer SJ, et al: The gastroesophageal flap valve: in vitro and in vivo observations. Gastrointest Endosc 44:541–547, 1996.
20. Ismail T, Bancewicz J, Barlow J: Yield pressure, anatomy of the cardia and gastroesophageal reflux. Br J Surg 82:943–947, 1995.
21. Iwakiri K, Kobayashi M, Kotoyari M, et al: Relationship between postprandial esophageal acid exposure and meal volume and fat content. Dig Dis Sci 41:926–930, 1996.
22. Johnson LF, DeMeester TRP: Development of the 24-hour intraesophageal pH monitoring composite scoring system. J Clin Gastroenterol 8(Suppl 1):52–58, 1986.
23. Johnson LF, DeMeester TR: Twenty-four hour pH monitoring of the distal esophagus: a quantitative measure of gastroesophageal reflux. Am J Gastroenterol 62:325–332, 1974.
24. Johnson LF, Lin YC, Hong SK: Gastroesophageal dynamics during immersion in water to the neck. J Appl Physiol 38:449–454, 1975.
25. Kahrilas PJ, Shi G, Manka M, Joehl RJ: Increased frequency of transient lower esophageal sphincter relaxation induced by gastric distention in reflux patients with hiatal hernia. Gastroenterology 118:688–695, 2000.
26. Kuster E, Ros E, Toledo-Pimentel V, et al: Predictive factors of the long term outcome in gastro-oesophageal reflux disease: six year follow up of 107 patients. Gut 35:8–14, 1994.
27. Liebermann-Meffert D, Duranceau A: Embryology, anatomy and physiology of the esophagus. In Orringer MB, Zuidema GD (editors): Shackelford's Surgery of the Alimentary Tract. The Esophagus, ed 3. Philadelphia: Saunders, 1991, pp. 3–39.
28. Liebermann-Meffert D, Luescher U, Neff U, et al: Esophagectomy without thoracotomy: is there a risk of

intramediastinal bleeding? A study on blood supply of the esophagus. Ann Surg 206:184–192, 1987.

29. Liebermann-Meffert D, Walbrun B, Hiebert CA, Siewert JR: Recurrent and superior laryngeal nerves: a new look with implications for the esophageal surgeon. Ann Thorac Surg 67:217–223, 1999.

30. Marchand P: The gastro-oesophageal "sphincter" and the mechanism of regurgitation. Br J Surg 42:504–513, 1955.

31. Mason RJ, Lund RJ, DeMeester TR, et al: Nissen fundoplication prevents shortening of the sphincter during gastric distention. Arch Surg 132:719–726, 1997.

32. McLaughlan G, Rawlings JM, Lucas ML, et al: Electrodes for 24-hour pH monitoring: a comparative study. Gut 28:935–939, 1987.

33. Meyer GW, Austin RM, Brady CE, Castell DO: Muscle anatomy of the human esophagus. J Clin Gastroenterol 8:131–137, 1986.

34. Miller FA: Utilization of inlying pH-probe for evaluation of acid peptic diathesis. Arch Surg 89:199–203, 1964.

35. Öberg S, Peters JH, DeMeester TR, et al: Inflammation and specialized intestinal metaplasia of cardiac mucosa is a manifestation of early gastroesophageal reflux disease. Ann Surg 226:522–532, 1997.

36. O'Sullivan GC, DeMeester TR, Joelsson BE, et al: The interaction of the lower esophageal sphincter pressure and length of sphincter in the abdomen as determinants of gastroesophageal competence. Am J Surg 143:40–47, 1982.

37. Pellegrini CA, DeMeester TR, Skinner DB: Response of the distal esophageal sphincter to respiratory and positional maneuvers in humans. Surg Forum 27:380–382, 1976.

38. Peters JH, DeMeester TR, Crookes P, et al: The treatment of gastroesophageal reflux disease with laparoscopic Nissen fundoplication. Ann Surg 228:40–50, 1998.

39. Pettersson GB, Bombeck CT, Nyhus LM: The lower esophageal sphincter: mechanisms of opening and closure. Surgery 88:307–314, 1980.

40. Pouderoux P, Lin S, Kahrilis PJ: Timing, propagation, coordination, and effect of esophageal shortening during peristalsis. Gastroenterology 112:1147–1154, 1997.

41. Pouderoux P, Shi G, Tatum RP, et al: Esophageal solid bolus transport: studies using concurrent videofluoroscopy and manometry. Am J Gastroenterol 94:1457–1463, 1999.

42. Salo JA, Kivilaakso EO, Kiviluoto TA, et al: Cytokeratin profile suggests metaplastic epithelial transformation in Barrett's oesophagus. Ann Med 28:305–309, 1996.

43. Sawney RA, Shields HM, Allan CH, et al: Morphological characterization of the squamocolumnar junction of the esophagus in patients with and without Barrett's epithelium. Dig Dis Sci 41:1088–1098, 1996.

44. Schwizer W, Hinder RA, DeMeester TR: Does delayed gastric emptying contribute to gastroesophageal reflux disease? Am J Surg 157:74–81, 1989.

45. Seaman WB: Roentgenology of pharyngeal disorders. In Margulis AR, Burhenne JH (editors): Alimentary Tract Roentgenology, ed 2, vol I. St. Louis: Mosby, 1973, pp. 305–336.

46. Singh P, Adamopoulos A, Taylor RH, Colin-Jones DG: Oesophageal motor function before and after healing of oesophagitis. Gut 33:1590–1596, 1992.

47. Stein HJ, Barlow AP, DeMeester TR, Hinder RA: Complications of gastroesophageal reflux disease: role of the lower esophageal sphincter, esophageal acid and acid/alkaline exposure, and duodenogastric reflux. Ann Surg 216:35–43, 1992.

48. Stein HJ, DeMeester TR, Naspetti R, et al: Three-dimensional imaging of the lower esophageal sphincter in gastroesophageal reflux disease. Ann Surg 214:374–384, 1991.

49. Theisen J, Oberg S, Peters JH, et al: Gastro-esophageal reflux disease confined to the sphincter. Dis Esophagus 14:235–238, 2001.

50. Zaninotto G, DeMeester TR, Bremner CG, et al: Esophageal function in patients with reflux-induced strictures and its relevance to surgical treatment. Ann Thorac Surg 47:362–370, 1995.

51. Zaninotto G, DeMeester TR, Schwizer W, et al: The lower esophageal sphincter in health and disease. Am J Surg 155:104–111, 1988.

52. Zhuang Z, Vortmeyer AO, Mark EJ, et al: Barrett's esophagus: metaplastic cells with loss of heterozygosity at the APC gene locus are clonal precursors to invasive adenocarcinoma. Cancer Res 56:1961–1964, 1996.

Surgery for Congenital Lesions of the Esophagus

A. Alfred Chahine and Kurt D. Newman

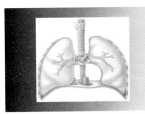

▶ EMBRYOLOGY

At about Day 18 or 19 of fetal life, the notochord, the anlage of the vertebral column, starts to form, first in close association with endodermal cells, then separating from them. The foregut develops from the endodermal cells as they are separating from the notochord. At about 3 weeks of embryonic development, the tracheal primordium appears as a ventral diverticulum in the cephalad portion of the foregut. Over the next few weeks, growth and elongation of the diverticulum and the foregut along the tracheoesophageal groove contribute to the separation of the esophagus and the trachea, which is complete by about 5–6 weeks of fetal life. During the seventh and eight week, the esophageal epithelium proliferates and fills the lumen almost completely.

Vacuoles appear in the lumen and eventually coalesce to recanalize it by the tenth week.[85]

The major anomalies of the esophagus are a result of some aberration in the orderly development as just described. Failure of separation of the trachea and esophagus may result in esophageal atresia (EA) with or without a tracheoesophageal fistula (TEF) and laryngotracheoesophageal clefts. Tracheobronchial elements including cartilage can be left behind in the distal esophagus causing congenital esophageal stenosis. Failure of recanalization of the esophageal lumen may contribute to the pathogenesis of EA and esophageal webs. Intramural esophageal duplication cysts may result from failure of the esophageal vacuoles to completely coalesce and disappear. Aberrations in the orderly separation of endodermal cells, and the notochord may explain the formation of duplication cysts in the posterior mediastinum and vertebral defects associated with EA.

Recently, an Adriamycin-induced murine model of EA was described.[17] Using this model, investigators are studying the role that patterning genes and proteins like Sonic hedgehog (*Shh*) might play in the morphogenesis of EA.[37,38] Utilizing the same rat model, as well as neonates with EA/TEF, Spilde et al studied the molecular expression of foregut-patterning genes to shed a light on the origin of the TEF. The distal esophagus seems to arise as a diverticulum of the trachea, which elongates and joins the stomach rather than from the foregut itself.[17,87,88] They speculate that this might explain the well-known poor motility of the esophagus.

▶ ESOPHAGEAL ATRESIA

Historical Aspects

The historical background relevant to EA is very thoroughly reviewed by Harmon and Coran.[31] Durston in 1670 and Gibson in 1697 described the first cases of EA. It took about 250 years before the first reported cases of survivors by Leven and Ladd independently in 1939. Both were able to achieve success by performing a series of operations including gastrostomy, ligation of fistula, marsupialization of the upper pouch, and final reconstruction with an antethoracic skin tube. The early attempts at primary repair were all unsuccessful. It was not until 1941 that Haight reported the first survivor of a primary repair. In the decade that followed, it became evident that the mortality in infants of lower birth weights, those with severe associated anomalies, and those who are critically ill from aspiration pneumonia was very

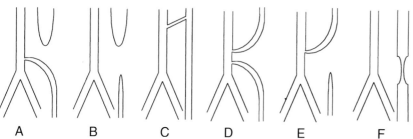

Figure 34–1 Classification of types of esophageal anomalies. **A,** EA with distal TEF. **B,** EA without TEF. **C,** TEF without EA ("H-type" fistula). **D,** EA with proximal and distal TEF. **E,** EA with proximal TEF. **F,** esophageal stenosis. EA, esophageal atresia. TEF; tracheoesophageal fistula.

high.[35,48,96] There followed a shift toward staging the operation for sick babies, with a gastrostomy, followed by division of the TEF and the esophageal reconstruction performed as a third stage.[35,48,96] In 1962, Waterston proposed a classification based on birth weight, presence of pneumonia, and associated anomalies.[96] The 1970s and 1980s witnessed major advances in respiratory, neonatal, anesthetic, and surgical care, as well as introduction of more effective antibiotics. These advances included endotracheal intubation, which made it easier to prevent aspiration from the esophageal pouch and to deal with its sequelae. As a result, multiple groups started recommending either direct primary anastomosis (anastomosis shortly after birth) or delayed primary anastomosis (anastomosis delayed for the treatment of other life-threatening anomalies or stabilization of the patient) regardless of the patient's weight but based on physiological criteria.° The end of the twentieth century ushered in the application of thoracoscopy to the repair of EA/TEF and other congenital anomalies of the esophagus.†

Epidemiology

The average rate of EA is reported to be about 2.4 per 10,000 births.[32] There is no significant, described sex predilection. Other congenital anomalies occur in patients with EA frequently, ranging from 30–76%.[14,16,20,27,94] This might be due to the fact that the malformation in EA occurs early in the first trimester when there is active organogenesis. As a result, the developmental cause of EA/TEF might also affect other organ systems at the same time. The number of associated anomalies (AAs) occurring in each patient increases with decreasing birth weight.[11,27,79] With the improvement in anesthetic, respiratory, and neonatal techniques over the last few decades, the AAs are now the major contributor to mortality in patients with EA.[20] The most common AA, is congenital heart disease present in some form in about 20% of the patients.‡ About 20% of patients will have some combination of the constellation of anomalies referred to as VATER or VACTERL association: Vertebral, Anorectal, Cardic, Tracheo Esophageal, Renal or Radial, and Limb anomalies.[18,68]

Babies born with EQ often have low birth weight and are premature.[11,74] In one study, 90% of the patients with EA were below the 50th percentile for gestational age, and 40% were below the 10th percentile, or small for gestational age (SGA).[41] The growth retardation might be secondary to decreased absorption of the amniotic fluid protein or from a mechanical factor.[41] Sever intrauterine growth retardation increases the mortality rate of the SGA neonate by 5 to 20 times that of

appropriate-for-gestational age neonates of the same gestational age.[2]

Anatomy

There are five types of EA with or without TEF. Different classification schemes have numbered them differently so it is preferred to describe the actual anomaly rather than assign it a number or letter: EA with distal TEF, EA without TEF, EA with proximal TEF, EA with proximal and distal fistula, and isolated TEF ("H-type TEF") (Figure 34-1). The distribution of the different types in large series has been relatively uniform across different decades and countries with the most common being EA with distal TEF (Table 34-1).[27,36,58,62,91] The fistula is usually small and most of the time arises from the midline of the membranous portion of the trachea just above the bifurcation, but there are significant variations.

Presentation

A significant number of cases of EA are now suspected on prenatal ultrasonography with polyhydramnios, absent or small stomach bubble, and visualization of an esophageal pouch in the neck being the most prominent features.[30,83] Suspecting the diagnosis prenatally is invaluable in preparing the family. Prenatal counseling with a pediatric surgeon and a neonatologist and planning for appropriate delivery

Table 34-1		
Distribution of Types of Esophageal Atresia°		
Type of anomaly	*Number*	*Percentage*
EA with distal TEF	1024	87.1
EA	82	7.0
H-type TEF	37	3.1
EA with proximal TEF	11	0.9
EA with double TEF	22	1.9

°Compiled from references 27, 36, 58, 62, 91.
EA, esophageal atresia; TEF, tracheoesophageal fistula.

°References 1, 33, 39, 49, 55, 62, 68, 70, 73.
†References 6, 47, 56, 61, 75–77, 97.
‡References 11, 18, 27, 60, 79, 94.

arrangements are extremely helpful. Postnatally, most patients with EA are diagnosed in the first few hours after birth. Choking with feeding, regurgitation of saliva and feeds, and respiratory distress from aspiration of saliva or gastric contents through the TEF are the most common signs and symptoms. Inability to pass a feeding tube confirms the diagnosis.

Patients with isolated TEF ("H-type" TEF) may not be diagnosed until later in life. Recurrent episodes of aspiration pneumonia and choking and coughing with feedings should raise the suspicion. Contrast esophagogram and rigid bronchoscopy are complementary in making the diagnosis.[7]

Patients with isolated EA often have a scaphoid abdomen because of the absence of gas in the intestines. If EA is sus-pected, always look for other physical signs of the VATER **569** association: anorectal malformations, limb anomalies, and vertebral defects (Figure 34-2).

Workup

A chest radiograph showing a curved catheter in the proximal esophageal pouch is often all that is required to make the diagnosis (Figure 34-3). In patients with isolated EA, the radiograph reveals absence of intestinal air (Figure 34-4). If there is still a doubt, a small amount of air injected into the pouch accentuates it on a plain radiograph and confirms the presence of EA (Figure 34-5). The use of barium to look for an upper pouch fistula should be discouraged

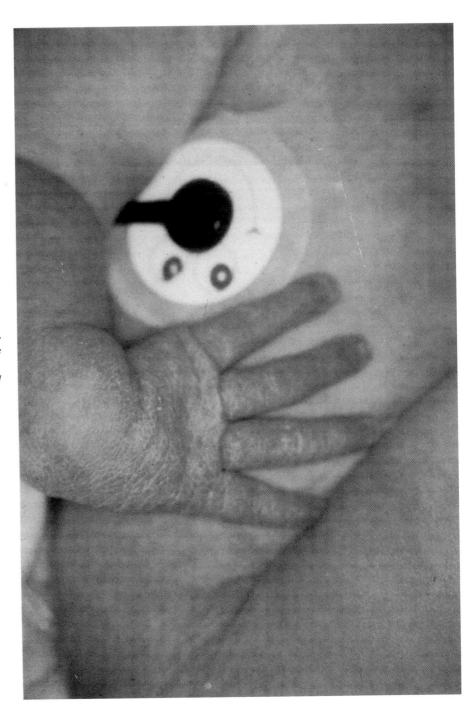

Figure 34–2 Radial aplasia, one component of the VATER association. (See color plate.) *(Courtesy of Dr. R. Ricketts, Emory University Medical Center.)*

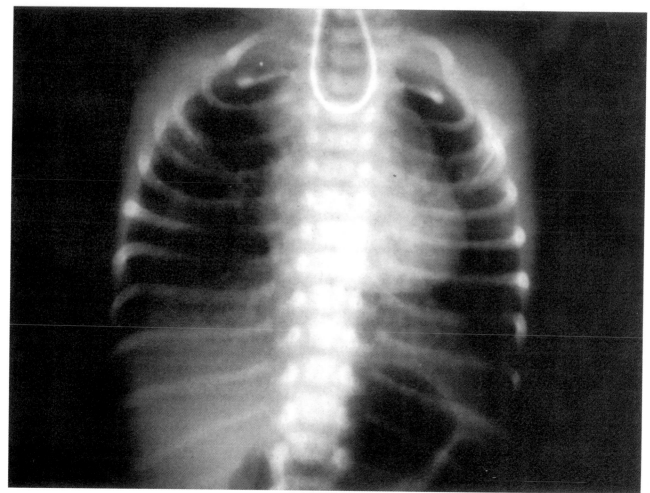

Figure 34–3 Chest radiograph of a patient with esophageal atresia and tracheoesophageal fistula. Note the catheter curved in the upper pouch and the presence of air in the intestinal tract. (*Courtesy of Dr. R. Ricketts, Emory University Medical Center.*)

because it may potentially lead to aspiration. Upper pouch fistulas are rare and are usually found at the time of repair by either bronchoscopy and/or a careful dissection of the proximal pouch. An esophagogram performed via a catheter being pulled up along the esophagus while the patient is prone is invaluable in making the diagnosis of "H-type" fistula (Figure 34-6).

An echocardiogram, renal ultrasound, and vertebral films should be performed to rule out major cardiac, renal, and vertebral anomalies as part of the VATER association. The echocardiogram is also helpful in determining the location of the aortic arch and of any aberrant central vessels, which might alter the surgical approach.

Initial Management

Patients born with EA are at risk for aspiration of saliva or gastric contents into the tracheobronchial tree. A Replogle-type soft sump suction catheter with the holes all close to the tip should be placed in the upper pouch and put on continuous suction. In the presence of a TEF, the patient should be placed in the reverse Trendelenburg position with the head up to minimize reflux of gastric contents into the trachea. Having the patient prone might also help in keeping the gas-

troesophageal junction at a less dependent position and decrease gastric reflux. With isolated EA, the Trendelenburg position facilitates the passive drainage of the hypopharynx and complements the active suction of the catheter. Even with a drainage catheter in place, frequent suctioning of the hypopharynx helps in decreasing the risk of aspiration. If there is any evidence of aspiration pneumonitis on a radiograph, broad-spectrum antibiotics should be started.

Positive-pressure ventilation should be avoided in a patient with a TEF if at all possible to minimize shunting through the TEF and abdominal distention. Because the majority of the fistulas are located just proximal to the carina, the tip of the tube should be kept high in the trachea to prevent the tip of the tube from getting lodged in the TEF. Sometimes, the TEF is significant enough that adequate ventilation cannot be maintained, especially in the face of respiratory distress syndrome (RDS) of the premature with its attendant high intraparenchymal pressures. In that case emergent ligation of the TEF might be warranted.[92] A more difficult way to control the TEF emergently is obliteration of the TEF with a Fogarty balloon introduced via bronchoscopy.[22] A hazardous situation can occur when a patient with significant steal through a TEF also has a very high intestinal obstruction, such as duodenal

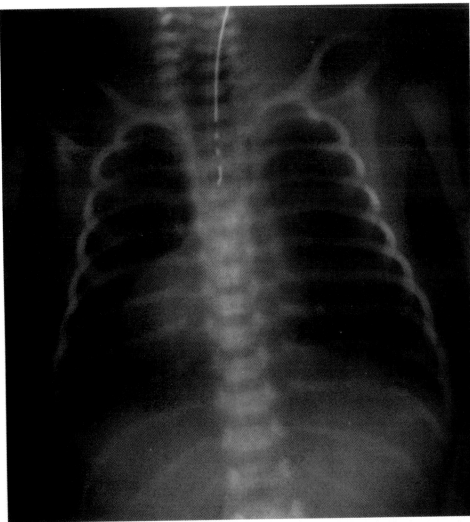

Figure 34–4 Chest radiograph of a patient with isolated esophageal atresia. Note the absence of air in the intestinal tract. *(Courtesy of Dr. C. Leftridge, Georgetown University Medical Center.)*

atresia. The massive gastric distention exacerbates the respiratory compromise and could lead to perforation of the stomach. Emergent gastric decompression has to be performed, sometimes at the bedside with a needle.

Operative Principles

Rigid bronchoscopy is helpful at the beginning of the procedure to identify the exact location of the TEF, recognize rare variants like double fistulas or H-type fistula and laryngotracheoesophageal clefts, identify the presence of tracheomalacia, and help in placement of the endotracheal tube to avoid dislodgement into the TEF[23,26,67] (Figure 34-7).

Primary repair of EA with division of the TEF and end-to-end anastomosis is the ideal goal (Figure 34-8). The standard approach is a right posterolateral thoracotomy. If the patient has a right-sided aortic arch, it might be easier to approach the esophagus from the left thorax. Having the patient tilted forward in the near prone position facilitates access to the posterior mediastinum. For reduction of some of the complications reported with thoracotomy in neonates, namely winged scapula and scoliosis, an axillary skin crease thoracotomy has been reported by Bianchi et al[9] and used with good results.[42] Traditionally, an extrapleural approach has been advocated to decrease the risk of empyema if an esophageal leak occurs. With the introduction of more pow-

erful antibiotics in the 1970s and 1980s, the importance of a retropleural approach with the potential increase in operative time has been questioned.[58,81]

The posterior mediastinum is exposed by dividing the parietal pleura. The azygous vein is divided to allow access to the TEF, which is usually located behind it. The fistula is circumferentially controlled and occluded. The fistula is divided, leaving about 1 mm of esophageal tissue on the tracheal side to avoid narrowing the tracheal lumen. Leaving more than a minimal amount of esophageal rim might create a pouch, which could accumulate secretions and cause repeated aspirations. The tracheal defect is closed in an airtight manner usually with an absorbable monofilament suture.

Gentle pressure by the anesthesiologist on the pouch catheter helps identify the upper pouch, which is usually high in the thoracic inlet. A transmural suture placed through the fistula and incorporating the catheter makes the manipulation of the upper esophagus less traumatic. The upper pouch and the trachea are very intimately juxtaposed, often sharing a common wall. The dissection between the esophageal pouch and the trachea is very delicate. Extreme caution should be applied to avoid injury to both vagus and recurrent laryngeal nerves. The pouch is mobilized as high as possible to minimize the tension of the anastomosis. The blood supply of the upper esophagus is intramural allowing for minimal ischemia even after extensive mobilization.

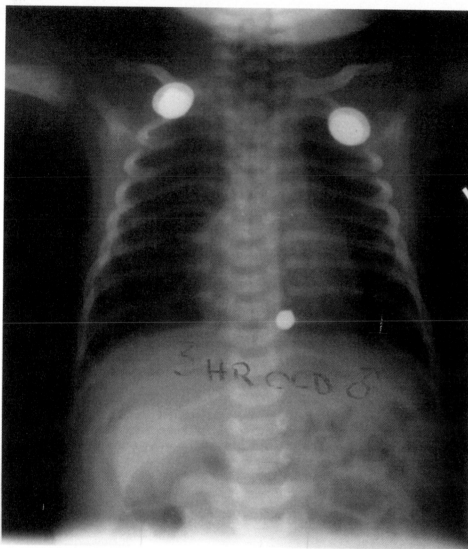

Figure 34–5 Air contrast esophagram in patient with esophageal atresia showing the distended proximal pouch. *(Courtesy of Dr. C. Leftridge, Georgetown University Medical Center.)*

In contrast, the lower esophagus is supplied by segmental branches from the aorta; therefore its mobilization should be minimized to prevent ischemia. The ends of the esophagus are trimmed and an end-to-end anastomosis is built in a single layer fashion with a fine monofilament absorbable sutures. The knots are tied extraluminally if possible. It is crucial to identify the mucosa of both the upper and lower esophagus and incorporate it in the sutures. If there is significant tension, it is helpful to leave the sutures untied and approximate all at the same time as the knots are tied to take some of the tension off. The esophageal and tracheal suture lines must be separated to avoid fistula formation. This is usually accomplished by the interposition of a pleural flap, but sometimes a pericardial flap is required. The routine use of gastrostomy and transanastomotic feeding tubes remains controversial.[31] Prior to constructing the anastomosis, congenital esophageal stenosis (CES) needs to be ruled out by passing a tube through the distal esophagus into the stomach.[95] At the completion of the procedure, a small chest tube is placed and secured to the endothoracic fascia away from the anastomosis. At about 5 or 7 days postoperatively, a contrast study is obtained to assess the anastomosis. The disparity in size between the distended proximal pouch and the small distal esophagus gives the appearance of a narrowing, but usually prompt emptying of contrast attests to the wide patency of the anastomosis (Figure 34-9A). With time, the size discrepancy becomes less pronounced (Figure 34-9B). If there is no leak, the chest tube is removed and feedings are started. Because of the frequent occurrence of gastroesophageal reflux (GER) and the deleterious effects acid can have on a fresh anastomosis, serious consideration should be made to keep the patient on acid-suppressing and promotility drugs until the anastomosis is well healed.

Repair of EA in patients with significant gaps between the two ends of the esophagus can be challenging. The magnitude of the challenge is reflected in the number of innovative techniques described to save the native esophagus. Rehbein and Schweder proposed approximating the two ends as much as possible and waiting for a fistula to develop around the sutures then dilating that fistula.[71] Staging the operation with initial ligation of the TEF and delayed primary anastomosis has been advocated.[69] The growth of the esophagus can be spontaneous or active with serial bougienage of the upper pouch. Delayed primary anastomosis is certainly a safe and effective strategy in patients with very low birth weight in whom the tissues are friable or in patients who are unstable.[11,73] Livaditis and Eklof described performing a circular

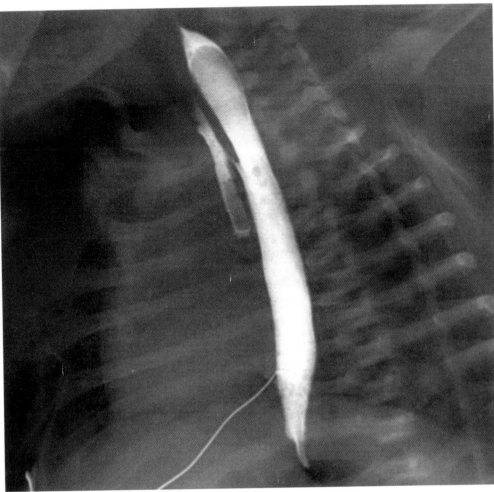

Figure 34–6 Contrast esophagram showing an isolated tracheoesophageal fistula ("H-type") with contrast delineating the trachea. *(Courtesy of Dr. C. Leftridge, Georgetown University Medical Center.)*

myotomy on the upper esophagus to gain length.[55] This has been used with good results by multiple groups.[54,72,86] Delayed ballooning and diverticulum formation are two described long-term complications of circular myotomy.[40,65] A second circular myotomy can be added via a cervical incision if more length is still needed. Kimura et al advocate elongating the esophagus by performing a series of cervical esophagostomies with gradual elongation.[44] Foker et al proposed the application of tension on the two ends through sutures brought out of the skin and tightened sequentially.[24] Elongating the distal esophagus by performing a Collis–Nissen fundoplication at the time of repair of EA has been described.[43] Schärli advocates division of the lesser curvature of the stomach to elongate it and partial gastric transfer to gain as much as 6 cm in length in the treatment of long gap atresia and pure EA.[82] Tubularization of the upper pouch after creation of a U-shaped flap is an attractive technique described by Bar-Maor et al.[5]

The repair of pure EA without a TEF is even more challenging. The distal esophagus is usually very short and the gap very significant. All of the aforementioned techniques can be tried in this situation. Most series report the most success with either delayed primary anastomosis or esophageal replacement.[19] Colonic interposition, jejunal interposition, creation of a gastric tube, and gastric transposition are well-established techniques for esophageal replacement in children.[66,89,90]

The approach to an H-type fistula is usually through a right cervical incision since the majority of them are in the neck. Direct division of the fistula and repair of the esophagus and tracheal components are the goal (Figure 34-10). Placement of a wire through the fistula via bronchoscopy and retrieving it from the mouth assist in the identification of the fistula and offer the opportunity to apply cephalad traction on the fistula to bring it up from the thorax if it is more distal than usual.[46]

In 1999, Lobe and Rothenberg performed the first thoracoscopic repair of isolated EA.[56] Since then, multiple groups have reported the successful thoracoscopic repair of EA with TEF[59,76,77] (Figure 34-11A and B). The thoracoscopic experience is still nascent and long-term results are not available. But the advantages seem to be better visualization secondary to the magnification and the avoidance of a thoracotomy. One of the drawbacks is the inability to take the tension off individual sutures by pulling the sutures all together and tying them one at a time.

Complications

Complications of EA repair can be thought of as short term (leak, stricture) and long term (tracheomalacia, GER, nutritional, recurrent fistula, foreign body impaction).

Most large series report the rate of anastomotic leak to be between 15% and 20%.[52,58,60] Most leaks are small and can

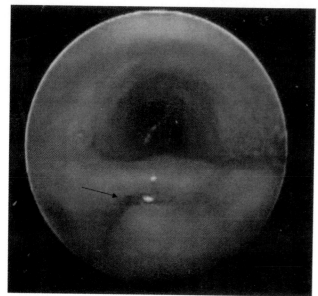

Figure 34–7 Bronchoscopic appearance of a tracheo-esophageal fistula in the membranous portion of the trachea proximal to the carina. (See color plate.)

the stenosis (whether it requires dilations, the number of dilation, and the need for resection). Singh et al proposed spatulating the distal esophagus, creating a wider anastomosis, as a way to decrease the rate of stricture formation.[84] Symptoms include choking, apnea, near-death spells, and food impaction. Most strictures are adequately treated with dilations. Strictures that are refractory to dilations should prompt a diligent search for and control of GER, often with a fundoplication. Recalcitrant strictures can also be secondary to the occurrence of ectopic tissues, tumors, or tracheobronchial remnants near the anastomosis.[15,51,95] The standard approach to refractory strictures has been a resection and reanastomosis. Recently, the application of interventional radiological techniques has allowed the recanalization of impassable strictures that could not be dilated.[13,28]

Gastroesophageal reflux is a major concern in patients with EA, occurring in as many as 54% of patients.[52,60] It is a significant contributor to the rate of occurrence of leaks and strictures as well as to respiratory complications including aspiration pneumonia and cyanotic, near-death spells.[52] The majority of patients with significant GER eventually require a fundoplication to control their symptoms. The short-term morbidity of fundoplication in patients with EA is higher than in the general population perhaps because of the dysmotility of the distal esophagus. A partial fundoplication, like the Toupet 270-degree wrap, could be considered in patients with severe dysmotility or small stomachs.

Recurrent TEF occurs in as many as 10% of the patients following EA repair.[21,52,58,60] Symptoms include coughing, gagging, cyanotic and apneic spells, and recurrent respiratory

be managed nonoperatively with broad-spectrum antibiotics and thoracic drainage. Very rarely, suture repair or cervical diversion is required for a major leak.

The rate of esophageal stricture following repair is variable ranging from 4% to about 50%.[52,58,60] The wide range probably reflects the variability in the criteria for defining

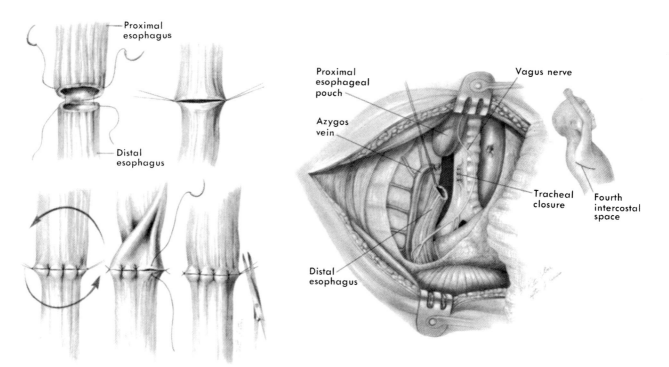

Figure 34–8 Construction of the anastomosis in a patient with esophageal atresia and tracheoesophageal fistula. End sutures are placed to draw the ends of the esophageal segments together. A single row of simple sutures completes the front presenting portions of the anastomosis, with the knots tied on the outside. One of the corner sutures is passed behind the esophagus, which is then rotated 180 degrees. The anastomosis is completed with simple sutures in the presenting posterior surface, which has been rotated into view. It is essential that the sutures are full thickness because the mucosa has a tendency to retract.

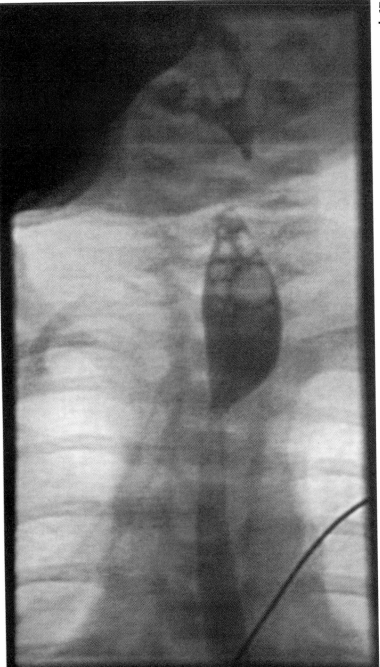

Figure 34–9 A, Postoperative esophagram at 1 week revealing a patent anastomosis and a size discrepancy between the proximal and distal esophagus.

A

infections. The diagnosis is difficult to make and relies heavily on contrast studies. Most will require a repeat resection, but a few reports of bronchoscopic obliteration with fibrin glue, laser, or tissue adhesives have been published.[8,10,29,34,57]

Tracheomalacia is common in patients with EA and is thought to be secondary to the prolonged compression of the developing trachea by the enlarged esophageal pouch. Patients with EA and severe tracheomalacia often have a characteristic barking cough. Severe symptoms include stridor, choking, apnea, and near-death spells. The diagnosis is confirmed by bronchoscopy performed while the patient is spontaneously breathing and more recently by cinecomputed tomography and magnetic resonance imaging.[45,98] Symptomatic patients usually benefit from aortosternopexy. Sutures are placed in the adventitia of the aorta and fixed anteriorly to the sternum, therefore suspending the trachea and increasing its diameter. The improvement in diameter is monitored bronchoscopically (Figure 34-12A and B). This can be accomplished via a left thoracotomy, an anterior thoracotomy, or more recently, thoracoscopically.[45,80,98]

Andrassy et al have studied the long-term nutritional status of patients with EA.[3] They found that even though the patients suffered from malnutrition in the first few years after repair, they seem to "catch up" in the later years, especially after the age of 13 years.

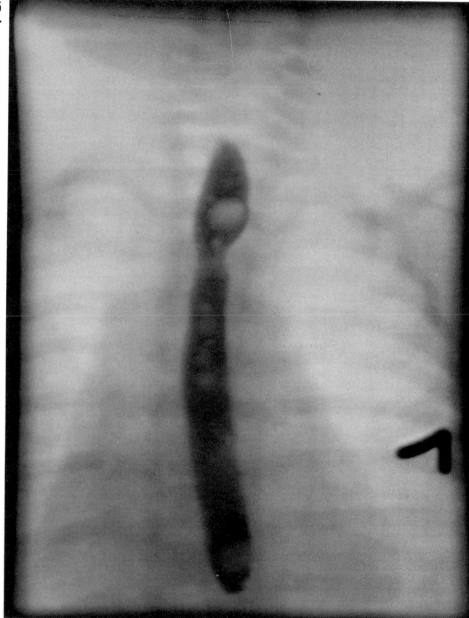

Figure 34–9 cont'd B, Esophagram at 2 months postoperatively showing a decrease in the size discrepancy.

B

Foreign body impaction in the esophagus after EA repair occurs in at least 13% of patients.[99] Often esophagoscopy is needed to clear the esophagus, evaluate for a stricture, and potentially dilate the esophagus. No specific predisposing factors were identified but the incidence of food impaction decreases after 5 years of age.

ESOPHAGEAL DUPLICATIONS

Anatomy and Embryology

The nomenclature of esophageal duplications is confusing. They have been referred to as enterogeneous cysts, esophageal duplication cysts, neuroenteric cysts, and gastrocytomas among others. In addition, there has been some confusion with bronchogenic cysts when these occur in the mediastinum between the esophagus and the trachea. Because the foregut and the notochord originate in direct continuity to each other and because both trachea and esophagus arise from the primitive foregut, it is helpful to view all these cysts as part of a continuum of foregut duplication cysts.[64] The duplications can be lined by alimentary or tracheobronchial mucosa, regardless of where they are located. About 50% of the cysts will contain ectopic gastric mucosa. They can be located in the posterior mediastinum or between the trachea and the esophagus. Cysts located in the posterior mediastinum are often associated with vertebral defects. Intramural duplications probably originate from a failure of vacuolization of the esophageal lumen.[85]

Most esophageal duplications do not communicate with the lumen, but they can be tubular with one or more openings into the lumen. They can be localized to the chest or extend into the abdomen with extensive thoracoabdominal compo-

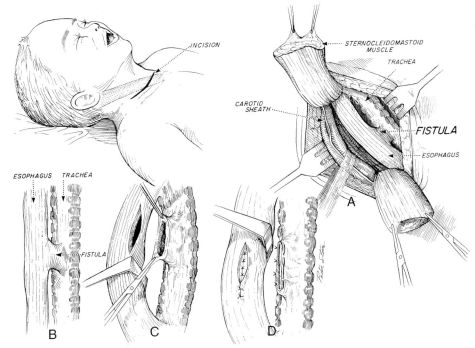

Figure 34–10 Repair of H-type fistula. An incision is made in the neck. The sternocleidomastoid is retracted or severed. The fistula is divided, flush with the esophagus to ensure closure of the trachea without narrowing the lumen.

nents. The majority are located in the distal esophagus, but they can occur anywhere along the length of the esophagus.[4,23]

Incidence

Esophageal duplications are rare with an incidence of 1 in 8200.[4] Only 10–22% of alimentary duplications are esophageal.[25]

Presentation

About a third of patients with esophageal duplications are asymptomatic. Symptomatic patients present with a variety of respiratory and intestinal symptoms: dyspnea, wheezing, recurrent infections and pneumonias, dysphagia, anorexia, and bleeding if they have ectopic gastric mucosa.[64] If the cyst has a fistula to the spinal canal, meningitis can be the presenting symptom.

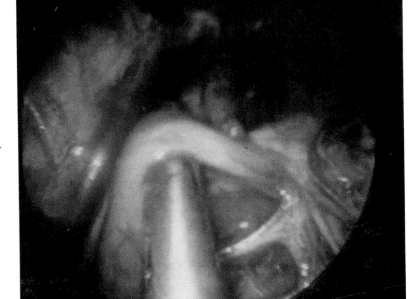

Figure 34–11 A, Thoracoscopic mobilization of the tracheoesophageal fistula. (See color plate.)

A

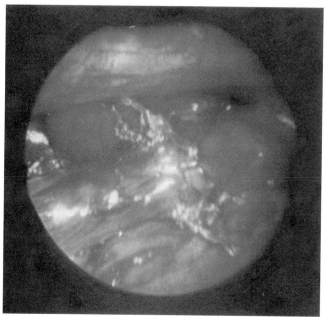

Figure 34–11 cont'd B, Thoracoscopic view of completed esophageal anastomosis.
(Courtesy of Dr. C. Albanese, Stanford University Medical Center.)

Diagnosis

Plain chest radiographs often show a mediastinal mass. These are also helpful to detect any associated vertebral anomalies. A computed tomography scan will delineate the mass further and allow an exact anatomic localization. If there are any vertebral anomalies, magnetic resonance

imaging is helpful to rule out intraspinal pathology. Contrast esophagogram can show extrinsic or intrinsic compression.

Treatment

Complete resection is the preferred method of treatment, traditionally via a thoracotomy. Marsupialization and simple aspiration have a high recurrence rate. If the cyst shares a common wall with either the tracheobronchial tree or the esophagus, part of the wall can be left behind but the mucosa has to be stripped to prevent recurrence. Intramural cysts are enucleated without violating the esophageal lumen. A bougie inserted into the esophagus might make the dissection easier. Posterior mediastinal cysts are usually easily excised unless they have an intraspinal component. Cysts located between the esophagus and the trachea can be challenging to remove because of the close association with the trachea. Long tubular thoracoabdominal duplications might require a combined thoracoabdominal approach.

Recently, thoracoscopy and minimal access techniques have been used to resect a significant number of these cysts.[47,53,61,75,97] As these techniques gain more acceptance and popularity, undoubtedly more and more of these lesions will be treated thoracoscopically.

► CONGENITAL ESOPHAGEAL STENOSIS

Congenital esophageal stenosis (CES) is a rare anomaly.

Anatomy

Three types of CES have been described: fibromuscular, membranous, and those secondary to tracheobronchial rem-

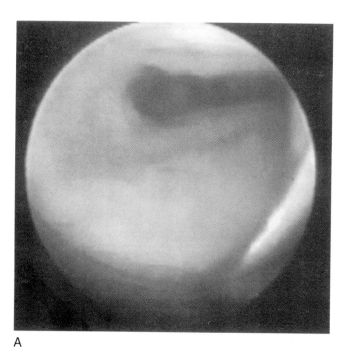

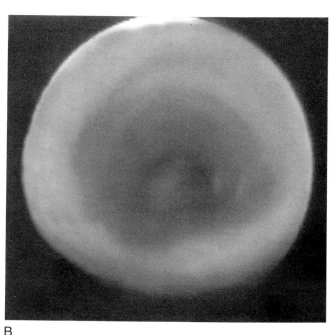

Figure 34–12 A, Bronchoscopic appearance of tracheomalacia in a patient with esophageal atresia with tracheoesophageal fistula. Note that the anterior and posterior walls of the trachea are almost touching. **B,** Bronchoscopic appearance of the same patient after aortosternopexy. The anterior wall is now stented open by the suspension of the aorta. (See color plate for part **A**.)
(Courtesy of Dr. D. Powell, Children's National Medical Center.)

nants. The latter two are usually refractory to dilations and require surgical relief. These lesions can coexist with EA and should be ruled out at the time of EA repair by inserting a catheter into the distal esophagus.[95]

Presentation

Patients with CES usually present with progressive feeding intolerance and regurgitation. Often the symptoms do not manifest themselves until the patient starts solid foods.

Diagnosis

An esophagogram is frequently diagnostic, showing the tapered narrowing in the distal esophagus similar to achalasia. Recently, endoscopic ultrasonography has been employed to differentiate stenosis secondary to tracheobronchial remnants from those associated with fibromuscular hyperplasia.[50,93]

Treatment

Stenosis due to tracheobronchial remnants and intraluminal membranes do not respond to dilation and require resection with end-to-end anastomosis. One of the complications is esophageal shortening and gastroesophageal reflux. Nihoul-Fékété et al recommended the addition of a Nissen fundoplication to the management of distal esophageal stenoses to prevent this complication.[63] The combined Collis gastroplasty and Nissen fundoplication have been proposed to prevent both the shortening and the reflux.[12]

LARYNGOTRACHEOESOPHAGEAL CLEFT

Laryngotracheoesophageal cleft (LTEC) is a rare anomaly arising from the failure of orderly separation of the trachea and esophagus.

Anatomy

There are four subtypes of LTEC[78]:

> Type I: Cleft present to, but not below, the vocal cords.
> Type II: Cleft extends into, but not through, the posterior cricoid cartilage.
> Type III: Cleft extends though the cricoid cartilage.
> Type IV: Cleft extends to the trachea.

Presentation

There is a wide spectrum of presenting symptoms. Patients with types I to III can have subtle symptoms: chronic cough, wheezing, and repeated chest infections. Patients with type IV often have severe symptoms similar to those of patients with TEF: choking with feeding, severe aspiration pneumonia, and respiratory distress.

Diagnosis

Rigid bronchoscopy and esophagoscopy are essential in making the diagnosis. Other associated anomalies including TEF, GERD, congenital heart disease, and cleft lip and palate should be sought.

Treatment

Observation of asymptomatic patients with type I clefts is often warranted. If they are symptomatic, they could be repaired endoscopically or open. Types II to IV clefts need to be repaired. The lateral pharyngotomy approach has been abandoned because of the high risk of recurrent laryngeal nerve injury and poor access to longer defects. The standard method is a transtracheal approach splitting the airway and trachea in the midline to expose the LTEC, which is then repaired. Long type IV clefts can be challenging to repair and might require cardiopulmonary bypass or extracorporeal membrane oxygenation. A multidisciplinary collaboration between pediatric surgeons, otorhinolaryngologists, and cardiac surgeons is often required.

If GERD is significant, aggressive therapy with fundoplication enhances the chances of success of LTEC repair.

REFERENCES

1. Abrahamson J, Shandling B: Esophageal atresia in the underweight baby: A challenge. J Pediatr Surg 7:608–613, 1972.
2. Anderson MS, Hay WW Jr: Intrauterine growth restriction and the small-for-gestational-age infant. In Avery GB, Fletcher MA, MacDonald MG, editors: Neonatology: pathophysiology and Management of the Newborn, 5th ed. Philadelphia, PA: Lippincott, Williams & Wilkins, 1999, pp. 411–445.
3. Andrassy RJ, Patterson RS, Ashley J, et al: Long-term nutritional assessment of patients with esophageal atresia and/or tracheoesophageal fistula. J Pediatr Surg 18:431–435, 1983.
4. Arbona JL, Fazzi JG, Mayoral J: Congenital esophageal cysts: Case report and review of literature. Am J Gastroenterol 79:177–182, 1984.
5. Bar-Maor JA, Shoshany G, Sweed Y: Wide gap esophageal atresia: A new method to elongate the upper pouch. J Pediatr Surg 24:882–883, 1989.
6. Bax KM, van Der Zee DC: Feasibility of thoracoscopic repair of esophageal atresia with distal fistula. J Pediatr Surg 37:192–196, 2002.
7. Benjamin B, Pham T: Diagnosis of H-type tracheoesophageal fistula. J Pediatr Surg 26:667–671, 1991.
8. Bhatnagar V, Lal R, Sriniwas M, et al: Endoscopic treatment of tracheoesophageal fistula using electrocautery and the Nd:YAG laser. J Pediatr Surg 34:464–467, 1999.
9. Bianchi A, Sowande O, Alizai NK, et al: Aesthetics and lateral thoracotomy in the neonate. J Pediatr Surg 33:1798–1800, 1998.
10. Brands W, Joppich I, Lochbuhler H: Use of highly concentrated human fibrinogen in paediatric surgery—a new therapeutic principle. Z Kinderchir 35:159–162, 1982.
11. Chahine AA, Ricketts RR: Esophageal atresia in infants with very low birth weight. Semin Pediatr Surg 9:73–78, 2000.
12. Chahine AA, Campbell AB, Hoffman MA: Management of congenital distal esophageal stenosis with combined Collis gastroplasty-Nissen fundoplication. Pediatr Surg Int 10:23–25, 1995.
13. Chahine AA, Poplausky M, Rozenblit G, et al: Recanalization of an esophageal atresia anastomosis by an interventional radiologic technique. Pediatr Endosurg Innov Tech 7:71–77, 2003.

580

14. Cozzi F, Wilkinson AW: Low birthweight babies with oesophageal atresia or tracheo-oesophageal fistula. Arch Dis Child 50:791–795, 1975.

15. De La Hunt MN, Jackson CR, Wright C: Heterotopic gastric mucosa in the upper esophagus after repair of atresia. J Pediatr Surg 37:E14, 2002.

16. Depaepe A, Dolk H, Lechat MF: The epidemiology of tracheo-oesophageal fistula and oesophageal atresia in Europe. EUROCAT Working Group. Arch Dis Child 68:743–748, 1993.

17. Diez-Pardo JA, Baoquan Q, Navarro C, et al: A new rodent experimental model of esophageal atresia and tracheo-esophageal fistula: Preliminary report. J Pediatr Surg 31:498–502, 1996.

18. Driver CP, Shankar KR, Jones MO, et al: Phenotypic presentation and outcome of esophageal atresia in the era of the Spitz classification. J Pediatr Surg 36:1419–1421, 2001.

19. Ein SH, Shandling B and Heiss K: Pure esophageal atresia: Outlook in the 1990s. J Pediatr Surg 28:1147–1150, 1993.

20. Ein SH, Shandling B, Wesson D, et al: Esophageal atresia with distal tracheoesophageal fistula: Associated anomalies and prognosis in the 1980s. J Pediatr Surg 24:1055–1059, 1989.

21. Ein SH, Stringer DA, Stephens CA, et al: Recurrent tracheoesophageal fistulas: A seventeen-year review. J Pediatr Surg 18:436–441, 1983.

22. Filston HC: The Fogarty balloon catheter as an aid to management of the infant with esophageal atresia and tracheoesophageal fistula complicated by severe RDS or pneumonia. J Pediatr Surg 17:149, 1982.

23. Filston HC, Rankin JS, Grimm JK: Esophageal atresia. Prognostic factors and contribution of preoperative telescopic endoscopy. Ann Surg 199:532–537, 1984.

24. Foker JE, Linden BC, Boyle EM Jr, et al: Development of a true primary repair for the full spectrum of esophageal atresia. Ann Surg 226:533–541; discussion 541–543, 1997.

25. Fowler CL: Esophageal duplications. In Ziegler MM, Azizkhan RG, Weber T, editors: Operative Pediatric Surgery. New York: McGraw-Hill, 2003, pp. 355–365.

26. Garcia NM, Thompson JW, Shaul DB: Definitive localization of isolated tracheoesophageal fistula using bronchoscopy and esophagoscopy for guide wire placement. J Pediatr Surg 33:1645–1647, 1998.

27. German JC, Mahour GH, Woolley MM: Esophageal atresia and associated anomalies. J Pediatr Surg 11:299–306, 1976.

28. Gilchrist BF, Scriven R, Sanchez J, et al: The application of vascular technology to esophageal and airway strictures. J Pediatr Surg 37:47–49, 2002.

29. Gutierrez C, Barrios JE, Lluna J, et al: Recurrent tracheoesophageal fistula treated with fibrin glue. J Pediatr Surg 29:1567–1569, 1994.

30. Haeusler MC, Berghold A, Stoll C, et al: Prenatal ultrasonographic detection of gastrointestinal obstruction: Results from 18 European congenital anomaly registries. Prenat Diagn 22:616–623, 2002.

31. Harmon CM, Coran AG: Congenital anomalies of the esophagus. In O'Neill JA, Rowe MI, Grosfeld JL, et al, editors: Pediatric Surgery, 5th ed. St. Louis: Mosby, 1998, pp. 941–967.

32. Harris J, Kallen B, Robert E: Descriptive epidemiology of alimentary tract atresia. Teratology 52:15–29, 1995.

33. Hays DM, Snyder WH: Results of conventional operative procedures for esophageal atresia in premature infants. Am J Surg 106:19–23, 1963.

34. Hoelzer DJ, Luft JD: Successful long-term endoscopic closure of a recurrent tracheoesophageal fistula with fibrin glue in a child. Int J Pediatr Otorhinolaryngol 48:259–263, 1999.

35. Holder TM, McDonald VG, Woolley MM: The premature or critically ill infant with esophageal atresia: Increased success with a staged approach. J. Thorac Cardiovasc Surg 44:344–358, 1962.

36. Holder TM, Ashcraft KW, Sharp RJ, et al: Care of infants with esophageal atresia, tracheoesophageal fistula, and associated anomalies. J Thorac Cardiovasc Surg 94:828–835, 1987.

37. Ioannides AS, Chaudhry B, Henderson DJ, et al: Dorsoventral patterning in oesophageal atresia with tracheo-oesophageal fistula: Evidence from a new mouse model. J Pediatr Surg 37:185–191, 2002.

38. Ioannides AS, Henderson DJ, Spitz L, et al: Role of Sonic hedgehog in the development of the trachea and oesophagus. J Pediatr Surg 38:29–36, 2003.

39. Ito T, Sugito T, Nagaya M: Delayed primary anastomosis in poor-risk patients with esophageal atresia associated with tracheoesophageal fistula. J Pediatr Surg 19:243–247, 1984.

40. Janik JS, Filler RM, Ein SH, et al: Long-term follow-up circular myotomy for esophageal atresia. J Pediatr Surg 15:835–841, 1980.

41. Jolleys A: An examination of the birthweights of babies with some abnormalities of the alimentary tract. J Pediatr Surg 16:160–163, 1981.

42. Kalman A, Verebely T: The use of axillary skin crease incision for thoracotomies of neonates and children. Eur J Pediatr Surg 12:226–229, 2002.

43. Kawahara H, Imura K, Yagi M, et al: Collis-Nissen procedure in patients with esophageal atresia: Long-term evaluation. World J Surg 26:1222–1227, 2002.

44. Kimura K, Nishijima E, Tsugawa C, et al: Multistaged extrathoracic esophageal elongation procedure for long gap esophageal atresia: Experience with 12 patients. J Pediatr Surg 36:1725–1727, 2001.

45. Kimura K, Soper RT, Kao SC, et al: Aortosternopexy for tracheomalacia following repair of esophageal atresia: Evaluation by cine-CT and technical refinement. J Pediatr Surg 25:769–772, 1990.

46. Ko BA, Frederic R, DiTirro PA, et al: Simplified access for division of the low cervical/high thoracic H-type tracheoesophageal fistula. J Pediatr Surg 35:1621–1622, 2000.

47. Koizumi K, Tanaka S, Haraguchi S, et al: Thoracoscopic enucleation of a submucosal bronchogenic cyst of the esophagus: Report of two cases. Surg Today 28:446–450, 1998.

48. Koop CE, Hamilton JP: Atresia of the esophagus: Increased survival with staged procedures in the poor-risk infant. Ann Surg 162:389–401, 1965.

49. Koop CE, Schnaufer L, Broennie AM: Esophageal atresia and tracheoesophageal fistula: Supportive measures that affect survival. Pediatrics 54:558–564, 1974.

50. Kouchi K, Yoshida H, Matsunaga T, et al: Endosonographic evaluation in two children with esophageal stenosis. J Pediatr Surg 37:934–936, 2002.

51. Lee H, Morgan K, Abramowsky C, et al: Leiomyoma at the site of esophageal atresia repair. J Pediatr Surg 36:1832–1833, 2001.

52. Leenderste-Verloop K, Tibboel D, Hazebroek FWJ, et al: Postoperative morbidity in patients with esophageal atresia. Pediatr Surg Int 2:2–5, 1987.

53. Lewis RJ, Caccavale RJ, Sisler GE: Imaged thoracoscopic surgery: A new thoracic technique for resection of mediastinal cysts. Ann Thorac Surg 53:318–320, 1992.

54. Lindahl H, Louhimo I: Livaditis myotomy in long-gap esophageal atresia. J Pediatr Surg 22:109–112, 1987.

55. Livaditis A, Eklof O: Esophageal atresia with tracheoesophageal fistula: Results of primary anastomosis in premature infants. Z. Kinderchir 12:32–39, 1973.

56. Lobe TE, Rothenberg SS, Waldschmidt J, et al: Thoracoscopic repair of esophageal atresia in an infant: A surgical first. Pediatr Endosurg Innov Tech 3:141–148, 1999.

57. Lopes MF, Pires J, Nogueria Brandao A, et al: Endoscopic obliteration of a recurrent tracheoesophageal fistula with enbucrilate and polidocanol in a child. Surg Endosc 17:657, 2003.

58. Louhimo I, Lindahl H: Esophageal atresia: Primary results of 500 consecutively treated patients. J Pediatr Surg 18:217–229, 1983.

59. Lovvorn HN, Rothenberg SS, Reinberg O, et al: Update on thoracoscopic repair of esophageal atresia with and without tracheoesophageal fistula. Pediatr Endosurg Innov Tech 5:135–139, 2001.

60. Manning PB, Morgan RA, Coran AG, et al: Fifty years' experience with esophageal atresia and tracheoesophageal fistula. Beginning with Cameron Haight's first operation in 1935. Ann Surg 204:446–453, 1986.

61. Merry C, Spurbeck WE, Lobe TE: Resection of foregut-derived duplications by minimal-access surgery. Pediatr Surg Int 15:224–226, 1999.

62. Myers NA: Oesophageal atresia: The epitome of modern surgery. Ann R Coll Surg Engl 54:277–287, 1974.

63. Nihoul-Fékété C, De Backer A, Lortat-Jacob S, et al: Congenital esophageal stenosis: A review of 20 cases. Pediatr Surg Int 2:86–92, 1987.

64. Nobuhara KK, Gorski YC, La Quaglia MP, et al: Bronchogenic cysts and esophageal duplications: Common origins and treatment. J Pediatr Surg 32:1408–1413, 1997.

65. Otte JB, Gianello P, Wese FX, et al: Diverticulum formation after circular myotomy for esophageal atresia. J Pediatr Surg 19:68–71, 1984.

66. Pedersen JC, Klein RL, Andrews DA: Gastric tube as the primary procedure for pure esophageal atresia. J Pediatr Surg 31:1233–1235, 1996.

67. Pigna A, Gentili A, Landuzzi V, et al: Bronchoscopy in new-borns with esophageal atresia. Pediatr Med Chir 24:297–301, 2002.

68. Pohlson EC, Schaller RT, Tapper D: Improved survival with primary anastomosis in the low birth weight neonate with esophageal atresia and tracheoesophageal fistula. J Pediatr Surg 23:418–421, 1988.

69. Puri P, Ninan GK, Blake NS, et al: Delayed primary anastomosis for esophageal atresia: 18 months' to 11 years' follow-up. J Pediatr Surg 27:1127–1130, 1992.

70. Randolph JG, Newman KD, Anderson KD: Current results in repair of esophageal atresia with tracheoesophageal fistula using physiologic status as a guide to therapy. Ann Surg 209:526–530; discussion 530–531, 1989.

71. Rehbein F, Schweder N: Reconstruction of the esophagus without colon transplantation in cases of atresia. J Pediatr Surg 6:746–752, 1971.

72. Ricketts RR, Luck SR, Raffensperger JG: Circular esophagomyotomy for primary repair of long-gap esophageal atresia. J Pediatr Surg 16:365–369, 1981.

73. Rickham PP: Infants with esophageal atresia weighing under 3 pounds. J Pediatr Surg 16:595–598, 1981.

74. Robert E, Mutchinick O, Mastroiacovo P, et al: An international collaborative study of the epidemiology of esophageal atresia or stenosis. Reprod Toxicol 7:405–421, 1993.

75. Rothenberg SS: Thoracoscopy in infants and children. Semin Pediatr Surg 3:277–282, 1994.

76. Rothenberg SS: Thoracoscopic repair of a tracheoesophageal fistula in a newborn infant. Pediatr Endosurg Innov Tech 4:289–294, 2000.

77. Rothenberg SS: Thoracoscopic repair of tracheoesophageal fistula in newborns. J Pediatr Surg 37:869–872, 2002.

78. Rutter MJ, Azizkhan RG, Cotton RT: Posterior laryngeal cleft. In Ziegler MM, Azizkhan RG, Weber T, editors: Operative Pediatric Surgery. New York: McGraw-Hill, 2003, pp. 313–32034.

79. Saing H, Mya GH, Cheng W: The involvement of two or more systems and the severity of associated anomalies significantly influence mortality in esophageal atresia. J Pediatr Surg 33:1596–1598, 1998.

80. Schaarschmidt K, Kolberg-Schwerdt A, Bunke K, et al: A technique for thoracoscopic aortopericardiosternopexy. Surg Endosc 16:1639, 2002.

81. Schaarschmidt K, Willital GH, Jorch G, et al: Delayed primary reconstruction of an esophageal atresia with distal esophagotracheal fistula in an infant weighing less than 500 g. J Pediatr Surg 27:1529–1531, 1992.

82. Schärli AF: Esophageal reconstruction in very long atresias by elongation of the lesser curvature. Pediatr Surg Int 7:101–105, 1992.

83. Shulman A, Mazkereth R, Zalel Y, et al: Prenatal identification of esophageal atresia: The role of ultrasonography for evaluation of functional anatomy. Prenat Diagn 22:669–674, 2002.

84. Singh SJ, Shun A: A new technique of anastomosis to avoid stricture formation in oesophageal atresia. Pediatr Surg Int 17:575–577, 2001.

85. Skandalakis JE, Gray SW, Ricketts R: The esophagus. In Skandalakis JE, Gray SW, editors: Embryology for Surgeons, 2nd ed. Baltimore: Williams & Wilkins, 1994, pp. 65–112.

86. Slim MS: Circular myotomy of the esophagus: Clinical application in esophageal atresia. Ann Thorac Surg 23:62–66, 1977.

87. Spilde TL, Bhatia AM, Marosky JK, et al: Complete discontinuity of the distal fistula tract from the developing gut: Direct histologic evidence for the mechanism of tracheo-esophageal fistula formation. Anat Rec 267:220–224, 2002.

88. Spilde TL, Bhatia AM, Miller KA, et al: Thyroid transcription factor-1 expression in the human neonatal tracheoesophageal fistula. J Pediatr Surg 37:1065–1067, 2002.

89. Spitz L: Gastric transposition for esophageal substitution in children. J Pediatr Surg 27:252–259, 1992.

90. Spitz L: Esophageal atresia: Past, present, and future. J Pediatr Surg 31:19–25, 1996.

91. Spitz L, Kiely E, Brereton RJ: Esophageal atresia: five year experience with 148 cases. J Pediatr Surg 22:103–108, 1987.

92. Templeton JM, Jr, Templeton JJ, Schnaufer L, et al: Management of esophageal atresia and tracheoesophageal fistula in the neonate with severe respiratory distress syndrome. J Pediatr Surg 20:394–397, 1985.

93. Usui N, Kamata S, Kawahara H, et al: Usefulness of endoscopic ultrasonography in the diagnosis of congenital esophageal stenosis. J Pediatr Surg 37:1744–1746, 2002.

94. van Heurn LW, Cheng W, de Vries B, et al: Anomalies associated with oesophageal atresia in Asians and Europeans. Pediatr Surg Int 18:241–243, 2002.

95. Vasudevan SA, Kerendi F, Lee H, et al: Management of congenital esophageal stenosis. J Pediatr Surg 37:1024–1026, 2002.

96. Waterston DJ, Bonham Carter RE, Aberdeen E: Oesophageal atresia: Tracheo-oesophageal fistula. A study of survival in 218 infants. Lancet 1:819–822, 1962.

97. Watson DI, Britten-Jones R: Thoracoscopic excision of bronchogenic cyst of the esophagus. Surg Endosc 9:824–825, 1995.

98. Weber TR, Keller MS, Fiore A: Aortic suspension (aortopexy) for severe tracheomalacia in infants and children. Am J Surg 184:573–577; discussion 577, 2002.

99. Zigman A, Yazbeck S: Esophageal foreign body obstruction after esophageal atresia repair. J Pediatr Surg 37:776–778, 2002.

Surgical Treatment of Benign Esophageal Diseases

Thomas W. Rice and Sudish C. Murthy

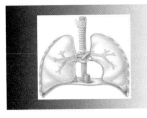

▷ INTRODUCTION

The esophagus actively transports solids and liquids from the pharynx to the stomach. It has no digestive, absorptive, metabolic, or endocrine functions. A muscular tube subtended by two sphincters performs this rudimentary transfer task. Despite simplicity in esophageal function and form, surgical treatment of benign esophageal disorders is challenging. Few options are available to repair damaged sphincters; disorders of the esophageal body are rarely amenable to surgical correction. Often progressive disease and/or failed surgical therapy result in a nonrepairable esophagus. The only treatment option is resection and replacement. Successful surgical therapy requires a sound understanding of esophageal anatomy, physiology, investigative techniques, and disease processes.

▷ ESOPHAGUS AND ITS SURROUNDINGS

Esophageal Wall

The esophagus is lined with stratified, nonkeratinizing squamous epithelium (Figure 35-1), separated from the remainder of the esophageal wall by a basement membrane. Immediately beneath the basement membrane is the lamina propria, a loose matrix of collagen and elastic fibers that forms a superficial undulating surface. The muscularis mucosae supports the lamina propria. This continuous muscle layer pleats the inner layers of the esophagus into a series of folds that disappear with distention. The epithelium, lamina propria, and muscularis mucosae comprise the esophageal mucosa.

The submucosa is composed of connective tissue that contains a rich network of blood vessels and lymphatics. Elastic fibers and collagen combine to make this the strongest esophageal layer. Submucosal glands are mixed types, producing a combination of serous and mucous secretions. These submucosal glands are unique to the esophagus and allow differentiation of the esophagus from the stomach in instances of glandular epithelial metaplasia. Ducts from these glands pierce the mucosa to drain into the esophageal lumen.

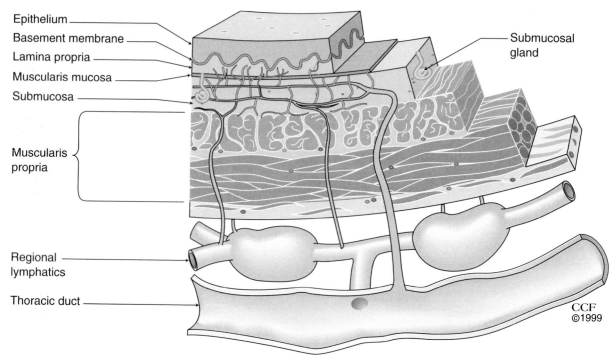

Epithelium
Basement membrane
Lamina propria
Muscularis mucosa
Submucosa

Muscularis propria

Regional lymphatics

Thoracic duct

Submucosal gland

CCF
©1999

Figure 35–1 Esophageal wall.

The muscularis propria is the muscular sleeve that provides the propulsive force necessary for swallowing. There are two layers of muscle: an inner circular layer and an outer longitudinal layer. The first 1–6 cm of the cervical esophagus is composed entirely of striated muscle. Smooth muscle first appears in the anterior circular layer. A gradual transition occurs within muscle bundles and by the junction of the upper and mid-third of the esophagus, close to the tracheal bifurcation, it is entirely smooth muscle.

The cricopharyngeus (upper esophageal sphincter, UES) is a continuous transverse band of muscle originating from the cricoid cartilage (Figure 35-2). Superiorly, the muscle of the cricopharyngeus blends with the inferior pharyngeal constrictor muscle. A posterior defect, Killian's triangle, is an inverted fan-shaped weakness in the inferior constrictor at the superior border of the cricopharyngeus. Inferiorly, the cricopharyngeus merges with the inner, circular layer of the muscularis propria. The longitudinal muscle layer of the muscularis propria originates from the lateral aspect of the cricoesophageal tendon. Posteriorly, these anterior and lateral components converge to meet at the midline. Thus, the proximal 1–2 cm of the posterior cervical esophagus is composed only of inner, circular muscle, creating a potential for a mirror-image triangular area of weakness called Laimer's triangle.

Contraction of the longitudinal muscle fibers of the esophageal body produces esophageal shortening. The inner circular muscle is arranged in incomplete rings producing a helical pattern. Contraction of the circular muscle produces corkscrew-type propulsion. Muscle layers are equal and uniform in thickness until the distal 3–4 cm of the esophagus. Here, the inner circular layer thickens and divides into incomplete horizontal muscular clasps on the lesser curve aspect of the distal esophagus and oblique

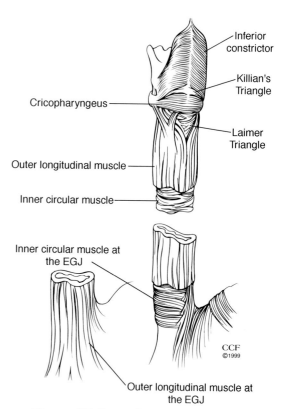

Inferior constrictor
Killian's Triangle
Cricopharyngeus
Laimer Triangle
Outer longitudinal muscle
Inner circular muscle
Inner circular muscle at the EGJ
Outer longitudinal muscle at the EGJ

CCF
©1999

Figure 35–2 Esophageal musculature.

fibers on the greater curve aspect. These become gastric sling fibers (Figure 35-2). Although no complete circular bands exist at the lower esophageal sphincter (LES), it is this area of rearranged circular fibers that corresponds to the high-pressure zone of the lower esophageal sphincter.

Because the esophagus lacks a serosal covering, esophageal adventitia or periesophageal tissue is in direct contact with the outer layer of the muscularis propria. This layer of loose connective tissue surrounding the esophagus contains lymphatics and regional lymph nodes, blood vessels, and nerves.

Lymphatics begin as blind endothelial lined saccules in the lamina propria just below the epithelium and basement membrane. The lymphatic anatomy is peculiar to the esophagus. In the body of the stomach and small and large intestines, lymphatics commence in the submucosa. Lymphatics of the mucosa drain into a rich submucosal plexus that runs the length of the esophagus and allows rapid drainage of lymph along the esophagus. The muscularis propria lymphatic network is rudimentary compared to the submucosal complex. Lymphatic channels intermittently pierce the muscularis to drain into lymphatic trunks that parallel the esophagus.[76] These trunks have valves that direct lymph flow toward regional lymph nodes. Direct connections between the submucosal plexus and thoracic duct are seen in up to 10% of autopsy specimens.[76,94,113] These connections allow early and rapid systemic spread of esophageal carcinoma.

The arterial supply of the esophagus is parasitic. It is derived from blood vessels supplying other organs in the neck, chest, and abdomen. Generally, these vessels divide at a distance from the esophagus and send small segmental branches to that segment of the esophagus. Esophageal blood supply has three principal sources. The superior and inferior thyroid arteries supply the cervical esophagus. The proximal and middle thoracic esophagus receives blood from branches of the bronchial arteries. The only dedicated esophageal arteries are one or two branches that arise from the anterior aspect of the aorta below the tracheal carina. These esophageal arteries directly supply the lower thoracic esophagus. The lower thoracic esophagus and abdominal esophagus receive arterial branches from the left gastric and, occasionally, the splenic arteries. The combination of a segmented arterial supply derived from multiple sources and a rich intramural vascular plexus ensures an excellent esophageal blood flow and permits extensive esophageal mobilization without esophageal arterial insufficiency or ischemia. Because esophageal arteries branch from larger arteries some distance from the esophagus, stripping of the esophagus from its bed during transhiatal (blunt) esophagectomy is possible without direct ligation of the esophageal arterial supply. Arterial spasm provides adequate hemostasis, so significant bleeding does not complicate this procedure.

Subepithelial esophageal venules drain into a substantial submucosal venous plexus that extends the length of the esophagus. There are venous connections between the lower thoracic and abdominal esophagus and the portal venous system. Venules pierce the muscularis propria, which drain into veins on the surface of the esophagus. Regional drainage is directed to the inferior thyroid and brachiocephalic veins in the neck, the azygous and hemiazygous veins in the chest, as well as the left gastric and splenic veins in the abdomen.

Both parasympathetic and sympathetic nerves innervate the esophagus. Branches of the vagus nerve supply parasympathetic fibers that are motor to the muscle coat and secretomotor to the submucosal glands. The cervical and thoracic sympathetic chain and the celiac plexus provide sympathetic fibers that promote contraction of sphincters and relaxation of the esophageal body muscle, increase peristaltic and glandular activity, and cause vasoconstriction. These fibers enter the esophageal wall with the blood supply and form fibers and ganglia within it. The myenteric, Auerbach's plexus, is positioned between the longitudinal and circular layers of the muscularis propria and controls these muscles. The submucosal, Meissner's plexus, controls the muscularis mucosa and submucosal glands.

Regional Anatomy

The esophagus spans the lower neck, thoracic cavity, and upper abdomen (Figure 35-3). The anatomy of the esophagus is best divided into fifths: cervical, upper thoracic, middle thoracic, lower thoracic and abdominal esophagus. The anterior wall of the cervical esophagus is in intimate contact with posterior membranous trachea. The recurrent laryngeal nerves course anteriorly and laterally in the tracheoesophageal groove. The carotid sheaths bind the cervical esophagus laterally. The posterior wall of the cervical esophagus lies on the vertebral bodies.

The thoracic esophagus occupies the posterior mediastinum and passes anteriorly to the vertebral bodies. The upper thoracic esophagus lies posteriorly to the trachea and is bound laterally by the mediastinal pleura. In its lower left aspect, it is sandwiched between the azygous vein on the right and the aortic arch on the left. The middle thoracic esophagus lies behind the pulmonary hilum and between the azygous vein and the descending aorta. The lower thoracic esophagus has the same lateral and posterior boundaries, but lies behind the pericardium. The thoracic duct is situated between the azygous vein and the descending thoracic aorta and posteriorly and to the right of the lower and midthoracic esophagus. At approximately the level of the fourth thoracic vertebra it crosses the midline to become a left-sided structure.

The abdominal esophagus is cradled in the muscular esophageal hiatus. The inferior vena cava is on the right posterolateral aspect; the abdominal aorta is on the left posterolateral aspect. Superiorly, the left lateral segment of the liver overlies the esophagus and esophagogastric junction.

▶ ESOPHAGEAL FUNCTION

Swallowing has three phases: oral, pharyngeal, and esophageal. The action of swallowing is voluntarily initiated and is followed by a cascade of involuntary muscle activities that propels the swallowed bolus aborally (Figure 35-4). The esophageal phase of swallowing commences with the relaxation of the UES during the initiation of pharyngeal contraction. Food is pushed by pharyngeal contraction and pulled by the pressure differential between the hypopharynx (atmospheric pressure) and the thoracic esophagus (intrathoracic pressure) into the cervical esophagus. The duration of UES relaxation is between 0.5 and 1 s. After passage of the bolus, the UES contracts, reaching twice resting pressure. This pressure overshoot is the beginning of esophageal peristalsis.

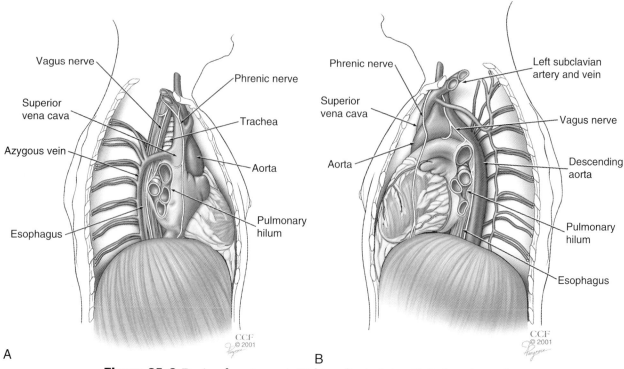

Figure 35–3 Regional anatomy. **A,** Right mediastinal view. **B,** Left mediastinal view.

The primary peristaltic wave is a progressive contraction activated by voluntary swallowing. With a conduction speed of 2–5 cm/s, this wave carries the bolus into the stomach in 4–8 s. The strength of the primary peristaltic contraction increases with propagation along the esophagus. In > 95% of wet swallows, a primary wave normally follows. If impaction occurs, esophageal distention produces closure of the upper esophageal sphincter and a secondary peristaltic wave begins at the site of obstruction and passes distally. Tertiary contractions are isolated contractions that have no function but can occur spontaneously between swallows. Tertiary waves that occur during or immediately after swallowing are abnormal.

Resting pressure of the LES exceeds intragastric pressure and prevents reflux of gastric contents into the distal esophagus. Upon pharyngeal contraction, the LES relaxes until the swallowed bolus passes into the stomach. The LES then contracts, overshooting resting pressure by two to three times before returning to resting pressure. Transient relaxation of the LES normally occurs following meals lasts 5–30 s and may play a role in belching.

▶ **EVALUATION OF THE ESOPHAGUS**

History and Physical Examination

Symptoms of esophageal dysfunction are heartburn, regurgitation, dysphagia and odynophagia. Other symptoms such as bad taste, sore throat, hoarseness, cough, globus, hiccup, aspiration pneumonia, asthma, chest pain, nausea, vomiting, bloating, hematemesis, and melena may be associated with esophageal diseases. Physical examination of the esophagus is indirect and focuses on head and neck, thoracic, and abdominal findings. History and physical examination should concentrate on uncovering systemic diseases with esophageal manifestations (Box 35-1).

Investigations

Barium Esophagram

Typically, barium esophagram is the initial screening examination for most patients with esophageal symptoms and suspected disorders of esophageal structure or function. Three phases of a multiphasic study assess the mucosa, contour, and function of the esophagus. The double-contrast phase, conducted with the patient ingesting high-density barium and CO_2 tablets in the upright position, examines the mucosa (Figure 35-5). Next, esophageal function is assessed in the right anterior oblique (RAO) position with the ingestion of low-density barium in single swallows at 20- to 30-s intervals (Figure 35-6). The examination is video taped. The value of attempting to elicit reflux in this phase is questionable because 20% of normal individuals will have radiological reflux.[100] Barium tablets, barium-coated marshmallows, or solids may demonstrate abnormalities not visualized by liquid barium studies. The final phase, the full-column technique, is performed with the patient in a semiprone RAO position with low-density barium. Multiple quick swallows produce a column of barium that fully distends the esophagus. This optimizes imaging of the distal esophagus and can demonstrate small hiatal hernias, subtle strictures, or distal rings (Figure 35-7). The esophagus is allowed to empty; the remaining barium coating of the collapsed esophagus provides a mucosal relief study, now rarely used.

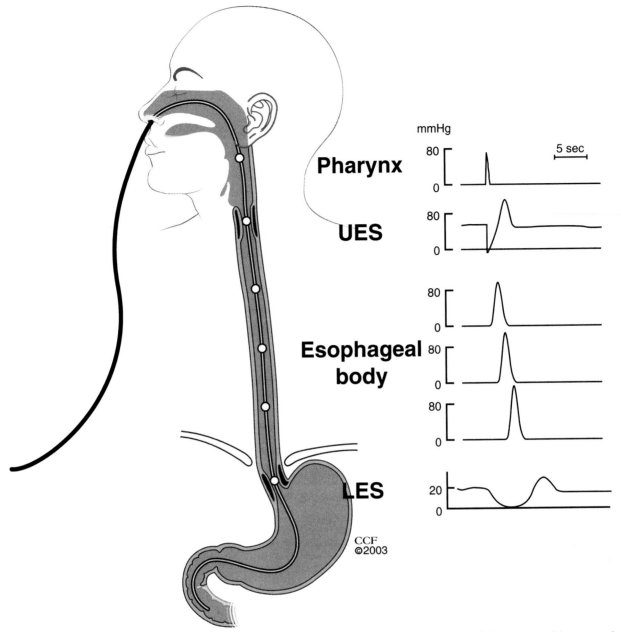

Figure 35–4 Esophageal function. Swallowing requires coordinated relaxation and contraction of the upper and lower esophageal sphincters (UES, LES) and adequate peristalsis of the esophageal body. On the right are the pressure profiles obtained by esophageal manometry in the pharynx, UES, three positions in the esophageal body, and LES during a swallow.

Timed barium esophagram is a simple test of esophageal function (Figure 35-8). After ingestion of a premeasured amount of barium, usually 250 ml, spot films are taken at 1-, 2-, and 5-min intervals and if necessary at 10 and 20 min after barium ingestion. This allows simple quantification of esophageal emptying and is useful for evaluations of both motility disorders and the results of therapy.[32,75]

Esophageal Manometry

Esophageal manometry is the primary evaluation of esophageal function. Water-perfused fine capillary tubes with side holes or solid-state microtransducers are used to study pressure profiles at rest and during swallowing. LES resting pressure, completeness, and duration of LES relaxation and LES length are measured (Figure 35-9 and Table 35-1). Theoretically, UES can be studied similarity, however, major differences between these two sphincters make UES evaluation less reliable. The UES is composed of striated muscle that has rapid contractions compared to the slow contractions of the LES smooth muscle. The pressure profile of the UES is asymmetric, with higher pressure in the anterior–posterior direction than in the lateral direction. Despite multiple techniques for measurement, assessment of the UES is less dependable and, thus, less useful than LES assessment. Morphology, amplitude, duration, and progression of esophageal peristalsis are evaluated in the esophageal body (Figure 35-9 and Table 35-1).

Box 35–1. Systemic Diseases of the Esophagus.

Connective tissue disorders
  Scleroderma
  Systemic lupus erythematosus
  Polymyositis
  Dermatomyositis
  Mixed connective tissue disorder
  Rheumatoid arthritis
  Sjögren's syndrome
  Raynaud's disease
Metabolic diseases
  Amyloidosis
  Diabetes mellitus
  Hypothyroidism
  Hyperthyroidism
Dermatological diseases
  Epidermolysis bullosa
  Phemphigus vulgaris
  Phemphigoid
  Erythema multiforme
  Lichen planus
  Behçet's disease
Infectious diseases
  Histoplasmosis
  Tuberculosis
  Actinomycosis
  Immunocompromised host
    Fungal
      Candida species
    Viral
      Herpes simplex
      Cytomegalovirus
    Mycobacterial
    Bacterial
      Streptococcus viridans
      Staphylococcus
      Bacilli
      Treponema pallidum
    Protozoal
Miscellaneous disorders
  Sarcoidosis
  Crohn's disease

Twenty-Four-Hour pH Monitoring

Ambulatory 24-h pH monitoring detects and quantifies gastroesophageal reflux. Therefore, this test is performed without acid suppression medication. Typically discontinued prior to testing are proton pump inhibitors at 1 week, H-2 blockers at 24 h, and antacids at 2 h. A pH probe, connected by a fine catheter passed through the nostril connected to a portable data logger, is placed 5 cm above the esophagogastric junction. Patients are instructed to have a "typical day" regarding activity and eating. Because symptom correlation is an important component of this test, the patient keeps a diary to record symptoms. After 24 h, the probe is removed and the data are transferred to a computer for data analysis. Dual probes record pH in the distal thoracic and cervical esophagus. Patients unable to tolerate the standard 24-h transnasal catheter receive the Bravo probe, a pH capsule with radio transmission capabilities. Placed by endoscopy it is temporarily "pinned" to the mucosa. It provides prolonged monitoring

and is not recovered after being sloughed from the mucosa and passed through the gastrointestinal (GI) tract.

A pH measurement below 4 has arbitrarily been chosen to define a reflux episode. The normal parameters for 24-h pH monitoring, based on this reference, have been defined (Table 35-2). Total acid exposure time, expressed as a percentage of study time, is the best discriminator between normal and abnormal; total number of reflux episodes is the most unreliable measure of excessive acid exposure.[85,141] Composite scores, such as the DeMeester score and frequency-duration index, are no better than the simple measured parameters in the identification of abnormal reflux. Indices assessing the relationship of symptoms to reflux episodes have also been proposed. However, these scores have not been prospectively studied in large groups.

Esophagoscopy and Endoscopic Esophageal Ultrasound

Esophagoscopy is used to visually assess mucosal and structural esophageal abnormalities. Biopsies of epithelial abnormalities such as esophagitis, mucosal nodules, columnar-lined segments, and strictures are an intricate part of flexible fiberoptic esophagoscopy. However, the biopsies are limited to the mucosa. Indirect evidence of deeper mural abnormalities or extraesophageal lesions may be appreciated by extrinsic compression or displacement of the overlying epithelium.

Endoscopic esophageal ultrasound (EUS) is an extension of fiberoptic esophagoscopy that provides further definition of the esophageal wall and periesophageal tissue. It is indispensable in the evaluation of abnormalities of the esophageal wall and for the diagnosis of nonmucosal esophageal tumors. Ultrasound endoscopes scan the wall with ultrasound waves of 7.5 and 12 MHZ. Probes, which can be passed through the biopsy channel of flexible endoscopes, can evaluate esophageal strictures that prevent passage of standard ultrasound equipment. The esophagus and periesophageal tissues are viewed as five alternating layers of different echogenicity (Figure 35-10). This examination also images periesophageal structures including regional lymph nodes. Both the layer of origin and ultrasound characteristics of a mass are critical in diagnosis of benign esophageal tumors. Periesophageal masses and regional lymph nodes can also be studied. EUS directed fine-needle aspiration (FNA) provides cytological and pathological assessment of esophageal tumors, periesophageal masses, and regional lymph nodes.

New Investigations

Bilitech 2000

Nonacid reflux can be detected using the Bilitec 2000 ambulatory bilirubin monitor.[133] This fiberoptic spechtrophotometer detects the presence of bilirubin, the principal component of bile by the absorption of the band of light (450 nm) characteristic for bilirubin. The probe is placed similarly to the 24-h pH probe and monitored in a similar fashion. The reflux of duodenodenal contents, duodenogastroesophageal reflux (DGER), mirrors that of acid and has a graded increase producing increasing esophageal injury. In the absence of acid, DGER can produce symptoms, but not esophageal injury. Therefore, the Bilitec probe is usually not of benefit in the evaluation of the patient with gastroesophageal reflux disease

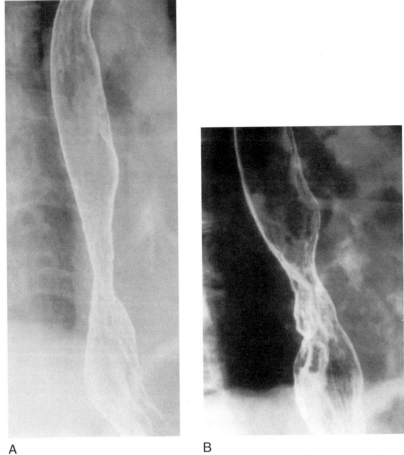

A   B

Figure 35–5 **Barium esophagram: mucosa.** Double contrast phase of the barium esophagram provides mucosal definition in (**A**) a patient with a hiatal hernia and peptic stricture. No significant ulceration is seen. (**B**) A patient with a columnar-lined esophagus, distal peptic stricture, ulcers, and nodules.

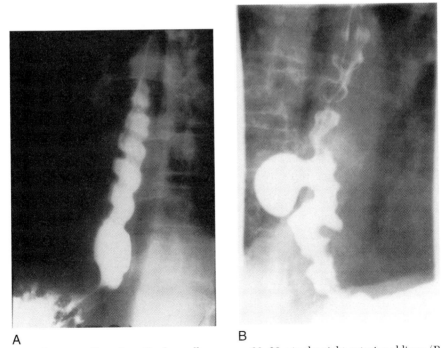

A   B

Figure 35–6 **Barium esophagram: function.** Single swallows every 20–30 s in the right anterior oblique (RAO) semiprone position assess esophageal function in (**A**) a patient with diffuse esophageal spasm (cork-screw esophagus) and in (**B**) a patient with a nonspecific motility disorder and a midthoracic diverticulum.

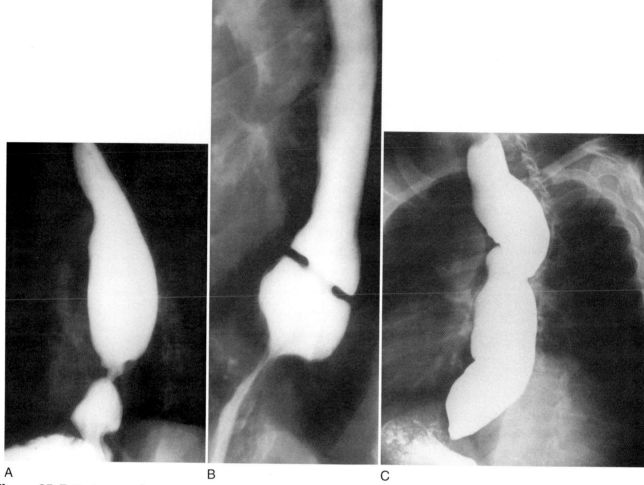

A   B   C

Figure 35–7 **Barium esophagram: contour.** The full column phase of the barium esophagram fills and fully distends the esophagus providing an examination of esophageal contour in (**A**) a patient with an obstructed esophagus due to a peptic stricture and associated nonreducible hiatal hernia, (**B**) a patient with a Schatzki's ring, and (**C**) a patient with achalasia.

(GERD). However, it is useful in the patient with previous esophagogastric surgery or the achlorhidric patient in whom symptoms are suggestive of reflux.

Esophageal Impedance

Multichannel intraluminal (MII) esophageal impedance is a new technique for assessment of esophageal function and GERD.[67,119,131] The measurement of impedance (resistance) to alternating current between two intraluminal electrodes allows detection of both the character and direction of a bolus. During swallowing, the baseline impedance of the esophageal mucosa rises abruptly as air, which has high impedance, precedes the bolus. As the bolus follows, impedance decreases because food has high ionic content and, thus, high electrical conductivity. Esophageal impedance remains low until the bolus passes out of the segment. There is an overshot of impedance above baseline. This is an artifact, the result of baseline mucosal impedance and the decreased esophageal cross-sectional area during peristalsis.

The combination of manometry and MII and 24-h pH monitoring and MII has allowed in-depth evaluation of motility disorders and the characterization of the refluxate in complicated GERD patients.

▶ BENIGN ESOPHAGEAL DISEASES AND THEIR TREATMENT

Hiatal Hernia

Herniation of abdominal contents through the esophageal hiatus is a common occurrence. With provocative maneuvers that increase intraabdominal pressure, 55% of patients undergoing barium esophagram were found to have herniation of the stomach into the chest.[126] Symptoms are secondary to reflux, incarceration or strangulation of herniated organs, or compression of thoracic structures. There are four types of hiatal hernia, each with its own symptom presentation. Type I, or sliding hiatal hernia, is the most common type (Figures 35-7A and 35-11). Herniation of the esophagogastric junction into the posterior mediastinum occurs because of thinning and elongation of the phrenoesophageal ligament. There is no potential for incarceration.

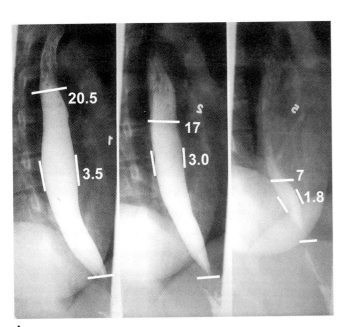

A

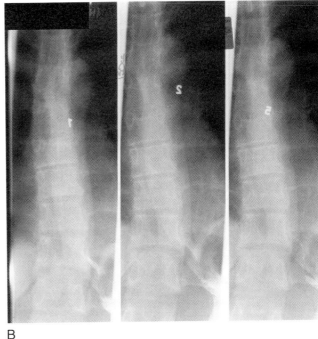

B

Figure 35–8 Timed-barium esophagram. A, Before Heller myotomy a patient was able to ingest only 70 ml of barium. The height (the barium-coated saliva is not included) and width of the column are measured at 1, 2, and 5 min after ingestion. Note markedly delayed esophageal emptying and incomplete emptying at 5 min. **B,** After Heller myotomy the ingestion of 70 ml of barium resulted in trace barium in the esophagus at 1 and 2 min and clearance by 5 min.

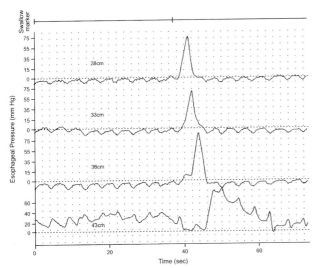

Figure 35–9 Normal esophageal manometry. The top three traces show normal esophageal peristalsis, both amplitude and conduction, after a 5-ml swallow. The bottom trace demonstrates a normal LES resting pressure, with relaxation to baseline on swallowing and overshoot on closing with return to normal resting pressure.
(Reproduced with permission from Adhami T, Shay SS: Esophageal motility in the assessment of esophageal function. Semin Thorac Cardiovasc Surg 13(3): 234–240, 2001.)

The majority of patients with type I hiatal hernias are asymptomatic. If symptoms occur they are GERD related. Type II hiatal hernias, or rolling hiatal hernias, are very uncommon (Figure 35-12). They result from a defect in or isolated weakness of the phrenoesophageal ligament, allowing a portion of the stomach to herniate through the hiatus while the esophagogastric junction remains anchored in the abdomen. Symptoms of gastric obstruction, strangulation, anemia, and, less commonly, shortness of breath and arrhythmia result from gastric herniation through the hiatus and the presence of the stomach in the chest. Type III, or mixed hiatal hernias, are the second most common type (Figure 35-13). Patients may present with either reflux or symptoms of type II hernias or both. As type III hernias increase in size, there may be organoaxial volvulus with the potential for strangulation. In many patients, these hernias may be a progression of type I hernias.[89] Type IV hiatal hernias contain the stomach and other abdominal contents such as colon, spleen, small bowel, and pancreas (Figure 35-14). The term paraesophageal hernia is sometimes used to describe any type II, III, or IV hiatal hernia.

Symptomatic hiatal hernias should be repaired. Repair of asymptomatic types II and III hernias is controversial. The potential for strangulation and gastric necrosis has been advocated as the prime reason to repair paraesophageal hernias in all patients, particularly since 50% mortality was initially reported when this complication occurred.[55] However, strangulation is an uncommon occurrence without antecedent symptoms; therefore this is an overestimate and careful follow-up of asymptomatic patients is a viable alternative to repair in all patients.

Repair follows the principles of surgical treatment of GERD. The addition of a fundoplication is controversial,

Table 35–1

Normal Values for Esophageal Manometry at The Cleveland Clinic Foundation[111]

	Normal[a]	High	Low
LES pressure (mm Hg)	24 ± 10	>45	<10
Contraction amplitude[b] (mm Hg)	99 ± 40	>180	<30
Contraction duration[b] (s)	3.9 ± .9	>7	<1.3

[a] Mean ± standard deviation.
[b] Mean of measurements at 3 and 8 cm above the LES.

Table 35–2

Normal Distal Values for 24-h pH Monitoring

Parameter	Johnson[65] 95th percentile	Richter[112] 95th percentile	Jamieson[64] Mean	Percentile
Total time (%)	4.45	5.78	4.5	95
Upright time (%)	8.42	8.15	7.1	93
Supine time (%)	3.45	3.45	1.5	86
No. of episodes	47	46	56	98
No. >5 min	3	4	3	94
Longest episode (min)	19.8	18.5	12	84
Composite score	14.7		16.7	96

From Adhami T, Richter JE: 24-hour monitoring in the assessment of esophageal function. Semin Thorac Cardiovasc Surg 13:241–253, 2001.

but is definitely indicated if symptomatic GERD is present. Laparoscopic repairs have been reported to have an earlier and increased rate of failure.[53] In most patients addition of a gastrostomy or gastropexy is not required.

Gastroesophageal Reflux Disease

Transient LES relaxation, a normal occurrence typically after meals, results in reflux of gastric contents into the esophagus that is rapidly cleared. However, failure of the antireflux barrier produces acid reflux of pathological proportions, GERD. The LES and diaphragmatic hiatal mechanism are the major components of the reflux barrier.[68,92] In patients with GERD there are LES abnormalities, including low resting pressures and inadequate length and a hiatal hernia in 50–90% of patients.[10,70,101,122] Rarely, there are demonstrable malfunctions of esophageal clearance, gastric emptying, or esophageal mucosal protection. Pathological reflux results in a progressive injury with inflammation, progressing to mucosal erosion, ulceration, and stricture. This injury can produce further abnormalities of esophageal peristalsis and LES function that perpetuates GERD. The mucosal response may produce metaplastic columnar lining (Barrett's esophagus) and the damage to the submucosa and muscularis propria can result in a short esophagus. The short columnar-lined esophagus with peptic stricture and the development of high-grade dysplasia or intramucosal carcinoma in a columnar-lined esophagus are the final phases of GERD (Figures 35-5 and 35-7A).

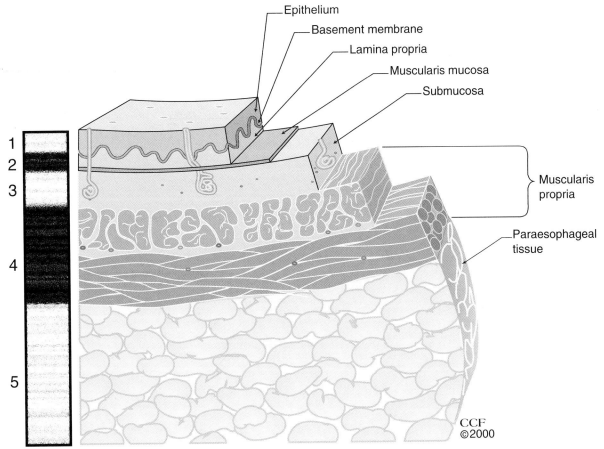

Figure 35–10 **The esophageal wall is visualized as five alternating layers of differing echogenicity by EUS.** The first (inner) layer is hyperechoic (white) and represents the superficial mucosa (epithelium and lamina propria). The second layer is hypoechoic (black) and represents the deep mucosa (muscularis mucosae). The third layer is hyperechoic and represents the submucosa. The fourth layer is hypoechoic and represents the muscularis propria. The fifth layer is hyperechoic and represents the paraesophageal tissue. The thickness of ultrasound layers does not equal the actual thickness of the anatomic layers.

The typical symptoms of GERD are acid reflux, regurgitation, and dysphagia. Other symptoms, such as chest-pain, asthma, and laryngitis, are termed atypical symptoms and are less likely to be attributable to acid reflux and are, thus, less likely to respond to treatment. Successful control of symptoms with proton pump inhibitors (PPIs) is an excellent clinical confirmation of suspected GERD. Investigation must confirm that abnormal reflux is present by 24-h pH monitoring and the presence of mucosal injury confirmed by esophagoscopy and biopsy. Further, it must define the structural and functional abnormalities via barium esophagram and manometry. In patients with suspected gastric drainage abnormalities, a nuclear medicine gastric emptying study is required. The presence of typical symptoms that respond to PPI therapy and the presence of abnormal acid exposure, determined by 24-h pH monitoring, are reliable predictors of successful surgical treatment of GERD.[22,121]

The mainstay of therapy for GERD is medical management. PPI can heal esophagitis in over 90% of patients. Indications for surgical management of uncomplicated GERD are volume regurgitation not controlled with PPI, the prospect of life-long therapy in a young patient, and side effects or tolerance of medical therapy. Atypical symptoms are less likely to respond to surgical therapy, particularly if they are not associated with typical GERD symptoms. That a patient has no symptomatic relief with medical management should alert the surgeon that GERD is probably not present and that this patient is unlikely to benefit from surgery. Initially, complicated GERD is usually managed with aggressive medical therapy; however, peptic esophageal stricture and chronic Barrett's ulcer may require surgery. The columnar-lined esophagus is not in itself an indication for surgery. It is debatable that surgery can reverse the changes of columnar lining. Partial reversal, although interesting, is not a compelling argument for surgical correction of GERD.[52] Effective reflux control may reduce the incidence of malignant degeneration in the columnar-lined esophagus. However, failure of antireflux repairs is frequently seen in patients with adenocarcinoma of the esophagus. Patients with columnar-lined esophagi have the most disordered physiology, largest hernias, and most disrupted hiatal mechanisms.[20] Therefore, either prevention of or halting malignant degeneration in a columnar-lined esophagus is not an indication for surgery. If a patient with a columnar-lined esophagus has antireflux surgery, the need for endoscopic surveillance is not eliminated. Therefore, the patient with a columnar-lined esophagus has the same indications for surgery as the patient with a squamous-lined esophagus.

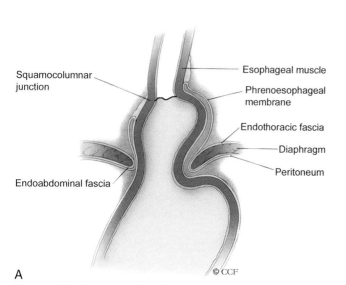

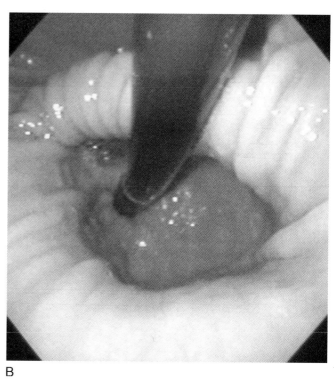

A   B

Figure 35–11 **Type I hiatal hernia. A,** Pictorial presentation. **B,** Retroflexed view from the intraabdominal stomach at esophagoscopy. The diaphragmatic impression and intrathoracic stomach can be seen.

The principles of antireflux surgery are the restoration of the intraabdominal length of esophagus, reconstruction of the esophageal hiatus, and reinforcement of the LES. These can be accomplished by a number of approaches and techniques. Possible approaches in descending order of morbidity are thoracoabdominal, thoracotomy, laparotomy, and laparoscopy. Facility with all of these approaches is necessary.

Restoration of the intraabdominal esophagus requires the reduction of the hiatal hernia and mobilization of the esophagus. This portion of the operation necessitates recognition of the short esophagus.[43] Failure to lengthen the short esophagus by extensive esophageal mobilization to the aortic arch or by the addition of a Collis gastroplasty will result in a repair under tension and early failure. The short esophagus should be suspected by a history of a stricture or previous dilation or the findings of a long segment columnar-lined esophagus, a large type I hiatal hernia (>4 cm), a type III hiatal hernia, or the failure of the hernia to reduce below the diaphragm on upright barium esophagram.

The importance of reconstruction of the hiatus cannot be underestimated. It plays a role in reflux prevention equal to that of the LES. The recent addition of mesh reinforcement of the hiatal closure ignores the past history of antireflux surgery and the dynamic nature of this structure. Complete mobilization of the hiatal crura and careful removal of the hernia sac will allow primary suture reconstruction of the hiatus. Failure to reconstruct the hiatus is a common cause of failure of laparoscopic antireflux surgery.[61] It is usually tension upon the repair, because of ignoring or not recognizing the short esophagus and not an unbutressed reconstruction of the hiatus that is the principal reason for reherniation after an otherwise adequate repair.

The final step in the surgical correction of GERD is the reinforcement of the LES by the construction of a fundoplication, which may be either a total or partial fundoplication. The Nissen fundoplication, which is a 360° total fundoplication, completely encircles the esophagus. Partial fundoplication is typically 270° and is either anteriorly placed, Belsey Mark IV, or posteriorly placed, Toupet. Theoretically, the trade-off is between better reflux control with a total fundoplication and less dysphagia with a partial fundoplication. Although some surgeons tailor the fundoplication to suit the peristaltic activity of the esophageal body,[140] in all but the patient with an aperistaltic esophagus will a total fundo-

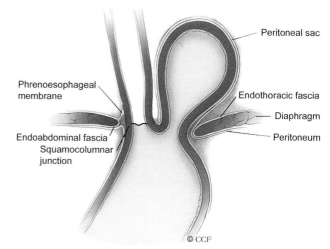

Figure 35–12 **Type II hiatal hernia.**

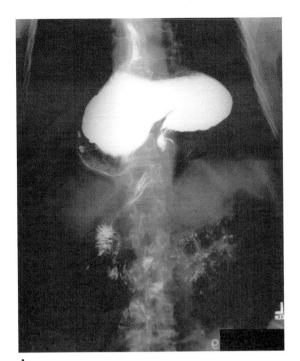
A

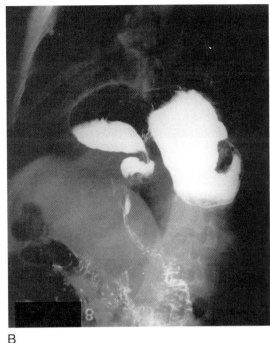
B

Figure 35–13 Type III hiatal hernia. A barium esophagram demonstrates a type III hiatal hernia with organoaxial rotation. **A,** Posteroanterior view. **B,** Lateral view.

plication be appropriate.[11,54,85,114,127] The use of a partial fundoplication in the face of complicated GERD is associated with increased incidence of failed repairs.[58] Dysphagia following surgery for GERD is usually transient with a properly constructed fundoplication. Prolonged dysphagia is an indication of a malformed fundoplication—a long, tight, or twisted fundoplication. Return of normal esophageal motility with resolution of GERD following fundoplication is hypothetically possible. It is more likely that the amplitude of the peristaltic wave will increase than failure of propagation will be corrected. Therefore any fundoplication should be constructed assuming the peristaltic abnormalities will not

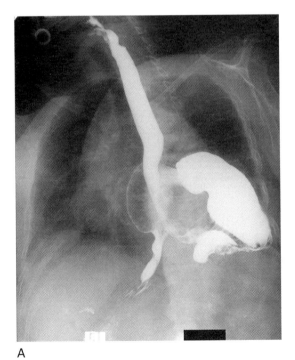
A

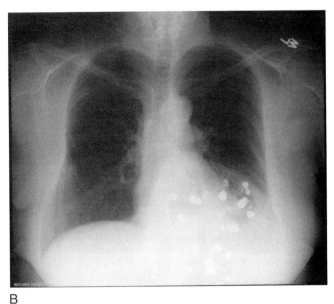
B

Figure 35–14 Type IV hiatal hernia. **A,** Barium esophagram demonstrates a type III hiatal hernia with organoaxial rotation. Three days later, barium is seen in colonic diverticulum on the preoperative chest X-ray. **B,** Posteroanterior view.

(Continued)

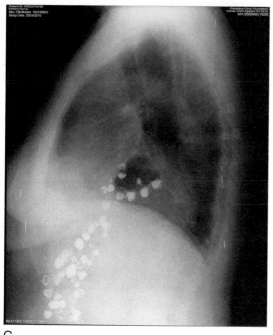

C

Figure 35–14 cont'd C, Lateral view. Therefore this is a Type IV hiatal hernia.

improve. Finally the potential for postprandial symptoms of gas bloat and early satiety must be mentioned to any patient being considered for fundoplication.

Antireflux operations are not infinitely durable. It is important that all patients are instructed in the avoidance of activities that excessively increase intraabdominal pressure and maintain their ideal weight. Unrealistic expectations of patients and the widespread application of laparoscopic fundoplication without careful patient selection in low volume centers by inexperienced surgical teams have produced poor results and have negatively impacted this operative approach.[56,110,135]

Motility Disorders

Achalasia

Achalasia is a degenerative esophageal disease culminating in aperistalsis of the esophageal body and abnormal relaxation of the lower esophageal sphincter. The underlying cause of this T cell-mediated destruction and eventual fibrous replacement of the esophageal myenteric neural plexus is unknown.[25,44,46] Patients complain of progressive dysphagia, regurgitation, and weight loss. Chest pain is reported more commonly in younger patients and manifests early on in the disease; however, it typically affects a minority of patients and, therefore is not a major complaint. Recurrent respiratory infection, aspiration pneumonia, and lung abscess may be initial presentations and herald advanced disease. Most patients seek medical attention only after significant and irreversible damage to the esophageal myenteric neural plexus has occurred.

Barium esophagogram is the single best diagnostic test for achalasia. Classic findings are esophageal dilation, aperistalsis, impaired esophageal emptying, and symmetrical tapering

at the esophagogastric junction (bird's beak or ace of spades appearance) (Figure 35-7C). Timed barium esophagogram allows quantification of esophageal obstruction and emptying (Figure 35-8). Manometry is the key diagnostic test. The diagnosis suggested by barium esophagram is confirmed by manometry. Achalasia is defined by incomplete or failed relaxation of the lower esophageal sphincter and aperistalsis of the esophageal body (Figure 35-15). Since the resting LES pressure is normal in 40% of patients, an elevated LES pressure is not required for diagnosis.[47,120] Esophagoscopy is essential to exclude pseudoachalasia (secondary esophageal obstruction secondary to malignancies), which may be clinically indistinguishable from primary achalasia. Biopsy during esophagoscopy is necessary to assess the esophageal mucosa.

Symptom relief is no longer the measure of successful outcome, since 30% of treated patients with symptom control have poor esophageal emptying by barium radiographs.[134] The treatment of achalasia is palliative and directed at reduction of lower esophageal sphincter pressure and improvement of esophageal emptying. Calcium channel blockers and long acting nitrates relax smooth muscle and provide transient, but incomplete, relief of symptoms. Unpleasant side effects may limit their use. The persistence of dysphagia, despite reduction of lower esophageal sphincter pressure in a placebo-controlled study of nifedipine, emphasizes the inadequacy of medical management of achalasia.[129]

Endoscopic injection of botulinum toxin has been used to treat achalasia. Palliation is temporary, lasting 6 months, with recurrent symptoms in more than 50% of patients.[130] Resistance to repeat injections is thought to be the result of antibody production against botulinum toxin. The use of botulinum toxin may complicate future surgery, because it causes inflammation and fibrosis in the plane between the submucosa and muscularis propria.[15,40,57] This therapy is reserved for patients who cannot tolerate definitive palliation.

Pneumatic dilation with modern instruments is successful in controlling symptoms. A summary of 13 studies (359 patients dilated with Rigiflex pneumatic dilators) demonstrated symptom palliation in 74% of patients dilated with a 3-cm balloon, 86% with a 3.5-cm balloon and 90% with a 4-cm balloon.[132] Esophageal perforation from individual series varied from 0 to 7% and averaged 2%.

Open modified Heller myotomy performed transabdominally or transthoracically has been successful in the treatment of achalasia. Two prospective studies have been reported comparing pneumatic dilation to myotomy.[33,38] After 4.8 years of follow-up, laparotomy and myotomy provided symptom control in 95% of patients while pneumatic dilation with the Mosher system provided symptom control in 65%.[33] In a small randomized study of 40 patients there was no difference between modalities, except myotomy was associated with a lower LES pressure and less reflux.[38]

Laparoscopic Heller myotomy results in shorter hospital stay, reduced morbidity, and more rapid return to work than either thoracotomy or laparotomy. These improvements have renewed interest in the surgical management of achalasia. With short follow-up (mean of 1 year) good to excellent symptom control is seen in 94% of patients, but 11% of patients reported reflux.[132] Preoperative pneumatic dilation has been reported to increase the risk of intraoperative esophageal perforation during laparoscopic Heller myotomy.[93]

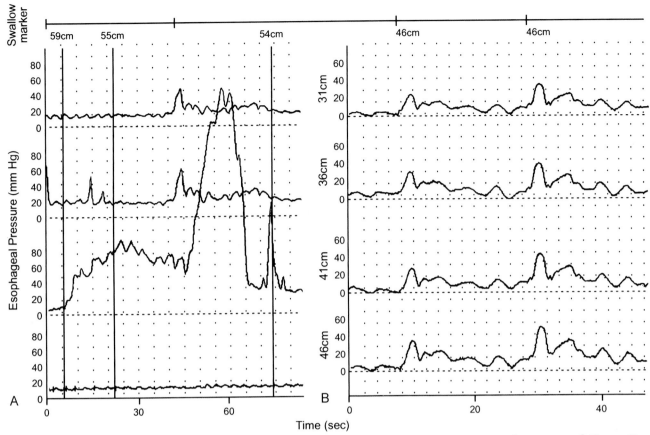

Figure 35–15 **Esophageal motility in achalasia. A,** LES pressure measured in the lower tracing has a mean of 60 mm Hg, no relaxation with wet swallow, and an exaggerated overshoot. **B,** Peristalsis is absent in the esophageal body. All traces show a simultaneous isobaric tertiary contraction (common cavity phenomena) of 30 mm Hg with the first swallow and 45 mm Hg with the second swallow. *[Reproduced with permission from Adhami T, Shay SS: Esophageal motility in the assessment of esophageal function. Semin Thorac Cardiovasc Surg 13(3):234–240, 2001.]*

Regardless of the surgical approach, the extent of myotomy is critical to good long-term outcome. A 3-cm extension of the myotomy onto the stomach is superior to a lesser myotomy for symptomatic and physiological effects.[97] Controversy continues over the need for fundoplication added to myotomy. A fundoplication has been reported to be less essential when a thoracotomy is used. This finding most likely reflects a lesser myotomy. However, with the adoption of longer extensions of the myotomy onto the stomach, it is prudent to add a partial fundoplication to reduce reflux.

Failure to reduce lower esophageal sphincter pressure or the production of acid reflux by either pneumatic dilation or Heller myotomy may produce a dilated sigmoid esophagus, which may require esophagectomy.[7,91,99,105,106]

Hypermotility Disorders

Diffuse esophageal spasm is characterized by simultaneous, nonperistaltic, repetitive high-amplitude contractions of the esophageal body. Contractions may occur spontaneously or with swallowing. The etiology of this rare motility disorder is unknown. Patients complain of chest pain, which frequently prompts an extensive cardiac evaluation. Dysphagia is a common accompanying symptom. Barium esophagram demonstrates a normal upper esophagus with a corkscrew pattern in the smooth muscle (distal two thirds) portion of the esophagus (Figure 35-6A). Esophageal manometry is diagnostic and shows uncoordinated esophageal motility. This disorder is defined by simultaneous contractions following >20% swallows with intermittent peristalsis and abnormalities of contraction that include repetitive, prolonged, and retrograde contractions. LES function is usually normal but both abnormal relaxation and hypertensive resting pressure have been reported.

Because this disorder is poorly understood, few treatment options exist. It is a dynamic disorder that uncommonly evolves into other motility disorders. Similarities to spastic bowel and associated psychiatric abnormalities in up to 80% of patients with esophageal contraction abnormalities have led to treatments aimed at removal of triggering stimuli or mild sedation.[26,27] Calcium channel blockers and nitrates have also been used for symptom control. Botulinum toxin injections have successfully controlled symptoms in selected patients. Pneumatic dilation has been used for patients with poor relaxation or hypertensive lower esophageal sphincter. A long myotomy extending from the aortic arch to the proximal stomach provides stomach pro-

598 vides good to excellent symptom control in 70% of patients refractory to medical therapy.[33]

Nutcracker esophagus is characterized by hyperperistalsis of the distal esophagus with contractions at least 2 standard deviations above normal. These patients have psychiatric disturbances similar to those with diffuse spasm. Chest pain and dysphagia are managed medically. However, therapeutic maneuvers that reduce hyperperistalsis are not necessarily associated with symptom amelioration. Myotomy has unpredictable results and surgical treatment should be avoided, if possible, in these patients.[39,128]

An LES resting pressure of more than 45 mm Hg accompanied by normal relaxation and normal peristalsis of the esophageal body characterizes hypertensive lower esophageal sphincter. Conservative medical therapy and bouginage are the treatments of choice of this rare motility disorder. Myotomy is rarely required.

Many abnormalities of the esophageal body or LES do not follow these patterns (Figure 35-6B). Despite all attempts to classify motility disorders, nonspecific motility disorders exist. These must remain classified as nonspecific to avoid incorrect categorization as part of a named abnormality, and, thus, prevent false diagnosis and incorrect therapy.

Secondary Esophageal Motility Disorders

Scleroderma or progressive systemic sclerosis is a systemic disease that commonly results in esophageal dysfunction. Fibrosis, collagen deposition, and patchy smooth muscle atrophy are histological hallmarks of esophageal involvement. Skeletal muscle is unaffected. Destruction of esophageal smooth muscle results in diminished peristalsis of the lower esophagus and a hypotensive lower esophageal sphincter. Reflux and dysphagia are common complaints. Therapy includes aggressive acid suppression with potent proton pump inhibitors and dilation of strictures. Surgery usually requires esophageal lengthening (Collis gastroplasty) and a partial fundoplication.[98] For extensive, unrepairable esophageal disease, resection may be required.

Neurological and muscular disorders such as stroke, amyotrophic lateral sclerosis, and muscular dystrophies may be accompanied by esophageal dysfunction. Esophageal involvement is also seen in patients with diabetes and/or alcoholic neuropathy. Metastatic carcinoma may mimic achalasia.

Diverticula

A diverticulum is an outpouching that protrudes from the gastrointestinal wall. True diverticula contain all layers of the gastrointestinal wall and are uncommon in the esophagus. Most esophageal diverticula consist of mucosa, submucosa, and strands of muscle fibers and are, therefore, false diverticula. The mechanisms by which diverticula develop are not completely understood. However, diverticula are termed pulsion, traction, or congenital, according to the suspected mechanism of formation. A pulsion diverticulum usually occurs at or proximal to an esophageal sphincter or proximal to areas of prolonged or increased pressure. They are assumed to be due to excessive outward pressure on the gastrointestinal wall. Generally, these are false diverticula. Traction diverticula result from forces arising outside the gastrointestinal wall and are usually true diverticula. They are far less common and are found adjacent to regions of periesophageal inflammation such as chronic lymphadenitis.

Diverticula of the esophagus are most commonly acquired pulsion and can be located anywhere along the esophagus. Traction and congenital diverticula are rare. There are three common anatomic sites of focal diverticula. Proximally, they occur in the hypopharyngeal or pharyngoesophageal region. Midesophageal diverticula are seen near the tracheal carina. Distal or epiphrenic diverticula appear within a few centimeters of the gastroesophageal junction.

Zenker's Diverticulum

Zenker's diverticulum is the most common esophageal diverticulum and occurs above the cricopharyngeus at Killian's triangle. Typically, it is located opposite the C6 or C7 vertebral body (Figure 35-16). Cook et al demonstrated incomplete upper esophageal sphincter opening in patients with Zenker's diverticula.[29] Over time, a permanent narrow-mouthed outpouching of the posterior pharynx and esophagus develops and enlarges inferiorly. As a result, saliva and ingested foodstuffs pool dependently in the sac and cannot empty easily into the esophagus.

Early on, patients may complain of a vague sensation or sticking in their throat, intermittent cough, excessive salivation, and intermittent solid food dysphagia. These minor symptoms may be dismissed as globus hystericus. As the sac enlarges, symptoms worsen as dysphagia becomes more frequent. This usually occurs in patients who are older than 50 years. Gurgling sounds during swallowing, regurgitation of undigested food ingested, halitosis, voice change, retrosternal pain, and respiratory problems may be accompanying

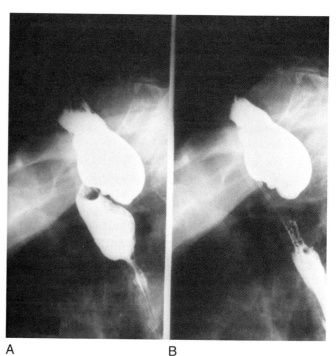

A   B

Figure 35–16 Zenker's diverticulum. Lateral view during barium esophagram shows (**A**) a large diverticulum that (**B**) does not clear with repeated swallowing.

symptoms. To aid swallowing, patients utilize unusual maneuvers such as throat clearing, coughing, or placing manual pressure on the neck. In rare cases, the diverticulum can become large enough to obstruct the esophagus. A neck mass may be observed in these patients. The most serious complication associated with a Zenker's diverticulum is aspiration that can lead to pneumonia or lung abscess. Perforation, hemorrhage or carcinoma may complicate Zenker's diverticula.

A Zenker's diverticulum is best identified and evaluated by barium esophagram. Endoscopy is rarely indicated. Manometric testing of the cricopharyngeal area should be reserved for clinical research subjects and atypical patients and, generally, is not necessary.

Treatment goals of Zenker's diverticula are to increase upper esophageal sphincter compliance and reduce the resting pressure in the cricopharyngeus. This can be accomplished endoscopically by creating an esophagodiverticulostomy with an endoscopic stapler.[28] Mid-term results with this technique are excellent.[103] An open surgical myotomy is adequate treatment for small diverticula. For large diverticula, a myotomy with suspension or excision of the diverticulum is indicated.[79] Both of these procedures provide similar outcomes with the same incidence of complications.[14,78]

Midthoracic Diverticula

Midthoracic diverticula usually develop within 4–5 cm of the tracheal carina. Until recently, these diverticula were commonly caused by traction secondary to mediastinal fibrosis and/or chronic lymphadenopathy from pulmonary tuberculosis or histoplasmosis. Many patients with these diverticula are found to have abnormal peristaltic waves from achalasia, diffuse esophageal spasm, or other nonspecific esophageal motor disorders (Figure 35-6B).[71,116]

Patients with midesophageal diverticula may be asymptomatic; however, a history of dysphagia, retrosternal pain, regurgitation, belching, epigastric pain, heartburn, and weight loss may be elicited. Although attributed to the diverticulum, these symptoms may be the result of the associated motor disorder. Complications are unusual, but spontaneous rupture, hemorrhage, aspiration, esophagobronchial fistula, and carcinoma have been reported.

Most patients with midthoracic diverticula require no treatment. Borrie and Wilson reported that although 80% of patients have a proven motility disorder, only 20% required surgery.[16] Diverticulectomy with esophageal myotomy is the preferred treatment for midthoracic diverticula associated with esophageal motility disorders. Right thoracotomy provides excellent exposure of the esophagus and airway at the tracheal bifurcation. Placing a bougie in the esophagus avoids compromise of the esophageal lumen and helps guide diverticulectomy. The mural defect should be repaired in two layers: the mucosal and submucosal layers closed with a continuous absorbable suture and the muscularis propria reapproximated with interrupted absorbable sutures. The esophageal repair may be buttressed with pleura, pleuropericardial fat pad, or omentum. A myotomy can be carried out on the esophageal wall opposite the diverticulectomy. Diverticulopexy with suspension of the diverticulum superiorly from the prevertebral fascia,[34] a myotomy alone,[37] and diverticulectomy alone[36] have been

successfully applied in the treatment of midthoracic esophageal diverticula. Treatment of true traction diverticulum, secondary to periesophageal inflammation, is often in the setting of an esophagobronchial fistula. Excision of the diverticulum, repair of the esophagus, removal of inflammatory nodes, closure of the airway fistula, and interposition of muscle are required.

Epiphrenic Diverticula

Epiphrenic diverticula occur in the distal third of the esophagus, usually within 10 cm of the gastroesophageal junction. There is an associated esophageal motor disorder; in general, a combination of abnormal peristalsis and anomalies in LES relaxation. These patients may have achalasia, diffuse esophageal spasm, or a nonspecific motility disorder. A hiatal hernia and associated esophageal dysmotility may be present with an epiphrenic diverticulum. Epiphrenic diverticula are occasionally asymptomatic, but those seen with motility disorders present with dysphagia, regurgitation, vomiting, chest and epigastric pain, anorexia, weight loss, cough, halitosis, or noisy swallowing. There is no apparent relationship between symptoms and the size of the diverticulum.

Barium esophagram best identifies epiphrenic diverticula and often characterizes the underlying motility disorder (Figure 35-17). Many patients show bizarre, nonpropulsive tertiary contractions during the examination. In addition to fixed, wide-mouthed diverticula, transient outpouchings can occur proximally in segments where peristalsis is absent. The timed barium esophagogram may be used in any patient in whom an emptying disorder is suspected, particularly in achalasia (Figure 35-8). Esophagoscopy generally yields little information about diverticula, but may rule out malignancy and assess associated esophageal problems. For the patient with a suspected motility disorder, esophageal motility is essential. Esophagoscopy may be required to pass the manometry catheter past the diverticulum into the stomach.

Although a good outcome has been achieved with diverticulectomy alone, the standard operation has become myotomy and diverticulectomy.[9,41] The addition of an antireflux procedure to diverticulectomy and myotomy is controversial. However, if added, a partial (nonobstructing) wrap, such as a Belsey, Toupet, or Dor fundoplication, may minimize postoperative dysphagia.

Benign Esophageal Tumors and Cysts

Benign esophageal tumors are uncommon and represent less than 1% of esophageal neoplasms. EUS is essential in the diagnosis. Thus, classification by layer of origin in the esophageal wall is the most clinically useful categorization of benign esophageal tumors (Box 35-2).

Tumors of the Mucosa

Squamous papillomas are small (<1 cm), solitary, sessile projections in the distal esophagus and are usually found incidentally.[109] Histological evaluation shows vascularized projections of the lamina propria covered by hyperplastic squamous epithelium. Biopsy differentiates squamous

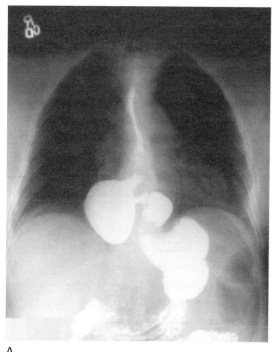

A

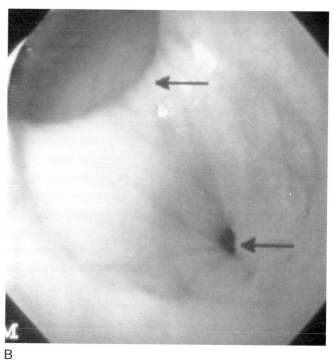

B

Figure 35–17 **Epiphrenic diverticulum. A,** Barium esophagram shows a large diverticulum. **B,** At esophagoscopy the wide mouth diverticulum *(upper arrow)* and the deviated distal esophageal lumen *(lower arrow)* are seen. The preferential filling of the diverticulum with swallowing can be appreciated from this examination.

papillomas from small superficial squamous cell carcinomas. Since progression to malignancy is rare, asymptomatic patients require no follow-up. Symptomatic papillomas or those with atypical histological features require excision, usually endoscopic. Although their cause is unknown, associations with human papilloma virus and gastroesophageal reflux have been reported.[107]

Fibrovascular polyps are collections of fibrous, vascular, and adipose tissue lined by normal squamous epithelium. These polyps, which usually arise in the cervical esophagus and extend into the esophageal lumen, may reach into the stomach. Most patients complain of dysphagia and respira-

tory symptoms.[80] Regurgitation into the hypopharynx with subsequent aspiration and asphyxia is possible. These lesions can be detected by either barium esophagram or esophagoscopy (Figure 35-18). Because fibrovascular polyps fill the esophageal lumen and have a composition similar to the mucosa, definition by esophagoscopy or EUS may be difficult or impossible.[117] Most polyps are surgically treated, although some have been removed endoscopically. Recurrence after resection is rare.

Tumors of the Submucosa

At esophagoscopy, lipomas are noted as a bulging of the overlying esophageal mucosa. They have a pale yellow appearance and soft or pillow-like texture when probed endoscopically. Esophagoscopic biopsies demonstrate only normal squamous epithelium because forceps rarely penetrate the submucosa. EUS demonstrates a hyperechoic homogeneous lesion that originates in and is confined to the submucosal layer. If asymptomatic, only observation is required.

Fibromas and neurofibromas are very uncommon. At endoscopy, unlike lipomas, they are firm "to the touch." These lesions, which arise from the submucosa, are less hyperechoic than lipomas by EUS. Symptomatic submucosal tumors have been enucleated with minimally invasive techniques.[115]

Granular cell tumors are of neural origin and arise from Schwann cells. The majority of patients with granular cell tumors are asymptomatic and rarely require surgery.[45] At endoscopy, these lesions are yellow, firm nodules, which can be diagnosed by routine endoscopic biopsies (Figure 35-19). On EUS, granular cell tumors arise from the submucosa and are hyperechoic but less so than lipomas.[102] Nests of cells with

---

Box 35–2. Classification of Benign Esophageal Tumors.

Mucosa (First and Second EUS layers)
    Squamous papilloma
    Fibrovascular polyp
    Retention cyst
Submucosa (Third EUS layer)
    Lipoma
    Fibroma
    Neurofibroma
    Granular cell tumor
    Hemangiomas
    Salivary gland-type tumor
Muscularis propria (Fourth EUS layer)
    Leiomyoma
    Duplication cyst
Periesophageal tissue (Fifth EUS layer)
    Foregut cyst

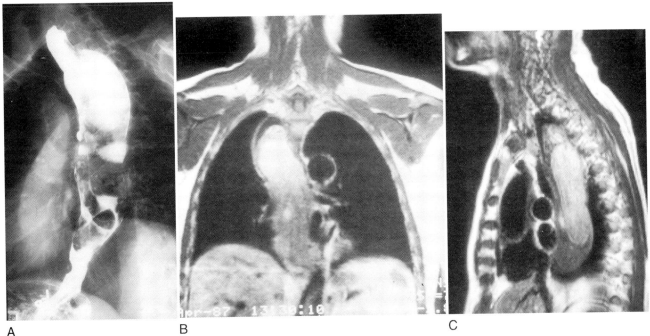

A   B   C

Figure 35–18 **Fibrovascular polyp. A,** A large polypoid filling defect of the intrathoracic esophagus is seen. **B, C,** MRI examination of the tumor demonstrates a large soft tissue mass filling the esophagus.

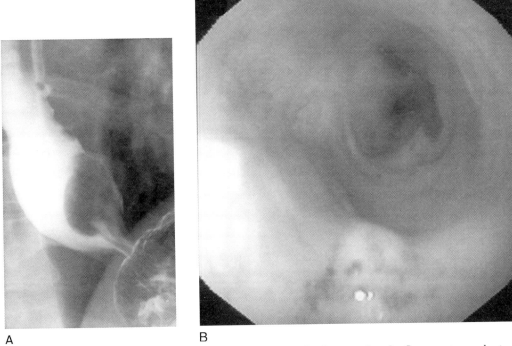

A   B

Figure 35–19 **Granular cell tumor. A,** In a patient with dysphagia and acid reflux symptoms a barium esophagram shows a polypoid filling defect in the distal esophagus. **B,** Esophagoscopy of another patient with a granular call tumor shows a tumor that is extraepithelial. Biopsy of this tumor was diagnostic for granular cell tumor.

pyknotic nuclei, abundant granular cytoplasm, absence of mitotic figures, and strong S-100 protein expression characterize these tumors. Malignant variants have been reported.[45,102]

Hemangiomas can present with dysphagia and bleeding. Most are found in the lower esophagus where they may be mistaken for esophageal varices. EUS examination reveals a hypoechoic mass with sharp margins arising from the second or third EUS layer.[6,84] Treatment options include observation, simple excision, fulgarization, or radiotherapy.[51] Salivary gland-type tumors have been rarely reported in the

602 esophagus and probably arise from submucosal esophageal glands.

Tumors of the Muscularis Propria

Leiomyomas are benign smooth muscle tumors of the muscularis propria. They are the most common benign esophageal tumors and account for more than 70% of these neoplasms. Most arise from the inner circular muscle layer of the distal and midthoracic esophagus. They have no gender preponderance and typically occur in younger patients (20–50 years old) than in esophageal cancer. Although frequently asymptomatic and discovered incidentally, leiomyomas can cause dysphagia, pain, or bleeding. In addition, distal esophageal leiomyomas are often associated with symptoms of GERD. Barium esophagram demonstrates smooth-contoured filling defects. At esophagoscopy and EUS, a normal overlying mucosa is seen over a hypoechoic tumor arising from the fourth ultrasound layer (Figure 35-20). Atypical EUS findings are a tumor 4 cm or larger, irregular margins, mixed internal echo characteristics, and associated regional lymphadenopathy. Definitive diagnosis is difficult to obtain since endoscopic biopsies do not reach the muscularis propria and EUS-directed FNA does not provide enough information to differentiate leiomyomas from leiomyosarcomas.

Symptomatic neoplasms should be resected. For asymptomatic tumors with typical EUS features expectant therapy and EUS observation are indicated. Leiomyosarcomas are exceedingly rare,[104] and malignant transformation of benign leiomyomas has been infrequently reported.[118]

Esophageal Cysts

Esophageal cysts are the second most common benign esophageal tumor accounting for 20% of these lesions. The minority are acquired epithelial cysts, arising in the lamina propria.[59] Submucosal glandular inflammation is the suspected cause. The majority of esophageal cysts are congenital foregut cysts.[96] They are lined with squamous, respiratory, or columnar epithelium and may contain smooth muscle, cartilage, or fat. An esophageal duplication is a type of foregut cyst; it is lined with squamous epithelium and its submucosal and muscularis elements interdigitate with the muscularis propria of the esophagus. Duplication cysts may be associated with vertebral and spinal cord abnormalities. Many foregut cysts present in the first year of life with life-threatening respiratory compromise due to mass effect. EUS can clearly define the intramural or extraesophageal nature of these tumors and further determine their anechoic, cystic nature (Figure 35-21).[12,35,82,87] Regardless, removal of all discovered cysts is suggested since most become symptomatic by adulthood.[125] In addition, transesophageal drainage has also been reported, but drainage of the cyst without destruction of its lining often results in recurrence.[77]

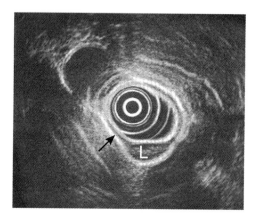

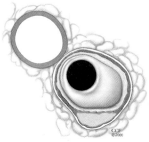

Figure 35–20 An esophageal leiomyoma (L). A, EUS of this most common benign tumor demonstrates a hypoechoic, homogeneous, well-demarcated tumor with no associated lymphadenopathy. EUS balloon overdistention blends the first three ultrasound layers into one hyperechoic layer. The tumor arises from and is confined to the fourth ultrasound layer (*arrow*). **B,** A benign leiomyoma arises from and is confined to the muscularis propria.

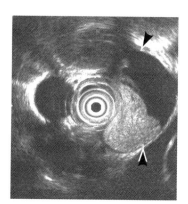

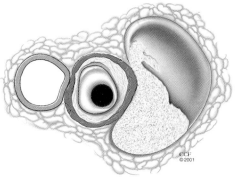

Figure 35–21 A foregut cyst. A, EUS demonstrates a mass (*arrows*) adjacent to the trachea and esophagus. The cyst has two components, one hyperechoic (white) representing proteinaceous material and one hypoechoic (black) representing fluid. **B,** A foregut cyst in close proximity to the esophagus and trachea.

Esophageal Injuries

Strictures

Erosive or corrosive injury, trauma, or malignancy can result in a fixed esophageal stenosis that subsequently restricts swallowing and produces dysphagia. Generally, the patient does not perceive difficulty swallowing until the esophageal lumen is one half its normal diameter. Since the obstruction is structural, dysphagia associated with esophageal stricture is unremitting and reproducible. Attempts to dislodge impacted food by dry swallowing or drinking water are frequently unsuccessful and regurgitation is then required before swallowing can resume. Regurgitation of saliva is the result of increased salivary production and distal obstruction. Dysphagia resulting from mechanical obstruction must be differentiated from motor dysphagia that accompanies esophageal dysmotility syndromes. With functional disorders, dysphagia is typically intermittent. Food impaction can be cleared by swallowing water and seldom requires regurgitation. For patients with oropharyngeal dysphagia, liquids are poorly tolerated and may cause drooling, gagging, aspiration, choking, or nasal regurgitation. In motor disorders of the esophageal body, both liquids and solids promote symptoms.

Congenital esophageal strictures, although rare, occur in the distal esophagus. They may be the result of the same developmental abnormalities that produce tracheoesophageal fistula or esophageal atresia.[124] Acquired esophageal strictures can be either benign or malignant (Box 35-3). Although most benign strictures result from chronic injury and resultant fibrous repair, they can occur after a single injury. Malignant strictures are usually primary esophageal adenocarcinomas or squamous cell carcinomas. Local invasion of a bronchogenic carcinoma or secondary involvement from breast, lung, or renal primary sites can produce a malignant stricture.

Barium esophagogram is the initial investigative tool in the evaluation of dysphagia and suspected esophageal stricture. Subtle strictures, not evident at esophagoscopy, and long, tight strictures are best evaluated by barium esophagram. Once the stricture anatomy is defined, esophagoscopy is crucial for tissue diagnosis of esophageal strictures. Endoscopic biopsy and dilation can be safely performed as one procedure.[8] Dilation allows examinations of the stricture and the distal GI tract. EUS is an important diagnostic adjunct following successful dilation.

Dilation is frequently required for diagnosis of esophageal stricture and in the majority of cases it is the initial treatment. A treatment algorithm is given in Figure 35-22. For benign dilatable strictures, the inciting agent must be identified and removed and the stricture treated by dilation as necessary. Nondilatable benign strictures and resectable malignant strictures are treated by excision and reconstruction. Inoperable malignant strictures are palliated.

Peptic esophageal stricture is a late complication of severe, poorly controlled GERD. Although initial damage is confined to the epithelium, with continued reflux exposure to upper gastrointestinal contents, the injury progresses to involve the submucosa, the esophageal musculature, and, eventually, periesophageal tissue. The components of this injury are spasm, inflammation, and fibrosis. Eventually, the injury–repair cycle ends in cicatricial fibrosis and obstructive

physiology of the distal esophagus. Most patients with peptic strictures present with dysphagia. It is less common for a patient to develop a symptomatic stricture during the treatment and follow-up of GERD. Though most patients do not have a prior diagnosis of GERD, more than 75% have symptoms of reflux.[138] Dysphagia is not a predominant symptom of GERD; more than 80% of GERD patients complaining of dysphagia do not have peptic strictures.[31] Peptic strictures can develop in 10–20% of patients with GERD.

Most peptic strictures are located in the distal esophagus, usually above a hiatal hernia (Figures 35-6 and 35-7A). They are smooth, tapered areas of concentric narrowing. Occasionally, asymmetrical peptic scarring may produce an eccentric stricture mimicking carcinoma. Peptic strictures are usually 1–4 cm in length and 2–20 mm in diameter.

Box 35–3. Causes of Esophageal Strictures.

Benign
  Congenital
    Esophageal atresia
    Tracheoesophageal fistula
    Web
  Acquired
    Peptic
      Gastroesophageal reflux
      Schatzki's ring
      Scleroderma
    Caustic ingestion
    Drug induced
      Anticholinergic medications
      Aspirin
      Clinitest
      Nonsteroidal antiinflammatory
      Potassium supplements
      Progesterone
      Quinidine
      Potassium supplements
      Theophylline
      Vitamin C
  Iatrogenic
    Sclerotherapy
    Postoperative (anastomotic)
    Radiation
    Postinstrumentation
    Nasogastric tube
  Infections
    Fungal
      Moniliasis
    Bacterial
      Syphilis
    Mycobacterial
      Tuberculosis
  Granulomatous
    Crohn's disease
  Dermatosis
    Epidemolysis bullosa dystrophica
    Pemphiod
    Behçet syndrome
Malignant
  Primary
  Secondary

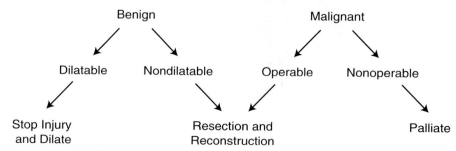

Figure 35–22 Treatment of esophageal strictures.

Advanced peptic strictures are 2 cm or greater in length and/or 9 mm or less in diameter. They may be difficult to dilate and often recur. Most peptic strictures occur at the squamocolumnar junction. Occurrence of the stricture well above the esophagogastric junction is suggestive of Barrett's mucosa. Barrett's mucosa has been reported in 44% of patients with peptic esophageal strictures.[123]

Associated abnormalities and complications (i.e., hiatal hernia, Schatzki's ring, and esophageal ulcer) are determined by esophagogram (Figure 35-7B). Esophagoscopy and biopsy are mandatory in the diagnosis of a benign peptic stricture. The initial therapy of peptic strictures is dilation and it is performed during diagnostic endoscopy.

Aggressive control of acid reflux should accompany successful dilation for long-term control of the disease. Both medical and surgical options are available for reflux control. Medical management should be started in all patients after dilation. The most potent acid suppression medications (proton pump inhibitors) are also the most successful in the medical treatment of peptic strictures.[86] Surgery should be considered for young patients who would require life-long medication and for patients who cannot tolerate medication. Early surgical correction provides better long-term results than late intervention because the esophageal injury is more likely to be reversible.

Scleroderma should be suspected in a patient who has refractory and complicated GERD. The disease affects the smooth muscle of the esophagus and results in an incompetent LES and poor motility of the esophageal body. Massive reflux and insufficient esophageal clearance cause severe GERD and peptic complications that are difficult to treat. The mainstay of treatment is acid suppression and repeated dilation. If antireflux surgery is required, an esophageal lengthening procedure and partial fundoplication are indicated. A total fundoplication may worsen the dysphagia as inadequate peristalsis and poor clearance may not overcome reconstructed LES. Peptic damage may be so severe it requires resection of the amotile strictured esophagus.

Schatzki's ring occurs precisely at the squamocolumnar junction (Figure 35-7B). These ring-like narrowings involve the mucosa and submucosa. They are thin, web-like constrictions, invariably associated with hiatal hernia and are best seen radiographically. These rings may be missed at esophagoscopy because of incomplete distention of the esophagus. Schatzki's rings, thought to be reflux related, are amenable to dilation.

Patients with pill-induced esophageal injury generally have no previous esophageal disease history. The initial injury is an ulcer and typically presents with chest pain and odynophagia.[73,90] Then, painless dysphagia heralds the onset of a pill-induced stricture. Many patients recall the initial episode of pill lodging, typically a rushed ingestion done without caution, often without liquids in a recumbent position. Pill injury is more common in women than in men.

Common locations of pill injury are in the cervical esophagus and in the thoracic esophagus at the aortic arch, however, other areas of anatomical or pathological narrowing may trap a pill. Potassium supplements administered because of heavy diuretic use in heart failure may stick in the distal esophagus because of extrinsic esophageal compression caused by cardiomegaly. Most medications produce superficial injuries. The most common findings seen at esophagogram or esophagoscopy are ulcers. Quinidine and potassium chloride produce severe esophagitis with deep ulceration. Healing of this injury may produce a short asymmetric stricture. Treatment of pill-induced stricture requires identification and cessation of the offending medication and substitution of an equivalent noninjurious drug. Pill injuries usually heal spontaneously without antacids, H_2 blockers, proton pump inhibitors, or sucralfate. Resolution of the edema and spasm of the acute injury is sufficient to relieve dysphagia. However, with a deep injury the subsequent stricture may require dilation.

Rarely an esophageal stricture can be caused by insertion of a nasogastric tube. Patients develop symptoms weeks to months after tube removal. The period of intubation can vary from days to weeks. The mechanism of injury is unknown but is postulated to be trauma from tube insertion, chronic irritation by the nasogastric tube, uncontrolled gastroesophageal reflux from an indwelling tube stenting the LES open, and/or impaired esophageal clearance secondary to the nasogastric tube. Typically, a barium esophagram demonstrates a long stricture with extensive ulceration in the mid and distal esophagus (Figure 35-23). Initially, the strictures are smooth, tapered concentric narrowings that mimic peptic strictures. Progression can be rapid with increased stricture length and severity that resembles caustic strictures. Treatment includes dilation, avoidance of esophageal intubation, and aggressive antireflux medication.

Radiation strictures may occur as soon as 3–8 months following radiation doses between 30 and 60 Gy.[24,95] They are smooth, concentric, and tapered and lie within the radiation portals. Low dose radiotherapy and concurrent adriamycin administration can also produce esophageal strictures. Other esophageal complications attributed to these therapies include esophagotracheal or esophagobronchial fistulas.

Anastomotic strictures will complicate as many as one-third of reconstructions following esophagectomy. Multiple

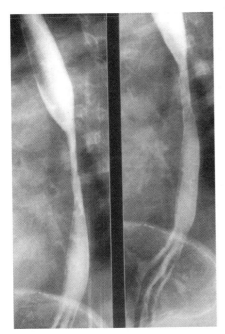

Figure 35–23 Nasogastric (NG) tube stricture. In a patient with a prolonged ICU stay and a protracted period of NG tube drainage a barium esophagram 1 month after discharge demonstrates a long smooth benign-appearing stricture of the midthoracic esophagus.

factors produce these strictures and include anastomotic tension, ischemia, infection, and radiation. Strictures are more common after anastomotic leaks, local infection, and/or adjuvant radiotherapy. Treatment is usually repeated dilation. Recurrent carcinoma may be difficult to detect by esophagoscopy and require endoscopic ultrasound.[23,81]

Corrosive Injuries

Corrosive injuries of the esophagus are caused by the ingestion of strong acid or alkali. There is a bimodal distribution of age and etiology. In children under 5 years of age, ingestion is usually accidental—the result of an inquisitive toddler ingesting improperly stored corrosive agents. The first swallow of the noxious substance usually stops further ingestion and injury. In adults, the ingestion of large volumes of caustic agents is a suicide attempt.

Early Management

Obtaining a history of the estimated amount and the nature of the ingested agent is critical to directing treatment.[48] Bleach and phosphate detergents are irritants that rarely produce significant injury. The ingestion of strong acid produces coagulation necrosis, which may limit the depth of injury. However, rapid passage and pooling in the stomach can promote gastric injury.[88] Ingestion of viscous alkali produces liquifaction necrosis and an increased depth of injury. Historically, most alkali agents were solids, generally restricting injuries to the mouth, oropharynx, hypopharynx, esophagus, and trachea. Significant solid corrosive ingestion may produce oral pain, drooling, excessive salivation, inability or refusal to swallow or drink, hoarseness, aphonia,

dyspnea, stridor, and ulceration of the mouth, pharynx, or larynx. Currently, the availability of liquid alkali has altered the pattern of injury. These agents pass rapidly through the upper GI tract producing severe injury to the esophagus at physiological points of narrowing (cricopharyngeus, upper thoracic esophagus at the tracheal bifurcation, and the distal thoracic esophagus) as well as the stomach and adjacent intraabdominal organs. Significant liquid caustic ingestion typically produces dysphagia, odynophagia, chest and abdominal pain, and signs of mediastinitis or peritonitis.

Patients should be admitted to the hospital and placed NPO. Because the injury is immediate, dilution or induction of emesis is not helpful. In fact, regurgitation of the alkali may worsen the injury by repeat exposure of the injured area to the agent. Fluid resuscitation and broad spectrum antibiotic therapy are essential. Early administration of corticosteroids does not limit the depth of injury or reduce the incidence of late strictures.[4,60] Intubation or tracheostomy and ventilation may be urgently required if there is significant laryngotracheal injury. Rapid evaluation of the upper GI tract with flexible fiberoptic esophagogastroduodenoscopy is important to identify location and extent of injury. This is facilitated by the smallest esophagoscope available with limited use of insufflation. The grading of caustic injury is similar to that of cutaneous burns.[142] First-degree injuries exhibit only mucosal edema and hyperemia. Second-degree injuries demonstrate blisters with vesicle and pseudomembrane formation. Third-degree injuries produce deep ulcers with eschar formation.

Patients with first-degree injuries require no specific treatments; the incidence of stricture is low. Patients with second- and third-degree burns are at increased risk of early mortality and late complications. The esophagus should be allowed to reepithelize; early dilation may increase stricture formation and increase the risk of perforation.[74] Frequent clinical assessment is necessary to detect and treat necrosis of the esophagus or stomach. Resection of the involved organ or organs with delayed reconstruction is recommended for transmural necrosis with mediastinitis or peritonitis. Tracheoesophageal fistula complicating caustic injury should be managed with esophageal resection and exclusion and tracheostomy.[19] Reconstruction is delayed for several months. Patients without acute complications should be placed on a bland liquid or mechanical soft diet and prophylactic acid suppression medication.

Ingestion of small alkali disc batteries presents a particular threat to small children. Severe esophageal injury may result within hours of ingestion. This results from current generation, seepage of extremely corrosive contents from damaged cases, and pressure necrosis. Careful endoscopic removal is aimed at preserving the integrity of the battery case.[83] Passage of batteries through the stomach or lower GI tract is uneventful.

Late Management

Dilation of caustic strictures should begin about 8 weeks after injury. Although retrograde dilation has been proposed as the safest technique, it requires gastrostomy. Prograde guided bouginage or balloon dilation has been successful. Short strictures not responding to initial dilation may benefit from local steroid injection followed by repeat

606 dilation.[42] Axial shortening of the esophagus results in hiatal hernia and GERD and may worsen the original corrosive injury. The need for excessive dilation and the inability to dilate to a sufficient diameter are indications for resection and reconstruction. Colonic interposition has been the organ of choice for replacement after resection of corrosive esophageal injuries, but the stomach, if not injured by the ingestion,[66] is at 1000 times the risk of the general population.[5,63]

Perforation

Perforation of the esophagus results in a chemical and infectious mediastinitis, which is lethal unless treated early and effectively. Iatrogenic injury is the most common cause of perforation.[66] The incidence of this complication is less than 0.05% during diagnostic endoscopy but increases with the complexity of the procedure and underlying esophageal pathology. A perforation rate up to 17% has been documented following dilation of caustic strictures.[69,108] In addition to instrumentation, the esophagus may be injured during any procedure performed in the vicinity of the esophagus. Trauma and spontaneous (barogenic) rupture are the next most common cause of perforation. The esophagus is normal in about 50% of perforations. Pathological changes in the remaining cases include benign strictures in 25% of patients, diverticula in 15%, carcinoma in 10%, and achalasia in 5%.[13,66]

A high index of suspicion is important for early recognition of injury. Symptoms of spontaneous rupture are often nonspecific and include acute chest and/or abdominal pain, odynophagia, dyspnea, and fever. A catastrophic presentation with acute sepsis may be seen. Any patient reporting symptoms following instrumentation of the esophagus should be considered to have a perforation until proven otherwise. Pleural effusion, pneumothorax, pneumomediastinum, and subcutaneous emphysema are nonspecific chest X-ray findings. However, chest X-rays are diagnostic in only 15% of patients and may be normal in 10%.[49] The clinical diagnosis of esophageal perforation is confirmed by barium esophagram (Figure 35-24). This is first performed with gastrograffin aqueous contrast material and, if negative, repeated with barium. Up to 22% of perforations will be missed if only aqueous contrast is used.[17]

Some injuries may be contained within the wall of the esophagus. In patients without fever or elevated white blood count, in whom the laceration is limited to the esophageal wall and there is free drainage of contrast material into the esophagus without distal esophageal obstruction, observation may be undertaken.[2,21] However, if a transmural injury with mediastinal soilage is identified, definitive surgical management is required after fluid resuscitation and administration of intravenous antibiotics. The principles of treatment are debridement of infected or necrotic tissue, closure of the perforation, treatment of underlying esophageal pathology, if present, and drainage of the mediastinum. A myotomy at the site of perforation allows the full extent of damage to the mucosa to be recognized and repaired. Reinforcement of the repair decreases mortality and fistula formation.[50] Delayed recognition of a perforation makes successful primary repair less likely. Therapy should be directed toward defunctioning, debridement, drainage, and

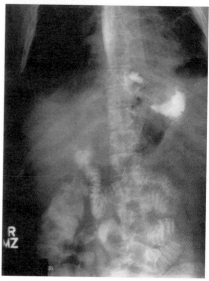

Figure 35–24 Perforation. Barium esophagram in a patient who has just undergone unguided esophageal dilation of a distal esophageal stricture shows extravasation of barium into the mediastinum.

resection.[3,18,136] Surgical drainage without repair is possible for most cervical perforations. Descending mediastinitis requires prompt treatment of the mediastinal component of a cervical perforation and may require the addition of a right thoracotomy to the cervical incision.[72] Palliation of perforated esophageal carcinoma has been successful with self-expanding, covered metallic stents.[137] One third of patients will experience dysphagia following repair of esophageal perforations and require either dilation or further surgery.[62] The best results are seen in patients with achalasia and other motor disorders who undergo a myotomy during perforation repair. In patients with strictures or diffuse esophageal disease, esophagectomy may produce the best long-term results.

Esophageal Foreign Bodies

The majority of ingested foreign bodies occur in toddlers.[139] In younger adults, ingested foreign bodies are usually associated with drug or alcohol use or psychiatric illness. In older adults, with either dentures or esophageal pathology, a food bolus may serve as the impacted foreign body. The site of impaction is invariably at a physiological or pathological area of narrowing. Plain film and contrast radiography are diagnostic in the majority of patients. Most small blunt objects pass into the distal GI tract without difficulty. Blunt impacted foreign bodies may be removed with a flexible esophagoscope and balloon catheters or baskets. Sharp or pointed objects, if the sharp edge is directed aborally, may be removed with flexible esophagoscopy; little damage is incurred from the sharp trailing edge. However, if the leading edge is sharp, rigid esophagoscopy with retraction of the sharp edge into the barrel of the rigid esophagoscope may be necessary. Surgical removal is rarely required for impacted foreign objects or those complicated by lacerations and mediastinitis.

CONCLUSION

The understanding of esophageal anatomy, function, and pathophysiology is essentially to correctly diagnose and successfully treat benign esophageal diseases. Esophageal conditions amenable to surgery are uncommon except for hiatal hernia and GERD. Restoration of esophageal function and the ability to swallow are essential. It is imperative that the first operation be successful. This success avoids leading the patient down the road to multiple reoperations that would ultimately culminate in esophagectomy for benign disease.

"It is preferable to bring your own esophagus to dinner"
Lucius D. Hill

REFERENCES

1. Adhami T, Shay SS: Esophageal motility in the assessment of esophageal function. Semin Thorac Cardiovasc Surg 13(3):234–240, 2001.
2. Altorjay A, et al: Nonoperative management of esophageal perforations. Is it justified? Ann Surg 225(4):415–421, 1997.
3. Altorjay A, et al: The role of esophagectomy in the management of esophageal perforations. Ann Thorac Surg 65(5):1433–1436, 1998.
4. Anderson KD, Rouse TM, Randolph JG: A controlled trial of corticosteroids in children with corrosive injury of the esophagus. N Engl J Med 323(10):637–640, 1990.
5. Appelqvist P, Salmo M: Lye corrosion carcinoma of the esophagus: A review of 63 cases. Cancer 45(10):2655–2658, 1980.
6. Araki K, et al: Esophageal hemangioma: A case report and review of the literature. Hepatogastroenterology 46(30):3148–3154, 1999.
7. Banbury MK, et al: Esophagectomy with gastric reconstruction for achalasia. J Thorac Cardiovasc Surg 117(6):1077–1084, 1999.
8. Barkin JS, Taub S, Rogers AI: The safety of combined endoscopy, biopsy and dilation in esophageal strictures. Am J Gastroenterol 76(1):23–26, 1981.
9. Benacci JC, et al: Epiphrenic diverticulum: results of surgical treatment. Ann Thorac Surg 55(5):1109–1113; discussion 1114, 1993.
10. Berstad A, et al: Relationship of hiatus hernia to reflux oesophagitis. A prospective study of coincidence, using endoscopy. Scand J Gastroenterol 21(1):55–58, 1986.
11. Bessel JR, et al: Chronic dysphagia following laparoscopic fundoplication. Br J Surg 87(10):1341–1345, 2000.
12. Bhutani MS, Hoffman BJ, Reed C: Endosonographic diagnosis of an esophageal duplication cyst. Endoscopy 28(4):396–397, 1996.
13. Bladergroen MR, Lowe JE, Postlethwait RW: Diagnosis and recommended management of esophageal perforation and rupture. Ann Thorac Surg 42(3):235–239, 1986.
14. Bonafede JP, et al: Surgical outcome in 87 patients with Zenker's diverticulum. Laryngoscope 107(6):720–725, 1997.
15. Bonavina L, et al: Previous endoscopic treatment does not affect complication rate and outcome of laparoscopic Heller myotomy and anterior fundoplication for oesophageal achalasia. Ital J Gastroenterol Hepatol 31(9):827–830, 1999.
16. Borrie J, Wilson RL: Oesophageal diverticula: principles of management and appraisal of classification. Thorax 35(10):759–767, 1980.
17. Buecker A, et al: Esophageal perforation: comparison of use of aqueous and barium-containing contrast media. Radiology 202(3):683–686, 1997.
18. Bufkin BL, Miller JI Jr, Mansour KA: Esophageal perforation: emphasis on management. Ann Thorac Surg 61(5):1447–1451; discussion 1451–1452, 1996.
19. Burrington JD, Raffensperger JG: Surgical management of tracheoesophageal fistula complicating caustic ingestion. Surgery 84(3):329–334, 1978.
20. Cameron AJ: Barrett's esophagus: prevalence and size of hiatal hernia. Am J Gastroenterol 94(8):2054–2059, 1999.
21. Cameron JL, et al: Selective nonoperative management of contained intrathoracic esophageal disruptions. Ann Thorac Surg 27(5):404–408, 1979.
22. Campos GM, et al: Multivariate analysis of factors predicting outcome after laparoscopic Nissen fundoplication. J Gastrointest Surg 3(3):292–300, 1999.
23. Catalano MF, et al: Postoperative screening for anastomotic recurrence of esophageal carcinoma by endoscopic ultrasonography. Gastrointest Endosc 42(6):540–544, 1995.
24. Chowhan NM: Injurious effects of radiation on the esophagus. Am J Gastroenterol 85(2):115–120, 1990.
25. Clark SB, et al: The nature of the myenteric infiltrate in achalasia: an immunohistochemical analysis. Am J Surg Pathol 24(8):1153–1158, 2000.
26. Clouse RE, Lustman PJ: Psychiatric illness and contraction abnormalities of the esophagus. N Engl J Med 309(22):1337–1342, 1983.
27. Clouse RE, et al: Low-dose trazodone for symptomatic patients with esophageal contraction abnormalities. A double-blind, placebo-controlled trial. Gastroenterology 92(4):1027–1036, 1987.
28. Collard JM, Otte JB, Kestens PJ: Endoscopic stapling technique of esophagodiverticulostomy for Zenker's diverticulum. Ann Thorac Surg 56(3):573–576, 1993.
29. Cook IJ, et al: Pharyngeal (Zenker's) diverticulum is a disorder of upper esophageal sphincter opening. Gastroenterology 103(4):1229–1235, 1992.
30. Csendes A, et al: Late results of a prospective randomised study comparing forceful dilatation and oesophagomyotomy in patients with achalasia. Gut 30(3):299–304, 1989.
31. Demeester TR, et al: Patterns of gastroesophageal reflux in health and disease. Ann Surg 184(4):459–470, 1976.
32. de Oliveria JM, et al: Timed barium swallow: a simple technique for evaluating esophageal emptying in patients with achalasia. Am J Roentgenol 169(2):473–479, 1997.
33. Ellis FH Jr, Crozier RE, Shea JA: Long esophagomyotomy for diffuse esophageal spasm and related disorders. In Siewert JR, Holscher AH, editors: Diseases of the Esophagus. New York: Springer-Verlag. 1988, pp. 913–917.
34. Evander A, et al: Diverticula of the mid- and lower esophagus: pathogenesis and surgical management. World J Surg 10(5):820–828, 1986.
35. Faigel DO, et al: The role of endoscopic ultrasound in the evaluation and management of foregut duplications. Gastrointest Endosc 45(1):99–103, 1997.
36. Fegiz G, et al: Surgical management of esophageal diverticula. World J Surg 8(5):757–765, 1984.
37. Fekete F, Vonns C: Surgical management of esophageal thoracic diverticula. Hepatogastroenterology 39(2):97–99, 1992.
38. Felix VN, et al: Achalasia: a prospective study comparing the results of dilatation and myotomy. Hepatogastroenterology 45(19):97–108, 1998.
39. Ferguson MK, Little AG: Angina-like chest pain associated with high-amplitude peristaltic contractions of the esophagus. Surgery 104(4):713–719, 1988.
40. Ferguson MK, Reeder LB, Olak J: Results of myotomy and partial fundoplication after pneumatic dilation for achalasia. Ann Thorac Surg 62(2):327–330, 1996.
41. Feussner H, Kauer W, Siewert JR: The surgical management of motility disorders. Dysphagia 8(2):135–145, 1993.

42. Gandhi RP, Cooper A, Barlow BA: Successful management of esophageal strictures without resection or replacement. J Pediatr Surg 24(8):745–749; discussion 749–750, 1989.

43. Gastal OL, et al: Short esophagus: analysis of predictors and clinical implications. Arch Surg 134(6):633–636; discussion 637–638, 1999.

44. Goldblum JR, et al: Achalasia. A morphologic study of 42 resected specimens. Am J Surg Pathol 18(4):327–337, 1994.

45. Goldblum JR, et al: Granular cell tumors of the esophagus: a clinical and pathologic study of 13 cases. Ann Thorac Surg 62(3):860–865, 1996.

46. Goldblum JR, Rice TW, Richter JE: Histopathologic features in esophagomyotomy specimens from patients with achalasia. Gastroenterology 111(3):648–654, 1996.

47. Goldenberg SP, et al: Classic and vigorous achalasia: a comparison of manometric, radiographic, and clinical findings. Gastroenterology 101(3):743–748, 1991.

48. Goldman LP, Weigert JM: Corrosive substance ingestion: a review. Am J Gastroenterol 79(2):85–90, 1984.

49. Goldstein LA, Thompson WR: Esophageal perforations: a 15 year experience. Am J Surg 143(4):495–503, 1982.

50. Gouge TH, Depan HJ, Spencer FC: Experience with the Grillo pleural wrap procedure in 18 patients with perforation of the thoracic esophagus. Ann Surg 209(5):612–617; discussion 617–619, 1989.

51. Govoni AF: Hemangiomas of the esophagus. Gastrointest Radiol 7(2):113–117, 1982.

52. Gurski RR, et al: Barrett's esophagus can and does regress after antireflux surgery: a study of prevalence and predictive features. J Am Coll Surg 196(5):706–712; discussion 712–713, 2003.

53. Hashemi M, et al: Laparoscopic repair of large type III hiatal hernia: objective followup reveals high recurrence rate. J Am Coll Surg 190(5):553–560; discussion 560–561, 2000.

54. Heider TR, et al: Complete fundoplication is not associated with increased dysphagia in patients with abnormal esophageal motility. J Gastrointest Surg 5(1):36–41, 2001.

55. Hill LD: Incarcerated paraesophageal hernia. A surgical emergency. Am J Surg 126(2):286–291, 1973.

56. Hogan WJ, Shaker R: Life after antireflux surgery. Am J Med 108(Suppl. 4a):181S–191S, 2000.

57. Horgan S, et al: Does botulinum toxin injection make esophagomyotomy a more difficult operation? Surg Endosc 13(6):576–579, 1999.

58. Horvath KD, et al: Laparoscopic Toupet fundoplication is an inadequate procedure for patients with severe reflux disease. J Gastrointest Surg 3(6):583–591, 1999.

59. Hover AR, et al: Multiple retention cysts of the lower esophagus. J Clin Gastroenterol 4(3):209–212, 1982.

60. Howel, JM, et al: Steroids for the treatment of corrosive esophageal injury: a statistical analysis of past studies. Am J Emerg Med 10(5):421–425, 1992.

61. Hunter JG, et al: Laparoscopic fundoplication failures: patterns of failure and response to fundoplication revision. Ann Surg 230(4):595–604; discussion 604–606, 1999.

62. Iannettoni MD, et al: Functional outcome after surgical treatment of esophageal perforation. Ann Thorac Surg 64(6):1606–1609; discussion 1609–1610, 1997.

63. Isolauri J, Markkula H: Lye ingestion and carcinoma of the esophagus. Acta Chir Scand 155(4–5):269–271, 1989.

64. Jamieson JR, et al: Ambulatory 24-h esophageal pH monitoring: normal values, optimal thresholds, specificity, sensitivity, and reproducibility. Am J Gastroenterol 87(9):1102–1111, 1992.

65. Johnson LF, Demeester TR: Twenty-four-hour pH monitoring of the distal esophagus. A quantitative measure of gastroesophageal reflux. Am J Gastroenterol 62(4):325–332, 1974.

66. Jones WG 2nd, Ginsberg RJ: Esophageal perforation: a continuing challenge. Ann Thorac Surg 53(3):534–543, 1992.

67. Kahrilas PJ: Will impedance testing rewrite the book on GERD? Gastroenterology 120(7):1862–1864, 2001.

68. Kahrilas PJ, et al: The effect of hiatus hernia on gastrooesophageal junction pressure. Gut 44(4):476–482, 1999.

69. Karnak I, et al: Esophageal perforations encountered during the dilation of caustic esophageal strictures. J Cardiovasc Surg (Torino) 39(3):373–377, 1998.

70. Kaul B, et al: Hiatus hernia in gastroesophageal reflux disease. Scand J Gastroenterol 21(1):31–34, 1986.

71. Kaye MD: Oesophageal motor dysfunction in patients with diverticula of the mid-thoracic oesophagus. Thorax 29(6):666–672, 1974.

72. Kiernan PD, et al: Descending cervical mediastinitis. Ann Thorac Surg 65(5):1483–1488, 1998.

73. Kikendall JW: Pill-induced esophageal injury. Gastroenterol Clin North Am 20(4):835–846, 1991.

74. Knox WG, et al: Bouginage and steroids used singly or in combination in experimental corrosive esophagitis. Ann Surg 166(6):930–941, 1967.

75. Kostic SV, et al: Timed barium esophagogram: A simple physiologic assessment for achalasia. J Thorac Cardiovasc Surg 120(5):935–943, 2000.

76. Kuge K, et al: Submucosal territory of the direct lymphatic drainage system to the thoracic duct in the human esophagus. J Thorac Cardiovasc Surg 125(6):1343–1349, 2003.

77. Kuhlman JE, et al: Esophageal duplication cyst: CT and transesophageal needle aspiration. Am J Roentgenol 145(3):531–532, 1985.

78. Laccourreye O, et al: Esophageal diverticulum: Diverticulopexy versus diverticulectomy. Laryngoscope 104(7):889–892, 1994.

79. Lerut T, et al: Zenker's diverticulum: is a myotomy of the cricopharyngeus useful? How long should it be? Hepatogastroenterology 39(2):127–131, 1992.

80. Levine MS, et al: Fibrovascular polyps of the esophagus: clinical, radiographic, and pathologic findings in 16 patients. Am J Roentgenol 166(4):781–787, 1996.

81. Lightdale CJ, et al: Diagnosis of recurrent upper gastrointestinal cancer at the surgical anastomosis by endoscopic ultrasound. Gastrointest Endosc 35(5):407–412, 1989.

82. Lim LL, Ho KY, Goh PM: Preoperative diagnosis of a paraesophageal bronchogenic cyst using endosonography. Ann Thorac Surg 73(2):633–635, 2002.

83. Litovitz T, Schmitz BF: Ingestion of cylindrical and button batteries: an analysis of 2382 cases. Pediatrics 89(4 Pt. 2):747–757, 1992.

84. Maluf-Filho F, et al: Giant cavernous hemangioma of the esophagus: endoscopic and echo-endoscopic appearance. Endoscopy 31(4):S32, 1999.

85. Manifold DK, et al: Oesophageal dysmotility is not associated with poor outcome after laparoscopic Nissen fundoplication. Br J Surg 86(7):969, 1999.

86. Marks RD, et al: Omeprazole versus H2-receptor antagonists in treating patients with peptic stricture and esophagitis. Gastroenterology 106(4):907–915, 1994.

87. Massari M, et al: Endoscopic ultrasonography in the evaluation of leiomyoma and extramucosal cysts of the esophagus. Hepatogastroenterology 45(22):938–943, 1998.

88. Maull KI, Scher LA, Greenfield LJ: Surgical implications of acid ingestion. Surg Gynecol Obstet 148(6):895–898, 1979.

89. Maziak DE, Todd TR, Pearson FG: Massive hiatus hernia: evaluation and surgical management. J Thorac Cardiovasc Surg 115(1):53–60; discussion 61–62, 1998.

90. McCord GS, Clouse RE: Pill-induced esophageal strictures: clinical features and risk factors for development. Am J Med 88(5):512–518, 1990.

91. Miller DL, et al: Esophageal resection for recurrent achalasia. Ann Thorac Surg 60(4):922–925; discussion 925–926, 1995.

92. Mittal RK, Balaban DH: The esophagogastric junction. N Engl J Med 336(13):924–32, 1997.

93. Morino M, et al: Preoperative pneumatic dilatation represents a risk factor for laparoscopic Heller myotomy. Surg Endosc 11(4):359–361, 1997.

94. Murakami G, et al: Direct lymphatic drainage from the esophagus into the thoracic duct. Surg Radiol Anat 16(4):399–407, 1994.

95. Ng TM, et al: Management of strictures after radiotherapy for esophageal cancer. Gastrointest Endosc 43(6):584–590, 1996.

96. Nobuhara KK, et al: Bronchogenic cysts and esophageal duplications: common origins and treatment. J Pediatr Surg 32(10):1408–1413, 1997.

97. Oelschlager BK, Chang L, Pellegrini CA: Improved outcome after extended gastric myotomy for achalasia. Arch Surg 138(5):490–495; discussion 495–497, 2003.

98. Orringer MB: Surgical management of scleroderma reflux esophagitis. Surg Clin North Am 63(4):859–867, 1983.

99. Orringer MB, Stirling MC: Esophageal resection for achalasia: indications and results. Ann Thorac Surg 47(3):340–345, 1989.

100. Ott DJ, Gelfand DW, Wu WC: Reflux esophagitis: radiographic and endoscopic correlation. Radiology 130(3):583–588, 1979.

101. Ott DJ, et al: Predictive relationship of hiatal hernia to reflux esophagitis. Gastrointest Radiol 10(4):317–320, 1985.

102. Palazzo L, et al: Endosonographic features of esophageal granular cell tumors. Endoscopy 29(9):850–853, 1997.

103. Peracchia A, et al: Minimally invasive surgery for Zenker diverticulum: analysis of results in 95 consecutive patients. Arch Surg 133(7):695–700, 1998.

104. Perch SJ, et al: Esophageal sarcomas. J Surg Oncol 48(3):194–198, 1991.

105. Peters JH, et al: Esophageal resection with colon interposition for end-stage achalasia. Arch Surg 130(6):632–636; discussion 636–637, 1995.

106. Pinotti HW, et al: Resection for achalasia of the esophagus. Hepatogastroenterology 38(6):470–473, 1991.

107. Politoske EJ: Squamous papilloma of the esophagus associated with the human papillomavirus. Gastroenterology 102(2):668–673, 1992.

108. Quine MA, et al: Prospective audit of perforation rates following upper gastrointestinal endoscopy in two regions of England. Br J Surg 82(4):530–533, 1995.

109. Quitadamo M, Benson J: Squamous papilloma of the esophagus: a case report and review of the literature. Am J Gastroenterol 83(2):194–201, 1988.

110. Richter JE: Let the patient beware: the evolving truth about laparoscopic antireflux surgery. Am J Med 114(1):71–73, 2003.

111. Richter JE, et al: Esophageal manometry in 95 healthy adult volunteers. Variability of pressures with age and frequency of "abnormal" contractions. Dig Dis Sci 32(6):583–592, 1987.

112. Richter JE, et al: Normal 24-hr ambulatory esophageal pH values. Influence of study center, pH electrode, age, and gender. Dig Dis Sci 37(6):849–856, 1992.

113. Riquet M, et al: Lymphatic drainage of the esophagus in the adult. Surg Radiol Anat 15(3):209–211, 1993.

114. Rydberg L, et al: Tailoring antireflux surgery: a randomized clinical trial. World J Surg 23(6):612–618, 1999.

115. Salo JA, et al: Enucleation of an intramural lipoma of the oesophagus by videothoracoscopy. Ann Chir Gynaecol 82(1):66–69, 1993.

116. Schima W, et al: Association of midoesophageal diverticula with oesophageal motor disorders. Videofluoroscopy and manometry. Acta Radiol 38(1):108–114, 1997.

117. Schuhmacher C, et al: Fibrovascular esophageal polyp as a diagnostic challenge. Dis Esophagus 13(4):324–327, 2000.

118. Seremetis MG, et al: Leiomyoma of the esophagus. A report of 19 surgical cases. Ann Thorac Surg 16(3):308–316, 1973.

119. Shay SS, Bomeli S, Richter J: Multichannel intraluminal impedance accurately detects fasting, recumbent reflux events and their clearing. Am J Physiol Gastrointest Liver Physiol 283(2):G376–G383, 2002.

120. Sifrim D, Janssens J, Vantrappen G: Failing deglutitive inhibition in primary esophageal motility disorders. Gastroenterology 106(4):875–882, 1994.

121. So JB, Zeitels SM, Rattner DW: Outcomes of atypical symptoms attributed to gastroesophageal reflux treated by laparoscopic fundoplication. Surgery 124(1):28–32, 1998.

122. Sontag SJ, et al: The importance of hiatal hernia in reflux esophagitis compared with lower esophageal sphincter pressure or smoking. J Clin Gastroenterol 13(6):628–643, 1991.

123. Spechler SJ, et al: The prevalence of Barrett's esophagus in patients with chronic peptic esophageal strictures. Dig Dis Sci 28(9):769–774, 1983.

124. Spitz L: Congenital esophageal stenosis distal to associated esophageal atresia. J Pediatr Surg 8(6):973–974, 1973.

125. St-Georges R, et al: Clinical spectrum of bronchogenic cysts of the mediastinum and lung in the adult. Ann Thorac Surg 52(1):6–13, 1991.

126. Stilson WL, et al: Hiatal hernia and gastroesophageal reflux. A clinicoradiological analysis of more than 1,000 cases. Radiology 93(6):1323–1327, 1969.

127. Tew S, et al: A prospective study of the effect of fundoplication on primary and secondary peristalsis in the esophagus. Dis Esophagus 10(4):247–252, 1997.

128. Traube M, et al: Surgical myotomy in patients with high-amplitude peristaltic esophageal contractions. Manometric and clinical effects. Dig Dis Sci 32(1):16–21, 1987.

129. Traube M, et al: The role of nifedipine therapy in achalasia: results of a randomized, double-blind, placebo-controlled study. Am J Gastroenterol 84(10):1259–1262, 1989.

130. Tsui JK: Botulinum toxin as a therapeutic agent. Pharmacol Ther 72(1):13–24, 1996.

131. Tutuian R, et al: Multichannel intraluminal impedance in esophageal function testing and gastroesophageal reflux monitoring. J Clin Gastroenterol 37(3):206–215, 2003.

132. Vaezi MF, Richter JE: Current therapies for achalasia: comparison and efficacy. J Clin Gastroenterol 27(1):21–35, 1998.

133. Vaezi MF, Shay SS: New techniques in measuring nonacidic esophageal reflux. Semin Thorac Cardiovasc Surg 13(3):255–264, 2001.

134. Vaezi MF, Baker ME, Richter JE: Assessment of esophageal emptying post-pneumatic dilation: use of the timed barium esophagram. Am J Gastroenterol 94(7):1802–1807, 1999.

135. Vakil N, Shaw M, Kirby R: Clinical effectiveness of laparoscopic fundoplication in a U.S. community. Am J Med 114(1):1–5, 2003.

136. Wang N, et al: Delayed primary repair of intrathoracic esophageal perforation: is it safe? J Thorac Cardiovasc Surg 111(1):114–121; discussion 121–122, 1996.

137. Watkinson A, et al: Plastic-covered metallic endoprostheses in the management of oesophageal perforation in patients with oesophageal carcinoma. Clin Radiol 50(5):304–309, 1995.

138. Watson A: Reflux stricture of the oesophagus. Br J Surg 74(6):443–448, 1987.

139. Webb WA: Management of foreign bodies of the upper gastrointestinal tract. Gastroenterology 94(1):204–216, 1988.

140. Wetscher GJ, et al: Tailored antireflux surgery for gastroesophageal reflux disease: effectiveness and risk of postoperative dysphagia. World J Surg 21(6):605–610, 1997.

141. Wiener GJ, et al: Ambulatory 24-hour esophageal pH monitoring. Reproducibility and variability of pH parameters. Dig Dis Sci 33(9):1127–1133, 1988.

142. Zargar SA, et al: The role of fiberoptic endoscopy in the management of corrosive ingestion and modified endoscopic classification of burns. Gastrointest Endosc 37(2):165–169, 1991.

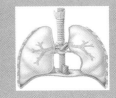

Staging Techniques for Carcinoma of the Esophagus

Whitney M. Burrows and Mark J. Krasna

Introduction
Esophageal Cancer Staging System
Staging Principles and Methodologies
Staging by Computed Tomography
Staging by Positron Emission Tomography
Staging by Endoscopic Ultrasonography
Staging by Minimally Invasive Surgery:
    Thoracoscopy and Laparoscopy
Adjunctive Staging Techniques and Future
    Directions

▶ INTRODUCTION

Theoretical and practical discord can exist among the separate phases of comprehensive cancer care. Initiated with diagnosis and culminating in treatment response, the possibility for correlative lapses is great. Cancer staging establishes a referential continuum, linking polar ends of cancer therapy. However, cancer staging is not only an instrument of organization. Staging enables prognostication. It furnishes a contextual framework within which therapeutic options can be compared. Scientific research and discourse also rely on staging for reference.

As in most solid tumors, accurate staging is fundamental to the management of esophageal carcinoma. Beginning in the late 1990s, moreover, the implications for esophageal cancer staging have increased markedly. Three forces are principally responsible for this rapid change. First, the incidence of esophageal cancer is increasing in the United States. There has been a dramatic increase in the incidence of adenocarcinoma of the distal esophagus in North America and Europe since 1976, complementing the overall rise. Although the squamous cell histological subtype remains more prevalent worldwide, the incidence of esophageal adenocarcinoma in North American white men has increased from 10% to nearly 60% over the last 2 decades.[2] A definitive etiopathological correlation has been established between adenocarcinoma and the epidemic—gastroesophageal disease. Second, the historical

view that esophageal cancer in the absence of visceral metastases is best treated surgically has been amended, if not definitively abandoned. Presently the potentially resectable but locally advanced esophageal cancer is treated with neoadjuvant chemoradiotherapy. This evolution in approach mandates refinements in pretreatment staging assessments. Third, both radiological and other limited invasive staging techniques have matured. With the approval of positron emission tomography (PET) in esophageal cancer staging by the Health Care Financing Administration in 2000, the standardization of endoscopic ultrasonography (EUS) and EUS-guided fine needle aspiration (EUS–FNA), and the acceptance of minimal access surgical staging techniques, the staging armamentaria has proliferated. Reproducible and accurate preresection esophageal cancer staging has developed into a realistic construct.

▶ ESOPHAGEAL CANCER STAGING SYSTEM

In 1987 the American Joint Committee on Cancer/ International Union against Cancer (AJCC/UICC) first defined the staging system for esophageal cancer using tumor–node–metastasis (TNM) subclassifications. In 1997 the present staging system was created (Table 36-1). Although it is a genesis for continual debate, this 1997 revision differs from the 1987 version only in its description of metastatic disease. Appropriate emphasis remains on depth of wall invasion by tumor (T_1–T_4) and node status (N_0–N_1). In patients whose esophageal cancer remains confined to the esophageal wall, given the absence of nodal spread, the 5-year survival rate is approximately 40%. The 5-year survival rate drops to approximately 4% if a patient's node-negative cancer violates the esophageal adventitia (the radial boundary of the wall). The probability of nodal spread increases with increasing tumor depth. The likelihood of nodal spread in tumors confined to the mucosa is less than 1%. With penetration of the submucosa, the chance of nodal metastases increases to nearly 50%. The 5-year survival rate for esophageal cancer patients who have no nodal disease approximates 40%. A decrease to 3% is observed for patients who have node-positive cancers.[34]

Table 36–1

Stage Grouping

Stage	Tumor	Node	Metastasis
Stage 0	T_{is}	N_0	M_0
Stage I	T_1	N_0	M_0
Stage IIA	T_2	N_0	M_0
	T_3	N_0	M_0
Stage IIB	T_1	N_0	M_0
	T_2	N_0	M_0
Stage III	T_3	N_0	M_0
	T_4	N_0	M_0
Stage IV	Any T	Any N	M_1
Stage IVA	Any T	Any N	M_{1a}
Stage IVB	Any T	Any N	M_{1b}

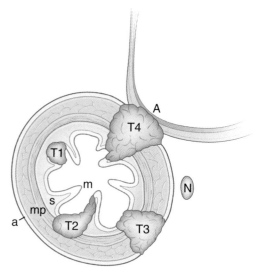

Figure 36–1 Stages of esophageal malignancy. T_1 lesions involve mucosa (m) or submucosa (s). A T_2 lesion invades the muscularis propria (mp), a T_3 lesion invades the adventitia (a), and a T_4 lesion involves adjacent organ (A). N indicates the metastatic lymph node.

T_{is} lesions are intraepithelial cancers confined to the esophageal epithelium without invasion of the basement membrane. T_1 cancers penetrate the basement membrane to invade the lamina propria, muscularis mucosa, or submucosa, but do not invade beyond the submucosa. T_2 cancers involve the muscularis propria, but are confined to the esophageal wall. T_3 cancers penetrate the esophageal wall into the paraesophageal space, but do not invade other mediastinal structures. T_4 cancers directly invade these structures and thereby are not amenable to surgical extirpation (Figure 36-1). With the advent of EUS and further elucidation of nodal pathophysiology, a clinical subdivision of the T_1 subdivision has been proposed. A T_{1a} subset has been defined for intramucosal cancers that invade, at most, through to the muscularis mucosa. An intramucosal cancer that penetrates into the submucosa has been designated as T_{1b}. Of the three mucosal layers deep to the epithelial basement membrane, the submucosa contains lymphatic channels vulnerable to seeding.

Involvement of *regional* lymph nodes is signified using a binary code of N_0 versus N_1. The N_0 descriptive reflects the absence of metastatic lymph node involvement. The presence of lymph node metastasis carries the N_1 designation. The present staging system offers no insight into the difference between regional and *nonregional* lymph nodes. The authors of the most recently published AJCC Cancer Staging Manual (6th edition) provide no additional clarification.[11] Partitioning of the thoracic esophagus into three anatomical segments (upper, middle, lower) is clearly defined by the authors. Therefore it is inferred that lymph node metastasis recognized in any paraesophageal bed remote from the esophageal segment in which the primary cancer arises is nonregional in characterization. Regardless, a lymph node map (Figure 36-2) is included in the AJCC manual. Again, distinct regions within this map are not drawn. Although further clues pertaining to node locality are offered in the subcategorization of distant metastasis (M), the clinical relevance of node region remains limited. Finally, the present staging system also has been criticized for not having a subclassification of N_1.[31] Investigators have demonstrated the prognostic significance of metastatic lymph node number. Kawahara and colleagues[15] have shown a four-node threshold as a negative predictor of survival. Integrating these data into the current staging system has not yet occurred.

Distant metastatic disease is also noted using binary designations: absent (M_0) or present (M_1). The 1997 revision of the initial staging system subdivides M_1 into M_{1a} (distant, nonregional lymph node metastases) and M_{1b} (extranodal [visceral] metastases). The M_{1a} subset is further broken down into two distribution patterns based on esophageal *anatomy;* no distinct symbol is given to indicate these anatomical subcategories. M_{1a} cancers of the upper thoracic esophagus have metastasized to cervical nodes. M_{1a} cancers of the lower thoracic esophagus have metastasized to the celiac lymph node basin. Metastatic *midthoracic* esophageal cancers to nodes or viscera, however, are *all* classified as M_{1b}. This intrastage lack of uniformity reflects the statistically significant observation that M_1 midesophageal cancers have marginal survival irrespective of nonregional lymph node metastasis or visceral organ disease spread; therefore the *a* or *b* identifiers are meaningless for this anatomical segment (see Table 36-1).

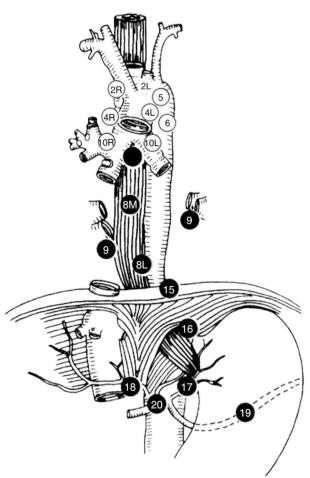

Figure 36–2 Regional lymph node stations for staging esophageal cancer.

ment stage. In esophageal carcinoma, this single-minded approach can have serious and potentially deleterious consequences. Fortunately, continued advances are anticipated in regard to staging techniques for esophageal cancer whereby clinical and pathological data should coincide. For now, little overlap exists and a broad net is usually cast in order to catch this essential information.

On the most elemental level, clinical and pathological staging techniques differ in respect to their degree of invasiveness. On the clinical end of the spectrum, purely noninvasive measures scarcely require patient contact. On the pathological end, general anesthesia is required and an overnight hospitalization is routine. Midway between these extremes, semiinvasive procedures necessitate instrumentation with minimal but definite risks, including perforation and hemorrhage. Clinical staging of esophageal carcinoma takes the form of computed tomography (CT) and PET. Of historical interest only, reference is made to barium swallow; it is not discussed further. The amalgamation of these technologies (CT–PET) is just now being evaluated. In the near future it is presumed that this combined examination will subsume both individual modalities, particularly CT (alone). More invasive techniques are needed to define pathological stage. Although commonly termed *minimally* invasive, surgical staging techniques are only minimal in reference to other surgeries; a more appropriate description would be *minimal access* surgical staging. Bridging the clinical and pathological staging gap is EUS and its potent counterpart, EUS–FNA. Finally, all three TNM subclassifications cannot be accurately assessed by one staging technique, regardless of its position along the spectrum of invasiveness. Rather, only the integration of at least two modalities' data conclusively stages an esophageal cancer.

The clinical distinction between N_1 (regional) and M_{1a} (nonregional) lymph node metastases seems particularly arbitrary. A proximal intrathoracic esophageal cancer that metastasizes to low cervical nodes (or even supraclavicular nodes) likely represents *regional* spread. Similarly, a distal esophageal cancer with celiac node involvement can easily reflect malignant progression by way of regional lymphatics. The staging methodology for metastatic midesophageal cancers is likewise incongruous. In summary, criticism of the current staging system is perpetuated by this ambiguity concerning $M_{1a,b}$ disease.

STAGING PRINCIPLES AND METHODOLOGIES

The pretreatment stage in esophageal carcinoma can be determined on the basis of clinical or pathological information. These data sources are critically different, both in the manner in which they are acquired and to the extent to which they can be therapeutically used. It is common practice to clinically stage a malignancy and await pathological confirmation of that stage *after* treatment. If treatment takes the form of surgery, confirmation is prompt. Nonetheless, this process completely undermines the concept of *pretreat-*

STAGING BY COMPUTED TOMOGRAPHY

Before the advent of PET and EUS, CT scanning served as the principal preresection staging technique for esophageal cancer. Today CT plays a more adjunctive role in staging. It remains the key instrument used in radiotherapy planning, a valuable tool for follow-up surveillance, and an expedient method of assessing tumor response to neoadjuvant treatment. Although it lacks accuracy and comprehensiveness, CT maintains characteristics important in screening; it is noninvasive, inexpensive, and widely available. Currently CT is used chiefly as an elemental technique for identifying distant metastatic disease; it is a convenient and rapid means of confirming occult, but more than subtle, M_{1b} or stage IVB esophageal cancer.

There has been no study to date comparing spiral and conventional CT for the purposes of esophageal cancer staging; a study likely never to be undertaken because the results would have no impact. Imaging technology aside, the typical examination consists of 7- to 10-mm contiguous cuts extending from the lower neck or thoracic inlet through the level of the kidneys, providing visualization of the thoracic esophagus, stomach, celiac axis, liver, and adrenal glands. In conventional CT, scanning is initiated at the time of inspiration. The posterior tracheal wall consequently distends,

614 improving the yield of detecting airway (T_4) involvement.[33] All CT images should be acquired after the administration of intravenous contrast (a dynamic bolus is employed in conventional CT). Vascular contrast permits differentiation of mediastinal structures, which is not as critical as in the radiological staging of lung cancer, but can be rewarding should typical mediastinal lymphadenopathy exist in an esophageal cancer. In the absence of obstructive dysphagia and history of aspiration, water-soluble oral contrast agents are given.

Esophageal wall thickness varies with the degree of luminal distension. Intraluminal air causes distension and enhances the assessment of wall thickness. Although the presence of intraluminal air is commonly associated with a distal obstructive carcinoma, it also can be recognized in 60% of normal subjects.[12] Regardless, the well-distended esophageal wall is less than 3 mm thick, and thickness greater than 5 mm is considered abnormal.[37] Often a cancer can cause mural eccentricity—an equally nonspecific, but notable, abnormal finding. In contrast to EUS, CT cannot distinguish among the layers of the esophageal wall; differentiating among T_{is}, T_1, and T_2 cancers is impossible, and T_3 penetration cannot be defined consistently. Prediction of T_4 disease by CT is slightly more reliable, but still vastly imprecise. Loss of the fat planes between the esophagus and the aorta, the pericardium, elements of the tracheobronchial tree, or the lung may suggest transmural cancer growth and imply invasion of these mediastinal structures. The normal presence of these fat planes, however, cannot be assumed. Mediastinal fat stores also are vulnerable to catabolic destruction from malnutrition associated with advanced esophageal cancer. Fat planes therefore do not necessarily function as reliable radiological clues. CT evidence for aortic invasion, specifically, includes the amount of circumferential contact between the aorta and esophageal cancer mass. An arc interface greater than 90 degrees suggests invasion, arcs between 45–90 degrees are indeterminate, and a contact arc less than 45 degrees relatively excludes invasion.[26] These criteria are reportedly 100% sensitive and 86% specific.[35] Findings correlating with tracheobronchial invasion include thickening of the tracheal or bronchial wall, indentation or displacement of the adjacent airway by an esophageal mass (the membranous tracheobronchial wall is normally flat or convex, especially on inspiration), and the obvious presence of tumor within the airway lumen or airway–esophageal fistula formation. Finally, a pericardial effusion is an unusual but ominous finding, especially when the pericardium adjacent to an esophageal cancer is pronounced and irregularly contoured.

An intrathoracic or abdominal lymph node measuring larger than 1 cm in short-axis dimension on CT is considered abnormally enlarged. CT determination of N and M_{1a} status in esophageal cancer staging relies on this standard criterion for lymphadenopathy. In the supraclavicular and retrocrural regions, the upper limits of normal are slightly lower: 0.5 and 0.6 cm, respectively.[37] As noted in other thoracic malignancies, however, lymph node enlargement is not necessarily commensurate with *metastatic* node involvement. Micrometastatic nodal spread is commonly confirmed in subcentimeter lymph nodes, and, likewise, benign lymphadenopathy is a well-recognized phenomenon

in obstructing esophageal cancers. In addition, CT can underestimate bulky pathologically malignant paraesophageal nodes (level 8), particularly if these enlarged nodes are contiguous with the primary cancer itself. In general, CT evaluation of metastatic lymph nodes is less than optimal and peculiarly dependent on anatomical zone. Pooled data for regional (mediastinal) lymphatic spread show sensitivities ranging from 34–61% and accuracies ranging from 51–70%. Marginally better rates have been described for abdominal nodal disease, with sensitivities of 50–76% and accuracies of 83–87%.[33] Interestingly, in patients with distal esophageal adenocarcinomas, Reed and coworkers[29] have found the CT identification of celiac node disease (M_{1a}) to be particularly dissatisfying.

Although metastatic spread of esophageal carcinoma most commonly occurs by way of a rich network of locoregional lymphatics, hematogenous spread to distant visceral sites is not unusual. At presentation, metastases are found in the liver of 35% of patients, in the lungs of 20%, in the bones of 9%, in the adrenal glands or brain of 2%, and in the pericardium, pleura, stomach, pancreas, or spleen of 1%.[27] With the obvious exception of the brain and extrathoracic skeleton, a staging CT scan for esophageal cancer should image all of these sites. As mentioned, a staging CT is probably most valuable in its capacity to reveal true metastatic disease (stage IVB). From the surgical perspective, whether curative or palliative in therapeutic intent, this capacity is keenly realized (Figure 36-3).

On CT, hepatic metastases are recognized as low-density lesions of variable size with ill-defined margins. Lung metastases generally present as small, well-circumscribed peripheral nodules.

Adrenal metastases cause the gland to become heterogeneously enlarged. Scanning with vascular enhancement renders the nonpathological lung and liver parenchyma contrastingly dense, and washout images with delayed contrast administration provide further characterization of adrenal masses. In the liver the size of the metastatic lesion is important, and 2 cm has been established as a relative

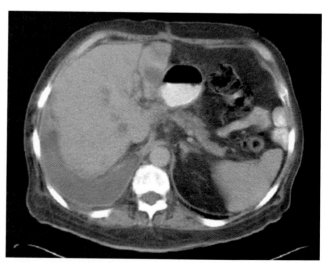

Figure 36–3 CT scan demonstrating esophageal cancer with lever metastases (stage IVB).

threshold. Sensitivities of 70–80% are reported for the detection of hepatic metastases 2 cm or larger in diameter.[37] In the era of PET and certainly CT–PET, the disappointingly high false-negative rate for subcentimeter liver metastases will likely be offset. The overall low sensitivity rates ranging from 27–66% for CT screening of *all* distant metastasis sites are expected to improve also, using the combination of these radiological technologies.

STAGING BY POSITRON EMISSION TOMOGRAPHY

The efficacy of PET in clinical esophageal cancer staging has become firmly established. This nuclear medicine study takes advantage of differential glycolytic activity in malignant and benign tissues. Trapped in glycogen processing pathways, radiolabeled 2-[^{18}F]fluoro-2-deoxy-D-glucose (FDG) preferentially accumulates in neoplastic cells with active glucose metabolism. Previously exploited in bronchogenic carcinoma, heightened FDG uptake is now recognized in 92–100% of esophageal cancers.[9] Spatial resolution on PET imaging, however, is limited. Although the primary malignant lesion is readily identified, local staging of disease is incomplete at best and not possible in a significant majority. Conversely, PET is a *whole-body* staging tool and is ideally suited to detect occult distant metastatic disease in sites not imaged by other esophageal cancer clinical staging techniques. This is particularly relevant in esophageal cancer metastatic to bone, and it seems to be reasonable to assume that PET will soon replace nuclear bone scanning in the staging of thoracic malignancies.

PET fails to provide any information pertaining to the layers of the esophageal wall and the immediate peritumoral area. Therefore PET cannot assist in the assigning of T stage. Similarly, PET does not distinguish the paraesophageal mediastinum to any appreciable degree, rendering staging on the basis of N impractical also. Nodal assessment is particularly poor for nodal metastases adjacent to the primary tumor (regional N_1 disease and a significant portion of M_{1a} spread). However, in contrast to CT's nodal assessment based on anatomy (e.g., size, location), FDG–PET's predictions are based on disease function. A malignant lymph node's ability to concentrate sufficient FDG to appear hypermetabolic on PET accounts for PET's disheartening identification of micrometastatic esophageal cancer in nodes measuring less than 1 cm on CT. As in lung cancer, PET can reveal esophageal cancer metastases in subcentimeter lymph nodes, although lymphatic invasion is trophically different in these two thoracic malignancies. The radiological appearance of a stage III lung cancer is typified by a distinct lung-based mass in conjunction with mediastinal lymphadenopathy; a discrete region of normal-seeming tissue more often than not separates these two areas of malignant disease. In a regionally metastatic esophageal cancer, this distinguishing space between the esophageal cancer itself and its corresponding infiltrated nodes is generally much more finite. Accordingly, the accuracy rates for PET detection of esophageal cancer lymph node metastases vary considerably, from 37–90%.[30]

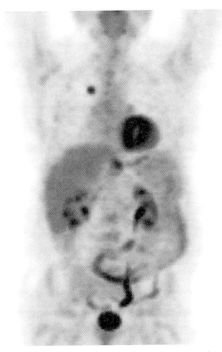

Figure 36–4 Solitary pulmonary metastases (stage IVB) as demonstrated by positron emission tomography.

PET's major strength in the clinical staging of esophageal carcinoma rests in its ability to accurately define, and occasionally uncover, distant metastatic disease (M_{1b}, particularly) (Figure 36-4). PET's superiority to CT in this capacity has been demonstrated, but also challenged. In one study from Pittsburgh,[23] 91 patients with esophageal cancer were evaluated for all distant metastases ($M_{1a,b}$) using 100 consecutive, prospectively collected FDG–PET scans. PET was found to be 69% sensitive, 93% specific, and 84% accurate. By comparison, CT was statistically less sensitive, specific, and accurate, with rates of 46%, 74%, and 63% ($p < .01$). All PET-missed metastatic foci were less than 1 cm in diameter. In 21 false-negative CT scans, PET realized 11 metastases; in 12 false-negative PET scans, CT showed 4 unrecognized metastases. More recently, we published data comparing PET and CT detection of pathologically confirmed M_1 disease. The sensitivity, specificity, and positive and negative predictive values for PET were 89%, 89%, 80%, and 94% versus 33%, 85%, 46%, and 77% for CT, respectively.[20] A smaller study from Stanford in 2002 showed no benefit to PET versus CT in the initial staging of esophageal cancer with respect to metastatic disease. Interestingly, in this particular study CT was a more sensitive indicator of distant metastases, whereas PET was more specific. A proposed explanation provided by its authors concerns the definition of metastatic disease *extent* and questions the statistical validity of comparing metastatic lesion number at each metastatic site versus the simple existence of distant disease (M_1) or not (M_0).[40] Closing to accrual in 2004, the prospective American College of Surgeons Oncology Group–sponsored trial (Z0060) should ultimately provide

616 the definitive answer regarding PET staging in esophageal cancer.

► STAGING BY ENDOSCOPIC ULTRASONOGRAPHY

In the locoregional assessment of esophageal cancer, EUS is arguably the most potent clinical staging tool available. Using high-frequency ultrasound (7.5 or 12 MHz is standard), it defines the layers of the esophageal wall. Endoscopy facilitates appropriate localization of the EUS transducer within the esophageal lumen at the level of the cancer. Guided dilation is occasionally required to properly position the standard 13-mm tipped echoprobe, but malignant stricture formation can render EUS problematic. Newer, miniaturized 20-MHz probes, however, fit through the biopsy channel of an endoscope and sometimes circumvent this size issue.

The sonographic depiction of the normal esophageal wall consists of five concentric rings of alternating echogenicity; each ring correlates with an established histological mural layer. The innermost layer is hyperechoic and corresponds to the superficial mucosa. A hypoechoic circular shadow immediately outside this first ring corresponds to the deep mucosa and muscularis mucosae. The middle hyperechoic ring represents the submucosa and submucosa–muscularis mucosae interface. The fourth visualized ring is hypoechoic and corresponds to the full thickness of the muscularis propria. The outermost ring appears hyperechoic and defines the limit of the esophageal wall or its adventitia. Malignant invasion through the layers of the esophageal wall or depth of penetration directly relates to the qualification of these five sonographic signals: Inability to enumerate a ring or loss of the characteristic concentric patterning indicates cancer invasion through the wall to that depth. In its ability to precisely view the individual layers of the esophageal wall,

EUS is the only clinical staging instrument that reliably determines an esophageal cancer's T status (Figure 36-5). Although rare, EUS overstaging and understaging of tumor depth does occur. Peritumoral edema and obscuration of tissue planes may suggest deeper tumor penetration than that which exists. Similarly, very superficial tumors with limited penetration may not be detected using most sonographic transducers.

Special emphasis is placed on the fourth ultrasound ring, where T_3 and cancers less than T_3 are differentiated. Sonographic distortion limited to the inner three rings defines a T_1 lesion. A T_2 cancer extends up to the fourth ring, but not beyond. Once the fifth ring becomes violated, the interface between the radial extent of the cancer and the images of the adjacent extraesophageal structures is analyzed; absence of this interface indicates T_4 invasion.

EUS also provides useful information pertaining to regional and nonregional lymph node status (Figure 36-6). Characteristic echographic texture and nodal morphology are the key elements used to predict metastatic lymph node involvement. Specifically, four features are considered most important: overall echogenicity, bordering, shape, and size. In order of diagnostic significance, malignant nodes are (1) hypoechoic, (2) distinctly bordered, (3) round and as in CT imaging, and (4) larger than 1 cm. The internal substance of an N_1 (or M_{1a}) node is subtly heterogeneous in its sonographic appearance. By contrast, a benign node is typically homogeneously hyperechoic, not sharply demarcated, ovoid, and small.[4] Realizing that only 25% of involved nodes possess all four characteristic malignant features, EUS accuracy for nodal spread exceeds 80%, and approaches 100%, should all four features be present.[1] Primary tumor and node proximity also has relevance in the EUS assessment of nodal spread; a positive correlation is noted for close proximity. In EUS-directed node evaluation, the cancer's T stage has even greater predictive significance. With deeper tumor penetration or increasing T stage, the incidence of nodal metastases increases parabolically. The probability of node involvement in T_1 tumors is 17%; in T_2 tumors it is 55%, in T_3 tumors it is 83%, and in T_4 tumors it is a marked 88%.

In a meta-analysis of 21 series, the overall clinical determination of N status was 77% accurate; higher accuracy was noted for defining nodal disease or N_1 (89%) than its absence or N_0 (69%).[32] In our series, clinical node staging by PET, CT, and EUS were compared. The sensitivity, specificity, positive predictive value, and negative predictive value were, respectively, 50.0%, 87.0%, 85.0%, and 55.6% for PET, 27.3%, 91.3%, 81.8%, and 46.7% for CT, and 94.1%, 50.0%, 74.4%, and 84.6% for EUS.[20] Other EUS studies have demonstrated improved accuracy, sensitivity, and specificity rates for the assessment of the celiac node basin as opposed to mediastinal node groupings. At the celiac axis (level 20), these previous values were 95%, 83%, and 98%; in the mediastinum (levels 2, 4, 7, 8, and 9), rates were lower—73%, 79%, and 63%.[4]

EUS–FNA provides cytopathological proof of nodal metastases. Biopsy confirmation is the only means of assuring nodal (N) staging. All forms of clinical node assessment (CT, PET, and EUS) have limited means of differentiating

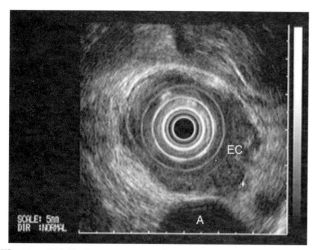

Figure 36–5 **Stage T_3 esophageal carcinoma as determined by endoscopic ultrasonography.** Obliteration of all ultrasonic layers indicates penetration through the entire esophageal wall. The interface between the aorta (A) and cancer (EC) is intact.

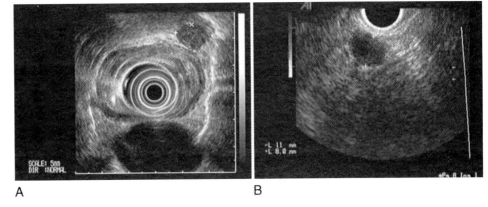

Figure 36–6 Malignant involvement of regional (A) and nonregional lymph nodes (B) by esophageal cancer, as depicted by endoscopic ultrasonography.

A   B

benign from malignant lymphadenopathy. Although it is more prevalent in lung cancer, nonpathological lymphoid proliferation with heightened cellular metabolic activity and benign lymph node enlargement is a well-recognized phenomenon in esophageal cancer also. This is particularly true in instances of luminal obstruction despite its common neoplastic cause. Tissue sampling of the radiologically positive lymph node can minimize this confounding of the data (Figure 36-7).

Two large studies of EUS–FNA included FNA of lymph nodes in esophageal cancer; the technique of EUS–FNA was first advanced in other gastrointestinal malignancies, particularly rectal carcinoma. In a large multicenter trial, EUS–FNA was evaluated in 457 patients.[38] One hundred seventy-one patients underwent FNA of a lymph node, including 32 patients with esophageal cancer. Ultimate diagnosis was obtained at resection or through clinical follow-up. EUS–FNA was found to be 92% sensitive, 93% specific, and 92% accurate. In a similar study of 333 patients, Williams and colleagues[39] analyzed node staging by EUS–FNA in a 39-patient cohort with esophageal cancer. In this particular subset, EUS–FNA proved to be 85% sensitive, 100% specific, and 89% accurate. Integrating clinical findings provided by EUS with pathological information acquired with EUS–FNA, Eloubeidi, Reed, and coinvestigators[7] reported on 51 patients with esophageal cancer who had celiac lymph nodes staged with EUS–FNA. FNA confirmed positive EUS M_{1a} disease in 88%. More impressively, the sensitivity of this tool in this nodal area (celiac axis) was 98%, the specificity was 100%, the accuracy was 98%, and the positive and negative predictive values were 100% and 83%, respectively.

EUS–FNA also has been used to document M_{1b} or visceral (nonnodal) metastases. Experience is limited and technically only possible in rare circumstances. EUS can evaluate only distant organs or sites that lie adjacent to the upper intestinal tract (esophagus, stomach, proximal duodenum). Portions of the retroperitoneum, including the left adrenal gland, and the left lateral segment of the liver draped over the esophageal–diaphragmatic hiatus are regions that are potentially assessed using this powerful clinical and pathological staging modality.

STAGING BY MINIMALLY INVASIVE SURGERY: THORACOSCOPY AND LAPAROSCOPY

In our view, esophageal cancer stage assessment is most definitively made on the basis of data obtained with thoracoscopy and laparoscopy. Despite advances offered by PET and EUS, the typical staging of esophageal cancer is often incomplete, if not inexact. Failure to integrate these modalities into a comprehensive staging routine culminates in clinical and pathological staging disparity. Furthermore, and perhaps more commonly an issue, these nonsurgical investigations have inherent technical limitations that undermine the quest for reliable pretreatment evaluation. For example, EUS cannot faithfully distinguish T_4 invasion of the respiratory airway because air in the tracheobronchial tree interferes with sonographic resolution. Also, a suspicious lymph node targeted for EUS–FNA may lie beyond the reach of an endoscopically guided needle (i.e., AP window node). Alternatively, the questionable node is reachable but lies just outside an esophageal wall

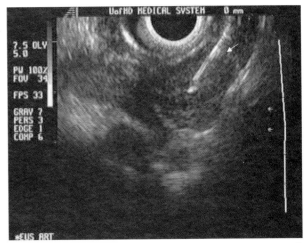

Figure 36–7 Endoscopic ultrasonographically-guided fine needle aspiration (*arrow*) of a radiologically malignant lymph node.

618 invaded by cancer; contamination is unavoidable as the sampling needle traverses this same wall. Similarly, miliary-type hepatic or small pulmonary metastases, parietal peritoneal or pleural studding, or minute omental implants all may contain metabolically active tumor, but in amounts unrecognizable by PET. All of these challenges can potentially be overcome through surgical staging. Thoracoscopic or laparoscopic staging, moreover, remains the only staging modality that can consistently offer pathological confirmation of N, M_{1a}, and, occasionally, M_{1b} disease.

The surgical approach to esophageal cancer staging has roots that predate the minimal access revolution. In 1977 Murray and associates[25] performed preresection mediastinoscopy and limited laparotomy in 30 patients with esophageal cancer. At mediastinoscopy, metastatic lymph node involvement was identified in five patients, or 17%, and minilaparotomy revealed malignant celiac nodes in 16 of 26 patients, or 62%. In 1986 Dagnini and colleagues[5] used primitive laparoscopy and local anesthesia to stage 369 patients with carcinoma of the esophagus and gastric cardia. Clinically unsuspected M_{1b} disease was discovered in 52 patients, or 14%. In 156 patients with cancers of the lower esophagus, liver metastases were found in 9.6%, peritoneal implants were found in 3.2%, and omental deposits were found in 1.9%. In 1992 Fiocco and Krasna[8] replaced the Chamberlain procedure with left thoracoscopy, heralding the marriage of videoscopy and thoracic surgery. One year later, Krasna and McLaughlin[18] described their technique of thoracoscopic lymph node staging (right and left) in 19 esophageal cancer patients; thoracoscopic lymph node assessment proved correct in 14 patients subsequently undergoing thoracotomy. Ultimately in 1999, a prospective intergroup NCI trial (CALGB 9380) confirmed thoracoscopic or laparoscopic esophageal cancer staging to be feasible in 77 of 107 evaluable patients, or 73%.[19] Compared with conventional (noninvasive) staging techniques, this trial also showed that malignant lymph node detection at staging was increased twofold using minimally invasive methods.

As depicted in Figure 36-8, our staging algorithm mandates thoracoscopy if EUS–FNA cannot establish N stage or fails to pathologically confirm N_1 spread; cytologically negative aspirates are not recognized as sufficient proof of N_0 disease. Findings on EUS primarily dictate which side of the chest is explored. Reference is commonly made to a specific node station, location, or other suspicious mediastinal process. A unilateral lung or pleural space abnormality recognized on CT or PET also may determine which side of the body is explored thoracoscopically. Right thoracoscopy is undertaken to assess ipsilateral paratracheal (2R), tracheobronchial angle (4R), subcarinal (7), paraesophageal (8R), and inferior pulmonary ligament (9R) lymph nodes and respective stations defined in parentheses. Left thoracoscopy provides access to the aortopulmonary window (5), preaortic (6), paraesophageal (8L), or inferior pulmonary ligament (9L) nodes; left-sided station 2 and 4 nodes are difficult to examine thoracoscopically, and level 7 nodes are more readily sampled from the right. Left thoracoscopy also can assist in the evaluation of T_4 aortic invasion.

Thoracoscopic staging is performed under general anesthesia. Lung isolation is facilitated with the use of a double-lumen endotracheal tube. The patient is turned in lateral decubitus and rotated slightly forward. Video monitors are placed at the head and foot to minimize parallax or mirror imaging when changing views from two opposing regions of the chest: apex and base or anterior and posterior. Intrapleural carbon dioxide insufflation augments lung deflation if air trapping prevents spontaneous collapse. A thoracotomy instrument set should be opened at the case's beginning and remain available until its completion. Typically two, but up to four, operating ports are established; proper port orientation and spatial arrangement are essential. Triangulating the object of interest enhances depth perception and encourages stereotactic two-handed operating. We routinely use a dual-channel working thoracoscope; with practice this instrument invariably eliminates at least one port or incision (Figure 36-9). Regardless of body side, the chest is first bluntly entered in the seventh or eighth intercostal space just posterior to the anterior axillary line. The pleural cavity is explored, and obvious M_{1b} disease is excluded. Additional sharp trocars are placed under vision. In general, the second port is placed in the approxi-

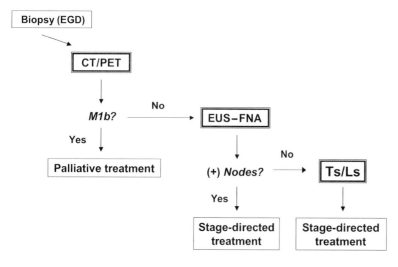

Figure 36–8 Esophageal cancer staging: The University of Maryland Algorithm Thoracoscopic (Ts), Laparoscopic (Ls).

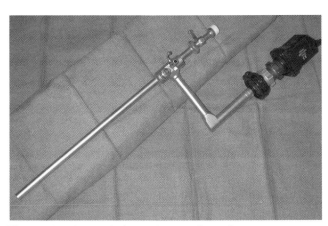

Figure 36–9 Dual-channel or working thoracoscope.

mate sixth space directly below or slightly posterior to the scapula's inferior tip.

In the right side of the chest, the mediastinal pleura overlying the upper esophagus is incised and carried inferiorly to the azygos arch. The paratracheal (level 2R) and tracheobronchial angle (level 4R) node basins are unroofed. The nodes are dissected circumferentially, and just before their complete mobilization, the node's lymphovascular pedicle is

clipped endoscopically. Endoscopic cotton-tipped dissectors (endoscopic kittners) are particularly useful when separating a node from its mediastinal attachments. The sampled node, like all tissue, is removed from the chest without excessive trocar sheath contamination or pleural soilage. Further dissection behind and below the azygos vein exposes the right main stem bronchus and its associated lymph nodes at 10R. Extending the parietal pleural opening down over the subcarinal space and along the inferior pulmonary ligament exposes station 7 and 9R nodes. Finally, representative paraesophageal nodes (station 8) are biopsied. Although they are located throughout the full length of the posterior mediastinum, these nodes are more conveniently sampled from the paraesophageal space alongside the *lower* thoracic esophagus. Level 2, 4, 7, and 10 nodes cooccupy this space in the upper chest; below the plane of the inferior pulmonary vein, only level 8 and 9 nodes are found.

Left-sided lymphadenopathy or intrathoracic phenomena remaining elusive after other staging techniques prompts left thoracoscopy. A questionable periaortic shadow seen on EUS (Figure 36-10A) is indisputably recognized as tumor encasement, or T_4 disease, on thoracoscopic inspection (Figure 36-10B). At Maryland, level 5 or aortopulmonary (window) nodes and level 6 or anterior mediastinal (paraaortic) nodes are routinely staged by left thoracoscopy. As mentioned, these nodal stations are outside the range of EUS–FNA and defy even the most talented bronchoscopists using transbronchial needle aspiration. After reflecting the left upper lobe off the mediastinal pleura, a triangular region

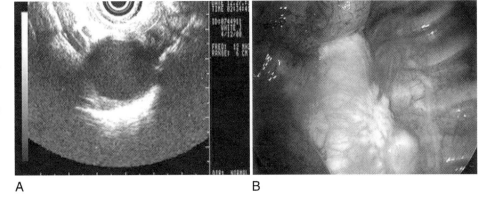

Figure 36–10 Aortic invasion by esophageal carcinoma (stage T_4) as suggested by endoscopic ultrasonography (A) and confirmed at thoracoscopy (B).

A   B

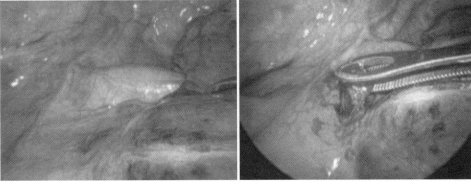

Figure 36–11 Thoracoscopic (A) staging of aortopulmonary window (level 5) lymph nodes.

A   B

620 framed by the phrenic nerve anteriorly and the vagus nerve posteriorly defines the aortopulmonary window (Figure 36-11). The parietal pleura between the superior border of the left main pulmonary artery trunk and underside of the aortic arch is judiciously incised. Level 5 nodes are exposed and sampled. Care is taken to protect the posterior aspect of the window where the left recurrent laryngeal nerve branches from its vagal trunk; electrocautery is avoided in the region to prevent both vascular and neuronal injury. Level 6 nodes can be uncovered by incising the parietal pleura overlying the lateral wall of the ascending aorta, anterior to the phrenic nerve. Invariably, level 6 nodes number far fewer than level 5 nodes. Right lung ventilation can be intermittently suspended to minimize mediastinal movement when dissecting these nodal basins. Finally, the rare left-sided paraesophageal node or left inferior pulmonary ligament node can be sampled as done during right thoracoscopy. After thoracoscopic staging, the pleural space is drained with a single straight chest tube brought through the most inferior (eighth intercostal space) thoracoscopy port site. Typically, the chest tube is removed the next morning and the patient is discharged.

Laparoscopic staging generally follows its thoracoscopic counterpart under the same anesthetic. The patient is (re)positioned in modified lithotomy with his or her lower legs cradled in padded stirrups. The operating surgeon stands between the patient's legs facing a single video monitor at the head of the bed. An orogastric tube is placed to decompress the stomach, and a urinary catheter is used to empty the bladder. These are removed at the end of the procedure. Four abdominal ports are employed. In the abdomen that has no upper midline scar, a point is selected two thirds of the distance from the xiphoid tip to the umbilicus. The proper selection of this point for insertion of the laparoscope is critical. A point too far from the epigastrium could prevent close viewing of the hiatus, and a point too close to the xiphoid likely leads to swordfighting among endoscopic instruments. Carbon dioxide pneumoperitoneum is slowly established to a maximal pressure of 15 mm Hg using a Veress needle. The Veress needle is exchanged for a 10- to 12-mm trocar equipped with a protective governing shield. A 30-degree laparoscope is introduced. After excluding malignant ascites, omental or peritoneal implantations, hepatic masses, and other forms of advanced disease, three additional ports are inserted under vision. A 5-mm trocar is placed in the right lower middle abdomen, through which a foldable liver retractor is used to displace the left lateral segment of the liver off the esophageal hiatus and esophagogastric junction. A second 5-mm trocar is inserted at the epigastrium, and a second 10- to 12-mm port is established beneath the middle left subcostal margin. With the pneumoperitoneum evacuated, this subcostal port should lie approximately 1 cm below the costal fold. The two trocars in the midline and the left abdominal port should be evenly spaced. Specimens are retrieved mainly through the left subcostal port.

Nodal metastases located below the diaphragm are commonly recognized in three principal basins. Level 16 or paracardial nodes can be found within or adjacent to the characteristic fat pad covering the esophagogastric junction. Level 17 nodes cluster along the left gastric artery. Level 20 nodes lie adjacent to the celiac artery trunk, close to its origin. If lymphatic flow is viewed as a centripetal process, metastatic spread from level 16 through level 20 could reflect disease progression from regional (level 16 involvement only) to nonregional (level 20) nodes. Alternatively, locoregional disease may still exist despite malignant celiac nodes if the primary cancer arises just proximal to the esophagogastric junction. To expose level 17 and 20 nodes, the lesser sac should be entered through an opening in the gastrohepatic ligament. In many patients this is an avascular plane. Dissection is continued along the stomach's lesser curvature up toward the right crural pillar. The lymphatics of suspicious nodes or malignant nodes proven positive at frozen section are clipped to better define radiotherapy fields. Laparoscopy also can expose occult nonnodal stage IVB disease. Microhepatic metastases (Figure 36-12A) or other unsuspected nonregional, nonnodal metastatic spread (Figure 36-12B) can be seen at laparoscopy; both of these examples were not recognized by clinical (noninvasive) staging methods. Bulky specimens may require endoscopic bags for their removal to minimize port site implantation or other forms of tumor fragmentation upon extraction. We have had only one "port site" metastasis in over 160 laparoscopic staging procedures, with an average of more than three ports placed per procedure. Furthermore, this presumed implant arose at the site of a jejunostomy tube's exit; the feeding tube was placed after laparoscopic staging that incidentally revealed diffuse intraabdominal metastases.

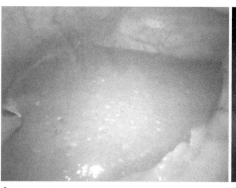

A

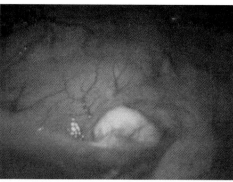

B

Figure 36–12 Metastatic disease (stage IVB) discovered at laparoscopy in the liver (A) and greater omentum (B). Clinical staging techniques (non-invasive) were unable to recognize such small metastatic deposits.

In our last report on 111 patients, thoracoscopic and laparoscopic staging again proved superior to nonsurgical (clinical) staging methods in patients with esophageal cancer.[17] Thoracoscopic staging was successfully performed in 96.2% of the patients studied, and laparoscopic staging could be accomplished in 98.7%; adequate exploration was prevented chiefly by pleural and peritoneal adhesions. Thirteen of 19 patients with clinical T_4 disease were downstaged to T_3, whereas eight patients with clinical T_3 disease were upstaged to T_4 at thoracoscopy or laparoscopy. Clinically positive mediastinal adenopathy was proven thoracoscopically in 18.8% of patients, and clinically positive abdominal node metastasis was confirmed laparoscopically in 63.2%. Clinically negative mediastinal nodes were pathologically proven positive in 8.8% of patients, and clinically negative abdominal nodes were recognized as positive in 18.6%. Thoracoscopic or laparoscopic biopsy in 17 patients suspected to have stage M_{1b} disease clinically confirmed distant disease in five patients (29.4%) and excluded M_{1b} disease in the remaining 12 (70.6%). Compared with true pathological results (obtained at either thoracoscopy, laparoscopy, or final resection), the clinical staging of mediastinal lymph node metastases was 63.6% sensitive, 56.9% specific, and 57.9% accurate, with positive and negative predictive values of 21.9% and 89.2%, respectively; clinical staging of abdominal lymph node metastases was 25.9% sensitive, 95.2% specific, and 68.1% accurate, with positive and negative predictive values of 77.8% and 66.7%, respectively. Compared with 69 evaluable patients undergoing definitive esophagectomy, a 100% specificity and positive predictive value was achieved by thoracoscopic or laparoscopic staging of lymph nodes, with an accuracy of 90.8% for malignant chest nodes and 96.4% for abdominal nodal metastases. As shown in Table 36-2, thoracoscopic and laparoscopic staging furnish a significantly better estimation of lymph node stage than that provided by clinical staging methods.

▶ ADJUNCTIVE STAGING TECHNIQUES AND FUTURE DIRECTIONS

Because of their proximity, the lower trachea and main stem bronchi are vulnerable to direct invasion by upper and midthoracic esophageal cancers. This pattern of regional growth is particularly characteristic of squamous cell carcinoma but can be seen in an adenocarcinoma whose behavior is atypical. Occasionally, metastatic paraesophageal or other mediastinal lymph nodes may secondarily involve the tracheobronchial lymphatics, or bulky nodes may erode into the airway itself. As described, CT and EUS cannot reliably stage T_4 involvement of the tracheobronchial tree. Similarly, as utile as a staging thoracoscopy can be, it can only provide further evidence of this particular form of T_4 disease, not pathological proof. Fiberoptic bronchoscopy is a simple tool that can confirm malignant invasion of the upper respiratory tract. A suspicion raised by CT (Figure 36-13A) is corroborated through EUS (Figure 36-13B) and proven on endobronchial biopsy at bronchoscopy (Figure 36-13C). We routinely add bronchoscopy to the staging of middle- and upper-third esophageal cancers that appear deeper than T_1

on EUS. This quick and straightforward procedure can be performed immediately before a planned thoracoscopic staging. In the rare circumstance that occult T_4 airway disease is recognized, scheduled thoracoscopy has been deferred.

Despite the miraculous evolution of molecular science, TNM staging in esophageal cancer remains a *supramolecular*, if not a multicellular, process. Independent of staging technique and irrespective of its methodology (clinical, pathological, or combined), the mere detection of malignant disease is difficult with any tumor focus smaller than 1 g or 1 cm^3. Definitive stage determination, moreover, can require additional tissue using today's usual analytical tools. Although significant strides have been achieved in the manner with which a suspicious node is sampled and increasingly sensitive means of recognizing nonregional cancer spread have been developed, confirmation of these suggestions still necessitates the comparatively crude (and historical) hematoxylin and eosin staining of biopsied tissue. This soon may change. The advent of monoclonal antibodies directed against epithelial cell–associated antigens and the refinement of related immunohistochemical and cytochemical techniques have enabled identification of a *single* disseminated tumor cell. This technology has been readily applied to breast, gastric, colon, and lung cancer; new staging subcategories such as pM1*i* have been proposed in these cancers to designate the most minimal of metastatic disease—the isolated tumor cell in a secondary organ. The existence of *micrometastatic* phenomena has recently been discovered in esophageal cancer as well. Occult pleural dissemination after lavage, bone marrow micrometastasis, lymph node micrometastasis, and even circulating tumor cells have been documented in both esophageal adenocarcinoma and squamous cell carcinoma.

In 1996 Thorban and colleagues[36] reported on the utility of iliac crest bone marrow aspirates in 90 patients with squamous cell esophageal cancer. At least 41.1%, or 37 patients, were found to have cytokeratin-positive tumor cells in their sampled bone marrow. As few as *one* tumor cell could be detected per 10^5 mononuclear bone marrow cells assayed (range 1–83). Only 3.2% of specimens examined after Giemsa staining showed morphologically identified tumor cells. Given the supreme importance of lymph node involvement in esophageal cancer—it being *the* most significant independent poor prognostic indicator—the existence and clinical significance of micrometastatic lymph nodes has been well investigated. As published in the *New England Journal of Medicine*, Izbicki and coworkers[14] found Ber-EP_4-positive tumor cells in 17% of patients already believed to have "tumor-free" lymph nodes. This form of upstaging was shown to be predictive of significantly reduced relapse-free survival and overall survival. Similar findings were reported by Komukai and associates.[16] Fourteen of 37 patients (38%) with esophageal squamous cell carcinoma were found to have nodal micrometastases using monoclonal antibody (AE_1/AE_3) directed against cytokeratin. Not only was survival (relapse-free and overall) negatively affected by node-positive micrometastatic disease, tumor recurrence was significantly more frequent in patients with micrometastatic tumor than in those without (50 versus 9%, $p = .008$). A completely different conclusion was reached

Table 36–2

Staging of Esophageal Cancer Mediastinal Lymph Node Metastases by Thoracoscopy and Laparoscopy Compared to Clinical (Non-Invasive) Methodologies

	Sensitivity [% (no.)]	p value	Specificity [% (no.)]	p value	PPV [% (no.)]	p value	NPV [% (no.)]	p value	Accuracy [% (no.)]	p value
Thoracic N$_1$										
CT/MRI/EUS	63.6	.7	56.9	<.001	21.9	.003	89.2	.9	57.9	<.001
Ts	45.5		100.0		100.0		90.0		90.8	
Abdominal N$_1$										
CT/MRI/EUS	25.9	<.001	95.2	.6	77.8	.02	66.7	.002	68.1	<.001
Ls	90.9		100.0		100.0		94.3		96.4	

Adapted from Krasna et al, 2002.

PPV, positive predictive value; NPV, negative predictive value; Ts, thoracoscopy; Ls, laparoscopy.

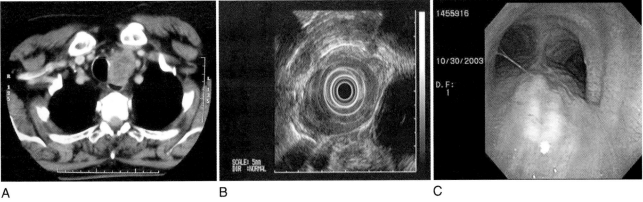

Figure 36–13 Tracheal invasion by esophageal carcinoma (stage T_4) as suggested by computer tomography (A) and endoscopic ultrasonography (B); pathologically proven by biopsy obtained at bronchoscopy (C).

by Glickman and fellow Harvard researchers.[10] Cytokeratin histochemical staining showed occult lymph node metastasis in 31% of patients with adenocarcinoma and 17% of patients with squamous cell carcinoma of the esophagus. These occult micrometastases, however, did not statistically correlate with poorer survival rates.

Gene amplification using reverse transcription–polymerase chain reaction (rt–PCR) coupled with various markers, including carcinoembryonic antigen (CEA) messenger ribonucleic acid, p53 tumor suppression gene, and epidermal growth factor, has enabled even *sub*cellular material to be analyzed for micrometastatic potential. In a pilot study, Luketich and associates[22] have identified lymph node metastases by rt–PCR in 49% of histologically node-negative (N_0) patients with esophageal cancer; lymph nodes from patients with benign esophageal diseases such as gastrointestinal reflux disease (GERD) and achalasia demonstrated no CEA-specific activity. Applying rt–PCR techniques for the detection of circulating tumor cells, Mori

and co-investigators[24] have reported on a limited subset of esophageal cancers within a group of gastrointestinal carcinomas and related nonhematological malignancy. In one esophageal cancer patient with stage I disease, according to conventional clinicopathological data, sampled blood tested positive for CEA mRNA. Despite timely and complete resection of the esophageal primary, lung metastases were noted at a particularly early time after esophagectomy.

In an attempt to further advance the pretreatment staging of esophageal cancer, we recently were granted preliminary approval by the Cancer and Leukemia Group B (CALGB) executive committee to investigate the applicability of the *sentinel* lymph node concept to the staging of esophageal cancer (Figure 36-14). Based on the nonrandom flow of tumor drainage, the sentinel node model was first established in melanoma and subsequently applied to breast cancer. It has changed the staging paradigm, refined risk stratification, and led to improved treatment allocation in both of these malignancies. A primary objective in our study

Figure 36–14 Sentinel lymph node (SLN) for staging of esophageal carcinoma. Study design proposed by the University of Maryland and granted preliminary approval by the Cancer and Leukemia Group B (CALGB). GI, gastrointestinal; SPECT, single photon emission computed tomography; Ts, thoracoscopy; Ls, laparoscopy; LN, lymph node; H&E, hematoxylin and eosin; IHC, immunohistochemistry; rt–PCR; reverse transcription–polymerase chain reaction.

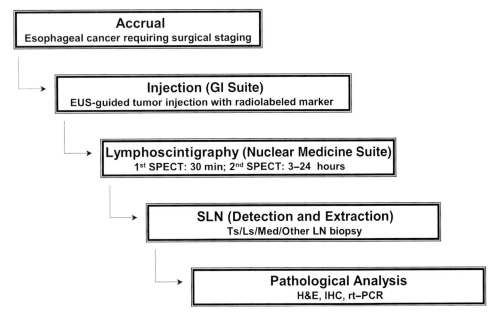

624 is to use minimally invasive staging techniques (thoracoscopy or laparoscopy) to identify the postulated sentinel node. Our current protocol in lung cancer employs an elongated Geiger counter that can be inserted through a standard 10- to 12-mm trocar at thoracoscopy; a similar instrument will be used in this proposed study. To assess the impact of occult micrometastases, all candidate nodes sampled will be subjected to both conventional pathological review and complete immunohistochemical and molecular analysis. We are hopeful that this concept will be tested on a multi-institutional basis soon.

REFERENCES

1. Bhutani MS, Hawes RH, Hoffman BJ: A comparison of the accuracy of echo features during endoscopic ultrasound (EUS) and EUS-guided fine needle aspiration for diagnosis of malignant lymph node invasion. Gastrointest Endosc 45:474, 1997.
2. Blot WJ, McLaughlin JK: The changing epidemiology of esophageal cancer. Semin Oncol 26:2, 1999.
3. Catalano MF, Sivak MV Jr, Rice TW, et al: Endoscopic features predictive of lymph node metastases. Gastrointest Endosc 40:442, 1994.
4. Catalano MF, Alcocer E, Chak A, et al: Evaluation of metastatic celiac lymph nodes in patients with esophageal carcinoma: Accuracy of EUS. Gastrointest Endosc 50:352, 1999.
5. Dagnini G, Caldironi MW, Marin G, et al: Laparoscopy in abdominal staging of esophageal carcinoma. Gastrointest Endosc 32:400, 1986.
6. Devessa SS, Blot WJ, Fraumeni JF Jr: Changing patterns in the incidence of esophageal and gastric carcinoma in the United States. Cancer 15:2049, 1998.
7. Eloubeidi MA, Wallace MB, Reed CE, et al: The utility of EUS and EUS-guided fine needle aspiration in detecting celiac lymph node metastasis in patients with esophageal cancer: A single-center experience. Gastrointest Endosc 54:714, 2001.
8. Fiocco M, Krasna MJ: Thoracoscopic lymph node dissection in the staging of esophageal disease. J Laparoendosc Surg 2:111, 1992.
9. Flanagan FL, Dehdashti F, Siegel BA, et al: Staging of esophageal cancer with ^{18}F-fluorodeoxyglucose positron emission tomography. AJR Am J Roentgenol 168:417, 1997.
10. Glickman JN, et al: The prognostic significance of lymph node micrometastasis in patients with esophageal carcinoma. Cancer 85:770, 1990.
11. Greene FL, Page DL, Fleming ID, et al, editors: American Joint Committee on Cancer Staging Manual, 6th ed. New York: Springer-Verlag, 2002.
12. Halber MD, Daffner RH, Thompson WM: CT of the esophagus: Normal appearance. AJR Am J Roentgenol 133:1047, 1979.
13. Iyer RB, Silverman PM, Tamm EP, et al: Imaging in oncology from the University of Texas M.D. Anderson Cancer Center. Diagnosis, staging, and follow-up of esophageal cancer. AJR Am J Roentgenol 181:78, 2003.
14. Izbicki JR, Hosch SB, Pichlmeier U, et al: Prognostic value of immunohistochemically identifiable tumor cells in lymph nodes of patients with completely resected esophageal cancer. N Engl J Med 337:1188, 1997.
15. Kawahara K, Maekawa T, Okabayashi K, et al: The number of lymph node metastases influences survival in esophageal cancer. J Surg Oncol 67:160, 1998.
16. Komukai S, Nishimaki T, Watanabe H, et al: Significance of immunohistochemically demonstrated micrometastases to lymph nodes in esophageal cancer with histologically negative nodes. Surgery 127:40, 2000.
17. Krasna MJ, Jiao X, Mao YS, et al: Thoracoscopy/laparoscopy in the staging of esophageal cancer: Maryland experience. Surg Laparosc Endosc Percutan Tech 12:213, 2002.
18. Krasna MJ, McLaughlin JS: Thoracoscopic lymph node staging for esophageal cancer. Ann Thorac Surg 56:671, 1993.
19. Krasna MJ, Reed CE, Nedzwiecki D, et al: CALGB 9380: A prospective trial of the feasibility of thoracoscopy/laparoscopy in staging esophageal cancer. Ann Thorac Surg 71:1073, 2001.
20. Kwong KF, Chalabi I, Beck S, et al: Comparison of FDG-PET, CT, and esophageal ultrasound imaging versus tissue diagnosis in pre-resection esophageal cancer patients. J Nucl Med 44:375, 2003 (abstract).
21. Lau LL, Moore MB, Brooks KR, et al: Molecular staging of lung and esophageal cancer. Surg Clin North Am 82:497, 2002.
22. Luketich JD, Kassis ES, Shriver SP, et al: Detection of micrometastases in histologically negative lymph nodes in esophageal cancer. Ann Thorac Surg 66:1715–1718, 1998.
23. Luketich JD, Friedman DM, Weigel TL, et al: Evaluation of distant metastases in esophageal cancer: 100 consecutive positron emission tomography scans. Ann Thorac Surg 68:1133–1136; discussion 1136–1137, 1999.
24. Mori M, Mimori K, Ueo H, et al: Clinical significance of molecular detection of carcinoma cells in lymph nodes and peripheral blood by reverse transcription-polymerase chain reaction in patients with gastrointestinal or breast carcinomas. J Clin Oncol 16:128, 1998.
25. Murray GF, Wilcox BR, Stared P: The assessment of operability of esophageal carcinoma. Ann Thorac Surg 23:393, 1977.
26. Picus D, Balfe DM, Koehler RE, et al: Computed tomography in the staging of esophageal carcinoma. Radiology 146:433, 1983.
27. Quint LE, Hepburn LM, Francis IR, et al: Incidence and distribution of distant metastases in newly diagnosed esophageal carcinoma. Cancer 76:1120, 1995.
28. Rankin S. Oesophageal cancer. In Husband JES, Reznek RH, editors: Imaging in Oncology. Oxford, UK: Isis Medical Media, 1998.
29. Reed CE, Mishra G, Sahai AV, et al: Esophageal cancer staging: Improved accuracy by endoscopic ultrasound of celiac lymph nodes. Ann Thorac Surg 67:319, 1999.
30. Rice TW: Clinical staging of esophageal carcinoma. Chest Surg Clin N Am 10:471, 2000.
31. Rice TW, Blackstone EH, Rybicki LA, et al: Refining esophageal cancer staging. J Thorac Cardiovasc Surg 125:1103, 2003.
32. Rosch T: Endosonographic staging of esophageal cancer: A review of literature results. Gastrointest Endosc Clin N Am 5:537, 1995.
33. Saunders HS, Wolfman NT, Ott DJ: Esophageal cancer. Radiologic staging. Radiol Clin North Am 35:281, 1997.
34. Steup WH, De Leyn P, Deneffe G, et al: Tumors of the esophagogastric junction. Long-term survival in relation to the pattern of lymph node metastasis and a critical analysis of the accuracy or inaccuracy of pTNM classification. J Thorac Cardiovasc Surg 111:85, 1996.
35. Takashima S, Takeuchi N, Shiozaki H, et al: Carcinoma of the esophagus: CT vs MRI imaging in determining respectability. Am J Roentgenol 156:297, 1991.
36. Thorban S, Roder JD, Nekarda H, et al: Immunocytochemical detection of disseminated tumor cells in the bone marrow of patients with esophageal carcinoma. J Natl Cancer Inst 88:1222, 1996.
37. Van Overhagen H, Becker CD: Diagnosis and staging of carcinoma of the esophagus and gastroesophageal junction,

and detection of postoperative recurrence by computer tomography. In Meyers MA, editor: Neoplasms of the Digestive Tract: Imaging, Staging, and Management. Philadelphia: Lippincott-Raven, 1998.

38. Wiersema MJ, Vilmann P, Giovannini M, et al: Endosonography-guided fine-needle aspiration biopsy; diagnostic accuracy and complication assessment. Gastroenterol 112:1087, 1997.

39. Williams DB, Sahai AV, Aabakken L, et al: Endoscopic ultrasound guided fine needle aspiration biopsy: A large single centre experience. Gut 44:720, 1999.

40. Wren SM, Stijns P, Srinivas S: Positron emission tomography in the initial staging of esophageal cancer. Arch Surg 137:1001, 2002.

Esophageal Resection and Replacement

Philip A. Linden and Scott J. Swanson

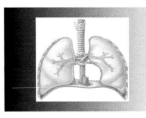

▶ INTRODUCTION

The first esophageal resection was performed over 125 years ago, yet it remains one of the most formidable operations, carrying the highest morbidity of any commonly performed resection. It remains the only means to cure esophageal cancer, yet the overall cure rate following esophagectomy is only 20%. The perioperative mortality has decreased from 40% to less than 3% in selected academic centers, largely because of advances in surgical technique, intensive care, and management of complications. With average mortality rates at 10%, and complication rates exceeding 50%, careful patient selection, thoughtful surgical planning, meticulous technique, and timely management of complications are essential to ensure good patient outcome. The esophageal surgeon must be familiar with the anatomy of the neck, chest, and abdomen, and be skilled in surgery of the entire alimentary tract to provide complete care of the patient requiring esophageal resection. Only with this knowledge can the surgeon fit the operation to the patient, and not the patient into the operation. These issues are detailed in this chapter.

▶ HISTORY OF ESOPHAGEAL RESECTION

The first esophageal resection is credited to Czerny, who, in 1877, resected a cervical esophageal tumor without reestablishing intestinal continuity. Resection of gastroesophageal

628 junction tumors via laparotomy with esophagogastric anastomosis was not uncommonly performed in the years following; however, surgeons were unwilling to operate on the esophagus through the chest because of concerns over respiratory impairment. It was not until 1911 that Torek performed the first resection of the thoracic esophagus.[71] He performed a transthoracic resection of the esophagus without reconstruction, leaving the patient with a cervical esophagostomy and gastrostomy. A 3-foot-long external rubber tube was used to "reconstruct" the esophagus, connecting the esophagostomy and gastrostomy; the patient lived for over 10 years following the operation. Turner, in 1933, performed the first resection of the thoracic esophagus with reconstruction in what was the first transhiatal esophagectomy. Resection and reconstruction via thoracotomy were first done in Japan in 1933 by Oshawa who performed the operation in 19 patients, half of whom survived.[52] His success rate in an era of primitive general anesthesia was remarkable; however his achievements did not receive the same publicity as that of Adams and Phemister, who were the first to describe transthoracic resection and reconstruction in the Western literature in 1938.[1]

Ivor Lewis, writing in 1946, is credited with popularizing transthoracic resection of the esophagus. He initially performed the operation in two stages, first mobilizing the stomach via laparotomy and second several days later resecting the esophagus and performing an intrathoracic anastomosis via right thoracotomy. Dr. Lewis showed a sophisticated understanding of the challenges involved in esophageal surgery when he stated that "the oesophagus is a difficult surgical field for three reasons: its inaccessibility; its lack of a serous coat, and its enclosure in structures where infection is especially dangerous and rapid."[39] The Ivor Lewis and transhiatal approaches are the most commonly employed techniques of esophageal resection used today. In 1962, McKeown described a three-stage esophagectomy, with the addition of a cervical incision and anastomosis to allow for better margins for proximal tumors.[44] It is now called the three-hole or triincisional esophagectomy. Recently, totally endoscopic approaches have been developed and performed successfully in a few centers across the nation.[40,48,67] It has yet to be seen whether these minimally invasive approaches represent advances in patient outcome.

▶ TECHNIQUES OF ESOPHAGEAL RESECTION

Modified McKeown or Triincisional Technique

Indications

The triincisional esophagectomy (modified McKeown) is a versatile technique that can be employed for tumors at any level and for a variety of benign and malignant conditions. It combines the advantages of the Ivor Lewis approach with those of a transhiatal technique. These include complete lymph node dissection in the chest, direct visualization of the intrathoracic dissection, avoidance of an intrathoracic anastomosis, maximal margins, and diminution of chances for postoperative gastroesophageal reflux disease (GERD). It is especially useful for tumors of the mid and upper

esophagus and for tumors arising in a long Barrett's segment where near total excision of the esophagus is required.

Contraindications

Fusion of the right pleural space or inability to support ventilation with the left lung would make an approach via right thoracotomy difficult.

Preparation

A detailed history and physical examination are necessary to evaluate for coexistent comorbid disease. Computed tomography (CT) of the chest and abdomen should be obtained to evaluate for metastatic disease, anatomical abnormalities, and location of the tumor adjacent to vital structures. Pulmonary function tests (PFTs) should be obtained. Poor FEV_1 is not a contraindication to a muscle-sparing limited thoracotomy, though increased risk of pulmonary complications may be expected. A video-assisted thoracic surgery (VATS) approach may be used in most circumstances if pulmonary function is a concern. Bowel preparation is not needed for gastric transposition. Head CT and positron emission tomography (PET) scan are useful in ruling out metastatic disease.

Technique

After intubation, bronchoscopy is performed to rule out tracheal or bronchial invasion and to mobilize any secretions from the left lung that will be used to support ventilation during right thoracotomy. Esophagogastroduodenoscopy is performed to identify the location of the tumor and to rule out disease of the stomach or duodenum. A double lumen tube is placed and the patient is positioned in a left lateral decubitus position. A right posterolateral thoracotomy incision is made wide enough to insert the surgeon's hand (approximately 10 cm). A portion of the latissimus is divided; the serratus is spared (Figure 37-1). Division of the intercostal muscle from the vertebral bodies posteriorly to the mammary vessels anteriorly will usually provide enough working space without division of a rib. The chest is entered through the fifth or sixth interspace depending on the location of the tumor. The lung is retracted anteriorly, and the inferior pulmonary ligament is divided using cautery. Alternatively, as experience with thoracoscopy increases, a VATS or minimally invasive approach may be employed.

In a region away from the tumor and away from any scarring, the pleura overlying the esophagus is incised anteriorly and posteriorly and the esophagus is surrounded with a penrose. With traction on the penrose, the esophagus is retracted both anteriorly and posteriorly and is dissected using electrocautery, including all adjacent lymph node tissue. Arterial branches supplying the esophagus from the aorta are clipped before being divided. Any cautery performed in the region of the carina must be at low settings to avoid thermal injury to the trachea. The azygous vein is typically divided, although this is not essential. At the level of the azygous vein, the vagus nerves are identified on the esophagus and divided between clips. Further cranial dissection proceeds with the vagus nerves away from the

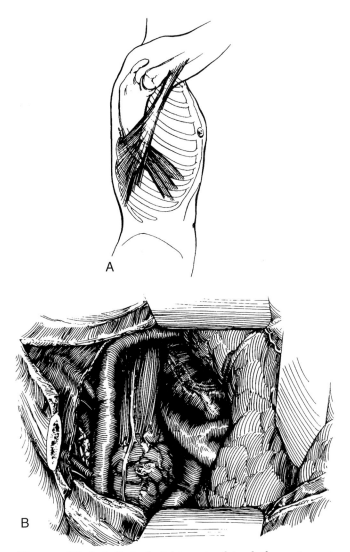

Figure 37–1 A limited right posterolateral thoracotomy is performed, dividing latissimus.
(*Reprinted with permission from Swanson S, Grondin S, Sugarbaker D: Total esophagectomy: The Brigham and Women's Hospital approach. Oper Tech Thorac Cardiovasc Surg 4:197–209, 1999.*)

esophagus, to avoid recurrent nerve injury. Blunt dissection is useful high in the right chest (Figure 37-2). A knotted penrose is placed around the cervical esophagus and pushed into the neck for retrieval during the cervical portion of the case (Figure 37-3). This penrose drain, positioned inside the vagus nerves relative to the esophagus, permits isolation of the cervical esophagus without traction on the recurrent nerve. A sponge is packed high in the chest to assist in hemostasis and is removed prior to closure.

The lower portion of the esophagus is encircled with a second penrose drain and the remaining distal esophagus is dissected, including in the specimen all tissue lateral to the pericardium and medial to the aorta and spine. If the tumor is near the gastroesophageal (GE) junction, a 2-cm rim of diaphragm is resected with the esophagus (Figure 37-4). The penrose is knotted and left in the abdomen for retrieval during the abdominal portion of the operation. Mass ligature of the thoracic duct at the level of the hiatus is per-

formed by encircling all tissue between the aorta and spine with a 0 silk suture. The chest is inspected for hemostasis, the sponge previously placed is removed, and a 28F straight chest tube is inserted through a separate stab incision and directed to the apex of the chest. The ribs are approximated with interrupted #2 vicryl sutures. The latissimus is closed with running 0 vicryl suture. The subdermal fascia is closed with a running 2-0 vicryl suture. The skin is closed with staples or suture.

The patient is repositioned in the supine position and is reintubated with a single lumen tube. A transverse roll is placed under the scapula and the head is turned 45° to the right. An upper midline laparotomy is performed from the umbilicus to the junction of the costal margin and the left side of the xyphoid. The abdomen is explored for metastatic disease. The left lobe of the liver is mobilized. The penrose surrounding the GE junction is grasped and the remaining phrenoesophageal ligament is divided (Figure 37-5). The gastroepiploic pulse is palpated. Assuming systemic pressure is adequate, the pulse should be easily palpable. At a point 2 cm away from the gastroepiploic artery on the greater curvature of the stomach, the lesser sac is entered. Dissection along the greater curvature of the stomach toward the spleen proceeds with division of vascular branches using double clips, silk ties, or the harmonic scalpel. Short gastric vessels are taken in identical fashion; large vessels should be tied. Displacement of the spleen anteriorly by placing lap pads behind the spleen may aid in dissection of the short gastric vessels. Dissection extends to the hiatus. Additional dissection toward the pylorus is also performed

The stomach is then lifted anteriorly and any adhesions between the stomach and pancreas are divided using electrocautery. The left gastric artery is identified and skeletonized, sweeping lymph node tissue onto the specimen. With a 30-mm vascular stapler, the base of the left gastric artery is clamped. A continued strong pulse in the gastroepiploic artery is confirmed and the left gastric artery is divided (Figure 37-6). The gastrohepatic ligament is divided using a combination of cautery and the stapler. Next, the duodenum is kocherized, bringing the pylorus to the midline. Either a pyloromyotomy or pyloroplasty may be performed. If a pyloroplasty is performed, it should be a single layer performed with interrupted 3-0 silk sutures, carefully incorporating mucosa and muscular wall.

Attention is then turned to the neck, and a 6-cm incision is made from the sternal notch along the anterior border of the sternocleidomastoid muscle. The platysma is divided, and dissection proceeds between the carotid sheath laterally and the strap muscles medially. The omohyoid muscle may be divided. The knot of the penrose should be palpable on the spine. The penrose is grasped and the esophagus is gently mobilized. The nasogastric tube is partially withdrawn, and the cervical esophagus is divided with a 75-mm linear stapler (Figure 37-7). A #2 silk suture ligature is fastened to the distal end of the divided esophagus, and the specimen is drawn into the abdomen with the attached silk suture. The cervical end of the silk suture is fastened to a clamp.

A gastric tube is fashioned by resecting the GE junction and the lesser curve of the stomach with a series of 75-mm thick tissue staplers (Figure 37-8). A narrow gastric tube aids in gastric emptying. A diameter of less than 6 cm, however, can compromise venous and arterial blood supply. The line

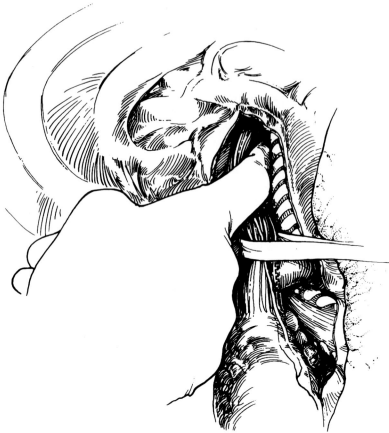

Figure 37–2 Blunt finger dissection close to the esophagus is used to free the esophagus up into the neck.
(*Reprinted with permission from Sugarbaker D, DeCamp M, Liptay M: Surgical procedures to resect and replace the esophagus. In Zinner M, Schwartz S, Ellis H, et al, editors: Maingot's Abdominal Operations. Stanford, CT: Appleton & Lange, 1997, pp. 885–910.*)

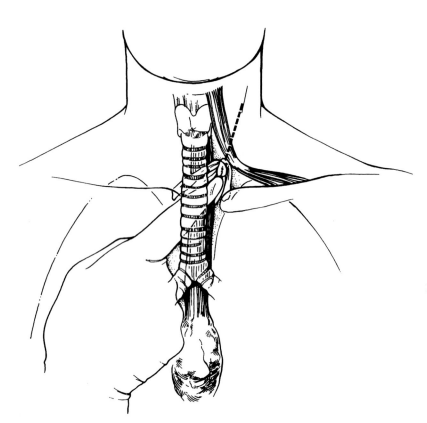

Figure 37–3 A knotted Penrose is placed into the left neck for later retrieval during the cervical dissection. This helps ensure isolation of the esophagus without injury to the recurrent nerves.
(*Reprinted with permission from Sugarbaker D, DeCamp M, Liptay M: Surgical procedures to resect and replace the esophagus. In Zinner M, Schwartz S, Ellis H, et al, editors: Maingot's Abdominal Operations. Stanford, CT: Appleton & Lange, 1997, pp. 885–910.*)

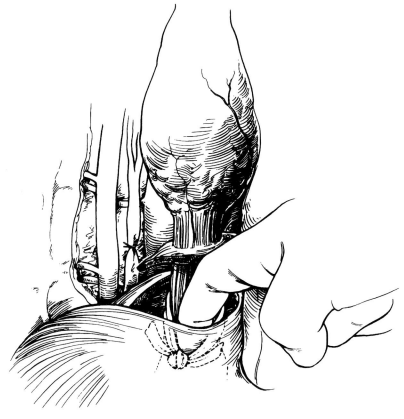

Figure 37–4 A rim of diaphragm is incorporated into the specimen for all GE junction tumors. A knotted penrose is placed into the abdomen to aid dissection of the esophagus at the GE junction during the abdominal phase of the operation.
(Reprinted with permission from Sugarbaker D, DeCamp M, Liptay M: Surgical procedures to resect and replace the esophagus. In Zinner M, Schwartz S, Ellis H, et al, editors: Maingot's Abdominal Operations. Stanford, CT: Appleton & Lange, 1997, pp. 885–910.)

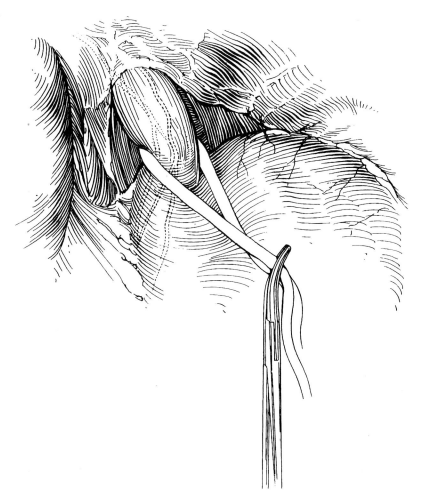

Figure 37–5 The phrenoesophageal ligament is divided fully after retrieval of the penrose.
(Reprinted with permission from Swanson S, Grondin S, Sugarbaker D: Total esophagectomy: The Brigham and Women's Hospital approach. Oper Tech Thorac Cardiovasc Surg 4:197–209, 1999.)

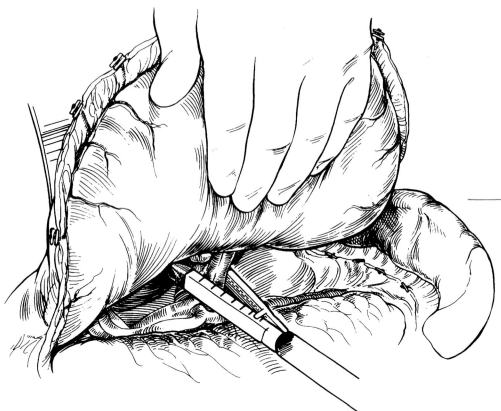

Figure 37–6 Following complete mobilization of the greater curvature of the stomach, and division of the gastrohepatic ligament, the left gastric vessels are identified. An endoscopic vascular stapler is used to divide these vessels with care not to impinge on the celiac axis.
(Reprinted with permission from Sugarbaker D, DeCamp M, Liptay M: Surgical procedures to resect and replace the esophagus. In Zinner M, Schwartz S, Ellis H, et al, editors: Maingot's Abdominal Operations. Stanford, CT: Appleton & Lange, 1997, pp. 885–910.)

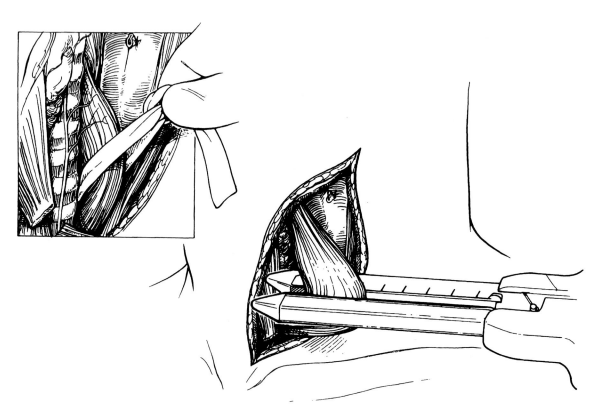

Figure 37–7 Retrieval of the Penrose placed around the esophagus inside the recurrent nerves during chest dissection. This aids in the prevention of recurrent nerve injury. The esophagus is divided after removal of the nasogastric tube.
(Reprinted with permission from Sugarbaker D, DeCamp M, Liptay M: Surgical procedures to resect and replace the esophagus. In Zinner M, Schwartz S, Ellis H, et al, editors: Maingot's Abdominal Operations. Stanford, CT: Appleton & Lange, 1997, pp. 885–910.)

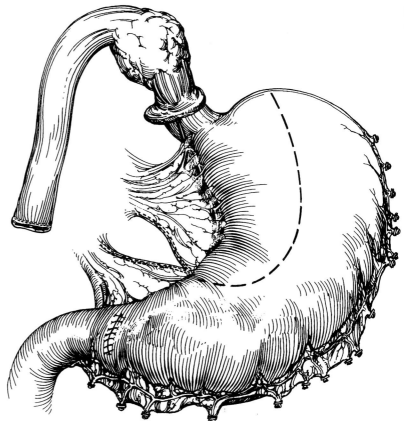

Figure 37–8 The gastric tube is created after complete dissection of the stomach and after the cervical esophagus is divided and brought into the abdomen. The gastric tube should be kept at least 5 cm in diameter. This also allows for longer margins for GE junction tumors. A pyloroplasty has been performed.
(Reprinted with permission from Swanson S, Grondin S, Sugarbaker D: Total esophagectomy: The Brigham and Women's Hospital approach. Oper Tech Thorac Cardiovasc Surg 4:197–209, 1999.)

of division ends at a point on the lesser curve near the crows feet of veins. At this point along the lesser curve, the right gastric artery and associated tissue can be divided to maximize conduit length.

With the specimen removed, a final check for hemostasis is made in the bed of the stomach and spleen. Prior to pulling the conduit into the neck, the esophageal hiatus should be dilated to four fingers. The gastric conduit may be pulled to the neck in relatively atraumatic fashion by the use of an endoscopic camera bag attached to a Foley catheter. The heavy silk tie that traverses the mediastinum from the neck is tied to the valved end of a 30-cm³ three-way Foley urinary catheter. The endoscopic bag is secured to the Foley balloon. The conduit is placed in the bag, and the valved end is drawn into the neck (Figure 37-9). The assistant must guide the conduit through the hiatus and up the lower mediastinum, ensuring that there is no torsion. The bag is cut away from the conduit in the neck, and the conduit is grasped with a babcock instrument. The pylorus should sit at the hiatus.

The neck anastomosis can be performed hand sewn with interrupted circumferential full thickness 3-0 silk sutures (Figure 37-10). Alternatively a side-to-side, functional end-to-end stapled anastomosis may be performed. The anastomosis is created with a 75-mm linear stapler followed by a 30-mm endoscopic stapler. The nasogastric tube (NGT) is advanced across the anastomosis and positioned just proximal to the pylorus prior to closing the remaining anastomotic defect. (Figure 37-11). A drain is placed along the spine posterior to the anastomosis and the

platysma is run closed using 2-0 vicryl sutures. The skin is closed with staples. A J-tube is inserted in the abdomen at a point 40 cm distal to the ligament of treitz. The abdominal fascia is closed using a running #2 monofilament suture and the skin is closed with staples.

Transhiatal Esophagectomy

Indications

Some believe that transhiatal esophagectomy is ideally suited for benign esophageal disease and possibly Barrett's with high-grade dysplasia where complete lymphadenectomy may not be necessary. Other factors such as poor pulmonary function (FEV_1 <800 or <35% predicted) or pleural symphasis would favor a technique that avoids a thoracotomy.

Contraindications

Bulky tumors of the midthoracic esophagus are difficult to visualize from the transhiatal approach and injury to adjacent structures may occur. Scarring after neoadjuvant treatment of esophageal tumors may also make the transhiatal approach difficult. The need to perform a complete lymphadenectomy is a contraindication to this approach.

The presence of severe coronary or valvular disease makes the episodic drops in blood pressure associated with blunt dissection behind the heart especially treacherous; a transthoracic approach may be preferable in these instances.

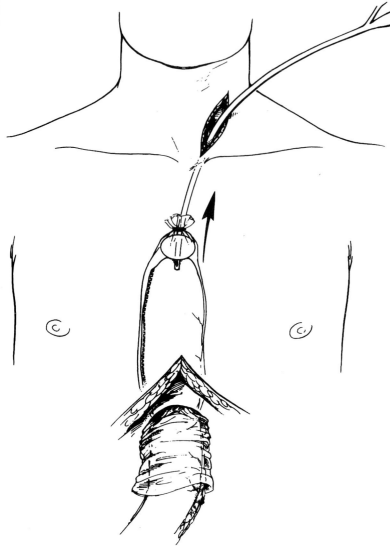

Figure 37–9 An endoscopic camera bag is used as an atraumatic means of drawing the conduit into the neck for anastomosis. Suction is applied to the Foley catheter as it is pulled into the neck. *(Reprinted with permission from Sugarbaker D, DeCamp M, Liptay M: Surgical procedures to resect and replace the esophagus. In Zinner M, Schwartz S, Ellis H, et al, editors: Maingot's Abdominal Operations. Stanford, CT: Appleton & Lange, 1997, pp. 885–910.)*

Preparation

The preparation is identical to that for a triincisional esophagectomy.

Technique

Bronchoscopy and esophagogastroduodenoscopy are performed as previously described. The abdominal portion of the procedure is performed as described in the previous section. An upper hand retractor aids in raising the xyphoid and sternum for visualization of the mediastinum. The esophagophrenic attachments are divided with cautery, the GE junction is separated from the crura, and the distal esophagus is encircled with a penrose. The hiatus is dilated to allow entry of the surgeon's hand. Various handheld malleable retractors may be used in dissection of the mediastinum through the hiatus. With the use of the penrose to retract the lower esophagus, the lower esophagus is dissected through the hiatus. Arterial branches supplying the lower esophagus from the aorta are clipped under direct vision.

With the fingertips against the esophagus, the esophagus is dissected off the vertebral plane bluntly into the upper chest. The palmar aspect of the fingertips is kept directly against the esophagus. Arteries supplying the esophagus branch approximately 1 cm away from the esophagus, and dissection close to the esophagus disrupts only the smaller arterial branches directly entering the esophagus. Close dissection of the esophagus also avoids injury to adjacent structures.

A cervical incision is made along the lower border of the left sternocleidomastoid muscle. Dissection proceeds as described in the previous section with the exception that the esophagus must be identified and encircled from the neck. An approach from the left neck aids in avoiding injury to the right recurrent laryngeal nerve, which is farther from the esophagus than the left recurrent nerve at this level. Dissection is kept immediately on the esophagus to avoid recurrent nerve injury. Metal retractors should not be placed near the tracheoesophageal groove. A penrose is placed around the cervical esophagus.

Dissection caudally is performed with two fingers against the esophagus in the posterior plane. Depending on the

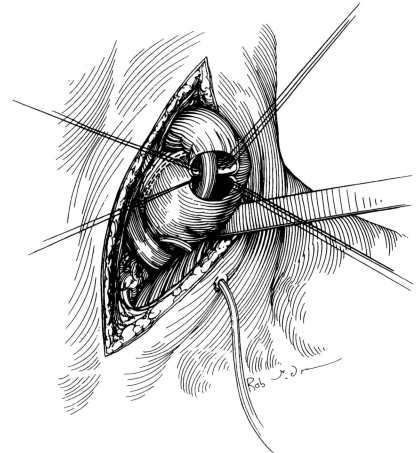

Figure 37–10 The cervical anastomosis may be hand sewn with interrupted silk sutures over a nasogastric tube.
(Reprinted with permission from Swanson S, Grondin S, Sugarbaker D: Total esophagectomy: The Brigham and Women's Hospital approach. Oper Tech Thorac Cardiovasc Surg 4:197–209, 1999.)

length of the surgeon's fingers and the width of the abdominal surgeon's hand, it should be possible for the two hands to contact directly. There always remains a thin plane of tissue that must be torn for the two hands to touch. Alternatively, a sponge stick can be advanced posteriorly from the neck to touch the dissecting hand from the abdomen (Figure 37-12). Dissection then proceeds in a similar fashion on the anterior surface of the esophagus. Extreme care must be taken in the region of the trachea and especially the carina to avoid injury to the membranous trachea. (At this point in the operation any difficulty dissecting the esophagus from the trachea or any concern of adhesion to or invasion of the trachea should result in repositioning the patient in the left lateral decubitus position, and a right thoracotomy should be performed for direct visualization and dissection.) The fingers from above and below should meet in the region of the carina (Figure 37-13).

As much dissection as possible should be performed under direct vision from the neck and from the abdomen. Portions of the lateral dissection near the lower aspect of the trachea often cannot be visualized, and lateral dissection must be performed bluntly. The surgeon's right hand is advanced from the abdomen high up in the chest to the point where circumferential dissection has been completed from the neck. The first and second fingers surround the esophagus, and, with a "raking" motion, the lateral attachments are avulsed as the hand is drawn back into the abdomen. Care must be taken near the region of the azygous vein (Figure 37-14). After complete mobilization of the esophagus, it is divided in the neck and the specimen is

brought out into the abdomen. The mediastinum is packed for hemostasis. Prior to drawing the gastric tube up into the neck, the mediastinal packing is removed and both pleural spaces are inspected for integrity. Entry into the pleural space is managed by chest tube placement prior to removing the drapes.

Ivor Lewis Esophagectomy

Indications

The indications are similar to that for a triincisional approach.

Contraindications

Tumors located in the upper third of the thoracic esophagus, above the carina, are better approached with resection of the cervical esophagus and anastomosis in the neck to ensure adequate margins. Long segment Barrett's esophagus with extension into the cervical esophagus is also a contraindication to an anastomosis in the right chest. A fused pleural space or severely compromised lung function should lead to reconsideration of a thoracotomy.

Technique

The patient is positioned supine. Preoperative bronchoscopy and esophagogastroduodenoscopy are performed.

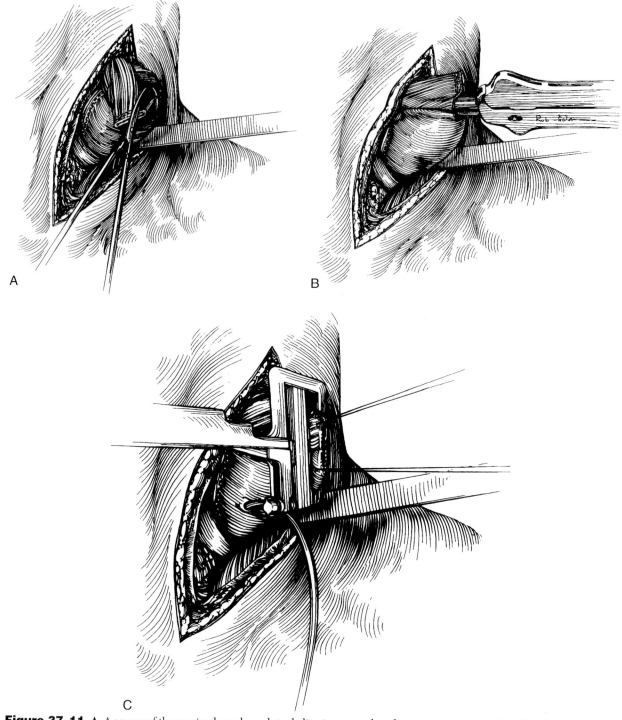

Figure 37–11 A, A corner of the proximal esophageal staple line is trimmed, and an enterotomy is made in the proximal gastric conduit away from the staple line. **B,** A GIA stapler is used to create the back wall of the cervical anastomosis. Additional length may be obtained with an additional fire of an endoscopic 30-mm stapler. **C,** The anterior wall of the anastomosis is closed with a TA stapler. In this figure a gastric drainage tube exits through the neck. These tubes can be used in place of a nasogastric tube and are more comfortable for the patient.
(Reprinted with permission from Swanson S, Grondin S, Sugarbaker D: Total esophagectomy. Oper Tech Thorac Cardiovasc Surg 4:197–654, 1999.)

An upper midline incision is made extending from the umbilicus to the xyphoid. The abdominal portion of the operation is identical to that described for a triincisional esophagectomy, with complete mobilization of the stomach, kocherization of the duodenum, pyloroplasty, construction of the gastric tube, and placement of a J-tube. The conduit is advanced into the chest as far as possible prior to closing the abdomen.

After placement of a double lumen endotracheal tube, the patient is repositioned in the left lateral decubitus

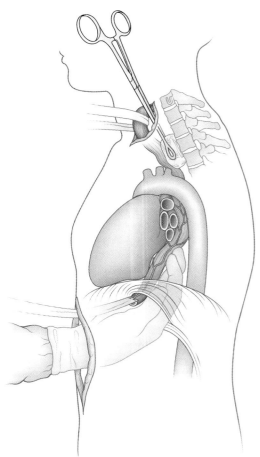

Figure 37–12 Posterior dissection is performed with the fingertips adjacent to the esophagus. Dissection from the cranial aspect may be performed with a sponge stick if the surgeon's upper hand cannot reach the lower hand.
(Modified with permission from Orringer MB, Sloan H: Esophagectomy without thoracotomy. J Thorac Cardiovasc Surg 76:643–654, 1978.)

position and a standard right posterolateral thoracotomy is performed. Entry into the chest is through the fourth or fifth interspace. The azygous vein is divided and the intrathoracic esophagus is dissected, including all adjacent areolar and lymphatic tissue. A margin of at least 5 cm and, ideally, 10 cm, is desirable, and thus the anastomosis is usually performed high in the right chest. The esophagus is dissected free to a point only several centimeters above the proposed line of transection to preserve blood supply to the anastomosis. The esophagus is divided and the stomach is pulled up and the gastric conduit is fashioned using a GIA stapler. A variety of techniques may be used to perform the anastomosis including a single-layer hand-sewn, double-layer hand-sewn, EEA stapled, and side-to-side functional end-to-end stapled anastomosis. With all techniques, wrapping the anastomosis with omentum and passage of the NGT prior to completion of the final portion of the anastomosis are advised.

If a hand-sewn anastomosis is to be performed, the proximal esophagus is divided with a knife after clamping the esophagus proximally with a noncrushing bowel clamp. A single-layer anastomosis is performed with interrupted 3-0 silk stitches with full thickness bites of the mucosa and

637

muscularis and careful approximation of tissues. Knots on the posterior row may be tied inside the lumen[66] (Figure 37-15). A double-layer anastomosis was described by Churchill and Sweet in 1942.[13,42] At a point at least 2 cm beyond the staple line, a 2-cm-diameter area of gastric serosa is scored. Underlying vessels are ligated with interrupted silks. The posterior layer of the anastomosis is created using interrupted 3-0 silks stitches. An inner, full-thickness layer is performed with a fine 4-0 absorbable suture, either catgut or monocryl, using a running Connell stitch to invert the mucosa. Prior to completion of the inner layer the NGT is passed to the hiatus. An anterior outer layer is then performed with interrupted 3-0 silk. Omentum is used to wrap the anastomosis. The distal portion of the stomach is reduced into the abdomen to avoid excess redundancy of the stomach in the chest, which might impair conduit emptying. Stitches are placed anchoring the conduit to the diaphragmatic hiatus. Some use additional stitches anchoring the intrathoracic conduit to the pleura, though the effectiveness of these stitches is debated.

If a stapled anastomosis is performed, it may be performed in a side-to-side, functional end-to-end manner with creation of the anastomosis with a GIA 75 or sequential 30-mm endoscopic staples, and closure of the defect with a TA 30- or 60-mm stapler. The anastomosis can also be performed with an EEA stapler, though anastomosis created with EEA staplers smaller than 33 carry a significant risk of stricture.[80] With the EEA stapler, passage of the NGT tube is, of course, performed after completion of the anastomosis.

Left Thoracoabdominal Approach

Indications

The indications for a left thoracoabdominal approach are limited. A distal esophageal tumor beyond 30–35 cm in a patient with compromised physiological status may be a suitable candidate, although some would argue that a transhiatal approach is preferable.

Contraindications

The presence of tumor at or above 30 cm makes an approach from the left chest much more difficult, as the anastomosis must be placed above the aortic arch or in the neck. A distal esophageal peptic stricture is considered by many to be a contraindication to limited distal esophagectomy as GE reflux is often a severe problem following distal esophagectomy and placement of the anastomosis low in the chest.

Technique

The left thoracoabdominal approach can be performed in a variety of ways. Isolation with a double lumen tube is necessary in all of the approaches. In the supine position, an upper midline laparotomy can be extended across the costal margin into the left chest via the seventh interspace and the diaphragm taken down in circumferential fashion. This position is least versatile and is generally used only when extension into the chest is unanticipated, as with proximal

638

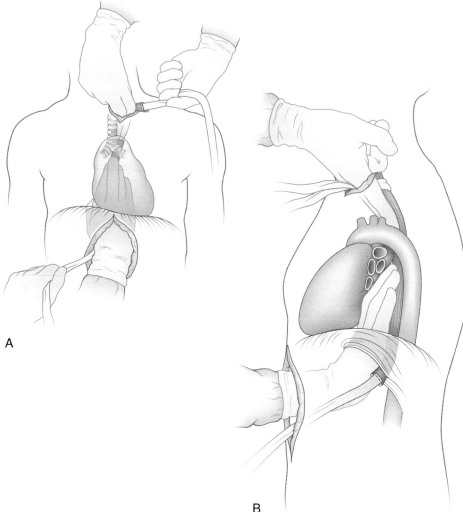

A

B

Figure 37–13 A–B, Blunt dissection of the esophagus off of the trachea is performed with the fingertips immediately against the esophagus. The fingertips are united. The fingertips from above should be able to reach near the carina, as they do during cervical mediastinoscopy.
(*Modified with permission from Orringer MB: Transhiatal esophagectomy without thoracotomy. In Cohn LH, editor: Modern Techniques in Surgery. Futura Publishing, 1983.*)

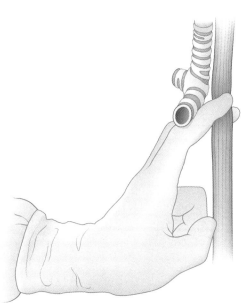

Figure 37–14 After dissection of the anterior and posterior planes, the lateral stalks can be torn between the first and second fingers in a "raking" motion.
(*Modified with permission from Orringer MB: Transhiatal esophagectomy without thoracotomy. In Cohn LH, editor: Modern Techniques in Surgery. Futura Publishing, 1983.*)

extension of certain tumors of the gastric cardia. Conversely, the patient may be placed in the full lateral position, and a complete esophagectomy may be performed through a thoracic incision. Abdominal dissection can be performed, though with some difficulty, through an enlarged hiatus or through a circumferential peripheral incision in the diaphragm (Figure 37-16).

The most versatile thoracoabdominal approach involves positioning the patient in the right lateral decubitus position with the abdomen rolled back 45 degrees. The abdomen is readily accessible for extension of the distal aspect of the thoracotomy across the costal margin and across the rectus muscle. The neck is prepped in the field if extension to the cervical esophagus is a possibility. An incision is made from a point behind the tip of the scapula along the seventh interspace across the costal margin to the middle of the abdomen. The inferior pulmonary ligament is divided using cautery. The esophagus is encircled with a penrose drain at a point away from the tumor where there is minimal scarring. Complete dissection of the esophagus and all surrounding lymphatic and connective tissue is performed up, including all tissue in between the aorta and the pericardium in the specimen. Dissection proceeds cranially posterior to the left pulmonary veins. Cranial dissection should be performed only to a point approximately 3 cm above the proposed line of transection to preserve blood supply to the anastomosis.

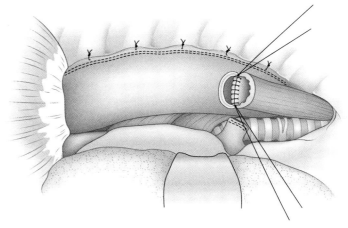

Figure 37–15 The Ivor Lewis anastomosis is performed at the level of the azygous vein, in two layers, after creating a circular enterotomy in the proximal conduit. The edges of the conduit are shown here tacked to the pleura, although it is debatable whether this effectively reduces tension on the anastomosis.
(Modified with permission from Sugarbaker D, DeCamp M, Liptay M: Surgical procedures to resect and replace the esophagus. In Zinner MJ, Schwartz SI, Ellis H, et al, editors: Maingot's Abdominal Operations. New York: Appleton & Lange, 1997, pp. 885–910.)

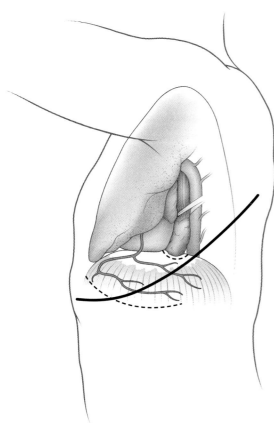

Figure 37–16 The left thoracoabdominal approach. The abdomen can be entered through incisions in the diaphragm as delineated by the dotted lines. Alternatively, the incision can be taken across the costal margin onto the abdomen, and the diaphragm taken down circumferentially from the costal margin incision.
(Modified with permission from Sugarbaker D, DeCamp M, Liptay M: Surgical procedures to resect and replace the esophagus. In Zinner MJ, Schwartz SI, Ellis H, et al, editors: Maingot's Abdominal Operations. New York: Appleton & Lange, 1997, pp. 885–910.)

At the diaphragmatic hiatus, a 2-cm rim of diaphragm is included with the specimen. Although it is at times possible to continue dissection of the short gastric vessels and gastrohepatic ligament through the hiatus, exposure is improved by taking the diaphragm down circumferentially at a point 2–3 cm away from its insertion on the chest wall.

Dissection proceeds from the GE junction along the greater curvature dividing all short gastric vessels. Dissection of the remainder of the gastric conduit is performed as detailed in the section on triincisional esophagectomy. Complete dissection of the stomach may not be required if only a very limited portion of distal esophagus is resected. Minimizing dissection at the expense of an entirely tension-free anastomosis, however, is unwise. Kocherization of the duodenum and either pyloroplasty or pyloromyotomy are performed. The conduit is lifted into the chest. The anastomosis can be performed hand sewn in either a single-layer or double-layer anastomosis. It may also be performed with a large (33) EEA stapler or side-to-side, functional end-to-end anastomosis. An NGT is positioned prior to completion of the anastomosis. The conduit should be tacked to the diaphragm and may also be tacked to the adjacent pleura. Buttressing the anastomosis with available omentum is recommended. The diaphragmatic rim is reattached to the chest wall with interrupted horizontal mattress 0 silk stitches. The costal margin is reattached with a single figure-of-eight wire or heavy prolene stitch. The abdominal fascia is closed in layers. Prior to closure of the thoracotomy a soft drain may be inserted dependently near the anastomosis, and an apical chest tube should be placed, each through separate stab incisions. The thoracotomy incision is closed with #2 vicryl paracostal sutures, a 0 vicryl latissimus layer, a 2-0 subdermal layer, and a 3-0 subcuticular stitch.

En Bloc Resection

The long-term survival rate following esophagectomy for esophageal cancer remains approximately 20% despite recent advances in surgical technique, instrumentation, and perioperative care. A large percentage of esophageal cancers present with invasion through the esophageal wall (T3) or nodal involvement (N1 or N2). Because radial margins are very difficult to assess grossly and even microscopically, ensuring complete removal of all invasive and nodal disease is difficult. To ensure complete margins and removal of all adjacent nodal tissue, several surgeons have advocated en bloc resection of the esophagus, including all adjacent tissues in the resected specimen. Demeester and Skinner recommend en bloc esophagectomy for all patients in whom the cardiopulmonary morbidity is not prohibitive.[6,29] In one of these studies, an FEV_1 <1.5 liters was considered prohibitive. In their

640 nonrandomized series, long-term survival was significantly better in the en bloc resection group vs. the conventional approach.

Technique

Although an en bloc resection may be performed through either the left or right chest, only very distal esophageal tumors may be resected with ease and with adequate margins via left thoracotomy. Because of the high incidence of postoperative reflux esophagitis, an approach via a right thoracotomy is advised. Entry into the chest is via the right sixth interspace. Two parallel incisions are made in the pleura. An incision is made anteriorly, entering the pericardium and posteriorly, behind the azygous vein. Intercostal veins draining into the azygous are ligated individually, and the thoracic duct and azygous vein are included in the specimen. Some surgeons do not resect the azygous vein. The left pleura bordering the specimen is harvested and included in the specimen. This plane of dissection is continued cranially to the carina. Above the carina, the margins are limited by the proximity of the trachea anteriorly and the spine posteriorly.

At the hiatus, a 2-cm rim of diaphragm is included with the specimen. In the abdomen, the lesser curvature of the stomach and all nodal tissue along the left gastric artery are taken. All tissue posterior to the stomach and superior to the border of the pancreas is removed. Nodes along the celiac axis, splenic artery, and superior mesenteric artery are dissected. The gastric tube is then pulled up to the neck for esophageal replacement. Demeester and his group routinely resect the proximal two thirds of stomach, greater omentum, spleen, and its associated nodes. They replace the esophagus with isoperistaltic colon.

Results

Retrospective trials comparing en bloc resection with conventional resection have been associated with heavy selection and staging bias. Patients with poor cardiopulmonary reserve are typically excluded from en bloc resection. Moreover, conventional resection patients are commonly understaged, as a limited nodal dissection is performed. Both factors would favor stage per stage improved survival in the en bloc group. In Skinner's series of 128 patients, 78 underwent en bloc resection and the remainder underwent a simpler resection, most via the transthoracic route. Perioperative mortality was similar at 4–5% in each group. The incidence of pneumonia, leak, and recurrent nerve injury was similar. Four-year survival in stage III patients was 37% after en bloc resection and 0% after transhiatal resection. Survival was also better in early stage patients after en bloc resection as compared with non–en bloc resection. In Demeester's series 69 patients with GE junction tumors were studied. Patients in good health with resectable disease underwent en bloc resection, whereas those in poor health or with apparently unresectable disease underwent a transhiatal resection. Five-year survival was significantly better in the en bloc resection group (41%) as compared to the transhiatal group (14%). The complication rate was not mentioned in this study.

Three-Field Lymph Node Dissection

Three-field lymph node dissection is a term applied to the addition of a cervical nodal dissection to the traditional thoracic and abdominal nodal dissections that are performed during esophagectomy for cancer. Ten to thirty percent of patients with lower esophageal cancers have cancers that spread to cervical nodal areas, and the same is true of celiac nodes in patients with cervical esophageal cancers.[3,5,9] Proponents of this technique argue that cervical nodes should be considered resectable even in lower esophageal cancers and should routinely be resected with the specimen.

The abdominal and thoracic phases of the operation are nearly identical to that performed during a triincisional en bloc resection of the esophagus. Attention is paid to dissect the recurrent nerve lymph node chain in the thorax. The neck is incised bilaterally with a U-shaped incision. The sternocleidomastoid muscles are divided. The deep cervical nodes deep and lateral to the jugular vein are dissected, dissection of the recurrent nerve nodes in the neck is continued, and the supraclavicular nodes are also removed.

In experienced hands, the incidence of recurrent nerve injury is no higher than with any other esophagectomy requiring a cervical incision. Altorki and Skinner described a recurrent nerve injury rate of 6%.[5] In their series there was only one perioperative death from their only case of pneumonia. Although the benefit of three-field lymph nodes dissections is not clear, several older studies suggested an improved survival.[4,49] More recently, a Japanese study by Ando et al and a U.S. study by Altorki et al have been published showing 5-year survival rates in the range of 40–50% following en-bloc esophagectomy with three-field lymph node dissection.[7,9] The Ando et al study was limited to squamous carcinoma patients while the U.S. study included patients with adenocarcinoma and squamous cell carcinoma. Perioperative mortality was 5–8% in both studies. There was a 20–25% pulmonary complication rate in each study. The recurrent nerve injury rate was 9% in Altorki et al, and was not mentioned in Ando et al. In these selected studies the perioperative morbidity is comparable to other studies, although perioperative mortality in the study by Ando et al is higher than the quoted rate of 3–4% from several recent large academic studies of esophagectomy without en-bloc or three-field dissections.[51,66] Long-term survival is impressive, although it is not clear if selection factors or differences in tumor biology between the Japanese and U.S. populations might account for some of the difference.

Techniques of Alternate Conduits: Colon and Jejeunum

Colon

Indications

The stomach is the preferred conduit for esophageal replacement. It has several advantages over the colon including a reliable blood supply that is usually free of atherosclerotic disease, low intraluminal bacterial burden, and the need for only a single anastomosis. In those instances

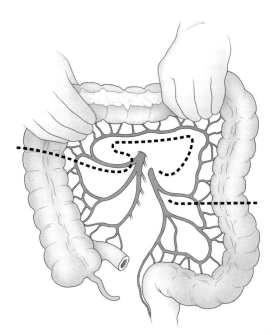

Figure 37–17 The mesentery of the mobilized colon is transilluminated, revealing the mesenteric vessels. The dotted lines are the lines of division for a conduit based on the left colic artery.
(Modified with permission from Sugarbaker D, DeCamp M, Liptay M: Surgical procedures to resect and replace the esophagus. In Zinner MJ, Schwartz SI, Ellis H, et al, editors: Maingot's Abdominal Operations. New York: Appleton & Lange, 1997, pp. 885–910.)

where stomach is not available, usually because of previous abdominal or gastric surgery or involvement of the stomach with tumor, the colon becomes the preferred conduit. The left colon differs from the right in that its lumen is smaller and more closely approximates that of the esophagus. Its usable length is usually greater than the right colon. The vascular anatomy of the left is more consistent than on the right; however, involvement by atherosclerotic disease of the inferior mesenteric artery is more common than in any other mesenteric vessel. In general, isoperistaltic orientation is preferred and can be achieved without tension.

Contraindications

Intrinsic disease of the colon by neoplasia, stricture, or extensive diverticulosis precludes its use as an esophageal replacement. In addition, prior abdominal surgery that may have interrupted either the arterial blood supply or venous drainage of the colon may render a segment of the colon unusable. The inferior mesenteric vein drains into the splenic vein, and prior severe pancreatitis or other causes of splenic vein thrombosis may render the left colon unusable as a conduit because of inferior mesenteric vein thrombosis.

Preparation

The patient should be screened for cardiopulmonary disease as for esophagectomy with gastric reconstruction. In addition, preoperative mesenteric angiography should be performed on any patient over 40 years of age or otherwise

with risk factors for atherosclerotic disease. A barium enema or colonoscopy should be performed to rule out a coexistent neoplasia or extensive diverticular disease. A mechanical and antibiotic bowel prep is administered.

641

Left Colon

As stated previously, the left colon has several advantages over the right including longer length, less vascular anatomical variation, and a caliber more similar to that of the esophagus. A midline laparotomy is performed and the abdomen is explored. The peritoneal attachments of the left colon to the retroperitoneum are divided along the white line of Toldt. The length of the conduit that is needed should be estimated by passing an umbilical tape from the proposed proximal line of transection of the esophagus via the proposed route of placement of the conduit to the point of proposed anastomosis to the stomach. The umbilical tape can then be used to measure an appropriate length of colon

The vessels supplying the left colon are visualized via transillumination. The middle colic artery should be test clamped with a noncrushing bulldog clamp. A palpable pulse should still be present in the marginal artery. If there is any question, a Doppler probe may be used, or the bulldog clamp should be left in place and the conduit inspected for adequate perfusion. Only after it is determined that the conduit is of satisfactory quality should the esophagectomy be completed. The left colon should then be prepared. The omentum is separated from the left colon and splenic flexure that is to be used as conduit. The middle colic artery is divided, and the mesentery is divided near its root, away from the marginal artery of Drummond (Figure 37-17). The colon is reanastomosed and the mesenteric defect is closed.

Either the proximal or distal anastomosis may be done first; however, we believe that construction of the proximal anastomosis first allows better determination of conduit length and ensures that the conduit will sit properly in the neck. The proximal end of the conduit may be drawn up into the neck utilizing an atraumatic method, such as an endoscopic camera bag (see triincisional technique). The posterior mediastinal (*in situ*) route is preferred as this is the shortest route between the stomach and esophagus (Figure 37-18). If the posterior mediastinal route is unavailable because of prior infection or scarring, as occurs with a prior gastric conduit leak, then the substernal or transpleural route is an option. These routes, however, result in more conduit angulation and may impair emptying. Routine resection of the manubrium or a portion of manubrium is necessary to prevent obstruction and allow adequate space for the colon if the substernal route is used. Excess length is taken out of the conduit. If there is significant excess length, the proximal end may be trimmed as needed. The proximal anastomosis is typically constructed with a single- or two-layer hand-sewn anastomosis of the end of the esophagus to the side of the antimesenteric tenia. A stapled technique may also be used as detailed in the section on triincisional esophagectomy. The anastomosis should be constructed over an NGT with its tip positioned in the center of the stomach. The conduit should be monitored for arterial insufficiency or venous engorgement. The gastrocolic anastomosis is performed using a large EEA stapler or in a side-to-side functional end-to-end stapled manner. Prior to

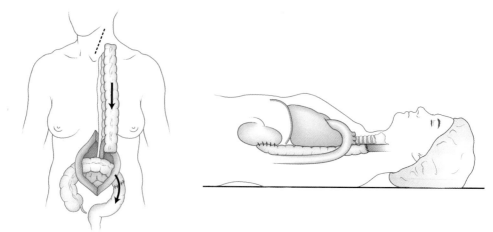

Figure 37–18 The posterior mediastinal (*in situ*) route is the shortest route between the stomach and esophagus.
(*Modified with permission from Sugarbaker D, DeCamp M, Liptay M: Surgical procedures to resect and replace the esophagus. In Zinner MJ, Schwartz SI, Ellis H, et al, editors: Maingot's Abdominal Operations. New York: Appleton & Lange, 1997, pp. 885–910.*)

closure the conduit should be sutured to the crus to prevent migration of the colon into the chest or herniation of abdominal viscera into the chest.

Right Colon

A variety of conditions may make the left colon unusable as a conduit. These include extensive diverticular disease, stricture secondary to ischemia or prior diverticular infection, atherosclerotic occlusion of the inferior mesenteric artery, and splenic vein thrombosis with thrombosis of the inferior mesenteric vein. The right colon is an acceptable conduit and will readily reach the esophagus in the neck.

The right colon is inspected for any pathology, and its retroperitoneal attachments are lysed. The mesentery of the right colon may be transilluminated showing the ileocolic, right colic, marginal, and middle colic arteries. Soft clamps are placed on the ileocolic and right colic arteries and the right colon is inspected for adequate perfusion via the marginal artery. The right colon is then harvested, leaving the marginal artery intact. An appendectomy is performed. Whether the ileocecal valve and short segment of ileum should be included in the conduit for esophageal anastomosis is controversial. The ileum does provide a better size match for anastomosis with the esophagus, and, in theory, the ileocecal valve should guard against reflux in the neck. Opponents argue that despite the size mismatch, a hand-sewn anastomosis of the end of esophagus to side of colon is quite easy, reflux esophagitis is rare high in the neck, and the ileocecal valve may contribute to antegrade obstruction.

Appropriate lengths of right colon are divided using a GIA 75-mm stapler and the colocolonic anastomosis is performed. From the surgeon's perspective, the right colon conduit is rotated counterclockwise and the proximal end is drawn up into the neck in atraumatic fashion. The proximal anastomosis is created most easily using a single-layer end of esophagus to the side of the colon along a tenia. Excess length is brought out into the abdomen and the conduit is tacked to the hiatus. At this point excess length in the distal conduit can be managed by excising colon at the end of the vascular conduit. The cologastric anastomosis is usually constructed with either EEA staplers or a side-to-side stapled technique. The colon may be brought into the anterior aspect or posterior aspect of the stomach.

Jejeunum

Indications

Jejunum may be used to replace a portion of the esophagus as a free graft, pedicled graft, or Roux-en-Y replacement.[14,43] Replacement of the esophagus with jejunum is indicated when the stomach is not available because of prior surgery or intrinsic disease. When limited distal esophagectomy is planned, jejunum or colon is preferred to stomach as the former two conduits are more resistant to the effects of gastroesophageal reflux. Replacement of a distal esophageal peptic stricture should be performed with colon or jejunum in preference to stomach. Interposing an isoperistaltic segment of intestine is preferable to gastric pull up, which has a very high incidence of recurrent severe reflux. Free jejunal graft is indicated in limited reconstruction of the cervical esophagus. Roux-en-Y jejunal replacement may be used to replace the stomach and distal esophagus after total gastrectomy including distal esophagectomy.

Contraindications

Intrinsic disease of the small bowel, whether due to inflammatory bowel disease or previous surgery, may prevent its use as a conduit. Generally, total esophageal replacement cannot be accomplished with jejunum alone, as the length is insufficient to reach the neck.

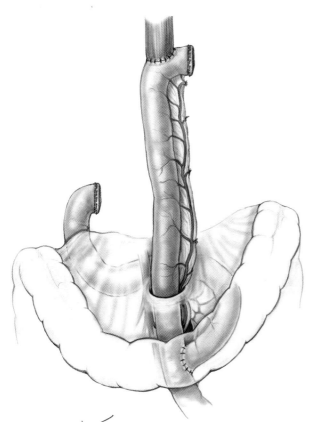

Figure 37–19 Roux-en-Y replacement with jejunum is useful for reconstruction following esophagectomy with gastrectomy as with proximal gastric tumors.

Preparation

Although mechanical bowel preparation is not necessary for jejunal interposition, it is advisable so that colon is available if the jejunum is found to be unacceptable as a conduit, or if the blood supply to the jejunum is damaged during harvest rendering it unusable as a conduit. Antibiotics (a cephalosporin and an anaerobic antibiotic) should be administered preoperatively.

Roux–en-Y Replacement

Roux-en-Y replacement (Figure 37-19) may be used for reconstruction following total gastrectomy and distal esophageal resection as indicated in proximal gastric tumors, or for esophageal resection into the upper chest. Occasionally a Roux-en-Y replacement may reach the neck, but this is variable, and, unlike the stomach, it will not reliably reach the cervical esophagus. When used following total gastrectomy, jejunum is divided approximately 20–30 cm beyond the ligament of treitz. The jejunum is elevated outside the abdomen, and the vascular arcade is transilluminated. The proposed point of division is identified and the line of division of the mesentery is also identified along with the proposed division of several vessels of the mesentery, which will allow movement of the jejunum up into the chest. The proposed feeder vessel is identified and preserved. The serosal surface of the mesentery is scored and

the vessels to be transected are clamped with a soft bulldog clamp. The conduit is observed over several minutes for evidence of ischemia or congestion. Sixty centimeters of jejunal conduit can be mobilized using this technique. A hole in the transverse mesocolon is made to the left of the middle colic vessels large enough for the jejunum and its mesentery to pass through. For replacement following total gastrectomy, the proximal anastomosis is to the very distal esophagus in the upper abdomen. If distal esophagectomy is also performed as for a malignant lesion of the cardia extending to the GE junction, the abdominal incision must be brought across the costal margin into the left sixth or seventh interspace. If, after division of the esophagus and mobilization of the Roux-en-Y limb into the lower chest, additional length of jejunum is needed, the next vessel in the mesenteric arcade is test clamped and then divided.

The esophagojejunal anastomosis can be performed by stapled or hand-sewn techniques. The stapled anastomosis is most easily performed with an EEA stapler. Ideally a size 33-mm EEA stapler should be used to protect against the development of strictures. The distal esophagus may be gently dilated with a lubricated dilator. A full thickness suture 2-0 prolene suture is used to create a pursestring in the distal esophagus. The shaft of the EEA stapler can be introduced via the stapled end of the proximal jejunum. Care must be taken not to occlude the ongoing lumen of the jejunum with the stapler. Two full thickness anastomotic doughnuts should be verified. After removal of the EEA stapler, the jejunal end can be closed with a TA 60 stapler. A hand-sewn anastomosis in two layers may also be performed. The outer layer is seromuscular on the jejunum to muscular esophagus using 3-0 silk and the inner layer is full thickness using interrupted 3-0 or 4-0 chromic gut.

The jejunum should be tacked to the hiatus at several points using interrupted silk sutures. This prevents herniation of abdominal contents into the chest and limits tension on the esophagojejunal anastomosis. Likewise, the defect in the colonic mesentery should be closed to prevent an internal hernia. The distal anastomosis can be performed hand sewn or with a side-to-side functional end-to-end stapled anastomosis.

Pedicled Jejunal Interposition

A left thoracoabdominal incision is used with a left seventh interspace incision extended across the costal margin and across the rectus muscle. As with the harvest of a Roux-en-Y loop, the jejunum is transilluminated and an appropriate length of jejunum is selected from a point 20 cm distal to the ligament of treitz. A single large vessel is used as a feeding vessel for the conduit. The jejunum is transected proximally and distally using a GIA stapler, and the mesentery is divided down each side to the origin of the vessel. The remaining jejunum is reconnected using a side-to-side functional end-to-end stapled technique. The pedicled jejunum is tunneled through the mesocolon and brought into the left chest. The proximal anastomosis is constructed as with the Roux-en-Y esophagojejunal anastomosis. The jejunogastric anastomosis may be hand sewn in two layers or stapled using an EEA stapler (Figure 37-20).

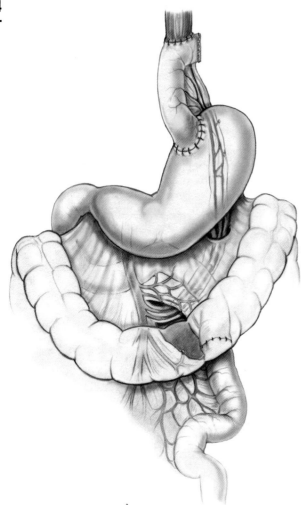

Figure 37–20 Pedicled jejunum is ideally suited for distal esophageal replacement. An appropriate length of jejunum is harvested beginning 20 cm beyond the ligament of treitz.

Free Jejunal Interposition

Free jejunal graft may reach portions of the upper esophagus that pedicled grafts may not. It is not clear whether the use of a short jejunal interposition is preferable to total esophageal replacement with a normal gastric conduit. The use of jejunum does carry a lower incidence of gastroesophageal reflux; however, the increased risk of life-threatening graft ischemia and necrosis is significant. Moreover, two anastomosis are required, increasing the risk of anastomotic leak.

As with the pedicled jejunal graft, a short segment of jejunum is chosen for harvest. A left cervical incision is made and the esophagus and carotid and jugular vessels are isolated. Soon after division of the jejunal vessels with scalpel, the artery and vein are flushed with heparinized saline. The proximal hand-sewn anastomosis is constructed first, an operating microscope and fine 9-0 or 10-0 suture is used to anastomose the jejunal vessels to the carotid and jugular vessels, and the distal anastomosis is then constructed (Figure 37-21). The graft is covered with a meshed split thickness skin graft to monitor graft viability in the postoperative period.

► CONSIDERATIONS IN ESOPHAGEAL RESECTION

Perioperative Mortality

Historically, esophagectomy has been associated with the highest perioperative mortality of any commonly performed resection. The combination of a long operation traversing three body compartments in an elderly, potentially malnourished individual and the potential for overwhelming mediastinal sepsis has produced perioperative mortality rates that were initially quoted at 15–40%.[19,24] Reports published after 1980 showed improvement in the mortality rates to approximately 15%, with a large meta-analysis of papers published between 1986 and 1996 showing mortality rates averaging 6–10%.[47,60] Several large academic centers have published large series with mortality rates ranging from 3 to 4%.[20,51,66]

It is clear that advances in surgical technique, anesthesia, and intensive care have markedly improved the safety of esophagectomy over the past several decades. In older series the greatest contributor to perioperative mortality was intrathoracic sepsis caused by either an anastomotic or a conduit leak. The mortality rate from a clinically overt intrathoracic leak may be greater than 50%.[75] Aggressive, early management of an intrathoracic esophageal leak is essential in limiting its possible fatal effects.

In the more recent, larger series published with mortality rates below 5%, the most common cause of perioperative death is not conduit leak but is rather pulmonary in etiology: respiratory insufficiency, pneumonia, or pulmonary embolus.[20,51,66] The combination of a low incidence of leak with early, aggressive management has made the intrathoracic enteric leak less of a factor in perioperative mortality.

Perioperative Complications

Anastomotic Leak

The incidence of intrathoracic leak following Ivor Lewis esophagectomy is typically 5–10%.[42,60] The incidence of leak after a cervical anastomosis is higher, generally in the 10–15% range.[51,60] Older studies have quoted cervical leak rates at 25–26%, while a recent large study described a leak rate of 8%.[24,56,66] A retrospective evaluation of anastomotic leaks revealed that albumin level below 3 g/dL, positive margins, and cervical anastomosis were risk factors for anastomotic leak following esophagectomy.[56] Several factors are believed to be responsible for the increased incidence of leak in the cervical position. The increase in length needed may cause increased tension on the anastomosis. Blood supply to the anastomosis may be compromised as it is further away from the origin of the gastroepiploic artery, and arterial inflow and venous drainage may be compromised by a tight thoracic inlet. In a randomized trial of hand-sewn versus stapled anastomosis in 102 patients undergoing Ivor Lewis esophagectomy, no significant difference was seen in the incidence of leaks between the two groups. The incidence of leak following a single hand-sewn monofilament anastomosis was 5% and after stapled anastomosis was 2%.[37] Clearly, the incidence of leak following hand-sewn anastomosis is more operator dependent than with stapled

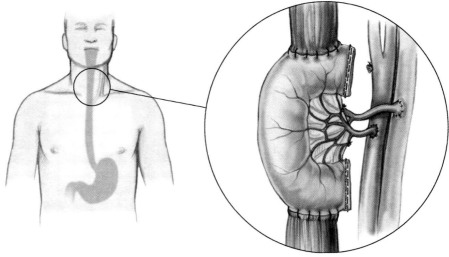

Figure 37–21 Free jejunal interposition may be used where pedicled graft will not reach, such as in the proximal esophagus. The arterial and venous supplies are anastomosed to the carotid and jugular vessels under the operating microscope. A split thickness skin graft covers the graft to allow for inspection of graft viability in the perioperative period.

anastomosis, and the reproducibility of the stapled anastomosis is its main advantage.

An intrathoracic leak is a life-threatening event that usually requires immediate operative intervention. Although the mortality rate from this complication has been lowered at large centers over the last few decades, the cost in ICU and hospital stay and delayed recovery remains high. The intervention required may range from repair and drainage of a limited leak, to placement of a T-tube, to complete diversion via spit fistula and reduction of viable gastric conduit into the abdomen. The more critically ill the patient is as a result of the leak, the more aggressive and definitive the treatment required. In rare instances (a clinically silent, small contained leak draining back into the conduit not near vital structures such as the trachea or aorta) such a leak may be treated conservatively with antibiotics and maintaining strict NPO status.

Leak following a cervical anastomosis, though more frequent, is uncommonly a life-threatening event. Older series have described mortality from a cervical leak as high as 20%, though recent series have described mortality rates that are much lower.[66,75] Cervical anastomotic leak occurs, in general, later than intrathoracic leaks, with many diagnosed only on routine postoperative barium swallow or upon commencement of oral feeds after a negative barium swallow.[76] Cervical leaks may present with low-grade fevers, localized redness, or wound discharge. Treatment usually entails limited opening of the neck incision and placement of a wick. Larger leaks resulting from anastomotic necrosis may be treated with a Silastic stent or T-tube. Leaks into the chest after cervical anastomosis, due to either retraction of the anastomosis into the chest or dependent drainage of enteric contents into the chest, must be treated in the same manner as any intrathoracic leak. The main long-term sequela of a cervical anastomotic leak without signs of systemic sepsis is an increased incidence of delayed stricture formation.

Anastomotic Stricture

Although anastomotic stricture is never life threatening, it is not uncommon and, if severe, negates the primary benefit of intestinal continuity following esophageal replacement. A large retrospective meta-analysis concluded that the incidence of symptomatic stricture was somewhat higher following anastomosis in the cervical position (28%) than after Ivor Lewis resection (16%).[60] This is in part due to the higher incidence of leak following cervical anastomosis. In an examination of risk factors of benign stricture following transhiatal esophagectomy, the use of a stapled anastomosis, anastomotic leak, and the presence of cardiac disease were the only risk factors identified for the development of stricture.[31] Earlier studies had identified intraoperative blood loss and poor vascularization of the gastric conduit as risk factors.[17,57] From these studies it is apparent that there are three factors influencing the development of postoperative stricture: infection, ischemia, and mechanical issues.

Anastomotic leak is a well-known risk factor for the development of a delayed stricture. Curiously, Honkoop et al found no difference in the incidence of delayed stricture between clinically overt leaks and those detected by swallow only.[31] Preemptive bougienage (7–10 days following operation) dilatation has been advocated by some to prevent the development of stricture following cervical leak.[50] Ischemia is one of the major contributors to anastomotic leak, and it is difficult to determine what effect this alone has on the development of postoperative stricture. Certainly all efforts in avoiding ischemia (adequate blood supply, systemic oxygen delivery, avoidance of congestion) should be made to avoid both leak and stricture. It is also evident that mechanical factors influence the development of stricture. Law et al performed a randomized trial of hand-sewn vs. EEA-stapled Ivor Lewis anastomosis. The incidence of stricture following the hand-sewn anastomosis was 9%, whereas that following stapled anastomosis was 40%. Strictures were not seen with the 33-mm EEA stapler, but had a 12.5% incidence with the 29-mm stapler and a 43% incidence when a 25-mm stapler was used.[37] Not every esophagus will allow a 33-mm stapler, but it should be used whenever possible. Otherwise, a hand-sewn anastomosis or different stapling technique should be considered.

Postoperative stricture is usually managed by repeat bougie dilation. In Honkoop's study, three dilations, on average, were needed to achieve normal swallowing. Perforation occurred in 2 of 519 episodes of dilation. Both

646 of these perforations resulted in patient deaths. In the study by Law et al, 53% were treated by one dilation, 20% by two, 12% by three, and 8% by four. No patient in either study was treated by reoperation.

Recurrent Laryngeal Nerve Injury

The incidence of recurrent nerve injury and vocal cord dysfunction following esophagectomy is higher with a cervical anastomosis than with an intrathoracic anastomosis. Malfunction of a single vocal cord, though seemingly a minor complication resulting in hoarseness, can lead to a series of life-threatening complications if not recognized early and treated. The lack of vocal cord apposition makes an effective cough and clearance of pulmonary secretions difficult. This is exacerbated by the loss of airway protection during swallowing and repeated episodes of overt or microaspiration.

As expected, the incidence of recurrent nerve injury is higher with a cervical anastomosis (11%) than with an intrathoracic anastomosis (5%).[60] In the right thorax, the recurrent nerve may be injured by traction on the vagus nerves, or by cautery near the nerve as it recurs around the subclavian artery. In addition, a neck dissection may result in direct injury to the recurrent nerves as the esophagus is dissected away from the tracheoesophageal groove. In the neck, dissection must be performed immediately against the esophagus with care to recognize and avoid the recurrent nerve. Dissection close to the recurrent nerves does not necessarily place them at risk; one series of three-field lymph node dissection with direct dissection of all lymph nodes adjacent to both recurrent nerves resulted in a recurrent nerve injury rate of only 6%.[5]

Early recognition and treatment of a recurrent nerve injury (in itself a non-life-threatening condition unless both cords are simultaneously injured) are essential in preventing the potentially lethal complications of aspiration and pneumonia. Any patient who presents with hoarseness and an ineffective cough following esophagectomy should undergo fiberoptic laryngoscopy. Unilateral paralyzed vocal cords should be medialized by either injection or prosthesis implantation. Early intervention can lead to a low incidence of pulmonary complications.[66]

Respiratory Complications

Pneumonia, atelectasis, and respiratory failure, in the modern era, are probably the most serious complications following esophagectomy when one takes into account their relatively high incidence and potentially life-threatening consequences. The incidence of pneumonia following esophagectomy ranges from 2% to 47%.[34,51] Respiratory failure following esophagectomy occurs in 4% of patients.[60] The assumption that avoidance of thoracotomy results in fewer pulmonary complications than a transthoracic esophagectomy has not conclusively been supported by the literature. In Goldminc et al's randomized trial comparing transhiatal to Ivor Lewis esophagectomy the incidence of pneumonia was 20% for both groups.[25] In Chu et al's randomized trial of 39 patients comparing transhiatal to Ivor Lewis esophagectomy the incidence of pneumonia was 10% after transhiatal and 0% after Ivor Lewis resection (no significant difference).[12]

A recent European randomized trial comparing transhiatal to en bloc triincisional esophagectomy did show a difference in the rate of pulmonary complications (pneumonia or lobar atelectasis) in the triincisional (57%) vs. the transhiatal group (27%).[34] The unusually high incidence of pulmonary complications in both groups of this series should be questioned. Typically rates of pulmonary complications are in the 20% range.[33] Previous series involving en bloc resections have described pneumonia rates of 5%.[6]

A muscle-sparing, limited thoracotomy, epidural anesthesia, and early ambulation are essential in limiting postthoracotomy respiratory complications. In most esophagectomy series, an FEV_1 <1 liter is a contraindication to thoracotomy. A thoracoscopic esophageal dissection may allow for a safe intrathoracic esophageal dissection in these high-risk patients.

Bleeding

The incidence of bleeding following esophagectomy is approximately 5% and does not vary according to the techniques used.[60] In a meta-analysis, average blood loss was slightly higher for the transthoracic approach, averaging 1000 ml, than for the transhiatal approach, averaging 728 ml.[33] Anticoagulants and antiplatelet agents should be stopped in advance of esophagectomy. Low-dose subcutaneous heparin does not increase the incidence of bleeding following esophagectomy. Direct arterial branches from the aorta to the esophagus usually found in the lower thorax should be clipped, and not simply cauterized. Larger arteries supplying the esophagus branch into a fine plexus of arterioles at a point 1–2 cm away from the esophagus. If blunt dissection of the esophagus is used, it should be kept immediately adjacent to the esophagus with disruption of only the smaller arterioles.

Chyle Leak

The thoracic duct drains the cisterna chyli in the abdomen beginning at the L2 level. It enters the chest through the aortic hiatus and ascends through the right chest behind the esophagus along the vertebral bodies between the azygous vein and the aorta. Occasionally, more than one channel exists in the lower chest at the level of the hiatus. At approximately the T6 level, it crosses to the left side behind the aorta and ascends along the left side of the esophagus posterior to the left subclavian artery. Above the clavicle, the duct descends behind the carotid sheath and anterior to the anterior scalene muscle and phrenic nerve to empty into the junction of the left internal jugular and subclavian vein.

The duct can be injured at any point along dissection of the esophagus. The incidence of chyle leak following esophagectomy ranges from 2% to 10%.[34,60] The incidence is higher following transthoracic resection, probably as a result of an extended radial dissection of the esophagus and associated nodal tissue. Prophylactic mass ligation of the duct at the hiatus may help decrease the incidence of postoperative leak. If chest tube output is 1000 ml/day or greater 48 h following esophagectomy, chylothorax should be suspected. Diagnosis can be difficult as the classic milky appearance of chyle is apparent only in a fed patient. Gram stain will exclude the presence of polymorphonuclear cells. Fluid should be sent for triglyceride level, cholesterol level, and cell count. A triglyceride level of greater than 1 mmol/liter is highly suggestive of a chyle leak, as is a lymphocyte count of greater than 90%. A cholesterol/triglyceride ratio of <1 and confirmation of chylomicrons on electrophoresis have also been suggested to be diagnostic of a chyle leak. Perhaps the best and simplest test is feeding cream at 30 ml/h via the J-tube for 3–4 h watching for a change from serous pleural fluid to a milky fluid.

There is no role for conservative management of a high-output chyle leak following esophagectomy. Continued loss of lymphocytes, protein, fats, and fluid at a rate of 1 liter/day or greater in a malnourished patient healing from a major operation invites disaster. Once the diagnosis is confirmed, or even if the diagnosis is highly suspected, the patient should be brought back to the operating room for ligation of the duct at the level of the hiatus. Cream should be instilled via the J-tube for several hours prior to reoperation. Approach to ligation of the duct should be via right thoracotomy or thoracoscopy. Often the exact site of injury can be located after the patient has been given cream enterally. It may be repaired with pledgeted 4-0 or 5-0 monofilament sutures. If there is any doubt about the integrity of the repair, the duct should be mass ligated at the level of the hiatus. The pleura is incised and a 0 silk mass ligature is used to encompass all tissue between the azygous vein and aorta along the spine. A pledgeted suture should be used if tissue integrity is poor. A careful search to confirm cessation of the leak should be performed prior to closure.

Recently, noninvasive methods for closure of thoracic duct leaks have been proposed. The thoracic duct can be cannulated percutaneously via puncture into the cisterna chyli and embolized with coils or fibrin glue. In a trial of 42 patients (nine of whom were postesophagectomy), the thoracic duct could be embolized in 26 patients, and 16 of these were cured.[15] This technology is in evolution, and at this point should be reserved for complex patients who either have failed surgical repair or are not candidates for surgical repair.

Postresection Reflux

Reflux of duodenal contents into the conduit occurs to some degree after esophagectomy in virtually all patients. It is not clear that preservation of the integrity of the pylorus protects against bile reflux. In fact, a study by Romagnoli et al involving 24-h bile monitoring of the denervated gastric conduit in 16 patients showed elevated concentrations of bile in the stomach irrespective of the presence or absence of a drainage procedure.[61]

The incidence of severe postoperative reflux requiring intervention following distal esophagectomy with esophagogastric anastomosis low in the chest approaches 20%.[73] For this reason, when esophageal replacement is contemplated for a distal peptic stricture, colon or jejunal interposition should be employed. These conduits, in the isoperistaltic position, are more resistant to the effects of gastric reflux and provide active peristalsis that allows for clearance of bile.

Impaired Conduit Emptying

Several factors have been implicated in delayed conduit emptying following esophagectomy including truncal vagotomy,

absence of pyloric drainage procedure, swelling at the pyloroplasty site, kinking of redundant conduit in the lower chest, and a conduit that is too wide and patulous. Some of these variables are difficult to assess, whereas others have been carefully studied. Following truncal vagotomy for ulcer disease there is a 25% incidence of impaired gastric emptying.[18] Whether this applies to transposed stomach following esophagectomy is not clear. One study showed that delayed emptying following esophagectomy with gastric replacement was less in those undergoing pyloroplasty (the time of emptying of radiolabeled water was 378 min in the no pyloroplasty vs. 161 min in patients undergoing pyloroplasty).[26] Other studies showed no objective difference in gastric conduit emptying.[32] In any event, there is often poor correlation between gastric emptying tests and symptoms.

Fok et al conducted a prospective randomized trial of pyloroplasty vs. no pyloroplasty in 200 patients undergoing Ivor Lewis esophagectomy with gastric reconstruction.[21] There were no complications from the pyloroplasty procedure. Thirteen of the 100 patients who had no drainage procedure had symptoms of delayed gastric emptying. Two of these patients died as a result of aspiration pneumonia, one required reoperation, and three others had prolonged symptoms. The daily postoperative nasogastric drainage was not significantly different between the two groups. Gastric emptying measured at 6 months was 6 min in the pyloroplasty group and 24 min in the patients without pyloroplasty. The patients without pyloroplasty also had more symptoms attributable to impaired gastric emptying at 6 months than the pyloroplasty patients. The authors strongly advocate a routine pyloric drainage procedure. The same group conducted a randomized trial of pyloroplasty to pyloromyotomy and found both to be effective and safe procedures.[36] Six months following the procedure, gastric emptying was twice as fast in the pyloroplasty groups vs. the pyloromyotomy group; however, the incidence of symptoms appeared to be no different.

The width of the gastric conduit is also believed to influence the rate of emptying. The gastric tube should be kept narrow, with the width not significantly exceeding that of the antrum. A retrospective study examined the relationship between conduit emptying and size and found that patients with a narrow gastric tube had a far lower incidence of symptoms attributable to delayed gastric emptying (3%) than patients with whole stomach (38%) or distal two-thirds stomach (14%) conduits.[10] A conduit that is too narrow, however, may become ischemic from a compromised arterial inflow and venous congestion. In the authors' opinion, conduit diameter should not be less than 5 cm. Proper length of the gastric conduit is also important as excess conduit can fold over into the right chest and has been associated with impaired emptying.

Local Recurrence

Factors involved in local recurrence include resection margins and clearance of adjacent nodal disease. Tam et al found a correlation between the incidence of local recurrence and the lateral spread of tumor outside the esophageal wall (T3), but no correlation with tumor differentiation or lymph node metastasis.[68] The importance of complete clearance of nodal tissue is debated among

648 proponents of complete lymphadenectomy (via transthoracic or en bloc dissection) and proponents of simple transhiatal dissection. This is discussed in a later section.

The issue of recurrence after incomplete linear margin is better understood. The palpable intraoperative *in situ* resection margin will be larger than the contracted gross postresection margin, which in turn is longer than the final fixed margin. Siu et al estimated that margins after removal of the esophagus were only about 50% of the *in situ* margin.[63] Descriptions of margin length must take this factor into account. Tam et al examined the *in situ* resection margins of 100 patients with squamous cell carcinoma of the esophagus. When the *in situ* margin was less than 5 cm there was a 20% incidence of anastomotic recurrence, between 5 and 10 cm there was an 8% chance, and when the margin was greater than 10 cm there were no anastomotic recurrences.[68] Wong[80] further points out that achieving a 10-cm margin is difficult to obtain, as the length of the average esophageal tumor was 6 cm. Assuming the average esophagus is 25 cm in length, only distal esophageal tumors can, on average, be resected with a 10-cm margin if the larynx is to be conserved. Another author suggests that an adequate distal margin after resection of adenocarcinoma of the GE junction should be 6 cm.[55]

Long-Term (5-Year) Survival

Long-term survival remains an elusive goal for the medical and surgical oncologist caring for a patient with esophageal cancer. Despite advances in perioperative care reducing the perioperative mortality rate to 7% and below, 5-year survival has not changed appreciably over the past two decades. The 5-year survival described by Cunh-Melo and associates between 1953 and 1978 (18%) is similar to that described in the recent meta-analysis by Hulscher et al[34] between 1990 and 1999 (22%). It remains to be seen whether the introduction of neoadjuvant treatment for advanced esophageal cancers (invading through the esophageal wall or with positive nodes) will change the overall survival of patients with esophageal cancer. Three randomized trials employing neoadjuvant chemoradiation prior to esophagectomy have been performed. A trial randomizing 100 esophageal cancer patients to preoperative chemoradiation followed by transhiatal esophagectomy vs. transhiatal esophagectomy alone showed that survival in the neoadjuvant group was 30% at 3 years vs. 16% in the surgery alone group—the difference was not statistically significant.[74] A European study randomizing 282 squamous cell cancer patients to neoadjuvant followed by en bloc transthoracic esophagectomy to esophagectomy alone found no difference in 5-year survival.[11] Walsh et al randomized 113 patients with adenocarcinoma to surgery alone vs. chemoradiation followed by surgery.[78] Five-year survival was approximately 50% in the neoadjuvant group, and was unusually poor in the surgery-alone group, 8%—the difference was statistically significant. Larger trials have been attempted; however, they have encountered difficulty enrolling patients in a randomized fashion, and the true benefit of neoadjuvant chemoradiation may never be measured.

A few isolated series in selected centers employing radical en bloc dissection of the esophagus with three-field lymph node dissection have described 5-year survival rates

in the 40–50% range.[7,9] These results are discussed in the sections entitled en bloc resection and three-field lymph node dissection.

► TRIALS COMPARING TRANSHIATAL TO TRANSTHORACIC RESCTION

Numerous nonrandomized, retrospective trials have been performed in an attempt to define differences in either perioperative complication rate or long-term survival between the transhiatal and transthoracic approaches (Table 37–1).[30,53,64] Most of these were limited by small study size and selection bias. A large meta-analysis review was performed by Rindani et al in 1999.[60] Forty-four trials published in the English literature between 1986 and 1996 consisting of 5483 patients undergoing either Ivor Lewis or transhiatal esophagectomy were reviewed. The overall incidence of pneumonia was 25% and was not appreciably different between the two techniques. The incidence of bleeding and cardiac complications was also not different. The most significant differences were seen in the anastomotic leak rate (16% transhiatal vs. 10% Ivor Lewis), stricture (28% transhiatal vs. 16% Ivor Lewis), and recurrent nerve injury (11% transhiatal vs. 5% Ivor Lewis). Perioperative

Table 37–1

Comparison of Transthoracic and Transhiatal Approaches to Esophagectomy: Perioperative Complications[a]

Complication	Transthoracic	Transhiatal
Blood loss (ml)	1001	728
Operative time (h)	5.6	4.0
Cardiac complications (%)	6.6	19.5
Pulmonary complications (%)	18.7	12.7
Anastomotic leak (%)	7.2	13.6
Vocal cord paralysis (%)	3.5	9.5
Chyle leak (%)	2.4	1.4
In-hospital mortality (%)	9.2	5.7

[a]Adapted from Hulscher J, Tijssen J, Lanschot J: Transthoracic versus transhiatal resection for carcinoma of the esophagus. A meta-analysis. Ann Thorac Surg 72:306–313, 2001. Cumulative review of all English literature (searched via MEDLINE) publications between 1990 and 1999 comparing transhiatal vs. transthoracic esophageal resection.

mortality was higher in the Ivor Lewis population (9.5%) than in the transhiatal population (6.3%). Overall long-term (5-year) survival was similar in the two groups—25%.

Hulscher et al also recently performed a meta-analysis of trials between 1990 and 1999 published in English language journals.[33] Fifty publications were identified, some randomized, some comparing transthoracic to transhiatal approaches, and some evaluating only one technique. Overall, cardiac complications (20% vs. 7%), anastomotic leakage (14% vs. 7%), and vocal cord paralysis (10% vs. 4%) were higher in the transhiatal versus the transthoracic groups. Pulmonary complications (19% vs. 13%), in-hospital mortality (9% vs. 6%), and operative time (5 vs. 4.2 h) were higher in the transthoracic versus the transhiatal group. Overall 5-year survival was similar among all the studies and patients evaluated (23% for transthoracic resections and 21.7% for transhiatal resections). These reviews are of historical and factual interest only, and little can be concluded about the relative merits of each technique in matched populations.

Three randomized prospective trials have been performed comparing transhiatal resection to transthoracic resection. Aside from demonstrating that either technique may be performed safely in skilled hands, no clear differences have been shown between the two techniques. This is in large part due to an inadequate number of patients enrolled in the trials. Extrapolating from their retrospective meta-analysis, Rindani et al estimated that 2360 patients would have to be randomized to show a significant difference in perioperative mortality, and 6400 patients would be needed to show a difference in long-term survival.[60] Clearly, this is beyond the capacity of any prospective esophagectomy trial.

The first randomized, prospective trial was published in 1993 by Goldminc et al.[25] They randomized 67 patients younger than 70 years with squamous cell cancer of the esophagus to Ivor Lewis esophagectomy or transhiatal esophagectomy. Operative time was longer (6 vs. 4 h) in the transthoracic group. There was no difference in incidence of pneumonia (20%), anastomotic leak, recurrent nerve injury, bleeding, perioperative mortality, or length of hospitalization. At a mean follow-up of 3 years, survival was not statistically different between the two groups. For those patients with nodal disease, however, none of the transhiatal patients was alive at 18 months, while 30% of the transthoracic patients were alive at 18 months.

Wong and colleagues reported a prospective, randomized series of 39 patients with lower third esophageal cancers treated with either an Ivor Lewis resection or a transhiatal resection.[12] The study was limited by the small size, short follow-up (mean 15 months), and patient exclusions. Patients undergoing neoadjuvant therapy or those with an $FEV_1 < 70\%$ were excluded from the study. There were no perioperative (30 day) deaths in either group, although the in-hospital mortality was 15% for the transhiatal group and 0% for the transthoracic group (not significantly different). Intraoperative hypotension occurred in 60% of transhiatal patients but only in 5% of transthoracic patients. There was no difference in blood loss, pneumonia, or recurrent nerve injury. Operating time was longer for the transthoracic group. The mean proximal margin was 3 cm longer in the transhiatal group. No significant difference was seen in tumor recurrence or survival.

More recently a randomized study was completed in the Netherlands comparing transhiatal resection vs. extended transthoracic en bloc resection for distal adenocarcinomas of the esophagus or cardia.[34] One hundred six patients had a transhiatal resection and 114 patients had a transthoracic resection. In-hospital mortality was 2–4% in each group. Respiratory complications including atelectasis and pneumonia were higher in the transthoracic group (57% vs. 27%) as was the incidence of chyle leak (10% vs. 2%). The high incidence of respiratory complications in the transthoracic group (57%) should be questioned, as it is much higher than that quoted in many prior transthoracic resection series.[60] Although statistical significance was not reached, there was a trend toward improved survival at 5 years in the transthoracic group (39% vs. 29%).

SUMMARY

The reduction in perioperative mortality from esophagectomy from over 40% over the past 50 years to as low as 3% as described in several large academic centers is attributable to improvements in patient selection, operative technique, intensive care, and early recognition and aggressive management of perioperative complications. Minimizing complications and optimizing chances at cure require that the skilled esophageal surgeon be familiar with the anatomy of the neck, chest, and abdomen, and be well trained in and ready to utilize a variety of routes of esophageal resection and methods of reconstruction.

REFERENCES

1. Adams W, Phemister D: Carcinoma of the lower thoracic esophagus; report of a successful resection and esophagogastrectomy. J Thorac Surg 7:621–632, 1938.
2. Ahmed ME: The surgical management and outcome of oesophageal cancer in Khartoum. J R Coll Surg Edinb 38:16–18, 1993.
3. Akiyama, H, Tsurumaru M, Ono Y: Principles of surgical treatment for carcinoma of the esophagus. Ann Surg 194:438–446., 1981.
4. Akiyama, H, Tsurumaru M, Kajiyama Y: Radical lymph node dissection for cancer of the thoracic esophagus. Ann Surg 220:364–372, 1994.
5. Altorki N, Skinner D: Occult cervical nodal metastasis in esophageal cancer: Preiliminary results of three-field lymphadenectomy. J Thorac Cardiovasc Surg 113:540–544, 1997.
6. Altorki N, Girardi L, Skinner D: En bloc esophagectomy improves survival for stage III esophageal cancer. J Thorac Cardiovasc Surg 114:948–956, 1997.
7. Altorki N, Kent M, Port J: Three-field lymph node dissection for squamous cell and adenocarcinoma of the esophagus. Ann Surg 236:177–183, 2002.
8. Altorki NK, Skinner DB: En bloc esophagectomy: The first 100 patients. Hepatogastroenterology 37:360–363, 1990.
9. Ando N, Ozawa S, Kitajima M: Improvement in the results of surgical treatment of advanced squamous esophageal carcinoma during 15 consecutive years. Ann Surg 232:225–232, 2000.
10. Bemelman W, Taat C, Slors F: Delayed postoperative emptying after esophageal resection is dependent on the size of the gastric substitute. J Am Coll Surg 180:461–464, 1995.

650

11. Bossett J, Gignoux M, Triboulet J: Chemoradiotherapy followed by surgery compared with surgery alone in squamous-cell cancer of the esophagus. N Engl J Med 337:161–167, 1997.

12. Chu K, Law S, Wong J, et al: A prospective randomized comparison of transhiatal and transthoracic resection for lower-third esophageal carcinoma. Am J Surg 174:320–324, 1997.

13. Churchill EaSR: Transthoracic resection of tumors of the stomach and esophagus. Ann Surg 115:897, 1942.

14. Coleman J, Searless J, Jurkiewicz M, et al: Ten years experience with the free jejujnal autograft. Am J Surg 154:394–398, 1987.

15. Cope C, Kaiser L: Management of unremitting chylothorax by percutaneous embolization and blockage of retroperitoneal lymphatic vessels in 42 patients. J Vasc Interv Radiol 13:1139–1148, 2002.

16. Daniel TM, Fleischer KJ, Flanagan TL, et al: Transhiatal esophagectomy: A safe alternative for selected patients. Ann Thorac Surg 54:686–689; discussion 689–690, 1992.

17. Dewar L, Gelfand G, Finley R: Factors affecting cervical anastomotic leak and stricture formation following esophagogastrectomy and gastric tube interposition. Am J Surg 163:484–489, 1992.

18. Dragstedt L, Camp E: Follow up of gastric vagotomy alone in the treatment of peptic ulcer. Gastroenterology 11:460–465, 1948.

19. Earlam R, Cunha-Melo J: Oesophageal squamous cell carcinoma: I. A critical review of surgery. Br J Surg 67:381–390, 1980.

20. Ellis H, Krasna M: Esophagogastrectomy for carcinoma of the esophagus and cardia: A comparison of findings and results after standard resection in three consecutive eight-year intervals with improved staging criteria. J Thorac Cardiovasc Surg 113:836–846, 1997.

21. Fok M, Cheng S, Wong J: Pyloroplasty versus no drainage in gastric replacement of the esophagus. Am J Surg 162:447–452, 1991.

22. Gelfand GA, Finley RJ, Nelems B, et al: Transhiatal esophagectomy for carcinoma of the esophagus and cardia. Experience with 160 cases. Arch Surg 127:1164–1167; discussion 1167–1168, 1992.

23. Gillinov AM, Heitmiller RF: Strategies to reduce pulmonary complications after transhiatal esophagectomy. Dis Esophagus 11:43–47, 1998.

24. Giuli R, Gignoux M: Treatment of carcinoma of the esophagus. Retrospective study of 2400 patients. Ann Surg 192:44–52, 1980.

25. Goldminc M, Maddern GBL, et al: Oesophagectomy by a transhiatal approach or thoracotomy: A prospective randomized trial. Br J Surg 80:367–376, 1993.

26. Gupta M, Chattopadhyay T, Sharma L: Emptying of the intrathoracic stomach with and without pyloroplasty. Am J Gastroenterol 84:921–923, 1989.

27. Gupta NM: Oesophagectomy without thoracotomy: First 250 patients. Eur J Surg 162:455–461, 1996.

28. Gurkan N, Terzioglu T, Tezelman S, et al: Transhiatal oesophagectomy for oesophageal carcinoma. Br J Surg 78:1348–1351, 1991.

29. Hagen J, Peters J, DeMeester T: Superiority of extended en bloc esophagogastrectomy for carcinoma of the lower esophagus and cardia. J Thorac Cardiovasc Surg 106:850–859, 1993.

30. Hankins J, Attar S, McLaughlin J, et al: Carcinoma of the esophagus: A comparison of the results of transhiatal vs. transthoracic resection. Ann Thorac Surg 47:700–705, 1989.

31. Honkoop P, Siersema P, van Blankenstein M, et al: Benign anastomotic strictures after transhiatal esophagectomy and cervical esophagogastrotomy: Risk factors and management. J Thorac Cardiovasc Surg 111:1141–1146, 1996.

32. Huang G, Zhang D, Zhang D: A comparative study of resection of carcinoma of the esophagus with and without pyloroplasty. In DeMeester T, Skinner D, editors: Esophageal Disorders: Pathophysiology. New York: Raven Press, 1985, pp. 383–388.

33. Hulscher J, Tijssen J, Lanschot J: Transthoracic versus transhiatal resection for carcinoma of the esophagus: A meta-analysis. Ann Thorac Surg 72:306–313, 2001.

34. Hulscher J, Van Sandick J, Van Lanschot J: Extended transthoracic resection compared with limited transhiatal resection for adenocarcinoma of the esophagus. N Engl J Med 347:1662–1669, 2002.

35. Junginger T, Dutkowski P: Selective approach to the treatment of oesophageal cancer. Br J Surg 83:1473–1477, 1996.

36. Law S, Cheung M, Wong J: Pyloroplasty and pyloromyotomy in gastric replacement of the esophagus after esophagectomy: A randomized controlled trial. J Am Coll Surg 184:630–636, 1997.

37. Law S, Fok M, Wong J, et al: Comparison of hand-sewn and stapled esophagogastric anastomosis after esophageal resection for cancer. A prospective randomized controlled trial. Ann Surg 226:169–173, 1997.

38. Lerut T, De Leyn P, Coosemans W, et al: Surgical strategies in esophageal carcinoma with emphasis on radical lymphadenectomy. Ann Surg 216:583–590, 1992.

39. Lewis I: The surgical treatment of carcinoma of the esophagus with special reference to a new operation for growths of the middle third. Br J Surg 34:18–31, 1946.

40. Luketich J, Schauer P, Christie N: Minimally invasive esophagectomy. Ann Thorac Surg 70:906–912, 2000.

41. Mannell A, Becker PJ: Evaluation of the results of oesophagectomy for oesophageal cancer. Br J Surg 78:36–40, 1991.

42. Mathisen D, Grillo H, Hilgenberg A, et al: Transthoracic esophagectomy: A safe approach to carcinoma of the esophagus. Ann Thorac Surg 45:137, 1988.

43. McConnel F, Hester R, Jurkiewicz M, et al: Free jejunal grafts for reconstruction of pharynx and cervical esophagus. Arch Otolaryngol 107:476–481, 1981.

44. McKeown K: Total three-stage oesphagectomy for cancer of the oesophagus. Br J Surg 63:259, 1976.

45. Millikan KW, Silverstein J, Hart V, et al: A 15-year review of esophagectomy for carcinoma of the esophagus and cardia. Arch Surg 130:617–624, 1995.

46. Moreno GE, Garcia GI, Pinto GA, et al: Results of transhiatal esophagectomy in cancer of the esophagus and other diseases. Hepatogastroenterology 39:439–442, 1992.

47. Muller J, Erasmi H, Pichlmaier H, et al: Surgical therapy of oesophageal carcinoma. Br J Surg 77:845–857, 1990.

48. Nguyen N, Schauer P, Luketich J: Combined laparoscopic and thoracoscopic approach to esophagectomy. J Am Coll Surg 188:328–332, 1999.

49. Nishimake T, Tanaka O, Suzuki T, et al: Patterns of lymphatic spread in thoracic esophageal cancer. Cancer 74:4–11, 1994.

50. Orringer M, Lemmer J: Early dilatation in the treatment of esophageal disruption. Ann Thorac Surg 42:536–539, 1986.

51. Orringer M, Marshall B, Iannettoni M: Transhiatal esophagectomy: Clinical experience and refinements. Ann Surg 230:392–403, 1999.

52. Oshawa T: The surgery of the esophagus. Arch Jpn Chir 10:605, 1933.

53. Pac M, Basoglu A, Keles M, et al: Transhiatal versus transthoracic esophagectomy for esophageal cancer. J Thorac Cardiovasc Surg 106:205–209, 1993.

54. Page RD, Khalil JF, Whyte RI, et al: Esophagogastrectomy via left thoracophrenotomy. Ann Thorac Surg 49:763–766, 1990.

55. Papachristou D: Histologically positive esophageal margin in the surgical treatment of gastric cancer. Am J Surg 139:711, 1980.

56. Patil P, Patel S, Desai P: Cancer of the esophagus: Esophagogastric anastomotic leak — a retrospective study of predisposing factors. J Surg Oncol 49:163–167, 1992.

57. Pierie J, de Graaf P, Poen H, et al: Incidence and management of benign anastomotic stricture after cervical oesophago-gastrostomy. Br J Surg 80:471–474, 1993.

58. Putnam JB Jr, Suell DM, McMurtrey MJ, et al: Comparison of three techniques of esophagectomy within a residency training program. Ann Thorac Surg 57:319–325, 1994.

59. Rahamim J, Cham CW: Oesophagogastrectomy for carcinoma of the oesophagus and cardia. Br J Surg 80:1305–1309, 1993.

60. Rindani R, Martin C, Cox M: Transhiatal versus Ivor-Lewis oesophagectomy: Is there a difference? Aust N Z J Surg 69:187–194, 1999.

61. Romagnoli R, Bechi P, Salizzoni M: Combined 24-hour intraluminal pH and bile monitoring of the denervated whole stomach as an esophageal substitute. Hepatogastroenterology 46:86–91, 1999.

62. Sharpe DA, Moghissi K: Resectional surgery in carcinoma of the oesophagus and cardia: What influences long-term survival? Eur J Cardiothorac Surg 10:359–363; discussion 363–364, 1996.

63. Siu K, Cheung H, Wong J: Shrinkage of the esophagus after resection for carcinoma. Ann Surg 203:173–176, 1986.

64. Stark S, Romberg M, Thomas J, et al: Transhiatal versus transthoracic esophagectomy for adenocarcinoma of the distal esophagus and cardia. Am J Surg 172:478–482, 1996.

65. Sutton DN, Wayman J, Griffin SM: Learning curve for oesophageal cancer surgery. Br J Surg 85:1399–1402, 1998.

66. Swanson SJ, Batirel HF, Bueno R, et al: Transthoracic esophagectomy with radical mediastinal and abdominal lymph node dissection and cervical esophagogastrostomy for esophageal carcinoma. Ann Thorac Surg 72:1918–1924; discussion 1924–1925, 2001.

67. Swanstrom L, Hansen P: Laparoscopic total esophagectomy. Arch Surg 132:943–949, 1997.

68. Tam P, Cheung H, Wong J, et al: Local recurrences after subtotal esophagectomy for squamous cell carcinoma. Ann Surg 205:189–194, 1987.

69. Thomas P, Doddoli C, Lienne P, et al: Changing patterns and surgical results in adenocarcinoma of the oesophagus. Br J Surg 84:119–125, 1997.

70. Tilanus HW, Hop WC, Langenhorst BL, et al: Esophagectomy with or without thoracotomy. Is there any difference? J Thorac Cardiovasc Surg 105:898–903, 1993.

71. Torek F: The operative treatment of carcinoma of the esophagus. Ann Surg 61:385, 1915.

72. Tsutsui S, Moriguchi S, Morita M, et al: Multivariate analysis of postoperative complications after esophageal resection. Ann Thorac Surg 53:1052–1056, 1992.

73. Turnball A, Ginsberg R: Options in the surgical treatment of esophageal carcinoma. Chest Surg Clin North Am 4:315–329, 1994.

74. Urba S, Orringer M, Turrisi A: Randomized trial of preoperative chemoradiation versus surgery alone in patients with locoregional esophageal carcinoma. J Clin Oncol 19:305–313, 2001.

75. Urschel J: Esophagogastrostomy anastomotic leaks complicating esophagectomy: A review. Am J Surg 169:634–639, 1995.

76. Vigneswaran W, Trastek V, Pairolero P: Transhiatal esophagectomy for carcinoma of the esophagus. Ann Thorac Surg 56:838–846, 1993.

77. Vigneswaran WT, Trastek VF, Pairolero PC, et al: Transhiatal esophagectomy for carcinoma of the esophagus. Ann Thorac Surg 56:838–844; discussion 844–836, 1993.

78. Walsh T, Noonan N, Hennessy T: A comparision of multi-modal therapy and surgery for esophageal adenocarcinoma. N Engl J Med 335:462–467, 1996.

79. Wang LS, Huang MH, Huang BS, et al: Gastric substitution for resectable carcinoma of the esophagus: An analysis of 368 cases. Ann Thorac Surg 53:289–294, 1992.

80. Wong J: Esophageal resection for cancer: The rationale of current practice. Am J Surg 153:18–24, 1987.

Combined Modality Therapy for Esophageal Cancer

Kelli R. Brooks and David H. Harpole, Jr.

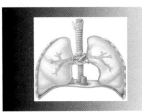

CHAPTER 38

INTRODUCTION

The incidence of carcinoma of the esophagus is rapidly increasing in Western populations, accounting for more than 13,000 cases per year.[10] Squamous cell carcinoma (SCC) has been the prominent histology; however, adenocarcinoma (AC) is steadily increasing, with a rise in carcinomas of the distal esophagus. Although the incidence of esophageal carcinoma continues to rise, controversy exists regarding the optimal therapy. In 1993 a review of the National Cancer Data Base by Daly et al[6] demonstrated the utilization of the various treatment strategies of surgery alone (18%), radiotherapy alone (12%), combined chemoradiotherapy (30%), and trimodality therapy (9%). Surgery has long been considered the standard of care for localized disease, with excellent survival rates in stage 1 disease. Most patients, however, have stage 2 or 3 tumors, and although surgery remains the best single-modality therapy for these stages, combined 5-year survival is approximately 20%.

Attempts at increasing survival from esophageal cancer have included the addition of preoperative chemotherapy and radiotherapy. Chemotherapy may downstage the primary tumor and thus increase resectability and may eliminate or delay the appearance of micrometastatic disease. Radiotherapy is used for improved local control. Early results from nonrandomized studies predicted a survival advantage for patients who underwent neoadjuvant treatment. A number of randomized trials have now been conducted in an attempt to identify optimal therapy for esophageal cancer, with a primary focus on neoadjuvant therapies.

CHEMOTHERAPY AND SURGERY

In the management of esophageal cancer there have been at least nine randomized trials conducted into the use of chemotherapy and surgery versus surgery alone. The vast majority of these trials consist of a cisplatin-based chemotherapy regimen. A concern exists over an increase in perioperative mortality with the addition of neoadjuvant chemotherapy. However, in none of the four recent trials discussed in the following does preoperative chemotherapy increase perioperative mortality.

In 1997 Law et al[14] randomized 147 patients with scc to receive chemotherapy with cisplatin and 5-fluorouracil (5-FU) followed by surgery (CT-S) or surgery alone (S). There was no significant survival advantage for those receiving combined therapy, with a median survival of 17 months (CT-S) versus 13 months (S).

In 1998 the North America Intergroup Trial (INT 0113) was published by Kelsen et al.[13] The trial randomized 467 patients and included both AC and SCC. Chemotherapy consisted of 5-FU and cisplatin and was repeated postoperatively in those patients who were pathological responders (R_0). Once again there was no improvement in overall survival in the group treated with neoadjuvant chemotherapy. Furthermore, there was no effect on the pattern of recurrence between the two groups.

In 2001 Ancona et al[1] in Italy published their series randomizing 96 patients with SCC to preoperative chemotherapy with 5-FU and cisplatin followed by surgery or surgery alone. There was no significant survival advantage in those patients treated with chemotherapy. There was a significant survival advantage in the 12.8% of patients who demonstrated complete pathological response to neoadjuvant therapy.

The largest trial conducted to date has been published only in abstract form. In 2001 Clark et al[5] reported the results of the UK Medical Research Council Group (MRC OE02). This trial randomized 802 patients with either SCC or AC to neoadjuvant chemotherapy with 5-FU and cisplatin followed by surgery or surgery alone. This trial did demonstrate a survival advantage for those who underwent neoadjuvant treatment. The median survival increased from 13.3 to 17.2 months, and the 2-year survival rate rose to 43% from 34%.

Although early nonrandomized studies suggested a survival advantage with the addition of chemotherapeutic agents in the treatment of esophageal cancers, this has not been established conclusively to date. However, those patients who have a pathological complete response (pCR) demonstrate an improved overall survival.

CHEMORADIOTHERAPY AND SURGERY

Preliminary nonrandomized studies suggested a survival advantage with combined modality therapy. The addition of chemotherapy for downstaging and control of micro-metastatic disease and radiotherapy for control of local disease theoretically should improve outcomes. Seven prospective randomized trials have been conducted examining the differences between surgery and chemoradiotherapy and surgery (CMT) in the outcomes of patients with esophageal carcinoma. There has been considerable discussion over the implications of these trials. Six of the seven trials have demonstrated no significant differences in survival. The results of these trials are summarized in Table 38-1.

The first study, by Nygaard et al[17] in 1992, consisted of four arms that randomized patients to surgery alone, preoperative chemotherapy (cisplatin and bleomycin), preoperative radiotherapy (35 Gy), and preoperative CMT (sequential). There was no significant difference in overall survival between the arms of the study. However, those patients who received preoperative radiotherapy had an improved survival over those who did not.

In 1994 Le Prise et al[15] randomized 86 patients with SCC to trimodality therapy versus surgery alone with no advantage. This trial was limited by low radiation dose (20 Gy) and sequential, not concurrent, chemoradiotherapy. Apinop et al[2] randomized 69 patients in the first randomized trial to use concurrent chemoradiotherapy and that consisted of 40 Gy with cisplatin- and 5-FU-based chemotherapy. Again there was no survival advantage.

In 1997 Bosset et al[3] randomized 282 patients with SCC to cisplatin-based chemotherapy and radiation therapy (37 Gy) delivered concurrently in two cycles versus surgery alone in a European organization treatment of cancer trial (EORTC). Median survival, at 18.6 months, was no different between the two groups. However, a complete pathological response was noted in 26% of patients undergoing combined modality therapy. These patients had a significant improvement in disease-free survival ($p = .003$). This trial also noted a significant increase in the postoperative mortality in patients who were treated with CMT.

Urba et al[19] reported in 1995 and again in 2001 the results of the Michigan series of 100 patients treated with cisplatin, 5-FU, and vinblastine and 45 Gy of concurrent hyperfractionated radiotherapy. The trial included patients with both AC and SCC. Once again there was no difference in median survival (17.6 versus 16.9 months). However, there was a trend in the CMT arm, although not statistically significant ($p = .15$), toward improved survival (30% versus 16%).

The Australian series was reported by Burmeister et al[4] in 2002 at the Annual Meeting of the American Society of Clinical Oncology in abstract form. The study randomized 205 patients with AC and SCC to chemotherapy with cisplatin and 5-FU and 35 Gy of concurrent radiotherapy. There was no significant difference in overall survival between groups. There was, however, a significant increase in disease-free survival in patients with SCC treated with CMT ($p = .04$), although this did not translate into an increase in overall survival.

Table 38-1

Preoperative Chemoradiotherapy and Esophageal Cancer

Author	Year	Number of patients		Histology	Chemo	Preoperative RT		pCR (%)	Median survival (mo)		3-yr survival (%)	
		S	CMT			Gy	Administration		S	CMT	S	CMT
Nygaard et al	1992	47	41	SCC	cis, bleo	35	Sequential	NS	6	7	9	17
Le Prise et al	1994	41	45	SCC	cis, 5-FU	20	Sequential	10	10	11	14	19
Apinop et al	1994	35	34	SCC	cis, 5-FU	40	Concomitant	20	7	10	20	26
Walsh et al	1996	58	55	AC	cis, 5-FU	40	Concomitant	22	11	16	6	32
Bosset et al	1997	143	139	SCC	cis	37	Concomitant	20	18	19	34	36
Urba et al	2001	50	50	SCC/ AC	cis, vinbl 5-FU	45	Concomitant	28	18	17	16	30
Burmeister et al	2002	205[a]		SCC/ AC	cis, 5-FU	35	Concomitant	15	19	22	NS	NS

S, Surgery; CMT, combined modality therapy; SCC, squamous cell carcinoma; AC, adenocarcinoma; cis, cisplatin; bleo, bleomycin; 5-FU, 5-fluorouracil; vinbl, vinblastine; pCR, pathological, complete response; NS, not stated.

[a]Breakdown not reported.

In 1996 Walsh et al[20] reported the only trial to demonstrate a survival advantage with CMT. A total of 113 patients with AC were treated with cisplatin, 5-FU, and concurrent 40 Gy of radiotherapy. The median survival significantly ($p = 0.01$) increased in the CMT arm, 16 versus 11 months, as did the 3-year survival rate, 32% versus 6% ($p = 0.01$). The extremely low 3-year survival rate of 6% in the surgery-alone arm compares to an average of 20–30% 3-year survival rate in the surgery arm of comparable trials and has brought the results of this trial under a great deal of scrutiny.

In 2003 a meta-analysis of 11 randomized trials, including 2311 patients, was performed to determine differences in patient mortality and survival in those treated with combined modality therapy versus surgical resection alone. Seven trials addressed the question of chemotherapy and surgery versus surgery alone. Two-year survival was improved with chemotherapy and surgery compared with surgery alone by 4.4% (95% confidence interval [CI], 0.3–8.5%). Combined chemoradiotherapy increased survival by 6.4%, although this was not statistically significant (95% CI, −0.1 to 7.3%). Overall treatment-related mortality increased by 2.3% over surgery alone and was greater in patients treated with chemoradiotherapy (3.4%) than in those with chemotherapy (1.7%).[12] Although the results of this meta-analysis revealed a modest advantage for patients treated with combined modality therapy, this has yet to be confirmed in a large randomized trial. The recent Cancer and Leukemia Group B study designed to compare surgery and CMT was closed because of limited accrual.

PREDICTORS OF RESPONSE

Although there has been no definitive evidence that combined modality therapy improves overall survival, there is significant evidence that those who respond to therapy demonstrate prolonged disease-free intervals and improved overall survival. For this reason, recent efforts have focused on identifying those patients most likely to respond to a chemotherapeutic regimen in order to maximize therapeutic benefit while limiting toxicity from neoadjuvant regimens. Clinicopathological features such as TNM status have been investigated with conflicting results.[7,11] Nodal status has been identified as a potential predictor of response when determined by thoracoscopic and laparoscopic staging techniques ($p = 0.006$).[15] Molecular techniques to predict tumor response and patient outcomes are currently being studied. In 2001 Harpole et al[7] identified high-level expression of the platinum resistance markers glutathione S-transferase-π and P-glycoprotein, as well as the 5-FU marker thymidylate synthase, to be associated with early recurrence and death in patients treated with CMT using cisplatin and 5-FU. Other investigators have found high levels of metallothionein (MT) to be associated with cisplatin resistance and poor survival.[8] Continued investigation in this area allows therapy to be designated based on the molecular profile of an individual tumor.

FUTURE AGENTS

The current chemotherapy regimen for esophageal cancer consists of cisplatin and 5-FU and results, in a combined chemoradiotherapy protocol, in a complete response rate of 17–30% in the majority of trials. Because the complete response rate is the most important predictor of improved outcomes after CMT therapy, additional agents are being studied in order to improve the pCR rate. The most actively studied agents currently are irinotecan (CPT-11) and the taxanes, docetaxel (Taxotere), and paclitaxel. Phase II evaluations combining cisplatin and irinotecan have demonstrated response rates of 30–50%.[9] Meluch et al[16] have demonstrated a 41% 3-year survival rate in patients treated with CMT, including the chemotherapy regimen paclitaxel, carboplatin, and 5-FU, with acceptable toxicities. Other investigators have demonstrated no significant improvements in patients treated with taxanes with increased toxicities.[18] Continued investigation with varied treatment regimens and dosing strategies may allow the benefit of taxanes to be realized while decreasing the toxicity profile. Additional agents such as Xeloda, COX-2 inhibitors, and gemcitabine offer additional promise.

SUMMARY

Esophageal cancer is among the most rapidly increasing malignancies as a result of a dramatic increase in adenocarcinomas of the esophagus. The overall survival rate remains poor. Thus recent research efforts have focused on identifying the optimal treatment strategy for this disease. In spite of numerous trials into the use of neoadjuvant therapy, there remains no conclusive evidence of its efficacy. Large intergroup trials to investigate this question have closed because of limited accrual. Emerging chemotherapeutic agents have revealed encouraging, albeit early, results. The clear advantage to neoadjuvant therapy is seen in those patients who demonstrate a complete response to treatment. Continued research efforts to identify those patients with tumors most likely to respond allows treatment regimens to be tailored in order to maximize benefit while limiting risks of therapy.

REFERENCES

1. Ancona E, Ruol A, Santi S, et al: Only pathologic complete response to neoadjuvant chemotherapy improves significantly the long-term survival of patients with resectable esophageal squamous cell carcinoma: Final report of a randomized, controlled trial of preoperative chemotherapy versus surgery alone. Cancer 91:2165–2174, 2001.

2. Apinop C, Puttisak P, Precha N: A prospective study of combined therapy in esophageal cancer. Hepatogastroenterology 41:391–393, 1994.

3. Bosset JF, Gignoux M, Triboulet JP, et al: Chemoradiotherapy followed by surgery compared with surgery alone in squamous cell cancer of the esophagus. N Engl J Med 337:161–167, 1997.

4. Burmeister BH, Smithers B, Fitzgerald L, et al: A randomized phase III trial of preoperative chemoradiation followed by surgery (CR-S) versus surgery alone (S) for localized respectable cancer of the esophagus. Proc Am Soc Clin Oncol 21:130a (abstract 518), 2002.

5. Clark P: Surgical resection with or without pre-operative chemotherapy in oesophageal cancer: an updated analysis of a randomised controlled trial conducted by the UK Medical

656

Research Council Upper GI Tract Cancer Group. Proc Am Soc Clin Oncol 20:126a (abstract 502), 2001.

6. Daly JM, Karnell LH, Menck HR: National Cancer Data Base report on esophageal carcinoma. Cancer 78:1820–1828, 1996.

7. Harpole DM Jr., Moore MB, Herndon JE 2nd, et al: The prognostic value of molecular marker analysis in patients treated with trimodality therapy for esophageal cancer. Clin Canc Res 7:562–569, 2001.

8. Hishikawa Y, Abe S, Kinugasa S, et al: Overexpression of metallothionein correlates with chemoresistance to cisplatin and prognosis in esophageal cancer. Oncology 54:342–347, 1997.

9. Ilson DH, Minsky B: Irinotecan in esophageal cancer. Oncology 17(9 suppl 8):32–36, 2003.

10. Jemal A, Thomas A, Murray T: Cancer statistics 1999. CA Cancer J Clin 52:23–47, 2002.

11. Jiao X, Krasna MJ, Sonnet J, et al: Pretreatment surgical lymph node staging predicts results of trimodality therapy in esophageal cancer. Eur J Cardiothorac Surg 19:880–886, 2001.

12. Kaklamanos IG, Walker GR, Ferry K, et al: Neoadjuvant treatment for resectable cancer of the esophagus and the gastroesophageal junction: A meta-analysis of randomized clinical trials. Ann Surg Oncol 10(7):754–761, 2003.

13. Kelsen DP, Ginsberg R, Pajak TF, et al: Chemotherapy followed by surgery compared with surgery alone for localized esophageal cancer. N Engl J Med 339:1979–1984, 1998.

14. Law S, Fok M, Chow S, et al: Preoperative chemotherapy versus surgical therapy alone for squamous cell carcinoma of the esophagus: A prospective randomized trial. J Thorac Cardiovasc Surg 114:210–217, 1997.

15. Le Prise E, Etienne PL, Meunier B, et al: A randomized study of chemotherapy, radiation therapy, and surgery vs. surgery for localized squamous cell carcinoma of the esophagus. Cancer 73:1779–1784, 1994.

16. Meluch AA, Greco FA, Gray JR, et al: Preoperative therapy with concurrent paclitaxel/carboplatin/infusional 5-FU and radiation therapy in locoregional esophageal cancer: Final results of a Minnie Pearl Cancer Research Network phase II trial. Cancer J 9:251–260, 2003.

17. Nygaard K, Hagen S, Hansen HS, et al: Pre-operative radiotherapy prolongs survival in operable esophageal carcinoma: A randomized multicenter study of pre-operative radiotherapy and chemotherapy: The second Scandinavian trial in esophageal cancer. World J Surg 16:1104–1110, 1992.

18. Thirion P, Piedbois Y: Preoperative chemoradiotherapy using taxanes for locally advanced esophageal carcinoma. J Clin Oncol 19:1880–1882, 2001.

19. Urba S, Orringer M, Turrrisi A, et al: Randomized trial of preoperative chemoradiation versus surgery alone in patients with locoregional esophageal carcinoma. J Clin Oncol 19:305–313, 2001.

20. Walsh TN, Noonan N, Hollywood D, et al: A comparison of multimodal therapy and surgery for esophageal adenocarcinoma. N Engl J Med 335:462–467, 1996.

Mediastinum

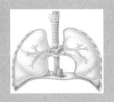

CHAPTER 39

Mediastinal Anatomy and Mediastinoscopy

Daniel P. Raymond and Thomas M. Daniel

MEDIASTINAL ANATOMY

The mediastinum is the thoracic space bounded superiorly by the thoracic inlet, inferiorly by the diaphragm, anteriorly by the sternum, and posteriorly by the spine. Laterally it is bounded by the pleural spaces and includes the mediastinal pleura. Numerous, arbitrary divisions of the mediastinum, ranging from three compartments to six, have been proposed for convenience in localizing pathology. Unfortunately the lack of consensus regarding these subdivisions has led to a certain amount of confusion in the literature.

The most classic description as described in Gray's Anatomy[3] divides the mediastinum into four compartments: superior, anterior, middle, and posterior (Figure 39-1). The superior mediastinum includes all structures from the thoracic inlet superiorly to a line drawn from the lower edge of the manubrium to the lower edge of the fourth thoracic vertebrae, inferiorly. Inferior to this line is the inferior mediastinum, which is subsequently divided into the anterior, middle, and posterior compartments that are bounded inferiorly by the diaphragm. The boundary between the anterior and middle compartments is the anterior pericardium; between the middle and posterior compartments is the posterior aspect of the tracheal bifurcation, pulmonary vessels, and pericardium. A revision of the four-compartment system combines the anterior and superior compartments into an anterosuperior compartment, thus creating three compartments. These two schemes, however, have been criticized because structures can be contained within two separate compartments. For example, in the four-compartment model the upper portions of the trachea and esophagus are contained within the superior mediastinum, while the lower portions are contained within the middle and posterior mediastinum, respectively.

An alternative model proposed by Shields in 1972[5] is perhaps the most straightforward (Figure 39-2). This describes a three-compartment model consisting of an anterior compartment, middle (or visceral) compartment, and a posterior compartment (paraventral sulcus). All three compartments are bounded inferiorly by the diaphragm, laterally by the pleural space, and superiorly by the thoracic inlet. The anterior compartment is bounded anteriorly by the sternum and posteriorly by the great vessels and pericardium. It contains the thymus, internal mammary vessels, fat, connective tissue, and potentially structures such as ectopic parathyroid tissue or a substernal goiter. Dorsal to the anterior compartment is the visceral compartment or middle mediastinum, which is bounded posteriorly by the ventral surface of the thoracic spine. The visceral compartment occupies the entire thoracic inlet and contains the great vessels, heart, pericardium, trachea, proximal mainstem bronchi, vagus nerves, phrenic nerves, esophagus, thoracic duct, descending aorta, and azygous venous system. The posterior compartment of the mediastinum or paraventral sulcus consists of potential spaces along the thoracic vertebrae that contain the sympathetic chain, proximal portions of the intercostal neurovascular bundles, thoracic spinal ganglia, and the distal azygous vein. The paraventral sulci are not technically in the mediastinum but contain structures that give rise to pathology that is classically considered in the posterior mediastinum (neurogenic tumors).

A detailed view of mediastinal anatomy as seen from the right side of the mediastinum is illustrated in Figure 39-3. A similar view of mediastinal anatomy as seen from the left side of the mediastinum is illustrated in Figure 39-4.

658

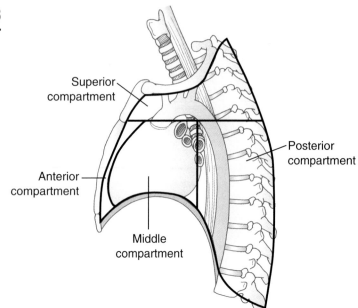

Figure 39–1 Four-compartment model of the mediastinum.

POTENTIAL SPACES IN THE MEDIASTINUM

When mediastinal anatomy is discussed, several potential spaces are described, most often in conjunction with staging lung cancer. The pretracheal space is a triangular space bounded anterolaterally by the superior vena cava and right brachiocephalic vein on the right, the aorta and pericardium on the left, and posteriorly by the trachea. This is the space explored by standard mediastinoscopy and is contiguous inferiorly with the subcarinal space. The subcarinal space is bounded superiorly by the carina, laterally by the mainstem bronchi, anteriorly by the pulmonary artery, and posteriorly by the esophagus (Figure 39-3). The aortopulmonary window is the space bounded superiorly by the aortic arch, medially by the trachea and esophagus, inferiorly by the pulmonary artery, and laterally by the pleura. This space contains lymph nodes, the ligamentum arteriosum, and the left recurrent laryngeal nerve (Figure 39-4) and can be accessed by an anterior mediastinotomy, extended cervical mediastinoscopy, or thoracoscopy/thoracotomy.

MEDIASTINAL LYMPH NODE ANATOMY

In 1997 the American Joint Committee and the Union Internationale Contre le Cancer adopted a regional lymph node classification in order to unify two previously utilized systems and provide a consistent, reproducible means of classifying thoracic lymph nodes.[4] This system, used primarily for staging lung cancer, classifies lymph nodes into 14 different stations based on anatomical position. Node stations 1 through 9 are contained within the mediastinal pleura and thus are mediastinal lymph nodes. Lymph node stations 2, 4, and 7 are depicted in Figure 39-3 and are the only nodal stations accessible by standard mediastinoscopy. Lymph node stations 5 and 6 are depicted in Figure 39-4 and are not accessible by routine mediastinoscopy. Chapter 16 discusses the role of the 14 lymph node stations in the diagnosis and management of lung malignancies.

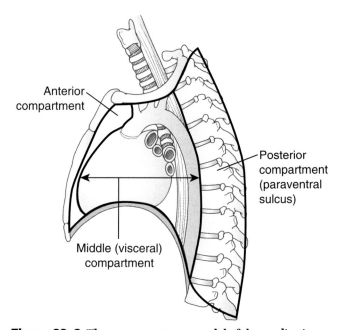

Figure 39–2 Three-compartment model of the mediastinum.

MEDIASTINOSCOPY

Mediastinoscopy is a surgical procedure requiring general anesthesia in which a small anterior cervical incision is made to permit the introduction of a mediastinoscope into the pretracheal space in order to evaluate the middle compartment of the mediastinum. The most common indication for mediastinoscopy is preoperative staging for lung cancer, which includes assessment of mediastinal lymph nodes for possible metastatic tumor and identification of possible direct invasion by the primary tumor into mediastinal struc-

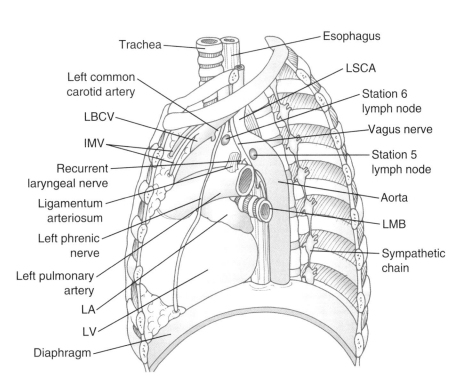

Figure 39–3 Right mediastinal view.
RBCV, right brachiocephalic vein; LBCV, left brachiocephalic vein; SVC, superior vena cava; RPA, right pulmonary artery; RMB, right main bronchus.

Figure 39–4 Left mediastinal view.
LSCA, left subclavian artery; LMB, left main bronchus; LA, left atrium; LV, left ventricle; IMV, internal mammary vessels; LBCV, left brachiocephalic vein.

tures. Lymph node stations accessible to mediastinoscopy include station 2 (high paratracheal), station 4 (low paratracheal), and station 7 (subcarinal). Since the redefinition of the 4R lymph node station in 1997 as extending below the azygous vein to the origin of the right upper lobe bronchus, it is not felt that mediastinoscopy can be used to reach and stage 10R lymph nodes. Although station 7 lymph nodes in the anterior subcarinal space (also called precarinal nodes) are accessible to mediastinoscopic biopsy, those located in the posterior subcarinal space are often not. Evaluation of nodes in this area can be attempted with esophageal ultrasound–directed transesophageal needle biopsy[7] or transcarinal needle biopsy during bronchoscopy. Other less common indications for mediastinoscopy include evaluation of primary lymphadenopathy (e.g., lymphoma, sarcoid), drainage of bronchogenic cysts, abscess drainage, identification of

660 ectopic parathyroid tissue, and tissue sampling for causes of superior vena cava syndrome.

PREOPERATIVE EVALUATION

Standard preoperative evaluation must include a thorough history and physical examination. Special considerations in a patient being evaluated for mediastinoscopy include any history of neck or chest surgery such as permanent tracheostomy, which may prevent access to the pretracheal space. Prior neck or sternal incisions, including prior mediastinoscopy, may complicate the initial dissection but are not absolute contraindications to the procedure. A large goiter may additionally preclude access to the pretracheal space. Another special consideration is vascular pathology, specifically innominate artery and aortic arch aneurysms or severe atherosclerosis. Significant vascular calcification increases the risk of embolic events as these vessels are manipulated during the procedure. In addition, total atherosclerotic occlusion of the left common carotid artery may predispose patients to stroke if their innominate artery supplying the right common carotid artery is compressed by the mediastinoscope. Aneurysmal disease may additionally produce a barrier to safe dissection of the pretracheal space.

SURGICAL TECHNIQUE

Once patients are intubated, they are placed in the supine position with their neck hyperextended by a support placed behind the shoulders (see Figure 39-5 and bottom inset). The endotracheal tube is brought out to the patient's right and kept as lateral and low in profile as possible in order to allow the surgeon to insert the mediastinoscope directly over the patient's chin. Care must be taken to avoid turning the patient's chin to the side as this results in an off-center incision, which makes subsequent dissection more difficult and also produces a suboptimal cosmetic result. Placement of a pulse oximeter on the patient's right upper extremity is useful as it allows the surgeon to be alerted to significant innominate artery compression by the mediastinoscope.

The entire sternum and anterior cervical areas are prepped and draped in order to facilitate a sternotomy if massive bleeding is encountered. A 3-cm-wide incision is made transversely 2 cm above the sternal notch, the platysma is divided transversely, and then a vertical plane is developed between the strap muscles down to the level of the trachea. Rarely, to reach this level, the surgeon may have to divide a low-lying thyroid isthmus or a thyroidea ima artery. The pretracheal fascia is subsequently divided and blunt finger dissection is undertaken to develop a plane anterior to the trachea in a caudal direction. Knowledge of the position of the innominate artery by evaluation of a CT scan preoperatively is beneficial to avoid injury to a high-riding innominate artery during the initial dissection. This cephalic displacement of the artery is most frequently seen in the setting of massively enlarged station 2 right paratracheal lymph nodes and should alert the surgeon to the elevated innominate artery. The surgeon can obtain useful information during initial finger dissection of the pretracheal space including the exact location of the ascending

aorta and the angle and level that the innominate artery crosses the field. Additionally, firm pathological lymph nodes alongside the distal trachea may be identified and partially dissected free of surrounding tissue. The mediastinoscope is then inserted in the pretracheal plane that has been created (Figure 39-5).

A standard mediastinoscope permits only one individual to visualize the operative field directly down the lumen of the mediastinoscope. Recently, videomediastinoscopy (Figure 39-5 and central inset) has permitted all members of the operative team including the surgeon, assistants, anesthesiologist, and scrub nurse to visualize the operative field and therefore enhance participation in the procedure, including anticipation of the surgeon's needs, as well as provide an educational benefit. In addition, magnification, improved optics, and superior lighting have improved anatomical visualization and, in the authors' opinion, enhanced the safety of the procedure.

HIGH PARATRACHEAL DISSECTION

The major anatomical landmark of the high paratracheal level is the innominate artery (Figures 39-6 and 39-7), which is seen as a pulsatile structure crossing anterior to the trachea. Level 2 lymph nodes lie to the left and right of the trachea at this level. Correlation of the endoscopic view at

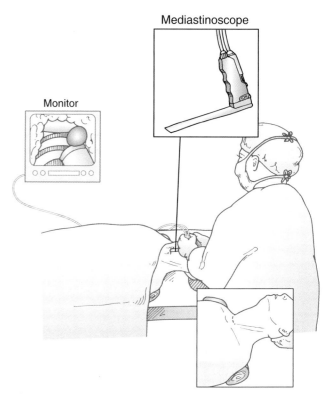

Figure 39–5 Patient and equipment positioning for videomediastinoscopy. The surgeon is shown looking across the operative field at the video monitor. Diagram of a video mediastinoscope (*top inset*). View of the patient's neck in extension, the incision site, and the support behind the patient's shoulders (*bottom inset*).

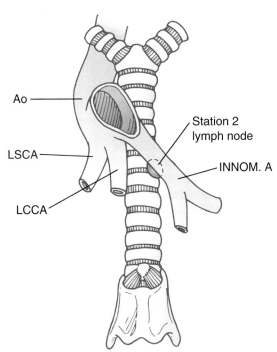

Figure 39–6 Anatomical structures at the high paratracheal level as seen from the surgeon's position standing at the patient's head. Ao, aorta; INNOM. A, innominate artery; LCCA, left common carotid artery; LSCA, left subclavian artery.

the station 2 lymph node level with anatomic structures as seen from the right chest is shown in Figure 39-8. Correlation of the endoscopic view with a transverse view of the mediastinal structures at this high paratracheal level is seen in Figure 39-9.

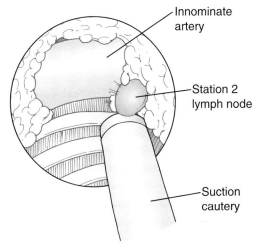

Figure 39–7 View through the mediastinoscope at the high paratracheal level. Note the tracheal rings posteriorly, the innominate artery anteriorly, and the use of the suction cautery to dissect through the pretracheal fascia and allow the underlying station 2 lymph node located to the right of the trachea to bulge into the operative field.

The operator's initial view of the paratracheal tissue to the right and left of the trachea may show no obvious nodal tissue. Subsequent blunt dissection through the pretracheal tissue plane, assisted by careful use of the suction cautery tip, will usually expose the underlying lymph nodes. Recognition of lymph nodes is often facilitated by their dark pigmentation. It is prudent, however, to dissect sufficiently to see the lymph node bulge (Figure 39-7) into the operative field as this technique helps prevent inadvertent biopsy of other dark paratracheal structures such as the vena cava or the right brachiocephalic vein, which do not "bulge" into the field.

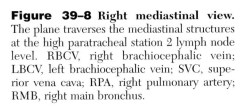

Figure 39–8 Right mediastinal view. The plane traverses the mediastinal structures at the high paratracheal station 2 lymph node level. RBCV, right brachiocephalic vein; LBCV, left brachiocephalic vein; SVC, superior vena cava; RPA, right pulmonary artery; RMB, right main bronchus.

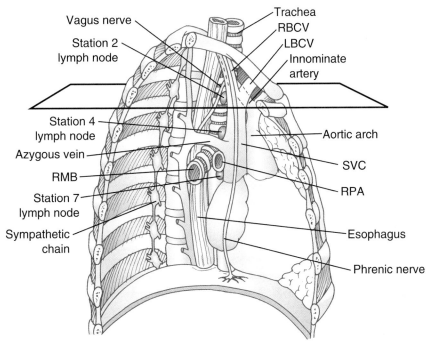

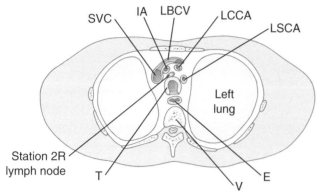

Figure 39–9 Transverse view of mediastinal structures at the high paratracheal level. LBCV, left brachiocephalic vein; LCCA, left common carotid artery; LSCA, left subclavian artery; E, esophagus; V, vertebra; T, trachea; SVC, superior vena cava; IA, innominate artery.

LOWER PARATRACHEAL DISSECTION

Dissection inferior to the innominate artery reaches the lower paratracheal area and station 4 lymph nodes, which lie on the right and left of the trachea superior to the carina (Figure 39-10). After blunt dissection of the paratracheal tissue permitting the level 4 nodes to bulge into the operative field, if there is any question about whether the tissue to undergo biopsy is a lymph node or not it is wise to aspirate the tissue first with a small bore needle to rule out a vascular structure (Figure 39-11). This maneuver may also alert the operator to the presence of a major blood vessel lying immediately beneath the node to be biopsied. It is necessary to be aware of the structures lying to the right of the trachea at this level. These structures include—in addition to the lymph nodes—the azygous vein, the superior vena cava, the mediastinal pleura, and the adjacent right upper lobe of the lung. The lung pleura is often pigmented like a node but characteristically is seen to move up and down behind the pleura with respiration. Structures lying to the left of the trachea at this level are the aortic arch, the left recurrent laryngeal nerve, a bronchial artery branch from the aorta, and the esophagus. The esophagus lies posterior and to the left of the trachea at this level and can be mistaken for a white tumor-filled lymph node. It may be recognized by the longitudinal muscle fibers of its outer muscular layer. When dissecting in the left lower paratracheal region, judicious use of electrocautery is recommended to avoid inadvertent injury not only to the esophagus but also the rarely visualized left recurrent laryngeal nerve lying in the tracheoesophageal groove. If esophageal injury is identified, the esophagus should immediately be repaired via a right or left thoracotomy. Most surgeons would prefer a right thoracotomy to repair the esophagus at this level. However, if preexisting lung pathology exists in the left chest a left thoracotomy may be used to address both. The site of esophageal injury usually lies directly medial to the aortic arch.

Correlation of the endoscopic view at the station 4 lymph node level (Figure 39-11) with anatomical structures as seen from the right chest is shown in Figure 39-12 with a plane traversing the structures at the lower paratracheal level. Correlation of the endoscopic view with a transverse view of

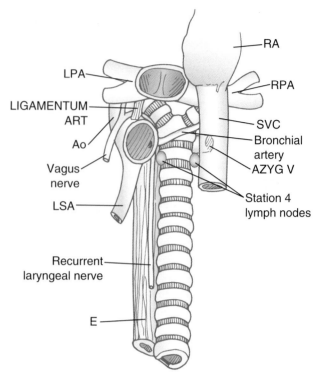

Figure 39–10 Anatomical structures at the lower paratracheal level as seen from the surgeon's position standing at the patient's head. RA, right atrium; RPA, right pulmonary artery; SVC, superior vena cava; AZYG V, azygous vein; E, esophagus; LSA, left subclavian artery; Ao, aorta; LIGAMENTUM ART, ligamentum arteriosum; LPA, left pulmonary artery.

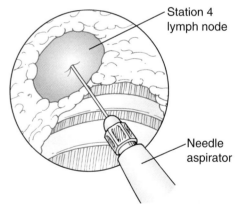

Figure 39–11 View through the mediastinoscope at the lower paratracheal level. Note the use of an aspirating needle to rule out a vascular structure before biopsy of the suspected lymph node.

the mediastinal structures at the lower paratracheal level is illustrated in Figure 39-13.

CARINAL DISSECTION

The major anatomical landmarks of the carinal area are the widening of the trachea, the proximal left main bronchus, and the right pulmonary artery passing anteriorly (Figure

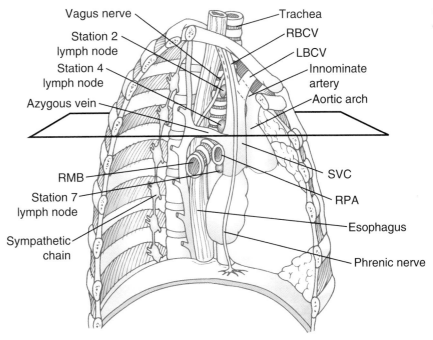

Figure 39-12 Right mediastinoscopic view with plane passing through the mediastinal structures located at the lower paratracheal level. RBCV, right brachiocephalic vein; LBCV, left brachiocephalic vein; SVC, superior vena cava; RPA, right pulmonary artery; RMB, right main bronchus.

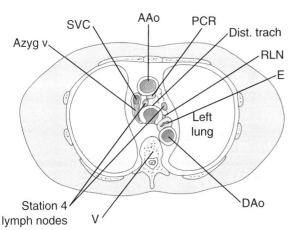

Figure 39-13 Transverse view of mediastinal structures at the lower paratracheal level. AAo, ascending aorta; PCR, pericardial recess. This is a fluid-containing structure often mistaken for a lower mediastinal lymph node. The attenuated conformation of the structure along the outer wall of the ascending aorta is a clue to it being a fluid-filled structure and not a node. RLN, recurrent laryngeal nerve; E, esophagus; DAo, descending aorta; V, vertebra; Azyg v, azygous vein; SVC, superior vena cava; Dist. trach, distal trachea.

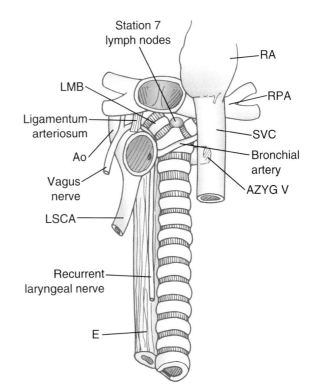

Figure 39-14 Anatomical structures at the carinal level as seen from the surgeon's perspective standing at the patient's head. RA, right atrium; RPA, right pulmonary artery; SVC, superior vena cava; AZYG V, azygous vein; E, esophagus; LSCA, left subclavian artery; Ao, aorta; LMB, left main bronchus.

39-14). The proximal right main bronchus is often difficult to identify as it commonly rises at a more posterior angle to the distal trachea than the left main bronchus. The mediastinoscopic view of structures at the carinal level is depicted in Figure 39-15. The most critical paratracheal structure to avoid during precarinal nodal biopsy is the right pulmonary artery. Extensive blunt dissection of the suspected nodal tissue followed by needle aspiration before biopsy is vital (Figure 39-15). It is easy during this part of the operation to mistake the proximal left main bronchus for the distal trachea, or vice versa, and therefore misidentify the node station undergoing biopsy. A helpful observation is

to identify the triangular cartilaginous ring of the distal trachea that is present just proximal to the carina (Figure 39-15). Also, recognition of the pulsatile right pulmonary artery passing immediately anteriorly suggests that dissection is at the proximal bronchial level and not the distal tracheal level.

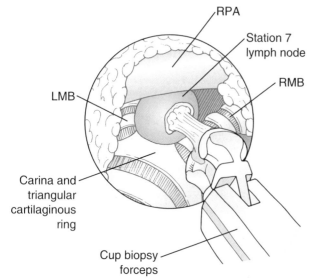

Figure 39–15 **View through the mediastinoscope at the carinal level.** Note the widened tracheal diameter and the triangular-shaped tracheal cartilage just proximal to the subcarinal tissue containing station 7 lymph nodes. After blunt dissection and needle aspiration, as described earlier, a nodal biopsy is illustrated with a cup biopsy forceps. RPA, right pulmonary artery; RMB, right main bronchus; LMB, left main bronchus.

Correlation of the endoscopic view at the carinal station 7 lymph node level with anatomical structures as seen from the right chest is shown in Figure 39-16. A plane traverses the structures at the carinal level. Correlation of the endoscopic view at the carinal level with a transverse view of the mediastinal structures at this level is seen in Figure 39-17.

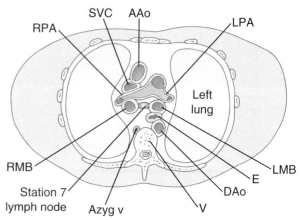

Figure 39–17 **Transverse view of mediastinal structures at the subcarinal level.** LPA, left pulmonary artery; LMB, left main bronchus; E, esophagus; DAo, descending aorta; V, vertebra; Azyg v, azygous vein; RMB, right main bronchus; RPA, right pulmonary artery; SVC, superior vena cava; AAo, ascending aorta.

NODE BIOPSY TECHNIQUE AND CLOSURE OF THE INCISION

As previously described, mediastinal node biopsy is initiated by first dissecting through the pretracheal fascia using a blunt suction cautery instrument (Figure 39-7). Next the suspected lymph node is aspirated with a 23-gauge needle to confirm that it is not a vascular structure (Figure 39-11). Finally, a biopsy is taken using a biopsy forceps (Figure 39-15). Often the first biopsy attempt removes only the outer capsule of the node and exposes the underlying parenchyma, which can then be further sampled. If no

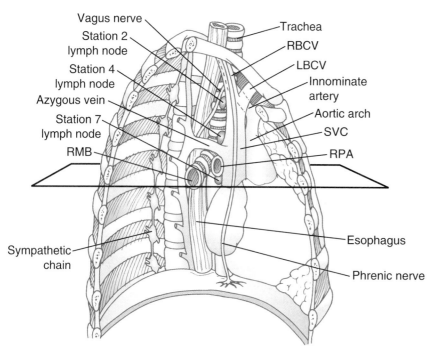

Figure 39–16 **Right mediastinal view with a plane passing through the structures located at the subcarinal level.** RBCV, right brachiocephalic vein; LBCV, left brachiocephalic vein; SVC, superior vena cava; RPA, right pulmonary artery; RMB, right main bronchus.

node is seen at the desired station, it is often helpful to withdraw the mediastinoscope slightly and even rotate it to see tissue lying more anterior or anterolateral to the trachea. These areas may reveal nodal tissue with further dissection. Following biopsy hemostasis can be achieved with electrocautery or with temporary packing with a gauze pledget attached to a string for later removal. Withdrawing the mediastinoscope a short distance and waiting will often achieve hemostasis as a result of simple tissue apposition. Rarely, an endoscopic clip applier may be utilized to address a visible bleeding vessel.

Once hemostasis has been achieved at all levels, the mediastinoscope is removed and the wound is closed in several layers. First, the strap muscles are reapproximated with interrupted sutures vertically in the midline. Subsequently, the platysma muscle is closed horizontally and the skin is closed with a subcuticular suture. It is our practice to obtain postprocedure chest X-rays on all patients to ensure the absence of a pneumothorax or other visible abnormality. The patient can subsequently be discharged to home after standard postanesthesia care. Alternatively, following mediastinoscopy the patient may be repositioned for tumor resection under the same anesthesia after frozen section evaluation of the lymph nodes by a pathologist.

MANAGEMENT OF MAJOR BLEEDING

It is important to have a plan ahead of time for managing major bleeding as blood loss and hypotension can occur very quickly. The first thing that is likely to happen is a complete loss of visualization. We recommend leaving the mediastinoscope in place and immediately packing the operative field with gauze pledgets attached to strings. These pledgets should always be instantly available. This maneuver will temporarily contain most hemorrhage except that from systemic arteries. Attention is then turned to volume resuscitation and blood replacement if necessary. Waiting several minutes and then removing the packing often accomplishes hemostasis. If not, repeat packing preceded by placement of a thrombogenic agent such as oxidized cellulose has, based on 25 years of experience, controlled all venous and minor arterial bleeding without having to resort to median sternotomy or thoracotomy. Aortic, innominate artery, bronchial artery injury adjacent to the aorta, and major pulmonary artery injuries will not be contained with packing. Management should start with compression of the vessel with the mediastinoscope or removing the mediastinoscope and compressing with one's finger the vessel against the sternum until either a median sternotomy (preferably in most situations) or a thoracotomy can be performed to allow direct vascular control.

LOCALIZATION TECHNIQUE

The introduction of positron emission tomography (PET) scanning in the staging of lung cancer[6] has placed a premium on accurate directed biopsy of a PET-positive node in addition to the usual sampling of node levels 2, 4, and 7. An awareness of the surrounding anatomical structures as previously described and illustrated in the text will permit accurate localization in most cases. However, occasions arise where confirmation of an exact anatomical site remains elusive in spite of extensive mediastinal dissection. A useful technique under these circumstances is to pass a flexible bronchoscope through the endotracheal tube, reduce its light source to a minimum, then observe the site of transtracheal illumination (see Figure 39-18 and inset).

EXTENDED CERVICAL MEDIASTINOSCOPY

A common misconception is that routine mediastinoscopy permits evaluation of the anterior mediastinum. However, a variation of mediastinoscopy known as extended cervical mediastinoscopy[1] has been described that can access the anterior mediastinum, as well as station 5 and 6 nodes in the aortopulmonary window (Figure 39-4). This procedure is begun through the same cervical incision, but the surgeon subsequently creates a plane anterior to the innominate artery and posterior to the left brachiocephalic vein. It is rarely done, however, because of the inherent difficulty of the procedure, the easy accessibility to the aortopulmonary window using an anterior mediastinotomy or thoracoscopy, and the belief among many thoracic surgeons that tumors of the left upper lobe with involvement of nodes in station 5 and 6 (if limited to intracapsular spread and in the absence of other mediastinal node involvement) have a better prognosis with surgical resection than tumors in other lobes with

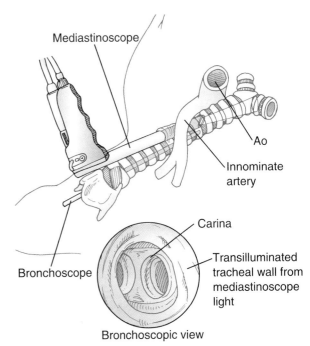

Figure 39–18 View of the mediastinoscope light transilluminating the right lower paratracheal region through the tracheal wall. Note the bronchoscope, which has been passed through the endotracheal tube, lying within the tracheal lumen. Inset shows a bronchoscopic view of the distal trachea and carina with bright transillumination of the right lower paratracheal wall from the mediastinoscope confirming the location of the mediastinal node station as that of 4R. Ao, aorta.

666 mediastinal node involvement and therefore do not have to be staged before lung resection.

▶ COMPLICATIONS

Mediastinoscopy is a safe procedure when performed by experienced surgeons with a knowledge of the surrounding mediastinal structures and a systemic deliberate method of tissue biopsy. A recent large series[2] of over 2000 procedures described a morbidity rate of 0.6% and a mortality rate of 0.2%. Possible major complications include major vessel hemorrhage (aorta, innominate artery, pulmonary artery, bronchial artery, vena cava, azygous vein), esophageal perforation, or stroke secondary to innominate artery compression in the setting of severe atherosclerosis. Other complications include left recurrent laryngeal nerve injury, pneumothorax, wound infection, and, rarely, tumor seeding of the neck incision.

REFERENCES

1. Ginsberg R, Rice TW, Goldberg M, et al: Extended cervical mediastinoscopy: A single staging process for bronchogenic carcinoma of the left upper lobe. J Thorac Cardiovasc Surg 94:673–678, 1987.

2. Hammond ZT, Anderson RC, Meyers BF, et al: The current role of mediastinoscopy in the evaluation of thoracic disease. J Thorac Cardiovasc Surg 118:894–899, 1999.
3. Mediastinum. In Gray's Anatomy: The Anatomical Basis of Medicine and Surgery, 38th ed. New York: Churchill Livingstone, 1995.
4. Mountain CF, Dresler CM: Regional lymph node classification for lung cancer staging. Chest 111:1718–1723, 1997.
5. Shields TW: The mediastinum, its compartments and the mediastinal lymph nodes. In General Thoracic Surgery, 5th ed. Philadelphia: Lippincott Williams & Wilkins, 2000.
6. Vesselle H, Pugsley JM, Valliers E, et al: The impact of fluorodeoxyglucose F18 positron-emission tomography on the surgical staging of non-small cell lung cancer. J Thorac Cardiovasc Surg 124:511–519, 2002.
7. Wallace MB, Silvestri GA, Sahai AV, et al: Endoscopic ultrasound-guided fine needle aspiration for staging patients with carcinoma of the lung. Ann Thorac Surg 72:1861–1867, 2001.

Anterior Mediastinal Masses

John C. Kucharczuk and Joseph B. Shrager

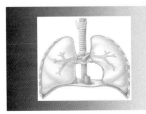

ANATOMY

The anatomy of the mediastinum is reviewed in detail in Chapter 39. Nevertheless, since a number of radiographic and surgical anatomical subdivisions of the mediastinum have been proposed, it is important to briefly review the anatomy from a thoracic surgical perspective. The simplest and most commonly used description is the three-compartment model proposed by Shields.[46] He divided the mediastinum into (1) the anterior compartment, (2) the middle or "visceral compartment," and (3) the posterior or "paravertebral" compartment. The anatomical limits of each compartment are shown in Figure 40-1, and the structures contained within each compartment are listed in Table 40-1. Locating a mass in the anterior mediastinum allows a differential diagnosis to be generated based on the knowledge of the normal structures within that compartment. From a thoracic surgical perspective, this approach allows the most appropriate diagnostic and therapeutic procedures to be selected.

INTRODUCTION TO ANTERIOR MEDIASTINAL MASSES

Box 40-1 is an extensive list of the varied pathologies that can present as a mass in the anterior mediastinal compartment. By far, the four most common are thymoma, lymphoma, teratoma, and germ cell tumor.

THYMIC TUMORS

Introduction

Lesions of the thymus account for approximately 50% of anterior mediastinal masses in adults and are thus of great importance. Although lymphomas and germ cell tumors of

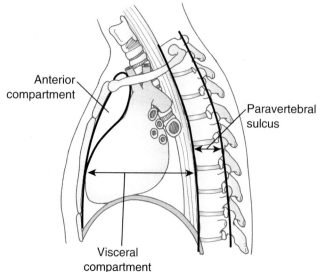

Figure 40–1 Three-compartment division of the mediastinum as proposed by Shields.
(Modified from Shields TW: General Thoracic Surgery, 2nd ed. Philadelphia: Lea & Febiger, 1983, with permission.)

the anterior mediastinum often involve the thymus and/or actually arise from cells within the thymus, these are most appropriately discussed as a separate group from thymic tumors per se and are usually classified separately. The thymic masses discussed in this section, then, are listed in Box 40-2.

Thymoma

Thymomas represent the most common thymic tumor, and approximately 95% are located in the anterior mediastinum. They are of surgical interest both because excision is the primary therapy and because of the interesting association with myasthenia gravis (MG), a disease the clinical course of which can be favorably influenced by thymectomy.

Thymomas may be completely encapsulated or invasive. Large series have demonstrated the incidence of encapsulated lesions to be between 40% and 70% and that of microscopic or grossly invasive lesions to be between 30% and 60%. Although local invasion is usually limited to the capsule or immediately adjacent structures, spread to more distant sites within the chest does occur, particularly to the pleura, diaphragm, and mediastinal lymph nodes. Aggressive thymomas can be associated with distant metastases in as high as 30% of patients at high-level referral centers,[2] but most broad studies report distant metastasis to be rare (<5%).

Pathology

Thymomas are derived from thymic epithelial cells, but most contain varying mixes of epithelial cells and lymphocytes.[33] Traditional histological classifications have therefore grouped thymomas according to cytological make-up: (1) predominantly lymphocytic, (2) predominantly epithelial, and (3) mixed.[24] There is also a recognized spindle cell

Table 40–1		
Components of Mediastinal Compartments as Proposed by Shields[a]		
Anterior	*Visceral (middle)*	*Paravertebral (posterior)*
Thymus	Pericardium/heart	Sympathetic chain
Internal thoracic vessels	Great vessels	Proximal intercostal nerve, artery, and vein
Internal thoracic lymph nodes	Trachea	Posterior paraesophageal lymph nodes
Prevascular lymph nodes	Proximal right and left mainstem	Intercostal lymph nodes
Fat and connective tissue	Esophagus Phrenic nerve Thoracic duct Proximal azygos vein Paratracheal and subcarinal lymph nodes (levels 2, 4, and 7) Pleuropericardial lymph nodes Fat and connective tissue	

[a]The nodal basin draining the anterior chest wall and female breast lies in the anterior compartment while the majority of those draining the lung and important in lung cancer staging lie in the visceral compartment.

Box 40–1.   Differential Diagnosis of a Mass Lesion in the Anterior Mediastinal Compartment.

Neoplastic
  Thyroid
    Substernal goiter
    Ectopic thyroid tissue
  Thymus
    Thymic hyperplasia
    Thymoma
    Thymic carcinoma
    Thymic carcinoid
    Thymic small-cell carcinoma
    Thymic cysts
    Thymolipoma
  Teratoma
    Mature teratoma
    Immature teratoma
    Teratoma with malignant component
  Lymphoma
  Ectopic parathyroid with adenoma
  Germ cell tumors
    Seminoma
    Nonseminoma
      Yolk sac tumors
      Embryonal carcinoma
      Choriocarcinoma lymphangioma
  Hemangioma
  Lipoma
  Liposarcoma
  Fibroma
  Fibrosarcoma
  Cervicomediastinal hygroma
Infectious
  Acute descending necrotizing mediastinitis
    Extension of deep cervical bacterial infection into the
      anterior compartment with abscess formation and sepsis
  Subacute mediastinitis
    Fungal, mycobacterial, actinomycosis or histoplasmosis
      infection causing an inflammatory mass in the anterior
      mediastinum
Vascular
  Aneurysm of the aortic arch with projection in the anterior
    mediastinum
  Innominate vein aneurysm
  Superior vena cava aneurysm
  Dilation of the superior vena cava (with anomalous
    pulmonary venous return)
  Persistent left superior vena cava

Box 40–2.   Thymic Masses.

Thymic hyperplasia
Thymoma
Thymic carcinoma
Thymic neuroendocrine tumors
  Carcinoid
  Small-cell carcinoma
Thymic cysts (nonthymomatous)
Thymolipoma
Metastases to the thymus

thymoma versus the other subtypes because of its microscopic similarity to lymphoma. Immunohistochemical staining for cytokeratin often helps to make the diagnosis, as antibodies to this protein are present in 95–100% of thymomas.[18] Chromogranin staining allows differentiation between thymoma and thymic carcinoid (the former being negative and the latter positive for chromogranin).

Classification (Table 40-2)

No TNM classification has been found to be of value for staging thymomas.

The most widely used clinical classification scheme has been that proposed by Masaoka et al in 1981.[30] This scheme takes into account the gross presence or absence of encapsulation and fixation/invasion into adjacent structures as identified at the time of surgery. It also recognizes the fact that a grossly well-encapsulated tumor may be found to have invasion through the capsule at microscopic examination. The Masaoka system itself or later variations on it have been found to have prognostic significance by numerous authors in the years since it was originally proposed.

In 1985, Marino and Muller-Hermelink[29] proposed a histological classification that has come to be known as the Muller-Hermelink (MH) classification. This scheme divides thymomas into cortical, medullary, and mixed types. The cortical type contains medium to large epithelial cells of characteristic appearance and usually abundant lymphocytes. The medullary type contains small to medium cells with different features and less lymphocytes. The former tend to be of higher clinical stage, while the latter tend to be of lower invasiveness. Many investigators have generated data in support of the prognostic significance of the MH classification,[41–44,57] showing that the medullary type has the best and the cortical type the least favorable prognosis. The World Health Organization (WHO) recently adopted a classification system based upon the MH criteria.[40] It has been suggested that such histological systems be used in combination with a Masaoka-type staging system to provide more precise prognostic information.

Presentation

Most thymomas present in patients beyond age 40 years, with no major predominance in men or women. About 50%

variant of the epithelial subtype. Approximately 50% of the tumors are of the mixed variety, with the remainder split between the epithelial and lymphocytic subtypes. Unfortunately, these subtypes have little prognostic significance, other than the generally better prognosis of the spindle cell variant, and thus more recent investigators have proposed alternative histological classification schemes (see later).

Of clinical significance is the fact that it may be more difficult to establish the diagnosis of thymoma from a small sample (e.g., needle biopsy) of a lymphocyte predominant

670

Table 40–2

Classification Schemes for Thymoma

Stage	Masaoka	WHO[a]
I	Encapsulated, tumor may invade into, but not through capsule microscopically	
II		
IIi	Microscopic transcapsular invasion	
IIii	Macroscopic invasion into thymus or fat or adherent to but not through pleura or pericardium	
III	Macroscopic invasion of neighboring organs, i.e., pericardium, great vessels, lung	
IV		
IVA	Pleural or pericardial dissemination	Type A (spindle cell, medullary)
IVB	Lymphogenous or hematogenous mets	Type AB (mixed)
		Type B
		B1 (lymphocyte-rich, predominantly cortical)
		B2 (cortical)
		B3 (epithelial, well-differentiated thymic carcinoma)
		Type C (thymic carcinoma)

[a]Terms in parentheses represent nomenclature from previous histological classifications that most closely approximate that WHO classification category.

of patients are asymptomatic, with the remaining presenting with either local symptoms (pain, dyspnea, cough, hoarseness), resulting from locally invasive tumors, or systemic symptoms of one of the associated systemic diseases.

Association with Myasthenia Gravis

Thymomas may present with a number of associated diseases, largely autoimmune in etiology, but the most common associated illness is MG. Accumulated experience suggests that 5–15% of patients with MG are found to have thymomas, while 30–50% of thymomas are associated with clinical MG. Notably, the disease may develop later, even following thymoma resection, if it is not present at the time of discovery of the thymic tumor. For this reason, it is essential that a complete thymectomy be performed as part of resection of any anterior mediastinal tumor that may represent a thymoma. As MG is an autoimmune disease caused by antiacetylcholine receptor (anti-achr) antibodies, its relationship to thymoma and treatment by thymectomy appear to be related to the role of the thymus in the creation of these antibodies.[15,49]

This association has a long and very interesting history that is largely beyond the scope of this chapter. Highlights, however, include the first description by Schumacher and Roth in 1912 of improvement in MG after thymectomy,[45] the more systematic evaluation of this concept by Blalock et al in the late 1930s,[5] and the subsequent controversy over

whether the morbidity and mortality of the procedure justified the chances of a remission from MG. Only in the late 1960s and 1970s did thymectomy for MG in the absence of thymoma gain wide acceptance as improvements in perioperative care reduced the morbidity of the procedure and the benefits became more clear. Although convincing data suggest that MG patients treated with thymectomy have a dramatically higher remission rate than historical controls treated by medication alone, it should be noted that there has never been a randomized study to definitively establish this concept. Further, such a study is unlikely to ever be carried out.

Association with Other Diseases

Box 40-3 lists MG and the other systemic, autoimmune disorders most commonly associated with thymoma. Two to fifteen percent of patients with thymoma suffer from a type of cytopenia. The most common of these is pure red cell aplasia, thought to be due to an abnormal IgG antibody that inhibits red cell synthesis. Most patients with this disease have the favorable, spindle cell type of thymoma.[3] Approximately one third of patients with aplasia are improved by thymectomy.[60] Hypogammaglobulinemia occurs in less than 5% of thymoma patients, principally the elderly. This disease generally does not respond to thymectomy, and the prognosis is poor. Of the other autoimmune

Box 40–3. Systemic Diseases Most Commonly Associated with Thymoma.

Myasthenia gravis
Cytopenias (most commonly, red cell hypoplasia)
Nonthymic malignancies
Hypogammaglobulinemia
Systemic lupus erythematosus
Polymyositis
Rheumatoid arthritis
Thyroiditis
Sjögren's syndrome
Ulcerative colitis

disorders that occur in association with thymoma in lower frequencies, lupus appears to be the most common; again, resection does not appear to impact the clinical course.

Approach to the Patient with Anterior Mediastinal Mass Suspicious for Thymoma

Imaging

Radiological studies play a central role in the evaluation of thymoma. Since many patients are asymptomatic at presentation, a widened mediastinum or loss of the normal anterior clear space on the lateral film of a routine chest radiogram may be the first sign of disease. In such a patient, a computed tomogram (CT) of the chest with intravenous contrast should be obtained as the next step. Patients who present with MG or another of the disorders that may be associated with thymoma should also have a chest CT.

Although no CT appearance is diagnostic of thymoma, a well-circumscribed, solid anterior mediastinal mass in an adult over 40 years old, without low-density areas that suggest the cystic and fatty components of a teratoma, is very likely to be a thymoma (Figures 40-2 and 40-3). The presence of calcification is not particularly helpful, as both thymomas and teratomas may contain calcium. In some cases, lymphoma will be the obvious diagnosis on the basis of adenopathy outside the anterior mediastinum, but in the absence of this finding, differentiating a thymoma from a lymphoma may be difficult. It is often possible to suspect one over the other only on the basis of the thymoma patient's typically more advanced age. Magnetic resonance imaging (MRI) provides useful additional information only in the setting in which the fluid or fatty nature of a component of the tumor is not clearly defined by CT, or when a vascular structure (e.g., aneurysm) is suspected and has not been clearly ruled out by the contrast CT study.

The chest CT also provides information about a putative thymoma's local and regional spread. Loss of planes between the tumor and normal structures may suggest direct invasion, and visceral or parietal pleural deposits may be visible as well. The presence of such signs of local aggressiveness might steer the surgeon toward biopsy rather than resection

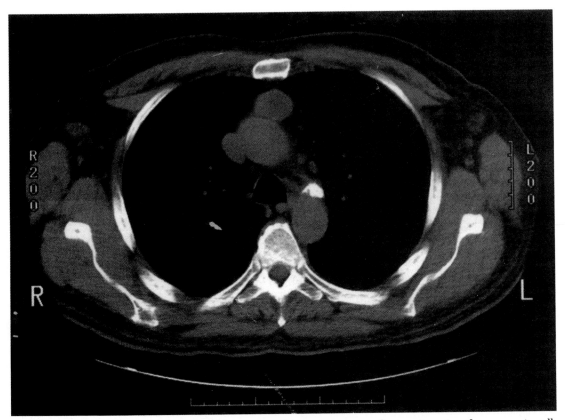

Figure 40–2 Characteristic computed tomographic appearance of a noninvasive thymoma. A well-circumscribed, solid anterior mediastinal mass.

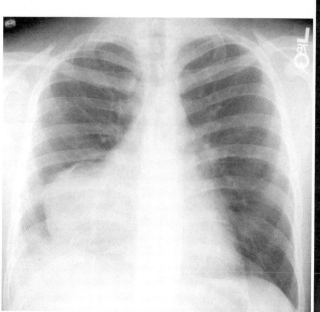

A

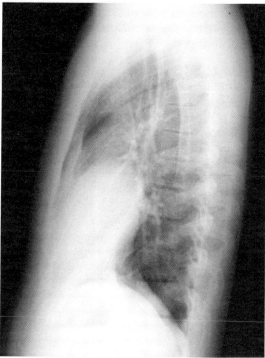

B

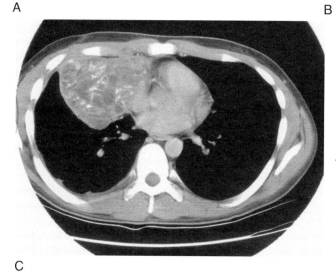

C

Figure 40–3 Characteristic radiographic appearance of a mediastinal teratoma in a 21-year-old male. The PA and lateral chest X-ray (**A** and **B**) show a large mediastinal mass adjacent to the right cardiac boarder. The CT scan (**C**) shows a complex cystic mass with solid components including fat and calcification consistent with a diagnosis of teratoma. In the absence of metastatic disease, the final differentiation between teratoma and teratocarcinoma can be made only by pathological review.
(Radiographs courtesy of Wallace T. Miller, Jr., M.D., Hospital of the University of Pennsylvania, Philadelphia, PA.)

given the data suggesting improved results with neoadjuvant chemoradiotherapy prior to operation in aggressive thymoma and thymic carcinoma.[4,27,55] The role of positron emission tomography (PET) in thymic tumors is not well defined, but it has been reported that thymomas have abnormal uptake and that invasive thymomas and thymic carcinomas have higher uptake than noninvasive tumors.[23]

Serum Studies

All male patients with an anterior mediastinal mass should have serum testing for α-fetoprotein (AFP), β-human chorionic gonadotropin (β-hCG), and lactic dehydrogenase (LDH). Although these levels are normal in mature teratoma, malignant germ cell tumors will have significant elevations and thus establish this diagnosis and rule out thymoma.

Evaluation for Myasthenia Gravis

All patients with suspected thymoma should be carefully questioned regarding the presence of muscle weakness or ocular signs of MG. The diagnosis of MG requires a characteristic history and/or physical findings as well as two positive diagnostic tests. Diagnostic testing for MG includes pharmacological, serological, and electrodiagnostic studies. Unfortunately, no single diagnostic test can rule out MG with certainty in patients with thymoma. If there is the slightest suggestion of MG on initial presentation the patient should undergo additional testing preoperatively under the direction of an experienced neurologist.

Patients with MG, depending upon disease severity, may require medical optimization prior to surgery by some combination of cholinesterase inhibitors, steroids, γ-globulin, and/or plasmapheresis. Additionally, avoidance of drugs that may exacerbate the symptoms of MG is critical (e.g., aminoglycosides, certain inhalation anesthetics, and iodinated radiographic contrast). Obtaining a preoperative forced vital capacity (FVC) for comparison postoperatively can be useful in determining the appropriateness of extubation in MG patients following general anesthesia. We generally require a minimum FVC of 10 ml/kg prior to extubation.

Biopsy

Typically, one would proceed directly to resection of a discrete anterior mediastinal mass in the following situations: (1) the CT or MR shows features consistent with teratoma; (2) the patient is over 40 years of age, without clinical signs or symptoms of lymphoma, and with normal AFP and β-hCG; or (3) the mass is associated with MG. In most other instances, since despite the history, physical examination, imaging, and serum studies, one is still left with a mass that could represent thymoma, lymphoma, or teratoma, biopsy is indicated.

The optimal approach for biopsy is controversial. Options include thin or core-needle biopsy, anterior mediastinotomy (Chamberlain procedure), transcervical mediastinotomy, and video-assisted thoracoscopy (VATS) (see later for technical details of these procedures). Needle biopsy has the disadvantage that optimal tissue may not be obtained, and the availability of pathologists adept at differentiating lymphoma from thymoma and among the various types of lymphoma by cytology and flow cytometry is required. Although mediastinotomy almost always provides adequate tissue for diagnosis, there exists a theoretical risk (unproven) that thymoma cells may be spread, rendering a previously contained tumor less clearly resectable (an even greater concern at VATS). *The authors favor mediastinotomy for situations in which lymphoma is the leading clinical diagnosis, but needle biopsy for tumors felt more likely to represent thymoma or germ cell tumor for which biopsy is felt to be required* (i.e., aggressive thymoma in which neoadjuvant protocols might be considered).

Treatment

Surgery

Complete surgical resection including complete thymectomy is the optimal management of thymoma that is not known preoperatively to be invasive. The technique of these procedures will be detailed later in this chapter.

Adjuvant Therapies

As noted above, aggressive thymomas should be considered for neoadjuvant chemotherapy prior to resection. The response rate to these regimens, which generally contain cisplatin, is high, and the rate of complete resection appears to be improved by such an approach. These patients should probably also receive postoperative radiotherapy.

Postoperative radiation therapy is certainly indicated in cases of incomplete resection and following complete resection of Masaoka stage III thymomas. Since the rate of recurrence of completely resected stage I tumors is less than 5%, these patients are generally not considered for adjuvant radiation. Adjuvant radiotherapy for completely resected

stage II thymoma is more controversial. We[50] and others[28] have recently presented data that strongly suggest that postoperative radiotherapy is not indicated in stage II disease.

Outcome

The outcome for patients with thymoma is stage specific. Patients with completely resected Masaoka stage I thymomas have an excellent prognosis with an expected recurrence rate of less than 5%. Their 10- and 20-year survival rates are 99% and 90%, respectively.[39] As the stage increases, the recurrence rates increase and the survival rates decrease. Patients with stage II thymomas treated by complete resection with or without postoperative radiation therapy have recurrence rates as high as 20%.[28,36] The 5- and 10-year survival rates are 70–90% and 55–85%, respectively.[6,36] Newer long-term data from Japan show improvement in the 10- and 20-year survival rates to 94% and 90%, respectively.[39] The 5-year survival rates for patients with stage III tumors drop to about 50%.[11] It is uncertain whether patients with advanced stage III and IV disease who undergo tumor debulking have an improved prognosis compared with those who undergo biopsy alone. Reports from M.D. Anderson on advanced stage thymoma treated with multimodality treatment including induction chemotherapy, resection, and postoperative consolidation therapy have been encouraging, but the number of treated patients remains small.[47]

Historically, the presence of thymoma was felt to adversely affect the outcome following thymectomy for MG. Several recent studies, however, suggest that this is not the case. A review from the Toronto General Hospital revealed no significant difference in the complete response rate or postoperative Osserman grade of MG patients undergoing thymectomy with and without thymoma.[13] The complete remission rate of MG at 5 years following thymectomy was 36% with or without thymoma.

Thymic Carcinoma

Thymic carcinomas are rare invasive epithelial malignancies. A clinicopathological study of 60 cases of thymic carcinoma revealed an overall 5-year survival of 33%.[52] Histologically, this group consists of a number of different cell types. They are unified, however, by their unequivocal malignant appearance on light microscopy. Although there is no formalized staging system, division of patients into those with low-grade histology and those with high-grade histology does have prognostic significance. Low-grade tumors include squamous, mucoepidermoid, and basaloid carcinomas. The high-grade tumors include sarcomatoid and clear cell carcinoma. The median survival time for patients with low-grade histology is 29 months compared to 11 months for patients with high-grade histology.[38] Effective therapy of thymic carcinoma requires a multimodality approach. This includes complete resection followed by postoperative radiation therapy with or without the addition of chemotherapy. Unfortunately, most patients have recurrence either locally or at distant sites and die of their disease. Multiple neoadjuvant chemotherapy protocols have been proposed for patients presenting with clearly unresectable disease. To date the numbers are too small and the

674 results too variable to determine if this approach converts these patients into operative candidates or affects their overall outcome.[26]

Neuroendocrine Tumors of the Thymus

Neuroendocrine tumors of the thymus include thymic carcinoid and small cell carcinoma of the thymus. These tumors are related biochemically by the presence of APUD (amine precursor uptake and decarboxylation) cells and may actually represent a spectrum of the same abnormality.

Thymic carcinoid occurs more frequently in men than woman. One third of patients present with Cushing's syndrome due to ectopic ACTH production. This portends a very poor prognosis. The treatment of thymic carcinoid is complete excision, and the overall cure rate is very low. The role of multimodality therapy is undefined.

Small cell carcinoma of the thymus is very uncommon. A 20-year review of extrapulmonary small cell carcinoma at the Mayo Clinic revealed only 3 cases out of a total of 54 patients.[16] This tumor, however, is very aggressive. It is treated with chemotherapy alone or in combination with radiation. Like small-cell carcinoma of the lung it is usually responsive to initial chemotherapy, but the response is often not durable.

Other Abnormalities of the Thymus

Hyperplasia

The infant thymus is a large triangular shaped gland that occupies a significant portion of the anterior mediastinum. In contrast, the adult thymus is an involuted organ consisting mostly of adipose tissue surrounded by a capsule. In true thymic hyperplasia, the gland is enlarged in both size and weight for the patient's age. Histologically the gland appears normal. Thymic hyperplasia presents along a spectrum ranging from the incidentally discovered mass to one causing respiratory compromise due to massive enlargement with tracheal compression. It can be seen in association with other disorders such as MG and can occur following severe illness, so-called thymic rebound.

Thymolipoma

Thymolipomas are distinguished from simple mediastinal lipomas by their location within the thymic capsule. Histologically, these neoplasms contain mature adipose cells as well as normal thymic components. Interestingly, thymolipomas can be associated with thymic paraneoplastic syndromes such as red cell aplasia, aplastic anemia, and hypogammaglobulinemia (see above). The treatment of thymolipoma is excision.

Thymic Cysts

Mediastinal thymic cysts account for less than 0.2% of anterior mediastinal masses.[58] They are often asymptomatic and are usually discovered incidentally. Most are unilocular and must contain thymic tissue within the cyst wall to confirm the diagnosis. As a unique entity they are inconsequential and completely benign. Removal is indicated to rule out other entities such as thymoma with cystic components and Hodgkin's disease. Excision yields a definitive diagnosis and completes treatment.

▶ GERM CELL TUMORS

Germ cell tumors comprise a group of neoplasms usually arising in gonadal tissue. The anterior mediastinum is the most common location for the occurrence of extragonadal germ cell tumors, which account for 15–20% of all anterior mediastinal masses. These tumors are divided into benign and malignant lesions.

Benign Mediastinal Teratoma

Benign mediastinal teratoma accounts for 60% of mediastinal germ cell tumors. It is usually asymptomatic in the adult. Children are more likely to present with symptoms due to airway compression. On CT scan the mass is well circumscribed and may or may not contain calcification. It usually shows variable enhancement due to the presence of different tissue types including fat, muscle, bone, and cystic components (Figure 40-3). Curative treatment consists of complete excision via median sternotomy or thoracosternotomy. Differentiation from teratocarcinoma can be made only by resection.

Malignant Mediastinal Germ Cell Tumors

The malignant mediastinal germ cell tumors are divided into seminomatous and nonseminomatous tumors. Seminomas account for 40% of these tumors while the nonseminomas account for 60%. The nonseminomas include embryonal cell carcinoma, choriocarcinoma, yolk sac tumors, and teratocarcinomas. These generally present as diffuse, not discrete, anterior mediastinal masses.

The malignant germ cell tumors are much more common in males but they have been reported in females.[32] The preoperative evaluation of these patients includes a complete physical examination and testicular examination in the male. Radiographic studies should include a chest X-ray as well as a CT scan of the chest, abdomen, and pelvis. Serum AFP, β-hCG, and LDH levels should be obtained. Patients with pure seminoma have normal AFP. Those with any elevation in AFP or marked elevation in β-hCG have mixed tumors containing both seminomatous and nonseminomatous elements. The differentiation between the seminomatous and nonseminomatous germ cell tumors has important prognostic and therapeutic implications. As with testicular seminomas, the pure mediastinal germ cell seminomas are extremely radiosensitive and are treated with radiation therapy. Following radiation, about 80% of patients with pure seminoma will be cured.[12] Residual masses greater than 3 cm should be resected.

Patients with nonseminomas have elevated AFB, β-hCG, and LDH. Following confirmation by biopsy they are usually treated with three-drug chemotherapy (bleomycin, etoposide, and cisplatin). Traditionally, surgical resection is reserved for residual mass following treatment with normalization of serum markers. A large series (31 patients) of treated mediastinal nonseminomatous germ cell tumors was reported from Indiana University in 1990.[37] Using cisplatin-based chemotherapy combined with adjunctive surgery for residual masses they project a 50% cure rate. Data from Memorial Sloan-Kettering suggest that all patients with postchemotherapy residual mass should undergo resection even if their markers remain elevated.[56]

LYMPHOMAS

Both Hodgkin's disease and non-Hodgkin's lymphomas can present as anterior mediastinal masses. The diagnosis is usually suspected on clinical history and CT scan. We recommend surgical biopsy over needle biopsy as the most efficient method of obtaining a precise diagnosis when lymphoma is suspected (see above). Surgical approaches to biopsy include cervical mediastinoscopy, anterior mediastinotomy, and, less commonly, thoracoscopy. It is imperative that the surgeon work in conjunction with the pathologist at the time of surgery to ensure adequate tissue has been obtained. The diagnosis of Hodgkin's disease is confirmed by the presence of Reed-Sternberg cells. The diagnosis and characterization of the non-Hodgkin's lymphoma relies on both light microscopy and cell surface markers. Flow cytometry requires fresh (unfixed) tissue, so it is important that the surgeon ensures that not all of the biopsy tissue is placed in formalin.

Controversy persists over the sensitivity and specificity of CT scan, gallium scan, and PET scan in determining the composition of residual masses following chemotherapy and/or radiotherapy for lymphomas. Some advocate multiple core needle biopsies in this setting, but this is sensitive to sampling error. The only definitive method of determining the composition of a residual mass is resection, and this may rarely be indicated.

SUBSTERNAL THYROID

Substernal thyroid and ectopic thyroid tissue can present as an anterior mediastinal mass. In most cases of substernal thyroid an enlarged thyroid gland is palpable in the neck. Often a chest radiograph will show deviation of the trachea. We have found a CT scan without contrast to be the single most useful test in differentiating substernal thyroid from other mediastinal masses. Because of its iodine content, substernal thyroid tissue shows enhancement on a noncontrast CT scan and usually confirms the diagnosis. The majority of substernal thyroids are goiters, but a benign process and a malignant one cannot be differentiated radiographically. The vast majority of substernal goiters are removed via a cervical approach. This is possible because the blood supply through the superior and inferior thyroid arteries originates in the neck. In some instances, a partial sternal split is required to provide adequate room for delivery of the gland from its substernal location. Infrequently, tracheal resection with primary anastomosis is required to correct tracheomalacia caused by compression or direct tracheal invasion in the case of malignant substernal thyroid neoplasms. This should be performed as a single-stage operation at the time of thyroid resection.

HYPERFUNCTIONING MEDIASTINAL PARATHYROID ADENOMA

Ectopic parathyroid glands can be located in the mediastinum. These patients often present with primary hyperparathyroidism after an unsuccessful neck exploration. Prior to proceeding with mediastinal exploration, localizing studies are utilized. Technitium-99m-sestamibi scintigraphy is the single most useful study to localize hyperfunctioning ectopic parathyroid adenomas in the mediastinum. This study can also be performed as a subtraction study with iodine-123. Nonfunctional, anatomical studies such as MRI may reveal a well-defined mass, however, they are usually small (<3 cm).

Treatment for an ectopic mediastinal parathyroid adenoma is resection. This is performed via a transcervical approach or mediasternotomy. Resection involves removal of the thymus and surrounding fat to include the adenoma. Intraoperative use of rapid parathormone levels confirms the successful localization and removal of the adenoma. The presence of parathyroid tissue should also be confirmed by frozen section examination. If the transcervical approach is selected and there is no normalization of intraoperative parathyroid hormone or parathyroid tissue cannot be confirmed pathologically, one should convert to mediasternotomy for complete evaluation.

SURGICAL APPROACHES TO BIOPSY

Chamberlain Procedure (Anterior Mediastinotomy)

This procedure is usually performed under general anesthesia, but it can be performed under local anesthesia if required. The patient is placed in a supine position with arms tucked. A 5-cm horizontally oriented incision is made just lateral to the sternomanubrial joint over the second costal cartilage. The pectoralis muscle fibers are split from the sternochondral to the costochondral junction. The second cartilage is removed subperichondrially and the pleura is gently swept laterally to avoid inadvertent pneumothorax. Care is taken to avoid injury to the internal thoracic artery and vein, but sometimes they must be divided to gain sufficient exposure. Biopsy is performed under direct vision with a scalpel or biopsy forceps. During closure, we feel it is important to reapproximate the perichondrium to promote regrowth of a normally shaped cartilage.

Transcervical Biopsy (Cervical Mediastinotomy)

Transcervical biopsy is performed through a transcervical collar type incision. The technique is identical to that describe below for transcervical thymectomy and is facilitated by use of the Cooper retractor. Once exposure is obtained, tissue can be procured directly with biopsy forceps or scalpel. The authors have found this approach to be particularly useful to biopsy lesions directly beneath the sternum that would be difficult to reach by a Chamberlain procedure and thus might otherwise require a sternotomy.[14]

676   Thoracoscopic Biopsy

VATS can be utilized for biopsy of anterior mediastinal masses, however, in most situations there are easier and more direct approaches. The anterior mediastinum can be reached from either the left or right thorax and the side should be selected based on the predominate location of the mass. Although we usually perform VATS with a standard 0° thoracoscope, a 30° scope can facilitate visualization of the anterior mediastinum. The thoracoscope is introduced through the fourth intercostal space in the posterior axillary line. Following this, one or two working ports are created somewhat more anteriorly. Port placement is important while working in the anterior mediastinal compartment. Significant experience is required to avoid "clashing" of instruments by inappropriately placed port sites.

From the right thorax, the anterior compartment can be reach by incising the pleura anterior to the phrenic nerve as it runs along the superior vena cava. The connective tissue is gently swept away and the anterior mediastinal compartment entered. The lesion should be identified both visually and by tactile sensation prior to biopsy. Working on the left side can be more difficult because of the proximity to the major vessels of the visceral compartment (the aorta and its branches). Nevertheless, the technique of incision anterior to the phrenic allows access.

In our opinion, the VATS approach is more cumbersome and associated with greater risks than either the anterior mediastinotomy or the transcervical approaches. Dissection around the phrenic nerves can result in temporary or permanent dysfunction. Spillage of tumor during biopsy may cause inadvertent contamination of the pleural space. Finally, this approach requires single lung ventilation, which adds an additional level of complexity to the anesthetic management, especially in patients with large masses and tracheal compression.

Extended Mediastinoscopy

In 1987 Ginsberg and colleagues reported the use of extended cervical mediastinoscopy in the staging of lung cancer.[17] This advanced technique allows for placement of a mediastinoscope into the anterior compartment through a standard cervical mediastinoscopy incision. This involves the creation of a tunnel between the origin of the innominate artery and the left carotid. The tunnel is created by careful digital dissection, and the mediastinoscope is then reinserted and advanced anteriorly toward the left into the tunnel, and the target lesion is clearly identified prior to biopsy. This technique requires considerable experience and carries the risk of significant bleeding because of the proximity of the aorta and pulmonary artery. We feel that unless one has been specifically trained in this technique, most anterior mediastinal masses are more safely and easily approached via anterior or cervical mediastinoscopy as described above.

▶ THERAPEUTIC SURGICAL PROCEDURES: TECHNIQUES OF THYMECTOMY

The main surgical procedure carried out for tumors of the anterior mediastinum is thymectomy, as thymoma is the most common tumor of this area and demands complete thymectomy. Only if there is a preoperative suspicion of a tumor other than thymoma (generally teratoma) might one set out to explore the anterior mediastinum and resect the tumor alone without the adjoining thymus. In this circumstance, a frozen section should always be obtained to confirm the preoperative diagnosis so as not to inadvertently perform less than a complete thymectomy for thymoma.

Thymectomy by Median Sternotomy

This is the most widely employed approach to thymectomy. Although full sternotomy is typical, partial upper sternotomy with extension of the bony incision into the third or fourth intercostal space also has its advocates.[54] Adjacent structures to which the tumor is adherent must be resected en bloc. This often includes pleura, pericardium, and in more aggressive tumors the innominate vein (which may be resected without reconstruction), superior vena cava (requiring reconstruction), and/or lung. Although classically it has been recommended that both pleural spaces be widely opened, the authors feel that this should be performed only on the side on which the tumor is adherent to the pleura, as opening an uninvolved hemithorax likely increases the risk of spread to that pleural space with no obvious benefit. In all procedures, the upper and lower thymic poles are traced as far into the neck and down toward the diaphragm as necessary to ensure complete resection, and all fatty tissue between the phrenic nerves is included in the resection.

Transcervical Thymectomy

We recently reported that noninvasive thymomas less than 4 cm in diameter may be completely resected along with the thymus by a transcervical approach.[14] However, one must have a low threshold with this approach to convert to sternotomy if any suggestion of gross invasion is encountered. In any case, longer-term follow-up should be examined before this approach is widely applied for even small thymomas. Strong evidence exists, on the other hand, that in the absence of thymoma, transcervical thymectomy (TCT) provides results very similar to more aggressive approaches to thymectomy in the treatment of MG.[48] Table 40-3 lists results of recent, large studies of the various approaches to thymectomy for MG. Note that there is no dramatic difference in complete MG remission rates between the proposed approaches to thymectomy.

TCT and transcervical approaches to other masses in the anterior mediastinum are performed through a 5-cm curvilinear incision in the jugular notch. Details of the procedure have been described elsewhere.[21] In brief, after dissection of the two cervical poles, they are each tied with a silk suture and used for traction to aid in dissection of the remainder of the gland. After branches from the innominate vein to the gland are ligated and divided, a Cooper thymectomy retractor (Pilling Instruments) is used to maximally lift the sternum as an inflatable bag beneath the shoulders is deflated. Extracapsular removal of the entire gland then proceeds by primarily blunt dissection within the mediastinum by the operator, seated at the head of the table, using a headlight (Figure 40-4). The resection includes the bulk of the extrathymic mediastinal fat between the phrenic nerves and

Table 40–3

Recent Large Studies of Myasthenia Gravis Response Rates following Thymectomy by Three Surgical Approaches[a]

	Reference	Crude complete remission rate	Mean follow-up (year)	Kaplan–Meier 5-year remission rate (%)
Maximal transcervical/ transsternal	Ashour et al[1]	35	1.7	N/A[b]
	Jaretzki et al[19]	46	3.4	50
Maximal transsternal	Budde et al[8]	21	4.3	N/A
	Busch et al[9]	19	7.7	N/A
	Klein et al[22]	40	5.0	N/A
	Masaoka et al[31]	40/45	5.0/20.0	N/A
	Mulder et al[35]	36	3.6	N/A
	Stern et al[51]	50	6.8	N/A
Extended transcervical[c]	Bril et al[7]	44	8.4	N/A
	Calhoun et al[10]	35	5.0	N/A
	Shrager et al[48]	40	4.6	43

[a]Includes only studies in the past 20 years in the English language literature, representing a pure series of one type of procedure, in adults, with at least 48 patients, that report complete remission rates and mean follow-up.

[b]N/A, not applicable.

[c]Includes only studies representing pure series of extended TCT using the Cooper thymectomy retractor.

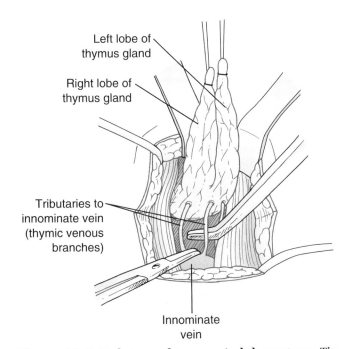

Left lobe of thymus gland

Right lobe of thymus gland

Tributaries to innominate vein (thymic venous branches)

Innominate vein

Figure 40–4 **Technique of transcervical thymectomy.** The surgeon's view from the head of the table as the ligated upper thymic poles are retracted anteriorly while the branches into the thymus from the innominate vein are controlled. (*Modified from Kaiser LR: Atlas of General Thoracic Surgery. St. Louis: Mosby-Year Book, 1997, with permission.*)

down to the diaphragm. The procedure does not remove the pleurae or fat directly apposed to the pleurae, tissue posterior to the phrenic nerves, or other areas where ectopic thymic tissue has been described. No drains are left in place. Patients are generally discharged late on the day of surgery.

"Maximal" Transcervical–Transsternal Thymectomy

Jaretzki and a few others have for many years advocated "maximal thymectomy" for MG, involving a cervical incision in addition to mediasternotomy, and requiring extensive neck and mediastinal dissection in the search for all areas where aberrant thymic tissue has been described.[20] Although Jaretzki has argued vehemently in favor of this approach, the data that this extensive operation provides significantly improved control of MG beyond that obtained by even the least invasive transcervical approach are controversial (Table 40-3) and have not convinced many to adopt this procedure.

Thoracoscopic Thymectomy

A number of thoracoscopic approaches to thymectomy have been described that appear to allow complete thymectomy to be performed.[34,59] Approaches that combine the thoracoscopic and transcervical techniques with sternal lifting have also been reported.[53] However, there is no doubt that intercostal, thoracoscopic port incisions are more painful than a small incision in the jugular notch as performed for TCT. Thus, there would appear to be little reason to use thoracoscopy in lieu of or in addition to the transcervical approach unless it can be demonstrated that this allows more complete resection of thymic tissue and results in higher complete responses in MG. This is very unlikely when even "maximal" thymectomy does not result in markedly higher response rates than TCT.

▶ SUMMARY

We have reviewed the various anterior mediastinal masses with particular regard to their presentation, diagnosis, and

678 management. The association of thymic disease and myasthenia gravis has been emphasized. Surgical approaches to biopsy and resection of anterior mediastinal masses, including their potential advantages and disadvantages, have been described. The appropriate management of anterior mediastinal masses requires flexibility and versatility on the part of the surgeon with regard to the method selected in each patient for biopsy or resection.

REFERENCES

1. Ashour MH, Jain SK, Kattan KM, et al: Maximal thymectomy for myasthenia gravis. Eur J Cardiothorac Surg 9:461–464, 1995.
2. Batata MA, Martini N, Huvos AG, et al: Thymomas: Clinicopathologic features, therapy and prognosis. Cancer 34:389–396, 1974.
3. Beard ME, Krantz SB, Johnson SA, et al: Pure red cell aplasia. Q J Med 47:339–348, 1978.
4. Berruti A, Borasio P, Roncari A, et al: Neoadjuvant chemotherapy with adriamycin, cisplatin, vincristine and cyclophosphamide in invasive thymomas: Results in six patients. Ann Oncol 4:429–431, 1993.
5. Blalock A, Harvey AM, Ford FR, et al: The treatment of myasthenia gravis by removal of the thymus gland. JAMA 117:1529–1533, 1941.
6. Blumberg D, Port JL, Weksler B, et al: Thymoma: A multivariate analysis of factors predicting survival. Ann Thorac Surg 60(4):908–914, 1995.
7. Bril V, Kojic J, Else WK, et al: Long-term clinical outcome after transcervical
8. Budde JM, Morris CD, Gal AA, et al: Predictors of outcome in thymectomy for myasthenia gravis. Ann Thorac Surg 72:197–202, 2001.
9. Busch C, Machens A, Pichlmeier U, et al: Long-term outcome and quality of life after thymectomy for myasthenia gravis. Ann Surg 224:225–232, 1996.
10. Calhoun RF, Ritter JH, Guthrie TJ, et al: Results of transcervical thymectomy for myasthenia gravis in 100 consecutive patients. Ann Surg 230(4):555–559, 1999.
11. Ciernik, IF, Meier U, Lutolf UM, et al: Prognostic factors and outcome of incompletely resected invasive thymoma following radiation therapy. J Clin Oncol 12(7):1484–1490, 1994.
12. Clamon G: Management of primary mediastinal seminoma. Chest 83(2):263–267, 1983.
13. de Perrot M, Liu J, et al: Prognostic significance of thymomas in patients with myasthenia gravis. Ann Thorac Surg 74(4):1658–1662, 2002.
14. Deeb M, Brinster C, Kucharczuk J, et al: Expanded indications for transcervical thymectomy in the management of anterior mediastinal masses. Ann Thorac Surg 72:208–211, 2001.
15. Drachman DB: Myasthenia gravis. N Engl J Med 330: 1797–1810, 1994.
16. Galanis E, Frytak S, et al: Extrapulmonary small cell carcinoma. Cancer 79(9):1729–1736, (1997).
17. Ginsberg R, Rice T, et al: Extended cervical mediastinoscopy: A single stagin procedure for bronchogenic carcinoma of the left uppper lobe. J Thorac Cardiovasc Surg 94:673–678, 1987.
18. Hirokawa K, Utsuyama M, Moriizumi E, et al: Immunohistochemical studies in human thymomas. Localization of thymosin and various cell markers. Virch Arch B 55:371–380, 1988.
19. Jaretzki A III, Penn A, Younger D, et al: Maximal thymectomy for myasthenia gravis: Results. J Thorac Cardiovasc Surg 95:747–757, 1988.
20. Jaretzki A III, Wolff M: Maximal thymectomy for myasthenia gravis: Surgical anatomy and operative technique. J Thorac Cardiovasc Surg 96:711–716, 1988.
21. Kaiser LR: Transcervical thymectomy. In Kaiser LR: Atlas of General Thoracic Surgery. St Louis: Mosby-Year Book, 1997, pp. 152–157.
22. Klein M, Heidenreich F, Madjlessif F et al: Early and late results after thymectomy in myasthenia gravis: a retrospective study. Thorac Cardiovasc Surg 47(3):170-173, 1999.
23. Kubota K, Yamade S, Kondo T, et al: PET imaging of primary mediastinal tumors. Br J Cancer 73:882–886, 1996.
24. Lewis JE, Wick MR, Scheithauer BW, et al: Thymoma: A clinicopathologic review. Cancer 60:2727–2743, 1987.
25. Liu RS, Yeh SH, Huang MH, et al: Use of fluorine-18 fluorodeoxyglucose positron emission tomography in the detection of thymoma: A preliminary report. Eur J Nucl Med 22:1402–1407, 1995.
26. Lucchi M, Mussi A, et al: The multimodality treatment of thymic carcinoma. Eur J Cardiothorac Surg 19:566–569, 2001.
27. Machiarini P, Chella A, Ducci F, et al: Neoadjuvant chemotherapy, surgery, and postoperative radiation therapy for invasive thymoma. Cancer 68:706–713, 1991.
28. Mangi AA, Wright CD, Allan JS, et al: Adjuvant radiation therapy for stage II thymoma. Ann Thorac Surg 74:1033–1037, 2002.
29. Marino M, Muller-Hermelink HK: Thymoma and thymic carcinoma. Relation of thymoma epithelial cells to the cortical and medullary differentiation of the thymus. Virch Arch A 407:119–149, 1985.
30. Masaoka A, Monden Y, Nakahara K, et al: Followup study of thymomas with special reference to their clinical stages. Cancer 48:2485–2492, 1981.
31. Masaoka A, Yamakawa Y, Niwa H, et al: Extended thymectomy for myasthenia gravis patients: A 20 year review. Ann Thorac Surg 62:853–859, 1996.
32. Mayordomo J, Paz-Ares L, et al: Ovarian and extragonadal malignant germ-cell tumors in females: A single institution experience with 43 patients. Ann Oncol 5(3):225–231, 1994.
33. McKenna WG: Malignancies of the thymus. In Roth JA, Ruckdeschel JC, Weisenburger TH, editors: Thoracic Oncology. Philadelphia: W.B. Saunders, 1989.
34. Mineo TC, Pompeo E, Lerut TE: Thoracoscopic thymectomy in autoimmune myasthenia: Results of a left-sided approach. Ann Thorac Surg 69:1537–1541, 2000.
35. Mulder DG, Graves M, Hermann C Jr: Thymectomy for myasthenia gravis: Recent myasthenia gravis in 100 consecutive patients. Ann Surg 230:555–561, 1999.
36. Nakahara K, et al: Thymoma: Results with complete resection and adjuvant postoperative irradiation in 141 consecutive patients. J Thorac Cardiovasc Surg 95:1041, 1988.
37. Nichols C, Saxman S, et al: Primary mediastinal nonseminomatous germ cell tumors. A modern single institution experience. Cancer 65(7):1641–1646, 1990.
38. Ogawa K, Toita T, et al: Treatment and prognosis of thymic carcinoma. Cancer 94:3115–3119, 2002.
39. Okumura M, Miyoshi S, Takeuchi Y, et al: Results of surgical treatment of thymomas with special reference to the involved organs. J Thorac Cardiovasc Surg 117(3):605–613, 1999.
40. Okumura M, Ohta M, Tateyama H, et al: The World Health Organization histologic classification system reflects the oncologic behavior of thymoma: A clinical study of 273 patients. Cancer 94:624–632, 2002.
41. Pescarmona E, Giardinia R, Brisigotti M, et al: Thymoma in childhood: A clinicopathological study of 5 cases. Histopathology 21:65–68, 1990.
42. Quintillo-Martinez L, Wilkins EW Jr, Choi N, et al: Thymoma. Histologic subclassification is an independent prognostic factor. Cancer 74:606–617, 1994.

43. Rendina EA, Pescarmona EO, Venuta F, et al: Thymoma: A clinicopathologic study based on newly developed morphologic criteria. Tumori 74:79–84, 1988.

44. Ricci C, Rendina EA, Pescarmona EO, et al: Correlations between histological type, clinical behaviour, and prognosis in thymoma. Thorax 44:455–460, 1989.

45. Schumacher ED, Roth P: Thymectomie bei einem fall von morbus basedowi mit myasthenia. Mitteil Grenzgebieten Med Chir 25:746, 1912.

46. Shields T: Primary tumors and cysts of the mediastinum. In Shields T, editor: General Thoracic Surgery. Philadelphia: Lee & Febiger, 2000, pp. 927–954.

47. Shin DM, Walsh GL, Komaki R et al: A multidisciplinary approach to therapy for unresectable malignant thymoma. Ann Intern Med 129(2):100–104, 1998.

48. Shrager JB, Deeb ME, Mick R, et al: Transcervical thymectomy for myasthenia gravis achieves results comparable to thymectomy by sternotomy. Ann Thorac Surg 74:320–327, 2002.

49. Simpson JA: The thymus in the pathogenesis and treatment of myasthenia gravis. In Satoyoshi E, editor: Myasthenia Gravis Pathogenesis and Treatment. Tokyo: University of Tokyo Press, 1981, pp. 301–307.

50. Singhal S, Shrager JB, Rosenthal DI, et al: Comparison of stages I-II thymoma treated by complete resection with and without postoperative irradiation. Presented at the Meeting of the Society of Thoracic Surgeons, San Diego, CA, 2003.

51. Stern LE, Nussbaum MS, Quinlan JG, et al: Long-term evaluation of extended thymectomy with anterior mediastinal dissection for myasthenia gravis. Surgery 130(4):774–778, 2001.

52. Suster S, Rosai J: Thymic carcinoma: A clinicopathologic study of 60 cases. Cancer 67:1025–1032, 1991.

53. Takeo S, Sakada T, Yano T: Video-assisted extended thymectomy in patients with thymoma by lifting the sternum. Ann Thorac Surg 71:1721–1723, 2001.

54. Trastek VF: Thymectomy. In Kaiser LR, Kron IL, Spray TL, editors: Mastery of Cardiothoracic Surgery. Philadelphia: Linpincott-Ravin, 1998, pp. 105–111.

55. Venuta F, Rendina EA, Pescarmona EO, et al: Multimodality treatment of thymoma: A prospective study. Ann Thorac Surg 64:1585–1591, 1997.

56. Vuky J, Vains M, Bacik J, et al: Role of postchemotherapy adjunctive surgery in the management of patients with nonseminoma arising from the mediastinum. J Clin Oncol 19:662–668, 2001.

57. Wilkins EW Jr: Discussion of Blumberg D, et al: Thymoma: a multivariate analysis of factors predicting survival. Ann Thorac Surg 60:908, 1995.

58. Wychulis A, Payne W, et al: Surgical treatment of mediastinal tumors: A 40 year experience. J Thorac Cardiovasc Surg 62:379–392, 1971.

59. Yim AP, Kay RL, Ho JK: Video-assisted thoracoscopic thymectomy for myasthenia gravis. Chest 108:1440–1443, 1995.

60. Zeok JV, Todd EP, Dillon M, et al: The role of thymectomy in red cell aplasia. Ann Thorac Surg 28(3):257–260, 1979.

Middle Mediastinum

Zane T. Hammoud and Michael J. Liptay

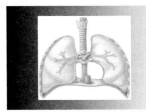

INTRODUCTION

The mediastinum is defined as that space that lies between the two pleural cavities. Within this space lies many vital structures. Superiorly, the mediastinum is bordered by the thoracic inlet; inferiorly, it is bordered by the thoracic surface of the diaphragm. The sternum comprises the anterior border while the spine comprises the posterior border. Traditionally, the mediastinum has been divided into three imaginary compartments: anterior, middle (or visceral), and posterior (Figure 41-1). Although such a division is convenient from an anatomical and surgical standpoint, it should be noted that structures located predominantly in one com-

partment may encroach upon, or involve, another compartment. For instance, the thymus, located in the anterior mediastinum, may extend into the middle mediastinum in certain pathological states.

The three imaginary compartments are defined by anatomical borders. The anterior compartment comprises that space inferior to the innominate vein, posterior to the sternum, and anterior to the anterior surfaces of the pericardium and of the great vessels. The middle, or visceral, compartment, extends from the anterior surfaces of the vertebral bodies to the posterior aspect of the anterior compartment (i.e., the anterior surface of the pericardium). The posterior compartment consists of the paravertebral sulci or costovertebral regions; although this is not truly a mediastinal space per se, it is nonetheless convenient to classify it as such because the pathological conditions that may arise from structures located in this compartment, (e.g., paraganglioma). This chapter shall limit its focus to the structures within the middle mediastinum and to the variety of pathological conditions that may affect, or may arise from, these structures.

ANATOMY/CONTENTS OF MIDDLE MEDIASTINUM

Lymph Nodes

The entire mediastinum is rich in lymphatics and in lymph node groups that drain a variety of organs and/or regions. The major lymph node groups in the middle mediastinum are those that drain the lungs and esophagus. In addition, there are minor lymph node groups located on the diaphragmatic aspect of the pericardium.

Trachea

The entire intrathoracic portion of the trachea, as well as the proximal portions of the right and left mainstem bronchi, is located in the middle mediastinum.

Esophagus

The major portion of the intrathoracic esophagus courses through the middle mediastinum en route to the gastro-esophageal junction.

Heart and Great Vessels

The heart, pericardium, and ascending aorta and proximal aortic arch are all located within the middle mediastinum.

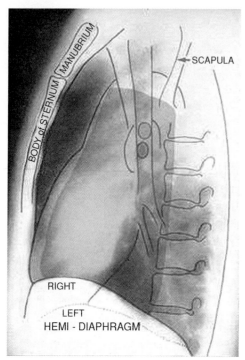

Figure 41–1 Lateral view of the middle mediastinum (grey). It extends to the anterior surface of the pericardium anteriorly and the posterior border is the anterior surface of the vertebral bodies.
(Used with permission of the University of Iowa Virtual.)

As will be discussed in detail in this chapter, all of these structures may develop pathological states that can warrant surgical attention.

▶ INVESTIGATION AND DIAGNOSIS

Noninvasive Investigations

Chest X-Ray

The chest radiograph (CXR) is one of the most common noninvasive diagnostic investigative tools. Often, an abnormality suspected on CXR leads to further investigation by other means. Such abnormalities include, but are not limited to, enlargement of the mediastinum suggestive of a mass, narrowing of the trachea suggestive of stenosis, and prominence of the pulmonary hila suggestive of adenopathy. However, the CXR is insensitive for the precise delineation of most mediastinal pathology. Mediastinal and hilar lymphadenopathy, subtle abnormalities of the trachea, and most esophageal pathology are often underappreciated on CXR views. Abnormalities of the heart or great vessels, when apparent on CXR, are implied only by the location of mediastinal widening or by the presence of a mediastinal mass. Although the CXR is sometimes helpful in suggesting a mediastinal abnormality, it is rarely, if ever, sufficient in the attempt to further define that abnormality.

Computed Tomography

Computed tomography (CT) is currently the most useful imaging modality by which most mediastinal structures are evaluated.[1] High-resolution CT scans, with cross-sectional imaging of structures at as low as 1-mm intervals, have been essential in the visualization of mediastinal structures. The addition of intravenous as well as oral contrast agents only adds to the information that may be obtained on CT. All structures located within the middle mediastinum may be visualized. Masses located within any mediastinal compartment may be precisely located, defined, and their extent further delineated.

Other Techniques

Ultrasonography, sometimes performed with endoscopic guidance, may be used to characterize a middle mediastinal mass.[17] However, this technique rarely provides information not provided by CT. Rarely, magnetic resonance imaging (MRI) may provide additional information. However, it is more likely to be useful in the evaluation of masses located in the posterior mediastinum, such as neurogenic tumors of the paravertebral sulci. Positron emission tomography (PET) scanning, with its ability to distinguish metabolically active tissues, is becoming increasingly useful in the noninvasive staging of the mediastinum in malignancies such as lung cancer.[11,12] However, it is limited by the fact that it is often difficult to distinguish metabolic activity that is secondary to inflammation and activity that is secondary to malignancy. Furthermore, PET is not an anatomical scan, so that the precise location of any abnormality seen on PET may be difficult to determine. The development of CT-PET scanning may overcome this limitation. Other modalities, such as leukocyte scintigraphy, iodine radionuclide imaging, lymphoscintigraphy, and *meta*-iodobenzylguanidine (MIBG) scanning may be utilized on rare occasions.

Invasive Procedures

Percutaneous Transthoracic Fine Needle Biopsy

If a tissue diagnosis is deemed necessary prior to a therapeutic decision, it may be possible to obtain such a diagnosis by performing a percutaneous biopsy. Commonly, this is performed under either ultrasound or CT guidance using local anesthesia, with or without a small amount of intravenous sedation. Fine needle biopsy of middle mediastinal masses is usually carried out transthoracically with passage of the needle through the lung, most commonly under CT guidance. A successful biopsy is obtained in a majority of cases, and the complication rate is acceptable. However, when the technique proves unsuccessful, a more invasive surgical approach is required. Thus, this technique has the potential of requiring a patient to undergo two procedures, making the technique less cost-effective, especially when potential complications are considered. Furthermore, depending on the specific disease process, the cytological diagnosis may be imprecise. For these and other reasons, we tend to use this technique on a very limited basis.

Recently transsternal core needle biopsy of mediastinal masses has been reported with success and minimal morbidity.[6] The advantage of core biopsy over fine needle aspiration affords the pathologist the histological architecture over the cell suspension of cytology. Nonetheless, for a variety of reasons surgical access and biopsy are often required.

Mediastinoscopy/Anterior Mediastinotomy

A standard cervical mediastinoscopy may be used to obtain tissue from masses located in the middle mediastinum. This is particularly true of enlarged lymph nodes, or masses suspected of being lymph nodes, that are located in the middle mediastinal compartment. In some instances, particularly when a mass is predominantly located on one side or the other in the middle mediastinum, an anterior mediastinotomy may be used to obtain a tissue diagnosis. With the use of one of these techniques, and at times both, a tissue diagnosis may be obtained in a majority of cases (Tables 41-1 and 41-2).

Table 41–1

Histological Diagnosis of Benign Mediastinal Lymphadenopathy (N = 206)

Diagnosis	Number (%)
Noncaseating granuloma	130 (63%)
Follicular-reactive hyperplasia	20 (10%)
Caseating granuloma	16 (8%)
Anthracosis	11 (5%)
Other	29 (14%)

From Hammoud ZT, Anderson RC, Meyers BF, et al: The current role of mediastinoscopy in the evaluation of thoracic disease. J Thorac Cardiovasc Surg 118(5):894–899, 1999.

Table 41–2

Pathological Diagnosis of Mediastinoscopy Identified Nonbronchogenic Cancer (N = 161)

Diagnosis	Number (%)
Non-Hodgkin's lymphoma	81 (50%)
Hodgkin's lymphoma	28 (17%)
Melanoma	10 (6%)
Sarcoma	9 (6%)
Other	33 (20%)

From Hammoud ZT, Anderson RC, Meyers BF, et al: The current role of mediastinoscopy in the evaluation of thoracic disease. J Thorac Cardiovasc Surg 118(5):894–899, 1999.

Video-Assisted Thoracoscopic Surgery (VATS)

The VATS approach to the diagnosis and management of mediastinal masses has gained widespread acceptance.[3,20] The technique permits good exposure of nearly the entire mediastinum, provides the surgeon various maneuvers of dissection, allows visualization of the anatomical relationship of the various mediastinal structures, and reduces surgical trauma compared to the traditional thoracotomy. Biopsy procedures of unresectable masses and resections of benign masses, such as benign cysts, are easily performed by VATS. Because of all of these attributes, the VATS approach is being used with increasing frequency in the management of various mediastinal lesions.

Other Techniques

Rarely, thoracotomy or full sternotomy may be necessary to establish a tissue diagnosis. Most commonly, however, such techniques are reserved for the possible management of a particular mediastinal mass. Some authors have also reported the use of endoscopic ultrasound guided fine needle aspiration biopsy in the diagnosis of mediastinal masses. Bronchoscopy, both flexible and/or rigid, is particularly helpful in the evaluation of tracheal diseases, whereas esophagoscopy is useful in the evaluation of esophageal pathology.

► SPECIFIC DISEASES

Adenopathy

The most common cause of malignant mediastinal lymphadenopathy is metastatic lung cancer. Although it has been suggested that the morphology of hilar lymph nodes may help to determine benign versus malignant lymphadenopathy,[18] this is often difficult in clinical practice. Based on the location and type of primary lung cancer, mediastinal lymph nodes at any station may be involved. Most commonly, lymph nodes located in the subcarinal, in the tracheobronchial angle, or in the paratracheal region appear enlarged on imaging studies when involved by an advanced lung cancer.

Other primarily thoracic malignancies, such as esophageal and tracheal carcinomas, may metastasize to mediastinal lymph nodes. Cancers located primarily in other body cavities, such as the abdomen, may, on rare occasion, also metastasize to mediastinal lymph nodes.

Lymphoma is one of the most common mediastinal tumors (Figure 41-2). Lymphoma may manifest as a primary mediastinal tumor or, more commonly, as generalized disease. Both Hodgkin's disease and non-Hodgkin's lymphoma may present as mediastinal lymphadenopathy. Hodgkin's disease is the most common mediastinal lymphoma.[24] Although they are usually located in the anterior mediastinum, when generalized these tumors may involve lymph nodes located throughout the mediastinum.

A wide variety of inflammatory conditions may also cause enlargement of mediastinal lymph nodes. Sarcoidosis is one of the most common causes of benign mediastinal lymphadenopathy (Figure 41-3). Radiographically, sarcoidosis

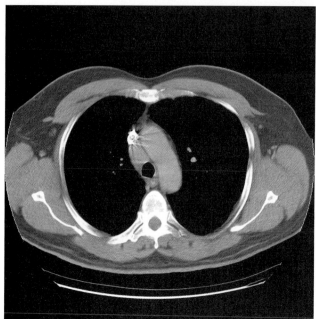

Figure 41–2 Chest CT scan demonstrating right paratracheal (level 4R) lymphadenopathy. This patient had non-Hodgkin's lymphoma.

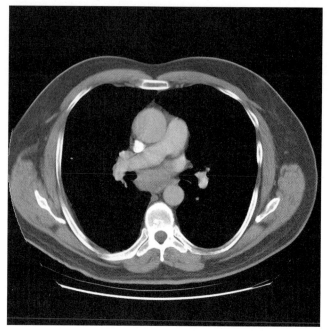

Figure 41–3 Chest CT scan demonstrating subcarinal (level 7) lymphadenopathy. This patient had sarcoidosis.

usually presents as bilateral hilar lymphadenopathy or as diffuse mediastinal lymphadenopathy. Bacterial as well as viral pneumonias, interstitial lung disease, and many other nonspecific inflammatory lung diseases may lead to mediastinal lymphadenopathy. Mycobacterial infections, such as tuberculosis, may present with unilateral hilar or mediastinal adenopathy, or both. Fungal infections, such as histoplasmosis and cryptococcosis, may also involve mediastinal lymph nodes. These latter infections are being seen more commonly as opportunistic infections in patients with the human immunodeficiency virus as well as in transplant recipients.

There are several other rare causes of mediastinal lymphadenopathy. Congestive heart failure may be associated with diffuse mediastinal lymphadenopathy. Castleman's disease, or giant lymph node hyperplasia, may present as a benign lymphoid mass in the chest in 70% of the cases.[25] Most of the lymph nodes in this disease are located along the tracheobronchial tree or hilum of the lung in the middle mediastinum.

Diseases of the Trachea

The adult trachea averages 11 cm in length from the cricoid cartilage to the carina. The majority of the trachea, as well as the mainstem bronchi, are located in the middle mediastinum. A variety of conditions, benign and malignant, may involve the trachea. Patients with tracheal stenosis due to benign lesions, as may be seen postintubation or during a tracheostomy, may present with wheezing or stridor; radiographically, these lesions appear as circumferential narrowing of the intrathoracic trachea. Tracheal compression and/or involvement by other tumors, such as thyroid cancer, may also manifest with respiratory symptoms and be evident radiographically.

The two most common primary tracheal tumors are squamous cell carcinoma and adenoid cystic carcinoma, occurring with approximately equal frequency.[7] Symptoms caused by these tumors include respiratory symptoms as well as hemoptysis. Although most tracheal lesions may be seen on imaging studies, bronchoscopic evaluation is nearly always mandatory. Most lesions are amenable to tracheal resection and reconstruction.

Other rare conditions may also be noted on examination of the trachea in the mediastinum. Malacia of some or of all of the intrathoracic trachea may be seen as flattening of the normal C-shaped trachea. Involvement of the tracheal lumen by systemic disease, such as amyloidosis, is also seen.

Diseases of the Esophagus

The esophagus begins in the neck at the level of the cricopharyngeus muscle and ends at the gastroesophageal junction, usually located in the abdomen. Within the middle mediastinum, it is intimately associated with the trachea anteriorly and with the aorta posteriorly. Esophageal masses, whether benign or malignant, may cause dysphagia and may be visible on imaging studies.[14,15] Leiomyoma, the most common benign esophageal tumor, may appear as an extraluminal esophageal mass in the middle mediastinum; treatment is by simple enucleation of the tumor. Malignant lesions, such as squamous cell carcinoma and adenocarcinoma, may present as a mediastinal mass or may cause compression of other mediastinal structures if the tumor is discovered at an advanced stage.

Tracheoesophageal fistulas, most commonly secondary to malignancy, usually present with recurrent pneumonias and may be visible on imaging of the mediastinum. Perforation of the esophagus, whether iatrogenic or spontaneous, is one of the most common causes of mediastinitis. Depending on the time to diagnosis, patients may be relatively asymptomatic or critically ill upon presentation. Radiographically, esophageal perforation may be first suspected by the presence of air in the mediastinum. Mediastinitis, from this as well as a myriad of other causes, may ensue and presents radiographically as diffuse inflammation, with loss of the normal fat planes and, on occasion, gas bubbles.

Cysts

A wide variety of cystic lesions may be found in the mediastinum. These lesions are encountered in children and in adults. They include cysts that originate from the tracheobronchial tree, the esophagus, the pericardium, the thymus, as well as numerous other organs within the mediastinum. Only the most common lesions will be discussed here.

Foregut Cysts

Foregut cysts are most commonly spherical and have thin walls, and they almost never communicate with either the tracheobronchial tree or the esophagus. They are most commonly discovered in the fourth decade of life with an equal prevalence in males and females. Two thirds of patients will ultimately develop symptoms, most commonly dyspnea, dysphagia, and pain.[22]

Bronchogenic Cysts

These are believed to result from sequestration of cells during embryonic development of the respiratory tree. They are rarely in communication with the tracheobronchial tree, are usually unilocular, and are lined by ciliated columnar epithelium. Most often, they are located in the region of the carina (Figure 41-4). They account for 50–60% of all mediastinal cysts and are usually discovered in adults. Although these cysts may be asymptomatic, a significant proportion will produce symptoms due to airway compression or to the presence of infection within the cyst.

Simple aspiration of these cysts has been advocated.[6,15] This approach has yielded unacceptable recurrence rates and in some cases can make the subsequent attempted resection more challenging.

Treatment is by complete surgical excision of the cyst, with the surgical approach dictated by the location of the cyst; for the commonly located subcarinal cyst, a standard right posterolateral thoracotomy has been the classic approach. Over the past decade numerous reports of thoracoscopic (VATS) approaches have been reported with successful results.[3,10] Ginsberg et al reported the first use of cervical mediastinoscopy to treat bronchogenic cysts in 1972.[5] A small series of three patients reported good results with outpatient partial resection of the cyst wall via mediastinoscopy.[19]

Regardless of the approach the primary goal is to completely resect the cyst wall to avoid recurrence and address the rare but significant incidence of malignant degeneration. Thoracoscopic complete resection when possible is our preferred approach for most uncomplicated bronchogenic cysts.

Esophageal Cysts

These cysts are less common than bronchogenic cysts. They are believed to arise embryologically from persistence of

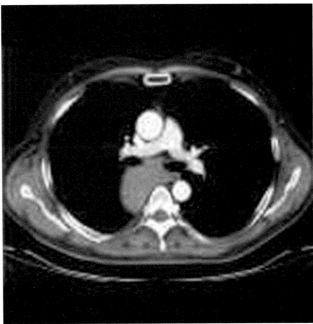

Figure 41–4 Chest CT scan of a 25-year-old female with a bronchogenic cyst in the subcarinal area. The patient had symptoms of substernal chest pain and cough.

foregut vacuoles. They do not usually communicate with the esophageal lumen, but they may be embedded entirely within the esophageal wall. At times, it may be difficult to distinguish an esophageal cyst from a bronchogenic one because of the close relationship that these cysts may have with both the esophagus and the tracheobronchial tree. When symptomatic, they usually present with pain and/or dysphagia. Treatment is by surgical excision, with care taken to avoid any esophageal mucosal injury.[2] Thoracoscopic resection is often possible.

Pleuropericardial Cysts

These are rare lesions felt to arise during embryonic development of the pericardium (Figure 41-5). They rarely are in communication with the pericardium and are most commonly found in the right cardiophrenic angle. These cysts are symptomatic in only a minority of patients; when symptomatic, the most common symptoms are dyspnea and chest pain. Radiology-guided needle aspiration of these has been recommended as a first step.[13,16,23] If the cysts recur, if symptoms develop, or if the diagnosis is in doubt, our preferred treatment is thoracoscopic surgical resection.[10,21]

Mediastinal Infections

Infections of the mediastinum, with resultant mediastinitis, may be due to several causes. The majority of these infections are secondary to esophageal perforation or to postoperative sternal infections after sternotomy. Perforation of the thoracic esophagus, whether iatrogenic (endoscopy) or spontaneous, leads to immediate contamination of the middle mediastinum by oropharyngeal secretions. The clinical manifestations of esophageal perforation are dependent on the timing of the

686

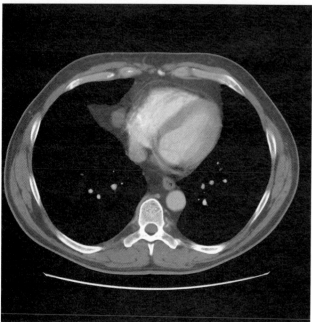

Figure 41–5 Chest CT scan of a 53-year-old male with an asymptomatic pericardial cyst located in the right lower medial diaphragmatic pericardial recess.

diagnosis. This represents a true surgical emergency, though the diagnosis may sometimes be made several days or even weeks after the event. Treatment centers around surgical debridement of nonviable tissues, primary repair if possible, adequate drainage, and systemic antibiotics.

Postoperative sternal infections after sternotomy, usually for cardiac procedures, may lead to significant morbidity and/or mortality. In cardiac surgery, some risk factors for this complication include diabetes, redo operations, and harvesting of bilateral internal mammary arteries. Treatment centers around prompt diagnosis, aggressive surgical debridement, and possible early muscle flap closure.

Descending necrotizing mediastinitis is a rare condition caused by progressive spread of an infectious process from an odontogenic abscess. Oropharyngeal bacteria may gain access to the mediastinum via the pretracheal or retrovisceral spaces or along the carotid sheaths. When it occurs, mediastinal involvement is generally seen within 48 h of the onset of the cervical infection. Diagnosis is often delayed secondary to the nonspecific nature of the presenting symptoms and is most commonly made when mediastinal air is seen on CT scan. Treatment consists of systemic antibiotics; surgical drainage of the neck and mediastinum; and, when appropriate, tracheostomy. In most cases, a cervical approach is sufficient to obtain surgical drainage with placement of drains into the mediastinum. Occasionally a thoracotomy or VATS approach is required to attain full debridement and wide drainage.[4,9]

Chronic fibrosing mediastinitis is a rare condition that results in the deposition of dense fibrous tissue throughout the middle mediastinal compartment. Most commonly, this condition is caused by chronic fungal infections, primarily histoplasmosis. The fibrous tissue may encase structures in the middle mediastinum, such as the vena cava, and lead to entrapment of these structures. Treatment, when necessary, is directed at relief of symptoms. On rare occasions, a thoracotomy may be necessary to relieve compression of the trachea or esophagus.

REFERENCES

1. Aquino SL, Duncan G, Taber KH, et al: Reconciliation of the anatomic, surgical, and radiographic classifications of the mediastinum. J Comput Assist Tomogr 25(3):489–492, 2001.
2. Cioffi U, Bonavina L, De Simone M, et al: Presentation and surgical management of bronchogenic and esophageal duplication cysts in adults. Chest 113(6):1492–1496, 1998.
3. Cirino LM, Milanez DC Jr, Fernandez A, et al: Diagnosis and treatment of mediastinal tumors by thoracoscopy. Chest 117(6):1787–1792, 2000.
4. Freeman RK, Vallieres E, Verrier ED, et al: Descending necrotizing mediastinitis: An analysis of the effects of serial surgical debridement on patient mortality. J Thorac Cardiovasc Surg 119(2):260–267, 2000.
5. Ginsberg RJ, Atkins RW, Paulson DL: A bronchogenic cyst successfully treated by mediastinoscopy. Ann Thorac Surg 13(3):266–268, 1972.
6. Gupta S, Wallace MJ, Morello FA Jr, et al: CT-guided percutaneous needle biopsy of intrathoracic lesions by using the transsternal approach: Experience in 37 patients. Radiology 222(1):57–62, 2002.
7. Hammoud ZT, Grillo HC, Mathisen DJ: Tumors of the cervical trachea. In Myers EN, Suen JY, Myers J, Hanna Ee, editors: Cancer of the Head and Neck, 4th ed. Philadelphia: W.B. Saunders, 2000.
8. Hammoud ZT, Anderson RC, Meyers BF, et al: The current role of mediastinoscopy in the evaluation of thoracic disease. J Thorac Cardiovasc Surg 118(5):894–899, 1999.
9. Hasegawa T, Endo S, Sohara Y: Classification of descending necrotizing mediastinitis. Ann Thorac Surg 69(4):1296, 2000.
10. Hazelrigg SR, Landreneau RJ, Mack MJ, Acuff TE: Thoracoscopic resection of mediastinal cysts. Ann Thorac Surg 56(3):659–660, 1993.
11. Kernstine KH, Mclaughlin KA, Menda Y, et al: Can FDG-PET reduce the need for mediastinoscopy in potentially resectable nonsmall cell lung cancer? Ann Thorac Surg 73(2):394–401, 2002.
12. Kiernan PD, Sheridan MJ, Lamberti J, et al: Mediastinal staging of non-small cell lung carcinoma using computed and positron-emission tomography. South Med J 95(10):1168–1172, 2002.
13. Kinoshita Y, Shimada T, Murakami Y, et al: Ethanol sclerosis can be a safe and useful treatment for pericardial cyst. Clin Cardiol 19(10):833–835, 1996.
14. Maerz LL, Deveney CW, Lopez RR, McConnell DB: Role of computed tomographic scans in the staging of esophageal and proximal gastric malignancies. Am J Surg 165(5):558–560, 1993.
15. Nath PH, Sanders C, Holley HC, McElvein RB: Percutaneous fine needle aspiration in the diagnosis and management of mediastinal cysts in adults. South Med J 81(10):1225–1228, 1988.
16. Okubo K, Chino M, Fuse J, Yo S, et al: Life-saving needle aspiration of a cardiac-compressing pericardial cyst. Am J Cardiol 85(4):521, 2000.
17. Panelli F, Erickson RA, Prasad VM: Evaluation of mediastinal masses by endoscopic ultrasound and endoscopic ultrasound-guided fine needle aspiration. Am J Gastroenterol 96(2):401–408, 2001.
18. Shimoyama K, Murata K, Takahashi M, Morita R: Pulmonary hilar lymph node metastases from lung cancer: Evaluation based on morphology at thin-section, incremental, dynamic CT. Radiology 203(1):187–195, 1997.

19. Smythe WR, Bavaria JE, Kaiser LR: Mediastinoscopic subtotal removal of mediastinal cysts. Chest 114(2):614–617, 1998.

20. Solaini L, Bagioni P, Campanini A, Poddie BD: Diagnostic role of videothoracoscopy in mediastinal diseases. Eur J Cardiothorac Surg 13(5):491–493, 1998.

21. Song J, Costic JT, Seinfeld FI, Laub GW: Thoracoscopic resection of unusual symptomatic pericardial cysts. J Laparoendosc Adv Surg Tech A 12(2):135–137, 2002.

22. St Georges R, Deslauriers J, Duranceau A, et al: Clinical spectrum of bronchogenic cysts of the mediastinum and lung in the adult. Ann Thorac Surg 52(1):6–13, 1991.

23. Stoller JK, Shaw C, Matthay RA: Enlarging, atypically located pericardial cyst. Recent experience and literature review. Chest 89(3):402–406, 1986.

24. Strollo DC, Rosado-de-Christenson ML, Jett JR: Primary mediastinal tumors: Part II. Tumors of the middle and posterior mediastinum. Chest 112(5):1344–1357, 1997.

25. Wright CD, Mathisen DJ: Mediastinal tumors: Diagnosis and treatment. World J Surg 25(2):204–209, 2001.

The Posterior Mediastinum

Dhruv Singhal and Larry R. Kaiser

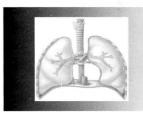

CHAPTER **42**

INTRODUCTION

The posterior mediastinum is an anatomically diverse region with visceral organs, major vessels, large neural structures, and important lymphatic vessels. Lesions that originate in the mediastinum are rare compared to diverse lesions that can involve the mediastinum secondarily. Lesions contained within it are primarily tumors of neurogenic origin. Less common is a potpourri of lesions including vascular tumors, mesenchymal tumors, and lymphatic lesions.

ANATOMY

The posterior mediastinum, also called the paravertebral compartment, is a defined space between the posterior pericardium and the anterior spinal ligament including the paravertebral gutters. According to the traditional four-compartment model, the mediastinum is divided into an anterior, middle, posterior, and superior division. The posterior mediastinum is bounded superiorly by the inferior border of the T4 vertebral body.[12,51]

In the traditional three-compartment model without a superior division, the entire length of the spine is included in the posterior mediastinum.[51] The diaphragm is the com-

mon inferior border for all three compartments. Within these boundaries, the posterior mediastinum houses the esophagus, descending aorta, sympathetic chain and vagus nerves, thoracic duct, azygous and hemiazygous veins, fat, and lymph nodes[12] (Figure 42-1).

EPIDEMIOLOGY

Great differences exist between children and adults with respect to the location of mediastinal masses.[52] In adults, 65% of the lesions arise in the anterosuperior, 10% in the middle, and 25% in the posterior compartments; this distribution is reversed in children, where 25% of lesions arise in the anterosuperior, 10% in the middle, and 65% in the posterior compartments. In general, the incidence of posterior mediastinal lesions is higher in children, whereas anterior lesions predominate in adults.

DIAGNOSIS

Approximately 50% of posterior mediastinal lesions are asymptomatic and are detected on chest radiographs taken for unrelated reasons. As a rough guideline, the absence of symptoms suggests that a lesion is benign, whereas the presence of symptoms suggests malignancy.

The percentage of patients with symptoms from mediastinal masses precisely parallels, or equals, the percentage of malignant lesions. In adults, 50–60% of lesions are symptomatic, whereas the percentage of symptomatic lesions is higher in children—60–80%. Since the incidence of symptoms parallels the incidence of malignancy, a child with a mediastinal mass is considerably more likely to have a malignancy than is an adult with a mediastinal mass.

When a posterior mediastinal mass is discovered, a detailed history and physical examination are useful, particularly in patients with rarer symptoms (e.g., hoarseness and Horner's syndrome). The age of the patient can also narrow the diagnostic possibilities.

Computed tomography (CT) is the imaging modality of choice for the posterior mediastinum because of its ability to localize masses and to determine somewhat the extent of invasion. CT can often distinguish among the various masses and identify their origin, allowing correct diagnosis based on radiographic imaging.[26] Although magnetic resonance imaging (MRI) has been cited as useful in particular circumstances such as with dumbbell tumors, cysts and extramedullary hematopoiesis, CT remains the superior imaging

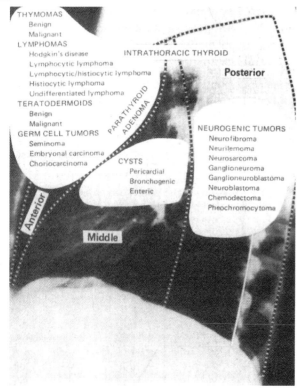

THYMOMAS
  Benign
  Malignant
LYMPHOMAS
  Hodgkin's disease
  Lymphocytic lymphoma
  Lymphocytic/histiocytic lymphoma
  Histiocytic lymphoma
  Undifferentiated lymphoma
TERATODERMOIDS
  Benign
  Malignant
GERM CELL TUMORS
  Seminoma
  Embryonal carcinoma
  Choriocarcinoma

INTRATHORACIC THYROID

Posterior

PARATHYROID ADENOMA

Anterior

Middle

CYSTS
  Pericardial
  Bronchogenic
  Enteric

NEUROGENIC TUMORS
  Neurofibroma
  Neurilemoma
  Neurosarcoma
  Ganglioneuroma
  Ganglioneuroblastoma
  Neuroblastoma
  Chemodectoma
  Pheochromocytoma

Figure 42–1 Lateral chest film divided into three anatomical subdivisions with the most common location of the tumors and cysts.
(From Davis RD Jr, Sabiston DC Jr: Primary mediastinal cysts and neoplasms. In Sabiston DC Jr, editor: Essentials of Surgery. Philadelphia: W.B. Saunders, 1987.)

modality for most posterior mediastinal masses.[31] Mediastinal sonography, although less expensive and comparable to CT in the diagnosis of many mediastinal masses, is not useful in the posterior mediastinum.[63]

The decision to biopsy a mediastinal mass is not straightforward. Biopsy before resection is not necessary in some cases and potentially harmful in others. The likelihood of a positive biopsy depends on the presence of local symptoms and the location and extent of the lesion. Lesions in the posterior mediastinum require either fine-needle aspiration (FNA) (CT-guided) or a thoracoscopic approach.[4,27] If these procedures are not possible because of their location in the paravertebral gutters, a limited posterolateral thoracotomy should be used to obtain adequate tissue for diagnosis.[10,43]

SURGICAL APPROACHES TO THE POSTERIOR MEDIASTINUM

Multiple standard approaches to reach the posterior mediastinum have been described including a cervical approach, paravertebral approach, thoracotomy, transabdominal approach, and thoracoscopy. The cervical approach is accomplished through an incision along the anterior border of the sternocleidomastoid muscle. For lesions that are in the superior portion of the posterior mediastinum, incising the buccopharyngeal fascia allows one to enter the peripharyngoesophageal space. When lower posterior mediastinal masses need to be reached, the paravertebral approach is utilized by resecting posterior segments of one or more ribs and entering the retropleural plane that leads to the posterior mediastinum. Standard posterolateral thoracotomy provides excellent access to the posterior mediastinum with the location of the lesion determining the intercostal space to be entered.

The mediastinum can also be accessed transabdominally through the esophageal hiatus in various antireflux operations, hiatal hernia repairs, and during the transhiatal esophagectomy. A combined cervical approach with transabdominal mobilization allows the surgeon to remove the esophagus extrapleurally without traversing the pleural cavities or bony thorax.[6]

Currently, the decision to perform thoracoscopic surgery for posterior mediastinal lesions remains dependent on the surgeon's experience and comfort with video-assisted devices but for biopsy this should be the procedure of choice[27,29,47] (Figure 42-2). Zierold and Halow[68] conducted a retrospective review that described use of thoracoscopic approaches for posterior mediastinal neurogenic masses. A total of 29 patients (13 men, 16 women), aged 26 to 68 years, who underwent a thoracoscopic resection were identified. Preoperative imaging included chest radiography and CT in all patients and MRI in 15 of 29 patients (52%). All tumors were located in the posterior mediastinum without preoperative evidence of invasion or malignancy. Conversion to an open procedure was required in 12 of 29 (41%) patients ("minithoracotomy" in 11, posterolateral thoracotomy in 1). Tumor size necessitating conversion to an open procedure (mean = 4.79 cm) and tumor size amenable to thoracoscopy alone (mean = 3.84 cm) were not significantly different (p <0.09). They concluded that thoracoscopic resection could be performed successfully, regardless of tumor type or size; however, malignancy, local invasion, and tumors greater than 5 cm may require an open procedure.

The standard surgical approach involves a posterolateral thoracotomy incision and exposure of the posterior mediastinum. The tumor is always in a paravertebral location and the exposure involves first incising the overlying pleura and then dissecting the lesion from the surrounding structures. Rarely is there any invasion of vertebral bodies but it is important to recognize any involvement at the level of a neural foramen manifest by widening of the foramen and an inability to recognize a discrete nerve root. Tumors arising from the sympathetic chain require segmental resection of the chain. Care should be taken to avoid unnecessary resection of segmental vessels that course along the vertebral bodies.

Once the pleura overlying the lesion has been incised, mobilization of the tumor proceeds expeditiously with a combination of sharp and blunt dissection. Complete resection can always be accomplished. Often the procedure may start with video thoracoscopic visualization of the tumor and if mobilization is feasible the tumor can be removed through a small incision. However, if mobilization proves difficult by the video thoracoscopic approach, there should be no hesitation in converting to an open procedure. This is especially important with lesions located at the apex of the chest.

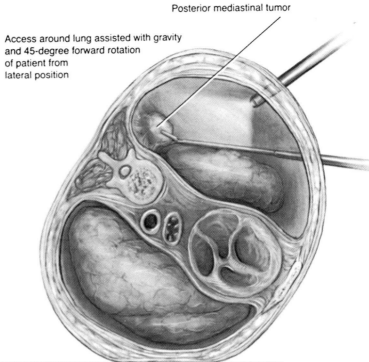

Posterior mediastinal tumor

Access around lung assisted with gravity
and 45-degree forward rotation
of patient from
lateral position

Figure 42–2 Thoracoscopic resection of a posterior mediastinal tumor.
(Reprinted with permission from Davis RD Jr, Sabiston DC Jr: Textbook of Surgery. Philadelphia: W.B. Saunders, 1997, p. 1915.)

LESIONS OF THE MEDIASTINUM

Neurogenic Tumors

Neurogenic tumors of the thorax commonly occur in the posterior mediastinum and primarily affect young adults and children.[49] In recent decades, although these tumors continue to be the most common malignancy in children, in adults they have become less common than tumors of the anterior mediastinum (thymomas or lymphomas). They now represent approximately 15% of all mediastinal masses in adults. Furthermore, in adults, the malignancy rate of neurogenic tumors is less than 10%. In children, fully 50% of these lesions are malignant.[49]

Neurogenic tumors originate from embryonic neural crest cells around the spinal ganglia and from either sympathetic or parasympathetic components (Box 42-1). The differential diagnosis for neurogenic tumors arising from the intercostal nerves includes neurofibroma, neurilemoma, and neurogenic sarcoma. Sympathetic ganglia tumors include ganglioneuroma, ganglioneuroblastomas, and neuroblastoma. Pheochromocytomas can occur from paraganglia cells. Neurogenic tumors rarely arise from the phrenic or vagus nerves.

Neurogenic tumors can be benign or malignant. Benign lesions are classified as either neurilemoma (schwannoma) or neurofibromas. Neurilemomas are more common than neurofibromas. Of patients with nerve sheath tumors 25–40% have multiple neurofibromatosis (von Recklinghausen's disease). Malignant tumors (neurogenic sarcomas or malignant schwannomas) are unusual. The incidence of malignancy is greater in tumors in patients with von Recklinghausen's disease (10–20%).

Patients with benign lesions are often asymptomatic as opposed to patients with malignant tumors, who frequently manifest symptoms of spinal cord compression or have cough, dyspnea, chest wall pain, and hoarseness. Horner's syndrome due to involvement of the superior cervical ganglion of the sympathetic chain is an unusual presentation. Most patients with neurogenic tumors are asymptomatic, so the initial diagnosis is usually made incidentally on chest radiographs. A rare patient may present with a pheochromocytoma or a chemically active neuroblastoma or ganglioneuroma. In all symptomatic patients, especially those with a history of significant hypertension or hypermetabolism, serum catecholamine levels and 24-h urine levels of homovanillic acid and vanillylmandelic acid should be determined. If these levels are elevated suggesting pheochromocytoma, preoperative adrenergic blockers need to be administered to avoid perioperative complications from episodic catecholamine release during tumor manipulation.

Neurogenic tumors that arise from intercostal nerves are typically neurilemomas or neurofibromas[35] (Box 42-1). Neurilemomas (schwannomas) are the most common neurogenic tumors.[48,56] Histologically, they appear as well

Box 42–1. Origin of Neurogenic Tumors in the Posterior Mediastinum.

Intercostal nerve tumors	Sympathetic ganglia tumors	Paraganglia cell tumors
Neurofibroma	Ganglioma	Paraganglioma (pheochromocytoma)
Neurilemoma	Ganglioneuroblastoma	
Neurofibrosarcoma Neurosarcoma	Neuroblastoma	

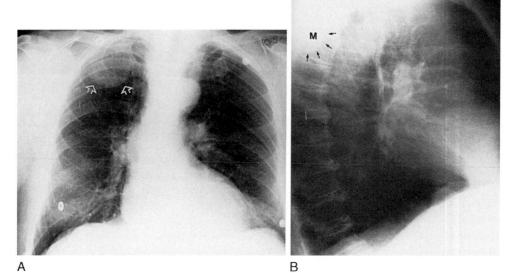

A   B

Figure 42–3 Posteroanterior and lateral chest radiographs: Neurofibroma. **A,** A large mass projects in the right apex (*open arrows*). It has a smooth, sharp inferior margin. The superior margin makes broad contact with the chest wall, forming obtuse angles. These findings suggest that the mass did not arise in the lung parenchyma. **B,** The lateral chest view demonstrates a barely perceptible mass projecting far posterior behind the anterior margin of the vertebra (*M with arrows*). The location suggests a neurogenic mass.
(*Reprinted with permission from Meholic A, Ketai L, Lofgren R: Hilum and mediastinum. In Meholic A, Ketai L, Lofgren R, editors: Fundamentals of Chest Radiology. Philadelphia: W.B. Saunders, 1996, p. 217.*)

encapsulated, firm, gray-tan masses.[2] Morphologically, they tend to resemble two patterns: organized architecture with a cellular palisading pattern of growth (Antoni's Type A) or a loose reticular pattern (Antoni's Type B).[32] These tumors tend to have a poor prognosis. Neurofibromas are poorly encapsulated with a random arrangement of spindle-shaped cells.[37] Associated with neurofibromatosis type 1, these tumors tend to form in the paravertebral gutters (Figure 42-3). Both of these tumors can occur as manifestations of von Recklinghausen's disease and can degenerate into neurosarcoma if left untreated.

Neuroblastoma, ganglioneuroblastoma, and ganglioneuroma are tumors of the sympathetic nervous system that arise from primitive sympathetic ganglia and are referred to collectively as neuroblastic tumors.[34] They arise wherever sympathetic tissue exists and may be seen in the neck, posterior mediastinum, adrenal gland, retroperitoneum, and pelvis. The three tumors differ in their degree of cellular and extracellular maturation; immature tumors tend to be aggressive and occur in younger patients (median age, just under 2 years), whereas mature tumors occur in older children (median age, approximately 7 years) and tend to behave in a benign fashion.[34]

The most benign tumor is the ganglioneuroma, which is composed of gangliocytes and mature stroma. They are present at an early age in the paravertebral region and are the most common neurogenic tumors occurring in childhood. Ganglioneuroblastoma is composed of both mature gangliocytes and immature neuroblasts and has intermediate malignant potential.[1]

Neuroblastomas also develop in children; greater than 75% of the cases are in children under 4 years. Histologically, these tumors are composed of small, round immature cells organized in a rosette pattern. They are highly invasive and by the time diagnosis is made, they often metastasize to the regional lymph nodes, bone, brain, liver, and lung. Neuroblastoma, however, may have a relatively benign course, even when metastatic. Symptoms at time of diagnosis typically included cough, dysphagia, chest pain, and occasionally paraplegia. At times, they may present with paraneoplastic syndromes such as profuse watery diarrhea secondary to vasoactive intestinal protein syndrome, opsoclonus-polymyoclonus syndrome, and pheochromocytoma-like syndrome. Features such as DNA content, tumor protooncogenes, and catecholamine synthesis influence prognosis, and their presence or absence aids in categorizing patients with neuroblastoma as high, intermediate, or low risk. Treatment consists of resection and, usually, chemotherapy. Despite recent advances in treatment, including bone marrow transplantation, neuroblastoma remains a relatively lethal tumor, accounting for 10% of pediatric cancers but 15% of cancer deaths in children.[34]

A CT scan can help elucidate the tumor type and extent of tumor involvement.[31,34] Neurogenic tumors from peripheral nerves will appear as well-defined round or oval masses that are noncalcified in the paravertebral gutter. Neurilemomas have variable enhancement with either homogeneity or heterogeneity.[38] With enhanced CT, these tumors demonstrate variable attenuation depending on their histology. Neurofibromas are usually homogeneous, low attenuation lesions on unenhanced CT. Enhanced CT will demonstrate homogeneous enhancement or early central blush. Malignant nerve sheath tumors show variable attenuation.[32]

Tumors arising from the sympathetic chain expand along the spinal axis making them difficult to detect on a lateral

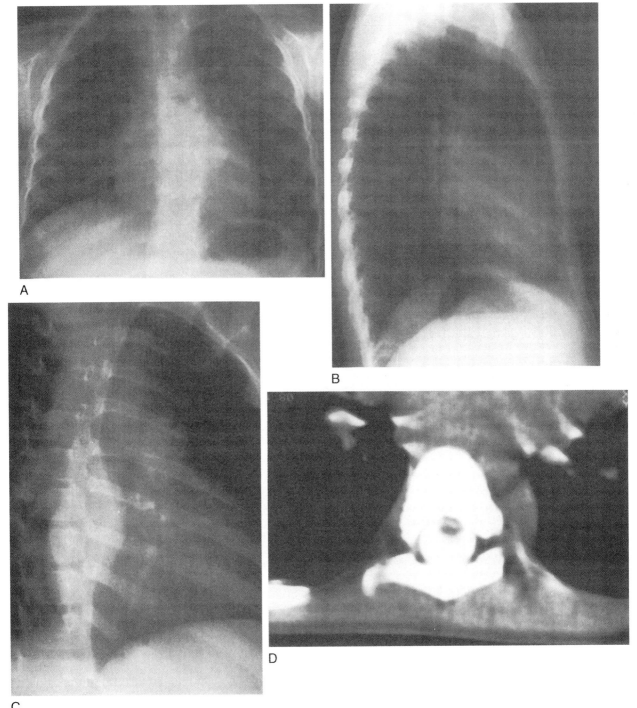

Figure 42–4 **A–C,** Chest films of a ganglioneuroblastoma. **D,** CT image of tumor extension into the spinal column.

view. Sympathetic chain tumors do not demonstrate calcification or bony changes. Characteristic radiographic findings of ganglioneuromas include oblong homogeneous low attenuation lesions on both enhanced and unenhanced CT. Neuroblastomas appear as aggressive soft tissue lesions with calcification (Figure 42-4). Ganglioneuroblastomas appear with combined radiographic features of both ganglioneuromas and neuroblastomas. On CT, paragangliomas characteristically appear in the aortopulmonary window with high

enhancement following administration of contrast medium (Figure 42-5).[32]

Tumors located in posterior mediastinum that extend into the spinal canal via the intervertebral foramen are referred to as dumbbell or sand-glass tumors. With a greater incidence in the number of cases of dumbbell neurogenic tumors in the posterior mediastinum, preoperative determination of intraspinal involvement of a neurogenic tumor is critical as surgical intervention mandates a combined

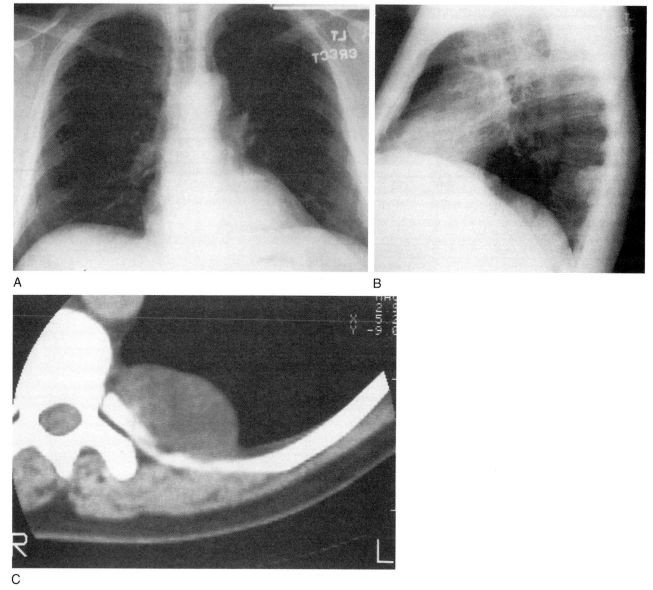

Figure 42–5 **A, B,** Chest films of a neurofibroma occurring in the posterior mediastinum. **C,** CT imaging better delineates the anatomical location of the mass and shows the absence of widening of the spinal foramen. This indicates that an intraspinal component to this tumor is unlikely.

surgical-neurosurgical procedure to avoid bleeding within the spinal canal that could lead to spinal cord compression.[5,18,33,66] This can be addressed by obtaining an MRI study. These patients may rarely present with symptoms of spinal cord compression. About 10% of patients with neurogenic tumors have extension through a vertebral foramen. Although the vast majority of these lesions are benign, approximately 1–2% are malignant. MRI typically shows a smoothly rounded homogeneous density abutting the vertebral column.

If a decision is made to obtain tissue, percutaneous FNA biopsy is an appropriate modality to confirm a diagnosis of a neurogenic tumor. A biopsy that reveals a spindle cell neoplasm with characteristic radiographic findings is diagnostic for a neurogenic tumor. Biopsies that demonstrate a combination of spindle cells and ganglion cells are diagnostic for ganglioneuromas. Immunohistochemical analysis can cinch the diagnosis, particularly with new emerging molecular markers such as S100 tumor antigen.[9,39]

Surgical intervention is the standard of care for neurogenic tumors, thus biopsy should be performed only if the results will alter therapy. Traditionally, surgical resection of a posterior mediastinum neurogenic tumor was accomplished through a posterolateral thoracotomy. Recent improvements in video-assisted thoracoscopic surgery have allowed minimally invasive approaches to diagnosis and treatment of many tumors in the posterior mediastinum.[41] Advantages of thoracoscopic surgery compared to the classic thoracotomy operation include decreased operative time, decreased average length of postoperative hospitalization, and more cosmetically acceptable results.[61] Benign intrathoracic tumors are ideal lesions for resection using a video-assisted technique.

Thoracoscopic resection of posterior mediastinal neurogenic tumors can be performed successfully regardless of tumor type or size. However, malignancy, local invasion, and tumors size greater than 5 cm are characteristics that will increase the likelihood of requiring an open incision.[68]

The standard cervical approach involves a posterolateral thoracotomy incision and exposure of the posterior mediastinum. The tumor is always in a paravertebral location and the exposure involves first incising the overlying pleura and then removing the lesion from the surrounding structures. Rarely is there any invasion of the bony vertebral body but it is important to recognize any involvement of a neural foramen. This is usually manifest by widening of the foramen and visualization of tumor going into the foramen along the nerve root. Some of these tumors may arise from the sympathetic chain and it is important to recognize this and resect that portion of the sympathetic chain. Usually a nerve root also will have to be sacrificed. Care should be taken to avoid resection of segmental vessels.

Once the pleura has been incised, it usually is easy to mobilize these lesions with a combination of sharp and blunt dissection. Complete resection can always be accomplished. Often the procedure may start with video thoracoscopic visualization of the tumor and mobilization. If this can be accomplished, the tumor can be removed through a small incision in the skin. However, if mobilization proves difficult by the video thoracoscopic approach, there should be no hesitation about conversion to an open procedure. This is especially important with lesions at the apex of the chest.

A well-described approach to dumbbell resection is a one-stage removal of the tumor performed through a posterolateral thoracotomy and transthoracic partial laminectomy.[57] This surgical approach avoids complications, notably from traction on the spinal cord.[59] Alternatively a posterior approach to the spine with laminectomy and removal of that portion of tumor within the canal can be immediately followed by thoracotomy and resection of the paravertebral tumor.

A more recently described procedure avoids a thoracotomy and invasion of the parietal pleura and uses a dorsal approach to perform a laminectomy with resection of a small portion of the neighboring rib root.[45] In either case, once a dumbbell tumor has been recognized, a combined two-team approach with thoracic and neurosurgeons working together to perform a one-stage removal is the procedure of choice.[60,66]

The prognosis of primary neurogenic mediastinal tumors varies with their histopathology. Patients with benign neurogenic tumors have an excellent prognosis with complete surgical resection while patients with malignant neurogenic tumors still have poor long-term survival prospects.[49] Recurrence of a benign lesion is unusual.[54]

With regard to neuroblastomas, spontaneous regression has been reported. Stage I (noninvasive) neuroblastomas are managed by resection alone while stage II lesions (locally invasive on same side of midline) require postoperative radiation. Stage III lesions (invasive across the midline) and stage IV lesions (systemic metastasis) require multimodality treatment including debulking, radiation, chemotherapy, and a second-look operation. Children under 1 year of age tend to have an excellent prognosis while in older children poorer prognosis is directly proportional to age.

Esophageal Masses

Esophageal-related posterior mediastinal masses include neoplasms, esophageal cysts,[16] diverticula, hiatal hernias, megaesophagus, and esophageal varices.[3]

Esophageal pathology rarely appears on chest roentograms. Plain chest radiography is frequently normal in patients with esophageal carcinoma. Subtle abnormalities are sometimes present including a retrocardiac mass, abnormal azygoesophageal recess interface, widened mediastinum, widened retrotracheal stripe, and esophageal air–fluid level. Hiatal hernia is the most common esophageal pathology detected on chest radiograph. As with other posterior mediastinal pathology, CT is reliable in predicting tumor size and assessing invasion of the mediastinum and tracheobronchial tree as well as spread to the liver, adrenals, and upper abdominal lymph nodes of esophageal carcinoma.

Endoscopic ultrasound (EUS) has become the most accurate imaging modality for locoregional cancer staging of the esophagus. FNA capabilities have added a whole new level of accuracy in nodal staging with reported numbers in the 90% range for luminal disease.[62] Transesophageal echocardiography (TEE) is effective at detecting mediastinal masses, though it should be used in conjunction with CT and/or MRI for more thorough evaluation. TEE can demonstrate impingement of the left atrium or ventricle, which is a common occurrence with posterior masses. Echocardiographers need to be aware of a type of posterior mediastinal encroachment that is common where there is gastric or esophageal pathology. These typically have two-dimensional echo features that may simulate a left atrial mass.[7]

Upper gastrointestinal barium examinations identify some type of hiatal hernia in as many as 15% of symptomatic patients.[17] This is discussed in detail in the following chapters. The barium swallow also remains the most useful study to clarify the nature of a retrocardiac mass such as a pseudotumoral venous collateral.[40] A complete discussion of esophageal cancer can be found in subsequent chapters.

Cysts of the Posterior Mediastinum

Mediastinal cysts form a group of uncommon benign lesions of congenital origin. Cystic lesions of the posterior mediastinum are relatively rare and include bronchogenic, hydatid,[25] enteric, intramural esophageal, and neuroenteric cysts. Thoracic CT is the most effective method for preoperative diagnosis of posterior mediastinal cysts.[67]

The significant controversy regarding these cysts is whether to manage them with observation or surgical resection. They are benign lesions in which surgery can be performed with a low morbidity and mortality rate, enabling the surgeon to rule out malignancy and offer a definitive cure.[67] Reports of uneventful operative courses without recurrence for mediastinal cysts are readily available.[30,53]

Bronchogenic Cysts

Mediastinal cysts constitute 20% of all mediastinal masses, and bronchogenic cysts make up 60% of all mediastinal cysts.[10,22,36,65,67] They are part of the spectrum of bronchopulmonary foregut abnormalities that include extralobar and intralobar sequestration and congenital cystic adenomatoid malformations.

They can be located in the lung parenchyma or mediastinum. Histologically, bronchogenic cysts demonstrate a lining covered with ciliated columnar epithelium. The wall consists of cartilage, mucous glands, and smooth muscle. They rarely communicate with the tracheobronchial tree.

Symptoms are present in the occasional patient, usually from compression of adjacent structures. Paraesophageal bronchogenic cysts have been pointed out incidentally during routine chest X-rays of the left posterior mediastinum (Figure 42-6). If the diagnosis of a bronchogenic cyst is made preoperatively and patients are asymptomatic, observation is an appropriate course. If there is any question of malignancy—based on radiographic appearance, positive cytology, or evidence of enlargement or recurrence—the lesion should be resected. The presence of symptoms—especially pain, cough, or hemoptysis—suggests the advisability of resection. Barium swallow may identify the source of dysphagia due to external compression. The presence of an air–fluid level indicates connection with the bronchopulmonary tree (rare) and the likelihood of recurrent infection and indicates that resection is in order. Once a bronchogenic cyst has become infected, the infection is difficult to eradicate and the lesion should be resected.[50]

Symptoms tend to develop with time, and resection at an asymptomatic stage may be best in healthy subjects. Video-assisted techniques provide ideal methods for resecting these benign lesions. Depending on location, many of these may be resected through the mediastinoscope.[55] Martinod et al reported their 3–7 year experience with thoracoscopic resection of 10 patients with posterior mediastinal bronchogenic. The average cyst size was 4.9 cm, and the largest diameter was 10 cm. There were no operative deaths and no postoperative complications. Long-term follow-up (range, 4.5–7.5 years) showed no late complications and no recurrence. This study found encouraging results for thoracoscopic excision of mediastinal bronchogenic cysts in selected patients.[36]

Gastroenteric Cysts

Gastroenteric, or duplication, cysts are periesophageal lesions that form from the posterior division of the primitive foregut. They may cause a middle or posterior mediastinal mass, particularly in the young. They occur within or adjacent to the wall of the esophagus. Communication with the upper gastrointestinal tract is uncommon.

Histologically, duplication cysts are lined by nonkeratinizing squamous, ciliated columnar, gastric, or small intestinal epithelium. In distinguishing bronchogenic from esophageal cysts, the lining epithelium is not helpful, but the presence of two muscle layers in esophageal cysts and bronchial glands or bronchial cartilage in bronchogenic cysts enables categorization in the majority of cases.[53]

Patients may present with a variety of symptoms but usually these lesions are asymptomatic. Respiratory compromise with cough, dyspnea, recurrent pulmonary infections, and chest pain is not that uncommon. If gastric mucosa is present, perforation into the esophagus can cause hematemesis or erosion into the adjacent lung parenchyma can develop into an abscess.

Diagnosis is facilitated by with esophageal ultrasound, chest CT scan, or contrast studies of the upper gastrointestinal tract[16] (Figure 42-7).[99] Tc scanning can be used to look for ectopic gastric mucosa. Resection is the therapy of choice, whether by thoracoscopic or open technique. Many of these lesions are amenable to a minimally invasive thoracoscopic approach that still allows for complete resection. Posterolateral thoracotomy is the procedure of choice when greater exposure is required. The question always arises as to whether it is necessary to resect these benign lesions. Certainly if the lesion is producing compressive symptoms or is infected resection is indicated; it is the asymptomatic lesion discovered accidentally that begs the question as to whether resection is indicated. Often it is unclear if the lesion is truly cystic because the cyst contents become so inspissated as to appear solid. When the cystic nature of the lesion is unclear a case can be made for resection, especially through a minimally invasive approach. Observation may be the approach chosen for those asymptomatic lesions that are clearly cystic.

Neuroenteric Cysts

Neuroenteric cysts make up 5–10% of foregut lesions. They present in infants under 1 year of age and are uncommon in adults.[30] They have a connection to the meninges usually by a stalk and are associated with congenital defects of the thoracic spine. Neuroenteric cysts possess endodermal and ectodermal or neurogenic elements. They develop because of failure of separation of the notochord from the primitive gut. A CT scan showing a cystic mediastinal lesion associated with a vertebral abnormality such as congenital scoliosis, hemivertebrae, and spina bifida should prompt consideration of neuroenteric cysts.

Other Masses of the Posterior Mediastinum

Primary or metastatic tumors of the thoracic spine may also appear as a posterior mediastinal paravertebral mass. Lymphomas, particularly Hodgkin disease, may involve the posterior parietal group of lymph nodes and produce a fusiform paravertebral soft tissue mass. Infections, such as tuberculosis, can result in a paravertebral mass as can a post-traumatic hematoma. A descending thoracic aortic aneurysm is an important lesion that can masquerade as a mediastinal neoplasm.

Extramedullary hematopoiesis, a compensatory response to insufficient bone marrow blood cell production, is a rare cause of a paravertebral mass.[15] The preferred sites of extramedullary hematopoietic involvement are the spleen, liver, and lymph nodes.[15] However, in hereditary spherocytosis, for example, the posterior paravertebral mediastinum is also commonly involved. It should be noted that extramedullary hematopoietic tumors can occur without severe chronic hemolytic anemia. Therefore, this lesion must be considered in the differential diagnosis of a posterior mediastinal mass in patients even without clinical evidence of anemia.[8] Earlier reports demonstrated the utility of a conventional chest radiograph and CT scan of the thorax for diagnosis without biopsy or thoracotomy.[13] Later reports clarify the superiority of MRI in identifying intrathoracic extramedullary

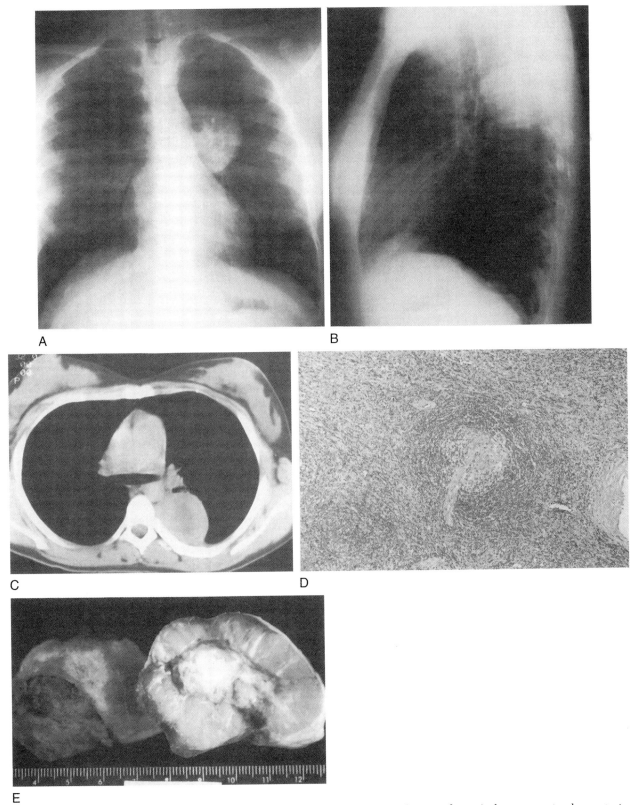

Figure 42–6 **A, B,** Chest films of a giant lymph node hyperplasia (Castleman's disease) that occurs in the posterior mediastinum. **C,** CT image of the tumor is similar to a neurogenic tumor. **D,** Photomicrograph of the tumor shows the small hyaline follicles and interfollicular capillary proliferation that are characteristic of the hyaline vascular form. **E,** Photograph of a gross specimen.

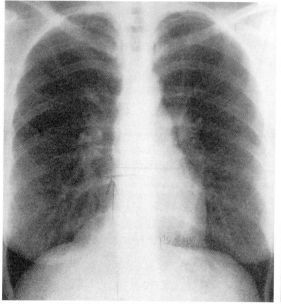

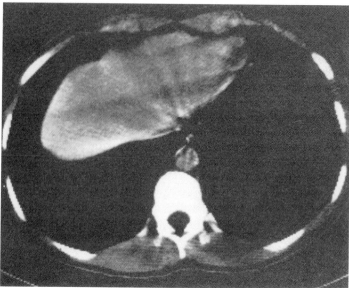

A B

Figure 42–7 A, Chest film of a pericardial cyst in the right pericardiophrenic angle. **B,** CT image shows the characteristic nearer attenuation of the mass and the typical anatomical location.

hematopoiesis though it usually is used in conjunction with CT because of specific limitations.[15,58]

Castleman's disease (giant lymph node hyperplasia) is characterized by mass lesions that are vascular tumors often surrounded by lymphadenopathy.[21,44] This arrangement makes CT useful diagnostically, since CT may reveal lymphadenopathy surrounding an encapsulated mass that enhances brightly and is distinct from the aorta (Figure 42-8). The term is applied to three lesions that are histologically distinct: hyaline vascular, plasma cell, and generalized. The first two represent localized disease, whereas the third refers to multicentric (generalized) disease.

Hyaline vascular Castleman's disease comprises 90% of cases. It is a localized lesion usually found incidentally in asymptomatic patients. Castleman's disease presenting as a spinal epidural mass lesion with cord compression has been reported.[23] Surgical excision is the treatment of choice; radiotherapy has not been effective. The plasma cell variant, also localized, is much less common. Patients are much more likely to have symptoms and present with fever, fatigue, weight loss, and hemolytic anemia. The sedimentation rate is often high and associated with hypergammaglobulinemia, which results from the production of interleukin-6 by the hyperplastic lymph nodes. Resection is the treatment of choice to prevent malignant degeneration.

Generalized, or multicentric, Castleman's disease has the histological features of both localized forms. The disease occurs in older patients, who typically present with severe systemic symptoms, generalized lymphadenopathy, and hepatosplenomegaly. The mortality from this disease is 50%, and the median survival is 27 months. Progression to lymphoma is common. The diagnosis of lymphoma is made from biopsy, and treatment is directed at managing the lymphoma.

Other rare causes of a primary posterior mediastinal mass usually presenting in the paravertebral sulci include angiomyolipoma,[14,28] extralobar pulmonary sequestration,[24] neuroendocrine carcinoma,[20] mediastinal ependymomas,[64] cellular hemangiomas,[46] melanotic paraganglioma,[19] and mediastinal extension of a pancreatic pseudocyst.

▶ INFECTIONS OF THE MEDIASTINUM

Descending necrotizing mediastinitis is a potentially fatal condition in its acute or chronic form that can involve the posterior mediastinum.[11] Acute mediastinitis most commonly occurs following postoperative infection or esophageal perforation. The organism most commonly isolated is *Staphylococcus*. In acute mediastinitis, the patient will present with the typical signs of infection including fever, tachycardia, and a leukocytosis. Subcutaneous emphysema may be another clue to an infectious source.[11,42] In chronic mediastinitis, the etiology is a granulomatous infection. When the granulomas rupture, the contents lead to a fibrotic reaction.

The posterior mediastinum is more susceptible to infection than the other compartments of the thorax. Anatomically, this is explained by the relative accessibility of the posterior mediastinum to the neck and abdomen. Inferiorly, the hiatus for the inferior vena cava and aorta crossing the diaphragm are well sealed. However, the esophageal hiatus, which is most posterior, is not closed as well and provides a tract between the posterior mediastinum and the abdominal cavity. Similarly, the infections from the head and neck have easier access to the posterior mediastinum. The more anterior fascial planes that come down from the neck terminate before reaching the mediastinal compartments. There are two posterior spaces that are direct connections between the pharynx and neck and

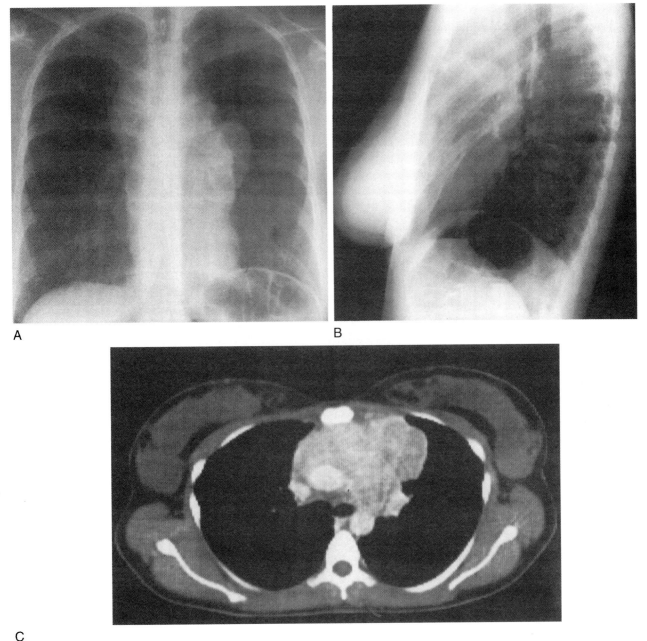

Figure 42–8 A, B, Chest films of a large B cell non-Hodgkin's lymphoma that involves the anterosuperior mediastinum. **C,** CT image shows the involvement of the mediastinal structures by the lymphoma.

mediastinum. The first space is located between the visceral fascia and the alar fascia and is termed the "danger space" because of its direct communication with the posterior mediastinum. The second space is located between the prevertebral fascia and the vertebral bodies allowing communication of vertebral infections.[11]

Not surprisingly, abscesses in the posterior mediastinum are more frequent than those in the anterior compartment. Although primary infection is possible, most infections are secondary and the source usually is readily apparent. Most common signs of posterior mediastinal abscess are pain, dysphagia, cough, and dyspnea. The pain occurs most often on swallowing and coughing, and it is felt posteriorly in the interscapular region or may radiate anteriorly. The symptoms are due to encroachment on the esophagus and tra-

chea in the upper part of the chest. Esophageal perforation is the most common cause of a posterior mediastinum abscess. Other causes of a posterior mediastinal abscess include extension of infection from the oropharynx, spine, lung pleura, or abdominal cavity.

CT scan may demonstrate an air–fluid level or mediastinal air (Figure 42-9). Nonsurgical management includes intravenous antibiotics, but surgical intervention usually is required on an urgent basis. Surgical intervention includes widely opening the mediastinal compartment by incising the pleura followed by debridement, irrigation, drainage, and wound closure with or without a muscle flap. In diffuse mediastinitis involving the posterior mediastinum, pericarditis and/or bilateral exudative pleuritis are often present.

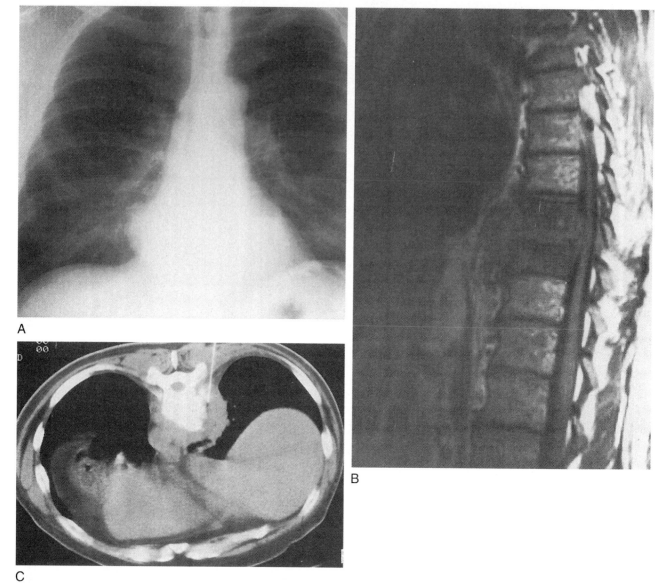

Figure 42–9 Paraspinous abscess in a 45-year-old male with AIDS and a systemic infection. **A,** Frontal chest radiograph demonstrates a mass behind the right side of the heart. **B,** Spinal MRI demonstrates reduced intensity in two vertebral bodies with posterior and anterior masses. **C,** CT-guided aspiration of the mass demonstrated a paraspinous *Staphylococcus aureus* infection. (*Reprinted with permission from Gamsu G: The mediastinum. In Moss AA, Gamsu G, Genant, HK, editors: Computed Tomography of the Body, 2nd ed., Vol. 1. Philadelphia: W.B. Saunders, 1992, p. 83.*)

▶ SUMMARY

Lesions of the posterior mediastinum most commonly are neurogenic in origin and usually are benign in adults. Despite this recognition, surgical intervention commonly is required. Minimally invasive surgical approaches may provide additional justification for removing these lesions before they become symptomatic.

REFERENCES

1. Adam A, Hochholzer L: Ganglioneuroblastoma of the posterior mediastinum: A clinicopathologic review of 80 cases. Cancer 47:373–381, 1981.

2. Al Refai M, Brunelli A, Fianchini A: Giant schwannoma of the posterior mediastinum. Chest 115:907–908, 1999.

3. Basheda SG, O'Donovan P, Golish JA: Giant esophageal varices. An unusual cause of a posterior mediastinal mass. Chest 103:1284–1285, 1993.

4. Bressler EL, Kirkham JA: Mediastinal masses: Alternative approaches to CT-guided needle biopsy. Radiology 191:391–396, 1994.

5. Buchfelder M, Nomikos P, Paulus W, et al: Spinal-thoracic dumbbell meningioma: A case report. Spine 26:1500–1504, 2001.

6. Chowbey PK, Vashistha A, Khullar R, et al: Laparoscopic excision of a lower posterior mediastinal paraspinal mass: Technique and feasibility of the laparoscopic approach. Surg Laparosc Endosc Percutan Tech 12:378–81; discussion 381–382, 2002.

7. D'Cruz IA, Feghali N, Gross CM: Echocardiographic manifestations of mediastinal masses compressing or encroaching on the heart. Echocardiography 11:523–533, 1994.

8. De Montpreville VT, Dulmet EM, Chapelier AR, et al: Extramedullary hematopoietic tumors of the posterior mediastinum related to asymptomatic refractory anemia. Chest 104:1623–1624, 1993.

9. Dillon KM, Hill CM, Cameron CH, et al: Mediastinal mixed dendritic cell sarcoma with hybrid features. J Clin Pathol 55:791–794, 2002.

10. Divisi D, Battaglia C, Crisci R, et al: Diagnostic and therapeutic approaches for masses in the posterior mediastinum. Acta Biomed Ateneo Parmense 69:123–128, 1998.

11. Endo S, Murayama F, Hasegawa T, et al: Guideline of surgical management based on diffusion of descending necrotizing mediastinitis. Jpn J Thorac Cardiovasc Surg 47:14–19, 1999.

12. Esposito C, Romeo C: Surgical anatomy of the mediastinum. Semin Pediatr Surg 8:50–53, 1999.

13. Falappa P, Danza FM, Leone G, et al: Thoracic extramedullary hematopoiesis: Evaluation by conventional radiology and computed tomography. Diagn Imaging 51:19–24, 1982.

14. Fukuzawa J, Shimizu T, Sakai E, et al: [Case report of angiomyolipoma of the posterior upper mediastinum]. Nihon Kyobu Shikkan Gakkai Zasshi 30:464–467, 1992.

15. Granjo E, Bauerle R, Sampaio R, et al: Extramedullary hematopoiesis in hereditary spherocytosis deficient in ankyrin: A case report. Int J Hematol 76:153–156, 2002.

16. Hara M, Arakawa T, Ogino H, et al: A case of isolated esophageal cyst in the posterior mediastinum. Radiat Med 19:161–164, 2001.

17. Hashemi M, Sillin LF, Peters JH: Current concepts in the management of paraesophageal hiatal hernia. J Clin Gastroenterol 29:8–13, 1999.

18. Heltzer JM, Krasna MJ, Aldrich F, et al: Thoracoscopic excision of a posterior mediastinal "dumbbell" tumor using a combined approach. Ann Thorac Surg 60:431–433, 1995.

19. Hofmann WJ, Wockel W, Thetter O, et al: Melanotic paraganglioma of the posterior mediastinum. Virchows Arch 425:641–646, 1995.

20. Horie Y, Kato M: Neuroendocrine carcinoma of the posterior mediastinum: A possible primary lesion. Arch Pathol Lab Med 123:933–936, 1999.

21. Hummel P, Benjamin V, Zagzag D: March 2002: 28-year-old woman with neck and back pain. Brain Pathol 12:395–397, 2002.

22. Itoh H, Shitamura T, Kataoka H, et al: Retroperitoneal bronchogenic cyst: Report of a case and literature review. Pathol Int 49:152–155, 1999.

23. Kachur E, Ang LC, Megyesi JF: Castleman's disease and spinal cord compression: Case report. Neurosurgery 50:399–402; discussion 402–403, 2002.

24. Kamiyoshihara M, Kawashima O, Sakata S, et al: Extralobar pulmonary sequestration in the posterior mediastinum. Scand Cardiovasc J 35:157–158, 2001.

25. Karnak I, Ciftci AO, Tanyel FC: Hydatid cyst: An unusual etiology for a cystic lesion of the posterior mediastinum. J Pediatr Surg 33:759–760, 1998.

26. Kawashima A, Fishman EK, Kuhlman JE, et al: CT of posterior mediastinal masses. Radiographics 11:1045–1067, 1991.

27. Kelemen JJ 3rd, Naunheim KS: Minimally invasive approaches to mediastinal neoplasms. Semin Thorac Cardiovasc Surg 12:301–306, 2000.

28. Kim YH, Kwon NY, Myung NH, et al: A case of mediastinal angiomyolipoma. Korean J Intern Med 16:277–280, 2001.

29. Kumar A, Kumar S, Aggarwal S, et al: Thoracoscopy: The preferred approach for the resection of selected posterior mediastinal tumors. J Laparoendosc Adv Surg Tech A 12:345–353, 2002.

30. Kumar R, Nayak SR: Unusual neuroenteric cysts: Diagnosis and management. Pediatr Neurosurg 37:321–330, 2002.

31. LeBlanc J, Guttentag AR, Shepard JA, et al: Imaging of mediastinal foregut cysts. Can Assoc Radiol J 45:381–386, 1994.

32. Lee JY, Lee KS, Han J, et al: Spectrum of neurogenic tumors in the thorax: CT and pathologic findings. J Comput Assist Tomogr 23:399–406, 1999.

33. Liu HP, Yim AP, Wan J, et al: Thoracoscopic removal of intrathoracic neurogenic tumors: A combined Chinese experience. Ann Surg 232:187–190, 2000.

34. Lonergan GJ, Schwab CM, Suarez ES, et al: Neuroblastoma, ganglioneuroblastoma, and ganglioneuroma: Radiologic-pathologic correlation. Radiographics 22:911–934, 2002.

35. Marchevsky AM: Mediastinal tumors of peripheral nervous system origin. Semin Diagn Pathol 16:65–78, 1999.

36. Martinod E, Pons F, Azorin J, et al: Thoracoscopic excision of mediastinal bronchogenic cysts: Results in 20 cases. Ann Thorac Surg 69:1525–1528, 2000.

37. Mondal A: Cytopathology of neuroblastoma, ganglioneuroblastoma and ganglioneuroma. J Indian Med Assoc 93:340–343, 1995.

38. Moon WK, Im JG, Han MC: Malignant schwannomas of the thorax: CT findings. J Comput Assist Tomogr 17:274–276, 1993.

39. Moran CA, Suster S, Fishback N, et al: Mediastinal paragangliomas. A clinicopathologic and immunohistochemical study of 16 cases. Cancer 72:2358–2364, 1993.

40. Moult PJ, Waite DW, Dick R: Posterior mediastinal venous masses in patients with portal hypertension. Gut 16:57–61, 1975.

41. Naunheim KS: Video thoracoscopy for masses of the posterior mediastinum. Ann Thorac Surg 56:657–658, 1993.

42. Nomori H, Horio H, Kobayashi R: Descending necrotizing mediastinitis secondary to pharyngitis. A case report. Scand Cardiovasc J 31:233–235, 1997.

43. Nordenstrom B: Paravertebral approach to the posterior mediastinum for mediastinography and needle biopsy. Acta Radiol Diagn (Stockh) 12:298–304, 1972.

44. Olscamp G, Weisbrod G, Sanders D, et al: Castleman disease: Unusual manifestations of an unusual disorder. Radiology 135:43–48, 1980.

45. Osada H, Aoki H, Yokote K, et al: Dumbbell neurogenic tumor of the mediastinum: A report of three cases undergoing single-staged complete removal without thoracotomy. Jpn J Surg 21:224–228, 1991.

46. Parker JR, Knott-Craig C, Min KW, et al: Cellular hemangioma of the posterior mediastinum: Unusual presentation of a rare vascular neoplasm. J Okla State Med Assoc 90:7–9, 1997.

47. Partrick DA, Rothenberg SS: Thoracoscopic resection of mediastinal masses in infants and children: An evaluation of technique and results. J Pediatr Surg 36:1165–1167, 2001.

48. Penkrot RJ, Bolden R: Thoracic neurilemmoma: Case report and review of the world literature. J Comput Tomogr 9:13–15, 1985.

49. Reeder LB: Neurogenic tumors of the mediastinum. Semin Thorac Cardiovasc Surg 12:261–267, 2000.

50. Roberts JR, Smythe WR, Weber RW, et al: Thoracoscopic management of descending necrotizing mediastinitis. Chest 112:850–854, 1997.

51. Ronson RS, Duarte I, Miller JI: Embryology and surgical anatomy of the mediastinum with clinical implications. Surg Clin North Am 80:157–169, x–xi, 2000.

52. Saenz NC, Schnitzer JJ, Eraklis AE, et al: Posterior mediastinal masses. J Pediatr Surg 28:172–176, 1993.

53. Salyer DC, Salyer WR, Eggleston JC: Benign developmental cysts of the mediastinum. Arch Pathol Lab Med 101:136–139, 1977.

54. Schmezer A, Reinosch W, Laqua D, et al: [Thoracic neurinoma: A rare tumor of the posterior mediastinum]. Chirurg 67:90–92, 1996.

702

55. Smythe WR, Bavaria JE, Kaiser LR: Mediastinoscopic subtotal removal of mediastinal cysts. Chest 114:614–617, 1998.

56. Strollo DC, Rosado-de-Christenson ML, Jett JR: Primary mediastinal tumors: Part II. Tumors of the middle and posterior mediastinum. Chest 112:1344–1357, 1997.

57. Suganuma H, Nakamura H, Sugiyama N, et al: [A case of dumbbell neurogenic tumors of the mediastinum]. Kyobu Geka 42:827–830, 1989.

58. Tamburrini O, Della Sala M, Mancuso PP, et al: [The diagnostic imaging of intrathoracic extramedullary hematopoiesis]. Radiol Med (Torino) 84:582–586, 1992.

59. Vasilakis D, Papaconstantinou C, Aletras H: Dumb-bell intrathoracic and intraspinal neurofibroma. Report of a case. Scand J Thorac Cardiovasc Surg 20:171–173, 1986.

60. Viard H, Sautreaux JL, Cougard P, et al: [Dumbbell neurogenic tumors of the posterior mediastinum. Apropos of five cases]. Ann Chir 45:699–703, 1991.

61. Watanabe M, Takagi K, Aoki T, et al: [Thoracoscopic resection of mediastinal tumors]. Nippon Kyobu Geka Gakkai Zasshi 42:1016–1020, 1994.

62. Waxman I, Dye CE: Interventional endosonography. Cancer J 8 (Suppl I):S113–123, 2002.

63. Wernecke K, Diederich S: Sonographic features of mediastinal tumors. AJR Am J Roentgenol 163:1357–1364, 1994.

64. Wilson RW, Moran CA: Primary ependymoma of the mediastinum: A clinicopathologic study of three cases. Ann Diagn Pathol 2:293–300, 1998.

65. Yang SW, Linton JA, Ryu SJ, et al: Retroperitoneal multilocular bronchogenic cyst adjacent to adrenal gland. Yonsei Med J 40:523–526, 1999.

66. Yuksel M, Pamir N, Ozer F, et al: The principles of surgical management in dumbbell tumors. Eur J Cardiothorac Surg 10:569–573, 1996.

67. Zambudio AR, Lanzas JT, Calvo MJ, et al: Non-neoplastic mediastinal cysts. Eur J Cardiothorac Surg 22:712–716, 2002.

68. Zierold D, Halow KD: Thoracoscopic resection as the preferred approach to posterior mediastinal neurogenic tumors. Surg Laparosc Endosc Percutan Tech 10:222–225, 2000.

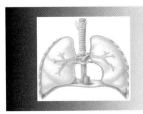

Surgical Treatment of Hyperhidrosis

Steven M. Keller and Chien-Chih Lin

CHAPTER **43**

▶ INTRODUCTION

Hyperhidrosis is commonly defined as sweating in excess of physiological requirements. Perhaps the earliest recognition of this disorder was by Charles Dickens, whose description of Uriah Heep in *David Copperfield* is an accurate clinical presentation of palmar hyperhidrosis[1,3]: "I saw Uriah Heep shutting up the office, and, feeling friendly towards everybody, went in and spoke to him, and at parting, gave him my hand. But oh, what a clammy hand this was! As ghostly to the touch as to the sight! I rubbed mine afterwards, to warm it, and to rub his off."

Patients are referred to a thoracic surgeon because of inordinate sweating of the palms, face, or axilla. Less commonly, patients complain of severe facial sweating. Multiple prior evaluations by internists and dermatologists are common.

The earliest sympathectomy undertaken specifically for treatment of hyperhidrosis was performed in Europe by Kotzareff in 1920.[14] The first sympathectomy for treatment of hyperhidrosis in the United States was accomplished in 1932 by Adson.[2] The earliest thoracoscopic sympathectomy was performed in 1939 for treatment of hypertension.[12] The first thoracoscopic sympathectomy for treatment of hyperhidrosis was reported in 1978.[16] Paravertebral, supraclavicular, transaxillary, and transthoracic approaches have also been utilized to gain access to the sympathetic chain. Interest and large volumes of cases did not occur until the availability of video-assisted thoracic surgery.

▶ CLINICAL PRESENTATION

The typical patient gives a history of palmar and plantar sweating since early childhood. Parents may report that excessive wetness of the hands and feet was present during infancy. Patients commonly report having been teased by other children who would not want to hold their hands and berated by teachers for submitting assignments that were wet and smudged. Puddles are left on computer and piano keyboards. As patients enter adulthood their wet hands adversely affect social interaction and influence career choice.

Sweating is intermittent and occurs both at times of apparent calm and obvious stress. It is usually worse during the summer months. Though the degree of hyperhidrosis varies, sweating is much greater than the dampness associated with stress. A dry hand may become soaking wet within minutes. Perspiration forms on the volar surface of the fingers, thenar, and hypothenar eminences and fills the palmar skin folds (Figure 43-1). Sweat may actually run down the arm and drip to the floor.

Virtually all patients with palmar hyperhidrosis also suffer from plantar hyperhidrosis, the degree and timing of which parallel that manifested in the hands. When walking barefoot, tracks similar to those seen after exiting a swimming pool are left. Footwear are ruined by the constant moistness. Open toe sandals are impossible to wear due to slippage of the wet foot. Despite the frequent moistness, fungal infections are rare. As many as 50% of patients with palmar and plantar hyperhidrosis also suffer from concomitant axillary hyperhidrosis that causes garment staining and odor (bromhidrosis).*

In addition to altering their lifestyle to avoid direct or indirect hand contact, sufferers from hyperhidrosis have developed a number of coping mechanisms. A handkerchief or tissue is always on hand. They frequently wipe their hands on their clothing. In social situations, a cold drink is ever present to provide a reason for their cold wet hand or an excuse for the need to wipe their hand prior to performing a handshake.

---

*References. 1, 11, 16, 21, 29, 36, 44.

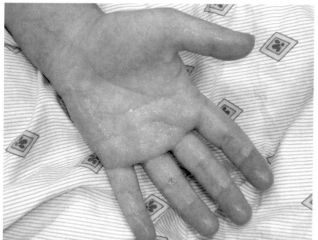

Figure 43–1 Typical appearance of palmar hyperhidrosis. Note wetness on thenar and hypothenar eminences as well as on the palmar surface of distal phalanges.

EPIDEMIOLOGY

The prevalence of palmar and plantar hyperhidrosis is estimated as 0.6–1%[1] and affects all racial groups. Investigators from Asia claim a prevalence as great as 2%, but no rigorous studies have been conducted. Though generalized hyperhidrosis may be associated with thyrotoxicosis, neurological diseases, and rare inherited disorders, patients with classic palmar and plantar hyperhidrosis do not have concomitant illnesses.

A familial history of hyperhidrosis has been obtained in as many as 65% of patients who have undergone thoracoscopic sympathectomy.[1,11,36,38] Detailed kindred information provided by 49 affected individuals has led to the conclusion that the disease allele is actually present in 5% of the population and that one or two copies of the allele will result in hyperhidrosis in 25% of carriers.[38]

AUTONOMIC NERVOUS SYSTEM

Anatomy and Function

The autonomic nervous system is responsible for thermoregulation. Though both the sympathetic and parasympathetic components may contribute to sweating, the sympathetic nervous system primarily controls extremity sweating. Impulses originating in the hypothalamus reach preganglionic fibers located in the lateral horn of the ventral root of the spinal column.[9] These myelinated fibers exit the ventral root and travel a brief distance through the spinal nerve before exiting as the white rami communicantes to join the paravertebral ganglia of the sympathetic chain. The nerve may immediately establish a synapse with an unmyelinated postganglionic fiber that returns to the spinal nerve as the gray ramus communicantes or may ascend a variable distance within the sympathetic chain before synapsing with a postganglionic fiber. The postganglionic nerve often travels a great distance before arriving at its target organ.

Sympathetic fibers originating from spinal levels T1–T6 ascend in the sympathetic chain and reach the hand via con-

nections of the stellate ganglia to the brachial plexus. The precise spinal levels responsible for palmar sweating have not been defined though T2 has been thought to be the common pathway. Release of acetylcholine from the postganglionic neurons stimulates the eccrine sweat glands.

The sympathetic chain descends vertically within the thorax over the rib heads (Figure 43-2); rarely it is found between the medial border of the rib head and the callus longus muscle.[45] The sympathetic ganglia are located approximately 2 mm cranial to the mid-portion of the underlying vertebral body.[46] For example, the T2 ganglia is located between the heads of the second and third ribs. In addition to the orderly arrangement of the sympathetic nerves, Kuntz identified inconstant sympathetic branches from the second intercostal nerve to the first intercostal nerve (and hence brachial plexus) that bypassed the stellate ganglia.[15] The physiological function of these nerves is unclear.

Whether hyperhidrosis represents focal dysfunction of the autonomic nervous system or is emblematic of a more global abnormality remains unknown. Resting palmar sweat production at room temperature is twice normal[41] (Figure 43-3A). The sudomotor skin response is enhanced due to shortened nerve recovery time.[27] Palmar sweat production in response to stress is greatly increased (Figure 43-3B). When compared with unaffected controls, pulmonary function and resting cardiac function in the supine position are normal.[30,31,33,43] Circulating plasma catecholamine levels are within normal limits.[32] However, peak exercise heart rate and resting heart rate in the standing position are increased.[30,31]

TREATMENT

Nonoperative

Aluminum chloride hexahydrate 20% anhydrous ethyl alcohol solution (Drysol) has been utilized as initial therapy of

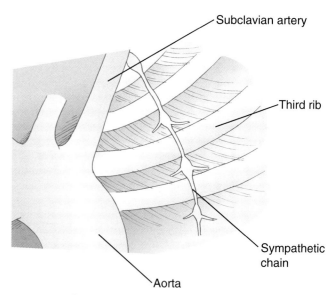

Figure 43–2 Left sympathetic chain.

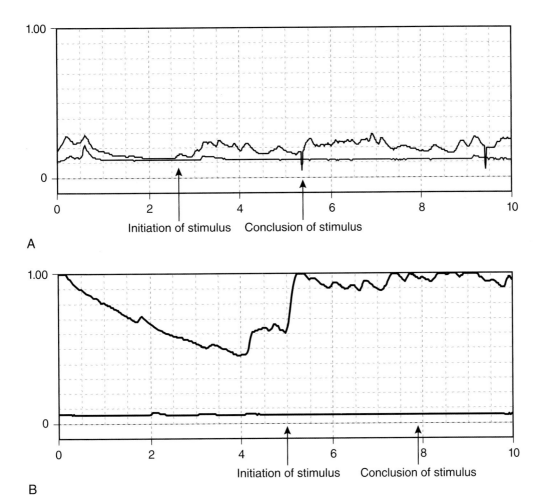

A

B

Figure 43–3 A, Normal sweat response. Following attachment of the measuring device (Skin Moisture Meter SKD 2000, Skinos Co., LTD, Japan), the patient reaches baseline. Sweating increases as autonomic stimulation begins. The subject never returns to baseline. The ordinate is minutes and the abscissa is cubic centimeters of moisture. Upper line—thenar eminence. Lower line—forehead. **B,** Abnormal sweat response. Attachment of the measuring device causes anxiety and the baseline never reaches normal. The response to the stimulus is many times greater than the normal subject. The ordinate is minutes and the abscissa is cubic centimeters of moisture. Upper line—thenar eminence. Lower line—forehead.

palmar and plantar hyperhidrosis. The solution is applied daily prior to sleep to the affected area and is covered in plastic wrap to prevent damage to clothing or bedding. Application frequency is decreased once the desired anhidrosis is obtained. Side effects include rash and paradoxical hyperhidrosis. Efficacy has not been assessed in a controlled trial and many patients report therapeutic failure.

Iontophoresis, placement of the hands or feet in a tap water solution through which an electric current flows, has been utilized as treatment of hyperhidrosis. The precise mechanism responsible for the elimination of sweat production is unknown. A battery-operated device is commercially available (Drionic). Control of palmar hyperhidrosis was reported in 82% of 112 patients who underwent eight daily 15-min treatments.[13] The mean remission was 35 days. Tingling, erythema, and vesicle formation were undesirable side effects.

The neurotoxin botulinum toxin A (Botox) stops sweat production by blocking the release of acetylcholine from the postganglionic nerve end. A randomized trial has

demonstrated efficacy of this treatment for axillary hyperhidrosis.[10] Other investigators have reported success for palmar hyperhidrosis utilizing 20–30 intradermal injections.[28,39] Median duration of sweat control varies between 6 and 9 months. Weakness of the intrinsic muscle of the hand manifested by a decrease in the thumb–index finger pinch strength has been reported in 25–60% of patients.

Oral anticholinergic medications such as glycopyrrolate and oxybutynin have been employed to block the stimulation of the sweat gland caused by the release of acetylcholine from the postganglionic sympathetic nerve fiber. No published reports have confirmed the efficacy of this treatment approach. Dry mouth, blurry vision, and constipation are common side effects.

Surgery

The goal of surgery is to interdict the sympathetic nerve innervation to the hand, axilla, or face. This may be accomplished by transecting or clipping the sympathetic chain;

706

resection of ganglia is not necessary. The thoracic level at which interruption is necessary to achieve the desired anhidrosis while simultaneously minimizing systemic side effects is not precisely known. Traditionally, palmar hyperhidrosis has been treated by transecting the sympathetic chain over the second and third ribs. If concomitant axillary hyperhidrosis is present, the sympathetic chain is also transected over the fourth rib. In the absence of palmar hyperhidrosis, axillary sweating is treated by transecting the sympathetic chain over the third and fourth ribs. Palmar hyperhidrosis may be effectively treated by limiting the transection to the level of the third rib.[35] Regardless of the surgical technique, correct identification of the anatomical level is crucial.

The second rib is generally the most proximal rib that can be seen within the thorax and can reliably be identified by a vertical, descending, arterial branch that crosses the rib 1 cm lateral to the sympathetic chain.[5] This arterial branch originates from the subclavian artery and forms the second intercostal artery (Figure 43-4A). The first intercostal space is covered by a fatpad and the first rib is generally not visible from within the thorax. Additional landmarks are the azygos vein, which lies at the level of the fifth interspace and the aortic arch, which reaches to the fourth interspace. The rib number can be determined with certainty by obtaining an intraoperative X-ray after a metallic marker has been introduced into the chest and placed over a rib.

Bilateral endoscopic thoracic sympathecotomy is the procedure of choice for the surgical treatment of palmar hyperhidrosis. Hospitalization is not necessary and the results are uniformly excellent. Virtually all patients will have dry warm hands. Axillary and facial sweating may also be treated in a similar fashion. The details of the operation are determined by the level at which the sympathetic chain is clipped or transected.

Operative Procedure for Hyperhidrosis

Following induction of general anesthesia, the arms are abducted 90°. The head of the operating table is elevated or the table flexed into the semi-Fowler's position to help the lungs fall away from the apex (Figure 43-5). A double-lumen endotracheal tube is not necessary. A 1-cm incision is made over the third interspace in the anterior axillary line just lateral to the pectoralis major muscle. CO_2 gas (600–1200 cm³) is insufflated, a 10-mm trocar is introduced, and the operating thoracoscopic (Karl Storz 26037 AA) is inserted. The sympathetic chain is visualized crossing the rib heads and the ribs correctly numbered. A cautery device is introduced via the operating thoracoscope.

Isolated palmar hyperhidrosis is treated by transecting the sympathetic chain over the second and third ribs (Figure 43-4B). Concomitant axillary hyperhidrosis is treated by transecting the sympathetic chain over the second, third, and fourth ribs. Isolated axillary hyperhidrosis may be treated by transecting the sympathetic chain over the third and fourth ribs. Craniofacial hyperhidrosis is treated by transecting the sympathetic chain over the second rib.[23] Hemostasis is ascertained and the lung inflated under direct vision as the trocar is withdrawn. The wound is closed and the identical procedure is repeated in the contralateral thorax. A chest X-ray is obtained in the recovery room. Small apical pneumothoraces that do not require chest tubes are common. The patient is discharged when awake and comfortable.

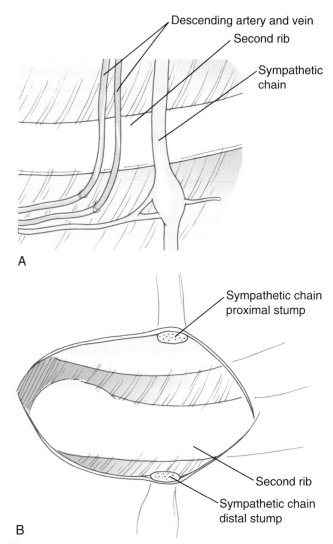

Figure 43-4 A, Descending vessels crossing the right second rib lateral to the sympathetic chain. **B,** Appearance following transection of the sympathetic chain. The proximal and distal stumps of the sympathetic chain are visible.

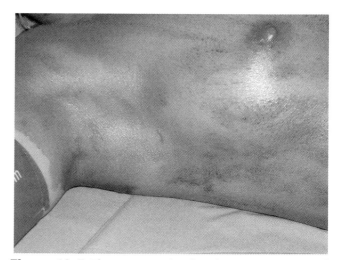

Figure 43-5 The patient is placed in the supine position with both arms perpendicular to the torso. A 1-cm incision is made lateral to the pectoralis major muscle at the level of the axillary hairline.

Variations of the procedure include the use of intermittent apnea instead of CO_2 gas and the harmonic scalpel in place of electrocautery. If clips are utilized, two 5-mm clips are necessary, the first for the 5-mm thoracoscope and the second for the automatic clip applier. Investigators who have access to millimeter diameter scopes and cautery instruments have described smaller incisions.[17] Intraoperative palmar skin temperature monitoring provides documentation of successful operation.[40] The author (S.M.K.) regularly obtains a 2° C increase.

Results of Endoscopic Thoracic Sympathecotomy

Virtually all patients report cure of palmar hyperhidrosis.[*] Recurrence during the next few years is reported as 1–3%.[11,22,26,36] Patient satisfaction as measured with quality of life questionnaires consistently demonstrates that >90% of patients are satisfied with the results of the surgery.[†] Treatment of axillary and craniofacial hyperhidrosis is somewhat less successful. Common reasons for dissatisfaction include compensatory sweating and recurrence.

Plantar sweating frequently abates following interruption of the T2–T3 ganglia. An increase in plantar skin temperature and decrease in the sympathetic skin responses are measurable.[4] The anatomical basis for this unexpected, but desirable response is unexplained.

Early treatment failures result from the inability to visualize the sympathetic chain due to extensive pulmonary–chest wall adhesions, the inability to access the sympathetic chain due to overlying vessels, and misidentification of the sympathetic chain.[25] The role of the Kuntz nerves is uncertain. Recurrent palmar hyperhidrosis may result from incomplete nerve interruption and nerve regeneration. Endoscopic reoperation is feasible, though the surgeon must be familiar with distorted intrathoracic anatomy and be prepared to perform a thoracotomy.[25]

Complications and Sequelae of Surgery

Immediate

Following surgery, patients commonly complain of incisional and retrosternal pain that is exacerbated by cough or deep breathing. Narcotic analgesics are generally necessary, but the most severe pain abates within 48 h. Patients return to work or school 3–7 days following surgery. Anhidrosis occurs over the upper chest and face.

Postoperative bleeding is a rare complication of endoscopic thoracic sympathecotomy and can occur from injury to either intrathoracic or extrathoracic structures. The former include the intercostal vasculature and venous branches that occasionally cross the sympathetic chain. Rarely, injury to a major arterial or venous vessel is caused by misplacement of the trocar or cautery. Bleeding from the chest wall musculature or vessel may track into the pleural space and cause an unsuspected hemothorax. Repeat chest X-ray is necessary in the presence of unexplained hypotension. Infection is exceedingly uncommon.

Horner's syndrome (ptosis, miosis, and anhidrosis) occurs in <1% of patients and results from damage to the sympathetic nerves that pass through the stellate ganglia.[26,29,36,37]

Nerve injury may occur as the result of misidentification of the nerve level or the proximal transmission of cautery heat. Ptosis is immediate and frequently permanent.

Chronic

Compensatory Sweating

Following successful operation, as many as 75% of patients report sweating on regions of the torso that had been previously dry.[*] Though usually no more than an annoyance, as many as 3% of patients are plagued by sweating of the chest, thighs, and legs that is as severe as the original palmar sweating. This "compensatory sweating" represents the most serious sequela of thoracic sympathecotomy. Unfortunately, the cause remains obscure. Gustatory sweating has been reported in as many as 73% of patients.[†]

Postoperative truncal and lower extremity sweating has been explained as the thermoregulatory response to the anhidrosis of the rostral chest and upper extremities. Attempts to ameliorate compensatory sweating by transecting only the rami and leaving the sympathetic chain intact resulted in an increased recurrence of palmar sweating and no change in the incidence of compensatory sweating.[7] Interruption of the sympathetic chain at fewer levels, thus sparing some of the sympathetic sweating, has been proposed. However, limiting the sympathecotomy to the T2 ganglia appears to have no demonstrable affect on the occurrence of compensatory sweating[17,22,26,36,37] when compared to interruption of both T2 and T3.[8,11,16,29]

Though interruption of the T2 ganglia has been thought necessary to achieve dry palms, this concept may not be correct. Sympathetic fibers to the hand originate from T2–T10,[35] but the relative contribution to sweating from each spinal level is not known. Twenty-eight patients who underwent interruption of only the T3 ganglia achieved dry hands and none developed compensatory sweating.[44] Interruption of the T4 ganglia was performed in 165 patients who suffered from palmar and axillary hyperhidrosis. Compensatory sweating was rare and mild, with only one patient reporting persistent palmar sweating.[20]

If the success of a more caudal sympathecotomy is confirmed, the current understanding of upper extremity sympathetic innervation and activity will require reassessment. Though sympathetic fibers from T2 and T3 spinal levels contribute fibers to the upper extremity, palmar sweating may be determined by sympathetic input originating distal to T4. Interruption at the T4 level would eliminate palmar sweating, while leaving the remaining upper extremity sympathetic innervation intact without the need for thermoregulatory compensation.[19]

Cardiopulmonary

Sympathetic fibers to the heart pass through the upper thoracic ganglia. Following T2 sympathecotomy, the heart rate at rest and with peak exercise is reduced 13% and 7%, respectively.[30] However, exercise capacity and the cardiorespiratory response to exercise remain unchanged.[31] Shortening of the QTc interval has been reported.[34]

---

*References 8, 11, 16–18, 20, 22, 29, 36, 37.
†References 11, 16, 17, 29, 36, 37.

*References 1, 4, 11, 16, 17, 21, 24, 26, 36, 37, 41.
†References 1, 11, 16, 29, 36, 37.

708

The lungs also receive sympathetic innervation via the thoracic ganglia. Interruption of the T2 ganglia has been reported to result in a subclinical decrease in carbon monoxide diffusion capacity.[33] Minor decreases in expiratory flow have been documented and attributed to small airway obstruction resulting from pulmonary sympathetic denervation.[43]

Other

Circulating epinephrine is secreted by the adrenal medulla in response to sympathetic stimulation. Systemic norepinephrine is produced by the postganglionic sympathetic fibers and reflects the activity of the sympathetic nervous system. Both catecholamines are normal in patients with hyperhidrosis. However, following T2–T3 interruption, norepinephrine levels are decreased while epinephrine levels are unchanged.[32] The decrease in norepinephrine levels may explain some of the aforementioned cardiopulmonary changes.

Treatment of Complications

The occurrence of severe compensatory sweating spurred the development of a potentially reversible procedure, interruption of the sympathetic chain by application of nerve compressing clips.[18] Clips placed on the sympathetic chain cranial to consecutive ribs will isolate the intervening ganglia. Palmar hyperhidrosis is controlled as effectively as with sympathetic chain transection.[18,24,36] Removal of the clips at a second operation has resulted in return of palmar sweating and decrease of compensatory sweating in as many as 60% of patients.[18,36] Successful reconstruction of the severed sympathetic chain with a sural nerve graft has been reported.[42]

▶ FUTURE INVESTIGATIONS

Compensatory sweating remains the most serious undesired consequence of thoracic sympathecotomy. A more detailed understanding of the autonomic nervous system is crucial to eliminate this potentially debilitating side effect. Clinical trials utilizing standardized operative procedures and outcomes measurements are required to document the results of novel surgical approaches. The recently formed International Society for Sympathetic Surgery (http://www.isss.net/) conducts regular meetings to promote interchange of ideas and techniques.

A National Institutes of Health–funded study to improve the understanding of the hyperhidrosis phenotype and inheritance as well as to identify the gene(s) that confer susceptibility to the disorder has been initiated. Hyperhidrosis patients, family members, and control subjects are included. DNA for genetic analysis is isolated from peripheral blood. Sweat production is measured at rest and under conditions of autonomic stimulation.

REFERENCES

1. Adar R, Kurchin A, Zweig A, Mozes M: Palmar hyperhidrosis and its surgical treatment: A report of 100 cases. Ann Surg 186:34–41, 1977.

2. Adson AW, Craig WM, Brown GE: Essential hyperhidrosis cured by sympathetic ganglionectomy and trunk resection. Arch Surg 31:794–806, 1935.

3. Amir M, Arish A, Weinstein Y, Pfeffer M, Levy Y: Impairment in quality of life among patients seeking surgery for hyperhidrosis (excessive sweating): Preliminary results. Isr J Psychiatry Relat Sci 37:25–31, 2000.

4. Chen H-J, Liang C-L, Lu K: Associated changes in plantar temperature and sweating after transthoracic endoscopic T2-3 sympathectomy for palmar hyperhidrosis. J Neurosurg (Spine 1) 95:58–63, 2001.

5. Chiou TSM, Liao K-K: Orientation landmarks of endoscopic transaxillary T-2 sympathectomy for palmar hyperhidrosis. J Neurosurg 85:310–315, 1996.

6. Drott C, Claes G, Olsson-Rex L, et al: Successful treatment of facial blushing by endoscopic transthoracic sympathecotomy. Br J Dermatol 138:639–643, 1998.

7. Gossot D, Toledo L, Fritsch S, Celerier: Thoracoscopic sympathectomy for upper limb hyperhidrosis: Looking for the right operation. Ann Thorac Surg 64:975–978, 1997.

8. Gossot, D, Kabiri H, Caliandro R, et al: Early complications of thoracic endoscopic sympathectomy: A prospective study of 940 procedures. Ann Thorac Surg 71:1116–1119, 2001.

9. Hamill RW: Peripheral autonomic nervous system. In Robertson D, Low PA, Polinsky RJ, editors: Primer on the Autonomic Nervous System. San Diego: Academic Press, 1996, pp. 12–25.

10. Heckmann M, Ceballos-Baumann AO, Plewig G for the Hyperhidrosis Study Group: Botulinum toxin A for axillary hyperhidrosis (excessive sweating). N Engl J Med 344: 488–493, 2001.

11. Herbst F, Plas EG, Fugger R, Fritsch A: Endoscopic thoracic sympathectomy for primary hyperhidrosis of the upper limbs. Ann Surg 220:86–90, 1994.

12. Hughes J: Endothoracic sympathectomy. Proc Soc Med 35: 585–586, 1942.

13. Karakoç Y, Aydemir EH, Kalkan T, Ünal G: Safe control of palmoplantar hyperhidrosis with direct electric current. Int J Dermatol 41:602–605, 2002.

14. Kotzareff A: Résection partielle du trone sympathique cervical droit pour hyperhidrose unilatérale. Rev Med Susse Rom 40:111–113, 1920.

15. Kuntz A: Distribution of the sympathetic rami to the brachial plexus. Arch Surg 15:871–877, 1927.

16. Kux M: Thoracic endoscopic sympathectomy in palmar and axillary hyperhidrosis. Arch Surg 113:264–266, 1978.

17. Lee DY, Yoon YH, Shion HK, et al: Needle thoracic sympathectomy for essential hyperhidrosis: Intermediate-term follow-up. Ann Thorac Surg 69:251–253, 2000.

18. Lin C-C, Mo L-R, Lee L-S, et al: Thoracoscopic T2-sympathetic block by clipping—a better and reversible operation for treatment of hyperhidrosis palmaris: Experience with 326 cases. Eur J Surg 164(Suppl 580):13–16, 1998.

19. Lin C-C, Telaranta T: Lin-Telaranta classification: The importance of different procedures for different indications in sympathetic surgery. Ann Chirurg Gyn 90:161–166, 2001.

20. Lin C-C, Wu H-H: Endoscopic T4 sympathetic block by clamping (ESB4) in treatment of hyperhidrosis palmaris et axillaries—experiences of 165 cases. Ann Chirurg Gyn 90:167–169, 2001.

21. Lin T-S: Transthoracic endoscopic sympathectomy for palmar and axillary hyperhidrosis in children and adolescents. Pediatr Surg Int 15:475–478, 1999.

22. Lin T-S, Fang H-Y: Transthoracic endoscopic sympathectomy in the treatment of palmar hyperhidrosis—with emphasis on perioperative management (1,360 case analyses). Surg Neurol 52:453–457, 1999.

23. Lin T-S, Fang H-Y: Transthoracic endoscopic sympathectomy for craniofacial hyperhidrosis: Analysis of 46 cases. J Lapareo-endoscop Adv Surg Tech 10:243–247, 2000.

24. Lin T-S, Huang L-C, Wang N-P, Lai C-Y: Video-assisted thoracoscopic T2 sympathetic block by clipping for palmar hyperhidrosis: Analysis of 52 cases. J Laparoendosc Adv Surg Tech 11:59–62, 2001.

25. Lin T-S: Video-assisted thoracoscopic "resympathecotomy" for palmar hyperhidrosis: Analysis of 42 cases. Ann Thorac Surg 72:895–898, 2001.

26. Lin T-S, Kuo S-J, Chou M-C: Uniportal endoscopic thoracic sympathectomy for treatment of palmar and axillary hyperhidrosis: Analysis of 2000 cases. Neurosurgery 51(Suppl 2):84–87, 2002.

27. Manca D, Valls-Solé J, Callejas MA: Excitability recovery curve of the sympathetic skin response in healthy volunteers and patients with palmar hyperhidrosis. Clin Neurophysiol 111:1767–1770, 2000.

28. Naver H, Swartling C, Aquilonius S-M: Palmar axillary hyperhidrosis treated with botulinum toxin: One-year clinical follow-up. Eur J Neurol 7:55–62, 2000.

29. Neumayer C, Bischof G, Fugger R, et al: Efficacy and safety of thoracoscopic sympathectomy for hyperhidrosis of the upper limb. Ann Chirurg Gyn 90:195–199, 2001.

30. Noppen M, Herregodts P, Dendale P, et al: Cardiopulmonary exercise testing following bilateral thoracoscopic sympathicolysis in patients with essential hyperhidrosis. Thorax 50:1097–1100, 1995.

31. Noppen M, Dendale P, Hagers Y, et al: Changes in cardiocirculatory autonomic function after thoracoscopic upper dorsal sympathicolysis for essential hyperhidrosis. J Autonom Nerv Sys 60:115–120, 1996.

32. Noppen M, Sevens C, Gerlo E, Vincken W: Plasma catecholamine concentrations in essential hyperhidrosis and effects of thoracoscopic D2-D3 sympathicolysis. Eur J Clin Invest 27:202–205, 1997.

33. Noppen MP, Vincken WG: Partial pulmonary sympathetic denervation by thoracoscopic D2-D3 sympathicolysis for essential hyperhidrosis: Effect on the pulmonary diffusion capacity. Respir Med 91:537–545, 1997.

34. Papa MZ, Schneiderman J, Tucker E, et al: Cardiovascular changes after bilateral upper dorsal sympathectomy. Ann Surg 204:715–718, 1986.

35. Ray BS, Hinsey JC, Geohegan WA: Observations on the distribution of the sympathetic nerves to the pupil and upper extremity as determined by stimulation of the anterior roots in man. Ann Surg 118:647–655, 1943.

36. Reisfeld R, Nguyen R, Pnini A: Endoscopic thoracic sympathectomy for hyperhidrosis. Surg Laparosc Endosc Percutan Tech 12:255–267, 2002.

37. Rex LO, Drott C, Claes G, et al: The Borås experience of endoscopic thoracic sympathecotomy for palmar, axillary, facial hyperhidrosis and facial blushing. Eur J Surg 164(Suppl 580):23–26, 1998.

38. Ro KM, Cantor RM, Lange KL, Ahn SA: Palmar hyperhidrosis: Evidence of genetic transmission. J Vasc Surg 35:388–386, 2002.

39. Saadia D, Voustianiouk A, Wang AK, Kaufmann H: Botulinum toxin type A in primary palmar hyperhidrosis. Neurology 57:2095–2099, 2001.

40. Sáiz-Sapena N, Vanaclocha V, Panta F, et al: Operative monitoring of hand and axillary temperature during endoscopic superior thoracic sympathectomy for the treatment of palmar hyperhidrosis. Eur J Surg 166:65–69, 2000.

41. Shih CJ, Lin MT: Thermoregulatory sweating in palmar hyperhidrosis before and after upper thoracic sympathectomy. J Neurosurg 50:88–94, 1979.

42. Telaranta T: Secondary sympathetic chain reconstruction after endoscopic thoracic sympathecotomy. Eur J Surg Suppl 580:17–18, 1998.

43. Tseng M-Y, Tseng J-H: Thoracoscopic sympathectomy for palmar hyperhidrosis: Effects on pulmonary function. J Clin Neurosci 8:539–541, 2001.

44. van't Riet M, De Smet AAEA, Kuiken H, et al: Prevention of compensatory hyperhidrosis after thoracoscopic sympa-thectomy for hyperhidrosis. Surg Endosc 15:1159–1162, 2001.

45. Wang Y-C, Sun M-H, Lin C-W, Chen Y-J: Anatomical location of T2-3 sympathetic trunk and Kuntz nerve determined by transthoracic endoscopy. J Neurosurg (Spine 1) 96:68–72, 2002.

46. Yarzebski JL, Wilkinson HA: T2 and T3 sympathetic ganglia in the adult human: A cadaver and clinical-radiographic study and its clinical application. Neurosurgery 21:339–342, 1987.

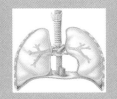

The Use of Genetic Science in Thoracic Disease

CHAPTER 44

Jonathan D'Cunha, Chuong D. Hoang, and Michael A. Maddaus

INTRODUCTION

A revolution in biotechnology is underway: the days of predicting cancer recurrence risk and mortality risk based on microscopic observations (such as degree of atypia, number of observed mitoses) are veering toward the realm of history. Although molecular diagnostic and analytic technologies are in their infancy, their application to the detection of occult cancer cells and to the analysis of tumor genetics is being assessed in many current studies. This chapter begins with a brief review of pathogenic and metastatic mechanisms, and then highlights six prominent areas of molecular diagnosis in lung cancer and other thoracic cancers: (1) molecular detection of occult micrometastases, (2) detection of molecular markers in blood, (3) microarray analysis of tumor genetics, (4) proteomics (the analysis of tumor protein expression profiles), (5) tumor marker panels, and (6) the "molecular frozen section."

MECHANISMS OF CARCINOGENESIS AND METASTASIS

The process of tumorigenesis and progression to metastasis is incompletely understood. Despite this, certain insights have served to guide investigators in developing our current understanding of the overall process as a normal cell devel-

ops into a malignant cell. These current concepts provide the basis and rationale for the molecular diagnosis of thoracic cancers.

Progression of normal bronchial or esophageal epithelium to overt carcinoma is the end result of a series of acquired genetic alterations that are under the influence of multiple environmental, biological, and molecular processes. Non-small-cell lung cancer (NSCLC) illustrates many features of this complex relationship. NSCLC pathogenesis is clearly influenced by carcinogens such as those contained in tobacco smoke. The critical control points in this sequence of malignant degeneration include various protooncogenes and tumor suppressor genes. Several studies have demonstrated that genetic abnormalities occur early in the process and remain persistent despite the cessation of smoking or limiting exposure to carcinogen.[41,56] In fact, the development of tumors may occur with either the activation or deletion of these critical regulatory genes. A number of genetic abnormalities have been identified frequently in early-stage lung cancers, such as mutations in the p53 tumor suppressor gene, mutations in the K-*ras* protooncogene, hypermethylation of the p16 tumor suppressor gene promoter, and loss of heterozygosity in chromosomal regions of importance.[41] These genetic events set the stage for the development of metastatic deposits of tumor.

Tumor metastasis is an equally complex series of molecular events. The fundamental steps required for metastasis include ongoing local tumor proliferation, angiogenesis,[16,17] invasion, dissemination, and implantation.[53,59] According to the prevailing model of tumor dissemination, this capability is acquired relatively late in a stepwise process of tumor progression. Initially, certain cells of the nascent tumor that possess advantageous growth characteristics are further selected to become the progenitors of successor cells that may predominate the tumor mass. These advantageous phenotypes must include self-sufficiency in growth signals, resistance to antigrowth signals, limitless replication, sustained angiogenesis, and evasion of apoptosis.[27] Subsequently, individual cells in these large populations acquire additional unique mutations conferring the rare capability to undergo the metastatic cascade. Only a subset of cells within the primary tumor will attain this phenotype after successive genetic aberrations.[14,47] Thus, any primary tumor mass is comprised of heterogeneous cell populations diverse in genotype and biological behavior. At the molecular level, a number of genes have been implicated in each of the distinct steps of metastasis, but the precise mechanism(s) remains poorly understood. Through this general understanding of carcinogenesis and metastasis, rational approaches to the genetic analysis of thoracic malignancies can be developed and interpreted.

▶ MOLECULAR DETECTION OF OCCULT MICROMETASTASES

The detection of regional thoracic lymph node metastases by routine histopathological analysis portends a significantly diminished survival rate, usually secondary to the later development of systemic metastases. However, even with N_0 status, the 5-year survival of patients with T_1 and T_2 tumors combined is about 60–70%, indicating the undetected presence of "occult micrometastases" (OM) in either lymph nodes or other systemic sites. The ability to accurately detect OM would allow better prediction of tumor recurrence and death risk as well as the use of targeted adjuvant therapy in high-risk patients.

Two techniques are primarily used to detect OM: immunohistochemistry (IHC) and the polymerase chain reaction (PCR) (Figure 44-1). Several groups have investigated the utility of antibodies (Abs) to various tumor markers in detecting OM within the lymph nodes of surgically resected stage I NSCLC. Such Abs include, for example, anti-cytokeratin monoclonal Abs (mAbs) (MNF116, CAM5.2, and AE1/AE3), Ber-Ep4 (an epithelial cell-specific mAb), and anti-p53 mAb. Detection rates have varied widely, with a change in nodal status occurring in 4–58% of lymph nodes. Of six recent studies, four showed a direct correlation between positive IHC results and an increased risk of cancer relapse (Table 44-1). Cancer and Leukemia Group B (CALGB) 9761 and the American College of Surgeons Oncology Group are two current clinical trials that are in the process of defining, in a prospective, multiinstitutional manner, the relationship between lymph node OM detected by IHC and systemic tumor recurrence.

Using IHC to detect OM has two main drawbacks: (1) the need for visual detection of OM deposits by a human operator and (2) the inability to test the entire nodal specimen, unless it is available for processing into slides that can then be stained and reviewed. The use of PCR-based

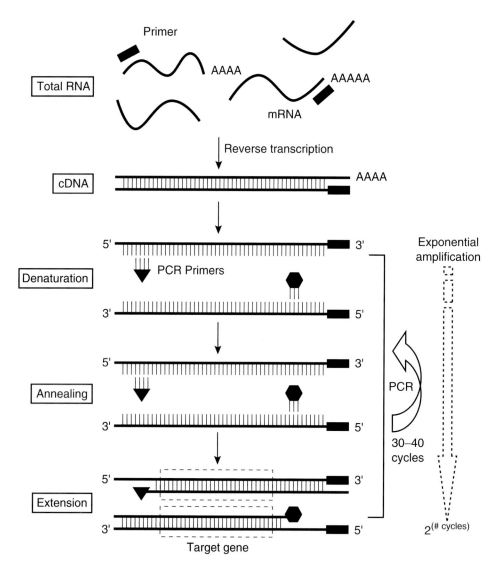

Figure 44–1 Schematic of the principles involved in RT-PCR. RNA from an experimental source is converted to cDNA. PCR amplification proceeds in three steps resulting in the identification of a gene of interest.

Table 44–1

Review of Studies Using IHC to Detect NSCLC Micrometastases

Study	Antibody	Total number of patients	Number (%) of patients with positive results	Statistically significant survival impact
Chen et al[9]	Polyclonal anticytokeratin	65	38 (58%)	Yes
Nicholson et al[44]	MNF116 mAb	49	3 (6%)	No
Maruyama et al[42]	CAM5.2 mAb	44	31 (70%)	Yes
Passlick et al[46]	Ber-Ep4 mAb	70	11 (16%)	Yes
Goldstein et al[23]	AE1/AE3 mAb	80	3 (4%)	No
Dobashi et al[13]	Anti-p53 mAb	31	14 (45%)	Yes

assays to detect tumor cell molecules, most typically tumor-related mRNA, overcomes those two drawbacks. To date, most NSCLC studies have focused on identifying which markers would serve as suitable surrogates for the presence of viable tumor cells and on defining the application of the technique.

Carcinoembryonic antigen (CEA) has emerged as a potentially suitable NSCLC tumor marker from a number of reverse transcriptase-PCR (RT-PCR)–based studies.[4,18,34,58] Collectively, those studies demonstrated that CEA has relatively high specificity (mRNA transcripts were detectable in almost all epithelial cells, including cancer cells, but not in nonepithelial cells) and relatively high sensitivity (it detected $10-10^3$ malignant cells in up to 10^7 normal cells). A recent study of ours, within the CALGB 9761 trial, examined the potential of CEA as a marker of OM in lymph nodes of patients with early-stage NSCLC by RT-PCR; our results further validated previous findings.[11] Of 53 stage I primary tumors that we analyzed, 39 (73.6%) were positive by CEA. Of the 232 associated lymph nodes, 38 (16.4%) were positive. Those 38 nodal specimens were distributed among 23 (43.4%) stage I patients as follows: 1 in 13 patients, 2 in 7 patients, 3 in 1 patient, 4 in 1 patient, and 5 in 1 patient. CEA analysis would have resulted in the molecular upstaging of 43.4% of stage I patients.

A potential shortcoming of OM detection by both IHC and RT-PCR is the binary yes or no result regarding OM presence or absence. Although predictive of increased tumor recurrence risk, simple yes or no results fail to further stratify risk. Studies of N_2 disease detected by hematoxylin and eosin (H&E) staining revealed significant survival differences between patients with lymph nodes replaced by tumor and patients with microscopic disease found incidentally after surgical resection.[38] Similarly, tumor recurrence and survival rates in patients with lymph nodes negative by

H&E that harbor OM may also be related to the number of micrometastatic tumor cells present.

A possible solution may be the use quantitative real-time RT-PCR (QRT-PCR), a technology now broadly available.[21] QRT-PCR, unlike other approaches to quantification of PCR products, requires no post-PCR product manipulation (such as gel electrophoresis of PCR products). Moreover, QRT-PCR enables rapid processing of many samples (96 reactions in 3–4 h). QRT-PCR uses a target molecule-specific oligonucleotide probe (in this case to CEA mRNA) with a covalently attached fluorescent reporter and quencher dye. When the probe is intact, the quenching dye absorbs the fluorescent energy of the reporter dye. If the target molecule of interest (in this case, CEA mRNA) is present, the specific oligonucleotide probe will anneal to it. During the PCR extension phase, the fluorescent probe is cleaved by the $5' \rightarrow 3'$ exonuclease activity of Taq DNA polymerase, thus increasing the reporter dye's emission. Curves plotting relative fluorescence change against PCR cycle number are constructed, and the point of increase in fluorescence above background is calculated; from this calculation, the C_T or threshold cycle is determined. Because C_T values decrease linearly with increasing target molecule quantity in the input sample, they provide quantitative measurement. Figure 44-2 shows a representative amplification plot from a patient with stage I NSCLC.

The potential application of QRT-PCR was demonstrated in the same group of 53 patients in our recent CALGB 9761 study cited previously: of 232 lymph nodes, 59 (25.4%) were positive by QRT-PCR for CEA mRNA. Estimates of the quantity of micrometastatic cells in those 59 nodes ranged from 1.07×10^3 to 3.24×10^5 cells per lymph node station (median, 7190 tumor cells per lymph node station). The increased sensitivity of this novel molecular approach (vs. standard

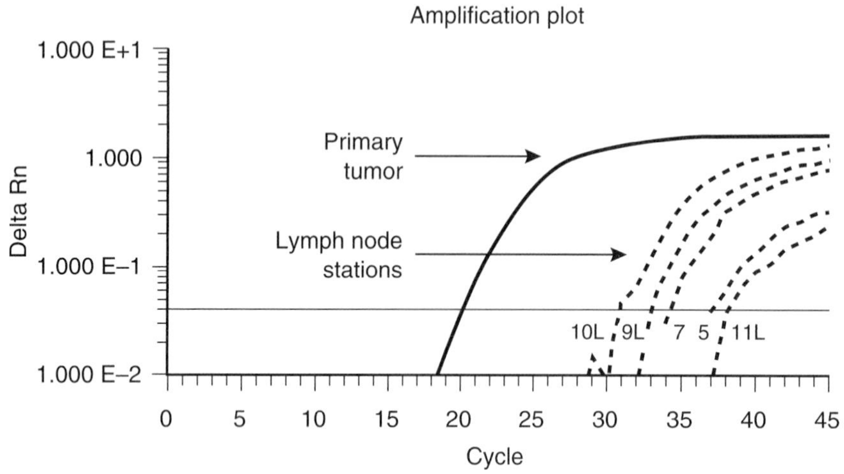

Amplification plot

Figure 44–2 Representative QRT-PCR amplification plot from a patient with stage I NSCLC. Change in normalized reporter signal (Rn, y-axis) plotted versus cycle number (x-axis). Amplification curves for primary tumor and lymph node stations are shown. Amplification curves are labeled as follows: primary tumor and lymph node stations 5, 7, 9L, 10L, and 11L.

H&E analysis) accounted for the additional seven patients whose tumors were upstaged. The prognostic importance of this analysis awaits the conclusion of CALGB 9761.

The same approach has been used to detect OM in the lymph nodes of patients with esophageal cancer. Godfrey et al used QRT-PCR for CEA mRNA to detect OM in 387 lymph nodes from 30 histologically node-negative patients.[22] Of the 30 patients, 11 harbored OM by this analysis; of the 11, 9 suffered disease recurrence. Kaplan–Meier analysis demonstrated that lymph nodes positive by QRT-PCR correlated with significantly lower disease-free ($p < .0001$) and overall survival rates ($p < .0006$).

► DETECTION OF MOLECULAR MARKERS IN BLOOD

The use of genetic science in thoracic cancers has raised the potential for finding an appropriate, clinically useful screening test. Screening peripheral blood is appealing: it is easily accessible, and the minimal overall change in blood volume may enable quantitative measurement. It has been known for years that circulating tumor cells are detectable in patients with very early-stage NSCLC, although detection is more frequent in patients with advanced disease.[40] A number of investigators have used RT-PCR to detect circulating tumor cells in patients with NSCLC; such assays have focused on a number of tumor-derived mRNA molecules, such as epidermal growth factor receptor (EGFR)[12] and CEA.[34]

Kurusu et al used RT-PCR to detect CEA mRNA in blood samples taken from patients with NSCLC preoperatively and then 2–3 weeks after surgical resection.[34] Preliminary *in vitro* studies demonstrated that the sensitivity of their assay for tumor cell detection was 10 NSCLC cancer cells in 10^6 peripheral blood leukocytes. Of 103 preoperative blood samples, 62 (60%) were positive by CEA mRNA analysis; of those 62 samples, 27 (44%) remained positive postoperatively, whereas 35 (56%) became negative. No difference in the rate of detection was seen between adenocarcinomas and squamous cell carcinomas. Of great interest were the postoperative results from patients with a positive preoperative blood test, stratified by postoperative

pathological stage (Table 44-2). Of 41 patients with a negative preoperative blood test, only two had a positive postoperative blood test. Important features of the Kurusu study include the following: (1) the clear correlation between a positive preoperative blood test and postoperative pathological stage, (2) the high rate of positive preoperative blood tests among patients with "early" stage IA and IB disease postoperatively, and (3) the correlation between persistent postoperative blood positivity and postoperative stage, suggesting persistent but undetected systemic disease. Detection of tumor markers in blood is not limited to nucleic acids. For a number of years, there has been interest in identifying abnormal proteins, peptides, and autoantibodies. Despite a large initiative to identify a suitable protein marker, no study has yet identified promising

Table 44–2

Results of RT-PCR for CEA in Peripheral Blood of NSCLC Patients

	CEA RT-PCR				
Postoperative stage	IA	IB	IIA	IIB	IIIA
Total number of patients	32	25	4	15	27
Positive preoperatively (n)	13	9	2	11	27
Positive preoperatively (%)	41	36	50	73	100
Positive postoperatively (n)/negative postoperatively (n)	3/10	3/6	1/1	4/7	16/11

results using existing markers.[15,31,50,54] However, efforts to detect serum autoantibodies have been more promising. Abnormally expressed and structurally altered proteins may elicit the production of autoantibodies in patients with lung cancer. Anti-p53 Abs have been found in the sera of patients with lung cancer containing p53 mutations.[30] Mitsudomi et al identified anti-p53 Abs in more than 20% of 188 patients with NSCLC.[43] In addition, several other autoantibodies have been recently identified as potential markers in lung cancer detection, including antiglycosylated annexins I and II (28) and anti-p40 Abs.[57] Brichory et al[3] found that antibodies to glycosylated annexins I and II were present in 60% of patients with lung adenocarcinomas and in 33% of patients with squamous cell carcinomas. Such studies have served as the basis for the development of biochips that may provide molecular profiles of the Ab response to tumor antigens in thoracic cancers.[5]

MICROARRAY ANALYSIS OF TUMOR GENETICS

The exact molecular basis for tumorigenesis and metastasis in thoracic cancers is unknown. Much of the control for this complex process takes place at the level of transcription, so significant insight into cellular function (of either tumor cells or normal cells) may be gained by global assessment of gene expression. Until recently, investigators were limited to the analysis of a finite number of genes in any particular experiment. The sequencing of the human genome, however, has heralded a new era in the investigation of cancer biology. Advanced tools have rapidly evolved to analyze complex genomes in a comprehensive way. A principal technology in this new era is the DNA microarray, which enables simultaneous analysis of the entire population of cellular genetic transcripts (gene expression profiling) in a given physiological or pathological state. Although the full potential of the DNA microarray has yet to be realized, it has shown promise in deciphering the biological complexities of cancer. The following section discusses the biological and clinical impact of microarray profiling studies in human lung and esophageal cancers.

Briefly, a DNA microarray comprises multiple, gene-specific polynucleotides (probes) arranged along exact coordinates of a two-dimensional grid (array), individually immobilized to a single substrate.[52] Total RNA pools from experimental or reference specimens are reverse transcribed to fluorescence-labeled complementary DNA (cDNA) before incubation with the microarray (Figure 44-3A). This process allows for simultaneous quantitation of the relative (experimental versus reference) amount of messenger RNA (mRNA) transcripts. The number of immobilized microarray probes—which may number in the hundreds of thousands—determines the amount of gene expression information returned from each microarray experiment. This method depends on the highly sensitive and specific hybridization between complementary strands of nucleic acids.

Microarray platforms are of two general types: cDNA and oligonucleotide. Typically, the cDNA microarray contains hundreds to tens of thousands of long PCR-derived representations of specific genes (about 600–2400 base pairs). In contrast, the oligonucleotide microarray (GeneChip Array, Affymetrix, Santa Clara, CA) contains tens of thousands to hundreds of thousands of 25-mer oligonucleotides complementary to unique gene sequences, directly deposited by light-directed chemical synthesis.[37] Currently, no consensus exists as to the ideal type of microarray platform. Each has distinct advantages and drawbacks that are beyond the scope of this discussion. In general, the data sets derived from each platform are identical; each allows for large-scale analysis of gene expression in biological specimens from a single experiment.

The vast amounts of data generated by microarray analyses have necessitated evolution in bioinformatics—a field concerned with the acquisition, storage, display, and analysis of genome-wide expression data. So many options are now available for analysis or "data mining" that choosing among them is challenging. The predominant analytic method in current use is a family of algorithms referred to as "cluster analysis." For example, one specific type of algorithm is hierarchical clustering. The term "cluster analysis" generally applies to methods for organizing multivariate data into groups with similar patterns, such that they may impart additional information about certain genes and the study specimens[48] (Figure 44-3B). Overall, data analysis can be divided into four common themes: detection of differen-

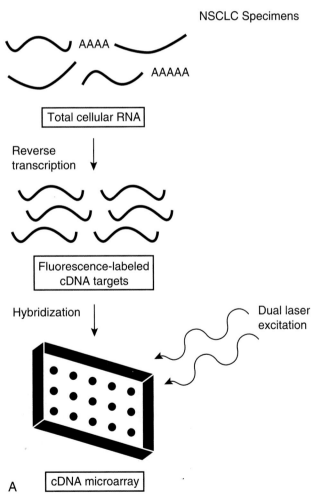

Figure 44–3 **Schematic of the principles involved in cDNA microarray processing. A,** The main components of a microarray experiment are outlined. Refer to text for specific details.

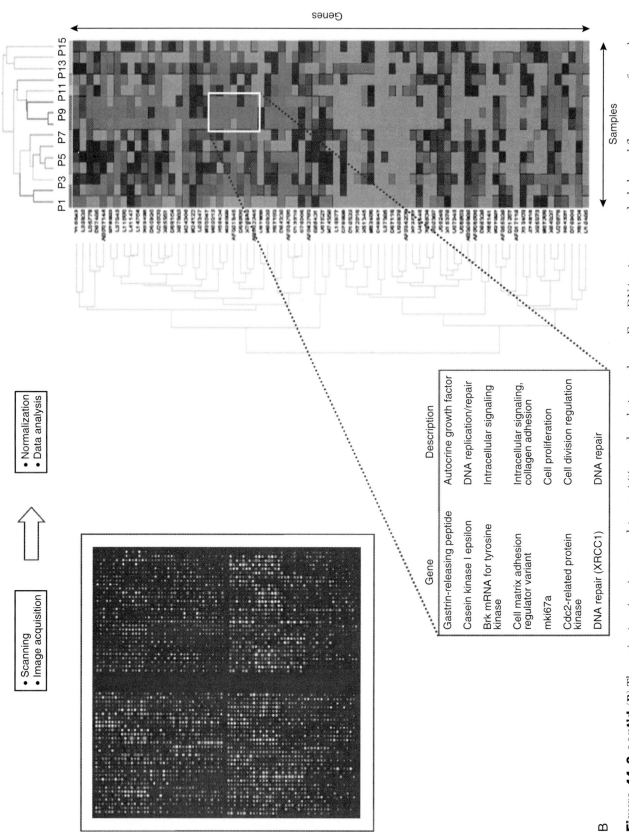

Gene	Description
Gastrin-releasing peptide	Autocrine growth factor
Casein kinase I epsilon	DNA replication/repair
Brk mRNA for tyrosine kinase	Intracellular signaling
Cell matrix adhesion regulator variant	Intracellular signaling, collagen adhesion
mki67a	Cell proliferation
Cdc2-related protein kinase	Cell division regulation
DNA repair (XRCC1)	DNA repair

Figure 44–3 cont'd (**B**) The main steps in microarray data acquisition and analysis are shown. For cDNA microarrays, dual-channel fluorescence for each gene spotted onto the microarray is detected by a confocal scanning microscope. Computer software merges and converts these data into a graphic image. Gene expression data are analyzed with sophisticated algorithms. Shown is an example of a two-dimensional hierarchical cluster analysis. Gene expression ratios are color coded (red, overexpression; green, underexpression; black, no change) to reflect relative mRNA transcript abundance. Further details are provided in the text. (See color plate.)

tial gene expression, pattern discovery, prediction of specimen characteristics, and inference of molecular pathways and networks. The existing microarray literature on lung and esophageal cancers has addressed the first three of these themes of analysis.

Initial NSCLC microarray profiling studies were conducted either on cell culture systems[8,19] or on matched tumor versus nontumor specimens[24,29,55] to identify genes with significantly altered expression levels. Many of the genes differentially expressed in tumor specimens were involved in cell cycle regulation, cell metabolism and signaling, or apoptosis; the findings of these initial NSCLC microarray profiling studies were consistent with those in the broader cancer literature. However, some genes were identified that were not commonly associated with NSCLC: they suggest previously unrecognized mechanisms in tumorigenesis, or perhaps represent novel therapeutic targets (or both). Recently, Bhattacharjee et al studied 186 NSCLC tumors using a clustering technique specialized for gene pattern discovery; they identified four distinct, novel subgroups of adenocarcinomas based on gene expression profiles,[2] and concluded that lung cancer diagnosis could be improved by integrating expression profile data.

Beer et al constructed a risk index based on a set of 50 genes identified by hierarchical clustering and univariate Cox analysis that could predict survival in early-stage lung adenocarcinoma patients.[1] Members of the gene set included genes not previously associated with survival, suggesting novel therapeutic targets. Beer et al stated that a gene set predictive of survival in early-stage adenocarcinoma might identify a high-risk subgroup of patients who could benefit from adjuvant therapy. Kikuchi et al microdissected individual cancer cells from 37 NSCLC tumors before performing microarray analysis to identify novel tumorigenesis genes as well as those related to chemosensitivity.[33] Their subset cluster analysis of 18 specimens identified 40 genes whose expression levels could discriminate gross, pathological, lymph node metastasis. Kikuchi et al speculated that such gene profile-based characteristics of NSCLC tumors could eventually guide personalized therapies.

Microarray studies of esophageal tumors have been generally small in terms of numbers of tumors analyzed, but some early insights have been noteworthy. Selaru et al used hierarchical cluster analysis in an attempt to classify esophageal tumor specimens by expression profiles. As predicted, they found that specimens from patients with Barrett's esophagus and from patients with esophageal cancer clustered separately.[51] In addition, Selaru et al were able to accurately subgroup squamous cell carcinomas and adenocarcinomas by comparing cluster analysis findings with histopathological subtypes.

Other investigators have used microarray analysis to gain insight into the progression of esophageal tumors from dysplasia to metastasis. Using a cancer gene-specific microarray of 588 genes, Zhou et al identified sets of differentially expressed genes in normal esophageal mucosa, basal cell hyperplasia, high-grade dysplasia, carcinoma *in situ*, and overt cancer.[60] Their analysis showed that two genes (P160ROCK and JNK2) in particular may play an important role in carcinogenesis. Their results are potentially powerful, because they evaluated gene expression across different

stages of carcinogenesis. In their analysis, the P160ROCK gene (a member of the family of Rho-associated serine/threonine kinase isoenzymes that regulate cell motility and morphological changes) was dramatically upregulated in the tissues with high-grade dysplasia. Thus, its activation may be one of the early events in carcinogenesis of esophageal tumors.

Additionally, Kihara et al analyzed the expression profiles of 20 surgically resected esophageal tumors in patients treated with adjuvant therapy.[32] They identified a profile of 52 genes correlated with prognosis and found that the gene set accurately predicted the chemosensitivity and chemoresistance of the tumors to various agents. From this gene set, they obtained a "drug response score" that correlated significantly with patient prognosis.

Clearly, genomic expression profiling has the potential to be applied clinically on small biopsy samples, and gene profiles may someday be used to guide treatment decisions. DNA microarrays and bioinformatics show promise in refining our approach to prognosis and to targeted therapies. Ultimately, understanding tumor cell function will require the direct merging of microarray data with other sources of genomic and biomedical information or techniques.

PROTEOMICS: THE ANALYSIS OF TUMOR PROTEIN EXPRESSION PROFILES

The sequencing of the human genome paved the way for the biological revolution now underway. Understanding the functionality of complex biological systems, in particular genomics, will no doubt lead to major advances in medicine and cancer biology in the near future. Proteomics holds promise for providing powerful tools to study translational lung cancer research.

Proteomics encompasses many platform technologies for protein separation and identification. Its major challenge is the vast increased complexity of the human proteome, as compared with the genome. Proteomic analysis of cancer specimens entails a number of variations. Analysis of tissue biopsies is far more complicated and challenging, given the heterogeneous nature of the samples. Most proteomic approaches to date have employed homogenization of the particular sample of interest, with subsequent separation of proteins by two-dimensional polyacrylamide gel electrophoresis (2-D PAGE).[45] Particular proteins of interest are identified as "spots" on these gels and then eluted from the gel using various techniques. The particular protein identity is then determined using mass spectrometry and proteomic databases.[39]

In contrast to other molecular approaches, studies in lung cancer have led the way among investigations of solid-organ tumors.[34] With lung cancer as the backdrop for translational investigations using proteomic approaches, Hanash et al[28] analyzed more than 1000 lung cancer-related samples using 2-D PAGE in combination with mass spectroscopy. They compiled a lung cancer proteomic database that integrates protein and gene expression data. Their ultimate goals are to identify novel biomarkers for the early detection of lung cancer, to develop novel classification of tumors, and to reveal targets for future therapeutic intervention.[7,20,28] Analysis of the gene expression and protein expression patterns in paral-

718 lel allowed them to directly compare gene and protein expression in the same tumor set.[6] They analyzed 165 protein spots representing protein products of 98 genes in 76 lung adenocarcinomas using 2-D PAGE. On essentially the same set of samples, they performed microarray analysis. Interestingly, of the 98 genes, only 21 showed a significant correlation between protein and mRNA levels. As an extension of their studies, they identified specific cytokeratin isoforms that were predictive of survival in lung cancer.[20]

TUMOR MARKER PANELS

Thoracic malignancies, like many tumors, cannot be characterized in full by a single molecular marker. Each tumor may have its own "molecular fingerprint." As we move to refining staging and treatment based on molecular markers, a panel of molecular markers for specific tumors (and possibly tumor subtype) will likely be routinely analyzed, allowing refinement of the sensitivity and specificity of risk prediction.

Kwiatkowski et al evaluated 244 patients with stage I NSCLC to identify variables predicting risk of tumor recurrence.[35] Variables included the following: adenocarcinoma solid tumor with mucin subtype, tumor diameter ≥4 cm, lymphatic invasion, p53 expression, K-*ras* mutation, and the absence of H-*ras* p21 expression. Based on their data, they proposed a molecular tumor subclassification. Five-year survival rates correlated inversely with the number of prognostic variables as follows: one or two factors, 87% 5-year survival; three factors, 58% 5-year survival; and four or more factors, 21% 5-year survival.

D'Amico et al proposed a molecular model system consisting of five biological markers involved in various parts of the metastatic process: growth regulation, cell cycle regulation, apoptosis, angiogenesis, and metastatic adhesion factor.[10] In a multivariable analysis of 408 stage I NSCLC patients, they found that five biological factors were predictive: erbB-2, RB, p53, factor VIII staining for angiogenesis, and CD-44. Using their system, patients were substratified by 5-year survival as follows: zero to one marker, 77%; two markers, 62%; three to five markers, 49%.

Recently, Gordon et al[25] expanded on this concept by demonstrating the diagnostic superiority of a small panel of tumor-associated genes whose expression levels can be used to calculate a set of gene expression ratios for any particular sample. The significant genes were identified by microarray analysis of 150 NSCLC tumors compared against 31 malignant mesothelioma samples. Using six genes to calculate three sets of gene expression ratios (calretinin/claudin-7, VAC-β/TACSTD1, and MRC OX-2/TITF-1), they were able to correctly classify 99% of tumors according to type. After refining their methodology, they identified a panel of eight genes and calculated a set of four gene expression ratios that accurately predicted treatment-related clinical outcome ($p = .0035$) for 29 patients with malignant mesothelioma.[26]

THE "MOLECULAR FROZEN SECTION"

The use of intraoperative frozen sections is fraught with the same drawbacks as all standard histopathological analysis—the need for human visualization (introducing errors and limits of detection) and the limited degree of sampling of a given specimen. Ideally, an assay would enable rapid processing of an entire specimen and provide a highly reliable yes or no answer as to the presence or absence of tumor cells in the specimen, perhaps with quantitation. Such an assay would have several ideal attributes: (1) an assay time of less than 20 min, (2) high sensitivity for genes with a low number of transcripts (500–1000), (3) the ability to analyze a number of biomarkers simultaneously, (4) automation, and (5) the ability to archive specimens for future analyses.

Raja et al[49] proposed an approach that fulfills some of these ideal assay attributes. Using a rapid RT-PCR format on node-negative esophageal carcinoma samples, they were able to discriminate between patients with or without a high risk of recurrence. The total time required for completion of their assay was about 30 min. In their frozen tissue analysis, rapid QRT-PCR correlated with the final pathological report for 11 of 12 patients. In the one discordant case, the quantitative RT-PCR result was positive; that test may have detected microscopic metastases, because that patient did have disease recurrence. Rapid QRT-PCR was more sensitive than intraoperative frozen section analysis in detecting metastatic disease. Their data suggested that rapid QRT-PCR may have a prognostic role and could guide intraoperative decisions.

Another alternative, yet equally interesting, approach employed by our laboratory is to eliminate the need for RT-PCR and, instead, analyze RNA directly. This novel approach is known as the Invader assay (Third Wave Technology Inc., Madison, WI). The principle of this method relies on the formation of a unique structure formed by the complementary hybridization of the RNA target to two oligonucleotide probes that are sequence specific. One probe is oriented upstream and must overlap or "invade" the second downstream fluorescent signal probe. This unique structure is recognized and only cleaved by a special class of enzymes (Cleavases).[36] These stringent assay elements ensure both accuracy and high analytic sensitivity. Using this system, Kwiatkowski et al demonstrated that glyceraldehyde-3-phosphate dehydrogenase (GAPDH) mRNA can be detected in as few as 500 cells.[36] We are currently working on modifying this platform to analyze lung and esophageal cancer specimens.

Regardless of the approach, we believe that multiple lines of investigation will likely yield the fastest, most accurate assay in the future. Such an assay could serve as a "molecular frozen section" and potentially replace standard frozen section histopathological assessment of tissues for metastatic cancer cells. Our model of the ideal assay is shown in Figure 44-4. It incorporates the five ideal attributes listed above, with the major advantage of a solid-phase platform that could be stored indefinitely and reinterrogated as future advances are made.

SUMMARY

It is becoming clear that translational research in thoracic cancers will make use of the entire armamentarium of molecular biology, including genomics and proteomics. Currently, the TNM stage is the most important predictor of survival. In the new era of molecular analysis of solid-

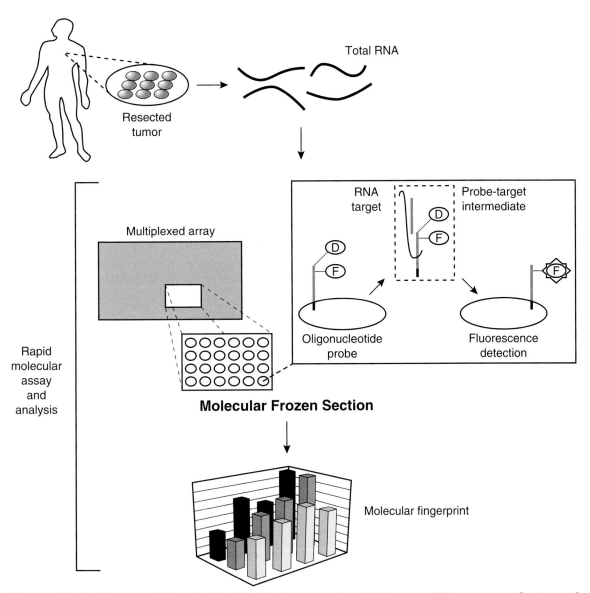

Figure 44–4 Schematic of the ideal "molecular frozen section." Advantages of this system are direct use of RNA, rapid running time, scalability to include multiple tumor markers, and high sensitivity and specificity. The inset describes the Invader assay. Complete details are described in the text.

organ tumors, it is highly likely that molecular subclassification strategies will add depth and refinement to our predictive ability. Many studies to date have suggested important molecular markers, but the challenge is to test these markers in large prospective studies with homogeneous groups of patients, so that clinicians can make better sense of the overall predictive ability of individual markers. Such studies would also serve as the framework for what is even more important: the rational design of molecularly targeted therapies. The future of genetic science in thoracic cancers lies in the ability to use assays and their markers to identify patients at risk for early recurrence. In addition, markers must ideally be used as molecular handles, so that novel compounds can target their functional pathways. A targeted approach is likely to result in a dramatic, positive impact on prognosis and survival.

REFERENCES

1. Beer DG, Kardia SLR, Huang CC, et al: Gene-expression profiles predict survival of patients with lung adenocarcinoma. Nat Med 8:816–824, 2002.
2. Bhattacharjee A, Richards WG, Staunton J, et al: Classification of human lung carcinomas by mRNA expression profiling reveals distinct adenocarcinoma subclasses. Proc Natl Acad Sci USA 98:13790–13795, 2001.
3. Brichory FM, Misek DE, Yim AM, et al: An immune response manifested by the common occurrence of annexins I and II autoantibodies and high circulating levels of IL-6 in lung cancer. Proc Natl Acad Sci USA 98:9824–9829, 2001.
4. Castaldo, G, Tomaiuolo, R, Sanduzzi A, et al: Lung cancer metastatic cells detected in blood by reverse transcriptase-polymerase chain reaction and dot-blot analysis. J Clin Oncol 15:3388–3393, 1997.

5. Celis JE, Gromov P: Proteomics in translational cancer research: Toward an integrated approach. Cancer Cell 3:9–15, 2003.

6. Chen G, Gharib TG, Huang CC, et al: Discordant protein and mRNA expression in lung adenocarcinomas. Mol Cell Proteomics 1:304–313, 2002.

7. Chen G, Gharib TG, Huang CC, et al: Proteomic analysis of lung adenocarcinoma: Identification of a highly expressed set of proteins in tumors. Clin Cancer Res 8:2298–2305, 2002.

8. Chen JJ, Peck K, Hong TM, et al: Global analysis of gene expression in invasion by a lung cancer model. Cancer Res 61:5223–5230, 2001.

9. Chen ZL, Perez S, Holmes EC, et al: Frequency and distribution of occult micrometastases in lymph nodes of patients with non-small-cell lung carcinoma. J Natl Cancer Inst 85:493–498, 1993.

10. D'Amico TA, Massey M, Herndon JE 2nd, et al: A biologic risk model for stage I lung cancer: Immunohistochemical analysis of 408 patients with the use of ten molecular markers. J Thorac Cardiovasc Surg 117:736–743, 1999.

11. D'Cunha J, Corfits AL, Herndon JE 2nd, et al: Molecular staging of lung cancer: Real-time polymerase chain reaction estimation of lymph node micrometastatic tumor cell burden in stage I non-small cell lung cancer—preliminary results of Cancer and Leukemia Group B Trial 9761. J Thorac Cardiovasc Surg 123:484–491; discussion 491, 2002.

12. De Luca A, Pignata S, Casamassimi A, et al: Detection of circulating tumor cells in carcinoma patients by a novel epidermal growth factor receptor reverse transcription-PCR assay. Clin Cancer Res 6:1439–1444, 2000.

13. Dobashi K, Sugio K, Osaki T, et al: Micrometastatic P53-positive cells in the lymph nodes of non-small-cell lung cancer: Prognostic significance. J Thorac Cardiovasc Surg 114:339–346, 1997.

14. Fidler IJ, Poste G: The cellular heterogeneity of malignant neoplasms: Implications for adjuvant chemotherapy. Semin Oncol 12:207–221, 1985.

15. Foa P, Fornier M, Miceli R, et al: Preoperative CEA, NSE, SCC, TPA and CYFRA 21.1 serum levels as prognostic indicators in resected non-small cell lung cancer. Int J Biol Markers 14:92–98, 1999.

16. Folkman J: Tumor angiogenesis: Therapeutic implications. N Engl J Med 285:1182–1186, 1971.

17. Folkman J: Angiogenesis in cancer, vascular, rheumatoid and other disease. Nat Med 1:27–31, 1995.

18. Fujita J, Ueda Y, Bandoh S, et al: A case of leptomeningeal metastasis from lung adenocarcinoma diagnosed by reverse transcriptase-polymerase chain reaction for carcinoembryonic antigen. Lung Cancer 22:153–156, 1998.

19. Gemma A, Takenaka K, Hosoya Y, et al: Altered expression of several genes in highly metastatic subpopulations of a human pulmonary adenocarcinoma cell line. Eur J Cancer 37:1554–1561, 2001.

20. Gharib TG, Chen G, Wang H, et al: Proteomic analysis of cytokeratin isoforms uncovers association with survival in lung adenocarcinoma. Neoplasia 4:440–448, 2002.

21. Gibson UE, Heid CA, Williams PM: A novel method for real time quantitative RT-PCR. Genome Res 6:995–1001, 1996.

22. Godfrey TE, Raja S, Finkelstein SD, et al: Prognostic value of quantitative reverse transcription-polymerase chain reaction in lymph node-negative esophageal cancer patients. Clin Cancer Res 7:4041–4048, 2001.

23. Goldstein NS, Mani A, Chmielewski G, et al: Immuno-histochemically detected micrometastases in peribronchial and mediastinal lymph nodes from patients with T1, N0, M0 pulmonary adenocarcinomas. Am J Surg Pathol 24:274–279, 2000.

24. Goodwin LO, Mason JM, Hajdu SI: Gene expression patterns of paired bronchioloalveolar carcinoma and benign lung tissue. Ann Clin Lab Sci 31:369–375, 2001.

25. Gordon GJ, Jensen RV, Hsiao LL, et al: Translation of microarray data into clinically relevant cancer diagnostic tests using gene expression ratios in lung cancer and mesothelioma. Cancer Res 62:4963–4967, 2002.

26. Gordon GJ, Jensen RV, Hsiao LL, et al: Using gene expression ratios to predict outcome among patients with mesothelioma. J Natl Cancer Inst 95:598–605, 2003.

27. Hanahan D, Weinberg RA: The hallmarks of cancer. Cell 100:57–70, 2000.

28. Hanash S, Brichory F, Beer D: A proteomic approach to the identification of lung cancer markers. Dis Markers 17:295–300, 2001.

29. Hellman S, Devita VT, Rosenberg SA: Cancer: Principles and Practice of Oncology. Philadelphia: Lippincott-Raven, 2001.

30. Iizasa T, Fujisawa T, Saitoh Y, et al: Serum anti-p53 autoantibodies in primary resected non-small-cell lung carcinoma. Cancer Immunol Immunother 46:345–349, 1998.

31. Karnak D, Ulubay G, Kayacan O, et al: Evaluation of Cyfra 21-1: A potential tumor marker for non-small cell lung carcinomas. Lung 179:57–65, 2001.

32. Kihara C, Tsunoda T, Tanaka T, et al: Prediction of sensitivity of esophageal tumors to adjuvant chemotherapy by cDNA microarray analysis of gene-expression profiles. Cancer Res 61:6474–6479, 2001.

33. Kikuchi T, Daigo Y, Katagiri T, et al: Expression profiles of non-small cell lung cancers on cDNA microarrays: Identification of genes for prediction of lymph-node metastasis and sensitivity to anti-cancer drugs. Oncogene 22:2192–2205, 2003.

34. Kurusu Y, Yamashita J, Ogawa M: Detection of circulating tumor cells by reverse transcriptase-polymerase chain reaction in patients with resectable non-small-cell lung cancer. Surgery 126:820–826, 1999.

35. Kwiatkowski DJ, Harpole DH Jr, Godleski J, et al: Molecular pathologic substaging in 244 stage I non-small-cell lung cancer patients: Clinical implications. J Clin Oncol 16:2468–2477, 1998.

36. Kwiatkowski RW, Lyamichev V, de Arruda M, Neri B: Clinical, genetic, and pharmacogenetic applications of the Invader assay. Mol Diagn 4:353–364, 1999.

37. Lipshutz RJ, Fodor SP, Gingeras, TR, Lockhart DJ: High density synthetic oligonucleotide arrays. Nat Genet 21:20–24, 1999.

38. Luke WP, Pearson FG, Todd TR, et al: Prospective evaluation of mediastinoscopy for assessment of carcinoma of the lung. J Thorac Cardiovasc Surg 91:53–56, 1986.

39. MacCoss MJ, Wu CC, Yates JR 3rd: Probability-based validation of protein identifications using a modified SEQUEST algorithm. Anal Chem 74:5593–5599, 2002.

40. Mao L: Recent advances in the molecular diagnosis of lung cancer. Oncogene 21:6960–6969, 2002.

41. Mao L, Lee JS, Kurie JM, et al: Clonal genetic alterations in the lungs of current and former smokers. J Natl Cancer Inst 89:857–862, 1997.

42. Maruyama R, Mitsudomi T, Ishida T, et al: Aggressive pulmonary metastasectomies for synovial sarcoma. Respiration 64:316–318, 1997.

43. Mitsudomi T, Suzuki S, Yatabe Y, et al: Clinical implications of p53 autoantibodies in the sera of patients with non-small-cell lung cancer. J Natl Cancer Inst 90:1563–1568, 1998.

44. Nicholson AG, Graham AN, Pezzella F, et al: Does the use of immunohistochemistry to identify micrometastases provide useful information in the staging of node-negative non-small cell lung carcinomas? Lung Cancer 18:231–240, 1997.

45. O'Farrell PH: High resolution two-dimensional electrophoresis of proteins. J Biol Chem 250:4007–4021, 1975.

46. Passlick B, Izbicki JR, Kubuschok B, et al: Detection of disseminated lung cancer cells in lymph nodes: Impact on staging and prognosis. Ann Thorac Surg 61:177–182; discussion 183, 1996.

47. Poste G, Fidler IJ: The pathogenesis of cancer metastasis. Nature 283:139–146, 1980.

48. Quackenbush J: Computational analysis of microarray data. Nat Rev Genet 2:418–427, 2001.

49. Raja S, Luketich JD, Kelly LA, et al: Rapid, quantitative reverse transcriptase-polymerase chain reaction: Application to intraoperative molecular detection of occult metastases in esophageal cancer. J Thorac Cardiovasc Surg 123:475–482; discussion 482–473, 2002.

50. Salgia R, Harpole D, Herndon JE 2nd, et al: Role of serum tumor markers CA 125 and CEA in non-small cell lung cancer. Anticancer Res 21:1241–1246, 2001.

51. Selaru FM, Zou T, Xu Y, et al: Global gene expression profiling in Barrett's esophagus and esophageal cancer: A comparative analysis using cDNA microarrays. Oncogene 21:475–478, 2002.

52. Southern E, Mir K, Shchepinov M: Molecular interactions on microarrays. Nat Genet 21:5–9, 1999.

53. Stetler-Stevenson WG, Kleiner DE Jr: Molecular Biology of Cancer: Molecular Mechanism of Cancer Invasion and Metastasis, pp. 123–136. Philadelphia: Lippincott, Williams & Wilkins, 2000.

54. Tas F, Aydiner A, Topuz E, et al: Utility of the serum tumor markers: CYFRA 21.1, carcinoembryonic antigen (CEA), and squamous cell carcinoma antigen (SCC) in squamous cell lung cancer. J Exp Clin Cancer Res 19:477–481, 2000.

55. Wang KK, Liu N, Radulovich N, et al: Novel candidate tumor marker genes for lung adenocarcinoma. Oncogene 21:7598–7604, 2002.

56. Wistuba II, Montellano FD, Milchgrub S, et al: Deletions of chromosome 3p are frequent and early events in the pathogenesis of uterine cervical carcinoma. Cancer Res 57:3154–3158, 1997.

57. Yamaguchi K, Patturajan M, Trink B, et al: Circulating antibodies to p40(AIS) in the sera of respiratory tract cancer patients. Int J Cancer 89:524–528, 2000.

58. Yamashita JI., Kurusu Y, Fujino N, et al: Detection of circulating tumor cells in patients with non-small cell lung cancer undergoing lobectomy by video-assisted thoracic surgery: A potential hazard for intraoperative hematogenous tumor cell dissemination. J Thorac Cardiovasc Surg 119:899– 905, 2000.

59. Yokota J: Tumor progression and metastasis. Carcinogenesis 21:497–503, 2000.

60. Zhou J, Zhao LQ, Xiong MM, et al: Gene expression profiles at different stages of human esophageal squamous cell carcinoma. World J Gastroenterol 9:9–15, 2003.

Innovative Therapy and Technology

Neil A. Christie, Hiran C. Fernando, and James D. Luketich

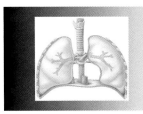

CHAPTER 45

Introduction
Radiofrequency Ablation (RFA)
Stereotactic Radiosurgery
Chemoperfusion of the Pleural Cavity
Summary

▶ INTRODUCTION

In this chapter, we review several innovative therapies for treatment of lung tumors. Application of these new therapies continues to evolve, and in most cases, surgical resection remains the mainstay of therapy. These new alternatives to traditional surgical treatment allow additional options when surgery is not clearly of benefit or when the patient is not a candidate for traditional surgery. As with other recent advances, such as video-thoracoscopy, these new less invasive approaches may allow surgeons to treat patients with thoracic malignancies even in the setting of marginal pulmonary reserve. Two new therapies currently being investigated in clinical trials, which may expand our nonoperative options, are radiofrequency ablation and lung stereotactic radiosurgery. The main goal of these less invasive therapies is to locally destroy the pulmonary or thoracic neoplasm while preserving the surrounding normal tissues. Another innovative therapy discussed in this chapter is hyperthermic pleural chemoperfusion for malignancies with a propensity for local pleural recurrence. It is important that thoracic surgical oncologists stay abreast of these new therapies, design clinical trials, and critically evaluate and report the results. We do not believe that the introduction of new technology should change the paradigm of who treats thoracic malignancies. Failure of surgeons to adapt to this new technology will lead to fragmentation in the care of the patient with a thoracic malignancy. In addition, most localized thoracic malignancies should still be treated surgically, and failure to involve an experienced thoracic surgical oncologist in the design of clinical trials will lead to compromise of patient care.

▶ RADIOFREQUENCY ABLATION (RFA)

After the widespread application of RFA for the ablation of unresectable liver tumors, this technique has been considered as an alternative therapy for the destruction of other solid tumors. RFA has largely replaced cryotherapy for the treatment of liver metastases as clinical trials have demonstrated a lower rate of complications with RFA.[6,9] Although

experience in the treatment of lung tumors is limited, the technique appears to be to be safe and feasible for ablation of peripheral lung nodules. The goal of RFA of lung tumors is coagulation necrosis of the lesion of interest with a small rim of extension into adjacent normal lung parenchyma. The technique uses radiofrequency energy to generate ionic vibration, which increases tissue temperature to over 60°C causing protein denaturation, thermal coagulation, and tissue necrosis.[14]

Animal models have been used to investigate the efficacy and feasibility of this technique in lung tissue. In a study by Goldberg et al,[16] a model of lung tumors prepared by infiltrating the pulmonary parenchyma of 11 rabbits with VX2 sarcoma cell suspensions was used. Seven lesions were treated with RFA for 6 min at 90° C, and the remaining four control tumors were left untreated. The authors noted computerized tomographic evidence of coagulation necrosis surrounding the tumor, manifested by increased opacity enveloping the lesion. This was followed by central tissue attenuation with peripheral hyperattenuation surrounding the treated site. Histological analysis revealed that at least 95% of the tumor nodules were necrotic, although some rabbits (43%) had residual tumor nests at the periphery of the tumor. Pneumothorax was the only procedure-related complication, and occurred in 29% of treated rabbits. In another study, Miao and colleagues implanted VX2 tumor cells in the lung of 18 rabbits (12 treated and 6 controls), and the lesions were then treated with RFA using a cooled tip electrode for 60 s.[29] Efficacy of therapy was followed up with magnetic resonance imaging (MRI), microangiography, and histopathology. Absolute tumor eradication was achieved with RFA in 33% and a partial response in 42% of rabbits that survived longer than 3 months. MRI evaluation of the lesion post-RFA demonstrated an early hyperintense peritumoral rim on T1- and T2-weighted MRI images, which subsequently turned into a homogeneous signal associated with decreased lesion size. Microangiography revealed no perfusion to the ablated lesions. On histological evaluation, the ablated lesions retained their tissue architecture, but showed coagulation necrosis with edema and inflammation of the normal surrounding lung. After 1–3 months of treatment, the ablated tumor became an atrophied nodule of coagulative necrosis within a fibrotic capsule.

Putnam and colleagues studied the effects of RFA on lung tumors 2–3.5 cm in size in a porcine model.[35] The authors used LeVeen electrodes to treat the lesions, and performed gross and histological evaluations at different time points of 3, 7, and 28 days post-RFA. There were no complications from the procedure, and histological evaluation demonstrated successful destruction of the lesion with minimal damage to surrounding parenchyma. Characteristic changes in the lesion consisted of a central coagulum surrounded by a hyperemic rim early after therapy. This was followed by organization of the lesion with surrounding inflammation and scar formation with eventual decrease in size by 28 days. The authors also noted some postprocedure pneumonitis and obstructive atelectasis adjacent to the treated lesion with some cases of limited intraparenchymal hemorrhage.

Experience with animal models that demonstrated feasibility and safety of pulmonary application, together with the success of RFA in the treatment of other solid tumors in humans, led to the clinical application of this technique in the lung. The clinical experience of RFA in the treatment of pulmonary malignancies is limited and consists of pilot projects, but preliminary results suggest it can be applied successfully. The initial Chinese experience in 22 patients (eight primary lung cancers, seven metastatic breast cancers, and five colorectal metastases) treated with RFA was recently reported.[21] Complications included five patients with pneumothorax and six with postprocedure fever. Lesion assessment with PET scans following RFA indicated nonviability in lesions smaller than 3.5 cm. Lesions larger than 3.5 cm had a partial response only, with residual uptake in the tumor periphery.

Dupuy and colleagues reported their initial experience with RFA of lung tumors in three patients with lung malignancies.[12] All treatments were performed percutaneously under computed tomography (CT) guidance with either sedation or general endotracheal anesthesia as an outpatient procedure. Only one pneumothorax developed on follow-up radiographs, which did not require intervention. All three patients developed pleural effusion and postprocedure fever. Follow-up of the ablated nodules with CT scans at 6 weeks and 3 months postoperatively in one patient revealed no residual disease, but a biopsy of the fibrotic nodule revealed atypical cells, prompting a second RFA treatment. The second patient died of unknown causes 5 weeks post-RFA and 3 weeks after external beam radiation. The third patient is alive, and positron emission tomography (PET) scan at 3 months post-RFA revealed no residual disease. Sewell and colleagues reported on 10 patients who were considered to be nonsurgical candidates who were treated with RFA under CT guidance using local anesthesia.[37] Procedure-related complications included four pneumothoraces and pain at the treated site. Follow-up PET scans revealed no significant fluorodeoxyglucose (FDG)-18 tracer uptake at the treated sites.

Yang reported the results of intraoperative RFA of 14 tumors in 13 patients who underwent immediate resection after RFA. Two patients did not undergo treatment because of bleeding at the RFA site and extensive tumor calcification in a metastatic sarcoma. Device placement was done under direct vision without image guidance. Median tumor kill was 70% and seven patients had 100% ablation. Partial ablation was attributed to suboptimal device placement, and with experience, 100% tumor kill was achieved in five of the last six cases.[43]

At the University of Pittsburgh we treated 33 lung tumors in 18 patients between September 2000 and March 2002. All patients had failed prior nonoperative therapies or were not candidates for surgical resection because of poor physiologic reserve. Patients had primary lung cancer or

pulmonary metastases with disease localized to the lungs. Treatment was performed with intent to cure or locally control the tumor. The RFA procedure was performed in the operating room with patients under general anesthesia and approached by either minithoracotomy (five patients) or CT-guided percutaneous technique (13 patients). Treatment in the operating room allows for complete anesthesia support as well as rapid access to instruments and easy placement of pigtail or chest tubes for pneumothoraces. After placement of a small finder-needle into the center of the lung nodule under CT guidance, a LeVeen needle electrode (Figure 45-1) (Radiotherapeutics Corporation, Sunnyvale, CA), which is sized according to the diameter of the target lesion, is then placed. The needle electrode has a diameter of 14 gauge with a 12–15 cm shaft length and is also placed under CT guidance. Several applications in different locations within the lesion may be required for larger masses. We use the Radio Therapeutics RF current generator (Radiotherapeutics Corporation, Sunnyvale, CA). Chest tubes were placed in all open procedures and in 55% ($n = 7$) of percutaneous procedures for procedure-related pneumothoraces. This complication was treated with placement of pleural pigtail catheters using Seldinger's technique. Evacuation of the pneumothoraces allowed for complete lung expansion and better targeting of the RFA electrode to the lesion. Radiological response was evaluated with a modified Response Evaluation Criteria in Solid Tumors (RECIST),[33] which included PET analysis. This evaluation was based on objective measurements of the lesion before and after treatment by CT scan size, mass quality, and FDG uptake on PET (Table 45-1). Mean size of the lesions was 5.3 cm (range 2–16 cm). Complete or partial response was seen in 9 of 18 (50%) patients, stable disease in 6 of 18 (35%), and tumor progression in 3 of 18 (15%) (Table 45-2). The best results were seen in smaller tumors, less than 4 cm in diameter. Representative CT scans prior to, and 3 months after, RFA are shown in Figures 45-2 and 45-3, respectively. One major complication occurred in a patient who had received RFA for a nodule near the superior segment artery who subsequently died of massive hemoptysis 21 days after RFA. After this case, only peripheral tumors were treated and no other bleeding complications were noted.

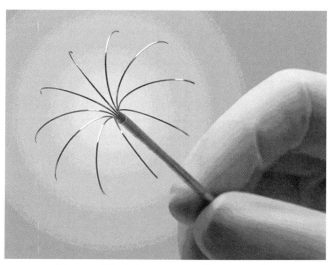

Figure 45–1 LeVeen needle electrode.

Table 45–1

RFA Response Criteria According to the Radiographic Appearance of the Treated Lesion[a]

Response[b]	CT mass size (RECIST)	CT mass quality	PET[c]
Complete (two of the following)	Lesion disappearance (scar) or less than 25% original size	Cyst cavity formation; low density	SUV <2.5
Partial (one of the following)	More than 30% decrease in the sum LD of target lesions	Mass central necrosis or central cavity with liquid density	Decreased SUV or area of FDG uptake
Stable lesion (one of the following)	Less than 30% decrease in the sum LD of target lesions	Mass solid appearance, no central necrosis or cavity	Unchanged SUV or area of FDG uptake
Progression (two of the following)	Increase of more than 20% in sum LD of target lesions	Solid mass, invasion adjacent structures	Higher SUV or larger area of FDG uptake

[a]Target lesions, tumors treated with RFA; sum LD, sum of the largest diameter (LD) of all target (RFA-treated) lesions; SUV, standard uptake value of 18-FDG in PET scan.
[b]Modified from the RECIST criteria (12;13).
[c]PET scan was used selectively in lesions with unclear response by CT imaging.

Table 45–2

Response to RFA and Survival[a]

Tumor type (number of patients)	Lesions (n)[b]	CR (%)	PR (%)	SD (%)	PD (%)	Alive NED (%)	Alive WD (%)	Died (%)
NSCLC (5)	5	0	2 (40)	3 (60)	0	3 (60)	1 (20)	1 (20)
Mets (13)	23	1 (7.7)	5 (38.5)	4 (30.8)	3 (23.1)	2 (15.4)	5 (38.4)	6 (46.2)
Size >5 cm (6)	10	0	2 (33.3)	2 (33.3)	2 (33.3)	1 (17)	1 (17)	4 (66)
Size <5 cm (12)	18	1 (8.3)	7 (58.3)	3 (25)	1 (8.3)	5 (41.7)	3 (25)	4 (33.3)

[a]NSCLC, non–small cell lung cancer; Mets, metastatic; CR, complete response; PR, partial response; SD, stable disease; PD, progressive disease; NED, no evidence of disease; WD, with disease.
[b]Data from three patients who underwent second RFA treatment (five tumors) are excluded from response and survival analysis.

These studies demonstrate the feasibility of RFA for lung tumors not amenable to surgical resection. More central RFA treatments run the potential of damage to larger branches of the pulmonary artery with delayed hemorrhage and should be approached cautiously. Tumors greater than 4 cm should not be considered ideal targets using the current technology. Clinical trials will be needed for continued assessment of safety and impact on long-term tumor control and survival.

▶ STEREOTACTIC RADIOSURGERY

Conventional radiation offers a relatively poor chance of cure for primary lung tumors and is generally considered palliative rather than curative treatment. Standard radiation techniques also lead to significant damage to surrounding nonneoplastic tissue. Radical radiotherapy with conventional techniques shows long-term survival rates of 3–13%.[17,22,41] One study of radical radiotherapy (44–52 Gy) showed 1-, 2-,

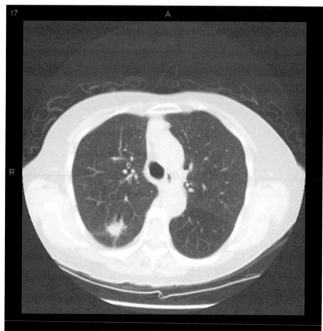

Figure 45–2 CT scan of right lung tumor prior to RFA.

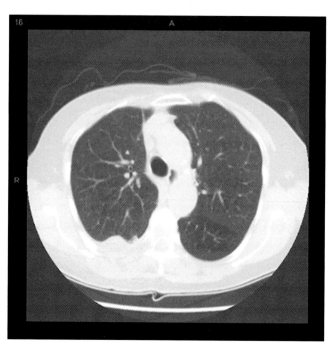

Figure 45–3 CT scan of right lung tumor 3 months after RFA showing a decrease in size and pleural reaction.

and 3-year survival rates of 43, 16, and 3%, respectively.[41] Another study of 53 patients with non–small cell lung carcinoma treated with definitive radiation (mean dose of 63 Gy) showed a 3-year survival rate of 19% and a 6-year survival rate of only 5%.[22] Smaller tumors may have a more favorable prognosis with primary radiotherapy with T-status being an independent predictor of survival following radiotherapy.[17,20,22,41] In subset analyses, patients with small tumors (T1) 5-year survival rates of 30–50% have been reported.[17,20]

The poor long-term survival with conventional radiation is associated with poor local control.* A meta-analysis of patients with stage I and II non–small cell lung cancers that were medically inoperable and treated by conventional radiation showed local failure to be the predominant mode of failure.[20] In 53 patients treated with primary radiation, local primary tumor progression was seen in 22 of 53 patients.[22]

Higher radiation doses appear to enhance local tumor control.[5,30] In one study, patients receiving greater than 70 Gy had better local control and cancer-specific survival than those treated with lower doses.[7] Another study demonstrated that doses greater than 65 Gy appeared to result in a decreased proportion of patients dying of lung cancer.[22] Many have suggested that intensified local treatment with higher doses of radiation is required to prevent local recurrence, which is the major cause of failure after conventional radiation therapy. Increased doses of radiation result in increased toxicity and damage to surrounding pulmonary parenchyma, however, which can limit dose escalation. The major toxicity encountered in treatment of lung tumors is pulmonary toxicity.[1,3,8,26] Dose–volume histogram data show a correlation between risk of pulmonary toxicity and indices of dose to lung parenchyma. The risk of toxicity increases as the area of adjacent normal lung irradiated increases. Grade III or higher pulmonary toxicity occurred in 38% (3 of 8) patients in whom greater than 30% of their lung volume received 25 Gy or more versus only 4% (1 of 23) patients with less than 30% of their lung volume receiving doses of 25 Gy or greater.[3] In another study of hyperfractionated accelerated radiotherapy, doses greater than 72 Gy were associated with a 17% rate of grade III or higher pulmonary toxicity.[26] Radiation fibrosis seems to depend on the volume of lung radiated above a threshold of 20–30 Gy.[1]

Poor local control with conventional radiation may also result from inaccurate tumor targeting and failure to satisfactorily conform the dose distribution to the tumor target volume. Three-dimensional conformal treatment planning is a radiotherapy technique that provides more accurate dose targeting via the direct transfer of three-dimensional anatomic information from diagnostic scans into the planning process. Three-dimensional conformal radiotherapy (3D-CRT) holds promise because it allows higher doses to be delivered to the target by improved shaping of the radiation portals with the conformal avoidance of normal structures.[34] 3D-CRT planning selects optimal treatment parameters to increase dose to tumor and to reduce normal tissue dose, permitting dose escalation while minimizing associated pulmonary radiation toxicity. A correlation exists between lung dose–volume histogram data and the risk of severe pulmonary toxicity.

Dose escalation in non–small cell lung cancer has been safely accomplished in patients using 3D-CRT, limiting target volumes, and segregating patients by the volume of normal lung irradiated.[19] 3D-CRT can result in improved survival with primary radiotherapy for lung cancer. Two hundred and seven patients treated with 3D-CRT to a median dose of 70 Gy showed a 1-year survival of 59% and 2-year survival of 45%. Patients treated with doses greater than 70 Gy had better local control and cause-specific

*References 2, 3, 5, 13, 20, 22, 26, 28.

survival than those treated with lower doses.[7] In two other studies using 3D-CRT with median doses of 60–70 Gy, 5-year survival was still limited at 12% in both studies. Local progression remained the cause of death in 30% of patients, indicating that local failure rates remain substantial despite 3D-CRT for stage I non–small cell lung cancer.[2,25]

Further improvement in local control may need to take into account issues of tumor mobility. Respiratory motion is significant and results in an increased field requiring radiation, limiting overall maximum dose to the tumor. Conformal radiotherapy beams are defined on the basis of static CT acquisitions by taking into account setup errors and organ tumor motion during breathing. In the absence of precise data, the size of the margins for treatment is estimated arbitrarily. One study evaluated the amplitude of maximum intrathoracic organ motion during breathing. CT scan images were taken during different phases of respiration (free breathing, deep breath-hold inspiration, and deep breath-hold expiration) in treatment positions and with patient immobilization. Greatest displacements were observed just above the diaphragm and smallest displacements were observed for the lung apices and adjacent to the carina. The use of personalized immobilization devices reduced lateral thoracic movements and lung apex movements. It was concluded that intrathoracic movements during extreme phases of breathing are considerable and quantification of organ motion is necessary for definition of the safety margins.[15]

In another study, radiologically implanted lung markers were followed with real-time lung imaging. Motion was seen of 5.5–10.0 mm laterally, 6.8–15.9 mm in the craniocaudal direction, and 8.1–14.6 mm in the ventrodorsal direction.[38] Twenty-two patients with stage I non–small cell lung carcinoma were treated with hypofractionated 3D-CRT after radiological evaluation of respiratory excursion. CT scans were taken during three respiratory phases and carefully analyzed to determine the planning target volume (which included the primary tumor and allowances for respiratory movement). Radiation doses of 48 or 60 Gy were administered at the edge of the moving tumor during normal breathing with 80% of the prescribed dose being confined to the target volume. Of 17 patients available for follow-up, 5 showed a complete response, 11 a partial response, and 1 progression. Sixteen (94%) were controlled locally. Lung cancer survival rate at 1 year was 94% and at 2 years was 73%. The treatments were well tolerated, and although focal radiation pneumonitis was demonstrated on CT, patients were asymptomatic and parameters of pulmonary function (vital capacity, total lung capacity, and diffusion capacity) did not change significantly.[13] It was demonstrated that small volume image-guided hypofractionated radiotherapy is feasible with increased potential for curative treatment for stage I non–small cell lung cancer with a high local tumor control rate and low morbidity.

To address the issue of lung mobility during breathing, some authors have evaluated the benefit of radiation only during periods of breath hold. One group studied deep-inspiration breath hold with the goals of tumor immobilization and expansion of normal lung tissue out of the high-dose region. They found that deep-inspiration breath hold was feasible in a clinical setting. Consistent lung inflation levels were achieved in patients as judged by both spirometry and verification radiographs. Breathing-induced tumor motion was significantly reduced using deep-inspiration breath hold compared to free breathing, enabling better target coverage.[27] In three-dimensional conformal radiation treatment with deep-inspiration breath hold, the estimated normal tissue complication probabilities decreased in all patients at their prescribed dose compared to free breathing. The dose to which patients could be treated with deep-inspiration breath hold increased on average from 69 to 88 Gy without increasing the risk of toxicity. The deep-inspiration breath-hold technique produced an advantage to conventional free-breathing treatment by decreasing lung density, reducing normal safety margins, and enabling more accurate treatment. These improvements contribute to the effective exclusion of normal lung tissue from the high-dose region and permit the use of higher treatment doses without increased risks of toxicity.[36] Another group evaluated the dosimetric benefit of self-gated radiotherapy at deep-inspiration breath hold in the treatment of patients with non–small cell lung cancer. In this study, the relative contributions of tumor immobilization at breath hold and increased lung volume at deep inspiration in sparing high-dose lung irradiation (greater than 20 Gy) were examined. Compared with free-breathing conditions, at deep-inspiration breath hold, the mean reduction in patient lung volume receiving greater than 20 Gy was 14% with the increase in lung volume alone, 22% with tumor immobilization alone (using deep-inspiration breath hold instead of free-breathing target volume), and 33% with the combined effect.[4]

Respiratory gating techniques are relatively new and potentially useful therapeutic additions to external-beam radiotherapy when applied to regions affected by intrafraction motion. During the imaging of dynamically moving spheres, gating reproduced the static volume to within 1% whereas errors of over 20% were observed when gating was not used. Respiratory gating may allow a reduction in treatment margins, an improvement in image quality, and an improvement in the positional and volumetric accuracy of gross tumor volume.[23] Others have described a gate pulse-controller that starts and stops the irradiation at a chosen phase of the respiratory cycle by using a laser displacement sensor for detection of respiratory motion, which controls a linear accelerator radiation source. Radiation delivery can be administered between 50% inspiration and 50% expiration or 70% inspiration and 30% expiration.[39]

Another approach to the issue of lung tumor mobility is the use of body-immobilization devices. The use of personalized immobilization devices can reduce lateral thoracic movements and lung apex movement. The use of a body frame immobilization device decreased tumor movement from a 8–20 to a 2–11 mm range. Immobilization consisted of a personalized body shell shaped to the patient's contour and application of external upper-abdominal pressure.[32] Clinical outcomes were reported using three-dimensional conformal hypofractionated single high-dose radiotherapy using a stereotactic body frame. There were 40 patients followed for more than 10 months. Thirty-one had primary lung carcinoma (T_1 19; T_2 8; T_3 4) and nine had metastatic lesions. All patients were irradiated using a stereotactic body frame and received four high-dose fractions of 10–12 Gy during a period of 5–13 days. The initial three patients received 40 Gy and the remaining 37 received 48 Gy. Of the

33 tumors followed for more than 6 months, 6 tumors (18%) disappeared completely, and 25 tumors (76%) decreased in size by 30% or more. Overall, 94% showed a local response. During the follow-up of 4–37 months (median 19 months) no complications greater than grade II lung toxicity were noted. Of the 16 patients with histologically confirmed T_1 N_0 primary lung carcinoma who received 48 Gy all tumors were locally controlled during the follow-up of 6–36 months (median 19 months). Of the nine metastatic tumors to the lung, seven responded and two did not. Three of the initial responders relapsed locally at a median of 7 months later.[31]

Dynamic real-time tracking of the tumor position during radiation therapy represents a more sophisticated method of conformal radiation delivery. One study reports fluoroscopic real-time tumor tracking during radiation therapy. Gold markers were inserted in the lung using fiberoptic bronchoscopy, and the three-dimensional position of a 1.0- to 2.0-mm gold marker was detected by fluoroscopy every 0.03 s. The treatment beam was gated to irradiate the tumor only when the position of the marker coincided with its planned position using the gated system. Twenty tumors were treated in 18 patients with high-dose hypofractionated focal irradiation (35–48 Gy in four to eight fractions administered over 4–10 days). Tumor markers were successfully implanted and maintained at the inserted position during and after the radiotherapy in 14 (88%) of 16 peripheral lung tumors and in 0 (0%) of 4 central lung tumors. Tracking of the tumor marker was successful in one of two tumors with a 1.0-mm marker and all 12 patients with a 2.0-mm marker. Overall, 13 (65%) of the 20 tumors were successfully treated with gated therapy using real-time radiological tracking. Local tumor control was achieved and maintained for all 12 patients (13 tumors) successfully treated with a median follow-up of 9 months (range 5–15 months). While localized radiation pneumonitis was found radiographically at the lung volume that was irradiated with above 20 Gy, 11 of 12 patients were asymptomatic. It was demonstrated that insertion of gold markers into or near peripheral type tumors

using fiberoptic bronchoscopy is a feasible and safe technique with excellent initial response and low incidence of clinical complications.[18]

The CyberKnife is a commercially available radiation delivery system that was initially developed for frameless radiosurgical ablation of brain tumors. The device has the capability, however, to image and treat within the thoracic and abdominal cavity. It is the only FDA-approved device for extracranial stereotactic radiosurgery. The CyberKnife system consists of a linear accelerator radiation source mounted on a robotic arm (Figure 45-4). Through the use of image-guidance cameras that image implanted gold fiducial tumor markers adjacent to the tumor, the CyberKnife system precisely localizes the tumor in space. The linear accelerator attached to the robotic arm is then used to deliver multiple highly focused beams of radiation that converge at the tumor site. In a recent study by Whyte et al, the experience with stereotactic radiosurgery with the CyberKnife system was reported in 23 patients. Nine patients were treated with a breath-holding technique and 14 with a respiratory-gated automated robotic technique. All tumors were deemed unresectable either by radiological criteria (T_4 lesion) or by patient unsuitability for surgery based on medical comorbidity or patient refusal. Radiation was delivered in a single fraction of 15 Gy. Procedural complications consisted of pneumothorax in three patients, only one of whom required a chest tube. There was no radiation esophagitis or clinically apparent radiation pneumonitis. Radiological response at follow-up at 1–3 months was complete in 2 patients, partial in 15, stable in 4, and progressive in 2.[40]

At the University of Pittsburgh, we treated six patients with either stage I lung cancer who are medically inoperable or patients with limited metastatic disease who were not felt to be good operative candidates with the CyberKnife at a dose of 20 Gy delivered in a single fraction. Although our experience does not yet allow assessment of long-term efficacy, early responses have been encouraging and toxicity is minimal. Representative CT scans prior to, and 3 months

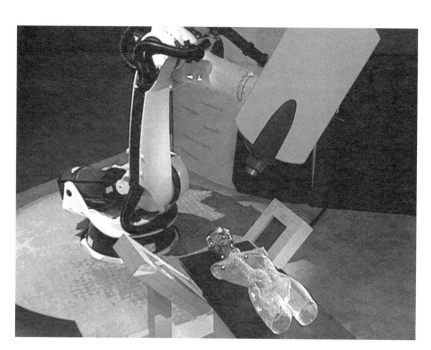

Figure 45–4 CyberKnife radiation delivery system with linear accelerator mounted on a robotic arm.

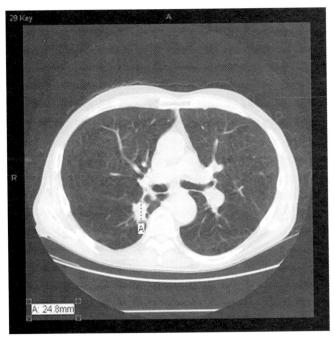

Figure 45–5 CT scan of right lung squamous cell carcinoma prior to CyberKnife treatment.

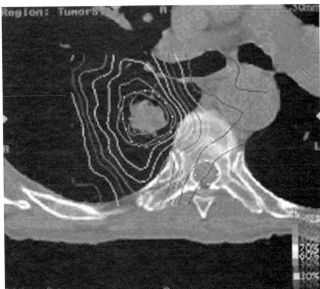

Figure 45–7 Radiation plan generated with CyberKnife radiation delivery system with radiation doses superimposed on the image of the tumor. (See color plate.)

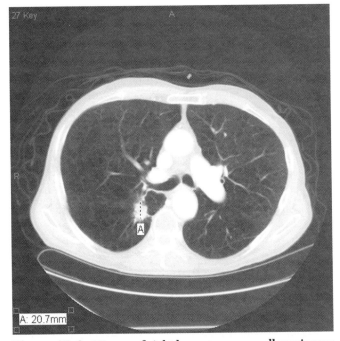

Figure 45–6 CT scan of right lung squamous cell carcinoma 3 months after CyberKnife radiosurgery (20 Gy to the 80th isodose line in one fraction) showing a decrease in size.

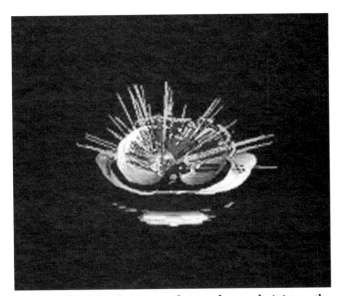

Figure 45–8 Radiation paths used to administer the radiation plan. (See color plate.)

after, CyberKnife radiosurgery are shown in Figures 45-5 and 45-6, respectively. The treatment plan isodose curves are shown in Figure 45-7, and the beam paths used to administer the radiation are shown in Figure 45-8. These early results with the CyberKnife radiosurgery system have demonstrated the safety and feasibility of stereotactic radiosurgery to the lung. Further studies with dose escalation and evaluation of optimal fractionation are needed to determine the full potential of stereotactic radiosurgery in the treatment of lung tumors.

▶ CHEMOPERFUSION OF THE PLEURAL CAVITY

The results of surgical therapy alone or combined with traditional chemotherapy or radiation therapy have been disappointing for patients with malignant pleural extension from malignant mesothelioma, thymic malignancies, and non–small cell lung cancer. The standard of care for most of these malignancies continues to evolve. One strategy is to surgically remove all gross disease and follow this with chemoperfusion of the pleural cavity. The advantage of this approach is a direct exposure of any residual microscopic disease to higher drug concentrations while minimizing the toxic systemic side effects. Adding hyperthermia to this strategy has been shown in some studies to increase the local tissue and cellular concentrations of the chemotherapy compared to normothermic perfusion. The drug most commonly reported for use in intrapleural hyperthermic chemoperfusion is cisplatinum. Additional proposed mechanisms of synergy between cisplatinum perfusion and hyperthermia include a significant enhancement of the DNA cross-linking effect of the drug and heat-induced inhibition of DNA repair.[24]

Most of the experience with intraoperative hyperthermic chemoperfusion has been for the treatment of intraperitoneal malignancies.[42] Recently, there have been a few nonrandomized trials of cytoreductive surgery followed by intraoperative hyperthermic intrathoracic perfusion chemotherapy. Although a cautionary note must be added regarding any efficacy, these reports have demonstrated feasibility and some enthusiasm that local control and, in some cases, survival may be better compared to historic controls.

The optimal temperature of the perfusate is unknown, but temperatures higher than 43° C may lead to an increased risk of pulmonary edema if the ipsilateral lung remains in place, for example, after pleurectomy alone. In the case of extrapleural pneumonectomy, perfusion at the same operative setting as the resection may lead to an increased risk of postpneumonectomy pulmonary edema due to the extra hydration that is given routinely to minimize the renal toxicity of the cisplatin. In our own protocol, if extrapleural pneumonectomy is performed, we delay the hyperthermic chemoperfusion with cisplatinum for 4 days. If the contralateral lung is functioning well at that point and there is minimal oxygen requirement, we return to the operating room and hydrate the patient aggressively to induce a diuresis and then perform the hyperthermic chemoperfusion at 43° C for 2 h using videothoracoscopic access. In most centers, this application is limited to clinical trials, with the majority of the experience being reported in patients with malignant mesothelioma and thymic malignancies, with fewer data in the treatment of stage IIIB non–small cell lung cancer. In one report, Yellin et al described the results of hyperthermic pleural perfusion with cisplatin in a heterogeneous group of patients with malignant pleural involvement.[44] This group of 26 patients included seven with malignant mesothelioma, seven with stage IVA thymoma, four with thymic carcinoma, one with chest wall sarcoma, three with non–small cell lung cancer, two with metastatic sarcoma, and two with metastatic carcinoma (one ovarian, one squamous of unknown origin). Surgical resection of all gross disease was attempted with resection and pleurectomy in 10, extrapleural pneumonectomy in 8, and incomplete resections in the other patients. Hyperthermic chemoperfusion was performed with cisplatin at various concentrations at an infusion temperature of 42° C for 1 h. Intrapleural temperatures ranged from 40.1 to 41.5° C with a maximal systemic temperature of 38° C. Creatinine clearance remained unchanged in all patients and no significant hematological toxicities were reported. The most notable postoperative complication was empyema, which occurred in 4 of 26 patients (15%). There was one postoperative death from a gastric herniation,

apparently unrelated to the chemoperfusion. Complete ipsilateral pleuropulmonary control of disease was reported in 17 of 24 (71%) evaluable patients. Overall 3-year survival was 44% in this group of patients, which, as noted, was better than the expected survival compared to historic controls.

In a report by de Bree et al, cytoreductive surgery was performed for 11 patients with malignant mesothelioma and 3 patients with pleural thymoma metastases followed by hyperthermic chemoperfusion of the pleural cavity with a combination of Adriamycin and cisplatin.[10] In the thymoma group, four perfusions were performed for three patients. Complications included one grade 2 nephrotoxicity and one wound dehiscence. At an early follow-up of 18 months, all three patients were alive and free of disease. In a follow-up comment, however, two of the patients suffered disease recurrence.[11] In the mesothelioma group, at a mean follow-up of 7 months, there were three recurrences with two of the patients dying of contralateral and peritoneal disease.

The role of intracavitary chemotherapy with or without hyperthermia for thoracic malignancies with pleural involvement remains unclear. Further clinical trials will be required to determine the ideal candidates, optimal chemotherapy, and the timing and temperature of the perfusate. Logical requirements for inclusion of patients in these treatment protocols include disease confined to one pleural cavity with no extrathoracic metastases and that gross removal of all local disease is achievable.

▶ **SUMMARY**

Although surgical resection remains the gold standard for local control of pulmonary malignancies, newer technologies such as radiofrequency ablation and stereotactic radiosurgery hold the potential for less invasive treatment in the future. We anticipate that these newer less invasive techniques will complement existing minimally invasive surgical treatments and may further ease the burden of treatment and also ultimately improve the survival in selected high-risk patients with pulmonary tumors. Critical appraisal of these techniques over the next decade will establish their role.

REFERENCES

1. Abratt RP, Morgan GW: Lung toxicity following chest irradiation in patients with lung cancer. Lung Cancer 35(2):103–109, 2002.
2. Armstrong J, Raben A, Zelefsky M, et al: Promising survival with three-dimensional conformal radiation therapy for non-small cell lung cancer. Radiother Oncol 44(1):17–22, 1997.
3. Armstrong J, Zelefsky M, Leibel SA, et al: Strategy for dose escalation using 3-dimensional conformal radiation therapy for lung cancer. Ann Oncol 6(7):693–697, 1995.
4. Barnes EA, Murray BR, Robinson DM, et al: Dosimetric evaluation of lung tumor immobilization using breath hold at deep inspiration. Int J Radiat Oncol Biol Phys 50(4):1091–1098, 2001.
5. Baumann M, Appold S, Petersen S, et al: Dose and fractionation concepts in the primary radiotherapy of non-small cell lung cancer. Lung Cancer 33(Suppl 1):S35–S45, 2001.

6. Bilchik AJ, Wood TF, Allegra DP: Radiofrequency ablation of unresectable hepatic malignancies: Lessons learned. Oncologist 6(1):24–33, 2001.

7. Bradley JD, Ieumwananonthachai N, Purdy JA, et al: Gross tumor volume, critical prognostic factor in patients treated with three-dimensional conformal radiation therapy for non-small cell lung carcinoma. Int J Radiat Oncol Biol Phys 52(1):49–57, 2002.

8. Byhardt RW, Martin L, Pajak TF, et al: The influence of field size and other treatment factors on pulmonary toxicity following hyperfractionated irradiation for inoperable non-small cell lung cancer: Analysis of a Radiation Therapy Oncology Group protocol. Int J Radiat Oncol Biol Phys 27(3):537–544, 1993.

9. Curley SA, Izzo, F, Delvio P, et al: Radiofrequency ablation of unresectable primary and metastatic hepatic malignancies: Results in 123 patients. Ann Surg 230(1):1–8, 1997.

10. de Bree E, van Ruth S, Baas P, et al: Cytoreductive surgery and intraoperative hyperthermic chemotherapy in patients with malignant pleural mesothelioma or pleural metastases of thymoma. Chest 121:480–487, 2002.

11. de Bree E, van Ruth S, Rutgers EJ, et al: Reoperation combined with intraoperative hyperthermic intrathoracic perfusion chemotherapy for pleural recurrence of thymoma. Letter to the editor. J Surg Oncol 80:224–225, 2002.

12. Dupuy DE, Zagoria RJ, Akerley W, et al: Percutaneous radiofrequency ablation of malignancies in the lung. AJR Am J Roentgenol 174:57–59, 2000.

13. Fukumoto S, Shirato H, Shimzu S, et al: Small-volume image-guided radiotherapy using hypofractionated coplanar and non-coplanar multiple fields for patients with inoperable stage I non-small cell lung carcinomas. Cancer 95(7):1546–1553, 2002.

14. Gazelle GS, Goldberg SN, Solbiati L, et al: Tumor ablation with radiofrequency energy. Radiology 217:633–646, 2000.

15. Giraud P, De Rycke Y, Dubray B, et al: Conformal radiotherapy planning for lung cancer: Analysis of intrathoracic organ motion during extreme phases of breathing. Int J Radiat Oncol Biol Phys 51(4):1081–1092, 2002.

16. Goldberg SN, Gazelle GS, Compton CC, et al: Radiofrequency tissue ablation of VX2 tumor nodules in the rabbit lung. Acad Radiol 3:929–935, 1996.

17. Graham PH, Gebski VJ, Langlands AO: Radical radiotherapy for early non-small cell lung cancer. Int J Radiat Oncol Biol Phys 31(2):261–266, 1995.

18. Harada T, Shirato H, Ogura S, et al: Real-time tumor-tracking radiation therapy for lung carcinoma by the aid of insertion of a gold marker using bronchofiberoscopy. Cancer 95(8):1720–1727, 2002.

19. Hayman JA, Martel MK, Ten Haken RK, et al: Dose escalation in non-small cell lung cancer using three-dimensional conformal radiation therapy: Update of a phase I trial. J Clin Oncol 19(1):127–136, 2001.

20. Jeremic B, Classen J, Bamberg M: Radiotherapy alone in technically operable, medically inoperable, early stage (I/II) non-small cell lung cancer. Int J Radiat Oncol Biol Phys 54(1):119–130, 2002.

21. Kang S, Luo R, Liao W, et al: Effect of radiofrequency ablation on lung cancer. Proceedings of the 37th Annual Meeting of the American Society of Clinical Oncology, 2001.

22. Kaskowitz L, Graham MV, Emami B, et al: Radiation therapy alone for stage I non-small cell lung cancer. Int J Radiat Oncol Biol Phys 27(3):517–523, 1993.

23. Keall PJ, Kini VR, Vedam SS, et al: Potential radiotherapy improvements with respiratory gating. Australas Phys Eng Sci Med 25(1):1–6, 2002.

24. Kodama K, Doi O, Tutsuda M, et al: Development of postoperative intrathoracic chemothermotherapy for lung cancer with objective of improving local cure. Cancer 64:1422–1428, 1989.

25. Lagerwaard FJ, Senanb S, van Meerbeeck JP, et al: Has 3-D conformal radiotherapy improved local control for stage I non-small cell lung cancer? Radiother Oncol 63(2): 151–157, 2002.

26. Maguire PD, Marks LB, Sibley GS, et al: 73.6 Gy and beyond: Hyperfractionated, accelerated radiotherapy for non-small cell lung cancer. J Clin Oncol 19(3):705–711, 2001.

27. Mah D, Hanley J, Rosenzweig KE, et al: Technical aspects of deep inspiration breath-hold technique in the treatment of thoracic cancer. Int J Radiat Oncol Biol Phys 48(4):1175–1185, 2000.

28. Marks LB, Sibley G: The rationale and use of three-dimensional radiation treatment planning for lung cancer. Chest 116(Suppl 6):539S–545S, 1999.

29. Miao Y, Ni Y, Bosmans H, et al: Radiofrequency ablation for eradication of pulmonary tumor in rabbits. J Surg Res 99:265–271, 2001.

30. Movsas B: Innovative treatment strategies in locally advanced and/or unresectable non-small cell lung cancer. Cancer Control 7(1):13–14, 2000.

31. Nagata Y, Negoro Y, Aoki T, et al: Clinical outcomes of 3D conformal hypofractionated single high-dose radiotherapy for one or two lung tumors using a stereotactic body frame. Int J Radiat Oncol Biol Phys 52(4):1041–1046, 2002.

32. Negoro Y, Nagata Y, Aoki T, et al: The effectiveness of an immobilization device in conformal radiotherapy for lung tumor: Reduction of respiratory tumor movement and evaluation of the daily setup accuracy. Int J Radiat Oncol Biol Phys 50(4):889–898, 2001.

33. Padhani AR, Ollivier L: The RECIST (Response Evaluation Criteria in Solid Tumors) criteria: Implications for diagnostic radiologists. Br J Radiol 74(887):983–986, 2001.

34. Patel RR, Mehta M: Three-dimensional conformal radiotherapy for lung cancer: Promises and pitfalls. Curr Oncol Rep 4(4):347–353, 2002.

35. Putnam JB, Thomsen SL, Siegenthale M: Therapeutic implications of heat-induced lung injury. Crit Rev Opt Sci Technol 75:139–160, 2000.

36. Rosenzweig KE, Hanley J, Mah D, et al: The deep inspiration breath-hold technique in the treatment of inoperable non-small cell lung cancer. Int J Radiat Oncol Biol Phys 48(1):81–87, 2000.

37. Sewell PE, Jackson, Vance RB, et al: Assessing radiofrequency ablation of non-small cell lung cancer with positron emission tomography. Radiology 217(Suppl 3):334, 2000.

38. Shimizu S, Shirato H, Ogura S, et al: Detection of lung tumor movement in real-time tumor tracking radiotherapy. Int J Radiat Oncol Biol Phys 51(2):304–310, 2001.

39. Tada T, Minakuchi K, Fujioka T, et al: Lung cancer intermittent irradiation synchronized with respiratory motion: Results of a pilot study. Radiology 207(3):779–783, 1998.

40. Whyte RI, Crownover R, Murphy MJ, et al: Stereotactic radiosurgery for lung tumors: Preliminary report of a phase I trial. Ann Thorac Surg 75:1097–1101, 2003.

41. Wigren T, Kellokumpu-Lehtinen P, Ojala A: Radical radiotherapy of inoperable non-small cell lung cancer: Irradiation techniques and tumor characteristics in relation to local control and survival. Acta Oncol 31(5):555–561, 1992.

42. Witkamp AJ, de Bree E, Zoetmulder FA: Rationale and techniques of intraoperative hyperthermic intraperitoneal chemotherapy. Cancer Treat Rev 27:365–375, 2001.

43. Yang S, Whyte R, Askin F, et al: Radiofrequency ablation of primary and metastatic lung tumors: Analysis of an ablate and resect study. The American Association for Thoracic Surgery 82nd Annual Meeting, 2002 (abstract).

44. Yellin A, Simansky DA, Paley, M, et al: Hyperthermic pleural perfusion with cisplatin: Early clinical experience. Cancer 92:2197–2203, 2001.

Adult cardiac

SECTION 2

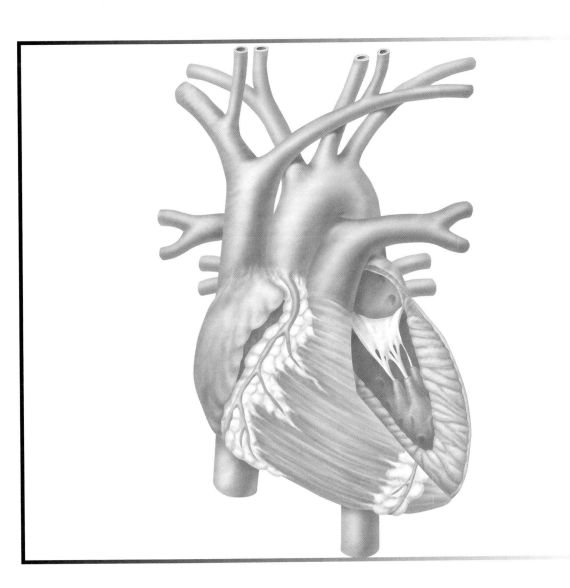

Basic Science

Diagnostic Procedures

Medical- and Catheter-Based Treatment of Cardiac Disease

Perioperative and Intraoperative Care of the Cardiac Surgical Patient

Surgical Management of Aortic Disease

Surgical Management of Valvular Heart Disease

Management of Cardiac Arrhythmias

Surgical Treatment of Coronary Artery Disease and its Complications

Surgical Management of Heart Failure

733

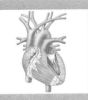
Surgical Anatomy of the Heart

Robert H. Anderson, Benson R. Wilcox, and Andrew C. Cook

▶ INTRODUCTION

It is axiomatic that safe surgery requires a thorough understanding of cardiac anatomy. In this chapter, we will attempt to provide a brief overview of cardiac structure as we consider it pertinent for the surgeon. When describing the heart, we will consider it as arranged within the body in its anatomical position.[8] Whenever possible, however, we will illustrate the cardiac components as they might be viewed by the surgeon during an operative procedure, irrespective of whether the pictures themselves were taken in the operating room or are photographs of autopsied hearts.[20] In some instances, nonetheless, the information discussed is best presented with the heart photographed in a nonsurgical orientation. When this occurs, it will be clearly stated.

▶ LOCATION OF THE HEART

Regardless of the surgical approach, having entered the mediastinum, the surgeon will be confronted by the heart enclosed in its pericardial sac. The sac is freestanding around the atrial chambers and the ventricles, but becomes adherent to the adventitial coverings of the great arteries and veins at their entrances to and exits from the heart, these attachments closing the pericardial cavity. The pericardial cavity is contained between the two layers of the serous pericardium, this being a thin-walled sack folded on itself within the fibrous cavity. The inner layer, or epicardium, is firmly attached to the myocardium, whereas the outer layer is adherent to the fibrous pericardium. The peri-

cardial cavity, therefore, is the space between the inner lining of the fibrous pericardium and the surface of the heart (Figure 46-1). By virtue of the shape of the cardiac chambers and great arteries, there are two recesses within this cavity that are lined by serous pericardium. The first is the transverse sinus, which occupies the inner curvature of the heart (Figure 46-2). Laterally, on each side, the ends of the transverse sinus are in free communication with the rest of the pericardial cavity. The second pericardial recess is the oblique sinus, a blind-ending cavity behind the left atrium (Figure 46-3).

Most of the cardiac surface facing the surgeon is occupied by the so-called right chambers, which in reality are anterior. Thus, the surgeon is confronted by the extensive appendage of the right atrium, receiving the superior caval vein at its superior border. To the left are the pulmonary trunk and aorta, exiting from the base of the heart and extending in a superior direction, with the aortic root in a posterior and rightward position. Should the aortic root not be in this "normal" relationship, then the ventriculoarterial connections will almost always be abnormal. The morphologically right appendage has a characteristic shape, being triangular and possessing a broad junction with the atrial cavity (Figure 46-4). The morphologically left appendage may not be seen immediately. If searched for, it will be found as a tubular structure at the left border of the pulmonary trunk (Figure 46-5), having a narrow junction with the rest of the atrium.

The ventricular mass then extends to the cardiac apex, which normally reaches into the left hemithorax. The overall cardiac silhouette is usually positioned with one third of its bulk to the right and two thirds to the left of the midline (Figure 46-6). An anomalous position of either the ventricular mass or the apex is again highly suggestive of the presence of congenital cardiac malformations. In shape, the ventricular mass is a three-sided pyramid, having diaphragmatic, anterior or sternocostal, and left or pulmonary surfaces. The margin between the first two surfaces is sharp, so it is called the acute margin. The transition between the sternocostal and pulmonary surfaces is more gradual and rounded. For the surgeon, it is the pulmonary surface that is considered to represent the obtuse margin, this being irrigated by the obtuse marginal arteries (Figure 46-7). The greater part of the anterior surface of the ventricular mass is occupied by the morphologically right ventricle. Its left

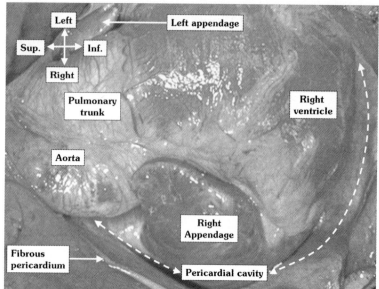

Figure 46–1 The heart is shown as seen by the surgeon through a median sternotomy. The pericardial cavity has been opened and is between the fibrous pericardium and the epicardium. The "compass" shows the orientation. (See color plate.)
(Copyright in the original illustration from which this figure was prepared belongs to Robert H. Anderson, Benson R. Wilcox, and Andrew C. Cook.)

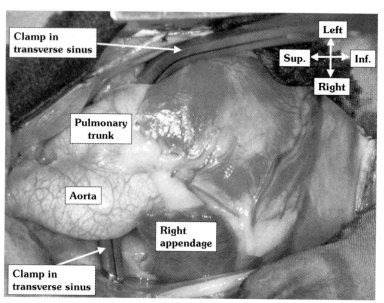

Figure 46–2 With the pericardium opened in the operating room, the surgical clamp has been passed through the transverse sinus of the pericardium, which is between the back of the arterial trunks and the front of the atrial chambers. (See color plate.)
(Copyright in the original illustration from which this figure was prepared belongs to Robert H. Anderson, Benson R. Wilcox, and Andrew C. Cook.)

border is marked by the anterior interventricular, or descending, branch of the left coronary artery, and its right border is marked by the right coronary artery, which runs obliquely in the atrioventricular groove.

The surface anatomy of the heart is helpful in determining the most appropriate site for an incision to gain access to a given cardiac chamber.[20] For example, the relatively bloodless outlet portion of the right ventricle just beneath the origin of the pulmonary trunk affords ready access to the ventricular cavity. The important landmark for the right atrium is the terminal groove, or sulcus terminalis, which marks the border between the appendage and the venous component (Figure 46-8). The sinus node is typically located within this groove, usually laterally within the superior cavoatrial junction inferior to the crest of the appendage. Posterior, and parallel, to the terminal groove is a second, deeper, groove between the right atrium and the right pulmonary veins. Dissections into

this deep interatrial groove, also known as Waterston's or Sondergaard's groove, permit incisions to be made into the left atrium (Figure 46-9).

MORPHOLOGICALLY RIGHT ATRIUM

The right atrium has three components, the appendage, the venous sinus receiving the systemic venous return, and the vestibule. It is separated by the septum from the left atrium. As already discussed, the junction between the appendage and the venous sinus is marked externally by the prominent terminal groove. Internally, the groove corresponds with the position of the terminal crest (crista terminalis), which gives origin to the pectinate muscles of the appendage (Figure 46-10). Significantly, the pectinate muscles within the appendage encircle the full extent of the third component,

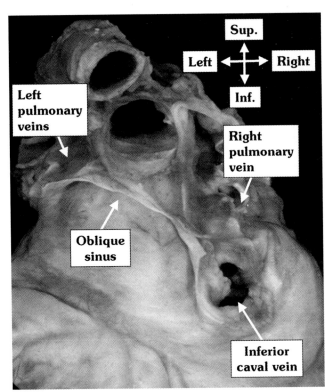

Figure 46–3 This anatomical specimen has been removed from the body and is viewed from behind, with the apex pointing down. The oblique sinus of the pericardium is seen between the pericardial reflections around the pulmonary veins and the inferior caval vein. (See color plate.)
(Copyright in the original illustration from which this figure was prepared belongs to Robert H. Anderson, Benson R. Wilcox, and Andrew C. Cook.)

summit of the terminal groove, and that continues in the transverse sinus behind the aorta across the interatrial groove as Bachman's bundle (Figure 46-12). The sinus node lies within the terminal groove in an immediately subepicardial position. It is a spindle-shaped structure that usually lies to the right of the crest, that is, lateral to the superior cavoatrial junction. In about one tenth of cases, the node extends across the crest into the interatrial groove, draping itself across the cavoatrial junction in horseshoe fashion.[1] For the surgeon, the artery to the sinus node is also of significance. This is a branch of the right coronary artery in about 55% of individuals and a branch of the circumflex artery in the remainder.[14] Irrespective of its origin, it usually courses through the anterior interatrial groove toward the superior cavoatrial junction, frequently running within the atrial myocardium. Having reached the cavoatrial junction, the artery may cross the crest of the appendage, course retrocavally, or even divide to form an arterial circle around the junction.

On first sight, when inspecting the internal morphology of the right atrium, there appears to be an extensive septal surface between the orifices of the caval veins and the orifice of the tricuspid valve. The apparent extent of this septum is spurious.[6,17] The true septum between the right and left atrial chambers is formed by the floor and the antero-inferior muscular rim of the oval fossa.[6] The extensive superior rim, the so-called septum secundum, is formed by the deep interatrial groove extending between the tributaries of the systemic venous sinus and the pulmonary veins (Figure 46-13). The larger part of the anterior atrial wall overlies the aortic root. These limited margins of the true atrial septum are of major surgical importance, since it is easy to pass outside the heart when attempting to gain access to the left atrium through a right atrial approach.

In addition to the position of the sinus node, and the extent of the atrial septum, the other major area of surgical significance within the right atrium is the site of the atrioventricular node. This is contained within the triangle of Koch (Figure 46-14). This important landmark is bounded by the tendon of Todaro, the attachment of the septal leaflet of the tricuspid valve, and the orifice of the coronary sinus.[5]

the vestibule, which is the muscle encircling the orifice of the tricuspid valve (Figure 46-11). This extensive array of pectinate muscles serves to identify an atrium as being morphologically right even when abnormally located, or duplicated as in isomerism.[18] Superiorly and anteriorly, the appendage terminates in a prominent crest that forms the

Figure 46–4 This picture of the heart, as seen in the operating room through a median sternotomy, shows the typical triangular appearance of the morphologically right atrial appendage. (See color plate.)
(Copyright in the original illustration from which this figure was prepared belongs to Robert H. Anderson, Benson R. Wilcox, and Andrew C. Cook.)

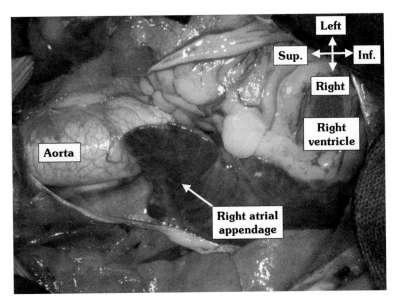

738

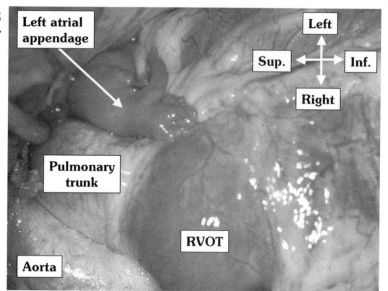

Figure 46–5 In this picture, with the pericardium opened through a median sternotomy, the heart has been rotated slightly to show the typical tubular configuration of the morphologically left atrial appendage. RVOT, right ventricular outflow tract. (See color plate.)
(Copyright for the original illustration from which this figure was prepared belongs to Robert H. Anderson, Benson R. Wilcox, and Andrew C. Cook.)

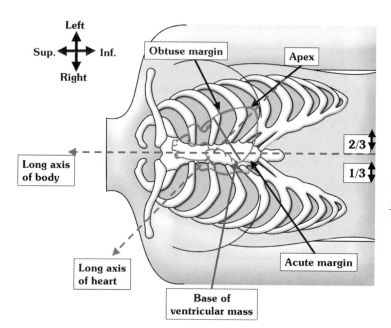

Figure 46–6 The cardiac structure placed in the context of the chest as would be seen by a surgeon standing on the right side of the operating table. Note that in the usual situation, two thirds of the cardiac silhouette are positioned to the left of the midline.
(Copyright for the original diagram from which this figure was prepared belongs to Robert H. Anderson, Benson R. Wilcox, and Andrew C. Cook.)

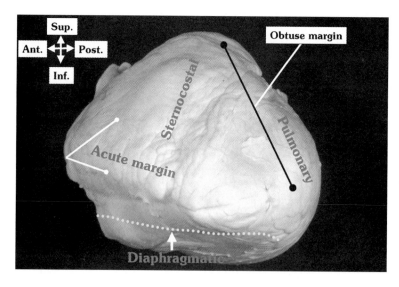

Figure 46–7 This heart has been removed from the thorax and is viewed from the apex, looking toward the base of the ventricular mass. It shows the surfaces of the ventricular mass and the locations of the acute and obtuse margins. (See color plate.)
(Copyright for the original illustration from which this figure was prepared belongs to Robert H. Anderson, Benson R. Wilcox, and Andrew C. Cook.)

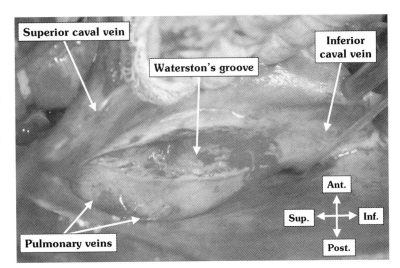

Figure 46–8 In this picture, taken in the operating room, the surgeon has reflected the atrial appendage to show the location of the terminal groove and the crest of the appendage. Note the site of the sinus node, which is shown by the *dotted lines*. (See color plate.)
(Copyright in the original illustration from which this figure was prepared belongs to Robert H. Anderson, Benson R. Wilcox, and Andrew C. Cook.)

Figure 46–9 In this picture, showing the view through a median sternotomy, the surgeon has incised through the epicardium covering Waterston's groove, showing the base of the deep fold between the systemic venous tributaries and the right pulmonary veins. (See color plate.)
(Copyright in the original illustration from which this figure was prepared belongs to Robert H. Anderson, Benson R. Wilcox, and Andrew C. Cook.)

Figure 46–10 Opening the right atrial appendage in this patient with a defect within the oval fossa reveals the markedly different configuration of the endocardial surfaces of the pectinated appendage as opposed to the smooth-walled systemic venous sinus. The pectinate muscles originate from the terminal crest, marked externally by the terminal groove (see Figure 46-7). (See color plate.)
(Copyright in the original illustration from which this figure was prepared belongs to Robert H. Anderson, Benson R. Wilcox, and Andrew C. Cook.)

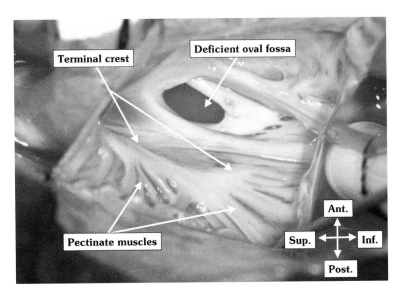

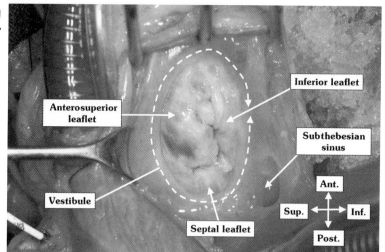

Figure 46–11 The right atrium has been opened to show the smooth vestibule of the tricuspid valve. Note that the three leaflets of the valve are positioned septally, anterosuperiorly, and inferiorly. Note also the extensive subthebesian sinus, often described as subeustachian when the heart is viewed in attitudinally incorrect fashion. (See color plate.)
(Copyright in the original illustration from which this figure was prepared belongs to Robert H. Anderson, Benson R. Wilcox, and Andrew C. Cook.)

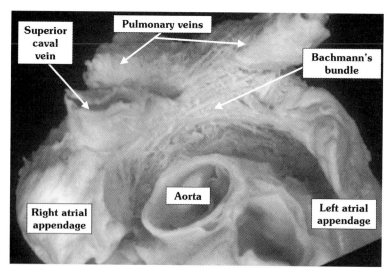

Figure 46–12 The heart has been photographed from in front, having removed the epicardium from the surface of the anterosuperior interatrial groove. Note the broad sweep of parallel fibers that extend from the crest of the atrial appendage in front of the superior caval vein toward the left atrial appendage. This is Bachmann's bundle. (See color plate.)
(Copyright in the original illustration from which this figure was prepared belongs to Robert H. Anderson, Benson R. Wilcox, and Andrew C. Cook.)

The tendon of Todaro is a fibrous structure formed by union of the eustachian valve and thebesian valves. The fibrous extension of these two valvar remnants buries itself in the tissue separating the oval fossa from the mouth of the coronary sinus, and runs medially as the tendon of Todaro, which inserts into the central fibrous body. The entire atrial component of the axis of atrioventricular conduction tissues is contained within the confines of the triangle of Koch. If, in hearts with normal segmental connections, this area is scrupulously avoided during surgical procedures, the atrioventricular conduction tissues will not be damaged. The node itself, located within the atrial musculature of the triangle, is some distance above the hinge point of the septal leaflet of the tricuspid valve. The atrioventricular bundle, however, penetrates more or less directly at the apex of the triangle of Koch.

Much has been written in recent years concerning the role of "specialized" pathways of tissue in conduction of the sinus impulse to the atrioventricular node.[12,13] It can now be stated with certainty that there are no insulated or isolated tracts of specialized conduction tissue extending between the nodes that can be avoided surgically as is possible with

the penetrating and branching atrioventricular bundles.[15] The major muscle bundles of the atrial chambers serve as preferential pathways of conduction, but the course of these preferential pathways is dictated by the overall geometry of the chambers. Ideally, prominent muscle bundles, such as the terminal crest or the superior rim of the oval fossa, should be preserved during atrial surgery. But, even if they cannot be preserved, the surgeon can be sure that internodal conduction will continue as long as some strand of atrial myocardium connects the nodes, providing that the arterial supply to the nodes, or the nodes themselves, are not traumatized. The key to avoidance of postoperative atrial arrhythmias, therefore, is the fastidious preservation of the sinus and atrioventricular nodes and their arteries.[20]

The central fibrous body touches on three of the four cardiac chambers, but it is in the right atrium that it becomes first and, perhaps most clearly, evident to the surgeon (Figure 46-14). Rather than being a specific body, it is better conceptualized as an area within the heart where the membranous septum and the leaflets of the atrioventricular and aortic valves join in fibrous continuity. When viewed from the left heart (Figure 46-15), it is possible to assess its

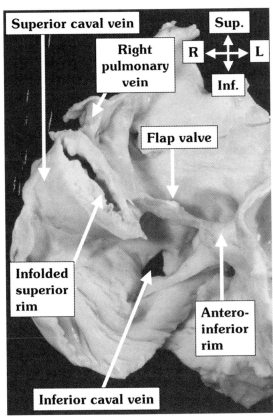

Figure 46-13 This heart has been sectioned in "four-chamber" fashion through the oval fossa. The section shows that the so-called septum secundum is no more than the infolded atrial walls between the tributaries of the systemic venous sinus and the right pulmonary veins. The true septal structures are the floor of the oval fossa and its hingepoint from the anteroinferior rim.
(Copyright in the original illustration from which this figure was prepared belongs to Robert H. Anderson, Benson R. Wilcox, and Andrew C. Cook.)

proximity to the aortic and mitral valves and to the left bundle branch of the conduction axis. Because of this intimate relationship to so many important structures within the heart, the central fibrous body acts as an anatomical focal point for the cardiac surgeon.[20]

The vestibule of the atrium, surrounding the orifice of the tricuspid valve, is continuous with both the venous component and the appendage of the right atrium. Its anterosuperior part overlies the anteroseptal commissure of the tricuspid valve and continues along the supraventricular crest of the right ventricle. The posteroinferior component extends beneath the orifice of the coronary sinus, where there is usually an extensive trabeculated diverticulum found behind the sinus, the so-called post-Eustachian sinus of Keith.

MORPHOLOGICALLY LEFT ATRIUM

Owing to its position, only the appendage of the left atrium may be immediately evident to a surgeon on exposing the heart. As with the right atrium, the left atrium has a venous component, an appendage, and a vestibule, and is separated from its partner by the septum. In addition, the left atrium possesses a well-formed body, forming the dome of the atrium when the veins are connected anomalously as in totally anomalous pulmonary venous connection. Unlike the right atrium, however, the venous component of the left atrium is considerably larger than the appendage, and the narrow junction between these two parts is not marked either by a terminal groove or crest (Figure 46-16). The pectinate muscles are confined within the appendage, and again, unlike the right side, do not extend around the vestibule.[18] This difference in the extent of the pectinate muscles always permits the morphologically right appendage to be distinguished from the morphologically left structure. Because of its posterior position, and its firm anchorage by the four pulmonary veins, direct access to the left atrium can be difficult, so surgeons must use their knowledge of anatomy to gain best exposure of the cavity. Probably the most popular route is an incision made just posterior to the interatrial groove. As described above, this extensive infolding between the right pulmonary veins and the venous sinus of the right atrium produces the superior rim of the oval fossa. A posteriorly directed incision along this groove takes the surgeon directly into the left atrium. Because the infolding of the interatrial groove also forms the superior border of the oval fossa, much the same access

Figure 46-14 The right atrium has been opened via a median sternotomy to show the landmarks of the triangle of Koch. In this patient, the continuation of the eustachian valve through the tendon of Todaro is clearly seen, with the tendon inserting into the atrioventricular component of the central fibrous body. (See color plate.)
(Copyright in the original illustration from which this figure was prepared belongs to Robert H. Anderson, Benson R. Wilcox, and Andrew C. Cook.)

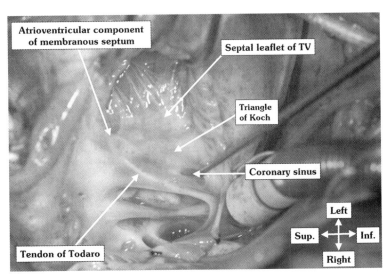

742

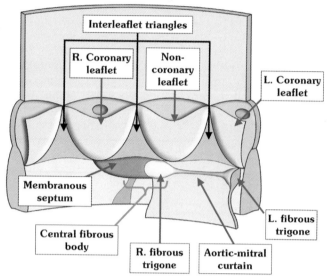

Figure 46–15 The left ventricular aspect of the aortic root, illustrating the various components of the fibrous skeleton. The area of fibrous continuity between the leaflets of the aortic and mitral valves is thickened at both ends to form the so-called fibrous trigones. As can be seen, the right trigone is then continuous with the membranous septum these structures forming the central fibrous body. Note that the membranous septum itself continues upward to the sinotubular junction as one of the fibrous interleaflet triangles of the aortic root. Note also the location of the left bundle branch. See also Figure 46-27.
(Copyright in the original diagram from which this figure was prepared belongs to Robert H. Anderson, Benson R. Wilcox, and Andrew C. Cook.)

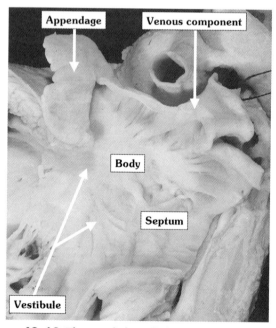

Figure 46–16 The morphologically left atrium is photographed from its left side to show the component parts. Note the extensive body, which also receives the septal aspect of the chamber. (See color plate.)
(Copyright in the original illustration from which this figure was prepared belongs to Robert H. Anderson, Benson R. Wilcox, and Andrew C. Cook.)

can be gained by approaching through the right atrium and incising just superiorly within the fossa. A further approach to the left atrium is the so-called superior approach, incising directly through the roof.

Once access is gained to the left atrium, the small size of the opening of the appendage is apparent, lying to the left of the mitral orifice as viewed by the surgeon. The greater part of the pulmonary venous atrium will usually be located inferiorly, away from the operative field, and the vestibule of the mitral orifice will dominate the picture (Figure 46-17). The septal aspect will be anterior, exhibiting the typically roughened flap-valve aspect of its left side (see Figure 46-16). The large sweep of tissue between the flap-valve of the septum and the opening of the appendage is the internal aspect of the deep anterior interatrial groove.

▶ MORPHOLOGICALLY RIGHT VENTRICLE

Understanding ventricular morphology is greatly aided by considering the ventricles in terms of three components (Figure 46-18), rather than the traditional "sinus" and "conus" parts. The three portions are the inlet, trabecular, and outlet parts, respectively.[3] The inlet portion of the right ventricle contains, and is limited by, the tricuspid valve and its tension apparatus. The leaflets of the valve are positioned septally, inferiorly or murally, and anterosuperiorly. The most constant distinguishing feature of the valve is the direct attachments to the septum of the cords of its septal leaflet (Figure 46-19). The trabecular component of the right ventricle extends out to the apex, where its wall is particularly thin and is especially vulnerable to perforation by cardiac catheters and pacemaker electrodes. The outlet component of the right ventricle is a complete muscular structure, the infundibulum, which supports the pulmonary valve. The three leaflets of the pulmonary valve do not have a ring or an annulus. Instead, they are attached to the infundibular musculature in semilunar fashion (Figure 46-20), the semilunar hingepoints crossing the anatomical ventriculoarterial junction, which does form a complete ring, as does the sinotubular junction.[2] The basal attachments of the leaflets are attached within the ventricle, upstream relative to the anatomical ventriculoarterial junction, while the peripheral attachments are to the arterial sinotubular junction. The overall valvar structure, therefore, takes the form of a three-pointed coronet (Figure 46-21). A distinguishing feature of the right ventricle is the prominent muscular shelf separating the tricuspid and pulmonary valves, the supraventricular crest. Although at first sight it has the appearance of a large muscle bundle, much of the crest is no more than the infolded inner heart curve. Incisions, or deep sutures through this part, run into the transverse sinus and right atrioventricular groove, and can jeopardize the right coronary artery.[16] The distal part of the crest is continuous with the free-standing subpulmonary infundibulum, the presence of this muscular sleeve permitting the valve to be removed and used as an autograft in the Ross procedure (Figure 46-22). The body of the supraventricular crest inserts between the limbs of a prominent and important right ventricular septal trabeculation. This structure, which we term the septomarginal trabeculation, has anterior and posterior limbs that clasp the crest. The anterior limb runs

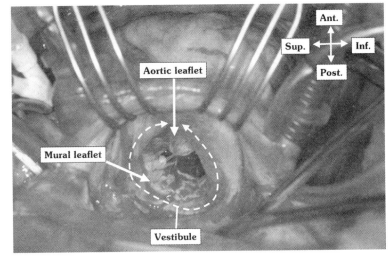

Figure 46–17 The left atrium is photographed in the operating room through an incision made in the dome. Note the vestibule of the mitral valve, which has aortic and mural leaflets. (See color plate.)
(Copyright in the original illustration from which this figure was prepared belongs to Robert H. Anderson, Benson R. Wilcox, and Andrew C. Cook.)

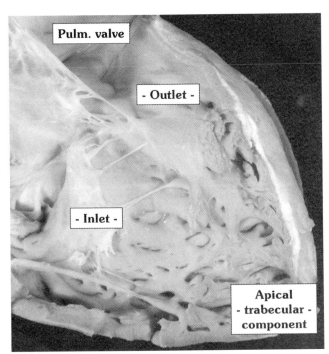

Figure 46–18 The morphologically right ventricle is opened in clam-like fashion and the septal surface is photographed to show its three component parts.
(Copyright in the original illustration from which this figure was prepared belongs to Robert H. Anderson, Benson R. Wilcox, and Andrew C. Cook.)

up to the attachment of the leaflets of the pulmonary valve, while the posterior limb extends backward inferior to the interventricular component of the membranous septum. The characteristic medial papillary muscle (Figure 46-22) usually arises from this posterior limb, and a line extending from the muscle to the apex of the triangle of Koch marks the location of the atrioventricular conduction axis. The body of the septomarginal trabeculation runs to the apex of the ventricle, where it breaks up into a sheath of smaller trabeculations. Some of these mingle into the trabecular portion, and some support tension apparatus of the tricuspid valve. Two trabeculations may be particularly prominent. One becomes the anterior papillary muscle of the tricuspid

valve, while the other extends from the septomarginal trabeculation to the papillary muscle, forming the so-called moderator band. Other significant right ventricular trabeculations are usually found in the transitional zone to the infundibulum. Variable in number, these are the septoparietal trabeculations (Figure 46-23).

It is the coarseness of the apical trabeculations that serve as the most constant feature of the morphologically right ventricle when the chamber is malformed. In the normal heart, there are a number of morphological differences between the two ventricles, including the arrangement of the leaflets of the atrioventricular valves and their tension apparatus, their shape, the thickness of their walls, and the configuration of the outflow tracts. These features, however, can be altered or lacking in the congenitally abnormal heart. When making the final arbitration, therefore, it is important to follow the "Morphological method" introduced by Van Praagh and his colleagues.[19] This states that one variable feature should not be defined on the basis of another feature that is itself variable. When distinguishing ventricular morphology, therefore, it is necessary to rely on the contrast between the coarse trabeculations of the right ventricle and those that are much finer in the apical part of the left ventricle.

MORPHOLOGICALLY LEFT VENTRICLE

The left ventricle is also conveniently considered in terms of inlet, trabecular, and outlet components (Figure 46-24), although in contrast to the right ventricle, the inlet and outlet components overlap considerably in the morphologically left ventricle. The inlet component surrounds, and is limited by, the mitral valve and its tension apparatus. The two leaflets of the mitral valve, supported by two prominent papillary muscles and their commissural cords, and closing along a solitary zone of apposition, have widely differing appearances (Figure 46-25). The anterosuperior leaflet is short, squat, and relatively square. This leaflet, which is in fibrous continuity with two of the leaflets of the aortic valve, is best termed the aortic leaflet, since it is not strictly in either an anterior or superior position. The other leaflet is much shallower, and its junctional attachment more extensive, being connected to the parietal part of the left atrioventricular

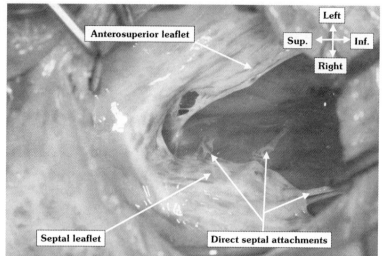

Figure 46–19 The tricuspid valve is seen through the right atrium in the operating room. Note the tendinous cords that attach the septal leaflet directly to the septum. This is the most characteristic morphological feature of the tricuspid valve. (See color plate.)
(Copyright in the original illustration from which this figure was prepared belongs to Robert H. Anderson, Benson R. Wilcox, and Andrew C. Cook.)

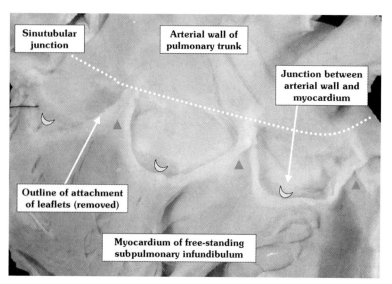

Figure 46–20 The pulmonary outflow tract has been opened and the leaflets of the pulmonary valve removed, showing their initial semilunar attachment. Note that the most distal attachment is to the sinutubular junction (*dotted line*), and proximally, the hingepoint incorporates right ventricular musculature into the base of each pulmonary valvar sinus (*gray crescents*). Fibrous triangles made up of the wall of the pulmonary trunk (*red triangles*) are incorporated within the ventricular outflow tract. (See color plate.)
(Copyright in the original illustration from which this figure was prepared belongs to Robert H. Anderson, Benson R. Wilcox, and Andrew C. Cook.)

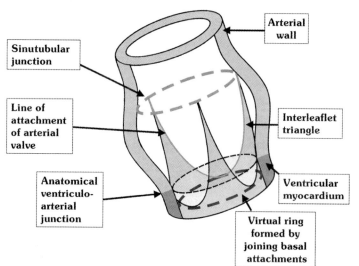

Figure 46–21 The idealized three-dimensional arrangement of the arterial valves. There is no ring-like "annulus" supporting the valvar leaflets. Instead, the leaflets are attached within the arterial root in crown-like fashion.
(Copyright in the original diagram from which this figure was prepared belongs to Robert H. Anderson, Benson R, Wilcox, and Andrew C. Cook.)

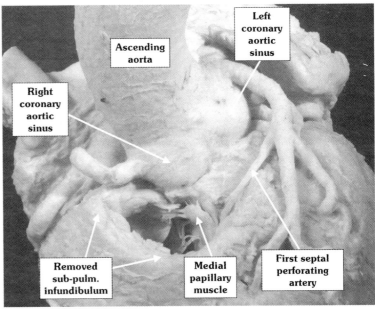

Figure 46–22 The free-standing sleeve of sub-pulmonary infundibular musculature has been removed in this anatomical specimen, as the surgeon would remove the pulmonary valve during the Ross procedure. Note that the dissection has not impinged on the cavity of the left ventricle. Note also the location of the medial papillary muscle and the first septal perforating artery. *(Copyright in the original illustration from which this figure was prepared belongs to Robert H. Anderson, Benson R. Wilcox, and Andrew C. Cook.)*

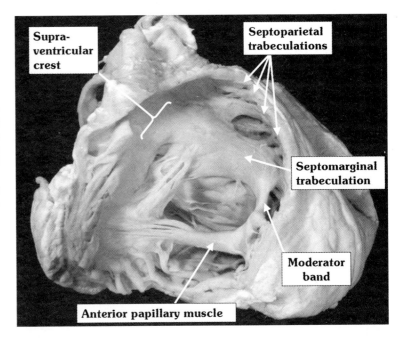

Figure 46–23 This heart, seen in anatomical orientation, has been prepared by windowing the anterior wall of the right ventricle. The dissection reveals the continuation of the septomarginal trabeculation through the moderator band to the anterior papillary muscle, and shows well the multiple septoparietal trabeculations. *(Copyright in the original illustration from which this figure was prepared belongs to Robert H. Anderson, Benson R. Wilcox, and Andrew C. Cook.)*

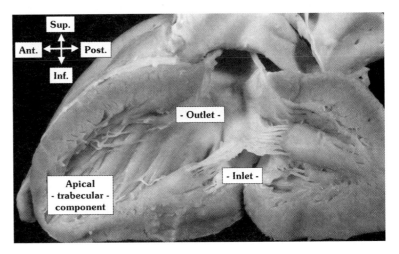

Figure 46–24 The morphologically left ventricle is opened in clam-like fashion to show its three component parts. *(Copyright in the original illustration from which this figure was prepared belongs to Robert H. Anderson, Benson R. Wilcox, and Andrew C. Cook.)*

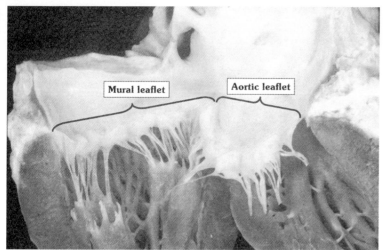

Figure 46–25 The heart has been opened through the left atrioventricular junction, and spread to show the difference in structure between the aortic and mural leaflets of the mitral valve.
(Copyright in the original illustration from which this figure was prepared belongs to Robert H. Anderson, Benson R. Wilcox, and Andrew C. Cook.)

junction. It is accurately termed the mural leaflet. Because the aortic leaf of the mitral valve also forms part of the outlet of the left ventricle (Figure 46-26), the distinction of inlet and outlet is somewhat blurred. The papillary muscles of the valve, located in anteroinferior and posterosuperior positions, are close to each other at their origin. The muscles are usually described as being posteromedial and anterolateral,

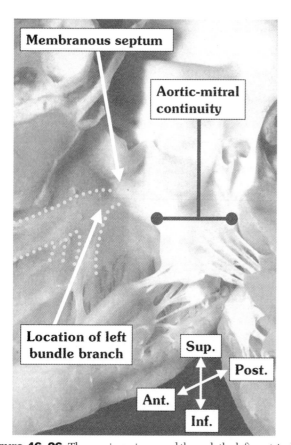

Figure 46–26 The specimen is opened through the left ventricular outflow tract, showing the relationship of the left bundle branch to the membranous septum and the aortic root. Note also the region of aortic to mitral valvar fibrous continuity. (See color plate.)
(Copyright in the original illustration from which this figure was prepared belongs to Robert H. Anderson, Benson R. Wilcox, and Andrew C. Cook.)

but this is wrong, reflecting the penchant of the morphologist to describe the heart as though positioned on its apex.[8] Unlike the tricuspid valve, the leaflets of the mitral valve have no direct septal attachments, the deep posterior diverticulum of the subaortic outflow tract displacing the aortic leaflet of the mitral valve away from the septum (Figure 46-26). The trabecular component of the left ventricle extends to the ventricular apex and has characteristically fine trabeculations (Figure 46-24). As in the right ventricle, the apical myocardium is surprisingly thin. This feature is important to the cardiac surgeon who has reason to place catheters and electrodes in the right ventricle or drainage tubes in the left side.[20] .Immediate perforation, or delayed rupture, may occur. The outlet component of the left ventricle supports the aortic valve. Unlike its right ventricular counterpart, it is not a complete muscular structure. The septal wall is largely composed of muscle, but the membranous septum forms part of the subaortic outflow tract. The posterior portion of the outflow tract is composed of the fibrous curtain joining the apparatus of the aortic valve to the aortic leaflet of the mitral valve (Figure 46-26). As with the pulmonary valve, the leaflets of the aortic valve are hinged in semilunar fashion, with the peripheral attachments supported at the sinotubular junction, while the most basal parts take origin from ventricular structures. The overall arrangement is crown-like (Figure 46-21), rather than forming an "annulus."[2,4]

The muscular septal surface of the outflow tract is characteristically smooth, and down this surface cascades the fan-like left bundle branch. The landmark of the descent of the left bundle branch is the membranous septum immediately beneath the zone of apposition between the right coronary and noncoronary leaflets of the aortic valve (Figure 46-15). The bundle descends, initially, as a relatively narrow solitary fascicle, but soon divides into three interconnected fascicles that radiate into anterior, septal, and posterior divisions. The interconnecting radiations do not fan out to any degree until the bundle itself has descended to between one third and one half the length of the septum.

AORTA

The ascending aorta begins at the distal extremity of the three aortic sinuses, the sinotubular junction, which lies at the line of opening of the free edge of the leaflets of the aortic valve. It runs its short course passing superiorly, obliquely to the right, and slightly forward toward the sternum. It is contained within the fibrous pericardial sack so its surface is covered with serous pericardium. Its anterior surface abuts directly on the pulmonary trunk, which is also covered with serous pericardium. The two vessels together make up the so-called vascular pedicle of the heart. The ascending aorta is related anteromedially to the right atrial appendage, and posterolaterally to the right ventricular outflow tract and the pulmonary trunk. Extrapericardially, the thymus gland lies between it and the sternum. The medial wall of the right atrium, the superior caval vein, and the right pleura relate to its right side. On the left, its principal relationship is with the pulmonary trunk. Posterior to the ascending aorta is the transverse sinus of the pericardium, which separates it from the "roof" of the left atrium and the right pulmonary artery.

The arch of the aorta begins at the superior attachment of the pericardial reflection just proximal to the origin of the brachiocephalic artery (Figure 46-27). It continues superiorly briefly before coursing posteriorly and to the left, crossing the lateral aspect of the distal trachea and finally terminating on the lateral aspect of the vertebral column. Here it is tethered by the parietal pleura and the

arterial ligament. During its course, it gives off the brachiocephalic, the left common carotid, and the left subclavian arteries. Bronchial arteries may arise from the arch, and can be particularly troublesome if not carefully identified in the presence of aortic coarctation. The left phrenic and vagus nerves run over the anterolateral aspect of the arch just beneath the mediastinal pleura. The left recurrent laryngeal nerve takes origin from the vagus and curls superiorly around the arterial ligament before passing on to the posteromedial side of the arch. Here, the arch relates to the tracheal bifurcation and esophagus on its medial border, but also to the left main bronchus and the left pulmonary artery inferiorly.

The descending, or thoracic, aorta continues from the arch, running an initial course lateral to the vertebral bodies and reaching an anterior position at its termination. It gives off many branches to the organs of the thorax throughout its course, as well as the prominent lower nine pairs of intercostal arteries. These latter vessels are of critical concern for the cardiac surgeon. In coarctation of the aorta, they serve as primary collateral vessels to bypass the obstructed aorta, accounting for the rib notching seen in older children with this lesion. These vessels, and their branches to the chest wall, can be a source of troublesome bleeding if not properly secured when operating on such patients. Also, the surgeon must remember that the dorsal branches of the intercostal vessels contribute a spinal branch that is important in supplying blood to the spinal cord. Because it is difficult to predict exactly from where these vital branches will arise, the surgeon must make every attempt to protect their origin from permanent occlusion. The important bronchial arteries (Figure 46-28) also arise from the descending segment of the thoracic aorta. These vessels can become dilated in the presence of pulmonary atresia, when they serve as a source of pulmonary vascular supply.

▶ PULMONARY ARTERIES

The pulmonary trunk is a short vessel, usually less than 5 cm in length in the adult (Figure 46-29). It is completely contained within the pericardium and, similar to its running mate, the ascending aorta, is covered with a layer of serous pericardium except where the two vessels abut each other in the vascular pedicle. It takes origin from the most anterior aspect of the heart, lying just behind the lateral edge of the sternum and the second left intercostal space. Initially, the pulmonary trunk overlies the aorta and left coronary artery, but it soon moves to a side-by-side relationship with the ascending aorta. The left coronary artery turns abruptly anteriorly to lie between the left atrial appendage and the pulmonary trunk. The arterial ligament extends from the aorta to the very end of the pulmonary trunk as the latter divides into left and right pulmonary arteries. The left pulmonary artery courses laterally in front of the descending aorta and the left main stem bronchus before it sends branches to the hilum of the lung. The right pulmonary artery is somewhat longer than the left, having to traverse the mediastinum beneath the aortic arch, and then behind the superior caval vein, to reach the hilum of the lung. It lies in a posteroinferior position relative to the azygos vein, and is anterior to the left main bronchus. The right pulmonary

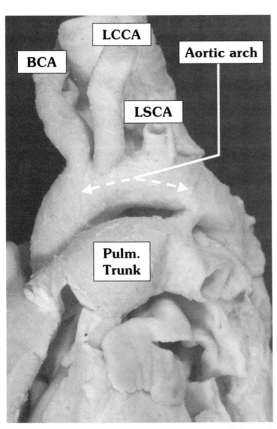

Figure 46–27 The heart has been photographed from the left side in anatomical position to show the normal structure of the great arteries and the arterial duct. BCA, brachiocephalic artery; LCCA, left common carotid artery; LSCA, left subclavian artery. *(Copyright in the original illustration from which this figure was prepared belongs to Robert H. Anderson, Benson R. Wilcox, and Andrew C. Cook.)*

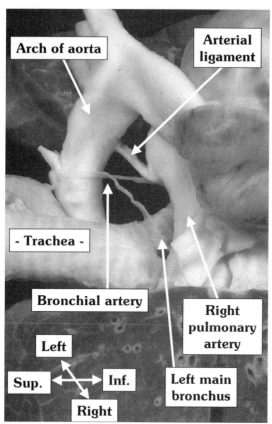

Figure 46–28 This heart is positioned as it might be seen by the surgeon working through a median sternotomy. The aortic arch is deflected forward, and has been dissected to show the origin of the bronchial arteries. Note that the arterial duct in this specimen has become ligamentous.
(Copyright in the original illustration from which this figure was prepared belongs to Robert H. Anderson, Benson R. Wilcox, and Andrew C. Cook.)

artery often branches before reaching the lateral wall of the superior caval vein posterior to the transverse sinus of the pericardium. In this situation, a large upper lobar branch may be mistaken for the right pulmonary artery itself.

► CORONARY ARTERIES AND VEINS

The coronary circulation is made up of the coronary arteries and veins together with the lymphatics of the heart. Because the lymphatics are of very limited significance to operative anatomy, they will not be discussed further. The coronary arteries are the first branches of the ascending portion of the aorta, arising from the aortic root immediately above its attachment to the heart. Normally, there are three sinuses at the aortic root, but only two coronary arteries. The sinuses can be named, therefore, according to whether they give rise to an artery, the normal arrangement being a right coronary, left coronary, and noncoronary sinus (Figure 46-30). In this respect, the terms "right" and "left" refer to the coronary sinuses giving rise to the right and left coronary arteries, rather than to the position of the sinuses relative to the right–left coordinates of the body. This is important because in the normal heart, the aortic root is obliquely situated, whereas in malformed hearts, the root is frequently abnormally situated. Whatever the position of the aortic root, however, the two coronary arteries, when two are present, almost always take origin from those aortic sinuses that face the sinuses of the pulmonary trunk. Because of this, it is more convenient, and more accurate, to term these sinuses the left-hand and right-hand facing sinuses, taking as the point of reference the observer standing within the nonfacing sinus and looking toward the pulmonary trunk (Figure 46-31). This convention, introduced by the group from Leiden,[9] holds true irrespective of the relationships of the arterial trunks.

The coronary arteries usually arise from the aortic sinuses beneath the sinotubular junction. Deviations of origins relative to the junction are not uncommon and are considered abnormal only when they deviate by a distance greater than one centimetre. According to Bader,[7] this occurs in 3.5% of hearts. The arterial opening can be deviated either toward the ventricle, so that the artery arises deep within the aortic sinus, or toward the aortic arch, so that the origin is outside the sinus. Such displacement may lead to the artery taking an oblique course through the aortic wall, a so-called intramural course, which introduces the

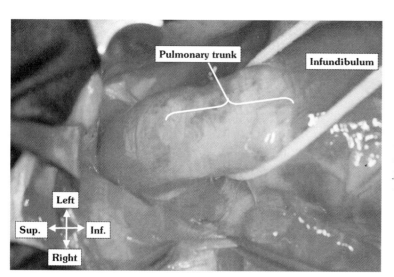

Figure 46–29 This view of the heart through a median sternotomy shows the extent of the pulmonary trunk, the surgeon having encircled the trunk with a tape. Note the circular ventriculoarterial junction. (See color plate.)
(Copyright in the original illustration from which this figure was prepared belongs to Robert H. Anderson, Benson R. Wilcox, and Andrew C. Cook.)

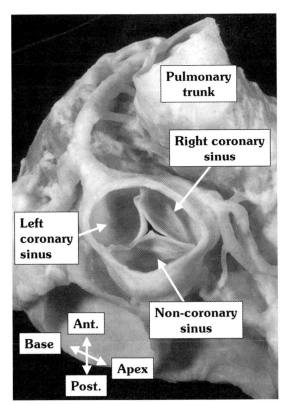

Figure 46–30 The aorta has been removed at the level of the sinotubular junction, and the heart photographed from above and from the right. The dissection shows the origin of the coronary arteries from the two aortic sinuses adjacent to the pulmonary trunk. Note again the circular anatomical ventriculoarterial junction between the pulmonary trunk and the right ventricular infundibular musculature (compare with Figure 46-29).
(Copyright in the original illustration from which this figure was prepared belongs to Robert H. Anderson, Benson R. Wilcox, and Andrew C. Cook.)

in about half of all hearts, there are two orifices within the right-hand facing sinus. In such instances, the orifices are unequal in size, the larger giving rise to the main trunk of the right coronary artery, while the considerably smaller second orifice usually gives rise to an infundibular artery, or rarely to the artery supplying the sinus node. The coronary arteries can also arise, though rarely, from a solitary orifice, usually within the right-hand facing sinus.

The epicardial course of the major coronary arteries follows the atrioventricular and interventricular grooves. The right coronary artery emerges from the right-hand facing aortic sinus and immediately enters the right atrioventricular groove (Figure 46-32). In approximately 90% of cases, this artery gives rise to the so-called posterior descending artery at the crux, the artery in reality being positioned inferiorly rather than posteriorly. In a good proportion of these cases, the artery then continues beyond the crux, and supplies downgoing branches to the diaphragmatic surface of the left ventricle. This is called right coronary arterial dominance (Figure 46-33). As the artery encircles the tricuspid orifice, it is most closely related to the origin of the valvar attachments near the take-off of its acute marginal branch. Other important branches also take origin from this encircling segment of the artery. Immediately after its origin, the artery gives rise to downgoing infundibular branches, one of which may also arise by a separate orifice. In just over half the cases, the right coronary artery also gives rise to the artery to the sinus node. Very rarely, but of major significance when present, the nodal artery can arise laterally from the right coronary artery, coursing over the lateral margin of the appendage to reach the terminal groove.[20]

The main stem of the left coronary artery emerges from the left-hand facing sinus between the pulmonary trunk and the left atrial appendage. It is a very short structure, rarely extending beyond 1 cm before branching into its anterior interventricular and circumflex branches (Figure 46-34). In some hearts, the main stem trifurcates, with an intermediate branch present between the two main branches. The intermediate branch supplies the obtuse margin of the left ventricle. The anterior interventricular artery runs within the anterior interventricular groove, giving off diagonal branches to the obtuse margin, and the

potential for luminal narrowing and disturbances in myocardial perfusion, particularly when the deviated origin is intimately related to a valvar commissure[10].

The left coronary artery almost always takes origin from a single orifice within the left-hand facing sinus. In contrast,

Figure 46–31 From the stance of the surgeon, the two aortic sinuses supporting the coronary arteries are to the right- and left-hand sides. The right-hand sinus, conventionally, is considered "Sinus #1." In the normal heart, this sinus gives rise to the right coronary artery. The convention of naming the sinuses holds good irrespective of the interrelationships of the arterial trunks.
(Copyright in the original diagram from which this figure was prepared belongs to Robert H. Anderson, Benson R. Wilcox, and Andrew C. Cook.)

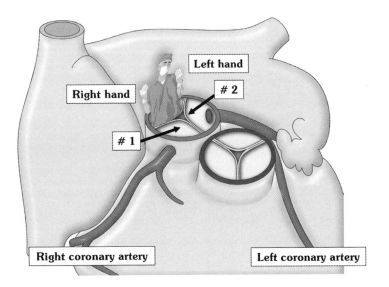

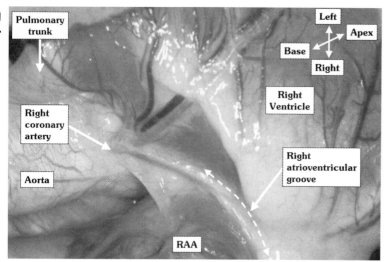

Figure 46–32 This picture, taken in the operating room through a median sternotomy, shows the aortic origin of the right coronary artery. (See color plate.) *(Copyright in the original illustration from which this figure was prepared belongs to Robert H. Anderson, Benson R. Wilcox, and Andrew C. Cook.)*

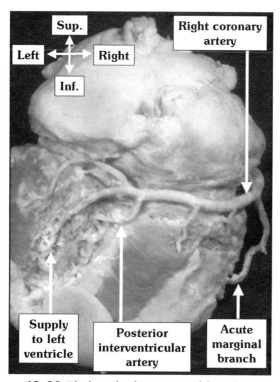

Figure 46–33 The heart has been removed from the thorax and is positioned on its apex. The dissection shows a right dominant coronary artery.
(Copyright in the original illustration from which this figure was prepared belongs to Robert H. Anderson, Benson R. Wilcox, and Andrew C. Cook.)

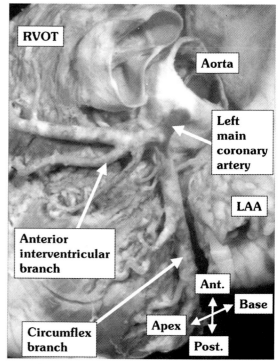

Figure 46–34 This dissection, with the heart positioned in anatomical position and photographed from the left side, shows the branches of the mainstem of the left coronary artery. RVOT, right ventricular outflow tract; LAA, left atrial appendage. (See color plate.)
(Copyright in the original illustration from which this figure was prepared belongs to Robert H. Anderson, Benson R. Wilcox, and Andrew C. Cook.)

important perforating branches that pass inferiorly into the septum. The first septal perforating branch is particularly important (Figure 46-22), since it is at major risk when the pulmonary valve is removed for use as a homograft.[11] The interventricular artery then continues toward the apex, and frequently curves under the apex onto the diaphragmatic surface of the ventricles. The circumflex branch of the left coronary artery passes backward to run in relationship with the mitral orifice. It is most closely related to the orifice

when it gives rise to the inferior interventricular artery at the crux, a so-called dominant left coronary artery (Figure 46-35). A dominant left coronary artery, however, is found in only about 10% of cases. When the left coronary is not dominant, the circumflex artery usually terminates by supplying downgoing branches to the pulmonary surface of the left ventricle. In roughly 45% of normal individuals, the circumflex artery also gives rise to the artery that supplies the sinus node.

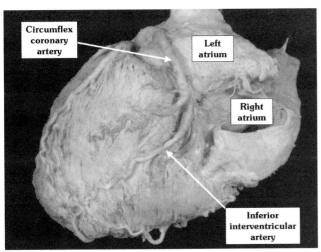

Figure 46–35 In this heart, which is positioned in anatomical orientation but photographed from its diaphragmatic aspect, it is the circumflex coronary artery that is dominant (compare with Figure 46-33).
(Copyright in the original illustration from which this figure was prepared belongs to Robert H. Anderson, Benson R. Wilcox, and Andrew C. Cook.)

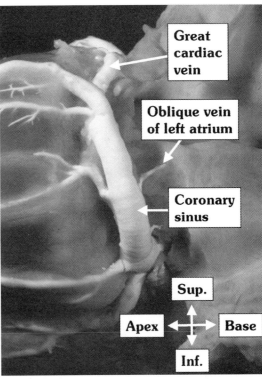

Figure 46–36 This specimen has been prepared by filling the coronary sinus with Silastic. The heart is positioned to show its diaphragmatic aspect. The coronary sinus is formed at the union of the great cardiac vein with the oblique vein of the left atrium. (See color plate.)
(Copyright in the original illustration from which this figure was prepared belongs to Robert H. Anderson, Benson R. Wilcox, and Andrew C. Cook.)

Child Health and Great Ormond Street Hospital for Children NHS Trust benefits from R&D funding received from the NHS Executive.

Throughout much of their epicardial course, the arteries and their accompanying veins are encased in epicardial adipose tissue. In some hearts the myocardium itself may form a "bridge" over segments of the artery. The role of these "bridges" in the development of coronary arterial disease is not clear. They certainly can be an impediment to surgeons in their effort to isolate the artery.

The coronary veins drain blood from the myocardium to the right atrium. The smaller veins, namely the anterior and the so-called smallest cardiac veins, drain directly to the cavity of the atrium. They are not of surgical significance. The larger veins accompany the major arteries and are the tributaries of the coronary sinus. The great cardiac vein runs alongside the anterior interventricular artery. It encircles the mitral orifice to enter the posterior and leftward margin of the atrioventricular groove, becoming the coronary sinus as it receives the oblique vein of the left atrium (Figure 46-36). The coronary sinus then runs within the groove, lying between the left atrial wall and the ventricular myocardium, before draining into the right atrium. At the crux, the sinus receives the middle cardiac vein, which has ascended with the inferior interventricular artery, and the small cardiac vein, which has encircled the tricuspid orifice in company with the right coronary artery. Occasionally, these latter two veins drain directly to the right atrium. The orifice of the coronary sinus is guarded by the Thebesian valve, which, on very rare occasions, may be imperforate. Valves are also found within the cardiac veins. That found in the great cardiac vein where it turns round the pulmonary surface is most constant, and is called the valve of Vieussens.

ACKNOWLEDGMENTS

The research on which this review is based was supported by grants from the British Heart Foundation together with the Joseph Levy Foundation. Research at the Institute of

REFERENCES

1. Anderson KR, Ho SY, Anderson RH: The location and vascular supply of the sinus node in the human heart. Br Heart J 41:28–32, 1979.
2. Anderson RH: Clinical anatomy of the aortic root. Heart 84:670–673, 2000.
3. Anderson RH, Becker AE: Cardiac Anatomy. An Integrated Text and Colour Atlas, 1st ed. London: Gower Medical Publishing, 1980, pp. 3.2–3.3.
4. Anderson RH, Devine WA, Ho SY, et al: The myth of the aortic annulus: The anatomy of the subaortic outflow tract. Ann Thorac Surg 52:640–646, 1991.
5. Anderson RH, Ho SY: Architecture of the sinus node, the atrioventricular conduction axis, and the internodal myocardium. J Cardiovasc Electrophysiol 9:1233–1248, 1998.
6. Anderson RH, Webb S, Brown NA: Clinical anatomy of the atrial septum with reference to its developmental components. Clin Anat 12:362–374, 1999.
7. Bader G: Beitrag zur Systematic und Haufigkeit der Anomalien der Coronararterien des Menschen: Virch Arch Pathol Anat 337:88–96, 1963.
8. Cook AC, Anderson RH: Editorial. Attitudinally correct nomenclature. Heart 87:503–506, 2002.

752

9. Gittenberger-de Groot AC, Sauer U, Oppenheimer-Dekker A, Quaegebeur J: Coronary arterial anatomy in transposition of the great arteries: A morphologic study. Pediatr Cardiol 4(Suppl I):15–24, 1983.

10. Gittenberger-de Groot AC, Sauer U, Quaegebeur J: Aortic intramural coronary artery in three hearts with transposition of the great arteries. J Thorac Cardiovasc Surg 91:566–571, 1986.

11. Hosseinpour AR, Anderson RH, Ho SY: The anatomy of the septal perforating arteries in normal and congenitally malformed hearts. J Thorac Cardiovasc Surg 121:1046–1052, 2001.

12. Isaacson R, Titus JL, Merideth J, et al: Apparent interruption of atrial conduction pathways after surgical repair of transposition of the great arteries. Am J Cardiol 30:533–535, 1972.

13. James TN: The connecting pathways between the sinus node and the A-V node and between the right and the left atrium in the human heart. Am Heart J 66:498–508, 1963.

14. James TN: Anatomy of the Coronary Arteries. New York: Hoeber, 1961, pp. 103–106.

15. Janse MJ, Anderson RH: Internodal atrial specialised pathways—fact or fiction? Eur J Cardiol 2:117–137, 1974.

16. McFadden PM, Culpepper WS, Ochsner JL: Iatrogenic right ventricular failure in tetralogy of Fallot repairs: Reappraisal of a distressing problem. Ann Thorac Surg 33:400–402, 1982.

17. Sweeney LJ, Rosenquist GC: The normal anatomy of the atrial septum in the human heart. Am Heart J 98:194–199, 1979.

18. Uemura H, Ho SY, Devine WA, et al: Atrial appendages and venoatrial connections in hearts from patients with visceral heterotaxy. Ann Thorac Surg 60:561–569, 1995.

19. Van Praagh R, David I, Wright GB, Van Praagh S: Large RV Plus small LV is not single RV. Circulation 61:1057–1058, 1980.

20. Wilcox BR, Anderson RH: Surgical Anatomy of the Heart, 2nd ed. London: Gower Medical Publishing. 1992.

Physiology of the Coronary Circulation

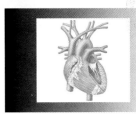

David G. Harrison, Abdul R. Doughan, and Frank W. Sellke

INTRODUCTION

Myocardial perfusion is regulated by a complex array of influences intrinsic and extrinsic to the vasculature and may also be influenced by obstructive atherosclerotic lesions, and in some cases, nonatherosclerotic occlusions within the large coronary arteries. An understanding of how coronary flow is regulated under normal circumstances and in disease states is critical for optimal intraoperative and postoperative management of the surgical patient. Whereas most operative decisions are made based on the anatomy of the large, epicardial coronary arteries, the vasomotor state of these vessels can also have a significant role in the regulation of perfusion to the myocardium. Most of the control of myocardial blood flow, however, lies in the microcirculation invisible to the angiographer. Because of its obvious impor-

tance in terms of delivery of blood and nutrients to the myocardium, there has been long-standing interest in the properties of the resistance circulation of the heart. Prior to the mid-1980s, it was difficult to directly study the coronary microcirculation either *in situ* or *in vitro*. Therefore, studies of coronary vasomotor regulation and of the coronary microcirculation had been limited to indirect assessments using measurements of coronary flow and calculations of coronary resistance. These investigations provided much insight into the properties of the intact coronary circulation. Significantly more has been learned in the past 20 years as new analytical methods have been developed for direct investigation of coronary vascular regulation. Furthermore, methods have recently been developed for study of the coronary circulation in humans that have increased our understanding of coronary pathophysiology.

Blood vessels are composed of several types of cells. The endothelium comprises the inner most cell layer and is surrounded by a variable number of layers of smooth muscle cells. The vascular smooth muscle is in turn surrounded by the adventitia, which provides structural integrity, especially in larger arteries. For many years, the endothelium was thought to serve as a barrier to diffusion of macromolecules. In the past 20 years, however, an enormous amount has been learned about the role of the endothelium as a major regulator of vascular function. In the early 1980s, Furchgott and Zawadzki[19] discovered that the endothelium plays a critical role in modulation of vasomotor tone, and, hence, control of blood flow to the myocardium and other organs. The smooth muscle layer regulates vascular tone in response to paracrine factors (locally released from endothelium, activated platelets, or leukocytes, etc.), circulating vasoactive stimuli, or neuronally released mediators (Figure 47-1).

In the coronary vasculature and in other vascular beds, the microcirculation is composed of resistance arterioles, capillaries, and venules. There are unique features of the coronary microcirculation that allow it to function in the setting of a contracting support structure, to interact with the surrounding tissue, and to respond to rather dynamic changes in requirements for nutrients. These features of the coronary microcirculation have been presented previously in review articles[17,22] and entire books.[33,49] In this chapter, we intend to briefly discuss and emphasize some of the more critical aspects of the physiology of the coronary circulation. In particular, we will emphasize regulation of myocardial perfusion as it relates to the coronary microcirculation. Finally, we will discuss new information regarding the physiology and pharmacology of the coronary circulation in disease states.

754

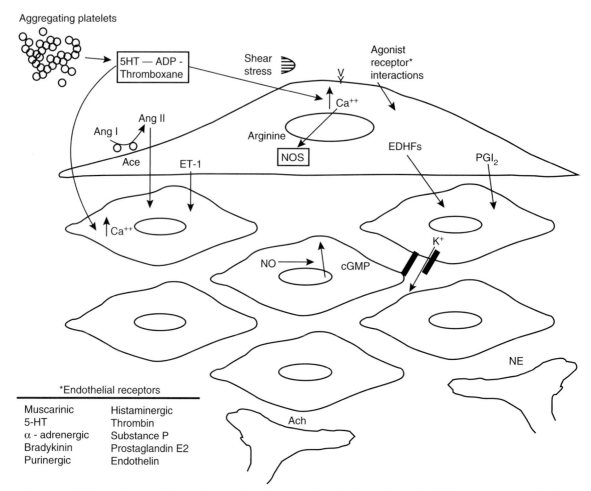

Figure 47–1 **Regulation of vascular tone by factors released from the endothelium, activated platelets and leukocytes, neuronally released factors and circulating substances.** Ang, angiotensin; 5HT, 5-hydroxytryptamine (serotonin); ET, endothelin; ADP, adenosine diphosphate; EDHF, endothelium-derived hyperpolarizing factor; PGI$_2$, prostaglandin I$_2$; Ach, acethylcholine; NE, norepinephrine.

THE CORONARY RESISTANCE CIRCULATION AS DEFINED BY PRESSURE GRADIENTS

By definition, resistance vessels are vessels over which pressure losses occur. Traditionally, resistance vessels were considered to be precapillary arterioles (25–50 μm) and it was thought that vessels larger than this had little, if any, role in the regulation of myocardial perfusion. This concept was radically altered in the early 1980s when first Nellis et al,[42] and subsequently Chilian and co-workers,[9] demonstrated that approximately 50% of total coronary vascular resistance is present in vessels larger than 100 μm in diameter. These investigators determined that pressure decreases could be observed in vessels as large as 300 μm. As illustrated in Figure 47-2, the distribution of vascular resistance is not constant, but rather depends on many factors including vascular tone. The intravenous administration of dipyridamole and other vasodilators causes a significant redistribution of microvascular resistance such that larger arteries and veins account for a greater proportion of resistance under conditions of vasodilation. Ischemia results in a similar redistribution of resistance.[10] Up

to 30% of resistance may reside in the venous circulation under conditions of maximal vascular dilatation. This is in contrast to that predicted by older traditional theories of vascular regulation that considered veins merely collection vessels and passive conduits for the return of blood to the heart.

In the coronary circulation, pressure losses occur not only as vessel size decreases. There are additional losses in pressure in vessels as they penetrate from the epicardium to the endocardium.[7] In fact, during maximal vasodilation, this pressure gradient may increase from a few (8–10) mm Hg to greater than 20 mm Hg. Importantly, in the setting of cardiac hypertrophy, this transmural pressure gradient is further increased[18] (Figure 47-3). This causes a reduction of perfusion pressure in the subendocardium and may explain, in part, the susceptibility of hypertrophied hearts to develop subendocardial ischemia or infarction. This susceptibility of the subendocardium and its lower perfusion pressure in the setting of cardiac hypertrophy almost certainly has implications for the distribution of cardioplegic solution in patients with aortic stenosis and other diseases associated with cardiac hypertrophy.

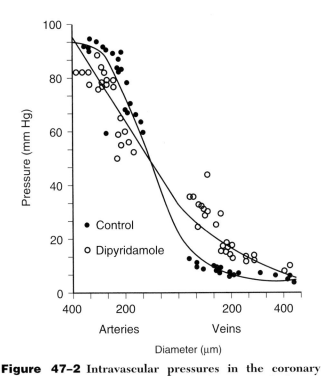

Figure 47–2 Intravascular pressures in the coronary microcirculation under basal conditions and during vasodilation with dipyridamole. The distribution of vascular resistance is not static. Rather the size of the vessels regulating vascular tone depends on the tone of the vasculature.
(Adapted from Chilian WM, Layne SM, Klausner EC, et al: Redistribution of coronary microvascular resistance produced by dipyridamole. Am J Physiol 256:H383–H390, 1989.*)*

Endogenous and Exogenous Control

Vasomotor tone results from complex interactions between circulating and locally derived substances, properties intrinsic to the vessel wall, influences from surrounding parenchymal tissue, neuronal influences, and extravascular factors. Properties intrinsic to the vessel wall and interactions with adjacent tissues work together to promote metabolic regulation and autoregulation. Endothelial regulation of vasomotor tone is also critically involved in regulation of vasomotor tone and hence myocardial perfusion. All of these factors play a role in setting the tone of the microvessels. These are summarized in Figure 47-4.

Endothelial Regulation of the Coronary Circulation

During the past 20 years, it has become clear that the endothelium plays a major role in modulation of vasomotor tone. Numerous neurohumoral stimuli modulate coronary vascular tone via their effect on the endothelium. As in all other circulations, the endothelium releases a variety of substances in the coronary circulation that modulate tone of the resistance vessels. These substances include nitric oxide (NO•), prostaglandins, a hyperpolarizing factor, endothelin, and reactive oxygen species (Figure 47-1). Among these various factors, NO• plays a predominant role. The enzyme responsible for production of NO• is a 133-kDa protein constitutively expressed by endothelial cells that is known as the endothelial nitric oxide synthase (eNOS or NOS-3). The biochemical mechanisms responsible for function of the NO synthases have recently been elucidated. For all isoforms, an electron donor, NADPH, binds to a site at the carboxyl terminus of the protein. Electrons are then transferred from NADPH to the flavins flavin adenine dinucleotide (FAD)

Figure 47–3 Transmural losses of coronary perfusion pressure in normal and hypertrophied hearts. Pressures were measured using micropuncture-servo null techniques in hearts perfused via the left main coronary artery at 100 mm Hg.
(Adapted from Fujii M, Nuno DW, Lamping KG, et al: Effect of hypertension and hypertrophy on coronary microvascular pressure. Circ Res 71:120–126, 1992.*)*

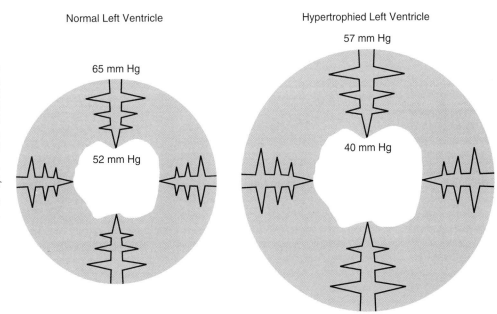

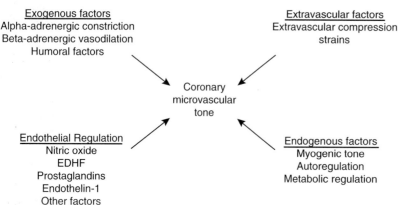

Exogenous factors
Alpha-adrenergic constriction
Beta-adrenergic vasodilation
Humoral factors

Extravascular factors
Extravascular compression
strains

Coronary
microvascular
tone

Endothelial Regulation
Nitric oxide
EDHF
Prostaglandins
Endothelin-1
Other factors

Endogenous factors
Myogenic tone
Autoregulation
Metabolic regulation

Figure 47–4 Major factors contributing to regulation of coronary microvascular tone (myogenic tone and autoregulation, endothelium, neurogenic influences). EDHF, endothelium-derived hyperpolarizing factor.

and flavin mononucleotide (FMN), which are bound within the reductase domain. For the neuronal NOS and eNOS, electrons are stored on the flavins until the enzyme is activated by calcium/calmodulin (Ca/CaM). When calmodulin binds to the enzyme, electrons are transferred to a prosthetic heme group in the oxygenase domain. Upon heme reduction, catalysis of arginine to citrulline and nitric oxide occurs. The NO• formed diffuses to underlying vascular smooth muscle, where it (among other actions) stimulates soluble guanylate cyclase, increasing cGMP and prompting vasodilation via activation of cyclic guanosine monophosphate (cGMP)-dependent protein kinase.[39] There is substantial evidence that NO• may undergo reactions with other molecules, such as thiol-containing compounds, to form biologically active nitroso intermediates.[40] Although binding of calcium/calmodulin is a prerequisite for activity of the enzyme, there is evidence that other phenomena, such as phosphorylation,[12] membrane binding,[59] binding of eNOS with heat shock protein 90, and association with the integral membrane protein caveolin,[37] can also modulate NOS activity. The eNOS is constitutively expressed, however, its expression is subject to modest and yet likely important degrees of regulation. Thus, factors such as shear stress,[58] the state of endothelial cell growth,[2] hypoxia,[36] exposure to oxidized low-density lipoprotein, and exposure to cytokines have been shown to affect expression of eNOS. In some instances, factors known to decrease eNOS expression are associated with decreases in eNOS mRNA half-life rather than changes in the rate of its transcription. In the coronary circulation, the release of NO• confers a state of basal vasodilation, and administration of NO synthase antagonists produces an increase in resting coronary resistance. When substances such as acetylcholine and bradykinin are administered, coronary microvessels of all sizes dilate. In a variety of common disease states, endothelial nitric oxide production is reduced because of a variety of mechanisms. These are discussed more fully below.

Nitric oxide mediates its cellular effects via several signaling pathways. The best characterized and probably most important of these involves activation of soluble guanylate cyclase, which in turn catalyzes the formation of cGMP from guanidine triphosphate. cGMP serves as an allosteric regulator of the enzyme cGMP-dependent protein kinase (PKG). PKG phosphorylates contractile proteins and ion channels decreasing intracellular calcium and the sensitivity of contractile proteins to intracellular calcium. Oxidation

products of nitric oxide can bind to sulfhydryl groups and protein tyrosines to form nitrosothiols and nitrotyrosines, which may modulate enzyme function and form stable nitrosocompounds. Nitric oxide also binds to cytochrome oxidase in the mitochondria and regulates oxygen consumption. This may have a very important effect in terms of modulating myocardial oxygen demand. The organic nitrates and sodium nitroprusside release nitric oxide and mediate their effects via identical signaling pathways. Importantly, receptors for the atrial (ANP) and brain (BNP) natriuretic peptides are also particulate forms of guanylate cyclases, and these substances produce vasodilation via similar pathways. Recombinant BNP has proven a useful treatment for heart failure.

There is also abundant evidence, particularly in smaller vessels both in the coronary and peripheral circulations, that factors other than NO• can modulate endothelium-dependent vascular relaxation. One such factor is the endothelium-derived hyperpolarizing factor (EDHF). Even before the endothelium was found to be critical in modulating vascular tone, it was known that certain relaxing substances would hyperpolarize vascular smooth muscle. It was subsequently shown that this phenomenon was endothelium dependent. The hyperpolarization is mediated by opening of a calcium-dependent potassium channel, and in some cases by activating an Na^+-K^+-ATPase. When the vascular smooth muscle is hyperpolarized, voltage-sensitive calcium channels are closed, leading to a reduction in intracellular calcium. There are probably several different EDHFs. One is almost certainly the cytochrome P-450 metabolite of arachidonic acid, epoxyeicosatrienoic acid (EET). Another EDHF is likely hydrogen peroxide. It has also been suggested that potassium may be the EDHF. The role of the various EDHFs probably varies depending on the vessel size, the species studied, and the vascular bed studied.

Prostaglandin synthesis by the endothelium also contributes to modulation of tone in the coronary microcirculation. The predominant prostaglandin produced by endothelial cells is prostacyclin or PGI_2. There is substantial interaction between nitric oxide, EDHF, and prostacyclin. A major stimulus for release of prostacyclin, NO, and the EDHF is shear stress, or the tangential force of fluid as it flows over the endothelium, resulting in flow-dependent vasodilation. Interestingly, in eNOS knockout mice, flow-dependent vasodilation is not altered, but is mediated by PGI_2 and EDHF. Thus the loss of nitric oxide may be compensated by an increase in prostacyclin and EDHF production. As blood vessels decrease in size, the importance of nitric oxide seems to decline and the role of the EDHF increases. This may allow the production of EDHF to increase when nitric oxide is absent.

Metabolic Regulation and Autoregulation

The tone of the coronary microcirculation, and consequently levels of myocardial perfusion, is tightly coupled to the state of myocardial oxygen consumption. When myocardial oxygen needs are increased, coronary flow rises accordingly. In part, this is due to the fact that myocardial oxygen extraction is near maximum even under resting conditions. Thus, the ability of the myocardium to extract additional oxygen to meet increased demand is limited.

Autoregulation refers to the ability of a vascular bed to constrict and dilate to maintain flow constant during changes in perfusion pressure. In the coronary circulation, autoregulation is most effective between pressures of 40 and 160 mm Hg. The range of pressures over which autoregulation can be observed is different for the subendocardium as compared to the subepicardium. Thus, flow will begin to decrease at pressures <70–75 mm Hg in the subendocardium, as opposed to substantially lower pressures in the more superficial layers of the heart.[5] Importantly, chronic hypertension shifts the range of pressures over which autoregulation occurs in the subendocardium such that flow will begin to decline at even higher pressures. This may be related to changes in subendocardial perfusion pressure and thus may also explain the propensity of the subendocardium to develop ischemia in the setting of myocardial hypertrophy. Of note, during both autoregulation and metabolic regulation, studies using direct observations of the coronary microcirculation indicate that the predominant changes in vasomotion occur in vessels <100 μm in diameter.

The signaling molecule(s) linking flow to demand and participating in the autoregulation process has been the subject of extensive investigation. It now appears that autoregulation is mediated by the concerted actions of several paracrine factors. These include nitric oxide, the EDHF, and adenosine. Blockade of one of these is insufficient to abolish autoregulation, as the loss of one factor seems to be compensated by the presence of others. Recently, it has been suggested that hydrogen peroxide serves as a hyperpolarizing factor, released by the endothelium and opening a calcium-dependent potassium channel in the vascular smooth muscle. Adenosine also causes hyperpolarization of vascular smooth muscle. The idea that several factors work together to mediate autoregulation and metabolic regulation was first suggested by Duncker et al,[14] and has recently been confirmed in studies by others. This redundancy of control of such important processes as coronary metabolic and autoregulation is extremely important because it allows appropriate regulation of coronary tone even when one or more of these pathways is inhibited or abnormal.

Myogenic Tone

Myogenic tone is a property of the vascular smooth muscle in most vessels, including coronary microcirculation.[26] Myogenic contraction is defined as an increase in wall tension, or a decrease in vessel diameter, in response to an increase in vascular transmural pressure. Myogenic mechanisms importantly contribute to regulation of blood flow and maintenance of basal vascular tone and have been postulated to be one mechanism whereby autoregulation occurs. Increases in myogenic tone, which occur during stretch of vascular smooth muscle, are associated with an increase in inositol 1,4,5-trisphosphate, presumably due to activation of phospholipase C.[26,41,43,44] An important mediator of myogenic tone may be 20-hydroxeicosatetraenoic acid (20-HETE), a cytochrome P-450 metabolite of arachidonic acid that is synthesized in response to increases in intracellular calcium in cerebral and renal arterioles. Once formed, 20-HETE seems to produce vascular smooth muscle constriction and causes vasoconstriction by inhibiting large conductance Ca^{2+}-activated K^+ (BK) channels, inducing depolarization and further increasing $[Ca^{2+}]_i$, an effect likely caused by activation of L-type Ca^{2+} channels and/or the activation of PKC and inhibition of Na^+-K^+-ATPase. Mitogen-activated protein (MAP) kinases have also been suggested to be involved in regulation of myogenic tone, but this is controversial. It has been shown that 20-HETE stimulates endothelial production of thromboxane in coronary arterioles, and thus stimulates endothelium-dependent vasoconstriction in vivo. Recently, the small g protein Rho has been recognized to be important in modulation of vasomotor tone. It appears that its down stream mediator in this role is Rho kinase, and that Rho kinase may modulate myogenic tone by regulation of the actin cytoskeleton. There is substantial interest in the use of Rho kinase inhibitors as potential therapeutic agents for treatment of hypertension and coronary spasm. Myogenic responses to increases in pressure are greater in coronary microvessels from the subepicardium than in vessels from the subendocardium.[26] Myogenic tone may be reduced after cardiopulmonary bypass, sepsis, and other inflammatory states in which the expression of iNOS is increased. This may lead to altered distribution of myocardial perfusion.

Neurohumoral Control of the Circulation

There has been an enormous amount of research devoted to understanding the role of the sympathetic and parasympathetic nervous systems in regulation of coronary perfusion.[64] In vivo, the vascular response to sympathetic stimulation is mediated by both α-adrenergic and β-adrenergic receptors. In the coronary circulation, the predominant receptor subtype seems to be the β-adrenergic receptor. For example, direct sympathetic nerve stimulation stimulates coronary vasodilation and an increase in coronary flow occurs. If β-adrenergic antagonists are administered, a transient vasoconstriction can be observed. When coronary microvessels are studied in vitro, α-adrenergic stimulation has minimal contractile effects.[61] When selective $α_2$-adrenergic stimulation is applied using pharmacological stimuli, there is rather potent vasodilation of all sized coronary microvessels, predominantly due to a release of endothelium-derived nitric oxide (NO•). β-Adrenergic stimulation produces a potent relaxation of all coronary arteries, but especially small resistance vessels.[61] It appears that the $β_2$-adrenergic receptor subtype predominates in vessels less than 100 μm in diameter in in vitro studies,[61] whereas a mixed $β_1$- or

758 β₂-adrenergic receptor population controls vascular resistance in *in vivo* studies. Larger coronary vessels are regulated by a mixed β₁- and β₂-adrenoceptor subtype population.

Activation of cholinergic receptors by either vagal stimulation or the infusion of acetylcholine produces uniform vasodilation of coronary vessels.[28] This vasodilation is predominantly mediated by endothelium-derived NO[•] although release of EDHF,[20] and the release of prostaglandin substances,[51] may contribute.

Effects of Humoral Agents on the Coronary Microcirculation

The response of the coronary microcirculation to a variety of humoral agents is very heterogeneous. For example, serotonin constricts vessels greater than 100 μm in diameter, whereas it causes potent vasodilation of smaller arteries.[30] In contrast, vasopressin produces greater constriction of microvessels less than 100 μm in diameter than it produces in larger microvessels.[30,53] In the larger epicardial coronary arteries, vasopressin causes predominantly vasodilation. Endothelin-1 produces vasoconstriction when administered to the adventitial surface of coronary microvessels. The degree of constriction produced by endothelin-1 is inversely related to the size of the vessels. Paradoxically, when endothelin-1 is administered intraarterially, vasodilation occurs presumably via release of nitric oxide.[29] Activation of other receptors, such as the thromboxane receptor,[51] results in uniform constriction of all coronary arterioles and veins.

Extravascular Forces

The coronary circulation is particularly unique in that it is exposed to a large number of extravascular forces produced by contraction of adjacent myocardium and intraventricular pressures. Extravascular influences may become more evident during ischemia or in the setting of other pathological processes leading to decreased tissue compliance or increased tissue edema. For example, collateral perfusion is particularly sensitive to changes in heart rate (more frequent extravascular compression) and ventricular diameter (stretch).[11,49] Of relevance to the concept of extravascular forces is the idea that these might collapse coronary vessels under certain circumstances. In 1978, Bellamy reported that flow through the epicardial coronary arteries halted when aortic pressure fell to values ranging from 25 to 50 mm Hg.[4] This observation, and others like it, raised the possibility that extravascular forces might be sufficiently high to collapse vessels when intraluminal pressures declined to values below this "critical closing pressure." It soon became apparent, however, that flow in the coronary microcirculation continued even when the arterial driving pressure was minimally higher than coronary venous pressure. Based on modeling and various experimental interventions, it was determined that the decrease of antegrade blood flow in larger upstream vessels associated with continued forward flow in microvessels was likely due to capacitance in the coronary circulation.[15] Kanatsuka and colleagues used a floating microscope to visualize epicardial capillaries and were able to show that red cells continued to flow, even after perfusion had stopped in the more proximal vessels. Using this approach, they were able to show that the "stop-flow"

pressure in the epicardial coronary microvessels was only a few mm Hg higher than right atrial pressure.[24] Furthermore, they did not observe closure of epicardial coronary microvessels at any pressure. It therefore seems likely that the concept of "critical closing pressure" is not applicable to all vessels in the coronary circulation. It is conceivable, however, that vessels deeper in the subendocardium might be made to collapse by pressure transmitted from the ventricular chamber, particularly when left ventricular diastolic pressure is very high.

Contribution of Coronary Venules in Overall Vascular Resistance

Although the arterial microcirculation is considered to be the predominant regulator of coronary blood flow, venules may have considerable importance under conditions of vascular dilation, as noted above,[10] such as during exercise, metabolic stress, or reperfusion after myocardial ischemia. The venous circulation may also influence myocardial stiffness and diastolic properties of the heart. Veins may respond differently to agonists and neuronal stimulation compared to arteries in the same vascular bed.[25,51] Thus, a consideration of the venous circulation apart from the arterial circulation may be warranted under certain physiological and clinical conditions.

Not only is vasomotor regulation differentially controlled between the venous and arterial microcirculations, but certain reactions to pathological stimuli occur preferentially on one side of the capillary bed. For example, postcapillary venules are the initiating site of neutrophil adherence and transmigration,[66] whereas arterioles seldom manifest these initial changes in the inflammatory response. In addition, complement fragment C5a causes neutrophil adherence in venules but not in arterioles, suggesting that different mechanisms mediate neutrophil-endothelial adherence in the two vessel types. However, although ischemia-reperfusion has been determined to cause endothelial dysfunction in veins,[31] under similar conditions, arterioles appear to be more susceptible to a reduction in endothelium-dependent relaxation than are coronary venules,[46] despite the fact that leukocytes preferentially adhere to venular as compared to arterial endothelial cells.

▶ THE ROLE OF ENDOTHELIAL FACTORS IN VASCULAR GROWTH, DEVELOPMENT, AND RESPONSE TO INJURY

Relevant to a role of endothelial mediators in the coronary microcirculation is the recent interest in the role of nitric oxide and nitric oxide–related factors on the growth of vascular cells and blood vessels (Figure 47-5). Nitric oxide is a potent inhibitor of vascular smooth muscle proliferation and promotes vascular smooth muscle apoptosis, and therefore has an important role in inhibiting vascular lesion formation. In rabbits, treatment with L-nitroarginine methyl ester (L-NAME, which inhibits NO[•] formation) markedly increases the neointimal development following vascular balloon injury.[6] Likewise, local transfection of the rat carotid artery with the eNOS cDNA reduces the intimal prolifera-

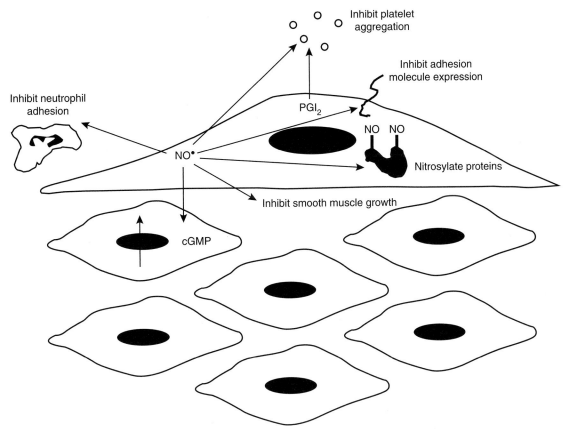

Figure 47–5 Schematic representation of endothelium and vascular smooth muscle demonstrating the multifaceted roles of nitric oxide released from the endothelium in the modulation of vascular function, structure, and the response to injury. cGMP, cyclic guanidine monophosphate.

tion that follows balloon injury.[60] The vascular response to injury is enhanced in mice deficient in eNOS.[38] This effect of NO• on vascular smooth muscle growth is mediated by cGMP and can be mimicked by cGMP analogs.[65] Interestingly, atrial natriuretic factor (which increases cGMP via activation of a particulate guanylate cyclase) shares this property of nitric oxide.[23]

Although NO• and cGMP-elevating agents inhibit the growth of fibroblasts and vascular smooth muscle, they promote growth of endothelial cells and enhance formation of new blood vessels, and thus NO seems extremely important in modulation of angiogenesis. The effect of the vascular endothelial cell growth factor (VEGF-1) is mediated by NO, and the effects of VEGF are absent in mice lacking eNOS. Interestingly, proliferating endothelial cells express about six-fold as much eNOS mRNA as confluent cells.[2] This is associated with a three-fold increase in eNOS protein and nitric oxide production by the proliferating cells as compared to nongrowing cells. If this is considered in terms of the ability of the vessel to respond to injury, it makes teleological sense. This seems to represent a feedforward condition that promotes vascular growth. Although endothelial cells are proliferating to form new blood vessels, the production of high levels of NO promotes tube formation. Likewise, following endothelial denudation, the proliferating endothelial cells produce large amounts of nitric oxide as they grow back to recover the exposed intima to make up for the paucity of endothelial cells in this area. This would tend

to minimize platelet adhesion and vascular smooth muscle proliferation in the area. It is also advantageous that endothelial cells do not seem to be sensitive to the growth-inhibitory effects of nitric oxide. This would permit rapid reendothelialization of a denuded region, even while producing large quantities of nitric oxide.

Recently, it has been recognized that bone marrow-derived endothelial progenitor cells (EPC) contribute to new vessel development and likely to reendothelialization of denuded regions of the vasculature. The biology of these cells is only now being elucidated, but it appears that the number of EPCs from one individual to the next is highly variable, and affected by classic risk factors for atherosclerosis. Thus, subjects with diabetes, hypertension, and cigarette smoking have fewer EPCs that those without risk factors. Further, the ability of EPCs to transmigrate is impaired by these risk factors. Importantly, the HMG-CoA reductase inhibitor atorvastatin has been shown to triple the circulating level of EPCs.

► REGULATION OF THE CORONARY CIRCULATION IN DISEASE STATES

A variety of systemic and cardiac diseases affect the coronary microcirculation. These may be considered functional alterations involving changes in responsiveness of the coronary vasculature, and structural effects, such as alterations

760 in the number and diameter of the coronary microvessels. A particularly important aspect of endothelial regulation of vasomotion is that endothelial-mediated vasodilation is abnormal in a variety of pathological conditions. These include atherosclerosis (Figure 47-6), hypercholesterolemia, diabetes, hypertension, cigarette smoking, and aging. The mechanisms underlying these abnormal endothelium-dependent responses are likely multifactorial. Factors responsible include abnormalities of G-protein signaling, resulting in reduced activation of eNOS in response to endothelial cell receptor activation, an alteration of levels of the critical cofactor for eNOS tetrahydrobiopterin, and an overproduction of the asymmetrical dimethylarginine (ADMA), which acts as an antagonist for the eNOS substrate L-arginine. A substantial body of data suggests that in some of these conditions (hypercholesterolemia, hypertension, and diabetes), increased production of vascular superoxide ($O_2^{\bullet-}$) occurs. Superoxide reacts very rapidly with $NO^{\bullet}$, leading to the formation of the toxic peroxynitrite anion. Interestingly, tetrahydrobiopterin is potently oxidized by peroxynitrite. Oxidized tetrahydrobiopterin is incapable of sustaining eNOS NO production and in the absence of tetrahydrobiopterin the electron flow in the nitric oxide synthases are diverted to molecular oxygen to form superoxide. Thus oxidation of tetrahydrobiopterin could not only reduce nitric oxide production, but also increase superoxide production by the NO synthase enzyme. The ultimate effect is to diminish endothelium-dependent vasodilation and dramatically increase endothelial oxidant stress.

The initial studies demonstrating abnormal endothelium-dependent vascular relaxation in various disease models were performed in larger vessels. Subsequent experiments demonstrated that most, if not all, of these disease processes also affect the coronary microcirculation in a similar fashion. This is of particular interest in the case of hypercholesterolemia and atherosclerosis. One of the first examples of

an alteration in coronary microvessels in atherosclerosis was made in vessels from monkeys fed a high cholesterol diet for 18 months.[50] These animals develop advanced atherosclerotic lesions in larger vessels, and had previously been shown to have abnormal vasodilation in response to acetylcholine, the calcium ionophore A23187, and thrombin in larger vessels. In coronary microvessels from monkeys fed a high cholesterol diet for 18 months, relaxations to the same acetylcholine, bradykinin, and the calcium ionophore A23187 were dramatically impaired, and, in some cases, these agents produced paradoxical constrictions. Similar findings have been made in other animal models of diet-induced atherosclerosis. Subsequent studies performed using *in vivo* techniques showed that vasoconstriction caused by serotonin and ergonovine (both known to be modulated by the endothelium) was markedly enhanced in the coronary microcirculation of hypercholesterolemic monkeys.[8] These findings are striking because the coronary microcirculation is spared from the development of overt atherosclerosis. Thus, vessels that have been exposed to a high cholesterol milieu, even in the absence of atherosclerosis, develop abnormal vasomotion. Although it is difficult to perform such studies in human vessels, investigators have used Doppler techniques to measure coronary flow in humans. Diminished flow responses to acetylcholine have been demonstrated in humans with hypercholesterolemia.[13] Importantly, this abnormality of vascular function has been corrected by reduction of serum cholesterol. Similar observations have been made in either humans or experimental models of hypertension,[57] ischemia followed by reperfusion,[46,47] and diabetes.[35] Indeed, altered endothelial regulation of vasomotion has been found in the coronary arteries of patients with chest pain and normal coronary arteries, and it is thought that, at least in some instances, this might contribute to their clinical symptoms.

The loss of NO in cardiovascular disease not only leads to a decrease in vasodilation, but also predisposes to atherosclerotic lesion formation and vascular smooth muscle proliferation. NO also has antioxidant properties and prevents adhesion molecule expression by endothelial cells. The clinical relevance of this has been brought to light by a series of studies showing that impaired endothelium-dependent vasodilation is associated with a dramatic increase in subsequent cardiovascular events. A very important recent study has shown that an improvement in forearm endothelium-dependent vasodilation caused by vitamin C infusion forebears a poor prognosis in terms of major cardiovascular events during subsequent follow-up. An improvement in endothelium-dependent vasodilation in response to the vitamin C can be interpreted as indicating high levels of oxidative stress, and this study seems in keeping with the notion that oxidative stress is a common mechanism leading to atherosclerosis and altered endothelium-dependent vasodilation.

A particularly important clinical setting in which endothelial function is altered in the coronary microcirculation is following cardioplegic arrest and extracorporeal circulation.[54] This abnormality persists for some time after cardiopulmonary bypass and normalizes thereafter. Obviously, such a deficit in endothelial function may have important clinical implications, because of the frequency in which cardioplegia is used in cardiovascular surgery. It is not

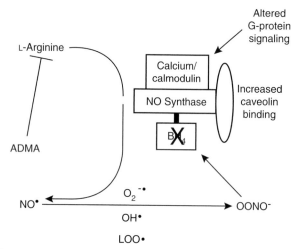

Figure 47–6 Reduced production/bioreactivity of endothelium-derived NO in the setting of atherosclerosis, diabetes, and many other pathological conditions. ADMA, asymmetrical dimethylarginine, acts as an antagonist of L-arginine. Superoxide and other oxygen free radicals may interfere with NO availability in conditions of increased oxidant stress. OONO•, peroxynitrite radical may inhibit tetrahydrobioterin, a cofactor for nitric oxide synthase (NOS).

uncommon for patients undergoing coronary artery bypass grafting, with seemingly complete coronary revascularization, to exhibit signs of myocardial ischemia during the hours following surgery. It is conceivable that alterations of endothelial function may contribute to this alteration in cardiac function. In addition, it is likely that the arteriopathy often observed after cardiac transplantation is in part related to endothelial injury as a result of inadequate vascular preservation.

A condition that rather strikingly alters coronary vascular reactivity is the development of collateral vessels. When a coronary artery is gradually occluded, flow to the subtended myocardium does not cease, but persists via perfusion through collateral vessels. When these vessels fully develop, they are capable of providing normal resting perfusion to the region previously served by the occluded vessel, albeit at a lower perfusion pressure. Because collateral vessels represent "new" vessels, and because of their obvious pathophysiological importance, there has been interest in factors that might modulate their reactivity. Interestingly, the coronary arterioles nourished by collaterals develop markedly abnormal vascular reactivity characterized by impaired endothelium-dependent vascular relaxations and enhanced constrictions to vasopressin.[53] These observations were originally made in vitro in microvessels from a canine model of collateral development, but have since been repeated in a porcine model of chronic ischemia.[21,55] The mechanism of the impaired microvascular endothelium-dependent relaxation in the collateral-dependent region is not known. However, changes in shear stress or pulsatile flow in the collateral-dependent microvasculature may contribute to the altered vascular reactivity.[58] Another explanation involves changes in intracellular calcium mobilization that have been observed in collateral vessels,[48] which may impact on changes in vascular tone and responses. Finally, altered expression of syndecan-4 and other heparan sulfate extracellular matrix proteins has been documented after ischemia, which may affect signal transduction leading to NO release from the endothelium.[32]

Recent studies have addressed the possibility that collateral growth and coronary microvessel function might be altered by the direct perivascular application or infusion of angiogenic growth factors such fibroblast growth factor (FGF)-1 or FGF-2, or VEGF. Indeed, such studies have shown that these therapeutic interventions are not only associated with improved myocardial function and improved perfusion in chronic ischemic models, but also with normalization of endothelium-dependent relaxation in the collateral-dependent vasculature.[3,21,55] The cause of this enhancement of endothelium-dependent relaxation is not fully understood but several mechanisms may be involved. Both FGF-2 and VEGF release nitric oxide,[56] which may improve collateral perfusion and decrease tissue ischemia. The expression of receptors for both FGF-2 and VEGF is selectively increased in chronically ischemic myocardium,[56] suggesting that these growth factors are functionally upregulated. This may also explain why enhanced endothelium-dependent relaxation occurs only in the collateral-dependent region and not in the normally perfused myocardium after the perivascular exogenous administration of VEGF or FGF-2. Alternatively, FGF-2 and VEGF may counteract the effects of substances detrimental to vascular function or stabilize nitric oxide or NOS. Another possibility is that the growth factors induce enough collateral formation to prevent a reduction in myocardial blood flow or in pulsatile perfusion. Finally, these growth factors may stimulate the release of bone marrow-derived EPCs, which then enhance collateral regrowth and endothelial function at these sites. In summary, treatment of collateral-dependent vessels with angiogenic growth factors may enhance endothelium-dependent relaxation, in addition to improving other aspects of cardiac performance. This may, at least in theory, be the basis for a clinical improvement in patients after therapeutic angiogenesis suffering inoperative myocardial ischemia.

STRUCTURAL CHANGES IN THE CORONARY MICROCIRCULATION

For years it has been observed that patients with cardiac hypertrophy due to a variety of causes have chest pain suggestive of myocardial ischemia. This has led to an extensive body of research examining potential alterations of structure of the coronary microcirculation in a variety of conditions associated with cardiac hypertrophy. In both experimental animals and humans with cardiac hypertrophy, there is a reduction in the maximal capacity of the coronary circulation to dilate in response to either reactive hyperemia or pharmacological stimuli.[33,34,57] Two hypotheses have been proposed to explain this defect in vasodilator function. One is that as the myocardium hypertrophies, the coronary resistance circulation does not increase to keep pace with the larger myocardial mass. Thus, peak flow normalized to myocardial mass is reduced because of this relative paucity of coronary arterioles.

It has been assumed that these studies examining a loss of maximal vasodilator reserve reflect a structural alteration of the coronary microcirculation, because they are observed during maximal pharmacological stimulation, and thus the resultant flow must reflect the driving pressure for perfusion and the cross-sectional area of the coronary resistance circulation. It is also likely that some impaired vasodilator responses attributed to losses of vascular cross-sectional area are due to changes in endothelial function. Many of the diseases associated with myocardial hypertrophy are also associated with a loss of endothelial nitric oxide production. As discussed above, shear stress imparted by flowing blood is a major stimulus for activation of the endothelial nitric oxide synthase and it is likely that the loss of nitric oxide production in response to shear could decrease the maximal vasodilator response to supposedly endothelium-independent vasodilators.

Related to these perturbations of the coronary microcirculation is that the larger epicardial coronary arteries do not enlarge appropriately as the myocardium hypertrophies. In normal hearts there is a linear relationship between the diameter of an epicardial coronary artery and the mass of myocardium perfused. In hypertrophied hearts from dogs with experimental hypertension, this linear relationship is shifted upward such that for any diameter coronary artery, the amount of myocardium perfused is approximately doubled. This results in a functional 50% stenosis even in the absence of a coronary stenosis. Thus the superimposition of

762 a coronary lesion that would otherwise be considered insignificant may be flow limiting in the presence of cardiac hypertrophy.

PHARMACOLOGY OF THE CORONARY MICROCIRCULATION

The response of the coronary microcirculation to a variety of neurohumoral stimuli is not constant, but rather is heterogeneous. Similarly, a variety of pharmacological agents such as organic nitrates, adenosine, dipyridamole, and certain inhalation anesthetics exert heterogeneous effects on the coronary microcirculation that may have an influence on the distribution of blood flow to the heart and other organs (Figure 47-7).

The organic nitrates (e.g., nitroglycerin) represent diverse groups of compounds that contain a nitrate ester moiety. Unlike many other nitrovasodilators, the organic nitrates do not spontaneously release nitric oxide, but must undergo a three electron reduction of the nitrogen atom that eventually is released as NO•. Both enzymatic and nonenzymatic mechanisms for this "biotransformation" have been implicated; it is thought that enzymatic processes predominate *in vivo*. Recently the mitochondrial enzyme aldehyde dehydrogenase has been shown to be responsible for this biotransformation of nitroglycerin. The importance of this is that it appears that only certain tissues are capable of this enzymatic process. This is true in the coronary circulation. It was noted as early as the 1960s[16,63] that the organic nitrates produced prolonged vasodilation of the larger

epicardial coronary arteries, while producing only minimal and short-lived increases in coronary flow. In keeping with these findings, *in vitro* and *in vivo* studies have shown that coronary microvessels >200 μm in diameter are potently dilated in response to nitroglycerin, while vessels <100 μm in diameter are dilated only minimally by suprapharmacological concentrations (>1 μmol/liter) of the drug.[27,52] This property of nitroglycerin is shared by other organic nitrates and is likely related to the common requirement for biotransformation of the nitrate ester. In contrast to the organic nitrates, other nitrovasodilators, such as S-nitrosocysteine (a nitrosothiol) or sodium nitroprusside, yield nitric oxide upon a simple one-electron reduction. These agents potently dilate all size coronary microvessels to an equal extent, probably because they do not require enzymatic biotransformation. Thus, it seems that the smaller coronary microvessels (<100 μm in diameter) can respond to nitric oxide, but are simply incapable of biotransforming nitroglycerin to the free NO• gas. Subsequent studies have shown that this biotransformation process likely requires glutathione, and that differences in the ability of large but not small coronary microvessels to respond to nitroglycerin may be related to variations in intracellular glutathione levels in different sized microvessels.[62]

This pharmacological property of the organic nitrates to preferentially dilate larger coronary arteries, while having minimal effect on the smaller coronary microvessels, is extremely important in terms of their antianginal properties. Drugs that dilate the smaller (<100 μm) coronary microvessels have been implicated in producing the coronary steal phenomenon. Thus, by sparing coronary microvessels

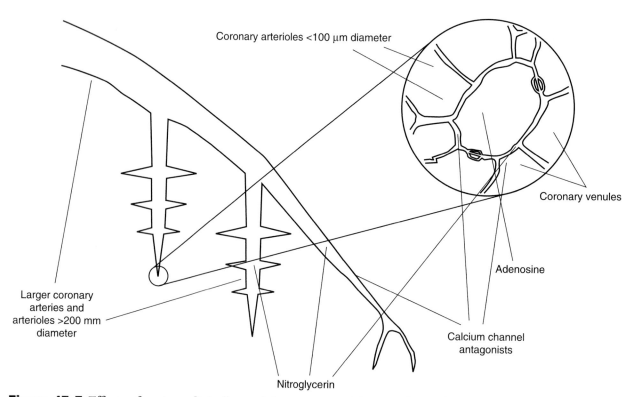

Figure 47-7 Effects of various clinically used drugs on arterial, arteriolar, and venular tone. Note nitroglycerin selectively dilates large arteries, and calcium channel blockers dilate vessels of all classes and size, whereas adenosine preferentially relaxes microvessels.

<100 μm in diameter, the organic nitrates avoid this untoward effect while having the beneficial effects of dilating venous capacitance vessels (reducing cardiac preload), epicardial coronary arteries (sites of coronary stenoses), and coronary collateral vessels. This profile of vascular activity may explain the tremendously beneficial effect these drugs and other agents that have a similar heterogeneous vasomotor effect[45] have in the treatment of myocardial ischemia.

Adenosine has an effect on the coronary microvessels that is precisely the opposite of that caused by organic nitrates. Although adenosine is not generally considered a pharmacological agent, it is worth mentioning here because it is used therapeutically for treatment of arrhythmias and diagnostically to induce myocardial ischemia. Dipyridamole is also often used for this latter purpose, and its effect is mediated by its ability to both enhance adenosine's release and inhibit its degradation. Adenosine produces potent vasodilation of coronary microvessels <100 μm in diameter and only modest dilation of larger vessels.

The dihydropyridine-type calcium channel antagonists produce uniform vasodilation of all classes of coronary microvessels. There has not been a reported comparison of the effect of the other subtypes of calcium channel antagonists.

As indicated in the section entitled "Metabolic Regulation and Autoregulation" in this chapter, there is a great deal of interest in the role of potassium channels in modulating coronary flow. A variety of potassium channel opening agents, principally those that affect the K_{ATP} channel, have been studied in terms of their ability to alter coronary hemodynamics. These agents, which include drugs such as cromakalim, Lemakalim, and Bemikalim, are potent vasodilators of all vessels, and markedly increase coronary flow when administered *in vivo*. The profile of coronary microvessels dilated by these agents does not seem to have been examined, but they are capable of hyperpolarizing smooth muscle of very small coronary arterioles. A potentially useful therapeutic agent is nicorandil, an organic nitrate with potassium channel opening properties. Not surprisingly, nicorandil dilates all sized coronary microvessels under normal conditions; however, it becomes selective for vessels larger than 100 μm in diameter when K_{ATP} channels are blocked by glibenclamide.[1]

▶ SUMMARY

In this review, we have summarized some of the newer concepts regarding physiological, pathophysiological, and pharmacological control of the coronary microcirculation. Whenever possible, we have focused on studies that have directly examined the coronary microvessels using some of the newer technology (*in vitro* preparations or *in situ* observations). It is not possible, however, to understand these studies without consideration of some of the more classic studies of the intact coronary circulation performed in intact animals or isolated hearts. Although these older approaches, in general, employed indirect techniques, they provided a wealth of insight and understanding of coronary blood flow regulation. In reviewing this literature, it is clear that many of the methods used in the past three decades for study of the coronary circulation and microcirculation have largely been abandoned, or are being used in relatively few laboratories. In part, this is due to the fact that the research questions that have arisen regarding vascular function have necessitated the use of more basic techniques, including cell culture and molecular biological approaches. Another reason for this is the difficulty of these studies and the expense of larger animals used in many of the physiological experiments. A relatively recent development has been the ability to make many *in vivo* measurements of coronary hemodynamics in human subjects in the catheterization laboratory, bypassing the absolute need for large animal studies of flow. Nevertheless, as vascular biology research examines more fundamental questions, it will be important not to lose sight of the need to take basic observations back to the intact circulation. As emphasized in this chapter, properties of peripheral vessels cannot be extrapolated to the coronary circulation, and properties of one size or class of coronary microvessel may not be present in another size or class of coronary microvessel. Future studies will be most successful when fundamental observations can be tested in intact vessels and circulations, including the coronary circulation.

REFERENCES

1. Akai K, Wang Y, Sato K, et al: Vasodilatory effect of nicorandil on coronary arterial microvessels: its dependency on vessel size and the involvement of the ATP-sensitive potassium channels. J Cardiovasc Pharmacol 26:541–547, 1995.
2. Arnal J-F, Yamin J, Dockery S, Harrison DG: Regulation of endothelial nitric oxide synthase mRNA, protein and activity during cell growth. Am J Physiol (Cell Physiol) 267:C1381–C1388, 1994.
3. Bauters C, Asahara T, Zheng L, et al: Recovery of disturbed endothelium-dependent flow in the collateral-perfused rabbit ischemic hindlimb after administration of vascular endothelial growth factor. Circulation 91:2802–2809, 1995.
4. Bellamy RF: Diastolic coronary artery pressure-flow relations in the dog. Circ Res 43:92–101, 1978.
5. Boatwright RB, Downey HF, Bashour FA, Crystal GJ: Transmural variation in autoregulation of coronary blood flow in hyperperfused canine myocardium. Circ Res 47:599–609, 1980.
6. Cayatte AJ, Palacino JJ, Horten K, Cohen RA: Chronic inhibition of nitric oxide production accelerates neointima formation and impairs endothelial function in hypercholesterolemic rabbits. Arterioscler Thromb 14:753–759, 1994.
7. Chilian WM: Microvascular pressures and resistances in the left ventricular subepicardium and subendocardium. Circ Res 69:561–570, 1991.
8. Chilian WM, Dellsperger KC, Layne SM, et al: Effects of atherosclerosis on the coronary microcirculation. Am J Physiol 258:H529–H539, 1990.
9. Chilian WM, Eastham CL, Marcus ML: Microvascular distribution of coronary vascular resistance in beating left ventricle. Am J Physiol 251:H779–H788, 1986.
10. Chilian WM, Layne SM, Klausner EC, et al: Redistribution of coronary microvascular resistance produced by dipyridamole. Am J Physiol 256:H383–H390, 1989.
11. Conway RS, Kirk ES, Eng C: Ventricular preload alters intravascular and extravascular resistances of coronary collaterals. Am J Physiol 254:H532–H541, 1988.
12. Corson M, James N, Latta S, et al: Phosphorylation of endothelial nitric oxide synthse in response to fluid shear stress. Circ Res 79:984–991, 1996.

764

13. Drexler H, Zeiher AM, Meinzer K, Just H: Correction of endothelial dysfunction in coronary microcirculation of hypercholesterolaemic patients by L-arginine. Lancet 338:1546–1550, 1991.

14. Duncker DJ, van Zon NS, Ishibashi Y, Bache RJ: Role of K+ ATP channels and adenosine in the regulation of coronary blood flow during exercise with normal and restricted coronary blood flow. J Clin Invest 97:996–1009, 1996.

15. Eng C, Jentzer JH, Kirk ES: The effects of the coronary capacitance on the interpretation of diastolic pressure-flow relationships. Circ Res 50:334–341, 1982.

16. Fam WM, McGregor M: Effect of nitroglycerin and dipyridamole on regional coronary resistance. Circ Res 22:649–659, 1968.

17. Feigl EO: Coronary physiology. Physiol Rev 63:1–205, 1983

18. Fujii M, Nuno DW, Lamping KG, et al: Effect of hypertension and hypertrophy on coronary microvascular pressure. Circ Res 71:120–126, 1992.

19. Furchgott RF, Zawadzki JV: The obligatory role of endothelial cells in the relaxation of arterial smooth muscle by acetylcholine. Nature 288(5789):373–376, 1980.

20. Hammarstrom AK, Parkington HC, Coleman HA: Release of endothelium-derived hyperpolarizing factor (EDHF) by M3 receptor stimulation in guinea-pig coronary artery. Br J Pharmacol 115:717–722, 1995.

21. Harada K, Friedman M, Lopez J, et al: Vascular endothelial growth factor administration in chronic myocardial ischemia. Am J Physiol 270:H1791–H1802, 1996.

22. Hoffman JI: Transmural myocardial perfusion. Prog Cardiovasc Dis 29(6):429–464, 1987.

23. Itoh H, Pratt RE, Ohno M, Dzau VJ: Atrial natriuretic polypeptide as a novel antigrowth factor of endothelial cells. Hypertension 19:758–761, 1992.

24. Kanatsuka H, Ashikawa K, Komaru T, et al: Diameter change and pressure-red blood cell velocity relations in coronary microvessels during long diastoles in the canine left ventricle. Circ Res 66:503–510, 1990.

25. Klassen G, Armour J: Epicardial coronary venous pressure measurements: Autonomic responses. Can J Physiol Pharmacol 60:698–706, 1982.

26. Kuo L, Davis MJ, Chilian WM: Myogenic activity in isolated subepicardial and subendocardial coronary arterioles. Am J Physiol 255:H1558–H1562, 1988.

27. Kurz MA, Lamping KG, Bates JN, et al: Mechanisms responsible for the heterogeneous coronary microvascular response to nitroglycerin. Circ Res 68:847–855, 1991.

28. Lamping KG, Chilian WM, Eastham CL, Marcus ML: Coronary microvascular response to exogenously administered and endogenously released acetylcholine. Microvasc Res 43:294–307, 1992.

29. Lamping KG, Clothier JL, Eastham CL, Marcus ML: Coronary microvascular response to endothelin is dependent on vessel diameter and route of administration. Am J Physiol 263:H703–H709, 1992.

30. Lamping KG, Kanatsuka H, Eastham CL, et al: Nonuniform vasomotor responses of the coronary microcirculation to serotonin and vasopressin. Circ Res 65:343–351, 1989.

31. Lefer D, Nakanishi K, Vinten-Johansen J, et al: Cardiac venous endothelial dysfunction after myocardial ischemia and reperfusion in dogs. Am J Physiol:H850–H856, 1992.

32. Li J, Parovian C, Li J, et al: Modulation of microvascular signaling by heparan sulfate matrix: Studies in syndecan-4 transgenic mice. Microvasc Res 65:38–46, 2002.

33. Marcus M: The Coronary Circulation in Health and Disease, 1st ed. New York: McGraw-Hill, 1983.

34. Marcus ML, Harrison DG, Chilian WM, et al: Alterations in the coronary circulation in hypertrophied ventricles. Circulation 75:I19–I25, 1987.

35. Matsunaga T, Okumura K, Ishizaka H, et al: Impairment of coronary blood flow regulation by endothelium-derived nitric oxide in dogs with alloxan-induced diabetes. J Cardiovasc Pharmacol 28:60–67, 1996.

36. McQuillan LP, Leung GK, Marsden PA, et al: Hypoxia inhibits expression of eNOS via transcriptional and posttranscriptional mechanisms. Am J Physiol 267:H1921–H1927, 1994.

37. Michel J, Feron O, Sacks D, Michel T: Reciprocal regulation of endothelial nitric-oxide synthase by Ca2+-calmodulin and caveolin. J Biol Chem 272:15583–15586, 1997.

38. Moroi M, Gold H, Yasuda T, et al: Mice mutant in endothelial nitric oxide synthase: Vessel growth and response to injury (abstract). Circulation 94:890, 1996.

39. Murad F: Cyclic guanosine monophosphate as a mediator of vasodilation. J Clin Invest 78:1–5, 1986.

40. Myers PR, Minor RL Jr, Guerra R Jr, et al: The vasorelaxant properties of the endothelium-derived relaxing factor more closely resemble S-nitrosocysteine than nitric oxide. Nature 345:161–163, 1990.

41. Narayanan J, Imig M, Roman RJ, Harder DR: Pressurization of isolated renal arteries increases inositol trisphosphate and diacylglycerol. Am J Physiol 266:H1840–H1845, 1994.

42. Nellis SH, Liedtke AJ, Whitesell L: Small coronary vessel pressure and diameter in an intact beating rabbit heart using fixed-position and free-motion techniques. Cir Res 49:342–353, 1981.

43. Osol G, Laher I, Cipolla M: Protein kinase C modulates basal myogenic tone in resistance arteries from the cerebral circulation. Circ Res 68:359–367, 1991.

44. Osol G, Laher I, Kelley M: Myogenic tone is coupled to phospholipase C and G protein activation in small cerebral arteries. Am J Physiol 265:H415–420, 1993.

45. Park KW, Dai H-B, Lowenstein E, et al: Heterogeneous vasomotor responses of rabbit microvessels to isoflurane. Anesthesiology 81:1190–1197, 1994.

46. Piana RN, Wang SY, Friedman M, Sellke FW: Angiotensin-converting enzyme inhibition preserves endothelium-dependent coronary microvascular responses during short-term ischemia-reperfusion. Circulation 93:544–551, 1996.

47. Quillen JE, Sellke FW, Brooks LA, Harrison DG: Ischemia-reperfusion impairs endothelium-dependent relaxation of coronary microvessels but does not affect large arteries. Circulation 82:586–594, 1990.

48. Rapps J, Jones A, Sturek M, et al: Mechanisms of altered contractile responses to vasopressin and endothelin in canine collateral arteries. Circulation 95:231–239, 1997.

49. Schaper W: The Pathophysiology of Myocardial Perfusion, 1st ed. Amsterdam, The Netherlands: Elsevier/North Holland Biomedical Press, 1979.

50. Sellke FW, Armstrong ML, Harrison DG: Endothelium-dependent vascular relaxation is abnormal in the coronary microcirculation of atherosclerotic primates. Circulation 81:1586–1593, 1990.

51. Sellke FW, Dai HB: Responses of porcine epicardial venules to neurohumoral substances. Cardiovasc Res 27:1326–1332, 1993.

52. Sellke FW, Myers PR, Bates JN, Harrison DG: Influence of vessel size on the sensitivity of porcine microvessels to nitroglycerin. Am J Physiol 258:H515–H520, 1990.

53. Sellke FW, Quillen JE, Brooks LA, Harrison DG: Endothelial modulation of the coronary vasculature in vessels perfused via mature collaterals. Circulation 81:1938–1947, 1990.

54. Sellke FW, Shafique T, Schoen FJ, Weintraub RM: Impaired endothelium-dependent coronary microvascular relaxation after cold potassium cardioplegia and reperfusion. J Thorac Cardiovasc Surg 105:52–58, 1993.

55. Sellke FW, Wang SY, Friedman M, et al: Basic FGF enhances endothelium-dependent relaxation of the collateral-perfused

coronary microcirculation. Am J Physiol 267:H1303–1311, 1994.

56. Sellke FW, Wang SY, Stamler A, et al: Enhanced microvascular relaxations to VEGF and bFGF in chronically ischemic porcine myocardium. Am J Physiol 271:H713–720, 1996.

57. Treasure CB, Klein JL, Vita JA, et al: Hypertension and left ventricular hypertrophy are associated with impaired endothelium-mediated relaxation in human coronary resistance vessels. Circulation 87:86–93, 1993.

58. Uemetsu M, Ohara Y, Navas JP, et al: Regulation of endothelial cell nitric oxide synthase mRNA expresiion by shear stress. Am J Physiol 269:C1371–C1378, 1995.

59. Venema RC, Sayegh HS, Arnal J-F, Harrison DG: Role of the enzyme calmodulin-binding domain in membrane association and phospholipid inhibition of endothelial nitric oxide synthase. J Biol Chem 270:14705–14711, 1995.

60. von der Leyen HE, Gibbons GH, Morishita R, et al: Gene therapy inhibiting neointimal vascular lesion: In vivo transfer of endothelial cell nitric oxide synthase gene. Proc Natl Acad Sci USA 92:1137–1141, 1995.

61. Wang SY, Friedman M, Johnson RG, et al: Adrenergic regulation of coronary microcirculation after extracorporeal circulation and crystalloid cardioplegia. Am J Physiol 267:H2462–H2470, 1994.

62. Wheatley RM, Dockery SP, Kurz MA, et al: Interactions of nitroglycerin and sulfhydryl-donating compounds in coronary microvessels. Am J Physiol 266:H291–H297, 1994.

63. Winbury MM, Howe BB, Weiss HR: Effect of nitrates and other coronary dilators on large and small coronary vessels; an hypothesis for the mechanism of action of nitrates. J Pharmacol Exp Ther 168:70–95, 1969.

64. Young MA, Knight DR, Vatner SF: Autonomic control of large coronary arteries and resistance vessels. Prog Cardiovasc Dis 30:211–234, 1987.

65. Yu SM, Hung LM, Lin CC: cGMP-elevating agents suppress proliferation of vascular smooth muscle cells by inhibiting the activation of epidermal growth factor signaling pathway. Circulation 95:1269–1277, 1997.

66. Yuan Y, Mier R, Chilian W, et al: Interaction of neutrophils and endothelium in isolated coronary venules and arterioles. Am J Physiol (Heart Circ Physiol) 268:H490–H498, 1995.

Physiology of the Myocardium

R. John Solaro and Margaret V. Westfall

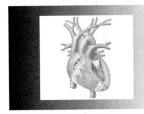

CHAPTER 48

INTRODUCTION: THE INTEGRATIVE BIOLOGY OF THE MYOCARDIUM

The essence of the function of the muscles that make up the myocardium is to precisely transfer the volume of blood added to the ventricular chambers during diastole to the arteries.[3] This transfer must occur within narrow limits of end-diastolic pressures and must produce a flow of materials to the organs that matches the needs of the cells. By "needs" we mean matching the flow of oxygen, which is consumed by the cells at a rate greater than all other materials, to the demand for oxygen. By supplying the tissue oxygen needs, the demand for all other substances in blood is met. An inevitable consequence of the work done during exercise is an increase in oxygen consumption, and with linear incremental increases in oxygen consumption there are linear incremental increases in cardiac output (CO) to match the increases in venous return (VR). The tight coupling of oxygen demand to CO and VR indicates a regulatory system that is able to sense the tissue oxygen needs, and to engage control mechanisms that adjust the cardiac output. In this chapter we are concerned with the role of the myocardium in the task of the cardiovascular system to couple oxygen demand to oxygen supply.

In accomplishing this task, the activity of the myocardium must vary over a wide range in short-term regulation over seconds, minutes, and hours and in long-term regulation over days, weeks, and years. In the short term, during the course of a normal day as tissue oxygen demands and hence cardiac output changes from sleep to strong exercise, variations in activity of the myocardium occur by both intrinsic and extrinsic control mechanisms. The major intrinsic regulator is the Frank–Starling mechanism in which the pressure developed by the ventricle increases as the end–diastolic volume increases. Extrinsic regulators of the myocardium include autonomic nerves of the sympathetic and parasympathetic system, and humeral factors including catecholamines, thyroid hormone, and insulin. In long-term regulation, the activity of the myocardium is also more permanently changed in response to chronic changes in oxygen demand associated with frequent bouts of chronic exercise and altered state of the pump and vascular system associated with aging and various long-standing pathologies. In this long-term regulation, the size of the cells making up the ventricular myocardium changes (hypertrophy or atrophy without a change in cell number). The cells are remodeled by alterations in subcellular mechanisms regulating contraction and relaxation. This long-term regulation occurs physiologically with normal development of the heart from the immature to the mature myocardium, with normal physiological aging, and with acquired or inherited pathologies that directly or indirectly affect the function of the myocardium.[4,11] In this chapter, we focus on current concepts and theories of the cellular, subcellular, and molecular mechanisms for short-term regulation of the myocardium. These mechanisms are constrained to account for the dynamic and steady-state functional properties of the heart. Changes in flow and ventricular volumes during an episode of exercise reveal these functional properties.

CARDIAC DYNAMICS IN EXERCISE

Figure 48-1 displays changes in heart rate (HR), CO, stroke volume (SV), and ventricular volumes of a young healthy adult during a bout of exercise on a stationary bike. The measurements were made before and after administration of propranolol, a β-adrenergic blocking agent. Note that in the control condition CO increased with work load but end-diastolic volume (EDV) remained rather constant even though CO nearly tripled. SV increased and end-systolic volume (ESV) decreased. These data show that the increased VR that occurs in exercise is handled by the heart largely by increases in HR and decreases in ESV. Elevations in EDV as a mechanism to increase CO are not favorable owing to the increase energy cost according to the law of LaPlace.[3] A decrease in ESV provides an important mechanism for matching CO to increased VR without increases in EDV. As we will develop, this reduction in ESV at constant EDV can be one measure of the contractile ability of the cells of the hearts, i.e., the contractility or inotropic state of the heart. Following blockade of adrenergic β-receptors with

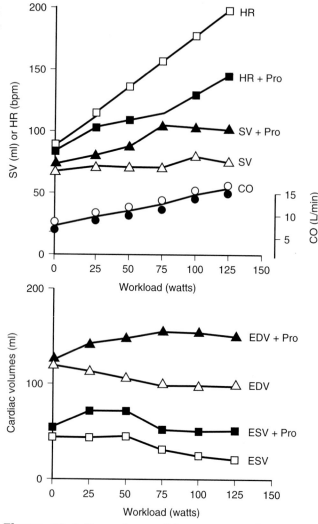

Figure 48–1 Dependence of heart rate, cardiac output, and left ventricular volumes on work load in a bout of exercise. The experiments were carried on a normal young healthy male before and after the administration of propranolol, a β-adrenergic blocking agent. See text for description. *(Data courtesy of Dr. Edward Lakatta.)*

propranolol, there is a blunting of the ability of the sympathetic nervous system to influence the heart. However, CO still increased about three-fold. This is testimony to the ability of the cardiovascular system to match the CO to the increased tissue oxygen needs without sympathetic nervous system control mechanisms. Yet, the increase in CO in the presence of propranolol occurred with a cost. One cost was that the increase in HR was reduced. With a decrease in HR and constant CO, the SV had to be elevated (CO = SV × HR). The increase in SV occurred largely because of an increase in EDV. Increases in EDV present a threat to the economy of contraction, and also may stimulate hypertrophic signaling pathways as a result of cell stretch.[4,11] These effects of propranolol indicate an important role of the β-receptors and the sympathetic nervous system in regulation of the ability of the heart to maintain CO with little or no change in EDV. Figure 48-2 depicts the dynamics of cardiac function with data relating time dependence of left ventricular volume before and after an episode of exercise. These data demonstrate not only the decrease in ESV with little change in EDV, but also enhanced dynamics and abbreviation of the contraction/relaxation cycle. The abbreviation of cardiac cycle time is critical for the maintenance of cardiac filling during the fast HR that occurs with exercise. Figure 48-2 also illustrates that the volume changes are associated with shortening of the cells making up the left ventricular chamber and that the changes in cell length reflect changes in sarcomere length. We discuss next the molecular and cellular mechanisms responsible for maintenance of CO with elevations of VR with minimal change in EDV.

▶ MOLECULAR CELLULAR BIOLOGY

Figure 48-3 depicts cellular structures involved in excitation, contraction, and relaxation. Tight junctions of low electrical resistance connect heart cells.[1,12] When one cell is activated (depolarized), all cells become activated. Therefore, in contrast to the case with skeletal muscle, the heart *does not* recruit motor units to regulate contraction. Instead, regulation is at level of the cells themselves. We will see that there are mechanisms that permit regulation of the activity

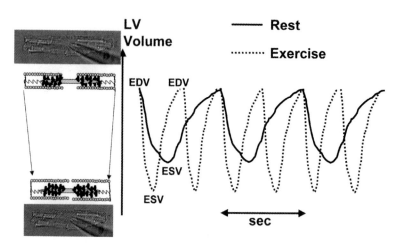

Figure 48–2 Time dependence of left ventricular volume before and during exercise. Note the reduction in cycle time associated with the increased HR. The left panel depicts how the change in volume reflects a change in sarcomere (SL) and cell length (CL) of ventricular myocytes making up the ventricular chamber.

Figure 48–3 Microscopic view of a portion of a myocardial cell illustrating structures critical to excitation–contraction coupling. The T-tubule-containing channels and transporters are shown as an invagination of the surface membrane or sarcolemma, which contains surface α- and β-receptors for norepinephrine, epinephrine, and muscarinic receptors for acetylcholine. Also shown is the sarcoplasmic reticulum (SR), an internally enclosed network of tubules in which high concentrations of Ca^{2+} are stored in diastole. With electrical excitation of the cell, Ca^{2+} channels open and the small release of Ca^{2+} into the cytoplasm induces Ca^{2+} release from the SR through ryanodine receptors (RyR2; SR Ca^{2+} release channels). Ca^{2+} moves to the myofilaments (shown as a half-sarcomere) and activates contraction (see Figure 48-4). Ca^{2+} is removed from the cytoplasm by an SR Ca^{2+}-activated Mg-ATPase (SERCA2a) and exchanged for Na^+ by the action of the Na^+, Ca^{2+} exchange protein (NCX) in the sarcolemma. Phospholamban (PLB) inhibits transport of Ca^{2+} by SERCA2a, and the inhibition is released when PLB becomes phosphorylated. See the text for details.

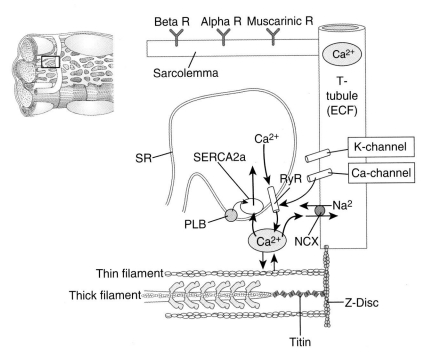

of each cell to meet varying demands on the circulation. We will therefore concentrate now on understanding overt left ventricular cardiac function in terms of the properties of the cardiac myocytes. The objectives are to understand the following:

- The molecular and cellular mechanisms responsible for the changes in wall tension and ventricular volume that occur in the transition from diastole to systole.
- The regulatory devices used by the heart to ensure ejection of an SV equal to the LV at optimal EDV during basal physiological states and during exercise.
- The mechanisms that ensure that dynamics of the heart beat are tuned to match the prevailing frequency, the HR.

SARCOMERE MECHANICS

Sarcomeres are fundamental structural units responsible for the ability of myocardial cells to shorten and generate forces (Figures 48-3 and 48-4). Side arms of the myosin molecules (cross-bridges) that make up the thick filament are molecular motors that also hydrolyze ATP. Light chains on the myosin head, which are different in ventricles and atria, appear to regulate the rate of the ATP hydrolysis. A thick filament associated protein, myosin-binding protein C, or C-protein may be important in regulating the radial movement of the cross-bridge. C-protein also binds to titin, a long structural protein that extends from the center of the sarcomere to the Z-line. This interaction is of significance in cross-bridge function and in generation of passive tension. The reaction of the myosin cross-bridges with the actins of the thin filaments generates active cellular force, shortening, and power.[6,16] The basic reaction cycle includes an attachment step, a movement of the lever arm of the myosin head, which impels the thin filament in each half-sarcomere

to slide toward the center, and a detachment step, which completes the cycle.[6] Figure 48-4 displays the cross-bridge in diastole (left) and at the end of the power stroke (right). The energy for these movements comes from the hydrolysis of one Mg-ATP during each cycle. In diastole, the cross-bridges contain bound Mg-ADP and P_i, which has been generated from Mg-ATP splitting on the surface of the head, poising it for reaction with actin. As actin sites become available, the cross-bridge attaches and enters into a catalytic cycle in which the release of P_i and Mg-ADP together with isomerization of the cross-bridge induce a progressive change in mechanical state of the cross-bridge leading to thin filament sliding. The terminal state is a strongly bound rigor cross-bridge that is free of P_i and nucleotide. Detachment requires binding of Mg-ATP, which is quickly split, without release of products, so that the cycle may begin again if actins remain accessible. Each actin–cross-bridge reaction cycle therefore is powered by the hydrolysis of Mg-ATP.

Ca^{2+} binding triggers conformational changes and movements of the thin filament proteins troponin (Tn; a heterotrimeric protein complex) and tropomyosin (Tm) that switch on the actin–cross-bridge reaction.[10,11] Figures 48-4 and 48-5 illustrate the steps in this process. In diastole, Tn and Tm are situated on the thin filament in positions that hinder the actin–cross-bridge reaction. Tn and Tm are held in this position largely through the tethering action of troponin I (TnI). TnI is an inhibitory protein of the Tn complex, which binds tightly to actin through a highly basic peptide, to the C-terminal end of TnT, the Tm binding unit of Tn, and the C-terminal lobe of TnC, the Ca^{2+} receptor protein. This inhibitory property of TnI is amplified by virtue of these multiple protein–protein interactions to immobilize the long α-helical Tm in a blocking position that encompasses many actins along the thin filament. When released into the myofilament space by mechanisms

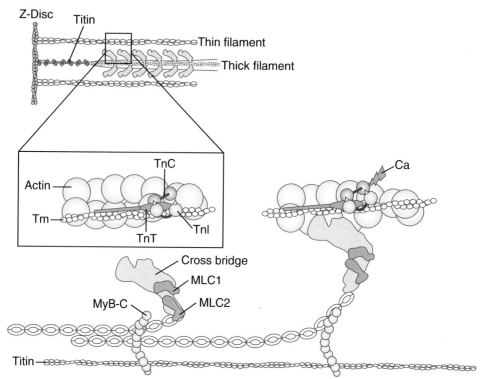

Figure 48–4 Illustration of a cardiac myocyte half sarcomere illustrating a regulatory unit in diastole and systole. Microscopic view shows a regulatory unit consisting of seven actins, one tropomyosin (Tm), and one heterotrimeric troponin complex, which consists on a Ca^{2+} binding protein (TnC), an inhibitory protein (TnI), and a Tm-binding protein (TnT). Although not shown in this depiction the thin filament in a half sarcomere contains approximately 30 regulatory units. The action of cross-bridges, discussed further in the text, in each half sarcomere impels the thin filaments toward the center of the sarcomere in reaction with actin powered by ATP hydrolysis. Cross-bridges are impeded from reacting with the thin filament by tropomyosin and troponin. Ca^{2+} binding to a regulatory lobe of troponin C releases the thin filament from this inhibition. See the text for a further description. Myosin-binding protein C (MyB-C) and myosin light chains (MLC1 and MLC2) modulate cross-bridge activity. Titin is a major structural protein responsible for passive tension.

summarized below, Ca^{2+} binds to a single regulatory site on the N-terminal lobe of troponin C (TnC), the Ca^{2+} receptor protein in the heterotrimeric Tn complex. Ca^{2+} binding to the C-lobe exposes a "sticky patch" of hydrophobic amino acids that promotes binding of TnC to the inhibitory peptide and C-terminal regions of TnI. This reaction releases the inhibitory peptide from actin, and leads to a pivoting of the Tn complex on the thin filament with TnT acting as a lever to move Tm from its blocking position on the thin filament. An important aspect of the transition from diastole to systole is that the reaction of cross-bridges with the thin filament can itself promote more actin–cross-bridge reactions by cooperative, feedback mechanisms. It is apparent that cross-bridge binding may enhance the affinity of TnC for Ca^{2+} as well as move Tm further away from the region of actin that reacts with the cross-bridges. At this stage it is important to understand that the number of cross-bridges reacting with the thin filaments determines the force generated by the sarcomere. An important determinant of the number of cross-bridges reacting with the thin filaments is the amount of Ca^{2+} released to the myofilaments and, thus, the relative occupation of sarcomeric TnC proteins with Ca^{2+} (in the basal state this is about 20–25% of the total

TnC).[10] Other important determinants of the number of cross-bridges reacting with the thin filaments are the sarcomere length[5] and the load (velocity of shortening).[6] We discuss below the mechanisms by which each of these variables affects the number of cycling cross-bridges.

Molecular springs interlaced with the thin and thick filaments form elastic elements in the sarcomere that determine passive elastic properties of the cell and have a possible role in active contraction of the cells.[2] A major elastic element is the giant protein, titin, which is shown in Figure 48-3 as a long and flexible protein extending from Z-line to the midline of the sarcomere. As illustrated in Figure 48-3, titin has a region near the Z-line that is coiled much like a spring. There is accumulating and solid evidence that when the sarcomere is stretched, titin elongates giving rise to passive tension. Moreover, there is evidence that when the sarcomere shortens the titin spring imposes a restoring force that is likely to be important in early diastole. Regions of titin in the thin filament–thick filament overlap zone also interact with myosin-binding protein C, a thick filament associated protein that binds to the head/neck region of myosin. Thus, the conformational changes in titin may also affect cross-bridge disposition. Although not depicted

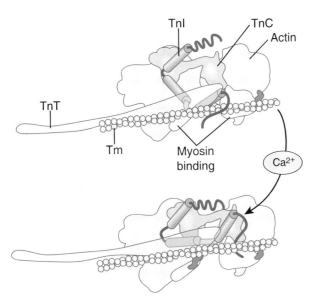

Figure 48–5 Molecular mechanism of thin filament activation by Ca²⁺. In diastole, tropomyosin (Tm) and troponin (Tn) act to impede the thin filament–cross-bridge reaction by steric and allosteric effects on the actin sites that react with myosin. TnI, the inhibitory protein, binds tightly to actin through an inhibitory peptide (Ip). With Ca²⁺ binding to TnC, a strong attraction between the Ip and C-terminal regions of Tn is promoted resulting in movement of Ip of TnI away from the actin binding site, a release of TnT, and a movement of Tm exposing regions of actin that react with myosin cross-bridges also. See the text for a further discussion.

in detail Figure 48-3, the Z-disc of the sarcomere not only anchors the thin filaments, but also links sarcomeres in series by titin and thin filament interactions. There are also lateral connections linking the sarcomere to the surface membrane. In addition to its role in force transmission, the Z-disc is emerging as a locus of communication in the cells. The Z-disc appears as a crossroad for interactions among many diverse proteins including channels, kinases, and phosphatases, and cytoskeletal elements that connect to the nucleus as well as to a network of cytoskeletal proteins and membrane proteins at focal adhesion complexes.[2]

Figure 48-6 relates the circumferential shortening associated with the heartbeat to sarcomeric activity. We will use Figure 48-6 to discuss the cellular and sarcomeric correlates of preload, afterload, and contractility. Thus, in Figure 48-6, we relate the contraction relaxation cycle of the heart beat to events in a single sarcomere; mechanical changes that occur in the active and passive elements of the sarcomere are related to the beat of the heart. The sarcomere is depicted as a contractile element in series with a passive spring that is a lumped elastic element (collagen, titin, and cytoskeletal proteins). A load attached to the end of the sarcomere establishes the sarcomere length before activation and is termed the preload. The preload stretches the sarcomere to its diastolic length; the correlate of the preload in the ventricle is the EDV. In the ventricle, an end-diastolic pressure (EDP) develops as the passive springs are stretched. Figure 48-6 also illustrates the sarcomere with an attached afterload. This is a load that the sarcomere does not "see" until after activation. The correlate of afterload in

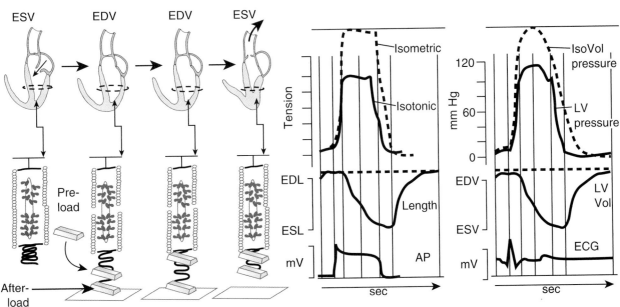

Figure 48–6 Relations between ventricular states in the cardiac cycle and the mechanics of isolated muscle preparations. The cycle begins on the left at an ESV and ES sarcomere length. In the linear muscle setup the analogue of EDV is a weight, the preload, added prior to activation. The addition of the preload establishes sarcomere length. The load the sarcomere discovers it must lift is not seen until after activation and is the afterload, which is supported on the platform. With activation as trigged by the action potential and measured as the ECG, force-generating cross-bridges react with actin, develop tension isometrically until the tension developed matches the afterload. At that point the sarcomere shortens with a velocity appropriate to match the number of reacting cross-bridges to the load. This sarcomeric activity is reflected in the ventricle as an increase in wall tension, isovolumic pressure development followed by opening of the aortic valve and ejection of blood against the rising pressure in the aorta. Dashed lines in the figure represent measurements in which muscle length was held constant or in which the aorta was clamped to produce an isovolumic beat. The peak amplitude of pressure or tension provides a measure of contractility.

772 the ventricle is the aortic pressure. With cellular excitation, Ca^{2+} is released into the myofilament space, the cross-bridges in the sarcomere react with actin sites on thin filaments, and the cell develops tension, shortens, and stretches the elastic element. As tension increases, the afterload is lifted, as the muscle cell shortens. The sarcomere will shorten as long as it can develop tension equal to the afterload. As excitation wanes the cell returns to the diastolic state, ready for another cycle. Figure 48-6 also shows records of the isotonic twitch (the load is constant) and the ventricular pressure. The correlate of cellular tension is the pressure (by the law of LaPlace, where wall tension = pressure × radius of curvature/2 × wall thickness), and the correlate of cellular length is the ventricular volume. In fact, the aortic pressure is increasing during ejection, and, thus, strictly speaking, afterload is not constant. This is referred to as an auxotonic twitch.

The concept of contractility is illuminated by repeating the above sequence of events but with the sarcomere held isometric (dashed lines in Figure 48-6). In this case the sarcomere cannot lift the load and develops the maximum isometric tension possible at the particular length established by the preload and the extent of availability of thin filament sites for reaction with cross-bridges. The peak amplitude of isometric tension is a measure of contractility, one definition of which is maximum tension when the sarcomeres are neither lengthening nor shortening. The peak tension in the isometric twitch reflects in part the amount of Ca^{2+} delivered to the myofilaments, and in part the sarcomere length. As we will see the amount of Ca^{2+} is a regulated variable in heart muscle cells; thus, peak tension or contractility in the isometric twitch could increase or decrease. In animal experiments, this measure of contractility can be determined in beating hearts as well.[3] The approach is to transiently cross-clamp the aorta, which in effect makes resistance and therefore afterload infinite. Dashed lines in the right panel of Figure 48-6 show an isovolumic beat of the ventricle. The peak pressure in this isovolumic beat is a measure of the contractility in the same way that peak tension is a measure of contractility in the sarcomere.

How can contractility be measured in humans without doing the drastic invasive procedure of clamping the aorta? And how does this present definition of contractility relate to the previous indication that contractility is related to end-systolic length and thus end-systolic (ESP) pressure of the sarcomeres? The answers to both these questions are couched in terms of the pressure–volume loop (P–V loop) of the left ventricular beat. Figure 48-7 shows the dependence of ventricular pressure on ventricular volume during cardiac cycles occurring at three different afterloads. The figure also illustrates that the cross-sectional area of the ventricles at the ESV and the EDV is associated with changes in sarcomere length of the cells. In a beat, the volume added during diastole (loading volume) stretches the sarcomeres from the ESV to establish the end-diastolic cell length and EDV. With electrical activation, Ca^{2+} is released into the myofilament space. The sarcomeres develop tension isometrically (isovolumic pressure development) until the cell tension produces a pressure greater than the aortic pressure (the afterload); the valve opens and blood is ejected from the ventricle. The ejection continues with shortening of the sarcomeres to a point at which the pressure developed in the

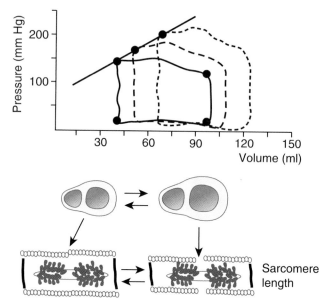

Figure 48–7 Pressure volume (P–V) relations of the left ventricle at varying end-diastolic volumes generated by infusion of blood or saline into the circulation. The P–V loops represent data obtained in human subjects in a resting condition. End-systolic pressure (ESP) points are designated with filled circles. These points represent a state in which the ventricle is neither lengthening nor shortening and developing the peak pressure (tension) at that particular ventricular volume (sarcomere length). Thus points on the volume–ESP relation reflect the length tension properties of the muscle cells. The relation between these points and a circumferential array of ventricular cells and the length of the sarcomere is schematically shown to illustrate that the P–V loop is rooted in a complex relation between sarcomere length and ventricular geometry. See the text and Covell and Ross[3] for a further discussion.

ventricle no longer exceeds the afterload. At this ESP point, the valve closes with the waning of electrical activation and restoration of diastolic Ca^{2+} and pressure falls isovolumically. The ESP is thus a point in which the sarcomeres are no longer shortening or lengthening. ESP is, in effect, a point essentially reflecting isometric tension, i.e., a measure of contractility. The ESP points can be varied by varying afterload as displayed in Figure 48-7 with the dashed P–V loops. Afterload was increased in this example by rapidly increasing the loading volume through an increase in VR. As discussed below, these ESP points reflect isovolumic pressure or isometric cellular tension and are points on the sarcomere length tension relation. It is important to realize that a line connecting these points represents a constant state of contractility. The pressure or tension is different at each of the points because the muscle and sarcomere length has changed not because the contractility has changed. Each beat depicted in Figure 48-7 thus occurred with essentially the same amount of Ca^{2+} released to the myofilaments. The increase in ESP with increases in ventricular volume is the essence of Starling's law of the heart, also known as the Frank–Starling relation.[3,5]

Note that the ESP also reflects the extent of shortening as previously discussed. Imagine, as we will consider below, that the contractility increases. The ESP–volume relation will shift up and to the left and thus at a given afterload the sarcomere will be able to shorten further than at the previous level. Circumferential shortening will occur to a greater extent, and the SV will be increased for a given afterload. We take this concept up again after describing the cellular mechanisms by which contractility can be altered.

EXCITATION–CONTRACTION COUPLING

With the realization that Ca^{2+} ions trigger and regulate the number of actin–cross-bridge reactions, it is easy to understand that switching the heart beat on and off must involve cellular mechanisms that provide and remove Ca^{2+} ions to and from troponin C. Figure 48-8 shows evidence that during a beat of the cells there is transient increase in intracellular Ca^{2+}. Adult mammalian myocardial cells have evolved elaborate membranous structures and membrane proteins to keep Ca^{2+} away from the myofilaments during diastole and to provide Ca^{2+} to the myofilaments during systole.[1,13,15] The myofilaments are surrounded by a reticulum of tubular membranes, called the sarcoplasmic reticulum (SR). These tubules form an internally enclosed compartment that is not contiguous with the extracellular fluid and that contains a number of proteins that regulate the storage, release, and reuptake of Ca^{2+}. As illustrated in Figure 48-3, the surface membrane or sarcolemma of ventricular myocytes plunges into the cellular interior and forms the T-tubules. These invaginations occur along the length of the cell in register with each of the sarcomeres. The T-tubules serve to bring the extracellular fluid as well membrane ion channels, transporters, and exchangers into the depths of the cell interior. The T-tubules are in proximity to the terminal swellings of the SR that are the main storage depots for Ca^{2+} during diastole.

Integrated activity of proteins and protein complexes in the sarcolemma (SL), T-tubules, the SR, and the myofilaments makes up the essential elements of a process known as excitation–contraction coupling, whereby electrical impulses arising at the cell are coupled to a release of Ca^{2+} and to the promotion of the actin–cross-bridge reaction.[1,13,15] Measurements of cellular processes of membrane potential, intracellular Ca^{2+}, and tension are displayed in Figure 48-8. The triggering event is action potential depolarization of the SL and the ensuing depolarization of the sarcolemmal T-tubule. This excitatory process initiates activation of voltage-dependent, L-type Ca^{2+} channels (also known as dihydropyridine receptors), which are primarily clustered within the T-tubules at the sarcolemmal–SR junction. The transverse tubules of the SR contain Ca^{2+} release channels. These channels are also known as ryanodine receptors (RyR2, cardiac isoform) owing to their ability to bind this alkaloid. Depolarization-induced influx of Ca^{2+} current (I_{Ca}) through the L-type channels contributes approximately 20–25% of the free Ca^{2+} in a cardiac twitch. Equally important, I_{Ca} is proposed to act locally to trigger the release of SR Ca^{2+} via the SR Ca^{2+} release channels. The release of Ca^{2+} through the RyRs contributes the remaining 75–80% of Ca^{2+} necessary for cardiac contraction. The process of coupling between the influx of Ca^{2+} via I_{Ca} and Ca^{2+} release from the RyR2 is known as Ca^{2+}-induced Ca^{2+} release (CICR). The gating of the RyR2 by I_{Ca} is the essence of CICR. Experiments employing fluorescent indicators that sense Ca^{2+} have revealed the activity of local clusters of

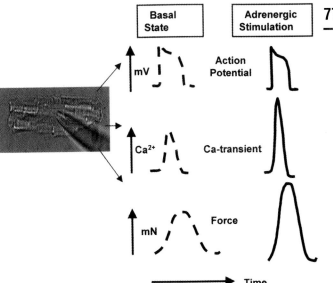

Figure 48–8 Schematic of action potential, intracellular transient change in Ca^{2+}, and isometric tension of a single cardiac myocyte in a basal state and during stimulation with an adrenergic agonist. The effects of adrenergic stimulation are to abbreviate the action potential and to increase the amplitude and dynamics of both the Ca^{2+} transient and the twitch tension.

RyR receptors. These experiments demonstrate elementary events known as Ca^{2+} sparks that reflect the activity of small groups of RyRs. Enhanced I_{Ca} influx increases localized Ca^{2+} accumulation, which increases Ca^{2+} spark frequency, and produces a graded stimulation of RyR Ca^{2+} release from the SR. Release into the cytosol increases the local concentration of Ca^{2+} surrounding the myofilaments and promotes Ca^{2+} binding to TnC on the thin filaments. The reaction of Ca^{2+} with TnC triggers the protein–protein interactions that release regulatory units of the thin filament from an inhibited state (Figures 48-4 and 48-5). It is important to understand that during a beat of the heart in a basal physiological state the amount of Ca^{2+} delivered to the myofilaments is sufficient to activate only about 20–25% of the regulatory units. The 75% of actin–cross-bridge reactions that remain available for increases in contractility form a molecular basis for what is commonly referred to as "cardiac reserve."

As illustrated in Figure 48-8, the elevation in Ca^{2+} levels observed during systole is transient, with SL and SR proteins working to sequester and return Ca^{2+} to baseline levels in the return to diastole.[1,13,15] In the steady-state contraction/relaxation cycle, an equal efflux must match the influx of Ca^{2+}. In human hearts, this sequestration process involves two major cellular pumps. The majority of Ca^{2+} (70%) is resequestered into the SR via Ca^{2+} pumps (sarcoendoplasmic reticulum Ca^{2+} pump; SERCA2a isoform) present on the longitudinal tubules of the SR. SERCA2a is a Ca^{2+}-activated Mg-ATPase that couples Mg-ATP hydrolysis to the active transport of Ca^{2+} from the cytoplasmic space into the SR. A high-capacity, low-affinity Ca^{2+} binding protein, known as calsequestrin, serves as a sink for Ca^{2+} in the interior of the SR. Most of the remaining Ca^{2+} is removed from the cell via the SL Na^+/Ca^{2+} exchanger (NCX) operating in the inward mode (inward $I_{Na/Ca}$). Relatively small and slow processes for Ca^{2+} efflux from the cytosol include

774

transport via a sarcolemmal Ca²⁺ pump and transport into the mitochondrial space.[5] The proportion of Ca²⁺ flux through the NCX and these slow processes is species dependent, with a lower proportion of Ca²⁺ handled by these mechanisms in rodents compared to humans. This species difference requires consideration when applying results obtained in rodent studies to human cardiac function.[1]

▶ MODULATION OF EC COUPLING BY PHOSPHORYLATION

The autonomic nervous system is the major regulator of the amount of Ca²⁺ delivered to the myofilaments.[1,13,15] The myocardium has evolved an elaborate signaling cascade to link adrenergic and cholinergic neural activity as well as blood levels of neurohumors such as epinephrine and acetylcholine to modulation of cellular Ca²⁺ fluxes. As illustrated in Figure 48-9, binding of neurotransmitters, neurohumors, or pharmacological agonists to adrenergic or cholinergic receptors triggers the cascade. GTP-binding proteins, known collectively as G-proteins, transduce receptor binding to an alteration of the enzyme activity of adenylyl cyclase, which is responsible for the generation of cyclic AMP (cAMP) from ATP. Stimulatory G-proteins (G$_s$) linked to adrenergic β-receptors promote the formation of cAMP, whereas inhibitory G-proteins (G$_i$) inhibit adenylyl cyclase and may also activate phosphatases. cAMP activates protein kinase A (PKA), which phosphorylates key proteins that regulate the entry and exit of Ca²⁺ from the myofilament space. In the case of SR, the PKA substrate is phospholamban (PLB), a small proteolipid that, when dephosphorylated, inhibits the activity of SERCA2a (Figures 48-3 and 48-9). PLB is also a substrate for Ca²⁺-activated calmodulin-dependent kinase (CAMK).[1,13] This Ca²⁺-dependent phosphorylation appears important in a "staircase" effect in which force generated by the myocardium increases with HR. With the increased frequency there is a higher Ca²⁺ influx because of increased amplitude and delayed inactivation of I_{Ca}. Phosphorylation of PLB by either PKA or CAMK depresses the PLB–SERCA2a interaction and releases Ca²⁺ pumping activity from inhibition; Ca²⁺ affinity of the pump increases, without changes in the maximum Ca²⁺ transport velocity. This increase in Ca²⁺ uptake increases Ca²⁺ loaded into the SR and induces an accelerated relaxation of the myocytes. This increase in rate of Ca²⁺ removal from the cytoplasm and myofilaments accounts in large part for the enhanced relaxation and abbreviated contraction/relaxation cycle during adrenergic stimulation. The enhanced relaxation also depends on PKA-dependent phosphorylation of TnI.[10,11,17] The phosphorylation of TnI at PKA sites enhances Ca²⁺ release from TnC and speeds up cross-bridge cycling rate.[10] These consequences of PLB and TnI phosphorylation are critical to the ability of the heart to tune its activity cycle to the fast heart rates during adrenergic stimulation and to accommodate the increasing VR without a significant change in EDV (see Figures 48-1 and 48-2). A subunit in the oligomeric assembly of proteins that makes up the L-type Ca²⁺ channel of the heart is also a substrate for PKA.[1] Phosphorylation enhances the probability that the channel will open upon depolarization, but does not affect the unitary conductance. This increase in the trigger for

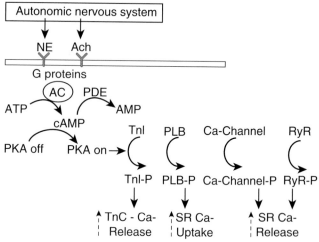

Figure 48–9 Schematic representation of autonomic signal transduction and signaling in cardiac muscle cells. With binding of neurotransmitters (acetylcholine (ACH) and nor-epinephrine (NE)) to the receptors indicated, there is an activation on adenylyl cyclase (AC), elaboration of cAMP, and activation of protein kinase A (PKA). Levels of cAMP are also regulated by the activity of phosphodiesterases (PDE) that convert cAMP to AMP. PKA phosphorylates troponin I (TnI), phospholamban (PLB), Ca²⁺ channel subunits, and ryanodine receptors (RyR) as well as K channels (not shown). These phosphorylations elicit effects on Ca²⁺ uptake and release into the cytoplasmic space with a net result of increased contractility and dynamics of contraction and relaxation. Separate enzymes called phosphatases catalyze dephosphorylation. See the text for a further discussion.

Ca²⁺ release together with the increased Ca²⁺ loading associated with PLB phosphorylation essentially accounts for the increase in the systolic Ca²⁺ transient (Figure 48-8). Regulation of the release of Ca²⁺ through SR RyRs by PKA and by CAMK also provides a mechanism to control delivery of Ca²⁺ to the myofilaments and thus to control contractility by an increase in the open probability of the Ca²⁺ release channel. The amount of Ca²⁺ loaded within the SR lumen is a critical factor influencing RyR Ca²⁺ release. Increases in SR Ca²⁺ content generally stimulate the frequency and amplitude of Ca²⁺ sparks and decreases in content reverse these trends. The duration of the cardiac action potential is also abbreviated with adrenergic stimulation (Figure 48-8). This appears because of PKA-dependent phosphorylation of one form of the K channel important in determination of the duration of the action potential.[14] Separate enzymes called phosphatases, which are controlled by a poorly understood regulatory pathway, catalyze dephosphorylation and restoration of the basal state.

▶ CROSS-BRIDGES AND STROKE VOLUME

In connecting the molecular and cellular properties of the heart to cardiac output, we use the premise that the stroke volume ultimately depends on the actin–myosin interaction. Up to now we have discussed the determinants of SV in terms of contractility, afterload, and preload. We now discuss the relations between contractility, afterload, and preload as determinants of the number and rate of cycling of force generating cross-bridges reacting with the thin filaments. The following equation serves to illustrate the progression of this analysis from active cross-bridges, which determine the systolic change in cell length and tension, to SV and to CO:

$$CO = HR \times SV \leftarrow \text{(change in LV volume and pressure)}$$
$$\leftarrow \text{(change in cell tension and length)}$$

The cellular properties of length and tension are related in a highly complex manner to LV pressure and volume.[3] Yet an understanding of how systolic cross-bridges determine cell tension and shortening sets the stage for understanding the geometric considerations that relate these properties to the ventricular chamber.[3,9]

CELLULAR BIOLOGY OF CONTRACTILITY

Changes in the amount of Ca^{2+} delivered to the myofilaments, which recruit spare actin–cross bridge reactions, may occur by the following:

- Changes in the intracellular Ca^{2+} and activity of the autonomic nervous system that releases neurohumors, which alter the state of phosphorylation of the regulatory proteins in the cells as described above.
- Changes in the chemical environment of the cells. One example is the accumulation of metabolic wastes that occurs during a reduction in coronary flow and that results in acidosis.
- Changes in HR. With increases in HR, it is known that the SR fills to a greater extent with Ca^{2+}, through phosphorylations involving Ca^{2+} calmodulin-dependent kinases.
- Administration of pharmacological agents. Drugs that affect contractility are known as inotropic agents. Some agents such as dobutamine mimic adrenergic neurotransmitters, and some agents such as digitalis indirectly increase Ca^{2+} loading into the SR by inhibiting Na^+, K^+-ATPase, reducing the Na gradient, and thus inhibiting Ca^{2+} extrusion through the Na^+, Ca^{2+} exchanger. There are inotropic agents that inhibit breakdown of cAMP by an inhibition of phosphodiesterase

activity, whereas other agents known as Ca^{2+} sensitizers **775** activate the sarcomere directly.[8]

Figure 48-10 shows a record of ventricular pressure and of tension developed by ventricular papillary muscles. In precise determinations of contractility, it is important that afterload and preload remain constant. Both of these constraints are met if the pressure is developed at constant LV volume or the tension is developed at constant muscle length. In this case, peak pressure or tension would be expected to vary with the amount of Ca^{2+} delivered to the myofilaments as would occur with variations in sympathetic nervous system stimulation, for example. Note that the rate of increase in the pressure also varies with contractility. The time derivative of the pressure trace gives the maximum rate of pressure rise ($+dp/dt$) and fall ($-dp/dt$), both of which are useful indices of contractility in the clinic, even though afterload and preload are not strictly controlled. Ejection fraction (SV/EDV) is also an index of contractility, as is the ratio of end-systolic to end-diastolic dimensions obtained from echo-cardiographic assessment of cardiac function.

▶ CELLULAR BIOLOGY OF AFTERLOAD

Cardiac muscle cells lift light loads faster than heavier loads according to a general characteristic property of striated muscle known as the force–velocity relation.[6] The velocity of shortening approaches a maximum value (V_{max}) as the load approaches zero, velocity is zero at the maximum load, and the cells develop maximum isometric tension under the particular conditions. As load increases between these extremes, the rate of thin filament sliding decreases permitting a longer time for the cross-bridges to react. By this mechanism, the number of cycling cross-bridges is matched to the load the muscle discovers it must lift. As discussed in the context of Figure 48-6, at the isometric extreme (zero velocity), the level of Ca^{2+} activation determines maximum tension. It is also apparent that Ca^{2+} also increases V_{max} by increasing the rate that the cross-bridges enter the

Figure 48–10 Comparison of isovolumic beats and isometric twitches at three levels of contractility. Peak amplitude of tension or pressure under these conditions provides a measure of contractility or inotropic state of the heart. Maximum rates of pressure development ($+dp/dt_{max}$) also provide a measure of contractility. Even though pressures are not developed isovolumically during normal beats, $+dp/dt_{max}$ remains a useful index of contractility.

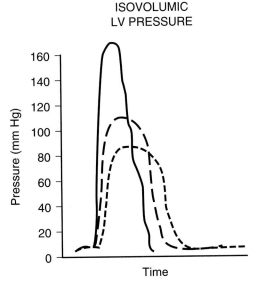

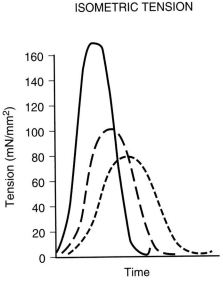

force-generating state. Thus, the force–velocity relation shifts with increases or decreases in contractility.

CELLULAR BIOLOGY OF CELL LENGTH

We now explicitly relate the sarcomere length tension properties of the cardiac muscle cells to the pressure–volume relation. Figure 48-11 displays the entire relation between sarcomere length and the active and passive (resting) tension. Active tension rises and falls from an optimum value, whereas passive tension rises exponentially. The rise in passive tension, which would elevate diastolic LV pressure, is so steep in heart cells as to disallow filling of the ventricle to sarcomere lengths greater than 2.2 μm. In other words, during diastole atrial pressures cannot rise high enough to fill the ventricles to a volume that produces sarcomere lengths exceeding 2.2 μm. Thus, in the physiological state, considerations of the length–tension relations, and therefore the volume pressure relations of the heart, are restricted to the operating range illustrated in Figure 48-11. To measure the length–tension relation, the muscle cells are stretched at rest to various sar-

comere lengths and held isometric. The cells develop a passive tension as they are stretched. At each length, the cells are stimulated to give a measure of the total isometric tension at that particular sarcomere length. Two such lengths are illustrated in Figure 48-11. At the shorter length, there is no passive tension and maximum developed tension is essentially zero owing to double overlap of thin filaments. At the optimum sarcomere length, active tension (the difference between total and passive tension) is at an optimum. Some resting tension exists at this sarcomere length as passive elements (notably titin) in the sarcomere and extracellular matrix are stretched. At the optimum sarcomere length of 2.2 μm, there is maximal overlap between the thick filament cross-bridges and the thin filaments.

In Figure 48-12, we show how the working range of the length–tension relation relates to the pressure–volume relation of the left ventricle. The basic premise is that cell and sarcomere length track the change in ventricular volumes and ventricular pressure tracks changes in cell tension. Thus, one can imagine the generation of the volume–pressure relation by an approach similar to that for generation of the length–tension relation. In this case though EDV is incrementally increased, EDP is measured at each volume, as is peak systolic isovolumic pressure. Figure 48-12 indicates an association of each ventricular volume with a particular sarcomere length. Important points are the following:

- Measurements of the relation between cell length and tension relation and ventricular volume and isovolumic peak systolic pressure are made at constant contractility. The basal inotropic state represents about 20–25% of the maximum inotropic state.
- A line connecting the peak systolic pressure points determined at constant volumes is a measure of contractility. These systolic pressure points are essentially the same ESP points inscribed by variations in afterload as described in Figure 48-7. Recall we mentioned that the ESP represents a point at which the cells are neither lengthening nor shortening.
- The position of the ESP–volume relation is a critical determinant of ESV and thus the ability of the ventricle to eject blood.
- Figure 48-12 indicates that this position changes with an increase in contractility, which we now picture as an increase in Ca^{2+} activation of the cells that results in an increase in peak systolic pressure at a particular ventricular volume. This relation between ventricular volume and pressure was recognized by Otto Frank and Ernest Starling over 100 years ago and is commonly referred to as the Frank–Starling relation or Starling's law of the heart.

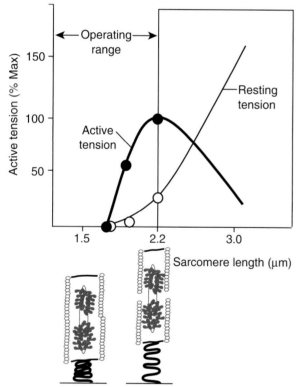

Figure 48–11 Dependence of tension on sarcomere length.
Three measurements are shown in which a linear muscle preparation (papillary muscle or trabecula) was stretched from its equilibrium length and determinations of resting (passive) and total active force made. Active tension is the difference between total tension and passive tension. Beyond a sarcomere length of 2.2 μm, resting tension rises to high levels that are nonphysiological as discussed in the text. Thus, the cells never operate beyond the working range into the shaded panel. Two sarcomeres, depicted at the extremes of the length–tension relation, illustrate the stretching of passive springs in titin and the change in overlap of the thin and thick filaments.

Despite this long-standing knowledge of Starling's law, the molecular mechanism responsible for the shape of the ESP–volume relation remains unclear.[5] The relation is steeper than one would expect from simple geometric considerations of filament overlap. There is excellent evidence that this relatively steep relation is due to a length dependence of Ca^{2+} activation.[5] Measurement of myofilament response to Ca^{2+} demonstrated a decrease in Ca^{2+} sensitivity as the sarcomere become shorter. Thus, at a constant level of systolic Ca^{2+}, we would expect the sarcomeres to be more sensitive to Ca^{2+} as their length increases. This results in a steeper length–tension relation that would occur with no

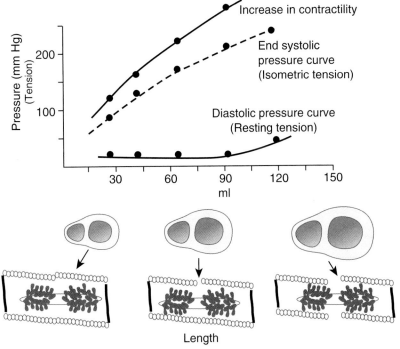

Figure 48–12 Generation of systolic and diastolic pressure curves from steady-state measurements of isovolumic pressure development over a range of end-diastolic volumes. Points on curves were generated by plotting the peak diastolic and systolic pressures at each ventricular volume in hearts with cross-clamped aortas as in Figure 48-6. The correlation of ventricular volume with sarcomere length and pressure with tension emphasizes that the dependence of pressure on volume is rooted in the length–tension relation of cardiac sarcomeres.

change in Ca^{2+} sensitivity. Length-dependent changes in interfilament spacing, radial movements of cross-bridges away from the thick filament proper, and cross-bridge-dependent activation of the myofilaments have all been invoked as mechanisms for length-dependent activation.[5]

CARDIAC FUNCTION CURVES

So far we have depicted regulation of CO as relations between work load, HR, and ventricular volumes (Figure 48-1), as relations between time and ventricular volume changes (Figure 48-2), and as a relation between ventricular volume and ventricular pressure (Figure 48-7). We now consider another view of regulation of cardiac output as so-called "Starling curves" or "the Starling relation" or simply "cardiac function curves." These curves relate some measure of ventricular filling such as EDV or EDP to some measure of ejection, SV, or CO. Figure 48-13A depicts the transition from determinations of SV from pressure–volume loops at constant contractility and afterload to a relation between EDV and SV. Three beats are shown at different preloads. The function curve thus provides a relation between EDV and SV at constant afterload and contractility. Figure 48-13B indicates the shift in cardiac function curve as a result of an elevated afterload. In this case, the pressure–volume loops show the same SV, which is achieved at an elevated EDV. Figure 48-13C indicates the shift in the cardiac function curve as a result of increased contractility. The pressure–volume loops show the same SV, which is achieved at a lower EDV and ESV. One imagines the same shift for all the preloads indicated in Figure 48-13A. With knowledge of the HR, it is possible to convert the EDV–SV

relation to a relation between EDV and CO. Effects of increases and decreases in afterload and contractility on the relation between EDV and CO and SV are illustrated in Figure 48-14.

The exact cardiac function that is operative in the heart at any particular time reflects the integrated effects of many factors. These include the determinants of afterload (blood pressure) and of contractility, changes in HR, level of autonomic nervous system activity and circulating neurohumors, the intracellular and cellular chemical environment (anoxia, hypoxia, acidosis, hypercapnia, metabolites), and the presence of pharmacological agents that affect afterload or contractility. The EDV is determined by the flow of blood back to the heart, which in turn is determined by the total blood volume, the venous tone, resistance to flow, pumping actions of muscle, and the intrathoracic pressure. The integrated effects of these determinants of cardiac function in the physiological state are revealed in the exercise episode depicted in Figure 48-1. Pathophysiological states may be understood in terms of a breakdown of these physiological control mechanisms.[7,8] For example, in heart failure the SR Ca^{2+} load may be diminished by reduced expression of SERCA2a. There may also be alterations in myofilament response to Ca^{2+}. The ultimate effect of these changes is a reduction in contractility, much like that simulated by β-adrenergic blockade in the data shown in Figure 48-1. With elevations in EDV, heart cells are stimulated to grow but the growth becomes maladaptive and failure ensues as remodeling occurs. Detailed discussion of these events is beyond the scope of this chapter, but it is clear that understanding of cardiac pathophysiology begins with an understanding of the physiology of the myocardium.[7,8]

EFFECT OF INCREASED EDV
AT CONSTANT AFTERLOAD
AND CONTRACTILITY

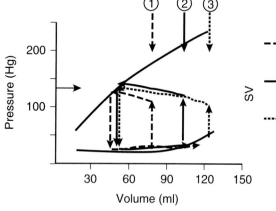

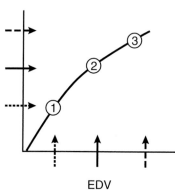

A

GENERATION OF STARLING
CARDIAC FUNCTION CURVES

EFFECT OF INCREASED
AFTERLOAD AT CONSTANT
CONTRACTILITY

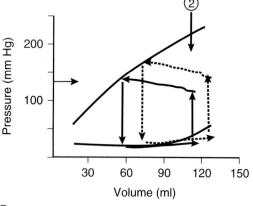

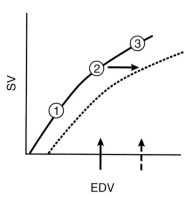

B

Figure 48–13 Generation of Starling cardiac function curves from pressure–volume relations. A, Three beats are shown with increases in preload at constant contractility and afterload. A plot of stroke volume (SV) at each of the end-diastolic volumes (EDV) associated with each beat generates a common form of the cardiac function curve or Starling relation. **B,** Change in steady-state pressure–volume loop after an increase in afterload. Only beat 2 from **A** is shown for illustrative purposes, but a similar shift in the cardiac function would occur at all EDVs. **C,** Change in steady-state pressure–volume loop after an increase in contractility. Only beat 2 from (**A**) is shown for illustrative purposes, but a similar shift in the cardiac function would occur at all EDVs.

EFFECT OF INCREASED
CONTRACTILITY AT
CONSTANT AFTERLOAD

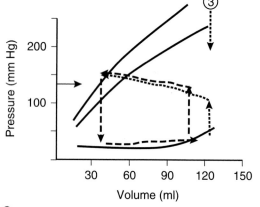

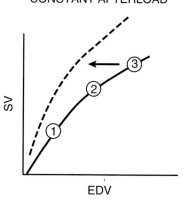

C

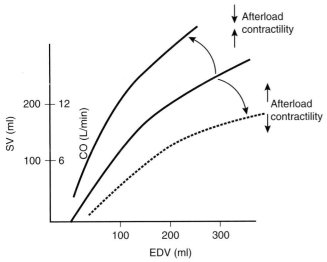

Figure 48–14 **Effect of alterations in afterload and contractility on the cardiac function curve.** The figure emphasizes that each curve represents a state of constant contractility and afterload. Shifts in the cardiac function curve from a physiological basal state (solid line) as indicated occur with changes in afterload and contractility

REFERENCES

1. Bers DM: Excitation-Contraction Coupling and Cardiac Contractile Force, 2nd ed. Boston: Kluwer Academic Publishers, 2001.
2. Clark KA, Mittal B, Sanger JM, Sanger JW: Striated muscle cyto-architecture: An intricate web of form and function. Annu Rev Cell Dev Biol 18:637–706, 2002.
3. Covell JW, Ross J Jr: Systolic and diastolic function (mechanics) of the intact heart. In Page E, Fozzard H, Solaro RJ, editors: Handbook of Physiology: Section 2: The Cardiovascular System, Vol. 1, The Heart. New York: Oxford University Press, 2002, pp. 741–785.
4. Frey N, Olson E: Cardiac hypertrophy: The good, the bad, and the ugly. Annu Rev Physiol 65:45–79, 2003.
5. Fuchs F: The Frank-Starling relationship: Cellular and molecular mechanisms. In Solaro RJ, Moss RL, editors: Molecular Control Mechanisms in Striated Muscle Contraction. Boston: Kluwer Academic Publishers, 2002, pp. 379–416.
6. Homsher E: Determinants of unloaded shortening velocity in striated muscle. In Solaro RJ, Moss RL, editors: Molecular Control Mechanisms in Striated Muscle Contraction. Boston: Kluwer Academic Publishers, 2002, pp. 417–442.
7. Katz AM: A modern view of heart failure: Practical applications of cardiovascular physiology. In Page E, Fozzard H, Solaro RJ, editors: Handbook of Physiology: Section 2: The Cardiovascular System, Vol. 1, The Heart. New York: Oxford University Press, 2002, pp. 786–804.
8. Rice CL, Solaro RJ: Support of the failing heart. In Wilmore DW, Cheung LY, Harken AH, et al, editors: ACS Surgery Principals and Practice. New York: WebMD Corp, 2002, pp. 1391–1400.
9. Solaro RJ: Integration of myofilament response to Ca^{2+} with cardiac pump regulation and pump dynamics. Adv Physiol Ed 22:S155–S163, 1999.
10. Solaro RJ: Modulation of cardiac myofilament activity by protein phosphorylation. In Page E, Fozzard H, Solaro RJ, editors: Handbook of Physiology: Section 2: The Cardiovascular System, Vol. 1, The Heart. New York: Oxford University Press, 2002, pp. 264–300.
11. Solaro RJ, Wolska BM, Arteaga G, et al: Modulation of thin filament activity in long and short term regulation of cardiac function. In Solaro RJ, Moss RL, editors: Molecular Control Mechanisms in Striated Muscle Contraction. Boston: Kluwer Academic Publishers, 2002, pp. 291–327.
12. Spray DC, Suadicani SO, Srinivas M, et al: Gap junctions in the cardiovascular system. In Page E, Fozzard H, Solaro RJ, editors: Handbook of Physiology: Section 2: The Cardiovascular System, Vol. 1, The Heart. New York: Oxford University Press, 2002, pp. 169–212.
13. Tada M, Toyofuku T: Cardaic sarcoplasmic reticulum Ca^{2+}-ATPase. In Page E, Fozzard H, Solaro RJ editors: Handbook of Physiology: Section 2: The Cardiovascular System, Vol. 1, The Heart. New York: Oxford University Press, 2002, pp. 301–334.
14. Thomas D, Zhang W, Karle C, et al: Deletion of protein kinase A phosphorylation sites in the HERG potassium channel inhibits activation shift by protein kinase A. J Biol Chem 274:27457–27462, 1999.
15. Trafford AW, Eisner DA: Excitation-contraction coupling in cardiac muscle. In Solaro RJ, Moss RL, editors: Molecular Control Mechanisms in Striated Muscle Contraction. Boston: Kluwer Academic Publishers, 2002, pp. 48–89.
16. Walker JW: Kinetics of the actin-myosin interaction. In Page E, Fozzard H, Solaro RJ, editors: Handbook of Physiology: Section 2: The Cardiovascular System, Vol. 1, The Heart. New York: Oxford University Press, 2002, pp. 240–263.
17. Westfall MV, Metzger JM: Troponin I isoforms and chimeras: Tuning the molecular switch of cardiac contraction. News Physiol Sci 16:278–281, 2001.

Ventricular Mechanics

Leon Axel

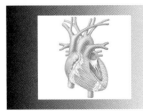

Introduction
Ventricular Structure
Basic Continuum Mechanics Review
Cardiac Cycle
Function Measures
Mechanical Effects of Disease
Summary

▶ INTRODUCTION

Chapter 48 (Physiology of the Myocardium) considered the dynamics of the heart both from a global level, through the use of pressure–volume loops, and at the cellular and subcellular level. In this chapter, we will look at the mechanics of the ventricle, focusing on the intermediate scale between these two extremes and using a physics-based approach. After a review of the structural elements of the ventricle and some of the basic principles of fluid and solid mechanics, we will consider mechanical events in the cardiac cycle and how they are affected by common physiological alterations. We will also review some frequently used methods for assessing ventricular mechanics. We will then consider how these mechanical factors can play a role in common clinical conditions, as a background for later chapters on topics such as failure.

▶ VENTRICULAR STRUCTURE

It is assumed that the reader is already familiar with basic anatomy and physiology of the heart. For completeness, we will review some aspects relevant to our subsequent discussion.

As indicated in Chapter 48, the active forces generated by activation of the contractile elements of the myocytes are transmitted to the rest of the cell through the cytoskeleton. The myocytes are mechanically coupled together, in turn, through the fibrous elements of the extracellular matrix (ECM). The ECM is composed of strands of collagen, fibronectin, and other long-chain proteins that tie the myocytes together at a hierarchy of scales.[1] It provides some of the passive stiffness of the heart, as well as serving to couple the active forces generated in the myocytes to the rest of the heart. The ECM is produced by the fibroblasts; it is regulated in response to mechanical loading of the heart, and apparently plays a role in the development of heart failure. The ECM invests the myocytes in a complex weave and helps define the fiber and sheet architecture of the heart wall (described below).

The myocytes are joined together tightly end to end through intercalated discs. Electrical excitation can be transmitted from cell to cell through these connections, effectively forming an electrical syncytium between the cells. Although they are locally well aligned with each other, branching of the muscle cells helps form a woven sort of structure with a dominant local direction. The cells are further tied together into bundle-like fibers by the fibers of the ECM. The muscle fibers have consistent regional variations in orientation, varying from an oblique orientation in the subepicardial region, through circumferential orientation around the ventricle in the midwall, to an oblique orientation in the opposite direction in the subendocardial region.[8]

In addition to the primary organization of the myocytes into fibers, there is a secondary organization of the fibers into sheets. These sheets are a few cell layers thick. Small potential spaces form thin clefts between the sheets; these are more apparent in dried specimens because of shrinkage. As with the fibers, the sheets split and merge over scales of a few cell lengths, forming a woven sort of structure rather than long coherent strands. These sheets also have a consistent pattern of organization within the wall.[6] The asymmetry of the wall structure due to the fibers and sheets leads to an asymmetry in the passive stiffness properties of the wall and a greater ease of shearing along the plane of the sheets.

Although the myocytes can have spontaneous electrical activation and can propagate electrical activation from one cell to the next along their length, electrical activation of the myocytes is normally initiated by impulses carried through a specialized conducting network and originating in specialized pacemaker tissue in the sinoatrial node. After spreading rapidly over the atria, initiating atrial contraction, there is a delay while the activation propagates more slowly through the atrioventricular (AV) node before propagating rapidly again through the bundle of His and the right and left bundle branches and their subsequent branches (Purkinje fibers) along the endocardium to initiate a coordinated ventricular contraction. Subsequent relaxation of the myocytes is locally initiated and not directly coordinated by the conduction system. The depolarization and repolarization of the myocardial cells, associated with their contraction and relaxation, result in weak voltage (on the order of millivolts) on the surface of the body, which can be detected as the electrocardiogram (ECG).

The right and left ventricles (RV and LV, respectively) supply separate parallel circulations (the pulmonary and systemic, respectively), which are ultimately connected in series; they share a common wall, the interventricular septum. Although the output of both ventricles must balance over a short time scale (unless there is a shunt between the circulations), the lower resistance of the pulmonary

782 circulation means that the pressure in the right ventricle is normally lower than the left. Thus, the right ventricular free wall is normally thinner than that of the left, and the interventricular septum bulges toward the right side.

To keep the blood moving forward through the heart during the cardiac cycle, there are valves at both the inlets to the ventricles (the AV valves, the mitral and tricuspid) and the outlets (the semilunar valves, the aortic and pulmonary). During systole, the AV valves are closed and the semilunar valves are open, permitting forward flow of the pressurized blood from the ventricles into the great arteries, while during diastole the semilunar valves are closed and the AV valves are open, permitting filling of the ventricles with blood from the atria. The papillary muscles connect the edges of the AV valves to the more apical portions of the ventricular cavities through the chordae tendineae. They help prevent inversion and insufficiency of these valves during systole. The AV valves are surrounded by fibrous rings of tissue; these may reinforce their periphery.

The purpose of the left and right ventricles is to pressurize the blood to propel it out into their corresponding circulatory beds, the systemic and pulmonary circuits, respectively. Thus the LV is connected to the aorta and the RV is connected to the pulmonary artery. The RV differs from the LV in having a longer tubular section of outflow tract, the infundibulum, below the pulmonary valve. The pumping of the blood into the great arteries is intermittent; the distensibility of the arterial walls helps smooth out the blood flow, with energy stored in the proximal great vessels during systole being recovered during diastole (the "windkessel" effect). The ventricles must refill between systolic contractions. The blood that accumulates in the atria during systole, as well as additional return during diastole, can be passed across the AV valves into the ventricle during diastole. Active contraction of the atrium at the start of the next cardiac cycle helps further charge the ventricle for the next ventricular contraction.

The ventricles and much of the atria are invested by the pericardium. This is a double-layered fibrous sac that is flexible but not stretchy. The inner ("visceral") layer is effectively part of the epicardial aspect of the heart, whereas the outer ("parietal") layer fits closely around it with a potential space between them. Normally, the layers are separated only by a thin film of fluid; this serves to lubricate them so that they can slide freely over each other. The pericardium is, in turn, surrounded by the intrathoracic cavity, which is normally at subatmospheric pressure; this may help with venous return to the right side of the heart.

▶ BASIC CONTINUUM MECHANICS REVIEW

Blood and cardiac tissue are both continuous materials, subject to mechanical forces. Although blood is a fluid and tissue is a solid, they have some mechanical aspects in common. Although they are actually composed of discrete cells and subcellular components, it is convenient for our purposes to consider them as if they were a smooth, locally homogeneous material, or a "continuum." We will first consider some of the basic underlying aspects of continuum mechanics, and then some more specific aspects of solid and fluid mechanics relevant to the heart. There are many texts on continuum mechanics,[3] but the series of books by Y.C. Fung is particularly focused on biomedical applications.[4] Glass et al[5] also provide an overview of the continuum mechanics of the heart. We will use some mathematical notation to express the mechanical relations, but will seek to provide more intuitive qualitative explanations as well.

Any mechanical system, including the heart and the blood within it, is subject to forces that determine its motion and change of configuration. Contraction of the heart, initiated by activation of the contractile elements within the muscle cells, results in generation of active forces along the direction of these contractile elements. The magnitude of the force generated will depend on factors such as the length of the muscle at the initiation of the contraction, as described elsewhere in this book. The distributed active forces within the heart wall, in turn, result in deformation of the heart wall and an increase in pressure of the blood within the ventricles. The deformation will result in the development of passive forces (due to stretching or compression of the muscle cells and associated connective tissue elements) within the wall that oppose the active contraction; the pressure rise in the blood within the chamber will exert an outward force on the wall that will also tend to oppose the contraction. The pressurized intracavitary blood will tend to flow toward any lower pressure regions with which it is connected, normally toward the peripheral circulation, but also across any abnormal interventricular connections or across any incompetent valves that may be present. The rate of this flow will be determined by a combination of the pressure difference driving it and the resistance to the flow. The net combination of the forces within the heart wall and blood determines the temporal evolution of the cardiac shape and the amount of blood ejected from the heart during systole; the energy added to the system during systole and the tissue properties of the cardiovascular system determine the time course of the cardiac shape and the ventricular filling during diastole.

At a discrete point within the heart, at a given time, there will be a net vector of force, acting to accelerate the material at the point in a corresponding direction. However, when we consider a small region of material around the point, there will be a net distribution of forces acting on the region and tending to deform it, which we call stress. The stress can be defined as the force acting on a surface, divided by the area of the surface. Stresses acting perpendicular to the surface are called normal stresses, whereas stresses acting tangentially to the surface are shear stresses. Stress is characterized by a higher order quantity than a vector, the stress tensor. At a given location in the heart wall at a given time, forces may be acting to stretch the myocardium in one direction, for example, radially, while simultaneously acting to compress the tissue in another direction, for example, circumferentially. The corresponding resulting deformation of the material is called strain, and is also characterized by a tensor quantity. Again, at a given location, the tissue may have undergone stretching in one direction, relative to a reference state such as end diastole, whereas at the same time it may have undergone compression in another direction. At each location, there will be a direction in which the shortening is greatest and an orthogonal direction in which the lengthening is greatest. The strains along these directions (and the remaining orthogonal direction) are the principal strains. In general, the angle between two material line elements within the tissue will change due to the deformation of the material, reflecting local shear. However, line elements along the principal directions will remain mutually perpendicular during the motion. The principal strains provide a reference system-independent way to describe the deformation. A general motion of a given portion of the wall can be described as a combination of rigid body motion (displacement and rotation) and deformation (strain) (Figure 49-1).

It can be useful for some purposes to approximate the heart wall as a thin curved membrane surrounding the pressurized blood. In this case, the relationship between the pressure difference across the wall and the tension in the wall that contains this pressure is given by the LaPlace law. The LaPlace law states that force balance across a curved membrane means that the wall tensions needed to balance the pressure difference across the membrane at a given location depend on the principal curvatures of the membrane:

$$\Delta P = \frac{T_1}{r_1} + \frac{T_2}{r_2} \tag{1}$$

where r_1 and r_2 are the greatest and least (principal) radii of curvature of the membrane and T_1 and T_2 are the tensions in the membrane along the corresponding directions. Specifically, the higher the pressure difference, the greater the tension must be (which is intuitively obvious), whereas the smaller the radius of curvature, the lower the tension needs to be (which is not quite as intuitively obvious). For a cylinder at a given pressure difference, the tension will be proportional to the radius of curvature, whereas for a more general shape, approximated locally by an ellipsoid, the mean tension will be proportional to the reciprocal of the sum of the reciprocals of the principal radii of curvature. This relationship will be modified for a thick wall composed of tissue with anisotropic material properties, but the qualitative features will still hold. Another modifying factor is the presence of residual forces in the heart wall even in the absence of external loading of the heart.[7] These residual stresses have the effect of helping restore the heart to its expanded state during diastole, and may help equalize stresses across the heart wall.

We can consider motion of a continuous material from two conventional points of view, commonly called the Lagrangian and Eulerian reference frames. In the Lagrangian approach, we follow the motion of individual material points, for example, relative to a reference configuration such as at end diastole. The Lagrangian approach is particularly useful for describing the deformation of solid materials, like the muscle of the heart wall. The Eulerian approach considers the motion of material passing through fixed locations in space. The Eulerian approach is particularly useful for describing the flow of fluids, such as the distribution of the velocity of the blood within the ventricular chambers. We can transform the description of motion from one reference frame to the other.

The stiffness of the heart wall is generally a complex quantity, best described by a matrix rather than a simple scalar quantity (like the stiffness of a simple spring). In addition to directional nonuniformity, or anisotropy, that is, different degrees of stiffness in different directions, the material of the heart wall demonstrates significant nonlinearity, that is, the forces tending to oppose deformation of the heart wall are not simply proportional to the deformation, but can increase dramatically with increasing deformation. The tissue properties of the heart wall also reflect viscoelastic material properties. For example, after a sustained stretch (as with prolonged dilatation), a viscoelastic material tends to not fully recover to its initial configuration, even when the forces that maintained the stretch are removed, a phenomenon called "stress relaxation."

Force generation in the myocardium is produced by the active contraction of the myocytes, reflecting the interaction of the contractile proteins initiated by excitation. Although the force is only directly generated along the length of the cells, reflecting the local alignment of the contractile proteins along the cell axis, the mechanical coupling between the cells via the collagen and other connective tissue elements in the extracellular matrix results in transmission of the forces across the wall. As the tissue deforms under the influence of the active forces, the resulting deformation produces passive forces that tend to oppose the deformation. The compression of the blood within the cardiac chambers by the contracting heart wall produces a rise in pressure that pushes outward, tending to locally expand the wall. There are also residual forces within the heart wall that tend to restore it to its end-diastolic configuration. The residual stresses within the heart wall can be demonstrated by the tendency of the heart wall to spring open when it is incised. The heart also tends to return to its expanded configuration even in the absence of pressurized blood within it. The magnitude of these forces and their origin and significance, reflecting the residual stresses, are still the subject of ongoing investigation. The net result is that the local forces within the wall reflect a combination of these active and passive forces. Thus, there is generally greatest systolic shortening along the local direction of the fibers within the heart wall, which are aligned in oppositely oriented oblique directions in the subepicardium and subendocardium, but there is also a significant component of cross-fiber shortening during systole in the subendocardium. The degree to which this reflects the geometry of the fiber and sheet organization of the heart wall is also the subject of ongoing investigation.

Fluid flow reflects the response of the material of a fluid (such as blood) to the forces acting on it. These include forces acting along pressure gradients (so that fluid tends to

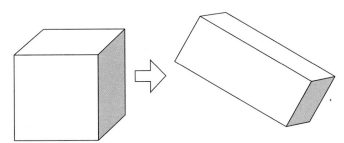

Figure 49–1 A general motion of a portion of the heart wall can be considered as a combination of rigid body motion (translation and rotation) and deformation (here, side-to-side stretching combined with top-to-bottom shortening).

784 flow from regions of higher pressure to regions of lower pressure) and internal forces due to the viscosity of the fluid in the presence of shears or gradients in velocity (the viscous forces act to oppose and reduce such shears), as well as external forces such as gravity. Because the fluid is continuous and its material is conserved, that is, it is neither created nor destroyed in the circulating system, in regions where the area available to the fluid to flow is increased or decreased, the velocity of the flow in those regions must correspondingly decrease or increase inversely proportionally to the area of the flow, so that the volume rate of the flow is preserved. For incompressible material, such as the blood in the lumen of blood vessels or the ventricular cavity, the continuity equation can be expressed as

$$\nabla \cdot \mathbf{v} = 0 \qquad (2)$$

where $\mathbf{v}$ is the velocity vector. Within the wall of the ventricle, the entry or exit of blood into or from the heart wall during the cardiac cycle will be reflected in a corresponding change in the local volume of the wall. The motion of the blood will be determined by a combination of the external (e.g., gravity) and internal (e.g., pressure and viscosity) forces acting on it. This is expressed as the Navier–Stokes equation. There is no slip of the blood relative to the surface of the endocardium (or any other such fluid–solid interface) right at the contact between the blood and the wall. The resulting velocity shear within the fluid between the more freely moving blood near the middle and the stationary blood right at the edge of the lumen results in a frictional drag due to the viscosity of the blood; this contributes to the resistance to flow that the ventricle must overcome in order to pump the blood through the circulation. This no-slip condition provides a boundary condition for the Navier–Stokes equation.

The conservation of energy in the flowing fluid means that the change in kinetic energy reflected in the changes in velocity predicted by the continuity equation can come about only by acceleration along pressure gradients. This is expressed as the Bernoulli equation, which can be written in simplified form for steady flow of an incompressible fluid, neglecting viscosity and gravitational forces, as

$$p_1 - p_2 = \frac{1}{2} \rho \left(\mathbf{v}_1^{\,2} - \mathbf{v}_2^{\,2} \right) \qquad (3)$$

where p_i and $\mathbf{v}_i$ are the pressure and velocity, respectively, at two locations along a streamline in the fluid, and ρ is the density of the fluid. We can see that as the velocity increases, the pressure decreases. This can be used to estimate the pressure gradient across a short stenotic region (or across an incompetent valve) from the corresponding increased velocity of the jet, through the approximate "modified Bernoulli formula,"

$$p = 4\,\mathbf{v}^2 \qquad (4)$$

where $\mathbf{v}$ is the magnitude of the peak velocity in the jet in m/s and p is the pressure drop in mm Hg.

The tendency of the flow of fluid to break up into swirls or turbulence through its momentum will be opposed by the tendency of the viscosity of the fluid to dampen out such motions, especially in combination with the no-slip condition

at the walls. The relative magnitudes of these opposing tendencies can be expressed through the Reynolds number, R,

$$R = \frac{VL\rho}{\mu} = \frac{VL}{\nu} \qquad (5)$$

where V is a characteristic velocity of the flow, L is a characteristic length of the region in which it is flowing, ρ is the density, and μ is the coefficient of viscosity; ν is the "kinematic viscosity," μ/ρ. For example, for flow in a blood vessel, V could be the average velocity and D could be the diameter of the vessel. For steady flow in long straight tubes, the transition to turbulence takes place for Reynolds numbers on the order of or above 2000. For pulsatile flow, we can also consider the Womersley number, α,

$$\alpha = L \sqrt{\frac{\omega}{\nu}} \qquad (6)$$

where ω is the characteristic frequency of the pulsation. The Reynolds number expresses the ratio of the convective flow inertia to the shear force, whereas the Womersley number expresses the ratio of the oscillatory inertia force to the shear force. A large Reynolds number or Womersley number implies a dominant convective or oscillatory flow inertia force, respectively, while a small number implies a dominant viscous shear force.

CARDIAC CYCLE

The cardiac cycle is schematically illustrated in Figure 49-2. As indicated above, the cardiac cycle is normally initiated by spontaneous depolarization of the sinoatrial (SA) node. This initiates contraction of the atria, resulting in a rise in atrial pressure (and a voltage spike, the P wave, in the ECG). This, in turn, causes increased forward flow of blood across the AV valves from the atria into the ventricles. The delay in the conduction of the electrical excitation due to passage through the AV node allows the ventricles to fill a bit more from the atrial contraction as well, before the ventricles contract. The excitation of the ventricles results in a bigger set of voltage spikes, the QRS complex, in the ECG. The resulting rise in intraventricular pressure causes the AV valves to close (associated with the "first heart sound" audible with a stethoscope, S1). At this point, both the AV and semilunar valves are closed, and the heart is in the "isovolumic contraction" phase of the cardiac cycle. The pressure continues to rise in the ventricle because of the contraction of the wall; the semilunar valves will open when the intraventricular pressure exceeds the pressure on the other side, in the great arteries. At this point, blood starts to flow out into the great arteries, raising the pressure in the arteries. The ejection phase of systole will continue until the myocytes repolarize and start to relax. This is associated with the T wave in the ECG. As the myocytes relax, the pressure drops in the ventricle. As the intraventricular pressure falls below the pressure in the great arteries, the semilunar valves close (associated with the "second heart sound" audible with a stethoscope, S2). At this point, both the AV and semilunar valves are closed, and the heart is in the "isovolumic relaxation" phase of the cardiac cycle. As the intraventricular pressure continues to fall, it drops below the pressure in the atria and the AV valves open, again permitting flow of blood

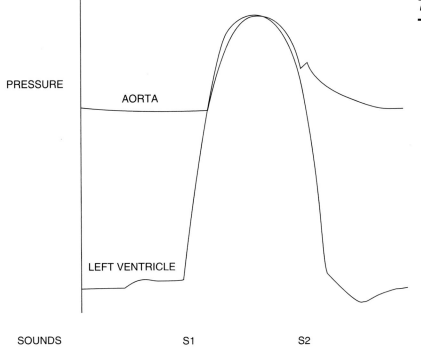

Figure 49–2 Schematic diagram of the cardiac cycle. The time course of pressure in the pulmonary artery and right ventricle is similar to that in the aorta and left ventricle, but at a smaller scale.
(Adapted from Hurst JW, Logue RB: The Heart, 2nd ed. New York: McGraw-Hill, 1970, p. 76.)

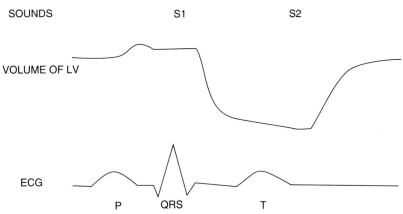

across the AV valves from the atria into the ventricles. There is rapid ventricular filling in the early phase of diastole, but it slows down as the ventricle fills, until another cardiac cycle starts at the end of diastole, as described above.

Activation of the ventricle is synchronized through rapid propagation of the activating wave of depolarization through the specialized conduction system of the ventricle. The timing of the initiation of ventricular contraction is delayed relative to that of the aria because of slower passage of the wave of depolarization through the AV node (giving the atrial contraction some time to contribute to ventricular filling). However, the internal delays within the ventricle are normally much shorter, so that the ventricular myocardium effectively all contracts together.

Force generation within the myocardium is initiated by the electrical depolarization of the cell membrane. Unlike skeletal muscle, which must be depolarized by an impulse from a nerve, cardiac muscle cells are normally depolarized by an exciting impulse from the cardiac conduction system (derived from specialized myocytes, although nerve-like in their action), by depolarization of an adjacent muscle cell with which it is in intimate contact, or even spontaneously, if

no external stimulus arrives. This depolarization results in release of intracellular calcium into the cytosol, from internal stores in the sarcoplasmic reticulum. The resulting increase in cytosolic calcium concentration initiates the interaction of the contractile proteins, actin and myosin, which generates force acting along their length. The many parallel bundles of these contractile protein units lined up within the length of the myocyte thus produce a force tending to shorten the myocyte. This force is transferred to the rest of the myocyte through internal connections to the cytoskeleton and then to the rest of the myocardial tissue through connections of the myocytes to the ECM.

The magnitude of the force generated by the myocytes is dependent on their initial length at the time of initiation of the contraction, as described by the Frank–Starling law. This provides a feedback mechanism to help regulate the output of the heart according to the needs of the rest of the circulatory system. For example, if the ventricle empties insufficiently in one cycle, it will be relatively more stretched at the initiation of the next beat, and will contract more vigorously, thus tending to return to the normal operating state.

786

The active contraction of the ventricle results in compression of the blood within the ventricular chamber. This, in turn, raises the pressure of the blood within the chamber (without significantly changing its volume). When the pressure in the chamber exceeds that in the great vessels, the semilunar valves open and the pressurized blood flows down the pressure gradient into the lower pressure arterial and more distal portions of the circulation. The rate of the resulting flow depends on the resistance presented by the circulation. The resistance to flow out of the ventricle is collectively determined by the whole of the branching vessels in the circulation. The resistance of each tubular segment of the circulation depends on its length and diameter; these add together in series and parallel much like electrical resistances. Normally, much of the total resistance comes from the small arterioles just upstream from the capillaries of the microcirculation. The tension in the wall (and thus the diameter and corresponding resistance) of these vessels can be regulated, for example, in response to local metabolic needs, providing another mechanism for adjusting cardiac output.

The flow into the microcirculation of most organs is greatest during systole, or whenever the local arterial pressure (and thus driving force for the blood) is highest. However, the myocardium is in the unique situation of having elevated pressure surrounding the tissue capillaries during myocardial contraction, thus decreasing the net driving force for forward arterial blood flow during systole (although augmenting venous drainage from the tissue). Thus, most blood flow into the myocardium takes place during diastole, when the interstitial pressure drops within the heart wall. The perfusion of the myocardium is thus particularly dependent on the smoothing of the diastolic time course of the blood pressure provided by the windkessel effect of the elastic aorta (and thus may be adversely affected by the stiffening of the aorta associated with aging, which can result in a more rapid drop in arterial pressure during diastole).

There are four principal filling mechanisms that have traditionally been proposed to explain the refilling of the ventricle during diastole. First, there will be some elastic recoil of the myocardium back toward its original shape, before it was deformed by the active forces of contraction. These passive forces tending to reexpand the wall of the ventricle will help draw blood into the chamber across the AV valve. Second, the pressure wave created by prior ventricular contraction will be propagated across the circulation to the atrial blood and will help push the blood across into the now relaxed ventricle. Third, the increased blood flowing into the heart wall during diastole may contribute an erectile effect to the wall, augmenting the tendency of the heart wall to return to its expanded end-diastolic configuration. Finally, as mentioned above, the atrial contraction near the end of ventricular diastole helps the final filling of the ventricle before the next ventricular contraction. The ability of the heart wall to relax during diastole, so as to permit proper filling, is an important aspect of the cardiac cycle. Abnormal stiffness leading to diastolic dysfunction can result in cardiac failure, even in the absence of abnormality in the heart's ability to contract.

The performance of the heart as a pump will depend not only on its intrinsic ability to generate force to pressurize the blood ("contractility") but also on the resistance into which it is pumping ("afterload") and the amount of blood with which it is charged at the start of the cycle ("preload"). The interpretation of the state of myocardial contractility from functional measures must thus also assess the loading conditions. The greater the afterload (resistance to flow), the lower the cardiac output will be, other things being held constant. Such an increase in afterload could be dynamic, (e.g., due to increased arteriolar tone), or fixed (e.g., due to pulmonary embolization). The effect of preload is manifested through the Frank–Starling mechanism, with the myocardial contractile force depending on the degree of initial stretch of the myocardium. As a relatively load-independent measure of contractility, it has been proposed to use the slope of the line relating end-systolic pressure and volume. However, these data are not readily obtained in human subjects.

Although it is frequently convenient to consider the function of the LV and RV separately, there can be significant interaction between them. In addition to the common wall shared by the LV and the RV, the interventricular septum, their circulations are connected in series. Thus, elevations in pressure in the RV can have an impact on the ability of the LV to contract, because of increased stiffening of the septum, and elevated pulmonary venous pressures backing up before a failing LV can present an increased load to the RV. Respiratory effects are another way in which the LV and RV may indirectly interact. With inspiration, the intrathoracic pressure drops, augmenting the return to the right side of the heart from the systemic veins. On the other hand, the return to the left side of the heart through the pulmonary veins will be diminished. In expiration, the reverse will hold. Although this is normally a small effect, in pathological states such as pericardial diseases these effects may be more pronounced. The pericardium invests the ventricles in a sac that is flexible but is very resistant to stretching on short time scales, so that increased filling of one side of the heart tends to come at the expense of the filling of the other side. Thus these respiratory effects are exaggerated ("pulsus paradoxus") in conditions such as cardiac tamponade that further interfere with cardiac filling.

When there is an acute need for increased cardiac output, as with exercise, this is in large part supplied by increasing the heart rate. In tachycardia, it is primarily the diastolic phase of the cardiac cycle that is shortened, with the duration of systole relatively less affected. Although this is normally well tolerated, extreme elevations of the heart rate will not permit adequate filling of the ventricle and thus will have a negative effect on cardiac output.

Physical conditioning, as in athletes participating in endurance sports such as long distance running or rowing, can result in several adaptations in the athlete, including an increase in cardiac size and a decrease in resting heart rate, with the ability to increase their heart rate over a much larger range than unconditioned subjects.

There are many feedback and regulatory mechanisms that serve to keep the mechanics of the heart in balance with the body's needs. Feedback control is an important aspect of the design of many human-engineered systems. Typically, some aspect of the system or its output is monitored; if the monitored value drifts away from the desired range a signal is sent to the system to adjust it so that it returns back toward the desired state. The heart is similarly subject to such regulation over several time scales and by several different mechanisms.

Humoral (hormonal) influences can work over different time scales to adjust cardiac output to meet the body's needs. Epinephrine is released into the circulation as part of the body's "fight or flight" acute reaction to danger or other stress. Epinephrine acts on the SA node to increase the heart rate; it also acts on the myocytes to increase their contractility. Both effects serve to increase cardiac output. Epinephrine also affects the arteriolar tone in various organs differently, acting to redistribute the relative blood flow to the organs through their relative peripheral resistances. The heart itself acts as an endocrine organ to help regulate cardiac function over a longer time scale, for example, through the release of atrial natriuretic peptide in response to stretch of the atrial wall related to failure. Atrial natriuretic peptide is a hormone that affects the handling of water and electrolytes so as to help maintain the intravascular volume. Steroid hormones also affect the regulation of intravascular volume, and thus blood pressure. Hormonal changes in pregnancy also affect the circulation (e.g., leading to an increase in the circulating volume), and thus cardiovascular mechanics. The nervous system also influences cardiac function. Activation of the sympathetic nervous system effectively results in the release of epinephrine directly at the SA node, increasing the heart rate. Release of acetylcholine from the parasympathetic nervous system has the opposite effect, slowing the heart rate.

Changes in the resistance of the peripheral circulation (afterload) will have corresponding reciprocal changes in cardiac output, in the absence of any other compensatory changes. Thus, increased resistance (e.g., due to increased arteriolar tone or pulmonary embolization) would result in decreased cardiac output, whereas decreased resistance (e.g., in gram-negative sepsis) would result in increased cardiac output. In general, other compensating mechanisms, such as changes in heart rate or blood pressure, would moderate the effects of such altered resistance. On the other hand, variations in resistance are one of the compensatory mechanisms the body can employ when needed to maintain a steady cardiac output or to adjust it to meet the body's needs. Changes in the circulating volume or the venous return to the heart will alter the end-diastolic volume of the heart (preload) and thus the contractile state of the heart. This will, in turn, alter cardiac output in a similar manner. Handling of water and electrolytes by the kidney plays a major role in the regulation of the circulating blood volume. Thus, it can be used to compensate for changes in cardiac output on time scales of hours to days.

Alterations in the contractile state of the heart through neurohumoral mechanisms can be used to help adjust cardiac output to meet demand, such as with exercise, as described above. On the other hand, loss of normal contractility can result in systolic heart failure if other compensatory mechanisms are inadequate.

Pregnancy and delivery can lead to dramatic changes in circulating volume as well as peripheral resistance. Although normally well suited for the needs of gestation and labor, these increased demands on the heart can lead to decompensation in patients with decreased ability to adjust to them, such as with mitral stenosis.

▶ FUNCTION MEASURES

The function of the heart can be characterized globally or locally. Global measures of cardiac function are the most familiar and widely used, and their use has had the largest scale clinical trials. Global function measures primarily include measures relating to the volume of the ventricular chamber, although other global function measures can also be useful.

Values of the ventricular chamber volumes at different phases of the cardiac cycle can be used to assess global cardiac function. The difference between the volume at end diastole (ED) and end systole (ES) is the stroke volume (SV); the ratio of the SV to the ED volume is the ejection fraction (EF):

$$EF = (ED - ES) / ES \qquad (7)$$

The stroke volume multiplied by the heart rate (HR) gives the cardiac output (CO):

$$CO = (SV)(HR) \qquad (8)$$

To account for the differences to be expected in the values of the cardiac output for different sized subjects, we can use the cardiac index (CI), which scales the cardiac output for body surface area (BSA):

$$CI = CO / BSA \qquad (9)$$

The rates of change in ventricular volume can also provide useful measures of cardiac function. In particular, the rates of early ejection from and early filling of the ventricle can be used as measures of the contractility and stiffness of the ventricle, respectively, although they will also depend on other factors.

Pressures in the blood are dependent on the contractile force generated by the heart wall. Although blood pressure is normally closely regulated, changes in the contractile state of the heart will be reflected in the pressure. Thus, an inability to generate sufficient arterial pressure is a sign of cardiac decompensation. The filling pressures upstream of the ventricles (e.g., central venous pressure for the RV and capillary wedge pressure for the LV) provide a measure of the preload; as the heart fails, these pressures will rise as part of the compensatory mechanisms used to help maintain normal cardiac output.

Peripheral resistance is very important in the regulation of blood flow, both global and regional. However, it cannot be readily measured directly. Rather, we infer it from the ratio of blood flow and blood pressure. It can be expressed in standardized units, such as Wood units, but these are not commonly used clinically.

Myocardial mass is another measure of the mechanical state of the heart. It can be calculated from the volume of the ventricular walls (which can be measured from tomographic images), multiplied by an assumed value for the density of myocardium, such as 1.05 g/cm³. Myocardial mass will be increased in either concentric (primarily thickening) or eccentric (primarily dilation) hypertrophy. Note that it can also be increased in infiltrative disease of the heart wall, which, however, does not contribute working muscle to the mass.

788

Measurement methods for these global functional measures include noninvasive imaging and invasive catheter-based approaches. Projection imaging of the ventricular cavity can be used to calculate its volume and the related measures described above. Projection nuclear imaging with radioisotope-labeled red cells can be used to calculate the ejection fraction by measuring the integrated radioactivity in the image of the ventricle, and then finding the ratio of the difference in end-diastolic and end-systolic activity to the end-diastolic value (correcting for background activity); however, the absolute values of the respective volumes cannot be found with this technique. Projection images of the ventricular cavities obtained by contrast injection during cardiac catheterization can be used to estimate corresponding ventricular volumes by assuming the form of the geometric relations between the two-dimensional (2D) projection and the underlying three-dimensional (3D) shape, although these formulas may be unreliable in the presence of disease.

Tomographic imaging methods can be more reliable for the measurement of ventricular volumes, as there may be no need to make any assumptions about the ventricular geometry. The tomographic imaging method most widely used for studying the heart is echocardiography. Although this does provide good quality tomographic images of the heart wall, the lack of spatial registration between images obtained with conventional echocardiography limits the reliability of volume estimates. An additional kind of data that can be obtained with echocardiography is the measurement of flow velocities (or at least the component of velocity along the line of the ultrasound beam), through the Doppler effect. This can be used to estimate corresponding pressure gradients in jets across valves or other obstructions using the modified Bernoulli formula. Tomographic radionuclide imaging with single-photon emission computed tomography (SPECT) or positron emission tomography (PET) can provide spatially registered image data that can be used to calculate absolute volumes, but the relatively low resolution of such imaging lessens its value. Magnetic resonance imaging (MRI) with cardiac synchronization of the imaging can provide high-quality spatially registered images that can be used to calculate volumes; this is the current "gold standard" method for cardiac global function volume measurements. X-ray computed tomography (CT) has made recent advances in imaging quality and speed, and can also provide global function volume measures, although it is still poorer in temporal resolution than MRI and has the additional disadvantages of involving radiation exposure and the use of potentially harmful contrast agents.

Invasive catheter-based methods for assessing cardiac function include the use of pressure-measuring catheters to directly measure pressures in the cardiac chambers and across obstructing lesions, and they are commonly used in the cardiac catheterization laboratory. Catheters with ultrasound transducers at their tips can be used to measure local blood flow velocities through the Doppler effect. Thermodilution catheters can be used to directly measure cardiac output, and they are commonly used in intensive care settings. Conductance catheters provide a different invasive method for monitoring cardiac output, but are more suitable for research purposes.

Regional measures of cardiac function can also be obtained from imaging. Projection imaging gives information only about the motion of the portion of the wall at the edge of the heart in the particular projection used to make the image. Tomographic imaging provides wall motion information all around the heart, although it will be less reliable where the plane of the image intersects the wall obliquely (e.g., near the apex or base of the heart in short-axis imaging). Although imaging of the ventricular cavity provides information only about the motion of the endocardial surface of the wall, tomographic imaging provides images of both endocardial and epicardial surfaces, permitting measurement of wall thickening. A limitation of both approaches is the uncertainty of how to account for the contribution of the motion of the heart as a whole to the local wall motion. The motion in the imaging plane may be approximately compensated for by subtracting the motion of the centroid of the ventricle, but the through-plane motion of the curved heart wall can still lead to apparent changes in wall motion or thickening that are just reflections of the changing location of the intersection of the heart with the spatially fixed imaging plane.

The lack of recognizable features that can be tracked within the heart wall means that conventional imaging is limited to assessing the radial component of the heart wall motion, and that only at the surfaces of the wall. Using invasive techniques, we can imbed material markers within the wall, such as small metal beads or ultrasound crystals, whose position can be tracked as the heart moves. However, in addition to the invasive nature of these procedures, which pose some risk and can alter the local motion of the wall, only a limited number of such markers can be tracked in the heart of a given subject, limiting the sampling density of tracked points within the wall.

Echocardiography can provide some information on intramural motion through the use of the Doppler effect to track the velocity (or the component of velocity along the line of the ultrasound beam) of the tissue of the wall. The gradient of the velocity gives the rate of tissue deformation or one-dimensional (1D) component of the strain rate along the ultrasound beam. It would be necessary to integrate this over time to estimate the total deformation over the cardiac cycle. In addition to the limited spatial component information available from the Doppler effect, there is still the uncertainty of how to account for the through-plane motion.

MRI has several advantages as a method for noninvasive assessment of within-wall cardiac motion, including the potential to recover the full 3D motion pattern within the heart wall. There are two approaches that have been used to study intramural motion with MRI, magnetization tagging and phase shifts. Magnetization tagging uses the ability of modified MR imaging techniques to noninvasively create localized perturbations of the tissue magnetization, e.g., with spatial modulation of magnetization (SPAMM),[9] to noninvasively produce MR-visible landmarks within the heart wall. These will persist for times on the order of the tissue T1 relaxation times, so that they can be tracked over the cardiac cycle; we can produce a new set of such tags at a consistent phase of each cardiac cycle. The tags provide a direct marker for the displacement of the underlying tissue in the image plane, as they move exactly the same way. For tags created as sheets of altered magnetization initially perpendicular to the image plane, the intersection of these sheets with the image plane will look like dark lines in the images of the heart wall; motion of these lines shows the local 1D component of the motion perpendicular to the originally tagged plane, even in the presence of through-plane motion. Phase shift approaches to studying the intra-mural motion use the phase shift of the received signal that can be produced by motion along modified magnetic field gradients used in MRI. The phase shift is typically dependent on the motion between two times, effectively giving a measure of the velocity if those times are close together, or a measure of the interval displacement if they are further apart. In using the velocity mode, the results must be integrated to find the net displacement, whereas in the interval displacement mode, the results for different intervals must still be combined to find the full motion over the cardiac cycle. In either case, additional reference images must also be obtained to correct for other (nonmotion) possible sources of phase shifts.

From a suitable set of data on the regional motion within the heart wall, derived from either multiplanar tagged MRI or phase-shift MRI sensitized to motion in multiple directions, we can reconstruct the full 3D motion of the heart wall. This will generally require some sort of interpolation to fill in the gaps in the image-derived data, because of the finite density of spatial sampling of the motion in the images. Finite element methods provide one way to carry out this 3D motion reconstruction.

Given 2D or 3D data on the motion of (and within) the heart wall, there are several ways we can quantitatively characterize the motion. The material-point correspondence data provided by tagged MRI permit us to map the serial displacements of each point within the wall; this can be considered as a set of vectors over time linking corresponding locations of each material point (a "Lagrangian" representation of the motion). The velocity data provided by phase-shift MRI could be used to follow the serial evolution of velocity vectors at each spatial location in the images (an "Eulerian" representation of the motion). The velocities must be integrated over time to recover the displacements, a process that is subject to cumulative error because of the integration of noise or other errors in the measurements.

Although the displacement and velocity are useful to describe the motion of material points, we are also interested in characterizing the motion of the material neighborhood around each such point. In addition to the "rigid body" components of the motion, its average displacement and rotation, we can characterize its deformation (or strain). Strain is defined as the fractional change in length, due to the motion, of a material line segment initially oriented along a given direction in the tissue. Strain is a more complex quantity than the displacement and cannot be adequately described by a vector, but rather must be described with a tensor. For example, at a given location in the wall, the tissue may be lengthening in the radial direction while at the same time it is shortening in the circumferential and longitudinal directions. The local radial, circumferential and longitudinal strains provide a useful intuitive way to characterize the deformation. Another potential choice of strains would be along and perpendicular to the local muscle fiber orientation within the wall. In general, for a given set of initial orientations of material line segments in the tissue, the angle between the segments will also change due to the motion ("shear"); the shears between each pair of initial

directions will also be needed to fully characterize the deformation. For example, the shear between the longitudinal and circumferential directions is a measure of the local torsion of the heart wall around the long axis of the ventricle. However, there will always be a set of three mutually orthogonal initial directions in the tissue at each location that will remain orthogonal after the motion, the "eigenvectors" or principal directions of the deformation. One of these directions will lie along the direction of the greatest lengthening and another will lie along the direction of the smallest lengthening or greatest shortening; the strains along these directions of the eigenvectors are called the principal strains. The principal strains and their directions provide a description of the deformation that is independent of the choice of reference frame.

It would be of interest to know what forces (stresses) within the heart wall are associated with the observed deformation. These also need to be described with tensors. However, these forces cannot be directly measured, even in an experimental setting, due to the inevitable perturbation of the state of the wall by the invasive nature of the process of mechanically coupling to the wall in an attempt to measure the stress within the wall. Alternatively, we can try to estimate the force within the wall by theoretical models. The simplest approach considers the wall as a curved membrane and uses the force balance implied by the LaPlace law to estimate the total force within the wall through the local curvature and the pressure difference across the wall. Assuming the force to be uniformly distributed across the wall, we can calculate the corresponding stress of force per unit area perpendicular to each direction considered. More sophisticated formulas try to take the finite thickness of the wall into explicit account. However, such approximations generally neglect the anisotropy of the material properties of the heart wall. In addition, they generally neglect the presence of significant residual stresses in the wall even in the absence of pressure differences (the unloaded state), as manifested experimentally by the springing open of an incision into the heart wall even in the absence of contraction or pressurized blood within the chamber.[7] Computer modeling with the finite element approach can potentially include such effects, but it is still subject to the uncertainty of what values to use for the mechanical properties of the material of the heart wall.

MECHANICAL EFFECTS OF DISEASE

There are many diseases that can affect the function of the heart.[2] However, the presence of pathological conditions potentially affecting the function of the heart does not necessarily lead to symptomatic disease. There are many potential compensatory mechanisms that can be activated to overcome the deleterious effects of such conditions, at least in part. It is when the capacities of these mechanisms are exceeded or when increased demands exceed their reserve that the alterations in function become clinically manifest. Thus, although the symptoms may appear relatively quickly, the disease may have been present for some time, but adequately compensated for until the compensatory mechanisms were exceeded. Similarly, it may be clinically sufficient if a therapeutic intervention can get the effects of the disease into a range that the body's compensatory mechanisms can manage, even if the underlying condition is not fully corrected.

In addition to the neurohumoral compensatory mechanisms described above, chronically increased hemodynamic load can lead to cardiac hypertrophy. Hypertrophy can take two forms, a "concentric" thickening of the ventricular wall in response to an increased pressure demand (afterload) (e.g., due to obstruction to aortic outflow at or near the aortic valve or to chronically elevated arterial pressure) or an "eccentric" dilation of the cardiac chamber in response to an increased volume to be pumped (e.g., due to valvular insufficiency or a septal defect). In both cases, in the mature heart there is an increase in the size (diameter or length) of the myocytes, but not their number. The concentrically hypertrophied heart can generate greater pressure because of the greater number of contractile elements per cell; the force per unit thickness of wall can still be similar to the normal heart. However, the associated fibrosis that may be present in the wall can lead to increased stiffness and slower diastolic filling. There can also be an increased distance for oxygen and nutrients to diffuse from the capillaries into the center of the hypertrophied myocytes, potentially placing them at greater risk of ischemia. In eccentric hypertrophy, the increased ventricular diameter means that the myocytes must generate increased tension in the wall even for the same pressure in the blood, as predicted by the LaPlace law. This increased demand on the myocytes can lead to progressive dysfunction if it is not compensated for. This has led to interest in the development of surgical approaches to effectively decrease the diameter of the heart in intractable failure.

Ischemia and infarction of the myocardium due to atherosclerotic vascular disease are major public health problems in the Western world, and increasingly elsewhere as well. Ischemia (inadequate blood supply to meet the metabolic needs of the tissue) leads to impairment or loss of the ability of the affected muscle to contract. This may be transient or reversible, as in stunning or hibernation. Sustained ischemia can lead to infarction, with irreversible loss of contractile function. Acute infarction is characterized by necrosis of the myocytes; chronic infarction is characterized by healing with fibrous replacement or scarring of the affected portion of the wall. The loss of contractile function due to ischemia or infarction of the heart wall is manifested by reduced or absent active motion of the wall, or even by dyskinetic motion with thinning or bulging of the affected wall during systole. In the extreme, the affected portion of the wall may become aneurysmally dilated, effectively acting as "dead space" in the ventricle. The potentially normal tissue adjacent to the infarct may also show reduced motion, presumably due to mechanical "tethering" by the infarct. The more remote normal myocardium may undergo some degree of hypertrophy to compensate for the loss of function in the infarcted portion of the wall. However, in some cases there may be a progressive dilatation of the heart wall, leading to failure, a deleterious "remodeling."

There can be significant interaction between the LV and RV because of the common wall they share, the interventricular septum, and their circulations that are connected in series. Thus, for example, in right ventricular hypertension due to pulmonary hypertension there is flattening or even reverse bowing of the septum during systole (it is normally convex to the right side); the increased stiffness of the interventricular septum may also affect the motion of the remainder of the LV.

Valve disease can lead to two different types of increased hemodynamic load on the ventricles: valvular stenosis increases the resistance to flow through the valve, tending to lead to concentric hypertrophy in the case of stenosis of the semilunar valves, whereas valvular insufficiency increases the volume to be pumped, tending to lead to eccentric hypertrophy. A valve can be both stenotic and insufficient, leading to mixed effects. The turbulence associated with the flow through abnormal valves also contributes another source of energy dissipation that effectively increases the demand on the heart. The effects of an acute change in valvular function, such as with acute mitral insufficiency due to infarction, may be more poorly tolerated than a comparable amount of chronic dysfunction that has developed more slowly, as there is less opportunity to utilize compensatory mechanisms. Shunts can increase the volume to be pumped in a manner similar to valvular regurgitation. As with valvular regurgitation, an acutely acquired shunt may be more poorly tolerated than a chronic one. A chronic left-to-right shunt can lead to the development of secondary pulmonary hypertension, with the potential for reversal of the shunt direction (Eisenmenger syndrome) and cyanosis.

In addition to the mechanical dysfunction of the myocardium associated with ischemic disease and hypertrophy, there are a variety of other diseases that can affect the myocardium, including the cardiomyopathies. These can also lead to progressive dilatation of the ventricles. Although in some cases there is an association with an inciting episode of myocarditis or toxic exposure, or an underlying muscle dystrophy, in many cases the dysfunction is just "idiopathic." The final common pathway is often a steadily worsening cycle of increased preload leading to dilatation, leading to greater demand for the development of active wall tension, thus leading to still greater dilatation. In restrictive cardiomyopathies, there may be an apparent concentric hypertrophy, but this may just represent infiltrative replacement of the working myocardium with material such as amyloid. This can result in an impairment of the ability of the ventricle to fill during diastole. In hypertrophic cardiomyopathy, there is focal or diffuse hypertrophy in the absence of an increased pressure load; the hypertrophied muscle typically has a disordered muscle fiber structure and variable amounts of fibrosis. This presumably is associated with decreased contraction efficiency of the affected myocardium. In addition, encroachment on the left ventricular outflow tract, in the common asymmetrical septal hypertrophy form of the condition, can lead to subaortic stenosis, because of both the bulging muscle itself and the resulting systolic anterior motion of the anterior leaflet of the mitral valve due to the pressure drop associated with the local acceleration of the blood.

The pericardium encloses the heart, particularly the ventricles, and thus can affect their filling. When there is scarring and thickening of the pericardium due to prior inflammation, the resulting constriction of the ventricles can result in abrupt cessation of diastolic filling as the stiffened pericardium starts to be stretched. The stiffened pericardial sac surrounding the ventricles results in equalization of the diastolic pressures between the LV and RV. The fixed total volume available within the pericardium, combined with the differing effects of respiration on venous return to the right and left sides of the circulation, causes a characteristic decrease in systemic cardiac output with inspiration. The accumulation of a pericardial effusion can result in similar compromise of cardiac venous return and ventricular filling. This is particularly seen with relatively rapid fluid accumulation that does not leave enough time for stretching of the pericardium to accommodate the effusion, leading to pericardial tamponade. Emergency drainage of the effusion may be necessary in cases of tamponade.

Pneumothorax can also lead to impaired venous return to the chest, with resulting decreased cardiac output, especially with the development of positive intrathoracic pressure, a "tension pneumothorax." Emergency evacuation of the pneumothorax may be necessary in this situation.

Pulmonary embolism leads to an increase in the resistance to pulmonary outflow, and thus a decrease in inflow to the left side of the heart. An acute embolus can present an immediate abruptly increased load on the right ventricle, while chronic embolization can lead to secondary pulmonary hypertension and RV hypertrophy.

Rhythm disturbances can affect the rate or regularity of the heart beat. A rate that is too rapid does not allow enough time for proper filling of the ventricle between contractions, and thus diminishes the effectiveness of the contractions, whereas a rate that is too slow may result in insufficient output because of the limited stroke volume available from each beat (especially in an unconditioned heart). The effects of irregular heart rhythms mostly depend on the corresponding average heart rate, although prolonged asystole can lead to syncope. Conduction abnormalities can lead to problems through the development of different degrees of heart block, whereas intraventricular bundle branch blocks can lead to uncoordinated and thus less efficient ventricular contraction. The loss of coordination of atrial and ventricular contraction can also result in less efficient cardiac contraction cycles. Pacemaker therapy can help avoid excessive bradycardia or prolonged asystole by initiating ventricular contraction from the site of the pacemaker lead implantation. Sequential atrial/ventricular or multisite pacing may be needed for most efficient cardiac contractions.

SUMMARY

The principles of continuum mechanics can be used to better understand the function of the heart in health and disease and provide a rational basis for the diagnosis and management of heart disease.

REFERENCES

1. Borg TK, Caulfield JB: The collagen matrix of the heart. Fed Proc 40:2037–2041, 1981.
2. Braunwald E, editor: Heart Disease, 3rd ed. Philadelphia: W.B. Saunders, 1988.
3. Fung YC: A First Course in Continuum Mechanics, 3rd ed. Englewood Cliffs, NJ: Prentice-Hall, 1993.
4. Fung YC: Biomechanics: Circulation, 2nd ed. New York: Springer-Verlag, 1997.
5. Glass L, McCulloch A, Hunter P: Theory of Heart. New York: Springer-Verlag, 1991.
6. LeGrice IJ, Smail BH, Chai LZ, et al: Laminar structure of the heart: Ventricular myocytes arrangement and connective tissue architecture in the dog. Am J Physiol 269:H571–H582, 1995.
7. Omens JH, Fung YC: Residual strain in the rat left ventricle. Circ Res 66:37–45, 1989.
8. Streeter D Jr: Gross morphology and fiber geometry of the heart. In Berne RM, Sperelakis N, editors: Handbook of Physiology, Sec. 2, Cardiovascular System. Vol. 1. The Heart. Bethesda, MD: American Physiologic Society, 1979, pp. 61–112.
9. Axel L, Dougherty L: MR imaging of motion with spatial modulation of magnetization. Radiology 171:841–845, 1989.

Shock and Sepsis

Mitchell P. Fink and Kyle J. Gunnerson

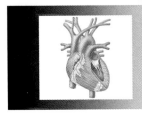

▶ DEFINITION OF SHOCK

The first century Roman savant Aulus Cornelius Celsus made the following observation: "When much blood is lost, the pulse becomes feeble, the skin extremely pale, the body covered with a malodorous sweat, the extremities frigid, and death occurs speedily." Although a French surgeon, Le Dran, introduced the term *choc* to describe a severe impact or jolt, an English physician, Clarke, later applied the term *shock* to describe the rapid physiological deterioration of a badly injured trauma victim. When blood pressure measurement was introduced into medical practice, the term shock was used to denote arterial hypotension associated with hemorrhage. Great physiologists of the first part of the twentieth century, including Keith, Cannon, Blalock, and Cournard, introduced the notion that tissue hypoperfusion rather than simply arterial hypotension was the key feature of hemorrhagic shock. Currently, shock is generally regarded as a syndrome precipitated by a systemic derangement of perfusion leading to widespread cellular dysoxia and vital organ dysfunction. Indeed, because of increasing recognition that acquired derangements in mitochondrial function can impair cellular energetics, shock can be even more broadly defined as acute physiological derangements prompted by inadequate production of adenosine triphosphate (ATP) by cells in many organs of the body.

▶ CLASSIFICATION OF SHOCK

Blalock proposed that shock can be categorized into one of four major types: neurogenic, cardiogenic, hypovolemic, or vasogenic.[24] A still simpler classification scheme will be used here.

Hypovolemic Shock

The primary derangement in hypovolemic shock is loss of circulating volume. Blood loss (hemorrhage) is the most

794

common cause of hypovolemic shock, but hemodynamically significant hypovolemia also can result from inadequate replacement of asanguinous fluids. The diagnosis of hemorrhagic shock is fairly straightforward when the site of bleeding is identified. Common causes of hemorrhagic shock include trauma, gastrointestinal bleeding, bleeding during or after surgical procedures, rupture of aortic or other arterial aneurysms, and peripartum catastrophes (e.g., placental abruption or postpartum uterine bleeding). When bleeding is internal, the diagnosis may be less obvious. Often the history is helpful. Special studies including computed tomography, angiography, abdominal ultrasonography, diagnostic paracentesis or peritoneal lavage, or chest tube placement can be helpful. Time-consuming diagnostic studies (e.g., computed tomography), however, should not be performed if the patient is very unstable. In any case, diagnostic studies should not delay treatment with intravenous asanguinous fluids, packed red blood cells, and (if indicated) platelet transfusions and coagulation factors. Prompt surgical intervention, when indicated, is crucial.

Nonhemorrhagic hypovolemic shock can be caused by severe dehydration secondary to massive urinary or gastrointestinal fluid losses due, for example, to diabetic ketoacidosis or cholera. Massive insensible losses of water or perspiration can precipitate shock in patients with major burn injuries or heat stroke. Another form of nonhemorrhagic hypovolemic shock is caused by the sequestration of asanguinous fluid in the extravascular compartment as a result of surgery, bowel obstruction, hepatic failure, systemic inflammation, acute pancreatitis, or thermal injuries. This phenomenon is often referred to as "third spacing."

Cardiogenic Shock

The primary problem in cardiogenic shock is an acute profound deterioration in the pumping function of the heart. The most common causes are acute myocardial ischemia and/or infarction, impaired myocardial contractility due to toxins or medications, valvular disease, dysrhythmias, ventricular septal rupture, myocardial contusion, and myocarditis.

Since the introduction of thrombolytic therapy, angioplasty, and stenting, the incidence of cardiogenic shock complicating acute coronary syndromes has decreased to 4–7% from as high as 20% previously.[80] Two recent trials suggest that early angioplasty improves survival among patients with cardiogenic shock complicating acute myocardial infarction.[18,90]

Underlying causes for acute mitral insufficiency and cardiogenic shock include papillary muscle rupture secondary to acute myocardial infarction, endocarditis, blunt chest trauma, or sudden failure of a previously implanted mechanical valve. Without surgical correction, shock associated with acute mitral insufficiency carries a very high risk of mortality.[211] Acute aortic insufficiency is usually a complication of endocarditis but also can be related to acute aortic dissection or mechanical valve failure. Acute ventricular septal defects typically lead to cardiogenic shock a few days after an acute myocardial infarction.

The clinical picture in cases of cardiogenic shock secondary to right ventricular infarction is somewhat different from other forms of cardiogenic shock, being characterized by increased right atrial pressure and normal or low pulmonary artery wedge (occlusion) pressure (PAOP). Completely isolated right ventricular infarction is uncommon; involvement of a portion of the left ventricular wall is usually present as well.[49,170] Treatment consists of intravascular volume loading with or without infusion of inotropic agents. An unusual cause of shock due to right heart failure is compression of the right atrium by an isolated intrapericardial clot after cardiac surgery. This diagnosis typically is made by transesophageal echo or at reoperation.

Obstructive Shock

Extracardiac obstructive shock is caused by a lesion or process interfering with the forward flow of blood. In some cases, the major problem is impaired diastolic filling. Conditions in this category include cardiac tamponade, tension pneumothorax, obstruction of the large veins by a mediastinal mass, and constrictive pericarditis. In other cases, the main problem is impaired ventricular ejection as a result of an acute increase in afterload. A classic example of this process is a massive pulmonary embolus,[196] although aortic dissection leading to aortic occlusion also can lead to occlusive shock on this basis.

Other Causes of Shock

This miscellaneous category includes shock due to sepsis, anaphylaxis, spinal cord injury, and adrenal insufficiency. A detailed discussion of each of these conditions is beyond the scope of this chapter, although sepsis will be reviewed in more detail later.

Anaphylactic reactions are commonly triggered by insect stings, food antigens, and medications and can be mediated by both immunoglobulin E (IgE)-dependent and IgE-independent pathways.[38] In addition to arterial hypotension, other common features of anaphylaxis include airway obstruction due to angioedema and generalized urticaria. Cardiac output typically decreases dramatically, and calculated vascular resistance increases during anaphylactic shock.[145] The primary pathophysiological problems in this condition are functional hypovolemia secondary to increased microvascular permeability combined with decreased myocardial contractility. The treatment of severe anaphylaxis and shock begins with removing the offending agent if possible. The next step, often carried out simultaneously, is to protect the airway. Intravenous epinephrine and intravenous fluids should be administered to support blood pressure and cardiac output. Supplemental oxygen should be provided. Antihistamines, corticosteroids, glucagon, albuterol, and aminophylline are secondary medications that are mostly useful as prophylactic interventions to decrease the risk of a recurrence.[76]

Neurogenic shock is characterized by hypotension and paradoxical bradycardia associated with an acute injury to the spinal cord that disrupts sympathetic outflow leaving unopposed vagal tone.[220] The term neurogenic shock should not be confused with the term "spinal shock"; the latter term is used to denote a temporary loss of spinal reflex activity below the level of a spinal cord injury. Blunt trauma accounts for over 85% of all spinal cord injuries.[179,220] In addition to the standard management of any trauma victim, neurogenic shock is managed by infusing intravenous crystalloid or colloid volume expanders and vasopressors as needed. A mean arterial pressure (MAP) of 70 mm Hg is a reasonable target to minimize the risk of secondary injury to the cord on the basis of inadequate perfusion.[68] The value of administering methylprednisolone in cases of acute spinal cord injury is debatable,[32,95] but data are lacking to support the notion that intervention is of particular value in cases of neurogenic shock.

Glucocorticoids are required by the cardiovascular system to maintain responsiveness to epinephrine, norepinephrine, and angiotensin II. Inadequate circulating levels of cortisol are associated with the development of hypotension. The hypothalamic–pituitary–adrenocortical (HPA) axis is suppressed in patients taking a corticosteroid medication for the management of a chronic underlying condition, such as inflammatory bowel disease or rheumatoid arthritis. If treatment with the corticosteroid medication is abruptly discontinued, for example, because of nausea and vomiting secondary to a gastrointestinal viral syndrome, then acute adrenal insufficiency can develop rapidly. Indeed, if so-called "stress doses" of hydrocortisone or an equivalent agent are not provided to patients with a suppression of the HPA axis, then symptoms of acute adrenal insufficiency also can occur. The clinical findings that are associated with acute adrenal insufficiency are nonspecific, and can include unexplained fever, hypotension refractory to fluid resuscitation, and eosinophilia.[6] Controversy exists regarding the best way to establish the diagnosis of adrenal insufficiency in critically ill patients. Some experts advocate using the cosyntropin stimulation test.[6] Marik and Zaloga, however, have presented convincing data in support of the idea that a random serum cortisol level less than 25 μg/dl in a patient with critical illness it is sufficient to establish the presence of adrenal insufficiency.[137] In such cases, administration of hydrocortisone is warranted.[137] If adrenal insufficiency is strongly suspected in the setting of critical illness, then treatment with stress doses of hydrocortisone or a synthetic corticosteroid should be instituted. Dexamethasone can be given without altering circulating levels of immunoreactive cortisol or interfering with the cosyntropin stimulation test. The starting regimen for corticosteroid therapy in this setting should be equivalent to 300 mg of hydrocortisone per day in divided doses.

▶ DETERMINANTS OF OXYGEN DELIVERY

With the exception of selected cases of septic shock, a common feature of all forms of shock is a decrease in the delivery of oxygen (DO_2) to tissues such that the transport of oxygen to cells is inadequate to meet their metabolic demands. Under these conditions, oxygen utilization ($\dot{V}O_2$) is determined by its availability not by the intrinsic demand associated with the metabolic work performed by cells. This state of affairs is called "supply-dependent oxygen uptake" (see Figure 50-1). Systemic DO_2 (i.e., the amount of oxygen delivered to tissues in arterial blood per unit time) is determined by four factors (Figure 50-2): the concentration hemoglobin in the blood, the fractional saturation of the hemoglobin with oxygen, cardiac output, and (to a relatively minor extent) the amount of oxygen dissolved in the blood:

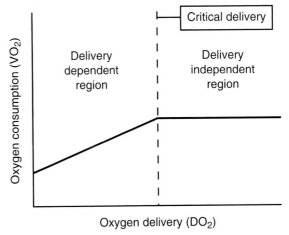

Figure 50–1 The relationship between oxygen delivery and oxygen consumption in shock. When DO_2 decreases to less than the value for critical delivery, oxygen consumption ($\dot{V}O_2$) is linearly dependent on the delivery of oxygen to the tissues (DO_2). In the delivery-dependent region, the oxygen extraction ratio is maximal and anaerobic metabolism increases.

$$
\begin{aligned}
\text{Systemic } DO_2 \\ (\text{ml O}_2/\text{min})
&= \text{cardiac output (ml blood/min)} \\
&\quad \times \text{arterial oxygen content} \\
&\quad (\text{ml O}_2/\text{ml blood}) \\
&= \text{cardiac output (liters/min)} \\
&\quad \times 10 \ (\text{dl/liter}) \times \{[\text{arterial hemoglobin} \\
&\quad \text{concentration (g/dl)} \times 1.36 \ \text{ml O}_2/\text{g} \\
&\quad \text{hemoglobin} \times \text{fractional arterial} \\
&\quad \text{hemoglobin saturation}] + [\text{arterial} \\
&\quad \text{partial pressure of oxygen (mm Hg)} \\
&\quad \times 0.003 \ (\text{ml O}_2/\text{dl blood})]\}
\end{aligned}
$$

In the absence of regurgitant flow, cardiac output is determined by left ventricular stroke volume (LVSV) times heart rate. As noted in Chapters 3 and 4, LVSV is determined by ventricular preload, afterload, and contractility.

Strictly speaking, "preload" is a parameter used in *in vitro* studies to specify the degree of stretch imposed on a strip of myocardial tissue prior to a contraction. End-diastolic volume (EDV) is the *in vivo* correlate of preload. Clinicians frequently use end-diastolic pressure (EDP) as a surrogate for EDV, but EDP is determined not only by volume, but also by the diastolic compliance of the ventricular chamber. Ventricular compliance is altered by various pharmacological agents and pathological conditions. For example, diastolic compliance decreases when the ventricle is ischemic or hypertrophied. Thus, measuring a "normal" central venous pressure or pulmonary artery wedge pressure may not rule out inadequate preload as a cause of shock.

Increased intrathoracic pressure decreases venous return. This phenomenon is the primary mechanism responsible for the development of shock in patients with tension pneumothorax. Increased intrathoracic pressure also can decrease cardiac output in patients receiving positive pressure ventilation especially when intravascular volume is low or positive end-expiratory pressure (PEEP) is applied. The magnitude of the effect of positive pressure mechanical ventilation on cardiac output is determined, in part, by pulmonary compliance. Thus, when the lungs are

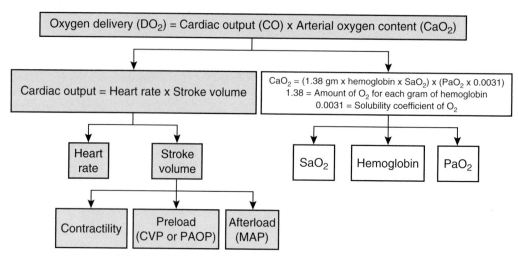

Figure 50–2 Determinants of oxygen delivery Do$_2$.

relatively noncompliant, as is typically the case in patients with the acute respiratory distress syndrome (ARDS), high airway pressures may not be transmitted to the pleural and mediastinal spaces. Even if extrinsic PEEP is not applied, positive pressure mechanical ventilation can still generate PEEP if air is trapped within the lung at the end expiration because of high airway resistance, short expiratory times, or both. This phenomenon is sometimes called intrinsic PEEP or auto-PEEP. Intrinsic PEEP can further embarrass venous return and thereby compromise cardiac output.[20]

"Afterload" is another term used in clinical practice that has been borrowed from studies of myocardial function carried out using isolated muscle strips studied *in vitro*. Afterload is the force resisting contraction. The *in vivo* correlate of afterload is the input impedance of the arterial tree. Because vascular input impedance is difficult to measure, systemic vascular resistance (SVR), calculated as MAP/cardiac output, is often used by clinicians as a proxy for afterload. SVR is primarily determined by the degree of vasomotor tone in the precapillary smooth muscle sphincters. Other factors such as hematocrit and plasma fibrinogen concentration also contribute.

Contractility refers to the ability of the myocardial fibers to shorten at constant preload and afterload. Numerous factors can compromise myocardial contractility. These factors include loss of ventricular mass due to infarction, ischemia or ischemia/reperfusion injury, various drugs, and certain proinflammatory cytokines.

▶ COMPENSATORY RESPONSES TO SHOCK

Stages of Shock

The progression of shock is usually divided into three stages. The first stage has been called early, reversible, or compensated shock. This stage is characterized by compensatory responses that help to minimize tissue injury. If the etiology of shock is recognized and treated early in this stage, full recovery with minimal residual morbidity is the likely outcome. The second stage of shock is the beginning of cellular and microvascular injury. In this stage, shock can be treated, but recovery can be prolonged and complicated by organ failure. The third stage is late, irreversible, or decompensated shock. When shock reaches this point, cellular and tissue injury is extensive and largely irreversible. Progression to death is inevitable, regardless of therapy.

Autonomic Nervous System

Even minor decreases in arterial blood pressure activate the baroreceptor reflex via stretch receptors located in the carotid sinus, splanchnic vasculature, and aortic arch. Hypovolemia also activates stretch receptors located in the right atrium. Activation of these receptors increases outflow through the sympathetic nervous system. Compensatory responses mediated by the sympathetic nervous system include (1) redistribution of blood flow away from skeletal muscle beds and the splanchnic viscera;[46,167] (2) augmentation of myocardial contractility and heart rate;[46] (3) constriction of venous capacitance vessels, particularly in the splanchnic bed, augmenting venous return;[46,167] (4) release of adrenocortical and adrenomedullary hormones including hydrocortisone and epinephrine;[138] and (5) activation of the renin–angiotensin axis.[53]

Renin–Angiotensin System

The renin–angiotensin system is another important neurohumoral compensatory mechanism in shock.[53] When blood flow is decreased through the renal circulation, juxtaloglomerular cells in the kidney release renin. Renin is also released in response to decreased renal distal tubular sodium delivery and sympathetic activation.[78]

Angiotensinogen, which is produced by the liver, is cleaved by renin to yield the inactive decapeptide, angiotensin I. Angiotensin-converting enzyme (ACE) then converts circulating angiotensin I into angiotensin II (AII). ACE-dependent formation of AII occurs primarily in the lungs. ACE also converts the vasodilator, bradykinin, into an inactive peptide. AII can also be generated locally at its site of action, thus it can function as a paracrine mediator.[102]

In shock, AII acts to restore systemic arterial blood pressure by increasing arteriolar vasomotor tone, primarily in the mesenteric bed.[167] AII also stimulates the release of aldosterone from adrenal cortex and thereby promotes renal retention of sodium and water retention. In addition, AII stimulates the secretion of epinephrine from the adrenal medulla, increases myocardial contractility, and promotes the release of arginine vasopressin from the posterior pituitary.[78]

Arginine Vasopressin

Arginine vasopressin (AVP), a nonapeptide secreted by the posterior pituitary gland, is also known as antidiuretic hormone. In its role as an antidiuretic factor, AVP increases the permeability of the collecting ducts in the kidneys to water, thereby promoting the reabsorption of water driven by the osmotic gradient in the renal medulla. AVP also regulates gastrointestinal and uterine smooth muscle activity, platelet aggregation, liver glycogenolysis, and the secretion of adrenocorticotropic hormone (ACTH) and aldosterone.[150,219] AVP, of course, is also a vasoconstrictor albeit not a very potent one, under normal conditions. Whereas plasma AVP concentrations of 1–7 pg/ml (0.9–6.5 pmol/liter) are sufficient to increase renal reabsorption of free water, circulating AVP levels of 10–200 pg/ml (9–187 pmol/liter) are necessary to promote arteriolar vasoconstriction.[118] Although AVP plays at most a minor role in the normal minute-to-minute regulation of arteriolar vasomotor tone, during episodes of severe hypotension due to hypovolemia or sepsis, plasma concentrations of this hormone increase considerably.[27]

Transcapillary Refill

The movement of fluid into or out of the intravascular compartment is a function of several parameters and can be described by the Starling equation (Figure 50-3). The rate and direction of net fluid movement across the capillary wall are determined by the hydrostatic pressure gradient between the microvascular and the interstitial spaces. During the compensatory response to shock, precapillary vasoconstriction decreases microvascular blood pressure (Pmv), promoting the net movement of fluid from the interstitial compartment into the vascular compartment.[75]

▶ DECOMPENSATORY MECHANISMS IN SHOCK

When the shock state persists for a period of time, the syndrome eventually becomes refractory to treatment and multiorgan dysfunction ensues. Every organ is affected eventually.

Peripheral Vasomotor Decompensation

In animal models of hemorrhagic shock, the onset of irreversibility is signaled by vasodilation of precapillary sphincters despite persistent activation of the sympathetic nervous systems and high circulating levels of the vasoconstricting autocoids, AII and AVP.[27] Current hypotheses to explain the loss of vasomotor responsiveness to endogenous constrictors in irreversible shock include (1) excessive production of the potent vasodilator nitric oxide, secondary to induction of the enzyme inducible nitric oxide synthase (iNOS);[199] (2) energetic failure (i.e., inadequate ATP synthesis) in vascular smooth muscle cells as a result of activation of the enzyme poly(ADP-ribosyl) polymerase (PARP)-1;[199] (3) deleterious effects of lipid mediators;[163] and (4) opening of ATP-sensitive potassium channels in vascular smooth muscle cells.[176,200]

Inappropriate vasodilation and vasoplegia (i.e., reduced responsiveness to vasopressors) are key features of septic

Figure 50–3 Transcapillary refill. Several parameters affect the movement of fluid into and out of the intravascular space across the capillary walls. In the compensatory response to shock, precapillary sphincters contract more than postcapillary ones, causing a decreased P_{mv}. As a result, P_{mv} decreases promoting the net influx of fluid into the intravascular space. Q_f, flow across the capillary wall (volume/unit time); K_f, filtration coefficient; P_{mv}, microvascular (i.e., capillary hydrostatic) pressure; P_{pmv}, perimicrovascular (interstitial) fluid hydrostatic pressure, σ, osmotic reflection coefficient; π_{mv}, capillary colloid osmotic pressure; π_{pmv}, perimicrovascular (interstitial) colloid osmotic pressure.

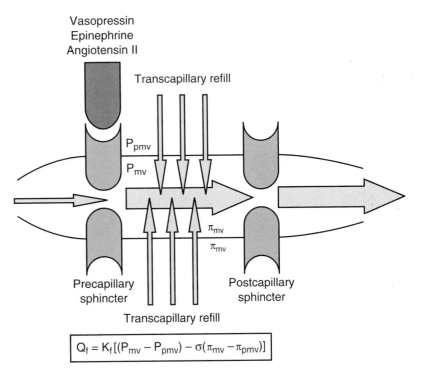

$$Q_f = K_f[(P_{mv} - P_{pmv}) - \sigma(\pi_{mv} - \pi_{pmv})]$$

798 shock. Although the pathophysiology of this phenomenon remains incompletely understood, several important mechanisms have been implicated, namely (1) activation of ATP-sensitive potassium channels in the plasma membranes of vascular smooth muscle cells;[117] (2) induction of iNOS expression in vascular smooth muscle cells, leading to excessive release of the endogenous vasodilator, nitric oxide;[154,198] (3) insufficient release of AVP;[118] and (4) energetic failure in vascular smooth muscle cells due to PARP-1 activation.[218]

Endothelial Activation and Leukosequestration

Activation of endothelial cells occurs in shock. Endothelial activation leads to increased expression of adhesion molecules, such as E-selectin and intracellular adhesion molecule (ICAM)-1, on the surface of these cells. Increased expression of these adhesion molecules promotes first rolling then adhesion and transudation of circulating polymorphonuclear neutrophils (PMNs). Sequestration of activated PMNs in the lungs, liver, and other organs has been implicated as being an important factor leading to the development of organ system dysfunction as a consequence of hemorrhage and resuscitation or sepsis.[84,156]

Decreased Erythrocyte Deformability

Normal human erythrocytes are 7 μm in diameter. The mean diameter of capillaries is 4.5 μm. Therefore, flow through the microcirculation depends on the deformability of erythrocytes, a characteristic that allows these cells to alter their shape and squeeze through small vessels to deliver oxygen. The deformability of erythrocytes is impaired during shock, leading to further embarrassment of Do_2.[9,191,206] The mechanism(s) responsible for this phenomenon are not clear, but may involve alterations in the synthesis of prostaglandins or nitric oxide.[110,114]

Cellular Depolarization

Hemorrhagic and septic shock are associated with decreases in the normal electrochemical potential gradient across the cytosolic membranes of cells. Cellular depolarization is associated with disturbances in the regulation of several intracellular ion concentrations, a factor that might contribute to cellular, and hence organ, dysfunction in shock. The molecular basis for cellular depolarization in shock is poorly understood, although diminished aerobic production of ATP is undoubtedly important.[45] Another factor contributing to attenuation of the transmembrane electrochemical potential gradient may be the release of a circulating depolarizing factor during shock.[29,62,67]

Mitochondrial Dysfunction

There is increasing evidence that the ability of cells to utilize available O_2 is compromised as a consequence of shock or sepsis due to acquired intrinsic derangements in mitochondria. This phenomenon has been termed "cytopathic hypoxia."[70] Until recently, the notion that mitochondrial dysfunction occurs in sepsis or shock was mostly derived from studies using animals or even cultured cells. Recently, however, clinical data are becoming available that lend credence to the idea that acquired mitochondrial dysfunction is an important determinant of patients with septic shock.[30,34]

A number of mechanisms might be responsible for the development of mitochondrial dysfunction as a consequence of shock or sepsis. Nitric oxide can compete with oxygen for binding to cytochrome oxidase, the terminal enzyme in the mitochondrial electron transport chain. Accordingly, iNOS induction leading to excessive production of nitric oxide might inhibit mitochondrial respiration on this basis. In addition, nitric oxide can react with superoxide radical anion, a reactive oxygen species (ROS) that is produced during and after resuscitation from shock, to form a potent oxidizing and nitrosating agent, peroxynitrite anion. This latter moiety can damage nuclear DNA, leading to activation of PARP-1. Activation of this enzyme depletes cellular levels of nicotinamide adenine dinucleotide (NAD^+), a vital redox-active enzymatic cofactor that is essential for converting fuels, such as glucose, into forms that can be used to support mitochondrial oxidative phosphorylation and ATP synthesis. Potent inhibitors of PARP-1 are being developed as potential therapeutic agents for treating patients with shock and sepsis.

▶ DIAGNOSIS AND DIFFERENTIAL DIAGNOSIS

When the clinician is confronted with a profoundly hypotensive patient with an obvious source of bleeding, making the diagnosis of hemorrhagic shock is fairly straightforward. Establishing the proper diagnosis can be considerably more difficult when bleeding is not obvious or the primary problem is an occult source of sepsis or blood pressure is normal because of intact compensatory mechanisms. Despite the difficulties inherent in diagnosing these occult forms of shock, it is of the utmost importance to identify these patients as early as possible. In patients with sepsis, early institution of therapy with appropriate antibiotics improves survival.[141] In patients with septic shock, very prompt "goal-directed" hemodynamic resuscitation also clearly improves survival.[169]

As in almost all aspects of clinical medicine, making an early diagnosis starts by a obtaining a thorough problem-directed history and performing a careful physical examination. Obtaining an accurate list of current medications is quite important, because many drugs (e.g., β-adrenergic antagonists or diuretics) can alter the physiological responses to shock. Physical examination can reveal an obvious source of infection or bleeding. Even in the absence of arterial hypotension, other findings on physical examination, such as tachycardia, tachypnea, diaphoresis, mental status changes, poor capillary refill, or cutaneous mottling, can suggest the presence of shock. However, even if these signs are absent, the clinician cannot rule out truly occult shock on the basis of clinical findings alone in certain groups of patients, such as those with trauma, gastrointestinal bleeding, or infection. Accordingly other adjunctive diagnostic studies are needed.

A number of adjunctive modalities are useful, or at least potentially useful, for identifying tissue hypoperfusion (a key feature of most forms of shock), sepsis (a risk factor for septic shock), or occult hemorrhage. Many of these adjunctive assays (e.g., measurement of blood lactate concentration and sublingual capnography) are also useful for assessing the adequacy of resuscitation and will be discussed in detail in that context below. Procalcitonin (PCT) is a 14-kDa, 116 amino acid polypeptide prohormone of calcitonin that is released by numerous cell types. Accumulating data suggest that measurements of PCT can be quite useful for distinguishing sepsis from other causes of systemic inflammation.[142] Abdominal ultrasonography is an efficient way to rule out or establish the presence of hemoperitoneum in patients with nonpenetrating trauma.[172]

TREATMENT OF SHOCK

Treatment begins during the initial assessment and primary survey. Resuscitation, as always, starts with "the ABC's": control of the *airway*, adequacy of *breathing*, and support of the *circulation*. All patients with known or suspected shock should receive supplemental oxygen. If any doubt exists about the patency of the airway or the adequacy of ventilation, endotracheal intubation should be performed and mechanical ventilation initiated. Mechanical ventilation may prevent damage to the respiratory muscles during shock or sepsis.[63]

In all forms of shock, circulatory support depends on obtaining intravenous access. Two large bore (16-gauge or larger) peripheral intravenous catheters should be placed and administration of a crystalloid solution (normal saline or Ringer's lactate solution) initiated. Percutaneous placement of an introducer sheath in a femoral vein using the Seldinger technique is an efficient and safe way to obtain intravenous access in order to infuse large volumes of fluids rapidly. Central venous access may also be necessary for hemodynamic monitoring and/or to infuse vasoactive drugs.

End Points of Resuscitation

Except for selected cases of septic shock, most cases of shock are characterized by impaired microcirculatory flow such that the transport of oxygen to tissues is inadequate to meet metabolic demand. The goal of resuscitation is to restore global and microvascular perfusion to levels that support normal aerobic cellular respiration. Although the fundamental concept is straightforward, deciding when resuscitation has achieved this goal is not. Indeed, considerable controversy surrounds the issue of what is the proper end point for resuscitation.[132,134,164]

Until fairly recently, clinicians resuscitated patients with shock, guiding their therapy solely by using easily measured clinical parameters, such as arterial blood pressure, heart rate, and urine output. These clinical parameters, although clearly useful, lack sensitivity; in other words, tissue hypoperfusion can persist despite normalization of blood pressure, urine flow, and heart rate. Prompted by the recognition that simple clinical parameters are not reliable indices for the adequacy of perfusion, clinicians sought to use more invasive means to assess oxygen delivery and uptake. One approach was championed by Shoemaker, who analyzed data collected from hundreds of patients with shock and noted that after resuscitation, survivors had significantly higher values than nonsurvivors for three key parameters related to oxygen transport: cardiac output, sys-

temic DO_2, and systemic $\dot{V}O_2$ (systemic oxygen consumption).[1,25,188] Based on these prospectively collected but retrospectively analyzed data, Shoemaker proposed the following hemodynamic and oxygen transport goals for resuscitation: cardiac index (i.e., cardiac output indexed to body surface area) greater than 4.5 liters/min/m², systemic DO_2 index greater than 600 liters/min/m², and a systemic oxygen consumption index greater than 170 liters/min/m².[23,186] These targets represent levels of cardiac output and systemic DO_2 and systemic $\dot{V}O_2$ that are considerably greater than normal. Shoemaker reasoned that these supranormal values were required to repay an "oxygen uptake deficit" that was accumulated during the period of shock.[187] A number of clinical trials attempted to validate Shoemaker's hypothesis with variable results. A meta-analysis that reviewed the literature regarding the use of supranormal targets for resuscitation of patients with shock concluded that this strategy fails to improve survival.[88]

One plausible interpretation to explain the negative results obtained in many trials of resuscitation to supranormal hemodynamic and oxygen transport end points is that the high levels of cardiac output observed by Shoemaker and co-workers in shock survivors were simply markers of greater physiological reserve in these patients. Another interpretation, however, is suggested by the observation that many of the patients enrolled in the negative trials of supranormal resuscitation had been in an ICU for as long as 24 h before being randomized to treatment with the control or goal-directed resuscitation regimen. Thus, it is possible that resuscitation to supranormal indices of oxygen transport is ineffective when started late in the course of shock, but might be effective if initiated earlier. This notion is supported by the results from one study that specifically targeted high-risk elective surgical patients for enrollment.[31] In this trial, treatment with a standard or "goal-directed" resuscitation regimen was initiated prior to the induction of general anesthesia, and mortality was significantly reduced among the patients randomized to receive therapy titrated to supranormal indices of oxygen transport. The notion that "early goal-directed" resuscitation is efficacious is further supported by results reported in 2001 by Rivers and colleagues.[169] In this study, patients with septic shock were randomized to conventional therapy or goal-directed resuscitation to "normal" physiological end points during the first 6 h after presentation to an emergency department. Rather than targeting specific values for cardiac output, systemic DO_2 or systemic $\dot{V}O_2$, the investigators sought to achieve "normal" systemic oxygen extraction as assessed by measuring the oxygen saturation of hemoglobin in the superior vena cava. The goal for resuscitation for patients randomized to the experimental arm of the trial was central venous oxygen saturation greater than 70%. Using this goal as well as a carefully planned algorithm for resuscitation, these investigators showed that early goal-directed resuscitation of septic shock improved 30-day mortality from 46.5 to 30.5%.

During glycolysis, the oxidized form of NAD$^+$ is used as an electron acceptor (oxidizing agent) in the reaction (catalyzed by glyceraldehyde-3-phosphate dehydrogenase) that converts glyceraldehyde-3-phosphate into 1,3-diphosphoglycerate. Under aerobic conditions, NAD$^+$ is regenerated in the cell when mitochondria oxidize the reduced form of

800 nicotinamide adenine dinucleotide (NADH) using molecular oxygen as the ultimate electron acceptor. However, under anaerobic conditions, this pathway for the regeneration of NAD$^+$ is not applicable. Accordingly, to maintain glycolysis as a source of ATP synthesis under anaerobic conditions, cells utilize an alternate reaction to regenerate NAD$^+$ that does not depend upon the availability of oxygen. In this reaction, pyruvate (the end product of glycolysis) is reduced to lactate while NADH is oxidized to NAD$^+$. Thus, glucose is converted to lactate by anaerobic glycolysis. Lactate is exported out of cells and, under conditions when many cells are supporting ATP synthesis by increasing anaerobic glycolysis (i.e., during shock), the lactate concentration in blood increases. Thus, measurements of blood lactate concentration are a useful way to detect increased anaerobic metabolism and monitor the adequacy of resuscitation.

Another factor contributes to the development of hyperlactatemia in shock. The most important organs for the clearance (metabolism) of lactate are the liver and renal cortex. Cells in these organs either convert lactate into glucose (gluconeogenesis) or oxidize lactate to pyruvate and then, ultimately, to carbon dioxide and water. When the splanchnic circulation is compromised in shock, hepatic lactate clearance is impaired, further contributing to the build-up of lactate levels in the circulation.

In a classic study, Broder and Weil demonstrated that blood lactate levels correlate with the risk of mortality in patients with shock.[36] They reported that only 11% of patients in circulatory shock survived with a lactate greater than 4 mmol/liter.[36] Other investigators obtained similar findings.[208] The rate that lactate concentration decreases following resuscitation also has prognostic significance. In a study of patients with shock resuscitated to predetermined goals for Do$_2$, V̇o$_2$, and cardiac index, Abramson et al reported that survival was 100% when the blood lactate concentration decreased to ≤2 mmol/liter within 24 h.[2] If the decrease in lactate concentration to this level required 24–48 h, then only 78% of the patients survived. If the reduction in lactate concentration required longer than 48 h, then survival was only 14%. Similar observations have been made by others.[61,130]

The interpretation of hyperlactatemia is straightforward in patients with hemorrhagic or cardiogenic shock. In sepsis, however, there is evidence that the rate of glycolysis increases, even in the absence of tissue hypoxia.[126,180] This phenomenon has been termed accelerated aerobic glycolysis and may reflect a change in the ratio of the active and inactive forms of the enzyme complex, pyruvate dehydrogenase, that is the rate-limiting step for the entry of substrate into the mitochondrial tricarboxylic acid cycle.[70] Despite the presence of this phenomenon, very high blood lactate concentrations in patients with septic shock (e.g., levels ≥5 mmol/liter) are probably evidence of underresuscitation and on-going tissue hypoxia and/or splanchnic hypoperfusion. Certainly, persistently high blood lactate levels portend a bad outcome for patients with septic shock.[12,13,190]

In addition to the production of lactate, acidosis is another consequence of anaerobic metabolism. Although the biochemical basis for the development of acidosis during anaerobiosis is remarkably complicated, the essential element is fairly easy to explain. When a molecule of ATP is hydrolyzed to adenosine diphosphate (ADP) and inorganic phosphate (P$_i$), the reaction also generates a proton. In mitochondria, ADP is phosphorylated to ATP by an enzyme, the F$_o$F$_1$ ATPase that uses the electrochemical protonic gradient across the inner mitochondrial membrane as the driving force to power the reaction. The ATP-generating reaction catalyzed by the F$_o$F$_1$ ATPase consumes a proton. Accordingly, the net yield of protons is zero when ATP is hydrolyzed in the cell and then regenerated through the process of mitochondrial oxidative phosphorylation. In contrast, protons are not consumed by the two ATP-generating substrate-level phosphorylation reactions that occur during glycolysis. Accordingly, the net yield of protons is positive when ATP is hydrolyzed in the cell and then regenerated only by the anaerobic breakdown of glucose. Thus, during anaerobic glycolysis, the utilization of ATP (to power cellular processes) coupled with the anaerobic production of ATP by substrate-level phosphorylation reactions results in the development of acidosis.[89]

Base excess (BE) is defined as the amount of base (in millimoles) that is required to titrate 1 liter of whole arterial blood to a pH of 7.40 with the sample fully saturated with oxygen at 37°C under an atmosphere with PCO_2 = 40 mm Hg. In trauma patients, repetitive measurements of calculated BE are commonly used to guide resuscitation. The data supporting this practice are retrospective.[17,55,98,108,189] It is important to note that BE can be influenced by the choice of resuscitation fluid. When patients are resuscitated using large volumes of normal saline, the large chloride load can induce the development of metabolic acidosis even in the absence of tissue hypoxia and anaerobic metabolism.[104]

Measures of Tissue Perfusion

Scvo$_2$, lactate, and BE are all global indices of tissue perfusion. It has been hypothesized that maldistribution of blood flow may be a greater problem in shock than is the decrease in total cardiac output. In hemorrhagic or cardiogenic shock, blood flow to the splanchnic organs decreases out of proportion to the decrease in cardiac output.[167] Thus, monitoring perfusion to the gastrointestinal (GI) tract might be an ideal way to titrate resuscitation of shock. Because tissue PCO_2 is increased in low flow states as a result of decreased clearance and increased release (from the reaction of bicarbonate anion with protons), measuring mucosal PCO_2 has been advocated as a way to monitor perfusion of the GI tract.[69] Results from several prospective studies suggest that the ability to normalize gastric mucosal PCO_2 or the closely related calculated parameter, gastric mucosal pH (pH$_i$), within 24 h of starting resuscitation portends a good outcome for trauma victims.[14,44,99,100,171] Moreover, several studies suggested that there is a poor correlation between pH$_i$ and global indices of perfusion, suggesting that tissue capnometry might be a more sensitive way to detect visceral hypoperfusion.[44,99,171] Small increases (5–15 mm Hg) in the difference between arterial and gastric mucosal PCO_2 become apparent before other signs of hemodynamic instability.[83,217] The converse is true as well; when normal perfusion is restored, the mucosal–arterial PCO_2 gap normalizes.[123,124] Although attractive on theoretical grounds, measurements of gastric P_{CO_2} have not gained much favor among clinicians. The currently available technique remains somewhat cumbersome and the reliability of the method can be confounded by factors such as enteral feeding and gastric acid secretion.[69]

Weil and colleagues extended the notion of monitoring gastric mucosal P_{CO_2} to measurements of esophageal and later sublingual mucosal P_{CO_2}.[178] The tongue is supplied by systemic vessels not mesenteric ones, and thus monitoring sublingual P_{CO_2} is probably not advantageous because it provides an index of hepatosplanchnic perfusion. Rather, this approach for monitoring is attractive because it represents a very simple and noninvasive way to assess global perfusion in almost any patient.[165,212] If the sublingual P_{CO_2}–arterial P_{CO_2} gap is within the normal range (<25 mm Hg), then the diagnosis of a low output form of shock can be excluded. If the sublingual P_{CO_2}–arterial P_{CO_2} gap is abnormally wide, then hypoperfusion is present and efforts to improve resuscitation, and possibly obtain more specific diagnostic information regarding the adequacy of cardiac filling and performance, are warranted.[207]

Future Approaches for Regional Tissue Perfusion Monitoring

Orthogonal polarization spectral (OPS) imaging uses polarized light to enable clinicians to visualize the flow of blood through the microcirculation at the bedside or in the operating room.* The microcirculation is easily visualized and individual blood cells can be identified as they flow through the vasculature. The currently available device that incorporates this technology has proven useful as a research tool, but its utility in clinical practice remains uncertain.

Near infrared spectroscopy (NIRS) permits monitoring of the redox state of the terminal enzyme, cytochrome oxidase, in the mitochondrial redox chain. Although quite expensive and difficult to use, this technology is attractive because it permits direct assessment of the adequacy of delivery of oxygen to the actual site where it is utilized in cells to support the synthesis of ATP. Although still largely an experimental tool, NIRS has been used to assess myocardial and cerebral oxygenation in patients.[148]

Monitoring the NADH content of cells represents another intriguing way to assess tissue perfusion. Reducing equivalents in the form of NADH (and the reduced form of flavin adenine dinucleotide, $FADH_2$) are generated during the metabolism of various substrates, including fats and sugars. These reducing equivalents are then oxidized by the electron transport chain in mitochondria, using molecular oxygen as the final electron acceptor and the energy thereby released to drive the phosphorylation of ADP to form ATP. During tissue dysoxia, NADH accumulates in cells and thus monitoring NADH levels is a way to assess the delivery of oxygen to cells. NADH, but not NAD^+, fluoresces following excitation with ultraviolet light. Very sensitive detectors can measure NADH autofluorescence and, hence, provide information about cellular bioenergics.[11,52,96,97] Whether this technology can be made sufficiently simple and robust to be useful in clinical practice remains to be determined.

Most clinicians assess the adequacy of cardiac preload during the resuscitation of patients with shock by inserting a central venous pressure (CVP) or Swan-Ganz catheter and determining CVP or pulmonary artery occlusion pressure (PAOP). However, neither CVP nor PAOP correlates well with the true parameter of interest, left ventricular end-diastolic volume (LVEDV).[79] Extremely high or low CVP or PAOP values, of course, are informative, but readings in a large middle zone, say from 5 to 20 mm Hg, are not very useful (Figure 50-4). Furthermore, changes in CVP or PAOP fail to correlate well with changes in stoke volume (Figure 50-5).[127] Echocardiography can be used to estimate LVEDV, but this approach is very dependent on the skill and training of the individual using it,[48,113,193,205] and isolated measurements of LVEDV fail to predict the hemodynamic response to alterations in preload.[82]

When intrathoracic pressure increases during the application of positive airway pressure in mechanically ventilated patients, venous return decreases, and, as a consequence, left ventricular stroke volume (LVSV) also decreases. Therefore, pulse pressure variation (PPV) during a positive pressure can be used to predict the responsiveness of cardiac output to changes in preload.[144] PPV is defined as the difference between the maximal pulse pressure and the minimum pulse pressure divided by the average of these two pressures (Figure 50-6).[144] Michard and colleagues validated this approach by comparing PPV, CVP, PAOP, and systolic pressure variation as predictors of preload responsiveness in a cohort of critically ill patients. They classified patients as being preload responsive if their cardiac index increased by at least 15% after rapid infusion of a standard volume of intravenous fluid.[143] Receiver-operating characteristic (ROC) curves

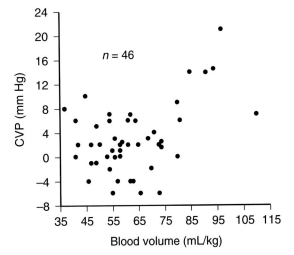

Figure 50–4 **Correlation between central venous pressure (CVP) and blood volume.** In 46 patients with shock, the correlation is statistically significant; however, CVP is not a clinically useful predictor of blood volume. *(Reprinted from Cohn JN: Central venous pressure as a guide to volume expansion. Ann Intern Med 66:1284, 1967, with permission.)*

*References 21, 43, 77, 85, 120–122, 140.

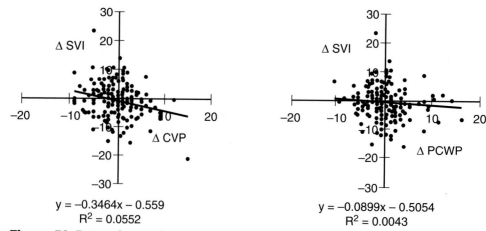

$$y = -0.3464x - 0.559$$
$$R^2 = 0.0552$$

$$y = -0.0899x - 0.5054$$
$$R^2 = 0.0043$$

Figure 50–5 Correlation of changes in central venous pressure (ΔCVP) and pulmonary artery capillary wedge pressure (ΔPCWP) as they relate in the changes in stroke volume index (ΔSVI). Note the poor correlation between ΔCVP or ΔPAOP (PCWP), on the one hand, and ΔSVI, on the other.
(Modified from Lichtwarck-Aschoff M: Intrathoracic blood volume accurately reflects circulatory volume status in critically ill patients with mechanical ventilation. Intensive Care Med 18:145, 1992, with permission.)

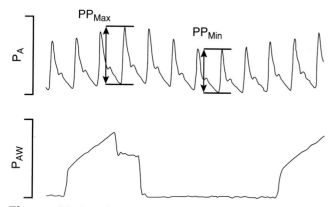

Figure 50–6 Pulse pressure variation with mechanical ventilation. The difference between the maximum pulse pressure (PP_{max}) and minimum pulse pressure (PP_{min}) before and after a positive pressure breath is delivered. P_{aw}, airway pressure; P_A, arterial pressure. A pulse pressure variation of >15% suggests that the patient's cardiac output will increase with an increase in preload (i.e., the patient will be volume responsive).
(Reprinted from Gunn, SR, Pinsky, MR: Implications of arterial pressure variation in patients in the intensive care unit. Curr Opin Crit Care 7:214, 2001, Lippincott Williams & Wilkins, Inc., with permission.)

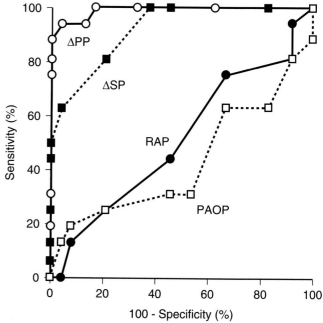

Figure 50–7 Receiver-operating characteristic curve for pulmonary artery occlusion pressure (PAOP), right atrial pressure or CVP (RAP), systolic pressure variation (ΔSP), pulse pressure variation (ΔPP), and their respective predictive values to detect volume responsiveness in a mechanically ventilated patient.
(Reprinted from Michard F, Boussat S, Chemla D, et al: Relationship between respiratory changes in arterial pulse pressure and fluid responsiveness in septic patients with acute circulatory failure. Am J Respir Crit Care Med 162:136, 2000, with permission.)

demonstrated that PPV was the best predictor of preload responsiveness (Figure 50-7). Although atrial arrhythmias can interfere with the usefulness of this technique,[82] PPV remains a very useful approach for assessing preload responsiveness in most patients because of its simplicity and reliability.

Asanguinous Intravenous Fluids

Numerous clinical trials have been carried out to address the question of whether patients with shock are better treated with colloid solutions or crystalloid solutions. Meta-analyses of the results from these trials suggest that outcome is not affected by the choice of fluid.[47,182]

The two most commonly used crystalloid solutions are 0.9% sodium chloride solution (normal saline; NS) and Ringer's lactate solution (LR). The composition of these two

Table 50–1

Composition of Common Resuscitation Fluids

Crystalloids	Na (mEq/l)	K (mEq/l)	Cl (mEq/l)	Ca (mEq/l)	Lactate (mEq/l)	Osmol (mOsm/l)
NaCl 0.9%	154		154			308
Ringer's lactate	130	4	110	3	27	275
Colloids						
Albumin 5% (50 g/l)	130–160		130–160			308
Albumin 25% (240 g + 10 g globulins per liter)	130–160		130–160			1500
Hydroxyethyl starch + NaCl 0.9% (Hespan)	154		154			310
Hydroxyethyl starch + balanced salt solution (Hextend)	143	3	124	5	28	307

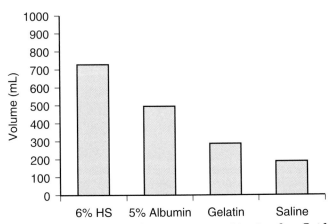

Figure 50–8 Plasma volume expansion 90 min after fluid administration in postoperative general surgical patients. HS indicates 6% hetastarch in normal saline.
(*Reprinted from Lamke LO, Liljedahl SO: Plasma volume changes after infusion of various plasma expanders. Resuscitation 5:96, 1976, with permission.*)

Table 50–2

Physical Properties of Colloids

	wMW × 10³	COPᵃ (mm Hg)	Molar substitution
5% albumin	69	19	None
20% albumin	69	78	None
Dextran 70	70	40	None
Pentastarch	280	40	0.5
6% hetastarch	450	30	0.7

COP, colloid osmotic pressure.

fluids is shown in Table 50-1. Although NS and LR have been regarded by many clinicians as being essentially interchangeable, accumulating data support the view that the use of large volumes of NS, but not LR, promotes the development of hyperchloremic metabolic acidosis[105,181,210] and coagulopathy.[209]

Per unit volume, colloid solutions are more efficient than crystalloid solutions for expanding intravascular volume (Figure 50-8). Colloids include the starches, hetastarch and pentastarch; human serum albumin (HSA); gelatin; and dextran. Colloids are dissolved in either NS or a balanced salt solution. In North America, the most commonly used colloids are HSA and hetastarch (Table 50-2). Recent reviews suggest that there are no clinically significant differences among the various colloid solutions when used for shock resuscitation.[3,40,41] When compared with the use of

804 saline-based solutions (Hespan), the use of hetastarch dissolved in a calcium-containing low-chloride balanced salt solution (Hextend) may be associated less acidosis and use of blood products.[74,214]

Blood Products

In hemorrhagic shock, the rapid administration of packed red blood cells (PRBC) and, if indicated, platelets and thawed fresh frozen plasma (FFP) can be lifesaving. Whenever possible, fully cross-matched PRBC are preferable. However, cross-matching is time-consuming, and when immediate therapy is warranted, type-specific blood can be given safely. In dire emergencies, type O Rh-negative blood can be administered to women of childbearing potential and type O Rh-positive blood can be given to men or postmenopausal females.

Vasoactive Agents

Table 50-3 lists the vasoactive and inotropic agents that are most commonly used for the management of critically ill patients. Infusion of a vasopressor to support blood pressure should never be used as a substitute for intravascular volume expansion when acute hypovolemia is the primary problem underlying the development of shock. When inappropriate vasodilation is a component of the pathophysiological process, as is often the case in patients with septic shock, then infusion of a vasopressor may be needed to restore MAP to a value, typically about 60 mm Hg, that is high enough to maintain adequate renal and cerebral perfusion. Diminished myocardial contractility is a primary problem of cardiogenic shock, and alterations in cardiac performance also occur in other forms of shock (notably sepsis) as well. When tissue perfusion is compromised because of impaired myocardial contractility, then agents with positive inotropic activity, such as dobutamine, epinephrine, or milrinone, should be employed.

▶ SHOCK AFTER CARDIAC SURGERY

Numerous factors can contribute to the development of shock after cardiac operations, including hypovolemia (inadequate preload); cardiac dysfunction secondary to myocardial stunning secondary to tissue ischemia and reperfusion, myocardial infarction, and the effects of cardiodepressant cytokines, such as tumor necrosis factor (TNF)-α, released during cardiopulmonary bypass; and inappropriate peripheral vasodilation, possibly secondary to acidosis-induced activation of ATP-sensitive potassium channels in vascular smooth muscle cells.[33] Coronary perfusion pressure is important to maintain flow through newly placed bypass grafts, and MAP should be maintained at about 70 mm Hg in the early postoperative period.

Hypovolemia, due to inadequately replaced operative losses, ongoing hemorrhage, or sequestration of "third-spaced" fluid, is a common cause of both low cardiac output after cardiac operations. Because ventricular compliance is often abnormal after these procedures, measurements of CVP or PAOP (or even left atrial pressure) may provide misleading information regarding preload responsiveness. Accordingly, measurements of pulse pressure variation, as described above, can be quite useful for guiding resuscitation of intravascular volume. Of course, this approach will not be useful in patients with atrial dysrhythmias or if an intraaortic balloon pump is in place. In these cases, transesophageal echocardiography can be used to provide information about ventricular filling and function.[103]

▶ SEPSIS AND SEPTIC SHOCK: DEFINITION AND PATHOPHYSIOLOGY

Approximately 750,000 people in the United States develop severe sepsis each year.[5] Despite advances in critical care medicine, the mortality rate for this condition remains about 30%.[5]

According to the results from a recent international consensus conference, sepsis is the clinical syndrome defined by the presence of both infection and a systemic inflammatory response.[125] Infection is defined as a pathological process caused by the invasion of normally sterile tissue or fluid or body cavity by pathogenic or potentially pathogenic microorganisms. Signs of a systemic inflammatory response are listed in Box 50-1. Severe sepsis is defined as the presence of sepsis plus organ dysfunction.

Pathogenesis

The pathophysiology of sepsis is extraordinarily complex and a thorough discussion of this topic, which by itself is the subject of whole textbooks, is beyond the scope of this chapter. In simple terms, sepsis is the consequence of excessive and disseminated activation of the innate immune system. Cells of the innate immune system, including monocytes, macrophages, and PMNs, are activated by microbes or microbial products, such as lipopolysaccharide (LPS; endotoxin), bacterial DNA, and peptidoglycans. Once activated, these cells secrete a variety of proinflammatory cytokines, including TNF, interleukin (IL)-1β, IL-6, IL-8, and IL-18. These mediators, in turn, activate endothelial cells and induce increased expression of iNOS and cyclooxygenase-2, an enzyme that catalyzes the formation of prostaglandins and thromboxane A_2. Excessive production of nitric oxide and possibly certain vasodilating prostaglandins, such as prostacyclin, leads to loss of vasomotor tone. In addition to the release of these mediators, activated monocytes, macrophages, and PMNs release proteolytic enzymes and ROS that can damage cytosolic membranes or even nuclear DNA. Microbial invasion and the release of proinflammatory mediators also lead to intravascular activation of the coagulation cascade, promoting microvascular thrombosis and impaired tissue perfusion. Cytokines and/or ROS also can impair mitochondrial function, leading to the development of cytopathic hypoxia, as noted previously.

Cardiovascular Manifestations

Heart rate is almost always increased in patients with sepsis. Prior to resuscitation, intravascular volume is commonly reduced in patients with sepsis and is a major factor leading to circulatory instability and collapse.[42,162,166,213] In patients who have been inadequately fluid resuscitated,

Table 50-3

Commonly Used Vasopressors and Inotropes, Dosages and Potency

Agent	Dose range	Peripheral vasculature		Cardiac effects			Typical use
		Vasoconstriction	Vasodilation	Heart rate	Contractility	Dysrhythmias	
Dopamine	1–1 µg/kg/min	0	1+	1+	1+	1+	Falling out of favor as first-line vasopressor; "renal dose" does not improve renal function; may be used with bradycardia and hypotension
(Dopaminergic activity 4+ all doses)	5–10 µg/kg/min	1–2+	1+	2+	2+	2+	
	11–20 µg/kg/min	2–3+	1+	2+	2+	3+	
Vasopressin	0.04–0.1 units/min	3–4+	0	0	0	1+	Septic shock, postcardiopulmonary bypass shock state
Phenylephrine	20–200 µg/min	4+	0	0	0	1+	Vasodilatory shock
Norepinephrine	2–20 µg/min	4+	0	2+	2+	2+	First line vasopressor for septic shock, vasodilatory shock
Epinephrine	1–8 µg/min	4+	0	4+	4+	4+	Refractory shock, shock with bradycardia, anaphylactic shock
Dobutamine	1–20 µg/kg/min	1+	2+	1–2+	3+	3+	Cardiogenic shock, septic shock
Milrinone	37.5–75 µg/min	0	2+	1+	3+	2+	Cardiogenic shock, right heart failure, dilates pulmonary artery; caution in renal failure

806

Box 50–1. Diagnostic Criteria for Sepsis.[c]

Infection[a] documented or suspected, and some of the
following[b]

General variables
  Fever (core temperature >38.3° C)
  Hypothermia (core temperature <36° C)
  Heart rate >90 bpm or >2 SD above normal value for age
  Tachypnea
  Altered mental status
  Significant edema or positive fluid balance (>20 ml/kg
    over 24 h)
  Hyperglycemia (plasma glucose) >120 mg/dl or
    7.7 mmol/liter in the absence of diabetes

Inflammatory variables
  Leukocytosis (WBC count >12,000 μl^{-1})
  Leukopenia (WBC count <4,000 μl^{-1})
  Normal WBC count with >10% immature forms
  Plasma C-reactive protein >2 SD above the normal value
  Plasma procalcitonin >2 SD above the normal value

Hemodynamic variables
  Arterial hypotension[b] (SBP <90 mm Hg, MAP <70, or
    an SBP decrease >40 mm Hg in adults or <2 SD
    below normal for age)
  Svo_2 >70%[b]
  Cardiac index >3.5 liters/min/m²

Organ dysfunction variables
  Arterial hypoxemia (Pao_2/Fio_2 <300)
  Acute oliguria (urine output <0.5 ml/kg/h or 45 mmol/liter
    for at least 2 h)
  Creatinine increase >0.5 mg/dl
  Coagulation abnormalities (INR >1.5 or aPTT >60 s)
  Ileus (absent bowel sounds)
  Thrombocytopenia (platelet count <100,000 μl^{-1})
  Hyperbilirubinemia (plasma total bilirubin >4 mg/dl or
    70 mmol/liter)

Tissue perfusion variables
  Hyperlactemia (>1 mmol/liter)
  Decreased capillary refill or mottling

Reprinted with permission from Levy M, Fink M, Marshall JC, et al: 2001
SCCM/ESICM/ACCP/ATS/SIS International Sepsis Definitions Conference.
Crit Care Med 31:1250–1256, 2003.

WBC, white blood cell; SBP, systolic blood pressure; MAP, mean arterial blood
pressure; Svo_2, mixed venous oxygen saturation; INR, international normalized
ratio; aPTT, activated partial thromboplastin time.

[a]Infection defined as a pathological process induced by a microorganism.

[b]Svo_2 sat >70% is normal in children (normally, 75–80%), and CI 3.5–5.5 is normal in
children; therefore, neither should be used as signs of sepsis in newborns or
children.

[c]Diagnostic criteria for sepsis in the pediatric population are signs and symptoms
of inflammation plus infection with hyper- or hypothermia (rectal temperature
>38.5 or <35° C), tachycardia (may be absent in hypothermic patients), and at
least one of the following indications of altered organ function: altered mental
status, hypoxemia, increased serum lactate level, or bounding pulses.

septic shock can present as a hypodynamic state with a low
cardiac output.[166,213] Multiple factors are responsible for
inadequate preload in patients with sepsis, including
increased venous capacitance, increased microvascular permeability, increased insensible losses secondary to fever,
and poor fluid intake.

Myocardial depression and low supraventricular rhythm
(SVR) are the characteristic hemodynamic features found

in patients with sepsis.[161] Decreased systolic function is
manifested by low left ventricular stroke work index
(LVSWI)[151,197] and decreased left ventricular ejection fraction.[157,158] Myocardial depression is reversible in patients
who recover from septic shock, whereas ventricular function remains depressed in nonsurvivors.[86,151,158] The
depression of cardiac function in sepsis is caused by
the presence of circulating myocardial depressant factors.[162] TNF-α, an important proinflammatory cytokine,
has been shown to impair myocardial performance.[153]
Studies suggest that TNF-α and another key proinflammatory cytokine, IL-1, act synergistically to cause myocardial depression in sepsis.[116] The mechanisms by which
these cytokines induce acute negative inotropic effects
include Ca^{2+} dyshomeostasis, oxidant stress, disruption
of excitation–contraction coupling, desensitization of the
β-adrenoreceptor, as well as myocardial edema and
myocyte necrosis.[91,115] These myocardial effects may be
mediated in part via the induction iNOS.[159,160]

Pulmonary Dysfunction

Peripheral stimulation of pulmonary J receptors, carotid
body chemoreceptors, as well as hypoperfusion of the
medullary respiratory center, results in tachypnea, hyper-
pnea, hypocapnia, and respiratory alkalosis. In addition,
dynamic compliance of the lung–chest wall unit typically
decreases, further adding to the work of breathing. The
increased work of breathing, possibly combined with
hypoperfusion of the diaphragm, can lead to respiratory failure. The inflammatory process that leads to shock in some
patients with sepsis also can injure the lung, leading to the
development of ARDS. Indeed, sepsis is the most common
cause of ARDS.[112,184] The mortality rate for patients with
sepsis complicated by ARDS approaches 60%.[112,184] The
pathophysiology and management of patients with ARDS
have been extensively reviewed in the literature and are
beyond the scope of this chapter.[37,146]

Renal Dysfunction

Acute renal failure (ARF) is a serious complication in
patients with sepsis and circulatory shock. Despite improvements in the support of these patients, the mortality rate
remains high (35–80%).[81] The pathogenic mechanisms leading to ARF in patients with sepsis are unclear; however,
cytokine- and/or oxidant-mediated damage to renal epithelial cells and alterations in renal perfusion probably play
important roles.

HPA Axis

IL-1, IL-6, and TNF-α stimulate ACTH secretion from
cultured pituitary preparations and IL-1α, IL-1β, and IL-6
stimulate glucocorticoid production in cultured adrenal
preparations.[202] Acute administration of recombinant TNF-α
to humans increases circulating ACTH and cortisol
levels.[149] Cortisol inhibits signaling via the proinflammatory
transcription factor, NF-κB, and down-regulates the
expression of TNF-α and other proinflammatory
cytokines.[10] Thus, cytokine-mediated activation of the HPA

axis represents a negative feedback loop that helps to prevent excessive inflammation. Interestingly, however, proinflammatory cytokines also can suppress the HPA axis and glucocorticoid receptor (GR) function. Persistent elevation of circulating IL-6 levels blunts the release of ACTH[139] and TNF-α impairs corticotrophin-releasing hormone-stimulated ACTH release.[15,73] Furthermore, inappropriately low ACTH and cortisol levels are common in patients with sepsis.[15,168,194]

Gastrointestinal Tract

Both structural changes and alterations in cellular function lead to increased intestinal mucosal permeability in sepsis. The changes in gastrointestinal permeability are postulated to play a major role in the development of multisystem organ dysfunction. It is likely that a number of mechanisms lead to intestinal mucosal injury, including ischemia, mediator-induced cytotoxicity, and the generation of reactive oxygen species that inhibits mitochondrial respiration (cytopathic hypoxia).[203,204]

Central Nervous System (CNS)

Blood flow through the CNS remains remarkably constant over a wide range of driving pressures; this phenomenon is called autoregulation. Because of autoregulation, CNS perfusion is typically maintained in patients with shock unless MAP is less 50 mm Hg. The biochemical basis for the development of encephalopathy in patients with serious infections is poorly understood, but most patients with sepsis develop alterations in mental status ranging from impaired attention and orientation to deep coma.[66,155] Septic encephalopathy is a diagnosis of exclusion, and other conditions, such as encephalitis, liver or renal failure, or adrenal insufficiency should be ruled out.

Multiple Organ Dysfunction Syndrome (MODS)

Although isolated dysfunction of a single organ system (usually the lungs) is common in patients with sepsis, many patients with serious infections develop a syndrome, MODS, that is characterized by dysfunction of multiple organs.[111,169] If MODS develops, survival is uncommon. The pathophysiological mechanism(s) responsible for MODS remain an active area of investigation. One key factor that must be considered in assessing the validity of any proposed theory is that the histopathology of human MODS is remarkably bland; widespread cell death, whether due to necrosis or apoptosis, certainly cannot be the explanation for the development of acute lung injury, hepatic dysfunction, and acute renal failure in patients with MODS.[93] Rather, MODS appears to be a syndrome caused by widespread cellular dysfunction. Why cells in multiple tissues and organs fail to function normally in patients with sepsis remains an open question. One theory proposes that failure of the gastrointestinal mucosal barrier permits systemic absorption of microbes and microbial products that promote ongoing inflammation and cytokine-mediated organ damage.[7] Indeed, Doig and colleagues demonstrated an excellent relationship between increased intestinal permeability on admission to the ICU and the subsequent development of MODS.[57] These data notwithstanding, it is undoubtedly too simplistic to characterize MODS as a syndrome caused by the deleterious effects of gut-derived toxins. Rather, it seems much more probable that one or more common cellular pathways (e.g., cytokine-induced alterations in the expression of key cellular proteins) are activated by the dysregulated systemic inflammatory response that underlies the development of sepsis and septic shock.

► MANAGEMENT OF SEPTIC SHOCK

In patients with sepsis or septic shock, antimicrobial therapy remains a cornerstone of care. The choice of antibiotics depends on the likely source of infection, whether the infection is community acquired or nosocomial, the patient's immunologic status, and antibiotic resistance patterns in the hospital or community. Empiric therapy should be started as soon as the diagnosis is suspected and then tailored for specific microorganisms. Initially, multiple antibiotics may be necessary, but once an organism is isolated, monotherapy is usually adequate. Multiple antibiotic coverage is recommended for *Pseudomonas aeruginosa*, febrile neutropenia (with shock), and severe intraabdominal infections.[175]

It is crucial to identify, if possible, the source of infection. If the infection is caused by a problem that can be corrected by a surgical or radiological intervention, then resuscitation should occur simultaneously with the necessary procedure. Efforts to "tune the patient up" prior to fixing an anastomotic leak or draining a large abscess are not advised; resuscitation can occur in the operating room or radiology suite as well as in the ICU.

Vasoactive Agents

Vasoactive agents (Table 50-3) are often required to maintain adequate perfusion pressure in patients with septic shock, even after aggressive resuscitation of intravascular volume. Failure to maintain adequate tissue perfusion increases the risk of MODS and death.

Guidelines published by the Society of Critical Care Medicine and the Third European Consensus Conference in Intensive Care Medicine recommend dopamine as a first-line agent.[92,201] Nevertheless, recent evidence suggests that dopamine may not be the ideal vasopressor for a number of reasons. In sepsis, chronotropic sensitivity to β-adrenergic stimulation is increased.[192] Tachycardia and tachydysrhythmias, therefore, frequently limit the value of this agent in patients with septic shock.[136,138,183] In addition, the positive chronotropic and inotropic effects of dopamine increase myocardial oxygen requirements, possibly promoting the development of cardiac ischemia (especially in the presence of coronary atherosclerosis).[183] Dopamine also can adversely affect mesenteric perfusion.[101,147,152,185] Although still widely used, so-called "renal-dose" dopamine (i.e., infusion of the drug at less 5 μg/kg/min) fails to decrease the incidence of acute renal failure in critically ill patients.[17,106,135,136]

808

Norepinephrine activates α- and β₁-adrenoreceptors. Many experts regard this agent as the first-line vasopressor for treating hypotension in septic patients with persistent hypotension despite adequate resuscitation of intravascular volume.[136,138]

Dobutamine, a racemic mixture of two stereoisomers of a synthetic catecholamine, increases myocardial contractility by activating cardiac α- and β₁-adrenoreceptors.[107,173] Dobutamine also causes some arteriolar vasodilation by activating β₂-adrenoreceptors on vascular smooth muscle cells. Evidence suggests that the α effects cause systemic venous constriction thereby increasing venous return and augmenting cardiac output. These effects may take place in the small capacitance vessels.[22,107,173] Dobutamine can be useful to treat septic shock when cardiac output is low. Because dobutamine-induced vasodilation can exacerbate hypotension, this agent is often combined with a vasoconstrictor, such as norepinephrine, for the management of septic shock.[60,123]

Epinephrine is a potent α-, β₁-, and β₂-adrenergic agonist. It increases peripheral arteriolar tone as well as cardiac contractility. It is the first-line agent for the treatment of anaphylactic shock and is used to support myocardial contractility following cardiac surgery. Unlike other commonly used inotropic agents or vasoconstrictors, epinephrine increases blood lactate concentration in patients with sepsis.[56,123,128] Increased blood lactate levels may reflect accelerated aerobic glycogenolysis and/or maldistribution of blood flow. However, in either event, exacerbation of lactic acidosis is undesirable, and, thus, epinephrine is not a front line agent for septic shock.

Phenylephrine is a synthetic catecholamine that is a selective α-adrenergic agonist. It is commonly used intraoperatively to counter the vasodilatory effects of anesthesia. There are limited data on the hemodynamic effects of phenylephrine in patients with sepsis.[72,216]

AVP has been studied as a vasoactive agent for the management of hypotension in patients with sepsis or other conditions associated with systemic inflammation. Vasopressin receptors are down-regulated in sepsis. This effect appears to be mediated by IL-1β, TNF-α, and interferon-γ in a nitric oxide-independent fashion.[39] Although AVP is not a potent vasopressor in normal subjects, very low doses of this agent (0.04 units/min) markedly increase arterial blood pressure in hypotensive septic patients with intractable hypotension.[119,129] In addition, AVP enhances the pressor response to catecholamines. Cardiopulmonary bypass, particularly if very prolonged, is associated with activation of a systemic inflammatory response that can lead to profound and refractory vasodilation.[109] AVP (0.1 units/min) reverses this vasodilatory shock state.[8,58] Because high doses of AVP are associated with mesenteric ischemia, this agent should be used with caution and doses should not exceed 0.04–0.1 units/min.[59]

Hemodynamic Goals

The primary aim of the initial phase of resuscitation should be to increase MAP to greater than 60 mm Hg in order to keep blood pressure within the autoregulatory range for the kidneys, CNS, and other organs. Many clinicians regard the necessity to use vasopressor agents or signs of poor tissue per-

fusion to be indications for placement of a pulmonary artery (Swan-Ganz) catheter for monitoring. Rigorous data supporting the value of this sort of monitoring, however, are lacking. Indeed, considerable controversy exists regarding this issue.° Currently, the best available evidence indicates that routine use of a pulmonary artery catheter fails to improve outcome and increases the risk of pulmonary embolization in high-risk surgical patients.[177] Data from a carefully performed single-center randomized clinical trial support the view that titrating resuscitation to achieve central venous oxygen saturation ≥70% within the first few hours after presentation improves the outcome for patients with septic shock.[169] The protocol employed in this study utilized red blood cell transfusions to increase hematocrit to 30% and infusion of dobutamine (titrated up to a maximum 20 μg/kg/min) to increase cardiac output (Figure 50-9). In the absence of strong data to support other strategies, the hemodynamic goals for the treatment of septic shock after the first 6 h should be maintenance of CVP between 10 and 15 mm Hg, blood hemoglobin concentration greater than 7 g/dl,[87] MAP greater than 60 mm Hg, and urine output greater than 0.5 ml/kg/min.

Specific Therapy

Sepsis is associated with profound decreases in plasma levels of the naturally occurring anticoagulant, protein C.[71] The risk of mortality is inversely correlated with circulating protein C concentration.[71] Recently, a large, randomized, placebo-controlled study demonstrated that treatment of patients with severe sepsis with a formulation of recombinant human activated protein C, called drotrecogin alfa (activated), is associated with a reduction in the relative risk of death by 19.4%.[19] The incidence of serious bleeding was higher in the treatment group (3.5 vs. 2.0%). The treatment effect was most apparent in the sickest subset of patients.[65] Although this agent is very expensive, two recent cost-effective analyses suggest that the cost of treating patients with drotrecogin alfa (activated) is comparable to other commonly employed interventions for serious diseases when the data are analyzed on a cost per life saved basis.[4,131] Based on these data, administration of drotrecogin alfa (activated) is indicated for patients with severe sepsis with a high risk of mortality, provided contraindications (e.g., high risk of bleeding) are absent.

Although very high doses of corticosteroids were previously advocated for the treatment of septic shock, the results from several large multicentric randomized clinical trials led clinicians to abandon this therapeutic approach.[28,64,195] Subsequently, findings from two small single-center randomized trials suggested that prolonged administration of physiological "stress doses" of hydrocortisone can improve hemodynamics and promote resolution of shock in patients with severe sepsis.[26,35] Recently, these findings were confirmed and extended by Annane and colleagues, who demonstrated a 10% absolute reduction in mortality when vasopressor-dependent septic shock patients with evidence of adrenal insufficiency were treated with hydrocortisone and a mineralocorticoid.[6] All patients with proven or suspected adrenal insufficiency and septic shock should be treated with stress doses of hydrocortisone.

°References 50, 51, 54, 94, 177, 215.

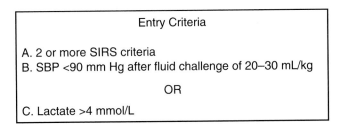

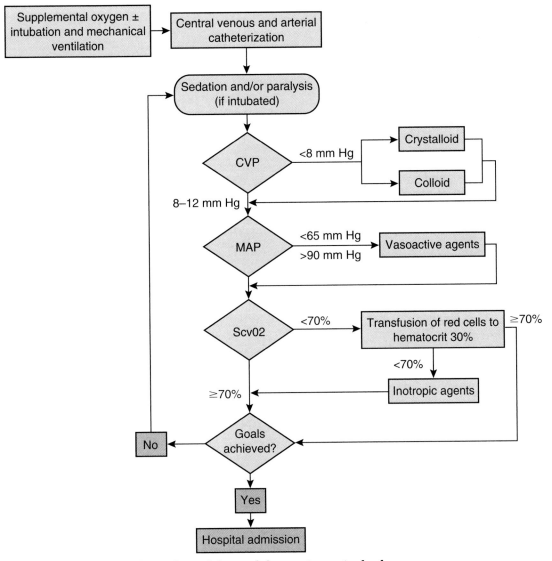

Figure 50–9 **Protocol for early goal-directed therapy in septic shock.**
(Reprinted with permission from Rivers E, Nguyen B: Early goal-directed therapy in the treatment of severe sepsis and septic shock. N Engl J Med 345:1371, 2001.)

REFERENCES

1. Abraham E, Shoemaker WC, Bland RD, et al: Sequential cardiorespiratory patterns in septic shock. Crit Care Med 11:799–803, 1983.
2. Abramson D, Scalea TM, Hitchcock R, et al: Lactate clearance and survival following injury. J Trauma 35:584–588, 1993.
3. Alderson P, Schierhout G, Roberts I, et al: Colloids versus crystalloids for fluid resuscitation in critically ill patients. Cochrane Database Syst Rev CD000567, 2000.
4. Angus DC, Linde-Zwirble WT, Clermont G, et al: Cost-effectiveness of drotrecogin alfa (activated) in the treatment of severe sepsis. Crit Care Med 31:1–11, 2003.
5. Angus DC, Linde-Zwirble WT, Lidicker J, et al: Epidemiology of severe sepsis in the United States: Analysis of incidence, outcome, and associated costs of care. Crit Care Med 29: 1303–1310, 2001.
6. Annane D, Sebille V, Charpentier C, et al: Effect of treatment with low doses of hydrocortisone and fludrocortisone on mortality in patients with septic shock. JAMA 288:862–871, 2002.

7. Aranow JS, Fink MP: Determinants of intestinal barrier failure in critical illness. Br J Anaesth 77:71–81, 1996.

8. Argenziano M, Chen JM, Choudhri AF, et al: Management of vasodilatory shock after cardiac surgery: Identification of predisposing factors and use of a novel pressor agent. J Thorac Cardiovasc Surg 116:973–980, 1998.

9. Astiz ME, DeGent GE, Lin RY, et al: Microvascular function and rheologic changes in hyperdynamic sepsis. Crit Care Med 23:265–721, 1995.

10. Auphan N, DiDonato JA, Rosette C, et al: Immunosuppression by glucocorticoids: Inhibition of NF-kB activity through induction of IkB synthesis. Science 270:286–290, 1995.

11. Avontuur JA, Bruining HA, Ince C: Inhibition of nitric oxide synthesis causes myocardial ischemia in endotoxemic rats. Circ Res 76:418–425, 1995.

12. Bakker J, Coffernils M, Leon M, et al: Blood lactate levels are superior to oxygen-derived variables in predicting outcome in human septic shock. Chest 99:956–962, 1991.

13. Bakker J, Gris P, Coffernils M, et al: Serial blood lactate levels can predict the development of multiple organ failure following septic shock. Am J Surg 171:221–226, 1996.

14. Barquist E, Kirton O, Windsor J, et al: The impact of antioxidant and splanchnic-directed therapy on persistent uncorrected gastric mucosal pH in the critically injured trauma patient. J Trauma 44:355–360, 1998.

15. Bateman A, Singh A, Kral T, et al: The immune-hypothalamic-pituitary-adrenal axis. Endocr Rev 10:92–112, 1989.

16. Baue AE, Durham R, Faist E: Systemic inflammatory response syndrome (SIRS), multiple organ dysfunction syndrome (MODS), multiple organ failure (MOF): Are we winning the battle? Shock 10:79–89, 1998.

17. Bellomo R, Chapman M, Finfer S, et al: Low-dose dopamine in patients with early renal dysfunction: A placebo-controlled randomised trial. Australian and New Zealand Intensive Care Society (ANZICS) Clinical Trials Group. Lancet 356: 2139–2143, 2000.

18. Berger PB, Holmes DR Jr, Stebbins AL, et al: Impact of an aggressive invasive catheterization and revascularization strategy on mortality in patients with cardiogenic shock in the Global Utilization of Streptokinase and Tissue Plasminogen Activator for Occluded Coronary Arteries (GUSTO-I) trial. An observational study. Circulation 96: 122–127, 1997.

19. Bernard GR, Vincent JL, Laterre PF, et al: Efficacy and safety of recombinant human activated protein C for severe sepsis. N Engl J Med 344:699–709, 2001.

20. Beyar, R, Halperin HR, Tsitlik JE, et al: Circulatory assistance by intrathoracic pressure variations: Optimization and mechanisms studied by a mathematical model in relation to experimental data. Circ Res 64:703–720, 1989.

21. Biberthaler P, Langer S, Luchting B, et al: In vivo assessment of colon microcirculation: Comparison of the new OPS imaging technique with intravital microscopy. Eur J Med Res 6:525–534, 2001.

22. Binkley PF, Murray KD, Watson KM, et al: Dobutamine increases cardiac output of the total artificial heart. Implications for vascular contribution of inotropic agents to augmented ventricular function. Circulation 84:1210–1215, 1991.

23. Bishop MH, Shoemaker WC, Appel PL, et al: Prospective, randomized trial of survivor values of cardiac index, oxygen delivery, and oxygen consumption as resuscitation endpoints in severe trauma. J Trauma 38:780–787, 1995.

24. Blalock A: Shock: Further studies with particular reference to the effects of hemorrhage. Arch Surg 29:837, 1937.

25. Bland RD, Shoemaker WC, Abraham E, et al: Hemodynamic and oxygen transport patterns in surviving and nonsurviving postoperative patients. Crit Care Med 13:85–90, 1985.

26. Bollaert PE, Charpentier C, Levy B, et al: Reversal of late septic shock with supraphysiologic doses of hydrocortisone. Crit Care Med 26:645–650, 1998.

27. Bond RF, Johnson G III: Vascular adrenergic interactions during hemorrhagic shock. Fed Proc 44:281–289, 1985.

28. Bone RC, Fisher CJ Jr, Clemmer TP, et al: A controlled clinical trial of high-dose methylprednisolone in the treatment of severe sepsis and septic shock. N Engl J Med 317:653–658, 1987.

29. Borchelt BD, Wright PA, Evans JA, et al: Cell swelling and depolarization in hemorrhagic shock. J Trauma-Injury Infect Crit Care 39:187–192, 1995.

30. Boulos M, Astiz ME, Barua RS, et al: Impaired mitochondrial function induced by serum from septic shock patients is attenuated by inhibition of nitric oxide synthase and poly(ADP-ribose) synthase. Crit Care Med 31:353–358, 2003.

31. Boyd O, Grounds RM, Bennett ED: A randomized clinical trial of the effect of deliberate perioperative increase of oxygen delivery on mortality in high-risk surgical patients. JAMA 270:2699–2707, 1993.

32. Bracken MB, Shepard MJ, Holford TR, et al: Administration of methylprednisolone for 24 or 48 hours or tirilazad mesylate for 48 hours in the treatment of acute spinal cord injury. Results of the Third National Acute Spinal Cord Injury Randomized Controlled Trial. National Acute Spinal Cord Injury Study. JAMA 277:1597–1604, 1997.

33. Brayden JE: Functional roles of KATP channels in vascular smooth muscle. Clin Exp Pharmacol Physiol 29:312–316, 2002.

34. Brealey D, Brand M, Hargreaves I, et al: Association between mitochondrial dysfunction and severity and outcome of septic shock. Lancet 360:219–223, 2002.

35. Briegel J, Forst H, Haller M, et al: Stress doses of hydrocortisone reverse hyperdynamic septic shock: A prospective, randomized, double-blind, single-center study. Crit Care Med 27:723–732, 1999.

36. Broder G, Weil MH: Excess lactate: An index of reversibility of shock in human patients. Science 143:1457, 1964.

37. Brower RG, Rubenfeld GD: Lung-protective ventilation strategies in acute lung injury. Crit Care Med 31(4 Suppl): S312–S326, 2003.

38. Brown AF: Therapeutic controversies in the management of acute anaphylaxis. J Accid Emerg Med 15:89–95, 1998.

39. Bucher M, Hobbhahn J, Taeger K, et al: Cytokine-mediated downregulation of vasopressin V(1A) receptors during acute endotoxemia in rats. Am J Physiol Regul Integr Comp Physiol 282:R979–R984, 2002.

40. Bunn F, Alderson P, Hawkins V: Colloid solutions for fluid resuscitation. Cochrane Database Syst Rev CD001319, 2000.

41. Bunn F, Lefebvre C, Li Wan PA, et al: Human albumin solution for resuscitation and volume expansion in critically ill patients. The Albumin Reviewers. Cochrane Database Syst Rev CD001208, 2000.

42. Carroll GC, Snyder JV: Hyperdynamic severe intravascular sepsis depends on fluid administration in cynomolgus monkey. J Physiol Regul Integr Comp Physiol 243:R131–R141, 1982.

43. Cautero N, Gelmini R, Villa E, et al: Orthogonal polarization spectral imaging: A new tool in morphologic surveillance in intestinal transplant recipients. Transplant Proc 34:922–923, 2002.

44. Chang MC, Cheatham ML, Nelson LD, et al: Gastric tonometry supplements information provided by systemic indicators of oxygen transport. J Trauma 37:488–494, 1994.

45. Chaudry IH, Clemens MG, Baue AE: Alterations in cell function with ischemia and shock and their correction. Arch Surg 116:1309–1317, 1981.

46. Chien S: Role of the sympathetic nervous system in hemorrhage. Physiol Rev 47:214–288, 1967.

47. Choi PT, Yip G, Quinonez LG, et al: Crystalloids vs. colloids in fluid resuscitation: A systematic review. Crit Care Med 27:200–210, 1999.
48. Clements FM, Harpole DH, Quill T, et al: Estimation of left ventricular volume and ejection fraction by two-dimensional transoesophageal echocardiography: Comparison of short axis imaging and simultaneous radionuclide angiography. Br J Anaesth 64:331–336, 1990.
49. Cohn JN, Guiha NH, Broder MI, et al: Right ventricular infarction. Clinical and hemodynamic features. Am J Cardiol 33:209–214, 1974.
50. Connors AF: Right heart catheterization: Is it effective? New Horiz 5:195–200, 1997.
51. Connors AF, Speroff T, Dawson NV, et al: The effectiveness of right heart catheterization in the initial care of critically ill patients. JAMA 276:889–897, 1996.
52. Coremans JM, Ince C, Bruining HA, et al: (Semi-)quantitative analysis of reduced nicotinamide adenine dinucleotide fluorescence images of blood-perfused rat heart. Biophys J 72: 1849–1860, 1997.
53. Cumming AD, Driedger AA, McDonald JW, et al: Vasoactive hormones in the renal response to systemic sepsis. Am J Kidney Dis 11:23–32, 1988.
54. Dalen JE, Bone RC: Is it time to pull the pulmonary artery catheter? JAMA 276:916–918, 1996.
55. Davis JW, Parks SN, Kaups KL, et al: Admission base deficit predicts transfusion requirements and risk of complications. J Trauma 41:769–774, 1996.
56. Day NP, Phu NH, Bethell DP, et al: The effects of dopamine and adrenaline infusions on acid-base balance and systemic hemodynamics in severe infection. Lancet 348:219–223, 1996.
57. Doig CJ, Sutherland LR, Sandham JS, et al: Increased intestinal permeability is associated with the development of multiple organ dysfunction syndrome in critically ill ICU patients. Am J Respir Crit Care Med 158:444–451, 1998.
58. Dunser MW, Mayr AJ, Ulmer H, et al: The effects of vasopressin on systemic hemodynamics in catecholamine-resistant septic and postcardiotomy shock: A retrospective analysis. Anesth Analg 93:7–13, 2001.
59. Dunser M, Wenzel V, Mayr AJ, et al: Arginine vasopressin in vasodilatory shock: A new therapy approach? Anaesthesist 51:650–659, 2002.
60. Duranteau J, Sitbon P, Teboul JL, et al: Compared effects of epinephrine, norepinephrine, norepinephrine-dobutamine on the gastric mucosal blood flow in patients with septic shock (abstract). Am J Respir Crit Care Med 153:A832, 1996.
61. Durham RM, Neunaber K, Mazuski JE, et al: The use of oxygen consumption and delivery as endpoints for resuscitation in critically ill patients. J Trauma 41:32–39, 1996.
62. Eastridge BJ, Darlington DN, Evans JA, et al: A circulating shock protein depolarizes cells in hemorrhage and sepsis. Ann Surg 219:298–305, 1994.
63. Ebihara S, Hussain SN, Danialou G, et al: Mechanical ventilation protects against diaphragm injury in sepsis: Interaction of oxidative and mechanical stresses. Am J Respir Crit Care Med 165:221–228, 2002.
64. Effect of high-dose glucocorticoid therapy on mortality in patients with clinical signs of systemic sepsis. The Veterans Administration Systemic Sepsis Cooperative Study Group. N Engl J Med 317:659–665, 1987.
65. Eichacker PQ, Natanson C: Recombinant human activated protein C in sepsis: Inconsistent trial results, an unclear mechanism of action, and safety concerns resulted in labeling restrictions and the need for phase IV trials. Crit Care Med 31(1 Suppl):S94–S96, 2003.
66. Eidelman LA, Putterman D, Putterman C, et al: The spectrum of septic encephalopathy. Definitions, etiologies, and mortalities. JAMA 275:470–473, 1996.
67. Evans JA, Darlington DN, Gann DS: A circulating factor(s) mediates cell depolarization in hemorrhagic shock. Ann Surg 213:549–556, 1991.
68. Fehlings MG, Louw D: Initial stabilization and medical management of acute spinal cord injury. Am Fam Physician 54:155–162, 1996.
69. Fink MP: Tissue capnometry as a monitoring strategy for critically ill patients: Just about ready for prime time. Chest 114:667–670, 1998.
70. Fink MP: Bench-to-bedside review: Cytopathic hypoxia. Crit Care 6:491–499, 2002.
71. Fisher CJ Jr, Yan SB: Protein C levels as a prognostic indicator of outcome in sepsis and related diseases. Crit Care Med 28 (9 Suppl):S49–S56, 2000.
72. Flancbaum L, Dick M, Dasta J, et al: A dose-response study of phenylephrine in critically ill, septic surgical patients. Eur J Clin Pharmacol 51:461–465, 1997.
73. Gaillard RC, Turnill D, Sappino P, et al: Tumor necrosis factor alpha inhibits the hormonal response of the pituitary gland to hypothalamic releasing factors. Endocrinology 127:101–106, 1990.
74. Gan TJ, Bennett-Guerrero E, Phillips-Bute B, et al: Hextend, a physiologically balanced plasma expander for large volume use in major surgery: A randomized phase III clinical trial. Hextend Study Group. Anesth Analg 88:992–998, 1999.
75. Gann DS, Carlson DE, Byrnes GJ, et al: Role of solute in the early restitution of blood volume after hemorrhage. Surgery 94:439–446, 1983.
76. Gavalas M, Sadana A, Metcalf S: Guidelines for the management of anaphylaxis in the emergency department. J Accid Emerg Med 15:96–98, 1998.
77. Genzel-Boroviczeny O, Strotgen J, Harris AG, et al: Orthogonal polarization spectral imaging (OPS): A novel method to measure the microcirculation in term and preterm infants transcutaneously. Pediatr Res 51:386–391, 2002.
78. Givertz MM: Manipulation of the renin-angiotensin system. Circulation 104:E14–E18, 2001.
79. Godje O, Peyerl M, Seebauer T, et al: Central venous pressure, pulmonary capillary wedge pressure and intrathoracic blood volumes as preload indicators in cardiac surgery patients. Eur J Cardiothorac Surg 13:533–539, 1998.
80. Goldberg RJ, Gore JM, Alpert JS, et al: Cardiogenic shock after acute myocardial infarction. Incidence and mortality from a community-wide perspective, 1975 to 1988. N Engl J Med 325:1117–1122, 1991.
81. Groeneveld ABJ, Tra DD, van der Meulen J: Acute renal failure in the medical intensive care unit: Predisposing, complicating factors and outcome. Nephron 59:602–610, 1991.
82. Gunn SR, Pinsky MR: Implications of arterial pressure variation in patients in the intensive care unit. Curr Opin Crit Care 7:212–217, 2001.
83. Hamilton-Davies C, Mythen MG, Salmon JB, et al: Comparison of commonly used clinical indicators of hypovolaemia with gastrointestinal tonometry. Intensive Care Med 23:276–281, 1997.
84. Harlan JM, Winn RK: Leukocyte-endothelial interactions: Clinical trials of anti-adhesion therapy. Crit Care Med 30:S214–S219, 2002.
85. Harris AG, Sinitsina I, Messmer K: Validation of OPS imaging for microvascular measurements during isovolumic hemodilution and low hematocrits. Am J Physiol Heart Circ Physiol 282:H1502–H1509, 2002.
86. Hayes MA, Timmins AC, Yau EH, et al: Oxygen transport patterns in patients with sepsis syndrome or septic shock: Influence of treatment and relationship to outcome. Crit Care Med 25:926–936, 1997.
87. Hebert PC, Wells G, Blajchman MA, et al: A multicenter, randomized, controlled clinical trial of transfusion requirements

in critical care. Transfusion Requirements in Critical Care Investigators, Canadian Critical Care Trials Group. N Engl J Med 340:409–417, 1999.

88. Heyland DK, Cook DJ, King D, et al: Maximizing oxygen delivery in critically ill patients: A methodologic appraisal of the evidence. Crit Care Med 24:517–524, 1996.

89. Hochachka PW, Mommsen TP: Protons and anaerobiosis. Science 219:1391–1397, 1983.

90. Hochman JS, Sleeper LA, Webb JG, et al: Early revascularization in acute myocardial infarction complicated by cardiogenic shock. SHOCK Investigators. Should We Emergently Revascularize Occluded Coronaries for Cardiogenic Shock. N Engl J Med 341:625–634, 1999.

91. Hoffmann JN, Werdan K, Hartl WH, et al: Hemofiltrate from patients with severe sepsis and depressed left ventricular contractility contains cardiotoxic compounds. Shock 12:174–180, 1999.

92. Hollenberg SM, Ahrens TS, Astiz ME, et al: Practice parameters for hemodynamic support of sepsis in adult patients in sepsis. Crit Care Med 27:639–660, 1999.

93. Hotchkiss RS, Swanson PE, Freeman BD, et al: Apoptotic cell death in patients with sepsis, shock, and multiple organ dysfunction. Crit Care Med 27:1230–1251, 1999.

94. Hoyt JW: Effectiveness of right heart catheterization: Time for a randomized trial. JAMA 277:112–114, 1997.

95. Hurlbert RJ: The role of steroids in acute spinal cord injury: An evidence-based analysis. Spine 26:S39–S46, 2001.

96. Ince C, Sinaasappel M: Microcirculatory oxygenation and shunting in sepsis and shock. Crit Care Med 27:1369–1377, 1999.

97. Ince C, Ashruf JF, Avontuur JA, et al: Heterogeneity of the hypoxic state in rat heart is determined at capillary level. Am J Physiol Heart Circ Physiol 264:H294–H301, 1993.

98. Ivatury RR, Sugerman H: In quest of optimal resuscitation: Tissue specific, on to the microcirculation. Crit Care Med 28:3102–3103, 2000.

99. Ivatury RR, Simon RJ, Islam S, et al: A prospective randomized study of end points of resuscitation after major trauma: Global oxygen transport indices versus organ-specific gastric mucosal pH. J Am Coll Surg 183:145–154, 1996.

100. Ivatury RR, Simon RJ, Havriliak D, et al: Gastric mucosal pH and oxygen delivery and oxygen consumption indices in the assessment of adequacy of resuscitation after trauma: A prospective, randomized study. J Trauma 39:128–134, 1995.

101. Jakob SM, Ruokonen E, Takala J: Effects of dopamine on systemic and regional blood flow and metabolism in septic and cardiac surgery patients. Shock 18:8–13, 2002.

102. Jan Danser AH: Local renin-angiotensin systems: The unanswered questions. Int J Biochem Cell Biol 35:759–768, 2003.

103. Joffe II, Jacobs LE, Lampert C, et al: Role of echocardiography in perioperative management of patients undergoing open heart surgery. Am Heart J 131:162–176, 1996.

104. Kellum JA: Determinants of blood pH in health and disease. Crit Care 4:6–14, 2000.

105. Kellum JA: Fluid resuscitation and hyperchloremic acidosis in experimental sepsis: Improved short-term survival and acid-base balance with Hextend compared with saline. Crit Care Med 30:300–305, 2002.

106. Kellum JA, Decker JM: Use of dopamine in acute renal failure: A meta-analysis. Crit Care Med 29:1526–1531, 2001.

107. Kenakin TP: An in vitro quantitative analysis of the alpha adrenoceptor partial agonist activity of dobutamine and its relevance to inotropic selectivity. J Pharmacol Exp Ther 216:210–219, 1981.

108. Kincaid EH, Chang MC, Letton RW, et al: Admission base deficit in pediatric trauma: A study using the National Trauma Data Bank. J Trauma 51:332–335, 2001.

109. Kirklin JK: Prospects for understanding and eliminating the deleterious effects of cardiopulmonary bypass. Ann Thorac Surg 51:529–531, 1991.

110. Kirschenbaum LA, Astiz ME, Rackow EC, et al: Microvascular response in patients with cardiogenic shock. Crit Care Med 28:1290–1294, 2000.

111. Knaus WA, Draper EA, Wagner DP, et al: Prognosis in acute organ-system failure. Ann Surg 202:685–672, 1985.

112. Kollef MH, Schuster DP: The acute respiratory distress syndrome. N Engl J Med 332:27–34, 1995.

113. Konstadt SN, Thys D, Mindich BP, et al: Validation of quantitative intraoperative transesophageal echocardiography. Anesthesiology 65:418–421, 1986.

114. Korbut R, Gryglewski RJ: The effect of prostacyclin and nitric oxide on deformability of red blood cells in septic shock in rats. J Physiol Pharmacol 47:591–599, 1996.

115. Krown KA, Yasui K, Brooker MJ, et al: TNF alpha receptor expression in rat cardiac myocytes: TNF alpha inhibition of L-type Ca2+ current and Ca2+ transients. FEBS Lett 376:24–30, 1995.

116. Kumar A, Haery C, Parrillo JE: Myocardial dysfunction in septic shock. Crit Care Clin 16:251–287, 2000.

117. Landry DW, Oliver JA: The ATP-sensitive K+ channel mediates hypotension in endotoxemia and hypoxic lactic acidosis in dog. J Clin Invest 89:2071–2074, 1992.

118. Landry DW, Oliver JA: The pathogenesis of vasodilatory shock. N Engl J Med 345:588–595, 2001.

119. Landry DW, Levin HR, Gallant EM, et al: Vasopressin presor hypersensitivity in vasodilatory septic shock. Crit Care Med 25:1279–1282, 1997.

120. Langer S, Biberthaler P, Harris AG, et al: In vivo monitoring of microvessels in skin flaps: Introduction of a novel technique. Microsurgery 21:317–324, 2001.

121. Langer S, Born F, Hatz R, et al: Orthogonal polarization spectral imaging versus intravital fluorescent microscopy for microvascular studies in wounds. Ann Plast Surg 48:646–653, 2002.

122. Langer S, Harris AG, Biberthaler P, et al: Orthogonal polarization spectral imaging as a tool for the assessment of hepatic microcirculation: A validation study. Transplantation 71:1249–1256, 2001.

123. Levy B, Bollaert PE, Charpentier C, et al: Comparison of norepinephrine and dobutamine to epinephrine for hemodynamics, lactate metabolism, and gastric tonometric variables in septic shock: A prospective, randomized study. Intensive Care Med 23:282–287, 1997.

124. Levy B, Bollaert PE, Lucchelli JP, et al: Dobutamine improves the adequacy of gastric mucosal perfusion in epinephrine-treated septic shock. Crit Care Med 25:1649–1654, 1997.

125. Levy MM, Fink MP, Marshall JC, et al: 2001 SCCM/ESICM/ACCP/ATS/SIS International Sepsis Definitions Conference. Crit Care Med 31:1250–1256, 2003.

126. L'Her E, Sebert P: A global approach to energy metabolism in an experimental model of sepsis. Am J Respir Crit Care Med 164:1444–1447, 2001.

127. Lichtwarck-Aschoff M, Zeravik J, Pfeiffer UJ: Intrathoracic blood volume accurately reflects circulatory volume status in critically ill patients with mechanical ventilation. Intensive Care Med 18:142–147, 1992.

128. Mackenzie S, Kapadia F, Immo G, et al: Adrenaline in the treatment of septic shock: Effects on hemodynamics and oxygen transport. Intensive Care Med 17:36–39, 1991.

129. Malay MB, Ashton RC Jr, Landry DW, et al: Low-dose vasopressin in the treatment of vasodilatory septic shock. J Trauma 47:699–703, 1999.

130. Manikis P, Jankowski S, Zhang H, et al: Correlation of serial blood lactate levels to organ failure and mortality after trauma. Am J Emerg Med 13:619–622, 1995.

131. Manns BJ, Lee H, Doig CJ, et al: An economic evaluation of activated protein C treatment for severe sepsis. N Engl J Med 347:993–1000, 2002.

132. Marik PE: The optimal endpoint of resuscitation in trauma patients. Crit Care 7:19–20, 2003.

133. Marik PE: Low-dose dopamine: A systematic review. Intensive Care Med 28(7):877–883, 2002.

134. Marik PE, Bankov A: Sublingual capnometry versus traditional markers of tissue oxygenation in critically ill patients. Crit Care Med 31:818–822, 2003.

135. Marik PE, Iglesias J: Low-dose dopamine does not prevent acute renal failure in patients with septic shock and oliguria. NORASEPT II Study Investigators. Am J Med 107:387–390, 1999.

136. Marik PE, Mohedin M: The contrasting effects of dopamine and norepinephrine on systemic and splanchnic oxygen utilization in hyperdynamic sepsis. JAMA 272:1354–1357, 1994.

137. Marik PE, Zaloga GP: Adrenal insufficiency in the critically ill: A new look at an old problem. Chest 122:1784–1796, 2002.

138. Martin C, Papazian L, Perrin G, et al: Norepinephrine or dopamine for the treatment of hyperdynamic septic shock? Chest 103:1826–1831, 1993.

139. Mastorakos G, Chrousos GP, Weber JS: Recombinant interleukin-6 activates the hypothalamic-pituitary-adrenal axis in humans. J Clin Endocrinol Metab 77:1690–1694, 1993.

140. Mathura KR, Vollebregt KC, Boer K, et al: Comparison of OPS imaging and conventional capillary microscopy to study the human microcirculation. J Appl Physiol 91:74–78, 2001.

141. Meehan TP, Fine MJ, Krumholz HM, et al: Quality of care, process, and outcomes in elderly patients with pneumonia. JAMA 278:2080–2084, 1997.

142. Meisner M: Pathobiochemistry and clinical use of procalcitonin. Clin Chim Acta 323:17–29, 2002.

143. Michard F, Boussat S, Chemla D, et al: Relation between respiratory changes in arterial pulse pressure and fluid responsiveness in septic patients with acute circulatory failure. Am J Respir Crit Care Med 162:134–138, 2000.

144. Michard F, Chemla D, Richard C, et al: Clinical use of respiratory changes in arterial pulse pressure to monitor the hemodynamic effects of PEEP. Am J Respir Crit Care Med 159:935–939, 1999.

145. Mink S, Becker A, Sharma S, et al: Role of autacoids in cardiovascular colapse in anaphylactic shock in anaesthetized dogs. Cardiovasc Res 43:173–182, 1999.

146. Morrison RJ, Bidani A: Acute respiratory distress syndrome epidemiology and pathophysiology. Chest Surg Clin North Am 12:301–323, 2002.

147. Neviere R, Mathieu D, Chagnon JL, et al: The contrasting effects of dobutamine and dopamine on gastric mucosal perfusion in septic patients. Am J Respir Crit Care Med 154:1684–1688, 1996.

148. Nollert G, Jonas RA, Reichart B: Optimizing cerebral oxygenation during cardiac surgery: A review of experimental and clinical investigations with near infrared spectrophotometry. Thorac Cardiovasc Surg 48:247–253, 2000.

149. Nolten WE, Goldstein D, Lindstrom M, et al: Effects of cytokines on the pituitary-adrenal axis in cancer patients. J Interferon Res 17:349–357, 1993.

150. Normon AW, Litwack G: Hormones, 2nd ed. San Diego: Academic Press, 1997.

151. Ognibene FP, Parker MM, Natanson C, et al: Depressed left ventricular performance: Response to volume infusion in patients with sepsis and septic shock. Chest 93:903–910, 1988.

152. Olson D, Pohlman A, Hall JB: Administration of low-dose dopamine to nonoliguric patients with sepsis syndrome does not raise intramucosal pH nor improve creatinine clearance. Am J Respir Crit Care Med 154:1664–1670, 1996.

153. Pagani FD, Baker LS, Hsi C, et al: Left ventricular systolic and diastolic dysfunction after infusion of tumor necrosis factor alpha in conscious dogs. J Clin Invest 90:389–398, 1992.

154. Palmer RMJ: The discovery of nitric oxide in the vessel wall: A unifying concept in the pathogenesis of sepsis. Arch Surg 128:396–401, 1993.

155. Papadopoulos MC, Davies DC, Moss RF, et al: Pathophysiology of septic encephalopathy: A review. Crit Care Med 28:3019–3024, 2000.

156. Parent C, Eichacker PQ: Neutrophil and endothelial cell interactions in sepsis. The role of adhesion molecules. Infect Dis Clin North Am 13:427–447, 1999.

157. Parker MM, Shelhamer JH, Bacharach SL, et al: Profound but reversible myocardial depression in patients with septic shock. Ann Intern Med 100:483–490, 1984.

158. Parker MM, Shelhamer JH, Natanson C, et al: Serial cardiovascular variables in survivors and nonsurvivors of human septic shock: Heart rate as an early predictor of prognosis. Crit Care Med 15:923–929, 1987.

159. Parratt JR: Nitric oxide. A key mediator in sepsis and endotoxaemia? J Physiol Pharmacol 48:493–506, 1997.

160. Parratt JR: Nitric oxide in sepsis and endotoxaemia. J Antimicrob Chemother 41(Suppl A):31–39, 1998.

161. Parrillo JE: Myocardial depression during septic shock in humans. Crit Care Med 18:1183–1184, 1990.

162. Parrillo JE, Burch C, Shelhamer JH, et al: A circulating myocardial depressant substance in humans with septic shock. Septic shock patients with a reduced ejection fraction have a circulating factor that depresses in vitro myocardial cell performance. J Clin Invest 76:1539–1553, 1985.

163. Patel JP, Beck LD, Briglia FA, et al: Beneficial effects of combined thromboxane and leukotriene receptor antagonism in hemorrhagic shock. Crit Care Med 23:231–237, 1995.

164. Porter JM, Ivatury RR: In search of the optimal end points of resuscitation in trauma patients: A review. J Trauma 44:908–914, 1998.

165. Povoas HP, Weil MH, Tang W, et al: Comparisons between sublingual and gastric tonometry during hemorrhagic shock. Chest 118:1127–1132, 2000.

166. Rackow EC, Kaufman BS, Falk JL, et al: Hemodynamic response to fluid repletion in patients with septic shock: Evidence for early depression of cardiac performance. Circ Shock 22:11–22, 1987.

167. Reilly PM, Wilkins KB, Fuh KC, et al: The mesenteric hemodynamic response to circulatory shock: An overview. Shock 15:329–343, 2001.

168. Richards ML, Caplan RH, Wickus GG, et al: The rapid low-dose (1 microgram) cosyntropin test in the immediate postoperative period: Results in elderly subjects after major abdominal surgery. Surgery 125:431–440, 1999.

169. Rivers E, Nguyen B, Havstad S, et al: Early goal-directed therapy in the treatment of severe sepsis and septic shock. N Engl J Med 345:1368–1377, 2001.

170. Roberts N, Harrison DG, Reimer KA, et al: Right ventricular infarction with shock but without significant left ventricular infarction: A new clinical syndrome. Am Heart J 110:1047–1053, 1985.

171. Roumen RM, Vreugde JP, Goris RJ: Gastric tonometry in multiple trauma patients. J Trauma 36:313–316, 1994.

172. Rozycki GS: Surgeon-performed ultrasound: Its use in clinical practice. Ann Surg 228:16–28, 1998.

173. Ruffolo RR Jr: The pharmacology of dobutamine. Am J Med Sci 294:244–248, 1987.

174. Rutherford EJ, Morris JA Jr, Reed GW, et al: Base deficit stratifies mortality and determines therapy. J Trauma 33:417–423, 1992.

814

175. Rybak MJ, McGrath BJ: Combination antimicrobial therapy for bacterial infections. Guidelines for the clinician. Drugs 52:390–405, 1996.

176. Salzman AL, Vromen A, Denenberg A, et al: K(ATP)-channel inhibition improves hemodynamics and cellular energetics in hemorrhagic shock. Am J Physiol Heart Circ Physiol 272:H688–H694, 1997.

177. Sandham JD, Hull RD, Brant RF, et al: A randomized, controlled trial of the use of pulmonary-artery catheters in high-risk surgical patients. N Engl J Med 348:5–14, 2003.

178. Sato Y, Weil MH, Tang W, et al: Esophageal PCO_2 as a monitor of perfusion failure during hemorrhagic shock. J Appl Physiol 82:558–562, 1997.

179. Savitsky E, Votey S: Emergency department approach to acute thoracolumbar spine injury. J Emerg Med 15:49–60, 1997.

180. Scharte M, Han X, Bertges DJ, et al: Cytokines induce HIF-1 DNA binding and the expression of HIF-1-dependent genes in cultured rat enterocytes. Am J Physiol Gastrointest Liver Physiol 284:G373–G384, 2002.

181. Scheingraber S, Rehm M, Sehmisch C, et al: Rapid saline infusion produces hyperchloremic acidosis in patients undergoing gynecologic surgery. Anesthesiology 90:1265–1270, 1999.

182. Schierhout G, Roberts I: Fluid resuscitation with colloid or crystalloid solutions in critically ill patients: A systematic review of randomised trials. BMJ 316:961–964, 1998.

183. Schreuder WO, Schneider AJ, Groenveld ABJ, et al: Effect of dopamine vs norepinephrine on hemodynamics in septic shock: Emphasis on right ventricular performance. Chest 95:1282–1288, 1989.

184. Schuster DP, Kollef MH: Acute respiratory distress syndrome. Dis Mon 42:265–328, 1996.

185. Segal JM, Phang PT, Walley KR: Low-dose dopamine hastens onset of gut ischemia in a porcine model of hemorrhagic shock. J Appl Physiol 73:1159–1164, 1992.

186. Shoemaker WC, Appel PL, Kram HB, et al: Prospective trial of supranormal values of survivors as therapeutic goals in high-risk surgical patients. Chest 94:1176–1186, 1988.

187. Shoemaker WC, Appel PL, Kram HB: Tissue oxygen debt as a determinant of lethal and nonlethal postoperative organ failure. Crit Care Med 16:1117–1120, 1988.

188. Shoemaker WC, Montgomery ES, Kaplan E, et al: Physiologic patterns in surviving and nonsurviving shock patients. Use of sequential cardiorespiratory variables in defining criteria for therapeutic goals and early warning of death Arch Surg 106:630–636, 1973.

189. Siegel JH, Rivkind AI, Dalal S, et al. Early physiologic predictors of injury severity and death in blunt multiple trauma. Arch Surg 125:498–508, 1990.

190. Silverman HJ: Lack of a relationship between induced changes in oxygen consumption and changes in lactate levels. Chest 100:1012–1015, 1991.

191. Simchon S, Jan KM, Chien S. Influence of reduced red cell deformability on regional blood flow. Am J Physiol Heart Circ Physiol 253:H898–H903, 1987.

192. Smith LW, Winbery SL, Barker LA, et al: Cardiac function and chronotropic sensitivity to beta-adrenergic stimulation is sepsis. Am J Physiol Heart Circ Physiol 251:H405–H412, 1986.

193. Smith MD, MacPhail B, Harrison MR, et al. Value and limitations of transesophageal echocardiography in determination of left ventricular volumes and ejection fraction. J Am Coll Cardiol 19:1213–1222, 1992.

194. Soni A, Pepper GM, Wyrwinski PM, et al: Adrenal insufficiency occurring during septic shock: Incidence, outcome, and relationship to peripheral cytokine levels. Am J Med 98:266–271, 1995.

195. Sprung CL, Caralis PV, Marcial EH, et al: The effects of high-dose corticosteroids in patients with septic shock. A prospective, controlled study. N Engl J Med 311:1137–1143, 1984.

196. Stein PD: Pulmonary embolism. Curr Opin Crit Care 1:23, 1995.

197. Suffredini AF, Fromm RE, Parker MM, et al: The cardiovascular response of normal humans to the administration of endotoxin. N Engl J Med 321:280–287, 1989.

198. Szabo C: Alterations in nitric oxide production in various forms of circulatory shock. New Horiz 3:2–32, 1995.

199. Szabo C, Billiar TR: Novel roles of nitric oxide in hemorrhagic shock. Shock 12:1–9, 1999.

200. Szabo C, Salzman AL: Inhibition of ATP-activated potassium channels exerts pressor effects and improves survival in a rat model of severe hemorrhagic shock. Shock 5:391–394, 1996.

201. Third European Consensus Conference in Intensive Care Medicine: Tissue hypoxia: How to detect, how to correct, how to prevent? Am J Respir Crit Care Med 154:1573–1578, 1996.

202. Turnbull AV, Rivier C: Regulation of the HPA axis by cytokines. Brain Behav Immun 9:253–275, 1995.

203. Unno N, Fink MP: Intestinal epithelial hyperpermeability. Mechanisms and relevance to disease. Gastroenterol Clin North Am 27:289–307, 1998.

204. Unno N, Menconi MJ, Fink MP: Nitric oxide-induced hyperpermeability of human intestinal epithelial monolayers is augmented by inhibition of the amiloride-sensitive Na(+)-H+ antiport: Potential role of peroxynitrous acid. Surgery 122:485–491, 1997.

205. Urbanowicz JH, Shaaban MJ, Cohen NH, et al: Comparison of transesophageal echocardiographic and scintigraphic estimates of left ventricular end-diastolic volume index and ejection fraction in patients following coronary artery bypass grafting. Anesthesiology 72:607–612, 1990.

206. Valensi P, Gaudey F, Parries J, et al: Glucagon and noradrenaline reduce erythrocyte deformability. Metabolism 42:1169–1172, 1993.

207. Vallet B, Tavernier B, Lund N: Assessment of tissue oxygenation in the critically-ill. Eur J Anaesthesiol 17:221–229, 2000.

208. Vincent JL, Dufaye P, Berre J, et al: Serial lactate determinations during circulatory shock. Crit Care Med 11:449–451, 1983.

209. Waters JH, Gottlieb A, Schoenwald P, et al: Normal saline versus lactated Ringer's solution for intraoperative fluid management in patients undergoing abdominal aortic aneurysm repair: An outcome study. Anesth Analg 93:817–822, 2001.

210. Waters JH, Miller LR, Clack S, et al: Cause of metabolic acidosis in prolonged surgery. Crit Care Med 27:2142–2146, 1999.

211. Wei JY, Hutchins GM, Bulkley BH: Papillary muscle rupture in fatal acute myocardial infarction: A potentially treatable form of cardiogenic shock. Ann Intern Med 90:149–152, 1979.

212. Weil MH, Nakagawa Y, Tang W, et al: Sublingual capnometry: A new noninvasive measurement for diagnosis and quantitation of severity of circulatory shock. Crit Care Med 27:1225–1229, 1999.

213. Weil MH, Nishijima H: Cardiac output in bacterial shock. Am J Med Sci 64:920–923, 1978.

214. Wilkes NJ, Woolf R, Mutch M, et al: The effects of balanced versus saline-based hetastarch and crystalloid solutions on acid-base and electrolyte status and gastric mucosal perfusion in elderly surgical patients. Anesth Analg 93:811–816, 2001.

215. Williams G, Grounds M, Rhodes A: Pulmonary artery catheter. Curr Opin Crit Care 8:251–256, 2002.

216. Yamazaki T, Shimada Y, Taenaka N, et al: Circulatory responses to afterloading with phenylephrine in hyperdynamic sepsis. Crit Care Med 10:432–435, 1982.

217. Yee JB, McJames SW: Use of gastric intramucosal pH as a monitor during hemorrhagic shock. Circ Shock 43:44–48, 1994.

218. Zingarelli B, Day BJ, Crapo JD, et al: The potential role of peroxynitrite in the vascular contractile and cellular energetic failure in endotoxic shock. Br J Pharmacol 120:259–267, 1997.

219. Zingg H, Bourque C, Bichet D: Vasopressin and Oxytocin: Molecular, Cellular and Clinical Advances. New York: Plenum Press, 1998.

220. Zipnick RI, Scalea TM, Trooskin SZ, et al: Hemodynamic responses to penetrating spinal cord injuries. J Trauma 35: 578–582, 1993.

Tissue Regeneration

Michael V. Sefton, Peter Zandstra, Céline Liu Bauwens, and William L. Stanford

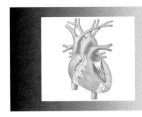

▶ INTRODUCTION

It has been proposed that disruptions of the normally precise cellular architecture in the heart can be corrected or reversed by tissue regeneration. In part because of the limited ability to repair itself, current treatments are restricted to addressing the sequelae of the primary defect and do not directly restore lost structure or function. The ability to reestablish cardiac tissue architecture and recover cardiac function through the implantation of biosynthetic constructs has great appeal.[3]

▶ BASIC IDEAS OF TISSUE ENGINEERING AND REGENERATION

Modes of Tissue Engineering

"Tissue engineering" and "regenerative medicine" are synonyms for the use of cells, soluble and matrix bound factors, and supporting structures to regenerate damaged tissue/organ structures and function. Almost every tissue has been reconstructed to at least a limited extent using some form of tissue engineering.[26,45] The list is expanding every month from "simple" tissues such as bone to complex internal organs such as liver and kidney.[34,75,107,111] One of the approaches to tissue engineering (Figure 51-1) involves the use of scaffold materials to control cell seeding.[112] In principle, scaffolds can be selected to bring cells together into the desired three-dimensional organization while providing a mechanically stable matrix for the cells to associate into tissue analogues. Scaffolds can also be selected to affect cell phenotype. In the case of cardiac cells this may be very important, as there is clear evidence that the structure of the extracellular environment affects cardiac cell phenotype.[101]

Regenerative medicine strategies can come in several other forms as well (Figure 51-1). For example, adult progenitor or stem cells are directly injected for *in situ* cell therapy (see Chapter 97) or can be genetically modified prior to seeding into a material scaffold that is then incubated further in a bioreactor prior to implantation. Alternatively, an implanted material induces a specific response such as tissue regeneration *in vivo*. There is also the self-assembly approach[48] where progenitor cells are coaxed into expressing their intrinsic capacities for regenerating a tissue structure. Regenerative medicine and tissue engineering encompass a number of synergistic approaches, combining engineered cells and/or stem cells, growth factors and biomaterial scaffolds, gene therapy, and other advanced biotechnologies. These have largely emerged independently and only recently has it been recognized that they are different facets of the same area. The field of "biomaterials" has become "tissue engineering," and "tissue engineering" has become "regenerative medicine." Modern approaches draw all these strategies under one umbrella so that the synergies can be fostered and exploited.

From Tissues to Organs: Key Goals and Issues

Regardless of the approach to regenerative medicine or the scope of the application (a vascular graft, a pediatric valve,

818

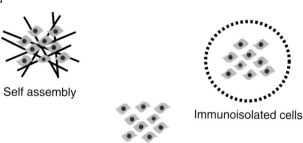

Figure 51–1 **Approaches to tissue regeneration.** Direct cell injection: cells are delivered directly to the target site for *in situ* therapy. Self-assembly: cells secrete their own matrix to produce a tissue equivalent *in vitro* without any external scaffold. Tissue replacement: cells are seeded into a biomaterial scaffold and incubated further in a bioreactor. Immunoisolation: cells are microencapsulated or otherwise placed behind a permselective membrane to isolate them from the host immune system. Tissue control: the material induces a particular host response upon implantation.

or an entire heart) there are three overlapping therapeutic goals—the three Rs:

- Make tissue and organ **replacement** safer, more effective and more widely available.
- **Repair** tissues and organs without having to replace them.
- Enable tissues and organs to **regenerate** so that repair and regeneration become one and the same.

Furthermore, the problems of reaching these goals can be summarized (Table 51-1) in three categories (here largely in the context of tissue engineering):

- **Cell number:** What is the source of cells to be used and how will large numbers be generated? How will they be supplied with nutrients, etc. within a device of reasonable volume?
- **Cell function:** How will the scaffold, extracellular matrix, and diffusible factors interact to generate the desired cell phenotype? How will the engineered tissue/organ function integrate with the host to ensure a functional outcome?
- **Cell durability:** What will happen over the long term as re-modeling and/or the host immune/inflammatory system responds to the new tissue?

For the replacement, repair, or regeneration of cardiovascular tissue, these central issues of regenerative medicine will need to be addressed. Some of these issues (Table 51-1) reflect the fundamental nature of how an organ is different from a tissue: the large size and three-dimensional structure and the presence of multiple cell types that work in unison. Beyond these largely scientific challenges, there are the no less critical, practical questions of manufacturing, steriliza-tion, storage, and distribution and the regulatory and public policy issues that will need to be addressed before such therapies can be made available to the patients who are expected to benefit. Furthermore we will also need new imaging or other noninvasive strategies to monitor the suc-cess (or not) of these therapies: to enable the translation into clinical practice.

► LESSONS FROM DEVELOPMENTAL BIOLOGY

The cardiovascular system is the first organ system to develop in the mammalian embryo, as it is immediately required to deliver oxygen and other nutrients from the placenta to the developing embryo before the embryo is too large and dense to permit nutrient diffusion. Approxi-mately, a third of null mutations generated in the mouse have resulted in embryonic lethality, with a high percentage due to cardiovascular failure. Not all of the lethal defects have been due to cell autonomous defects; rather, tissue-specific knockouts in the heart have demonstrated the exquisite sensitivity by the cardiovascular system to pertur-bations in the general patterning of the embryo and placen-tal functionality.

Regenerative medicine aims to utilize the lessons from developmental biology in two ways: first, to activate latent regenerative potential within an affected tissue rather than destructive remodeling and wound healing and second, to grow replacement tissues for the injured organ. Here, we will briefly overview the complexity of cardiovascular development, in particular cardiogenesis, highlighting the themes that will likely play critical roles in regenerative therapy of this system.

Cardiac Induction and Morphogenesis

Heart development is orchestrated in a dynamic fashion of coordinated differentiation, proliferation, and cell migra-tion leading to the induction of the precardiac mesoderm to form the cardiac crescent, the heart tube, looping, cham-ber, and, finally, remodeling of the heart (outlined in Figure 51-2). Microarray analysis suggests that at least one sixth of the mammalian genome is differentially expressed in the heart in a temporal fashion during mammalian develop-ment. The heart is composed of a number of specialized cell lineages, primarily of mesoderm derivation, with the exception of ectoderm-derived neural crest cells that migrate to the aorta during septation. The heart mesoderm and the foregut endoderm, which provide inductive signals for cardiac development, are closely associated throughout heart development.

The endocardial and myocardial cells are derived from the ventral splanchnic mesoderm of the lateral plate, which also gives rise to the dorsal aortae and associated vascular networks and the hematopoietic system. Members of the transforming growth factor (TGF)–β superfamily (e.g., BMP2, BMP4) and its signaling cascade are critical mor-phogenetic factors that induce cardiac mesoderm. BMP2 or BMP4 ectopically induces the homeobox protein Nkx2.5, which is required for heart formation. Furthermore, the BMPs induce FGF8 expression, which is also an important

Table 51–1

Critical Issues Associated with Tissue Engineering a Heart

	Objective	*Critical issues*
Cell number	~300 g of cells (3×10^{11} cells) ~200 ml O_2/h[a]	Cell source/purity Vascularization
Function	Cellular phenotype (multiple cell types) Coordinated muscle contraction Pump blood Connect to circulation	Microenvironment (soluble and insoluble factors) Pacemaker and electrical conduction Valves and conduits Biomechanical elasticity and strength Nonthrombogenicity
Durability	Fatigue resistance Hypoxia and disease tolerance Host tolerance	Biocompatibility Remodeling Innate/adaptive immune response
	Manufacturing and quality control	
	Ethical, legal, and social issues	
	Imaging and noninvasive diagnostics	
	Regulatory and public policy issues	

[a]Based on moderate activity.[13]

inducer of cardiac gene expression.[6] The zone of cardiac induction, known as the cardiac field, is defined not only by positive signals but also by negative regulators such as Wnt proteins secreted by the neural plate. The morphogenetic actions of these factors upon the cardiac field result in the formation of the first anatomically recognizable structure of the developing heart, the cardiac crescent. The activation of Nkx2.5 initiates expression of a wave of transcription factors that participate in a combinatorial fashion to finely regulate cardiac development. (Figure 51-2).

The heart tube develops from the cardiac crescent, as cells within the crescent migrate ventrally along a fibronectin gradient partitioning the mesodermal–endodermal interface. The coordinated differentiation of the endoderm and cardiac mesoderm is again critical for this stage of heart development. For example, Gata4 is required within the endoderm for the migration of cardiac crescent cells ventrally to form the heart tube.[71] A subpopulation down-regulates N-cadherin and delaminates from the epithelium to form the endocardium, while the migrating cardiogenic epithelial cells differentiate into the myocardium. The heart begins to contract rhythmically, pumping blood from the yolk sac into the atrium and through the ventricular outflow tract.

The looping of the heart converts the cranial–caudal polarity of the heart tube into the right–left polarity of the four-chambered heart and is mediated by asymmetrical expression of two paracrine factors expressed specifically in the left side of the lateral plate mesoderm, Nodal and Lefty2, along with the transcription factor Pitx2. The Notch signaling pathway is involved in maintaining left–right asymmetry with mutations in this pathway leading to human congenital heart defects. During looping, the endocardium and myocardium become separated by an expanded extracellular matrix known as the cardiac jelly secreted by the myocardium. Endocardial cells migrate into the cardiac jelly to form the endocardial cushions, which together with neural crest cells form the septa and valves. Abnormal development of the endocardial cushion is the primary cause of a number of congenital heart defects including septal defects and tetralogy of Fallot.

Cardiogenic Remodeling

After looping, myocardial trabeculation becomes evident along the inner myocardial layers. Trabeculation is driven by the mechanical forces imposed by looping, the shape of the

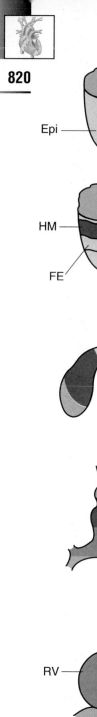

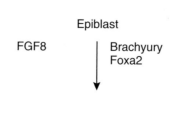

Epiblast

FGF8 | Brachyury
Foxa2

Heart mesoderm

BMP2 & 4
FGF8 | Nkx2.5
Wnt inhibitors
β–catenin

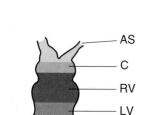

Cardiac crescent

FGF8 | Nkx2.5 | Mef2b
FGF10 | Tbx5 | Mef2c
VEGF | Gata4 | Hand1
Retinoic acid | Gata6 | Hand2

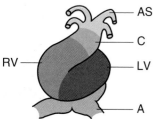

Linear heart tube

Nodal | Pitx
Lefty2 | Hand1 | Nkx2.5
Notch | Hand2 | Mef2c
Retinoic acid

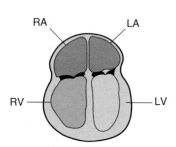

Looped heart tube

Retinoic acid | YB1 | Nkx2.5
VEGF | Carp | Mef2b
PDGF | Tbx5 | Pax3
TGFβ | Iroquois 1-5

Figure 51–2 An overview of heart development. The primary morphologically distinguishable stages of heart development are pictured as simple diagrams on the left. The epiblast (Epi) and the extraembryonic ectoderm (EE) that becomes the embryonic portion of the placenta are shown at the start of gastrulation with the primitive streak (PS) migrating distally. The future heart mesoderm (HM) and foregut endoderm (FE) move through the primitive streak to the anterior side of the epiblast driven by FGF8 signaling. Many of the inductive queues that specify the heart mesoderm into the cardiac crescent are secreted by the surrounding endoderm and ectoderm. Patterning of the heart begins at the cardiac crescent stage with the future conotruncus (C), ventricle (V), and atrium (A) becoming specified. Coordinated with the closure of the heart tube, in which a primitive endocardium is formed and the aortic sac (AS) and the left (LV) and right ventricles (RV) are specified, the heart begins to beat. During looping, the heart tube adopts a spiral shape, with the outer surface moving rightward, and the inflow tract (including the common atrium) being forced dorsally and cranially. Septation, trabeculation, and vasculogenesis of the coronary arteries are coordinated in the final stages of heart development.
(*Drawings courtesy of Leo Sin.*)

Chambered heart

ventricles, and muscle contraction. The finger-like projections of trabeculae are critical for compartmentalizing the blood in the heart prior to its septation and coordinating intraventricular conduction. The coordinated generation and transmission of electrical signals that control the precisely timed rhythmic contractions of the atrial and ventricular chambers that constitute the heartbeat are performed by the cardiac conduction system (CCS). The heart begins beating with the closure of the heart tube, at which point the pacemaker activity is found in the sinus venosus and the contraction is propagated up the muscle of the tubular heart. During the looping stage, the outflow tract is contractile, although the conduction through the outlet is slow and persists for much of the cardiac cycle suggesting that one role of the contraction is to prevent reflux of blood in the absence of valves. Molecularly, the propagation of the impulses is mediated through the gap junctions that are formed by connexins. Mutations in either Nkx2.5 or Tbx5 lead to dramatic down-regulation of connexins 40 and 43 and conduction defects,[12,40] demonstrating that these principle role players in early cardiac morphogenesis also act in the specification of the CCS.

Vascular Development

The coronary vessels arise through *de novo* vascular development known as vasculogenesis. Once the vessel connects to the aorta, the vascular smooth muscle cells (VSMC) migrate to the vessels and differentiate, leading to mature vessels. The intraembryonic vasculature is derived from two discrete mesodermal sources. The splanchnopleural mesoderm, which gives rise to the endocardium and myocardium, also gives rise to hemangioblasts that first form the major vessels of the embryo through vasculogenesis, then gives rise to the definitive hematopoietic stem cells that replace the first wave of primitive hematopoietic cells born in the yolk sac. Angioblasts derived from the somatopleural mesoderm give rise to the vascular networks of the body wall and kidney as well as the dorsal portion of the paired dorsal aortae.[80] As in the yolk sac, the vascular network of the embryo is rapidly remodeled by angiogenesis to form a continuum of larger and smaller vessels. Angiogenesis leads to capillary formation through sprouting and nonsprouting, or intussusception, mechanisms controlled by the Tie/angiopoietin receptor tyrosine kinase family, and their ligands. As the vessel matures, the endothelium secretes extracellular matrix proteins including fibronectin, laminin, collagen, and heparin sulfate proteoglycans, which are believed to regulate cell polarity adhesion, proliferation, and differentiation.[25] Surrounding the basement membrane maturing vessels develop a medial layer comprised largely of VSMC in response to platelet-derived growth factor (PDGF), although the source of the VSMC is unclear. TGF-β expression is activated by the interactions of the endothelium and VSMC, which then inhibits proliferation and migration of endothelial cells.

Hypoxia and hemodynamic forces play central roles in vascular remodeling during embryonic development as well as in the maintenance of cardiovascular homeostasis in the adult via triggering changes in transcriptional regulation that controls the development and remodeling of the vasculature. Hypoxia and pathogenic ischemia are potent inducers of the basic helix–loop–helix–PAS heterodimer HIF1,[117] which in turn induces a variety of molecules including erythropoietin (EPO) and vascular endothelial growth factor (VEGF) to increase red blood cell production and induce endothelial cell proliferation and vessel growth, respectively. Whereas changes in hemodynamic forces result in changes in PDGF fibroblast growth factor (FGF) and TGF-β factor expression among other genes, the lack of hemodynamic forces caused by blood flow stoppage in redundant vessels leads to pruning of the vessels, in which endothelial cells retract toward adjacent capillaries.

Growth of the heart continues through hyperplasia until shortly after birth when the cardiomyocytes and interstitial cells become postmitotic and further growth of the heart is due to hypertrophy. Following cardiovascular trauma, positive and negative feedback loops, activated to compensate for myocardial failure, reactivate developmental programs leading to cardiovascular remodeling but not regeneration. For example, while activation of c-Myc and c-Fos induces proliferation in the fetal heart, in the postmitotic adult heart, they induce cardiac hypertrophy and cell cycle reentry in postmitotic cardiomyocytes, which can lead to heart failure.

Implications for Tissue Engineering

The preceding overview highlights several key features that underscore hurdles that must be cleared to tissue engineer a cardiac patch, valve, or even a whole heart. First, the heart is made up of a number of different cell types, some of which are derived from a common mesenchymal progenitor, while neural crest cells are derived from a discrete ectodermal progenitor. Furthermore, many different types of temporally and spatially controlled inductive signals control heart development. Some of these signals are cell intrinsic, such as the temporal cascade of transcription factors that "turn on" transcription of one another or the extracellular matrix proteins that are secreted by cardiomyocytes, while other signals are cell extrinsic, such as the mechanical forces of adjacent tissues and hemodynamic flow or the temporally controlled release of cytokines by endodermal and ectodermal cells in neighboring tissues. Many of the intrinsic developmental programs are initiated or maintained by extrinsic signals. Thus, tissue engineering cardiovascular components will require sophisticated coculture techniques with cells that normally provide inductive and repressive signals or the staged release of soluble and/or matrix bound factors. Finally, new approaches will be needed to replicate the intricate control of oxygen gradients and hypoxia and mechanical force.

▶ BIOMATERIALS IN TISSUE ENGINEERING

In many modes of regenerative medicine, biomaterials are a central component. Unfortunately, for soft tissues, there are few biodegradable materials and few scaffold designs that have the requisite biomechanical properties and the capability to mimic the environmental conditions that support regeneration.

There are a wide variety of ways ranging from salt leaching to solvent precipitation[110] for preparing porous scaffolds with the roughly 100–300 μm pores suitable for cell seeding (Figure 51-3). In principle, any material can be converted into

822 a scaffold through at least one of these methods. However, some are more suited for one method rather than another because of questions regarding solubility, viscosity (molecular weight), or synthesis (cross-linking, available as a polymer or synthesized from monomers). Ready-made scaffolds are now becoming available commercially, at least for one or two materials. Various rapid-prototyping methods (e.g., three-dimensional printing[68]) are being converted from their use in manufacturing to the creation of scaffolds with biologically complex shapes. None of the standard biodegradable materials (e.g., polyanhydrides) (Figure 51-4) has the requisite elastomeric nature for cardiovascular constructs. New materials based on elastin,[41] acellular matrices (e.g., porcine small intestine submucosa, SIS[46]), polyurethanes,[102] or a glycerol-sebacic acid copolymer[118] are being developed, although all require further study and development before being readily available for use. A complexity of some biodegradable materials, such as the lactide-glycolides, is that many result in a lowering of the local pH so that there is an adverse effect on cell phenotype during biodegradation.[59]

An alternative approach worth noting is that of Niklason et al[74] who use a somewhat rigid scaffold (polyglycolic acid mesh) but allow it to degrade and be replaced by cell-produced extracellular matrix prior to implantation. Similarly the self-assembly approach[48] relies on the cells making their own matrix, and no biomaterial is used even before implantation: a sheet of cells in matrix is simply rolled up to form a tube Instead of a scaffold in some devices such as vascular grafts, collagen is used as an immobilization matrix for cells (e.g., smooth muscle cells) that contract the collagen, typically under mechanical tension to form an arterial substitute.[94] Multifunctional materials that combine biodegradability, elastomeric qualities, processability, and phenotype control (through immobilized ligands such as RGD peptides or controlled release strategies[90]) remain the goal of further research into new biomaterials.

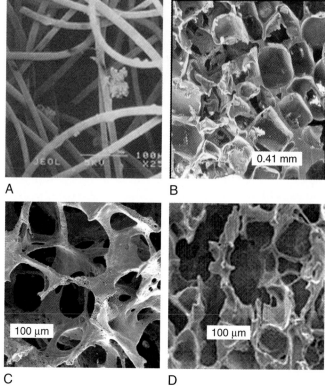

Figure 51–3 Typical scaffold structures. (**A**) Polyglycolic acid fiber mesh. (**B**) PLGA (75/25) scaffold prepared by salt leaching. (**C**) PLGA (75/25) scaffold with a trabecular structure prepared by particulate leaching and simultaneous phase inversion[32] for bone tissue engineering applications (Osteofoam). (**D**), Polyurethane[102] scaffold for cardiac application prepared by particulate (salt) leaching.
(**A** *from Lab-grown organs begin to take shape. Science 422, 1999.* **B** *and* **C** *courtesy of M. Shoichet.* **D** *courtesy of J. D. Fromstein and K. A. Woodhouse.*)

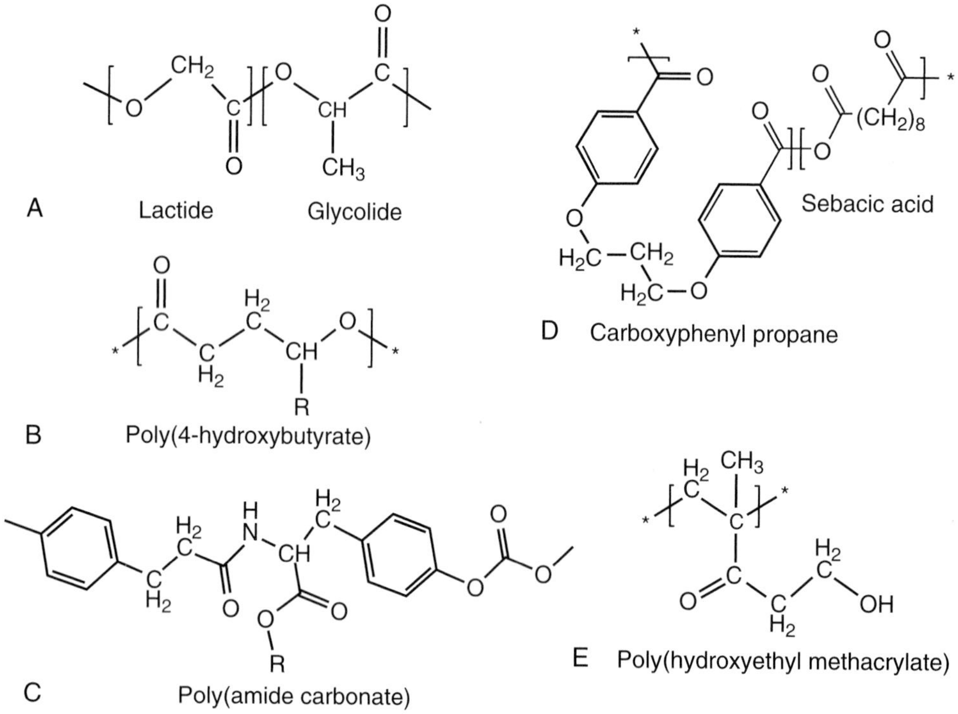

Figure 51–4 Chemical structures of biomaterials used in tissue regeneration. (**A**) Poly (lactide-glycolide) (PLGA). Changing the proportions of the two repeat units leads to differences in degradation rates as well as physical and biological properties. (**B**) Poly(4-hydroxybutyrate). R = hydrogen. Other variations on this structure (different R, more CH_2) are available. (**C**) A poly(amide carbonate) made from desaminotyrosine and tyrosine alkyl ester. (**D**) A polyanhydride. (**E**) PolyHEMA. All but polyHEMA are biodegradable. The degradability arises from the hydrolytic instability of the ester, amide, or anhydride linkages.

A   Lactide   Glycolide

B   Poly(4-hydroxybutyrate)

C   Poly(amide carbonate)

D   Carboxyphenyl propane   Sebacic acid

E   Poly(hydroxyethyl methacrylate)

Although the biomaterial is an important means of affecting cell phenotype, it is the local environment that dictates cell phenotype. With a biomaterial scaffold the cell must migrate into the scaffold and/or grow, become attached produce its own extracellular matrix, and adopt the desired phenotype. It must also make the critical connections with neighboring cells (e.g., intercalated disks) and with the host tissue where relevant. The biochemical and biomechanical cues (and the spatial and temporal control thereof) for all these have yet to be uncovered in the absence of a scaffold let alone in the context of a material that is being remodeled as the tissue develops. Cell adhesion and migration are typically greater on hydrophilic, positively charged rigid surfaces, but there are many exceptions to this.[89] The relationships among biomaterial surface structure, protein adsorbate and integrin binding, signal transduction, and cell phenotype, are largely unknown. Unfortunately most studies have used tissue culture polystyrene, and it is generally accepted that the understanding gleaned from these studies will not be relevant to the materials used in tissue engineering.

CELL SOURCES

One of the more controversial and more crucial aspects of tissue regeneration is the source of the cells to be used for *in situ* therapy (see also Chapter 97) or for tissue engineering. Whereas embryonic sources have greater proliferative potential, adult sources have fewer ethical concerns. It is not yet clear which will satisfy the clinical need; Table 51-2 provides a summary of the current status.

Adult Cells

Obtaining adult cardiomyocytes in sufficient quantities for effective transplantation into an injured heart has thus far been hindered by the limited proliferative capacity of these cells. The use of noncardiac cells that exhibit contractile properties, as well as other adult stem cells that may still have the potential to differentiate to cardiac cells, appears to be a practical alternative.

Several recent studies have investigated whether introducing skeletal satellite cells (a precursor cell with some, albeit limited, capacity for self-renewal) into the heart may promote regeneration of the injured myocardium, improving cardiac function.[35,108] This source of cells is relatively easy to culture, making them desirable candidates for clinical use. Furthermore, these cells have the potential for autologous transplantation thereby eliminating any immunological or ethical problems (see Chapter 97). In mice, the cells appear to mimic cardiac muscle,[18] including intercalated disks, and provide functional improvement. However the engrafted cells form skeletal muscle, never

Table 51–2

Cell Sources for Cardiac Tissue Engineering: Advantages and Disadvantages

Cell sources	Advantages	Disadvantages
Adult cardiac cells	Target cell source	Little proliferative or developmental potential, limited resource
Fetal cardiac cells	Some proliferative potential, appropriate developmental potential; demonstrated efficacy	Limited resource; ethical considerations
Endothelial progenitor cells	Some proliferative potential; may elicit *in vivo* healing through indirect mechanisms	Appropriate developmental potential yet to be demonstrated; may not be appropriate for larger tissue replacement or *in vitro* tissue engineering
Adult bone marrow-derived cells	Significant *in vitro* proliferative potential; some demonstration of efficacy	Appropriate developmental potential to be demonstrated; safety tolerance after *in vitro* culture to be determined
Embryonic stem cells	Significant *in vitro* proliferative potential; demonstration of efficacy; appropriate developmental potential; sustainable resource	*In vitro* culture may introduce genetic changes; safety tolerance after *in vitro* culture and differentiation to be determined

824 expressing cardiac specific markers.[70] In a separate transplantation study by Scorsin et al[92,93] no gap junctions were detected on the membranes of the skeletal cells, suggesting impaired electrical coupling and an inability to form cardiac-like syncytia with neighboring cells. Similar issues have been seen in the first clinical trials.[67,120]

Bone marrow-derived cells have the capacity for extensive proliferation[38,84] and, at least a subset of them, may be capable of developing into cells that resemble cardiomyocytes. Orlic et al[76,77] injected damaged myocardium with Lin c-kit[pos] bone marrow cells transfected to express green fluorescent protein. Within 9 days cells with morphological characteristics of cardiomyocytes, smooth muscle cells, and endothelial cells occupied the damaged site. Cardiac function improved, as assessed by hemodynamic parameters, and various myocyte specific genes were expressed. Despite these exciting results, identification of the cells in the regenerated tissue as true cardiomyocytes has been ambiguous, as the expression of skeletal markers has not been rigorously examined. Regardless of the molecular nature of the cells that integrate into cardiac muscle, clinical translation of this cell source has been difficult because no specific markers for progenitor identification have been identified, and technologies for the propagation of large numbers of appropriate cells are still under development.[11]

Embryonic Cells

Embryonic stem (ES) cells are pluri/totipotent[33] cells derived from the inner cell mass of the developing blastocyst. Cultured under specific conditions, ES cells are able to self-renew indefinitely while retaining their capacity to differentiate into cell lineages of all three primary germ layers *in vitro*. This characteristic of ES cells holds great promise for cell therapy, potentially providing a cell source in sufficient quantities for a variety of organs.

Protocols have been established for *in vitro* differentiation of mouse (m)ES cells into cardiomyocytes representing all specialized cell types of the heart (atrial-like, ventricular-like, sinus nodal–like, and Purkinje-like).[56a] During differentiation, cardiac-specific genes, proteins, receptors, and ion channels are expressed in a developmental pattern paralleling that of early cardiogenesis. *In vitro* differentiation of mES cells normally requires an initial aggregation step to form embryoid bodies (EBs). EB size, medium components (FBS, growth factors, additives), culture conditions (i.e., oxygen tension, glucose), and specific ES cell lines all affect ES cell differentiation to cardiomyocyte. The presence of cardiomyocytes can be observed by the appearance of spontaneous rhythmically contracting areas in EBs. With differentiation, the number of spontaneously beating areas increases. Beating cells are primarily mononucleated and rod-shaped, and contain cell–cell junctions consistent with those observed in cardiomyocytes developing in the heart.[11a]

Successful use of ES cell-derived donor cells requires the generation of relatively pure cardiomyocyte cultures, requiring the removal of other differentiated cell types as well as undifferentiated ES cells that may form teratomas upon engraftment.[23,31,116] For assistance in the generation of purified cultures of cardiomyocytes, a genetic selection technique[42,50,57] has been employed, whereby a fusion gene, encoding neomycin resistance driven by an MHC promoter, is stably transfected into ES cells.

Recent studies have determined that cardiomyocytes can be obtained from human ES cells (hES cells) using appropriate culture conditions. Although in-depth characterization is still underway, indications are that differences exist between mouse and human ES cell differentiation to cardiomyocytes. For example, Xu et al[124] observed cardiac differentiation in hES cells maintained for 260 population doublings (approximately 50 passages); late-passage mES cells may have difficulty differentiating to cardiomyocytes.

Phenotype Control

Human ES cells are a highly promising option as a source of transplantable cells. However, for achievement of an effective improvement in cardiac function in a damaged heart, it will be necessary to generate large numbers of functionally mature cells either *in vitro* or after transplantation. This in turn requires controlling ES cell differentiation. It is in this context that we are drawing on the lessons of developmental biology (outlined above) to influence *in vitro* cardiac development. For example, dimethyl sulfoxide (DMSO) promotes differentiation of mES cells to cardiomyocytes[62] and also induces the expression of GATA-4 and Nkx-2.5.[103] Also retinoic acid has been shown to specifically accelerate the differentiation of mES cells to ventricular cardiomyocytes, while affecting a decrease in the number of atrium and pacemaker-like cells.[122]

In addition to soluble factors, proteins in the extracellular matrix (ECM) play a role in regulation of ES cell-derived cardiac differentiation.[113] Studies in the EB system on β_1-integrin-deficient ES cells revealed that β_1-integrin is important for normal cardiogenesis.[23] Among other defects, electrophysiological studies revealed that specification of cardiac precursors into pacemaker, atrial, and ventricular cells was significantly impaired in β_1-integrin-deficient cells. Sarcomeric architecture was incomplete and disarranged in the absence of β_1-integrin. These findings indicate that heart muscle phenotypes may be modulated by controlling the interactions between differentiating cell and substrata, including biomaterials.

Effects of Physicochemical Parameters

Physicochemical parameters, like protein modulators of cell function, can influence cardiac development. Reduced medium oxygen tension results in the activation of HIF-1, one of a number[95] of genes involved in developmental processes that are directly or indirectly regulated by hypoxia.[47] Hypoxia is known to induce mRNA transcription for the VEGF protein.[83,95] VEGF may be working by enhancing cell survival of BMP-induced mesoderm formation, and thus also enhance the development of cardiac myocytes.

High glucose, supplemented medium has been shown to strongly increase and accelerate cardiac differentiation *in vitro*, enhance the mRNA levels of certain cardiac-specific contractile proteins, and improve the degree of structural organization of sarcomeres.[27] High glucose levels *in vitro* can up-regulate the expression of fibronectin, collagen, and laminin in several cell types,[8,15,53] as well as increase mRNA levels of integrin α_3, α_5, and β_1-subunits and their cognate proteins.[87]

Bioreactors

Bioreactor systems make it possible to generate scalable quantities of the cell type of interest by achieving high-density cultures and controlling key bioprocess parameters (Figure 51-5). A stirred culture vessel overcomes many of the limitations of static culture systems, eliminating spatial concentration gradients of physicochemical parameters that, as previously described, have important effects on both ES and adult cell-derived differentiation. In addition to eliminating oxygen and glucose concentration gradients, it is also important to monitor and control their levels. Therefore, another requirement for scale-up is a control system that allows us to monitor and optimize parameters, such as glucose and oxygen, to improve the efficiency of cardiomyocyte generation.

Bioreactor systems are currently under development for culturing adult bone marrow-derived multipotent cells. These cells are capable of cytokine-dependent proliferation, as individual cells in stirred suspension cultures, while maintaining their ability to form functional differentiated mesenchymal cell types.[11] Such a system would permit large-scale expansion of mesenchymal progenitors that have the potential to differentiate into cardiomyocytes.

Stirred suspension cultures pose a problem in ES cell differentiation because ES cells express surface molecules during the first 4 days of differentiation that make them prone to aggregation.[19] For application of the stirred culture system to ES cell differentiation, a strategy was developed whereby ES cells are encapsulated in agarose hydrogel microcapsules. Encapsulation permits the formation of uniform EB sizes, prevents EB aggregation, allows high cell densities in liquid suspension culture, and enables ES cell differentiation in a scalable, controlled environment. Currently, the effects of glucose and oxygen are being investigated as factors that may

increase the baseline frequency of mouse ES cell-derived cardiomyocytes. Preliminary studies suggest that culturing cells at higher glucose concentrations and under hypoxic conditions may improve the efficiency of ES cell differentiation to cardiomyocytes. Further investigations utilizing stirred suspension cultures with control of key bioprocess parameters show promise in the development of a process for large-scale production of viable, ES cell-derived cardiomyocytes for tissue engineering and/or implantation.

TISSUE AND ORGAN FUNCTION

Function of an engineered tissue with the host requires both maintenance of cellular phenotype and the integration of the construct within the host tissue. It will be necessary to ensure that engineered cardiac cells and tissue will not only contract in unison with the surrounding native myocardium to produce the desired force but that the biograft is electrically integrated with the host, to prevent arrhythmogenesis. The appearance of arrhythmias in 4 of 10 patients in the phase 1 clinical trial of skeletal muscle cell *in situ* cardiac repair[67] (see also Chapter 97) highlights this issue, which appears to be a major limitation of current cardiac cell therapy strategies.

Underlying such integration and the implicit control of the construct phenotype is the creation of the arborized networks (vessels, lymphatics, and nerves) needed to sustain large and complex tissue structures. Then there are the issues associated with blood compatibility, tissue remodeling, and, more generally, the immune and inflammatory responses to the new tissue or cells. Using autologous cells is an approach that is immunologically preferable, but it likely precludes the "off-the-shelf" concept behind much of the attraction of tissue engineering.

Mechanical Elasticity and Strength Development

A critical feature of the heart is its mechanical characteristics (Table 51-3). Simply speaking, the heart must pump

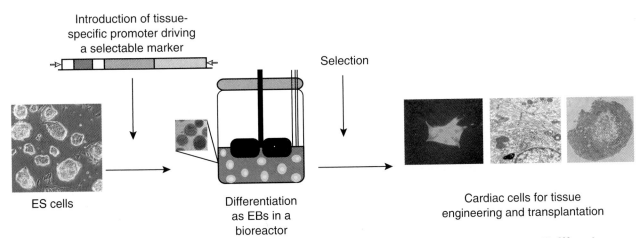

Figure 51–5 **The bioreactor-mediated generation of purified cardiac cells from embryonic stem cells.**[123] Embryonic stem cells are transduced with an appropriate selection cassette and grown in scalable stirred suspension bioreactors as embryoid bodies. Once cardiac commitment has begun, a selectable agent is added to the bioreactor to eliminate noncardiac cells. After selection, the purified cardiac cells can be used in tissue engineering or cardiac transplantation studies. (See color plate.)

Introduction of tissue-specific promoter driving a selectable marker

Selection

ES cells

Differentiation as EBs in a bioreactor

Cardiac cells for tissue engineering and transplantation

825

Table 51–3

Mechanical Attributes of the Heart as Drawn from a Simple Biophysical Approach[13]

Power requirements	Heart contracts 72 min^{-1} × 5 liters/min at 100 mm Hg = ~1.3 W (PV work) at rest; with exercise, power requirements are ~6 × higher
Total oxygen consumption	~10–20 × PV work (200 ml O$_2$/h at moderate activity)
Fatigue life	10 years of life = 3 × 10^8 cycles
Wall tension	3 × 10^4 N/m based on law of Laplace with radii of curvature (left ventricle) of 20–80 mm and thickness ~8 mm
Frank–Starling law	Cardiac output = venous return; stroke volume increases with circulatory filling pressure or myocardium stretch

blood at a mean pressure of roughly 100 mm Hg. Hence heart muscle must stretch in response to capillary filling pressure and eject a volume of blood that varies with demand. The latter requires a uniform and well-coordinated contraction that generates the required power. The mechanical fatigue limitations of a heart that must beat 3 × 10^8 times over 10 years must be compared with the flexural fatigue life of synthetic elastomeric materials that are typically much lower.

It will be a significant challenge to replicate the complex architecture of the myocardium and its nonlinear viscoelastic properties in both resting and activated states.[24] Although some constructs exhibit a significant burst strength[48] and some groups are very advanced in the use of the tools of biomechanics to advance vascular graft[72] or heart valve development, this area has received less attention than it deserves.[14]

Tissue Architecture and Electrical Conduction

The complexity of the electrical conduction pathways in the heart has received little attention in the tissue engineering literature. The cells need to form the appropriate intercellular connections and matrix arrangements to enable the directed beating of contracting cells to generate the forces required to pump blood.[2] The proper formation of the intercalated disks between myocytes is also critical in enabling electrical pulses to be transmitted in the correct direction at normal speeds and in allowing suitable force transmission. As noted previously, the heart also contains specialized cells that participate in the electrical conduction routes found throughout the heart. These specialized cells are crucial to the coordination of the heart's contrac-

tile effort, and including them in the proper places in a regenerated substitute may be critical. There are clear differences between the rhythmic twitching of cultured cardiac cells en mass and the organized, efficient, regulated beating of the heart; only the latter will generate the force required to pump blood at systolic pressure levels. It is not difficult to envision the problems yet to be faced. Given the variety of electrical conduction-related diseases in a normal myocardium, there is good reason to suspect that simple mimicry of heart muscle may fall short of the goal.

Thrombogenicity and Endothelialization

The need for blood compatibility is another crucial characteristic of cardiovascular constructs. All biomaterials lack the desired nonthrombogenicity and most extracellular matrices initiate thrombosis; endothelialization of the construct is another critical issue. Endothelial cells (EC) have a reversible plasticity,[7,54,85] and they can become activated (proliferative or adhesive to leukocytes) upon exposure to inflammatory cytokines (e.g., interleukin-1 [IL-1], tumor necrosis factor [TNF]) or to growth factors such as VEGF. Flow and the associated shear stress, normally in the range of 5–20 dyn/cm^2, elongate and align cells in the direction of flow,[21,37] and modify gene expression[63] as well as many other functions including markers of antithrombogenicity.

ECs provide a hemocompatible surface by production of molecules that modulate platelet aggregation (e.g., prostacyclin), coagulation (thrombomodulin[22,58]), and fibrinolysis[96] (e.g., tissue plasminogen activator). They can be transformed into a prothrombotic surface, for example, by the action of thrombin or through exposure to some biomaterials.[16,17,49,56] Blood compatibility has been a key issue in the development of vascular grafts. ECs have been seeded on a variety of biomaterials, with or without protein precoating with fibronectin, collagen, and other ECM proteins. Recent clinical success[66] has renewed enthusiasm for this approach. Factors identified as critical to the success of the EC seeding technique[121] are cell source and isolation technique, method of cell deposition, EC adhesion to the graft under flow conditions, and the thrombogenicity[30] of the EC. Many of the preseeded cells are lost on implantation because of insufficient adhesion[121], and thus the protection from thrombosis provided by the cells is limited because of the incomplete cell coverage. The potential to exploit the presence of circulating endothelial cell progenitors has only begun to be explored.[82]

It is also worth noting the effects of the endothelium on the neighboring tissue and the corresponding effects on EC phenotype. With VSMC, this bidirectional cross-talk is thought to be a critical regulator of vascular homeostasis[44]: secretion and expression of molecules such as nitric oxide,[78] prostacyclin,[69] and endothelin[61] act on VSMC to regulate vessel tone. Meanwhile, VSMC inhibits EC endothelin-1 (ET-1) production to increase EC NO and eNOS expression.[20] Many other relevant systems (e.g., MMP secretion and matrix remodeling) are also affected by the interactions between EC and other cell types.

Endothelial Cells and Vascularization

The intrinsic nature of large cell-based constructs and the corresponding difficulty of supplying cells deep within the construct with nutrients are other problems. Diffusion is fine for 100 μm or so, and low cell densities can extend this limit, but at the cost of making constructs too large to be useful. Thin or essentially two-dimensional (e.g., a tube) constructs are feasible without an internal blood/nutrient supply. However, it is hard to combine cells at tissue densities (10^9 cells/cm^3) into large tissues without some sort of prevascularization or its alternative. Thus, a capillary network (and a lymphatic network) needs to be "engineered" as part of the creation of a larger structure.

Approaches to create vascularized constructs are illustrated in Figure 51-6. Sheridan et al have incorporated an endothelial cell mitogen (VEGF) into three-dimensional porous poly(lactide-co-glycolide, PLG) scaffolds during fabrication[97] to promote scaffold vascularization. Sustained delivery of bioactive VEGF translated into a significant increase in blood vessel ingrowth in mice and the vessels appeared to integrate with the host vasculature. We are using microencapsulated VEGF$_{165}$-secreting cells (prepared by transfection of L929 cells) as a means of exploring this strategy, at least for microcapsules.[114] Of course VEGF is but one angiogenic factor[1] and issues associated with the functional maturity of the vessels and the need for multiple factors may limit this strategy. In a third approach, Kaihara et al micromachined a hierarchical branched network mimicking the vascular system in two dimensions. Silicon and

Pyrex surfaces were etched with branching channels ranging from 500 to 10 μm in diameter[39] that were then seeded with rat hepatocytes and microvascular endothelial cells. Finally we note that there are initial attempts at adapting endothelial seeding approaches in a modular approach to create scalable and vascularized tissue constructs.

Host Response and Biocompatibility

Questions related to the immune and inflammatory response to tissue constructs are starting to draw attention. The host response to a tissue engineered construct is manifested by the innate and adaptive immune systems, involving both plasma (e.g., complement) and cellular components (e.g., macrophages, T cells, etc.), that are directed against engineered cells and grafts or the materials used in tissue constructs. This potent immune response is most often mediated by MHC mismatches between donor and host tissue in allogeneic transplantations. This response can also be manifested in situations where autologous cells or tissues are engineered to express therapeutic but foreign factors or if these autologous cells are placed in tissue constructs that themselves negatively impact immune consequences.[9]

Immunosuppressants have enabled the successful transplantation of kidneys, hearts, and other organs. With the advent of tissue engineering, new configurations of tissues and

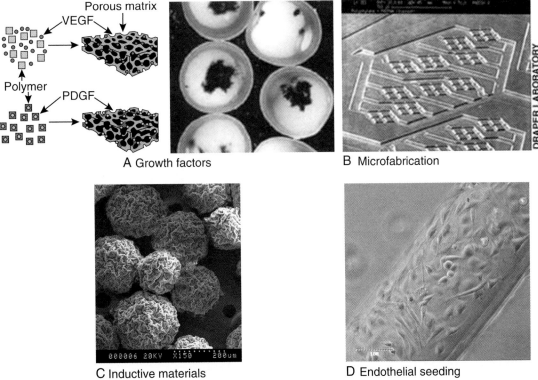

Figure 51–6 Vascularization strategies. (A) Growth factors such as VEGF (and PDGF) can be delivered by controlled release delivery systems such as microspheres[97] or cell-containing microcapsules.[114] **(B)**, Microchannel networks are fabricated into silicon chips; multiple layers are used to generate arborized networks with capacity for perfusion.[39] **(C)** Materials have been discovered that induce blood vessels to grow without exogenous growth factors. **(D)** Endothelial cells are seeded within tissue constructs to create a vascular network.
(**A** *adapted from Sheridan MH, Shea LD, Peters MC, Mooney DJ: Bioabsorbable polymer scaffolds for tissue engineering capable of sustained growth factor delivery. J Control Rel 64:91–102, 2000, and from the authors' own work.* **C** *courtesy of Rimon Therapeutics Inc.* **D** *courtesy of A. McGuigan.*)

828

organs (often with an added biomaterial component) are being developed, and our understanding of the immune and inflammatory response to these new therapies is being shown to be inadequate. For example, microencapsulation prevents the direct recognition of the transplanted cells but does not prevent indirect recognition, hence resulting in immune stimulation.[55] On the other hand, some xenogeneic cell transplants (mice to rat) survive in situations of cardiac repair despite the species differences,[88] although this may be specific to the animal model or to cardiac repair. The longevity of a transplant is also dependent on the ability of somatic cells to withstand and respond to the stresses of implantation, rejection, and other injuries.[29] The presence of a biomaterial scaffold and the oft-associated hypoxia may further exacerbate this situation. The classic "foreign body reaction" to biomaterials is well known, but the details of the molecular signals (complement regulatory proteins, MMPs) that accompany this phenomenon (in the context of biomaterials) are only beginning to be defined.

A variety of approaches have been undertaken or are in development to generate or to improve upon graft acceptance.[86] These approaches include methods to block the innate immune response such as by use of drugs or transferred genes to block NF-κB signaling pathways, for example. Other methods to block the innate response include the use of antibodies to IL-1 or TNF or the use of antiadhesion and antielastase antibodies. Perhaps nuclear transfer and therapeutic cloning strategies[65] may be necessary, assuming the various ethical issues can be resolved. We must better understand the mechanism of the host response itself so that we can design better biomaterials, select or engineer more suitable cells, devise better strategies for controlling both innate and adaptive immune responses, and enable a functional integration of the new tissue with the host.

► APPLICATIONS

There has been some, albeit limited, effort in translating the basics of tissue regeneration into cardiovascular constructs. The efforts directed to tissue engineered vascular grafts, cardiac valves, and cardiac patches are described briefly here. The use of cell therapy for *in situ* repair (see Chapter 97) is discussed more fully elsewhere.

The vascular graft, based on the work of Weinberg and Bell,[119] has received much attention for many years leading to some human experiments at least in the context of pulmonary artery transplantation.[100] It consists of smooth muscle cells (VSMCs) in a collagen scaffold, with an EC lining of the inner lumen.[73,94] Contraction of the collagen gel by the VSMC results in orientation of the VSMC and the development of robust (but perhaps not yet strong enough) grafts. VSMC cultured on type 1 collagen gel took on the synthetic phenotype, but this was inhibited when elastin was added to the gel.[36,125] The related topic of endothelial seeding of vascular grafts is discussed briefly above.[66]

Tissue-engineered heart valves grown *in vitro* using biodegradable poly-4-hydroxybutyrate-coated polyglycolic acid mesh and autologous cells (endothelial and carotid artery medial cells) functioned as pulmonary valves for 5 months in growing lambs.[99,104–106] The originally crude structures evolved over time to take on more of a natural, specialized layered structure and these valves "grew" as the animal grew. This remodeling was started in a bioreactor that used cyclical movement and nutrient flow to mimic physiological processes and then further remodeling occurred *in vivo*. With collagen sponges,[109] acellular matrices,[10] or intestinal submucosa[60] is another approach that builds on the extensive experience associated with porcine valve substitutes[91] (see Chapter 97).

To date, there have been only limited attempts at producing myocardium. In cases of congenital defect or severe disease (where the tissue structure is absent, disorganized, or unsuitable for *in situ* seeding of cells), *in situ* repair using a cell suspension may not be sufficient. It may be necessary to organize the cells prior to surgical implantation. In one set of studies, cardiac tissue structure and aspects of cardiac function were reestablished *in vitro* in the absence of three-dimensional cues from extracellular scaffolds.[4,5] These results suggest that cardiac cells possess an innate capacity to reestablish complex, three-dimensional, cardiac organization *in vitro*. Other investigators have used three-dimensional meshes or foams as culture scaffolds. Freed and co-workers have developed a model system using a biodegradable polymer mesh[79,81] that can be used for electrophysiological studies. Li and co-workers[51,52] have grown three-dimensional cardiac grafts and implanted them into host myocardia. Two critical observations from this work were the survival of functional grafts and the apparent vascularization of the implants by the host circulation. Current developments have highlighted the limitations of existing degradable biomaterials that are too rigid for this application. Several new materials and approaches are under development.[43,64,98,115]

► SUMMARY

Overall, the field of cardiac tissue engineering is very much in its infancy. Although the results to date are exceedingly encouraging, much remains to be done to develop clinically relevant approaches, let alone move toward a whole heart. Hence an NIH task force[123] has emphasized development of heart components such as a cardiac patch or a valve before "graduating" to whole heart engineering. This too is the view of the LIFE initiative.

The LIFE Initiative, a multiinstitutional affiliation of researchers, was created to use tissue engineering and regeneration to produce an endless supply of human vital organs for transplantation.[3] With an unlimited supply of vital organs, replacing a damaged or failed organ would become not substantially different than any other surgical procedure and there would be no wait for a suitably matched donor organ. Of more significance, a large number of patients may benefit from the implantation of smaller structures—heart muscle, valves, vascular grafts—so that the "spin-off" benefits of a tissue engineering effort may become even more important than the whole organ.

REFERENCES

1. Ahrendt G, Chickering DE, Ranieri JP: Angiogenic growth factors: A review for tissue engineering. Tissue Eng 4(2): 117–130, 1998.

2. Akins RE: Prospects for the use of cell implantation, gene therapy, and tissue engineering in the treatment of myocardial disease and congenital heart defects. In Sames K, editor: Medizinische Regeneration und Tissue Engineering. Landsberg, Germany: EcoMed, 2000.

3. Akins R, Sefton MV: Tissue engineering the human heart. New Surg 1:26–32, 2001.

4. Akins RE, Boyce RA, Madonna ML, et al: Cardiac organogenesis in vitro: Reestablishment of three-dimensional tissue architecture by dissociated neonatal rat ventricular cells. Tissue Eng 5(2):103–118, 1999.

5. Akins RE, Schroed NA, Gonda SR, Hartzell CR: Neonatal rat heart cells cultured in simulated microgravity. In Vitro Cell Dev Biol Anim 33:337–343, 1997.

6. Alsan BH, Schultheiss TM: Regulation of avian cardiogenesis by Fgf8 signaling. Development 129:1935–1943, 2002.

7. Augustin-Voss HG, Johnson RC, Pauli BU: Modulation of endothelial cell surface glycoconjugate expression by organ derived biomatrices. Exp Cell Res 192:346–351, 1991.

8. Ayo SH, Radnik RA Glass WF 2nd, et al: Increased extracellular matrix synthesis and mRNA in mesangial cells grown in high-glucose medium. Am J Physiol 260(2 Pt. 2):F185–191, 1991.

9. Babensee JE, Anderson JM, McIntire LV, Mikos AG: Host response to tissue engineered devices. Adv Drug Delivery Rev 33:111–139, 1998.

10. Bader A, Schilling T, Teebken OE, et al: Tissue engineering of heart valves—human endothelial cell seeding of detergent acellularized porcine valves. Eur J Cardiothorac Surg 14:279–284, 1998.

11. Baksh D, Davies JE, Zandstra PW: Adult human bone marrow derived mesenchymal progenitor cells are capable of adhesion independent survival and expansion. Exp Hematol 31:723–732, 2003.

11a. Boheler KR, Czyz J, Tweedie D, et al: Differentiation of pluripotent embryonic stem cells into cardiomyocytes. Circ Res 91:189–201, 2002.

12. Bruneau BG, Nemer G, Schmitt JP, et al: A murine model of Holt-Oram syndrome defines roles of the T-box transcription factor Tbx5 in cardiogenesis and disease. Cell 106:709–721, 2001.

13. Burton AC: Biophysical Basis of the Circulation. St. Louis: Yearbook Medical Publishers, 1972.

14. Butler DL, Goldstein SA, Guilak F: Functional tissue engineering: The role of biomechanics. J Biomech Eng 122:570–575, 2000.

15. Cagliero E, Roth T, Roy S, Lorenzi M: Characteristics and mechanisms of high-glucose-induced overexpression of basement membrane components in cultured human endothelial cells. Diabetes 40(1):102–110, 1991.

16. Cenni E, Ciapetti G, Cavedagna D, et al: Production of prostacyclin and fibrinolysis modulators by endothelial cells cultured in the presence of polyethylene terephthalate. J Biomed Mater Res 27(9):1161–1164, 1993.

17. Cenni E, Granchi D, Ciapetti G, et al: Cytokine expression in vitro by cultured human endothelial cells in contact with polyethylene terephthalate coated with pyrolytic carbon and collagen. J Biomed Mater Res 50(4):483–489, 2000.

18. Chiu RC, Zibaitis A, Kao RL: Cellular cardiomyoplasty: Myocardial regeneration with satellite cell implantation. Ann Thorac Surg 60(1):12–18, 1995.

19. Dang SM, Kyba M, Perlingeiro R, et al: Efficiency of embryoid body formation and hematopoietic development from embryonic stem cells in different culture systems. Biotechnol Bioeng 78(4):442–453, 2002.

20. Di Luozzo G, Bhargava J, Powell RJ: Vascular smooth muscle cell effect on endothelial cell endothelin-1 production. J Vasc Surg 4:781–789, 2000.

21. Eskin SG, Ives CL, McIntire LV, Navarro LT: Response of cultured endothelial cells to steady flow. Microvasc Res 1:87–94, 1984.

22. Esmon CT: Regulation of blood coagulation. Biochim Biophys Acta 1477(1–2):349–360, 2000.

23. Fassler R, Rohwedel J, Maltsev V, et al: Differentiation and integrity of cardiac muscle cells are impaired in the absence of beta 1 integrin. J Cell Sci 109(Pt. 13):2989–2899, 1996.

24. Fung YC: Biomechanics: Mechanical Properties of Living Tissues, 2nd ed. New York: Springer-Verlag, 1993, p. 433.

25. Grant DS, Kleinman HK, Martin GR: The role of basement membranes in vascular development. Ann NY Acad Sci 588:61–72, 1990.

26. Grikscheit TC, Vacanti JP: The history and current status of tissue engineering: The future of pediatric surgery. J Pediatr Surg 37(3):277–288, 2002.

27. Guan K, Furst DO, Wobus AM: Modulation of sarcomere organization during embryonic stem cell-derived cardiomyocyte differentiation. Eur J Cell Biol 78(11):813–823, 1999.

28. Gulbins H, Meiser BM, Reichenspurner H, Reichart B: Cell transplantation—a potential therapy for cardiac repair in the future? Heart Surg Forum 5(4):E28–34, 2002.

29. Halloran PF, Melk A: Renal senescence, cellular senescence, and their relevance to nephrology and transplantation. Adv Nephrol Necker Hosp 31:273–283, 2001.

30. Hedeman Joosten PP, Verhagen HJ, Heijnen-Snyder GJ, et al: Thrombogenesis of different cell types seeded on vascular grafts and studied under blood-flow conditions. J Vasc Surg 28:1094–1103, 1998.

31. Hilberg F, Wagner EF: Embryonic stem (ES) cells lacking functional c-jun: Consequences for growth and differentiation, AP-1 activity and tumorigenicity. Oncogene 7(12):2371–2380, 1992.

32. Holy CE, Shoichet MS, Davies JE: Engineering three-dimensional bone tissue in vitro using biodegradable scaffolds: Investigating initial cell-seeding density and culture period. J Biomed Mater Res 51(3):376–382, 2000.

33. Hubner K, Fuhrmann G, Christenson LK, et al: Derivation of oocytes from mouse embryonic stem cells. Science 300(5623):1251–1256, 2003.

34. Humes H, Buffington D, MacKay S, et al: Replacement of renal function in uremic animals with a tissue-engineered kidney. Nat Biotechnol 17:451–455, 1999.

35. Hutcheson KA, Atkins BZ, Hueman MT, et al: Comparison of benefits on myocardial performance of cellular cardiomyoplasty with skeletal myoblasts and fibroblasts. Cell Transplant 9(3):359–368, 2000.

36. Ito S, Ishimura S, Wilson S E: Inhibitory effect of type I collagen gel containing alpha-elastin on proliferation and migration of vascular smooth muscle and endothelial cells. Cardiovasc Surg 5(2):176–183, 1997.

37. Ives CL, Eskin SG, McIntire LV: Mechanical effects on endothelial cell morphology: in vitro assessment, In Vitro Cell Dev Biol 22(9):500–507, 1986.

38. Jiang Y, Vaessen B, Lenvik T, et al: Multipotent progenitor cells can be isolated from postnatal murine bone marrow, muscle, and brain. Exp Hematol 30(8):896–904, 2002.

39. Kaihara S, Borenstein J, Koka R, et al: Silicon micromachining to tissue engineer branched vascular channels for liver fabrication. Tissue Eng 6:105–117, 2000.

40. Kasahara H, Usheva A, Ueyama T, et al: Characterization of homo- and heterodimerization of cardiac Csx/Nkx2.5 homeoprotein. J Biol Chem 276:4570–4580, 2001.

41. Keeley FW, Bellingham CM, Woodhouse KA: Elastin as a self-organizing biomaterial. Use of recombinantly expressed human elastin polypeptides as a model for investigations of structure and self-assembly of elastin. Phil Trans R Soc Lond B Biol Sci 357(1418):185–189, 2002.

830

42. Klug MG, Soonpaa MH, Koh GY, Field LJ: Genetically selected cardiomyocytes from differentiating embryonic stem cells form stable intracardiac grafts. J Clin Invest 98(1):216–224, 1996.

43. Kofidis T, Akhyari P, Boublik J, et al: In vitro engineering of heart muscle: Artificial myocardial tissue. J Thorac Cardiovasc Surg 124(1):63–69, 2002.

44. Korff T, Kimmina S, Martiny-Baron G, Augustin HG: Blood vessel maturation in a 3-dimensional spheroidal coculture model: Direct contact with smooth muscle cells regulates endothelial cell quiescence and abrogates VEGF responsiveness, FASEB J 15(2):447–457, 2001.

45. Langer R, Vacanti J: Tissue engineering. Science 260:920–926, 1993.

46. Lantz GC, Badylak SF, Hiles MC, et al: Small intestine submucosa as a vascular graft: A review. J Invest Surg 3:297–310, 1993.

47. Le YJ, Corry PM: Hypoxia-induced bFGF gene expression is mediated through the JNK signal transduction pathway. Mol Cell Biochem 202(1–2):1–8, 1999.

48. L'Heureux N, Pâquet S, Labbé R, et al: A completely biological tissue-engineered human blood vessel. FASEB J 12:47–56, 1998.

49. Li JM, Menconi MJ, Wheeler HB, et al: Precoating expanded polytetrafluoroethylene grafts alters production of endothelial cell-derived thrombomodulators, J Vasc Surg 15(6):1010–1017, 1992.

50. Li M, Pevny L, Lovell-Badge R, Smith A: Generation of purified neural precursors from embryonic stem cells by lineage selection. Curr Biol 8(17):971–974, 1998.

51. Li RK, Jia ZQ, Weisel RD, et al: Survival and function of bioengineered cardiac grafts. Circulation 100(19 Suppl):II63–II69, 1999.

52. Li RK, Yau TM, Weisel RD, et al: Construction of a bioengineered cardiac graft. J Thorac Cardiovasc Surg 119(2):368–375, 2000.

53. Li W, Shen S, Khatami M, Rockey JH: Stimulation of retinal capillary pericyte protein and collagen synthesis in culture by high-glucose concentration. Diabetes 33(8):785–789, 1984.

54. Lipton BH, Bensch KG, Karaswek MA: Microvessel endothelial cell transdifferentiation: Phenotypic characterization. Differentiation 46:117–133, 1991.

55. Loudovaris T, Mandel TE, Charlton B: CD4+ T cell mediated destruction of xenografts within cell-impermeable membranes in the absence of CD8+ T cells and B cells. Transplantation 61:1678–1684, 1996.

56. Lu A, Sipehia R: Antithrombotic and fibrinolytic system of human endothelial cells seeded on PTFE: The effects of surface modification of PTFE by ammonia plasma treatment and ECM protein coatings. Biomaterials 22:1439–1446, 2001.

56a. Mattson VA, Rohwedel J, Hescheler J, Wobus AM: Embryonic stem cells differentiate in vitro into cardiomyocytes representing sinus nodal, atrial, and ventricular cell types. Mech Div 44:41–50, 1993.

57. Marchetti S, Gimond C, Iljin K, et al: Endothelial cells genetically selected from differentiating mouse embryonic stem cells incorporate at sites of neovascularization in vivo. J Cell Sci 115(Pt. 10):2075–2085, 2002.

58. Marcum JA, McKenney JB, Rosenberg RD: Acceleration of thrombin-antithrombin complex formation in rat hindquarters via heparinlike molecules bound to the endothelium. J Clin Invest 74(2):341–350, 1984.

59. Martin C, Winet H, Bao JY: Acidity near eroding polylactide-polyglycolide in vitro and in vivo in rabbit tibial bone chambers. Biomaterials 17:2373–2380, 1996.

60. Matheny RG, Hutchison ML, Dryden PE, et al: Porcine small intestine submucosa as a pulmonary valve leaflet substitute. J Heart Valve Dis 9:769–775, 2000.

61. Mawji IA, Marsden PA: Perturbations in paracrine control of the circulation: Role of the endothelial-derived vasomediators, endothelin-1 and nitric oxide. Microsc Res Tech 60:46–58, 2003.

62. McBurney MW, Jones-Villeneuve EM, Edwards MK, Anderson PJ: Control of muscle and neuronal differentiation in a cultured embryonal carcinoma cell line. Nature 299 (5879):165–167, 1982.

63. McCormick SM, Eskin SG, McIntire LV, et al: DNA microarray reveals changes in gene expression of shear stressed human umbilical vein endothelial cells. Proc Natl Acad Sci USA 98(16):8955–8960, 2001.

64. McDevitt T, Woodhouse KA, Murray CE, Stayton PS: Spatially organised layers of cardiomyocytes on biodegradable polyurethane films for myocardial repair. J Biomed Mater Res 66A(3):586–595.

65. McLaren A: Cloning: Pathways to a pluripotent future. Science 288(5472):1775–1780, 2000.

66. Meinhart JG, Deutsch M, Fischlein T, et al: Clinical autologous in vitro endothelialization of 153 infrainguinal ePTFE grafts. Ann Thorac Surg 71:S327–331, 2001.

67. Menasche P, Hagege AA, Vilquin JT, et al: Autologous skeletal myoblast transplantation for severe postinfarction left ventricular dysfunction. J Am Coll Cardiol 41(7):1078–1083, 2003.

68. Mironov V, Boland T, Trusk T, et al: Organ printing: Computer-aided jet-based 3D tissue engineering. Trends Biotechnol 21(4):157–161.

69. Moncada S: Biological importance of prostacyclin. Br J Pharmacol 76:3–31, 1982.

70. Murry CE, Wiseman RW, Schwartz SM, Hauschka SD: Skeletal myoblast transplantation for repair of myocardial necrosis. J Clin Invest 98(11):2512–2523, 1996.

71. Narita N, Bielinska M, Wilson DB: Wild-type endoderm abrogates the ventral developmental defects associated with GATA-4 deficiency in the mouse. Dev Biol 189:270–274, 1997.

72. Nerem RM: Role of mechanics in vascular tissue engineering. Biorheology 40(1–3):281–287, 2003.

73. Nerem RM, Seliktar D: Vascular tissue engineering. Annu Rev Biomed Eng 3:225–243, 2001.

74. Niklason LE, Gao J, Abbott VM, et al: Functional arteries grown in-vitro. Science 284:489–493, 1999.

75. Oberpenning F, Meng J, Yoo J, Atala A: De novo reconstitution of a functional mammalian urinary bladder by tissue engineering. Nat Biotechnol 17:149–155, 1999.

76. Orlic D, Kajstura J, Chimenti S, et al: Bone marrow cells regenerate infarcted myocardium. Nature 410(6829):701–705, 2001.

77. Orlic D, Kajstura J, Chimenti S, et al: Transplanted adult bone marrow cells repair myocardial infarcts in mice. Ann NY Acad Sci 938:221–229; discussion 229–230, 2001.

78. Palmer RM, Aston DS, Moncada S: Vascular endothelial cells synthesize nitric oxide from L-arginine. Nature 333, 664–666, 1988.

79. Papadaki M, Bursac N, Langer R, et al: Tissue engineering of functional cardiac muscle: Molecular, structural, and electrophysiological studies. Am J Physiol Heart Circ Physiol 280(1):H168–178, 2001.

80. Pardanaud L, Luton D, Prigent M, et al: Two distinct endothelial lineages in ontogeny, one of them related to hemopoiesis. Development 122:1363–1371, 1996.

81. Radisic M, Euloth M, Yang L, et al: High-density seeding of myocyte cells for cardiac tissue engineering. Biotechnol Bioeng 82(4):403–144, 2003.

82. Rafii S: Circulating endothelial precursors: Mystery, reality and promise. J Clin Invest 105:17–19, 2000.

83. Ramirez-Bergeron DL, Simon MC: Hypoxia-inducible factor and the development of stem cells of the cardiovascular system. Stem Cells 19(4):279–286, 2001.

84. Reyes M, Verfaillie CM: Characterization of multipotent adult progenitor cells, a subpopulation of mesenchymal stem cells. Ann NY Acad Sci 938:231–233; discussion 233–235, 2001.

85. Risau W: Differentiation of endothelium. FASEB J 9(10): 926–933, 1995.

86. Rossini AA, Greiner DN, Mordes JP: Induction of imunologic tolerance for transplantation. Physiol Rev 79(1):99–141, 1999.

87. Roth T, Podesta F, Stepp MA, et al: Integrin overexpression induced by high glucose and by human diabetes: Potential pathway to cell dysfunction in diabetic microangiopathy. Proc Natl Acad Sci USA 90(20):9640–9644, 1993.

88. Saito T, Kuang JQ, Bittira B, et al: Xenotransplant cardiac chimera: Immune tolerance of adult stem cells. Ann Thorac Surg 74:19–24, 2002.

89. Saltzman WM: Cell interactions with polymers. In Lanza RP, Langer R, Chick WL, editors: Principles of Tissue Engineering. Austin, TX: R. G. Landes, 1997, pp. 225–246.

90. Saltzman WM, Olbricht WL: Building drug delivery into tissue engineering. Nat Rev Drug Discov 1:177–186, 2002.

91. Schoen FJ: Future directions in tissue heart valves: Impact of recent insights from biology and pathology. J Heart Valve Dis 8:350–358, 1999.

92. Scorsin M, Hagege AA, Marotte F, et al: Does transplantation of cardiomyocytes improve function of infarcted myocardium? Circulation 96(9 Suppl):II-188–193, 1997.

93. Scorsin M, Hagege A, Vilquin JT, et al: Comparison of the effects of fetal cardiomyocyte and skeletal myoblast transplantation on postinfarction left ventricular function. J Thorac Cardiovasc Surg 119(6):1169–1175, 2000.

94. Seliktar D, Black RA, Vito RP, Nerem RM: Dynamic mechanical conditioning of collagen-gel blood vessel constructs induces remodeling in vitro, Ann Biomed Eng 28(4): 351–362, 2000.

95. Semenza GL: Regulation of hypoxia-induced angiogenesis: A chaperone escorts VEGF to the dance. J Clin Invest 108(1): 39–40, 2001.

96. Shen GX: Vascular cell-derived fibrinolytic regulators and atherothrombotic vascular disorders (Review). Int J Mol Med 1(2):399–408, 1998.

97. Sheridan MH, Shea LD, Peters MC, Mooney DJ: Bioabsorbable polymer scaffolds for tissue engineering capable of sustained growth factor delivery. J Control Rel 64: 91–102, 2000.

98. Shimizu T, Yamato M, Isoi Y, et al: Fabrication of pulsatile cardiac tissue grafts using a novel 3-dimensional cell sheet manipulation technique and temperature-responsive cell culture surfaces. Circ Res 90(3):e40, 2002.

99. Shinoka T, Breuer CK, Tanel RE, et al: Tissue engineering heart valves: Valve leaflet replacement study in a lamb model. Ann Thorac Surg 60(6 Suppl):513–516, 1995.

100. Shin'oka T, Imai Y, Ikada Y: Transplantation of a tissue-engineered pulmonary artery. N Engl J Med 344:532–533, 2001.

101. Simpson DG, Terracio L, Terracio M, et al: Modulation of cardiac myocyte phenotype in vitro by the composition and orientation of the extracellular matrix. J Cell Physiol 161(1):89–105, 1994.

102. Skarja G, Woodhouse KA: In vitro degradation and erosion of degradable, segmented polyurethanes containing an amino acid-based chain extender. J Biomater Sci Polymer Ed 12: 851–873, 2001.

103. Skerjanc IS, Sheffield WP, Silvius JR, Shore GC: Identification of hydrophobic residues in the signal sequence of mitochondrial preornithine carbamyltransferase that enhance the rate of precursor import. J Biol Chem 263(33): 17233–17236, 1988.

104. Sodian R, Hoerstrup SP, Sperling JS, et al: Tissue engineering of heart valves: In vitro experiences. Ann Thorac Surg 70(1):140–144, 2000.

105. Sodian R, Sperling JS, Martin DP, et al: Fabrication of a trileaflet heart valve scaffold from a polyhydroxyalkanoate biopolyester for use in tissue engineering. Tissue Eng 6(2): 183–188, 2000.

106. Stock UA, Vacanti JP, Mayer JE Jr, Wahlers T: Tissue engineering of heart valves—current aspects. Thorac Cardiovasc Surg 50(3):184–193, 2002.

107. Strain AJ, Neuberger JM: A bioartificial liver—state of the art. Science 295(5557):1005–1009, 2002.

108. Taylor DA, Atkins BZ, Hungspreugs P, et al: Regenerating functional myocardium: Improved performance after skeletal myoblast transplantation. Nat Med 4(8):929–933, 1998.

109. Taylor P, Allen SP, Dreger SA, Yacoub MH: Human cardiac valve interstitial cells in collagen sponge: A biological three-dimensional matrix for tissue engineering. J Heart Valve Dis 11:298–307, 2002.

110. Thomson, RC, Yaszemski MJ, Mikos AG: Polymer scaffold processing. In Lanza RP, Langer R, Chick WL, editors: Principles of Tissue Engineering. Austin, TX: R. G. Landes, 1997, pp. 263–272.

111. Vacanti CA, Langer R, Schloo B, Vacanti JP: Synthetic polymers seeded with chondrocytes provide a template for new cartilage formation. Plast Reconstr Surg 88(5):753–759, 1991.

112. Vacanti JP, Morse MA, Saltzman WM, et al: Selective cell transplantation using bioabsorbable artificial polymers as matrices. J Pediatr Surg 23(1 Pt. 2):3–9, 1988.

113. Valencik ML, McDonald JA: Cardiac expression of a gain-of-function alpha(5)-integrin results in perinatal lethality. Am J Physiol Heart Circ Physiol 280(1):H361–H367, 2001.

114. Vallbacka JJ, Sefton MV: Microencapsulation of VEGF-secreting cells for therapeutic angiogenesis. Ann Biomed Eng 29(Suppl 1): S-150, 2001.

115. van Luyn MJ, Tio RA, Gallego y van Seijen XJ, et al: Cardiac tissue engineering: Characteristics of in unison contracting two- and three-dimensional neonatal rat ventricle cell (co)-cultures. Biomaterials 23(24):4793–4801, 2002.

116. Wakitani S, Takaoka K, Hattori T, et al: Embryonic stem cells injected into the mouse knee joint form teratomas and subsequently destroy the joint. Rheumatology 42(1):162–165, 2003.

117. Wang GL, Jiang BH, Rue EA, Semenza GL: Hypoxia-inducible factor 1 is a basic-helix-loop-helix-PAS heterodimer regulated by cellular O_2 tension. Proc Natl Acad Sci USA 92: 5510–5514, 1995.

118. Wang Y, Ameer GA, Sheppard BJ, Langer R: A tough biodegradable elastomer. Nat Biotechnol 20(6):602–606, 2002.

119. Weinberg CB, Bell E: A blood vessel model constructed from collagen and cultured vascular cells. Science 231:397–400, 1986.

120. Weisel RD: Cellular approaches to preventing heart failure. Heart Surg Forum 6(2):121–122, 2003.

121. William SK: Endothelial cell transplantation. Cell Transplant 4(4):401–410, 1995.

122. Wobus AM, Kaomei G, Shan J, et al: Retinoic acid accelerates embryonic stem cell-derived cardiac differentiation and enhances development of ventricular cardiomyocytes. J Mol Cell Cardiol 29(6):1525–1539, 1997.

123. Working Group on Tissue Genesis and Organogenesis for Heart, Lung and Blood Applications, National Institutes of Health, August 13, 1999, www.nhlbi.nih.gov/meetings/workshops/tissueg1.htm.

124. Xu C, Police S, Rao N, Carpenter MK: Characterization and enrichment of cardiomyocytes derived from human embryonic stem cells. Circ Res 91(6):501–508, 2002.

125. Yamamoto M, Yamamoto K, Noumura T: Type I collagen promotes modulation of cultured rabbit arterial smooth muscle cells from a contractile to a synthetic phenotype. Exp Cell Res 204:121–129, 1993.

Blood Coagulation, Transfusion, and Conservation

D. Dean Potter, Jr., William C. Oliver, Jr., and Hartzell V. Schaff

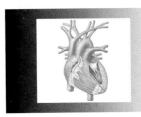

CHAPTER **52**

INTRODUCTION

Perioperative complications related to bleeding and thrombosis remain an important problem in cardiac surgery. Each year, as many as 5–25% of patients experience serious bleeding after cardiac surgery, and 2–3% of patients require reoperation to control hemorrhage.[12] Major advances have been made in understanding the mechanisms underlying normal coagulation, the effects of cardiopulmonary bypass on coagulation, and strategies to limit hemorrhage after cardiac surgery. This chapter focuses on normal blood coagulation, common abnormalities of coagulation, current recommendations for transfusion therapy, and blood conservation strategies.

PHYSIOLOGY OF HEMOSTASIS

The coagulation cascade is a combination of two separate, but linked, pathways (Figure 52-1) designed to form the prothrombinase complex that rapidly converts prothrombin to thrombin.[51] Thrombin then converts soluble fibrinogen into insoluble fibrin clot, stabilizing the fragile platelet plug. These pathways are multienzyme reactions that combine a serine protease and a nonenzymatically active protein cofactor on a cell membrane. These complexes catalyze the speed of reactions critical for clot formation by 10^4 to 10^5. The enzymes and cofactors of the coagulation system are numbered with Roman numerals in the order of discovery (Table 52-1), with activated forms designated with "*a.*"

The extrinsic pathway of coagulation is the most important pathway for the formation of thrombin *in vivo* and is initiated by exposure of plasma factor VIIa to the membrane-bound tissue factor protein.[118] Tissue factor is located in the subendothelium and does not contact the circulating blood when the endothelium is intact. Endothelial injury allows factor VIIa to complex with tissue factor, which activates factors X and IX.[111] Factors Xa and VIIa then catalyze the activation of additional factor VII, accelerating the cascade.

The intrinsic pathway of coagulation is initiated with exposure of factor XII to negatively charged surfaces.[56] Factor XIIa then activates factor XI, which in turn activates factor IX. The significance of factors XII and XI is unknown since deficiencies in either are not invariably associated with a bleeding diathesis.[51] Factor IXa and cofactor VIIIa form the "Xase" complex, which activates factor X.

The prothrombinase complex consists of factors Xa, Va, and calcium, which markedly amplifies the conversion of

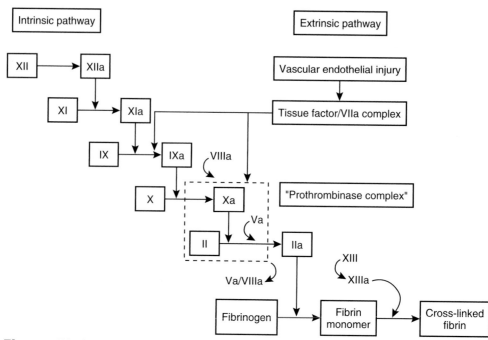

Figure 52–1 A representation of the intrinsic and extrinsic pathways of the coagulation cascade.
(*Reprinted with permission from Slaughter TF: The coagulation system and cardiac surgery. In Estafanous FG, Barash PG, Reves J G, editors: Cardiac Anesthesia: Principles and Clinical Practice: Philadelphia: Lippincott, Williams & Wilkins, 2001, p. 320.*)

prothrombin to thrombin. Thrombin formation is the key step in coagulation. First, thrombin catalyzes the activation of factors XI, VIII, VII, and V to promote the coagulation cascade. Second, thrombin activates platelets and amplifies platelet aggregate formation. Third, thrombin cleaves fibrinogen into fibrin.[158] Fibrin polymerizes into long strands[46] that are cross-linked with covalent bonds by factor XIIIa. This insoluble fibrin clot is the basis for the stable hemostatic plug. Formation of the stable hemostatic plug requires intricate interplay between both systems of blood coagulation. The intrinsic system acts as an amplifier of blood coagulation, while the extrinsic pathway of coagulation acts as the initiator.

PLATELET ADHESION AND AGGREGATION

Platelets play an important role in hemostasis via activation of prothrombin and propagation of the hemostatic plug.[155] Damage to the vascular wall allows platelets to anchor to the subendothelial matrix through the interaction of von Willebrand factor and platelet membrane glycoprotein Ib (GPIb).[98,128,130,136] Binding of von Willebrand factor to the membrane GPIb stimulates platelet contraction and pseudopod formation resulting in spreading of the platelets on the damaged vessel wall. Platelet glycoprotein IIb/IIIa (GPIIb/IIIa) also interacts with von Willebrand factor, and the binding of both GPIb and GPIIb/IIIa by von Willebrand factor results in release of storage granules, production of prostaglandin endoperoxides, and platelet activation.[23,132] Thrombin also activates platelets by several independent pathways.[147] The activated GPIIb/IIIa undergoes conforma-

tional change and serves as a binding site for fibrinogen.[8,93] In addition, the activated platelet membrane provides a procoagulant surface for formation of the "Xase" and prothrombinase complexes catalyzing the coagulation cascade.[55] Thus, platelets form the base that initially plugs the injured vessel wall, complexes factors and cofactors that rapidly catalyze clot formation, and approximate fibrinogen with thrombin, which leads to stabilization of the fragile platelet plug.

FIBRINOLYSIS AND DOWN-REGULATION OF COAGULATION

The fibrinolytic system (Figure 52-2) allows remodeling and removal of thrombus by a carefully balanced group of fibrinolytic and antifibrinolytic enzymes that maintain vascular patency by dissolving fibrin.[48,79] The principal enzyme of fibrinolysis is plasmin, which is cleaved from circulating plasminogen. Thrombin accelerates plasmin formation by stimulating the release of tissue plasminogen activator (tPA) from endothelial cells.[77] Tissue plasminogen activator binds tightly to fibrin, producing plasmin within the thrombus with minimal stimulation of circulating plasminogen.[102]

In addition, fibrin within a thrombus accelerates formation of plasmin by plasminogen activators. The localized formation of plasmin within the new thrombus allows for controlled clot formation by breakdown and remodeling of the fibrin matrix.[150] Plasminogen-activator inhibitor I and α_2-antiplasmin are the two major physiological inhibitors of fibrinolysis. Small amounts of α_2-antiplasmin are incorporated into the fibrin matrix of a fresh clot. When plasmin is generated within the clot, it must saturate all the binding

Table 52–1

Coagulation Factors and Cofactors

Factor	Name	Function
I	Fibrinogen	Structural zymogen
II	Prothrombin	Protease zymogen
III	Tissue factor	Cofactor/initiator
IV	Ionized calcium	Cofactor
V	Proaccelerin	Cofactor
VII	Proconvertin	Protease zymogen
VIII	Antihemophiliac factor	Cofactor
IX	Christmas factor	Protease zymogen
X	Stuart-Prower factor	Protease zymogen
XI	Plasma thromboplastin antecedent	Protease zymogen
XII	Hageman factor	Protease zymogen
XIII	Fibrin-stabilizing factor	Fibrin stabilization

sites of α_2-antiplasmin prior to clot lysis, preventing premature clot lysis. Plasminogen-activator inhibitor I is an acute phase reactant that is synthesized by endothelial cells and is subsequently released into the blood and extracellular matrix. Plasminogen-activator inhibitor I binds and inhibits tPA, preventing formation of plasmin and inhibiting fibrinolysis.

Endothelial cells secrete thrombomodulin, which binds to thrombin neutralizing its clotting activity by preventing the cleavage of fibrinogen to fibrin,[84,117] increases susceptibility to inactivation by antithrombin, and catalyzes activation of protein C by a factor of 20,000.[143] Activated protein C complexes with a cofactor, protein S, which inactivates factors Va and VIIIa.[117] An imbalance between the coagulation cascade, platelet function, fibrinolysis, and inactivation of the coagulation cascade may result in severe bleeding or thrombotic complications.

▶ COMMON DISORDERS OF COAGULATION

von Willebrand disease

von Willebrand disease (vWd) is the most commonly inherited clotting disorder (Table 52-2), affecting 1% of the population.[122] von Willebrand factor plays an essential role in platelet adhesion by binding platelet GPIb as well as GPIIb/IIIa receptors and acting as a carrier protein for factor VIII.

There are three subtypes of vWd (Table 52-3) that are characterized by quantitative and/or qualitative disorders of the von Willebrand factor protein.[67] Type 1 vWd is characterized by a partial quantitative deficiency of von Willebrand factor and is the most common, comprising 70–80% of all cases.[116] Type 2 is subdivided into four parts. Type 2A is the most common of the subtypes and is differentiated by reduced platelet function due to the loss of high-molecular-weight multimeric forms of von Willebrand factor. Type 2B

Figure 52–2 A schema of the fibrinolytic system. tPA, tissue plasminogen activator; PAI-1, plasminogen activator inhibitor type 1; FDP, fibrinogen degradation products.
(*Reprinted with permission from Bick RL: Thrombotic and hemorrhagic problems during cardiopulmonary bypass surgery and cardiovascular procedures. In Pifarré R, editor: Management of Bleeding in Cardiovascular Surgery. Philadelphia: Hanley & Belfus, Inc., 1999, p. 20.*)

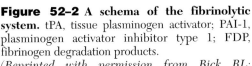
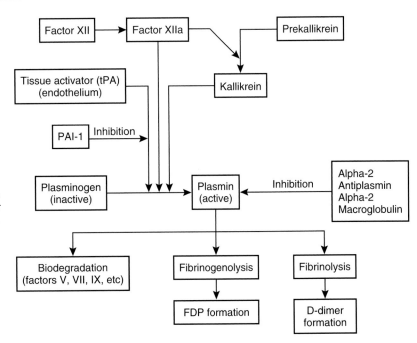

836

Table 52–2	
Common Inherited Clotting Disorders	
Deficient factor	*Incidence in general population*
von Willebrand factor	1/100–1/10,000
Fibrinogen	1/1,000,000
Prothrombin	1/2,000,000
Factor V	1/1,000,000
Factor VII	1/500,000
Factor VIII	1/10,000
Factor IX	1/60,000
Factor X	1/1,000,000
Factor XI	1/1,000,000
Factor XIII	1/1,000,000
Antithrombin	1/2000–1/5000
Factor V Leiden	1/100–1/1,000,00
Protein C	1/500–1/1000
Protein S	1/1000–3/10,000

of the ristocetin cofactor assay and further testing are best performed by a hematologist. Prevention of hemorrhage following major surgery in any patient with vWd requires factor VIII levels greater than 50 IU/dl intraoperatively and postoperatively for 10 days. Desmopressin (1-deamino-8-D-arginine vasopressin, DDAVP) has minimized blood loss associated with surgical procedures in patients with types 1 and 2N vWd that have demonstrated an excellent response to previous DDAVP treatments.[90,123] Patients with vWd who have not previously been treated with DDAVP require factor VIII concentrates postoperatively.

Desmopressin is a synthetic analog of vasopressin[87] that increases factor VIII and von Willebrand factor in patients with vWd and hemophilia. It is administered intravenously over 30 min in a dose of 0.3 µg/kg. More rapid infusion may cause significant hypotension. Plasma factor VIII and von Willebrand factor increase three to five times above the basal levels and persist for 6–8 h following administration. This therapy may be repeated every 48 h, but repeated treatments become less effective.[89] Thus, transfusions of blood products may be required to maintain adequate levels of von Willebrand factor perioperatively. Desmopressin is contraindicated in type 2B vWd because thrombosis may occur secondary to aggregation of platelets.[64] Side effects of DDAVP are usually mild, but volume overload and hyponatremia may occur due to its antidiuretic effect. Although extremely rare, myocardial infarction (MI) and stroke have occurred in hemophiliacs and uremic patients with significant atherosclerotic disease exposed to DDAVP.[17,21]

Hemorrhaging patients that are not responsive to DDAVP require blood products. Fresh frozen plasma (FFP) contains factor VIII and von Willebrand factor, but large volumes are required to achieve concentrations necessary to obtain adequate hemostasis. Cryoprecipitate contains 5–10 times more von Willebrand factor than FFP, and is effective in preventing or attenuating bleeding in vWd.[115] Replacement therapy for specific coagulation factor deficiencies have been recently developed. Classified according to purity, intermediate and high purity factor VIII concentrates contain large amounts of factor VIII and von Willebrand factor. Factor VIII concentrates are given in 50–100 IU/kg doses once or twice per day to maintain factor VIII levels. Adequate factor replacement is best monitored by factor VIII assay. Platelet transfusions provide additional von Willebrand factor that may lessen coagulopathy and excessive bleeding if cryoprecipitate or factor VIII concentrates are not effective.[22]

Patients with vWd undergoing cardiopulmonary bypass normally require transfusion of factor VIII concentrates, and repeated transfusions are needed to maintain factor VIII levels greater than 50 IU/dl for 10 days. Rarely, patients with vWd develop alloantibodies to von Willebrand factor that may cause anaphylactic reactions.[9] Treatment with recombinant factor VIII has been used in emergency situations but contains no von Willebrand factor. Because it has a very short half-life, a continuous intravenous infusion is necessary.

Hemophilia A and B

Hemophilia A and B are caused by inherited X-linked recessive deficiencies of clotting factors VIII and IX, respectively.[88] Hemophilia A affects 1:10,000 live births, and

has von Willebrand factor molecules that show increased affinity for platelet GPIb, which may cause thrombocytopenia and thrombosis in addition to hemorrhage. Type 2M is similar to type A with reduced platelet function despite normal multimeric forms of von Willebrand factor. Finally, in type 2N, there is normal von Willebrand factor quantity, function, and structure, with decreased binding to factor VIII. Type N is also known as autosomal hemophilia. Type 3 is the least common and most severe type of vWd because of a complete deficiency of von Willebrand factor.

Accurate diagnosis is essential to prevent hemorrhage after cardiopulmonary bypass in patients with vWd. The diagnosis is suspected when coagulation studies result in a prolonged activated partial thromboplastin time with a normal prothrombin time. The single best screening test, thereafter, is the ristocetin cofactor assay.[116] Interpretation

Table 52–3

Subtypes of von Willebrand Disease and Appropriate Treatments

Type	Disorder	Treatment	Treatment alternative
1	Decreased quantity and function of von Willebrand factor	Desmopressin	Antifibrinolytic estrogen
2A	Decreased plasma antigen, von Willebrand factor activity, and absence of multimeric forms	Factor concentrates	
2B	Increased affinity of platelet GPIb	Factor concentrates	Do not use desmopressin
2M	Decreased plasma antigen, von Willebrand factor activity, with presence of multimeric forms	Factor concentrates	
2N	Normal von Willebrand factor, decreased factor VIII activity	Desmopressin	Factor concentrates
3	Absent von Willebrand factor antigen and function	Factor concentrates Recombinant factor VIII	Desmopressin Platelet concentrates

Adapted from Mannucci PM: Treatment of von Willebrand's disease. J Intern Med 242 (Suppl 740): 130, 1997.
GPIb, glycoprotein Ib.

hemophilia B has an incidence of 1:60,000 live births making these disorders the most common of the inherited coagulation disorders. The severity of hemophilia is directly related to the level of circulating clotting factors (Table 52-4).

Prevention of hemorrhage in hemophiliacs after open heart surgery is based on replacement of the deficient coagulation factor with either plasma-derived or recombinant factors. Appropriate clinical management involves hematologists, cardiologists, cardiac anesthesiologists, and cardiac surgeons.[38,74,126,142,149] Specific discussion of factor replacement will be included in the transfusion therapy portion of this chapter.

Occasionally, mild cases of hemophilia may be treated with DDAVP; however, transfusion of blood products is

Table 52–4

Classification for Hemophilia A or B

Class of hemophilia	Level of factor VIII or XI (%)	Clinical state	Joint involvement
Very mild	25–50	Bleed only after surgery or major trauma	Rare
Mild	5–24	Bleed after any surgery or minor trauma; spontaneous bleed very rare	Rare
Moderate	2–4	Occasional spontaneous bleed; excessive bleed after any trauma	May have hemarthrosis
Severe	<2	Frequent spontaneous bleeds; bleeding after any trauma	Characterized by hemarthrosis

838 usually required. All platelet antagonists should be stopped for 10–14 days prior to any elective operation. Factor levels should approach 80–100% of normal factor levels for hemophilia A and 50–60% of normal factor levels for hemophilia B, prior to cardiopulmonary bypass (Table 52-5). Factor level activity should be determined by assay prior to initiation of cardiopulmonary bypass to establish the levels of factors VIII and IX required in the pump prime to prevent excessive dilution of the coagulation factors.[126] Standard heparinization protocols for cardiopulmonary bypass may be used followed by neutralization with protamine. To maintain adequate factor levels postoperatively, factor VIII or IX is infused continuously early after operation. Thereafter, adequate factor levels can be maintained by intermittent transfusion of isolated factor concentrates for 4–14 days. The half-life of factor VIII is 12 h versus 24 h for factor IX; thus, patients with hemophilia A require factor replacement twice per day.

Inhibitors to factor VIII or IX occur in 18–52% of patients with hemophilia A and 2–16% of patients with hemophilia B, potentially complicating therapy.[2,86,105] Mild responders may be treated by large and frequent infusions of factor VIII or IX to competitively bind to the inhibitor. High responders are best treated with recombinant products, induced immunosuppression, or intravenous immunoglobulin G.[15,105] To avoid factor VIII and IX concentrates, factors VIIa, IXa, and Xa in prothrombin-complex concentrates may be administered. More recently, recombinant factor VIIa has been used to avoid factor VIII or IX infusions in patients with inhibitors. Both substitute products are less effective at controlling hemorrhage (50–75%) than traditional therapy (85–90%) in patients without inhibitors. Recombinant factor VIIa, the more effective therapy in patients with inhibitors, may have a role in other patients to prevent excessive hemorrhage unresponsive to conventional therapy.[68,80–82,88,137]

Factor V Leiden

Factor V is an essential part of the prothrombinase complex that activates prothrombin to thrombin in the coagulation cascade. Activated protein C cleaves factor Va, thus inhibiting the coagulation cascade. Mutations in the factor V gene lead to a prothrombotic state. A point mutation (Arg 506 → Gln) is named factor V Leiden and accounts for 95% of all activated protein C resistance.[10] Patients with factor V Leiden have increased risk of developing a deep venous thrombo-

sis.[124] The risk of stroke or myocardial infarction in patients with activated protein C resistance is unclear.[37,92] Despite the increased risk of thrombosis in activated protein C, studies have not shown a relationship between bypass graft occlusion and activated protein C resistance.[39] Management of patients with factor V Leiden includes standard anticoagulation with heparin during cardiopulmonary bypass, followed by Coumadin for prevention of venous thrombosis.

Antithrombin Deficiency

Antithrombin is the most abundant inhibitor of the coagulation system. It binds to and inhibits thrombin and factor Xa. Heparin catalyzes the binding of antithrombin to thrombin and factor Xa, accounting for its anticoagulant properties. Deficiencies of antithrombin increase the risk of thromboembolism and can cause heparin resistance in patients undergoing cardiopulmonary bypass.[11,33,91] A 50% reduction in antithrombin concentration is clinically important, whether congenital or acquired. Acquired etiologies include sepsis, trauma, renal failure, nephrotic syndrome, and cirrhosis.[97]

Patients with antithrombin deficiency are at risk for major thrombosis if exposed to cardiopulmonary bypass. Antithrombin activity may reach 50–80% of normal with initiation of cardiopulmonary bypass because of dilution and antithrombin consumption.[70] Administration of heparin consumes antithrombin causing levels to fall critically low in antithrombin-deficient patients. Levels of antithrombin above 80% decrease the risk of thromboembolism.[95] Previously diagnosed patients with antithrombin deficiency who require cardiopulmonary bypass may be treated with large doses of heparin, FFP, cryoprecipitate, or antithrombin concentrates. Antithrombin concentrates (500–1000 U) are more effective and quicker than additional heparin or FFP in treating heparin-resistant patients. Subsequent heparin is more effective following antithrombin concentrate administration.[75,156] Antithrombin concentrates carry a lower risk of viral infection or allergic reaction than FFP or cryoprecipitate.[97]

Protein C and S Deficiencies

Protein C is activated by the thrombin–thrombomodulin complex. Activated protein C combined with its cofactor, protein S, proteolytically cleaves factors Va and VIIIa. Deficiencies of protein C or S predispose affected individuals

---

Table 52–5

Recommended Perioperative Factor Levels in Hemophiliacs Undergoing Cardiac Surgery

	Preoperative factor level (%)	*Postoperative factor level (%)*	*Duration of treatment (days)*	*Factor half-life (h)*
Hemophilia A	80–100	>50	7–14	12
Hemophilia B	50–60	>40	4–7	24

to thromboembolic disease.[144] There have been reports of intracardiac[104] or aortic[110] thrombi secondary to protein C deficiency. Acquired deficiencies of protein C or S may occur in severe liver disease, disseminated intravascular coagulation, nephrotic syndrome, acute respiratory distress syndrome, pregnancy, and human immunodeficiency virus infection.[30,139] Patients who have protein C or S deficiencies can undergo cardiopulmonary bypass with standard anticoagulation protocols. Postoperatively, long-term anticoagulation with Coumadin is recommended.

Heparin-Induced Thrombocytopenia

Heparin-induced thrombocytopenia (HIT) is a drug-induced immune thrombocytopenia that occurs in up to 30% of surgical patients.[14] Two types of HIT are classified based on severity of thrombocytopenia and thromboembolic events. Type I HIT has no symptoms, moderate thrombocytopenia ($<150 \times 10^9$/liter), develops 3–14 days after initiation of heparin therapy, and resolves spontaneously upon discontinuation of heparin. Type II HIT has severe, persistent thrombocytopenia ($<75 \times 10^9$/liter), may occur within hours to days of heparin administration, and is often associated with thromboembolic and hemorrhagic events.[152] Approximately 35% of patients with type I HIT will progress to type II HIT. Type II HIT carries a 30% mortality rate and a high morbidity (up to 80%) because of thrombosis of major vessels in the extremities, or cerebral, and mesenteric circulations. Heparin-induced thrombocytopenia has been reported after full-dose unfractionated heparin therapy, low-dose prophylactic therapy, exposure to heparin-containing arterial catheter flush solutions, and heparin-coated catheters. Low-molecular-weight heparins are less likely to induce thrombocytopenia and thrombosis than unfractionated heparin therapy, but cross-reactivity does occur.

The diagnosis of HIT is based on clinical suspicion and laboratory confirmation. Any patient who develops arterial or venous thrombosis despite heparin therapy should be evaluated for HIT. Thrombocytopenia may be the only sign of type I HIT. Early after cardiac surgery, many patients have mild thrombocytopenia. However, a 50% reduction early postoperatively is highly suggestive of HIT.[153] There are two tests to establish the diagnosis of HIT. At Mayo Clinic, we use the enzyme-linked immunosorbent assay (ELISA) for antibodies specific for the platelet factor 4/heparin complex, which has greater than 90% sensitivity and specificity. An alternative test, the heparin-induced platelet aggregation assay, has excellent sensitivity, but low specificity.[108] Once HIT has been confirmed or suspected clinically with a negative laboratory test, all heparin must be discontinued including heparin-flush solutions and heparin-coated catheters. Patients with HIT who require anticoagulation postoperatively should receive direct thrombin inhibitors (hirudin, argatroban) or Coumadin. Thrombotic complications in patients with previously unrecognized HIT are best treated with direct thrombin inhibitors.

Patients with a history of HIT who require cardiac surgery pose a difficult problem for the surgical and anesthetic team. Management of patients with HIT who require cardiopulmonary bypass is dependent on the type of previous HIT episode. Patients with previous type 1 HIT may undergo cardiopulmonary bypass with standard heparinization protocols without further evaluation. All heparin must be avoided postoperatively. In patients with antecedent type II HIT, the level of platelet factor 4/heparin complex antibodies should be known preoperatively. If this antibody test is negative, one may safely proceed with cardiopulmonary bypass utilizing standard heparin anticoagulation and neutralization methods. If the ELISA is positive for heparin antibodies, consideration should be given to postponing the procedure for 4–8 weeks. If delaying the operation is not possible, a direct thrombin inhibitor can be used for anticoagulation during cardiopulmonary bypass, and this is best accomplished with a multidisciplinary team involving hematologists and anesthesiologists.[34,72,108] Other approaches include the use of low-molecular-weight heparin, danaproid, ancrod, platelet GPIIb/IIIa antagonists alone,[71] or platelet aggregation inhibitors prior to heparinization.[3,47,49]

Direct thrombin inhibitors, r-hirudin and argatroban, do not require antithrombin and heparin cofactor II; thus, they do not cross-react with heparin antibodies. Dosing schedules for r-hirudin that prevent clot formation during cardiopulmonary bypass have been described (0.25 mg/kg bolus before cardiopulmonary bypass, 0.20 mg/kg in cardiopulmonary bypass pump prime, and continuous infusion of 0.5 mg/min after the bolus and throughout cardiopulmonary bypass),[108] and the ecarin clotting time (ECT) is probably the best marker for anticoagulation using r-hirudin (r-hirudin concentration greater than 3.5 µg/ml by ECT).[72,108] R-hirudin has a half-life of only 30–60 min in patients with normal renal function; thus, neutralization is not required. No clot formation or thrombotic episodes have been reported with r-hirudin. Excessive postoperative bleeding may be treated with transfusion of FFP and platelet concentrates. Return of cell salvaged blood is discouraged following separation from cardiopulmonary bypass to allow r-hirudin levels to fall. R-hirudin is eliminated by the kidneys; thus, other alternatives are required in patients with renal failure or insufficiency.

Antiphospholipid Thrombosis Syndromes

There are two varieties of antiphospholipid thrombosis syndromes: lupus anticoagulant and anticardiolipin antibody thrombosis syndromes.[13] Both are associated with thrombosis and thrombocytopenia; however, the anticardiolipin syndrome is commonly associated with arterial and venous thrombosis. Most patients with antiphospholipid syndromes are healthy with no underlying medical conditions and are classified as having primary syndromes. Secondary antiphospholipid syndromes are caused by malignancy, lymphoproliferative disorders, autoimmune diseases (systemic lupus erythematosus, rheumatoid arthritis), mixed connective tissue disease, viral infections (human immunodeficiency virus), and drug reactions.

In the antiphospholipid syndromes, intravascular thrombosis occurs despite a prolonged activated partial thromboplastin time and activated clotting time.[40,41] Management of anticoagulation during cardiopulmonary bypass is challenging, and direct heparin levels or anti-Xa concentrations are more accurate indications of heparinization than monitoring with activated partial thromboplastin time or activated clotting time. In one report, heparin-celite-activated partial thromboplastin time titration curves were used successfully

840 for monitoring anticoagulation in two patients who were receiving antifibrinolytic therapy.[41]

▶ PHARMACOLOGICAL ANTICOAGULANTS

Eighty years after its discovery, heparin remains the most widely available parenteral pharmacological anticoagulant. Heparin inhibits thrombin indirectly by catalyzing antithrombin binding to thrombin, factors IXa, Xa, XIa, and XIIa.[151,154] The level of anticoagulation by heparin is monitored by activated partial thromboplastin time, and heparin is reversed with protamine. Low-molecular-weight heparin contains only molecules that weigh an average of 8000 Da, causes increased anti-factor Xa activity compared to unfractionated heparin, and cannot be monitored by activated partial thromboplastin time. Factor replacement with blood products may be necessary for reversal of anticoagulation with low-molecular-weight heparin since protamine only partially reverses the anti-Xa activity of low-molecular-weight heparin.

Warfarin is an enteral anticoagulant that inhibits the γ-carboxylation of glutamic acid residues in vitamin K-dependent factors II, VII, IX, and X, thus inhibiting the generation of thrombin. The half-life of factor VII is 6 h and the half-life of factor II is 50–80 h,[83] and these two factors are reduced the most when stable anticoagulation is achieved. The extent of anticoagulation is monitored with prothrombin time/international normalized ratio. Anticoagulation with warfarin is reversed by vitamin K (0.5–1 mg vitamin K intravenously [IV] infused over 30 min) or replacement of clotting factors with FFP (2 units FFP IV infused over 2 h). The full effect of vitamin K requires approximately 6 h, while the effect of FFP is immediate. Depending on the initial prothrombin time, repeated transfusion of FFP may be required. Rapid reversal of anticoagulation by Coumadin with recombinant factor VIIa (15–90 µg/kg, one time intravenous dose) has been shown to be safe and effective in a small series of patients.[36]

▶ EFFECTS OF CARDIOPULMONARY BYPASS ON BLOOD COAGULATION

Excessive bleeding during or after cardiopulmonary bypass is related both to surgical trauma and acquired defects of coagulation. The incidence of reoperation for excessive bleeding has been reported as high as 4.2%, and in approximately 50% of patients, no specific site of surgical bleeding is identified.[103]

Hemorrhage after cardiac surgery is generally related to a combination of several alterations in the hemostatic system (Box 52-1). Hemodilution of clotting factors and platelets occurs because of the priming volume of the bypass circuit.[6,59] Contact of the blood with the extracorporeal circuit activates and consumes clotting factors and causes platelet dysfunction.[60,63] Primary fibrinolysis is activated by release of tPA from endothelial cells.[140] The concentrations of platelets, fibrinogen, thrombin, coagulation factors V, VII, IX, X, and plasminogen decrease during cardiopulmonary bypass because of dilution by the cardiopulmonary bypass prime or consumption (factor V).[59] In most patients, these levels of clotting factors do not fall below the level thought to maintain adequate hemostasis during or after cardiopulmonary bypass (concentrations above 30% are adequate for all factors except factor V, which requires only 10–15%).[129]

Box 52–1. Etiologies of Excessive Bleeding after Cardiopulmonary Bypass.

Acquired platelet dysfunction
Thrombocytopenia
Hemodilution
Consumption of clotting factors
Primary fibrinolysis
Poor surgical hemostasis
Heparin rebound or inadequate neutralization

Thrombocytopenia has been associated with excessive postbypass bleeding. Platelet counts decrease rapidly to about 50% of preoperative levels after initiating cardiopulmonary bypass because of dilution and loss in the extracorporeal circuit filters, but platelet counts often remain above 100,000/liter throughout cardiopulmonary bypass and return to normal levels days after operation. Prophylactic postoperative platelet transfusions do not reduce blood loss.[134]

More important than the decrease in coagulation factors and platelet count is the progressive loss of platelet function during cardiopulmonary bypass.[157] Bleeding time is significantly prolonged and platelet aggregation is impaired within minutes of initiating cardiopulmonary bypass. The bleeding time progressively increases to greater than 30 min when the duration of cardiopulmonary bypass is 2 h or more and shortens rapidly with the administration of protamine. Bleeding time normalizes by 2–4 h postbypass in most cases.[29] This acquired platelet dysfunction appears to be caused by contact of the blood to the synthetic surfaces of the extracorporeal oxygenator, regardless of whether bubble or membrane oxygenators are used.[42] In addition, hypothermia induces reversible platelet dysfunction by impairing platelet thromboxane synthesis.[146]

During extracorporeal circulation, activity of surface platelet receptors GPIb and GPIIb/IIIa is diminished, thereby inhibiting binding of von Willebrand factor and fibrinogen, respectively.[120] The loss of GPIb decreases platelet adhesion to the subendothelium and loss of GPIIb/IIIa decreases platelet plug formation.

Mechanical trauma to platelets due to shear stress, surface adherence, and turbulence within the extracorporeal circuit may cause fragmentation of platelet membranes and loss of platelet membrane receptors. Also, platelet dysfunction may be caused by the proteolytic removal of platelet membrane GPIb receptor by plasmin.[120] Despite these observations, no correlation between bleeding and loss of platelet membrane receptors has been established.

Abnormalities of platelet function have been attributed to transient platelet activation. Cardiopulmonary bypass increases plasma and urine levels of platelet factor 4, β-thromboglobulin, and thromboxane B_2, all indicators of platelet activation *in vivo*.[59,60] Depletion of α-granules occurs within 2 h of cardiopulmonary bypass, yet platelet function improves postbypass despite the reduced number of platelet α-granules. Thus, it is unlikely that depletion of α-granules is primarily responsible for the transient platelet dysfunction associated with cardiopulmonary bypass.

Primary fibrinolysis has been suggested as an etiology of postbypass bleeding because of the presence of fibrin-split products during and immediately following extracorporeal circulation.[12,141] The mechanism for activation of the fibrinolytic system during cardiopulmonary bypass is not completely understood. The levels of tPA increase throughout cardiopulmonary bypass and correspond with a decrease in the levels of plasminogen inhibitor.[141] Several factors may release tPA from the vascular endothelium including thrombin stimulation during cardiopulmonary bypass, contact activation with the circuit, or the action of heparin. Additionally, heparinization for cardiopulmonary bypass causes a marked increase in the level and activity of plasmin.[70] Yet, stimulation of the fibrinolytic system has not consistently correlated with postbypass hemorrhage. Fibrin degradation products are rapidly cleared from the blood with normal hepatic function; thus, many coagulopathies are transient and resolve with removal of the stimulus for primary fibrinolysis.

Other etiologies of postbypass bleeding include poor surgical hemostasis; rarely, heparin rebound; or inadequate heparin neutralization. Meticulous surgical technique and more accurate protamine dosing protocols have markedly reduced these causes of excessive bleeding. Thus, coagu-lopathies secondary to cardiopulmonary bypass are most likely the result of functional platelet defects and fibrinolysis.

BLOOD CONSERVATION STRATEGIES

Current studies suggest that 30–70% of patients undergoing primary coronary bypass procedures receive homologous blood transfusions,[32,53] placing a large strain on blood procurement and processing centers. Improved screening of donor blood has dramatically reduced the risk of transmission of infectious disease, but other potential complications of blood transfusions remain, including the risks of transfusion reactions, sensitization to blood products, and immunosuppression (Table 52-6). Thus, surgical teams should be thoroughly familiar with blood conservation strategies.[54]

Preoperative Autologous Donation

Preoperative autologous donation is an effective and safe technique to reduce transfusion requirements in patients undergoing cardiac surgery,[20,24,145] but this is used all too infrequently because many patients are scheduled for operation soon after surgical consultation. Consequently, timing to arrange and undergo preoperative autologous donation is difficult and the risk of exacerbating hypotension, arrhythmias, and unstable angina is also present. The American Association of Blood Banks' guidelines for preoperative autologous donation[4] suggest that no more than 450 ml or 12% of estimated

	Table 52–6			
Risks of Homologous Blood Transfusion				

	Estimated frequency		
Risk factor	**Per million units**	**Per actual unit**	**Number of deaths per million units**
Infection			
Viral			
Hepatitis A	1	1/1,000,000	0
Hepatitis B	7–32	1/30,000–1/250,000	0–0.14
Hepatitis C	4–36	1/30,000–1/150,000	0.5–17
HIV	0.4–5	1/200,000–1/2,000,000	0.5–5
HTLV I and II	0.5–4	1/250,000–1/2,000,000	0
Parvovirus B19	100	1/10,000	0
Bacterial contamination			
Red cells	2	1/500,000	0.1–0.25
Platelets	83	1/12,000	21
Acute hemolytic reactions	1–4	1/25,000–1/1,000,000	0.67
Delayed hemolytic reaction	1000	1/1000	0.4
Acute lung injury	200	1/5000	0.2

Adapted from Goodnough, LT, Brecher, ME, Kanter, MH, et al: Transfusion medicine—blood transfusion. N Engl J Med 340(6): 440, 1999.

blood volume should be withdrawn at one time, and the patient's hemoglobin concentration should be 11 g/dl or greater at the time of donation. Donations should not be performed more frequently than every third day. Erythropoietin (up to 300 units/kg, three times per week injected subcutaneously) may provide additional benefit to patients undergoing preoperative autologous donation, especially in anemic patients, because of its red blood cell–stimulating property.[24]

Acute Normovolemic Hemodilution

Autologous blood may be collected (15–20% of blood volume) in the operating room prior to operation with reinfusion of crystalloid or colloid for maintenance of intravascular volume. This technique preserves the blood in the freshest state and maintains platelet and clotting factor activity. In contrast to preoperative autologous donation, greater numbers of patients are eligible to undergo this technique because of the cardiovascular monitoring and personnel in the operative environment. Several reports have demonstrated a 20–58% reduction in homologous blood transfusion when autologous blood is retransfused after cardiopulmonary bypass.[58,109]

Platelet Plasmapheresis

Platelet-rich plasma (PRP) can be obtained by plasmapheresis.[16] Blood is collected via a large central venous catheter, separated by centrifugation, and the red blood cells are returned via this catheter. Autologous PRP is retransfused after cardiopulmonary bypass and heparin neutralization. Conservation of blood products by PRP remains controversial.[16,45,52,127]

Cell Salvage Autotransfusion

In addition to routine cardiotomy suction devices, intraoperative autotransfusion can be preformed with a cell salvage device that uses wall vacuum and a blood-processing system. Cell salvage may be used prior to and after neutralization of heparin. Blood is removed from the surgical field with wall suction and is mixed with an anticoagulant (heparin or citrate). Blood is separated from plasma and other formed elements by a centrifuge and washed with saline. Salvaged, processed blood has a hematocrit between 50 and 60%, but is largely devoid of clotting factors and platelets. Residual blood in the extracorporeal circuit may be transferred to the cell salvage system after discontinuation of cardiopulmonary bypass; this technique also reduces the use of homologous blood and is cost-effective.[19,96,100]

▶ PHARMACOLOGICAL INTERVENTIONS

Aprotinin

Aprotinin is a polypeptide isolated from bovine lung that is a broadly reactive serine protease inhibitor with antifibrinolytic and platelet-sparing activity. It has been shown to markedly reduce blood loss by 43–88% and blood transfusion requirements by 60–100% in patients undergoing cardiopulmonary bypass in a dose-dependent manner.[24] There are two dosing protocols for aprotinin; the high-dose (full Hammersmith) schedule involves 280 mg loading dose, 280 mg in the car-

diopulmonary bypass prime, and 70 mg/h infusion continued until the patient leaves the operating room. With the low-dose (half Hammersmith) schedule, 140 mg is given in the pump oxygenator as a priming dose, 140 mg loading dose is given to the patient intravenously, and a 35 mg/h infusion is continued until the patient leaves the operating room. Even though the high-dose schedule is more expensive, it appears to reduce blood loss more than the low-dose schedule.[76,78]

There is controversy as to whether the use of aprotinin or other antifibrinolytic drugs increases graft thrombosis.[28] In randomized, prospective studies, the risk of graft occlusion was similar to patients not treated with aprotinin, but perioperative infarction rates were slightly higher (17.5% for high-dose aprotinin, 14.3% for low-dose aprotinin, and 8.9% in the placebo group).[28,78] When aprotinin is administered, the activated partial thromboplastin time should be maintained above 750 s to minimize the risk of thrombosis.

The mechanism by which aprotinin reduces bleeding has not been completely elucidated. Aprotinin preserves platelet membrane receptors, increases von Willebrand factor expression, and alters the thromboxane:prostacyclin ratio. In addition, aprotinin reduces both plasmin activity secondary to decreased contact activation of the kallikrein system and the intrinsic coagulation pathway, along with a reduction in the level of fibrinolysis.[61,62,94]

Aprotinin and other antifibrinolytic agents, described below, are used selectively at Mayo Clinic. Approximately 15–20% of patients undergoing cardiopulmonary bypass are treated with aprotinin. High-dose aprotinin is used in patients who are at the highest risk of postoperative bleeding, which includes most reoperations, complex procedures, valvular operations for carcinoid heart disease, complex congenital operations, cardiac transplants, and placement of assist devices. Patients undergoing reoperative coronary artery bypass receive the low-dose schedule.

Tranexamic Acid and ε-Aminocaproic Acid

Tranexamic acid is a synthetic competitive inhibitor of plasmin. A combination of tranexamic acid (10 mg/kg bolus with 1 mg/kg/h infusion stopped 2 h postoperatively) and intraoperative autologous blood donation has been shown to reduce blood loss and blood transfusion similarly to aprotinin alone in patients undergoing cardiopulmonary bypass at high risk for bleeding.[106] Tranexamic acid is approximately 10 times more potent than ε-aminocaproic acid and has a more sustained activity.[44] It has been shown to be associated with significant decreases in blood loss and transfusion requirements when given prophylactically.[66] The optimal dosing schedule for tranexamic acid has not been determined but very high doses may increase the risk of perioperative myocardial infarction.[113]

ε-Aminocaproic acid is another synthetic competitive inhibitor of plasmin that decreases blood loss when administered prophylactically (5 g bolus with 1 g/h infusion stopped at 2 h postoperatively).[113,148]

Desmopressin

Desmopressin (DDAVP) is a synthetic analog of vasopressin that has no vasoconstrictor activity. It increases the plasma levels of factor VIII and von Willebrand factor, but does not increase synthesis of von Willebrand factor. Thus, patients with severe hemophilia A or vWd do not respond to DDAVP. Studies of routine use of DDAVP during cardiopulmonary bypass have shown conflicting results in regard to postoperative blood loss.[29,57,121,131] Desmopressin may be effective in reducing bleeding when thromboelastography (TEG) shows abnormal coagulation.[99]

Reinfusion of Shed Mediastinal Blood

Autotransfusion of shed mediastinal blood is one of the simplest methods of blood conservation. Blood is collected by a commercial device and directly reinfused into the patient with or without washing. Most studies suggest that autotransfusion of shed blood can decrease homologous blood requirements; however, routine use requires special equipment and does increase cost of patient care.[5,18,101] We do not use this method routinely. In addition, reinfusion of large amounts of shed blood may exacerbate platelet dysfunction because of fibrinolytic products (fibrin monomers, D-dimers, and tissue-type plasminogen activator) contained in the transfusion.[31,133]

TRANSFUSION THERAPY

Transfusion of blood products places the recipient at risk for transmission of viruses, hemolytic reactions, bacterial infections, acute lung injury, and immunomodulation.[54] Increased donor screening, new laboratory tests for bacterial and viral antigens, improved cross-matching of ABO antigens, and an increased vigilance in patient identification prior to blood transfusion have reduced the risks of transfusing blood products (Table 52-6).

Packed Red Blood Cells

Allogenic packed red blood cells (PRBCs) have had plasma components, plasma, and platelets separated after donation. Standard PRBCs contain leukocytes or may be leukocyte reduced by removing the leukocyte layer during the isolation procedure. No single criterion exists for determining when PRBCs should be transfused.[27] Patients with normal coronary anatomy tolerate hemoglobin levels as low as 4 g/dl;[55] however, patients with coronary artery disease may develop myocardial ischemia with hemoglobin levels less than 8 g/dl. Postoperative hemoglobin levels less than 8 g/dl may be tolerated in the absence of symptoms such as tachycardia, hypotension, or myocardial ischemia. Prophylactic transfusions for otherwise healthy patients with asymptomatic anemia or transfusions to replace intravascular volume in the absence of hemorrhage are not recommended.[27]

Fresh Frozen Plasma

Fresh frozen plasma contains all the factors in the coagulation cascade.[149] A 250-ml unit contains approximately 550 mg of fibrinogen, has a long shelf life, can be quickly prepared and transfused, and has a low risk of viral transmission if collected from a single donor. Indications for transfusions of FFP include prolonged prothrombin time (>15 s) or activated partial thromboplastin time (>40 s) due to coagulation factor deficiencies.[25] In the presence of ongoing bleeding, transfusion of FFP may decrease homologous blood requirements.[24] More recently, point-of-care testing of prothrombin time and activated partial thromboplastin time has been utilized to improve appropriateness of FFP infusions.[35]

Platelets

Platelets may be obtained from multiple donors in pooled concentrates or apheresed from one donor. Platelet transfusion may be useful with ongoing bleeding associated with thrombocytopenia or suspected platelet dysfunction.[107] Because platelet dysfunction occurs secondary to cardiopulmonary bypass, platelet transfusion may be indicated even with platelet counts within the normal range. Risks of viral transmission, hemolytic reaction, and bacterial infection are greater with pooled platelet concentrates than single apheresis units.[26]

Cryoprecipitate

Cryoprecipitate contains factor VIII, fibrinogen, von Willebrand factor, factor XIII, and fibronectin. Indications for transfusion include fibrinogen deficiency, hemophilia A, or vWd. This product is considered to have a significant risk of viral transmission because of the large number of donors required to produce it. In general, cryoprecipitate transfusions are used when there is evidence of fibrinogen deficiency not corrected by FFP. Laboratory confirmation of low fibrinogen concentration should precede cryoprecipitate transfusion.

Factor VIIa, Factor VIII, and Factor IX Concentrates

Recombinant factor VIIa is a new therapy that has been approved for the treatment of patients with hemophilia who have inhibitors to factor VIII or IX. Recombinant factor VIIa is also effective in reversing Coumadin rapidly, and has been shown to reduce coagulopathic bleeding after general surgical operations for trauma and in patients after cardiopulmonary bypass.[1,65] There are no studies addressing the prophylactic use of recombinant factor VIIa in cardiac surgery, but recombinant factor VIIa has been shown to decrease perioperative blood loss by nearly 60% and eliminate homologous blood transfusions in a prospective randomized trial of patients after radical retropubic prostatectomy.[50] Theoretically, recombinant factor VIIa binds to tissue factor that is exposed because of endothelial injury at the surgical site. Thus, recombinant factor VIIa enhances thrombin generation in a localized and time-limited manner, without causing systemic coagulation. In the future, this product may have wider use in cardiac surgery.

Factor VIII and IX concentrates were developed for the treatment of patients with hemophilia A and B, respectively. Recommended factor levels are described in Table 52-4. Factor VIII concentrates, available in the United States, include low purity (<50 U/mg protein), intermediate purity (1–10 U/mg protein), high purity (50–1000 U/mg protein), and very high purity (3000 U/mg protein, plasma-derived or recombinant products). Less immunomodulation occurs with administration of high-purity concentrates. Factor IX concentrates may be obtained from prothrombin complex concentrates, activated prothrombin complex concentrates, and porcine factor IX. In current practice at our clinic, high-purity and very high-purity factor VIII concentrates and factor IX concentrates are administered to maintain adequate factor levels perioperatively.

► SPECIAL CLINICAL SITUATIONS

Postoperative Bleeding

Excessive bleeding after cardiac surgery (≥2 ml/kg/min of chest tube drainage) can delay extubation and increase in-hospital mortality and length of stay. Assessment of postoperative bleeding involves quantitation of mediastinal chest tube drainage and clinical observation of hypovolemia or cardiac tamponade. Laboratory evaluation should start with hemoglobin concentration, platelet count, prothrombin time, activated partial thromboplastin time, and activated clotting time. If available, thromboelastography provides a qualitative analysis of coagulation and may differentiate a surgical from coagulopathic cause of excessive bleeding.[138] Point-of-care testing of coagulation parameters minimizes delay in diagnosis and treatment.[7,35] Based on the results of those tests and the clinical signs of a primary defect in hemostasis such as subcutaneous or mucous membrane bleeding, a simple algorithm (Figure 52-3) has been designed to reduce blood product exposure for patients with excessive bleeding after cardiopulmonary bypass.[107] Surgical reexploration is necessary when there is persistent bleeding despite normal coagulation and after empiric therapy.

Jehovah's Witnesses

Jehovah's Witnesses refuse blood transfusion based on religious beliefs, which complicate the management of their cardiac surgery. However, several studies have demonstrated that even complex cardiac procedures can be performed in Jehovah's Witnesses with low mortality and discharge hematocrits >30%.[112,125] To minimize postoperative anemia, a multimodal approach may include preoperative erythropoietin (up to 300 units/kg three times per week injected subcutaneously) and iron therapy, acute normovolemic hemodilution, cell salvage, aprotinin therapy, and postoperative autotransfusion of shed mediastinal blood. Clarification of each individual's wishes for handling of blood products and conservation measures is critical to planning the appropriate strategy. New surgical techniques such as endovascular stenting and coronary artery bypass grafting without cardiopulmonary bypass may be especially useful.

Emergency Surgery after Thrombolytic Therapy

Thrombolytic therapy and use of GPIIb/IIIa inhibitors during percutaneous interventions in the treatment of acute myocardial infarction are well established.[43,119] But these agents may exacerbate bleeding when urgent surgical procedures are necessary. Tissue-type plasminogen activator (tPA) has replaced streptokinase and urokinase as the thrombolytic of choice. Significant perioperative bleeding and increased transfusion requirements were reported in 8% of patients undergoing emergency coronary artery bypass grafting after unsuccessful thrombolysis with tPA.[69] If an operation cannot be delayed in patients who recently received tPA, antifibrinolytic drugs such as aprotinin may help counteract ongoing thrombolysis.

Abciximab is a monoclonal antibody specific for platelet GPIIb/IIIa receptor. It binds irreversibly and inhibits platelet function for up to 48 h after discontinuation of the drug. Several reports have documented increased bleeding when emergent coronary artery bypass is required early after abciximab therapy.[73,114,135] If coronary bypass grafting cannot be delayed 12 h or more from the time of exposure to abciximab, intensive treatment of the coagulopathy due

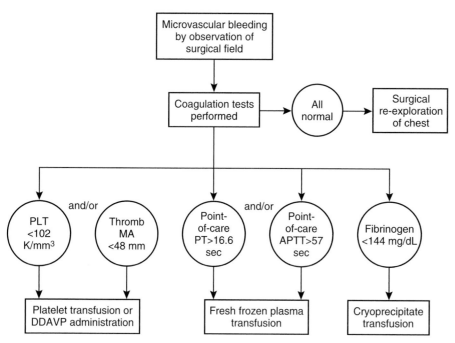

Figure 52–3 One treatment algorithm to minimize blood product exposure with excessive postoperative bleeding. PLT, platelet count; Thromb MA, thromboelastogram maximum amplitude; PT, prothrombin time; APTT, activated partial thromboplastin time; DDAVP, desmopressin.
(Reprinted with permission from Nuttall GA, Oliver WC, Santrach PJ, et al: Efficacy of a simple intraoperative transfusion algorithm for nonerythrocyte component utilization after cardiopulmonary bypass. Anesthesiology 94: 775, 2001.)

to abciximab with platelet transfusions reduces the in-hospital adverse events to those of patients who were not treated with abciximab.[135] Prophylactic platelet transfusions may minimize the bleeding diathesis in patients who were given abciximab within 12 h of the emergent operation, and antifibrinolytic therapy with aprotinin is recommended.

Tirofiban and eptifibatide are competitive antagonists of the GPIIb/IIIa receptor that inhibit platelet function up to 4 h after the drug's discontinuation. In these patients, platelet function returns rapidly, and excessive postoperative bleeding is less than that caused by abciximab. Delaying surgery for 2–4 h should be adequate to prevent excessive bleeding.

REFERENCES

1. Al Douri M, Shafi T, Al Khudairi D, et al: Effect of administration of recombinant activated factor VII (rFVIIa; NovoSeven) in the management of severe uncontrolled bleeding in patients undergoing heart valve replacement surgery. Blood Coagul Fibrin 2000. 11:S121–S127, 2000.
2. Aledort LM: Hemophilia: yesterday, today, and tomorrow. Mt Sinai J Med 63:225, 1996.
3. Aouifi A, Blanc P, Piriou V, et al: Cardiac surgery with cardiopulmonary bypass in patients with type II heparin-induced thrombocytopenia. Ann Thorac Surg 71:678–683, 2001.
4. Walker RH: Autologous transfusions. In American Association of Blood Banks (AABB) Technical Manual. Arlington, VA: American Association of Blood Banks, 1990, pp. 433–448.
5. Axford TC, Dearani JA, Ragno G, et al: Safety and therapeutic effectiveness of reinfused shed blood after open heart surgery. Ann Thorac Surg 57:615–622, 1994.
6. Bachman F: McKenna R, Cole ER, et al: The hemostatic mechanism after open-heart surgery. I. Studies on plasma coagulation factors and fibrinolysis in 512 patients after extracorporeal circulation. J Thorac Cardiovasc Surg 70:76–85, 1975.
7. Belisle S, Hardy J-F: Hemorrhage and the use of blood products after adult cardiac operations: myths and realities. Ann Thorac Surg 62:1908–1917, 1996.
8. Bennett JS, Vilare G: Exposure of platelet fibrinogen receptors by ADP and epinephrine. J Clin Invest 64:1393–1398, 1979.
9. Bergamaschini L, Mannucci PM, Federici AB, et al: Post-transfusion anaphylactic reaction in a patient with severe von Willebrand disease: role of complement and alloantibodies to von Willebrand factor. J Lab Clin Med 125:348–355, 1995.
10. Bertina RM, Koeleman BP, Koster T, et al: Mutation in blood coagulation factor V associated with resistance to activated protein C. Nature 369:64–69, 1994.
11. Bick RL: Clinical relevance of antithrombin III. Semin Thromb Hemost 8:276–287, 1982.
12. Bick, RL: Hemostasis defects associated with cardiac surgery, prosthetic devices, and other extracorporeal circuits. Semin Thromb Hemost 11:249–280, 1985.
13. Bick RL and Baker, WF: The antiphospholipid and thrombosis syndromes. Med Clin North Am 78:667–684, 1994.
14. Blakeman B: Management of heparin-induced thrombocytopenia: a cardiovascular surgeon's perspective. Semin Hematol 36:37–41, 1999.
15. Bloom AL: Management of factor VIII inhibitors: evolution and current status. Haemostasis 22:268–275, 1992.

16. Boldt J: Acute platelet-rich plasmapheresis for cardiac surgery. J Cardiothorac Vasc Anesth 9:79–88, 1995.
17. Bond L, Bevin D: Myocardial infarction in a patient with hemophilia A treated with DDAVP. N Engl J Med 318:121, 1988.
18. Bouboulis N, Kardara M, Kesteven PJ, et al: Autotransfusion after coronary artery bypass surgery: is there any benefit? J Card Surg 9:314–321, 1994.
19. Breyer RH, Engelman RM, Rousou JA, et al: Blood conservation for myocardial revascularization. Is it cost effective? J Thorac Cardiovasc Surg 93:512–522, 1987.
20. Britton LW, Eastlund DT, Dziuban SW, et al: Predonated autologous blood use in elective cardiac surgery. Ann Thorac Surg 47:529–532, 1989.
21. Byrnes JJ, Larcada A, Moake JL: Thrombosis following desmopressin for uremic bleeding. Am J Hematol 28:63–65, 1988.
22. Castillo R, Monteagudo J, Escolar G, et al: Hemostatic effect of normal platelet transfusion in severe von Willebrand disease. Blood 77:1901–1905, 1991.
23. Chow TW, Hellums JD, Moake JL, et al: Shear-stress-induced von Willebrand factor binding to glycoprotein Ib initiates calcium influx associated with aggregation. Blood 80:113–120, 1992.
24. Cooley DA: Conservation of blood during cardiovascular surgery. Am J Surg 170:53s–59s, 1995.
25. Anonymous: Consensus conference. Fresh-frozen plasma. Indications and risks. JAMA 253:551–553, 1985.
26. Anonymous: Consensus conference. Platelet transfusion therapy. JAMA 257:1777–1780, 1987.
27. Anonymous: Consensus conference. Perioperative red blood cell transfusion. JAMA 260:2700–2703, 1988.
28. Cosgrove III DM, Heric B, Lytle BW, et al: Aprotinin therapy for reoperative myocardial revascularization: a placebo-controlled study. Ann Thorac Surg 54:1031–1038, 1992.
29. Czer LS, Bateman TM, Gray RJ, et al: Treatment of severe platelet dysfunction and hemorrhage after cardiopulmonary bypass: reduction in blood product usage on cardiopulmonary bypass? J Am Coll Cardiol 9:1139–1147, 1987.
30. D'Angelo A, Vigan-D'Angelo S, Esmon CT, et al: Acquired deficiencies of protein S. Protein S activity during oral anticoagulation in liver disease and in disseminated intravascular coagulation. J Clin Invest 81:1445–1454, 1988.
31. de Haan J, Schonberger J, Haan J, et al: Tissue-type plasminogen activator and fibrin monomers synergistically cause platelet dysfunction during retransfusion of shed blood after cardiopulmonary bypass. J Thorac Cardiovasc Surg 106:1017–1023, 1993;
32. Deitrich W, Barankay A, Dilthey G, et al: Reduction of blood utilization during myocardial revascularization. J Thorac Cardiovasc Surg 97:213–219, 1989.
33. Demers C, Ginsberg JS, Hirsh J, et al: Thrombosis in antithrombin-III-deficient persons. Report of a large kindred and literature review. Ann Intern Med 116:754–761, 1992.
34. Despotis GJ, Hogue CW, Saleem R, et al: The relationship between hirudin and activated clotting time: implications for patients with heparin-induced thrombocytopenia undergoing cardiac surgery. Anesth Analg 93:28–32, 2001.
35. Despotis G, Santoro S, Spitznagel E, et al: Prospective evaluation and clinical utility of on-site monitoring of coagulation in patients undergoing cardiac operations. J Thorac Cardiovasc Surg 107:271–279, 1994.
36. Deveras RA, Kessler CM: Reversal of warfarin-induced excessive anticoagulation with recombinant human factor VIIa concentrate. Ann Intern Med 137:884–888, 2002.
37. Doggen CJM, Manger Cats V, Bertina RM, et al: Interaction of coagulation defects and cardiovascular risk factors. Increased risk of myocardial infarction associated with factor

846

V Leiden or prothrombin 20210A. Circulation 97:1037–1041, 1998.

38. Donahue BS, Emerson CW, Slaughtar T: Elective and emergency cardiac surgery on a patient with hemophilia B: J Cardiothorac Vasc Anesth 13:92–97, 1999.

39. Donaldson MC, Belkin M, Whittemore AD, et al: Impact of activated protein C resistance on general surgical vascular patients. J Vasc Surg 25:1054–1060, 1997.

40. Ducart AR, Collard EL, Osselaer JC, et al: Management of anticoagulation during cardiopulmonary bypass in a patient with a circulating lupus anticoagulant. J Cardiothorac Vasc Anesth 11:878–879, 1997.

41. East CJ, Clements F, Mathew J, et al: Antiphospholipid syndrome and cardiac surgery: management of anticoagulation in two patients. Anesth Analg 90:1098–1101, 2000.

42. Edmunds LH Jr, Ellison N, Colman RW, et al: Platelet function during cardiac operation. Comparison of membrane and bubble oxygenators. J Thorac Cardiovasc Surg 83:805–812, 1982.

43. The EPIC investigators: Use of monoclonal antibody directed against the platelet glycoprotein IIb/IIIa receptor in high-risk coronary angioplasty. N Engl J Med 330:956–961, 1997.

44. Ereth MH, Oliver WC, Santrach PJ: Perioperative interventions to decrease transfusion of allogenic blood products. Mayo Clin Proc 69:575–586, 1994.

45. Ereth MH, Oliver WC, Beynen FMK, et al: Autologous platelet-rich plasma does not reduce transfusion of homologous blood products in patients undergoing repeat valvular surgery. Anesthesiology 79:540–547, 1993.

46. Ferry JD: The mechanism of polymerization of fibrin. Proc Natl Acad Sci USA 38:566–569, 1952.

47. Follis F, Schmidt CA: Cardiopulmonary bypass in patients with heparin-induced thrombocytopenia and thrombosis. Ann Thorac Surg 70:2173–2181, 2000.

48. Francis CW, Marder VJ: Physiologic regulation and pathologic disorders of fibrinolysis. Hum Pathol 18:263–275, 1985.

49. Frederiksen JW. Cardiopulmonary bypass in humans: bypassing unfractionated heparin. Ann Thorac Surg 70:1434–1443, 2000.

50. Friederich PW, Henny CP, Messelink EJ, et al: Effect of recombinant activated factor VII on perioperative blood loss in patients undergoing retropubic prostatectomy: a double-blind placebo-controlled randomised trial. Lancet 361:201–205, 2003.

51. Furie B, Furie BC: Molecular and cellular biology of blood coagulation. N Engl J Med 326:800–806, 1992.

52. Giordano GF, Rivers SL, Chung GKT, et al: Autologous platelet-rich plasma in cardiac surgery: effect of intraoperative and postoperative transfusion requirements. Ann Thorac Surg 46:416–419, 1988.

53. Goodnough LT, Johnston MF, Toy PTC: The variability of transfusion practice in coronary artery bypass surgery. JAMA 265:86–90, 1991.

54. Goodnough LT, Brecher ME, Kanter MH, et al: Transfusion medicine—blood transfusion. N Engl J Med 340:438–447, 1999.

55. Gould SA, Rosen AL, Sehgal LR, et al: Fluosol-DA as a red cell substitute in acute anemia. N Engl J Med 314:1653–1656, 1986.

56. Griffin JH: The role of surface in the surface-dependent activation of Hageman factor (blood coagulation factor XII). Proc Natl Acad Sci USA 75:1998–2002, 1978.

57. Hackman T, Gascoyne RD, Naiman SC, et al: A trial of desmopressin (1-desamino-8-D-arginine vasopressin) to reduce blood loss in uncomplicated cardiac surgery. N Engl J Med 321:1437–1443, 1989.

58. Hallowell P, Bland JHL, Buckley MJ, et al: Transfusion of fresh autologous blood in open-heart surgery: a method for reducing bank blood requirements. J Thorac Cardiovasc Surg 64:941–948, 1972.

59. Harker LA: Bleeding after cardiopulmonary bypass. N Engl J Med 314:1446–1448, 1986.

60. Harker LA, Malpass TW, Branson HE, et al: Mechanism of abnormal bleeding in patients undergoing cardiopulmonary bypass: acquired transient platelet dysfunction associated with selective α-granule release. Blood 56:824–834, 1980.

61. Havel MP, Griesmacher A, Weigel G, et al: Aprotinin increases release of von Willebrand factor in cultured human umbilical vein cells. Surgery 112:573–577, 1992.

62. Havel MP, Griesmacher A, Weigel G, et al: Aprotinin decreased release of 6-keto-prostaglandin F1 alpha and increases release of thromboxane B2 in cultured human umbilical vein endothelial cells. J Thorac Cardiovasc Surg 104:654–658, 1992.

63. Heimark RL, Kurachi K, Fujikawa K, et al: Surface activation of blood coagulation, fibrinolysis and kinin formation. Nature 286:456–460, 1980.

64. Hemophilia of Georgia, USA: Protocols for the treatment of haemophilia and von Willebrand disease. Haemophilia 6:84–93, 2000.

65. Hendriks HGD, van der Maaten JMAA, de Wolf J, et al: An effective treatment of severe intractable bleeding after valve repair by one single dose of activated recombinant factor VII. Anesth Analg 93:287–289, 2001.

66. Horrow JC, Hlavacek J, Strong MD, et al: Prophylactic tranexamic acid decreases bleeding after cardiac operations. J Thorac Cardiovasc Surg 99:70–74, 1990.

67. Hoyer LW, Rizza CR, Tuddenham EG, et al: von Willebrand factor multimer patterns in von Willebrand's disease. Br J Haematol 55:493–507, 1983.

68. Ingerslev J, Freidman D, Gastineau, D, et al: Major surgery in haemphilic patients with inhibitors using recombinant factor VIIa. Haemostasis 26:118–123, 1996.

69. Kereiakes FJ, Topol EJ, George BS, et al: Emergency coronary artery bypass surgery preserves global and regional left ventricular function after intravenous tissue plasminogen activator therapy for acute myocardial infarction. J Am Coll Cardiol 11:899–907, 1988.

70. Kongsgaard UE, Smith-Erichsen N, Geiran O, et al: Changes in the coagulation and fibrinolytic systems during and after cardiopulmonary bypass surgery. Thorac Cardiovasc Surg 37:158–162, 1989.

71. Koster A, Kukucka M, Bach F, et al: Anticoagulation during cardiopulmonary bypass in patients with heparin-induced thrombocytopenia type II and renal impairment using heparin and the platelet glycoprotein IIb-IIIa antagonist tirofiban. Anesthesiology 94:245–251, 2001.

72. Latham P, Revelis AF, Joshi GP, et al: Use of recombinant hirudin in patients with heparin-induced thrombocytopenia with thrombosis requiring cardiopulmonary bypass. Anesthesiology 92:263–266, 2000.

73. Lee LY, DeBois W, Krieger KH, et al: The effect of platelet inhibitors on blood use in cardiac surgery. Perfusion 17:33–37, 2002.

74. Legget PL, Doyle D, Smith WB, et al: Elective cardiac operation in a patient with severe haemophilia and acquired factor VIII antibodies. J Thorac Cardiovasc Surg 87:556–560, 1984.

75. Lemmer JH, Despotis GJ: Antithrombin III concentrate to treat heparin resistance I patients undergoing cardiac surgery. J Thorac Cardiovasc Surg 123:213–217, 2002.

76. Lemmer Jr. JH, Stanford W, Bonney SL, et al: Aprotinin for coronary bypass operations: efficacy, safety, and influence on early saphenous graft patency. A multicenter, randomized, double-blind, placebo-controlled study. J Thorac Cardiovasc Surg 107:543–551, 1994.

77. Levin EG, Marzec U, Anderson J, et al: Thrombin stimulates tissue plasminogen activator release from cultured human endothelial cells. J Clin Invest 74:1988–1995, 1984.

78. Levy J, Pifarre R, Schaff H, et al: A multi-center, double-blind, placebo-controlled trial of aprotinin for reducing blood loss and the requirements for donor-blood transfusion in patients having repeat coronary artery bypass grafting. Circulation 92:2236–2244, 1995.

79. Loskutoff DJ, Curriden SA: The fibrinolytic system of the vessel wall and its role in the control of thrombosis. Ann NY Acad Sci 598:238–247, 1990.

80. Lusher JM, Blatt PM, Penner JA, et al: Autoplex vs proplex: a controlled, double-blind study of effectiveness in acute hemarthrosis in hemophiliacs with inhibitors to factor VIII. Blood 62:1135–1138, 1983.

81. Lusher J, Ingerslev J, Roberts H, et al: Clinical experience with recombinant factor VIIa. Blood Coagul Fibrinolysis 9:119–128, 1998.

82. Lusher JM, Shapiro SS, Palascak JE, et al: Efficacy of prothrombin-complex concentrates in hemophiliacs with antibodies to factor VIII: a multicenter therapeutic trial. N Engl J Med 303:421–425, 1980.

83. Makis M, Watson HG: The management of coumarin-induced over-anticoagulation. Br J Haematol 114:271–280, 2001.

84. Mann KG, Krishnaswamy S, Lawson JH: Surface-dependent hemostasis. Semin Hematol 29:213–226, 1992.

85. Mann KG, Neshim ME, Church WR, Haley P, Krishnaswamy S: Surface dependent reactions of vitamin K dependent enzyme complex. Blood 70:1–16, 1990.

86. Mannucci PM. Modern treatment of hemophilia: from the shadows towards the light. Thromb Haemost 70:17–23, 1993.

87. Mannucci PM: Treatment of von Willebrand's disease. J Int Med 242:129–132, 1997.

88. Mannucci PM: Tuddenham GD: The hemophilias—from royal genes to gene therapy. N Engl J Med 344:1773–1779, 2001.

89. Mannucci PM, Bettega D, Cattaneo M: Consistency of response to repeated DDAVP infusions in patients with von Willebrand disease and haemophilia A. Br J Haematol 82:87–93, 1992.

90. Mannucci PM, Ruggeri ZM, Pareti FI, Capitanio A: A new pharmacological approach to the management of hemophilia and von Willebrand disease. Lancet 1:869–872, 1977.

91. Marciniak E, Farley CH, DeSimone PA: Familial thrombosis due to antithrombin III deficiency. Blood 43:219–231, 1974.

92. Margaglione M, D'Andrea G, Giuliani N, et al: Inherited prothrombotic conditions and premature ischemic stroke. Sex difference in the association with factor V Leiden. Arterioscler Thromb Vasc Biol 19:1751–1756, 1999.

93. Marguerie GA, Edgington TS, Plow EF: Interaction of fibrinogen with its platelet receptor as part of a multistep reaction in ADP-induced platelet aggregation. J Biol Chem 255:154–160, 1980.

94. Marx G, Pokar H, Reuter H, et al: The effects of aprotinin on hemostatic function during cardiac surgery. J Cardiothorac Vasc Anesth 5:467–474, 1991.

95. Matsuo T, Yamada T, Yamanashi T, et al: Choice of anticoagulant in a congenital antithrombin III (AT III)-deficient patient with chronic renal failure undergoing regular haemodialysis. Clin Lab Haematol 11:213–219, 1989.

96. McCarthy PM, Popovsky MA, Schaff HV: Effect of blood conservation efforts in cardiac operations at the Mayo Clinic. Mayo Clin Proc 63:225–229, 1988.

97. Menache D: Antithrombin III concentrates. Hematol Oncol Clin North Am 6:1115–1120, 1992.

98. Meyer D, Girma JP: von Willebrand factor: structure and function. Thromb Haemost 70:99–104, 1993.

99. Mongan PD, Hosking MP: The role of desmopressin acetate in patients undergoing coronary artery bypass surgery. Anesthesiology 77:38–46, 1992.

100. Moran JM, Babka R, Silberman S: Immediate centrifugation of oxygenator contents after cardiopulmonary bypass: role in maximum blood conservation. J Thorac Cardiovasc Surg 76:510–517, 1978.

101. Morris JJ, Tan YS. Autotransfusion: is there a benefit in a current practice of aggressive blood conservation? Ann Thorac Surg 58:502–508, 1994.

102. Mosesson MW: Fibrin polymerization and it regulatory role in hemostasis. J Lab Clin Med 116:8–17, 1990.

103. Moulton MJ, Creswell LL, Mackey ME, et al: Reexploration for bleeding is a risk factor for adverse outcomes after cardiac operations. L Thorac Cardiovasc Surg 111:1037–1046, 1996.

104. Nair KS, Weerasinghe A, Dahdal M, et al: Cardiac intraventricular thrombus in protein C deficiency. J R Soc Med 94:641–642, 2001.

105. Nilsson IM: The management of hemophilia patients with inhibitors. Transfus Med Rev 6:285–293, 1992.

106. Nuttall GA, Oliver WC, Ereth MH, et al: Comparison of blood-conservation strategies in cardiac surgery patients at high risk for bleeding. Anesthesiology 92:674–682, 2000.

107. Nuttall GA, Oliver WC, Santrach PJ, et al: Efficacy of a simple intraoperative transfusion algorithm for nonerythrocyte component utilization after cardiopulmonary bypass. Anesthesiology 94:773–781, 2001.

108. Nuttall GA, Oliver, Jr WC, Santrach PJ, et al: Patients with a history of type II heparin-induced thrombocytopenia with thrombosis requiring cardiac surgery with cardiopulmonary bypass: a prospective observational case series. Anesth Analg 96:344–350, 2003.

109. Ochsner JL, Mills NL, Leonard GL, et al: Fresh autologous blood transfusions in extracorporeal circulation. Ann Surg 177:811–817, 1973.

110. Onwuanyi A. Sachdeva R. Hamirani K, et al: Multiple aortic thrombi associated with protein C and S deficiency. Mayo Clinic Proc 76:319–322, 2001.

111. Osterud B, Rapaport SI: Activation of factor IX by the reaction product of tissue factor and factor VII: additional pathway for initiating blood coagulation. Proc Natl Acad Sci USA 74:5260–5264, 1977.

112. Ott DA, Cooley DA: Cardiovascular surgery in Jehovah's Witnesses. JAMA 238:1256–1258, 1977.

113. Ovrum E, Am Holen E, Abdelnoor M, et al: Tranexamic acid (Cyklokapron) is not necessary to reduce blood loss after coronary artery bypass operations. J Thorac Cardiovasc Surg 105:78–83, 1993.

114. Pang JT, Fort S, Della Siega A, et al: Emergency coronary artery bypass surgery in the era of glycoprotein IIb/IIIa receptor antagonist use. J Card Surg 17:425–431, 2002.

115. Perkins HA: Correction of the hemostatic defects in von Willebrand disease. Blood 30:375–380, 1967.

116. Phillips MD, Santhouse A: von Willebrand disease: recent advances in pathophysiology and treatment. Am J Med Sci 316:77–86, 1998.

117. Preissner KT: Anticoagulant potential of endothelial cell membrane components. Haemostatis 18:271–306, 1988.

118. Rao LV, Rapaport SI: Activation of factor VII bound to tissue factor: a key early step in the tissue factor pathway of blood coagulation. Proc Natl Acad Sci USA 85:6687–6691, 1988.

119. The RESTORE Investigators: Effects of glycoprotein IIb/IIIa blockade with tirofiban on adverse cardiac events in patients with unstable angina or acute myocardial infarction undergoing coronary angioplasty. Circulation 96:1445–1453, 1997.

120. Rinder CS, Mathew JP, Rinder HM, et al: Modulation of platelet surface adhesion receptors during cardiopulmonary bypass. Anesthesiology 75:563–570, 1991.

848

121. Rocha E, Llorens R, Paramo JA, et al: Does desmopressin acetate reduce blood loss after surgery in patients on cardiopulmonary bypass? Circulation 77:1319–1323, 1988.

122. Rodeghiero F, Castaman G, Dini E: Epidemiological investigation of the prevalence of von Willebrand's disease. Blood 69:454–459, 1987.

123. Rodeghiero F, Castaman G, Mannucci PM: Clinical indications for desmopressin (DDAVP) in congenital and acquired von Willebrand disease. Blood Rev 5:155–161, 1991.

124. Rosendaal FR, Koster T, Vandenbroucke JP, et al: High risk of thrombosis in patients homozygous for factor V Leiden (activated protein C resistance). Blood 85:1504–1508, 1995.

125. Rosengart TK, Helm RE, DeBois WJ, et al: Open heart operations without transfusion using a multimodality blood conservation strategy in 50 Jehovah's Witness patients: implications for a "bloodless" surgical technique. J Am Coll Surg 184:618–629, 1997.

126. Rosko RR, Gilchrist GS, Kazmier FJ, et al: Management of haemophilia A and B during cardiac surgical correction of transposition of the great arteries. Mayo Clin Proc 58:182–186, 1983.

127. Rubens FD, Fergusson D, Wells PS, et al: Platelet-rich plasmapheresis in cardiac surgery: a meta-analysis of the effect on transfusion requirements. J Thorac Cardiovasc Surg 116:641–647, 1998.

128. Ruggeri ZM, Ware J: The structure and function of von Willebrand factor. Thromb Haemost 67:594–599, 1992.

129. Rush B, Ellis H: The treatment of patients with factor V deficiency. Thromb Diath Haemorrh 14:74–82, 1965.

130. Sakariassen KS, Bolhuis PA, Sixma JJ: Human platelet adhesion to artery subendothelium is mediated by factor VIII-von Willebrand factor bound to the subendothelium. Nature 279:636–638, 1979.

131. Salzman EW, Weinstein MJ, Weintraub RM, et al: Treatment with desmopressin acetate to reduce blood loss after cardiac surgery: a double-blind randomized trial. N Engl J Med 314:1402–1406, 1986.

132. Savage B, Shattil SJ, Ruggeri ZM: Modulation of platelet function through adhesion receptors—a dual role of glycoprotein IIb-IIIa mediated by fibrinogen and GPIbl-vWF. J Biol Chem 267:11300–11306, 1992.

133. Shonberger JPAM, van Oeveren W, Bredee JJ, et al: Systemic blood activation during and after autotransfusion. Ann Thorac Surg 57:1256–1262, 1994.

134. Simon TL, Akl BF, Murphy W: Controlled trial of routine administration of platelet concentrates in cardiopulmonary bypass surgery. Ann Thorac Surg 37:359–364, 1984.

135. Singh M, Nuttall GA, Ballman KV, et al: Effect of abciximab on the outcome of emergency coronary artery grafting after failed percutaneous coronary intervention. Mayo Clin Proc 76:784–788, 20013.

136. Sixma JJ, Pronk A, Nievelstein PFEM, et al: Platelet adhesion to extracellular matrices of cultured cells. Ann NY Acad Sci 614:181–192, 1991.

137. Sjamsoedin LM, Heijnen L, Mauser-Bunschoten EP, et al: The effect of activated prothrombin-complex concentrates (FEIBA) on joint and muscle bleeding in patients with hemophilia A antibodies to factor VIII: a double-blind clinical trial. N Engl J Med 305:717–721, 1981.

138. Spiess BD, Tuman KJ, McCarthy RJ, et al: Thromboelastography as an indicator of post-cardiopulmonary bypass coagulopathies. J Clin Monit 3:25–30, 1987.

139. Stahl CP, Wideman CS, Spira TJ, et al: Protein S deficiency in men with long-term human immunodeficiency virus infection. Blood 81:1801–1807, 1993.

140. Tabuchi N, de Haan J, Boonstra PW, et al: Activation of fibrinolysis in the pericardial cavity during cardiopulmonary bypass. J Thorac Cardiovasc Surg 106:828–833, 1993.

141. Tanaka K, Takao M, Yada I, et al: Alterations in coagulation and fibrinolysis associated with cardiopulmonary bypass during open heart surgery. J Cardiothorac Anesth 3:181–189, 1989.

142. Taper NM, Renisson F, Rickard K. Cardiac surgery and catheterization in patients with haemophilia. Haemophilia 6:84–88, 2000.

143. Thompson EA, Salem HH: The role of thrombomodulin in the regulation of hemostatic interactions. Prog Hematol 15:51–70, 1987.

144. Tollefson DF, Friedman KD, Marlar RA: Protein S deficiency. A cause of unusual or unexplained thrombosis. Arch Surg 123:881–884, 1988.

145. Toy PT, Strauss RG, Stehling LC, et al: Predeposited autologous blood for elective surgery. A national multicenter study. N Engl J Med 316:517–520, 1987.

146. Valeri CR, Cassidy G, Khuri S, et al: Hypothermia-induced reversible platelet dysfunction. Ann Surg 205:175–181, 1987.

147. Van Obberghen-Schilling E, Pouyssegur J: Signaling pathways of the thrombin receptor. Throm Haemost 70:163–167, 1993.

148. Vander Salm TJ, Ansell JE, Okike ON, et al: The role of epsilon-aminocaproic acid in reducing bleeding after cardiac operation: a double-blind randomized study. J Thorac Cardiovasc Surg 95:538–540, 1988.

149. Vander Woude JC, Milam JD, Walker WE, et al: Cardiovascular surgery in patients with congenital plasma coagulopathies. Ann Thorac Surg 46:283–288, 1988.

150. Vassalli JD, Sappino AP, Belin D: The plasminogen activator / plasmin system. J Clin Invest 88:1067–1072, 1991.

151. Villanueva GB, Danishefsky I: Evidence for a heparin-induced conformational change in antithrombin III. Biochem Biophys Res Commun 74:803–809, 1977.

152. Visentin GP, Aster RH: Heparin-induced thrombocytopenia and thrombosis. Curr Opin Hematol 2:351–357, 1995.

153. Walenga JM, Bick RL: Heparin-induced thrombocytopenia, paradoxical thromboembolism, and other side effects of heparin therapy. Med Clin North Am 82:635–658, 1998.

154. Warkentin TE, Kelton JG: Heparin and platelets. Hematol Oncol Clin North Am 4:243–264, 1990.

155. Weiss HJ: Platelet physiology and abnormalities of platelet function: parts 1 and 2. N Engl J Med 293:531–541, 580–588, 1975.

156. Williams WR, D'Ambra AB, Beck JR, et al: A randomized trial of antithrombin concentrate for treatment of heparin resistance. Ann Thorac Surg 70:873–877, 2000.

157. Woodman RC, Harker LA: Bleeding complications associated with cardiopulmonary bypass. Blood 76:1680–1697, 1990.

158. Wu KK: Platelet activation mechanisms and markers in arterial thrombosis. J Intern Med 239:17–34, 1996.

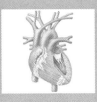
Coronary Angiography, Valve and Hemodynamic Assessment

Lawrence A. Garcia

INTRODUCTION

Since the first catheter was placed in the vascular tree by Forsmann[24], techniques to achieve vascular access have developed rapidly. Sones performed the first selective diagnostic coronary catheterization in 1956.[61,62] Later, Gruentzig performed the first coronary angioplasty in 1977.[28,29] Subsequently, angioplasty and the placement of intravascular stents have become the predominant forms of catheter-based intervention in all major vascular beds.

Recall that coronary artery disease remains the number one cause of death in the United States.[1] This has remained relatively unchanged over the past several decades despite improvements in acute coronary syndrome care, out of hospital treatments, and early access to invasive revascularizations. Coronary artery disease remains a major cause of morbidity in addition to its high end for mortality in the United States.

Right or left heart catheterizations can be performed via brachial, radial, or femoral (being the most common) access sites.[11,13,21,33,47] Other potential sites include direct cut-down (brachial or femoral) or in rare instances direct left ventricular (LV) puncture.[59]

DIAGNOSTIC CATHETERIZATION TECHNIQUES

Indications

The indications for coronary angiography are usually to confirm the presence of clinically suspected coronary artery occlusive disease.* Further, angiography is pursued in patients where a percutaneous intervention or surgical revascularization may be planned. Diagnostic angiography is also performed in patients in whom valve replacement/repair or percutaneous procedures are planned. The risk-to-benefit ratio should always be evaluated prior to angiography to identify those patients that might fully benefit from imaging.

Contraindications

The principal contraindications to coronary angiography include bleeding diathesis, renal failure (true or impending), fever, ongoing infection, or severe anemia (Box 53-1). Also, uncontrolled or uncorrected hypokalemia, hyperkalemia, digoxin toxicity, severe allergy to contrast dyes, and over anticoagulation with a PT (INR) over 1.8 (although access in the radial artery makes catheterization with INR

*References 10, 15, 38, 55, 65, 66.

849

850

over 1.8 possible) are considered relative contraindications to catheterization.

Complications

Complications of coronary angiography primarily involve the vascular access site. Catheter manipulation within atherosclerotic vessels may lead to emboli (both thrombus and air) or clot formation causing stroke, myocardial infarction, worsening renal function, or congestive heart failure (Table 53-1). Recall that pseudoaneurysm or vascular access complications may be as high as 3%[55] in patients with severe peripheral occlusive diseases.

Angiography

Beyond the first nonselective injection for coronary angiography, today all coronary angiography is performed by selective injection. In rare instances, nonselective coronary imaging may still be performed.

The most common access for coronary angiography is the femoral approach, although brachial, radial, and axillary approaches may also be performed. The most common method of cannulation of the vessel is the Seldinger technique,[57] in which the vessel is punctured and a guide wire, usually "J" tipped, is advanced into the vessel.[5,37] This wire then serves as a "rail" for the sheath and dilator to enter the vessel.

Once access is obtained, the sheath then acts as an entry point for passage and exchange of catheters and devices over

Table 53–1	
Possible Complications of Peripheral Catheterization	
Vascular access dissection or perforation	0.1–0.2%
Bleeding/hematoma	1.5–2.0%
Allergic reaction	0.5–2.0%
Vasovagal events	1.0–2.0%
Death	0.1–0.2%

the "J" wire. Various preshaped coronary catheters and graft catheters are available for coronary and graft or conduit angiography. Once a catheter is advanced into the aorta it is positioned either in the ascending aorta or in the descending aorta for clearing and flushing. The guidewire is withdrawn and the catheter is connected to a "manifold" system that in a "closed" system allows the pressure at the tip of the catheter to be transduced and allows contrast injections without reconnecting an apparatus or device. Once the catheter is "cleared" it is advanced with pressure monitoring into the ostia of the coronary artery. If the pressure waveform "dampens" this would suggest either an ostial coronary artery lesion or an unfavorable angle of the catheter. Care should always be taken with engagement and injection into any arterial conduit so as to avoid dissection or lifting of present lesion flaps. Contrast may be carefully injected to identify the lesion or problem with the dampened waveform. At times, the original catheter may be downsized (5 French for a 6 French diagnostic catheter); small volume contrast injection under cine or nonselective angiography may define the anatomy and allude to the current problem to complete the study.

Left Coronary Angiography

In cannulating the left main coronary ostium, care should always be taken to confirm that the pressure tracing is not damped or ventricularized to allow a complete and safe study. Normally, a preshaped catheter such as a Judkins left 4 catheter (JL4) is used as a default catheter for left coronary angiography. It is successful in engaging the left main ostia 80% of the time. If the root is dilated or narrow then a larger or shorter catheter may be needed (JL6 or JL3.5). Conversely, if the anatomy is altered with a left main origin that is posterior, an Amplatz catheter may be used to cannulate the left main (LM) ostia. The coronary anatomy is defined with contrast injections of 8–10 ml during cine runs. The angles taken during angiography allow the three-dimensional reconstruction of the anatomy using "orthogonal" views to see the arteries in multiple planes. The left system begins with the left main, which then terminally bifurcates into the left anterior descending (LAD) and left circumflex (LCX) coronary arteries. At times the LM may terminally trifurcate with the LAD, LCX, and an intermediate branch (ramus intermedius) supplying much of the left ventricular free wall. The LAD gives off septal arteries as it courses down the interventricular groove as well as various diagonal arteries supplying the anterolateral free wall of the left ventricle. The LCX gives off "marginal" arteries as it courses in the atrioventricular (AV) groove. The marginal arteries supply the lateral free wall of the left ventricle (Figure 53-1).

Right Coronary Angiography

The right coronary artery (RCA) is usually engaged with a Judkins right 4-cm catheter (JR4). The RCA courses in the interventricular groove and gives off acute marginal and right ventricular branches that supply the right ventricular (RV) free wall. The RCA terminally bifurcates at "the crux" to form the right posterior descending artery (RPDA) and right posterolateral coronary artery supplying the inferior and inferolateral segments of the left ventricle, respectively.

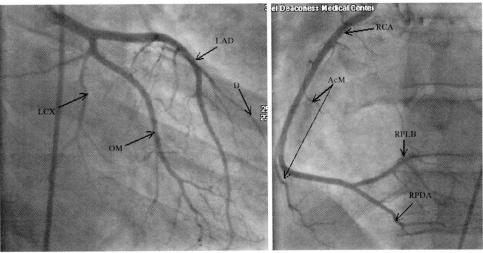

Figure 53–1 Coronary angiography of the left and right coronary arteries. LAD, left anterior descending artery; D, diagonal artery; LCX, left circumflex artery; OM, obtuse marginal artery; RCA, right coronary artery; AcM, acute marginal artery; RPDA, right posterior descending artery; RPLB, right posterolateral branch artery.

The RPDA courses in the interventricular septum supplying the interventricular septum as well (Figure 53-1).

The dominance of the coronary circulation is dependent upon which artery supplies the AV nodal artery. In over 90% of patients this artery is given by the RPDA from the RCA. In 8–10% of patients this artery is given from the left posterior descending artery (LPDA) from the LCX.

Coronary Anomalies

Several coronary anomalies can exist. Most are anatomical variants such as dual ostia for the LAD and LCX. Others may be congenital such as with the origin of the LCX from the right coronary artery° (Figure 53-2). Most congenital anomalies such as these have little impact on coronary circulation. In the case of the LAD from the RCA or right coronary cusp and coursing posteriorly there is an increased mortality with these patients secondary to arrhythmias and ischemia.[54,60]

Angiographic Projections

As with any angiography it is necessary to obtain multiple views in various orthogonal planes of a vessel to fully

°References 4, 50, 52, 54, 56, 60, 70.

define all its segments clearly. This dictum is no different with the coronary circulation. Clearly, without orthogonal angulation an inexperienced eye may not see a significant coronary lesion. Generally, all views are reported by convention with left or right angulation first followed by the cranial or caudal angulation. For example, a 30/25 left anterior oblique (LAO)/cranial is 30-degrees LAO with 25 degrees of cranial angulation.

Of note, all major coronary arteries lie in one of two planes: either the interventricular septum or along the AV groove (Figure 53-3). As such the image projections try to show the intended anatomy in profile. For example, the RPDA coursing along the interventricular septum along the inferior wall is best seen with the interventricular septum in its longest profile, the flat right anterior oblique (RAO) projection. Alternatively, the LCX coursing along the AV groove is best visualized in the anteroposterior (AP) or RAO caudal projection looking at the AV groove in profile.

Left Main

The LM is best seen in a shallow LAO with a little caudal for its mid and distal segment and some cranial angulation for its proximal or ostial segments. Another helpful view is the

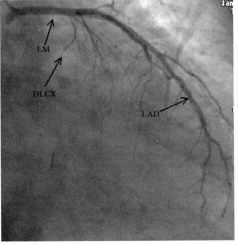

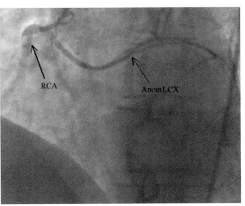

Figure 53–2 A, Long left main with a diminutive LCX. **B,** Anomalous left circumflex artery arising from the right coronary artery seen in an RAO view. LM, left main; DLCX, diminutive left circumflex artery; LAD, left anterior descending artery; RCA, right coronary artery; AnomLCX, anomalous left circumflex artery.

A   B

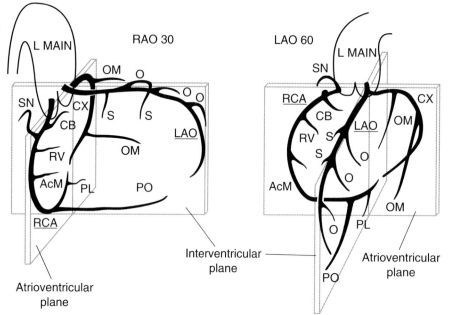

RAO 30

LAO 60

Figure 53–3 Representation of coronary anatomy in relation to the interventricular and atrioventricular valve planes. Coronary branches are as indicated. L Main, left main; LAD, left anterior descending; D, diagonal; S, septal; CX, circumflex; OM, obtuse marginal; RCA, right coronary; CB, conus branch; SN, sinus node; AcM, acute marginal; PD, posterior descending; PL, posterolateral left ventricular.
(Used with permission from Grossman's Cardiac Catheterization, Angiography, and Intervention, 6th ed. "Coronary Angiography." Philadelphia: Lippincott, Williams & Wilkins, 2000.)

steep LAO/caudal ("spider view") of the terminal LM bifurcation. This last view is not helpful with a horizontal positioned heart and may be best viewed for these patients with a steep RAO/caudal view.

Left Anterior Descending and Diagonal Arteries

The LAD has a course that is anterior and inferior from the LM. It then enters the interventricular groove and courses to the apex of the heart. The best view for the LAD comes in several views for the various segments of interest. The proximal LAD is best seen in the steep LAO projections with cranial angulation. The mid- and distal segments are generally best visualized with LAO and RAO with some caudal angulation. In some cases where the proximal LAD is not well seen (horizontal heart) an RAO/cranial of 30° each is sufficient to "open" the proximal LAD and bifurcation with the LCX.

The diagonal arteries, the major branches of the LAD, course off the LAD toward the lateral free wall of the LV. The best view for most of the diagonal arteries, their origin, and distal segments is usually a steep LAO with steep cranial angulation (50/45–50). In some cases the first diagonal artery is the only diagonal artery given by the LAD. This vessel then supplies the entire diagonal system and in our laboratory is called a "twin" LAD given the importance of this vessel to epicardial blood flow.

Left Circumflex Artery

The LCX is best seen in caudal projections. The proximal portion of the LCX is best seen in the RAO/caudal angulation. This angle also serves to show the marginal arteries as well. The alternative for the mid-segment of the LCX and marginal arteries is the steep LAO/caudal ("spider") view. Here the mid-segments of the LCX and marginal arteries

are usually visualized well. This view in large (obese) patients is usually challenging given the extra tissue the X-ray has to penetrate and, thus, much of the image may be distorted, dark, or hazy.

Right Coronary Artery

The RCA enters the anterior AV groove and courses distally as noted previously. The proximal segment of the RCA is best seen in the flat LAO angulation. If the ostium of the RCA is of interest then a steep (50°) LAO projection is best. The mid-segment of the RCA is best seen in the LAO and flat RAO projections. The "crux" or distal RCA and the proximal portions of the RPDA right posterolateral branch artery (RPLB) are best seen with an AP or slight LAO with 20–30° of cranial angulation. The RPDA mid- and distal segments are best visualized with a flat RAO projection.

Graft Angiography

Commonly, saphenous vein grafts to the right and left coronary circulations arise from the anterior surface of the aorta several centimeters from the sinus of Valsalva. The RCA grafts arise form the right anterior side of the aorta and the left system grafts arise from the left anterior side of the aorta with the LAD grafts usually being lower than the LCX grafts. In many cases the surgeon may place a ring at the origin of a graft that may greatly reduce the chance of missing a graft because one cannot cannulate or find it. The best views for the LAD/diagonal grafts are flat LAO and RAO projections to visualize the graft in its greatest profile. The distal (native) vessel is then imaged with some cranial or caudal projection to define all its segments after the distal anastomosis according to the vessel of interest (i.e., cranial for the LAD and caudal for the LCX). These images are usually easier to obtain and evaluate because there is less overlap of other coronary anatomy to deal with. However, the ability to "lay" out the origin or distal anastomosis may be challenging for some grafts. The RCA grafts are usually best seen with flat LAO and RAO projections. Again, after the graft has been imaged the distal vessel is imaged with some cranial or caudal angulation to fully define the anatomy after the distal anastomosis (Figure 53-4).

There has been an increasing use of the internal mammary artery (IMA) as the conduit of choice for the LAD and in some cases for the RCA given the high patency of these conduits over 10–15 years. Generally, the IMA is cannulated after the subclavian artery is engaged with the preformed catheter and "J" wire. The catheter is advanced and cleared. Then the catheter is withdrawn and gentle "counterclock" torque is applied until the

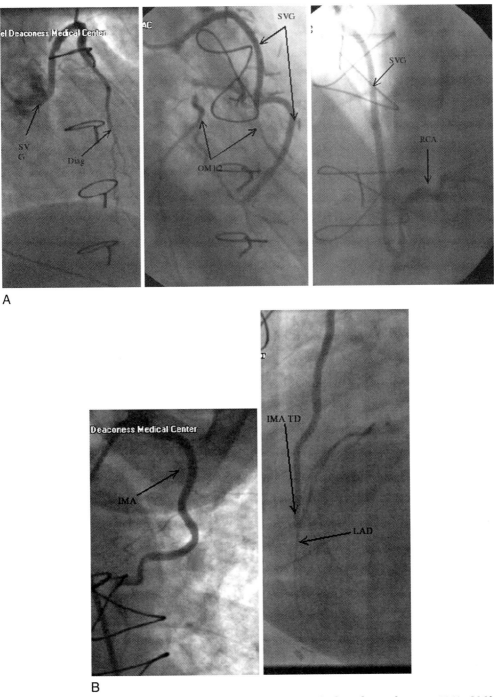

Figure 53–4 A, Graft angiography. SVG, saphenous vein graft; diag, diagonal artery; OM1, OM2, obtuse marginal arteries 1 and 2; RCA, right coronary artery. **B,** IMA angiography. IMA, internal mammary artery; IMA TD, internal mammary artery touch down; LAD, left anterior descending artery.

854 catheter engages the origin of the LIMA. Once the vessel is engaged the catheter is given a gentle "clockwise" torque to remove any excess tension on the catheter.[39] The views for angiography for the IMA are, generally, AP or slight RAO/cranial (0–20/40) for the proximal and mid-segments of the graft and steep flat LAO to lateral projection for the anastomosis of the IMA with the LAD. The RIMA conduit is similarly engaged from the right subclavian artery, as was the LIMA. The views for the mid-segment, origin, and anastomosis are, generally, flat LAO with some cranial and steep AP cranial, respectively (Figure 53-4).

► HEMODYNAMICS

Principles

The hemodynamic assessment performed during coronary angiography is as integral a part of the procedure as is the imaging of the coronary vasculature. At any given moment the hemodynamics reflect a culmination and interaction between various ongoing dynamic processes determining cardiac output, coronary artery disease, left ventricular function, systemic metabolic needs, and systemic and pulmonary pressures.[17,31] Hemodynamic measurements (vessel or ventricular pressures), cardiac outputs, and the evaluation of shunts are an integral part of any diagnostic coronary evaluation. All pressures should be measured with a transducer that will allow direct real-time measurements. A key element for this process is the establishment of a zero reference. The "zero" reference is usually accepted at the mid-chest level in the AP direction. Once "zeroed" the pressure evaluation may continue with accurate information being obtained.

Right Heart Catheterization

The measurement of right heart (RH) pressures and oxygen saturations allows a very good and easy method to obtain the current cardiovascular status. Recall, cardiac output (CO) is the flow of blood from the heart to the body and is reported in liters/min. To standardize this number for a patient's size these units are divided by the patients body surface area (BSA) to derive the cardiac index (CI) in liters/min/m² body area.

With the right heart catheter (RHC), oxygen saturations should be obtained from the superior vena cava, right atrium, right ventricle, pulmonary artery, and pulmonary capillary wedge pressure positions. When obtained with an arterial saturation the CO/CI can be calculated and possible shunts can be determined (see below).

Pressure tracings are obtained at each level of the advancement of the RHC. Normal values for the RH/arterial (LV) pressures are shown in Table 53-2 and Figure 53-5. Since the introduction of the balloon-tipped RH[64] catheter, RH catheterization has become very common in the cath lab and in the critically ill patient in the ICU.

Pressure Waveforms

Right atrial pressure: the A wave occurs with atrial systole, which occurs after the P wave on the surface electrocardiogram (ECG). With atrial diastole, there is a decline in the pressure waveform, which corresponds to the x descent. In the ventricle below as it initiates systole the x descent may be interrupted by an upward movement of the tricuspid valve, the "c" wave with the remainder of the x descent called x'. As ventricular systole progresses and forward flow occurs filling the atria against a closed tricuspid valve the v wave is the result. Ultimately, ventricular relaxation occurs

Table 53–2

Normal Cardiac Pressures and Values

	A wave	V wave	Mean	Systolic	End diastolic	Mean
RA	2–8	2–8	0–6			
RV				15–30	0–8	
PA				15–30	4–12	8–16
PCWP	3–15	3–10	1–10			
LV				100–140	3–12	
Aorta				100–140	60–90	70–110

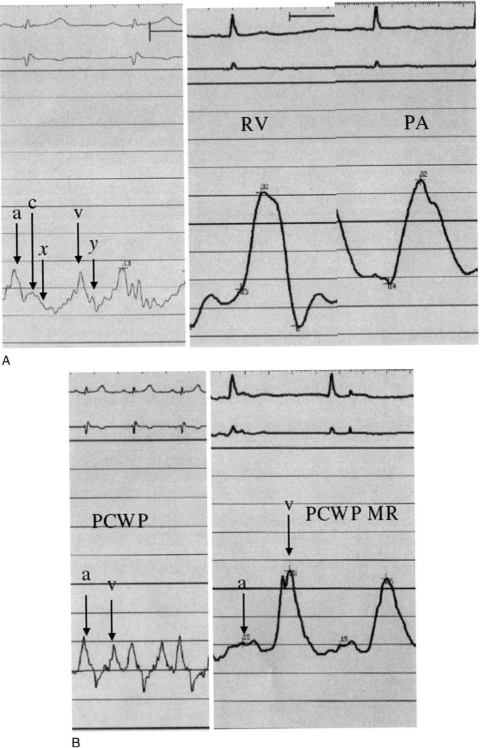

Figure 53–5 A, Right heart pressure tracings. RA, RV, and PA pressure tracings. RA, right atrium; RV right ventricle; PA, pulmonary artery; a, "a" wave from atrial systole; c, "c" wave from closed tricuspid valve and ventricular systole slightly pushing the valve into the atrium; v, "v" wave from ventricular systole; x, x descent with atrial diastole; y, y descent from atrial emptying after ventricular systole. **B,** Right heart pressure tracings. PCWP, pulmonary artery capillary wedge pressure; PCWP MR, pulmonary capillary wedge pressure tracing with substantial mitral regurgitation; "a", a wave; "v", v wave.

and the tricuspid valve opens and atrial pressure falls corresponding to the y descent.

Right ventricular pressure rises with ventricular systole. As diastole commences the pulmonic valve closes and a rapid decline in pressure is noted. After the tricuspid valve opens there is rapid filling of the ventricle and an increase in its pressure, though not to a great degree. With atrial systole, the final pressure recorded is the end diastolic pressure.

In the pulmonary artery after ventricular systole opens the pulmonic valve, there is a rise in the systolic pressure noted in the pulmonary artery. As diastole commences the pressure declines; with closure of the pulmonic valve, the diastolic pressure levels out to a higher degree than in the ventricle. The diastolic pressure of the pulmonary artery correlates closely with the left atrial and pulmonary capillary wedge pressures (PCWP).

With the use of balloon-tipped catheters, a "wedge" position, where the catheter is wedged into a distal vessel, can infer pressure from the downstream circulation,[41] namely, the left atrium. This maneuver is easy and allows an indirect measure of left atrial pressures without need for transseptal access into the left atrium. Many studies have proved the validity[3,41,48] of PCWP as a surrogate to left atrial access in evaluation of mitral disease (stenosis).

Lastly, the arterial pressure waveform begins with left ventricular systole. Once the aortic valve opens systolic pressure rises. As ventricular diastole begins and pressures fall the aortic valve closes and the aortic pressure declines. There is an interruption in the pressure tracing corresponding to the aortic valve closure called the "dicrotic notch." Depending on the patency of the aortic valve and the compliance of the aorta the usual pulse pressure is 45–50 mm Hg. In noncompliant aortic systems (elderly, calcified vessels) or in aortic regurgitation there is a wide pulse pressure of usually over 80 mm Hg (Figure 53-5).

Cardiac Output

Cardiac output, the amount of blood sent to deliver enough oxygen, glucose, and nutrients to the body, is expressed in liters per minute. This measurement can be obtained through several methods such as Fick, thermodilution, or dye methods.[3,19,22,40,63] The Fick[22] method is the most commonly used in our laboratory. This method is based on the hypothesis that the uptake of oxygen in the lungs is directly proportional to the blood flow in the pulmonary circulation. By measuring the oxygen extracted from the inspired air and the AV oxygen difference across the lungs, pulmonary blood flow and, subsequently, cardiac blood flow can be calculated. The calculation of CO is

$$CO \text{ (liters/min)} = \frac{O_2 \text{ consumption (ml/min)}}{AVO_2 \text{ difference}}$$

The normal oxygen consumption index is 110–150 ml/min/m². In our laboratory we assume an arteriovenous O_2 (AVO$_2$) index difference of 125 ml/min/m² (110 ml/min/m² for elderly females). This allows an estimation of the CI, understanding there is an inherent error assuming the oxygen consumption. By multiplying the BSA by the CI, CO is calculated. The more reliable way to determine O_2 consumption is to measure it directly. There are several ways to determine oxygen consumption: the Douglas bag where the oxygen content of expired air is compared with the O_2 content in the air and thus oxygen consumption is calculated, or the metabolic rate meter (MRM)[40] where the patient breaths into a container with O_2 and CO_2 sensors that measure the expired content of oxygen or carbon dioxide and oxygen consumption can then be calculated. Thus, to calculate the AVO$_2$ difference one needs the arterial saturation, the most mixed venous saturation (PA saturation, assuming no shunts), the hemoglobin, and the oxygen consumption. The equation then becomes

$$AVO_2 \text{ difference} = PA \text{ (\%sat)} - Pa \text{ (\% sat)} \text{ (Hgb) } (1.36)/10$$

where PA is the oxygen saturation in the pulmonary artery, Pa is the oxygen saturation in the systemic (left ventricular/pulmonary vein), Hgb is the hemoglobin content, and 1.36 is the correction factor for fully saturated hemoglobin's ability to carry oxygen.

The cardiac index (CI) can then be calculated as

$$CI = \frac{O_2 \text{ Consumption (assumed or directly measured)}}{AVO_2 \text{ difference}}$$

Once calculated the CI is multiplied by the BSA and the CO is determined. Tables 53-2 and 53-3 show the normal values for the right heart catheterization and left ventricular pressures with CO and CI.

Shunts

When the flow of blood in the heart enters another chamber without traversing a valve a shunt is present. Evaluation, detection, and localization of intracardiac shunts are an integral part of the diagnostic coronary catheterization and right heart catheterization.

Left-to-Right Shunts

The classic left-to-right shunt seen in the catheterization laboratory is an atrial septal defect (ASD). Other causes of left-to-right shunting include ASD (Figure 53-6), ventricular septal defect (VSD) (Figure 53-6), or patent ductus

Table 53–3	
Normal Indices	
Oxygen consumption index (ml/min/m²)	110–150
AVo$_2$ difference (ml/liter)	30–50
CO/CI	2.5–4.2/2.0–3.0
Resistances PVR SVR	20–130 700–1600

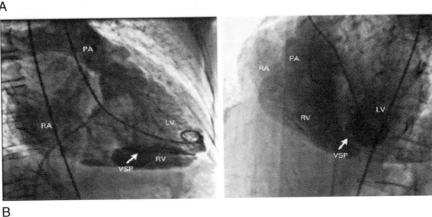

Figure 53–6 A, ASD noted from transesophageal echocardiography both 2-D and color flow Doppler images. LA, left atrium; RA, right atrium. **B,** VSD noted in ventriculography from RAO and LAO projections. RA, right atrium; RV, right ventricle; LV, left ventricle; PA, pulmonary artery; VSP, ventricular septal perforation.

arteriosus (PDA). In each of these there is a step-up in oxygen saturation at a different level of the right heart catheterization. For the ASD this occurs in the right atria, the VSD in the right ventricle, and the PDA in the right ventricle. The key element to understanding and quantifying the shunt is to determine where the most mixed venous sample can be obtained. In the case of the ASD it is a combination of the superior vena cava (SVC) and inferior vena cava (IVC); for a VSD it is the right atrium and for a PDA it is the right ventricle.

The oximetry run is the method by which the right heart chambers or vessels are evaluated during a shunt evaluation. Early work by Dexter and colleagues[16] defined what we use today for maximal changes in each right heart chamber for oxygen saturations. In general, a maximal change of 8% from the SVC to the PA is considered significant to evaluate further for the presence of an intracardiac shunt.

If a shunt is suspected, oximetry is performed. Once the data are collected, it is important to quantify the amount of the shunt. The pulmonary, systemic blood flows and the magnitude of the left-to-right shunt should be calculated. Pulmonary blood flow ($\dot{Q}_P$) is calculated by

$$\dot{Q}_P = \frac{O_2 \text{ Consumption (ml/min)}}{[PV_{O_2}] - [PA_{O_2}]}$$

Systemic blood flow ($\dot{Q}_S$) is calculated by

$$\dot{Q}_S = \frac{O_2 \text{ Consumption (ml/min)}}{[SA_{O_2}] - [MV_{O_2}]}$$

The $\dot{Q}_P/\dot{Q}_S$ or the ratio of the relative blood flows in the pulmonary and systemic circulations can then be reduced to

$$\dot{Q}_P/\dot{Q}_S = \frac{[SA_{O_2}] - [MV_{O_2}]}{[PV_{O_2}] - [PA_{O_2}]}$$

Again, the mixed venous sample (MV_{O_2}) is a value of the average from the right atrium for VSD, right ventricle for PDA, and a derived number from the Flamm[23] equation where MV_{O_2} is 3(SVC) + 1 (IVC)/4 for an ASD.

A $\dot{Q}_P/\dot{Q}_S$ over 2.0 is considered high and should be considered for surgical correction or percutaneous closure. A level between 1.5 and 2.0 is intermediate and surgical or percutaneous closure is pursued if there is low surgical risk or symptoms for percutaneous closure (Figure 53-7) are present (cryptogenic stroke for ASD or PFO). A ratio under 1.0 suggests a right-to-left shunt.

Right-to-Left Shunt

Usually, any significant right-to-left shunt is detected early without catheterization given that the patient usually has cyanosis or arterial hypoxemia. The oximetric evidence is a $\dot{Q}_P/\dot{Q}_S$ under 1.0. Usually a ratio under 0.7 in considered critical and under 0.3 not compatible with life.

Regardless of the cause, the basis for evaluation of the site of the right-to-left shunt may be analyzed if the pulmonary vein, left atrium, left ventricle, and aortic saturations can be obtained. When the shunt is extraanatomical from the pulmonary circulation the site of "step-down" is

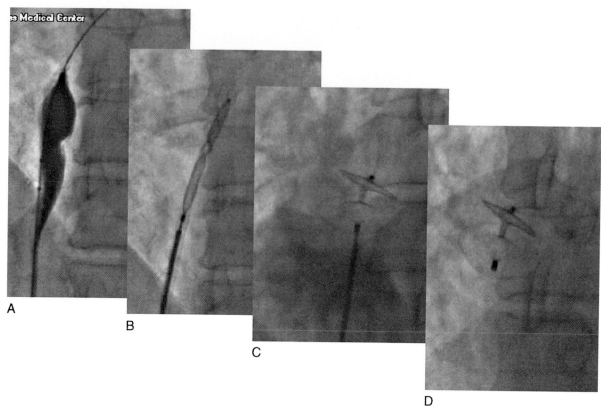

Figure 53–7 PFO/ASD closure device (Amplatzer, Amplazter Industries, Chicago, IL). **A,** Sizing balloon in the canal of the atrial defect. **B,** Constrained device in the Mullins sheath (Cordis Corporation, Miami, FL). **C,** Deployed device without release. **D,** Final release of device.

the site of the shunt. For example, if the step-down occurs in the left ventricle then there is a VSD. Unfortunately, this would require entering the left atrium, which may be problematic in some patients.

Bidirectional Shunts

If there is evidence of both a left-to-right and right-to-left shunting then a formula comparing the effective blood flow (Q_{eff}) is used. This flow rate is the hypothetical flow in the absence of any left-to-right or right-to-left shunting.

$$Q_{eff} = \frac{O_2 \text{ Consumption (ml/min)}}{[PVo_2] - [MVo_2]}$$

Then the left-to-right and right-to-left shunts are $\dot{Q}_P - \dot{Q}_{eff}$ and $\dot{Q}_{eff} - \dot{Q}s$, respectively.

Assessment of Vascular Resistance

Vascular resistance is calculated by dividing the pressure gradient across the vascular bed in question by the blood flow through it. In essence, there are two major vascular beds, systemic and pulmonary. For systemic vascular resistance (SVR)

$$SVR = \frac{MAP - R_A}{\text{Cardiac output (systemic blood flow)}}$$

For pulmonary vascular resistance (PVR)

$$PVR = \frac{PA - PCWP\ (LA)}{\text{Cardiac output (pulmonary blood flow)}}$$

Normal values for the SVR and PVR are listed in the Table 53-3. A high vascular resistance is seen in systemic hypertension, hypovolemia, significant blood loss, and congestive heart failure. A low SVR is seen with high fevers, sepsis, thyrotoxicosis or AV fistulas.

Valve Assessment

The assessment of valvular abnormalities is an integral part of any catheterization. During a routine right and left heart catheterization diagnostic information may be derived for all four valves in the heart. The principal valvular anomalies that would require interrogation and potential surgical repair would be aortic stenosis, aortic regurgitation, mitral stenosis, and mitral regurgitation and in some cases severe tricuspid regurgitation.

Aortic Stenosis

Generally, hemodynamically significant aortic stenosis (AS) is secondary to a primary valve problem (congenital bicuspid aortic valve) or from valve degeneration (calcific AS).[9,46,51,58] Patients referred for catheterization for evaluation of aortic stenosis generally have one of the following indications for the procedure: syncope, angina, or left ventricular dysfunction. The aortic valve area may decrease over time. The hemodynamic assessment of aortic stenosis in the catheterization laboratory is an important part of the overall evaluation of a patient with aortic stenosis. If done correctly, with attention to detail, it can define the hemodynamic stenosis and objectively help determine the timing for surgical repair.

To determine the significance of AS simultaneous measurements of pressure across the aortic valve must be performed. To best achieve this a catheter must be passed into the left ventricular cavity and this pressure compared with a simultaneous pressure measurement in the ascending aorta. Because it is difficult to place a long sheath at the level of the sinus of Valsalva to measure direct pressure differences from the LV to the ascending aorta, a catheter placed in the abdominal aorta and zeroed with a catheter placed in the ascending aorta will allow the determination of any pressure difference or augmentation for a "simultaneous" pressure recording from the LV and aorta.

Entering the left ventricle in a retrograde fashion can be quite challenging in some patients with AS. The deformities of the valve apparatus and calcific build-up may make "finding" the orifice of the aortic valve very difficult. It is usual to attempt to cross the aortic valve with the pigtail catheter in a retrograde fashion without the use of a wire. If this attempt fails then attempts with a straight wire extended from the tip of the pigtail catheter is used to "probe" the aortic valve while changing the orientation of the catheter to adjust the area probed by the wire and with gentle retraction of the catheter to adjust the anterior–posterior orientation of the wire. If the pigtail catheter does not provide an adequate orientation despite some of the maneuvers noted above then a Judkins right (JR4) or Amplatz left 1 (AL1) catheter, among others (Feldman), can then improve the orientation of the wire to eventually cross into the left ventricle.

Once the LV is entered, simultaneous pressures should be measured after being zeroed. These pressures then followed with a simultaneous cardiac output (either thermodilution or Fick) must be obtained. In our laboratory it is also routine to obtain a simultaneous PCWP tracing to evaluate the mitral valve at this time. Once the cardiac output is obtained the aortic valve may be calculated using the Gorlin equation.[27]

$$\text{Aortic valve area} = cm^2 = \frac{CO/(DFP \text{ or } SEP)(HR)}{C(\sqrt{\Delta P})}$$

where CO is cardiac output in ml/min, DFP/SEP is diastolic filling period or systolic ejection period, HR is heart rate in beats/min, C is an empirical constant (44.3 for aortic and tricuspid valves and 37.7 for the mitral valve), and P is the pressure gradient measured in mm Hg.

In the Gorlin equation, heart rate and systolic ejection periods are generally similar among most patients. Therefore, an alternative equation has been suggested called the Hakki formula.[31] Here the aortic valve area can be estimated by dividing the cardiac output in liters per minute by the square root of the peak-to-peak gradient.

$$\text{Valve area} = \frac{\text{cardiac output (liters/min)}}{\sqrt{\text{pressure gradient}}}$$

A severe valve area is considered when the valve area is under 1.0 cm² and is critical for valve areas under 0.7 cm². If aortic valve replacement is not an option for a particular patient given other comorbidities then an aortic valvuloplasty may be considered and is discussed elsewhere in this text. However, the long-term outcomes from aortic valve dilation are poor with recurrence being the rule and not the exception.

Aortic Regurgitation

Aortic regurgitation is the result of an incompetent aortic valve. This dynamic process allows blood to enter the left ventricular cavity in diastole in a retrograde fashion across the aortic valve. The consequences of the regurgitant fraction are an increased demand on the LV to maintain an adequate cardiac output in addition to the regurgitant volume. The magnitude of the regurgitant volume is dependent on the size of the orifice in the aortic valve and the pressure difference between the aorta and left ventricle in diastole. The principal causes of aortic regurgitation are primary disease of either the valve (rheumatic or endocarditis) or the aortic root (aneurysm, syphilis, ankylosing spondylitis).*

The clinical signs of chronic aortic regurgitation begin with a widened pulse pressure on noninvasive measurements. The patient with chronic aortic insufficiency (AI) will also have several clinical signs of their AI on physical examination: Quinckes pulses (nail bed capillary pulsations), Durrozier's sign (systolic murmur over the femoral artery when compressed proximally and diastolic murmur when compressed distally), Corrigan's pulse (water-hammer pulsation with early rise then collapse), the Austin-Flint murmur (early closure of the mitral valve from aortic regurgitation simulating mitral stenosis), or de Mussett's sign (head bobbing with each cardiac cycle).

The key for preoperative evaluation of patients with chronic aortic regurgitation is angiography for coronary artery disease and evaluation of the left ventricular function. If the patient is mildly symptomatic with any change in left ventricular function then there is consensus that an aortic valve replacement is warranted.[7,8,34] The key issue is to replace the valve before any irreversible changes to LV function occur.[8] In the catheterization laboratory the elements of a left heart catheterization with a right heart evaluation are necessary to fully define the function and anatomy of the heart.

Mitral Stenosis

Mitral stenosis is almost invariably a result of rheumatic fever. The fusion of the mitral apparatus is from the commissure, at the cusps, subvalvular at the cusps, or a combination of these.[7,12,32,68] In adults the normal valve area is between 4 and 6 cm². A valve area under 2 cm² is considered mild mitral stenosis and under 1 cm² is considered critical mitral stenosis. Given the hemodynamic results of chronic mitral stenosis, elevated pulmonary and capillary pressures, the typical feature of severe and critical mitral stenosis is dyspnea with exertion.

Determining the gradient across the mitral valve can be accomplished in one of two ways. First, there can be direct measurements of left atrial (LA) pressure through a transseptal

---

*References 8, 26, 34, 42, 43, 69, 71.

860 approach into the LA from the right atrium (RA). This is the most accurate method of determining the LA pressure compared with the left ventricular pressure. The most significant problem with this approach is the issue of performing a transseptal puncture with the inherent risks (aortic puncture, PA puncture). A more low-risk approach that has been validated is to obtain a confirmed PCWP through a right heart catheterization at the time of simultaneous LV tracings. With this method we can reliably evaluate the mitral valve and discern its hemodynamic significance of stenosis for valvuloplasty or surgical repair/replacement.

The procedure for hemodynamic assessment of mitral stenosis in the catheterization laboratory is generally to obtain access in both the femoral artery and vein. A right heart catheterization is performed with a confirmed PCWP obtained. Confirming the PCWP by "wedge" oxygen saturation confirms the pulmonary vein samples for the valve area cardiac output calculation. A pigtail catheter is placed into the left ventricular cavity and a simultaneous tracing of LV and PCWP is obtained. A gradient less than 5 mm Hg at the time of the catheterization may allow the Gorlin equation to have a significant error in the true valve area. As such the patient should have a hemodynamic stress, exercise, physical, or chemical, atrial pacing to increase the atrial gradient. Once the maximal gradient is confirmed, diastolic filling periods and the cardiac output obtained, the valve area can be calculated through the Gorlin equation. Likewise, as with aortic stenosis, the Hakki formula if calculated under adequate conditions of heart rate and cardiac output may approximate the mitral valve area by taking the cardiac output divided by the square root of the gradient.

Mitral Regurgitation

Mitral regurgitation (MR) may be the consequence of disruptions of the mitral leaflets, mitral annulus, or subvalvular apparatus to include the chordae or papillary musculature.[18,20,35,49] Generally, mitral leaflet abnormalities are from rheumatic processes, chronic mitral valve prolapse, or bacterial endocarditis. Other causes include systemic diseases such as systemic lupus erythematosus. When the mitral annulus becomes dilated, as a consequence of left ventricular dilation, the annulus may not allow a close coaptation of the mitral cusps and MR is the result. Further, if the annulus becomes calcified, the ability to constrict with ventricular constriction is impaired and thus MR is the result. Lastly, chordal and subchordal structures (papillary muscles) if congenitally short, long, or fibrotic may rupture; in addition, papillary dysfunction from ischemia or infarction may not allow the tethering of the valvular apparatus in systole, thus resulting in MR.

Ischemic MR is one special case of significant mitral regurgitation.[6,14,36] Recall that the posterior papillary musculature has a single blood supply (usually the left circumflex coronary artery). Thus with an acute coronary syndrome involving the marginal circulation of the LCX, potentially significant MR complicating congestive heart failure may result.

In the catheterization laboratory, significant mitral regurgitation is assessed with left ventriculography. In the right anterior oblique projection the left ventricle and left atrium are seen in profile; thus any MR can be assessed and quantified. Trace to mild MR (1+) appears but promptly clears before the next cardiac cycle. Mild to moderate MR (2+) appears and clears after the next cycle or does not opacify as darkly as the left ventricle. Moderate to severe MR (3+) appears and does not clear with subsequent cardiac cycles and is opacified as deeply as the left ventricle. Lastly, severe MR (4+) appears and does not clear with subsequent cardiac cycles and is opacified more deeply than the left ventricle.

The clinical indication for repair or replacement is based on hemodynamic assessment, left ventricular size, and other comorbidities (atrial fibrillation, etc).

Pericardial Disease

The pericardium forms a cavity held firmly in place with its attachments to the sternum, vertebral bodies, and the diaphragm, which holds the heart in place in the chest in different body positions. The pericardium consists of two layers: an inner layer (visceral) intimately associated with the surface of the heart and an outer layer (parietal) that is a continuation of the visceral pericardium as it reflects on itself. The parietal pericardium is fibrous and the visceral pericardium is smooth, made up of a single layer of mesothelial cells. Within this pericardial space there is usually about 50 ml of clear ultrafiltrate fluid that act principally as a lubricant to reduce any friction between the heart and its surrounding pericardium. There are various pathophysiological processes that affect the pericardium.[*]

For this discussion, we will assume that the reader is familiar with normal pericardial pressures and its impact on normal cardiac function. In essence, normal pericardial pressures are zero or negative such that they impart only a small effect to cardiac distending pressures. We will discuss two relevant pericardial abnormalities that are encountered in the catheterization laboratory: acute pericarditis and constrictive pericarditis.

Acute pericarditis is a syndrome caused by inflammation of the pericardium reflected by chest pain, possible pericardial friction rub, and ECG abnormalities. The causes of acute pericarditis usually are infectious, idiopathic, uremic, secondary to neoplasm, or trauma. Without doubt the principal reason for evaluating a patient in the catheterization laboratory following acute pericarditis is the presence of an effusion requiring pericardial drainage (Figure 53-8).

Various ECG signs of acute pericarditis and a pericardial effusion are ST abnormalities, usually diffuse elevation up to 1–2 mm, with PR segment depression. Also, given that the heart "swings" with each cardiac cycle within the fluid space of the effusion, "electrical alternans" is very often seen. Pericardial effusion once suspected is readily detected with echocardiography. Clinical signs of a significant pericardial effusion are noted on the physical examination. The consequence of a large pericardial effusion is tamponade. In tamponade an increase in intrapericardial pressure within the pericardial space causes an elevation of intracardiac pressures (equalization of pressures), abnormalities of the jugular venous pressures, progressive limitation of ventricular diastolic filling, and ultimately a reduction of stroke volume and cardiac output. Given this constellation of hemodynamic effects the clinical findings of a patient in impending or fulminant tamponade are characterized by tachycardia,

---

[*]References 2, 25, 44, 53, 67, 72.

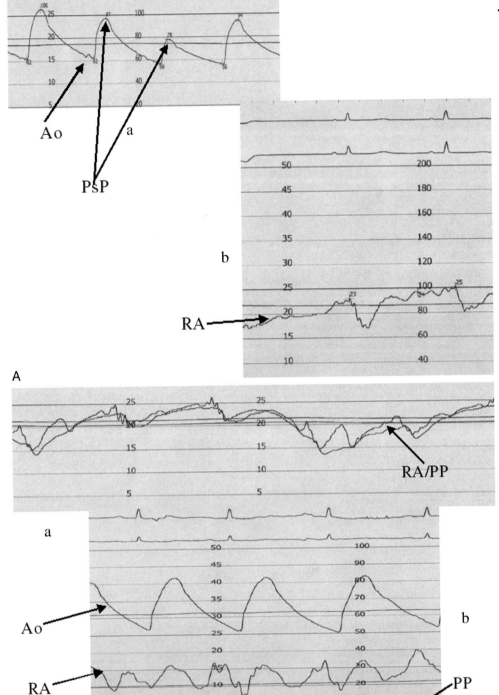

Figure 53–8 A, Hemodynamics of tamponade. (a) Aortic pressure. Arrows indicate "pulsus paradoxus" of over 20 mm Hg. (b) RA pressure prepericardiocentesis. Ao, central aortic pressure; PsP, pulsus paradoxus; RA, right atrium. **B,** (a) Pericardial and right atrial pressure prepericardiocentesis and drainage. Note the "tracking" of the RA with the PP. (b) Hemodynamics of aorta, right atrium, and pericardial space following evacuation of 400 ml of fluid. Note the loss of significant pulsus, the separation of the pericardial and right atrial pressure tracings. RA, right atrium; PP, pericardial pressure; Ao, central aortic pressure.

a large pulsus paradoxus, and abnormalities of the jugular venous pulsations. If clinical signs or echocardiographic findings indicate tamponade physiology, a pericardial drain should be placed.

In the catheterization laboratory, access to the pericardial space is usually from just left of the subxiphoid, with the needle directed toward the patient's left shoulder. In our laboratory it is our practice to begin with a right heart catheterization to PCWP then return the catheter to the right atrium and access an arterial system (usually the femoral artery). Right atrial (central venous) pressures reveal blunted *x* and prominent *y* descents. It has then been our practice to enter the pericardial space with an "alligator" clip attached to the needle to allow us to see if we come in

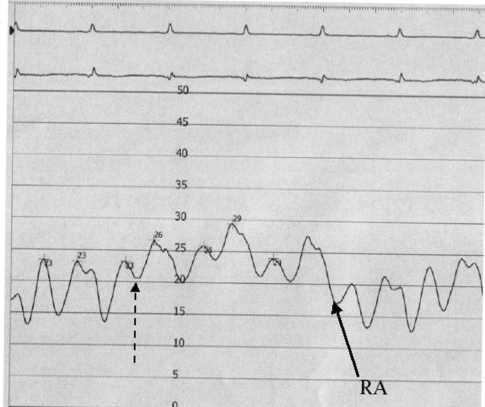

Figure 53–9 Right atrial pressure tracing in constrictive pericarditis with evident "Kussmaul's sign" during inspiration. RA, right atrium. Dashed arrow indicates inspiration.

contact with the epicardium (an injury current ST elevation will be seen). Once entered the needle is transduced with and compared to a catheter in the right atrium. If tamponade is present the pressures should be similar and track each other. At this time two quick syringes are aspirated to the various studies needed for effusion (various electrolytes and cultures). Once the pericardial space has been entered a "J" tipped wire is advanced into the space. Over this wire a dilator is advanced and ultimately a drain is placed. Aspiration of the effusion follows with intermittent hemodynamic assessments. As the effusion is drained the pericardial pressure should return to 0 or negative with a resultant decline in right atrial pressure. The drain should be left in place until the drainage falls below 30 ml for 24 h.

Specific forms of pericarditis include viral, tuberculous, bacterial, fungal, post-acute myocardial infarction, uremic, neoplastic, and radiation.

Constrictive pericarditis is usually a uniform scarring of the pericardium causing restriction of diastolic filling of the heart. The constriction usually follows acute pericarditis. After the initial event there is fibrin deposition and scarring of the pericardium, ultimately leading to the uniform restriction of diastolic filling.

The hemodynamics of constrictive pericarditis are that as the uniform scarring impairs cardiac filling there is an elevation and equalization of the diastolic pressure in all four cardiac chambers. The central venous pressures show prominent x and y descents appearing as a "**W**" waveform. Moreover, the right and left ventricular tracings will reveal diastolic equalization with the classic "dip and plateau" of ventricular filling. There is rapid ventricular fill-

ing in early diastole, hence the "dip" and slow to negligible filling in late diastole, and hence the "plateau" of ventricular filling. It is important to remember that if ventricular filling is low, such as in hypovolemia, the classic patterns may not be seen or missed. Therefore in our laboratory we recommend a volume load to raise the RA pressure to fully rule in or out the prospect of constrictive pericarditis. Another hemodynamic effect of a uniform constriction to cardiac filling is the lack of transmitted intrathoracic pressures to the pericardium and heart chambers. Thus, in constrictive pericarditis with inspiration, systemic venous and right atrial pressures do not fall and may actually increase,[45] which is known as "Kussmaul's sign" (Figure 53-9).

REFERENCES

1. AHA reference Brock R, Milstein BB, Ross DN: Percutaneous left ventricular puncture in the assessment of aortic stenosis. Thorax 11:163–169, 1956.
2. Aikat S, Ghaffari S. A review of pericardial diseases: clinical, ECG and hemodynamic features and management. Clev Clin J Med 67:903–914, 2000.
3. Alpert JS. The lessons of history as reflected in the pulmonary capillary wedge pressure. J Am Coll Cardiol 13: 830–831, 1989.
4. Angelini P. Normal and anomalous coronary arteries: definitions and classification. Am Heart J 117:418–434, 1989.
5. Barry WH, Levin DC, Green LH, et al: Left heart catheterization and angiography via the percutaneous femoral approach using an arterial sheath. Cathet Cardiovasc Diagn 5:401–409, 1979.

6. Birnbaum Y, Chamoun AJ, Conti VR, Uretsky BF: Mitral regurgitation following acute myocardial infarction. Coron Artery Dis 13:337–344, 2002.

7. Boon NA, Bloomfield P: The medical management of valvular heart disease. Heart 87:395–400, 2002.

8. Borer JS, Herrold EM, Hochreiter Ca, et al: Aortic regurgitation: selection of asymptomatic patients for valve surgery. Adv Cardiol 39:74–85, 2002.

9. Braunwald E, Goldblatt A, Aygen MM et al: Congenital aortic stenosis: clinical and hemodynamic findings in 100 patients. Circulation 27:426–433, 1963.

10. Braunwald E, Swan HJC, Gorlin R, McIntosh HD: Cooperative study on cardiac catheterization. Circulation 37(suppl):III93–101, 1968.

11. Brock R, Milstein BB, Ross DN: Percutaneous left ventricular puncture in the assessment of aortic stenosis. Thorax 11:163–169, 1956.

12. Bruce CJ, Nishimura RA: Clinical assessment and management of mitral stenosis. Cardiol Clin 16: 375–403, 1998.

13. Campeau L: Percutaneous radial artery approach for coronary angiography. Cathet Cardiovasc Diagn 16:3–7, 1989.

14. Cohn LH: Mitral valve repair for ischemic mitral regurgitation. Adv Cardiol 39:153–156, 2002.

15. Davies RF, Goldberg AD, Forman S, et al: Asymptomatic cardiac ischemia pilot (ACIP) study two-year follow-up; outcomes of patients randomized to initial strategies of medical therapy versus revascularization. Circulation 95: 2037–2043, 1997.

16. Dexter L, et al: Studies of congenital heart disease. II. The pressure and oxygen content of blood in the right auricle, right ventricle and pulmonary artery in control patients, with observations on the oxygen saturation and source of pulmonary capillary blood. J Clin Invest 26:554–558, 1947.

17. Dexter L, Whittenberger JL, Haynes FW, et al: Effect of exercise on circulatory dynamics of normal individuals. J Appl Physiol 3:439, 1951.

18. Enriquez-Saranao M, Orszulak TA, Schaff HV, et al: Mitral regurgitation: a new clinical perspective. Mayo Clin Proc 71: 1034–1043, 1997.

19. Fegler G: Measurement of cardiac output in anesthetized animals by a thermodilution method. Q J Exp Physiol 39:153, 1954.

20. Fenster MS, Feldman MD: Mitral regurgitation: an overview. Curr Probl Cardiol 20:193–280, 1995.

21. Fergusson DJG, Kamada RO. Percutaneous entry of the brachial artery for left heart catheterization using a sheath: further experience. Cathet Cardiovasc Diagn 12:209–211, 1986.

22. Fick A: Uber die Messung des Blutquantums in den Herzventrikeln. Sitz der Physik-Med ges Wurtzberg 1870.

23. Flamm MD, Cohn KE, Hancock EW: Measurement of systemic cardiac output at rest and exercise in patients with atrial septal defect. Am J Cardiol 23:258–265, 1969.

24. Forsmann W: Die Sondierung des rechten Herzens. Klin Wochenschr 8:2085, 1929.

25. Fowler NO: Pericardial disease. Heart Dis Stroke 1:85–94, 1992.

26. Giardi LN: Surgical approaches when arotic regurgitation is associated with aortic root disease. Adv Cardiol 39:86–92, 2002.

27. Gorlin R, Gorlin SG: Hydraulic formula for calculation of area of stenotic mitral valve, other cardiac values and central circulatory shunts. Am Heart J 41:1–29, 1951.

28. Gruentzig AR: Perkutane Dilatation von Coronarstenosen-Beschreibung eines neuen Kathetersystems. Klin Wochenschr 54:543, 1976.

29. Gruentzig AR, Turina MI, Schneider JA: Experimental percutaneous dilatation of coronary artery stenosis. Circulation 54:81, 1976.

30. Guyton AC, Jones EC, Coleman TG: In Circulatory Physiology: Cardiac Output and Its Regulation. Philadelphia: W. B. Saunders, 1973, p. 4.

31. Hakki AH, Iskandrian AS, Bemis CE, et al: A simplified valve formula for the calculation of stenotic cardiac valve areas. Circulation 63:1050–1055, 1981.

32. Hasegawa R, Kitahara H, Watanabe K, et al: Mitral stenosis and regurgitation with systemic lupus erythematosus and antiphospholipid antibody syndrome. Jpn J Thorac Cardiovasc Surg 49:711–713, 2001.

33. Hillis LD: Percutaneous left heart catheterization and coronary arteriography using a femoral artery sheath. Cathet Cardiovasc Diagn 5:393–399, 1979.

34. Hoit BD: Medical treatment of valvular heart disease. Curr Opin Cardiol 6:207–211, 1991.

35. Irving T, Li XK, Sahn DJ, Kenny A: Assessment of mitral regurgitation. Heart 88:iv11–19, 2002.

36. Iung B: Management of ischaemic mitral regurgitation. Heart 89:459–464, 2003.

37. Judkins MP, Kidd HJ, Frische LH, Dotter CT: Lumen-following safety J-guide for catheterization of rotuous vessels. Radiology 88:1127–1130, 1967.

38. Kadir S. Regional anatomy of the thoracic aorta. In Kadir S. editor: Atlas of Normal and Variant Angiographic Anatomy. Philadelphia: W. B. Saunders, 1991, p. 19.

39. Kuntz RE, Baim DS: Internal mammary angiography: A review of technical issues and newer methods. Cathet Cardiovasc Diagn 20:10–16, 1990.

40. Lange RA, Dehmer GJ, Wells PJ, et al: Limitations of the metabolic rate meter for measuring oxygen consumption and cardiac output. Am J Cardiol 64:783–786, 1989.

41. Lange RA, Moore DM, Cigarroa RG, Hillis LD: Use of pulmonary capillary wedge pressure to assess severity of mitral stenosis: is true left atrial pressure needed in this condition? J Am Coll Cardiol 13:825–831, 1989.

42. Lauterman D, Braun J: Ankylosing spondylitis—cardiac manifestations. Clin Exp Rheumatol 20:S11–115, 2002.

43. Levine AJ, Dimitri WR, Bonser RS: Aortic regurgitation in rheumatoid arthritis necessitating aortic valve replacement. Eur J Cardiothorac Surg 15:213–214, 1999.

44. Maisch B: Pericardial diseases, with a focus on etiology, pathogenesis, pathophysiology, new diagnostic imaging methods and treatment. Current Opin Cardiol 9:379–388, 1994.

45. Meyer TE, Sareli P, Marcus RH, et al: Mechanism underlying Kussmaul's sign in chronic constrictive pericarditis. Am J Cardiol 64:1069–1072, 1989.

46. Moller JH, Nakib A, Elliott RS, Edwards JE: Symptomatic congenital aortic stenosis in the first year of life. J Pediatr 67:728–734, 1966.

47. Nguyen T, Saito S, Grines C: Vascular access. J Interv Cardiol 15:163–166, 2002.

48. Nishimura RA, Rihal CS, Tajik AJ, Jolmes DR Jr: Accurate measurement of the transmitral gradient in patients with mitral stenosis: a simultaneous catheterization and Doppler echocardiographic study. J Am Coll Cardiol 24:152–158, 1994.

49. Otto CM. Timing of surgery in mitral regurgitation. Heart 89: 100–105, 2003.

50. Rapp AH, Hillis LD: Clinical consequences of anomalous coronary arteries. Coron Artery Dis 12:617–620, 2001.

51. Roberts WC: Valvular, subvalvular and supravalvular aortic stenosis. Morphologic features. Cardiovasc Clin 5:97–126, 1973.

52. Roberts WC, Kragel AH: Anomalous origin of either the right of left main coronary artery from the aorta without coursing of the anomalistically arising artery between aorta and pulmonary trunk. Am J Cardiol 62:1263–1267, 1988.

53. Roberts WC, Spray TL: Pericardial heart disease. Curr Probl Cardiol 2:1–71, 1977.

864

54. Roberts WC, Siegel RJ, Zipes DP: Origin of the RCA from the left sinus of Valsalva and its functional consequences: analysis of 10 necropsy patients. Am J Card 49:863–868, 1982.

55. Ross J, Brandenburg RO, Dinsmore RE, et al: Guidelines for coronary angiography, a report from the ACC/AHA Task Froce on assessment and diagnostic and therapeutic cardiovascular procedures. Subcommittee on Coronary Angiography. J Am Coll Cardiol 10:935–950, 1987.

56. Safi AM, Rachko M, Tang A, et al: Anomalous origin of the left main coronary artery from the right sinus of Valsalva: disabling angina and syncope with noninterarterial courses: case report of two patients. Heart Dis 3:24–27, 2001.

57. Seldinger SI: Catheter replacement of the needle in percutaneous arteriography, a new technique. Acta Radiol 39: 368, 1953.

58. Selzer A: Changing aspects of the natural history of valvular aortic stenosis. N Engl J Med 317:91–98, 1987.

59. Semple T, McGuiness JB, Gardner H: Left heart catheterization by direct ventricular puncture. Br Heart J 30: 402–406, 1968.

60. Serota H, Barth CW, Seuc CA, et al: Rapdi identification of the course of anomalous coronary arteries in adults: the "dot and eye" method. Am J Cardiol 65:891–898, 1990.

61. Sones FM Jr, Shirey EK: Cine coronary anteriography. Mod Concepts Cardiovasc Dis 31:735–738, 1962.

62. Sones FM Jr, Shirey EK, Proudfit WL, Wescott RN: Cine coronary arteriography. Circulation 20:773, 1959.

63. Stewart GN: Researches on the circulation time and on the influences which affect it: IV. The output of the heart. J Physiol 1897.

64. Swan HJC, Ganz W, Forrester J, et al: Catheterization of the heart in man with use of a flow directed balloon tipped catheter. N Engl J Med 283:447–451, 1970.

65. The TIMI IIIB Investigators: Effects of tissue plasminogen activator and a comparison of early invasive and conservative strategies in unstable angina and non-Q wave myocardial infarction: Results of the TIMI IIIB trial (Thrombolysis in Myocardial Ischemia). Circulation 89:1545–1556, 1994.

66. van Miltenburg-van Zijl AJM, Simoons ML, Veerhoek RJ, Bossuyt PMM: Incidence and follow-up of Braunwald subgroups in unstable angina pectoris. J Am Coll Cardiol 25:1286–1292, 1995.

67. Vasquez A, Butman SM: Pathophysiologic mechanisms in pericardial disease. Curr Cardiol Rep 4:26–32, 2002.

68. Waller BF: Rheumatic and nonrheumatic conditions producing valvular heart diseases. In Frankl WS, Brest AN editors: Cardiovascular Clinics. Valvular Heart Disease: Comprehensive Evaluation and Management. Philadelphia: F. A. Davis, 1986, pp. 3–104.

69. Ward C: Clinical significance of the bicuspid aortic valve. Heart 83:81–85, 2000.

70. Yamanaka O, Hobbs RE: Coronary artery anomalies in 126,595 patients undergoing coronary arteriography. Cathet Cardiovasc Diagn 21:28–40, 1990.

71. Yener N, Oktar GL, Erer D, et al: Bicuspid aortic valve. Ann Throac Cardiovasc Surg 8:264–267, 2002.

72. Zhang S, Kerins DM, Byrd BF 3rd: Doppler echocardiolgraphy in cardiac tamponade and constrictive pericarditis. Echocardiography 11:507–521, 1994.

Applications of Computed Tomography in Cardiovascular Disease

William Stanford

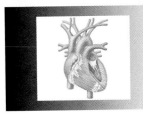

INTRODUCTION

With the technological explosion of computed tomography (CT) in the past few years, imaging of the heart and great vessels has dramatically changed. Less often is there dependence upon the plain film and interventional procedures and more often there is dependence on CT and magnetic resonance (MR) and especially CT angiographic (CTA) and MR angiographic (MRA) techniques. CT images, which initially took over 4 min to generate can now be generated in 500 ms with helical imaging and 50–100 ms with electron beam imaging. Since these improvements in temporal resolution are fast enough to essentially stop the heart, visualization of small structures such as calcium deposits within the coronary arteries is now possible. Not only has the temporal resolution increased but also the spatial resolution and now isotropic voxels of $0.5 \times 0.5 \times 0.5$ mm are obtainable. These advances, along with the increasing use of three-dimensional (3D) reconstruction, have revolutionized cardiovascular imaging. In addition, the ability to obtain these rapid temporal resolutions has moved CT from only anatomical visualization into the arena of functional and perfusion imaging. This chapter will review current applications of CT in imaging the heart and great vessels.

HISTORICAL ASPECTS

CT was first reported by Sir Godfrey Houndsfield in 1970. Houndsfield was an electrical engineer working for EMI, an electronics firm in England. While there, he conceived the idea of taking cross-sectional X-ray data and reformatting the data into images. For this, he and Alan M. Comack, a Tufts professor of mathematics, working independently, received the Nobel Prize in medicine in 1979.

The first images produced by Hounsfield were very crude and took 4.5 min to generate. With the technological advances of rotating X-ray tubes and solid state detector rings, image times rapidly decreased and by 1978, 2-s images with excellent resolution became the norm.

In the early 1980's, another important advance moved CT into the realm of cardiac imaging. This was the introduction of electron beam technology by Dr. Douglas Boyd of the University of California, San Francisco.[6] The electron beam scanner, while having an appearance similar to a conventional CT scanner, does not have an X-ray tube rotating around the patient. Instead, electrons are generated by a source and then bent electromagnetically to sweep tungsten target rings

866 located in the gantry beneath the patient. The X-rays produced by the electron sweep traverse the patient and are collected by solid-state detectors located in the gantry above the patient (Figure 54-1). This technology dramatically decreased scan times to 50–100 ms and essentially froze cardiac motion and for the first time made it possible to image cardiac contraction and to visualize small structures such as plaques within the walls of the coronary arteries.

A third major advance in CT imaging came in the early 1990s with the introduction of helical/spiral CT (HCT) with its slip ring technology. With this technology, the X-ray tube continuously rotates around the patient as the patient moves through the scanner gantry. These advances decreased scan times to 500 ms while producing volumetric data sets with spatial resolutions as small as 0.5 mm³. Further advances in HCT technology have now increased imaging platforms from a single detector to 4-row and now 16-row and in the future 32-row and 64-row detectors are expected. These advances have also shortened imaging time so that the entire heart can be scanned in a 20–30 s breath-hold.

SCANNER CHARACTERISTICS

Conventional CT

The design of conventional CT scanners is to rotate an X-ray source around the patient while continuously generating data that are collected by fixed detectors in the surrounding scanner gantry. The tube movement is limited by cables so that once the tube rotates around the patient, it has to stop and rewind. This constrained tube travel is a major limitation of conventional CT; however, the cross-sectional image detail is excellent and spatial detail of 9–12 line pairs (lp)/cm is possible.

Helical CT

Current generation HCT scanners have 4–16 detector rings; however, scanners should soon be available with 32–64 detector rings. With HCT technology, scan times have decreased from 2 s to 400 ms and now with partial reconstruction algorithms, scan times as low as 125 ms are possible. An additional advantage of the helical technology is that data are generated as a volumetric data set, and this permits later reformations of different slice thicknesses that are suitable for 3D reconstructions. Helical CT images are frequently ECG gated, and this further decreases motion artifact by allowing imaging during the quiet phase of the cardiac cycle. The latter is especially important in coronary calcification screening.

Electron Beam CT

The electron beam CT scanners (EBT) (GE-Imatron Inc., South San Francisco, CA) appear similar to conventional CT scanners but operate on a different principle. With this technology, electrons are generated and bent electromagnetically to sweep tungsten target rings that are located in the gantry beneath the patient. The X-rays generated from the tungsten target rings pass through the patient and onto solid-state detectors positioned in the gantry above the patient. Because there are no moving parts other than the patient table, images with temporal resolutions of 50–100 ms are possible and this becomes extremely important in cardiac imaging.

There are several EBT sequences that are used to image the heart. In the flow mode sequence eight 8-mm slices can be generated in 224 ms. It then takes 8 ms for the scanner to reset and then an additional eight 8-mm slices can be obtained in another 224 ms. The advantage of this sequence is that images can be generated sequentially and this allows the visualization of a contrast bolus as it enters, peaks, and washes out of a region of interest. This sequence is similar to the first pass images in nuclear medicine.

The second sequence is the movie (cine) sequence. In this sequence, images of the contracting heart are generated every 58 ms (17 images a second). These images can be acquired in systole and diastole and this allows visualization of cardiac contraction (Figure 54-2). The sequence, usually

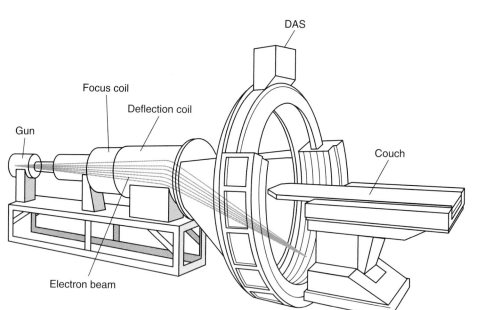

Figure 54–1 Diagram of the Imatron C-150 EBT scanner. The scanner uses a focused electron beam that sweeps across a tungsten target ring in 50 or 100 ms. There are four target rings, and each target can generate up to two fan beam images. In the flow mode there is an 8-ms lag to reset the electron beam. Consequently, eight transverse sections can be scanned in 244 ms. (*Courtesy of GE-Imatron Inc., South San Francisco, CA.*)

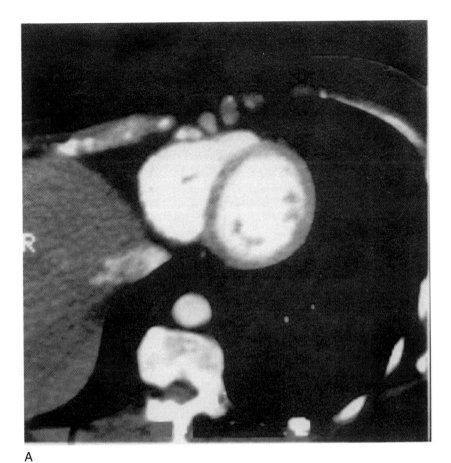

A

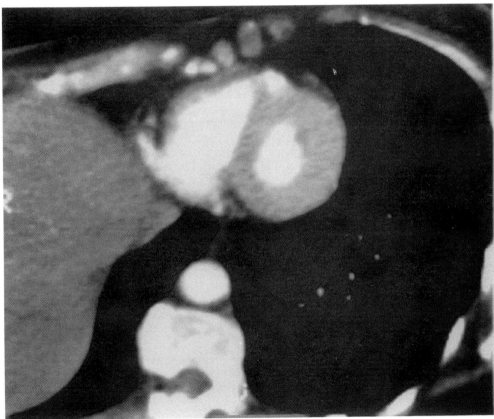

B

Figure 54–2 **Movie mode EBT images at the mid-left ventricular level.** The images show the ventricle in diastole (**A**) and in systole (**B**).

868 consisting of 10–12 same-level images, is triggered off the R wave of the ECG. Once completed, it then takes 8 ms for the scanner to reset and another data set at the same or usually a different level can be obtained. This cine sequence allows for 8–12 slices of up to 12 images per slice to be taken during cardiac contraction and thus imaging throughout diastole and systole is possible. The spatial resolution in the flow and movie modes is moderate at 4.5 lp/cm.

Lastly, in the step volume scan (SVS) and continuous volume scan (CVS) sequences 1.5-, 3-, or 6-mm single-slice thicknesses are possible. The temporal resolution is 100 ms, which equates to nine images per second and the pixel size can vary from 0.06 to 1 mm². A maximal resolution of 9.5 lp/cm is possible, dependent upon the field of view and the reconstructive algorithm selected. The SVS images are acquired in a manner similar to that of conventional CT scanners, i.e., a single target ring is swept to produce an image and then the table moves and a second image is generated. Multiple sweeps of the same target can be taken and volume averaged if additional resolution is required; however, this comes at the price of increased radiation exposure. The CVS mode is similar to spiral or helical CT scanning with up to 140 images on the C-150 and up to 280 images on the C-300 scanner possible during an acquisition period of up to 33 s. The minimal exposure time is 100 ms and the images can be contiguous or overlapped. This mode allows a complete 140-slice, 3-mm-thick data set to be acquired during a single breathhold. Scan widths of 1.5–10 mm are possible.

► ADVANTAGES OF CT

The main advantage of CT imaging is that cross-sectional images are generated. The images have excellent temporal and spatial resolution; however, because some organs such as the heart do not lie in conventional imaging planes, true short and longitudinal axis anatomical images may not be possible without reformatting. For the problem to be eliminated, some scanner couches and/or gantries can be tilted to position the heart into a more appropriate scanning plane. Generally, cardiac images are acquired in a short axis plane similar to "bread loafing" or in a longitudinal axis projection similar to the four chamber view of echocardiography. Because of the excellent resolution of CT, imaging of structures as small as 0.5 mm is possible. Additionally, tissues with different CT attenuations such as fat, myocardium, and calcium can be readily identified. An example is in imaging of the pericardium where the low attenuation epicardial and mediastinal fat lies adjacent to the higher attenuated fibrous pericardium. At times, the addition of contrast material allows further definition of the myocardium and functional imaging of the heart is possible if the movie mode sequence is selected.

EBT and helical scanner technology allows for the entire heart to be imaged within a single breathhold. Because the HCT images are acquired contiguously in a volumetric data set, later reformation is possible.

► DISADVANTAGES OF CT

The disadvantages of CT are the still somewhat long scan times, which, unfortunately, do not completely eliminate cardiac motion. Other disadvantages inherent in all scanners are that they are stationary and the patient has to be transported to the scanner and be subjected to radiation. Also, contrast administration is often necessary.

► CONTRAST CONSIDERATIONS

In cardiac imaging, it is important that contrast be administered for many of the studies. Contrast can be given as a bolus or as a continuous infusion, but because of the speed of the scanners, contrast and arrival times become critical. Commonly, volumes of 80–150 ml of contrast material varying from 240 to 370 mg of iodine/ml are administered. The contrast material is generally infused at a rate of 1–4 ml/s using a power injector.

Because of the importance of optimizing the contrast bolus, several timing methodologies are available. One is to administer a test bolus of 10 ml of contrast material and do repeated imaging over the area of interest to determine contrast arrival time. Another is to do a circulation time using either cardiogreen dye or a solution of 0.5% magnesium sulfate. All are injected at 4 ml/s. With magnesium sulfate, approximately 10 ml of a 0.5% solution is generally administered with the bolus arrival manifested by a warm sensation in the back of the tongue or throat. With cardiogreen dye an earlobe densitometer records the arrival of the cardiogreen dye bolus. Other techniques are the "sure start" technologies where the scanner monitors the rise in contrast attenuation over the area of interest. When the attenuation approaches the preselected threshold, the scanner is triggered automatically. Alternately, a fixed delay of 15–30 s may be used.

► POSITIONAL AND PATIENT CONSIDERATIONS

With all CT scanners, there remains the necessity for individuals to be transported to the scanner. Although it is important that the patient remain quiet and suspend respiration, it is often still possible with EBT and HCT scanners to obtain satisfactory images, even if the individual is unable to hold his or her breath.

► RADIATION DOSAGE

The effective dose is the overall radiation exposure to the patient. This is designated in millisieverts (mSv) and is frequently equated to months of background exposure. The effective dose for a chest sequence using a multislice helical CT is approximately 5.1 mSv in males and 8.1 mSv in females. For an EBT chest study, the exposure would be 5.2 mSv in males and 7.6 mSv in females. For a 50-ms cardiac cine sequence, the exposure would be 0.58 mSv per image and for a 10-image sequence this would give an exposure of 5.8 mSv. One additional advantage of the electron beam technology is that the radiation beam enters from beneath the patient, and therefore there is less exposure to breast and thyroid tissue.

For a multislice HCT prospectively triggered coronary calcification study, the effective male/female dose would be 2.9/3.6 mSv (12 and 14 months of background radiation) and for an EBT calcium study, the effective dose would be

1.0/1.4 mSv (4 and 6 months of background radiation). If a multislice HCT coronary calcium study was retrospectively triggered, this would increase the radiation exposure to 5.2/6.4 mSv, which would equate to 21 and 26 months of background radiation and if a CT angiographic study were done using retrospective gating, the radiation dose could reach as high as 10.9/13.0 mSv.[9,13] However, tube current modulation techniques have now been introduced that can ramp down the power of the scanner during noncritical times, and this can significantly decrease the radiation exposure.

CARDIAC ANATOMY

The axial images produced by CT can precisely define the cross-sectional anatomy of the great vessels, atria, and ventricles. A further advantage is that the images are displayed without the superimposition of overlying structures, and this allows calcifications, fluid collections, and myocardium and pericardium to be readily identified.

Although conventional CT, helical CT, and electron beam CT are able to identify cardiac anatomy, motion artifact can remain a problem. With contrast enhancement, conventional CT can visualize cardiac chambers and great vessel anatomy extremely well; however, HCT and EBT, because of their faster scan times, are better suited for imaging moving structures. In a typical cardiac sequence the superior vena cava, pulmonary arteries, and aorta are routinely visualized as are the right and left atria and ventricles, plus ventricular outflow tracts. With CT the interface between the contrast-enhanced cardiac chambers and myocardium is usually well defined, especially if the image is acquired during diastole; in systole, this interface may be partially degraded by motion. Overall, both HCT and EBT, because of their faster scan times, generally better define structural detail.

CHAMBER SIZE

Cardiac chamber size has been extensively evaluated by EBT. Comparisons have included radiopaque casts as well as volumetric comparisons from cardiac catheterization and echo data. Overall, these studies have confirmed that the volumes of all cardiac chambers can be accurately assessed within 2–5% of the cast volumes over a broad range.[19,20] Although there are few data to support the accuracy of HCT, similar accuracies would be expected.

CARDIAC FUNCTION

Studies in dogs involving chronically implanted aortic flow meters as well as thermodilution catheters have demonstrated that with EBT the stroke volumes (SV) of the left ventricle (LV) and right ventricle (RV) can be assessed with a high degree of accuracy over a reasonably broad range. Measurements have included, in addition to the stroke volume, the regurgitant volume, mass, and ejection fraction. With suspended respiration, the right and left ventricular stroke volumes have been shown to be virtually identical; therefore, any differences between the RV SV and the LV SV reflect the extent of valvular regurgitation.[21]

LV mass can also be measured with a high degree of accuracy using EBT.[10] Right ventricular mass is more difficult to assess because of its thinness, but if high-resolution 3-mm slice thicknesses are acquired, the correlations are very good.[12] In addition, the EBT scanner cine sequence has shown high accuracy in assessing regional and segmental ventricular wall motion.[11] In normal subjects, there is commonly heterogeneity of LV wall motion with the basal segments having a lower ejection fraction than the average of the entire ventricle. With altered loading conditions, this heterogeneity can be significantly reduced. In general, increases in stress result in a more homogeneous contraction pattern.

Also, the qualitative assessment of wall motion is very important. This is particularly true in patients with aneurysms or localized infarcts where there are often hypokinetic or akinetic areas of ventricular contraction. This is also true in individuals with cardiomyopathies in which there can be either a poor or very vigorous ventricular contraction. At the present time, helical CT, although very accurate in assessing cardiac function, is just starting to be used clinically in the measurement of ventricular function.[14,16]

INTRACARDIAC MASSES

Ventricular Thrombi

Ventricular thrombi present as filling defects within the opacified cardiac chambers and as such are relatively easy to identify on CT.[29] The thrombi may be sessile, convex, or pedunculated and at times calcified. They are often found in association with abnormalities of wall motion, especially in individuals with prior myocardial infarction or in individuals with an otherwise poorly contractile myocardium. In these instances, a filling defect adjacent to the akinetic area is very suggestive of a thrombus. Inferior wall thrombi are best visualized on short axis projections whereas apical thrombi are best seen on long axis projections (Figure 54-3). Although filling defects within the cardiac chambers are generally visualized on all scanners, the assessment of wall motion is possible only on the electron beam and the newer HCT scanners.

Left Atrial Thrombi

Left atrial thrombi also present as filling defects and are often present in patients where there is stagnation of blood flow within the left atrium, such as in mitral stenosis and/or atrial fibrillation. The left atrial appendage is a frequent site for the development of thrombi, and since CT shows the appendage in cross section, it often provides better information than transthoracic echocardiography (Figure 54-4). With transesophageal echocardiography thrombi within the left atrium are commonly identified, but there have been a number of instances in which transesophageal echocardiography has missed left atrial appendage thrombi.

CARDIAC TUMORS

Cardiac tumors also present as filling defects and their appearance is often characteristic (Figure 54-5). Left atrial

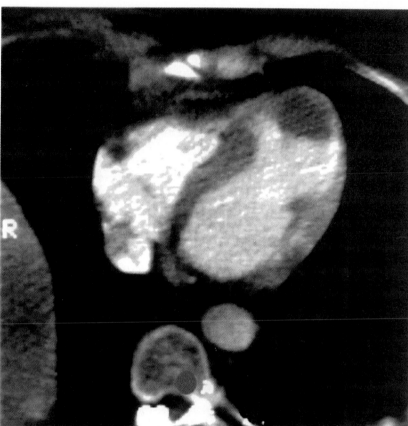

Figure 54–3 EBT study in a 58-year-old man showing a thrombus as a filling defect in an apical left ventricular aneurysm.

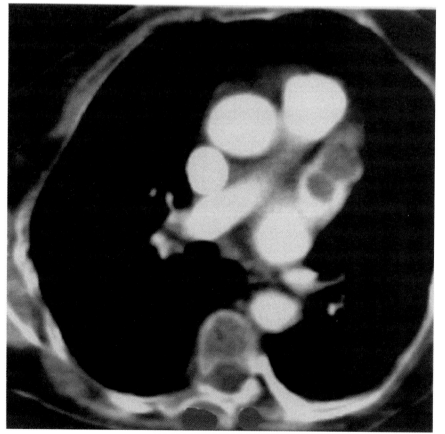

Figure 54–4 Atrial fibrillation in a 77-year-old woman. The examination was requested to rule out left atrial thrombus; the two-dimensional echocardiographic examination was negative. The EBT study shows a large dumbbell-shaped thrombus within the left atrial appendage.

myxoma is the most common cardiac tumor and these can vary greatly in size; however, the presence of a stalk that allows the tumor to move during ventricular contraction is helpful in their identification. Because these tumors can move back and forth between the ventricle and atrium, they can obstruct the mitral valve orifice and therefore result in a clinical presentation similar to mitral stenosis. Tumors lying within the myocardial wall often have calcifications and thus are readily identifiable on all CT scanners.

ISCHEMIC DISEASE

Cardiovascular ischemic disease is a major socioeconomic problem. In 1999, coronary artery disease affected more than 5.6 million Americans, and its economic impact was in excess of $326 billion dollars.[3] Thus, imaging methodologies to identify individuals with ischemic heart disease are of great importance.

CORONARY ARTERY DISEASE

The identification of coronary artery calcification as an indicator of the coronary atherosclerotic burden is becoming increasingly important. Both EBT and HCT are the major imaging modalities for evaluating coronary artery calcification (Figure 54-6). Along with the identification of calcium,

CTA can additionally evaluate associated stenosis and non-calcified plaque, and their identification now constitutes two of the major applications of helical and electron beam CT imaging.

CORONARY ARTERY CALCIFICATION

Coronary artery calcification is an accepted marker for atherosclerotic disease. Calcium forms early in the development of the atherosclerotic plaque, and frequently it can be seen before the lumen narrows sufficiently to be identified on cardiac catheterization or radionuclide studies. Thus, calcification can serve as an indicator of overall atherosclerotic plaque burden. In fact, Rumberger et al reported that the extent of calcification as determined by EBT scanning represents about one fifth of the total plaque volume.[22] With EBT, calcium score sensitivities of 92% and specificities of 51% as an indicator of significant (>75%) coronary artery stenoses have been reported.[17]

Helical CT also has a major application in evaluating coronary calcification and several studies have shown correlations of 0.97–0.98 as compared with EBT.[5,7] The differences between HCT and EBT appear more pronounced in individuals with calcium scores less than 10, but above scores of 10, the correlations may vary by less than 10%.[22] Calcification has also been shown to be important in identifying individuals at increased risk for coronary events. In

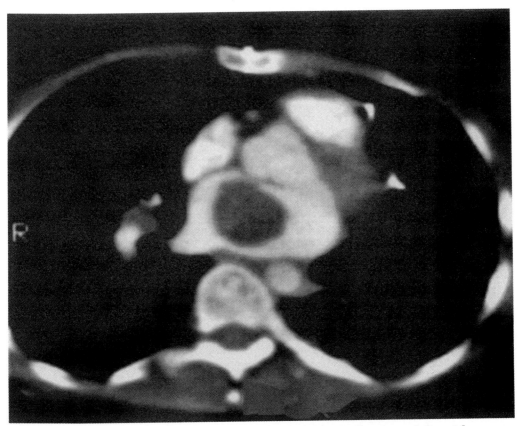

Figure 54–5 Short axis EBT study in a 33-year-old woman showing a left atrial myxoma presenting as a filling defect in the contrast-enhanced left atrium.

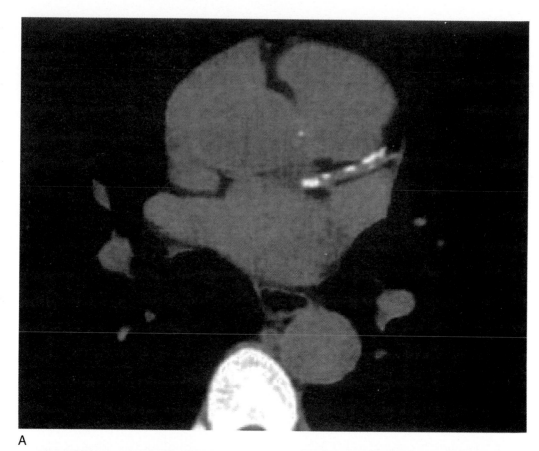

A

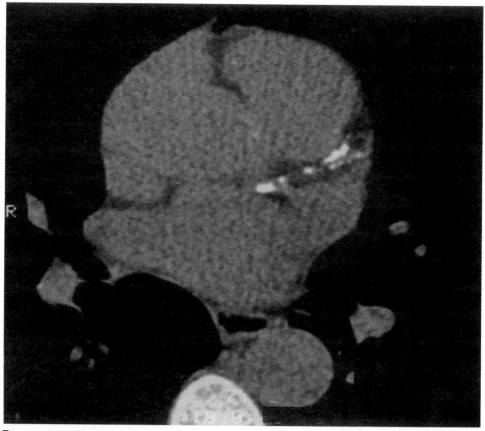

B

Figure 54–6 Fifty-five year old diabetic with left anterior descending coronary artery calcification. Helical 2.5-mm image (**A**) as compared with an EBT image (**B**).

fact, Arad et al have shown that a calcium score of 160 or greater has an odds ratio of 20 or greater in identifying individuals at risk for a cardiac event. Similarly, individuals with calcium scores greater than 400 are at even higher risk for coronary events.[4,15]

COMPLICATIONS OF ISCHEMIC HEART DISEASE

Both helical and electron beam scanners are currently being used to evaluate sequelae of cardiac events. Infarctions, ventricular aneurysms, thrombi, wall motion abnormalities, and pericardial thickening can all result from myocardial infarction (Figure 54-7). Not only can structural abnormalities be identified, but function can also be evaluated. Both EBT and HCT show potential in evaluating complications of coronary artery disease.[27]

VALVULAR HEART DISEASE

Although cardiac catheterization and echocardiography are the primary imaging modalities in evaluating valvular heart disease, CT also has significant applications. Leaflet thickening and calcification, as well as commissural fusion, can readily be identified as can ventricular hypertrophy and cardiac chamber enlargement as sequelae of valvular dysfunction. Functionally, electron beam can define leaflet motion. The application of HCT in the evaluation of cardiac function is just beginning to be reported.[14,16]

CONGENITAL HEART DISEASE

The cross-sectional imaging capabilities of EBT and HCT are excellent in identifying the arterial and venous relationships as seen in congenital abnormalities such as transposition of the great vessels, tetralogy of Fallot, etc. The poststenotic dilatations that may occur in aortic and pulmonic valve stenoses are readily identified as are aberrant superior vena cava and aberrant coronary arteries. Ventricular hypertrophy and chamber dilatation are also readily identified. EBT is useful in diagnosing and quantifying intracardiac shunts and in demonstrating flow through arteriovenous malformations. As yet, helical CT has only limited application in assessing cardiac function, but increasing reports demonstrate significant potential in this area.[14,16]

PERICARDIAL DISEASE

The lack of slice overlap and the excellent resolution make CT an extremely important modality in assessing pericardial disease.[22,23] Attenuation differences between the pericardium and the surrounding epicardial and mediastinal fat can readily distinguish pericardium. Calcifications are also easily identified.

Fluid collections may be more problematic. If the fluid collection is serous, it is usually readily identified. However, if the fluid has a high protein content or is bloody, this differentiation may become more problematic. Fluid collections can be free flowing or loculated, and thin section

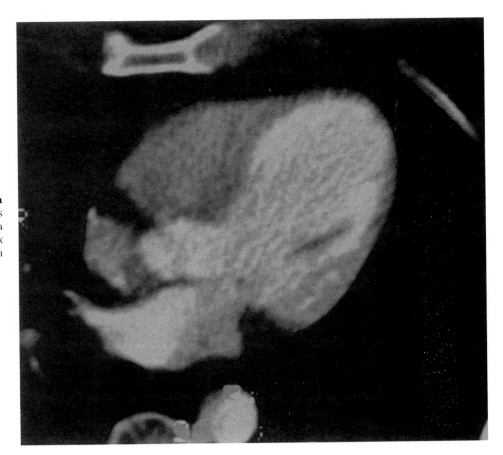

Figure 54–7 Anterior infarct in a 70-year-old woman. The long axis image taken in systole shows a thinned-out, bulging area in the apex of the left ventricle consistent with an aneurysm.

874 images are preferable in evaluating effusion configuration and content (Figure 54-8). In the assessment of pericardial disease, contrast is usually not administered but can be used to better define inflammation or to evaluate diastolic filling, which may be impaired in pericardial constrictive disease. In addition, pericardial thickening secondary to metastatic disease is readily assessed.

▶ CTA

A major application that is receiving considerable attention is CTA. Not only have HCT and EBT excellent sensitivity in defining coronary stenoses (Figure 54-9)[1,2], but with opacification of the vessel lumen, the presence of noncalcified plaque within the coronary arterial wall can also be identified. This application now makes it possible to differentiate noncalcified fibrous from soft plaque.[25] The latter differentiation is important in that soft plaque is now thought to have a greater potential to rupture and cause a cardiac event. For CTA, Achenbach et al have shown EBT sensitivities and specificities of 92–94% as compared to angiography in identifying significant stenoses.[1]

▶ EBT AND HCT IN EVALUATION OF BYPASS GRAFT PATENCY

Both HCT and EBT have shown potential in assessing coronary artery bypass graft (CABG) patency. The largest study evaluating CABG patency with CT was a multicenter study that reported an EBT sensitivity of 93.4% in documenting angiographically open grafts and an 88.9% specificity in documenting angiographically closed grafts. The overall accuracy was 92.1%.[30,31] In this study there were no significant differences in the identification of the left anterior descending artery (LAD), right coronary artery (RCA), or circumflex graft occlusions. Bypass graft reformation can also be helpful in documenting patency. HCT also has potential in this area with investigators reporting a sensitivity of 85.7% and a specificity of 100% in assessing CABG patency.[32]

▶ EBT AND MYOCARDIAL PERFUSION

Few studies are available reporting the use of CT in assessing myocardial perfusion. There are reports of EBT perfusion as compared with regional radiolabeled microspheres and the results have been moderately good.[23,33] At present, although the technique remains somewhat experimental, increasing interest is being shown in measuring myocardial perfusion.

▶ CT IMAGING OF AORTIC DISEASE

Aortic Aneurysms

The ability to image both the vessel wall and arterial lumen in axial planes and do so with excellent spatial and temporal

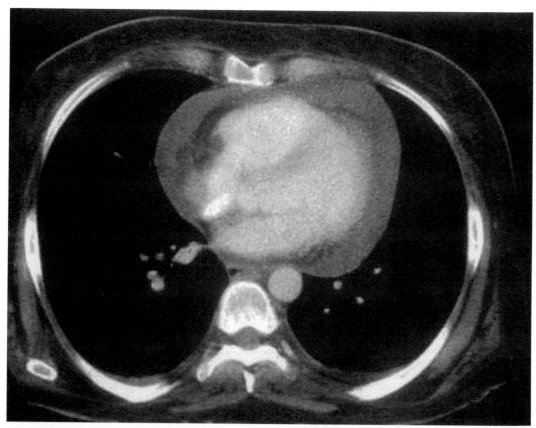

Figure 54–8 HCT image showing a large pericardial effusion surrounding the left and right ventricles. The effusion is of low attenuation.

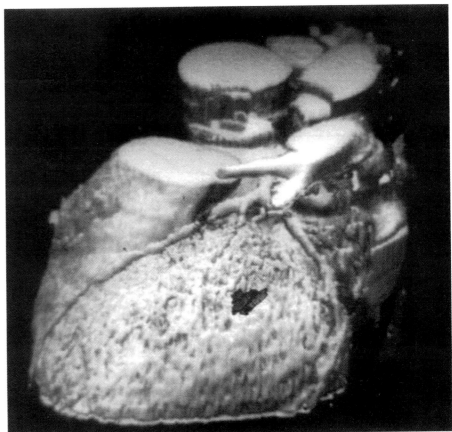

A

Figure 54–9 EBT 2.5-mm reformatted image of LAD stenosis pre- (**A**) and post-balloon angioplasty (**B**). *(Reproduced with permission from Moshage WEL: Coronary artery stenosis: three-dimensional imaging with electrocardiographically triggered, contrast agent-enhanced, electron-beam CT. Radiology 196:707–714, 1995.)*

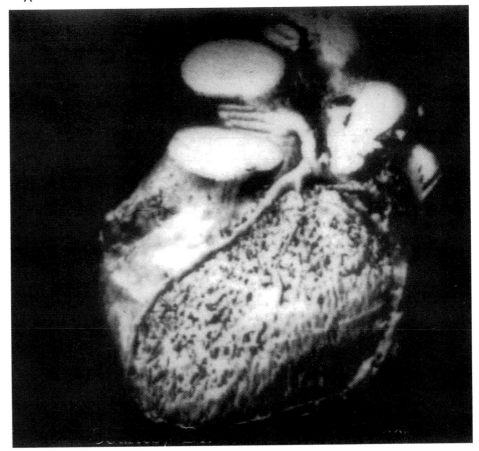

B

resolutions has made CT an important imaging modality in evaluating aortic aneurysms and dissections.[8] With both the helical and electron beam scanner, images from above the aortic arch to the iliac vessels can be acquired within a 20–30 s breathhold. Because these data are acquired as a continuous data set, excellent 3D reconstruction is possible.

The indications for CT imaging of the aorta are in patients with a widened or otherwise abnormal mediastinum, patients presenting to the emergency room with sudden onset chest pain where an aneurysm or dissection needs to be rapidly ruled out, patients with chest trauma to rule out aortic lacerations, and in the follow-up of postoperative complications (Figure 54-10).

Imaging Sequences

Patients with known or suspected aneurysms or dissections of the aorta usually undergo a helical or EBT study that produces either contiguous axial 3-mm-thick slices or a 2.5–3 mm volumetric data set. Imaging is generally begun approximately 2 cm cephalad to the top of the aortic arch so that any branch vessel involvement can be evaluated. The scans usually extend caudally to the iliac or femoral vessels. In evaluation of both dissections and aneurysms, attention is directed at documenting the location and extent of any tear and/or any associated periaortic leak or branch vessel involvement

In trauma the presence of blood within the mediastinum or contrast material outside the aortic lumen are indications for further evaluations including angiography. The visualization of a tear associated with extravasation is often diagnostic and this may obviate the need for further imaging.

The 3D reformatting capability of CT additionally allows for accurate evaluation of branch vessel involvement as well as the ability to obtain accurate measurements of vessel size and tortuosity for stent placement.

Pulmonary Emboli

Pulmonary emboli are identified as a filling defect or cutoff in the contrast-enhanced pulmonary arteries. Because CT is essentially noninvasive and produces axial images without overlapping structures, it is an ideal method for evaluating suspected pulmonary embolism (Figure 54-11). This is particularly true with the faster EBT and spiral CT scanners. The excellent resolution exquisitely details the vessel lumen and the aortic wall and with the continuous volumetric sets, vessels can be traced as far as the subsegmental branches. CT has a sensitivity of 74.1% and a specificity of 89.5%, as compared to pulmonary angiography or high probability V̇/Q̇ scan.[24] CT is particularly well suited in intensive care unit (ICU) patients who often have associated air space disease, effusions, or atelectasis.

Alternative Imaging Modalities

The diagnosis of cardiovascular disease previously has depended heavily upon cardiac catheterization supplemented by nuclear medicine and echocardiographic techniques. However, with the advent of CT and MR, increasing

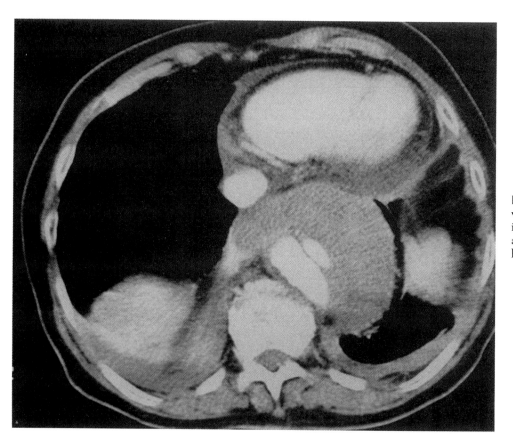

Figure 54–10 A 75-year- old woman with chest pain. The EBT image shows a leaking thoracic aortic aneurysm with surrounding hematoma.

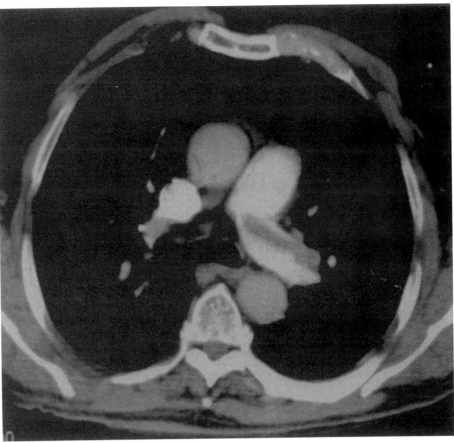

Figure 54–11 Pulmonary embolus in a 74-year-old man with sudden chest pain.

numbers of studies are being done in the evaluation of cardiovascular disease.

The gold standard against which all imaging modalities are measured is cardiac catheterization. This modality, while having superior spatial and temporal resolution, can also provide access for concomitant interventional manipulations. However, catheterization is invasive and often requires an overnight hospitalization. In addition, the radiation exposure may be significant and there is some morbidity from the contrast material and catheterization.

Imaging during cardiac catheterization can visualize only the blood pool and not the vessel wall, and therefore, structures lying outside of the blood pool are often not well seen. CT, on the other hand, can identify not only the vessel lumina but also the cardiac chamber and vessel wall anatomy. This ability, plus the ability of CT to obtain static cross-sectional and longitudinal images without overlying structures, is one of its major advantages.

► SUMMARY

CT has many applications in imaging cardiovascular disease. Its speed, excellent resolution, and cross-sectional capabilities are its major advantages. Its disadvantages are the necessity of administering contrast material and the exposure to radiation. Definition of cardiac structures, intracardiac thrombi/tumors, pericardial disease, and great vessel abnormalities are all major applications of CT, and the faster temporal resolutions of HCT and EBT also make these

modalities useful in evaluating cardiac function and coronary artery calcification. CT technology is additionally helpful in evaluating the complications of cardiovascular disease and in following up postoperative patients. Thus, CT, with its temporal and spatial resolution, is now becoming a major imaging modality in the assessment of cardiovascular disease.

REFERENCES

1. Achenbach S, Giesler T, Ropers D, et al: Detection of coronary artery stenoses by contrast-enhanced, retrospectively electrocardiographically-gated, multislice spiral computed tomography. Circulation 103:2535–2538, 2001.
2. Achenbach S, Moshage W, Ropers D, et al: Value of electron beam computed tomography for the noninvasive detection of high-grade coronary-artery stenoses and occlusions. N Engl J Med 339:1964–1971, 1998.
3. American Heart Association: 2001 Heart & Stroke Statistical Update. Dallas: American Heart Association, 2001, p 28.
4. Arad Y, Spadaro LA, Goodman K, et al: Prediction of coronary events with electron beam computed tomography. J Am Coll Cardiol 36:1253–1260, 2000.
5. Becker CR, Jakobs TF, Aydemir S, et al: Helical and single-slice conventional CT versus electron beam CT for the quantification of coronary artery calcification. AJR Am J Roentgenol 174:543–547, 2000.
6. Boyd DP, Lipton M: Cardiac computed tomography. Proc IEEE 71:298–307, 1983.
7. Carr JJ, Crouse JR 3rd, Goff DC Jr, et al: Evaluation of subsecond gated helical CT for quantification of coronary

artery calcium and comparison with electron beam CT. AJR Am J Roentgenol 174:915–921, 2000.

8. Cleverly JR, Barrie JR, Raymond GS, et al: Direct findings of aortic injury on contrast–enhanced CT in surgically proven traumatic aortic injury: a multicenter review. Clin Radiol 57: 281–286, 2002.

9. Cohnen M, Poll L, Puttmann C, et al: Radiation exposure in multi-slice CT of the heart. Forthschr. Rontgenstr 173: 295–299, 2001.

10. Feiring A, Rumberger JA, Reiter SJ, et al: Determination of left ventricular mass in dogs with rapid acquisition-cardiac computed tomographic scanning. Circulation 72:1355–1364, 1985.

11. Feiring AJ, Rumberger JA, Reiter SJ, et al: Sectional and segmental variability of left ventricular function: experimental and clinical studies using ultrafast computed tomography. J Am Coll Cardiol 12:415–425, 1988.

12. Hajduczok ZD, Weiss RM, Stanford W, et al: Determination of right ventricular mass in humans and dogs with ultrafast cardiac computed tomography. Circulation 82:202–212, 1990.

13. Hunold P, Vogt FM, Schmermund A et al: Radiation exposure during non-invasive coronary artery imaging: comparison multislice CT with electron beam CT. Radiology 221(P): 540, 2001.

14. Kapur V, Johnson PC, Smith DD, et al: Multi-slice cardiac CT left ventricular mass calculations. Radiology 225(P):152, 2002.

15. Keelan PC, Bielak LF, Ashai K, et al: Long-term prognostic value of coronary calcification detected by electron beam computed tomography in patients undergoing coronary angiography. Circulation 104:412–417, 2001.

16. Mochizuki T, Merose K, Higashino H, et al: Two and three dimensional CT ventriculography: a new application of helical CT. AJR Am J Roentgenol 174:203–208; 2000.

17. Nallamothu BK, Saint S, Bielak LF, et al: Electron beam computed tomography in the diagnosis of coronary artery disease: a meta-analysis. Arch Intern Med 161:833–838, 2001.

18. Oren RM, Grover-McKay M, Stanford W, et al: Accurate preoperative diagnosis of pericardial constriction using cine computed tomography. J Am Coll Cardiol 22:832–838, 1993.

19. Pietras RJ, Wolfkiel CJ, Veselik K, et al: Validation of ultrafast computed tomographic left ventricular volume measurement. Invest Radiol 26:28–34, 1991.

20. Reiter SJ, Rumberger JA, Fiering AJ, et al: Precision of measurements of right and left ventricular volume by cine computed tomography. Circulation 74:890–900, 1986.

21. Reiter SJ, Rumberger JA, Stanford W, et al: Quantitative determination of aortic regurgitant volumes in dogs by ultrafast computed tomography. Circulation 76:728–735, 1987.

22. Rumberger JA, Simons DB, Fitzpatrick LA, et al: Coronary artery calcium area by electron beam computed tomography and coronary atherosclerotic plaque area: a histopathologic correlative study. Circulation 92:2157–2162, 1995.

23. Rumberger JA, Feiring AJ, Lipton MJ, et al: Use of ultrafast computed tomography to quantitate regional myocardial perfusion: a preliminary report. J Am Coll Cardiol 9:59–69, 1987.

24. Safriel Y, Zinn A: CT pulmonary angiography in the detection of pulmonary emboli. A meta-analysis of sensitivities and specificities. Clin Imaging 26:101–105, 2002.

25. Schroeder S, Kopp AF, Baumbach A, et al: Noninvasive detection and evaluation of atherosclerotic coronary plaques with multislice computed tomography. J. Am. Coll. Cardiol. 37:1430–1435, 2001.

26. Stanford W: Computed tomography and ultrafast computed tomography in pericardial disease. In Elliott LP, editor: Cardiac Imaging in Infants, Children, and Adults. Philadelphia: J.B. Lippincott, 1991, pp. 415–420.

27. Stanford W: Electron beam computed tomography in the evaluation of ischemic heart disease. In Taveras JM, Ferrucci JT, editors: Radiology on CD ROM: Diagnosis – Imaging – Intervention. Philadelphia: Lippincott, Williams & Wilkins, 2002, Chapter 19:2.

28. Stanford W: Multidetector CT vs electron beam CT in the quantification of coronary artery calcification. Emphasis on lower calcium scores. Radiology 225(P):238, 2002.

29. Stanford W, Rooholamini SA, Galvin JR: Ultrafast computed tomography for detection of intracardiac thrombi and tumors. In Elliot LP, editor: Cardiac Imaging in Infants, Children, and Adults. Philadelphia: J.B. Lippincott, 2001, pp. 494–500.

30. Stanford W, Brundage BH, MacMillan R, et al: Sensitivity and specificity of assessing coronary bypass graft patency with ultrafast computed tomography: results of a multicenter study. J Am Coll Cardiol; 12:1–7, 1988.

31. Stanford W, Rooholamini M, Rumberger J, et al: Evaluation of coronary bypass graft patency by ultrafast computed tomography. J Thorac Imaging 3:52–55, 1988.

32. Tello R, Costello P, Ecker C, et al: Spiral CT evaluation of coronary artery bypass graft patency. J Comput Assist Tomogr 17:253–259, 1993.

33. Wang T, Ritman EL: Regional myocardial perfusion—quantitation with high speed volume scanning CT. Circulation 76 (Suppl):IV-5, 1987 (abstract).

Cardiovascular Magnetic Resonance in Cardiovascular Diagnosis

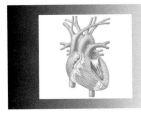

CHAPTER 55

Susan B. Yeon and Warren J. Manning

INTRODUCTION

Cardiovascular magnetic resonance (CMR) offers uniquely versatile imaging capabilities for the diagnosis and management of cardiovascular disease.[32,48] With adaptation of magnetic resonance (MR) technology to overcome the technical challenges posed by underlying cardiac and respiratory motion, information to aid in the diagnosis and management of a variety of cardiovascular disorders can be noninvasively acquired. In addition, CMR capabilities permit great flexibility, precision, and reproducibility in the acquisition and display of anatomical and functional data useful for surgical diagnosis, planning, and follow-up.

IMAGING PRINCIPLES AND APPROACHES

CMR entails exposure to static and dynamic magnetic fields without the application of ionizing radiation. Images are generated from spatially distributed induced radiofrequency signals arising from water and fat protons in the body. Differences in proton density, magnetic relaxation times (T1, or longitudinal relaxation time; T2, transverse relaxation time), blood flow, and other parameters produce intrinsic signal contrast among tissues. CMR approaches can be generally classified into spin-echo (black blood) and gradient-echo (bright blood) categories (though signal from the blood pool may also be modified by prepulses or flow properties). Spin-echo imaging is particularly useful for defining anatomical structure and tissue characterization (e.g., fat replacement or iron deposition). Gradient-echo techniques can produce single-shot (displaying a single phase during the cardiac cycle) or cine (displaying multiple phases at one level during the cardiac cycle) images. Cine images demonstrate motion of structures (such as cardiac chambers and valves) during the cardiac cycle, permitting qualitative and quantitative assessment of motion. Both spin-echo and gradient-echo CMR techniques are flow sensitive.

Because of the inherent contrast between the blood pool and surrounding tissue, administration of an exogenous CMR contrast agent is generally not required. However, administration of an extracellular MR-specific intravenous contrast agent, such as gadolinium-diethylenetriamine pentaacetic acid (Gd-DTPA), enables certain applications such as contrast-enhanced (CE), MR angiography (MRA), and assessment of myocardial perfusion and viability. Gadolinium induces T1 shortening, which is detected as increased signal in CE T1-weighted images (the signal enhancement is not linearly related to contrast agent concentration). Flow velocity encoding (also known as phase contrast) is an additional CMR modality that enables quantitation of blood flow. This method enables determination of regurgitant fraction and shunt flows.

IMAGING COMPARISONS

The advantages and limitations of CMR complement those of other imaging techniques such as echocardiography, computed tomography (CT), X-ray angiography, and radionuclide imaging. As compared to echocardiography and radionuclide imaging, CMR offers superior anatomical scope

880 and spatial resolution. CMR provides more reproducible measures of left ventricular (LV) cavity volumes and systolic function, thus enhancing noninvasive follow-up of disease processes.[8] In contrast to echocardiography and nuclear imaging, CMR permits unrestricted image acquisition orientation, which can be readily adjusted to particular patient and study requirements. On the other hand, retained advantages of echocardiography include portability; general availability, greater case of patient monitoring; and greater sensitivity for structures with chaotic motion, such as vegetations. Although CMR myocardial perfusion techniques have been shown to provide useful qualitative and quantitative data, they have not yet been clinically validated to provide the prognostic information proven for radionuclide techniques.

As noted earlier, CMR generally does not require the use of an exogenous contrast agent. When needed, however, gadolinium-containing CMR contrast agents have a much more favorable safety profile in regard to both nephrotoxity and anaphylaxis as compared with iodinated agents used in X-ray angiography and CT scanning.[60] Further comparisons between CMR and other techniques will be made in the sections below dealing with specific types of examinations.

▶ IMAGING PRECAUTIONS

Precautions generally applicable to general MR imaging are applicable to CMR. Prior to imaging, all patients must undergo detailed screening for any potential contraindications to MR scanning. In addition to general concerns of metallic implants and severe claustrophobia, patients should be screened for the presence of any MR-incompatible material. Excluded devices include some that are relatively common among those with cardiovascular disease, such as pacemakers, retained permanent pacemaker leads, and implantable cardioverters-defibrillators (ICDs). Bioprosthetic and mechanical heart valves, sternotomy wires, thoracic vascular clips, and intracoronary stents are generally considered MR safe at field strengths up to 1.5 T, although they may produce local artifacts that reduce image quality.[29]

Due to bulk cardiac motion during systole and diastole, most CMR protocols require electrocardiogram (ECG) triggering with images composed from data collected during multiple successive cardiac cycles. However, good functional image quality can frequently be obtained among patients with atrial fibrillation,[33] although image quality may be impaired among subjects with frequent and irregular premature beats. Among patients with irregular rhythms, non-ECG gated real-time imaging (which permits real-time image acquisition analogous to two-dimensional [2D] echocardiography but at lower spatial and temporal resolutions than that attained with a gated CMR technique) can provide useful information.[68]

All subjects require appropriate monitoring during their CMR studies. Basic monitoring modalities include ECG monitoring for rate and rhythm (magnetic fields distort ST segment appearance rendering it uninterpretable), intercom voice contact, and visualization (by direct view and/or camera). For patients requiring greater intensity of monitoring, automated cuff blood pressure monitoring and pulse oximetry can be added.

▶ CMR APPLICATIONS

Diseases of the Thoracic Aorta

CMR is widely used clinically for the assessment of aortic aneurysms and aortic dissection. The structure of the aorta is delineated by a combination of the following protocol components in the transverse, coronal, sagittal, and/or oblique planes: (1) ECG-gated spin-echo imaging that reveals the aortic wall with flowing blood appearing black; (2) ECG-gated steady-state free precession (SSFP) imaging that produces bright-blood images in single-shot as well as cine acquisitions; and (3) three-dimensional (3D) contrast-enhanced magnetic resonance angiography (CE-MRA) using a gradient echo acquisition. Temporally resolved CE-MRA is particularly useful to minimize motion artifacts that would otherwise result in nondiagnostic or false-positive results.

Aortic Dissection

CMR, along with CT and transesophageal echocardiography (TEE), is a primary method to diagnose and monitor patients with acute or chronic aortic dissection. Because each of these diagnostic modalities has been found to have high diagnostic accuracy for dissection, the selection among these methods is generally governed by patient condition, institutional access, and local expertise. Among these, CMR offers a comparable combination of sensitivity and specificity (sensitivity above 95% and specificity above 90%) for dissection.[72] CMR can assess aortic valve integrity and proximal coronary involvement. CMR and CT can provide information regarding involvement of major branch vessels and all segments of the aorta, unlike TEE, which is limited to the thoracic aorta and by the adequacy of acoustic windows (particularly for the segment of ascending aorta anterior to the trachea). All three methods provide useful information regarding pericardial involvement. The main disadvantages of CMR in the acute setting are potential obstacles to continuous monitoring and care of an unstable patient during transport and study and the requirement that the patient remain motionless during the examination. Thus CT (often located in the emergency department) is the most common initial imaging modality chosen to diagnose acute aortic dissection and echocardiography is next most common.[26] However, CMR is considered the imaging procedure of choice[69] for serial follow-up of the medically or surgically treated patient with dissection according to the Recommendations of the Task Force on Aortic Dissection of the European Society of Cardiology (which have been endorsed by the American College of Cardiology).[16] Follow-up is recommended following hospital discharge at 1, 3, 6, and 12 months and yearly thereafter.[16] Accurate interpretation of postoperative images requires knowledge of the surgical procedure performed and the expected range of routine postoperative sequelae including thickening around the graft and presence of thrombus outside the graft and within the native aortic wrap.[64]

CMR aortic assessment can often be completed within 30 min and can display the location and extent of dissection identified as an intimal flap separating true and false aortic lumina along with sites of intraluminal communication. CMR can readily assess involvement of the aortic root, arch vessels, and renal arteries. Spin-echo images may identify relatively bright regions within the true or false lumen attributable to stagnant blood flow or thrombus. Gradient echo images demonstrate flap motion and blood flow in the true and false lumina (Figure 55-1). The 3D CE-MRA is highly sensitive for dissection[43] and can be implemented with subsecond temporal resolution to obviate the need for a breath-hold.[21] However, steady-state free precession (SSFP) imaging without exogenous contrast can be accomplished within 4 min and may suffice.[57] Additional scans can be performed to assess the presence of aortic regurgitation (using cine imaging of the LV outflow tract), the size of the regurgitant fraction (using a phase velocity encoding acquisition at the base of the aortic root), LV function (cine MR), presence of any accompanying pericardial effusion (cine and spin-echo MR), and involvement of the proximal coronary arteries (coronary MRA).

Aortic Aneurysm

CMR is also a superior method for identification of true and false thoracic aortic aneurysms. In true aneurysms, the aneurysmal aortic wall is comprised of intima, media, and adventitia. False aneurysms represent a contained rupture of the intima and media with only the adventia and periadventitial connective tissue limiting the hemorrhage. Thus, false aneurysms generally have a narrow "neck" or communication with the main aortic lumen. True aneurysms are more commonly fusiform (bulge aligned along the long axis of the aorta; Figure 55-2) than saccular (sack-like bulge extending from a side of the aortic wall). CE-MRA reveals the presence and extent of these lesions as well as any associated thrombus. 3D CE-MRA is recommended as the imaging modality of choice for most patients with chronic disease.[27] As for aortic dissection, advantages of CMR assessment as compared with CT and X-ray angiography include the capability to evaluate for associated complications such as aortic regurgitation, hemopericardium, and left ventricular dysfunction as well as lack of requirement for a potentially nephrotoxic iodinated contrast agent. Following composite graft replacement of the ascending aorta, CMR is useful for detection of postoperative complications, such as leakage or hematoma formation.[18]

Aortic Intramural Hematoma

Intramural hematoma can be identified by the presence of a localized thickening, frequently crescentic or circular, within the wall of the aorta, interposed between intima and media, with characteristics of an acute or subacute collection of blood.[52] CMR has been found to be superior to CT in distinguishing acute intramural hematoma from atherosclerotic plaque and chronic intraluminal thrombus.[86] Acute hemorrhage appears isointense or more intense as compared with the aortic wall on T1-weighted images and displays high

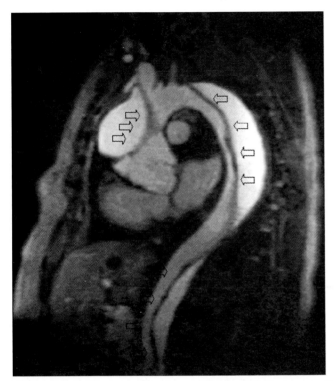

Figure 55–1 **3D contrast-enhanced MRA oblique image of the thoracic aorta demonstrating a DeBakey classification type 1 dissection (*at arrows*) involving the ascending and descending thoracic aorta.**

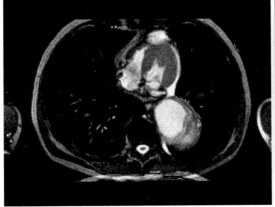
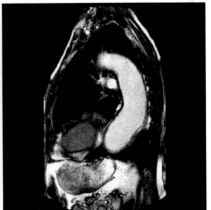

Figure 55–2 Transverse (A) and oblique sagittal (B) images of a patient with a descending thoracic aortic aneurysm (*at arrows*) partially filled with thrombus (at arrowhead). Each image was acquired in <1 sc with an SSFP sequence without the administration of exogenous contrast agent. (*Courtesy of Tim Leiner, MD, PhD.*)

A

B

882 signal intensity on T2-weighted images.[52,56] In contrast, sub-acute hemorrhage displays high signal intensity on T1 images and less signal intensity on T2 images. The layer of displaced calcified intima overlying the hematoma generally produces a relatively smooth surface concave to the lumen (crescentic shape), which may help distinguish this entity from protuberant, frequently irregularly shaped, atherosclerotic plaque.

Sinus of Valsalva Aneurysm

A sinus of Valsalva aneurysm can be readily visualized by CMR as an enlargement or outpouching (frequently creating a "windsock" appearance) of a sinus of the aortic root. In addition, the complication of rupture of the aneurysmal sinus into an adjacent chamber (most commonly the right ventricle) can be detected on cine images as a region of signal void produced by the turbulent jet emanating from the sinus via the rupture into the communicating chamber (Figure 55-3). Shunt flow through the rupture is generally present both in diastole and systole. The magnitude of the shunt may be calculated using flow velocity encoding data.

Atherosclerotic Plaque and Aortic Penetrating Ulcer

CMR can provide qualitative and quantitative information about the presence, thickness, and distribution of atherosclerotic plaque in the aorta.[11,20] Complex plaque is generally defined as protuberant plaque at least 4 mm in thickness or plaque with mobile elements (thrombus) since plaque with these characteristics is associated with embolic risk.[80] Plaque thickness can readily be ascertained by CMR, although overlying mobile elements may be obscured in images obtained over multiple cardiac cycles because of their chaotic motion and relatively small size.[44] Because ascending aortic plaque is a predictor of adverse cerebral outcomes following coronary artery bypass grafting with cardiopulmonary bypass, preoperative identification of such

plaque may prompt alteration in surgical strategy or technique.[24,80] However, the utility of CMR for preoperative assessment of aortic plaque location and burden has not yet been assessed.

Aortic ulceration occurs in regions of atherosclerotic plaque. Penetrating ulcers are described as those breaching the internal elastic lamina with associated hematoma formation in the media.[30,78] CMR images visualize the position and shape of such ulcers and accompanying adjacent intramural hematoma.[44,86] Penetrating ulcers are also frequently associated with aortic aneurysm formation.[77,78] The presence of associated chest or back pain is a significant risk factor for progression to pseudoaneurysm or free rupture.[78]

Takayasu Arteritis

Takayasu arteritis is a chronic idiopathic vasculitis that primarily affects the aorta and its branches. It is most prevalent among Asian women under 40 years of age.[4,36] The aortic arch (or distal aorta) and its branches, as well as the pulmonary arteries, have characteristically tapered narrowings or occlusions with fewer areas of dilation. The availability of noninvasive imaging is important among these patient who require long-term follow-up to guide medical and surgical therapy. These lesions have been traditionally detected by conventional X-ray angiography, but CMR (as well as CT) can accurately display these lesions and also provide information regarding a vessel wall abnormality.[84,85] CMR evidence of vessel wall edema is common among these patients and does not correlate well with subsequent lesion development.[79] Therefore the current role of CMR in this disease is to identify the characteristic angiographic lesions as can be identified by 3D CE-MRA.[84]

Congenital Aortic Anomalies

CMR can readily identify and characterize aortic coarctation, patent ductus arteriosus, and other congenital abnormalities involving the great vessels.

Aortic coarctation is characterized by a ridge of medial thickening and intimal hyperplasia along the posterolateral aortic wall. Coarctation most commonly presents just distal to the left subclavian, occurring more rarely just proximal to the left subclavian. An oblique sagittal view aligned with the descending and ascending thoracic aorta will reveal the location of the coarctation, as well as associated collaterals, using spin-echo, gradient-echo, or CE-MRA techniques.[25,63] In addition, CMR can identify cardiac lesions that frequently accompany coarctation including bicuspid aortic valve (imaged by a cine SSFP of the valve in cross section) and ventricular septal defect (imaged by a gradient-echo cine CMR of the interventricular septum in a horizontal long-axis or four-chamber view). CMR is also useful for follow-up after surgical repair or balloon angioplasty[63] and routine CMR follow-up has been recommended.[76] Potential complications that may be visualized include recoarctation, and aneurysm or pseudoaneurysm formation at repair site.

Whereas patent ductus arteriosus can usually be identified by transthoracic echocardiography, CMR may be useful when echocardiographic images are nondiagnostic because of poor acoustic windows.[12] For both patent ductus arteriosus and ventricular septal defects, CMR can provide an

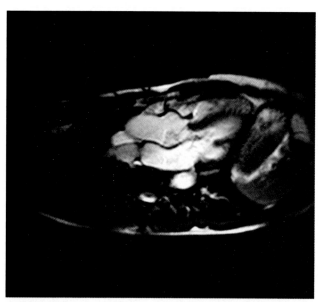

Figure 55–3 SSFP image of a ruptured sinus of Valsalva aneurysm with signal void in the right ventricle from associated turbulent shunt flow.

assessment of the pulmonic-to-systemic flow ratio ($\dot{Q}$P:$\dot{Q}$S) by applying the flow velocity encoding technique.[58]

Thoracic Trauma

Chest radiography and CT are generally the initial imaging modalities for assessment of acute thoracic trauma. CMR may provide useful supplemental information when other testing is indeterminate. CMR is particularly useful for assessment of diaphragmatic, mediastinal, and aortic injury if CT results are equivocal.[50] CMR is also helpful for characterizing posttraumatic masses such as hematomas.[50]

CMR may also be useful in identifying an aortic tear, occurring most commonly by rapid deceleration forces from a motor vehicle accident. The tear usually occurs in the region of the ligamentum arteriosus. Among those who survive to detection and repair, a pseudoaneurysm is found with associated surrounding hematoma. While this lesion can be rapidly identified by T1-weighted spin-echo CMR imaging, CT and TEE are more frequently used in acute settings. When surgical repair of traumatic aortic rupture is postponed pending stabilization of other injuries and medical problems, CMR can be used to monitor aneurysm progression[17] and selection of patients for treatment by endovascular stent placement.[19]

Cardiac Imaging

Ventricular Structure and Function

CMR provides a gold standard for the quantitative assessment of left and right ventricular chamber sizes, systolic function, and mass with greater reproducibility than available using other techniques.[8] Gender-specific normal reference values for CMR LV mass, volumes, and ejection fraction have been defined and may be sequence dependent.[1,67] A set of breath-hold short-axis cine images (acquired using a pulse sequence like SSFP) spanning the ventricles can be acquired within 10 mins. SSFP techniques provide superior endocardial border definition thereby enabling use of semiautomated techniques for image analysis. Regional systolic function can be assessed by examining segmental wall motion and thickening. A 17-segment model common to echocardiography and nuclear cardiology is recommended.[53,54] In addition, CMR tagging methods may be useful in characterizing focal abnormalities and myocardial twist.[61]

Similarly, CMR provides unsurpassed efficacy in assessment of right ventricular structure and function.[65] Whereas right ventricular function has been most commonly assessed clinically by echocardiography, echocardiographic assessment is limited by variability of views and suboptimal image quality and generally remains only qualitative.

Identification of Myocardial Scar and Ischemia

Among patients with resting regional LV systolic dysfunction, identification of the presence and distribution of scar and viable myocardium within dysfunctional regions has important prognostic and therapeutic implications. A delayed CE inversion-recovery CMR technique has proven highly sensitive for determining the presence and spatial extent of acute and chronic myocardial infarction identified as regions of hyperenhancement (Figure 55-4).[38,71,82] Among heart failure patients with ischemic heart disease, CMR identification of scar closely agrees with positron emission tomography (PET) data.[41] Among patients with stable coronary artery disease undergoing revascularization by coronary artery bypass graft surgery or percutaneous intervention, the transmural and segmental extent of LV scar detected by CMR is a strong negative predictor for regional and global recovery of systolic function following revascularization.[39]

MR stress testing is useful for assessment of ischemia by induction of either wall motion abnormalities or perfusion defects with pharmacological stress. MR perfusion techniques for assessment of myocardial ischemia using contrast enhancement show promise in preliminary clinical application.[2,34]

Congenital Heart Disease

CMR plays an important role in the diagnosis and management of simple and complex congenital heart disease.[55] Its capabilities are complimentary to those of echocardiography and cardiac catheterization in patients with congenital heart disease. CMR is particularly useful among children and adults with suboptimal acoustic windows[73] and those with

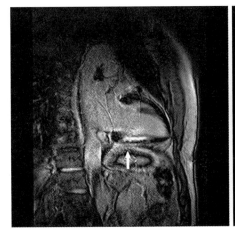
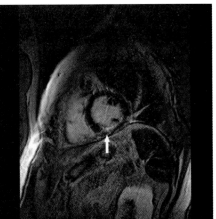

Figure 55–4 (A) Two-chamber and (B) mid-ventricular short-axis delayed contrast-enhanced inversion recovery image in a patient with an inferior myocardial infarction. The region of contrast hyperenhancement (*arrows*) corresponds to scar.

A

B

884 complex lesions. CMR can effectively identify the location, orientation, and relationships between the vena cavae, cardiac chambers, valves, great vessels, and pulmonary veins. Anatomical structure can be displayed in tomographic views and in 3D reconstructions, which are particularly helpful to delineate complex spatial relationships. In addition, phase-contrast scans can be used for measurement of flow and thus quantify the magnitude of shunts associated with atrial and ventricular septal defects (Figure 55-5).[7] Aortic forward and regurgitant flow can be quantified by phase-contrast imaging in an axial (or oblique) plane transverse to the long axis of the ascending aorta. Similarly, phase-contrast

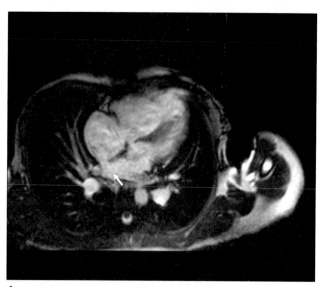

A

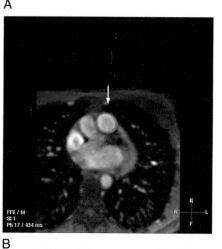

B

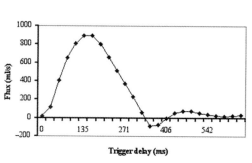

Figure 55–5 A, Four-chamber view of a sinus venosus atrial septal defect (*at arrow*). **B,** Main pulmonary artery (*arrow*) and **C,** aortic root (*arrow*) cross-sectional phase-contrast images (*left*) and corresponding flux contours (*right*) indicating a pulmonary-to-systemic shunt ratio ($\dot{Q}_P/\dot{Q}_S$) of 3.0.

C

imaging in a cross-sectional slice of the proximal main pulmonary artery (oblique, generally near coronal view) enables quantification of pulmonary artery forward and regurgitant flows. Thus the ratio of pulmonary and aortic (forward) flows ($\dot{Q}$P/$\dot{Q}$S) can be calculated to identify and quantify a significant ($\dot{Q}$P:$\dot{Q}$S >1.5) intracardiac shunt.[7] CMR is particularly helpful for quantitation of right ventricular size and function important for clinical assessment of many types of congenital heart disease.[31]

Cardiac and Paracardiac Masses

CMR can readily delineate cardiac and paracardiac masses such as tumors, myxomas, and thrombi. Intracardiac masses are usually initially detected by transthoracic echocardiography and frequently are effectively characterized by echocardiography alone. When echocardiographic images are suboptimal or do not adequately define the extent of the mass, CMR is useful to further define the characteristics and spatial extent of the mass within and beyond the cardiac borders. CMR may be more sensitive than echocardiography for detection of intracardiac and paracardiac involvement with lymphoma.[75] The 3D characterization of the mass by CMR is often helpful for surgical planning. Spin-echo images with and without administration of gadolinium contrast are useful for identifying the anatomical structure of the mass in relation to adjacent cardiac structures and vascularity. Gradient-echo CMR can demonstrate the phasic motion of the mass during the cardiac cycle.

Lipomatous hypertrophy of the interatrial septum can result in thickening of the septum with relative sparing in the region of the fossa ovalis. The diagnosis is generally made by echocardiography alone, but marked focal septal thickening may suggest an atrial mass (thrombus or tumor). Fatty deposits may extend beyond the septum to surrounding pericardial deposits and occasionally cause deformation of the adjacent superior vena cava (Figure 55-6). On T1-weighted images, the fatty tissue produces a characteristically high signal intensity (bright) that is selectively suppressed with a fat suppression sequence.

Thrombus is generally suspected by the appearance of a mass in a region of blood stasis (such as an aneurysmal or akinetic left ventricular apex). Early thrombus is seen as a region of high signal intensity on T1- and T2-weighted images. After 1–2 weeks, higher signal intensity may be noted on T1-weighted images and decreased signal intensity on T2-weighted images. Chronic thrombi have low signal intensity, with even greater signal loss in regions of calcification. Delayed CE imaging may also define thrombi as a signal void lining the LV cavity adjacent to hyperenhanced myocardial infarction and surrounding blood pool.[51]

Pericardial Disease

CMR imaging capabilities, including wide field of view, enable it to readily identify pericardial masses and cysts, pericardial effusion, and pericardial thickening. A pericardial effusion has low signal intensity (relatively dark) on T1-weighted images and high signal intensity (bright) on T2-weighted and gradient-echo scans. Like CT, CMR is particularly useful for identifying loculated effusions. CMR is also helpful in identifying accompanying pericardial masses or pericardial thickening.

CMR is a useful adjunct in the diagnosis of constrictive pericarditis (Figure 55-7). While the diagnosis requires clinical assessment for constrictive physiology, CMR can effectively identify focal regions of pericardial thickening characteristic of this disorder. On spin-echo CMR images, normal pericardial thickness is ≤3 mm. Among patients with pericardial constriction the CMR pericardial thickness is generally >6 mm[49] with 4–6 mm being intermediate. Pericardial thickening associated with constriction is frequently focal so identifying the location of thickening may be important to the surgical approach.[9,62] Spin-echo images

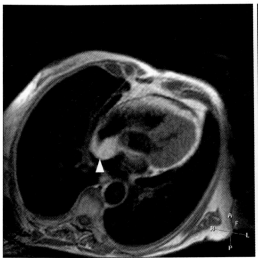
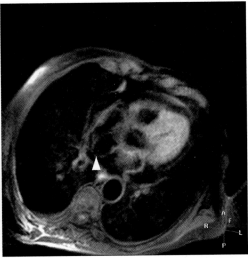

A   B

Figure 55–6 Lipomatous hypertrophy of the interatrial septum (*at arrow*) without (A) and with (B) a fat suppression prepulse. Note that the lipomatous mass is impinging upon the insertion of the superior vena cava into the right atrium. On the right, note signal nulling after fat saturation prepulse.

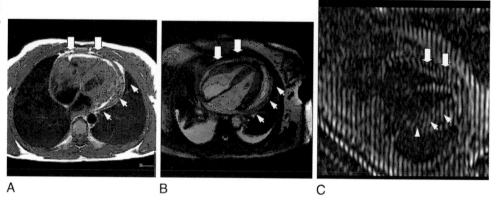

Figure 55–7 Axial dual inversion T1-weighted (**A**) and cine SSFP (**B**) images of a patient with effusive-constrictive pericarditis. Pericardial fluid appears relatively bright on the images while pericardium and organized material appear dark. The end-systolic tagged four-chamber image (**C**) demonstrates tethering of pericardial elements to right ventricular (block arrows) and left ventricular (arrowheads) walls.

rather than gradient-echo images should be used to assess pericardial thickness since the latter may overestimate pericardial thickness and fail to distinguish between patients with and without constriction.[28] However, cine acquisitions are useful to demonstrate abnormal early diastolic septal motion characteristic of constriction. CT is also useful for determination of pericardial thickness and is preferred for identification of pericardial calcifications (which lack signal by CMR). CMR tagging methods are useful in identifying regions of parietal to visceral pericardial adherence.[42] In these areas, lack of free sliding between the pericardial layers during the cardiac cycle is visualized as persistent continuity in tag lines crossing the pericardial interface (lines deform but do not break).

Valvular Heart Disease

Although echocardiography is the clinical "workhorse" for assessment of valvular morphology and stenosis, CMR offers specific advantages for the quantitative assessment of valvular regurgitation. The presence of valvular regurgitation can be detected as a flow disturbance (signal void) on cine images although the magnitude of the signal void is reduced with gradient-echo and SSFP images with shorter echo times. Importantly, flow velocity encoding is a powerful technique for quantifying the regurgitant volume (Figure 55-8). Flow velocity encoding (phase-contrast) scans of the aortic root in axial or oblique (near axial) cross-sectional views enable quantitation of aortic forward and

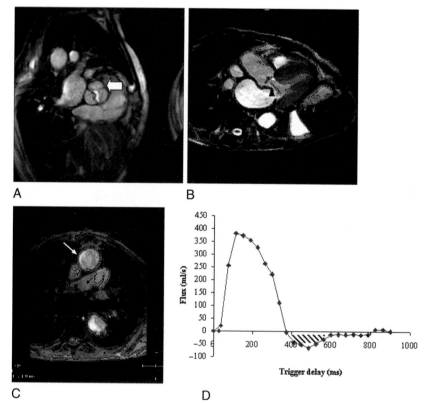

Figure 55–8 A, Systolic short-axis view of a functionally bicuspid aortic valve. Note the fused raphe between the left and right coronary cusps (*at block arrow*). **B,** Cine SSFP image demonstrating a small jet of turbulent flow of aortic regurgitation (*arrowhead*) directed into the left ventricular outflow tract. Phase contrast image at the aortic root (**C**) and associated flux contour (**D**) demonstrate a small volume of retrograde flow (*hatched area*) consistent with mild aortic regurgitation.

regurgitant flows. The difference between LV stroke volume (derived from modified Simpson's rule applied to a contiguous stack of short-axis images spanning the LV) and forward aortic flow is a quantitative measure of mitral regurgitation. The regurgitant fraction can be calculated as the ratio of the regurgitant volume to total stroke volume.

Cross-sectional and longitudinal views of the valves can be used to characterize valve deformities and stenoses (Figure 55-8). Flow velocity encoding techniques may be useful in estimating valve gradients, although this application has not yet been fully validated.[37]

Cardiomyopathies

CMR is useful in characterizing biventricular structure and function among patients with cardiomyopathy. The high reproducibility of CMR measures of ventricular size and function makes it a valuable tool for quantitative serial assessment among patients with dilated cardiomyopathy.

Among patients with hypertrophic cardiomyopathy, CMR can accurately delineate the distribution of hypertrophy among ventricular segments free of limitations (such as foreshortening of the apex and off-axis views) encountered by echocardiography. Thus, CMR is particularly helpful in identifying asymmetrical or apical hypertrophy (Figure 55-9).

Among patients with hypertrophic cardiomyopathy, delayed CE CMR frequently identifies regions of myocardial scarring that generally occurs at the junction of the interventricular septum with the right ventricular free wall.[13]

Finally, CMR provides unique information for certain specific types of cardiomyopathy. CE images may detect focal myocardial abnormalities associated with sarcoidosis.[70] Myocardial iron deposition associated with LV dysfunction is associated with a depressed $T2^*$.[3] CMR serves as a cornerstone for diagnosis of arrhythmogenic right ventricular dysplasia to determine right ventricular cavity size, to evaluate global and regional right ventricular free wall function, and to detect any fibrofatty infiltration of myocardium, although the specificity and sensitivity of these findings have not been fully defined.[14] CMR may also be useful for discriminating between cardiomyopathy due to ischemic and nonischemic causes since it has a high predictive value for excluding the presence of left main or three-vessel coronary disease.[40]

Coronary Artery imaging

Coronary MRA is currently among the most technically demanding CMR techniques. At experienced centers, coronary MRA can effectively identify significant stenoses

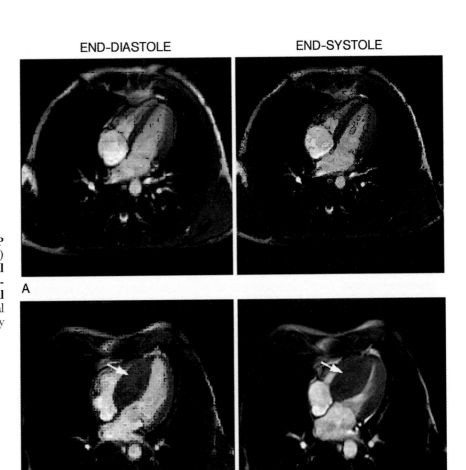

END-DIASTOLE   END-SYSTOLE

A

B

Figure 55–9 Comparison of cine SSFP four-chamber images at end-diastole (left) and end-systole (right) in (A) a normal subject and (B) in a patient with hypertrophic cardiomyopathy with asymmetrical septal hypertrophy. Note the marked septal hypertrophy (arrow) in (B) with near cavity obliteration in end-systole.

in the proximal to mid-native coronary arteries.[40] Current imaging protocols incorporate methodology to suppress the effects of cardiac motion and respiratory motion.[47] Cardiac motion is addressed via robust ECG signal detection to trigger gating and customized adjustment of the acquisition window. Respiratory motion artifacts are suppressed by MR navigators or prolonged breath-holds.[23] A 3D acquisition is employed to enhance the signal-to-noise ratio (SNR) although SNR is somewhat diminished by the prepulses required to optimize the contrast/noise ratio (CNR). To enhance contrast between blood in the coronaries and the surrounding myocardium and epicardial fat, a T_2-weighted preparation prepulse and a frequency-selective fat-saturation prepulse are applied. In a multicenter study of patients referred for elective X-ray coronary angiography, coronary MRA had a 72% accuracy in diagnosing coronary artery disease (defined as a ≥50% diameter stenosis on X-ray angiography) (Figure 55-10).[40] The accuracy of coronary MRA for diagnosis of left main coronary artery disease or three-vessel disease was 87%. Of note, the negative predictive value of MRA for left main or three-vessel disease was 97–100%.

MRA is also useful for assessment of coronary artery bypass graft patency. Reverse saphenous vein and internal mammary artery grafts are easier to image than native coronary arteries because they have a larger lumen, are relatively immobile, and have a less tortuous course than native arteries. However, local image artifacts due to associated implanted metallic objects (such as hemostatic clips, stainless steel graft markers, and sternal wires) may interfere with adequate graft visualization.[47] In spite of these limitations, various investigators have demonstrated a sensitivity of 88–98% and a specificity of 72–100% for coronary MRA detection of coronary artery bypass graft patency.° Recent work by Langerak and colleagues suggests a high-resolution navigator-gated 3D MRA approach can yield not only high sensitivity and specificity for graft occlusion (83% and 98–100%, respectively) but also fairly high sensitivity and specificity for graft stenosis ≥70% (73% and 80–87%, respectively).[45] These investigators have found an even higher sensitivity and specificity for graft stenosis ≥70% (87–100% and 84–100%, respectively) using a flow velocity encoding protocol.[46]

°References 5, 15, 22, 35, 66, 83.

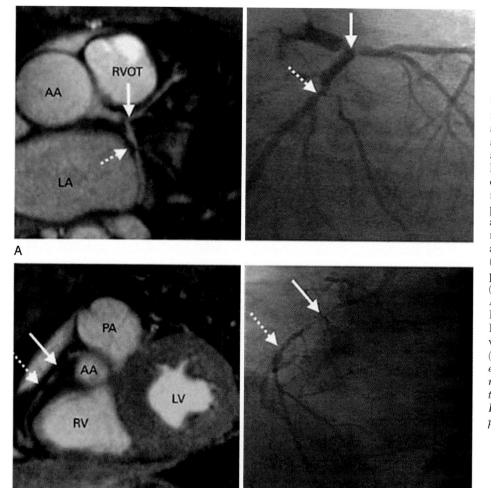

Figure 55–10 A, A coronary magnetic resonance angiogram using a 3D gradient echo sequence (left) and a corresponding X-ray coronary angiogram (right) indicating a severe lesion at the bifurcation of the left main coronary artery (*solid arrows*), and a more distal focal stenosis of the proximal left circumflex coronary artery (*broken arrows*). **B,** A coronary magnetic resonance angiogram (left) and a corresponding X-ray angiogram (right) indicating two stenoses of the proximal (*solid arrows*) and middle (*broken arrows*) right coronary artery. AA, ascending aorta; LA, left atrium; RVOT, right ventricular outflow tract; PA, pulmonary artery; RV, right ventricle; LV, left ventricle. (*From Kim WY, Danias PG, Stuber M, et al: Three-dimensional coronary magnetic resonance angiography for the detection of coronary stenoses. N Engl J Med 345:1863–1869, 2001, with permission.*)

Figure 55-11 3D coronary magnetic resonance angiograms reformatted from axial (A) and double oblique (B) imaging planes indicating anomalous origin of the left main coronary artery (*black block arrow*) from the right sinus of Valsalva. The left coronary artery courses between the aorta and the main pulmonary artery prior to bifurcating into the left anterior descending (*arrowhead*) and left circumflex (*arrow*) arteries. The right coronary artery (*white arrow*) originates normally from the right sinus of Valsalva.

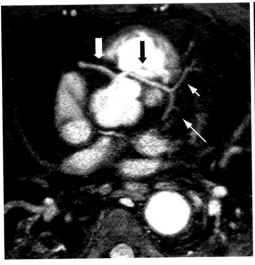
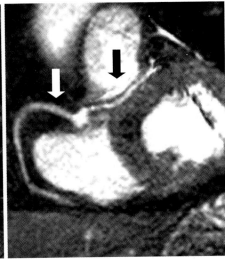

A   B

The most common clinical use of coronary MRA is for the identification and characterization of anomalous coronary arteries. Studies comparing MRA with conventional X-ray coronary angiography reveal equivalent to superior accuracy in the identification of anomalous coronary arteries.[10,59,74,81] Because coronary MRA demonstrates the origin and course of each coronary artery in 3D relation to the great vessels, it can resolve spatial ambiguity sometimes encountered when interpreting conventional projection X-ray coronary angiographic images.[10,59,81] Coronary MRA is particularly helpful in identifying whether the anomalous artery courses between the aorta and the pulmonary artery (Figure 55-11), a malignant configuration associated with sudden death and myocardial infarction among young adults.[6] In addition, among patients undergoing cardiac surgery for repair or palliation of other congenital defects it may be important to identify and define any coincident anomalous coronary arteries to avoid inadvertent iatrogenic injury.[74]

▶ THE FUTURE ROLE OF CMR

CMR technical capabilities and clinical applications are continuing to evolve. Areas under active investigation include use of targeted contrast agents and use of interventional CMR to guide percutaneous procedures. As technical advances continue and clinical experience broadens, CMR is expected to play an ever expanding role in the clinical diagnosis and management of cardiovascular disorders.

REFERENCES

1. Alfakih K, Thiele H, Plein S, et al: Comparison of right ventricular volume measurement between segmented k-space gradient-echo and steady-state free precession magnetic resonance imaging. J Magn Reson Imaging 16:253–258, 2002.
2. Al-Saadi N, Nagel E, Gross M, et al: Noninvasive detection of myocardial ischemia from perfusion reserve based on cardiovascular magnetic resonance. Circulation 101:1379–1383, 2000.
3. Anderson LJ, Holden S, Davis B, et al: Cardiovascular T2-star (T2°) magnetic resonance for the early diagnosis of myocardial iron overload. Eur Heart J 22:2171–2179, 2001.
4. Arend WP, Michel BA, Bloch DA, et al: The American College of Rheumatology 1990 criteria for the classification of Takayasu arteritis. Arthritis Rheum 33:1129–1134, 1990.
5. Aurigemma GP, Reichek N, Axel L, et al: Noninvasive determination of coronary artery bypass graft patency by cine magnetic resonance imaging. Circulation 80:1595–1602, 1989.
6. Basso C, Maron BJ, Corrado D, et al: Clinical profile of congenital coronary artery anomalies with origin from the wrong aortic sinus leading to sudden death in young competitive athletes. J Am Coll Cardiol 35:1493–1501, 2000.
7. Beerbaum P, Korperich H, Barth P, et al: Noninvasive quantification of left-to-right shunt in pediatric patients: phase-contrast cine magnetic resonance imaging compared with invasive oximetry. Circulation 103:2476–2482, 2001.
8. Bellenger NG, Burgess MI, Ray SG, et al: Comparison of left ventricular ejection fraction and volumes in heart failure by echocardiography, radionuclide ventriculography and cardiovascular magnetic resonance; are they interchangeable? Eur Heart J 21:1387–1396, 2000.
9. Breen JF: Imaging of the pericardium. J Thorac Imaging 16:47–54, 2001.
10. Bunce NH, Lorenz CH, Keegan J, et al: Coronary artery anomalies: assessment with free-breathing three-dimensional coronary MR angiography. Radiology 227:201–208, 2003.
11. Chan SK, Jaffer FA, Botnar RM, et al: Scan reproducibility of magnetic resonance imaging assessment of aortic atherosclerosis burden. J Cardiovasc Magn Reson 3:331–338, 2001.
12. Chien CT, Lin CS, Hsu YH, et al: Potential diagnosis of hemodynamic abnormalities in patent ductus arteriosus by cine magnetic resonance imaging. Am Heart J 122:1065–1073, 1991.
13. Choudhury L, Mahrholdt H, Wagner A, et al: Myocardial scarring in asymptomatic or mildly symptomatic patients with hypertrophic cardiomyopathy. J Am Coll Cardiol 40:2155–2164, 2002.
14. Corrado D, Fontaine G, Marcus FI, et al: Arrhythmogenic right ventricular dysplasia/cardiomyopathy: need for an international registry. Study Group on Arrhythmogenic Right

890

Ventricular Dysplasia/Cardiomyopathy of the Working Groups on Myocardial and Pericardial Disease and Arrhythmias of the European Society of Cardiology and of the Scientific Council on Cardiomyopathies of the World Heart Federation. Circulation 101:E101–106, 2000.

15. Engelmann MG, Knez A, von Smekal A, et al: Non-invasive coronary bypass graft imaging after multivessel revascularisation. Int J Cardiol 76:65–74, 2000.

16. Erbel R, Alfonso F, Boileau C, et al: Diagnosis and management of aortic dissection. Eur Heart J 22:1642–1681, 2001.

17. Fattori R, Celletti F, Descovich B, et al: Evolution of post-traumatic aortic aneurysm in the subacute phase: magnetic resonance imaging follow-up as a support of the surgical timing. Eur J Cardiothorac Surg 13:582–586; discussion 586–587, 1998.

18. Fattori R, Descovich B, Bertaccini P, et al: Composite graft replacement of the ascending aorta: leakage detection with gadolinium-enhanced MR imaging. Radiology 212:573–577, 1999.

19. Fattori R, Napoli G, Lovato L, et al: Indications for, timing of, and results of catheter-based treatment of traumatic injury to the aorta. AJR Am J Roentgenol 179:603–609, 2002.

20. Fayad ZA, Nahar T, Fallon JT, et al: In vivo magnetic resonance evaluation of atherosclerotic plaques in the human thoracic aorta: a comparison with transesophageal echocardiography. Circulation 101:2503–2509, 2000.

21. Finn JP, Baskaran V, Carr JC, et al: Thorax: low-dose contrast-enhanced three-dimensional MR angiography with subsecond temporal resolution—initial results. Radiology 224:896–904, 2002.

22. Galjee MA, van Rossum AC, Doesburg T, et al: Value of magnetic resonance imaging in assessing patency and function of coronary artery bypass grafts. An angiographically controlled study. Circulation 93:660–666, 1996.

23. Gay SB, Sistrom CL, Holder CA, et al: Breath-holding capability of adults. Implications for spiral computed tomography, fast-acquisition magnetic resonance imaging, and angiography. Invest Radiol 29:848–851, 1994.

24. Gillinov AM, Lytle BW, Hoang V, et al: The atherosclerotic aorta at aortic valve replacement: surgical strategies and results. J Thorac Cardiovasc Surg 120:957–963, 2000.

25. Godart F, Labrot G, Devos P, et al: Coarctation of the aorta: comparison of aortic dimensions between conventional MR imaging, 3D MR angiography, and conventional angiography. Eur Radiol 12:2034–2039, 2002.

26. Hagan PG, Nienaber CA, Isselbacher EM, et al: The International Registry of Acute Aortic Dissection (IRAD): new insights into an old disease. JAMA 283:897–903, 2000.

27. Hartnell GG: Imaging of aortic aneurysms and dissection: CT and MRI. J Thorac Imaging 16:35–46, 2001.

28. Hartnell GG, Hughes LA, Ko JP, et al: Magnetic resonance imaging of pericardial constriction: comparison of cine MR angiography and spin-echo techniques. Clin Radiol 51:268–272, 1996.

29. Hartnell GG, Spence L, Hughes LA, et al: Safety of MR imaging in patients who have retained metallic materials after cardiac surgery. AJR Am J Roentgenol 168:1157–1159, 1997.

30. Hayashi H, Matsuoka Y, Sakamoto I, et al: Penetrating atherosclerotic ulcer of the aorta: imaging features and disease concept. Radiographics 20:995–1005, 2000.

31. Helbing WA, Bosch HG, Maliepaard C, et al: Comparison of echocardiographic methods with magnetic resonance imaging for assessment of right ventricular function in children. Am J Cardiol 76:589–594, 1995.

32. Higgins CB, De Roos A, editors: Cardiovascular MRI and MRA. Lippincott, Williams & Wilkins, 2002.

33. Hundley WG, Meshack BM, Willett DL, et al: Comparison of quantitation of left ventricular volume, ejection fraction, and

cardiac output in patients with atrial fibrillation by cine magnetic resonance imaging versus invasive measurements. Am J Cardiol 78:1119–1123, 1996.

34. Ibrahim T, Nekolla SG, Schreiber K, et al: Assessment of coronary flow reserve: comparison between contrast-enhanced magnetic resonance imaging and positron emission tomography. J Am Coll Cardiol 39:864–870, 2002.

35. Jenkins JP, Love HG, Foster CJ, et al: Detection of coronary artery bypass graft patency as assessed by magnetic resonance imaging. Br J Radiol 61:2–4, 1988.

36. Kerr GS, Hallahan CW, Giordano J, et al: Takayasu arteritis. Ann Intern Med 120:919–929, 1994.

37. Kilner PJ, Manzara CC, Mohiaddin RH, et al: Magnetic resonance jet velocity mapping in mitral and aortic valve stenosis. Circulation 87:1239–1248, 1993.

38. Kim RJ, Fieno DS, Parrish TB, et al: Relationship of MRI delayed contrast enhancement to irreversible injury, infarct age, and contractile function. Circulation 100:1992–2002, 1999.

39. Kim RJ, Wu E, Rafael A, et al: The use of contrast-enhanced magnetic resonance imaging to identify reversible myocardial dysfunction. N Engl J Med 343:1445–1453, 2000.

40. Kim WY, Danias PG, Stuber M, et al: Coronary magnetic resonance angiography for the detection of coronary stenoses. N Engl J Med 345:1863–1869, 2001.

41. Klein C, Nekolla SG, Bengel FM, et al: Assessment of myocardial viability with contrast-enhanced magnetic resonance imaging: comparison with positron emission tomography. Circulation 105:162–167, 2002.

42. Kojima S, Yamada N, Goto Y: Diagnosis of constrictive pericarditis by tagged cine magnetic resonance imaging. N Engl J Med 341:373–374, 1999.

43. Krinsky GA, Rofsky NM, DeCorato DR, et al: Thoracic aorta: comparison of gadolinium-enhanced three-dimensional MR angiography with conventional MR imaging. Radiology 202:183–193, 1997.

44. Kutz SM, Lee VS, Tunick PA, et al: Atheromas of the thoracic aorta: a comparison of transesophageal echocardiography and breath-hold gadolinium-enhanced 3-dimensional magnetic resonance angiography. J Am Soc Echocardiogr 12:853–858, 1999.

45. Langerak SE, Vliegen HW, de Roos A, et al: Detection of vein graft disease using high-resolution magnetic resonance angiography. Circulation 105:328–333, 2002.

46. Langerak SE, Vliegen HW, Jukema JW, et al: Value of magnetic resonance imaging for the noninvasive detection of stenosis in coronary artery bypass grafts and recipient coronary arteries. Circulation 107:1502–1508, 2003.

47. Manning WJ, Stuber M, Danias PG, et al: Coronary magnetic resonance imaging: current status. Curr Probl Cardiol 27:275–333, 2002.

48. Manning WJ, Pennell DJ, editors: Cardiovascular Magnetic Resonance. London: Churchill Livingstone, 2002.

49. Masui T, Finck S, Higgins CB: Constrictive pericarditis and restrictive cardiomyopathy: evaluation with MR imaging. Radiology 182:369–373, 1992.

50. Mirvis SE, Shanmuganathan K: MR imaging of thoracic trauma. Magn Reson Imaging Clin North Am 8:91–104, 2000.

51. Mollet NR, Dymarkowski S, Volders W, et al: Visualization of ventricular thrombi with contrast-enhanced magnetic resonance imaging in patients with ischemic heart disease. Circulation 106:2873–2876, 2002.

52. Murray JG, Manisali M, Flamm SD, et al: Intramural hematoma of the thoracic aorta: MR image findings and their prognostic implications. Radiology 204:349–355, 1997.

53. Nagel E, Lehmkuhl HB, Bocksch W, et al: Noninvasive diagnosis of ischemia-induced wall motion abnormalities with the use of high-dose dobutamine stress MRI: comparison

with dobutamine stress echocardiography. Circulation 99:763–770, 1999.

54. Nagel E, Lorenz C, Baer F, et al: Stress cardiovascular magnetic resonance: consensus panel report. J Cardiovasc Magn Reson 3:267–281, 2001.

55. Nienaber CA, Rehders TC, Fratz S: Detection and assessment of congenital heart disease with magnetic resonance techniques. J Cardiovasc Magn Reson 1:169–184, 1999.

56. Nienaber CA, von Kodolitsch Y, Petersen B, et al: Intramural hemorrhage of the thoracic aorta. Diagnostic and therapeutic implications. Circulation 92:1465–1472, 1995.

57. Pereles FS, McCarthy RM, Baskaran V, et al: Thoracic aortic dissection and aneurysm: evaluation with nonenhanced true FISP MR angiography in less than 4 minutes. Radiology 223:270–274, 2002.

58. Petersen SE, Voigtlander T, Kreitner KF, et al: Quantification of shunt volumes in congenital heart diseases using a breath-hold MR phase contrast technique—comparison with oximetry. Int J Cardiovasc Imaging 18:53–60, 2002.

59. Post JC, van Rossum AC, Bronzwaer JG, et al: Magnetic resonance angiography of anomalous coronary arteries. A new gold standard for delineating the proximal course? Circulation 92:3163–3171, 1995.

60. Prince MR, Arnoldus C, Frisoli JK: Nephrotoxicity of high-dose gadolinium compared with iodinated contrast. J Magn Reson Imaging 6:162–166, 1996.

61. Reichek N: MRI myocardial tagging. J Magn Reson Imaging 10:609–616, 1999.

62. Reinmuller R, Gurgan M, Erdmann E, et al: CT and MR evaluation of pericardial constriction: a new diagnostic and therapeutic concept. J Thorac Imaging 8:108–121, 1993.

63. Riquelme C, Laissy JP, Menegazzo D, et al: MR imaging of coarctation of the aorta and its postoperative complications in adults: assessment with spin-echo and cine-MR imaging. Magn Reson Imaging 17:37–46, 1999.

64. Rofsky NM, Weinreb JC, Grossi EA, et al: Aortic aneurysm and dissection: normal MR imaging and CT findings after surgical repair with the continuous-suture graft-inclusion technique. Radiology 186:195–201, 1993.

65. Rominger MB, Bachmann GF, Pabst W, et al: Right ventricular volumes and ejection fraction with fast cine MR imaging in breath-hold technique: applicability, normal values from 52 volunteers, and evaluation of 325 adult cardiac patients. J Magn Reson Imaging 10:908–918, 1999.

66. Rubinstein RI, Askenase AD, Thickman D, et al: Magnetic resonance imaging to evaluate patency of aortocoronary bypass grafts. Circulation 76:786–791, 1987.

67. Salton CJ, Chuang ML, O'Donnell CJ, et al: Gender differences and normal left ventricular anatomy in an adult population free of hypertension. A cardiovascular magnetic resonance study of the Framingham Heart Study Offspring cohort. J Am Coll Cardiol 39:1055–1060, 2002.

68. Schalla S, Nagel E, Lehmkuhl H, et al: Comparison of magnetic resonance real-time imaging of left ventricular function with conventional magnetic resonance imaging and echocardiography. Am J Cardiol 87:95–99, 2001.

69. Schmidta M, Theissen P, Klempt G, et al: Long-term follow-up of 82 patients with chronic disease of the thoracic aorta using spin-echo and cine gradient magnetic resonance imaging. Magn Reson Imaging 18:795–806, 2000.

70. Shimada T, Shimada K, Sakane T, et al: Diagnosis of cardiac sarcoidosis and evaluation of the effects of steroid therapy by gadolinium-DTPA-enhanced magnetic resonance imaging. Am J Med 110:520–527, 2001.

71. Simonetti OP, Kim RJ, Fieno DS, et al: An improved MR imaging technique for the visualization of myocardial infarction. Radiology 218:215–223, 2001.

72. Sommer T, Fehske W, Holzknecht N, et al: Aortic dissection: a comparative study of diagnosis with spiral CT, multiplanar transesophageal echocardiography, and MR imaging. Radiology 199:347–352, 1996.

73. Task Force of the European Society of Cardiology, in collaboration with the Association of European Paediatric Cardiologists. The clinical role of magnetic resonance in cardiovascular disease. Eur Heart J 19:19–39, 1998.

74. Taylor AM, Thorne SA, Rubens MB, et al: Coronary artery imaging in grown up congenital heart disease: complementary role of magnetic resonance and x-ray coronary angiography. Circulation 101:1670–1678, 2000.

75. Tesoro-Tess JD, Biasi S, Balzarini L, et al: Heart involvement in lymphomas. The value of magnetic resonance imaging and two-dimensional echocardiography at disease presentation. Cancer 72:2484–2490, 1993.

76. Therrien J, Thorne SA, Wright A, et al: Repaired coarctation: a "cost-effective" approach to identify complications in adults. J Am Coll Cardiol 35:997–1002, 2000.

77. Tittle SL, Lynch RJ, Cole PE, et al: Midterm follow-up of penetrating ulcer and intramural hematoma of the aorta. J Thorac Cardiovasc Surg 123:1051–1059, 2002.

78. Troxler M, Mavor AI, Homer-Vanniasinkam S: Penetrating atherosclerotic ulcers of the aorta. Br J Surg 88:1169–1177, 2001.

79. Tso E, Flamm SD, White RD, et al: Takayasu arteritis: utility and limitations of magnetic resonance imaging in diagnosis and treatment. Arthritis Rheum 46:1634–1642, 2002.

80. Tunick PA, Kronzon I: Atheromas of the thoracic aorta: clinical and therapeutic update. J Am Coll Cardiol 35:545–554, 2000.

81. Vliegen HW, Doornbos J, de Roos A, et al: Value of fast gradient echo magnetic resonance angiography as an adjunct to coronary arteriography in detecting and confirming the course of clinically significant coronary artery anomalies. Am J Cardiol 79:773–776, 1997.

82. Wagner A, Mahrholdt H, Holly TA, et al: Contrast-enhanced MRI and routine single photon emission computed tomography (SPECT) perfusion imaging for detection of subendocardial myocardial infarcts: an imaging study. Lancet 361:374–379, 2003.

83. White RD, Pflugfelder PW, Lipton MJ, et al: Coronary artery bypass grafts: evaluation of patency with cine MR imaging. AJR Am J Roentgenol 150:1271–1274, 1988.

84. Yamada I, Nakagawa T, Himeno Y, et al: Takayasu arteritis: diagnosis with breath-hold contrast-enhanced three-dimensional MR angiography. J Magn Reson Imaging 11:481–487, 2000.

85. Yamada I, Numano F, Suzuki S: Takayasu arteritis: evaluation with MR imaging. Radiology 188:89–94, 1993.

86. Yucel EK, Steinberg FL, Egglin TK, et al: Penetrating aortic ulcers: diagnosis with MR imaging. Radiology 177:779–781, 1990.

Nuclear Cardiology and Positron Emission Tomography in the Assessment of Patients with Cardiovascular Disease

Brian G. Abbott and Barry L. Zaret

▶ INTRODUCTION

Nuclear cardiology involves the imaging of cardiac radiopharmaceutical distribution to characterize physiological and pathophysiological processes in the heart. The ability to image myocardial perfusion and metabolism noninvasively with nuclear techniques has led to the development of a field that has been validated extensively and provides powerful diagnostic and prognostic information in the management of patients with known or suspected coronary artery disease (CAD). Moreover, nuclear cardiology procedures have been employed widely in the evaluation of patients prior to cardiac and noncardiac surgery. This chapter provides an overview of the concepts and techniques used in nuclear cardiology and summarizes its role in the assessment of patients with stable coronary disease and acute coronary syndromes and in the determination of myocardial viability in patients considered for revascularization. As a complete discussion of the technical and procedural aspects of nuclear cardiology is beyond the scope of this chapter, the central focus will be on the utilization of nuclear cardiology in patients with known or suspected CAD, with an emphasis on patients undergoing cardiac surgery. For a more detailed discussion the reader is referred to other more comprehensive reviews.[16,122]

General Principles

Nuclear cardiology has been dominated by radionuclide myocardial perfusion imaging (MPI) as a means to evaluate patients with known or suspected coronary disease. MPI is performed to evaluate diagnostically patients with symptoms suggestive of myocardial ischemia and to risk stratify patients with known CAD. Radionuclide MPI plays a central role in the evaluation of the cardiac patient and is in widespread clinical use, with more than 5 million MPI procedures performed in the United States annually.[5]

Myocardial perfusion is governed during resting conditions by the coronary resistance vessels. During periods of increased work, such as during exercise, flow is increased to balance the metabolic demands of the myocardium. This is achieved by vasodilation of precapillary arterioles, which reduces vascular resistance in the coronary arterial bed. In stenotic, atherosclerotic coronary arteries, resting flow is maintained by decreasing downstream vascular resistance. While this compensation maintains flow under resting

894 conditions, a significant stenosis (>50–70% narrowing of the lumen) impairs coronary flow reserve, or the ability of the artery to increase flow appropriately during periods of increased demand.

Radioactive Tracers

Myocardial perfusion is imaged with the use of radiopharmaceuticals that accumulate rapidly in the myocardium in proportion to myocardial blood flow. The most commonly used radiotracers currently are the technetium-99m-labeled (^{99m}Tc) compounds sestamibi and tetrofosmin, and, to a lesser extent, thallium (^{201}Tl). When injected intravenously, these tracers are extracted from the blood pool and accumulate in cells, including myocytes, that have an intact cell membrane and are metabolically active. ^{99m}Tc sestamibi and tetrofosmin are lipophilic cationic complexes that are taken up by myocytes across mitochondrial membranes, but at equilibrium are retained within the mitochondria because of a large negative transmembrane potential. ^{201}Tl is transported like potassium across the myocyte sarcolemmal membrane, via the Na$^+$-K$^+$-ATPase transport system. Because the retention of radiotracer is proportional to myocardial flow, the amount of tracer uptake is a surrogate visualized representation of regional myocardial perfusion. The tracers used are radioactive isotopes that undergo radioactive decay over a short period of time.

Equipment and Procedures

As the accumulated radiotracer decays, photons are emitted that exit the body and can be detected using a specialized gamma camera. MPI employs the use of single-photon emission computed tomography (SPECT) techniques to acquire and ultimately display the perfusion distribution obtained from the radiotracer uptake. After the radiopharmaceutical is injected, the patient lies supine on the SPECT camera table and is positioned in the gantry of the camera. As the camera detector moves around the patient, emitted photons interact with the camera's crystal and produce scintillations of light that represent the spatial distribution of radioactivity in the patient. The emitted "counts" localized to each region of the myocardium are then stored digitally. This three-dimensional representation of myocardial perfusion is then processed and reconstructed using computer algorithms to display the acquired information in a series of slices, oriented in the short axis and horizontal and vertical long axes of the left ventricle. The slices are then displayed on a computer screen for visual inspection of regional myocardial perfusion as well as computer quantification of tracer uptake. The stress images, acquired after injection of radiotracer during exercise or pharmacological stress (described later in detail), are displayed adjacent to images acquired at rest, permitting direct comparison of perfusion in the two imaging states. The maximum uptake of radiotracer in the heart is used to represent normal perfusion, and the rest of the myocardial counts are considered as relative uptake to this maximum. A regional perfusion defect on the stress images that is not present on the resting study is considered to be "reversible" and consistent with stress-induced ischemia in that vascular territory. A defect that persists on stress and rest is deemed "fixed" and representative

of scar/prior myocardial infarction (Figure 56-1). Quantitative programs are commonly used to assess the extent and severity of each defect, which is then incorporated into the final interpretation of regional myocardial perfusion. The perfusion images are also obtained in concert with electrocardiographic (ECG) gating, which stores the counts with respect to the timing of the cardiac cycle. By gating the acquisition to the R-R interval of the ECG, images from each frame can be summed and displayed as a movie of the left ventricle contracting from diastole to systole. Performing gated SPECT facilitates measurement of left ventricular ejection fraction (LVEF) and LV volumes by automated computer algorithms, as well as visual inspection of the movie for regional wall motion and thickening[7,8] (Figure 56-2).

A typical SPECT MPI protocol involves the performance of exercise, typically on a treadmill or bicycle, or with a pharmacological stressor, such as adenosine, dipyridamole, or dobutamine in patients unable to perform physical exercise. The radiotracer is injected at peak stress and the stressor is then continued for an additional 1–2 min to maximize myocardial extraction of the circulating tracer. Imaging is performed 30–60 min later for sestamibi or tetrofosmin, since these agents have only minimal redistribution or washout from the myocardium. The initial imaging can be either at rest or at stress and both studies can be performed on the same day. Although ^{201}Tl is used less commonly for stress MPI, it is commonly used for rest imaging in a "dual isotope" protocol. In this protocol ^{201}Tl is injected for resting imaging, which is then followed immediately by stress perfusion imaging with ^{99m}Tc agent,[8] thus obviating the need to wait 2–3 h for the first dose to decay. As such, imaging time is reduced and patient throughput is increased.

▶ STABLE CORONARY ARTERY DISEASE (DIAGNOSIS AND RISK STRATIFICATION)

Stress Testing in the Detection of Coronary Artery Disease

Nuclear cardiology is a central part of the evaluation of patients with suspected or proven CAD. The ability of SPECT myocardial perfusion imaging to detect CAD in patients with symptoms suggestive of ischemic heart disease has been validated extensively.

Exercise Stress Testing

Exercise stress testing without adjunct noninvasive imaging is frequently used as the initial screening test in patients without known CAD who present with chest pain syndromes or symptoms suggestive of ischemia. The premise of exercise stress testing is that the increased myocardial oxygen demand during exercise will produce clinical signs of ischemia (angina, ECG changes) in the setting of a flow-limiting stenosis that impairs myocardial blood supply. The diagnostic performance of this test varies greatly depending on the pretest likelihood of the population being studied. In patients with an intermediate pretest probability of CAD on the basis of symptoms and risk factors, exercise treadmill testing is useful as an initial screening test. However, the overall sensitivity of treadmill exercise testing is approximately

70%. A meta-analysis of more than 24,000 patients undergoing exercise stress testing and coronary angiography observed a mean sensitivity of 68% and a mean specificity of 77%. Accuracy was greatest in patients with multivessel coronary disease and those with left main or three-vessel CAD.[35]

Exercise Stress Myocardial Perfusion Imaging

Because exercise treadmill testing relies on changes in the 12-lead ECG as a surrogate of ischemia, the accuracy of the test is highly dependent on the baseline electrocardiogram.

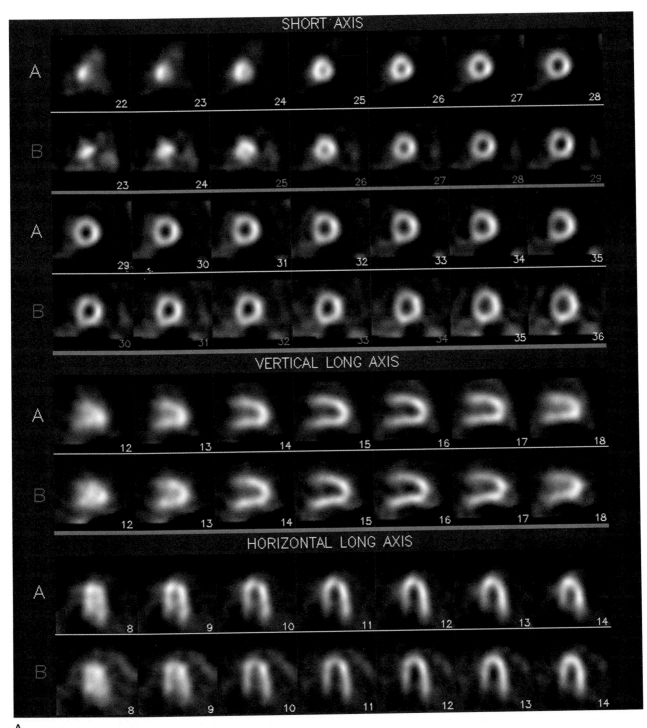

A

Figure 56–1 SPECT myocardial perfusion imaging. Visual display of SPECT myocardial perfusion imaging with stress study above the rest study for comparison. Each panel contains three representations of the same imaging procedure, each oriented differently: short-axis slices from apex to mid-ventricle and mid-ventricle to base (top), vertical long-axis slices from septum to lateral wall (middle), and horizontal long-axis slices from inferior to anterior wall (bottom). **A,** The first set of images is a normal study in grayscale with uniform uptake of radiotracer on stress and rest.

(Continued)

896 Abnormalities such as previous myocardial infarction (Q waves or left bundle branch block) or ST-T wave changes due to left ventricular hypertrophy or therapy with digoxin hamper the ability to interpret ischemic changes accurately during exercise. In patients with an abnormal ECG, myocardial perfusion imaging adds significant diagnostic accuracy to the treadmill test for detecting CAD.

Numerous studies have consistently shown that SPECT myocardial perfusion imaging with technetium-labeled agents, such as sestamibi, yields a >90% sensitivity for the detection of CAD.[11,16,31,81] False negative scans tend to occur in the setting of single-vessel disease, particularly in the left circumflex artery distribution, a mild degree of stenosis <70%, or when the patient is unable to achieve the

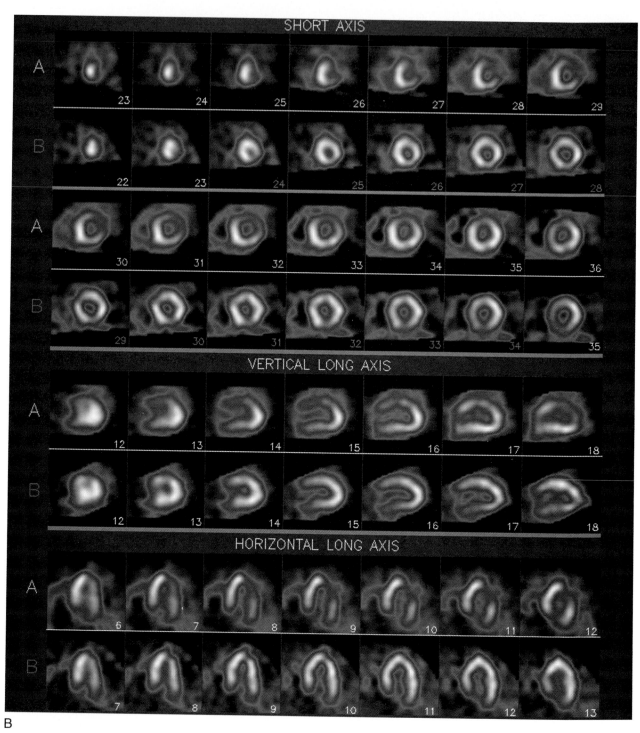

B

Figure 56–1 cont'd B, A color-enhanced study. Review of the stress images demonstrates a perfusion defect in the anterolateral wall as evidenced by less radiotracer accumulation relative to other regions of the left ventricle. As the corresponding rest images show normal perfusion throughout the myocardium, the perfusion defect is considered "reversible," consistent with ischemia.

Chapter 56 ■ Nuclear Cardiology and Positron Emission Tomography in the Assessment of Patients with Cardiovascular Disease

897

target heart rate or is taking antianginal therapy. These studies have also observed that the specificity of stress SPECT imaging is in the range of 68%. The less optimal specificity can be attributed to both referral bias (performing angiography in only those patients with abnormal scans), as well as false positive scans with defects due to artifacts produced by soft tissue attenuation (diaphragm, breast) or patient motion. Contemporary imaging techniques that employ ECG gating have facilitated the simultaneous assessment of myocardial perfusion and function. Examination of regional wall motion and thickening enhances the evaluation of a suspect area of hypoperfusion by providing the ability to distinguish true myocardial scarring from attenuation. More recent technical advances such as attenuation correction hold promise in further improving the specificity of SPECT MPI.

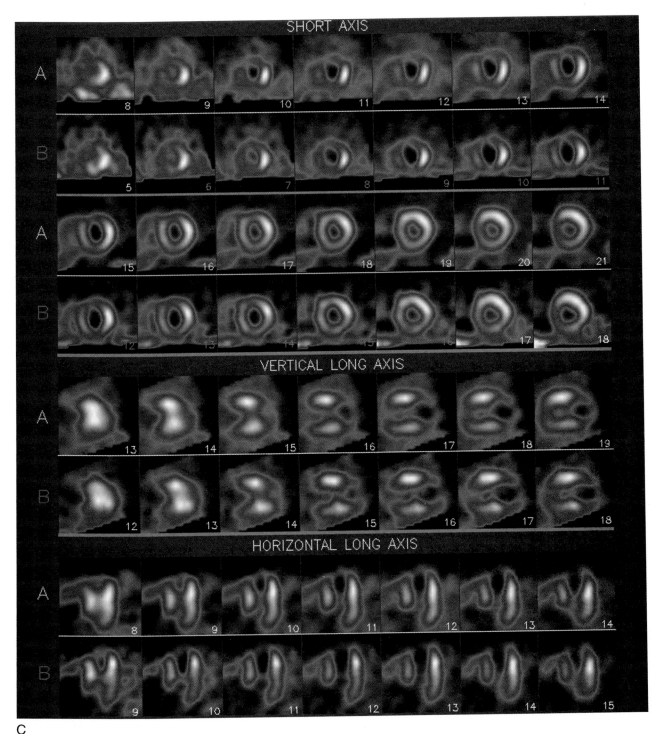

C

Figure 56–1 cont'd C, The SPECT images demonstrate large perfusion defects in the anteroseptal, inferoseptal, and apical regions, which are present on both the stress and rest images. Because these defects do not show any change from stress to rest, they are termed "fixed" defects, consistent with scar (prior myocardial infarction).

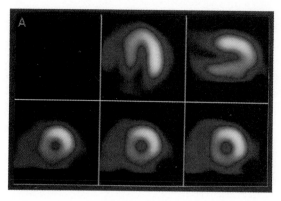

SYSTOLE

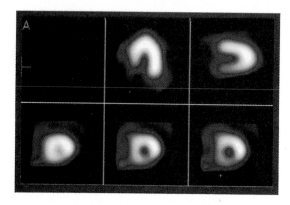

LEFT VENTRICULAR EJECTION
FRACTION AND VOLUMES

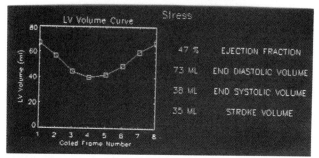

Figure 56–2 **Gated SPECT still frame images of diastole and systole.** During SPECT image acquisition, the acquired images can be stored in relation to the cardiac cycle using the R-R interval of the ECG. The resulting images that are "gated" to the cardiac cycle can then be viewed as a cine-loop from diastole to systole. Moreover, these data can be used to calculate left ventricular volumes during diastole and systole, as well as the corresponding left ventricular ejection fraction (diastole–systole).

Pharmacological Stress MPI

As many patients are unable to perform physical exercise to a workload adequate for a diagnostic exercise stress test, myocardial perfusion imaging performed after pharmacological stress is used frequently as an alternative.° This is typically performed after the intravenous infusion of a vasodilator, such as dipyridamole or adenosine, or with the

°References 56, 58, 71, 75, 79, 90.

inotrope dobutamine. Dipyridamole stimulates the release of endogenous adenosine in the distal coronary vasculature, which then binds adenosine receptors in the vasculature producing the desired effect of coronary artery vasodilation, as well as undesirable effects such as flushing, bronchospasm, headache, and even transient heart block. This vasodilation of the resistance vessels increases myocardial blood flow, mimicking the effects of physical exercise. Dipyridamole is typically administered intravenously as a bolus injection over 4 min with peak effect occurring at 8 min, at which time the radiotracer is injected.[81] A 4- to 6-min continuous infusion of intravenous adenosine is now used more commonly.[91] Both agents are equally effective in increasing myocardial blood flow 3- to 5-fold over rest, which is similar to that produced by exercise. However, adenosine tends to achieve maximal flow in more patients than dipyridamole; and short-lived side effects (i.e., hypotension, atrioventricular [AV] block, chest pain, and flushing) are more common with adenosine than dipyridamole.[58]

An intravenous infusion of dobutamine is also effective for pharmacological stress. It is typically used as an alternative to vasodilator stress in patients with bronchospasm and pulmonary disease. The dobutamine infusion produces increased myocardial oxygen demand by increasing heart rate, blood pressure, and myocardial contractility.

All of the currently used pharmacological stress agents have similar ability to produce flow heterogeneity and corresponding perfusion defects in the presence of a significant (>50–70%) stenosis of a coronary artery. A meta-analysis of dipyridamole SPECT imaging demonstrated a sensitivity of 89% and specificity of 65% for the detection of CAD. Dipyridamole and adenosine tests had essentially similar sensitivities and specificities. The sensitivity of dobutamine SPECT imaging to detect CAD is approximately 80%, which is slightly lower than that of the vasodilator agents.[62]

Several novel agents designed to bind specifically to the adenosine A_{2a} receptors responsible for coronary artery vasodilation are currently under investigation. Preliminary data suggest that these A_{2a} receptor agonists may selectively increase coronary blood flow without producing the side effects described previously.

Prognosis and Risk Stratification

Stable Angina

The goals of stress testing extend beyond the detection of CAD alone. For stress testing information to be useful, results must reliably identify patients of sufficiently low risk that further evaluation or intervention can be safely avoided, while also providing additional information to the clinical risk assessment when results are abnormal. The ability of both exercise and pharmacological MPI to add incremental prognostic information to the clinical risk assessment in patients with known CAD has been evaluated in thousands of patients.[54] Several large studies of patients with known or suspected CAD, including both men and women, have demonstrated the incremental prognostic value of a normal MPI.[43,44] Perhaps of greatest clinical utility is that these studies have consistently shown that patients with normal MPI have a subsequent annual rate of cardiac death and nonfatal MI of less than 1%, even in patients with known CAD.[41,42,44]

When the results are abnormal, the SPECT scan provides incremental prognostic information beyond that obtained by clinical, ECG, and stress testing combined. Moreover, the value of SPECT MPI in determining prognosis is such that the information obtained from subsequent coronary angiography does not provide any incremental prognostic information beyond that obtained by the SPECT results alone.[42,44,55,117] The increase in the risk of hard events increases in proportion to the severity and extent of the perfusion defect when assessed by semiquantitative methods or automated quantitative approaches. The degree of ischemia on SPECT is associated with an increase in the short-term incidence of nonfatal myocardial infarction (MI), while scar size is more predictive of cardiac death.[21,67,101] Other important stress MPI variables that are predictive of future cardiac events are listed in Box 56-1. The prognostic ability of stress MPI is also enhanced by inclusion of ECG-gated SPECT, which permits assessment of left ventricular global systolic performance, the most potent predictor of event-free survival, as well as analysis of regional wall motion.[76,101,102]

Medical Therapy vs. Revascularization

One of the most important contributions of stress MPI in the clinical evaluation of patients with known or suspected CAD is the ability to provide prognostic information that can be used to guide further testing and therapies. Because the extent and severity of ischemia on a stress MPI study is directly proportional to the risk of future cardiac events, this information can be incorporated into the decision-making process concerning medical or revascularization therapies for a given patient. Patients with mild ischemic defects that are not high risk generally can be safely treated medically, while those with high-risk findings should be strongly considered for more invasive evaluation with a lower threshold for revascularization. A 3-year follow-up study of patients with mild to moderate defects on stress SPECT MPI treated with medical therapy noted a 2% incidence of cardiac death or nonfatal infarction and <5% rate of revascularization, suggesting that SPECT imaging is highly useful in selecting patients with CAD at a sufficiently low risk for events such that revascular-

ization is not necessary.[92] In contrast, the benefit of revascularization over medical therapy has been characterized in patients with high-risk stress SPECT MPI findings. Hachamovitch and colleagues[44] followed up 5183 patients after stress MPI for a mean of 2 years and found that the rates of MI and cardiac death did not differ substantially between patients treated with medical therapy or revascularization after a normal or mildly abnormal scan. However, patients with severely abnormal scans had a significantly higher annualized cardiac death rate when treated medically (4.6%/year) compared to those referred for revascularization (1.3%/year) (Figure 56-3).[44] Patients with a greater ischemic burden on imaging were also found to benefit more from revascularization than medical therapy, with serial imaging studies showing a greater reduction in reversible defect size in those treated with revascularization.[17] Thus, revascularization can be employed selectively in patients with CAD based on the extent and severity of the ischemic burden. Patients with low-risk findings can be treated medically, while more extensive ischemia is best treated with more aggressive interventions.

These principles have been shown to impact favorably in terms of both patient outcomes and cost when applied clinically. Several large studies have focused on the clinical utilization of stress MPI to guide patient management and have shown that referral for coronary angiography is accordingly low (~3.5%) after a normal stress MPI, but increases to 60% when the stress MPI was moderately to severely abnormal.[14,42,44] This demonstrates that clinicians can incorporate MPI into their practice appropriately, particularly when deferring further invasive evaluation when the MPI is normal. The use of stress MPI to guide patient management has also been demonstrated to be cost effective. An "ischemia-guided" approach to managing patients with CAD has been shown to optimize utilization of angiography and subsequent revascularization procedures. The Economics of Noninvasive Diagnosis (END) study[104] compared differences in cost in 11,372 consecutive patients referred for either stress MPI or cardiac catheterization as the initial approach. Not only were the rates of subsequent MI the same in the two groups, costs were significantly higher for the direct cardiac catheterization group as compared to the MPI ischemia-guided approach. Moreover, patients sent directly to cardiac catheterization were more likely to be treated with coronary revascularization in all subsets of risk when compared to those undergoing stress MPI initially. The ischemia-guided approach to stable angina was found to be less costly, with less interventions and similar cardiac event rates. These cost differences can be directly attributed to a decrease in apparent unnecessary procedures in patients with negative MPI results.

Preoperative Evaluation for Noncardiac Surgery

Perioperative cardiac events are an important cause of morbidity and mortality during and after noncardiac surgery, and occur in more than 2% of patients undergoing these procedures. Much of this risk can be assessed preoperatively via clinical evaluation (presence of history of coronary artery or cerebrovascular disease, congestive heart failure, renal insufficiency, insulin-requiring diabetes, or high-risk surgical procedure) to identify patients at high risk for cardiac complications who might benefit from risk-reduction strategies (specific perioperative medical therapy or revascularization),

---

Box 56–1. Stress Testing Variables Associated with Worse Prognosis.

Perfusion parameters
    Multivessel disease pattern
    Large reversible (ischemic) defect
    Large scar >14% of left ventricle
    Transient left ventricular dilation with stress
    Right ventricular uptake
    Resting left ventricular dysfunction
    Pulmonary uptake of ^{201}Tl
Nonperfusion parameters
    Poor exercise capacity
    Angina at low workload
    Dynamic ST-segment depression ≥ 3 mm with exercise
    Exercise-induced ventricular arrhythmias
    Vasodilator stress-induced ST segment depression ≥ 1 mm
    Hypotensive blood pressure response

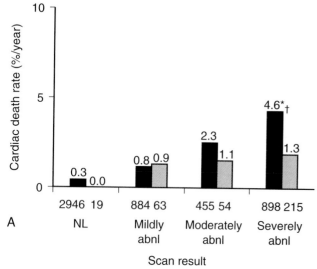

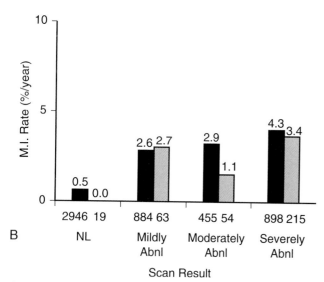

Figure 56–3 SPECT myocardial perfusion imaging and prognosis. This large retrospective analysis of patients undergoing stress SPECT myocardial perfusion imaging demonstrates the incremental prognostic information obtained with the imaging results. The annualized incidence of cardiac death (**A**) and myocardial infarction (**B**) is displayed for patients treated medically (solid columns) and those undergoing revascularization (gray columns) with respect to the myocardial perfusion imaging scan result. Annualized cardiac events were low (<1%) in both groups with normal SPECT studies. However, event rates increased with respect to the degree of SPECT abnormality. Survival was significantly improved in those with severely abnormal scans who underwent revascularization. (*$p < .01$ vs. patients undergoing revascularization early after nuclear testing; $^{†}p < .001$ within patients treated with medical therapy after nuclear testing; NL, normal; Abnl, abnormal.)
(Reprinted with permission from Hachamovitch R, Berman DS, Shaw LJ, et al: Incremental prognostic value of myocardial perfusion single photon emission computed tomography for the prediction of cardiac death: differential stratification for risk of cardiac death and myocardial infarction. Circulation 97:535–543, 1998.)

and subjects of sufficiently low risk that further evaluation prior to surgery is not necessary. However, patients with an intermediate risk for cardiac complications may benefit from further noninvasive testing to identify ischemia and provide further risk stratification prior to surgery.[30] Provocative testing for ischemia is typically performed in such patients. However, exercise testing is not always feasible in patients with pulmonary disease or low exercise capacity, and in particular those undergoing orthopedic or vascular surgery. Pharmacological stress MPI has been shown to add significant information to preoperative risk stratification. It is recommended for those patients with intermediate clinical risk predictors (prior MI, diabetes, renal insufficiency) who have poor functional capacity or those undergoing a high-risk surgical procedure (emergent surgery, aortic or peripheral vascular surgery, prolonged procedures with anticipated large blood loss or volume shifts).* When results of stress MPI are normal, the incidence of perioperative cardiac events has been shown to be approximately 1% for all procedures, including major vascular surgery. When abnormal, the severity and extent of ischemia are the most important predictors of adverse cardiac events during and after surgery.[30,32,109]

▶ ACUTE CORONARY SYNDROMES

Territory at Risk and Infarct Size

Resting MPI has been used to determine the territory at risk during an acute coronary syndrome and can be used to assess the extent of myocardial salvage achieved with reperfusion strategies.[46] ^{99m}Tc-labeled radiopharmaceuticals can be injected at rest in the setting of an acute ST-segment elevation MI upon presentation. After initial treatment and stabilization with either pharmacological or mechanical reperfusion, perfusion images can be acquired that represent the initial myocardial area at risk *during* the coronary occlusion. These images are then compared to those acquired at rest after a subsequent injection *after* reperfusion. The difference in the size of the defect is the "salvage index" (initial territory at risk—ultimate scar) between these two scans, which represents the degree of myocardium that was rescued by reperfusion. Although this methodology is not used widely in clinical practice, it is a useful tool in the evaluation of therapies used in the treatment of acute MI. The salvage index has been validated as a surrogate marker of patient outcome, and provides a quantitative means to compare the efficacy of therapeutic strategies.[23,37] The use of the infarct size, territory at risk, and the salvage index has played a central role in trials focusing on the efficacy of primary angioplasty[25,119] and thrombolysis.[23] This methodology can also assist in determining important clinical factors associated with reperfusion outcome such as time to reperfusion[48] and the significance of electrocardiographic changes.[119]

Myocardial infarct size can be measured quantitatively after MI and has been shown to be highly predictive of outcome.[37,52,83,84] The ischemic burden on cardiac stress SPECT imaging is associated with future nonfatal myocardial infarction, whereas fixed perfusion defects and a depressed ejection

---

*References 12, 30, 32, 103, 109, 115.

fraction are predictive of future cardiac death.[101] Quantification of the infarct size as a percentage of the left ventricle is an effective means to risk stratify a patient's risk for cardiac death over the near term. Studies using [99mTc] SPECT after acute MI have observed that mortality within the subsequent 24 months was approximately 8% if the infarct encompassed more than 12–14% of the left ventricle.[83,84]

Rest MPI for Acute Coronary Syndrome

The triage of patients presenting to the emergency department (ED) with acute chest pain is a substantial diagnostic challenge. Radionuclide myocardial perfusion imaging has been shown to have favorable diagnostic and prognostic value in this setting, with an excellent sensitivity to detect acute MI that is not recognized by other testing modalities (i.e., serum markers, ECG).[47,65,66,110,118] A major advantage of a triage protocol that employs rest SPECT MPI is that ischemia/infarction can be detected earlier than with serum markers. A patient with chest pain and an ECG that is normal or nondiagnostic for ischemia or infarction can be injected in the ED and then imaged within 30–60 min (Figure 56-4). Several observational and randomized studies have repeatedly shown that a normal resting perfusion imaging study has a negative predictive value > 99% to exclude MI and that defects at rest are associated with a higher incidence of death and MI at 30 days.[2,113,118] As such, a normal resting MPI in a patient with chest pain essentially excludes acute MI (AMI) and is predictive of a sufficiently low risk of near-term adverse cardiac events that the patient can be discharged home. Alternatively, an abnormal study is associated with a worse near-term outcome, and hospitalization is warranted. Once MI or unstable angina has been excluded, provocative testing can be performed, with or without MPI, to identify stress-induced ischemia. Protocols that utilize immediate rest MPI to exclude an acute coronary syndrome, and subsequent stress testing to evaluate for significant CAD, have demonstrated both reductions in unnecessary hospitalizations and cost savings compared to routine care.[1,95,118]

Post-Myocardial Infarction Risk Stratification

Stress MPI has been shown to have excellent diagnostic value in patients after an AMI. Dipyridamole vasodilator stress MPI early after AMI is highly predictive of future cardiac events. In fact, recent studies have found that the most important predictors of future cardiac death and recurrent MI are the extent and severity of degree of the reversible (ischemic) myocardial perfusion defect. Brown and colleagues[22] reported the results of a multicenter trial that randomized 451 patients after a first AMI to either early (hospital Days 2–4) dipyridamole stress MPI or routine predischarge (hospital Days 6–12) submaximal exercise MPI. The extent and severity of the stress defect and the degree of defect reversibility were found to be the most important predictors of cardiac death and recurrent MI. The early use of pharmacological stress perfusion imaging after AMI was more predictive of early and late cardiac events and provided greater incremental diagnostic and prognostic value than predischarge submaximal exercise perfusion imaging. One major advantage of this approach is that management decisions can be made much earlier in the hospital course after an uncomplicated AMI.

▶ ASSESSMENT OF MYOCARDIAL VIABILITY

Left Ventricular Ejection Fraction and Prognosis

Numerous studies have demonstrated that left ventricular systolic performance is a powerful and independent predictor

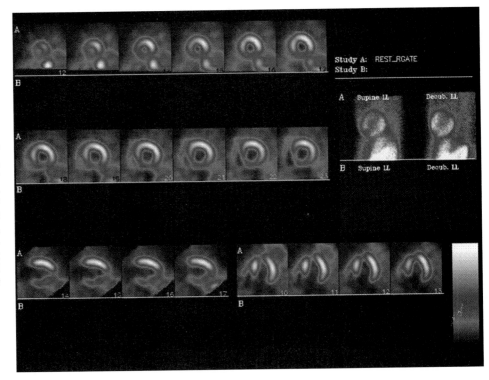

Figure 56-4 Rest SPECT myocardial perfusion imaging during ongoing chest pain in a patient with a normal electrocardiogram. Injection of radiotracer during ongoing chest pain and subsequent imaging 45 min later demonstrates a moderate-sized area of decreased perfusion in the inferior wall. The patient was brought directly to cardiac catheterization, and coronary angiography demonstrated a 95% stenosis of the right coronary artery that was treated with angioplasty and intracoronary stenting.

902 of mortality in patients both with and without CAD. When the left ventricular ejection fraction (LVEF) becomes depressed after MI or with chronic ischemic heart disease, the risk of sudden cardiac death increases substantially.[18,24,45,89]

Data from the Thrombolysis in Myocardial Infarction (TIMI) trials indicated the prognostic significance of LVEF assessment was also maintained after thrombolysis, although the overall mortality was lower than in the prethrombolytic era.[123] The powerful prognostic significance of resting LVEF assessed by radionuclide angiography is also important in patients treated with thrombolysis or primary angioplasty.[24,38] Resting LVEF not only is the strongest predictor of 6-month mortality, but is also predictive of ventricular arrhythmias and sudden death in a similar group of patients.[78] The prognostic significance of LVEF in patients with chronic CAD is also well established and is independent of the extent of anatomical disease.[86]

All of the available techniques used to assess left ventricular function, including nuclear techniques such as radionuclide angiography and gated SPECT, as well as two-dimensional echocardiography, contrast ventriculography, and magnetic resonance imaging, can provide similar prognostic information in patients with myocardial infarction and chronic CAD. Radionuclide angiography is the most accurate, widely validated, and reproducible technique, making it a useful tool when serial measurements of LVEF are required.[116] However, the more widespread utilization of two-dimensional resting echocardiography and gated SPECT MPI has led to these modalities replacing radionuclide angiography for the assessment of LVEF. Ejection fraction assessed during gated SPECT stress MPI provides incremental prognostic information beyond the perfusion imaging results. In a study of 1680 patients undergoing stress MPI, patients with a gated SPECT LVEF ≥45% had low mortality rates (<1%/year), even when associated with severe perfusion defects. However, patients with an LVEF <45% on gated SPECT had a mortality rate of 9.2%/year, even if only mild/moderate perfusion abnormalities were present.[102] This underscores the importance of LVEF in determining prognosis and the need to pursue aggressive medical and surgical strategies in patients with depressed LVEF.

PET and SPECT in Determining Myocardial Viability

Because LVEF is a major determinant of survival in patients with ischemic heart disease, therapeutic strategies that may improve systolic performance and thereby improve survival have been widely studied. Patients with chronic CAD and patients after AMI represent two important groups at risk for the development of left ventricular dysfunction. However, left ventricular systolic dysfunction is not always due to scarring and fibrosis of the myocardium and may be the result of the repetitive and/or chronic myocardial, ischemia. As such, left ventricular dysfunction at rest may not necessarily be irreversible. Thus the evaluation of patients with ischemic cardiomyopathies due to chronic CAD or MI becomes important in order to select which patients might have reversible dysfunction and potentially benefit from coronary revascularization.

Ischemic myocardial dysfunction may be produced by four pathophysiological processes. After MI, the myocardium within the vascular territory served by an acutely occluded culprit artery may undergo necrosis and scarring, leading to extensive fibrosis and subsequent regional dysfunction. With an acute coronary syndrome, if myocardial blood flow is restored either spontaneously or with a therapeutic reperfusion strategy such as angioplasty or thrombolysis, regional contractile dysfunction may occur even without myocardial necrosis, a state that has been termed "stunning." This postischemic dysfunction after a transient period of ischemia followed by reperfusion is characterized by normal flow but reduced function in the absence of myocardial scarring. Regional dysfunction may also be observed in chronic CAD, with reductions in blood flow presumably occurring more slowly. The contractile impairment is thought to be due to a compensatory down-regulation of function during prolonged periods of myocardial hypoperfusion, a concept termed "hibernation." Left ventricular dysfunction may also deteriorate due to "remodeling," characterized by histological and biochemical changes in the myocardium as a result of an ischemic insult.

Myocardial viability was initially defined as the ability to recover global and/or regional left ventricular function after revascularization. In this paradigm, treatment of repetitive or chronic ischemia, defined pathologically as stunning and hibernation, respectively, was deemed responsible for the improvement in contractility. As such the ability to identify dysfunctional but viable myocardium due to these pathological states became important when considering a patient for potential revascularization.

Although recovery of function may be an important goal of revascularization, the central goal of assessing myocardial viability is to predict outcome with therapy, e.g., differentiate patients with potentially reversible left ventricular dysfunction whose prognosis may be improved with revascularization from those with large areas of infarct/scar who may not benefit (or even do worse) with surgery. Thus, viability assessment provides better insight into the risk:benefit ratio in patients with ischemic left ventricular dysfunction by effectively stratifying those with a significant amount of viable myocardium who are at increased risk if treated medically from those who would be at high risk with either treatment.

At present, there exist a number of diagnostic approaches for assessing myocardial viability in patients with ischemic cardiomyopathy. The major nuclear cardiology modalities to determine viability include techniques that assess cell membrane integrity, regional perfusion, and/or myocardial metabolism.

Viability assessments are typically performed in a particular subset of patients, namely those with known CAD and left ventricular systolic dysfunction who are potential candidates for surgical revascularization. Most viability assessment is performed in patients with chronic ischemic cardiomyopathies, or after acute myocardial infarction, since as many as 50% of patients with prior MI will have residual viable myocardium.[20] The methods utilized for viability assessment are similar to those used for prognostic assessment in patients with CAD. As such, protocols used for stress MPI can be easily modified to obtain information regarding viability. However, if the assessment of viability is the principal clinical question, a protocol designed to assess viability specifically should be used. The nuclear cardiology techniques that have been validated extensively in the assessment of myocardial viability include the use of positron emission tomography (PET) imaging of myocardial metabolism, and resting SPECT perfusion imaging of ^{201}Tl and the ^{99m}Tc-labeled tracers sestamibi and tetrofosmin.

Positron Emission Tomography

PET is generally considered the noninvasive "gold standard" for viability assessment. PET viability studies involve the determination and comparison of both myocardial blood flow and the metabolic status of the myocardium.[9,100] Perfusion is usually assessed with ^{13}N-labeled NH$_3$, and glucose utilization is typically assessed with [^{18}F]fluorodeoxyglucose (FDG), which when taken up by the myocardium reflects glucose transport across the myocyte membrane. FDG accumulates in myocytes in proportion to glucose uptake, but undergoes phosphorylation by hexokinase to FDG-6-phosphate in the first step of glycolysis. FDG-6-phosphate is a form of deoxyglucose that becomes "trapped" in the myocyte and is not metabolized further. As such, FDG uptake indirectly reflects exogenous glucose utilization. Normal myocardium preferentially utilizes fatty acids for energy, but switches to increased glucose utilization during periods of ischemia. In myocardial regions with ischemic dysfunction, myocardial glucose uptake may be increased, and thus FDG uptake will be enhanced, reflecting viability. Conversely, FDG will not accumulate in areas of fibrosis or scar. FDG uptake is then compared to resting perfusion imaging. Perfusion metabolism is considered "matched" if areas of preserved flow show normal metabolic activity, and areas of reduced flow have diminished FDG uptake (scar). However, perfusion and metabolism may be discordant or "mismatched." In this scenario, FDG uptake will be present in areas of hypoperfusion, indicating that despite decreased blood flow, the myocardium is still metabolically active, hence viable. This mismatched defect is the most predictive of functional recovery after revascularization (Figure 56-5).

Quantitative Methods

The clinical assessment of myocardial viability using FDG is based predominantly on comparison of its qualitative or semiquantitative uptake relative to a myocardial perfusion tracer. Quantification of myocardial glucose uptake is possible but requires kinetic modeling of transmembrane transport and phosphorylation to adjust for the behavior of injected FDG in relation to endogenous glucose.[63,64,114] Another quantitative approach is the assessment of myocardial glucose utilization, using dynamic PET acquisitions and sequential arterial blood sampling to measure fractional [^{18}F]FDG uptake in relation to the delivered dose.

Perhaps of equal importance is the ability of cardiac PET to determine absolute myocardial blood flow using tracer kinetic models. Quantitative myocardial blood flow can be measured with dynamic imaging of ^{13}N-labeled ammonia, [82]Rb, or H$_2$[15]O. These agents can be used to determine regional myocardial blood flow. Flow can be measured at rest and after pharmacological vasodilation to determine the myocardial blood flow reserve (ratio of maximal flow:resting flow). This coronary flow reserve has been used in the assessment of stenosis severity (flow limitation) in CAD,[29,39] as well as the evaluation of changes in flow after medical treatment of CAD risk factors such as hyperlipidemia,[40] diabetes,[121] and smoking.[27]

Flow reserve is also useful in differentiating viable from nonviable myocardium, since a certain degree of myocardial blood flow is necessary to maintain myocyte viability. In the setting of a functionally significant coronary artery stenosis, the vasculature distal to the lesion may retain the ability to vasodilate and thus increase regional myocardial blood flow. As such, regions of myocardium that can achieve this must therefore be viable. Flow reserve has been studied as a surrogate for myocardial viability in patients with previous infarction and chronic CAD.[77]

Single-Photon Emission Computed Tomography

Thallium

[201]Tl has been used as a tracer to assess both regional blood flow and myocardial viability. [201]Tl is actively transported across the myocyte sarcolemmal membrane via the Na$^+$-K$^+$-ATPase similar to potassium and is extracted from the blood in proportion to myocardial blood flow. Cellular extraction is diminished only when there is irreversible injury to the myocyte, making ^{201}Tl an attractive agent for imaging pathophysiological conditions such as chronic hypoperfusion and postischemic dysfunction. Because retention of ^{201}Tl in the myocardium corresponds to cell membrane integrity, regional uptake corresponds to viable myocardium. As such, decreased myocardial uptake early after ^{201}Tl injection can be due to reduced regional blood flow or infarction. After injection, ^{201}Tl redistributes in the myocardium via continuous exchange between the myocardium and the extracardiac compartments (interstitium, blood pool), driven by the concentration gradient of the tracer and intact myocyte viability. Imaging after redistribution will show less regional heterogeneity of initial ^{201}Tl distribution, thereby reducing the relative difference between the ischemic and normal regions. An increase in regional ^{201}Tl activity on the redistribution images is indicative of myocardium that has reduced flow but more importantly intact cellular integrity, and thus viability. As such, ^{201}Tl redistribution has been used to distinguish viable from scarred myocardium. [201]Tl can be imaged at rest and again 4 h later to assess redistribution, or by using another injection if part of a stress MPI protocol. Viability can also be assessed quantitatively with [201]Tl. The presence of ^{201}Tl uptake >50–60% of maximum will be predictive of functional recovery in the majority of segments. Moreover, the final ^{201}Tl uptake with redistribution appears to be more important than the degree of change from rest to redistribution in predicting recovery.[15,19,112]

Technetium-Labeled Tracers

[99m]Tc agents currently are used more commonly than thallium for stress MPI, and these agents can still provide insight into the viability of the myocardium. The ability to determine viability from an initial stress-rest MPI study often obviates the need for further testing with PET or thallium protocols. Uptake and retention of the ^{99m}Tc perfusion tracers sestamibi and tetrofosmin require that the myocyte cell and mitochon-

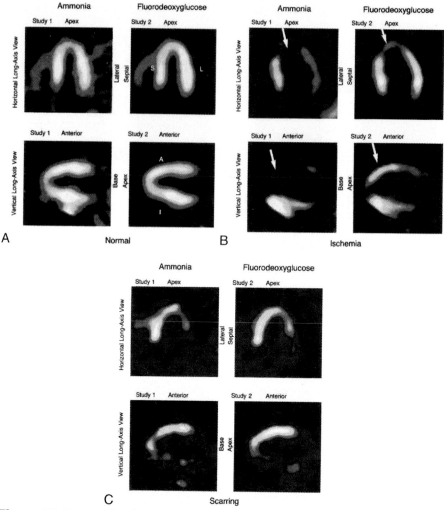

Figure 56–5 **Example of a positron emission tomography (PET) viability study.** For each panel, perfusion imaging with ^{13}N-labeled ammonia uptake is on the left, and metabolic imaging with [^{18}F]fluorodeoxyglucose (FDG) uptake on the right. The upper row of each panel is the horizontal long-axis slice with the apex at the top, and the lower row is a vertical long-axis slice with the apex pointing to the left. The yellow and white areas are sites of maximal activity and the blue areas are sites of minimal activity. The red areas indicate intermediate activity. (**A**) Normal images. (**B**) An example of ischemia and viable tissue. (**C**) An example of myocardial scarring. Note the homogeneous uptake of both ammonia and FDG in the normal study. In the presence of ischemia (**B**), there is a mismatch *(arrows)*, with decreased perfusion and augmented metabolic activity in the apex and the anterior wall. With scarring (**C**), there is equally decreased uptake of FDG and ammonia in the inferior and lateral walls. A, anterior wall; I, inferior wall; L, lateral wall; S, septum. *(Reprinted with permission from Zaret BL, Wackers FJ: N Engl J Med 329[12]:855–863, 1993.)*

drial membranes be intact. As such, tracer accumulation indicates cellular integrity, and thus reflects cellular viability.° Computer-assisted quantitative analysis of regional myocardial uptake of sestamibi has been shown to improve accuracy in predicting functional recovery after revascularization, and similar to ^{201}Tl, tracer uptake >50% of peak is suggestive of myocardial viability.[74] The administration of nitrates to enhance resting blood and hence tracer uptake has also been studied with ^{99m}Tc-labeled agents because of issues regarding the underestimation of viability with sestamibi compared to PET imaging.[13,72,99] Recently, assessment of metabolism for

viability has been performed using SPECT systems with special equipment (high-energy collimators or coincidence detection) or with hybrid SPECT–PET cameras.[26,33,98]

Prognostic Implications of Viability Assessment

Despite recent advances in medical and antiarrhythmic device therapy for heart failure, patients with ischemic cardiomyopathy and congestive heart failure continue to have a poor prognosis.[51,93] Although many of these patients would benefit from orthotopic heart transplant, donor organ supply is limited. In 2002, with almost 5000 transplant candidates, just over 2000 transplants were performed, and 25% of can-

°References 10, 59, 70, 73, 97, 107.

didates died waiting for a donor organ.[4,111] With such limited access to transplantation, surgical revascularization is often considered to improve survival in these patients. The selection of appropriate patients for surgical revascularization is largely based on early surgical survival studies that provided insight as to which patients obtain the most benefit from surgical revascularization. The Veterans Administration Cooperative Trial[6] and the Coronary Artery Surgery Study[61] both demonstrated that patients with significant left main or multivessel CAD and depressed ejection fraction (35–50%) have a better survival with revascularization than medical therapy. Not unexpectedly, these patients often have high perioperative mortality with coronary artery bypass grafting (CABG).[68,85] Assessment of viability may be useful in these patients to balance the potential benefits of revascularization with the risk of the procedure. The potential to improve ventricular function (and moreover survival) with revascularization necessitates an evaluation for hibernating myocardium in most patients with left ventricular dysfunction, especially those without angina. However, viability testing may not be necessary if the patient has angina pectoris or if initial testing reveals stress-induced ischemia.

The clinical end points commonly used in viability assessment include recovery of regional or global ventricular function and improvement in symptoms and/or survival. Most studies focusing on the assessment of myocardial viability have employed improvement in ventricular function with revascularization as the clinical end point. Although many studies have focused on the ability of viability assessment to predict functional recovery with revascularization, relatively few have used survival and outcomes as an end point. The prognostic implications of PET perfusion-metabolism mismatch and the presence of viability on imaging with thallium or sestamibi have been demonstrated in several studies.[3] These studies have consistently shown similar findings. Patients with perfusion-metabolism mismatch have a very high mortality when managed medically, and much lower mortality if revascularized. Conversely, those with matched defects, indicating scar, had no such difference in outcomes between medical and surgical management. Although the methods included a combination of techniques and outcomes used (death, non-fatal MI, unstable angina, need for transplant or revascularization), this distinction is not subtle. Patients with demonstrated viability had an annual event rate of 27% if treated medically compared to 6% in similar patients who underwent coronary revascularization.[53] On the other hand, patients with matched defects suggesting no viability had similar event rates with medical or surgical treatment. This dichotomy in outcomes underscores the prognostic implication of determining viability. A recent meta-analysis pooled data from 24 studies of viability using all currently used techniques encompassing over 3000 patients further illustrates this point.[3] In patients with ischemic cardiomyopathy (mean LVEF 32±8%) those with demonstrated viability had an annual mortality of 3.2% if treated with revascularization and 16% if treated medically. Those without viability had essentially similar outcomes (7.7 vs. 6.2% mortality, respectively). This analysis provides further evidence that the preoperative determination of viability yields important information regarding not only functional recovery, but improvement in survival as well.

It is unclear whether the improvement in outcome with revascularization is entirely due to improvement in LVEF after surgery. A recent study suggests that this may not be necessary. Samady et al[96] examined survival after CABG in 104 patients with an assessment of function before and after surgical revascularization. Outcome was similar in patients irrespective of whether the LVEF improved after CABG, suggesting that revascularization of ischemic myocardium, even without improvement in ventricular function, may prevent future infarction and death. Of note, no formal viability assessment was performed in the majority of these patients. Based on studies such as these, some have advocated revascularization for all patients with ischemic cardiomyopathy, asserting that hibernating myocardium should be suspected in all patients with CAD and LV dysfunction. However, others maintain that preoperative viability assessment provides an opportunity to balance the potential benefit from surgical revascularization against the risks of the procedure. The currently ongoing Surgical Treatments for Ischemic Heart Disease (STICH) trial, a randomized study of medical therapy, surgical revascularization, and/or ventricular restoration (aneurysmectomy) is designed to evaluate the best treatment approach for patients with ischemic cardiomyopathy and heart failure.[108]

▶ EVALUATION OF PATIENTS POSTREVASCULARIZATION

Despite technical advances, the effectiveness of both percutaneous and surgical revascularization procedures is limited by restenosis and vein graft closure, respectively. Progression of the underlying atherosclerosis or development of new stenoses can cause recurrent ischemia, manifesting as recurrence of symptoms, congestive heart failure due to left ventricular dysfunction, MI, or cardiac death.

Symptom status is not a reliable predictor of stenosis after coronary angioplasty, as evidenced by up to 25% of subjects having silent ischemia on treadmill testing.[36] However, routine exercise treadmill testing is not currently advocated after coronary angioplasty as it does not reliably detect restenosis.[34] SPECT imaging has been demonstrated to accurately detect restenosis, particularly in the 3–9 month window of greatest risk for restenosis, with positive and negative predictive values of ~90%.[80] A recent study demonstrated that[201]Tl stress defect size was predictive of cardiac death and MI even up to 3 years after percutaneous transluminal coronary angioplasty (PTCA).[49] Further study is necessary to evaluate if routine stress MPI after angioplasty indeed alters prognosis, particularly in asymptomatic patients, and in high-risk subsets of patients (i.e., decreased LV function, multivessel or proximal left anterior descending artery disease, diabetes, renal failure) after angioplasty.

The prognostic value of SPECT MPI after CABG surgery has been demonstrated in more than 2000 patients.° These studies are summarized in Table 56-1. These reports consistently demonstrate that the finding of reversible defects on stress SPECT MPI is a strong predictor of worse cardiac outcome in symptomatic subjects early (1–5 years)

°References 28, 69, 82, 87, 94, 124.

Table 56–1

Utility of Stress Myocardial Perfusion Imaging after Coronary Artery Bypass Surgery

Reference	Year	N	Tracer	Mean time to SPECT after CABG (years)	Follow-up after SPECT (years)	Cardiac death (%)	Nonfatal MI (%)	Late revascularization (%)	Findings
Palmas et al[94]	1995	294	^{201}Tl	≥5	2.6 ± 0.9	6.8	7.1	9.9	Summed stress score and ^{201}Tl lung uptake predictive of events
Desideri et al[28]	1997	75	^{201}Tl	3.1 ± 4.4	3.2 ± 2	5.3	9.3	10.7	Summed stress score significant predictor of events
Nallamothu et al[87]	1997	255	^{201}Tl	5	3.4 ± 2.3	9.4	3.9		Multivessel disease pattern and ^{201}Tl lung uptake 7.5% annualized mortality; if only one of these, 3.4%; if neither, mortality is 0.6%
Lauer et al[69]	1998	873	^{201}Tl	Median 6	3	6.5	8.2		Asymptomatic group, 58% with defects; death 9% with defects and 3% with no defects
Miller et al[84]	1998	411	^{201}Tl	<2	5.8	12.9	2.7	5.4	Number of abnormal ^{201}Tl segments strongest predictor of events
Zellweger et al[124]	2001	1544	^{201}Tl rest/ ^{99m}Tc stress	7.1 ± 5	≥1	3.4			Age, ischemia, and infarct size predictive of cardiac death; symptomatic patients ≤ 5 years and all patients >5 years post-CABG may benefit from testing

SPECT, single-photon emission computed tomography; MI, myocardial infarction; CABG, coronary artery bypass grafting.

after CABG, and in all subjects >5 years after surgical revascularization.

FUTURE DIRECTIONS

Although the cornerstone of nuclear cardiology has long been perfusion imaging, the field has seen significant advances in terms of new agents that target other biological processes. Interest in the concept of "hot spot" imaging with tracers that visualize infarction or ischemia has been renewed with the introduction of new radiopharmaceuticals that target these processes in the myocardium. These tracers localize in areas of ischemia or infarction and produce a positive signal for imaging. Examples include glucarate,[57,60,88] a metabolite of glucose metabolism that binds to nuclear histones that are exposed in recently damaged myocytes, annexin V,[50] which binds to the plasma membrane of cells undergoing apoptosis, or programmed cell death, and nitroimidazole compounds,[105,120] which localize in tissues experiencing low oxygen tension (i.e., ischemia, tumors). Although the clinical experience with these agents is currently limited, these agents hold promise for imaging acute coronary syndromes in the future.[2,106] Other molecular-based areas currently under investigation include imaging of atherosclerosis, angiogenesis, plaque vulnerability, and gene expression.[16] Such new approaches will no doubt enhance the future clinical viability of the field.

REFERENCES

1. Abbott BG, Abdel-Aziz I, Nagula S, et al: Selective use of single-photon emission computed tomography myocardial perfusion imaging in a chest pain center. Am J Cardiol 87: 1351–1355, 2001.
2. Abbott BG, Wackers FJ: Use of radionuclide imaging in acute coronary syndromes. Curr Cardiol Rep 5:25–31, 2003.
3. Allman KC, Shaw LJ, Hachamovitch R, et al: Myocardial viability testing and impact of revascularization on prognosis in patients with coronary artery disease and left ventricular dysfunction: a meta-analysis. J Am Coll Cardiol 39:1151–1158, 2002.
4. American Heart Association: Heart disease and stroke statistics. www.americanheart.org: accessed April 9, 2003.
5. American Society of Nuclear Cardiology/ IMV Technology Marketing Group S: AMR census data, 2001.
6. Anonymous: Eleven-year survival in the Veterans Administration randomized trial of coronary bypass surgery for stable angina. The Veterans Administration coronary artery bypass surgery cooperative study group. N Engl J Med 311: 1333–1339, 1984.
7. Anonymous: Imaging guidelines for nuclear cardiology procedures. American Society of Nuclear Cardiology. Myocardial perfusion SPECT protocols. J Nucl Cardiol 3: G34–46, 1996.
8. Anonymous: Imaging guidelines for nuclear cardiology procedures, part 2. American Society of Nuclear Cardiology. J Nucl Cardiol 6:G47–84, 1999.
9. Araujo LI, Maseri A: Whole heart distribution of myocardial perfusion, metabolism and myocardial viability by positron emission tomography. Br Med Bull 45:922–932, 1989.
10. Arrighi JA, Ng CK, Dey HM, et al: Effect of left ventricular function on the assessment of myocardial viability by technectium-99m sestamibi and correlation with positron emission tomography in patients with healed myocardial infarcts or stable angina pectoris, or both. Am J Cardiol 80: 1007–1013, 1997.
11. Azzarelli S, Galassi AR, Foti R, et al: Accuracy of 99mTc-tetrofosmin myocardial tomography in the evaluation of coronary artery disease. J Nucl Cardiol 6:183–189, 1999.
12. Baron JF, Mundler O, Bertrand M, et al: Dipyridamole-thallium scintigraphy and gated radionuclide angiography to assess cardiac risk before abdominal aortic surgery. N Engl J Med 330:663–669, 1994.
13. Baszko A, Blaszyk K, CieSlinski A, et al: 99mTc-sestamibi tomoscintigraphy at rest and after nitrate administration in predicting wall motion recovery after revascularization. Nucl Med Commun 19:1141–1148, 1998.
14. Bateman TM, O'Keefe JH, Jr., Dong V, et al: Coronary angiographic rates after stress single-photon emission computed tomographic scintigraphy. J Nucl Cardiol 2:217– 223, 1995.
15. Bax JJ, Wijns W, Cornel JH, et al: Accuracy of currently available techniques for prediction of functional recovery after revascularization in patients with left ventricular dysfunction due to chronic coronary artery disease: comparison of pooled data. J Am Coll Cardiol 30:1451–1460, 1997.
16. Beller GA, Zaret BL: Contributions of nuclear cardiology to diagnosis and prognosis of patients with coronary artery disease. Circulation 101:1465–1478, 2000.
17. Berman DS, Kang X, Schisterman EF, et al: Serial changes on quantitative myocardial perfusion SPECT in patients undergoing revascularization or conservative therapy. J Nucl Cardiol 8:428–437, 2001.
18. Bigger JT Jr, Fleiss JL, Kleiger R, et al: The relationships among ventricular arrhythmias, left ventricular dysfunction, and mortality in the 2 years after myocardial infarction. Circulation 69:250–258, 1984.
19. Bonow RO: Identification of viable myocardium. Circulation 94:2674–2680, 1996.
20. Bonow RO, Dilsizian V: Thallium 201 for assessment of myocardial viability. Semin Nucl Med 21:230–241, 1991.
21. Boyne TS, Koplan BA, Parsons WJ, et al: Predicting adverse outcome with exercise SPECT technetium-99m sestamibi imaging in patients with suspected or known coronary artery disease. Am J Cardiol 79:270–274, 1997.
22. Brown KA, Heller GV, Landin RS, et al: Early dipyridamole (99m)Tc-sestamibi single photon emission computed tomographic imaging 2 to 4 days after acute myocardial infarction predicts in-hospital and postdischarge cardiac events: comparison with submaximal exercise imaging. Circulation 100:2060–2066, 1999.
23. Bruce CJ, Christian TF, Schaer GL, et al: Determinants of infarct size after thrombolytic treatment in acute myocardial infarction. Am J Cardiol 83:1600–1605, 1999.
24. Burns RJ, Gibbons RJ, Yi Q, et al: The relationships of left ventricular ejection fraction, end-systolic volume index and infarct size to six-month mortality after hospital discharge following myocardial infarction treated by thrombolysis. J Am Coll Cardiol 39:30–36, 2002.
25. Castro PF, Corbalan R, Baeza R, et al: Effect of primary coronary angioplasty on left ventricular function and myocardial perfusion as determined by Tc-99m sestamibi scintigraphy. Am J Cardiol 87:1181–1184, 2001.
26. Cornel JH, Bax JJ, Fioretti PM, et al: Prediction of improvement of ventricular function after revascularization. 18F-fluorodeoxyglucose single-photon emission computed tomography vs low-dose dobutamine echocardiography. Eur Heart J 18:941–948, 1997.

908

27. Czernin J, Sun K, Brunken R, et al: Effect of acute and long-term smoking on myocardial blood flow and flow reserve. Circulation 91:2891–2897, 1995.

28. Desideri A, Candelpergher G, Zanco P, et al: Exercise technetium-99m sestamibi single-photon emission computed tomography late after coronary artery bypass surgery: long-term follow-up. Clin Cardiol 20:779–784, 1997.

29. Di Carli M, Czernin J, Hoh CK, et al: Relation among stenosis severity, myocardial blood flow, and flow reserve in patients with coronary artery disease. Circulation 91:1944–1951, 1995.

30. Eagle KA, Berger PB, Calkins H, et al: ACC/AHA guideline update for perioperative cardiovascular evaluation for noncardiac surgery—executive summary: a report of the American College of Cardiology/American Heart Association task force on practice guidelines (committee to update the 1996 guidelines on perioperative cardiovascular evaluation for noncardiac surgery). Circulation 105:1256–1267, 2002.

31. Fleischmann KE, Hunink MG, Kuntz KM, et al: Exercise echocardiography or exercise SPECT imaging? A meta-analysis of diagnostic test performance. JAMA 280:913–920, 1998.

32. Fleisher LA, Rosenbaum SH, Nelson AH, et al: Preoperative dipyridamole thallium imaging and ambulatory electrocardiographic monitoring as a predictor of perioperative cardiac events and long-term outcome. Anesthesiology 83:906–917, 1995.

33. Fukuchi K, Katafuchi T, Fukushima K, et al: Estimation of myocardial perfusion and viability using simultaneous ^{99m}Tc-tetrofosmin-FDG collimated SPECT. J Nucl Med 41:1318–1323, 2000.

34. Garzon PP, Eisenberg MJ: Functional testing for the detection of restenosis after percutaneous transluminal coronary angioplasty: a meta-analysis. Can J Cardiol 17:41–48, 2001.

35. Gianrossi R, Detrano R, Mulvihill D, et al: Exercise-induced ST depression in the diagnosis of coronary artery disease. A meta-analysis. Circulation 80:87–98, 1989.

36. Gibbons RJ, Balady GJ, Timothy Bricker J, et al: ACC/AHA 2002 guideline update for exercise testing: summary article. A report of the American College of Cardiology/American Heart Association task force on practice guidelines (committee to update the 1997 exercise testing guidelines). J Am Coll Cardiol 40:1531–1540, 2002.

37. Gibbons RJ, Miller TD, Christian TF: Infarct size measured by single photon emission computed tomographic imaging with (99m)Tc-sestamibi: a measure of the efficacy of therapy in acute myocardial infarction. Circulation 101:101–108, 2000.

38. Gosselink AT, Liem AL, Reiffers S, et al: Prognostic value of predischarge radionuclide ventriculography at rest and exercise after acute myocardial infarction treated with thrombolytic therapy or primary coronary angioplasty. The zwolle myocardial infarction study group. Clin Cardiol 21: 254–260, 1998.

39. Gould KL: Quantification of coronary artery stenosis in vivo. Circ Res 57:341–353, 1985.

40. Gould KL, Martucci JP, Goldberg DI, et al: Short-term cholesterol lowering decreases size and severity of perfusion abnormalities by positron emission tomography after dipyridamole in patients with coronary artery disease. A potential noninvasive marker of healing coronary endothelium. Circulation 89:1530–1538, 1994.

41. Hachamovitch R, Berman DS, Kiat H, et al: Effective risk stratification using exercise myocardial perfusion SPECT in women: gender-related differences in prognostic nuclear testing. J Am Coll Cardiol 28:34–44, 1996.

42. Hachamovitch R, Berman DS, Kiat H, et al: Exercise myocardial perfusion SPECT in patients without known coronary artery disease: incremental prognostic value and use in risk stratification. Circulation 93:905–914, 1996.

43. Hachamovitch R, Berman DS, Kiat H, et al: Incremental prognostic value of adenosine stress myocardial perfusion single-photon emission computed tomography and impact on subsequent management in patients with or suspected of having myocardial ischemia. Am J Cardiol 80:426–433, 1997.

44. Hachamovitch R, Berman DS, Shaw LJ, et al: Incremental prognostic value of myocardial perfusion single photon emission computed tomography for the prediction of cardiac death: differential stratification for risk of cardiac death and myocardial infarction. Circulation 97:535–543, 1998.

45. Hallstrom A, Pratt CM, Greene HL, et al: Relations between heart failure, ejection fraction, arrhythmia suppression and mortality: analysis of the cardiac arrhythmia suppression trial. J Am Coll Cardiol 25:1250–1257, 1995.

46. Haronian HL, Remetz MS, Sinusas AJ, et al: Myocardial risk area defined by technetium-99m sestamibi imaging during percutaneous transluminal coronary angioplasty: comparison with coronary angiography. J Am Coll Cardiol 22:1033–1043, 1993.

47. Heller GV, Stowers SA, Hendel RC, et al: Clinical value of acute rest technetium-99m tetrofosmin tomographic myocardial perfusion imaging in patients with acute chest pain and nondiagnostic electrocardiograms. J Am Coll Cardiol 31: 1011–1017, 1998.

48. Hirayama A, Kusuoka H, Adachi T, et al: Comparison of time of reperfusion during anterior wall acute myocardial infarction to left ventricular volume one month and 20 months later. Am J Cardiol 89:1335–1340, 2002.

49. Ho KT, Miller TD, Holmes DR, et al: Long-term prognostic value of Duke treadmill score and exercise thallium-201 imaging performed one to three years after percutaneous transluminal coronary angioplasty. Am J Cardiol 84: 1323–1327, 1999.

50. Hofstra L, Liem IH, Dumont EA, et al: Visualisation of cell death in vivo in patients with acute myocardial infarction. Lancet 356:209–212, 2000.

51. Hunt SA, Baker DW, Chin MH, et al: ACC/AHA guidelines for the evaluation and management of chronic heart failure in the adult: executive summary. J Heart Lung Transplant 21: 189–203, 2002.

52. Hurrell DG, Milavetz J, Hodge DO, Gibbons RJ: Infarct size determination by technetium 99m sestamibi single-photon emission computed tomography predicts survival in patients with chronic coronary artery disease. Am Heart J 140:61–66, 2000.

53. Iskander S, Iskandrian AE: Prognostic utility of myocardial viability assessment. Am J Cardiol 83:696–702, 1999.

54. Iskander S, Iskandrian AE: Risk assessment using single-photon emission computed tomographic technetium-99m sestamibi imaging. J Am Coll Cardiol 32:56–62, 1998.

55. Iskandrian AS, Chae SC, Heo J, et al: Independent and incremental prognostic value of exercise single-photon emission computed tomographic (SPECT) thallium imaging in coronary artery disease. J Am Coll Cardiol 22:665–670, 1993.

56. Iskandrian AS, Verani MS, Heo J: Pharmacologic stress testing: mechanism of action, hemodynamic responses, and results in detection of coronary artery disease. J Nucl Cardiol 1:94–111, 1994.

57. Johnson LL, Schofield L, Mastrofrancesco P, et al: Technetium-99m glucarate uptake in a swine model of limited flow plus increased demand. J Nucl Cardiol 7:590–598, 2000.

58. Johnston DL, Daley JR, Hodge DO, et al: Hemodynamic responses and adverse effects associated with adenosine and dipyridamole pharmacologic stress testing: a comparison in 2,000 patients. Mayo Clin Proc 70:331–336, 1995.

59. Kauffman GJ, Boyne TS, Watson DD, et al: Comparison of rest thallium-201 imaging and rest technetium-99m sestamibi imaging for assessment of myocardial viability in patients with

Chapter 56 ■ Nuclear Cardiology and Positron Emission Tomography in the Assessment of Patients with Cardiovascular Disease

909

coronary artery disease and severe left ventricular dysfunction. J Am Coll Cardiol 27:1592–1597, 1996.

60. Khaw BA, Nakazawa A, O'Donnell SM, et al: Avidity of technetium 99m glucarate for the necrotic myocardium: in vivo and in vitro assessment. J Nucl Cardiol 4:283–290, 1997.

61. Killip T, Passamani E, Davis K: Coronary artery surgery study (CASS): a randomized trial of coronary bypass surgery. Eight years follow-up and survival in patients with reduced ejection fraction. Circulation 72:V102–109, 1985.

62. Kim C, Kwok YS, Heagerty P, Redberg R: Pharmacologic stress testing for coronary disease diagnosis: a meta-analysis. Am Heart J 142:934–944, 2001.

63. Knuuti MJ, Nuutila P, Ruotsalainen U, et al: Euglycemic hyperinsulinemic clamp and oral glucose load in stimulating myocardial glucose utilization during positron emission tomography. J Nucl Med 33:1255–1262, 1992.

64. Knuuti MJ, Nuutila P, Ruotsalainen U, et al: The value of quantitative analysis of glucose utilization in detection of myocardial viability by PET. J Nucl Med 34:2068–2075, 1993.

65. Kontos MC, Jesse RL, Anderson FP, et al: Comparison of myocardial perfusion imaging and cardiac troponin in patients admitted to the emergency department with chest pain. Circulation 99:2073–2078, 1999.

66. Kontos MC, Jesse RL, Schmidt KL, et al: Value of acute rest sestamibi perfusion imaging for evaluation of patients admitted to the emergency department with chest pain. J Am Coll Cardiol 30:976–982, 1997.

67. Kroll D, Farah W, McKendall GR, et al: Prognostic value of stress-gated Tc-99m sestamibi SPECT after acute myocardial infarction. Am J Cardiol 87:381–386, 2001.

68. Kron IL, Flanagan TL, Blackbourne LH, et al: Coronary revascularization rather than cardiac transplantation for chronic ischemic cardiomyopathy. Ann Surg 210:348–352; discussion 352–354, 1989.

69. Lauer MS, Lytle B, Pashkow F, et al: Prediction of death and myocardial infarction by screening with exercise-thallium testing after coronary-artery-bypass grafting. Lancet 351:615–622, 1998.

70. Leoncini M, Sciagra R, Maioli M, et al: Usefulness of dobutamine Tc-99m sestamibi-gated single-photon emission computed tomography for prediction of left ventricular ejection fraction outcome after coronary revascularization for ischemic cardiomyopathy. Am J Cardiol 89:817–821, 2002.

71. Leppo JA: Dipyridamole myocardial perfusion imaging. J Nucl Med 35:730–733, 1994.

72. Li ST, Liu XJ, Lu ZL, et al: Quantitative analysis of technetium 99m 2-methoxyisobutyl isonitrile single-photon emission computed tomography and isosorbide dinitrate infusion in assessment of myocardial viability before and after revascularization. J Nucl Cardiol 3:456–463, 1996.

73. Maes A, Mortelmans L, Nuyts J, et al: Importance of flow/metabolism studies in predicting late recovery of function following reperfusion in patients with acute myocardial infarction. Eur Heart J 18:954–962, 1997.

74. Maes AF, Borgers M, Flameng W, et al: Assessment of myocardial viability in chronic coronary artery disease using technetium-99m sestamibi SPECT. Correlation with histologic and positron emission tomographic studies and functional follow-up. J Am Coll Cardiol 29:62–68, 1997.

75. Mahmarian JJ, Verani MS: Myocardial perfusion imaging during pharmacologic stress testing. Card Clin 12:223–245, 1994.

76. Mansoor MR, Heller GV: Gated SPECT imaging. Semin Nucl Med 29:271–278, 1999.

77. Marzullo P, Parodi O, Sambuceti G, et al: Residual coronary reserve identifies segmental viability in patients with wall motion abnormalities. J Am Coll Cardiol 26:342–350, 1995.

78. McClements BM, Adgey AA: Value of signal-averaged electrocardiography, radionuclide ventriculography, holter monitoring and clinical variables for prediction of arrhythmic events in survivors of acute myocardial infarction in the thrombolytic era. J Am Coll Cardiol 21:1419–1427, 1993.

79. McGuinness ME, Talbert RL: Pharmacologic stress testing: experience with dipyridamole, adenosine, and dobutamine. Am J Hosp Pharm 51:328–346, 1994.

80. Milavetz JJ, Miller TD, Hodge DO, Holmes DR, Gibbons RJ: Accuracy of single-photon emission computed tomography myocardial perfusion imaging in patients with stents in native coronary arteries. Am J Cardiol 82:856–861, 1998.

81. Miller DD, Younis LT, Chaitman BR, et al: Diagnostic accuracy of dipyridamole technetium 99m-labeled sestamibi myocardial tomography for detection of coronary artery disease. J Nucl Cardiol 4:18–24, 1997.

82. Miller TD, Christian TF, Hodge DO, et al: Prognostic value of exercise thallium-201 imaging performed within 2 years of coronary artery bypass graft surgery. J Am Coll Cardiol 31:848–854, 1998.

83. Miller TD, Christian TF, Hopfenspirger MR, et al: Infarct size after acute myocardial infarction measured by quantitative tomographic ^{99m}Tc sestamibi imaging predicts subsequent mortality. Circulation 92:334–341, 1995.

84. Miller TD, Hodge DO, Sutton JM, et al: Usefulness of technetium-99m sestamibi infarct size in predicting posthospital mortality following acute myocardial infarction. Am J Cardiol 81:1491–1493, 1998.

85. Mitropoulos FA, Elefteriades JA: Myocardial revascularization as a therapeutic strategy in the patient with advanced ventricular dysfunction. Heart Failure Rev 6:163–175, 2001.

86. Mock MB, Ringqvist I, Fisher LD, et al: Survival of medically treated patients in the Coronary Artery Surgery Study (CASS) registry. Circulation 66:562–568, 1982.

87. Nallamothu N, Johnson JH, Bagheri B et al: Utility of stress single-photon emission computed tomography (SPECT) perfusion imaging in predicting outcome after coronary artery bypass grafting. Am J Cardiol 80:1517–1521, 1997.

88. Narula J, Petrov A, Pak KY, et al: Very early noninvasive detection of acute experimental nonreperfused myocardial infarction with ^{99m}Tc-labeled glucarate. Circulation 95:1577–1584, 1997.

89. Nelson GR, Cohn PF, Gorlin R: Prognosis in medically-treated coronary artery disease: influence of ejection fraction compared to other parameters. Circulation 52:408–412, 1975.

90. Ogilby JD, Iskandrian AS, Untereker WJ, et al: Effect of intravenous adenosine infusion on myocardial perfusion and function. Hemodynamic/angiographic and scintigraphic study. Circulation 86:887–895, 1992.

91. O'Keefe JH, Jr, Bateman TM, Handlin LR, et al: Four-versus 6-minute infusion protocol for adenosine thallium-201 single photon emission computed tomography imaging. Am Heart J 129:482–487, 1995.

92. O'Keefe JH, Jr, Bateman TM, Ligon RW, et al: Outcome of medical versus invasive treatment strategies for non-high-risk ischemic heart disease. J Nucl Cardiol 5:28–33, 1998.

93. Packer M, Fowler MB, Roecker EB, et al: Effect of carvedilol on the morbidity of patients with severe chronic heart failure: results of the arvedilol prospective randomized cumulative survival (COPERNICUS) study. Circulation 106:2194–2199, 2002.

94. Palmas W, Bingham S, Diamond GA, et al: Incremental prognostic value of exercise thallium-201 myocardial single-photon emission computed tomography late after coronary artery bypass surgery. J Am Coll Cardiol 25:403–409, 1995.

95. Radensky PW, Hilton TC, Fulmer H, et al: Potential cost effectiveness of initial myocardial perfusion imaging for assessment of emergency department patients with chest pain. Am J Cardiol 79:595–599, 1997.

96. Samady H, Elefteriades JA, Abbott BG, et al: Failure to improve left ventricular function after coronary revascular-

910

ization for ischemic cardiomyopathy is not associated with worse outcome. Circulation 100:1298–1304, 1999.

97. Sawada SG, Allman KC, Muzik O, et al: Positron emission tomography detects evidence of viability in rest technetium-99m sestamibi defects. J Am Coll Cardiol 23:92–98, 1994.

98. Schinkel AF, Bax JJ, Sozzi FB, et al: Prevalence of myocardial viability assessed by single photon emission computed tomography in patients with chronic ischaemic left ventricular dysfunction. Heart 88:125–130, 2002.

99. Schneider CA, Voth E, Gawlich S, et al: Significance of rest technetium-99m sestamibi imaging for the prediction of improvement of left ventricular dysfunction after Q wave myocardial infarction: importance of infarct location adjusted thresholds. J Am Coll Cardiol 32:648–654, 1998.

100. Schwaiger M: Metabolism and blood flow as new markers of myocardial viability in the evolution of myocardial infarction. Eur J Nucl Med 12:S62–65, 1986.

101. Sharir T, Germano G, Kang X, et al: Prediction of myocardial infarction versus cardiac death by gated myocardial perfusion SPECT: risk stratification by the amount of stress-induced ischemia and the post-stress ejection fraction. J Nucl Med 42:831–837, 2001.

102. Sharir T, Germano G, Kavanagh PB, et al: Incremental prognostic value of post-stress left ventricular ejection fraction and volume by gated myocardial perfusion single photon emission computed tomography. Circulation 100:1035–1042, 1999.

103. Shaw LJ, Eagle KA, Gersh BJ, et al: Meta-analysis of intravenous dipyridamole-thallium-201 imaging (1985 to 1994) and dobutamine echocardiography (1991 to 1994) for risk stratification before vascular surgery. J Am Coll Cardiol 27:787–798, 1996.

104. Shaw LJ, Hachamovitch R, Heller GV, et al: Noninvasive strategies for the estimation of cardiac risk in stable chest pain patients. The economics of noninvasive diagnosis (END) study group. Am J Cardiol 86:1–7, 2000.

105. Shi CQ, Sinusas AJ, Dione DP, et al: Technetium-99m-nitroimidazole (BMS181321): a positive imaging agent for detecting myocardial ischemia. J Nucl Med 36:1078–1086, 1995.

106. Sinusas AJ: The potential for myocardial imaging with hypoxia markers. Semin Nucl Med 29:330–338, 1999.

107. Soufer R, Dey HM, Ng CK, et al: Comparison of sestamibi single-photon emission computed tomography with positron emission tomography for estimating left ventricular myocardial viability. Am J Cardiol 75:1214–1219, 1995.

108. The Stich Trial: http://www.stichtrial.org: accessed April 9, 2003.

109. Stratmann HG, Younis LT, Wittry MD, et al: Dipyridamole technetium 99m sestamibi myocardial tomography for preoperative cardiac risk stratification before major or minor nonvascular surgery. Am Heart J 132:536–541, 1996.

110. Tatum JL, Jesse RL, Kontos MC, et al: Comprehensive strategy for the evaluation and triage of the chest pain patient. Ann Emerg Med 29:116–125, 1997.

111. Transplant facts. www.ustransplant,org/facts: accessed April 10, 2003.

112. Udelson JE: Steps forward in the assessment of myocardial viability in left ventricular dysfunction. Circulation 97:833–838, 1998.

113. Udelson JE, Beshansky JR, Ballin DS, et al: Myocardial perfusion imaging for evaluation and triage of patients with suspected acute cardiac ischemia: a randomized controlled trial. JAMA 288:2693–2700, 2002.

114. Uren NG, Camici PG: Hibernation and myocardial ischemia: clinical detection by positron emission tomography. Cardiovasc Drugs Ther 6:273–279, 1992.

115. Van Damme H, Pierard L, Gillain D, et al: Cardiac risk assessment before vascular surgery: a prospective study comparing clinical evaluation, dobutamine stress echocardiography, and dobutamine Tc-99m sestamibi tomoscintigraphy. Cardiovasc Surg 5:54–64, 1997.

116. van Royen N, Jaffe CC, Krumholz HM, et al: Comparison and reproducibility of visual echocardiographic and quantitative radionuclide left ventricular ejection fractions. Am J Cardiol 77:843–850, 1996.

117. Vanzetto G, Ormezzano O, Fagret D, et al: Long-term additive prognostic value of thallium-201 myocardial perfusion imaging over clinical and exercise stress test in low to intermediate risk patients: study in 1137 patients with 6-year follow-up. Circulation 100:1521–1527, 1999.

118. Wackers FJ, Brown KA, Heller GV, et al: American Society of Nuclear Cardiology position statement on radionuclide imaging in patients with suspected acute ischemic syndromes in the emergency department or chest pain center. J Nucl Cardiol 9:246–250, 2002.

119. Watanabe J, Nakamura S, Sugiura T, et al: Early identification of impaired myocardial reperfusion with serial assessment of ST segments after percutaneous transluminal coronary angioplasty during acute myocardial infarction. Am J Cardiol 88:956–959, 2001.

120. Weinstein H, Reinhardt CP, Leppo JA: Direct detection of regional myocardial ischemia with technetium-99m nitroimidazole in rabbits. J Nucl Med 39:598–607, 1998.

121. Yokoyama I, Momomura S, Ohtake T, et al: Reduced myocardial flow reserve in non-insulin-dependent diabetes mellitus. J Am Coll Cardiol 30:1472–1477, 1997.

122. Zaret BL, Beller G: Nuclear Cardiology: State of the Art and Future Directions, 2nd ed. St Louis, MO: Mosby, 1999.

123. Zaret BL, Wackers FJ, Terrin ML, et al: Value of radionuclide rest and exercise left ventricular ejection fraction in assessing survival of patients after thrombolytic therapy for acute myocardial infarction: results of thrombolysis in myocardial infarction (TIMI) phase II study. The TIMI study group. J Am Coll Cardiol 26:73–79, 1995.

124. Zellweger MJ, Lewin HC, Lai S, et al: When to stress patients after coronary artery bypass surgery? Risk stratification in patients early and late post-CABG using stress myocardial perfusion SPECT: implications of appropriate clinical strategies. J Am Coll Cardiol 37:144–152, 2001.

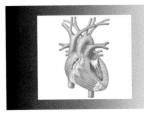

CHAPTER 57

Diagnostic Echocardiography

Rosario Freeman and Catherine M. Otto

Echocardiography is a vital tool for the diagnosis and management of cardiovascular disease with the advantages of relatively low cost as well as minimal patient risk and discomfort. Diagnostic applications of echocardiography include precise anatomical definition and physiological interrogation of cardiac and vascular structures, as well as direct real-time visualization of myocardial and valvular function.[12,33,34,48] Advances

in image quality and Doppler quantitation have expanded the utility of echocardiography. Current applications include routine screening for cardiac function, initial diagnosis of cardiac abnormalities, monitoring disease progression, and optimizing the timing of surgical intervention. Echocardiography is also used for screening potential donor hearts for transplantation.[49] Use of this technique now has expanded beyond the diagnostic laboratory to include the intensive care unit, the emergency department, the electrophysiology laboratory, and the operating room.[12]

▶ BASIC PRINCIPLES

Ultrasound images are generated from complex analyses of reflected ultrasound waves on internal structures. Audible sound waves are between 20 Hertz (Hz) and 20 kHz in frequency. Sound waves that are higher in frequency are termed ultrasound. Factors that can affect image generation include ultrasound beam refraction, beam attenuation due to absorption of ultrasound energy by intervening tissue, and disarrayed beam reflection, or scatter. Propagation of ultrasound waves is optimal through liquid medium. Air and bone cause significant acoustic impedance. Therefore, air-filled lungs or other intrathoracic air results in poor ultrasound penetration and suboptimal image generation. Image quality is also adversely affected when patient positioning is limited or when other intervening structures are present such as ribs or surface bandages.

▶ ULTRASOUND IMAGING MODALITIES

Echocardiographic examinations may include use of several ultrasound modalities, including M-mode, two-dimensional imaging, color flow imaging, and spectral Doppler displays with continuous-wave and pulsed Doppler ultrasound. M-mode (motion) is produced by displaying signals from a single ultrasound beam against the time dimension (Figure 57-1). M-mode is useful for measurement of cardiac dimensions and for timing of events, such as valve opening and closing. M-mode also displays rapid motion such as fluttering of the anterior mitral valve leaflet with aortic regurgitation and the independent mobility of valvular vegetations and aortic dissection flaps.

Transthoracic 2D Images

Two-dimensional (2D) echocardiographic images depict cardiac anatomy in real time using a simultaneous array of

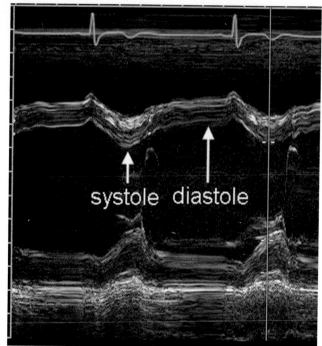

Figure 57–1 M-mode tracing from a normal individual depicting left ventricular wall thickness and chamber size during systole and diastole. The continuous ECG tracing along the top of the figure demonstrates the time dimension.

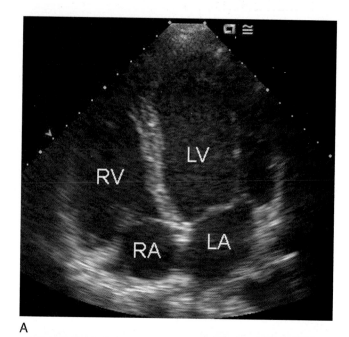

A

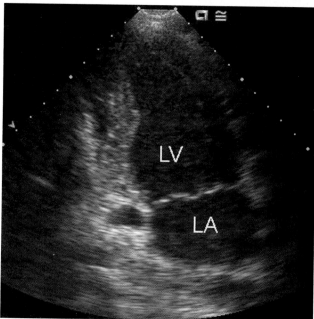

B

Figure 57–2 The apical four-chamber view shows the lateral and inferoseptal walls of the left ventricle (**A**). The apical two-chamber view shows the left ventricular anterior and inferior walls (**B**).

ultrasound beams across the tomographic plane. Transthoracic echocardiographic (TTE) examinations use transducer positions ("windows") that provide acoustic access to the heart: parasternal, apical, subcostal, and suprasternal. From these windows, tomographic image planes are aligned with respect to the cardiac anatomy in long-axis, short-axis, and four-chamber views (Figure 57-2). Standard 2D imaging utilizes reflection of the fundamental transmitted frequency. Suboptimal image quality due to poor ultrasound penetration can be improved by using harmonic imaging, which improves endocardial definition. However, planar subjects, such as valve leaflets, may appear thickened when using harmonic imaging. Acoustic shadowing from structures that block propagation of ultrasound waves, such as prosthetic valves or calcification, will block imaging distal to the shadowing structure. Alternative acoustic windows are then necessary to visualize the shadowed field. For example, with TTE, a mechanical mitral prosthesis creates acoustic shadowing of the left atrium, hindering evaluation of valvular and paravalvular regurgitation (Figure 57-3). Transducer placement posterior to the heart via transesophageal echocardiography (TEE) is then required for evaluation of prosthesis regurgitation in this setting. Recognition of ultrasound-created image artifacts is essential to correctly identify abnormal findings. Common ultrasound artifacts include reverberations, beam width artifacts, and beam refraction, as well as external artifacts generated from electronic effects on the ultrasound machine. An example of this is intraoperative electrocautery use during imaging.

Transesophageal Images

With TEE, the transducer is mounted on a flexible endoscope and positioned in the esophagus and stomach. TEE is performed in awake patients by a cardiologist using mild conscious sedation with appropriate monitoring during the procedure. TEE is also increasingly used in the operating room for intraoperative evaluation of complex cardiac disease. Image planes in TEE are similar to those used on TTE studies; however, manipulation of the esophageal probe is constrained by esophageal anatomy. Oblique image planes

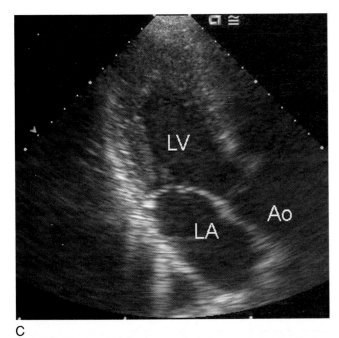

C

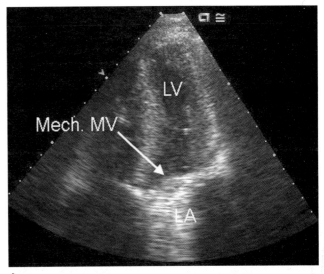

A

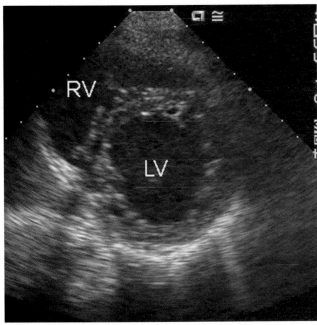

D

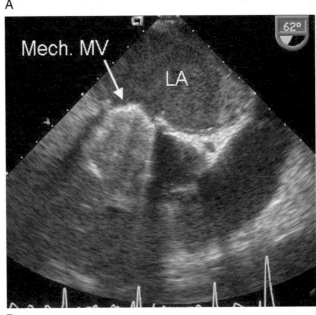

B

Figure 57–3 St. Jude mechanical prosthesis in the mitral position demonstrating acoustic shadowing of the left atrium when using TTE (**A**) and visualization of the left atrium when the same patient is imaged using TEE (**B**).

Figure 57–2 cont'd The apical long-axis view shows the left ventricular anteroseptum and posterior walls (**C**). And the short-axis view (**D**) shows a cross section through the midportion of the right and left ventricles.

often hinder acquisition of correct cardiac dimensions and may limit complete Doppler analysis by the inability to align the ultrasound beam in a parallel manner. Compared to TTE images, image resolution is significantly improved with TEE because of the lack of intervening air or bone. The placement of the transducer posterior to the heart allows for better visualization of posterior cardiac structures such as the mitral valve, left atrium, left atrial appendage, intraatrial septum, and thoracic aorta.

TEE is more accurate than TTE imaging for identification of valvular vegetations and complications of endocardi-

tis,[15,40,42,43] diagnosis of aortic dissection,[5,18,47] evaluation of mitral valve prostheses,[4] evaluation of complex congenital heart disease,[27] and intraoperative evaluation of mitral valve repair. TEE is used to identify left atrial thrombus as a potential cardiac source of distal embolic disease and to exclude thrombus presence prior to elective cardioversion for atrial fibrillation.[24] In the intensive care unit, TEE has been used in determining the etiology of unexplained hypotension[22]; TEE is particularly helpful in patients following cardiac surgery who are at increased risk for ischemia, hypovolemia, and pericardial tamponade.[21,37,39]

Doppler Echocardiography

Doppler echocardiography is based on the change in frequency (Doppler shift) of reflected, backscattered signals from moving red blood cells. Spectral analysis of the Doppler shift provides information on the direction and velocity of blood flow. By convention, frequency shifts toward the transducer are shown above the zero baseline, and frequency shifts away from the transducer are shown below. Doppler frequency shifts (Δf) are converted to blood flow velocities (V) using the Doppler equation, assuming a parallel intercept angle (θ) between the ultrasound beam and direction of blood flow:

$$V = [c(\Delta f)]/[2F_o(\cos \theta)]$$

where c is the speed of sound in blood and F_o is the transducer frequency.

Pulsed Doppler ultrasound samples blood velocities at a specified depth and thus has a limited maximum velocity, termed the Nyquist limit. Velocities above the Nyquist limit result in signal aliasing, with signal depicted on both sides of the baseline and no measurable peak velocity. In conjunction with a 2D diameter measurement for calculation of the cross-sectional area (CSA) of flow, velocity time integral (VTI) of the pulsed Doppler velocity curve allows calculation of stroke volume (SV) at various intracardiac sites as

$$SV = CSA \times VTI$$

This concept is used for calculation of stenotic valve areas using the continuity equation and for calculation of regurgitant volumes using the flow convergence proximal to the regurgitant valve.

Continuous-wave Doppler ultrasound samples velocities along the entire length of the ultrasound beam, allowing for measurement of high blood velocities. For both pulsed and continuous-wave Doppler techniques, detecting the maximum velocity relies on maintaining a parallel angle between the ultrasound beam and the flow of interest. A nonparallel intercept angle will result in velocity underestimation. Continuous-wave Doppler data allows calculation of pressure (P) differences across stenotic and regurgitant valves. When a blood flow stream narrows, (i.e., when traversing a valvular orifice), flow velocity (v) increases in proportion to the degree of narrowing as described by the simplified Bernoulli equation, which ignores viscous losses and acceleration:

$$\Delta P = 4v^2$$

The Bernoulli equation is used to calculate pressure gradients across stenotic valves, to evaluate left ventricular dP/dT, and to estimate pulmonary arterial systolic pressures using the tricuspid regurgitant jet velocity.

Color Doppler echocardiography is a specific application of pulsed Doppler echocardiography in which data from multiple pulsed Doppler velocity samples across a 2D image plane are combined and converted into images using a color scale. These images are superimposed onto a 2D image, providing real-time directional blood flow information. By convention, flow toward the transducer is depicted in red and flow away is depicted in blue, with the color transition occurring at the Nyquist limit.

Color Doppler echocardiography is used for qualitative evaluation of valvular regurgitation by examining the timing and extent of flow disturbance created by the regurgitant jet. Severity is usually rated on a scale of 1+ (mild) to 4+ (severe). A similar qualitative evaluation is used for intracardiac shunts.

Qualitative measurement of regurgitant flow can be performed utilizing data from Doppler ultrasound techniques.[34] Measurement of the narrowest jet width (vena contracta) from the long-axis view using color Doppler is a simple method, and is accurate even in the presence of eccentric jets. The proximal isovelocity surface area (PISA) method utilizes the concept that blood accelerates in a laminar fashion toward a regurgitant orifice, forming multiple "hemispheres" of isovelocity (Figure 57-4). The flow rate through any given hemisphere equals the regurgitant flow rate. Color Doppler analysis of the flow convergence region provides an accurate measurement of flow velocity at a given distance from the orifice; the regurgitant volume can then be calculated from flow velocities. A simplified calculation of the effective regurgitant orifice area ($EROA$) can be performed by setting the color Doppler aliasing velocity at 40 cm/s, assuming the mitral regurgitant peak velocity is 5 m/s and measuring the distance between the aliasing velocity to the valve orifice (r).[36]

$$EROA = r^2/4$$

Other markers of regurgitant severity include measurement of the peak E wave velocity for mitral regurgitation and spectral Doppler interrogation of the vascular structures connected to the cardiac chamber receiving the regurgitant flow. With moderate or greater regurgitation severity, flow reversal can be documented. Examples of this are systolic flow reversal in the pulmonary veins and hepatic veins in mitral and tricuspid regurgitation, respectively, and holodiastolic flow reversal in the proximal abdominal aorta with aortic regurgitation.

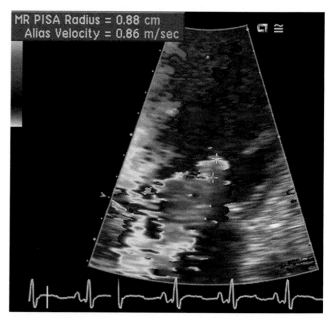

Figure 57–4 Severe mitral regurgitation imaged by TTE with color Doppler imaging of the proximal isovelocity surface area.

Other Imaging Modalities

Contrast echocardiography opacifies intracardiac chambers via intravenously introducing microbubble contrast agents. Contrast agents include agitated saline, used to opacify the right heart chambers for detection of intracardiac shunts (Figure 57-5), and commercially made products that traverse the pulmonary bed to provide left heart opacification. When image quality is suboptimal, opacification of the left-sided cardiac chambers allows for enhanced endocardial definition aiding in wall motion analyses[16] (Figure 57-6). Contrast agents have the potential to provide information on myocardial perfusion, although this methodology is still in development.[28]

Epicardial echocardiography is performed by placing the transducer directly on the epicardium intraoperatively in a sterile manner. This modality is utilized when anterior structures are suboptimally seen via a transesophageal approach. In intravascular ultrasound, imaging of vascular structures is performed from a transducer within a percutaneously placed catheter. Intravascular images obtained from intracoronary transducer placement assist in plaque characterization and assessment of stenosis severity.

Three-dimensional (3D) echocardiography can provide moving gray-scale images of cardiac structures and is being used clinically at some centers. Research applications of 3D echocardiography include tracing cardiac structures to analyze the 3D relationships associated with altered cardiac function, for example, in ischemic mitral regurgitation.

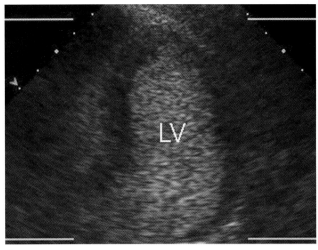

A

B

Figure 57–6 Representative comparison (A,B) of digital loop cine clips during a dobutamine echocardiogram at different dobutamine infusion doses to identify induced ischemia. Intravenous administration of microbubble contrast was used to enhance endocardial border definition for wall motion analysis.

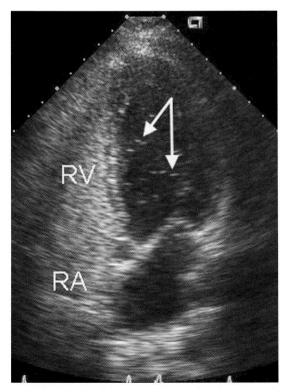

Figure 57–5 Opacification of the right atrium and right ventricle with intravenous agitated saline contrast. The presence of a patent foramen ovale is demonstrated by right-to-left shunting across the intraatrial septum with bubbles (*arrows*) identified in the left ventricle within three cardiac cycles.

► VENTRICULAR FUNCTION

Systolic Function

Assessment of left ventricular systolic function is the most common indication for echocardiography. 2D or M-mode measurements of internal chamber dimension at end systole and at end diastole are accurate and reproducible. Fractional shortening, the change in internal chamber dimension divided by the end-diastolic dimension, is an approximate measurement of systolic function with normal ranging between 25 and 45%. Left ventricular systolic function is more precisely described by ejection fraction (*EF*) derived from end-diastolic volume (*EDV*) and end-systolic volume (*ESV*) as

$$EF = (EDV - ESV)/EDV \times 100\%$$

where volumes are calculated from endocardial border tracings in two orthogonal views using geometric formulas, such as the summation of discs method (Figure 57-7). Because volume calculation is dependent on geometric assumptions of the left ventricle, accuracy depends on adequate endocardial definition and standard nonoblique imaging planes. Estimation of ejection fraction is more challenging with abnormal segmental wall motion and in the setting of underlying arrhythmia where variability in the cardiac cycle length affects beat-to-beat evaluation of left ventricular volume. Echocardiographic measures of ejection fraction are comparable to nuclear imaging and angiographic techniques.[12]

When image quality precludes tracing of endocardial borders, a qualitative assessment of ejection fraction is reliable when estimated by an experienced reader. Visual estimates of ejection fraction usually are reported in increments of 5 or 10 ejection fraction units (e.g., 50–55% or 20–30%).

Another measure of systolic function is derived from the early systolic rate of velocity increase in the mitral regurgitant jet, a relatively load-independent measure of contractility. The slope of the mitral regurgitant jet represents the rate of change in left ventricular pressure over time (*dP/dt*). This rate of change can be measured as shown in Figure 57-8. A normal *dP/dt* is >1000 mm Hg/s; a lower *dP/dt* is concordant with depressed left ventricular performance.

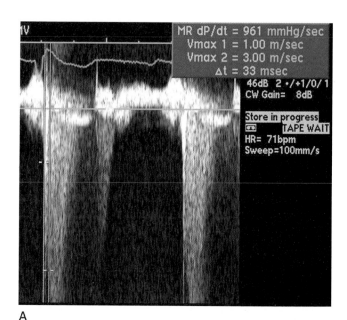

A

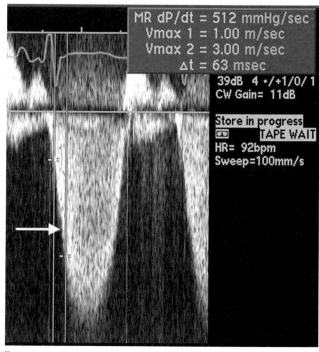

B

Figure 57–8 Compared with continuous Doppler tracings of the mitral regurgitant jet in an individual with only mildly reduced left ventricular systolic function (**A**), there is a decreased rate of rise to the peak left ventricular cavity pressure during early systole in a patient with severely reduced left ventricular systolic dysfunction (**B**) *(arrow)*.

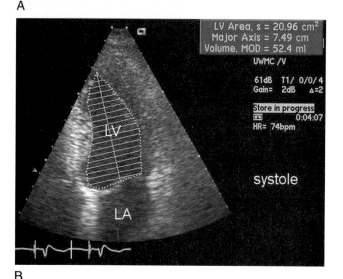

Figure 57–7 Endocardial border tracings of the left ventricle in the apical four-chamber view during diastole (**A**) and systole (**B**) are used to calculate end-diastolic and end-systolic left ventricular volumes. Using the same left ventricular volume calculation for the apical two-chamber view, the ejection fraction can then be calculated using the apical biplane method of disks algorithm.

Quantitative evaluation of right ventricular systolic function is difficult because of the complex geometry of the right ventricle. Right ventricular function is usually reported qualitatively on a scale of normal, mildly, moderately, or severely depressed. Evaluation of right heart function includes the noninvasive assessment of pulmonary artery pressures. The maximal velocity (V) obtained from continuous Doppler recording of the tricuspid regurgitant (TR) jet is used to calculate the right ventricular to right atrial systolic pressure difference, using the simplified Bernoulli equation (Figure 57-9). Right atrial pressure (RAP) is estimated from examination of the inferior vena cava (IVC) at rest and with inspiration. In the absence of pulmonary stenosis, which is rare in the general population, right ventricular systolic pressure equals pulmonary arterial systolic pressure. The pulmonary artery systolic pressure (PAP) is then

$$PAP = 4(V_{TR})^2 + RAP$$

This measurement is widely applicable as 90% of normal individuals have some degree of tricuspid regurgitation.

Diastolic Function

Diastole is composed of four phases: (1) isovolumic relaxation, (2) atrioventricular valve opening with passive early rapid ventricular filling, (3) diastasis, or deceleration of passive left ventricular filling due to equalization of atrial and ventricular pressures, and (4) late active ventricular filling

due to atrial contraction. Doppler evaluation of left ventricular filling demonstrates two peaks of flow, termed "E" and "A" waves, corresponding to the "early" and "atrial" contributions of ventricular filling.[14] In normal, young individuals, the E wave is dominant with atrial contraction contributing <20% to ventricular filling, and an E:A velocity ratio in the vicinity of 1.3. With aging, there is an expected, gradual increase in the relative contribution of atrial filling with reversal of the E and A velocities seen in the elderly (Figure 57-10). In addition to the age-related changes in the left ventricular filling pattern, other factors that can affect the pressure gradient between the atria and the ventricle, such as preload, heart rate, flow rate, and atrial contractile function, can also affect the filling pattern.

Diastolic dysfunction can be classified as "impaired relaxation" with impairment of early diastolic filling or "decreased compliance" with abnormalities in late diastolic filling. Impaired myocardial relaxation results in prolongation of isovolumic relaxation, a slower rate of decline in early diastolic velocity, and a lower early peak filling velocity with an E:A ratio less than 1. Conversely, decreased ventricular compliance, seen often in conjunction with increased left atrial pressure, leads to increased contribution of early diastolic filling with a steep deceleration slope and a shortened isovolumic relaxation time. In this scenario, because the ventricle fills rapidly in the early phase, the atrial contribution is

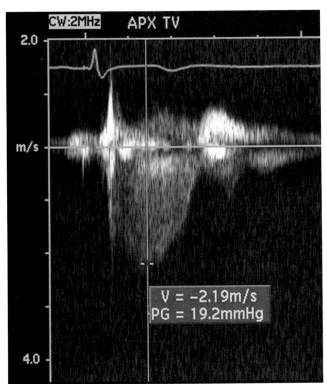

Figure 57-9 The peak pressure gradient (PG) is calculated using the peak velocity (V) from the continuous Doppler tracings of the tricuspid regurgitant jet utilizing the simplified Bernoulli equation. The pulmonary arterial systolic pressure is then obtained by adding the estimated right atrial pressure to the PG calculation.

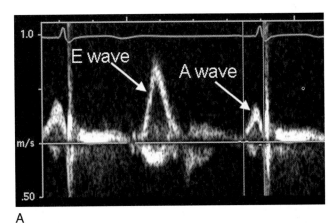

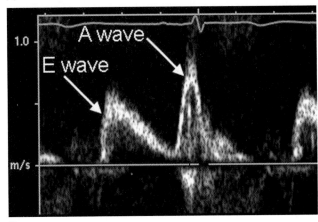

Figure 57-10 Transmitral pulsed Doppler ultrasound in a normal 19-year-old patient (A) and 86-year-old patient (B) showing the age-dependent reversal in the peak E to A velocity ratio over time.

918 relatively smaller, and the E:A ratio is >1 and termed a "restrictive pattern." Abnormalities in diastolic function can also be seen with extracardiac constraint of ventricular filling such as in constrictive pericarditis or tamponade. Doppler evaluation of diastolic function using the left ventricular filling pattern must be done in the context of understanding other conditions that affect the filling pattern as described previously. A more complete evaluation of diastolic function can be obtained by measurement of the isovolumic relaxation time, evaluation of mitral inflow with changes in loading conditions (e.g., with the Valsalva maneuver), assessment of pulmonary venous inflow patterns, and tissue Doppler analysis of mitral annular motion.[14]

Normal right ventricular filling demonstrates respiratory variation in transtricuspid velocities. On inspiration, there is an increase in systemic venous return resulting in a transient increase in velocities, with a normal magnitude increase of approximately 20%. In contrast, because left atrial filling is not respiratory dependent, left ventricular filling velocities do not normally express respiratory changes. The presence of respiratory variation in the transmitral Doppler images and exaggerated respiratory variation in the transtricuspid Doppler images can be seen with pericardial tamponade and chronic pulmonary disease (Figure 57-11). Other factors that can affect normal intrathoracic pressure generation and its effect on the heart will also affect the atrioventricular Doppler interrogation. Examples of this include concurrent positive pressure ventilation, pericardial constriction, and pulmonary hypertension.

ISCHEMIC HEART DISEASE

Direct visualization of coronary anatomy is not routinely possible with echocardiography and requires coronary angiography. However, 2D echocardiography allows for direct real-time visualization of endocardial motion and wall thickening from multiple echocardiographic views. In the presence of ischemic heart disease, segmental wall motion abnormalities can be detected, correlating with impaired coronary blood flow to a particular myocardial region. Typically, ventricular segments are described by the wall segment affected, which can be correlated with coronary anatomy. Myocardial function is graded as normal, hyperkinetic, hypokinetic, akinetic, or dyskinetic for each segment.

Myocardial Infarction

Wall motion abnormalities on a resting echocardiographic study may be due to an acute or old myocardial infarction, stunned myocardium, or myocardial hibernation. Both acute and old transmural infarcts result in severe hypokinesis or akinesis of the affected segments. However, an old transmural infarct typically appears thinned and scarred (Figure 57-12), whereas an acute infarction is associated with normal wall thickness. Resting echocardiographic assessment of the infarct zone correlates well with other derived measures of infarct burden[32] and, with ejection fraction estimation, offers long- and short-term prognostic information.[7]

Resting TTE has been utilized to evaluate patients presenting to the emergency room with chest pain[41] and in

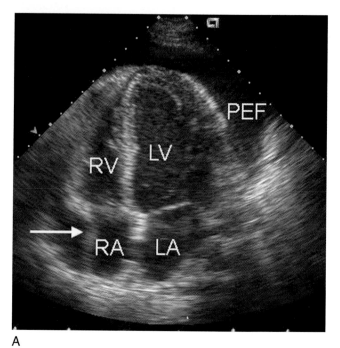

A

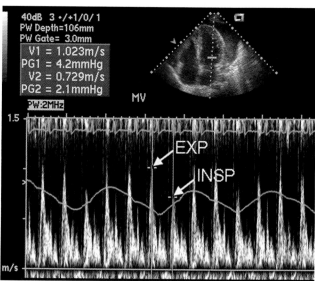

B

Figure 57–11 Circumferential pericardial effusion (PEF) in a patient presenting 2 weeks after aortic valve replacement with increasing dyspnea. There is right atrial systolic collapse seen on the apical four chamber view (**A**) *(arrow)*. The transmitral pulsed Doppler tracing demonstrates respiratory variation in flow (**B**). EXP, expiration; INSP, inspiration.

patients with recurrent pain following myocardial infarction or coronary revascularization procedures. The absence of regional wall motion abnormalities is an effective means of ruling out acute ischemia with a negative predictive accuracy approximating 95%.[12] In the operating room, intraoperative TEE allows for continuous monitoring of cardiac function and has been used during coronary revascularization, during valvular surgery, and to monitor patients undergoing noncardiac surgery at high risk of cardiac events. TEE has also proven useful to evaluate cardiac function in the hemody-

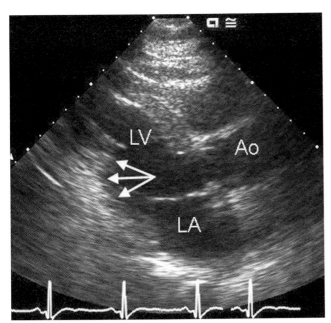

Figure 57–12 The basal posterior wall on the apical long-axis view is thinned, scarred, and akinetic *(arrows)*, consistent with prior myocardial infarction.

namically unstable patient where ischemia is suspected, but where transthoracic windows are suboptimal.[21,22]

After acute ischemia, myocardial stunning can occur with either hypokinesis or akinesis that may persist for days or weeks following successful coronary reperfusion. In the area of myocardial hibernation, akinesis is seen, even with myocardial viability, because of chronic severe impairment of coronary blood flow. With restoration of adequate coronary flow, hibernating segments may regain normal function. Dobutamine stress echocardiography can help differentiate hibernating myocardium from an area of irreversible infarction.[1]

Stress Testing for Coronary Disease

In the setting of coronary artery disease without prior infarction, there are no segmental wall motion abnormalities because coronary blood flow is adequate to supply oxygen demand at rest. However, with increased myocardial demand and resultant ischemia, segmental wall motion abnormalities become apparent. Stress echocardiography allows for diagnosis of induced myocardial ischemia in a controlled setting. There is a high correlation between abnormalities on stress echocardiography and demonstrable coronary artery disease by coronary angiography. Stress echocardiography is useful for identification of specific myocardial regions affected by flow-limiting coronary lesions, and to follow disease progression in patients with known coronary artery disease. Additionally, this technique is used to assess adequacy of coronary revascularization in patients with recurrent symptoms and to evaluate the functional significance of residual lesions to determine if further revascularization procedures are needed, and can offer prognostic information following revascularization.[2]

Stress echocardiography is most commonly performed with either treadmill exercise or dobutamine infusion. Exercise protocols using upright and recumbent bicycles also exist. The addition of echocardiographic imaging before and immediately following exercise increases both the sensitivity and specificity of the test compared to standard treadmill exercise stress testing. Compared to standard treadmill exercise stress testing, stress echocardiography is particularly useful when there are abnormalities in the baseline ECG and in women.

Stress-induced ischemia is identified with onset of hypokinesis or akinesis of a myocardial segment on the immediate poststress images that had normal wall motion at rest. Using standard views of the left ventricle, accuracy in detecting induced ischemia is increased by utilizing side-by-side comparison of the rest and immediately postexercise cine-loop digital images. Because ischemic segmental wall motion abnormalities may normalize once the oxygen supply deficit is restored, a submaximal test or any delay in obtaining the stress images after exercise lowers the sensitivity of the test.[12,29] Interpretation of stress echocardiography also incorporates data from the ECG, maximum workload achieved, and the hemodynamic response to exercise.

Pharmacological stress echocardiography is an alternative to exercise when testing cannot be performed because of physical limitations or with significant respiratory interference from exercise-induced tachypnea. This modality is also used when exercise response may be limited, such as in postcardiac transplant patients with denervated hearts where testing is done to monitor for transplant vasculopathy.[30]

Adrenergic-stimulating medications, typically intravenous dobutamine, are infused according to a protocol. Dobutamine typically starts at 5 µg/kg/min and is incrementally increased at intervals of 3–5 min to a maximum of 40 µg/kg/min. If the target heart rate (85% of the patient's maximum predicted heart rate) is not achieved, atropine can also be administered. Echocardiographic imaging is performed before dobutamine infusion and at each dose level. Ischemia is identified as a new wall motion abnormality (Figure 57-6).

In addition to diagnosis of the presence or severity of coronary disease, dobutamine stress echocardiography has also been used for the assessment of myocardial viability based on augmentation of myocardial function at low infusion rates of dobutamine (5–10 µg/kg/min) followed by worsening of myocardial function at higher doses of dobutamine, with the onset of ischemia.[1]

With stress echocardiography, diagnosis of inducible ischemia is dependent on accurate evaluation of segmental wall motion, which may be difficult in several situations. Resting segmental abnormalities in patients with preexisting coronary artery disease make the diagnosis of ischemia more difficult compared to patients with normal wall motion at rest. When endocardial definition is suboptimal, intravenous contrast agents that opacify the left ventricular cavity aid in endocardial border definition.[16] False interpretation of a wall motion abnormality may be observed if acoustic windows are oblique to the desired tomographic plane. Finally, provocation of inducible ischemia is dependent on reaching the workload that exceeds adequate coronary flow. A suboptimal workload may not adequately induce ischemia, leading to a nondiagnostic stress study.

Complications of Acute Myocardial Infarction

Echocardiography is the diagnostic tool of choice to evaluate complications of myocardial infarction.[12] New segmental

920

wall motion abnormalities can be detected when postinfarction angina occurs. In the setting of congestive heart failure, assessment of residual left ventricular systolic function and estimation of pulmonary pressures can be performed. When ischemic disease causes systolic dysfunction and left ventricular chamber enlargement, significant regurgitation can result from distortion of the mitral subvalvular apparatus. Mitral regurgitation as a direct result of ischemia on the papillary muscle can also be identified. These include papillary dysfunction from acute ischemia, rupture of a necrotic papillary muscle head, and scarring with retraction of the papillary muscle and subvalvular apparatus.

Myocardial necrosis with ventricular rupture can be identified both in the free wall and the interventricular septum using a combination of 2D and Doppler techniques. A ventricular septal defect is identified by characteristic color flow and continuous-wave Doppler flow across the defect. A ventricular free wall rupture that is contained is termed a pseudoaneurysm. Pseudoaneurysms have a typical echocardiographic appearance that includes an abrupt transition from normal myocardial tissue to the aneurysmal dilation, a narrow aneurysmal "neck," and thrombus within the pseudoaneurysm.

Other complications of myocardial infarction include ventricular aneurysm formation. Similar to pseudoaneurysms, these are at risk of developing thrombus within the aneurysmal cavity. Mural thrombi occur primarily in anterior and apical infarctions, and are less frequent with early revascularization. Right ventricular infarction is most often associated with inferior myocardial infarctions and is diagnosed on echocardiography by evaluation of right ventricular size and systolic function. A cause of hypoxemia following inferior myocardial infarction is increased right-sided pressures with resulting right-to-left shunting across a patent foramen ovale. This can be diagnosed by TEE evaluation of the intraatrial septum with a contrast study using agitated saline contrast. A similar phenomenon has been described in postoperative hypoxemic patients with increased right atrial pressure.[49]

► CARDIAC MASSES

Direct visualization of the heart and surrounding structures allows for detection of abnormal cardiac masses as small as 1–2 mm. Cardiac masses include normal structures, tumors, thrombi, and vegetations (Figures 57-13 and 57-14). These categories are not mutually exclusive (i.e., a lesion may consist of coexistent vegetations and thrombi). Initial echocardiographic diagnosis of structural abnormalities should be made after differentiation from ultrasound artifacts and normal structural variants. Additionally, interpretation of abnormalities should be made after correlation with clinical history such as with pacing wires, central venous catheters, and sutures in the postoperative patient (Figure 57-15).

Left ventricular thrombi occur most often in the setting of aneurysm formation after myocardial infarction. The sensitivity and specificity of TTE echocardiography are approximately 95% and 88%, respectively, for detection of apical thrombi, when careful apical imaging with a high-frequency transducer is used.[33] TEE is less sensitive for apical thrombi as the apex is in the far field of the image. Atrial thrombi occur most often in patients in atrial fibrillation (Figure 57-16),

but can also occur in patients in sinus rhythm and lower atrial blood velocities, such as when mitral stenosis is present. Left atrial thrombi are rarely visualized by TTE. Rather, TEE is indicated when a diagnosis of left atrial thrombus is suspected. The sensitivity and specificity of TEE for detection of left atrial thrombus are high (100% and 100%), but care is needed to visualize the appendage in at least two image planes for a definitive diagnosis.[33]

Valvular vegetations are identified on echocardiography as independently mobile masses attached to the upstream side of cardiac valves (e.g., the ventricular side of the aortic valve or the left atrial side of the mitral valve). Vegetations are most often due to infective endocarditis. However, the differential also includes nonbacterial thrombotic endocarditis and benign masses such as papillary fibroelastomas.

Tumors in the heart are 20 times more likely to be noncardiac in origin. The most common metastatic tumors in the heart are lung, breast, lymphoma, leukemia, stomach, and melanoma. Involvement includes direct invasion into the pericardium, distant metastasis with pericardial or intramyocardial masses, and, in rare cases, endocardial masses. In the case of renal cell carcinoma, direct extension via the inferior vena cava into the right atrium can be seen. Primary cardiac tumors in the heart are rare, and the majority of these are benign. Atrial myxomas present with constitutional symptoms, embolic events, and symptoms of functional mitral valve obstruction. Papillary fibroelastomas may be found incidentally on echocardiography (where they mimic a valve vegetation) or may present with embolic events.

In patients with a systemic embolic event, echocardiography may identify a potential cardiac source of the embolus in

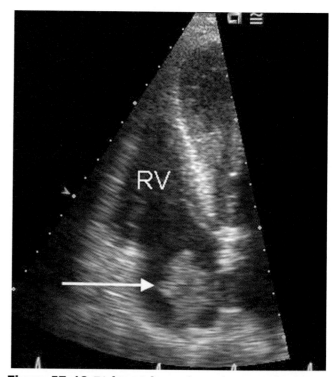

Figure 57–13 Right atrial mass (*arrow*) in a renal-pancreas transplant patient with transplant organ failure and a dialysis catheter in place as seen in the apical four-chamber view. Several fungal blood cultures were positive for *Candida glabrata*.

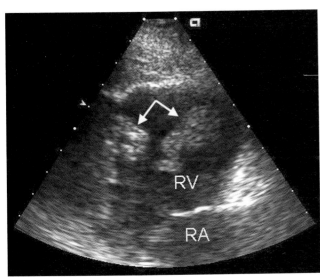

Figure 57–14 Mobile thrombus is identified in the right ventricle of a patient with increasing oxygen requirements and atrial fibrillation *(arrows)*. Subsequent diagnostic testing demonstrated acute deep venous thrombosis of the right peroneal and posterior tibial veins and massive bilateral pulmonary emboli with pulmonary infarct.

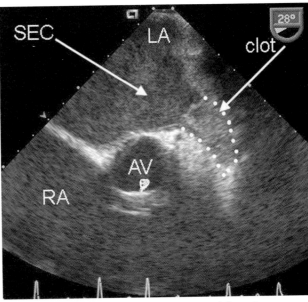

Figure 57–16 Imaged using TEE, an atrial thrombus is seen in the left atrial appendage outlined by dotted line *(arrow)* in a patient with atrial fibrillation and congestive heart failure undergoing evaluation for elective cardioversion. Low-velocity blood flow is evidenced by the spontaneous echo contrast (SEC) seen at the mouth of the left atrial appendage.

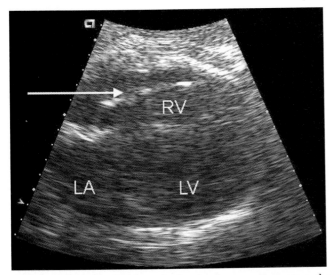

Figure 57–15 A bright echodensity is seen traversing the tricuspid valve *(arrow)* on the subcostal view in a patient with a right ventricular pacing lead.

patent foramen ovale is made with infusion of a contrast agent during imaging with contrast seen in the left atrium within three cardiac cycles after opacification of the right atrium (Figure 57-5). A Valsalva maneuver may be needed to transiently increase right atrial pressure during the contrast injection to make the diagnosis.

► CARDIOMYOPATHIES

Congestive Heart Failure

Useful diagnostic tools from echocardiography in the evaluation of patient with congestive heart failure include the assessment of left and right ventricular systolic and diastolic function, measurement of chamber size and wall thickness, visualization of valvular anatomy and function, and clinical evaluation of hemodynamic status. Ischemic heart disease is the most common cause of myocardial dysfunction and resultant congestive heart failure. Other causes of congestive heart failure include primary abnormalities of the myocardium, or cardiomyopathies, and the secondary effects of other cardiac disease processes on the myocardium, such as valvular heart disease and pulmonary hypertension. Significant chronic pulmonary hypertension leads to right ventricular chamber enlargement with resultant right-sided valvular regurgitation, hypertrophy, and right ventricular systolic dysfunction.[9] Serial echocardiographic studies assist in clinical monitoring of pulmonary pressures, intravascular volume status, valvular dysfunction, and guidance of medical therapy such as continuous vasodilator therapy. Echocardiography has low sensitivity for detecting acute pulmonary emboli.[31]

up to 30% of cases.[20] Findings associated with an increased risk of embolism include left-sided thrombi, right-to-left shunting across a patent foramen ovale, atrial septal aneurysms, aortic atherosclerotic disease, and findings suggesting low velocity blood flow such as systolic dysfunction and spontaneous echo contrast.[20,26] Other potential sources of distal embolic disease that can be identified by echocardiography include intracardiac tumors and valvular vegetations. A patent foramen ovale, present in approximately 20% of unselected patients at autopsy, is associated with an increased risk of systemic embolic events. Echocardiographic diagnosis of a

Dilated Cardiomyopathy

Dilated cardiomyopathies are characterized by cardiac chamber enlargement and systolic dysfunction (Figure 57-17). Systolic dysfunction is typically global in nature, but heterogeneity in regional function can be observed. Although anatomy and function of cardiac structures are readily described, etiology identification from the echocardiogram is usually not possible. Often, dilated cardiomyopathy is associated with distortion of the atrioventricular valvular apparatus, with resulting regurgitation. Systolic dysfunction and chronic volume overload can also lead to secondary pulmonary hypertension. Although systolic dysfunction is typically the dominant finding, with increased myocardial wall stress and intracardiac pressures, impaired diastolic filling is often present as well. A restrictive filling pattern on the transmitral Doppler interrogation has been correlated with clinical symptoms and has been shown to be a predictor of adverse outcome or need for transplantation.[35] In addition to standard evaluation of ventricular and valvular anatomy and function, echocardiographic studies include valvular annular measurements and quantification of regurgitant flow, left ventricular mass measurements, pulmonary pressure estimates, and visualization of thrombi if present. Measurements of left ventricular mass, Doppler derived dP/dT,[25] and ejection fraction can provide prognostic information on clinical outcome.

Hypertrophic Cardiomyopathy

Hypertrophic cardiomyopathy is manifested clinically by impaired diastolic function with preserved systolic function.[46] The classic hypertrophic pattern is asymmetrical septal hypertrophy (Figure 57-18), but several patterns of hypertrophy can also be seen. If the septum is significantly thickened, dynamic left ventricular outflow obstruction may be present with systolic anterior motion of the mitral valve leaflet against the interventricular septum. When this occurs, there is a late-peaking high-velocity jet at the site of obstruction on Doppler interrogation. The faulty systolic coaptation of the mitral valve also results in posteriorly directed mitral regurgitation. The severity of left ventricular outflow obstruction present can be altered by different loading conditions, with increased intracardiac volume decreasing the severity of obstruction.

In patients with hypertrophic cardiomyopathy, serial echocardiographic studies can demonstrate disease progression, assess the impact of medical therapy, evaluate the effects of atrioventricular sequential pacing, and assist in timing of surgical or percutaneous myomectomy intervention. Echocardiography is used in the cardiac catheterization laboratory to guide percutaneous septal ablation procedures. Intraoperatively, a combination of TEE and epicardial imaging is used to guide and evaluate the results of surgical myotomy/myectomy and to evaluate any procedural complications, such as a postoperative ventricular septal defect.[30]

Restrictive Cardiomyopathy

Restrictive cardiomyopathy is uncommon and is typically caused by one of several infiltrative disease processes, such as sarcoidosis and amyloidosis. Similar to hypertrophic cardiomyopathy, restrictive cardiomyopathy is characterized by normal systolic function and impaired diastolic function.[46] However, progression over time may lead to systolic dysfunction as well. Echocardiographic features of restrictive cardiomyopathy include increased myocardial wall thickness, biatrial enlargement, elevation in pulmonary arterial systolic pressures, and a transmitral diastolic filling consistent with impaired diastolic filling. However, these findings

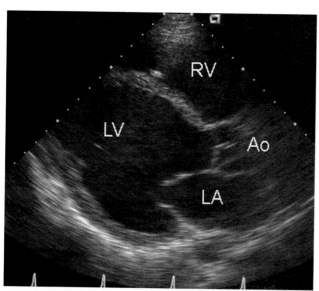

Figure 57–17 Left ventricular chamber enlargement in a patient with idiopathic dilated cardiomyopathy and severe systolic dysfunction seen on the parasternal long-axis view.

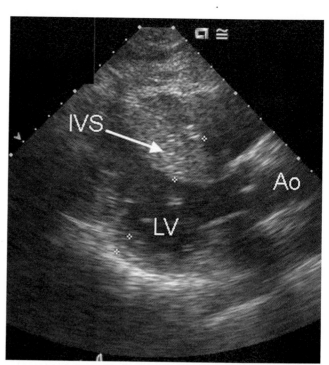

Figure 57–18 Asymmetrical hypertrophy of the interventricular septum (IVS) in a patient with hypertrophic cardiomyopathy seen on the parasternal long-axis view.

are not universal, making restrictive cardiomyopathy often difficult to definitively diagnose.

Cardiac Transplantation

With severe impairment of myocardial function, serial echocardiography is beneficial to reassess left ventricular function and optimize intravascular volume status. In end-stage disease, echocardiography is used in the decision-making process for placement of a left ventricular assist device (LVAD) or biventricular assist device. Echocardiographic identification of significant aortic regurgitation, severe mitral stenosis, or transatrial flow across either an atrial septal defect or a patent foramen ovale is important as their presence may adversely affect optimal LVAD performance. Functional issues including assessment for peridevice hematoma, leak, thrombus, and evaluation of right ventricular function can be made, but acoustic shadowing from the device may make a complete assessment difficult.

Following cardiac transplantation, acute complications identified by echocardiography include pericardial effusion, right ventricular dysfunction, and pulmonary hypertension. Organ rejection is evidenced by myocardial thickening and diastolic dysfunction in the initial stages, progressing eventually to systolic dysfunction.[10] Normal findings following cardiac transplantation include biatrial enlargement from the suturing of the residual native atria to the transplanted heart. The biatrial suture line is discerned as a linear echodensity along the midatrial wall. Aortic and pulmonary artery suture lines are typically difficult to identify. Pericardial effusions are common and not of concern unless hemodynamically significant. Posttransplantation, echocardiography is used to assist in biotome placement during cardiac biopsy when monitoring for organ rejection. In screening for development of transplant vasculopathy, dobutamine stress echocardiography has shown higher sensitivity than other stress testing modalities.[45] However, confirmatory testing for transplant vasculopathy is performed percutaneously in the cardiac catheterization laboratory using intravascular ultrasound.

▶ PERICARDIAL DISEASE

The pericardium is a thin, dense structure that forms an enclosed space around the heart with its superior aspect at the proximal great vessel level. Visual distinction of the pericardium is often difficult echocardiographically because of its position adjacent to other mediastinal structures. Pericarditis classically presents with chest pain, diagnostic changes on an electrocardiogram, and an auscultated rub. Concurrent pericardial effusion may or may not be present. Pericardial thickening can occur, but may not be readily identified because of localization of the thickening and its adjacent positioning to other mediastinal structures.

Constrictive Pericarditis

With recurrent pericarditis, the pericardium can become permanently thickened and adherent to the myocardium, causing impaired cardiac filling or "constriction." Constrictive pericarditis may also be caused by radiation therapy, prior trauma, or prior cardiac surgery. Doppler interrogation demonstrates rapid early diastolic filling with an abrupt cessation once the limit of the encased pericardial sac is reached, with equalization of diastolic pressures between the two ventricles. Left ventricular size and systolic function are typically normal. Echocardiographic diagnosis of constriction is supported with identification of inferior vena cava dilation, premature opening of the pulmonic valve, and characteristic changes in Doppler patterns, such as a prominent y descent on hepatic vein tracings and a restrictive filling pattern on transmitral Doppler interrogation.[11]

Differentiation between pericardial constriction and restrictive cardiomyopathy can be challenging.[3] Both conditions have increased central venous pressures with low cardiac output and preserved left ventricular systolic function. Echocardiographic findings that suggest constriction over restriction include exaggerated respiratory variation in right and left ventricular filling of greater than 25% in comparing inspiratory to expiratory velocities across the atrioventricular valves.[11] Additionally, pulmonary hypertension is less prominent in constriction compared to restrictive cardiomyopathy. Supplementary diagnostic tests that may be helpful include chest tomography or magnetic resonance imaging (MRI), which allow measurement of the thickened pericardial wall. Direct myocardial biopsy assists in detection of infiltrative myocardial disease. Simultaneous left- and right-sided pressure tracings with volume loading in the cardiac catheterization laboratory can also aid in the diagnosis.

Pericardial Effusion and Tamponade

A small amount of fluid in the pericardial space is a normal finding. Fibrinous stranding, tumors, or hematoma within the pericardial space can be readily identified by echocardiography. Larger amounts of fluid collection are abnormal and can cause external cardiac compression, or tamponade. Echocardiographic quantification and localization of pericardial fluid guide clinical decision making on timing of drainage procedures, assessment of feasibility for drainage, and selection on percutaneous versus surgical approaches.

When pericardial fluid accumulates slowly, a large volume (more that a liter) can be contained in the pericardial space at a low pressure and with few obvious clinical signs. When fluid accumulates more rapidly, intrapericardial pressures may exceed intracardiac pressure leading to hemodynamic compromise or tamponade physiology. Clinical findings of tamponade include increased jugular venous pressure, pulsus paradoxus, and systemic hypotension. Effects of increased intrapericardial pressure on thin myocardial free-walled chambers is invagination, or collapse. Because the atria are lower pressure cardiac chambers, they are affected before the ventricles. In tamponade, abnormal systolic collapse of the right atrial free wall (Figure 57-11) and abnormal diastolic collapse of the right ventricular free wall are seen on echocardiography.[11] If there is right ventricular hypertrophy or significantly increased right ventricular pressure from pulmonary hypertension, right ventricular diastolic collapse may not necessarily be seen. Other echocardiographic findings in tamponade include exaggerated septal motion during the cardiac cycle, vena caval dilation, and exaggerated respiratory variation in flows (>25%) across the atrioventricular valves. However, in the patient with clinical signs of tamponade and a large pericardial effusion, the absence of echocardiographic

924 signs of tamponade does not exclude the diagnosis. If clinical suspicion is high, pericardiocentesis may be needed to assess the effect of fluid removal on hemodynamics.

Focal tamponade due to a loculated fluid collection can also occur, particularly in the postoperative cardiac patient. Common locations of pericardial fluid collection following cardiac surgery include posteriorly and small hematomas adjacent to the right atrium, which may impede right atrial inflow. In these patients, suboptimal acoustic windows caused by limitations in patient positioning or surface bandages often limit image quality. The postoperative patient with hemodynamic instability may require TEE for complete evaluation.[21,22,37,39]

▶ VALVULAR DISEASE

Echocardiography is invaluable for the evaluation of valvular anatomy and function, delineating etiology of valvular dysfunction, and assessment of other valvular structures for concurrent disease.[8] In addition, echocardiography allows analysis of the effects of valvular disease on other structures, such as cardiac chambers and the pulmonary vascular bed, and provides a means for monitoring disease progression.[13] Other than coronary angiography in the preoperative patient, echocardiography has eliminated the need for invasive valvular diagnostics in the catheterization laboratory in most patients.

Aortic Stenosis

Aortic stenosis is most often caused by degenerative changes of a trileaflet valve. Characterized by progressive leaflet thickening and calcification, this slow disease process typically does not present clinically until the seventh or eighth decades of life (Figure 57-19). Other causes of aortic stenosis include secondary calcification of a bicuspid aortic valve and rheumatic valve disease with commissural fusion and retraction. Rheumatic valvular disease uniformly involves the mitral valve with concurrent aortic valve stenosis occurring in 5–10% of cases.

Aortic stenosis severity is evaluated using peak instantaneous transaortic velocities obtained from continuous Doppler ultrasound tracings (Figure 57-19). Several acoustic windows are used to obtain the maximal velocity. A velocity >4 m/s indicates severe stenosis, a velocity of 3–4 m/s indicates moderate stenosis, and a velocity of 2.5–3 m/s indicates mild stenosis. Both the maximum and mean transaortic pressure gradients are calculated using the simplified Bernoulli equation as described previously. Because transvalvular pressure gradients vary with volume flow rate, given a fixed valve area, higher pressure gradients and flow velocities would be present in the setting of increased stroke volume (i.e., aortic regurgitation), and lower pressure gradients and velocities would be present when flow rates are decreased (i.e., left ventricular systolic dysfunction).

Aortic valve area (AVA) is relatively independent of flow rate and is calculated using the continuity equation as

$$AVA = (CSA_{LVOT} \times VTI_{LVOT})/VTI_{aorta}$$

where the cross-sectional area (CSA) of the left ventricular outflow tract (LVOT) is calculated from the measured diam-

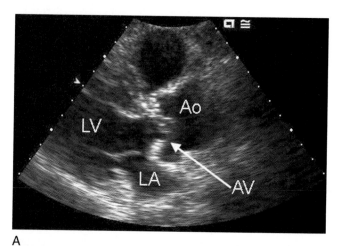

A

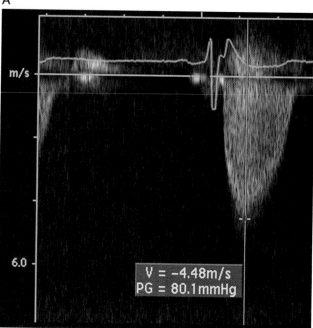

B

Figure 57–19 Severe aortic stenosis evidenced by thickened, calcified valve leaflets (**A**). On continuous Doppler imaging across the aortic valve, the peak velocity (V) is 4.5 m/s, corresponding to a peak gradient (PG) of 80 mm Hg using the simplified Bernoulli equation (**B**).

eter in the parasternal long-axis view, velocity time integrals (VTI) in the left ventricular outflow tract are obtained with pulsed Doppler from an apical view, and the aortic signal is recorded with continuous Doppler from whichever window yields the highest velocity signal. For routine clinical use, this equation can be simplified further by substituting peak velocities (V) in place of the VTI measurements:

$$AVA = (CSA_{LVOT} \times V_{LVOT})/V_{aorta}$$

A valve area <1.0 cm² indicates severe stenosis and a valve area of 1.0–1.5 cm² is consistent with moderate stenosis. This method for valve area estimation is concordant with other diagnostic measure techniques.[23]

The increased afterload from aortic stenosis causes an increase in myocardial wall stress with resulting left ventricular hypertrophy and impairment in diastolic filling. Systolic dysfunction typically occurs only in the late stages of the disease. With surgical disease, aortic stenosis severity should always be fully evaluated preoperatively by TTE. Although TEE may be used intraoperatively, quantitation of aortic stenosis severity by TEE is limited by the inability to optimally align the ultrasound beam for Doppler interrogation of the aortic valve. Direct planimetry of the valve orifice is limited by the nonplanar anatomy of the aortic valve, acoustic shadowing, and beam width artifact due to valve calcification. Limitations in echocardiographic evaluation of aortic stenosis include measurement variability, adequate alignment of the ultrasound beam to maximize transaortic velocities, and accurate measurement of the left ventricular outflow tract diameter and cross-sectional area.

Aortic Regurgitation

Causes of aortic regurgitation include a congenital bicuspid valve, endocarditis, and aortic root dilation with failure of leaflet coaptation. Echocardiography reliably identifies the cause of valvular regurgitation, which is important as the surgical approach for regurgitation due to aortic root disease differs substantially from the approach to primary valve dysfunction.

Doppler echocardiography has both a high sensitivity and specificity for detecting regurgitant flow and allows evaluation of regurgitant severity. Regurgitation is qualitatively evaluated as mild, moderate, or severe based on the size of the color flow jet relative to the left ventricular outflow tract in parasternal views (Figure 57-20). More quantitative evaluation from color flow images is possible by measurement of the vena contracta or calculation of regurgitant orifice areas based on the area of acceleration proximal to the valve as described previously. With moderate to severe aortic regurgitation, pulsed Doppler examination shows holodiastolic flow reversal in the descending thoracic and proximal abdominal aorta (Figure 57-20). The density of the continuous-wave Doppler signal is another measure of regurgitant severity with the diastolic deceleration slope of the regurgitant jet reflecting the aortic to left ventricular diastolic pressure difference. Acute regurgitation is characterized by a steep diastolic deceleration slope and, in severe cases, with equalization of aortic and left ventricular pressures, velocity approaches zero at end diastole. Eccentric regurgitant jets that are directed posteriorly toward the mitral valve may result in high-frequency fluttering and early closure of the anterior mitral valve leaflet, identified by M-mode tracings.

Even more important than Doppler evaluation of regurgitant severity is the effect of chronic volume overload on the left ventricle. Echocardiographic evaluation of left ventricular size and systolic function provide key data for timing of surgery in asymptomatic individuals with chronic aortic regurgitation.[13] Current guidelines recommend surgery when the end-systolic dimension is >50–55 mm or the end-diastolic dimension is >70–75 mm, and the ejection fraction is <50%.[8]

Mitral Stenosis

Mitral stenosis is nearly always caused by rheumatic valvular disease with commissural fusion and leaflet restriction. In severe cases, the subvalvular apparatus is also affected with chordal thickening, fusion, and calcification. Mitral annular

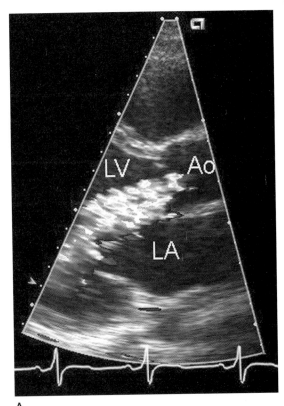

A

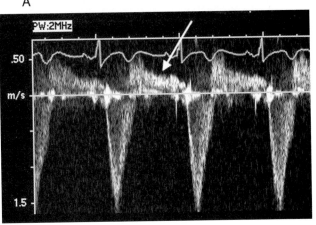

B

Figure 57–20 Moderate aortic insufficiency filling the left ventricular outflow tract, imaged using color Doppler imaging (**A**). Continuous Doppler ultrasound of the descending thoracic aorta demonstrates holodiastolic flow reversal (**B**) *(arrow)*.

calcification rarely causes significant functional mitral stenosis. The mean pressure gradient can be calculated from the transmitral velocity curve using the simplified Bernoulli equation. The mitral valve area (MVA) can be calculated based on the time interval between the peak pressure gradient and one half the peak gradient (or pressure half time) where

$$MVA = 220/\text{pressure half time}$$

Also, 2D planimetry of the mitral valve orifice in a parasternal short-axis view is very accurate and reproducible for measurement of mitral valve area. When the clinical symptoms seem discrepant with the severity of mitral stenosis at

926 rest, exercise testing with evaluation of the rise in pulmonary pressures with exercise may be helpful.[8]

The choice between percutaneous valvuloplasty and a surgical approach is based on echocardiographic evaluation of mitral valve morphology. A score is derived by assessing the degree of leaflet thickening, mobility, calcification, and the involvement of the subvalvular apparatus.[8] Patients with unfavorable morphology (a high score) do poorly with percutaneous balloon valvotomy and are referred for surgery. Other conditions that favor a surgical approach include the presence of mitral regurgitation, other valvular disease, concurrent coronary disease, and the presence of left atrial thrombi. TEE is required prior to a percutaneous procedure in all patients to exclude the presence of left atrial thrombus.

Mitral Regurgitation

Mitral regurgitation may be due to primary disease involving the valve leaflets or to distortion of the valvular apparatus secondary to another disease process. TTE allows identification of the cause and mechanism of mitral regurgitation in most cases, although TEE may be needed if transthoracic images are suboptimal. Primary causes of mitral regurgitation include myxomatous disease (Figure 57-21), rheumatic disease, and endocarditis. Secondary causes include dilated cardiomyopathy and ischemic cardiac disease.

Color Doppler has a very high sensitivity and specificity for detection of regurgitation. A small degree of mitral regurgitation is present in 80% of normal individuals. More severe degrees of regurgitation are graded as mild, moderate, or severe based on a combination of Doppler echocardiographic findings. As imaged with color Doppler, the regurgitant flow disturbances in the left atrium range from a small localized area adjacent to the valve to a large flow disturbance that fills the entire left atrium with severe regurgitation. The shape and direction of the regurgitant jet aid in establishing the mechanism of valve dysfunction. Posteriorly directed jets are typically due to anterior leaflet pathology and vice versa. Annular dilation leads to failure of leaflet coaptation and centrally directed jets. Eccentric jets that adhere to the atrial wall typically appear smaller than free jets in the left atrial chamber. Evaluation from at least two orthogonal views with careful adjustment of instrument settings is essential for color flow evaluation of mitral regurgitation.

Another simple measure of mitral regurgitant severity is the presence of systolic flow reversal in the pulmonary veins. Complete evaluation may require transesophageal imaging as flow reversal may be seen in some, but not all, pulmonary veins with an eccentric jet. Quantitative evaluation of regurgitation severity is possible by measurement of the regurgitant flow volume using the proximal isovolumic surface area, calculation of regurgitant orifice area, and measurement of the vena contracta. Although these measures are not yet routine, they are helpful in distinguishing moderate from severe regurgitation in difficult clinical cases.

The effects of chronic mitral regurgitation on the left ventricle and pulmonary vasculature can be evaluated with echocardiography and form the basis of clinical decision making for the timing of surgical intervention.[8,13] In the asymptomatic patient with severe mitral regurgitation, an end-systolic dimension >45 mm and an ejection fraction <60% are indications for surgical intervention. Mitral valve

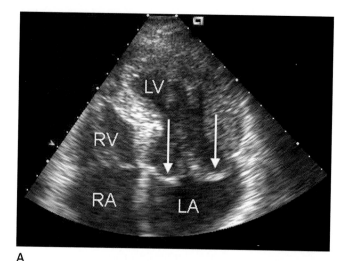

A

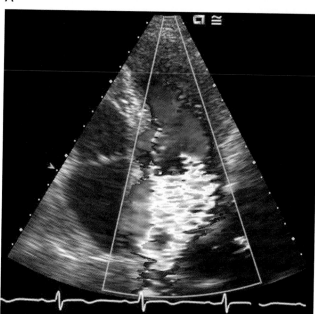

B

Figure 57–21 Myxomatous disease of the mitral valve with redundant, thickened mitral valve leaflets. There is bileaflet mitral valve prolapse during systole identified on the apical four-chamber view (**A**) (*arrows*) with severe mitral regurgitation filling the entire left atrium by color Doppler imaging (**B**).

repair is preferred over mitral valve replacement whenever possible. In patients referred for surgical intervention, close collaboration between the echocardiographer and cardiac surgeon is needed in evaluation of the likelihood of mitral valve repair. Intraoperatively, TEE is used to evaluate the adequacy of the repair and identify residual mitral regurgitation or other complications.

Right-Sided Valve Disease

Right-sided valvular disease occurs less frequently than left-sided lesions in adults. Trace to mild regurgitation of both the tricuspid and pulmonic valves can be seen in normal individuals. Tricuspid regurgitation most often is secondary to left-sided heart disease with pulmonary hypertension and consequent right ventricular dilation and systolic dysfunction. Tricuspid regurgitation is also seen with valvular destruction from endocarditis and rheumatic valve disease. Rare causes include carcinoid valvular disease, which causes leaflet thickening and retraction, and Ebstein's anomaly. Moderate to severe tricuspid regurgitation results in a large jet on color flow imaging and systolic flow reversal in the hepatic veins on subcostal views.

In adults, the most common cause of significant pulmonic regurgitation is residual disease years after repair of tetralogy of Fallot. Pulmonic regurgitation is diagnosed on echocardiography using color flow, pulsed, and continuous-wave Doppler similar to those described for aortic regurgitation. Pulmonic and tricuspid stenosis are rare and are evaluated using methods analogous to those described for left-sided stenoses.

Prosthetic Valves

Although the echocardiographic evaluation of prosthetic valves is similar to native valves, there are several added issues to address. Knowledge of the different valve types and the individual flow dynamics of each valve is important to discriminate normal from abnormal transvalvular flow and function. Optimal evaluation is often hindered by valve positioning and acoustic shadowing from artificial materials incorporated into the valves.

Prosthetic valves that are currently encountered fall into two main classes, bioprosthetic and mechanical valves. Because of the sewing ring and struts in traditional bioprosthetic valves, the functional valve area is smaller than with native valves with resulting normal higher antegrade velocities. In the mitral position, acoustic shadowing can limit visualization of the left atrium and evaluation of mitral regurgitation. Reverberations from the struts can also limit leaflet imaging. Newer stentless tissue valves for the aortic position are now available with a functional flow area and flow dynamics comparable to native valves.[19] Echocardiographically, it is not uncommon to see a small amount of regurgitant flow in these valve types. Because of the absence of prosthetic material, the appearance of homograft and stentless tissue aortic valves can be echocardiographically indistinguishable from native valves.

When a mechanical valve is present, reverberations from artificial materials limit complete evaluation, particularly when evaluating mitral prostheses because of the posterior position and acoustic shadowing of the left atrium (Figure 57-3). Thus both TTE and TEE[13] often are needed for evaluation of mechanical valves. Flow profiles differ between the different mechanical valve types and also vary by valve size. In the ball and cage valve, antegrade flow is seen around the ball with a small amount of regurgitant flow seen circumferentially around the ball during closure. With a single tilting disk valve, there is an asymmetrical flow profile with a major and minor anterograde flow identified. Bileaflet valves have complex fluid dynamics with anterograde flow seen via two minor orifices where the leaflets are positioned, and one central major orifice. During valve closure, two small intersecting regurgitant jets are normally seen. Expected valvular velocities, areas, and gradients are dependent on valve size, patient size, valve type, and valve position.[19,33,38]

Valve dysfunction of bioprosthetic valves includes time-dependent tissue degeneration and fibrocalcific changes that can be imaged by echocardiography. With mechanical

valves, pannus or thrombus formation may impair disk motion. For all valve types, paravalvular regurgitation from suture loss or infection can occur, although differentiation of paravalvular from valvular regurgitation may be difficult in the presence of a calcified annulus. For prosthetic valves placed in the aortic position, a rare complication is development of a pseudoaneurysm of the mitral-aortic intravalvular fibrosa. Because of its communication with the left ventricular cavity, flow into and out of the pseudoaneurysm can be demonstrated by color Doppler imaging (Figure 57-22).

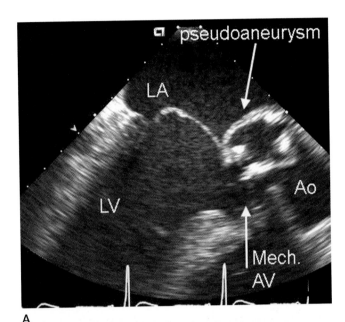

A

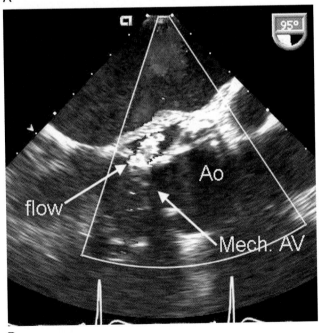

B

Figure 57-22 Pseudoaneurysm of the mitral-aortic intervalvular fibrosa (arrow) in a patient with a mechanical aortic valve placed 22 years ago for endocarditis (**A**). Systolic flow is seen by color Doppler imaging from the pseudoaneurysm to the left ventricular outflow tract (**B**).

928

Doppler interrogation can be used to assess valve gradients in patients with prosthetic valve stenosis, prosthesis undersizing, and anastomotic stenosis in valved conduits. Estimation of transvalvular gradients is relatively reliable for prosthetic valves with biological tissue leaflets. However, with mechanical valves, bileaflet valves in particular, flow is heterogeneous across the entire orifice face, and high local velocities at the smaller leaflet orifices may lead to overestimation of the transvalvular gradient.[33] Evaluation of regurgitant flow utilizes techniques similar to those with native valves. Serial echocardiographic examinations of prosthetic valves are typically not necessary unless valvular dysfunction is suspected. Because prosthetic valve hemodynamics vary depending on patient habitus and valve type, a baseline echocardiogram relatively soon (2–3 months) following surgery is essential to identify subsequent interval changes in function.

Endocarditis

Used in combination with clinical and bacteriological data, echocardiography provides invaluable information in the evaluation for endocarditis.[6,17,42] New criteria for the diagnosis of endocarditis (the Duke criteria) were published in 1994. Major echocardiographic diagnostic criteria include identification of mobile echodense masses adherent to valve leaflets or endocardial surfaces, paravalvular abscesses, and prosthetic valve dehiscence.[17] Vegetations typically appear as echodense, irregular masses of varying size attached to the upstream side point of the affected valve (Figure 57-23). The risk of endocarditis is highest in patients with valve prostheses, native valve disease, congenital heart disease, or a clinical risk factor, such as intravenous drug use. Although the specificity for TTE is adequate, ranging from 91–98%, the sensitivity of TTE for detection of valvular vegetations is relatively poor (ranging from 36–90%) with more studies at the lower end of the spectrum. For definitive detection of vegetations, TEE is both more sensitive and specific.[33] TEE also more readily diagnoses complications of endocarditis,[43] but carries the inherent risks of conscious sedation and the procedure itself.[40] In general, detection by TTE has improved as advents in technology have progressed.

Echocardiography also allows for visualization of complications of endocarditis including involvement of other valves, valvular dysfunction, leaflet perforation, paravalvular abscess, fistula development, and coronary embolization. Regurgitation is the typical manifestation of valve dysfunction. Stenosis is rare. Abscess usually occurs in the valve annulus, more commonly in the setting of a prosthetic valve and can be echolucent or echodense depending on the material within the abscess pocket. A paravalvular abscess in the aortic position may extend to the anterior mitral valve leaflet with involvement of the mitral-aortic intravalvular fibrosa. Other complications include involvement of the aortic sinuses with sinus of Valsalva aneurysm, identified as a dilated and distorted sinus. In a contained rupture, Doppler interrogation may demonstrate systolic flow into the cardiac chamber adjacent to the affected sinus.

Endocarditis of prosthetic valves manifests in a variety of ways. Vegetations can be identified on bioprosthetic valve leaflets or structures. In mechanical valves, valve instability,

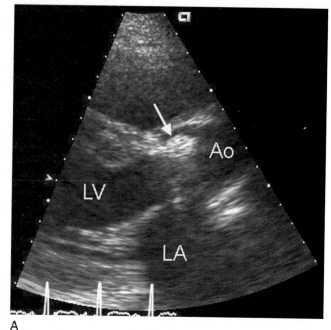

A

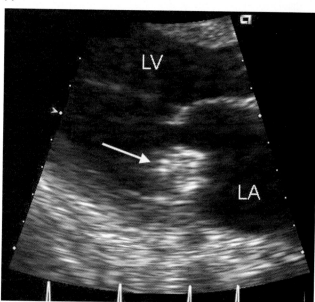

B

Figure 57–23 Endocarditis with large vegetations identified by TTE on the aortic valve (A) and mitral valve (B).

dehiscence, paravalvular leak, or an echogenic space adjacent to the prosthesis suggests infection and possible paravalvular abscess. Because of improved image resolution, TEE is particularly useful when assessing for paravalvular abscess.[40,43]

When endocarditis is suspected on the basis of predisposing factors, fever, sepsis, or embolic events, TTE is the initial procedure of choice because of its lower cost and patient risk. Additionally, TTE allows for better manipulation of the transducer to align the beam in a more parallel manner, useful when evaluating fistulas and abnormal communications. Limitations in the identification of endocarditis include the inability of distinguishing between acute and chronic lesions, reverberations from calcifications or prosthetic materials, and identification of nonbacterial thrombotic lesions, as can be seen in systemic lupus erythematosus. False-positive findings include normal leaflet thickening at a coaptation point, nodules of Arantius, Lambl's excrescences on the aortic valve, mitral leaflet redundancy resulting from myxomatous disease, partial flail leaflets, leaflet calcification, and degenerative changes. TEE may provide improved image quality in these cases. Regardless, if the echocardiographic evaluation for endocarditis is negative, but clinical suspicion remains high, a repeat study should be considered because a subsequent study may be abnormal if disease progression ensues.[6]

AORTIC DISEASE

Transthoracic echocardiography is the initial modality of choice when evaluating the aorta and, using several acoustic windows, is reasonably reliable in providing diameter measurements throughout most of the thoracic and proximal abdominal aorta. Standard measurements of aortic diameter at the aortic valve annulus, sinuses, sinotubular junction, ascending aorta, aortic arch, and descending thoracic aorta are typically performed on routine studies. Nonoblique imaging is essential for accurate measurement. Image resolution with TTE is often limited by overlying air-filled structures and the aorta's posterior position. An example is obscuration of the distal ascending aorta from the overlying trachea. Additionally, the distance from the transducer to the aorta hinders optimal image resolution of aortic wall and intraluminal abnormalities. Therefore, when clinically indicated, TEE is needed to complete a full evaluation of the aorta.[18,47] TEE is superior to TTE because of the shorter distance between the transducer and the aorta, use of a higher frequency transducer, and better ultrasound penetration.

Asymptomatic dilation of the ascending aorta is associated with poststenotic lesions, systemic hypertension, bicuspid aortic valves, and Marfan's disease. TEE can assist in the differentiation between a true aneurysm and a pseudoaneurysm, and can delineate aneurysmal diameter. As these lesions may rupture, serial echocardiography is used to monitor for progressive enlargement. Data from these studies are used for optimal time referral for prophylactic surgical repair. Aneurysmal dilation of the sinus of Valsalva can occur congenitally or as a complication of endocarditis or previous aortic valve surgery. Because of its anatomical location, Marfan's disease tends to involve all three sinuses with concurrent effacement of the sinotubular junction.

Atherosclerotic disease is difficult to diagnose with TTE. Using TEE, the severity and extent of atherosclerotic disease are readily imaged along the length of the thoracic and proximal abdominal aorta. Common findings include atherosclerotic plaques (Figure 57-24), ulceration, associated dilation, and adherent mobile thrombi, which are considered potential sources of distal embolic disease. Intraoperative use of TEE to localize atherosclerotic plaques directs optimal placement of the aortic cannula for the arterial bypass circuit and for aortic cross-clamping.

In aortic dissection, the dissection flap is recognized as a thin, often mobile echodensity within the aortic lumen. Although visualization with TTE is possible, ultrasound artifacts, beam width artifacts, and reverberations can cause

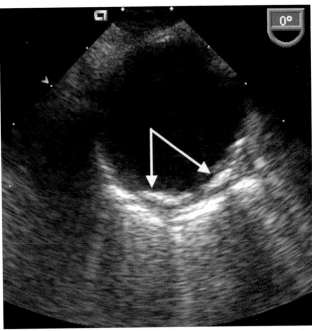

Figure 57–24 Mild atherosclerosis of the descending thoracic aorta imaged by TEE. Calcification within the atherosclerotic plaque causes acoustic shadowing distally in the far field.

false-positive findings. TEE is useful for improved image quality and more complete evaluation of the length of the thoracic aorta compared with TTE, especially for visualization of the ascending aorta and aortic arch.[5] The sensitivity of TTE ranges between 29% and 80% for detection of aortic dissection and is limited by artifacts that may be mistaken for dissection flaps. The specificity of TTE is also low, because of poor image quality of the posteriorly located aorta. Studies on the diagnostic quality of TEE demonstrate sensitivity and specificity approaching 100%.[33] Adequate visualization of the ascending aorta and aortic arch is crucial as their involvement determines surgical urgency. The false lumen, readily identified by TEE, may contain thrombus, may be localized, or may propagate distally. Color flow Doppler can be used to identify entrance and exit points to the false lumen.

Predisposing factors for aortic dissection that can be identified by echocardiography include congenital aortic valve disease, aneurysm, and atherosclerotic disease. In the hands of an experienced operator, TEE provides an efficient and accurate mechanism for diagnosing dissection. Associated findings with dissection can include intramural hematoma, extension of the dissection into the branch vessels or a coronary artery with resulting regional wall motion abnormalities, pericardial or pleural effusion, aortic root dilation, and flail aortic leaflet with aortic regurgitation.

TEE is also used intraoperatively to evaluate effectiveness of surgical repair and residual defects. Following surgical intervention, echocardiography is used to monitor for recurrent disease, to evaluate the proximal and distal graft anastomotic sites, and to assess prosthetic valvular function. As with TTE, limitations of TEE include ultrasound artifacts, beam width artifacts, and reverberations. Additional modalities of dissection detection include computed tomography (CT), MRI, and angiography with relatively comparable

930 sensitivity and specificity for detection. Both CT and angiography require exposure to radiation and contrast dye, which is a concern if concurrent renal dysfunction or dissection extension to the renal arteries is present. An intramural hematoma without a frank dissection flap may be missed by angiography. Although CT and MRI provide a wide field of view, both are not portable studies and provide still images, so evaluation of regional wall motion and aortic regurgitation is limited. Additionally, MRI cannot be used in patients with pacemakers or other metallic materials.

CONGENITAL HEART DISEASE

Echocardiography is the key diagnostic modality in patients with congenital heart disease.[27] Echocardiography accurately detects intracardiac shunts and can provide quantitation of the pulmonic to systemic shunt ratio. This is done by comparing the volume flow rates across the pulmonic and aortic valves. Echocardiography allows distinction between secundum, primum, and sinus venosus atrial septal defects with demonstration of the site of left-to-right flow across the atrial septum on color Doppler flow imaging. When TTE images are suboptimal, TEE provides improved visualization of the intraatrial septum. Other findings than can be associated with an atrial septal defect include right heart enlargement, hypertrophy, and pulmonary hypertension.

Ventricular septal defects typically are located in the perimembranous region adjacent to the aortic valve. In adults, ventricular septal defects are usually very small with high velocity left-to-right flow in systole, associated with a relatively small shunt volume. Larger ventricular septal defects result in more significant left-to-right shunting, manifest chronically as Eisenmenger's syndrome with equalization of right and left ventricular pressures. In this setting, Eisenmenger's physiology is recognized echocardiographically by right ventricular hypertrophy, low velocity to-and-fro flow across the large ventricular septal defect, and equal velocities in the tricuspid and mitral regurgitant jets.

A patent ductus arteriosus is associated with diastolic flow reversal in the descending thoracic aorta and a diastolic flow disturbance in the pulmonary artery. A large patent ductus results in left atrial and left ventricular enlargement due to chronic volume overload.

Congenital heart disease with previous surgical repair is increasingly encountered in adult patients. With knowledge of the previous surgical procedures and a careful and meticulous examination, the resultant anatomy and physiology can be demonstrated with echocardiography. However, in complex cases, other imaging procedures, including MRI and cardiac catheterization, may be needed for complete patient evaluation. Serial echocardiographic monitoring of repaired tetralogy of Fallot patients identifies the commonly encountered long-term complication of chronic pulmonic regurgitation with right heart enlargement. Adults with interatrial baffle repairs for transposition of the great arteries (TGA) may have identifiable baffle obstruction or leaks. Serial echocardiography in patients with TGA is most often performed to follow systemic (the anatomical right) ventricular systolic dysfunction. In patients with a Fontan procedure to direct systemic venous return directly to the pulmonary arteries, as occurs in patients with tricuspid atre-

sia, echocardiographic evaluation includes visualization of the Fontan conduit. In patients with aortic coarctation, Doppler examination of the descending thoracic aorta shows an increased antegrade flow velocity in systole with persistent flow into diastole. Prior operative reports often greatly assist the echocardiographer in interpreting the nature of congenital repair and in identifying complications. As is the case in general, when TTE images are suboptimal, TEE may provide improved image quality.

REFERENCES

1. Arnese M, Cornel JH, Salustri A, et al: Prediction of improvement of regional left ventricular function after surgical revascularization. A comparison of low-dose dobutamine echocardiography with 201T1 single-photon emission computed tomography. Circulation 91:2748–2752, 1995.
2. Arruda AM, McCully RB, Oh JK, et al: Prognostic value of exercise echocardiography in patients after coronary artery bypass surgery. Am J Cardiol 87:1069–1073, 2001.
3. Asher CR, Klein AL: Diastolic heart failure: restrictive cardiomyopathy, constrictive pericarditis, and cardiac tamponade: Clinical and echocardiographic evaluation. Cardiol Rev 10:218–229, 2002.
4. Bach DS: Transesophageal echocardiographic (TEE) evaluation of prosthetic valves. Cardiol Clin 18:751–771, 2000.
5. Banning AP, Masani ND, Ikram S, et al: Transoesophageal echocardiography as the sole diagnostic investigation in patients with suspected thoracic aortic dissection. Br Heart J 72:461–465, 1994.
6. Bayer AS, Bolger AL, Taubert KA, et al: Diagnosis and management of infective endocarditis and its complications. Circulation 98:1936–1948, 1998.
7. Bhatnagar SK, Moussa MA, Al-Yusuf AR: The role of prehospital discharge two-dimensional echocardiography in determining the prognosis of survivors of first myocardial infarction. Am Heart J 109:472–477, 1985.
8. Bonow RO, Carabello B, DeLeon AC, et al: ACC/AHA guidelines for the management of patients with valvular heart disease. A report of the American College of Cardiology/American Heart Association Task Force on Practice Guidelines (Committee on Management of Patients with Valvular Heart Disease). J Am Coll Cardiol 32:1486–1588, 1998.
9. Bossone E, Duong-Wagner TH, Paciocco G, et al: Echocardiographic features of primary pulmonary hypertension. J Am Soc Echocardiogr 12:655–662, 1999.
10. Burgess MI, Bhattacharyya A, Ray SG: Echocardiography after cardiac transplantation. J Am Soc Echocardiogr 15:917–925, 2002.
11. Chandrarratna PA: Echocardiography and Doppler ultrasound in the evaluation of pericardial disease. Circulation 84(Suppl. I): I-303–I-310, 1991.
12. Cheitlin MD, Alpert JS, Armstrong WF, et al: ACC/AHA guidelines for the clinical application of echocardiography. A report of the American College of Cardiology/American Heart Association Task Force on Practice Guidelines (Committee on Clinical Application of Echocardiography). Circulation 95:1686–1744, 1997.
13. Chen L, Otto CM: Longitudinal assessment of valvular heart disease by echocardiography. Curr Opin Cardiol 13:397–403, 1998.
14. Cohen GI, Pietrolungo JF, Thomas JD, Klein AL: A practical guide to assessment of ventricular diastolic function using

Doppler echocardiography. J Am Coll Cardiol 27:1753–1760, 1996.

15. Daniel WG, Mugge A, Martin RP, et al: Improvement in the diagnosis of abscesses associated with endocarditis by transesophageal echocardiography. N Engl J Med 324:795–800, 1991.

16. Dolan MS, Riad K, El-Shafei A, et al: Effect of intravenous contrast for left ventricular opacification and border definition on sensitivity and specificity of dobutamine stress echocardiography compared with coronary angiography in technically difficult patients. Am Heart J 142:908–915, 2001.

17. Durack DT, Lukes AS, Bright DK: New criteria for diagnosis of infective endocarditis: utilization of specific echocardiographic findings. Duke Endocarditis Service. Am J Med 96:200–209, 1994.

18. Goldstein SA, Mintz GS, Lindsay J Jr: Aorta: comprehensive evaluation by echocardiography and transesophageal echocardiography. J Am Soc Echocardiogr 6:634–659, 1993.

19. Grigg L, Fulop J, Daniel L, et al: Doppler echocardiography assessment of prosthetic heart valves. Echocardiography 7:97–114, 1990.

20. Gutterman DD, Ayres RW: Use of echocardiography in detecting cardiac sources of embolus. Echocardiography 10:311–320, 1993.

21. Heidenreich PA, Stainback RF, Redberg RF, et al: Transesophageal echocardiography predicts mortality in critically ill patients with unexplained hypotension. J Am Coll Cardiol 26:152–158, 1995.

22. Khoury AF, Afridi I, Quinones MA, Zoghbi WA: Transesophageal echocardiography in critically ill patients: Feasibility, safety, and impact on management. Am Heart J 124:1363–1371, 1994.

23. Kim CJ, Berglung H, Nishioka T, et al: Correspondence of aortic valve area determination from transesophageal echocardiography, transthoracic echocardiography, and cardiac catheterization. Am Heart J 132:1163–1172, 1996.

24. Klein AL, Grimm RA, Murray RD, et al: Assessment of Cardioversion Using Transesophageal Echocardiography Investigators. Use of transesophageal echocardiography to guide cardioversion in patients with atrial fibrillation. N Engl J Med 344:1411–1420, 2001.

25. Kolias TJ, Aaronson KD, Armstrong WF: Doppler-derived dP/dt and -dP/dt predict survival in congestive heart failure. J Am Coll Cardiol 36:1594–1599, 2002.

26. Leung DY, Black IW, Cranney GB, et al: Prognostic implications of left atrial spontaneous echo contrast in nonvalvular atrial fibrillation. J Am Coll Cardiol 24:755–762, 1994.

27. Linker DT: Practical Echocardiography of Congenital Heart Disease: From Fetus to Adult. Seattle: Churchill Livingstone, 2000.

28. Main ML, Magalski A, Morris BA, et al: Combined assessment of microvascular intergrity and contractile reserve improves differentiation of stunning and necrosis after acute anterior wall myocardial infarction. J Am Coll Cardiol 40:1079–1084, 2002.

29. Marwick TH, Nemec JJ, Pashkow FJ, et al: Accuracy and limitations of exercise echocardiography in a routine clinical setting. J Am Coll Cardiol 19:74–81, 1992.

30. Marwick TH, Stewart WJ, Lever HM, et al: Benefits of intraoperative echocardiography in the surgical management of hypertrophic cardiomyopathy. J Am Coll Cardiol 20:1066–1072, 1992.

31. Miniati M, Monti S, Pratali L, et al: Value of transthoracic echocardiography in the diagnosis of pulmonary embolism: results of a prospective study in unselected patients. Am J Med 110:528–535, 2001.

32. Oh JK, Gibbons RJ, Christian TF, et al: Correlation of regional wall motion abnormalities detected by two-dimensional echocardiography with perfusion defect determined by technetium 99m sestamibi imaging in patients treated with reperfusion therapy during acute myocardial infarction. Am Heart J 131:32–37, 1996.

33. Otto CM: Textbook of Clinical Echocardiography. Philadelphia: W. B. Saunders, 2000.

34. Otto CM: The Practice of Clinical Echocardiography. Philadelphia: W. B. Saunders, 2002.

35. Pinamonti B, Di Lenarda A, Sinagra G, Camerini F: Restrictive left ventricular filling pattern in dilated cardiomyopathy assessed by Doppler echocardiography: clinical, echocardiographic and hemodynamic correlations and prognostic implications. Heart Muscle Disease Study Group. J Am Coll Cardiol 22:808–815, 1993.

36. Pu M, Prior DL, Fan X, et al: Calculation of mitral regurgitant orifice area with use of a simplified proximal convergence method: initial clinical application. J Am Soc Echocardiogr 14:180–185, 2001.

37. Reichert CL, Visser CA, Koolen JJ, et al: Transesophageal echocardiography in hypotensive patients after cardiac operations. Comparison with hemodynamic parameters. J Thorac Cardiovasc Surg 104:321–326, 1992.

38. Reisner SA, Meltzer RS: Normal values of prosthetic valve Doppler echocardiographic parameters: a review. J Am Soc Echocardiogr 1:201–210, 1988.

39. Russo AM, O'Connor WH, Waxman HL: Atypical presentations and echocardiographic findings in patients with cardiac tamponade occurring early and late after cardiac surgery. Chest 104:71–78, 1993.

40. Ryan EW, Bolger AF: Transesophageal echocardiography (TEE) in the evaluation of infective endocarditis. Cardiol Clin 18:773–787, 2000.

41. Sabia P, Afrookteh A, Touchstone DA, et al: Value of regional wall motion abnormality in the emergency room diagnosis of acute myocardial infarction. A prospective study using two-dimensional echocardiography. Circulation 84(Suppl. i):I-85–I-92, 1991.

42. Sachdev M, Peterson GE, Jollis JG: Imaging techniques for diagnosis of infective endocarditis. Infect Dis Clin North Am 16:319–337, 2002.

43. Shapiro SM, Young E, DeGuzman S, et al: Transesophageal echocardiography in diagnosis of infective endocarditis. Chest 105:377–382, 1994.

44. Silver MT, Lieberman EH, Thibault GE: Refractory hypoxemia in inferior myocardial infarction from right-to-left shunting through a patent foramen ovale: a case report and review of the literature. Clin Cardiol 17:627–630, 1994.

45. Spes CH, Klauss V, Mudra H, et al: Diagnostic and prognostic value of serial dobutamine stress echocardiography for noninvasive assessment of cardiac allograft vasculopathy: a comparison with coronary angiography and intravascular ultrasound. Circulation 100:509–515, 1999.

46. Tam JW, Shaikh N, Sutherland E: Echocardiographic assessment of patients with hypertrophic and restrictive cardiomyopathy: imaging and echocardiography. Curr Opin Cardiol 17:470–477, 2002.

47. Tice FD, Kisslo J: Echocardiography in the diagnosis of thoracic aortic pathology. Int J Cardiovasc Imaging 9(Suppl. 2):27–38, 1993.

48. Weyman AE: Principles and Practice of Echocardiography. Philadelphia: Lea & Febiger, 1994.

49. Zaroff JG, Rosengard BR, Armstrong WF, et al: Maximizing use of organs recovered from the cadaver donor: Cardiac recommendations (1). March 28–29, 2001, Crystal City, VA. J Heart Lung Transplant 21:1153–1160, 2002.

Medical- and Catheter-Based Treatment of Cardiac Disease

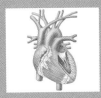

CHAPTER 58

Interventional Cardiology

Duane S. Pinto and Joseph P. Carrozza, Jr.

▶ INTRODUCTION

Interventional cardiology is a subspecialty of medicine that treats a variety of cardiovascular disorders using catheter-based therapeutics. Despite its humble beginnings in 1977, interventional cardiology now includes an array of procedures and techniques for the treatment of ischemic, valvular, and congenital heart disorders. The growth and maturation of the discipline have closely paralleled the rapid influx of new technologies and pharmacotherapeutics. This chapter will review the historical development in interventional cardiology, indications and techniques, as well as the evolution of the devices and medications used during these procedures.

▶ HISTORICAL PERSPECTIVE

After the refinement of diagnostic coronary angiographic catheters by Sones, Judkins, and Abrahms in the 1950s, the radiologist Charles Dotter performed the first endovascular dilation of a stenotic artery for therapeutic purposes in 1964.[34] Peripheral arterial lesions were treated with progressive coaxial catheter dilation to improve blood flow. Complications including hematoma formation and distal embolization were common, and this technique, referred to as "Dottering," did not gain favor in the United States. However, European investigators continued to study and modify the technique. One such physician, Andreas Gruentzig, modified the Dotter multiple catheter system and developed a double-lumen catheter with a distensible balloon on the end that provided circumferential rather than coaxial pressure on the atherosclerotic plaque. Gruentzig performed the first *peripheral* balloon angioplasty in 1974. After reducing the profile of the catheter, Gruentzig performed a series of preclinical studies in canines and human cadavers, culminating in the first human coronary angioplasty in the operating room during elective coronary artery bypass surgery. When Gruentzig performed the first *percutaneous* transluminal coronary angioplasty (PTCA) in September 1977, the discipline of interventional cardiology was born.[54]

Initially, balloon angioplasty was offered as an alternative to bypass surgery in symptomatic patients with focal, proximal stenoses. Dilation of these arteries was usually associated with significant improvement in angina and in objective measures of ischemia.[15] However, the application of PTCA was limited

934 to a small fraction of coronary lesions as first-generation fixed-wire balloons lacked the steerability and profile necessary to traverse distal and tortuous vessels. Easier to use over-the-wire and rapid-exchange systems began to replace the initial fixed balloon-on-wire system developed by Gruentzig. The development of conformable, low-profile balloons facilitated dilatation of distal lesions in tortuous and calcified vessels.

The major limitations of balloon angioplasty—abrupt vessel closure and restenosis—were addressed by the development of new devices in the late 1980s and early 1990s. With the introduction of atherectomy devices, laser balloon catheters, and endovascular stents, the more generic term *percutaneous coronary intervention* (PCI) replaced PTCA and referred to any catheter-based procedure intended to enlarge the lumen of a stenotic vessel. Atheroablative techniques such as directional and rotational atherectomy and excimer laser angioplasty were marketed initially as replacements for balloon angioplasty. Although these techniques improved technical success in certain high-risk subsets such as fibrocalcific and bifurcation stenoses, they were technically difficult to perform and did not have a major impact on restenosis.

The widespread use of endovascular prostheses, or stents, unequivocally improved the acute safety and long-term efficacy of catheter-based treatment. As such, by the end of the millennium, stenting became the default technology for catheter-based therapy, with 70–80% of all patients undergoing PCI receiving a stent. Despite the salutary effects of stenting, restenosis, or renarrowing of the stented segment, still occurs in 10–30% of patients, presenting usually as recurrent ischemia leading to repeat revascularization procedures. The use of adjunctive intravascular brachytherapy following balloon dilation of in-stent restenosis greatly reduced the need for subsequent revascularization procedures in patients who suffered restenosis despite stenting. Recently, several large randomized trials have demonstrated that stents that elute drugs such as sirolimus or paclitaxel have markedly reduced neointimal proliferation and restenosis. Drug-eluting stents will not only improve the long-term freedom from repeat revascularization, but may also extend the therapeutic armamentarium of the interventional cardiologist to allow treatment of lesions such as unprotected left main stenoses, previously treated only with bypass surgery. It is estimated that within 5 years, 20–30% of patients who would have required bypass surgery will be treated using catheter-based therapies such a drug-eluting stents.

PROCEDURE

As in diagnostic angiography, coronary intervention begins with placement of a vascular access sheath in the femoral, brachial, or radial artery. Although choice of the access site is at the discretion of the operator, over 95% of interventional procedures are performed via the femoral approach.[96] Radial or brachial arterial access may be preferable in certain circumstances such as iliofemoral occlusion, the presence of abdominal aortic aneurysm, recent femoral-popliteal bypass grafting, unfavorable body habitus, coagulopathy, or patient preference. Procedural success rates are comparable across all access sites, but radiation exposure and procedure times are slightly longer with brachial or radial procedures. Bleeding and vascular complications may be lower with brachial and radial access.[72]

Arterial access is obtained via percutaneous puncture of the anterior wall of the artery with a hollow needle.[69] A guidewire is advanced through the lumen of the needle to the aorta and the needle is removed. A vascular sheath is then inserted over this wire. Large-lumen guiding catheters are then advanced through the arterial sheath and over the guidewire to the ascending aorta. The guidewire is removed and selective cannulation of the coronary arteries or bypass conduits is undertaken.

PERCUTANEOUS TRANSLUMINAL CORONARY ANGIOPLASTY

Gruentzig's first balloon dilation procedure in 1977 heralded the dawn of interventional cardiology. First-generation catheters, guidewires, and balloons were quite rudimentary compared to contemporary devices, and operators often met with profound difficulty in treating stenotic arteries. Limitations included the inability to traverse lesions with the coronary guidewire due to poor steerability, and the failure to deliver balloons to the lesion for dilation. Advances such as improved radiological imaging, guidewires with steerable tips, lower profile and over-the-wire balloons, and better guiding catheters improved PTCA success rates to approximately 60%.[33]

Successful PTCA was limited also by an inability to expand balloons in fibrocalcific lesions. The mechanism of lumen enlargement with balloon dilation includes controlled plaque dissection, compression of the atheroma, stretching of the vessel wall, and plaque embolization (Figure 58–1). When adequate balloon expansion is prevented because of excessive plaque calcification or resilience, unsuccessful dilation may ensue resulting in a high residual stenosis. In addition, as a component of luminal enlargement from balloon angioplasty is due to vessel stretching, early elastic recoil may rapidly erode the initial gain.

In addition to these limitations, the barotrauma associated with dilation of stenotic lesions may lead to medial dissection and many of the complications of angioplasty. Abrupt vessel closure occurs in approximately 5% of cases and is due to a combination of factors including arterial dissection, vascular recoil, vasospasm, and thrombosis. Flow-limiting dissections and thrombosis were treated with prolonged balloon inflations and aggressive anticoagulation, but despite these treatments, emergency bypass surgery was required in almost 50% of cases of abrupt vessel closure. In the present era, emergency surgery was required in approximately 3–5% of procedures,[33] with significantly greater morbidity and mortality than elective bypass surgery.[6,13,104] Cardiac tamponade may develop on occasion because of vessel perforation with the coronary guidewire or with balloon dilation.

TECHNOLOGICAL ADVANCES

Atherectomy Devices

In the past two decades, technological advances have addressed the limitations of PTCA (Box 58–1). Atherectomy devices were designed to achieve luminal enlargement by

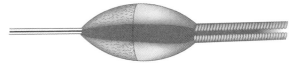

Figure 58–3 Rotational atherectomy catheter.
(Courtesy Boston Scientific Inc.)

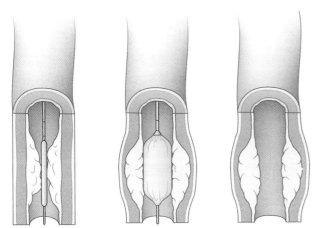

Figure 58–1 Mechanism of lumen enlargement with angioplasty. Inflation of the angioplasty balloon within the atherosclerotic plaque leads to fissuring and cracking of the intima with stretching of the media and adventitia.
(From Baim DS. In Grossman's Cardiac Catheterization, Angiography, and Intervention. 6th Ed. Philadelphia: Lippincott, Williams & Wilkins, 2000.)

Box 58–1. Devices Useful for Various Lesion Subsets.

Calcified lesions
 Rotational atherectomy
Thrombus-containing lesions
 Rheolytic thrombectomy
 Distal protection systems
Ostial lesions/eccentric lesions, bifurcation lesions
 Directional atherectomy
Restenosis
 Bare metal stents
 Drug-eluting stents

---

plaque removal rather than dissection and vascular stretching. Directional coronary atherectomy employs a cup-shaped cutter housed in a rigid cylinder in which a window is etched. A balloon is attached to the opposite wall of the cylinder (Figure 58–2). During balloon inflation, atheroma is directed into the housing, shaved by the rotating cutter, and compressed into the nosecone for removal. This device has been utilized successfully for treatment of bifurcation, ostial, eccentric, and ulcerated lesions. In addition, debulking of plaque prior to stenting theoretically could reduce the incidence of restenosis by improving stent expansion and reducing proliferation. Directional atherectomy was compared to PTCA in several multicenter trials that randomized patients with both native coronary and saphenous vein graft lesions. Atherectomy was associated with improved acute procedural outcomes compared to PTCA including larger

initial lumens and higher success rates, but the rates of periprocedural myocardial infarction were higher, without significant reduction in restenosis rates unless aggressive plaque debulking was performed.[9,59,125]

Rotational atherectomy (RA or PTCRA) incorporates a nickel-plated, brass burr coated with diamond chips on its leading edge (Figure 58–3). The burr is rotated at 140,000–200,000 revolutions per minute, and utilizing the principle of differential cutting, pulverizing plaque into 5- to 12-μm particles. These particles are cleared by the reticuloendothelial system. When RA was compared to laser angioplasty and PTCA, procedural success was greater with RA, but the need for repeat revascularization was higher with RA compared to PTCA.[105] Because RA has not been shown to impact restenosis favorably, it has been relegated to an "enabling device" used prior to PTCA or stenting to debulk heavily calcified plaque or improve vascular compliance in undilatable lesions.

Stents

Although Charles Dotter first proposed the concept of an endovascular prosthesis or "stent" in the 1960s, the development of coronary stents did not occur until the 1980s. Stents were originally approved to seal dissection flaps and reverse acute vessel closure following PTCA. The Gianturco–Roubin coil stent was the first stent approved in the United States based on its ability to stabilize dissections, reducing the incidence of abrupt vessel closure and early complications.[44] In 1994, the balloon-expandable Palmaz–Schatz slotted tube stent was approved for elective use after two randomized trials showed significant reductions in angiographic restenosis.[40,111] Several randomized comparisons of PTCA and stenting confirmed the superiority of stenting over balloon angioplasty alone. Large registries of "real-world stenting" found increased procedural success, reduced adverse cardiac events, less need for repeat revascularization at 6 months, and lower incidence of bypass surgery and mortality at 2 years.[40,55,111]

The remarkable improvement in procedural safety explains the rapid proliferation of stents from <1% of 270,000 interventions in 1994 to over 900,000 stents implanted in 700,000 procedures in 2001. In addition, stents effectively reduced the incidence of restenosis by allowing operators to safely achieve larger and more durable luminal enlargement. This can be explained by the "bigger is better"

Figure 58–2 Directional coronary atherectomy catheter.

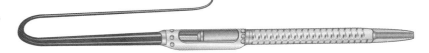

936 paradigm, which states that a larger posttreatment lumen diameter is associated with a lower risk of restenosis.

▶ COMPLICATIONS OF PCI

Death

Mortality from a variety of complications can occur during PCI including anaphylactoid reactions, acute myocardial infarction, pericardial tamponade, stroke, or vascular trauma. In the "stent era," mortality rates associated with elective coronary intervention have fallen to less than 0.3%.[18,30] Patients at higher risk include the elderly, those undergoing emergency PCI or PCI on saphenous vein grafts, and those with decompensated heart failure or reduced cardiac ejection fraction, cardiogenic shock, and acute myocardial infarction.[71,110]

Emergency Bypass Surgery

The widespread use of stents has led to an evolution of the role of the cardiac surgeon in managing acute complications of percutaneous coronary intervention. During the initial development of PTCA, immediate surgical back-up was necessary because of the not infrequent occurrence of acute vessel closure necessitating urgent surgical revascularization. The incidence of emergency cardiac surgery for failed PTCA was approximately 7% in the 1990s.[50,122] The need for emergency surgery has fallen dramatically in recent years paralleling improvements in stent technology and pharmacological therapy, and presently occurs in <1% of cases.[57,113]

Emergency bypass surgery is performed mainly for persistent abrupt vessel closure, extensive vessel dissection, unstable left main coronary artery stenosis or injury, uncontrolled vessel perforation, and cardiac tamponade. The Society of Thoracic Surgeons reported an operative mortality that exceeds 5% for patients requiring emergency bypass surgery within 6 h of PTCA.[106,113] Though the frequency of emergency surgery continues to fall, and surgical technique and postprocedure management continue to improve, patient outcomes continue to be significantly worse compared to elective surgery. The poor outcomes in this population are not unexpected since as PCI has improved, the patients who cannot be salvaged and require emergency surgery comprise a population with more unfavorable risk factors and comorbidities. Considerations such as conduit selection, myocardial protection, and the need for coronary artery repair make the surgical procedure technically demanding.

Though the incidence of emergency surgery is low, the American College of Cardiology and American Heart Association do not support the performance of elective PCI without surgical back-up[115]; however, the improvements in immediate PCI outcomes as well as the recognition of improved survival with PCI performed in the setting of acute myocardial infarction have led to the development of programs in which primary PCI is performed without surgical back-up. The C-PORT study confirmed the safety of primary PCI without surgical back-up.[8] It is well known that operator experience and hospital volume play important roles in these cases, since PCI for acute myocardial infarction is often more technically demanding than routine PCI. Various studies have correlated both limited operator experience (<75 cases/year) and low hospital volume (<200 cases/year) with less favorable outcomes for primary PCI.[22,85,90]

PCI for acute myocardial infarction at institutions without surgical back-up is currently performed, and guidelines have been published, consisting of requirements for operator and hospital volume, ready availability of necessary interventional and hemodynamic monitoring equipment, rigorous quality assurance, and a formalized protocol for immediate (<1 h) transfer for emergency coronary artery bypass grafting (CABG)[115] (Box 58-2). Certain lesion subsets that would

---

Box 58–2. Criteria for the Performance of Primary Angioplasty at Hospitals without On-Site Cardiac Surgery.

1. The operators must be experienced interventionalists who regularly perform elective intervention at a surgical center (≥75 cases/year). The institution must perform a minimum of 36 primary PCI procedures per year.
2. The nursing and technical catheterization laboratory staff must be experienced in handling acutely ill patients and comfortable with interventional equipment. They must have acquired experience in dedicated interventional laboratories at a surgical center. They participate in a 24-h, 365-day call schedule.
3. The catheterization laboratory itself must be well-equipped, with optimal imaging systems, resuscitative equipment IABP support, and must be well-stocked with a broad array of interventional equipment.
4. The cardiac care unit nurses must be adept in hemodynamic monitoring and IABP management.
5. The hospital administration must fully support the program and enable the fulfillment of the above institutional requirements.
6. There must be formalized written protocols in place for immediate (within 1 h) and efficient transfer of patients to the nearest cardiac surgical facility, which are reviewed/tested on a regular (quarterly) basis.
7. Primary intervention must be performed routinely as the treatment of choice around the clock for a large proportion of patients with AMI to ensure streamlined care paths and increased case volumes.
8. Case selection for the performance of primary angioplasty must be rigorous. Criteria for the types of lesions appropriate for primary angioplasty and for the selection for transfer for emergent aortocoronary bypass surgery are shown in Box 58-5.
9. There must be an ongoing program of outcomes analysis and formalized periodic case review.
10. Institutions should participate in a 3- to 6-month period of implementation during which time development of a formalized primary PCI program is instituted that includes establishing standards, training staff, detailed logistic development, and creation of a quality assessment and error management system.

AMI, acute myocardial infarction; IABP, intraaortic balloon pump; PCI, percutaneous coronary intervention.

ordinarily be attempted by operators with onsite surgical back-up are proscribed when surgical back-up is not available. Because of the risk of catheter injury to the left main artery, culprit stenoses that are downstream from a lesion in the left main coronary artery that is ≥ 60% should be avoided. When there is normal flow in the infarct artery, and either there is three-vessel disease or the culprit lesion is long or angulated, PCI should be avoided as well. High-grade left main coronary disease or hemodynamic instability should prompt rapid transfer to an institution equipped to perform bypass surgery, preferably after placement of an intraortic balloon counterpulsation device[115] (Box 58-3).

Myocardial Infarction

Although Q-wave myocardial infarction occurs in <1% of patients, the incidence of postprocedure myonecrosis (as measured by elevation of cardiac markers such as creatine phosphokinase [CPK]-MB and troponins) may be found in almost one third of patients and is more common following atherectomy procedures, and PCI is performed in thrombus-containing lesions, in the setting of acute coronary syndromes, or for treatment of saphenous vein graft disease.[60,73,74]

Periprocedural myocardial infarction may result from acute vessel closure, perforation, or, most commonly, embolization of thrombus or atheroma. Treatment of thrombus-containing lesions has always been a challenge for the interventional cardiologist.

Thrombectomy can be performed using an aspiration device, the Angiojet (Possis Medical, Minneapolis, MN) advanced over the coronary guidewire (Figure 58-4). With a high-speed saline injection at the tip of the catheter, an intense Venturi effect is created and thrombus can be macerated. The VEGAS-II trial compared intracoronary thrombolysis to thrombectomy and demonstrated a reduction in 30-day major adverse cardiac events with thrombectomy compared to prolonged infusion of urokinase.[75]

Despite effective thrombectomy with devices such as the Angiojet, distal embolization remains common during treatment of saphenous vein graft disease and in the setting of acute coronary syndromes. This observation is best explained by the finding that atheroembolism frequently occurs during manipulation of friable plaque. This has led to the development of other interventional devices aimed at reducing distal embolization of plaque and thrombus during intervention on high-risk lesions. The Percusurge Guardwire is a "balloon occlusion protection" device that uses a coronary guidewire with a hollow hypotube that allows for inflation of an occlusion balloon at the end of the wire (Figure 58-5). Inflation creates a static column of blood within the vessel, trapping any debris liberated during balloon inflation or stent deployment. A sump catheter is then advanced over the wire and used to aspirate the static column of blood and debris. The SAFER trial demonstrated a 50% reduction in periprocedural myocardial infarction for patients randomized to the Guardwire compared to conventional systems during intervention on saphenous vein bypass grafts. These devices are approved for use only during saphenous vein graft intervention.[10] A second class of embolic protection devices makes use of filters mounted at the end of the wire to trap embolized material rather than balloons (Figure 58-6). The latter have the theoretical advantage over the distal protection balloons in that antegrade blood flow can be preserved, limiting ischemic time due to occlusion.[119] Recently, the first filter device for use during PCI on saphenous vein grafts was approved in the United States. A randomized comparison of the filter device to the Percusurge Guardwire demonstrated equivalent outcomes.[118] Trials evaluating distal protection equipment in native coronary arteries are in development.

Box 58–3. Noninvasive Risk Stratification for Coronary Artery Disease.

High risk (>3% annual mortality rate)
1. Severe resting LV dysfunction (LVEF <0.35)
2. High-risk treadmill score (score ≤−11)
3. Severe exercise LV dysfunction (exercise LVEF <0.35)
4. Stress-induced large perfusion defect (particularly if anterior)
5. Stress-induced multiple perfusion defects of moderate size
6. Large, fixed perfusion defect with LV dilation or increased lung uptake (thallium-201)
7. Stress-induced moderate perfusion defect with LV dilation or increased lung uptake (thallium-201)
8. Echocardiographic wall motion abnormality (involving more than two segments) developing at a low dose of dobutamine (≤10 mg kg^{-1} min^{-1}) or at a low heart rate (<120 bpm)
9. Stress echocardiographic evidence of extensive ischemia

Intermediate risk (1–3% annual mortality rate)
1. Mild/moderate resting LV dysfunction (LVEF 0.35–0.49)
2. Intermediate-risk treadmill score (−11 < score < 5)
3. Stress-induced moderate perfusion defect without LV dilation or increased lung intake (thallium-201)
4. Limited stress echocardiographic ischemia with a wall motion abnormality only at higher doses of dobutamine involving upto two segments

Low risk (<1% annual mortality rate)
1. Low-risk treadmill score (score ≥5)
2. Normal or small myocardial perfusion defect at rest or with stress
3. Normal stress echocardiographic wall motion or no change of limited resting wall motion abnormalities during stress

LV, left ventricular; LVEF, left ventricular ejection fraction; bpm, beats per minutes

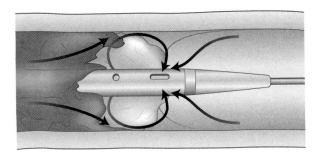

Figure 58–4 AngioJet rheolytic thrombectomy catheter. *(Courtesy Possis Medical.)*

938

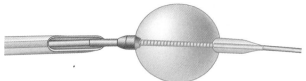

Figure 58–5 PercuSurge Guardwire Plus distal protection balloon.
(Courtesy Medtronic Inc.)

Other complications of coronary intervention include arrhythmias, stroke caused by spontaneous intracerebral hemorrhage with anticoagulation and embolism debris, or equipment from catheters, arteries, or cardiac chambers and valves.

Vascular Complications and Hemorrhagic Complications

The use of antithrombotic, fibrinolytic, antiplatelet agents, aggressive anticoagulation, and prolonged sheath placement is associated with an increase in vascular complications. Impaired coagulation, as well as the need for larger lumen catheters for coronary intervention (typically 6–8 French), leads to more frequent access site complications compared with simple diagnostic angiography. Complications include hematoma (1–5%), retroperitoneal hemorrhage, and pseudoaneurysm (1%) formation.[95] Patients with significant peripheral vascular disease are at higher risk for such complications. Infrequent (<1%) complications include arteriovenous fistula formation, infection, cholesterol embolization, and vascular occlusion. Femoral access site complications requiring surgical repair or transfusion occur in 2–5% of cases. Traditionally, surgery was performed to close pseudoaneurysms >2 cm because of significant risk of spontaneous rupture. Recently, ultrasound-guided injection of thrombin into the pseudoaneurysm has obviated the need for open surgical repair. Surgical exploration is undertaken for repair of fistulas and arterial lacerations, and in cases of arterial occlusion and uncontrolled bleeding leading to hemodynamic compromise.

The use of certain antiplatelet, antithrombotic, and fibrinolytic agents also translates into higher rates of bleeding in patients who may require emergency operation for unsuccessful or failed coronary intervention. Aspirin, a relatively weak inhibitor of platelet aggregation, has been shown to increase postoperative blood loss and the need for reexploration in some studies,[29,38,121] whereas other studies have found no increase in bleeding in patients without known coagulopathy undergoing their first bypass surgery, and an improvement in graft patency and survival with preoperative and early postoperative administration of aspirin.[48,49,86] Today, most cardiac surgeons routinely operate on patients treated with aspirin.

Operation within 12 h of thrombolytic therapy for acute myocardial infarction is associated with increased bleeding, transfusion, and a greater incidence of reoperation for peri-

operative bleeding.[11] Bypass surgery has been performed in patients treated with the antiplatelet medications known as glycoprotein IIb/IIIa receptor antagonists without an increase in bleeding complications or other adverse events.[78,81] Platelet transfusion may reverse the effect of the glycoprotein IIb/IIIa receptor antagonist, abciximab, and reduce the incidence of bleeding.

Clopidogrel, a member of the thienopyridine class of antiplatelet agents, has been shown to reduce ischemic cardiac events when administered early to patients with unstable angina or non-ST-segment elevation myocardial infarction.[117,124] It has also been shown to increase major bleeding and the need for reoperation 10-fold in patients undergoing CABG or who undergo PCI.[4,61] The Clopidogrel in Unstable Angina to Prevent Recurrent Events (CURE) trial showed that patients with unstable angina or non-ST-segment elevation myocardial infarction who discontinued clopidogrel less than 5 days before CABG surgery had increased major bleeding (9.6% clopidogrel group versus 6.3% placebo group; relative risk, 1.53; $p = .06$). Those who stopped taking clopidogrel more than 5 days before the procedure had no increase in bleeding within 7 days after surgery (4.4% clopidogrel group versus 5.3% placebo group).[124]

Contrast Nephropathy

Nephropathy induced by contrast media used for angiography is an important clinical concern. The occurrence of contrast-induced nephropathy is associated with poorer clinical outcomes.[53,89] Although most cases of contrast-induced nephropathy are self-limited, a fraction of patients will require short-term dialysis and some will require permanent dialysis. The risk of occurrence is less than 1% overall. Patients with baseline renal insufficiency, diabetes, or who receive large volumes of contrast are at highest risk. The risk in this population is more than 35%.[53,89] Additional risk factors include dehydration, advanced age, large contrast volume, multiple myeloma, exposure to nephrotoxic drugs, congestive heart failure, and liver disease.

The risk of contrast-induced nephropathy can be reduced with preprocedure and postprocedure hydration. Forced diuresis, calcium antagonists, dopamine, and atrial natriuretic peptide have not been shown to be beneficial.[116,123] The use of an isoosmolar contrast agent, iodixanol, was compared with a low-osmolar contrast agent, iohexol, in high-risk patients, and was shown to reduce the incidence of contrast-induced nephropathy.[7] There is evidence that acetylcysteine, selective dopamine-1 receptor agonists, and theophylline may be beneficial in some cases, but the role for these agents requires further study.[62,84,123]

Anaphylactoid Reactions

The term *anaphylaxis* typically has been reserved for allergic, IgE-mediated immediate hypersensitivity reactions.

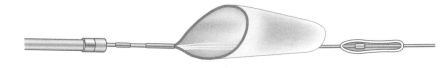

Figure 58–6 FilterWire EX distal protection system.
(Courtesy Boston Scientific Inc.)

Anaphylactoid reactions are clinically similar to anaphylaxis, but these reactions are not IgE mediated. Both anaphylaxis and anaphylactoid reactions can produce immediate, potentially life-threatening systemic reactions because of the massive release of mediators from mast cells and basophils.

The incidence of death from contrast media complications in the catheterization laboratory is estimated at 1 per 55,000. Mild cases may be associated with a variety of symptoms such as itching, urticaria, flushing, cough, sneezing, wheezing, abdominal cramps, diarrhea, headache, back and chest pain, nausea, vomiting, fever, and chills. More severe reactions lead to dyspnea, a sense of impending doom, and hypotension, potentially resulting in cardiovascular collapse and death. Depending on the severity of clinical findings, patients may require treatment with catecholamines, antihistamines, corticosteroids, or intravenous fluids. In patients with prior reactions, pretreatment with corticosteroids and diphenhydramine and the use of nonionic contrast media have significantly reduced the potential of recurrent reaction.[49]

Restenosis

Despite successful initial luminal dilation, the "Achilles heel" of balloon angioplasty has always been restenosis. It is important to remember that following the acute arterial injury that is prerequisite for luminal enlargement, a complex interaction between the vessel and blood elements occurs. Although these processes are often viewed as pathological, they actually recapitulate all of the elements of wound healing. Immediately following balloon dilation, 20–30% of the initial gain may be lost because of vascular recoil. Platelets, neutrophils, and macrophages adhere to the site of injury resulting in an inflammatory response and secretion of a variety of mitogens. Many of these growth factors, such as platelet-derived growth factor (PDGF), stimulate a change in smooth muscle cells from a contractile to a proliferative phenotype. Matrix metalloproteinases promote smooth muscle cell migration from the media to the intima. The combination of smooth muscle cell proliferation, matrix secretion, and vascular contraction (i.e., negative remodeling) is a ubiquitous process that in most vessel results in mild to moderate renarrowing, but in 20–50% of patients may result in a clinically significant restenosis.

This reparative process may continue for 6–12 months. Although angiographic restenosis may be silent clinically, many patients present with recurrent angina or provocable ischemia during functional testing. *Angiographic* restenosis (>50% stenosis) occurs in approximately 35–40% of patients,[111] while clinically significant restenosis requiring repeat revascularization occurs in approximately 15–20% of patients. Risk factors for restenosis following PTCA have been well documented (Box 58-4). Within large populations late lumen loss follows a near-gaussian distribution with approximately 50% of the initial gain in lumen diameter lost by 6–8 months.[76] The slope of the gain–loss relation is approximately 0.5 and is similar across all devices used for PCI. The reduction in restenosis rates observed following stenting is entirely explained by the ability of stents to safely maximize acute gain, thereby allowing greater tolerance for late loss.

Nevertheless, in-stent restenosis (ISR) continues to pose a problem in interventional cardiology. Despite

---

Box 58–4.   Risk Factors for Restenosis.

Patient factors	Lesion factors	Technical factors
Diabetes	Small vessels	High residual
End-stage	LAD location	posttreatment
renal disease	Long lesions	stenosis
Unstable coronary	Prior restenosis	
syndrome	Ostial location	
	Bifurcation	

---

advances in stent technology, clinically evident rates of restenosis in the current era range from 12% to over 50% in certain subgroups (see Box 58-4).[27,70] Randomized trials have shown that the use of intracoronary radiation therapy, termed brachytherapy, effectively reduces recurrence in patients with ISR.[79,102,129] The risk of recurrent ISR after repeat dilation alone exceeds 50% for the proliferative pattern of ISR, but with adjunctive γ-radiation the rate of revascularization of the target vessel was reduced from 66% in the placebo group to 16% for stents placed in saphenous vein grafts.[129] Likewise, β-radiation in the START trial was shown to reduce the need for repeat revascularization by 50% for ISR in native coronary arteries.[102] A higher incidence of late stent thrombosis was found in patients treated with intracoronary radiation, but this risk has been mitigated by prolonged antiplatelet therapy.[128]

Despite the benefits of vascular brachytherapy for treatment of restenosed stents, prevention is clearly a preferable strategy. Systemic pharmacotherapy has had little consistent effect in reducing restenosis, most likely because of the inability to deliver effective doses without incurring systemic toxicity. Stents serve as the ideal platform for *in situ* pharmacotherapy aimed at altering the proliferative response to vascular injury. Various antiinflammatory and antiproliferative, cell-cycle agents have been applied to stents and tested as antiproliferative agents. Stents provide an ideal platform for local drug delivery since they are located at the site of injury and remain in the vessel indefinitely. Polymer coatings on stents containing these medications allow for a slower controlled release. Presently, a variety of antiinflammatory, antiproliferative, and antimigratory agents are under investigation in a variety of drug-eluting stent platforms. Two agents, paclitaxel and sirolimus, have shown dramatic reductions in restenosis rates. The European RAVEL study compared sirolimus-coated stents to uncoated stents and demonstrated a 0% restenosis rate for drug-eluting stents when placed in lesions at low risk for restenosis.[91] In the larger United States SIRIUS trial that compared the sirolimus-eluting Cypher stent to a bare metal stent in a population at risk for restenosis, angiographic restenosis was reduced from 36.3 to 8.9%, and patients who received the drug-eluting stent had a significantly lower rate of repeat procedures than patients who received the control stent (4.2 versus 16.8%; $p < 0.05$).[92] Another agent that shows considerable promise is the paclitaxel-eluting stent. Preliminary data from the randomized TAXUS IV study demonstrated that angiographic restenosis was reduced

940 from 26.6 to 7.9% and repeat revascularization was reduced from 11.3 to 3%.[120]

▶ INDICATIONS FOR PCI

Catheter-based coronary revascularization can now be performed safely for a broad range of indications including elective treatment of coronary ischemia, urgent management of acute coronary syndromes, and emergency reperfusion during ST-segment elevation myocardial infarction. It is performed for a variety of clinical presentations to alleviate symptoms and reduce the risk of serious cardiac events.

Elective PCI

Although medical therapy is preferred in patients with minimal symptoms and only a small area of ischemic myocardium, patients with large amounts of ischemic but viable myocardium in jeopardy have better anginal control if coronary revascularization is performed. Patients who are asymptomatic or whose symptoms can be controlled with medications but have high risk noninvasive test findings (Box 58-5)[45] have been shown to have lower rates of death or myocardial infarction when treated with revascularization compared to medical therapy[30] (Figure 58-7). The American College of Cardiology/American Heart Association guidelines for Percutaneous Coronary Intervention suggest that asymptomatic or minimally symptomatic patients with coronary lesions that are 50% or greater in one or two arteries undergo PCI if there is a high likelihood of success and low risk of morbidity and mortality and the arteries supply moderate or large areas of viable myocardium.[115]

PCI for Acute Coronary Syndromes (Unstable Angina and Non-ST-Segment Myocardial Infarction)

Patients with moderate or severe stable angina that does not respond to medical therapy often require coronary revascularization to reduce myocardial infarction and to alleviate symptoms. Patients with unstable symptoms or non-Q-wave myocardial infarction have improved outcomes with early coronary revascularization. They should be treated with intensive medical therapy that includes antiplatelet and antithrombotic therapy and undergo risk-stratification and revascularization with either PCI or CABG early in the course of their illness. This "early-invasive" strategy has been shown to reduce death, refractory angina, and myocardial infarction.[21,43,65]

The decision regarding whether these patients can be treated medically or undergo revascularization is dependent upon the disease and the amount of myocardium at risk. Those in the lowest risk categories, such as those with disease in vessels that supply small areas of viable myocardium, may be treated medically, and conversely the patients with highest coronary risk, such as those with left main coronary artery stenosis, are most often treated with CABG.

A large number of patients with coronary disease are at intermediate risk. The decision of how best to treat those with multivessel disease, congestive heart failure, diabetes, or proximal left anterior descending (LAD) artery disease is often made collaboratively with the patient, cardiologist, and cardiac surgeon taking into account factors such as patient age, comorbidities, and preference, as well as angiographic appearance and technical factors. Retrospective analyses of various lesion subsets have demonstrated benefits of revascularization over medical therapy for those with at least one severe stenosis. These studies also show a survival benefit for CABG compared to PTCA that was most pronounced in the highest risk groups such as those with three-vessel disease or two-vessel disease with proximal LAD artery involvement. Lower-risk patients such as those with one- or two-vessel disease had similar outcomes with PTCA[68,87] (Figure 58-8).

PCI for Acute Myocardial Infarction

The benefits of mechanical or pharmacological reperfusion therapy in the setting of acute ST-segment elevation myocardial infarction are quite well established. PCI has been shown to effectively reestablish normal epicardial coronary perfusion in over 90% of patients. Long-term patency rates exceed 85% and both the risk of reinfarction and death are significantly reduced with PCI compared to thrombolytic therapy.[1,51,52,131] Even if transport to a facility equipped for immediate PCI is required, catheter-based revascularization has been shown to have superior outcomes when compared to thrombolytic therapy.[53] Patients who develop cardiogenic shock in the setting of acute myocardial infarction also seem to benefit from immediate revascularization with PCI or CABG. Improved survival at 6 months has been shown in a randomized trial comparing immediate revascularization, with either PCI or CABG, to initial medical stabilization with thrombolytic therapy and/or delayed revascularization. Reduced survival with immediate revascularization was noted, however, in the subset of acutely infarcting patients over 75 years of age compared to medical stabilization followed by delayed revascularization.[58] PCI may also be indicated as salvage therapy after failed thrombolytic administration for acute myocardial infarction, especially anterior infarction. Thrombolytic therapy fails to

---

Box 58–5. Patient Selection for Angioplasty and Emergency Aortocoronary Bypass at Hospitals without On-Site Cardiac Surgery.

Avoid intervention in hemodynamically stable patients with
  Significant (≥60%) stenosis of an unprotected left main (LM) coronary artery upstream from an acute occlusion in the left coronary system that might be disrupted by the angioplasty catheter
  Extremely long or angulated infarct-related lesions with TIMI grade 3 flow
  Infarct-related lesions with TIMI grade 3 flow in stable patients with three-vessel disease (189,239)
  Infarct-related lesions of small or secondary vessels
  Lesions in other than the infarct artery

Transfer for emergent aortocoronary bypass surgery for patients with
  High-grade residual left main or multivessel coronary disease and clinical or hemodynamic instability
  After angioplasty or occluded vessels
  Preferably with intraaortic balloon pump support

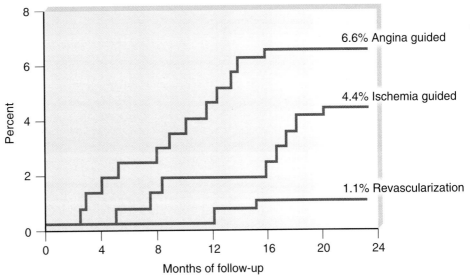

Figure 58–7 Two-year cumulative mortality rates for three treatment strategies in the Asymptomatic Cardiac Ischemia Pilot (ACIP) study. Two-year follow-up outcomes of patients randomized to initial strategies of medical therapy versus revascularization.
(From Davies RF, Goldberg AD, Forman S, et al: Asymptomatic cardiac ischemia pilot [ACIP] study two-year follow-up: outcomes of patients randomized to initial strategies of medical therapy versus revascularization. Circulation 95:2037–2043, 1997, with permission.)

restore normal blood in over 50% of patients. PCI for patients with persistent symptoms or persistent electrocardiographic evidence of ongoing infarction is termed "rescue PCI" and has been shown to result in improved arterial patency with reductions in infarct size, early heart failure, and mortality.[36]

Catheter-Based Therapy in the Postbypass Patient

In the first year after bypass surgery, approximately 8% of patients require repeat revascularization because of a recurrence of ischemia.[20] Over time, the number of patients who develop recurrences of symptoms increases substantially and is due to saphenous vein graft (SVG) attrition in most instances, although progression of native vessel disease also contributes to recurrent ischemia. Approximately 7% of grafts fail in the first week and another 15–20% in first year. Thereafter 1–2% per year fail during the first 5–6 years, and this increases to 3–5% per year in years 6–10 postoperatively.[67] At 10 years postoperatively, approximately half of all SVG conduits are occluded and only half of the remaining patent grafts are free of significant disease.[115] Arterial conduit grafts, especially the left internal mammary, are relatively resistant to atherosclerosis. Because of the increase in morbidity associated with repeat CABG,[88] PCI, if technically possible, is the preferred strategy. Graft failure within the first month of surgery is usually due to thrombosis,[41] while perianastomotic stenosis is usually the culprit 1–12 months after surgery and histologically resembles restenosis after PCI. The latter responds well to balloon dilation. When ischemia occurs more than 1 year after surgery, this may be due to progression of atherosclerotic disease in the native coronary vessels or accelerated atherosclerosis in bypass grafts.[101] As the disease in these grafts progresses the plaques become diffuse and are often degenerated, bulky, and thrombotic. PCI on these vessels is associated with substantial risk of distal embolization and periprocedural myocardial infarction.[82] This risk may be reduced by the use of thrombectomy devices and embolic protection devices.[10,75] Even if PCI of an SVG is performed success-

fully without adverse events, recurrent ischemic events are common because of restenosis, and rapidly progressive disease in the saphenous vein graft and native vessels.[101] Such patients, particularly those without a patent arterial conduit to the LAD artery should receive serious consideration for repeat surgical revascularization. Consensus guidelines have been published for PCI after CABG[115] (Box 58-6).

▶ MULTIVESSEL PCI

Several large, multicenter trials have compared outcomes following bypass surgery and multivessel PCI (Figure 58-9). The BARI trial was the only trial large enough to look at survival alone, and 5-year survival was not significantly different (86.3% PTCA versus 89.3% CABG; $p = .19$), and 5-year survivals free from Q-wave myocardial infarction were 78.7 and 80.4%, respectively.[25] After 5 years of follow-up, 54% of those assigned to PTCA had undergone additional revascularization procedures compared to only 8% of the patients assigned to CABG. CABG was avoided in 69% of PCI patients after 5 years and 45% required only a single repeat PCI.[42] Although the randomized trials did not show a mortality benefit in PCI versus CABG, the subgroup of diabetic patients with multivessel coronary disease had a 5-year mortality that was 19.4% in patients assigned to CABG and 34.5% among those assigned to PCI ($p < .003$).[63]

Overall, with the exception of treated diabetics, no significant mortality advantage has been demonstrated with CABG or PCI in numerous trials (Table 58-1). In general, CABG appears to be the superior choice in patients with diffuse coronary atherosclerosis, especially in the presence of diminished left ventricular function or diabetes. PCI appears to be more favorable in patients with discrete stenoses and normal heart function. Nevertheless, the group of patients that falls between these extremes is large and is currently the subject of much debate.

In a registry of patients who were screened but not randomized in the BARI trial, long-term follow-up demonstrated no significant difference in mortality between

942

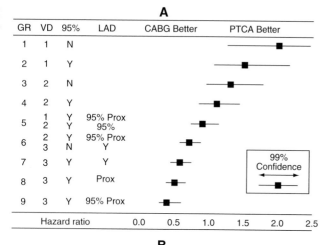

Figure 58-8 Adjusted hazard (mortality) ratios comparing coronary artery bypass grafting (CABG), percutaneous transluminal coronary angioplasty (PTCA), and medical therapy.
(From Jones RH, Kelsor K, Phillips HR, et al: Long-term survival benefits of coronary artery bypass grafting and percutaneous transluminal angioplasty in patients with coronary artery disease. J Thorac Cardiovasc Surg 111:1013, 1996.)

diabetic patients undergoing CABG compared with PCI.[37] In contrast to the randomized trial, patients in the BARI registry had their initial revascularization strategy chosen by their physicians. Patients with more extensive disease were usually treated with CABG, whereas those with more focal stenoses received PTCA. Despite the observation that patients with multivessel disease treated with PTCA or CABG have similar long-term prognoses, a consistent

---

Box 58-6.   Recommendations for Percutaneous Coronary Intervention with Prior Coronary Artery Bypass Graft Surgery.

Class I: Conditions for which there is evidence for and/or general agreement that the procedure or treatment is useful and effective.
1. Patients with early ischemia (usually within 30 days) after bypass surgery.

Class IIa: Conditions for which there is conflicting evidence, but weight of evidence/opinion is in favor of usefulness/efficacy.
1. Patients with ischemia occurring 1 to 3 years postoperatively and preserved left ventricular function with discrete lesions in graft conduits.
2. Disabling angina secondary to new disease in a native coronary circulation. (If angina is not typical, the objective evidence of ischemia should be obtained.)
3. Patients with diseased vein grafts >3 years following bypass surgery.

Class III: Conditions for which there is evidence and/or general agreement that the procedure/treatment is not useful/effective, and in some cases may be harmful.
1. Percutaneous coronary intervention to chronic total vein graft occlusions.
2. Patients with multivessel disease, failure of multiple saphenous vein grafts, and impaired left ventricular function.

From Smith SC Jr, Dove JT, Jacobs AK, et al: ACC/AHA guidelines of percutaneous coronary interventions (revision of the 1993 PTCA guidelines). *J Am Coll Cardiol* 37:2215–2239, 2001.

finding of all the trials is the significantly higher rate of repeat revascularization in patients treated with PTCA.

The treatment decisions for patients in the BARI registry more closely approximated "real-world practice," and nearly twice as many patients were selected for PTCA (1189) as CABG (625). Results were similar to the randomized trial. Mortality at 7 years was similar for PTCA (13.9%) and CABG (14.2%) (p = .66). Seven-year mortality was higher for patients undergoing PTCA in the randomized trial than in the registry (19.1% versus 13.9%, p < .01) but not for those undergoing CABG (15.6% versus 14.2%, p = .57).[37] The BARI registry data thus suggest that physicians are able to appropriately select patients with multivessel disease and/or treated diabetes for PTCA without compromising outcomes.

The idea that the routine use of stents would diminish the incidence of this complication and reduce the need for repeat revascularization led to the development of several trials comparing multivessel stenting with CABG. To date, three trials have reported results.[26,107,112] The ARTS trial randomized 1205 patients and showed that the combined end point of death/stroke or myocardial infarction was similar (12.5% CABG, 17% PCI; p = NS).[112] Revascularization rates after stent placement were lower than those seen with PTCA alone but remained higher than CABG (3.1% CABG versus 25% PCI; p < .01).

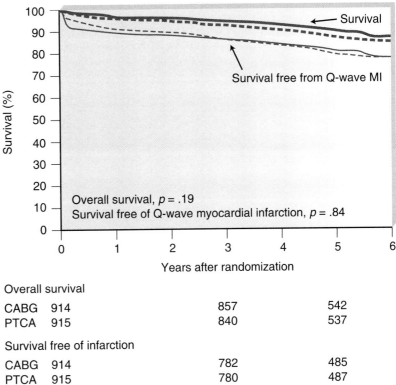

Figure 58–9 Survival and survival free from Q-wave myocardial infarction in the BARI Trial. No difference in advantage of CABG versus PTCA was found in overall survival or survival free from Q-wave MI was found in the BARI trial. *(From The Bypass Angioplasty Revascularization Investigation [BARI] Investigators: Comparison of coronary bypass surgery with angioplasty in patients with multivessel disease. N Engl J Med 335:217–225, 1996. Copyright 1996 Massachusetts Medical Society. All rights reserved.)*

Overall survival			
CABG	914	857	542
PTCA	915	840	537

Survival free of infarction			
CABG	914	782	485
PTCA	915	780	487

ENDOVASCULAR THERAPY FOR VALVULAR, MYOCARDIAL, AND CONGENITAL DISORDERS

Balloon Mitral Valvuloplasty

Inoue in 1984 and Lock in 1985 introduced percutaneous mitral balloon valvotomy (PMBV) for the treatment of selected patients with mitral stenosis.[64,83] A single deflated balloon or a double balloon is advanced from the venous access to the right atrium. With the use of a transeptal approach, the balloon is advanced across the interatrial septum to the left atrium and then across the stenotic mitral valve. The balloon is inflated and rapidly deflated fracturing calcifications of the leaflet tissue and separating fused commissures. Typically the valve area increases from a critically stenotic value of 1.0 cm² to approximately 2.0 cm², a change associated with a rapid reduction in left atrial pressure. This is smaller than the normal valve area of 3–5 cm², but it is sufficient to produce substantial hemodynamic improvements including a decrease in left atrial pressure and the transmitral pressure gradient, a reduction in pulmonary artery pressure, and an increase in cardiac output.

Patients are selected for PMBV on the basis echocardiographic and clinical criteria. Percutaneous mitral balloon valvotomy is a reasonable option for patients who are candidates for surgical commissurotomy. The salutary long-term results, lower costs, and the avoidance of thoracotomy make this procedure the treatment of choice in young patients with pliable, noncalcified mitral valves and no left atrial thrombus.[24] In addition, one may consider percutaneous valvotomy as a palliative procedure in patients with severe valve deformities, who are poor surgical candidates. Mitral valve repair or replacement is usually preferred in symptomatic patients with severe subvalvular or calcific disease, or in patients where left atrial thrombus or significant valvular regurgitation precludes safe balloon valvotomy. Closed commissurotomy is still performed in some developing nations where cost and lack of balloon catheters are continuing problems.

The ACC/AHA task force published recommendations for PMBV in 1998[3] and recommended consideration of PBMV in patients who have exercise intolerance or pulmonary hypertension, or in asymptomatic patients with a calculated effective mitral valve area 1.5 cm² or less with trace or mild mitral regurgitation and appropriate mitral anatomy as determined by echocardiography. Echocardiography is an essential screening procedure in patients being considered for PBMV.[24] The extent of valvular and subvalvular deformity can be evaluated and the likelihood of a successful result can be assessed. This can be accomplished by assigning a score of 0 to 4 for each of four factors including (1) the degree of leaflet rigidity, (2) the severity of leaflet thickening, (3) the amount of leaflet calcification, and (4) the extent of subvalvular thickening and calcification. The maximum score is 16; higher scores indicate more severe anatomical disease and a lower likelihood of a successful PBMV.[2]

The NHLBI Balloon Valvuloplasty Registry evaluated 736 patients treated with PBMV over the age of 18 who were followed for 4 years. The actuarial survival rate at 1, 2, 3, and 4 years was 93, 90, 87, and 84%, respectively. The event-free survival (freedom from death, mitral valve surgery, or repeat balloon valvotomy) at 1, 2, 3, and 4 years was 80, 71, 66, and 60%, respectively.[31] The clinical and hemodynamic results of PMBV have been compared with the different forms of surgical correction: closed surgical valvotomy and open and closed surgical commis-

Table 58–1

Randomized Comparisons of Coronary Artery Bypass Surgery to Percutaneous Coronary Transluminal Angioplasty

Trial[a]	Patients (n)	Primary end point (%)	Follow-up (years)	Comment
BARI	1792	D CABG:10.7 PTCA:3.7	5	Largest clinical trial to date comparing PTCA and CABG. Repeat revascularization was performed in 8% of CABG patients and 53% of PTCA patients. At 5 years, there was no difference in survival or survival or survival free of Q-wave MI. Of 25,000 patients with multivessel CAD who were screened, less than 2000 were randomized.
CABRI	1054	D CABG:2.7 PTCA:3.9	1	Chronic occlusions were treated and equivalent revascularization was not required. Atherectomy and stents were permitted in this trial.
RITA	1011	D + MI CABG:8.6 PTCA:9.8	2.5[b]	Forty-five percent of patients had one-vessel disease, 43% had two-vessel CAD, and 12% had three-vessel CAD. More patients in the surgical group had complete revascularization. 97% and 87% of two- and three-vessel disease patients had all diseased vessels by passed, compared to 81% and 63% for the PTCA group.
EAST	392	D+MI+T CABG:27.3 PTCA:28.8	3	Mean left ventricular ejection fraction was 61%. Confirmed findings of other randomized trials showing that residual angina and repeat revascularization were more common in the PTCA group.
GABI	359	A CABG:26 PTCA:29	1	Total occlusions excluded. In contrast to other studies, there was no difference in anginal status between the two groups. One-year death and nonfatal MI rates were higher in the CABG group. This may have been related to higher periprocedure MI rates in the CABG group.
ERACI	127	D + MI + RR CABG:23 PTCA53[c]	1	Only 17% of patients screened and 42% of eligible patients were randomized. Total occlusions were treated if the vessel supplied viable myocardium.

CABG, coronary artery bypass graft; PTCA, percutaneous transluminal coronary angioplasty; CAD, coronary artery disease; RR, repeated revascularization; BARI, Bypass Angioplasty Revascularization Investigation; EAST, Emory Angioplasty Surgery Trial; GABI, German Angioplasty Bypass-surgery Investigation; RITA, Randomised Intervention Treatment of Angina; ERACI, Estudio Randomizado Argentino de Angioplastia vs Cirugia; CABRI, Coronary Angioplasty versus Bypass Revascularization Investigation; MI, myocardial infarction; D, death; T, thallium defect; A, angina.

[a]References found in the complete guidelines published in Eagle KA, Guyton RA, Davidoff R, etc., J Am Coll Cardiol 34:1262–1341, 1999.

[b]Planned 5-year follow-up (interim results).

[c]$p < 0.05$ comparing CABG and PTCA cohorts.

surotomy. The outcome after PBMV was as good or better than after surgery in patients who are candidates for valvotomy.[12,126]

Mitral valve restenosis after previous commissurotomy can be treated with PBMV. The immediate hemodynamic results and the long-term hemodynamics appear to be identical to those seen with balloon valvotomy in unoperated mitral stenosis.[66] After PBMV, up to 21% of patients develop recurrent heart failure due to mitral restenosis. Although most of these patients undergo mitral valve replacement, repeat balloon valvuloplasty is an alternative approach,

especially in patients who are not good surgical candidates.[100]

Balloon Aortic Valvuloplasty

Percutaneous balloon dilation can also be performed for aortic stenosis. Typically, one or more balloons are advanced across a stenotic valve in a retrograde manner and inflated to dilate the valve.[108] This procedure has an important role in treating adolescents and young adults with congenital aortic stenosis. In patients with bicuspid or calcific valvular aortic stenosis, the mechanism of dilation is through fracture of calcific deposits within the valve leaflets as well as stretching of the annulus with separation of the calcified or fused commissures.[109] Although there is often immediate and significant reduction in the transvalvular pressure gradient, the postvalvotomy valve area rarely exceeds 1.0 cm^2. Despite only modest change in valve area, symptomatic improvement is usually seen.[16]

The role for this procedure is limited both by a high rate of serious complications and by poor durability.[16] Restenosis and clinical deterioration occur within 6–12 months in most patients. For these reasons, aortic valvuloplasty should not be considered a substitute for aortic valve replacement.[14,80,103] Aortic valvuloplasty can be performed in some cases as a "bridge" to surgery in hemodynamically unstable patients who are at high risk for AVR or in asymptomatic patients who require urgent noncardiac surgery. Aortic valvuloplasty may also be performed for palliation of congestive heart failure in patients with serious comorbid conditions and limited life expectancy.[14]

Ethanol Septal Ablation Hypertrophic Obstructive Cardiomyopathy (HOCM)

Nonsurgical septal reduction therapy, also called alcohol septal ablation, is a procedure whereby percutaneous obliteration of the first or second septal perforating coronary arteries is performed using absolute alcohol causing an iatrogenic septal infarct to reduce left ventricular outflow tract obstruction and thereby improve symptoms. Symptomatic patients with moderate to severe heart failure symptoms, and an interventricular septal thickness of 18 mm or greater, and a left ventricular outflow tract gradient at rest of at least 30 mm Hg, or an intraventricular gradient during provocation, are potential candidates for this procedure.[46]

This procedure has been shown to produce impressive reductions in outflow tract gradient and in symptoms. Significant reductions in pulmonary pressures, outflow tract gradient, left ventricular hypertrophy, and mass have been demonstrated.[93,99] Immediate hemodynamic results are comparable to those found with surgical myotomy/myectomy.[39,94,114] The most common complication of the procedure is the development of complete heart block requiring a permanent pacemaker in approximately 14% of patients.[23] Other complications include the development of coronary dissection or unwanted myocardial infarction. Reported results at 1-year follow-up continue to show benefit,[47,98] and long-term efficacy data are currently being collected.

Patent Foramen Ovale (PFO) and Atrial Septal Defect (ASD) Closure

PFO is a persistent flap-like opening between the remnants of the atrial septum primum and secundum and is present in roughly 25% of adults. It can be demonstrated in almost 50% of patients under age 55 years with cryptogenic stroke.[32,77] The presumed cause of stroke in these cases is "paradoxical embolism" whereby venous thrombus is allowed to access the systemic circulation through the PFO during physiological conditions when right atrial pressure exceeds left atrial pressure. Warfarin therapy is the current

standard of care for cryptogenic stroke in the patients with PFO, but despite its use the risk of recurrent stroke remains high. Patients with PFO and paradoxical embolism have an approximate 3.5% yearly risk of recurrent cerebrovascular events.[19] Surgical closure has been effective in preventing recurrent stroke, but adequate randomized studies comparing anticoagulation, surgical closure, and percutaneous closure have not been performed.[56] Because of the bleeding risks associated with chronic anticoagulant use, drug and monitoring costs, as well as the desire of physicians and patients to avoid prolonged recovery and open-heart surgery, percutaneous closure offers a less invasive option for stroke prevention in these patients. It has been employed in thousands of patients using a variety of occlusion devices. (Figures 58-10 and 58-11). Procedural outcomes are excellent, and the stroke recurrence rate is <1% at follow-up exceeding 1 year.[88,97,128] Presently, the Amplatzer PFO occluder (AGA Medical Corp., Golden Valley, MN) and the CardioSEAL (NMT Medical, Boston, MA) are approved under a Humanitarian Device Exemption by the Federal Drug Administration for PFO closure. At our institution, the procedure time is approximately 15–20 min using only

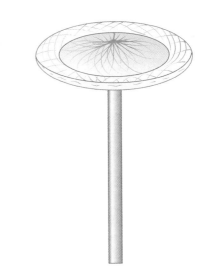

Figure 58–10 Amplatzer septal occlusion devices used for percutaneous closure.
(Courtesy AGA Medical Corporation.)

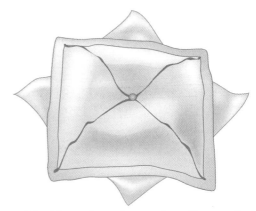

Figure 58–11 Cardioseal septal occlusion device for percutaneous closure.
(Courtesy NMT Medical, Inc.)

fluoroscopic guidance and transthoracic confirmation of appropriate positioning. Patients are required to take aspirin and clopidogrel as well as endocarditis prophylaxis at the time of dental procedures for 6–12 months. Long-term anticoagulation is not longer required thereafter. Randomized comparisons of percutaneous closure and anticoagulation have been initiated.

Although PFO represents a potential communication between the left and right atria, ASDs are congenital abnormalities characterized by a structural deficiency that leads to continuous, free communication between the atria. The defect is often asymptomatic until adulthood, but complications of an undetected lesion include irreversible pulmonary hypertension, right ventricular failure, atrial arrhythmias, paradoxical embolization, and cerebral abscess. These defects are generally repaired when the pulmonary:systemic flow ratio is 1.5 or greater, or in those where the defect leads to symptoms, embolism, or right ventricular dysfunction. Scuba divers with neurological compression sickness and ASD also may be considered for closure. Those with ostium primum defects, sinus venosus defects, or defects with <4 mm of surrounding tissue or stretched diameter >38 mm are better served by surgical rather than percutaneous closure. Percutaneous closure is usually performed using septal occlusion devices similar to those used for PFO closure. Adjunctive transesophageal echocardiographic or intracardiac echocardiography is often used to assist in sizing and placement. One multicenter, nonrandomized study compared 154 patients who underwent surgical closure and 442 who had closure with an Amplatzer septal occluder device. Both methods had equal success rates, but percutaneous closure was associated with fewer complications (7.2 versus 24.0%; $p < .0001$) and shorter duration of hospitalization (1 versus 3 days).[35]

REFERENCES

1. The Global Use of Strategies to Open Occluded Coronary Arteries in Acute Coronary Syndromes (GUSTO IIb) Angioplasty Substudy Investigators: A clinical trial comparing primary coronary angioplasty with tissue plasminogen activator for acute myocardial infarction. N Engl J Med 336:1621–1628, 1997.

2. Abascal VM, Wilkins GT, O'Shea JP, et al: Prediction of successful outcome in 130 patients undergoing percutaneous balloon mitral valvotomy. Circulation 82:448–456, 1990.

3. Task Force on Practice Guidelines (Committee on Management of Patients with Valvular Heart Disease): ACC/AHA guidelines for the management of patients with valvular heart disease. A report of the American College of Cardiology/American Heart Association. J Am Coll Cardiol 32:1486–1588, 1998.

4. Akowuah E, Shrivastava V, Cooper G: Coronary artery bypass graft surgery in patients with recent exposure to clopidogrel and aspirin therapy. J Am Coll Cardiol 41:1421–1422; author reply 1422–1423, 2003.

5. Andersen HR, Nielsen TT, Rasmussen K, et al, the DANAMI-2 Investigators: A comparison of coronary angioplasty with fibrinolytic therapy in acute myocardial infarction. N Engl J Med 349:733–742, 2003.

6. Andreasen JJ, Mortensen PE, Andersen LI, et al: Emergency coronary artery bypass surgery after failed percutaneous transluminal coronary angioplasty. Scand Cardiovasc J 34:242–246, 2000.

7. Aspelin P, Aubry P, Fransson S-G, et al, the NEPHRIC Study Investigators: Nephrotoxic effects in high-risk patients undergoing angiography. N Engl J Med 348:491–499, 2003.

8. Aversano T, Aversano LT, Passamani E, et al, for the Atlantic Cardiovascular Patient Outcomes Research Team: Thrombolytic therapy vs primary percutaneous coronary intervention for myocardial infarction in patients presenting to hospitals without on-site cardiac surgery: A randomized controlled trial. JAMA 287:1943–1951, 2002.

9. Baim DS, Cutlip DE, Sharma SK, et al: Final results of the Balloon vs Optimal Atherectomy Trial (BOAT). Circulation 97:322–331, 1998.

10. Baim DS, Wahr D, George B, et al: Randomized trial of a distal embolic protection device during percutaneous intervention of saphenous vein aorto-coronary bypass grafts. Circulation 105:1285–1290, 2002.

11. Barner HB, Lea JW 4th, Naunheim KS, Stoney WS Jr: Emergency coronary bypass not associated with preoperative cardiogenic shock in failed angioplasty, after thrombolysis, and for acute myocardial infarction. Circulation 79:I152–159, 1989.

12. Ben Farhat M, Ayari M, Maatouk F, et al: Percutaneous balloon versus surgical closed and open mitral commissurotomy: seven-year follow-up results of a randomized trial. Circulation 97:245–250, 1998.

13. Black AJ, Namay DL, Niederman AL, et al: Tear or dissection after coronary angioplasty. Morphologic correlates of an ischemic complication. Circulation 79:1035–1042, 1989.

14. Bonow RO, Carabello B, de Leon AC Jr, et al: Guidelines for the management of patients with valvular heart disease: Executive summary: A report of the American College of Cardiology/American Heart Association Task Force on Practice Guidelines (Committee on Management of Patients With Valvular Heart Disease). Circulation 98:1949–1984, 1998.

15. Bourassa MG, Wilson JW, Detre KM, et al: Long-term follow-up of coronary angioplasty: the 1977–1981 National Heart, Lung, and Blood Institute registry. Eur Heart J 10(Suppl. G):36–41, 1989.

16. Brady ST, Davis CA, Kussmaul WG, et al: Percutaneous aortic balloon valvuloplasty in octogenarians: morbidity and mortality. Ann Intern Med 110:761–766, 1989.

17. Braun MU, Fassbender D, Schoen SP, et al: Transcatheter closure of patent foramen ovale in patients with cerebral ischemia. J Am Coll Cardiol 39:2019–2025, 2002.

18. Bredlau CE, Roubin GS, Leimgruber PP, et al: In-hospital morbidity and mortality in patients undergoing elective coronary angioplasty. Circulation 72:1044–1052, 1985.

19. Bridges ND, Hellenbrand W, Latson L, et al: Transcatheter closure of patent foramen ovale after presumed paradoxical embolism. Circulation 86:1902–1908, 1992.

20. Cameron AA, Davis KB, Rogers WJ: Recurrence of angina after coronary artery bypass surgery: predictors and prognosis (CASS Registry). Coronary Artery Surgery Study. J Am Coll Cardiol 26:895–899, 1995.

21. Cannon CP, Weintraub WS, Demopoulos LA, et al: Invasive versus conservative strategies in unstable angina and non-Q-wave myocardial infarction following treatment with tirofiban: rationale and study design of the international TACTICS-TIMI 18 trial. Treat Angina with Aggrastat and determine Cost of Therapy with an Invasive or Conservative Strategy. Thrombolysis In Myocardial Infarction. Am J Cardiol 82:731–736, 1998.

22. Canto JG, Every NR, Magid DJ, et al, National Registry of Myocardial Infarction 2 Investigators: The volume of primary angioplasty procedures and survival after acute myocardial infarction. N Engl J Med 342:1573–1580, 2000.

23. Chang SM, Nagueh SF, Spencer WH 3rd, Lakkis NM: Complete heart block: determinants and clinical impact in patients with hypertrophic obstructive cardiomyopathy undergoing nonsurgical septal reduction therapy. J Am Coll Cardiol 42:296–300, 2003.

24. Cohen DJ, Kuntz RE, Gordon SP, et al: Predictors of long-term outcome after percutaneous balloon mitral valvuloplasty. N Engl J Med 327:1329–1335, 1992.

25. The Bypass Angioplasty Revascularization Investigation (BARI) investigators: Comparison of coronary bypass surgery with angioplasty in patients with multivessel disease. N Engl J Med 335:217–225, 1996.

26. Coronary artery bypass surgery versus percutaneous coronary intervention with stent implantation in patients with multivessel coronary artery disease (the Stent or Surgery trial): a randomised controlled trial. Lancet 360:965–970, 2002.

27. Cutlip DE, Chauhan MS, Baim DS, et al: Clinical restenosis after coronary stenting: perspectives from multicenter clinical trials. J Am Coll Cardiol 40:2082–2089, 2002.

28. Dacey LJ, Munoz JJ, Baribeau YR, et al: Reexploration for hemorrhage following coronary artery bypass grafting: incidence and risk factors. Northern New England Cardiovascular Disease Study Group. Arch Surg 133:442–447, 1998.

29. Dacey LJ, Munoz JJ, Johnson ER, et al: Effect of preoperative aspirin use on mortality in coronary artery bypass grafting patients. Ann Thorac Surg 70:1986–1990, 2000.

30. Davies RF, Goldberg AD, Forman S, et al: Asymptomatic Cardiac Ischemia Pilot (ACIP) study two-year follow-up: outcomes of patients randomized to initial strategies of medical therapy versus revascularization. Circulation 95:2037–2043, 1997.

31. Dean LS, Mickel M, Bonan R, et al: Four-year follow-up of patients undergoing percutaneous balloon mitral commissurotomy. A report from the National Heart, Lung, and Blood Institute Balloon Valvuloplasty Registry. J Am Coll Cardiol 28:1452–1457, 1996.

32. Di Tullio M, Sacco RL, Gopal A, et al: Patent foramen ovale as a risk factor for cryptogenic stroke. Ann Intern Med 117:461–465, 1992.

33. Dorros G, Cowley MJ, Simpson J, et al: Percutaneous transluminal coronary angioplasty: report of complications from the National Heart, Lung, and Blood Institute PTCA Registry. Circulation 67:723–730, 1983.

34. Dotter CT, Judkins MP: Transluminal treatment of arteriosclerotic obstruction: description of a new technique and preliminary report of its application. Circulation 30:654, 1964.

35. Du ZD, Hijazi ZM, Kleinman CS, et al: Comparison between transcatheter and surgical closure of secundum atrial septal defect in children and adults: Results of a multicenter nonrandomized trial. J Am Coll Cardiol 39:1836–1844, 2002.

36. Ellis SG, Da Silva ER, Spaulding CM, et al: Review of immediate angioplasty after fibrinolytic therapy for acute myocardial infarction: insights from the RESCUE I, RESCUE II, and other contemporary clinical experiences. Am Heart J 139:1046–1053, 2000.

37. Feit F, Brooks MM, Sopko G, et al: Long-term clinical outcome in the Bypass Angioplasty Revascularization Investigation Registry: Comparison with the randomized trial. BARI Investigators. Circulation 101:2795–2802, 2000.

38. Ferraris VA, Ferraris SP, Joseph O, et al: Aspirin and postoperative bleeding after coronary artery bypass grafting. Ann Surg 235:820–827, 2002.

39. Firoozi S, Elliott PM, Sharma S, et al: Septal myotomy-myectomy and transcoronary septal alcohol ablation in hypertrophic obstructive cardiomyopathy. A comparison of clinical, haemodynamic and exercise outcomes. Eur Heart J 23:1617–1624, 2002.

40. Fischman DL, Leon MB, Baim DS, et al: A randomized comparison of coronary-stent placement and balloon angioplasty in the treatment of coronary artery disease. Stent Restenosis Study Investigators. N Engl J Med 331:496–501, 1994.

41. Fitzgibbon GM, Kafka HP, Leach AJ, et al: Coronary bypass graft fate and patient outcome: angiographic follow-up of 5,065 grafts related to survival and reoperation in 1,388 patients during 25 years. J Am Coll Cardiol 28:616–626, 1996.

42. Writing Group for the Bypass Angioplasty Revascularization Investigation (BARI) Investigators: five-year clinical and functional outcome comparing bypass surgery and angioplasty in patients with multivessel coronary disease. A multicenter randomized trial. JAMA 277:715–721, 1997.

43. Fox KA, Poole-Wilson PA, Henderson RA, et al: Interventional versus conservative treatment for patients with unstable angina or non-ST-elevation myocardial infarction: The British Heart Foundation RITA 3 randomised trial. Randomized Intervention Trial of unstable Angina. Lancet 360:743–751, 2002.

44. George BS, Voorhees WD 3rd, Roubin GS, et al: Multicenter investigation of coronary stenting to treat acute or threatened closure after percutaneous transluminal coronary angioplasty: clinical and angiographic outcomes. J Am Coll Cardiol 22:135–143, 1993.

45. Gibbons RJ, Abrams J, Chatterjee K, et al: ACC/AHA 2002 guideline update for the management of patients with chronic stable angina—summary article: a report of the American College of Cardiology/American Heart Association Task Force on Practice Guidelines (Committee on the Management of Patients With Chronic Stable Angina). Circulation 107:149–158, 2003.

46. Gietzen FH, Leuner CJ, Obergassel L, et al: Role of transcoronary ablation of septal hypertrophy in patients with hypertrophic cardiomyopathy, New York Heart Association functional class III or IV, and outflow obstruction only under provocable conditions. Circulation 106:454–459, 2002.

47. Gietzen FH, Leuner CJ, Raute-Kreinsen U, et al: Acute and long-term results after transcoronary ablation of septal hypertrophy (TASH). Catheter interventional treatment for hypertrophic obstructive cardiomyopathy. Eur Heart J 20:1342–1354, 1999.

48. Goldman S, Copeland J, Moritz T, et al: Improvement in early saphenous vein graft patency after coronary artery bypass surgery with antiplatelet therapy: Results of a Veterans Administration Cooperative Study. Circulation 77:1324–1332, 1988.

49. Goss JE, Chambers CE, Heupler FA Jr: Systemic anaphylactoid reactions to iodinated contrast media during cardiac catheterization procedures: guidelines for prevention, diagnosis, and treatment. Laboratory Performance Standards Committee of the Society for Cardiac Angiography and Interventions. Cathet Cardiovasc Diagn 34:99–104; discussion 105, 1995.

50. Greene MA, Gray LA Jr, Slater AD, et al: Emergency aortocoronary bypass after failed angioplasty. Ann Thorac Surg 51:194–199, 1991.

51. Grines CL, Browne KF, Marco J, et al: A comparison of immediate angioplasty with thrombolytic therapy for acute myocardial infarction. The Primary Angioplasty in Myocardial Infarction Study Group. N Engl J Med 328:673–679, 1993.

52. Grines CL, Westerhausen DR Jr, Grines LL, et al: A randomized trial of transfer for primary angioplasty versus on-site thrombolysis in patients with high-risk myocardial infarction: The Air Primary Angioplasty in Myocardial Infarction study. J Am Coll Cardiol 39:1713–1719, 2002.

53. Gruberg L, Mintz GS, Mehran R, et al: The prognostic implications of further renal function deterioration within 48 h of

interventional coronary procedures in patients with pre-existent chronic renal insufficiency. J Am Coll Cardiol 36:1542–1548, 2000.

54. Gruentzig AR, Senning A, Siegenthaler WE: Nonoperative dilatation of coronary-artery stenosis: percutaneous transluminal coronary angioplasty. N Engl J Med 301:61–68, 1979.

55. Hannan EL, Racz MJ, Arani DT, et al: A comparison of short- and long-term outcomes for balloon angioplasty and coronary stent placement. J Am Coll Cardiol 36:395–403, 2000.

56. Harvey JR, Teague SM, Anderson JL, et al: Clinically silent atrial septal defects with evidence for cerebral embolization. Ann Intern Med 105:695–697, 1986.

57. Hasdai D, Berger PB, Bell MR, et al: The changing face of coronary interventional practice. The Mayo Clinic experience. Arch Intern Med 157:677–682, 1997.

58. Hochman JS, Sleeper LA, Webb JG, et al: Early revascularization in acute myocardial infarction complicated by cardiogenic shock. SHOCK Investigators. Should we emergently revascularize occluded coronaries for cardiogenic shock. N Engl J Med 341:625–634, 1999.

59. Holmes DR Jr, Topol EJ, Califf RM, et al: A multicenter, randomized trial of coronary angioplasty versus directional atherectomy for patients with saphenous vein bypass graft lesions. CAVEAT-II Investigators. Circulation 91:1966–1974, 1995.

60. Hong MK, Mehran R, Dangas G, et al: Creatine kinase-MB enzyme elevation following successful saphenous vein graft intervention is associated with late mortality. Circulation 100:2400–2405, 1999.

61. Hongo RH, Ley J, Dick SE, Yee RR: The effect of clopidogrel in combination with aspirin when given before coronary artery bypass grafting. J Am Coll Cardiol 40:231–237, 2002.

62. Huber W, Schipek C, Ilgmann K, et al: Effectiveness of theophyline prophylaxis of renal impairment after coronary angiography in patients with chronic renal insufficiency. Am J Cardiol 91:1157–1162, 2003.

63. Influence of diabetes on 5-year mortality and morbidity in a randomized trial comparing CABG and PTCA in patients with multivessel disease: The Bypass Angioplasty Revascularization Investigation (BARI). Circulation 96:1761–1769, 1997.

64. Inoue K, Owaki T, Nakamura T, et al: Clinical application of transvenous mitral commissurotomy by a new balloon catheter. J Thorac Cardiovasc Surg 87:394–402, 1984.

65. Invasive compared with non-invasive treatment in unstable coronary-artery disease: FRISC II prospective randomised multicentre study. FRagmin and Fast Revascularisation during InStability in Coronary artery disease Investigators. Lancet 354:708–715, 1999.

66. Iung B, Garbarz E, Michaud P, et al: Percutaneous mitral commissurotomy for restenosis after surgical commissurotomy: late efficacy and implications for patient selection. J Am Coll Cardiol 35:1295–1302, 2000.

67. Johnson WD, Kayser KL, Pedraza PM: Angina pectoris and coronary bypass surgery: patterns of prevalence and recurrence in 3105 consecutive patients followed up to 11 years. Am Heart J 108:1190–1197, 1984.

68. Jones RH, Kesler K, Phillips HR 3rd, et al: Long-term survival benefits of coronary artery bypass grafting and percutaneous transluminal angioplasty in patients with coronary artery disease. J Thorac Cardiovasc Surg 111:1013–1025, 1996.

69. Judkins MP: Selective coronary arteriography: a percutaneous transfemoral technique. Radiology 89:815–824, 1967.

70. Kastrati A, Schomig A, Elezi S, et al: Predictive factors of restenosis after coronary stent placement. J Am Coll Cardiol 30:1428–1436, 1997.

71. Keeley EC, Velez CA, O'Neill WW, Safian RD: Long-term clinical outcome and predictors of major adverse cardiac events after percutaneous interventions on saphenous vein grafts. J Am Coll Cardiol 38:659–665, 2001.

72. Kiemeneij F, Laarman GJ, Odekerken D, et al: A randomized comparison of percutaneous transluminal coronary angioplasty by the radial, brachial and femoral approaches: the access study. J Am Coll Cardiol 29:1269–1275, 1997.

73. Kini A, Marmur JD, Kini S, et al: Creatine kinase-MB elevation after coronary intervention correlates with diffuse atherosclerosis, and low-to-medium level elevation has a benign clinical course: implications for early discharge after coronary intervention. J Am Coll Cardiol 34:663–671, 1999.

74. Kugelmass AD, Cohen DJ, Moscucci M, et al: Elevation of the creatine kinase myocardial isoform following otherwise successful directional coronary atherectomy and stenting. Am J Cardiol 74:748–754, 1994.

75. Kuntz RE, Baim DS, Cohen DJ, et al: A trial comparing rheolytic thrombectomy with intracoronary urokinase for coronary and vein graft thrombus [the Vein Graft AngioJet Study (VeGAS 2)]. Am J Cardiol 89:326–330, 2002.

76. Kuntz RE, Gibson CM, Nobuyoshi M, Baim DS: Generalized model of restenosis after conventional balloon angioplasty, stenting and directional atherectomy. J Am Coll Cardiol 21:15–25. 1993.

77. Lechat P, Mas JL, Lascault G, et al: Prevalence of patent foramen ovale in patients with stroke. N Engl J Med 318:1148–1152, 1988.

78. Lemmer JH Jr, Metzdorff MT, Krause AH Jr, et al: Emergency coronary artery bypass graft surgery in abciximab-treated patients. Ann Thorac Surg 69:90–95, 2000.

79. Leon MB, Teirstein PS, Moses JW, et al: Localized intracoronary gamma-radiation therapy to inhibit the recurrence of restenosis after stenting. N Engl J Med 344:250–256, 2001.

80. Lieberman EB, Bashore TM, Hermiller JB, et al: Balloon aortic valvuloplasty in adults: failure of procedure to improve long-term survival. J Am Coll Cardiol 26:1522–1528, 1995.

81. Lincoff AM, LeNarz LA, Despotis GJ, et al: Abciximab and bleeding during coronary surgery: results from the EPILOG and EPISTENT trials. Improve long-term outcome with abciximab GP IIb/IIIa blockade. Evaluation of platelet IIb/IIIa inhibition in STENTing. Ann Thorac Surg 70:516–526, 2000.

82. Liu MW, Douglas JS Jr, Lembo NJ, King SB 3rd: Angiographic predictors of a rise in serum creatine kinase (distal embolization) after balloon angioplasty of saphenous vein coronary artery bypass grafts. Am J Cardiol 72:514–517, 1993.

83. Lock JE, Khalilullah M, Shrivastava S, et al: Percutaneous catheter commissurotomy in rheumatic mitral stenosis. N Engl J Med 313:1515–1518, 1985.

84. Madyoon H, Croushore L, Weaver D, Mathur V: Use of fenoldopam to prevent radiocontrast nephropathy in high-risk patients. Cathet Cardiovasc Interv 53:341–345, 2001.

85. Magid DJ, Calonge BN, Rumsfeld JS, et al: Relation between hospital primary angioplasty volume and mortality for patients with acute MI treated with primary angioplasty vs thrombolytic therapy. JAMA 284:3131–3138, 2000.

86. Mangano DT: Aspirin and mortality from coronary bypass surgery. N Engl J Med 347:1309–1317, 2002.

87. Mark DB, Nelson CL, Califf RM, et al: Continuing evolution of therapy for coronary artery disease. Initial results from the era of coronary angioplasty. Circulation 89:2015–2025, 1994.

88. Martin F, Sanchez PL, Doherty E, et al: Percutaneous transcatheter closure of patent foramen ovale in patients with paradoxical embolism. Circulation 106:1121–1126, 2002.

89. McCullough PA, Wolyn R, Rocher LL, et al: Acute renal failure after coronary intervention: incidence, risk factors, and relationship to mortality. Am J Med 103:368–375, 1997.

90. McGrath PD, Wennberg DE, Dickens JD Jr, et al: Relation between operator and hospital volume and outcomes follow-

ing percutaneous coronary interventions in the era of the coronary stent. JAMA 284:3139–3144, 2000.

91. Morice M-C, Serruys PW, Sousa JE, et al, the RAVEL Study Group: A randomized comparison of a sirolimus-eluting stent with a standard stent for coronary revascularization. N Engl J Med 346:1773–1780, 2002.

92. Moses JW: SIRollmUS-Coated Bx Velocity™ Balloon-Expandable Stent Trial. Data presented at Transcatheter Therapeutics, Washington, D.C., 2002.

93. Nagueh SF, Lakkis NM, Middleton KJ, et al: Changes in left ventricular diastolic function 6 months after nonsurgical septal reduction therapy for hypertrophic obstructive cardiomyopathy. Circulation 99:344–347, 1999.

94. Nagueh SF, Ommen SR, Lakkis NM, et al: Comparison of ethanol septal reduction therapy with surgical myectomy for the treatment of hypertrophic obstructive cardiomyopathy. J Am Coll Cardiol 38:1701–1706, 2001.

95. Nasser TK, Mohler ER 3rd, Wilensky RL, Hathaway DR: Peripheral vascular complications following coronary interventional procedures. Clin Cardiol 18:609–614, 1995.

96. Noto TJ Jr, Johnson LW, Krone R, et al: Cardiac catheterization 1990: a report of the Registry of the Society for Cardiac Angiography and Interventions (SCA&I). Cathet Cardiovasc Diagn 24:75–83, 1991.

97. Onorato E, Melzi G, Casilli F, et al: Patent foramen ovale with paradoxical embolism: mid-term results of transcatheter closure in 256 patients. J Interv Cardiol 16:43–50, 2003.

98. Oomman A, Ramachandran P, Subramanyan K, et al: Percutaneous transluminal septal myocardial ablation in drug-resistant hypertrophic obstructive cardiomyopathy: 18-month follow-up results. J Invasive Cardiol 13:526–530, 2001.

99. Park TH, Lakkis NM, Middleton KJ, et al: Acute effect of nonsurgical septal reduction therapy on regional left ventricular asynchrony in patients with hypertrophic obstructive cardiomyopathy. Circulation 106:412–415, 2002.

100. Pathan AZ, Mahdi NA, Leon MN, et al: Is redo percutaneous mitral balloon valvuloplasty (PMV) indicated in patients with post-PMV mitral restenosis? J Am Coll Cardiol 34:49–54, 1999.

101. Piana RN, Moscucci M, Cohen DJ, et al: Palmaz-Schatz stenting for treatment of focal vein graft stenosis: immediate results and long-term outcome. J Am Coll Cardiol 23:1296–1304, 1994.

102. Popma JJ, Suntharalingam M, Lansky AJ, et al: Randomized trial of 90Sr/90Y beta-radiation versus placebo control for treatment of in-stent restenosis. Circulation 106:1090–1096, 2002.

103. Rahimtoola SH: Catheter balloon valvuloplasty for severe calcific aortic stenosis: a limited role. J Am Coll Cardiol 23:1076–1078, 1994.

104. Reber D, Sendtner E, Tollenaere P, Birnbaum D: Emergency aortocoronary bypass grafting after failed percutaneous transluminal angioplasty versus elective bypass grafting. J Cardiovasc Surg (Torino) 37:71–73, 1996.

105. Reifart N, Vandormael M, Krajcar M, et al: Randomized comparison of angioplasty of complex coronary lesions at a single center. Excimer Laser, Rotational Atherectomy, and Balloon Angioplasty Comparison (ERBAC) Study. Circulation 96:91–98, 1997.

106. Reinecke H, Fetsch T, Roeder N, et al: Emergency coronary artery bypass grafting after failed coronary angioplasty: what has changed in a decade? Ann Thorac Surg 70:1997–2003, 2000.

107. Rodriguez A, Bernardi V, Navia J, et al: Argentine Randomized Study: coronary angioplasty with stenting versus coronary bypass surgery in patients with multiple-vessel disease (ERACI II): 30-day and one-year follow-up results. ERACI II Investigators. J Am Coll Cardiol 37:51–58, 2001.

108. Safian RD, Berman AD, Diver DJ, et al: Balloon aortic valvuloplasty in 170 consecutive patients. N Engl J Med 319:125–130, 1988.

109. Safian RD, Mandell VS, Thurer RE, et al: Postmortem and intraoperative balloon valvuloplasty of calcific aortic stenosis in elderly patients: mechanisms of successful dilation. J Am Coll Cardiol 9:655–660, 1987.

110. Schuhlen H, Kastrati A, Dirschinger J, et al: Intracoronary stenting and risk for major adverse cardiac events during the first month. Circulation 98:104–111, 1998.

111. Serruys PW, de Jaegere P, Kiemeneij F, et al: A comparison of balloon-expandable-stent implantation with balloon angioplasty in patients with coronary artery disease. Benestent Study Group. N Engl J Med 331:489–495, 1994.

112. Serruys PW, Unger F, Sousa JE, et al: Comparison of coronary-artery bypass surgery and stenting for the treatment of multivessel disease. N Engl J Med 344:1117–1124, 2001.

113. Seshadri N, Whitlow PL, Acharya N, et al: Emergency coronary artery bypass surgery in the contemporary percutaneous coronary intervention era. Circulation 106:2346–2350, 2002.

114. Sitges M, Shiota T, Lever HM, et al: Comparison of left ventricular diastolic function in obstructive hypertrophic cardiomyopathy in patients undergoing percutaneous septal alcohol ablation versus surgical myotomy/myectomy. Am J Cardiol 91:817–821, 2003.

115. Smith SC Jr, Dove JT, Jacobs AK, et al: ACC/AHA guidelines of percutaneous coronary interventions (revision of the 1993 PTCA guidelines)—executive summary. A report of the American College of Cardiology/American Heart Association Task Force on Practice Guidelines (committee to revise the 1993 guidelines for percutaneous transluminal coronary angioplasty). J Am Coll Cardiol 37:2215–2239, 2001.

116. Solomon R, Werner C, Mann D, et al: Effects of saline, mannitol, and furosemide on acute decreases in renal function induced by radiocontrast agents. N Engl J Med 331:1416–1420, 1994.

117. Steinhubl SR, Berger PB, Mann JT 3rd, et al: Early and sustained dual oral antiplatelet therapy following percutaneous coronary intervention: a randomized controlled trial. JAMA 288:2411–2420, 2002.

118. Stone GW, Rogers C, Hermiller J: A prospective randomized multicenter trial comparing distal protection during saphenous vein graft intervention with a filter-based device compared to balloon occlusion and aspiration: The FIRE Trial. J Am Coll Cardiol 41:43A, 2003.

119. Stone GW, Rogers C, Ramee S, et al: Distal filter protection during saphenous vein graft stenting: technical and clinical correlates of efficacy. J Am Coll Cardiol 40:1882–1888, 2002.

120. Stone GW: Preliminary results of the TAXUS IV trial. Presented at Transcatheter Therapeutics. Washington, DC, 2003.

121. Taggart DP, Siddiqui A, Wheatley DJ: Low-dose preoperative aspirin therapy, postoperative blood loss, and transfusion requirements. Ann Thorac Surg 50:424–428, 1990.

122. Taylor PC, Boylan MJ, Lytle BW, et al: Emergent coronary bypass for failed PTCA: a 10-year experience with 253 patients. J Invasive Cardiol 6:97–98, 1994.

123. Tepel M, van der Giet M, Schwarzfeld C, et al: Prevention of radiographic-contrast-agent-induced reductions in renal function by acetylcysteine. N Engl J Med 343:180–184, 2000.

124. The Clopidogrel in Unstable Angina to Prevent Recurrent Events Trial Investigators: Effects of clopidogrel in addition to aspirin in patients with acute coronary syndromes without ST-segment elevation. N Engl J Med 345:494–502, 2001.

125. Topol EJ, Leya F, Pinkerton CA, et: A comparison of directional atherectomy with coronary angioplasty in patients with coronary artery disease. The CAVEAT Study Group. N Engl J Med 329:221–227, 1993.

950

126. Turi ZG, Reyes VP, Raju BS, et al: Percutaneous balloon versus surgical closed commissurotomy for mitral stenosis. A prospective, randomized trial. Circulation 83:1179–1185, 1991.

127. Verheul HA, Moulijn AC, Hondema S, et al: Late results of 200 repeat coronary artery bypass operations. Am J Cardiol 67:24–30, 1991.

128. Waksman R, Ajani AE, Pinnow E, et al: Twelve versus six months of clopidogrel to reduce major cardiac events in patients undergoing gamma-radiation therapy for in-stent restenosis: Washington Radiation for In-Stent Restenosis Trial (WRIST) 12 versus WRIST PLUS. Circulation 106:776–778, 2002.

129. Waksman R, White RL, Chan RC, et al: Intracoronary {gamma}-radiation therapy after angioplasty inhibits recurrence in patients with in-stent restenosis. Circulation 101:2165–2171, 2000.

130. Wyman RM, Safian RD, Portway V, et al: Current complications of diagnostic and therapeutic cardiac catheterization. J Am Coll Cardiol 12:1400–1406, 1988.

131. Zijlstra F, Hoorntje JC, de Boer MJ, et al: Long-term benefit of primary angioplasty as compared with thrombolytic therapy for acute myocardial infarction. N Engl J Med 341:1413–1419, 1999.

Medical Management of Acute Coronary Syndromes

Robert M. Califf

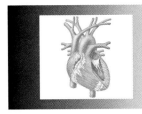

INTRODUCTION

Acute coronary syndromes (ACS) refer to the spectrum of conditions compatible with acute myocardial ischemia, from unstable angina to acute myocardial infarction (MI). These disorders are a major cause of morbidity and mortality around the world. In the United States, more than 650,000 people will have a new ACS event every year, and another 450,000 will have a repeat event.[1] Just under half of these people will die from their ACS event. These events also carry major financial costs; in 1998, Medicare paid $10.6 billion in hospital costs for ACS.[1]

One reason for the adverse clinical and financial consequences of ACS may be a lack of adherence to practice-guideline recommendations. Since 1980, the American College of Cardiology (ACC) and the American Heart Association (AHA) have published joint guidelines for the treatment of various cardiovascular diseases. In 2002, the ACC/AHA issued revised guidelines for the management of patients with unstable angina or non-ST-segment elevation acute MI (NSTEMI),[18] the two conditions that together make up non-ST-segment elevation (NSTE) ACS. For ST-segment acute MI, the remaining disorder of ACS, the guidelines were last updated in 1999.[80] Whenever possible, the recommendations given in this chapter will reflect these practice guidelines, representing a consensus of the relevant professional societies meant to assist physicians in making the most appropriate, evidence-based decisions about the management of their patients in specific circumstances.

PATHOPHYSIOLOGY OF ACS

The various manifestations of ACS share a pathophysiological origin. They begin with the disruption, through fissuring or rupture, of an atherosclerotic plaque within the wall of a coronary artery. This stimulates expression of tissue factor, which in turn stimulates platelet activation, the coagulation cascade, and thrombus formation within the arterial wall, partially or completely occluding the coronary artery. The resulting reduced or absent blood flow to the myocardium may or may not produce symptoms of ischemia. Increasingly, the importance of platelet-fibrin emboli and diffuse vascular inflammation with "downstream" smaller-vessel obstruction has been recognized.

Inflammatory Response to Injury

Many investigators have advanced the theory that atherosclerosis is an inflammatory response to injury within the vessel wall. The atherosclerotic lesions that form within the coronary vessels are products of this chronic inflammatory process.

Various risk factors cause inflammatory changes in the circulation and vessel wall, including excess low-density lipoprotein (LDL) cholesterol and oxidized LDL cholesterol, other sources of oxidative stress, cigarette smoking, hypertension, and diabetes. Recently, immune responses and viral infections have also been implicated, although these findings remain debated.[1,18,30,59] In a sense, some argue that atherosclerosis is the common response to combinations of these insults. Most recently, the concept that vascular progenitor cells from the marrow play a role in vessel repair has garnered intense interest. As this stem cell function becomes less effective with aging, the inability to repair vascular damage after inflammation may become a critical factor in the relationship between aging and atherosclerosis.

For patients who undergo percutaneous coronary intervention (PCI), the procedure itself can be traumatic for the vessel wall, and the response to this mechanical injury is more fibrotic. Therefore, ACS rarely occurs after PCI except in the immediate periprocedural period. In contrast, the lumen of saphenous vein grafts is prone to lipid-rich atheroma and superimposed diffuse thrombosis, so that vein grafts over time become sources of unstable atheromatous mass.

Plaque Rupture

The most dangerous kind of plaque is the nonobstructive, lipid-rich plaque that has a thin fibrous cap. This type of plaque, often called "vulnerable plaque," is most prone to rupture. There may be gender differences in plaque behavior, as women appear to be more prone to develop fissuring as opposed to rupture, with its corresponding higher risk of nonocclusive thrombus (Figure 59-1).

The degree of damage depends on the distribution of myocardium supplied by the artery affected; the degree of obstruction by the clot; the amount of small vessel obstructed from inflammation, thrombotic emboli, and vasoconstriction; and the extent of collateral flow. Even if the thrombus resulting from the original rupture does not obstruct the artery, smaller clots generated by the process (microemboli) can travel downstream to smaller arteries, occluding the microvasculature and causing myocardial necrosis.[79,93]

Most clinical signs of ACS reflect development of a clot large enough to cause ischemia, which can lead to myocardial necrosis with its ensuing risk of sudden death. Plaque rupture can cause no symptoms, exertion-related symptoms of ischemia (stable angina), unpredictable symptoms of ischemia without evidence of myocardial necrosis (unstable angina), signs of infarction without ST segment elevation on the electrocardiogram (ECG) (NSTEMI), signs of infarction with ECG changes such as ST-segment elevation (STEMI), or sudden death.

Angiographic and autopsy studies have shown that unstable angina and NSTEMI often reflect intermittent occlusion of coronary arteries with spontaneous recovery of blood flow to affected tissue (reperfusion).[38] The thrombotic occlusion is more persistent in ST-segment elevation MI because plaque damage is usually more severe or collateral flow is not present.

Role of Platelets in ACS

Plaque rupture leads to vessel-wall damage, which stimulates initiation of two pathways toward coagulation (Figure 59-2). The first, intrinsic pathway of the coagulation cascade ultimately results in the production of thrombin. Thrombin is an enzyme that splits fibrinogen into fibrin monomers, which, when cross-linked, stabilize a platelet-rich thrombus by forming a net. Thrombin also amplifies the coagulation process by stimulating further thrombin generation. In addition, fibrin-bound thrombin activates (1) factor XIII,

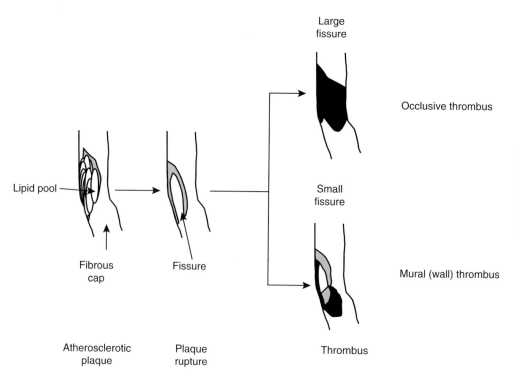

Figure 59–1 **Pathophysiology of acute coronary syndromes.** Rupture of an atherosclerotic plaque can lead to development of a mural (wall) thrombus or a partially or totally occlusive thrombus, resulting in ischemia.

Large fissure

Occlusive thrombus

Small fissure

Mural (wall) thrombus

Lipid pool

Fibrous cap

Fissure

Atherosclerotic plaque

Plaque rupture

Thrombus

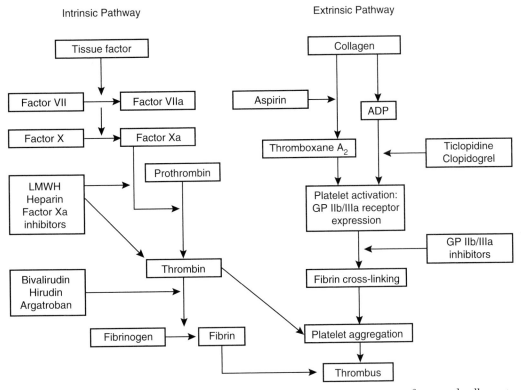

Figure 59–2 Role of platelets in thrombosis. Plaque rupture exposes tissue factor and collagen to the circulation, which stimulates intrinsic and extrinsic pathways to clotting. Medications that block various steps in these pathways are indicated in boxes.

a plasma enzyme that stabilizes the linked fibrin threads, and (2) carboxypeptidase B, another enzyme that reduces the body's intrinsic fibrinolytic process.

The second pathway leading from plaque rupture to thrombosis begins when injury to the endothelium of the vessel (caused by plaque rupture or PCI) exposes collagen and von Willebrand factor (vWF) to the bloodstream. Platelets in the bloodstream quickly bind to vWF, forming a protective layer over the injured vessel wall. The bound platelets are then activated by collagen and undergo a conformational change, spewing vasoactive substances into the circulation. During this change, glycoprotein (GP) IIb/IIIa receptors are expressed on the platelet surface. Simultaneously, platelets release adenosine diphosphate (ADP) and thromboxane, potent platelet stimulants, into the circulation. This release recruits and activates additional platelets. Fibrinogen in the bloodstream will cross-link platelets via their GP IIb/IIIa receptors. Platelets start to aggregate, and a thrombus forms. Aspirin, ticlopidine, and clopidogrel inhibit certain, but not all, portions of this pathway. The GP IIb/IIIa inhibitors block the final step in thrombus formation by occupying GP IIb/IIIa receptors on platelets, thus preventing cross-linking of fibrinogen and aggregation of platelets.

These complementary pathways result in clot formation. In simple terms, platelet activation leads to expression of the GP IIb/IIIa receptor. Fibrin cross-links multiple platelets by binding simultaneously to two molecules of GP IIb/IIIa. The coagulation cascade leads to the production of fibrin, which binds the platelet thrombus into a resistant net.

▶ DIAGNOSIS AND EPIDEMIOLOGY OF ACS SUBTYPES

Patients with possible ACS are categorized by the presence or absence of persistent ST-segment elevation on the ECG and the level of various biomarkers in the circulation (Figure 59-3). This nomenclature is critical because patients with persistent ST-segment elevation require life-saving, rapid reperfusion therapy, whereas no benefit of acute reperfusion therapy has been found in patients without ST-segment elevation. Patients with ACS but no persistent ST-segment elevation (and those with other ECG abnormalities) are retrospectively categorized as having unstable angina or NSTEMI, with or without Q waves, once the results of biomarker tests are available. This terminology is more descriptive than previous classifications, in that it reflects the need for clinicians to make immediate decisions about therapy once the medical history and ECG have been obtained. The epidemiology of ACS is changing, with more NSTE ACS and fewer STEMI cases. These changes in the ACS population seem to reflect the aging of society (older patients have a higher proportion of NSTE ACS than STEMI) in addition to the effectiveness of secondary prevention measures in precluding the complete vessel occlusion required to produce STEMI. The adoption of troponin measurement as a standard of care has further expanded the population of NSTEMI patients who previously would have been classified as having unstable angina.

Unstable coronary syndromes may be classified according to the Canadian Cardiovascular Society (CCS) classifications,

954

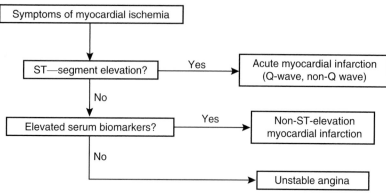

Figure 59–3 Categorization of patients with possible acute coronary syndromes. Adapted from the American Heart Association.[1]

which grade symptoms from class I through class IV (Table 59-1).[23] These classifications of angina are useful both prognostically and therapeutically. Patients with advanced CCS anginal symptoms have a higher risk of death from MI than patients with more stable symptoms. There also is some suggestion that more potent therapies may be best suited to patients with the most advanced disease.

INITIAL RISK STRATIFICATION

The information from the history, physical examination, ECG, and biomarker tests is used to assign patients to one of four categories: noncardiac disorders, chronic stable angina, possible ACS, and definite ACS. This chapter will focus on the latter two groups (Figure 59-4).

Figure 59-5 shows an algorithm by which patients with symptoms of cardiac ischemia are treated at Duke University Medical Center.° Patients with possible ACS are candidates for additional observation in a specialized facility (such as a chest pain unit).[69] Patients with definite ACS, as noted, are managed primarily according to the ECG pattern—those with ST-segment elevation are possible candidates for immediate reperfusion therapy and managed according to the ACC/AHA practice guidelines for acute STEMI,[80] and those without ST-segment elevation either undergo further observation or are admitted.[18] Patients with low-risk ACS and no transient ST-segment depression ≥0.05 or T-wave inversions ≥0.2 mV, no positive cardiac markers or hemodynamic abnormalities, and no positive stress test may be discharged and seen as outpatients.

The prognosis of patients with NSTE ACS with positive markers or ECG abnormalities, contrary to the conventional wisdom, actually is worse than that of patients with acute STEMI; those with ST-segment depression, for example, have a mortality rate at 6 months of 8.9% compared with 6.8% for those with ST-segment elevation.[82] The risks of death and of death or MI at 30 days can be calculated for the general ACS population without STEMI according to a predictive model developed from the large Platelet glycoprotein IIb/IIIa in Unstable angina: Receptor Suppression Using Integrilin Therapy (PURSUIT) trial database (Table 59-2).[17]

Perhaps not surprisingly, age, the ECG pattern, and the presence of heart failure represent most of the risk. What is particularly useful about this model, however, is that using these variables to determine early clinical risk also may allow prediction of which patients may derive more benefit from more aggressive treatment.

For acute MI, the risk of death at 30 days was 7.0% in the Global Utilization of Streptokinase and TPA for Occluded coronary arteries (GUSTO-I) trial, the largest trial of fibrinolysis in MI.[57] The rate had increased to 9.6% by 1 year.[22] Expected risk factors dominated among patients who died, the most powerful of which were age, heart rate, hemodynamics, prior MI, and location of current MI. Table 59-3 shows a nomogram for prediction of 1-year mortality after MI among 30-day survivors, using the three most predictive of the baseline clinical, ECG, and in-hospital variables.[22] The only unexpected finding regarding risk factors predictive of mortality at 1 year versus 30 days was the poor long-term prognosis of black patients.[22] After adjustment for other prognostic factors, including revascularization, black patients still had more than twice the risk of white patients for late mortality in GUSTO-I. Differential access to or use of secondary-prevention measures may explain some of this disparity.

Table 59–1

Canadian Cardiovascular Society Classification of Anginal Symptoms[23]

Class	Description
I	No angina with ordinary activity; pain with strenuous exertion
II	Slight limitation of ordinary activity
III	Marked limitations of ordinary activity
IV	Pain with any physical activity; symptoms may occur at rest

---

°This algorithm pertains to Duke University Medical Center only and should not be construed as presenting the definitive standard of care or containing diagnostic or therapeutic recommendations.

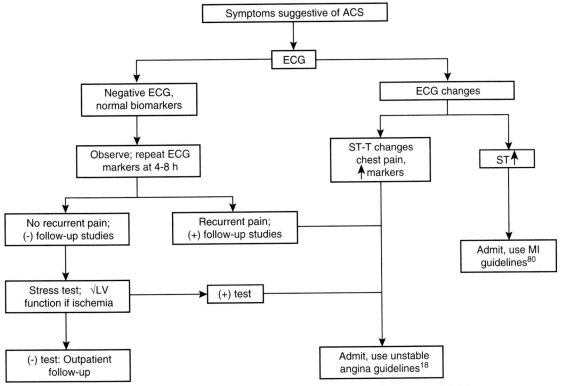

Figure 59–4 Evaluation and immediate management of patients with suspected ACS.

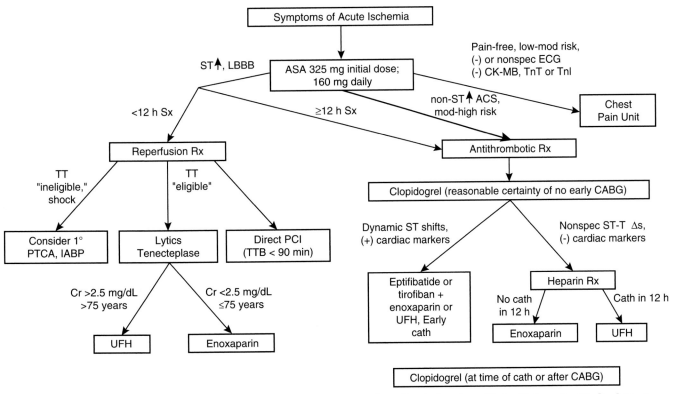

Figure 59–5 Algorithm for treatment of patients with symptoms of cardiac ischemia at Duke University Medical Center.

956

Table 59–2		
Prediction of Death or MI at 30 Days among Patients with NSTE ACS in the PURSUIT Trial[a]		
		Score
	Death	**Death or MI**
Age (years)		
50	0	8 (11)
60	2 (3)	9 (12)
70	4 (6)	11 (13)
80	6 (9)	12 (14)
Sex		
Female	0	0
Male	1	1
Worst CCS past 6 weeks		
0, I, II	0	0
III, IV	2	2
Heart rate (bpm)		
80	0	0
100	1 (2)	0
120	2 (5)	0
Systolic blood pressure (mm Hg)		
120	0	0
100	1	0
80	2	0
Heart failure		
No	0	0
Yes	3	2
ST depression at baseline		
No	0	0
Yes	3	1

Reprinted from Boersma et al[17] with permission.

[a]Separate points are assigned for the risk factors of age and heart rate, depending on whether the patient has unstable angina or MI (points for MI in parentheses).
CCS, Canadian Cardiovascular Society.

Cardiac biomarkers, especially the troponins, play an important role in risk stratification of patients with ACS, particularly those without ST-segment elevation. In the Global Use of Strategies To Open occluded coronary arteries (GUSTO-IIa), for example, a positive troponin T result at baseline was highly predictive of 1-year mortality.[71] At 1 year, mortality among patients who were troponin positive at arrival was 14% compared with 5% among those who were initially troponin negative. The TIMI group has shown a strong association between baseline troponin I level and 42-day mortality in NSTE ACS.[4] Moreover, a positive baseline troponin T can predict 1-year mortality in ACS,

even after adjustment for other baseline clinical and ECG characteristics.[66]

Troponin levels also add predictive information even in the presence of ST-segment elevation MI.[71] Among patients with MI in the GUSTO-IIa trial, those with a positive baseline troponin T had higher rates of death at 30 days (13% versus 4.7%), in-hospital repeat MI (91% versus 81%), and bypass surgery (16% versus 14%) compared with troponin-negative patients with STEMI.

Positive biomarkers predict not only which patients are at higher risk for adverse outcomes but also those who might benefit most from aggressive treatment. Lindahl and colleagues reported a greater benefit of dalteparin among baseline troponin T-positive patients (versus negative patients) in the FRagmin In unStable Coronary artery disease (FRISC) trial.[61] Other trials have shown preferential effects of platelet GP IIb/IIIa inhibitors among patients with NSTE ACS who are troponin positive at baseline.[47,48,68] Finally, the benefits of an invasive versus conservative mode of therapy may be greater for patients who are troponin positive at arrival.[51] The troponins appear to be a powerful tool for risk stratification and for selection of aggressive medical and interventional therapies.

A biomarker of more recent interest is C-reactive protein (CRP). Although generally recognized as a marker of systemic inflammation, and recently noted as a new risk marker for chronic coronary artery disease, the role of CRP in acute ACS has been less prominently discussed. In the recent GUSTO-IV ACS trial, elevated CRP was a potent predictor of recurrent vascular events.[51]

Even more recently, the TIMI group has shown the prognostic value of measurement of atrial natriuretic peptide (ANP) and brain natriuretic peptide (BNP) levels in patients with NSTE ACS.[73] This marker reflects atrial stretch, most often due to heart failure in this population. Patients with elevated ANP and BNP had a significantly increased risk of death during follow-up.

An approach gaining favor as the data increase is the "multimarker" strategy, initially introduced and recently confirmed in a randomized trial by Newby and colleagues,[69] which refers to the simultaneous use of troponin, creatine kinase-MB, and myoglobin. This approach might be further enhanced by including CRP and BNP in the mix of markers. In the future, arrays of protein biomarkers likely will be used to stratify prognosis, determine preferred treatment alternatives, and examine the biological impact of treatment for both research and clinical care.

▶ **MEDICAL- VERSUS CATHETERIZATION-BASED STRATEGIES**

Once a patient's risk has been estimated, the choices for management become split into two broad categories: medical management and catheter-based/surgical strategies. Table 59-4 details the definitive recommendations regarding early invasive approaches and procedures from the NSTE ACS and STEMI guidelines.[18,80] The bottom line for both STEMI and NSTE ACS is that for most patients with medium or high risk, the catheterization approach is the critical component of treatment, which should also include medical therapy. Thus, medical therapy is not seen as an

Table 59–3

Nomogram to Predict 1-Year Survival in Patients Receiving Fibrinolytic Agents for MI and Surviving to 30 Days, Using Baseline Clinical and ECG Factors and In-Hospital Factors

1. Find points for each marker		2. Sum points for all risk markers	3. Find risk for given point total	
	Points		*Total points*	*Predicated survival (%)*
Age (years)		Age _____	126	40
30	10	Prior MI _____	119	50
40	15	In-hospital CHF/PE _____	113	60
50	20	**Total** _____	105	70
60	32		94	80
70	46		77	90
80	59		75	91
90	73		72	92
100	86		69	93
			65	94
Prior MI			61	95
No	0		56	96
Yes	18		50	97
			40	98
In-hospital CHF/PE			25	99
No	0			
Yes	25			

Reprinted from Califf et al,[22] with permission.

alternative to invasive evaluation and management but rather as an adjunctive and critical component of the invasive strategy.

In general, for patients with NSTE ACS, medical management should be reserved only for those who are low risk, as evidenced by lack of ECG changes, hemodynamic abnormalities, or cardiac markers and those in whom procedures are contraindicated. Both the FRISC-II[37,53] and Treat angina with Aggrastat and determine the Cost of Therapy with Invasive or Conservative Strategies (TACTICS)–Thrombolysis In Myocardial Infarction (TIMI) 18 trials[25] have shown the superiority of an early invasive strategy versus a more conservative one. In FRISC-II, however, randomization occurred after ~5 days of treatment with dalteparin. Thus, although the catheterization-based strategy appeared to benefit patients, and dalteparin was beneficial during the waiting period, this approach is unlikely to be adopted because of the cost of prolonged observation. In the TACTICS–TIMI-18 trial, patients in the invasive arm underwent angiography much more rapidly than in FRISC-II (median, 24 h) with revascularization to follow. As with FRISC-II, the invasive strategy was associated with significantly improved clinical outcomes. Also, in agreement with the troponin substudy of FRISC II,[53] the troponin-positive patients in TACTICS–TIMI-18 derived particular benefit from more aggressive management, showing an absolute 10% reduction in the primary end point (compared with an absolute 3.5% reduction for the trial population as a whole). Most recently,

the British Randomised Intervention Trial of unstable Angina (RITA)-3 trial also showed a benefit of early, aggressive intervention in this population.[34]

For patients with STEMI, primary PCI has become the standard of care for eligible patients treated at experienced centers. Bypass surgery becomes an option for those who are not candidates for PCI, who have failed PCI, or who have persistent symptoms, unstable hemodynamics, or structural defects requiring concomitant cardiac surgery. Fibrinolysis remains the appropriate choice for patients who arrive at facilities with lesser procedural volumes or that lack expertise for the invasive approach. Among patients with STEMI, medical management (without fibrinolysis or direct PCI) should be considered only for patients with an absolute contraindication to both reperfusion approaches or those with comorbid disease leading to an expressed desire to avoid life-prolonging interventions.

Given the rapid evolution of these guidelines toward the invasive approach to management, several organizational issues have become important. Considerable information has accrued showing that volume and expertise are critical in delivering acute invasive care to patients with ACS of both types. These findings point to the possibility of developing "ACS centers" similar to currently used trauma centers, so that well-prepared facilities could provide the best coordinated care.[20] A subcomponent of this issue is the question of on-site surgery. The recently completed Cardiovascular Patient Outcomes Research Team (C-PORT) trial[8] found

Table 59–4

Guideline Class IA Recommendations for Early Invasive Strategy (vs. Medical Therapy Only) for Patients with NSTE ACS² and STEMI

Characteristic(s)	Treatment
ACS	
Angina that recurs; occurs at rest; occurs with HF symptoms, S3 gallop, pulmonary edema, worsening rales, or new or worsening MR; or occurs with low-level activity despite intensive antiischemic therapy; elevated troponin (T or I); new ST-segment depression; high-risk findings on noninvasive stress test; left ventricular systolic function (ejection fraction <40% on noninvasive study); hemodynamic instability; sustained ventricular tachycardia; PCI within 6 months; prior bypass surgery	Early angiography, possible intervention
Left main disease,ᵃ candidate for bypass	Bypass
Three-vessel disease with ejection fraction <50%	Bypass
Multivessel disease including proximal LAD, ejection fraction <50% or untreated diabetes	Bypass
Multivessel disease with ejection fraction >50%, no diabetesᵇ	PCI
MI	
If able to be performed <12 h after symptom onset, or >12 h if symptoms persist, if able to be performed <90 min at experienced centersᶜ	PCI
Persistent or recurrent symptomatic ischemia, spontaneous or induced, with or without ECG changes	PCI
Cardiogenic shock, severe pulmonary congestion, continuing hypotension, if able to be performed <18 h after onset	PCI
Failed angioplasty with persistent pain or hemodynamic instability; suitable anatomy	Bypass
Persistent, recurrent, or refractory ischemia; suitable anatomy; not a candidate for PCI	Bypass
Surgical repair of ventricular septal defect of mitral valve insufficiency	Bypass

Adapted from the ACC/AHA Guidelines.[18,80]
ᵃFifty percent diameter stenosis.
ᵇClass/level of evidence I/A if severe angina persists despite medical therapy.
ᶜOperators performing >75 PCI procedures per year; centers performing >200 procedures per year that have cardiac-surgery capability.

that direct PCI in sites without on-site surgery was superior to fibrinolysis with alteplase, although the trial was small and debate has arisen about whether these results are generalizable. Nevertheless, an increasing number of small hospitals are offering direct PCI for STEMI without on-site surgical back-up. Arrangements should be in place at these institutions for rapid transfer of patients who need surgery, although the number of such cases continues to increase.

The role of surgery in this invasive approach remains subjective and poorly defined. In general, current guidelines recommend surgery for patients with three-vessel disease, left main disease, or concurrent structural defects (e.g., mitral regurgitation, septal defect). Despite the finding in the Bypass Angioplasty Revascularization Investigation (BARI) of the superiority of surgery over PCI in patients with diabetes,[12] the referral patterns continue to favor PCI in diabetic patients unless the anatomy is considered to be technically prohibitive. Continuously emerging innovations such as drug-eluting stents, robotic surgery, and combined procedures make exact determination of the indication for PCI versus bypass surgery fluid at this time.

GUIDELINE-RECOMMENDED MEDICAL MANAGEMENT OF NSTE ACS

In an ideal world, every clinical decision would be backed by firm evidence from large, adequately powered, randomized clinical trials. Such data exist for few clinical decisions, however. Box 59-1 lists the class I, level A recommendations ("almost always do it") and class III, level A recommendations ("never do it") from the ACC/AHA guidelines for NSTE ACS.[18,21] For most therapeutic decisions, physicians treating patients with ACS will not be able to rely on solid evidence. Nevertheless, increasing support for the construct of "minimum necessary care" is accruing from ongoing studies; centers with excellent adherence to current guidelines have better patient outcomes.[21,74] It is also becoming clear that rates of adherence depend upon institutional and group systems rather than upon the memory of individual providers.

Antiischemic Agents

Several therapies are thought by consensus groups to be valuable for initial management of ACS. These include bedrest with continuous ECG for both arrhythmias and ongoing ischemia.[18] Also included is nitroglycerin, given sublingually, by spray, or intravenously. Patients should receive supplemental oxygen if they have evidence of respiratory distress or impaired oxygenation on pulse oximetry, and intravenous morphine can be valuable to relieve chest pain if nitroglycerin is ineffective.[18] Morphine also helps reduce anxiety, and therefore the catecholamine surge that accompanies acute chest pain. The third advantage of intravenous morphine is that it dilates blood vessels, which could benefit patients with pulmonary congestion that might be aided through preload reduction.

Antithrombotic Therapy

Given that the pathophysiology of ACS involves thrombosis in response to vascular injury, it makes sense that the cornerstone of its medical management involves antithrombotic therapy. The key antithrombotic treatment for ACS—and for atherosclerotic coronary disease generally—is oral **aspirin** therapy.[2] In four randomized trials of aspirin versus placebo in patients with unstable angina,[19,58,90,94] there was a ~51% reduction in the risk of death at ≥30 days and a 47% reduction in the risk of death or MI with aspirin versus placebo. Further, the effect of aspirin therapy appears to be greatest among the highest-risk patients, namely those with MI, estimating an aggregate benefit of ~24 fewer deaths for every 1000 patients treated with 5 weeks of aspirin therapy.[9] For patients with unstable angina, there are about 50 fewer ischemic events at 6 months (vascular death, nonfatal MI, or nonfatal stroke) for every 1000 patients treated with aspirin versus placebo.[9] Aspirin also may have more than just an antiplatelet effect. In a recent study, physicians with the highest plasma levels of C-reactive protein showed the greatest reduction in MI with aspirin treatment.[77] Another recent report noted that patients with chronic stable angina have increased levels of proinflammatory cytokines, which were reduced with aspirin treatment.[50]

Although the use of aspirin in ACS increases the risk of bleeding, there is a consensus that the benefits far outweigh the risks. Specifically, in patients undergoing bypass surgery, those treated throughout the procedure with aspirin have a dramatic reduction in postoperative ischemic events compared with those who did not receive aspirin throughout the procedure.[63]

For patients with either aspirin intolerance or true aspirin allergy, other oral antiplatelet agents may be valuable. In particular, a thienopyridine agent should be considered for this subgroup of patients. The recent Clopidogrel in Unstable Angina to Prevent Recurrent Ischemic Events (CURE) trial provided the basis for the use of the dual antiplatelet strategy among patients with ACS.[29] In this trial, 12,562 patients with NSTEMI were randomized to receive aspirin plus placebo therapy or aspirin plus **clopidogrel** therapy. The primary end point of the trial was the composite of cardiovascular death, MI, or stroke. The incidence of the primary end point at a mean follow-up of 9 months was reduced from 11.5% in the aspirin–placebo group to 9.3% in the aspirin–clopidogrel group (relative risk reduction, 0.80; $p < .001$). The effect was focused on the incidence of MI, reducing this component from 6.7–5.2%. The risks of both major bleeding and transfusion were increased with the combination therapy. The large CAPRIE trial supports the use of clopidogrel alone in high-risk patients.[26] This trial, which randomized 19,185 patients with vascular disease

---

Box 59–1. Guideline Recommendations for Medical Therapy in NSTE ACS.[18,21]

Class IA (Recommended) Therapies

Immediate, continued antiplatelet therapy with aspirin; add/substitute clopidogrel if aspirin not tolerated or as appropriate

Platelet glycoprotein IIb/IIIa inhibition (plus aspirin/clopidogrel and heparin) if continued ischemia or other high-risk features

Subcutaneous low-molecular-weight or intravenous unfractionated heparin (plus aspirin/clopidogrel)

Platelet glycoprotein IIb/IIIa antagonist (plus aspirin/clopidogrel and heparin) if angiography and percutaneous intervention planned

Lipid-lowering drugs (statin) and diet if low-density lipoprotein level >130 mg/dl

Hypertension control to <130/85 mm Hg

Angiotensin-converting enzyme inhibitor for patients with heart failure, ejection fraction <40%, hypertension, or diabetes

Class IIIA (Not Recommended) Therapies

Immediate-release dihydropyridine calcium antagonist without β-blockade

Thrombolytic therapy without ST-segment elevation, left bundle-branch block, or true posterior infarction

Abciximab, if percutaneous intervention is not planned

(ischemic stroke, MI, peripheral arteriolar disease), had a composite primary end point of vascular death, ischemic stroke, or nonfatal MI. With a mean follow-up of 1.9 years, the event rate was 5.32% with clopidogrel versus 5.83% for aspirin (relative risk reduction, 8.7%; 95% confidence interval, 0.3–16.5).

Bleeding in patients who undergo surgery after treatment with clopidogrel has been a contentious issue. As with aspirin, clopidogrel permanently impairs platelet function, but the effect on surgical bleeding (when used in conjunction with aspirin) appears to be more profound than with aspirin alone. This issue has caused many to withhold clopidogrel in patients with ACS until the anatomy has been defined, so that they would not undergo surgery after clopidogrel treatment unless PCI failed, whereas others have argued that the clear benefits of clopidogrel when added to aspirin outweigh the risk of surgery. Empirical analysis indicates that patients undergoing surgery more than 5 days after clopidogrel is discontinued no longer have an increased risk of bleeding.

Intravenous Antithrombin Therapy

With aspirin, intravenous or subcutaneous heparin has been a cornerstone of antithrombotic treatment of NSTE ACS, although the evidence is far from definitive.[72] Six randomized trials have been done, totaling only about 1300 patients. They showed a consistent trend toward a reduced incidence of death or MI during treatment with unfractionated heparin plus aspirin compared with aspirin alone ($p = .06$). The lack of statistical significance likely reflects the modest size of each individual trial and of the overall pooled population. This is partly why the ACC/AHA guideline recommendation for the use of heparin in NSTE ACS carries a grade of "B" for the supporting evidence.[18]

Heparin has several drawbacks as an antithrombotic agent. First, it binds to many plasma proteins present during atherosclerotic plaque rupture, making the drug less effective. Because the large size of the heparin molecule prevents deep penetration of thrombus, some thrombin in the ruptured plaque cannot be neutralized by heparin therapy. Heparin also requires an intermediary molecule, antithrombin III, making its pharmacodynamic effect less predictable. Adverse effects on platelets, including stimulation of platelet aggregation and development of the rare but sometimes fatal heparin-induced thrombocytopenia (HIT) syndrome, also make heparin suboptimal in acute situations. Finally, the apparent "rebound effect" after discontinuation of heparin infusion, evidenced by a cluster of clinical effects occurring within hours afterward, can have serious implications for patients with unstable coronary syndromes.[10]

The low-molecular-weight (LMW) heparins were developed to overcome some of the disadvantages of unfractionated heparin. They typically are given subcutaneously, appear to have a more stable dose–response, are less resistant to uptake by circulating plasma proteins, and may be less likely to cause HIT. Six moderate to large trials have randomized patients with ACS to receive one of three different LMW heparins or unfractionated heparin.[°] Together, the three trials of **enoxaparin** showed a clear advantage of this LMW heparin over standard heparin in reducing the composite end points of (1) death, MI, or recurrent ischemia and (2) death or MI.[3,15,32] The most recent trial, the Aggrastat to Zocor (A to Z) trial, showed that when combined with a platelet GP IIb/IIIa inhibitor, enoxaparin again trended toward superiority over unfractionated heparin.[15] The trial was a noninferiority trial by design, however, and a systematic overview of the entire enoxaparin experience shows substantial evidence of its superiority (Table 59-5).[†]

In the FRagmin In unstable Coronary artery disease (FRIC) study of **dalteparin**[52] and the FRAXiparine in Ischaemic Syndrome (FRAXIS) trial of **nadroparin**,[36] no benefit was shown over unfractionated heparin. Because the various LMW heparins have not been compared directly,

---

[°]References 3, 7, 11, 15, 32, 52, 89, 95, 96.
[†]References 3, 7, 11, 18, 32, 89, 95, 96.

Table 59–5

Clinical Efficacy of Enoxaparin in Randomized Trials of ACS

Study	N	Outcome measure	Time of measure (days)	Event rate Enoxaparin (%)	Control (%)
NSTE ACS					
ESSENCE[32]	3171	Death, infarction, recurrent ischemia	14	16.6	19.8
TIMI-11B[3]	3910	Death, infarction, urgent revascularization	43	17.3	19.7
STEMI					
ASENOX[89]	154	Death	30	7.1	8.2
Baird[5,11]	300	Death, reinfarction, readmission	90	26	36
ASSENT-3[7]	6116	Death, in-hospital reinfarction, in-hospital RI	30	11.4	15.4
ASSENT-3 Plus[95]	1639	Death, in-hospital reinfarction, in-hospital RI	30	14.2	17.4

RI, refractory ischemia.

this heterogeneity in results may reflect the trials or the specific agents, but it appears prudent to recommend the use of enoxaparin for patients with ACS when an LMW agent is chosen instead of standard heparin.

Because the LMW heparins have a prolonged half-life and they are given subcutaneously, surgical bleeding has been a concern. This issue has been particularly prominent in patients with renal dysfunction because the LMW heparins are eliminated by the kidneys. Although a significant part of the activity of LMW heparins is antagonized by protamine, recent studies have raised the issue of whether protamine has a detrimental effect on outcome.[87]

Three intravenous direct thrombin inhibitors—**argatroban, lepirudin,** and **bivalirudin**—have been approved for use in the United States. Argatroban and lepirudin are indicated for anticoagulant treatment of patients with HIT, whereas bivalirudin is indicated for anticoagulant use in patients with ACS undergoing PCI. None is specifically approved as a primary anticoagulant for treatment of ACS, but lepirudin has been studied extensively in this group of patients,[70] and the pivotal trials that led to bivalirudin approval[13,14] enrolled patients with unstable angina and recent MI. A systematic registry[42] is assessing improvements in clinical outcomes with the direct thrombin inhibitors among patients with ACS and those requiring PCI, but more work is needed before any of these can be considered a cornerstone of therapy for patients with NSTE ACS.

Intravenous Platelet Glycoprotein IIb/IIIa Inhibitors

Understanding the pivotal role that the platelet plays in the pathobiology of ACS led to development of the platelet GP IIb/IIIa inhibitors. These drugs have since become an important adjunctive therapy for patients with ACS. There are two basic categories of intravenous GP IIb/IIIa inhibitors: the monoclonal antibody and the small-molecule inhibitors. Three intravenous agents are approved for use in the United States: the monoclonal antibody fragment, abciximab; eptifibatide, a peptide inhibitor; and tirofiban, a peptidomimetic. These agents have many similarities but also many differences, including their sizes, ease and speed of reversibility, selectivity, and antigenic properties.[60]

The use of GP IIb/IIIa inhibitors in PCI or NSTE ACS has seen some of the most intense research in acute cardiac care in the last decade. At least 14 major clinical trials have compared these agents with placebo in these settings, and almost 50,000 patients have been randomized. This very large dataset allows us to draw inferences about the benefits and risks of this drug class.

There have been six moderate-to-large, placebo-controlled trials of GP IIb/IIIa inhibitors in patients with ACS.[16] In the aggregate, the 30-day incidence of death or MI was reduced by a modest, but statistically significant, relative 9% with the use of these agents. In each of the five trials that studied either a peptide or peptidomimetic GP IIb/IIIa inhibitor, the estimated effect always favored the platelet inhibitor, whereas in the single large trial of abciximab, the opposite was true. These trials differed in study design, however, making direct comparisons inappropriate and potentially misleading. For example, three trials measured a primary end point of death or MI at 30 days (PARAGON-A, PURSUIT, and GUSTO-IV); the other three also included refractory ischemia (PRISM and PRISM-PLUS) or severe recurrent ischemia (PARAGON-B). PARAGON-B had a 30-day primary end point, but the two tirofiban trials measured it much earlier (48 h in PRISM and 7 days in PRISM-PLUS). Nonetheless, it appears prudent to recommend only the small-molecule compounds for initial "upstream" GP IIb/IIIa inhibition in appropriate patients, specifically, those who are considered high risk at initial evaluation: those aged >65 years, those with prolonged or ongoing chest pain, those with chest pain at rest with ischemic ECG changes, those with hemodynamic instability (including evidence of heart failure), and those with elevated cardiac biomarkers (positive creatine kinase-MB or troponin).[18]

As with other antiplatelet agents, bleeding is increased with GP IIb/IIIa inhibitors, especially in the mucosal areas, including the gastrointestinal tract. There is no antidote to these agents, but the active half-life is relatively short, as the platelet is not irreversibly altered. Interesting data have emerged to indicate that patients undergoing bypass surgery may benefit from GP IIb/IIIa inhibition during the procedure.[75] Previous research has shown that platelets are activated during cardiopulmonary bypass, and a significant proportion of platelets sticks to the bypass conduits and membranes. The GP IIb/IIIa inhibitors reduce this effect. Furthermore, in patients who undergo urgent procedures after receiving GP IIb/IIIa inhibitors, clinical outcomes appear to be improved relative to those undergoing surgery without GP IIb/IIIa inhibition.[31] These findings must be examined in randomized clinical trials before routine treatment before surgery would be justified, but surgeons can at least be comfortable with proceeding when treatment already has occurred.

β-Blockers

All patients with ACS should be given a β-blocker if not contraindicated.[18] For patients in the acute phase of ischemia, an intravenous agent should be considered. Most of the data supporting β-blockade in ACS reflect literature on ST-segment elevation MI, most of which predates the reperfusion era. The largest experience with β-blockers was the first International Study of Infarct Survival (ISIS), which showed that mortality was reduced by ~15% with atenolol versus placebo treatment among 16,027 patients with suspected acute MI, many of whom did not have STEMI.[33] In a substudy of the TIMI-IIIB study, however, the rates of reinfarction and recurrent ischemia were lower with immediate use of metoprolol versus delayed use; the study did not have adequate statistical power to assess mortality.[91] Nonetheless, the bulk of the evidence supports use of β-blockade in all patients with ACS, unless there is an absolute contraindication, such as acute decompensated heart failure with various levels of bradycardia and heart block. Although other conditions, such as chronic lung disease, have been considered relative contraindications to β-blockers, a recent evaluation of the Medicare database provides supportive evidence for a major benefit of β-blockers even in patients with relative contraindications.[28]

Angiotensin-Converting Enzyme (ACE) Inhibitors

There are no data to support the use of ACE inhibitors as acute therapy for NSTE ACS, but substantial evidence supports their relatively early use in MI and their long-term

962 value in this population. A series of systematic overviews in which all known patient data have been combined into a single database provides definitive evidence of major benefit in patients with evidence of heart failure or left ventricular dysfunction.[56] Highly significant evidence for benefit in all MI patients was found in this overview, although the magnitude of the benefit was relatively small (5 lives saved per 1000 patients treated).

The Heart Outcomes Prevention Evaluation (HOPE) study, which compared ramipril and placebo in patients with vascular disease or high-risk characteristics such as diabetes, showed a significant improved clinical outcomes with ramipril.[49] The current guidelines therefore call for the use of ACE inhibitors in patients with ACS and heart failure, left ventricular dysfunction (ejection fraction <40%), hypertension, or diabetes. More large trials are underway evaluating ACE inhibitors in patients without left ventricular dysfunction, to determine whether the HOPE findings can be validated with other ACE inhibitors or angiotensin-receptor blockers (ARBs).

For patients unable to tolerate ACE inhibitors because of cough (a common side effect of ACE inhibitors), ARBs appear to produce similar benefits without the side effects. To date, ARBs cannot be recommended as substitutes for ACE inhibitors, because they have not been proven superior in head-to-head trials; rather, they should be reserved for patients with intolerance to ACE inhibitors.

Statins

Cholesterol-lowering therapy reduces vascular events and mortality in patients with coronary artery disease (CAD) and hypercholesterolemia[35] and patients with mild cholesterol elevation (209–218 mg/dl) after MI and unstable angina.[62,81] In the Myocardial Ischemia Reduction with Aggressive Cholesterol Lowering (MIRACL) study, 3086 patients were randomized to treatment with atorvastatin 80 mg daily or placebo 24–96 h after ACS.[83] At 16 weeks, only 14.8% of the treated patients had reached the primary end point of death, nonfatal MI, resuscitated cardiac arrest, or recurrent severe myocardial ischemia compared with 17.4% of the placebo-treated patients (p =.048). The risks of death, nonfatal MI, cardiac arrest, and worsening heart failure did not differ between the two groups, but the treated patients had fewer strokes and less severe recurrent ischemia. The Lipid-Coronary Artery Disease (L-CAD) study randomized patients with an ACS (n = 126) to early treatment with pravastatin, alone or combined with cholestyramine or niacin, or usual care. At 24 months, the early-aggressive treatment group had significantly fewer clinical events than the usual-care group (23% versus 52%; p = .005).[5] In a Swedish registry of ~20,000 patients, the adjusted relative risk of mortality was 25% lower in cardiac patients who started statin therapy before discharge.[88] However, several registries have not replicated these findings.[67] Nevertheless, the evidence for safety is substantial with early treatment, and continued long-term therapy is clearly much more likely when started in the hospital. The National Cholesterol Education Program 2 and the ACC/AHA guidelines for NSTE ACS therefore recommend a target LDL cholesterol level <100 mg/dl, a low-saturated-fat diet for people with an LDL cholesterol level >100 mg/dl, and the addition of lipid-lowering therapy for those with an LDL cholesterol level >130 mg/dl.[18,44,65]

▶ GUIDELINE-RECOMMENDED MEDICAL MANAGEMENT OF STEMI

General Management

For the most part, medical management in acute ST-segment elevation MI closely follows medical treatment in NSTE ACS, except when fibrinolytic agents are used. The primary difference is the withholding of platelet GP IIb/IIIa inhibitors if fibrinolytic agents are going to be given. Studies that have examined the use of such combination treatment in patients with MI have had disappointing results, although some role may be found in young patients at low risk of intracranial hemorrhage.[86,92]

Fibrinolytic Agents

The four most commonly used agents are streptokinase, alteplase, reteplase, and tenecteplase. Table 59-6 presents a brief comparison of these agents.* The incidence of TIMI grade 3 (or normal) blood flow at 90 min after treatment initiation ranges from 33% (with streptokinase) to 63% (with tenecteplase) when given with intravenous heparin. This knowledge is critical because early achievement of normal coronary blood flow has been linked with improved 30-day survival.[84] Tenecteplase has the added advantage of single-bolus dosing.

The most significant complications of fibrinolytic therapy relate to bleeding risk. The rate of in-hospital intracranial hemorrhage has ranged from 0.57% with streptokinase to 0.93% with tenecteplase (both given with intravenous heparin).[6,41,46] Rates of serious or major bleeding follow this basic pattern, but the use of transfusions in these patients has decreased over the years. For example, the rate of transfusion among alteplase-treated patients in GUSTO-I (enrollment completed in 1993) was 10%[45]; by 1997, when GUSTO-III completed enrollment, it had decreased to 6.3%[46]; and by 1998, when ASSENT-2 completed enrollment, it was only 5.5%.[6] Thus, although the incidence of serious bleeding has not decreased, physicians appear to have become more judicious in their use of transfusions, perhaps because of increasing knowledge of the risks of transfusion.[40]

▶ PREDISCHARGE RISK STRATIFICATION

Patients with ACS should undergo continuous risk stratification, from the initial assessment, to the initial response to treatment, to the hospital course after leaving the intensive or cardiac care unit. Once the patient has become stable, if a conservative approach to intervention has been chosen, noninvasive stress testing is recommended using radionuclide imaging, echocardiography, or exercise or pharmacological stress testing.[29,39,78] Such testing can detect ischemia in patients with a low likelihood of coronary disease, and, more importantly, an integrated estimate of risk,

---

*References 6, 21, 41, 45, 46, 76, 84.

Table 59–6

Fibrinolytic Agents for STEMI

Agent	Dose	90-min TIMI grade 3 flow (%)	30-day mortality	In-hospital events	
				Any stroke	Reinfarction
Streptokinase	1.5 MU[a]	33	7.4	1.4	4.0
Alteplase	100 mg, 15% as bolus[a]	54	6.3	1.6	4.0
Reteplase	2 10-U boluses[a]	59	7.5	1.6	4.2
Tenecteplase	30–40 mg[b]	55–63	6.2	1.8	4.1

[a]With intravenous heparin.
[b]Depending on weight.

including left ventricular function. With the results of noninvasive testing, other appropriate diagnostic and therapeutic measures can begin.

The choice of test should reflect patient characteristics, test availability, and expertise in interpretation. Because it is simple, inexpensive, and easy to perform and interpret, the standard low-level exercise ECG stress test remains the test of choice for patients able to exercise who have no confounding factors on the resting ECG. Otherwise healthy patients with confounding ECG factors should undergo exercise testing with imaging. Patients who cannot exercise should undergo pharmacological stress test with imaging. Low-risk patients without symptoms for 12–24 h can undergo a low-level exercise test (Bruce Stage II). Patients without ischemic signs for 7–10 days can undergo a symptom-limited test.

In general, induction of ischemia at a low workload (≤6.5 metabolic equivalents [METs]) or a high-risk treadmill score (≥11)[64] implies severe impairment in coronary blood flow. Such results are associated with increased risks for adverse outcomes or severe angina after discharge. Barring contraindications, such patients generally merit referral for early angiography and possible revascularization. Conversely, achievement of a higher workload (>6.5 METs) without evidence of ischemia (low-risk treadmill score ≥5) correlates with less coronary artery obstruction and a better prognosis. Such patients often can be safely managed conservatively. Ischemia developing at >6.5 METs may be associated with severe coronary artery obstruction, but unless patients have other high-risk markers (>0.2-mV ST-segment depression or elevation, decreased blood pressure, ST-segment shifts in multiple leads, or prolonged recovery of ST shifts), they also can be managed conservatively.

ACS in Patients with Previous Bypass Surgery

Although bypass surgery improves survival and quality of life, many patients return with acute ACS events, particularly after 5 years of follow-up. In general, patients with prior bypass surgery have a worse prognosis when an ACS event occurs than patients without prior surgery. Part of this increased risk accrues because of the advanced age of this population relative to patients without previous bypass grafting. Unfortunately, no clinical trials have specifically addressed the issue of management in postbypass patients with ACS. Most large trials have included these patients, however, offering some opportunity to look at potential differences in retrospect.

In NSTE ACS, no difference in benefit has been observed for any of the standard therapies as a function of previous bypass surgery.[54,55] In STEMI, outcomes after fibrinolysis trend in the same direction for postbypass patients as with others. When primary PCI is used as the method of reperfusion, identification of the infarct artery is difficult, and results of the procedure may be less successful.[43,85] When the bypass graft itself is the "culprit," the benefit of GP IIb/IIIa inhibitors is not clear.[85]

▶ SUMMARY

The field of ACS is now dominated by definitive, large clinical trials that have set a standard of care that is leading to better clinical outcomes. The criteria for surgical treatment of ACS continue to evolve, but the dominance of the invasive approach and the emerging technological improvements in both PCI and surgery likely will lead to more revascularization procedures. Invasive therapy still must be coupled with the best medical therapy, as outlined above.

REFERENCES

1. American Heart Association: Heart Disease and Stroke Statistics—2003 Update. Dallas: American Heart Association, 2003.
2. Antiplatelet Trialists' Collaboration: Collaborative overview of randomised trials of antiplatelet therapy, I: prevention of death, myocardial infarction, and stroke by prolonged

964

antiplatelet therapy in various categories of patients. Br Med J 308:81–106, 1994.

3. Antman EM, McCabe CH, Gurfinkel EP, et al: Enoxaparin prevents death and cardiac ischemic events in unstable angina/non-Q-wave myocardial infarction: results of the Thrombolysis In Myocardial Infarction (TIMI) 11B trial. Circulation 100:1593–1601, 1999.

4. Antman EM, Tanasijevic MJ, Thompson B, et al: Cardiac-specific troponin I levels to predict the risk of mortality in patients with acute coronary syndromes. N Engl J Med 335:1342–1349, 1996.

5. Arntz HR, Agrawal R, Wunderlich W, et al: Beneficial effects of pravastatin (+/− cholestyramine/niacin) initiated immediately after a coronary event (the randomized Lipid-Coronary Artery Disease [L-CAD] Study). Am J Cardiol 86:1293–1298, 2000.

6. The ASSENT-2 Investigators: Single-bolus tenecteplase compared with front-loaded alteplase in acute myocardial infarction: the ASSENT-2 double-blind randomised trial. Lancet 354:716–722, 1999.

7. The ASSENT 3 Investigators: Efficacy and safety of tenecteplase in combination with enoxaparin, abciximab, or unfractionated heparin: the ASSENT-3 randomised trial in acute myocardial infarction. Lancet 358:605–613, 2001.

8. Aversano T, Aversano LT, Passamani E, et al: Thrombolytic therapy vs primary percutaneous coronary intervention for myocardial infarction in patients presenting to hospitals without on-site cardiac surgery: a randomized controlled trial. JAMA 287:1943–1951, 2002.

9. Awtry EH, Loscalzo J: Aspirin. Circulation 101:1206–1218, 2000.

10. Bahit MC, Topol EJ, Califf RM, et al: Reactivation of ischemic events in acute coronary syndromes: results from GUSTO-IIb. J Am Coll Cardiol 37:1001–1007, 2001.

11. Baird SH, Menown IB, McBride SJ, et al: Randomised comparison of enoxaparin with unfractionated heparin following fibrinolytic therapy for acute myocardial infarction. Eur Heart J 23:627–632, 2002.

12. The BARI Investigators: Comparison of coronary bypass surgery with angioplasty in patients with multivessel disease. N Engl J Med 335:217–225, 1996.

13. Bittl JA, Chaitman BR, Feit F, et al: Bivalirudin versus heparin during coronary angioplasty for unstable or postinfarction angina: final report reanalysis of the Bivalirudin Angioplasty Study. Am Heart J 142:952–959, 2001.

14. Bittl JA, Strony J, Brinker JA, et al: Treatment with bivalirudin (Hirulog) as compared with heparin during coronary angioplasty for unstable or postinfarction angina. N Engl J Med 333:764–769, 1995.

15. Blazing MA. The Aggrastat to Zocor (A to Z) trial: preliminary results. Presented at the 52nd annual Scientific Sessions of the American College of Cardiology, March 30–April 1, 2003, Chicago, IL.

16. Boersma E, Harrington RA, Moliterno DJ, et al: Platelet glycoprotein IIb/IIIa inhibitors in acute coronary syndromes: a meta-analysis of all major randomised clinical trials (erratum published Lancet 359:2120, 2002). Lancet 359:189–198, 2002.

17. Boersma E, Pieper KS, Steyerberg EW, et al, for the PURSUIT Investigators: Predictors of outcomes in patients with acute coronary syndromes without persistent ST-segment elevation: results from an international trial of 9461 patients. Circulation 101:2557–2567, 2000.

18. Braunwald E, Antman EM, Beasley JM, et al: ACC/AHA 2002 Guideline update for the management of patients with unstable angina and non-ST-segment elevation myocardial infarction. Available at http://www.acc.org/clinical/guidelines/unstable/incorporated/index.htm. Accessed March 31, 2003.

19. Cairns JA, Gent M, Singer J, et al: Aspirin, sulfinpyrazone, or both in unstable angina. Results of a Canadian multicenter trial. N Engl J Med 313:1369–1375, 1985.

20. Califf RM, Faxon DP: Need for centers to care for patients with acute coronary syndromes. Circulation 107:1467–1470, 2003.

21. Califf RM, Peterson ED, Gibbons RJ, et al: Integrating quality into the cycle of therapeutic development. J Am Coll Cardiol 40:1895–1901, 2002.

22. Califf RM, Pieper KS, Lee KL, et al: Prediction of 1-year survival after thrombolysis for acute myocardial infarction in the GUSTO-I trial. Circulation 101:2231–2238, 2000.

23. Campeau L: Grading of angina pectoris. Circulation 54:522–523, 1976.

24. Cannon CP, Gibson CM, McCabe CH, et al: TNK-tissue plasminogen activator compared with front loaded alteplase in acute myocardial infarction: results of the TIMI 10B trial. Circulation 98:2805–2814, 1998.

25. Cannon CP, Weintraub WS, Demopoulos LA, et al: Comparison of early invasive and conservative strategies in patients with unstable coronary syndromes treated with the glycoprotein IIb/IIIa inhibitor tirofiban. N Engl J Med 344:1879–1887, 2001.

26. The CAPRIE Steering Committee: A randomised, blinded, trial of clopidogrel versus aspirin in patients at risk of ischaemic events (CAPRIE). Lancet 348:1329–1339, 1996.

27. Cheitlin MD, Alpert JS, Armstrong WF, et al: ACC/AHA guidelines for the clinical application of echocardiography. Developed in collaboration with the American Society of Echocardiography. Circulation 95:1686–1744, 1997.

28. Chen, J, Radford MJ, Wang Y, et al: Effectiveness of beta-blocker therapy after acute myocardial infarction in elderly patients with chronic obstructive pulmonary disease or asthma. J Am Coll Cardiol 37:1950–1956, 2001.

29. The CURE Trial Investigators: Effects of clopidogrel in addition to aspirin in patients with acute coronary syndromes without ST-segment elevation. N Engl J Med 345:494–502, 2001.

30. Danesh J: Coronary heart disease, Helicobacter pylori, dental disease, Chlamydia pneumoniae, and cytomegalovirus: meta-analyses of prospective studies. Am Heart J 138:S434–S437, 1999.

31. Dyke CM, Bhatia D, Lorenz TJ, et al: Immediate coronary artery bypass surgery after platelet inhibition with eptifibatide: results from PURSUIT. Ann Thorac Surg 70:866–871, 2000.

32. The ESSENCE Study Group: A comparison of low-molecular-weight heparin with unfractionated heparin for unstable coronary artery disease. N Engl J Med 337:447–452, 1997.

33. First International Study of Infarct Survival Collaborative Group: Randomised trial of intravenous atenolol among 16 027 cases of suspected acute myocardial infarction: ISIS-1. Lancet 2:57–66, 1986.

34. Fox KA, Poole-Wilson PA, Henderson RA, et al: Interventional versus conservative treatment for patients with unstable angina or non-ST-elevation myocardial infarction: the British Heart Foundation RITA 3 randomised trial. Lancet 360:743–751, 2002.

35. The 4S Study Group: Randomised trial of cholesterol lowering in 4444 patients with coronary heart disease: the Scandinavian Simvastatin Survival Study (4S). Lancet 344:1383–1389, 1994.

36. The FRAXIS Study Group: Comparison of two treatment durations (6 days and 14 days) of a low molecular weight heparin with a 6-day treatment of unfractionated heparin in the initial management of unstable angina or non-Q wave myocardial infarction. Eur Heart J 20:1553–1562, 1999.

37. FRISC II Investigators: Invasive compared with non-invasive treatment in unstable coronary-artery disease: FRISC II prospective randomised multicentre study. Lancet 354:708–715, 1999.

38. Fuster V, Badimon L, Badimon JJ, et al: The pathogenesis of coronary artery disease and the acute coronary syndromes. N Engl J Med 326:242–250, 1992.

39. Gibbons RJ, Balady GJ, Beasley JW, et al: ACC/AHA guidelines for exercise testing. J Am Coll Cardiol 30:260–311, 1997.

40. Goodnough LT, Brecher ME, Kanter MH, et al: Transfusion medicine. Blood transfusion. N Engl J Med 340:438–447, 1999.

41. Gore JM, Granger CB, Sloan MA, et al: Stroke after thrombolytic therapy: mortality and functional outcomes in the GUSTO-I trial. Circulation 92:2811–2818, 1995.

42. Granger CB: Strategies at patient care in acute coronary syndromes: rationale for the Global Registry of Acute Coronary Events (GRACE) Registry. Am J Cardiol 86: 4M–9M, 2000.

43. Grines CL, Westerhausen DR, Grines LL, et al: A randomized trial of transfer for primary angioplasty versus on-site thrombolysis in patients with high-risk myocardial infarction. J Am Coll Cardiol 39:1713–1719, 2002.

44. Grundy SM, Balady GJ, Criqui MH, et al: When to start cholesterol-lowering therapy in patients with coronary heart disease. Circulation 95:1683–1685, 1997.

45. The GUSTO Investigators: An international randomized trial comparing four thrombolytic strategies for acute myocardial infarction. N Engl J Med 329:673–682, 1993.

46. The GUSTO-III Investigators: A comparison of teteplase with alteplase for acute myocardial infarction [erratum published N Engl J Med 338:546–547, 1998]. N Engl J Med 337: 1118–1123, 1997.

47. Heeschen C, Hamm CW, Bruemmer J, et al: Predictive value of C-reactive protein and troponin T in patients with unstable angina: a comparative analysis. J Am Coll Cardiol 35: 1535–1342, 2000.

48. Heeschen C, Hamm CW, Goldmann B, et al: Troponin concentrations for stratification of patients with acute coronary syndromes in relation to therapeutic efficacy of tirofiban. Lancet 354:1757–1762, 1999.

49. The HOPE Study Investigators: Effects of ramipril on cardiovascular and microvascular outcomes in people with diabetes mellitus: results of the HOPE study and MICRO-HOPE substudy. Lancet 355:253–259, 2000.

50. Ikonomidis I, Andreotti F, Economou E, et al: Increased proinflammatory cytokines in patients with chronic stable angina and their reduction by aspirin. Circulation 100: 793–798, 1999.

51. James SK, Armstrong P, Barnathan E, et al: Troponin and C-reactive protein have different relations to subsequent mortality and myocardial infarction after acute coronary syndrome. A GUSTO-IV substudy. J Am Coll Cardiol 41: 916–1924, 2003.

52. Klein W, Buchwald A, Hillis SE, et al, for the FRIC Investigators: Comparison of low-molecular-weight heparin with unfractionated heparin acutely and with placebo for 6 weeks in the management of unstable coronary artery disease [erratum published Circulation 97:413, 1998]. Circulation 96: 61–68, 1997.

53. Kontny F: Improving outcomes in acute coronary syndromes: the FRISC II trial. Clin Cardiol 24:I3–I7, 2002.

54. Labinaz M, Kilaru R, Pieper K, et al: Outcomes of patients with acute coronary syndromes and prior coronary artery bypass grafting: results from the platelet glycoprotein IIb/IIIa in unstable angina: receptor suppression using integrilin therapy (PURSUIT) trial. Circulation 105:322–3277, 2002.

55. Labinaz M, Sketch MH Jr, Ellis SG, et al: Outcome of acute ST-segment elevation myocardial infarction in patients with prior coronary artery bypass surgery receiving thrombolytic therapy. Am Heart J 141:469–477, 2001.

56. Latini R, Maggioni AP, Flather M, et al: ACE inhibitor use in patients with myocardial infarction. Summary of evidence from clinical trials. Circulation 92:3132–3137, 1995.

57. Lee KL, Woodlief LW, Topol EJ, et al: Predictors of 30-day mortality in the era of reperfusion for acute myocardial infarction: results from an international trial of 41,021 patients. Circulation 91:1659–1668, 1995.

58. Lewis HD Jr, Davis JW, Archibald DG, et al: Protective effects of aspirin against acute myocardial infarction and death in men with unstable angina. Results of a Veterans Administration Cooperative Study. N Engl J Med 309:396–403, 1983.

59. Libby P, Ridker PM: Novel inflammatory markers of coronary risk: theory versus practice. Circulation 100:1148–1150, 1999.

60. Lincoff AM, Califf RM, Topol EJ: Platelet glycoprotein IIb/IIIa receptor blockade in coronary artery disease. J Am Coll Cardiol 35:1103–1115, 2000.

61. Lindahl B, Venge P, Wallentin L: Troponin T identifies patients with unstable coronary artery disease who benefit from long-term antithrombotic protection. J Am Coll Cardiol 29:43–48, 1997.

62. The LIPID Study Group: Prevention of cardiovascular events and death with pravastatin in patients with coronary heart disease and a broad range of initial cholesterol levels. N Engl J Med 339:1349–1357, 1996.

63. Mangano DT: Aspirin and mortality from coronary bypass surgery. N Engl J Med 347:1309–1317, 2002.

64. Mark DB, Shaw L, Harrell FE Jr, et al: Prognostic value of a treadmill exercise score in outpatients with suspected coronary artery disease. N Engl J Med 325:849–853, 1991.

65. National Cholesterol Education Program: Second report of the Expert Panel on Detection, Evaluation, and Treatment of High Blood Cholesterol in Adults (Adult Treatment Panel II). Washington, DC: U.S. Department of Health and Human Services. NIH publication No. 93-3096, 1993.

66. Newby LK, Christenson RH, Ohman EM, et al: Value of serial troponin T measures for early and late risk stratification in patients with acute coronary syndromes. Circulation 98: 1853–1859, 1998.

67. Newby LK, Kristinsson A, Bhapkar MV, et al: Early statin initiation and outcomes in patients with acute coronary syndromes. JAMA 287:3087–3095, 2002.

68. Newby LK, Ohman EM, Christenson RH, et al: Benefit of glycoprotein IIb/IIIa inhibition in patients with acute coronary syndromes and troponin T-positive status: the PARAGON-B troponin T substudy. Circulation 103: 2891–2896, 2001.

69. Newby LK, Storrow AB, Gibler WB, et al: Bedside multimarker testing for risk stratification in chest pain units: The chest pain evaluation by creatine kinase-MB, myoglobin, and troponin I (CHECKMATE) study. Circulation 103: 1832–1837, 2001.

70. The OASIS-2 Investigators: Effects of recombinant hirudin (lepirudin) compared with heparin on death, myocardial infarction, refractory angina, and revascularisation procedures in patients with acute myocardial ischaemia without ST elevation: a randomised trial. Lancet 353:429–438, 1999.

71. Ohman EM, Armstrong PW, Christenson RH, et al: Cardiac troponin T levels for risk stratification in acute myocardial ischemia. N Engl J Med 335:1333–1341, 1996.

72. Oler A, Whooley MA, Oler J, Grady D: Adding heparin to aspirin reduces the incidence of myocardial infarction and death in patients with unstable angina. A meta-analysis. JAMA 276:811–815, 1996.

73. Omland T, de Lemos JA, Morrow DA, et al: Prognostic value of N-terminal pro-atrial and pro-brain natriuretic peptide in patients with acute coronary syndromes. Am J Cardiol 89: 463–465, 2002.

74. Peterson ED, Pollack CV, Roe MT, et al: Early use of glycoprotein IIbIIIa inhibitors and outcomes in non-ST-elevation acute myocardial infarction: observations from NRMI-4. J Am Coll Cardiol 39:303A, 2002.

75. The PRISM-PLUS Study Investigators: Inhibition of the platelet glycoprotein IIb/IIIa receptor with tirofiban in unstable angina and non-Q-wave myocardial infarction. N Engl J Med 338:1488–1497, 1998.

76. The RAPID II Investigators: Randomized comparison of coronary thrombolysis achieved with double-bolus reteplase

966

(recombinant plasminogen activator) and front-loaded, accelerated alteplase (recombinant tissue plasminogen activator) in patients with acute myocardial infarction. Circulation 94:891–898, 1996.

77. Ridker PM, Cushman M, Stampfer MJ, et al: Inflammation, aspirin, and the risk of cardiovascular disease in apparently healthy men [erratum published N Engl J Med 337:356, 1997]. N Engl J Med 336:973–979, 1997.

78. Ritchie JL, Bateman TM, Bonow RO, et al: Guidelines for the clinical use of cardiac radionuclide imaging. Developed in collaboration with the American Society of Nuclear Cardiology. J Am Coll Cardiol 25:521–547, 1995.

79. Roe MT, Ohman EM, Maas AC, et al: Shifting the open-artery hypothesis downstream: the quest for optimal reperfusion. J Am Coll Cardiol 37:9–18, 2001.

80. Ryan TJ, Antman E, Brooks NH, et al: ACC/AHA guidelines for the management of patients with acute myocardial infarction. Available at http://www.acc.org/clinical/guidelines/nov96/1999/index.htm. Accessed March 31, 2003.

81. Sacks FM, Pfeffer MA, Moye LA, et al, for the Cholesterol And Recurrent Events Trial Investigators: The effect of pravastatin on coronary events after myocardial infarction in patients with average cholesterol levels. N Engl J Med 335:1001–1009, 1996.

82. Savonitto S, Ardissino D, Granger CB, et al: Prognostic value of the admission electrocardiogram in acute coronary syndromes. JAMA 281:707–713, 1999.

83. Schwartz GG, Olsson AG, Ezekowitz MD, et al: Effects of atorvastatin on early recurrent ischemic events in acute coronary syndromes. The MIRACL Study: a randomized trial. JAMA 285:1711–1718, 2001.

84. Simes RJ, Holmes DR Jr, Ross AM, et al: The link between the angiographic substudy and mortality outcomes in a large randomized trial of myocardial reperfusion: the importance of early and complete infarct artery reperfusion. Circulation 91:1923–1928, 1995.

85. Smith SC Jr, Dove JT, Jacobs AK, et al: ACC/AHA guidelines for percutaneous coronary intervention. Available at http://www.acc.org/clinical/guidelines/percutaneous/dirIndex.htm. Accessed March 31, 2003.

86. The SPEED Study Group: Trial of abciximab with and without low-dose reteplase for acute myocardial infarction. Circulation 101:2788–2794, 2000.

87. Stafford-Smith M: Protamine administration following CABG linked to worse outcomes. Presented at the 77th Clinical and Scientific Congress of the International Anesthesia Research Society, March 2003, New Orleans.

88. Stenestrand U, Wallentin L: Early statin treatment following acute myocardial infarction and 1-year survival. JAMA 285:430–436, 2001.

89. Tatu-Chitoiu G, Tatu-Chitoiu A, Bumbu A, et al: Accelerated streptokinase and enoxaparine: a new thrombolytic regimen in acute myocardial infarction (the ASENOX study). Eur Heart J 21 (Suppl):177, 2000 (abstract).

90. Theroux P, Ouimet H, McCans J, et al: Aspirin, heparin, or both to treat acute unstable angina. N Engl J Med 319:1105–1111, 1988.

91. The TIMI IIIB Investigators: Effects of tissue plasminogen activator and a comparison of early invasive and conservative strategies in unstable angina and non-Q-wave infarction: results of the TIMI IIIB trial. Circulation 89:1545–1556, 1994.

92. Topol EJ: Reperfusion therapy for acute myocardial infarction with fibrinolytic therapy or combination reduced fibrinolytic therapy and platelet glycoprotein IIb/IIIa inhibition: the GUSTO V randomised trial. Lancet 357:1905–1914, 2001.

93. Topol EJ, Yadav JS: Recognition of the importance of embolization in atherosclerotic vascular disease. Circulation 101:570–580, 2000.

94. Wallentin LC, for the Research Group on Instability in Coronary Artery Disease in Southeast Sweden: Aspirin (75 mg/day) after an episode of unstable coronary artery disease: long-term effects on the risk for myocardial infarction, occurrence of severe angina and the need for revascularization. J Am Coll Cardiol 18:1587–1593, 1991.

95. Wallentin L: ASSENT-3 PLUS: preliminary results. Presented at the 75th Scientific Sessions of the American Heart Association, Chicago, IL, November 17–20, 2002.

96. Wong GC, Giugliano RP, Antman EM: Use of low-molecular-weight heparins in the management of acute coronary artery syndromes and percutaneous coronary intervention. JAMA 289:331–342, 2003.

Nonatherosclerotic Coronary Heart Disease

Audrey Rosinberg, Roger J. Laham, and Donald S. Baim

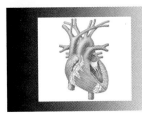

INTRODUCTION

Although myocardial ischemic syndromes (angina pectoris, myocardial infarction, and sudden cardiac death) are almost always caused by coronary atherosclerosis, they may occasionally result from one of a variety of nonatherosclerotic coronary artery diseases.[12,58,65] Less than 5% of all patients presenting with acute myocardial infarction do not have atherosclerotic disease as a cause of luminal narrowing as demonstrated at autopsy; however, this may be an overestimate when spontaneous reperfusion and lysis of acute coronary thrombosis on a ruptured nonocclusive atherosclerotic plaque are also considered.[19] These relatively uncommon diseases pose several problems to the clinician: (1) they often occur in patients in whom ischemic heart disease in uncommon, unsuspected, or masked by an underlying systemic disease; (2) they may require specialized techniques for diagnosis and treatment; and (3) their natural histories and optimal management are incompletely understood. Because specific and potentially life-saving therapies are often available, physicians and surgeons should have an overall familiarity with the diagnosis and treatment of these nonatherosclerotic coronary conditions.

CORONARY ARTERY ANOMALIES

Coronary artery anomalies (i.e., variations in the origin, course, or distribution of the coronary arteries) are present in 1–2% of the population.[20] These anomalies may make angiographic visualization of the coronary circulation more difficult, and they may increase the risk of coronary artery trauma during cardiac surgery.[58] Additionally, certain types of coronary anomalies may cause myocardial ischemia,[45] although most do so in a small fraction of the patients in whom they are present. Evaluation of each patient with a coronary anomaly should therefore include anatomical classification, recognition of the particular anomaly and its potential to result in myocardial ischemia, and documentation that ischemia is present using functional and perfusion imaging techniques. In the symptomatic patient with a coronary anomaly in whom ischemia has been documented by exercise testing, nuclear myocardial perfusion scanning, stress echocardiography, or transmyocardial metabolic testing, effective corrective treatment is generally possible. It is important to note that magnetic resonance imaging is emerging as a promising modality for the diagnosis of these anomalies.

Anomalous Origin from the Aorta

In normal coronary circulation, the right coronary artery originates from a single ostium within the right sinus of Valsalva, and the left coronary artery originates from a single ostium within the left sinus of Valsalva (Figure 60-1). Abnormally high or low locations of the coronary ostia and the presence within the appropriate sinus of Valsalva of separate ostia for the left anterior descending and circumflex coronary artery branches or for the right coronary artery and its conus branch are common minor variations that do not result in myocardial ischemia. Other anomalous patterns of coronary artery origin from the aorta are potential causes of myocardial ischemia, even in the absence of atherosclerosis.

Origin from the Contralateral Sinus of Valsalva

When one of the coronary arteries originates from the contralateral sinus of Valsalva, this anomalous vessel must traverse the base of the heart to reach its territory of distribution

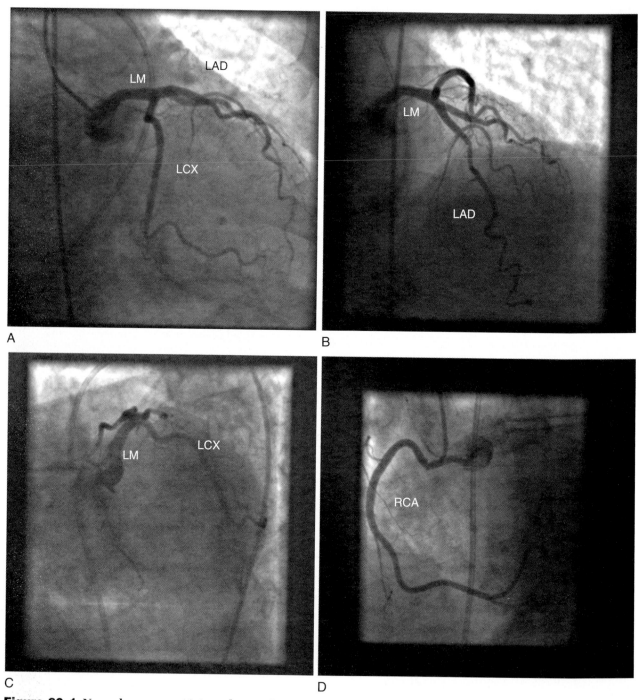

A

B

C

D

Figure 60–1 **Normal coronary origin and normal coronaries. A,** Right anterior oblique caudal projection of left coronary system showing the left main (LM), left anterior descending (LAD), and left circumflex artery (LCX). **B,** Right anterior oblique cranial projection of left coronary system. **C,** Left anterior oblique caudal projection of left coronary system. **D,** Right anterior oblique projection of right coronary artery.

by passing anterior to, posterior to, or between the aorta and the pulmonary artery (Figure 60-2).[40,46] Acute angulation at the origin of the artery from the aorta may result in anatomical or functional constriction of the proximal portion of the anomalous coronary artery. Increased cardiac output (e.g., as a result of exercise) causes aortic dilation and narrowing at the area of angulation at the abnormal coronary ostium. Anomalous vessels passing between the aorta and pulmonary artery seem to carry an additional risk of ischemia, possibly as a result of being compressed between the great vessels; however, this is unlikely at normal pulmonary artery pressures. Abnormal mechanical stresses or flow patterns may enhance the development of coronary atherosclerosis in the anomalous segment.

Origin of the left coronary artery from the right sinus of Valsalva with passage of the proximal left coronary artery between the aorta and pulmonary artery is associated with an increased incidence of exercise-related sudden cardiac death in young patients. In an autopsy study of 33 patients with this anomaly, sudden death occurred in 9 patients (27%), generally without prior warning symptoms. This is, however, a selected group of patients, because diagnosis at this age requires the presence of symptoms and exercise test abnormalities that lead to the diagnostic angiography.[12] In patients without coronary atherosclerosis, passage of the anomalous left coronary artery either anterior or posterior to both great vessels has been associated with pacing-induced myocardial lactate production and angina pectoris.[10,40] Thus, some recommend prophylactic coronary artery bypass surgery when this anomaly is detected in young patients.[45,46] In a study of 9 patients who underwent a modified unroofing procedure to move the coronary artery orifice to the appropriate sinus, all were free of symptoms and demonstrated no abnormalities on echocardiography suggestive of ischemia at 2-year follow-up.[69] Angina pectoris has also been reported in patients in whom the right coronary artery originates from the left sinus of Valsalva, but confirmation of myocardial ischemia has been less complete in these patients than in patients with anomalous origin of the left coronary artery.[40] The most common pattern of anomalous aortic origin—origin of the circumflex coronary artery from the right sinus of Valsalva or proximal right coronary artery—does not seem to impose independent ischemic risk.[40]

Single Coronary Artery

Derivation of the entire coronary circulation from a single ostium is a rare coronary anomaly. Approximately 40% of patients with this anomaly have an associated congenital cardiac defect (i.e., tetralogy of Fallot, transposition of the great vessels, improper division of the truncus arteriosis).[72] There is no clear sex predominance for this condition, and the frequency of occurrence of single left and single right coronary arteries is approximately equal.[36] As is also true in the case of anomalous origin from the contralateral sinus of Valsalva, one or more components of the coronary circulation system must cross the base of the heart to reach its territory of distribution by passing anterior to, posterior to, or between the great vessels. These transposed vessels may therefore be exposed to the risks of angulation, compression, and accelerated atherosclerosis. Because the entire

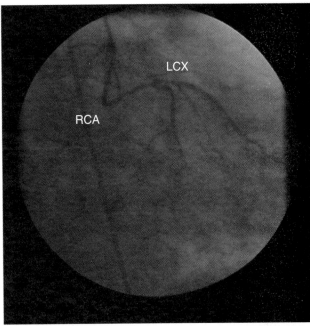

A

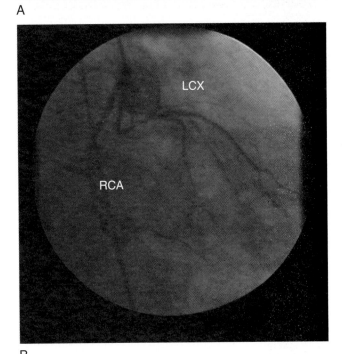

B

Figure 60–2 Anomalous origin of left circumflex (**LCX**) from right coronary artery (**RCA**) in shallow right anterior oblique (**A**) and right anterior oblique projections (**B**).

myocardium is supplied by way of the single coronary artery, proximal coronary atherosclerosis poses the risk of global myocardial ischemia.

Clinical manifestations of the single coronary artery anomaly depend in part on the associated cardiac defects and atherosclerosis, but up to 15% of patients with only this anomaly develop severe cardiac complications by age 40.[72] Angina pectoris and myocardial lactate production have been demonstrated in patients with a single coronary

970 artery in the absence of coronary atherosclerosis or vessel passage between the aorta and the pulmonary artery.[36]

Atresia of the Coronary Ostium

Atresia or severe stenosis of one of the coronary ostia (often associated with hypoplasia of the proximal coronary artery) is a rare congenital coronary anomaly, with only seven reported cases.[9,45] The absence of a second coronary ostium may lead to the incorrect diagnosis of a single coronary artery. Because the involved vessel is dependent on collateral flow from the contralateral coronary artery, myocardial ischemia or infarction may develop during infancy. In this sense, patients with ostial atresia bear an angiographic and clinical resemblance to patients with an anomalous origin of a coronary artery from the pulmonary artery (see below). Successful coronary artery bypass grafting has been reported in a 10-year-old male with ostial atresia.[9]

High Takeoff Coronary Ostia

The location of the coronary arteries within the sinuses of Valsalva allow for maximal diastolic filling. In some cases, the ostia have been reported to be located superior to the sinus (Figure 60-3) and associated with decreased coronary perfusion and myocardial ischemia. This theory has been challenged by the normal flow pattern seen in these arteries as well as in vein grafts and arterial conduits located well above the sinuses.[77]

Anomalous Origin from the Pulmonary Artery

Origin of a coronary artery from the pulmonary artery rather than from the aorta is a relatively uncommon but severe coronary anomaly that occurs in approximately 1 out of every 300,000 live births (0.25–0.5%). However, it is one of the most common causes of myocardial ischemia and infarction in children.[79] In more than 90% of cases, it is the left coronary artery that originates from the pulmonary artery, generally from the left posterior pulmonary sinus.[45] Origin of the right coronary artery, an accessory coronary artery, and both coronary arteries from the pulmonary artery have been described; the last of these is invariably fatal during the neonatal period.[44,45]

Edwards[18] first explained the pathophysiology of the hemodynamics that occur with the anomalous origin of the left coronary artery from the pulmonary artery. As the pulmonary artery pressure falls during the first weeks of life, perfusion of the anomalous coronary artery from the pulmonary artery decreases. Unless adequate collateral flow develops from the contralateral coronary artery, the territory of the anomalous vessel becomes ischemic. Angina pectoris or congestive heart failure with mitral regurgitation may then develop, and this is often accompanied by the electrocardiographic manifestation of myocardial ischemia or infarction. The clinical picture, called the *infantile syndrome*, develops in approximately 80% of affected patients, usually within the first 4 months of life.[45,79] The typical presentation in infants includes failure to thrive, profuse sweating, dyspnea, pallor, and atypical chest pain on eating or crying.[16] In the absence of surgical correction, this syndrome has an 85% first-year mortality, although the mortal-

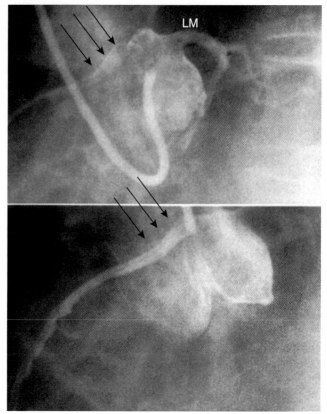

Figure 60–3 Anomalous origin of the right coronary artery (RCA, *arrows*) from the left cusp high in the aorta above the left main (LM) origin.

ity rate is somewhat lower with anomalous origin of the right coronary artery.[44] Those who do not develop the infantile syndrome may present during childhood or adult life with one of the following: asymptomatic murmur, mitral regurgitation, angina pectoris, or sudden death. In these patients, there is a greater than 80% incidence of sudden death at a mean age of 35 years.[79]

Patients who survive infancy tend to have extensive intercoronary collateral flow, with dilatation of both the normal and the anomalous vessels. This collateral flow reverses the direction of blood flow in the anomalous coronary artery, which constitutes a left-to-right shunt into the pulmonary artery. Despite extensive collateralization, electrocardiographic evidence of ischemia and pathological evidence of subendocardial fibrosis usually persist.

Diagnosis can generally be made on the basis of electrocardiographic and echocardiographic findings. In cases of uncertainty, angiography is warranted. Medical management is associated with a high mortality rate, and the current standard of care calls for immediate surgical repair at the time of diagnosis.[16] Surgical correction seeks to eliminate the left-to-right shunt and to establish an independent arterial blood supply to the anomalous vessel. A variety of techniques have been attempted since the earliest operative attempts by William J. Potts. Ligation of the anomalous vessel at its origin in combination with saphenous vein aortocoronary bypass grafting has been performed, but it is technically difficult in children who are less than 2 years old, and it is associated with a high rate of graft failure.[66]

Currently the most popular method reestablishes a two-coronary system via reimplantation of the anomalous vessel into the aortic root. Improvisation is sometimes necessary because of anatomical variations and insufficient coronary artery length. Overall, across a variety of series, the mortality rate of this procedure ranges from 0–16%.[16] Michielon and colleagues[53] followed 30 patients for an average of 15 years after surgery. They showed that the coronary transfer technique demonstrated the best freedom from long-term reoperation (92.3% ± 7.4%) as compared with subclavian interposition and intrapulmonary tunnel. Additionally, when surgery was performed before the patient was 6 months old, significantly improved left ventricular and mitral valve function was achieved, despite worse preoperative left ventricular function than that seen in older patients. Continued improvement in left ventricle function is seen up to 1 year after surgery. Because of the high morbidity and mortality rates of this coronary artery anomaly, aggressive early operative management that reestablishes a two-coronary system is warranted to achieve the best functional recovery. Most of these patients will recover normal mitral valve function after reperfusion alone. Despite the presence of preoperative mitral insufficiency, mitral valve repair at the time of initial repair is generally not recommended.

Coronary Artery Fistula

Direct precapillary anastomosis between a major coronary artery and a cardiac chamber or major vessel (e.g., superior vena cava, coronary sinus, pulmonary artery) is the most common hemodynamically significant coronary artery anomaly (see Figure 60-6).[45] These communications are often referred to as coronary-cameral fistulas and occur in approximately 1 out of every 50,000 patients with congenital heart disease. Fistulas from the right coronary artery are slightly more common than those from the left coronary artery, and bilateral fistulas are present in 4–5% of cases.[5] More than 90% of the fistulas drain into the venous circulation (right ventricle, 41%; right atrium, 26%; pulmonary artery, 17%; coronary sinus, 7%; superior vena cava, 1%); the remaining fistulas drain into the arterial circulation (left atrium, 5%; left ventricle, 3%).[45] Multiple patterns of anastomosis between the involved coronary artery and the recipient cardiac structure are possible. In addition to congenital fistulas, coronary artery fistulas can also be acquired as a result of trauma, angioplasty, transcutaneous catheter techniques for myocardial biopsies, and heart operations.[50] The involved coronary artery is usually markedly dilated proximal to the fistula, and flow through the fistula may be several times that delivered to the myocardium. When the fistula drains into the venous circulation, a significant left-to-right shunt may be present.[47] Runoff through a fistula may lower intracoronary diastolic pressure and produce myocardial ischemia in some patients by a "coronary steal" phenomenon.[45] Physical examination occasionally reveals a continuous heart murmur, which brings some patients with coronary artery fistulas to medical attention. The chest X-ray is usually normal, but it may show evidence of right ventricular overload and pulmonary prominence when a large left-to-right shunt is present, thereby mimicking a patent ductus arteriosus. Electrocardiographic abnormalities are uncommon. Diagnosis is best made by selective coronary angiography, particularly when catheterization to evaluate a continuous murmur has failed to disclose the expected anatomical abnormality. Similar fistulas may result from cardiac trauma.

Because the great majority of patients with coronary fistulas are asymptomatic, the decisions surrounding surgical correction are complex. Even in asymptomatic patients, clinical, electrocardiographic, and roentgenographic abnormalities are often present. Ischemia has been documented in some patients with coronary fistulas and no atherosclerosis,[45] and there is evidence that the majority of patients do become symptomatic with advancing age.[47] In addition to angina and myocardial infarction, congestive heart failure, bacterial endocarditis, and fistula rupture have been described. Antibiotic prophylaxis against bacterial endocarditis is recommended.[47] Because spontaneous fistula closure is rare and because the risk of surgical closure of the fistula is significantly lower in patients who are less than 20 years old, some have suggested elective fistula legation in young patients, including those patients who are asymptomatic.[47] Surgical closure is a safe and effective treatment. In a retrospective review over 28 years, Mavroudis and colleagues[50] demonstrated a 100% survival rate and a 100% closure rate after surgical ligation of the fistula.

A variety of transcatheter devices have been described to close coronary artery fistulas. These include coils, detachable balloons, and double-umbrella devices.[51,60] Criteria for transcatheter treatment include the absence of multiple fistulae, a single narrow drainage site, the absence of large branch vessels, and safe accessibility to the coronary artery that supplies the fistula.[50] Complications seen with transcatheter techniques include the migration of coils, transient arrhythmias, fistula dissection, and residual shunts.[50,51,60] Residual shunts pose a problem given the risk of bacterial endocarditis and the presence of a foreign body; repeat catheterization and occlusion are therefore recommended.[51] The exact role of surgical versus transcatheter therapy for coronary artery fistulas is still being debated. As transcatheter and imaging techniques improve, they will continue to obtain a greater role in treatment strategies.

Muscle Bridge

The coronary arteries normally course over the epicardial surface of the heart; occasionally, they may course through the myocardium, for varying lengths. The overlying muscle is referred to as a myocardial bridge, and the artery is called a *tunneled artery*. Intramyocardial segments of the large coronary arteries—particularly the left anterior descending artery—may be subject to systolic compression or "milking" (Figure 60-4). Although intramyocardial segments of the coronary arteries are present in approximately 20% of autopsied hearts,[27] angiographic evidence of systolic compression is reported in only 0.5% of patients who undergo coronary angiography for chest pain.[16] Angiographic diagnosis can be facilitated by the administration of nitroglycerin, which results in the accentuation of systolic narrowing.[38] In most cases, angiographic compression is a benign finding; however, when a long vessel segment demonstrates systolic compression to less than 25% of its diastolic diameter, ischemia may be revealed by exercise, by ^{201}Tl myocardial perfusion scanning, by exercise echocardiography, or by coronary sinus pacing/metabolic evaluation, even in the absence of coronary atherosclerosis.[59] Myocardial bridges

972 have been associated with myocardial ischemia and infarction, conduction disturbances, arrhythmias, and sudden death.[38] Because most coronary flow takes place during diastole, it is not clear how systolic compression alone results in myocardial ischemia. In some symptomatic patients, coronary compression may extend into early diastole, and excessive myocardial oxygen demand may be present as the result of associated left ventricular hypertrophy.[59] Although muscle bridges are a congenital anomaly, symptoms of ischemia may not develop until middle age.

Angina pectoris that results from systolic coronary artery compression may respond to therapy with beta-adrenergic blockers, calcium-channel blockers, and nitrates. When symptoms are refractory to medical therapy and when inducible ischemia has been unequivocally demonstrated, coronary stent placement, coronary bypass grafting, or simple unroofing of the bridged coronary segment has resulted in the relief of symptoms and the normalization of myocardial perfusion and metabolism.[30,59]

Coronary Artery Aneurysm

Coronary artery aneurysms, which are localized areas of coronary dilatation relative to adjacent normal arterial segments, occur in approximately 1.5% of patients studied by autopsy or coronary angiography.[28] The aneurysms are frequently multiple, may attain a diameter of several centimeters, involve the right coronary artery more frequently than the left,[6] and may be either congenital or acquired. Atherosclerosis either by stenosis with poststenotic dilatation or by primary destruction of the coronary intima and media accounts for approximately 50% of coronary aneurysms. Atherosclerotic damage may also produce diffuse coronary ectasia rather than focal coronary aneurysm.[65] Other pathological processes that damage the arterial wall (e.g., dissection, trauma, coronary angioplasty, vasculitis, mycotic emboli, syphilis, mucocutaneous lymph node syndrome) may also lead to aneurysm formation.[6,28] The remainder of coronary aneurysms are felt to be congenital in origin, although many of these may in fact be the residua of prior subclinical vasculitis.

There are no reliable clinical features of coronary artery aneurysm, although a diastolic or continuous heart murmur may occasionally be present.[28] The chest X-ray may show a paracardiac mass or calcification, and, although echocardiography may detect the largest and most proximal coronary aneurysms, coronary angiography is required for accurate diagnosis.

The clinical courses of patients with coronary artery aneurysms usually depend on the severity of the associated atherosclerotic stenoses. Even in the absence of stenosis, abnormal flow patterns within the aneurysm may lead to thrombus formation with subsequent vessel occlusion, distal thromboembolization, or myocardial infarction.[28] One case has been reported in which a large intramyocardial aneurysm resulted in angina by a coronary steal mechanism. Rupture of a coronary aneurysm is a rare but serious complication.

Surgical therapy of combined stenotic and aneurysmal atherosclerosis consists of ligation of the involved vessel immediately beyond the aneurysm (to eliminate subsequent emboli) and aortocoronary bypass grafting to the distal vessel. Similar surgery has been suggested in patients without stenotic lesions and even in asymptomatic patients with coronary aneurysms.[28] In patients with a single aneurysm, placement of a covered stent may exclude the aneurysm or pseudoaneurysm and restore normal laminar flow (Figure 60-5). Anticoagulant or antiplatelet therapy may also be of value in this condition.[65] Because aneurysmal changes are frequently present in other vessels (particularly the abdominal aorta), comprehensive arteriographic evaluation is recommended in patients with coronary artery aneurysms.[6,28]

▶ MECHANICAL INJURY TO CORONARY ARTERY

An acute mechanical insult to a previously normal coronary artery circulation may result in transient myocardial ischemia or myocardial infarction. Circumstantial evidence (e.g., recent chest trauma, intercurrent cardiac catheterization, predisposition to arterial embolization) often suggests that an ischemic event is the result of such an insult, but more commonly the clinical picture is indistinguishable from acute atherosclerotic myocardial infarction.

Coronary Artery Embolus

The coronary arteries may be partially protected from embolic events by the acute angulation of the coronary ostia relative to the aortic stream and by their position behind the aortic valve leaflets during systole. When coronary artery emboli do occur, the outcome is dictated by the size of the embolus and its position of impaction in the coronary circula-

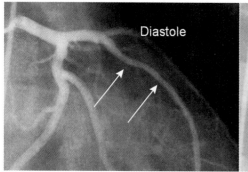
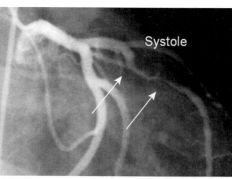

Figure 60–4 Muscle bridge *(arrow)* causing compression during systole.

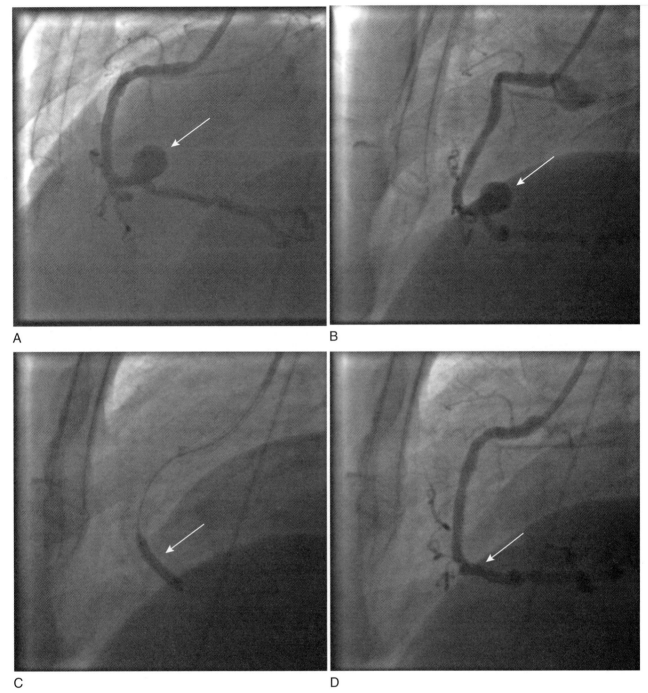

Figure 60–5 Right coronary artery pseudoaneurysm *(arrow)* in right anterior oblique projection (**A**) and left lateral projection (**B**). This is treated by the deployment of a balloon expandable covered stent (**C**), which leads to exclusion of the pseudoaneurysm (**D**).

tion. Small emboli tend to produce occlusion of a distal branch of one of the coronary arteries (most commonly the left anterior descending artery), thereby resulting in a small area of myocardial necrosis that may not be clinically evident.[64,68] These small emboli appear to be relatively frequent; in one autopsy series, they were found in 13% of patients with histologically evident myocardial necrosis.[64] Larger coronary artery emboli are relatively less frequent, but they generally result in clinically apparent myocardial infarction.

Coronary artery emboli should be considered in the differential diagnosis of acute myocardial ischemia in patients whose clinical condition predisposes them to arterial emboli, including patients with valvular heart disease (endocarditis, noninfected abnormal valve, prosthetic valve), mural thrombus (congestive cardiomyopathy, previous myocardial infarction, atrial fibrillation), left-sided cardiac catheterization, or the anatomical potential for paradoxical embolization (patent foramen ovale, atrial or ventricular septa defects with

974 continuous or intermittent right-to-left shunting).[64,68] Coronary emboli of a variety of materials, including tumor, myocardial or skeletal muscle, and materials used in cardiac surgery, have been reported. Extracardiac emboli may also be present. In patients sustaining coronary emboli, prompt coronary angiography may show occlusion of the involved vessel, but restudy as soon as 1 month after the acute event may show renewed vessel patency as the result of lysis or recanalization of the embolus.[68]

The role of cardiac surgery in the treatment of acute coronary emboli is yet to be established. When emboli occur during cardiac surgery, embolectomy is indicated to restore normal perfusion and abort myocardial infarction. Embolectomy performed for emboli associated with endocarditis[63] or cardiac catheterization seems to have less influence on the evolution of myocardial infarction. When embolization occurs spontaneously and patients present with an acute myocardial infarction, thrombolysis or primary angioplasty may be indicated. If primary angioplasty is performed, the use of thrombectomy catheters is recommended to minimize distal embolization. In addition, the use of anticoagulants and glycoprotein II_bIII_a antiplatelet therapy is indicated.

Coronary Artery Dissection

Hemorrhage into the coronary artery wall—with or without an associated intimal tear—forces the intima into the coronary lumen and may produce distal myocardial ischemia or infarction. Coronary artery dissections may occur by extension of aortic root dissection (secondary dissection), or they may be limited to the coronary artery (primary dissection). Primary coronary artery dissections may occur as the result of diagnostic coronary angiography, coronary angioplasty, cardiac surgery, or chest trauma (see below), or they may occur spontaneously. Angiographically evident localized coronary dissection occurs in at least 30% of patients undergoing coronary angioplasty and may progress to abrupt vessel reclosure during the first hour after the procedure in 2–3% of patients[4]; however, the use of stenting has all but eliminated this complication. Most spontaneous dissections occur in women, particularly during the peripartum period.[15,73] Hypertension and coronary atherosclerotic involvement are infrequent, but changes resembling cystic medial necrosis may be present.[15,73,74] The involved vessel is enlarged and ecchymotic, and it may rupture. The left anterior descending artery is involved in three fourths of the cases, usually within 2 cm of its origin.[74]

The diagnosis of coronary artery dissection during life relies on coronary angiography showing extravasation or delayed clearance of contrast, an intimal flap, or the presence of true and false lumina; however, dissection may present simply as occlusion of the involved vessel.[13,73] Although often treated by stenting, coronary artery dissections have been demonstrated to heal spontaneously.[70]

Coronary Artery Trauma

Nonpenetrating Blunt Trauma

Chest-wall impact, which is frequently the result of vehicular trauma, may lead to myocardial necrosis by direct myocardial contusion or by occlusive injury to the coronary arteries. This occlusive injury may be the result of coronary artery dissection, thrombosis, or rupture.[1,11] Coronary artery fistulas or aneurysms may develop as late sequelae.[3] The left anterior descending and right coronary arteries are more frequently involved. The electrocardiogram usually shows a pattern of acute myocardial infarction, but this finding does not distinguish between coronary occlusion and myocardial contusion. This distinction can be made by prompt coronary angiography, but it is of limited clinical utility unless immediate revascularization (bypass surgery, thrombolytic therapy, or angioplasty performed on an emergency basis) is contemplated. Recovery is the rule, although left ventricular aneurysm formation does occur.

Penetrating Trauma

Laceration of a coronary artery, such as that which may occur with a stab wound or a small-caliber gunshot wound, may cause acute myocardial ischemia, although the immediate presentation is generally that of acute pericardial tamponade. The left anterior descending and right coronary arteries are frequently involved. Laceration of small coronary artery branches may be treated with simple ligation without producing significant myocardial ischemia, but ligation of larger vessels often results in a large area of myocardial ischemia (manifested as immediate myocardial discoloration and hypokinesis), thereby necessitating coronary artery bypass grafting.[21] Development of a loud continuous murmur days to months after the original injury may signal the development of a coronary artery fistula. Surgical or percutaneous repair of these fistulas should be reserved for patients with evidence of hemodynamic compromise.[3]

Trauma during Cardiac Catheterization or Surgery

Catheterization of the left side of the heart and selective coronary angiography used to be associated with a 0.1–0.2% incidence of myocardial infarction as the result of coronary artery embolization (thrombus, dislodged plaque, air) or coronary artery dissection; however, improved catheter design and technique has brought that rate down to less than 0.01%.[39,71] Coronary artery dissection and embolization have been reported without ischemic sequelae, but, when they result in coronary occlusion, prompt reperfusion using percutaneous or surgical strategies is warranted. Laceration of a coronary artery is a potential but rare complication during pericardiocentesis.

Coronary Thrombosis

Coronary thrombosis clearly plays an important role in the evolution of myocardial infarction. When myocardial infarction develops in the setting of coronary atherosclerosis, superimposed coronary thrombosis is nearly always present. In certain disorders that involve thrombocytosis or platelet activation (including polycythemia vera, idiopathic thrombocytosis, thrombotic thrombocytopenia purpura, and multiple myeloma[67,76]), acute myocardial infarction has occurred in the absence of significant underlying atherosclerosis, and this necessitates prompt reperfusion therapy with thrombolysis or primary angioplasty and stenting. Although this circumstantial evidence points toward primary coronary thrombosis as the cause of infarction, the differentiation between in situ thrombosis and thromboembolus may be difficult.

PROGRESSIVE NONATHEROSCLEROTIC CORONARY OCCLUSIVE DISEASE

Progressive nonatherosclerotic coronary occlusion may result from coronary artery vasculitis,[62] intimal proliferation or fibrosis, abnormal accumulation of metabolic substances,[65] or extrinsic coronary artery compression.[25] When the large proximal coronary arteries are involved, angina pectoris or acute myocardial infarction may result, but clinical, angiographic, and even histological differentiation of progressive nonatherosclerotic coronary occlusion from atherosclerosis is often difficult. When the small coronary vessels (0.1–1.0 mm in diameter) are involved, as they may be in diabetes mellitus, collagen vascular disease, thrombotic thrombocytopenic purpura, homocystinuria, neuromuscular disorders, or cardiac transplantation, patients may develop cardiomyopathy arrhythmias, conduction defects, chest pain, or sudden death, despite angiographically normal epicardial coronary arteries.[35] The overall prevalence of small-vessel disease and the frequency with which it leads to clinical sequelae are not known.

Coronary Artery Vasculitis

Polyarteritis Nodosa

Polyarteritis nodosa is a systemic necrotizing vasculitis that affects medium and small arteries and that is most prevalent in males between the ages of 30 and 60 years. Some cases appear to be related to hepatitis B antigenemia, allergy, or amphetamine abuse. Approximately two thirds of affected patients have evidence of coronary artery involvement. In these patients, coronary aneurysm formation or occlusion may lead to myocardial infarction.[33,62]

Systemic Lupus Erythematosus

Systemic lupus erythematosus (SLE) is a chronic multisystem disease that most commonly affects women between the ages of 20 and 40 years. SLE is a connective tissue disease that is associated with the formation of autoantibodies and immune complexes; all organ systems can be involved. The prevalence of cardiovascular involvement is estimated to be more than 50%.[55] Pericarditis and myocarditis are common and may lead to chest pain and electrocardiographic abnormalities. On echocardiography, pericardial effusions can be seen in up to 50% of patients.[55] Symptoms of pericarditis include fever, tachycardia, and decreased heart sounds. Rarely, patients may develop tamponade or constrictive pericarditis with hypotension, increased jugular venous pressure, pulsus paradoxus, and a positive Kussmaul's sign. A pericardial friction rub may be heard.[17]

Treatment includes nonsteroidal antiinflammatory drugs, corticosteroids, and other immunosuppressants and immune modulators. Pericardiocentesis may be necessary to relieve pericardial tamponade.[55] Conduction abnormali-

ties can be seen in approximately 10% of patients with SLE. Congenital heart block may occur in children born to mothers with anti-SS-A antibodies. The heart block is usually irreversible and requires the placement of a permanent pacemaker.[55] The classic valvular abnormalities in patients with SLE are noninfective vegetations called Libman-Sacks endocarditis. These occur predominantly on the mitral valve, although any valve can be affected. Approximately 18% of these patients have significant valve dysfunction, and 8% will require surgical intervention.[24] Complications of valvular disease, including thromboembolic events, rupture of chordae, and infective endocarditis, have all been reported.[55] In addition, several studies have shown that patients with SLE are at a significantly higher risk of myocardial infarction as compared with the general population.[24,55] Atherosclerosis is the most common type of coronary artery involvement in patients with SLE, and premature and accelerated atherosclerosis are seen. Several young patients with SLE have developed acute myocardial infarction, despite the absence of conventional coronary atherosclerosis risk factors.[52,62] Pathological examination in these cases showed intimal fibrosis of the coronary arteries, but to what degree this was the result of coronary arteritis rather than atherosclerosis accelerated by the underlying disease or corticosteroid therapy is unclear. In one reported case, however, progressive coronary occlusion was observed on sequential coronary angiograms that were performed several days apart; this was attributed to coronary vasculitis.[31] Coronary vasculitis has also been reported in pathological studies of patients with rheumatoid arthritis and acute rheumatic fever.[62]

Wegener's Granulomatosis

Wegener's granulomatosis is a necrotizing vasculitis that most commonly affects the respiratory tract and kidneys. Cardiac involvement is not uncommon, occurring in up to 44% of patients with this condition.[32] Fibrinoid necrosis of the small and medium-sized coronary arteries has been described.[62] Pericarditis, coronary arteritis, and myocarditis are seen in up to 25% of patients with cardiac involvement.[32] One case of large-vessel coronary occlusion with myocardial infarction has been reported.[26] One small study found a high frequency of aortic valve abnormalities and thus recommends routine echocardiography of these patients.[56]

Takayasu's Disease (Pulseless Disease)

Takayasu's disease is predominantly a disease of young Asian women. Granulomatous panarteritis and fibrosis of the aorta and its large branches lead to stenosis and aneurysms of these vessels, which are associated with decreased pulse amplitude and vascular bruits. Clinical manifestations after the vessels become occlusive include limb ischemia, renovascular hypertension, and heart failure. Involvement of the coronary ostia and proximal coronary arteries may lead to angina pectoris or myocardial infarction.[62] Congestive heart failure and arrhythmia induced by a cardiac lesion are the most common causes of death in patients with Takayasu's arteritis.[54] Aortic regurgitation is also commonly reported in these patients. Although aortic valve replacement and repair of ascending aortic aneurysm has been performed, complications

976 such as valvular detachment, paravalvular leakage, and pseudoaneurysm formation are reported. Long-term studies are needed to determine the exact role and timing of cardiac surgery in patients with Takayasu's arteritis.[2]

Mucocutaneous Lymph Node Syndrome (Kawasaki's Disease)

Described by Kawasaki in 1967, this acute febrile illness affects infants and young children. Characterized by a variety of symptoms and signs that result from systemic vasculitis, it produces sterile conjunctivitis and oropharyngeal erythema and may lead to a desquamative reaction of the extremities and nonpurulent cervical adenopathy. In approximately 20% of patients, intense vasculitis of the coronary vasa vasorum leads to coronary artery aneurysm, thrombosis, or stenotic scarring. This is the most common cause of pediatric coronary disease in the world.[41] Death may result from myocardial ischemia or arrhythmia in 1–2% of patients, frequently during the recovery phase. Late presentation of myocardial ischemia as a result of coronary artery aneurysm or stenosis may occur (Figure 60-6). Coronary artery bypass grafting has been performed successfully for these patients.[23,61,62]

Infection

Syphilis is the most common infectious disease that affects the coronary arteries; however, it is rare in the Western hemisphere. Up to a fourth of patients with tertiary cardiovascular syphilis may have ostial stenosis of one or both coronary arteries, in addition to involvement of the ascending aorta or aortic valve. The right coronary artery is most frequently affected. Angina and myocardial infarction have resulted from syphilitic coronary disease.[34] Other infections that cause coronary arteritis include salmonella, tuberculosis, and leprosy, but these occur only rarely.[12] Viral infections have caused abnormalities of the coronary intima in experimental animals and have been proposed as a cause of myocardial infarction in young patients.[8] Recently, *Helicobacter pylori*, cytomegalovirus, and *Chlamydia pneumoniae* have gained attention with respect to restenosis, and they have been isolated from atherosclerotic lesions. However, their exact role in atherosclerosis and acute coronary syndromes remains unclear.[29,57]

Intimal Proliferation or Fibrosis

Fibrous hyperplasia of the coronary arteries may result in myocardial ischemia. This process is most frequently associated with fibromuscular hyperplasia of the renal arteries or the use of methysergide maleate (Sansert).[65] Intimal fibroblastic proliferation and medial calcification are distinct but idiopathic diseases of childhood that may lead to coronary artery obstruction.[45,58] In children with these disorders, other medium-sized arteries may be similarly involved.

Ionizing Radiation

Therapeutic doses of ionizing radiation delivered to the heart may cause pericarditis or myocardial fibrosis. Animal experimentation suggests that cardiac radiation may also injure capillary walls and enhance the development of lesions resembling atherosclerotic plaque in animals that are fed lipid-rich diets. In a small number of young patients

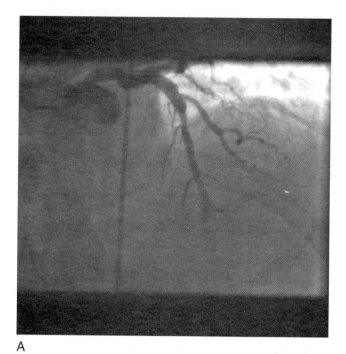

A

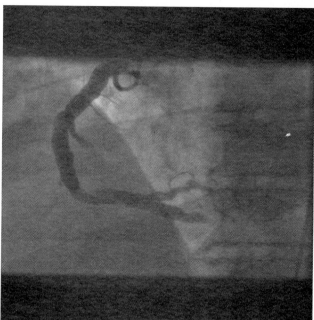

B

Figure 60–6 Coronary dilatation in Kawasaki disease seen in left coronary system (A) and right coronary system (B).

with no conventional risk factors for coronary atherosclerosis, acute myocardial infarction has been reported at varying intervals after therapeutic cardiac radiation.[43] The relationship between radiation and coronary atherosclerosis in these patients has not been established.[22]

▶ CARDIAC TRANSPLANTATION

Approximately 20% of patients develop significant coronary fibrosis or atherosclerosis within 3 years of cardiac transplantation. Angina pectoris is absent because of cardiac denervation, but myocardial infarction or sudden death may result. This process usually involves the epicardial coronary arteries and is therefore evident on coronary arteriography. Selective fibrosis of the smaller coronary vessels has also been reported. Intimal damage as a result of immunological rejection is believed to be the initiating injury that causes coronary artery disease after cardiac transplantation.[49] In patients who do not experience clinical or biopsy evidence for rejection, there is a lesser prevalence of coronary atherosclerosis.

ACCUMULATION OF METABOLIC SUBSTANCES

Specific metabolic substances may accumulate in various body tissues as the result of an inborn error of metabolism. Deposition of these substances in the walls of large and small coronary arteries may narrow the vessel lumen and lead to myocardial ischemia. These diseases include the mucopolysaccharidoses (Hunter's and Hurler's diseases),[7] gangliosidoses (Sandhoff's disease and G_{M1}), primary oxalosis, alkaptonuria, and Fabry's disease. Accentuated intimal proliferation of the coronary arteries has been reported in patients with homocystinuria and Friedreich's ataxia.[12,45,58,65]

In patients with systemic amyloidosis, amyloid may be deposited in the walls of both large and small coronary arteries, and this may lead to focal myocardial necrosis. The clinical importance of such small areas of necrosis in unclear, but they may contribute to the myocardial dysfunction that results from extensive deposits of amyloid in the myocardium. Cardiac involvement occurs in up to 50% of patients with primary amyloidosis, and it is associated with a poor prognosis.[75]

EXTRINSIC CORONARY ARTERY COMPRESSION

External compression of the coronary artery may cause progressive narrowing of the vessel lumen. This has been reported in patients with aneurysms of the sinus of Valsalva,[25] epicardial tumor metastases,[43] aortic root abscesses,[14] and dilated pulmonary arteries.[37] Systolic coronary compression by muscle bridges has been discussed previously.

SUBSTANCE ABUSE

Cocaine abuse is a major public health problem. During the hour after cocaine is used, the risk of myocardial infarction is 24 times the baseline risk.[78] Cocaine use has been linked with both acute and chronic cardiovascular diseases, including acute myocardial ischemia, cardiomyopathy, aortic dissection, arrhythmias, hypertension, acceleration of the development of atherosclerosis, and endocarditis. Myocardial infarction is secondary to increased myocardial oxygen demand because of α- and β-adrenergic stimulation in conjunction with coronary vasospasm and decreased oxygen delivery.[42] Patients with chest pain but without evidence of ischemia may simply be observed over a 12-hour period.[78] Those with evidence of infarction need to be treated aggressively with percutaneous coronary intervention. Vasospasm may respond to nitrates, calcium-channel blockers or α-blockers.[42]

REFERENCES

1. Allen RP, Liedtke AJ: The role of coronary artery injury and perfusion in the development of cardiac contusion secondary to nonpenetrating chest trauma. J Trauma 19:153–156, 1979.
2. Ando M, Kosakai Y, Okita Y, et al: Surgical treatment of aortic regurgitation caused by Takayasu's arteritis. J Card Surg 13:202–207, 1998.
3. Austin SM, Applefeld MM, Turney SZ, Mech KF Jr: Traumatic left anterior descending coronary artery to right ventricle fistula: report of two cases. South Med J 70:581–584, 1977.
4. Baim DS: Percutaneous transluminal coronary angioplasty: analysis of unsuccessful procedures as a guide toward improved results. Cardiovasc Intervent Radiol 5:186–193,1982.
5. Baim DS, Kline H, Silverman JF: Bilateral coronary pulmonary artery fistulae: report of five cases and review of the literature. Circulation 65:810–815, 1982.
6. Befeler B, Aranda JM, Embi A, et al: Coronary artery aneurysms: study of the etiology, clinical course and effect on left ventricular function and prognosis. Am J Med 62:597–607, 1977.
7. Brosius FC, Roberts WC: Coronary artery disease in the Hurler syndrome. Am J Cardiol 47:649, 1981.
8. Burch GE, Shewey LL: Viral coronary arteritis and myocardial infarction. Am Heart J 92:11–14, 1976.
9. Byrum CJ, Blackman MS, Schneider B, et al: Congenital atresia of the left coronary ostium and hypoplasia of the left main coronary artery. Am Heart J 99:354–358, 1980.
10. Chaitman BR, Lesperance J, Saltiel J, Bourassa MG: Clinical, angiographic, and hemodynamic findings in patients with anomalous origin of the coronary arteries. Circulation 53:122–131, 1976.
11. Cheitlin MD: Cardiovascular trauma—key references (Parts I and II). Circulation 65:1529–1532 and 66:244–247, 1982.
12. Cheitlin MD, McAllister HA, DeCastro CM: Myocardial Infarction without atherosclerosis. JAMA 231:951–959, 1975.
13. Ciraulo DA, Chesne RB: Coronary arterial dissection: an unrecognized cause of myocardial infarction, with subsequent coronary arterial patency. Chest 73:677–679, 1978.
14. Clarke NR, Forfar JC: Aortic root abscess presenting as unstable angina due to extrinsic compression of the left coronary artery. Postgrad Med J 78:168–169, 2002.
15. Claudon DG, Claudon DB, Edwards JE: Primary dissecting aneurysm of coronary artery. Circulation 45:259–266, 1972.
16. Dodge-Khatami A, Mavoudris C, Backer CL: Anomalous origin of the left coronary artery from the pulmonary artery: collective review of surgical therapy. Ann Thorac Surg 74:946–955, 2002.
17. Doherty NE, Siegel RJ: Cardiovascular manifestations of systemic lupus erythematosus. Am Heart J 110:1257–1265, 1985.
18. Edwards JE: The direction of blood flow in coronary arteries arising from the pulmonary trunk. Circulation 29:163–166, 1964.
19. Eliot RE, Baroldi G: Necropsy studies in myocardial infarction with minimal or no coronary reduction due to atherosclerosis. Circulation 49:1127–1131, 1974.
20. Engel HJ, Torres C, Page HL Jr: Major variations in anatomical origin of the coronary arteries: angiographic observations in 4,250 patients without associated congenital heart disease. Cathet Cardiovasc Diagn 1:157–159, 1975.
21. Espada R, Whisennand HH, Mattox KL, Beall AC Jr: Surgical management of penetrating injuries to the coronary arteries. Surgery 78:755–760, 1975.
22. Fajardo LF: Radiation-induced coronary artery disease [editorial]. Chest 71:563–564, 1977.

23. Fukushige J, Nihill MR, McNamara DG: Spectrum of cardiovascular lesions in mucocutaneous lymph node syndrome. Am J Cardiol 45:98–107, 1980.

24. Galve E, Candell-Riera J, Pigrau C, et al: Prevalence, morphologic types and evolution of cardiac valvular disease in systemic lupus erythematosus. N Engl J Med 319:817–823, 1988.

25. Garcia-Rinaldi R, Von Koch L, Howell JF: Aneurysm of the sinus of Valsalva producing obstruction of the left main coronary artery. J Thorac Cardiovasc Surg 72:123–126, 1976.

26. Gatenby PA, Lytton DG, Bulteau VG, et al: Myocardial infarction in Wegener's granulomatosis. Aust NZ Med 6: 336–340, 1976.

27. Geringer E: The mural coronary artery. Am Heart J 41: 359, 1951.

28. Glickel SZ, Maggs PR, Ellis FH Jr: Coronary artery aneurysm. Ann Thorac Surg 25:372–376, 1978.

29. Grahame-Clarke C, Chan NN, Andrew D, et al: Human cytomegalovirus seropositivity is associated with impaired vascular function. Circulation 108:678–683, 2003.

30. Grodin P, Bourassa MG, Noble J, et al: Successful course after supra-arterial myotomy for myocardial bridging and milking effect of the left anterior descending artery. Ann Thorac Surg 24:422, 1977.

31. Heibel RH, O'Toole JD, Curtiss EI, et al: Coronary arteritis in systemic lupus erythematosus. Chest 69:700–703, 1976.

32. Hoffman GS, Kerr GS, Leavitt RY, et al: Wegener's granulomatosis: an analysis of 158 patients. Ann Intern Med 116:488–498, 1992.

33. Holsinger DR, Osmundson PJ, Edwards JE: The heart in periarteritis nodosa. Circulation 25:610–618, 1962.

34. Holt S: Syphilitic ostial occlusion. Br Heart J 39:469, 1977.

35. James TN: Small arteries of the heart. Circulation 56:2–14, 1977.

36. Joswig BC, Warren SE, Vieweg WV, Hagan AD: Transmural myocardial infarction in the absence of coronary arterial luminal narrowing in a young man with single coronary arterial anomaly. Cathet Cardiovasc Diagn 4:297–304, 1978.

37. Kajita LJ, Martinez EE, Ambrose JA, et al: Extrinsic compression of the left main coronary artery by a dilated pulmonary artery: clinical, angiographic and hemodynamic determinants. Catheter Cardiovasc Interv 52:49–54, 2001.

38. Kalaria VG, Koradia N, Brell JA: Myocardial bridge: a clinical review. Cathet Cardiovasc Intervent 57:552–556, 2002.

39. Kennedy J: Symposium on catheterization complications. Complications associated with cardiac catheterization and angiography. Cathet Cardiovasc Diagn 8:5–11, 1982.

40. Kimbiris D, Iskandrian AS, Segal BL, Bemis CE: Anomalous aortic origin of coronary arteries. Circulation 58:606–615, 1978.

41. Kitamura S: The role of coronary bypass operation on children with Kawasaki disease. Coron Artery Dis 13: 437–447, 2002.

42. Kloner RA, Rezkalla SH: Cocaine and the heart. N Engl J Med 348:487–488, 2003.

43. Kopelson G, Herwig KJ: The etiologies of coronary artery disease in cancer patients. Int J Radiat Oncol Biol Phys 4:895–, 1978.

44. Lerberg DB, Ogden JA, Zuberbuhler JR, Bahnson HT: Anomalous origin of the right coronary artery from the pulmonary artery. Ann Thorac Surg 27:87, 1979.

45. Levin DC, Fellows KE, Abrams HL: Hemodynamically significant primary anomalies of the coronary arteries. Angiographic aspects. Circulation 58:25–34, 1978.

46. Liberthson RR, Dinsmore RE, Fallon JT: Aberrant coronary artery origin from the aorta. Report of 18 patients, review of literature and delineation of natural history and management. Circulation 59:748–754, 1979.

47. Liberthson RR, Sagar K, Berkoben JP, et al: Congenital coronary arteriovenous fistula. Report of 13 patients. Review of the literature and delineation of the management. Circulation 59:849–854, 1979.

48. Manzi S, Meilahn EN, Rairie JE, et al: Age-specific incidence rates of myocardial infarction and angina in women with systemic lupus erythematosus: comparison with the Framingham study. Am J Epidemiol 145:408–415, 1997.

49. Mason JW, Strefling A: Small vessel disease of the heart resulting in myocardial necrosis and death despite angiographically normal coronary arteries. Am J Cardiol 44:171–176, 1979.

50. Mavroudis C, Backer CL, Rocchini AP, et al: Coronary artery fistulas in Infants and children: a surgical review and discussion of coil embolization. Ann Thorac Surg 63:1235–1242, 1997.

51. McMahon CJ, Nihill MR, Kovalchin JP, et al: Coronary artery fistula: management and immediate-term outcome after transcatheter coil occlusion. Tex Heart Inst J 28:21–25, 2001.

52. Meller J, Conde CA, Deppisch LM, et al: Myocardial infarction due to coronary atherosclerosis in three young adults and systemic lupus erythematosus. Am J Cardiol 35:309–314, 1975.

53. Michielon G, Di Carlo D, Brancaccio G: Anomalous coronary artery origin from the pulmonary artery: correlation between surgical timing and left ventricular recovery. Ann Thorac Surg 76:581–588, 2003.

54. Miyata T, Sato O, Koyama H, et al: Long-term survival after surgical treatment of patients with Takayasu's arteritis. Circulation 108:1474–1480, 2003.

55. Moder KG, Miller TD, Tazelaar HD: Cardiac involvement in systemic lupus erythematosus. Mayo Clin Proc 74:275–284, 1999.

56. Morelli S, DiCastemenardo G, Conti F, et al: Cardiac involvement in patients with Wegener's granulomatosis. Rheumatol Int 19: 209–212, 2000.

57. Mulvihill NT, Foley JB: Inflammation in acute coronary syndromes. Heart 87:201–204, 2002.

58. Neufeld HN, Blieden LC: Coronary artery disease in children. Prog Cardiol 4:119, 1975.

59. Noble J, Bourassa MG, Petitclerc R, Dyrda I: Myocardial bridging and milking effect of the left anterior descending coronary artery: normal variant or obstruction. Am J Cardiol 37:993–,1976.

60. Okubo M, Nykanen D, Benson LN: Outcomes of transcatheter embolization in the treatment of coronary artery fistulas. Catheter Cardiovasc Interv 52:510–517, 2001.

61. Onouchi Z, Shinichiro S, Kiyosawa N, et al: Aneurysms in the coronary arteries in Kawasaki disease—an angiographic study of 30 cases. Circulation 66:6–13, 1982.

62. Parillo JE, Fauci AS: Necrotizing vasculitis, coronary angiitis and the cardiologist. Am Heart J 99:547, 1980.

63. Pfeifer JF, Lipton MJ, Oury JH, et al: Acute coronary embolism complicating bacterial endocarditis: operative treatment. Am J Cardiol 37:920–922, 1976.

64. Prizel KR, Hutchins GM, Bulkley BH: Coronary artery embolism and myocardial infarction. Ann Intern Med 85: 155–161, 1978.

65. Razavi M: Unusual forms of coronary artery disease. Cardiovasc Clin 7:25–46, 1975.

66. Richardson JV, Doty DB: Correction of anomalous origin of the left coronary artery. J Thorac Cardiovasc Surg 77:699–703, 1979.

67. Ridolfi RL, Hutchins GM, Bell WR: The heart and cardiac conduction system in thrombotic thrombocytopenia purpura. A clinicopathologic study of 17 autopsied patients. Ann Intern Med 91:357–363, 1979.

68. Roberts WC: Coronary embolism: a review of causes, consequences, and diagnostic considerations. Cardiovasc Med 3:699–704, 1978.

69. Romp RL, Herlong JR, Landolfo CK, et al: Outcome of unroofing procedure for repair of anomalous aortic origin of left or right coronary artery. Ann Thorac Surg 76:589–595, 2003.

70. Sarmento-Leite R, Machado PRM, Garcia SL: Spontaneous coronary artery dissection: stent it or wait for healing? Heart 89:164, 2003.

71. Sethi GK, Scott SM, Takaro T: Iatrogenic coronary artery stenosis following aortic valve replacement. J Thorac Cardiovasc Surg 77:760–767, 1979.

72. Sharbaugh AH, White RS: Single coronary artery. Analysis of the anatomic variation, clinical importance, and report of five cases. JAMA 230:243–246, 1974.

73. Shaver PJ, Carrig TF, Baker WP: Postpartum coronary artery dissection. Br Heart J 40:83–86, 1978.

74. Smith JC: Dissecting aneurysms of coronary arteries. Arch Pathol 99:117–121, 1975.

75. Smith RR, Hutchins GM: Ischemic heart disease secondary to amyloidosis of intramyocardial arteries. Am J Cardiol 44:413–417, 1979.

76. Virmani R, Popovsky MA, Roberts WC: Thrombocytosis, coronary thrombosis and acute myocardial infarction. Am J Med 67:498–506,1979.

77. Waller BF, Fry ETA, Hermiller JB, et al: Nonatherosclerotic causes of coronary artery narrowing: part I. Clin Cardiol 19:509–512, 1996.

78. Weber JW, Shofer FS, Larkin L, et al: Validation of a brief observation period for patients with cocaine associated chest pain. N Eng J Med 348:510–517, 2003.

79. Wesselhoeft H, Fawcett JS, Johnson AL: Anomalous origin of the left coronary artery from the pulmonary trunk. Its clinical spectrum, pathology and pathophysiology, based on a review of 140 cases with seven further cases. Circulation 38:403–425, 1968.

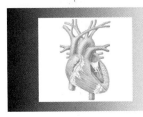

CHAPTER 61

The Pharmacological Management of Heart Failure

Eric H. Awtry and Wilson S. Colucci

result of the aging of the population and the improved survival of heart failure patients. In 2000, the most recent year for which statistics are available, the estimated prevalence of heart failure in the U.S. population was 5 million, with 550,000 new cases diagnosed in that year. In the same year, heart failure was listed as the primary diagnosis in almost 1 million hospital discharges, an increase of 165% since 1979. The economic impact is staggering, with a yearly cost of caring for these patients of over 22 billion dollars, more than half of which is accounted for by direct hospital costs. Despite improvement in therapies, one in five patients will die within 1 year of his or her initial diagnosis with heart failure, and in the United States, heart failure is listed as the principal cause for over 51,000 deaths each year and as a contributing cause in 262,000 deaths.

From a surgical standpoint, heart failure has significant impact on perioperative morbidity and mortality. Preoperative heart failure is a strong predictor of adverse outcome in patients undergoing noncardiac surgery, and a history of heart failure or depressed left ventricular systolic function is an independent predictor of mortality following coronary artery bypass surgery. A thorough understanding of the pathophysiology and treatment of heart failure is therefore essential for those physicians who manage patients in the perioperative period. Effective preoperative management of heart failure may prevent perioperative decompensation, and rapid recognition and treatment of postoperative heart failure are essential to prevent progressive pulmonary congestion and organ hypoperfusion. For the well-compensated patient, an understanding of the medical management of chronic heart failure ensures continuation of appropriate therapy both perioperatively and at the time of hospital discharge.

This chapter focuses primarily on the various pharmacological modalities available for the treatment of heart failure including their mechanisms of action, benefits as shown in clinical trials, and suggested utility in the management of patients with both acute and chronic heart failure. The use of many of these pharmacotherapies is based on our current understanding of the pathophysiological mechanisms underlying heart failure. Therefore, a brief mechanistic overview is provided in an effort to place these therapies in a pathophysiological context.

► INTRODUCTION

Heart failure has become an increasingly important cause of morbidity and mortality in the United States and in other industrialized nations. Despite improvement in heart failure treatment, its prevalence continues to rise, in large part as a

► PATHOPHYSIOLOGY OF HEART FAILURE

Our understanding of the pathophysiology of heart failure has evolved dramatically over the past two decades.[12] The traditional hemodynamic model, while still applicable in the

982 setting of acutely decompensated heart failure, is less relevant in the setting of chronic heart failure where the concepts of progressive ventricular remodeling and neurohormonal activation have come to the forefront.[43] These processes will be briefly discussed here as they relate to the pharmacological treatment of heart failure.

The term "heart failure" does not refer to a single entity; rather, it denotes a syndrome that is characterized by signs or symptoms of intravascular volume overload and/or manifestations of inadequate tissue perfusion. It is the end result of a variety of cardiac injuries and the ensuing pathological remodeling that impair the heart's ability to fill with or eject blood, and may originate from a wide range of disorders of the myocardium, pericardium, endocardium, or the intracardiac valves (Table 61-1). Pathophysiologically, heart failure can be categorized in several ways.

Left-sided heart failure is characterized by signs and symptoms of pulmonary congestion (dyspnea, orthopnea, pulmonary rales, pleural effusions), whereas *right-sided heart failure* is characterized by peripheral congestion (elevated jugular venous pressure, peripheral edema, hepatic congestion).

Systolic heart failure refers to heart failure that occurs in the setting of left ventricular systolic dysfunction (i.e., reduced ejection fraction), whereas *diastolic heart failure* refers to heart failure that results from impaired left ventricular diastolic filling despite normal left ventricular systolic function. These two abnormalities often coexist, although one usually predominates.

Acute heart failure denotes the sudden development of heart failure in the absence of preexisting cardiac dysfunction or the sudden decompensation in a patient with previously stable cardiac disease. This results from an abrupt alteration in cardiac structure or function (e.g., following an acute myocardial infarction or after valvular rupture) and is generally associated with clinical instability. *Chronic heart failure* results from a more indolent process of myocardial dysfunction and may be associated with less clinical severity owing to the development of compensatory mechanisms (see later).

Low-output heart failure results from a reduction in cardiac output (from either systolic or diastolic dysfunction) and is usually characterized by venous congestion and increased arterial resistance (i.e., vasoconstriction). *High-output heart failure* occurs in the setting of increased cardiac output (e.g., thyrotoxicosis, anemia, beriberi, Paget's disease, atrioventricular [AV] fistulas) and is characterized by venous congestion and normal or reduced arterial resistance.

Backward heart failure refers to the hypothesis that the manifestations of heart failure are primarily the result of an accumulation of fluid (and pressure) behind the failing ventricle. *Forward heart failure* proposes that heart failure results from a primary reduction in cardiac output with resultant organ hypoperfusion, sodium and water retention, and subsequent venous congestion. This is not as useful a distinction as both mechanisms likely operate in the majority of patients with heart failure.

Symptomatically, heart failure may be classified on the basis of its clinical severity (Table 61-2). Despite the varied etiologies and classifications of heart failure, the manifestations all reflect either intravascular volume overload, inadequate tissue perfusion, or a combination of both. A thorough explanation of all these forms of heart failure is beyond the scope of this chapter. The following discussion, therefore, will focus primarily on left ventricular systolic failure in both the acute and chronic setting.

Acute Heart Failure

The response of the cardiovascular system to the onset of myocardial dysfunction and the pathophysiological mechanisms underlying the subsequent progression to heart failure depend in large part on the acuity of the dysfunction. An acute cardiac insult results in a series of hemodynamic alterations that account for the clinical manifestations of left ventricular failure. This occurs irrespective of whether the initial insult depresses myocardial contractility (systolic dysfunction) or impairs ventricular filling (diastolic dysfunction). The cascade begins with a rise in left ventricular end-diastolic pressure (LVEDP). This elevated pressure is transmitted to the left atrium and subsequently to the pulmonary venous and capillary system. The increased intravascular pressure results in transudation of fluid into the pulmonary interstitium where it interferes with gas exchange resulting in hypoxemia and dyspnea. Additionally, there is often an associated reduction in cardiac output resulting in inadequate delivery of blood to the arterial system with resultant organ hypoperfusion.

The heart's response to these hemodynamic alterations is the activation of several compensatory mechanisms (Table 61-3).[4] A rapid, generalized activation of the adrenergic

---

Table 61–1

Common Causes of Heart Failure

Myocardial
 Ischemia/infarction
 Viral myocarditis
 Idiopathic cardiomyopathy
 Hypertrophic cardiomyopathy
 Hypertension
 Toxins (alcohol, cocaine, chemotherapeutic agents)
 Infiltrative diseases (amyloidosis, hemachromatosis)
 Infectious (Lyme disease, Chagas' disease)
 Peripartum cardiomyopathy
 Thyroid dysfunction
 Metabolic abnormalities (thiamine or selenium
  deficiency)

Valvular
 Aortic stenosis
 Aortic regurgitation
 Mitral stenosis
 Mitral regurgitation

Arrhythmic
 Tachycardia-mediated cardiomyopathy

Pericardial
 Constrictive pericarditis

Table 61–2	
Clinical Classifications of Heart Failure	

New York Heart Association Classification	
Class 1	Symptoms only with greater than usual activity
Class 2	Asymptomatic at rest but with symptoms during normal activities
Class 3	Asymptomatic at rest but with symptoms during minimal exertion
Class 4	Symptoms at rest

ACC/AHA Classification[a]	
Stage A	Patients with structurally normal hearts, asymptomatic, but at risk for the development of heart failure owing to the presence of risk factors (e.g., hypertension, coronary artery disease, diabetes)
Stage B	Patients with structurally abnormal hearts (e.g., LV systolic dysfunction, LVH, valvular dysfunction, prior myocardial infarction) but without symptoms of heart failure
Stage C	Patients with structurally abnormal hearts and current or prior symptoms of heart failure
Stage D	Patients with end-stage heart failure symptoms not responsive to standard therapy

[a]ACC/AHA, American College of Cardiology/American Heart Association.

system occurs and is associated with a withdrawal of parasympathetic tone.[21] Direct sympathetic stimulation of the heart as well as β-adrenergic-induced release of epinephrine and norepinephrine from the adrenal glands result in tachycardia and an increase in myocardial contractility, both of which serve to augment cardiac output. Catecholamine-induced peripheral arterial vasoconstriction redirects the available cardiac output away from relatively nonessential organs (e.g., skin, skeletal muscle, gut, kidney) and helps maintain sufficient blood pressure to ensure adequate perfusion of more vital organs (e.g., heart and brain). Furthermore, β-adrenergic stimulation of the juxtaglomerular apparatus in the kidneys results in the release of renin and activation of the renin-angiotensin system. The angiotensin II thus produced is a potent vasoconstrictor and acts in concert with the direct α-adrenergic stimulation of the vasculature to maintain blood pressure. The reduced renal blood flow resulting from depressed cardiac output and redistribution of blood volume results in activation of renal baroreceptors. This further stimulates renin release and augments sympathetic activation, thereby contributing to vasoconstriction.

In addition to producing the aforementioned hemodynamic alterations, acute heart failure is characterized by marked sodium and water retention. This occurs through a variety of mechanisms. Angiotensin II directly promotes the reabsorption of sodium in the proximal nephron and indirectly promotes the reabsorption of sodium from the distal nephron, this latter effect being mediated through angiotensin II-induced release of aldosterone from the adrenal cortex. Furthermore, angiotensin II and norepinephrine stimulate hypothalamic release of arginine vasopressin resulting in further vasoconstriction and free water reabsorption. These changes produce an expansion of intravascular volume and augmentation of venous return, thereby increasing ventricular end-diastolic volume (*preload*). The increased preload results in an increase in stroke volume by the Frank–Starling mechanism (Figure 61-1), and thereby helps support the cardiac output.

Chronic Heart Failure

In combination, the aforementioned mechanisms serve a compensatory role in acute heart failure, helping to maintain cardiac output and blood pressure to allow for adequate perfusion of vital organs. These compensatory mechanisms may initially be adequate to allow for clinical stability and the patient may subsequently go through a stage of asymptomatic ventricular dysfunction, maintained in part by chronic stimulation of the adrenergic and renin–angiotensin systems. As heart failure progresses, the hemodynamic overload induces changes in the shape and size of the ventricle, a process known as *ventricular remodeling*.[10] The specific changes that occur depend in part on the hemodynamic stressors facing the ventricle.[25] In predominantly pressure-overloaded conditions (e.g., hypertension, aortic stenosis), there is a rise in systolic wall stress that results in left ventricular hypertrophy. If this hypertrophy is insufficient to normalize the wall stress, dilation occurs. Under conditions of volume overload (e.g., aortic or mitral insufficiency) there is a rise in diastolic wall stress that induces ventricular dilation. This dilation in turn results in increased systolic wall stress (via the Laplace relationship) and subsequent hypertrophy. These hypertrophic changes help maintain systolic wall stress within a normal range and help preserve ventricular contractile function. However, with continued hemodynamic overload there is progressive ventricular dilation, eventuating in the development of a dilated, spherical heart. This altered ventricular morphology produces less efficient ventricular contraction, may induce mitral regurgitation owing to annular dilation and malcoaptation of the valve leaflets, and is associated with an adverse prognosis.

The stimuli that induce ventricular remodeling are varied and the mechanisms underlying the remodeling process are complex (Table 61-4).[10,22] It appears that increased wall stress (resulting from ventricular dilation and increased afterload) as well neurohormones (e.g., β-adrenergic and renin–angiotensin systems), vasoactive peptides (e.g., endothelin), and cytokines (e.g., tumor necrosis factor [TNF]-α) all mediate remodeling. These factors may have direct effects on the cardiac myocytes or may act indirectly via stimulation of second messenger systems, and thereby induce a variety of changes in myocyte structure and function. On a cellular level, myocyte hypertrophy results from the replication of sarcomeres either in parallel (producing ventricular hypertrophy) or in series (producing ventricular dilation). Alterations in the expression of various contractile proteins occur with reexpression of fetal genes and reduced

Table 61–3

Compensatory Mechanisms in Heart Failure

Compensatory response	Stimuli	Beneficial effects	Adverse effects	Potential pharmacological interventions
RAS activation	↓ CO/BP ↓ Renal blood flow ↑ β-Adrenergic activity	Maintain vital organ perfusion through vasoconstriction and sodium retention	↑ Afterload → worsened LV function Adverse LV remodeling (apoptosis, myocyte hypertrophy, etc.)	ACEIs ARB
Adrenergic activation	↓ CO/BP	↑ CO through ↑ in HR and contractility ↑ BP	↑ Ischemia ↑ Afterload → worsened LV function ↑ LVEDP → pulmonary congestion Adverse LV remodeling (apoptosis, myocyte hypertrophy, etc.)	β-Adrenergic-blocking agents
Renal salt and water retention	↑ ADH ↑ Norepinephrine ↑ Angiotensin II ↑ Aldosterone ↓ Renal blood flow	↑ Preload → ↑ SV and CO	Pulmonary and systemic congestion Adverse LV remodeling	Diuretics Aldosterone inhibitors ACEI/ARB β-Adrenergic blocking agents
↑ Natriuretic peptide secretion	Volume expansion (atrial stretch)	Diuresis Natriuresis Partial inhibition of RAS and norepinephrine	None known	Natriuretic peptide administration

ACEI, angiotensin-converting enzyme inhibitors; ADH, antidiuretic hormone; ARB, angiotensin receptor blocker; BP, blood pressure; CO, cardiac output; HR, heart rate; LV, left ventricular; LVEDP, left ventricular end-diastolic pressure; RAS, renin–angiotensin system; SV, stroke volume.

expression of adult contractile genes resulting in abnormalities of calcium handling and excitation–contraction coupling. Chronic stimulation of the sympathetic system is accompanied by a reduction in the density of β-adrenergic receptors in the myocardium and an uncoupling of the receptors from their intracellular mediators.[2] This results in a blunted response of the failing myocardium to either endogenous (e.g., exercise) or exogenous (e.g., dopamine or dobutamine) adrenergic stimulation.

In addition to these alterations of the contractile apparatus within the myocytes there is a progressive reduction in the number of myocytes, in part the result of apoptosis induced by the various stimuli of remodeling. Furthermore, changes in the extracellular matrix occur related to fibroblast proliferation, interstitial fibrosis, and increased expression of degrada-

tive enzymes such as matrix metalloproteinases. The latter factor results in the loss of mechanical coupling of myocytes and may contribute to the remodeling process by facilitating "myocyte slippage" and, thereby, ventricular dilation.

As the remodeling process develops, the neurohormonal effects of the β-adrenergic and renin–angiotensin systems on the peripheral vasculature and renal salt and water handling continue. The intense vasoconstriction, while maintaining flow to vital organs, contributes to hypoperfusion of the kidneys and progressive renal dysfunction. The augmented preload and cardiac output resulting from sodium and water retention help to maintain circulating blood volume and tissue perfusion. However, the associated increase in end-diastolic pressure and increased ventricular wall stress contribute to progressive ventricular remodeling, and

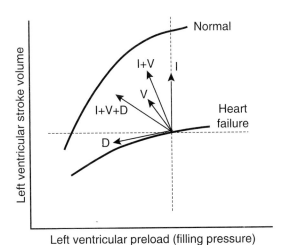

Figure 61–1 Frank–Starling curve with normal systolic function and with heart failure, and the hemodynamic effect of pharmacological therapy. In the normal setting, an increase in preload results in an increase in stroke volume. In heart failure this relationship is blunted, and at any given stroke volume the preload must be higher (horizontal dotted line). Similarly, for any given preload, the stroke volume is lower (vertical dotted line). Diuretic therapy (D) reduces preload without a significant effect on stroke volume whereas inotropic therapy (I) augments stroke volume without an appreciable effect on preload. Vasodilator therapy (V) has moderate beneficial effects on both preload and stroke volume; however, the greatest effects are seen with combination therapy (I + V, I + V + D).

result in pulmonary and systemic venous hypertension and precipitation of congestive symptoms. Thus, these initially compensatory changes become deleterious in the chronic setting. The inhibition of these processes offers not only a

mechanism for the treatment of heart failure but also the potential to reverse the adverse remodeling seen in the chronic state (Table 61-3).[29]

▶ PHARMACOLOGICAL AGENTS USED IN THE TREATMENT OF HEART FAILURE

The majority of pharmacological agents used for the treatment of heart failure effect benefit by either directly interfering with the hemodynamic alterations described above or through inhibition of the neurohormonal activation underlying these alterations (Figure 61-1). These medications fall into several categories: diuretics, vasodilators, inotropic agents, and neurohormonal inhibitors. Diuretics act to reduce preload (leftward shift on the Starling curve) resulting in decreased filling pressures and improved congestive symptoms. Although this fall in preload may be associated with a reduction in stroke volume, this effect is minimal in patients with elevated filling pressures. Pure venodilators similarly reduce filling pressures and congestive symptoms and have minimal effect on stroke volume. Arterial vasodilators and inotropic agents predominantly augment cardiac output and thereby improve organ perfusion; arterial vasodilators act indirectly via a reduction in vascular resistance whereas inotropic agents directly increase contractility and stroke volume. Although the increased cardiac output seen with these agents may result in a fall in filling pressures, the effect may be relatively modest. As a result of the differential effects of these agents, many patients with heart failure attain the greatest benefit from combination therapy. Neurohormonal inhibitors may have mixed hemodynamic effects. The blockade of adrenergic tone (β-blockers) and inhibition of the renin–angiotensin system (angiotensin-

Table 61–4

Factors Involved in Ventricular Remodeling

Stimulants of ventricular remodeling	Molecular and cellular events that mediate ventricular remodeling
Altered hemodynamic load (increased preload, afterload, wall stress)	Myocyte hypertrophy Myocyte loss (necrosis and apoptosis)
β-Adrenergic stimulation	Myocyte "slippage"
Activation of the renin–angiotensin system	Transition to fetal myocyte phenotype
Inflammatory cytokines (e.g., TNF-α, IL-1, IL-6)[a]	Neurohormonal activation
Vasoactive peptides (e.g., endothelin)	Fibroblast proliferation
Oxidative stress	Alterations in the interstitial matrix Alterations in excitation-coupling

TNF, tumor necrosis factor; IL, interleukin.

986 converting enzyme [ACE] inhibitors, angiotensin receptor blockers) result in vasodilation and augmented cardiac output. These agents may also decrease preload and reduce filling pressures via a reduction in neurohormonally mediated renal sodium and water retention.

Diuretics

Diuretics (Table 61-5) have long played an important role in the symptomatic treatment of heart failure.[5] The induced diuresis and natruresis reduce extracellular volume and ventricular filling pressures thereby ameliorating congestive symptoms. This effect occurs without a significant decrease in cardiac output or systemic blood pressure unless excessive diuresis and intravascular volume depletion occur. It should be noted that while diuretics are beneficial in controlling symptoms and improving exercise capacity in patients with heart failure, with the exception of spironolactone, diuretic use has not resulted in a decrease in mortality.[47]

Loop diuretics act in the thick ascending limb of the loop of Henle where they inhibit the Na^+-K^+-$2Cl^-$ transporter resulting in increased delivery of sodium and water to the distal nephron. They also decrease the tonicity of the medullary interstitium and thereby limit the osmotic reabsorption of free water from the collecting tubules. Currently available loop diuretics include furosemide, bumetanide, torsemide, and ethacrynic acid. There is an increased risk of ototoxicity with ethacrynic acid; therefore, this agent should be reserved for patients who are allergic/intolerant to other agents.

Furosemide is the most common loop diuretic used for the treatment of heart failure. For patients with mild to moderate congestive symptoms, it can be given orally at initial doses of 20–40 mg daily. Its bioavailability ranges from 40 to 70% and gradual dose titration is frequently required. Furosemide has a relatively short half-life. Once renal tubular levels of the drug decline avid sodium reabsorption occurs throughout the nephron, potentially limiting or preventing effective natruresis. A twice-daily dosing regimen may therefore be required to produce adequate salt and water loss. In patients with more severe volume retention or decompensated heart failure, intravenous administration of furosemide (20–100 mg) may produce a more rapid and effective diuresis. The maximum intravenous dose is 300 mg; however, the risk of ototoxicity increases at such high doses. For patients who require frequent, high doses of intravenous furosemide, a continuous infusion may produce a more effective diuresis and require a lower total daily dose.[19] The infusion is usually started at 5–10 mg/h and titrated as needed to obtain the desired effect. Bumetanide

Table 61–5

Diuretics Commonly Used in the Treatment of Heart Failure

Class/examples	Daily dose range	Duration of action (h)	Adverse effects (by class)
Loop diuretics			
Furosemide (Lasix)	20–480 mg po	4–6	Hypokalemia, hyperuricemia, metabolic alkalosis, ototoxicity at high doses
	20–300 mg iv		
Torsemide (Demadex)	5–40 mg po	12	
Bumetanide (Bumex)	0.5–5 mg po	4–6	
Ethacrynic acid (Edecrin)	25–100 mg po	12	
Thiazide diuretics			
Chlorothiazide (Diuril)	125–500 mg po	6–12	Hypokalemia, hyponatremia, hyperuricemia, hyperglycemia, hyperlipidemia
Hydrochlorothiazide (HydroDiuril)	12.5–50 mg po	12–18	
Chlothalidone (Hygroton)	25–100 mg po	24	
Thiazide-like diuretics			
Metalazone (Zaroxolyn)	0.5–10 mg po	24	Hypokalemia, hypomagnesemia
Aldosterone inhibitors			
Spironolactone (Aldactone)	25 mg po	8–12	Hyperkalemia, nausea, gynecomastia
Potassium-sparing diuretics			
Amiloride (Midamor)	5–10 mg po	24	Hyperkalemia when combined with ACEI/ARB
Triamterene (Dyrenium)	50–100 mg po	12	

po, orally; iv, intravenously; ACEI, angiotensin-converting enzyme inhibitor; ARB, angiotensin receptor blocker.

and torsemide have greater bioavailability than does furosemide (~80%) but have not demonstrated better efficacy and are significantly more expensive.

Thiazide diuretics act in the distal convoluted tubule where they inhibit the Na^+-Cl^- cotransporter.[5] Their efficacy is dependent on the delivery of sodium to the distal nephron; therefore, their diuretic effect is limited by sodium reabsorption from more proximal regions as occurs during intravascular volume depletion or in low flow states. Additionally, they are ineffective when glomerular filtration rates fall below 30 ml/min. Thiazides may be useful as the sole diuretic when treating mild congestive symptoms; however, their predominant role in the management of more advanced heart failure is as an adjunct to other diuretic therapy in patients who exhibit diuretic resistance. Although several thiazides are available, the most frequently used are hydrochlorothiazide (12.5–50 mg daily) and metalozone (2.5–10 mg daily). These agents exhibit synergism with loop diuretics and should be given approximately 30 min prior to administration of furosemide, bumetanide, or torsemide.

Spironolactone is a competitive inhibitor of aldosterone in the distal convoluted tubule and, as such, stimulates a mild natruresis and potassium reabsorption. It may be most effective in patients with advanced heart failure in whom marked activation of the renin–angiotensin–aldosterone system results in aldosterone levels as high as 20-fold normal. In a recent trial of patients with moderate to severe chronic heart failure (CHF) (New York Heart Association [NYHA] class III-IV), treatment with spironolactone (25–50 mg daily) reduced the risk of death by almost one third.[47] It also improved patients' symptoms and significantly reduced the rate of hospitalization for heart failure. The mechanism of benefit is unlikely to be related to a diuretic effect, as spironolactone is a weak diuretic. Rather, it likely reflects inhibition of aldosterone-induced myocardial fibrosis and ventricular remodeling.[56] The dose of spironolactone should not exceed 50 mg daily because of the risk of hyperkalemia, especially when used in conjunction with an ACE inhibitor or angiotensin receptor blocker for the treatment of heart failure.

Amiloride and triamterene inhibit the reabsorption of sodium in the distal convoluted tubule and proximal collecting duct resulting in a mild natruresis and reduction of the ionic gradient required for potassium secretion into the urine. These agents produce a mild diuresis without the potassium wasting seen with loop diuretics and thiazides, and may be effective for the control of mild congestive symptoms. However, when given alone they are not effective in maintaining a negative fluid balance in patients with advanced heart failure. In such patients, these agents may have benefit as part of a combination diuretic regimen, especially given their potassium-sparing properties.

Patients treated with diuretics require close monitoring of their renal function and serum electrolytes. Loop diuretics and thiazides can lead to profound hypokalemia and hypomagnesemia, especially when used in combination, while spironolactone may result in hyperkalemia. In contrast to loop diuretics, thiazides do not alter the tonicity of the renal medullary interstitium and may produce significant hyponatremia owing to the reabsorption of free water from the distal convoluted tubule in the face of a preserved interstitial gradient. In addition to these metabolic effects, thiazides may adversely affect serum lipid levels and spironolactone may induce gynecomastia.

Vasodilators

Nitrovasodilators

Nitric oxide is formed by normal endothelial and smooth muscle cells throughout the vasculature and functions in both a paracrine and an autocrine fashion. Its primary mechanism of action involves an induced increase in intracellular cyclic guanosine monophosphate, which results in vascular smooth muscle relaxation. Nitrosovasodilators such as sodium nitroprusside and organic nitrates (e.g., nitroglycerin) are metabolized to nitric oxide within the vasculature. They are potent vasodilators and, as such, are useful in the management of heart failure.

Nitroprusside is the sodium salt of nitric oxide and ferricyanide. It is a balanced vasodilator and produces both vasodilation and venodilation in both the systemic and pulmonary systems. These effects result in favorable hemodynamic changes including a decrease in right atrial and pulmonary capillary wedge pressures (i.e., decreased preload), a reduction in pulmonary and systemic resistance (i.e., decreased afterload), and an increase in stroke volume and cardiac output/index (Figure 61-2).[15] In contrast to other arterial vasodilators, nitroprusside does not cause a significant increase in heart rate and its use is usually associated with a decrease in myocardial oxygen demand. Nitroprusside is useful for the management of heart failure associated with elevated filling pressures, low cardiac output, and high vascular resistance, as occurs in patients with decompensated systolic failure. It is also ideally suited for the management of heart failure associated with profound hypertension, acute mitral regurgitation, acute aortic insufficiency, or acute ventricular septal defect.[7]

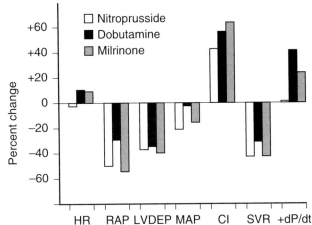

Figure 61–2 Comparative hemodynamic effects of maximally tolerated doses of nitroprusside, dobutamine, and milrinone in patients with severe heart failure. HR, heart rate; RAP, right atrial pressure; LVEDP, left ventricular end-diastolic pressure; MAP, mean arterial pressure; CI, cardiac index; SVR, systemic vascular resistance.
(Adapted from Colucci WS, Wright RF, Jaski BE, et al: Milrinone and dobutamine in severe heart failure: differing hemodynamic effects and individual patient responsiveness. Circulation 73; III-175, 1986.)

988

Nitroprusside is administered as a continuous infusion. Its onset of action is rapid (within 30 s), and it reaches peak effect within 2 min. Similarly, its effects completely resolve within 3 min of discontinuing its infusion. Owing to these rapid changes in hemodynamics it is best administered under the guidance of pulmonary (i.e., Swan-Ganz catheter) and systemic arterial monitoring. The usual starting dose is 0.1–0.25 µg/kg/min. The dose may be titrated up by 0.25 µg/kg/min every 5–10 min until the desired effect is achieved or the maximum dose is reached (10 µg/kg/min). The use of nitroprusside may be limited by the development of hypotension, especially in patients with normal left ventricular systolic function or low filling pressures. Rapid cessation of nitroprusside may result in rebound hypertension, likely reflecting neurohormonal activation. Nitroprusside is metabolized in the vasculature to nitric oxide and cyanide, the latter of which is further metabolized in the liver to thiocyanate, which is excreted by the kidneys. Accumulation of these toxic metabolites is more likely to occur when nitroprusside is infused at higher doses or for prolonged periods of time, especially in the setting of hepatic and/or renal dysfunction. Cyanide toxicity may manifest as abdominal pain, confusion, or seizure and is usually preceded by lactic acidosis. Thiocyanate toxicity usually presents as nausea, confusion, fatigue, psychosis, and, rarely, coma. If toxicity is suspected the infusion should be discontinued and serum levels of the metabolites measured. Cyanide toxicity can be treated with sodium nitrite (300 mg) or sodium thiosulfate (12.5 g), whereas thiocyanate toxicity may require hemodialysis.

Nitroglycerin, like nitroprusside, is a potent vasodilator; however, it has dose-dependent effects in the arterial and venous systems. At low doses it is a relatively selective venodilator resulting in increased venous capacitance and decreased left and right ventricular filling pressures. At higher doses, it is also an arterial dilator and results in a fall in pulmonary and systemic vascular resistance, although less predictably and to a lesser extent than nitroprusside. Intravenous nitroglycerin is an effective agent in the management of acute decompensated heart failure characterized by increased filling pressures and elevated vascular resistance. Additionally, nitroglycerin has a significant vasodilatory effect on epicardial coronary arteries and may indirectly improve left ventricular function by improving blood flow to ischemic myocardium. It is thus an agent of choice in managing heart failure associated with acute myocardial ischemia or infarction.

Intravenous nitroglycerin in usually initiated at 20 µg/min and titrated up by 10–20 µg/min every 5–10 min until the desired hemodynamic effect is achieved or the maximum dose is reached (400 µg/min). Its effects are immediate and resolve rapidly following discontinuation of the infusion. Nitroglycerin may result in hypotension, especially at high doses and in patients with low filling pressures. Its use is commonly associated with a headache, occasionally requiring down-titration or discontinuance of the infusion. Nitrate tolerance frequently develops but can usually be overcome by increasing the infusion rate.

Hydralazine

Hydralazine is a direct vasodilator that causes relaxation of arteriolar smooth muscle by an unknown mechanism. It does not cause venodilation or dilation of epicardial coronary arteries; thus, its hemodynamic effects are primarily limited to a reduction in vascular resistance. Hydralazine is an effective antihypertensive agent, especially when used in combination with other agents. When administered to patients with congestive heart failure, it is most effective when combined with venodilating agents (e.g., organic nitrates). The combination of hydralazine and oral nitrates, when added to a regimen of digoxin and diuretics, has been shown in randomized trials to reduce mortality, improve left ventricular systolic function, and reduce symptoms in patients with heart failure.[9] However, the benefit of this regimen on mortality and left ventricular (LV) function is less than that of ACE inhibitors.[11] In general, hydralazine is not a first-line agent for the treatment of heart failure. Nonetheless, it should be considered in patients who are intolerant of ACEI owing to allergy or renal insufficiency, and is the agent of choice for afterload reduction in pregnant patients. Additionally, it may offer further relief in patients with heart failure who remain symptomatic despite treatment with ACEI.

Hydralazine therapy is initiated at a dose of 10 mg four times daily and titrated upward as blood pressure tolerates to a maximum dose of 100 mg four times daily. Organic nitrates are given concurrently (e.g., isosorbide dinitrate 30–160 mg daily). Hydralazine-induced vasodilation is associated with a baroreceptor-mediated increase in sympathetic activity resulting in a reflex tachycardia, increased ventricular contractility, increased renin activity, and fluid retention. In patients with underlying coronary artery disease the arteriolar dilation may result in a coronary steal phenomenon and when combined with the tachycardia, may precipitate myocardial ischemia. Coadministration with β-adrenergic-blocking agents may prevent this complication; nonetheless, hydralazine should be used with caution in patients with an ischemia cardiomyopathy. Other side effects occur more frequently and include headaches, flushing, palpitations, nausea, and dizziness. A lupus-like syndrome occurs in 5–10% of patients and may require discontinuation of the drug.

Calcium Channel-Blocking Agents

In general, the use of calcium channel-blocking agents for the treatment of heart failure has been disappointing, despite the fact that they are relatively potent vasodilators. Verapamil and diltiazem have negatively inotropic effects and may worsen symptoms in patients with systolic heart failure. However, these agents may improve diastolic function owing to their rate slowing effects and induced alterations in calcium homeostasis and, thus, may be beneficial in the treatment of diastolic heart failure. The first-generation dihydropyridine, nifedipine, has been associated with an increase in adverse effects including a trend toward increased mortality in patients with systolic heart failure. This may relate to neurohormonal activation resulting from fluctuations in its hemodynamic effects, especially with short-acting formulations. Newer second-generation dihydropyridines, such as amlodipine and felodipine, appear to be safe in patients with heart failure but have not demonstrated significant benefit with regard to morbidity or mortality. Therefore, although these later agents could be considered for the treatment of hypertension or angina in patients with LV systolic dysfunction, calcium channel-blocking agents in general should not be used as a primary treatment for heart failure.

Neurohormonal-Inhibiting Agents

ACE Inhibitors

ACE inhibitors have a variety of beneficial effects on the pathophysiology of heart failure. Hemodynamically, ACE inhibitors are potent vasodilators and reduce both preload and afterload. The subsequent fall in intracardiac pressures and reduction in wall stress result in a decrease in myocardial oxygen demand potentially reducing ischemia, and a decrease in the activity of the sympathetic nervous system, thereby reducing electrical instability. Additionally, the ACE inhibitor-induced reduction in angiotensin, as well as the subsequent reduction in adrenal aldosterone release, may have direct effects on the extent of fibrosis and collagen deposition that characterize myocardial remodeling in heart failure. The effects of ACE inhibitors are primarily mediated by inhibition of the enzyme responsible for the conversion of angiotensin I to angiotensin II thereby decreasing production of the latter. However, some of the benefit of ACE inhibitors may result in part from their effects on the kinin system; ACE inhibitors decrease the degradation of kinins (e.g., bradykinin) and thereby enhance their vasodilatory effects and potentiate kinin-mediated synthesis of vasodilatory prostaglandins.

ACE inhibitors have been extensively studied in a wide variety of patients with heart failure and have almost universally demonstrated benefit in hemodynamics, symptoms, exercise capacity, hospitalization, and mortality.[20,23] In the Cooperative North Scandinavian Enalapril Survival Study (CONSENSUS), patients with severe (NYHA class IV) heart failure who were already treated with digoxin and diuretics had a 40% reduction in mortality at 6 months when treated with enalapril.[16] Patients with less severe heart failure (NYHA classes II–III and an ejection fraction of ≤35%) were studied in the treatment arm of the Studies Of Left Ventricular Dysfunction (SOLVD) trial.[51] In this trial, patients who were treated with enalapril had a 16% reduction in mortality and a 26% reduction in the risk of death or hospitalization for worsening heart failure. In the Acute Infarction Ramipril Efficacy study, patients with symptomatic heart failure, a recent myocardial infarction, and ejection fractions <40% demonstrated a 27% decrease in mortality after 30 days of treatment with ramipril.[1] Furthermore, several studies have demonstrated that asymptomatic patients with depressed ejection fractions (<35–40%) have reduced morbidity and mortality when treated with ACE inhibitors, although the magnitude of this benefit is less than that seen in patients with overt heart failure.[44,50] Thus, the results of clinical trials with ACE inhibitors reveal a consistent benefit in patients with symptomatic heart failure or asymptomatic LV dysfunction (Figure 61–3).

A variety of ACE inhibitors are currently available (Table 61-6). These agents differ in regard to their plasma half-life, dosing regimen, and ability to inhibit ACE at the tissue level. However, available data suggest that the beneficial effects of these agents are a class effect and not dependent upon individual pharmacological characteristics. Nonetheless, when selecting an ACE inhibitor for the treatment of heart failure,

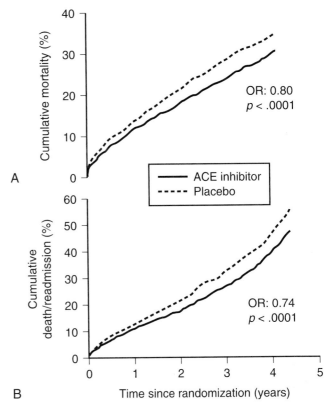

Figure 61–3 The effect of ACE inhibitors on the total mortality (A) and total mortality plus readmission for heart failure (B) in patients with heart failure and/or left ventricular systolic dysfunction.
(Modified from Flather MD, Yusuf S, Kober L, et al: Long-term ACE-inhibitor therapy in patients with heart failure or left-ventricular dysfunction: A systematic overview of data from individual patients. Lancet 355:1575–1581, 2000.)

preference should be given to those agents that have demonstrated efficacy in large-scale trials (enalapril, captopril, lisinopril, and ramipril). ACE inhibitors should be initiated at low doses, especially in patients with hypotension before treatment. If initial doses are tolerated hemodynamically, the dose should be gradually titrated upward over several days to several weeks. In general, these agents should be titrated upward to goal doses as determined by clinical trials or to the highest dose that can be tolerated. Although lower doses may offer mortality benefit similar to higher doses, higher doses are associated with augmented symptom control. In patients with decompensated heart failure who cannot receive oral agents intravenous enalaprilat can be used.[3] Enalaprilat is the active form of the oral ACE inhibitor enalapril. When given intravenously it is a balanced vasodilator resulting in a reduction in left and right ventricular filling pressures and vascular resistance.

Use of ACE inhibitors may be limited by the development of side effects. Hypotension is the most common adverse effect, occurs most frequently during the initiation of therapy, and is more common in patients who are volume depleted. It can usually be managed by reducing diuretic dosing and titrating the ACE inhibitor slowly. Moderate hypotension (systolic blood pressure >85 mm Hg) can frequently be tolerated as long as organ hypoperfusion is not present. ACE inhibitors produce vasodilation of renal effer-

Table 61–6

Oral Agents Commonly Used in the Treatment of Heart Failure

Class/examples	Starting dose	Target or maximum dose	Adverse effects (by class)
Nitrosovasodilators			
Isosorbide mononitrate (Imdur)	30 mg qd	120 mg qd	Headache; nitrate tolerance if continuous use
Isosorbide dinitrate (Isordil)	10 mg tid	30 mg tid	
Direct-acting vasodilators			
Hydralazine (Apresoline)	10 mg tid	100 mg tid	Reflex tachycardia, lupus-like syndrome
Angiotensin-converting enzyme inhibitors			
Captopril (Capoten)	6.25 mg tid	50 mg tid	Hypotension, cough, rash, angioedema, hyperkalemia; renal dysfunction (especially in patients with bilateral renal artery stenosis)
Enalapril (Vasotec)	2.5 mg bid	10–20 mg bid	
Lisinopril (Zestril, Prinivil)	2.5 mg qd	40 mg qd	
Ramipril (Altace)	2.5 mg qd	10 mg qd	
Quinapril (Accupril)	10 mg qd	40 mg qd	
Fosinopril (Monopril)	10 mg qd	40 mg qd	
Trandolapril (Mavik)	0.5 mg qd	8 mg qd	
Angiotensin receptor blockers			
Losartan (Cozaar)	50 mg qd	100 mg qd	Hyperkalemia, hypotension; renal dysfunction (especially in patients with bilateral renal artery stenosis)
Candesartan (Atacand)	4 mg qd	32 mg qd	
Valsartan (Diovan)	80 mg qd	320 mg qd	
β-Adrenergic-blocking agents			
Carvedilol (Coreg)	3.125 mg bid	25 mg bid	Bradycardia, hypotension, bronchospasm; may worsen HF during initiation and titration
Metoprolol (Toprol XL)	25 mg qd	200 mg qd	
Bisoprolol (Zebeta)	1.25 mg qd	10 mg qd	
Inotropic agents			
Digoxin (Lanoxin)	0.125 mg qd	Serum digoxin level: 0.5–0.8	Nausea, bradycardia, heart block, ventricular tachyarrhythmias
Calcium channel blockers[a]			
Amlodipine (Norvasc)	2.5 mg qd	10 mg qd	Amlodipine: pedal edema; verapamil and diltiazem: bradycardia, worsened systolic HF
Verapamil (Calan, Verelan)	120 mg qd	480 mg qd	
Diltiazem (Cardizem, Dilacor)	120 mg qd	540 mg qd	

[a]Calcium channel blockers should not be routinely used for the treatment of systolic heart failure (HF). Although amlodipine is safe in this setting, verapamil and diltiazem may worsen systolic HF, and their use is limited to the treatment of diastolic HF.

ent arterioles and thereby reduce glomerular filtration rate. Worsening renal function can be seen in 5–30% of patients treated with these agents; the risks are significantly higher in patients with more severe heart failure and in those with bilateral renal artery stenosis. Hypokalemia may also occur, even in the absence of declining renal function. At least 5–10% of patients treated with ACE inhibitors develop a dry, nonproductive cough. This likely results from the inhibition of bradykinin metabolism and resolves with cessation of the drug. Less than 1% of patients develop angioedema when treated with ACE inhibitors. This can be life-threatening and precludes further use of the drug. Both the efficacy and side effect profile of ACE inhibitors are affected by volume status, and careful monitoring of volume and appropriate diuretic dosing are important. Volume overload will blunt the therapeutic effects of ACE inhibitors, and whereas dietary sodium restriction may enhance the response to ACE inhibitors, volume depletion will exaggerate their hypotensive effects.

Angiotensin Receptor-Blocking Agents (ARBs)

Angiotensin receptor-blocking agents differ from ACE inhibitors in that they inhibit the binding of angiotensin to its receptor rather than blocking its production. Theoretically, ARBs should be more effective at inhibiting the renin–angiotensin–aldosterone system as they block angiotensin produced by both ACE and non-ACE pathways; however, clinical trials of ARB therapy in heart failure have not demonstrated consistent superiority over ACE inhibitors.[46] A meta-analysis of 17 trials comprising more than 12,000 patients demonstrated that ARBs were not superior to ACE inhibitors in reducing morbidity or mortality of patients with heart failure, although they appear to be beneficial in patients who are not already taking ACE inhibitors.[28] Recently, the results of the Candesartan in Heart Failure Assessment of Reduction in Mortality and Morbidity (CHARM) trials have shed more light on this subject.[45] These studies revealed that in patients with classes II–IV heart failure and LVEF ≤40%, treatment with the ARB candesartan results in clinically important reductions in mortality and hospitalization for heart failure. Importantly, the benefit was seen in patients who were intolerant with ACE inhibitors.[24] Furthermore, in patients who were already receiving an optimal dose of an ACE inhibitor, the addition of candesartan produced additive clinical benefit.[33]

ARBs have a similar risk of hypotension, renal dysfunction, and hyperkalemia as do ACE inhibitors, and combination ARB/ACEI therapy is associated with an increased incidence of these adverse effects. The risk of angioedema appears to be decreased with ARBs compared with ACE inhibitors. Additionally, because ARBs do not affect the kinin system, the incidence of cough is significantly less than that with ACE inhibitors. In general, ARBs are not yet considered first-line therapy for heart failure, although guidelines in this regard are evolving. ARBs are, however, a reasonable alternative in patients who are intolerant of ACE inhibitors owing to the development of a persistent cough or angioedema, and should be considered as additive therapy in patients with symptoms of persistent heart failure despite ACEI use.

β-Adrenergic-Blocking Agents

The recent understanding of heart failure not only as a hemodynamic syndrome related to LV systolic dysfunction, but as a state of adverse neurohormone-mediated remodeling, has prompted extensive investigation into the utility of β-blocking agents in the treatment of heart failure. Basic studies have shown that these agents can inhibit the adverse effects of norepinephrine on the myocardium and result in up-regulation of cardiac β-adrenergic receptors. The long-term administration of these agents is associated with a reversal of LV remodeling resulting in a decrease in LV volume and an increase in ejection fraction with concomitant improvement in hemodynamics.[6]

Large clinical trials encompassing more than 10,000 patients have demonstrated that these effects translate into significant clinical benefit.[8,14,34,39,41] Although the enrollment criteria and the specific β-blocking agent used varied between the trials, they all included patients with systolic heart failure (LV ejection fraction <35–45%) who were already being treated with a regimen of an ACE inhibitor and diuretic, with or without digoxin. In summary, these trials demonstrated an approximate 35% reduction in mortality and 40% reduction in hospitalization due to heart failure in patients treated with β-blocking agents.[30] Additionally, treatment with β-blockers reduces symptoms of heart failure and improves exercise capacity, although these effects may not be evident for several weeks or months after initiation of treatment (Figure 61-4).

Figure 61-4 The effect of β-blocker therapy on clinical end points in patients with heart failure. Data from trials using metoprolol, carvedilol, bucindolol, and nebivolol. HF indicates heart failure. End points D and E refer to patients who improved or deteriorated by at least one class. Left ventricular ejection fraction (LVEF) was measured after at least 5 months of therapy and reflects an unweighted mean increase of 29% with β-blocker therapy.
(Modified from Lechat P, Packer M, Chalon S, et al: Clinical effects of beta-adrenergic blockade in chronic heart failure: A meta-analysis of double-blind, placebo-controlled, randomized trials. Circulation 98:1184–1191, 1998.)

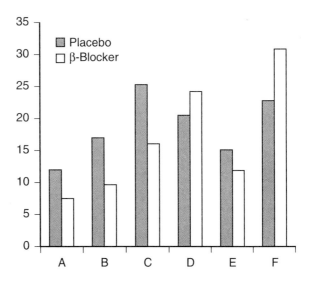

End point	Placebo	β-Blocker	OR	95% CI
A. All cause mortality	11.9%	7.5%	0.68	0.003
B. Hospitalization for HF	17.0%	9.6%	0.59	<0.001
C. Combined end point	25.4%	16.0%	0.63	<0.001
D. NYHA improvement	20.6%	24.3%	1.32	0.04
E. NYHA deterioration	15.3%	12.0%	0.70	0.03
F. LVEF (%)	23	31	–	$P < 10^{-9}$

992

Currently, three β-blocking agents are approved by the Food and Drug Administration (FDA) for the treatment of systolic heart failure: metoprolol, carvedilol, and bisoprolol. Metoprolol and bisoprolol are β₁-receptor specific, whereas carvedilol inhibits the β₁-, β₂-, and α₁-receptors and has both vasodilatory and antioxidant properties. The absolute magnitude of benefit is similar with these agents, and current trial data are inadequate to support use of one agent over another. β-Blocker therapy for heart failure should be initiated at lower doses than is routinely used for the treatment of hypertension or angina, and gradually titrated upward to doses that have demonstrated benefit in clinical trials (Table 61-6).

Use of β-blocking agents can be associated with significant adverse effects in patients with heart failure. The renal hemodynamic effect of these agents may result in volume retention, which, when combined with their negative inotropic effect, may cause an initial worsening of heart failure symptoms. This adverse effect is more common in patients who are volume overloaded prior to β-blocker therapy and usually responds to an increase in diuretic dose. Hypotension is frequently seen after the initiation of β-blockers and may limit use of these agents. This effect is more pronounced with carvedilol, owing to its peripheral vasodilating effects, and can usually be managed with a reduction in dose or changing to a β₁-receptor-specific agent. Other frequent side effects include fatigue and bradycardia, both of which can usually be managed with reduction of the dose of β-blocker and/or discontinuation of other AV nodal blocking agents (e.g., digoxin). Given the strength of the data supporting their use, β-blockers should be administered to all patients with systolic heart failure who do not have a contraindication to their use. Nonetheless, β-blockers should be avoided in patients with decompensated heart failure, symptomatic hypotension, or significant resting bradycardia or heart block in the absence of a permanent pacemaker.

Inotropic Agents

Digoxin

Digoxin is a cardiac glycoside and, as such, is a selective inhibitor of the membrane-bound Na⁺-K⁺-ATPase.[26] The binding of digoxin to this enzyme results in increased intracellular calcium with a resultant augmentation of myocardial contractility. In general the overall effect on global left ventricular systolic function is relatively small with an average absolute increase in ejection fraction of 1–2%. Digoxin also affects the cardiac conduction system through increases in vagal tone and decreases in sympathetic tone. This results in decreased automaticity of the atria and AV nodal tissues, and prolongation of the refractory period and reduction in conduction velocity of the AV node. The net result is a slowing of the atrial rate and blockade of the AV node.

Several clinical trials have evaluated the role of digoxin in the treatment of patients with heart failure. The Prospective Randomized study Of Ventricular failure and Efficacy of Digoxin (PROVED) and the Randomized Assessment of Digoxin on Inhibitors of Angiotensin Converting Enzyme (RADIANCE) trials studied the effects of withdrawal of digoxin from clinically stable patients with class II or III heart failure and systolic dysfunction.[42,53] They found that withdrawal

of digoxin was associated with a significant worsening of heart failure symptoms and deterioration of functional capacity. The Digitalis Investigation Group (DIG) trial evaluated the effect of starting digoxin in patients with systolic heart failure who were already receiving therapy with diuretics and ACE inhibitors.[18] In this trial, digoxin use was associated with a decrease in the risk of hospitalization for heart failure but no change in overall mortality. Thus, digoxin can no longer be considered a first-line therapy for patients with heart failure; however, it appears useful in patients who remain symptomatic despite therapy with other agents. In this setting, the serum digoxin level should be maintained at 0.5–0.8 ng/ml, as higher doses may be associated with adverse outcomes.

Digoxin may also be useful in the control of supraventricular arrhythmias in patients with depressed left ventricular systolic function. When used in this setting, digoxin may be given as an initial load (0.25 mg orally or intravenously every 8 h for 24 h) followed by a single daily dose of 0.125 or 0.25 mg. When used for the treatment of heart failure, there is little value in a loading dose, and once-daily dosing is appropriate. Digoxin is excreted unchanged by the kidney, and its dose must be adjusted in the setting of renal failure. It has a relatively narrow therapeutic window and intermittent monitoring of its serum level is required. Higher serum digoxin levels (>2.0 ng/ml) are associated with an increased risk of toxic side effects (Table 61-7), especially in the presence of hypokalemia or hypomagnesemia. Mild digoxin toxicity (ectopic beats, first-degree AV block, gastrointestinal symptoms) may require only withholding of the drug. More

Table 61–7
Signs and Symptoms of Digoxin Toxicity
Nausea, vomiting, abdominal pain
Anorexia
Fatigue, malaise
Confusion, delirium
Visual changes (yellow vision, halo around visual field)
First-, second-, and third-degree heart block
Excessively low ventricular rate in atrial fibrillation
Paroxysmal atrial tachycardia (classically with associated heart block)
Premature ventricular depolarizations
Ventricular tachycardia

severe toxicity (profound bradycardia, high-degree AV block, ventricular tachyarrhythmias) requires administration of digoxin-specific antibodies. Hemodialysis is ineffective for the treatment of digoxin toxicity.

Dopamine

Dopamine is the immediate metabolic precursor of epinephrine and norepinephrine. It is an endogenous catecholamine that functions as an essential neurotransmitter and is involved in the central regulation of movement and in the regulation of the cardiovascular system. Exogenously administered dopamine does not cross the blood–brain barrier, and thus, its effects are predominantly cardiovascular. The cardiovascular response to dopamine infusion is mediated by dopaminergic, β-adrenergic, and α-adrenergic receptors.[32] At low doses (e.g., 1–2 μg/kg/min) dopamine binds to dopaminergic receptors in the renal, mesenteric, and peripheral vasculature stimulating a rise in intracellular cyclic AMP and inducing vasodilation in these beds. Although it produces a mild fall in systemic vascular resistance (SVR), its main effect is to increase glomerular filtration rate, renal blood flow, and renal sodium excretion, thereby augmenting urine output. At intermediate doses (2–5 μg/kg/min), dopamine induces the release of norepinephrine from sympathetic nerve terminals in the heart and directly stimulates cardiac β_1-adrenergic receptors. This results in positive inotropic and chronotropic effects augmenting cardiac output and causing tachycardia. Although intermediate dose dopamine may be associated with increased systolic blood pressure, the SVR is usually unchanged owing to renal and splanchnic vasodilation. At high doses of dopamine (5–15 μg/kg/min), α-adrenergic stimulation occurs resulting in generalized vasoconstriction. A further rise in systolic blood pressure results; however, this occurs in association with an increase in SVR, which may suppress left ventricular systolic function owing to the increase in afterload. In addition, at high doses the α-adrenergic effects overcome the vasodilatory effects in the renal and splanchnic vessels, and renal blood flow and urine output may decline.

The varied hemodynamic effects of dopamine make it a potentially useful agent for the treatment of heart failure in a variety of clinical settings. In the patient with congestion and oliguria but with adequate blood pressure, low-dose dopamine increases renal blood flow thereby improving renal function, and augments urine output thereby decreasing ventricular filling pressures. In the patient with cardiogenic shock, higher dose dopamine is useful to maintain an adequate blood pressure. When used at the higher doses patients must be monitored closely for signs of worsening heart failure; placement of a pulmonary arterial catheter is helpful in this regard. Although the increased SVR may be partially offset by the increase in cardiac contractility, in many patients, the ventricular filling pressures rise as a result of increased afterload. In addition, the venoconstricting effects augment venous return, thereby increasing ventricular preload. For these reasons, dopamine is not routinely used alone for inotropic support of the failing heart. Rather, for the treatment of patients with CHF, dopamine is often combined with another inotrope (e.g., dobutamine) or vasodilator (e.g., nitroprusside).

Although dopamine may have beneficial effects in some patients with CHF, there are few data to suggest an improvement in long-term outcomes. The use of dopamine is often limited by the development of tachycardia, which may precipitate ischemia in patients with coronary artery disease. Both supraventricular and ventricular arrhythmias may occur. In addition, it may cause nausea, vomiting, and headaches, and may precipitate myocardial ischemia. Marked vasoconstriction may result in digital gangrene, especially in patients with peripheral vascular disease, and ischemic skin necrosis may occur at sites of cutaneous infiltration.

Dobutamine

Dobutamine is a synthetic catecholamine that acts by direct stimulation of α- and β-adrenergic receptors and is available as a racemic mixture of its (+) and (−) stereoisomers.[48] The (−) isomer is a potent α_1-receptor agonist and a relatively weak β_1-receptor agonist. The (+) isomer is a potent β_1- and β_2-receptor agonist and an α_1-receptor antagonist. The net effect is relatively selective β_1-receptor stimulation, resulting in augmentation of contractility and increased cardiac output. In contrast to the hemodynamic effects of dopamine, the inotropic effect of dobutamine is associated with relatively little increase in heart rate and with a modest reduction in left ventricular filling pressure and peripheral resistance. The latter effect results from β_2-receptor-mediated vasodilation. Dobutamine does not bind to dopamine receptors; thus, it does not result in renal or splanchnic vasodilation. Nonetheless, renal blood flow may increase as a reflection of increased cardiac output.

The hemodynamic effects of dobutamine make it an ideal agent for the treatment of decompensated heart failure, either alone or in combination with other inotropic or vasodilating agents. Dobutamine is usually started at a dose of 2.5 μg/kg/min and up-titrated in increments of 2.5 μg/kg/min as needed until an adequate therapeutic effect is obtained, adverse effects occur, or the maximum therapeutic dose is reached (15–20 μg/kg/min). Patients with more advanced heart failure may have a greater degree of β-receptor down-regulation and require higher initial doses of dobutamine. Patients on chronic β-blocker therapy may initially have relatively little inotropic response to dobutamine but a moderate vasopressor response resulting from the unmasking of α_1-adrenergic vasoconstriction in the presence of β-receptor blockade.

If an adequate therapeutic response is not achieved despite maximal doses of dobutamine, a second agent should be added. For patients with increased ventricular filling pressures and adequate systolic blood pressure, the addition of a diuretic and a vasodilator (such as nitroprusside) should be considered. Alternatively, a phosphodiesterase inhibitor such as milrinone (see later) may be of value in this setting by further augmenting cardiac output and vasodilation. Patients with CHF associated with hypotension may require the addition of a vasopressor (e.g., high-dose dopamine) to augment blood pressure and allow effective diuresis.

Dobutamine has proven an effective agent in the management of hospitalized patients with CHF. Additionally, intermittent administration of dobutamine to outpatients

994 with severe heart failure has resulted in an improvement in patients' symptoms and may reduce hospital admissions.[37] However, there has not been a demonstrable improvement in mortality in either setting. Continuous infusions of dobutamine are usually well tolerated for up to several days, although tolerance may develop and limit the efficacy of longer-term infusion. Dobutamine administration is occasionally limited by the development of excess tachycardia; however, it is not uncommon to see a slight fall in the heart rate after dobutamine infusion owing to withdrawal of sympathetic tone as the patient's hemodynamic status improves. Patients with a prior history of hypertension may have a marked hypertensive response to dobutamine, while those with volume depletion may become hypotensive as a result of mild vasodilation. As with dopamine, dobutamine, may precipitate atrial and ventricular arrhythmias and may aggravate myocardial ischemia.

Phosphodiesterase Inhibitors

Phosphodiesterase (PDE) is a membrane-bound enzyme that breaks down cyclic adenosine monophosphate (cAMP). It exists in several forms with type III PDE being the predominant isoform in cardiovascular issue. Milrinone and amrinone inhibit this enzyme and thereby result in increased cytosolic cAMP. This in turn results in increased myocardial contractility and augmentation of cardiac output. In the vasculature, these agents are potent vasodilators and venodilators resulting in reductions in systemic and pulmonary vascular resistance (afterload) and in right- and left-sided filling pressures (preload).

The mixed hemodynamic effects of PDE inhibitors distinguish them from other inotropes or vasodilators. When compared with dobutamine, milrinone produces a greater reduction in systemic vascular resistance for a given increase in cardiac output.[15] Similarly, when compared with nitroprusside, milrinone produces a greater increase in cardiac output for a given reduction in systemic vascular resistance (Figure 61-5).[36] Thus, PDE inhibitors may be useful for the management of patients with decompensated heart failure that is characterized by reduced cardiac output, elevated SVR, and elevated filling pressures. PDE inhibitors also have antiplatelet effects and cause dilation of epicardial coronary arteries and bypass grafts. These properties, combined with the previously noted reductions in pulmonary arterial pressure and pulmonary vascular resistance, have given these agents an important role in the hemodynamic support of patients following cardiac surgery.

Amrinone (now renamed inamrinone) is less selective for the PDE III isoenzyme, has a longer elimination half-life (2–3 h vs. 30–60 min), and is approximately 10-fold less potent than milrinone. Additionally, it has been associated with significant thrombocytopenia in 10% of patients in whom it is administered. For these reasons, amrinone has fallen out of favor and milrinone has become the PDE inhibitor of choice for the management of decompensated heart failure. Milrinone is given as an initial loading dose (50 μg/kg over 10 min) followed by a continuous infusion (0.25–1.0 μg/kg/min). It is excreted predominantly by the kidney; in patients with renal failure a 50% reduction in the infusion rate is required. Titration may be limited by the development of tachycardia and arrhythmias, both of which

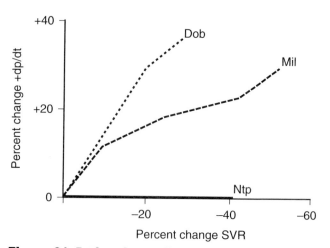

Figure 61–5 The relative effects of varying doses of nitroprusside (Ntp), dobutamine (Dob), and milrinone (Mil) on the peak positive dP/dt and systemic vascular resistance (SVR). *(Adapted from Colucci WS, Wright RF, Jaski BE, et al: Milrinone and dobutamine in severe heart failure: differing hemodynamic effects and individual patient responsiveness. Circulation 73; III-175, 1986.)*

are mediated by the increase in cAMP. Owing to the potent vasodilatory properties of PDE inhibitors, they should be used with care in patients who have normal or low vascular resistance and/or filling pressures. These patients may be intolerant of the vasodilation and marked hypotension may result.

Clinical trials have demonstrated the efficacy of intravenous milrinone in improving hemodynamics and reducing symptoms in hospitalized patients with decompensated heart failure.[17,49] However, a mortality benefit has not been demonstrated, and when administered routinely to patients with less severe CHF (i.e., no evidence of end-organ hypoperfusion), it does not appear to offer benefit over usual treatment with ACE inhibitors and diuretics.

Other Agents

Natriuretic Peptides

Natriuretic peptides are naturally occurring peptides that are produced in low levels in the normal heart. Atrial natriuretic peptide (ANP) is produced in the atria, whereas brain natriuretic peptide (BNP; originally isolated from porcine brain tissue) is produced in the ventricles. In patients with heart failure both ANP and BNP are secreted at high levels in response to increased intracardiac pressure and volume. These peptides act via a receptor-mediated guanosine monophosphate pathway in vascular smooth muscle cells and are degraded by neutral endopeptidase. They have potent balanced vasodilating actions resulting in decreased ventricular preload and afterload.[31] In the kidney these peptides cause vasodilation of the afferent arteriole thereby increasing glomerular filtration rate, and inhibit sodium reabsorption in the renal collecting ducts and aldosterone secretion by the adrenal glands thereby resulting in natriuresis and diuresis.

Nesiritide is a recombinant peptide that is identical to endogenous BNP and has both vasodilatory and natriuretic properties. In addition, it antagonizes the renin–angiotensin–aldosterone system. When administered to patients with heart failure, nesiritide reduces right atrial and pulmonary capillary wedge pressures, decreases systemic vascular resistance, increases cardiac output, and produces a diuresis and natriuresis.[13] Clinical studies have demonstrated persistent hemodynamic effects of prolonged (24–48 h) infusions and improvements in clinical status that may be greater than that seen with intravenous nitroglycerin.[35,54] Nesiritide is usually given as an initial bolus of 2 μg/kg followed by an infusion of 0.01 μg/kg/min. Its hemodynamic effects are apparent within 15 min and persist for up to 4 h after discontinuation of the infusion. Significant and prolonged hypotension can occur with this agent and is the most common limiting factor. It does not aggravate arrhythmias and has no toxic metabolites. Although it is not yet a first-line therapy for heart failure, nesiritide is a reasonable option in patients with decompensated CHF characterized by volume overload and increased filling pressures, especially for patients who are intolerant of inotropic agents and resistant to usual diuretics.

▶ APPROACH TO THE MANAGEMENT OF HEART FAILURE

Initial Approach/Clinical Assessment

The treatment of heart failure is dependent upon its recognition. Because heart failure may present in a variety of ways the clinician must maintain a high index of suspicion, especially in the patient with a prior history of heart failure or with risk factors for the development of heart failure. Acute heart failure usually presents dramatically with signs and symptoms of pulmonary and systemic congestion, at times associated with evidence of hypoperfusion (Table 61-8). In this setting the clinical examination is usually striking and the diagnosis is rarely overlooked. Conversely, chronic heart failure may have a more indolent course and the associated dyspnea, fatigue, and edema may be mistaken for other noncardiac conditions. Additionally, the physical examination of patients with chronic heart failure may be somewhat misleading in that they often have clear lung fields despite having significantly elevated filling pressures.

The initial evaluation of the patient with heart failure should include an assessment of the disease severity. The most common classification in this regard is that devised by the New York Heart Association (Table 61-2), which categorizes patients with symptomatic heart failure based upon their functional level. A broader classification scheme has recently been proposed by the American College of Cardiology/American Heart Association (ACC/AHA) and includes patients with structurally normal hearts but at risk for developing heart failure (Stage A), those with asymptomatic structural heart disease (Stage B), those with overt heart failure (Stage C), and those with severe heart failure that require specialized care such as mechanical assistance or transplantation (Stage D). Although the functional class may vary over time, these classifications remain useful because they provide an objective measure by which to follow disease progression and response to therapy. Additionally, the choice of specific therapies is, in part, dependent on disease sever-

ity. Patients with severe decompensated heart failure require the rapid administration of intravenous pharmacological therapy to reduce pulmonary congestion, augment perfusion of vital organs, and attain hemodynamic stability. Conversely patients with chronic compensated heart failure can frequently be treated with oral medications with the goal of controlling symptoms, improving functional capacity, and reducing long-term mortality.

In addition to the initiation of pharmacological therapy, the initial approach to the care of the patient with heart failure should always include a thorough evaluation of the etiology of heart failure and a careful search for aggravating or precipitating factors (Table 61-9). Although the history and physical examination may provide clues to the underlying cardiac abnormality, a formal assessment of cardiac function by echocardiography should be performed in all patients presenting with new or significantly worsened heart failure. This test permits identification and characterization of pericardial, myocardial, and valvular disease, and allows for the quantification of left ventricular systolic and diastolic function. Initial laboratory evaluation should also include a chest roentgenogram (to assess cardiac size, pulmonary congestion, and structural intrathoracic abnormalities), ECG (to evaluate for evidence of ischemic heart disease or ventricular hypertrophy), complete blood count, electrolytes, thyroid function tests, and assessment of renal function.

All patients with heart failure should be counseled regarding lifestyle modifications that may help to alleviate their symptoms. This includes moderate sodium restriction (≤2 g sodium daily); compliance with treatment regimens; and avoidance of alcohol, cigarettes, and nonsteroidal antiinflammatory agents. Most heart failure patients do not require fluid restriction, but close monitoring of their weight is essential for the early recognition of volume retention.

Table 61–8

Signs and Symptoms of Heart Failure

Evidence of congestion	Evidence of hypoperfusion
Symptoms	Symptoms
Orthopnea	Fatigue, weakness
Dyspnea on exertion	Confusion
Paroxysmal nocturnal dyspnea	Symptomatic hypotension
Anorexia, nausea	
Signs	Signs
Pulmonary rales	Cool extremities
Elevated jugular venous pressure	Mottled extremities
Hepatojugular reflux	Narrowed pulse pressure
Edema	Worsening renal insufficiency
Ascites	Progressive hyponatremia
Loud S_3	Cheyne–Stokes respirations

Table 61–9

Potential Aggravating Factors Contributing to Decompensation in Chronic Heart Failure

Myocardial ischemia or infarction

Systemic hypertension

Tachyarrhythmias (ventricular or supraventricular)

Superimposed valvular heart disease

Exacerbation of underlying lung disease

Pulmonary embolism

Infection

Thyroid disease

Anemia

Medication noncompliance

Dietary indiscretions (excessive salt and water intake)

Excessive alcohol use

Pharmacological Treatment of Chronic Compensated Systolic Heart Failure

Patients with chronic compensated heart failure represent a spectrum of patients ranging from those with asymptomatic LV dysfunction to those with previously decompensated heart failure who have responded to medical therapy. The goals of treatment in this population include maintenance of a symptom-free state, improvement in functional capacity, prevention of decompensation, and reduction of mortality. Several individual classes of medications have proven efficacy in this regard (Table 61-10), although in general, most patients with systolic heart failure require multidrug therapy.[27]

All patients with LV systolic dysfunction should receive treatment with an ACE inhibitor as these agents improve mortality of patients with all classes of heart failure and delay the onset of symptoms in patients with asymptomatic left ventricular dysfunction. Therapy should be initiated at low doses and slowly titrated upward if tolerated (i.e., systolic blood pressure > 90 mm Hg, no symptoms of hypotension) to doses that have been proven efficacious in randomized trials (Table 61-6). Renal function should be monitored closely, especially in patients with concomitant vascular disease. Other vasodilators should be considered in patients with symptomatic heart failure who are unable to tolerate ACE inhibitors owing to side effects. Although angiotensin receptor blocking agents should not be used as first-line therapy for heart failure, they are the preferred agents for patients who develop cough to ACE inhibitors. Patients who develop progressive renal insufficiency or hyperkalemia with ACE inhibitors are equally likely to develop these complications with ARBs; these agents should not be used in this setting. The combination of hydralazine and nitrates is a less effective regimen than ACE inhibitors, but is a reasonable alternative in patients who are intolerant of these agents or ARBs.

All patients with class II–IV heart failure should also receive a β-blocker, as these agents provide a marked mortality benefit. Care most be taken to ensure that patients are hemodynamically stable and euvolemic prior to starting β-blocker therapy as initiation of β-blockade may be associated with orthostatic hypotension and worsening of heart failure symptoms. These agents should always be started at low doses (see Table 61-6), titrated very slowly (increasing dose every 2 weeks), and should be avoided in patients who recently required intravenous diuretics or inotropic agents. They should also be avoided in patients with a heart rate <60 bpm, systolic blood pressure <100 mm Hg, or evidence of AV block, and should be used with care in patients with bronchospastic lung disease. Most patients with heart failure who receive β-blocker therapy should be concomitantly treated with diuretics, especially those patients with current or recent volume retention. If heart failure symptoms worsen after starting β-blockers, diuretic therapy should be increased and usually allows for continued β-blocker use. In general, β-blocker therapy should not be initiated during the hospitalization of patients with decompensated heart failure; rather, they should be started as an outpatient once a stable medical regimen has been established. It is generally preferable to initiate ACE inhibitor therapy prior to β-blocker therapy, as the former agents result in rapid relief of symptoms and may facilitate the initiation of the β-blocker.

Patients with symptoms or signs of congestion may respond to afterload reducing therapy alone; however, most require the addition of a diuretic. Loop diuretics such as furosemide are preferred as they are more effective than thiazide diuretics, especially in patients with renal insufficiency (serum creatinine >2.5 mg/dl). If volume overload persists despite upward titration of the loop diuretic, then addition of a thiazide (e.g., Zaroxolyn 2.5 mg orally given 30 min prior to the loop diuretic) should be considered and provides effective combination therapy. This combination can lead to profound potassium and magnesium wasting and requires close monitoring of serum electrolytes. Spironolactone 25–50 mg daily should be added to the regimen of patients with class IV heart failure as it provides a mortality benefit in this setting.

Digoxin should be considered in any patient who continues to have symptomatic heart failure despite treatment with ACE inhibitors and β-blockers. Although this agent has not demonstrated a mortality benefit in any class of heart failure, when used as part of a multidrug regimen it is useful for controlling symptoms and reducing hospital admissions. It may be particularly beneficial in patients with atrial

Table 61–10

Beneficial Effects of Oral Pharmacotherapy for Chronic Heart Failure

Medication	? Improves mortality	? Improves symptoms	? Reduces recurrent HF	Heart failure class for which treatment indicated
Angiotensin-converting enzyme inhibitors	Yes	Yes	Yes	Class I–IV[a]
β-Blockers	Yes	Yes	Yes	Class II–IV
Hydralazine	Yes	Yes	No	Class II—IV[b]
Spironolactone	Yes	Yes	No	Class III–IV
Diuretics	No	Yes	No	Class II–IV
Digoxin	No	Yes	Yes	Class II–IV

[a]Also indicated in patients with asymptomatic left ventricular systolic dysfunction.
[b]Not a first line drug but should be considered in patients who are intolerant of angiotensin-converting enzyme inhibitors.

fibrillation in whom improved heart rate control may lead to symptomatic improvement.

Treatment of Decompensated Systolic Heart Failure

Patients with chronic systolic heart failure may have periods of relative stability interrupted by periods of decompensation. These periods of decompensation may be precipitated by medication noncompliance, dietary indiscretion (e.g., excessive sodium or water intake), or progression of the underlying myopathic process. Often the patient will report a gradual worsening of symptoms or progressive weight gain over the course of several days, although the clinical presentation may appear relatively acute.

Patients with decompensated heart failure may present with hemodynamic instability and usually have evidence of systemic and pulmonary congestion with or without evidence of decreased organ perfusion. Although pulmonary arterial catheterization is sometimes necessary to precisely define the hemodynamic derangement, many patients with decompensated heart failure can be adequately evaluated on the basis of their clinical history and physical examination, specifically, whether or not they have evidence of pulmonary or systemic congestion and/or organ hypoperfusion. The presence of congestion may be evidenced by an elevation in the jugular venous pressure, the presence of pulmonary rales, or peripheral edema. These patients are usually dyspneic with minimal exertion or even at rest and often report increased orthopnea and paroxysmal nocturnal dyspnea. Hypoperfusion may be manifest as cold extremities, mottled skin, cyanosis, mental obtundation, or declining renal function. Measurement of the pulse pressure (the

difference between the systolic and diastolic blood pressures) may be quite helpful; in patients with heart failure, the pulse pressure narrows. A pulse pressure of less than 25% of the systolic blood pressure generally correlates with a cardiac index of less than 2.2 liters/min/m².

For patients in whom the hemodynamic profile needs to be more accurately defined or in whom initial therapy yields suboptimal results, direct measurement of hemodynamic parameters should be performed through the insertion of a Swan-Ganz catheter (Table 61-11). The information thus obtained may be used to guide the selection and titration of specific pharmacological therapy. Such "tailored therapy" should be undertaken with the goal of manipulating medications to achieve optimal hemodynamics, including a right atrial pressure <8 mm Hg, a pulmonary capillary wedge pressure <18 mm Hg, a cardiac index >2.2 liters/min/m², and a systemic vascular resistance of 800–1200 dynes-cm s⁻⁵.

When taken together, these findings can be used to classify the severity of hemodynamic impairment of a patient presenting with decompensated heart failure and help to make decisions regarding appropriate initial therapy (Figure 61-6).[52] Patients with LV dysfunction who are well compensated generally have acceptable filling pressures and adequate cardiac outputs, do not have congestion, and appear well-perfused. These patients require chronic heart failure therapy as outlined above for symptom control and mortality reduction. Patients with decompensated heart failure who have evidence of congestion without hypoperfusion have elevated filling pressures with adequate cardiac output. These patients may simply be volume overloaded and require aggressive diuresis. If the blood pressure is adequate, addition of a vasodilator (e.g., ACE inhibitor) may

Table 61–11

Potential Indications for Invasive Hemodynamic Assessment in Patients with Heart Failure

Assessment of volume status when clinical assessment is uncertain

Distinguishing heart failure from other etiologies of dyspnea (e.g., pulmonary disease)

Assessment of hemodynamic response to vasoactive medications

Guidance in achieving ideal hemodynamic goals ("tailored therapy")

Assessment of filling pressure in patients with persistent symptoms of heart failure despite aggressive medical therapy

Determination of appropriate therapy in patients with persistent congestion and progressive renal insufficiency following diuretic therapy

Assessment of pulmonary vascular resistance during evaluation for cardiac transplantation

Perioperative monitoring of volume status in patients with severe left ventricular dysfunction undergoing prolonged procedures associated with significant volume shifts or in patients with decompensated heart failure on preoperative assessment

---

further augment cardiac output and facilitate diuresis. Patients with signs of hypoperfusion but without congestion have acceptable filling pressures but decreased cardiac output. Therapy in this setting should be guided by the patient's blood pressure: patients with hypotension require inotropic therapy, whereas patients with adequate systolic blood pressure (>100 mm Hg) should receive vasodilators with or without inotropic agents to augment cardiac output. These patients do not generally require aggressive diuresis and, in fact, may be volume deplete and require gentle hydration. Patients with evidence of both congestion and hypoperfusion have both elevated filling pressures and decreased cardiac output and are the most difficult to manage. These patients frequently require combination therapy with inotropic agents, intravenous vasodilator therapy, and use of diuretics. Invasive hemodynamic monitoring may be most helpful in guiding therapy in this latter group of patients, especially in patients with associated hypotension.

A variety of intravenous agents are available for use in the treatment of patients with decompensated heart failure (Table 61-12). Initial management should be guided by the patient's specific hemodynamic alterations. In patients with severe hypotension leading to organ dysfunction, stabilization of the blood pressure is the primary goal, and the initial drug of choice is usually dopamine at moderate to high doses. Epinephrine or norepinephrine may be added if high doses of dopamine are inadequate; however, these agents are rarely required in the absence of pathological vasodilation (e.g., sepsis, postanesthesia). In general, vasoconstrictors should be avoided in patients with LV dysfunction as they may lead to further depression of cardiac output. In patients with adequate blood pressure whose predominant manifestation of heart failure is congestion, initial treatment with nitroprusside (or nitroglycerin or nesiritide) is usually effective. In patients whose predominant manifestation is hypoperfusion, dobutamine, milrinone, nitroprusside, or nesiritide may all be effective. The vast majority of patients with decompensated heart failure also require administration of intravenous diuretics and careful management of fluid balance.

Treatment of Diastolic Heart Failure

In contrast to the treatment of systolic heart failure, the treatment of diastolic heart failure has not been extensively studied and there are no large-scale, randomized trials by which to guide therapeutic recommendations. The general approach is aimed at treatment of the underlying cause and the relief of symptoms with medications that intuitively should reduce diastolic pressures.[57,58] The impairment in diastolic filling results in an increase in atrial pressure early in the course of this disease, with resultant pulmonary and venous congestion. Diuretics, therefore, play an important role in the management of this syndrome and help to control congestive symptoms. Care must be taken to avoid overdiuresis as these patients depend on an elevated filling pressure to maintain stroke volume. Calcium channel blockers (verapamil or diltiazem) and β-blockers slow the heart rate, prolong diastole, and allow increased time for left ventricular filling. Additionally, these agents may actually improve diastolic ventricular function (e.g., decrease LV stiffness and improve LV relaxation), owing to improvement

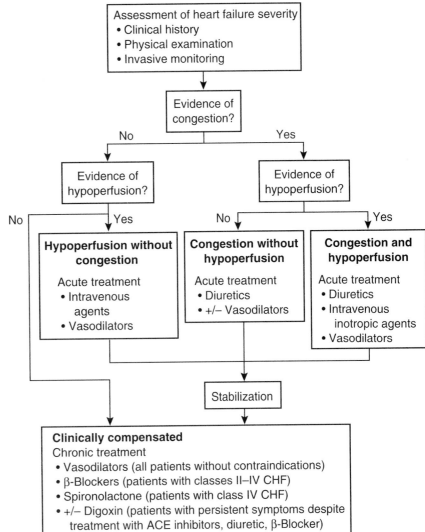

Figure 61–6 An approach to treatment of acute or decompensated heart failure.

in calcium homeostasis. In patients who are intolerant of these medications or have continued symptoms despite their use, ACE inhibitors may offer further benefit. Recent data suggest that ventricular hypertrophy is associated with stimulation of the renin–angiotensin system and that chronic activation of this system results in fluid retention as well as myocardial fibrosis and increased ventricular stiffness. Inhibition of this system with ACE inhibitors or ARBs may, therefore, offer further treatment of the underlying pathophysiological changes characteristic of diastolic heart failure.[55] Inotropic therapy, including digoxin, should be avoided in diastolic heart failure; these agents are unlikely to be beneficial in the face of preserved systolic function and may worsen diastolic function leading to further elevation of filling pressures and progressive heart failure.

Nonpharmacological therapies for diastolic heart failure are aimed at treating the underlying cause of the dysfunction and correcting associated abnormalities that may worsen this dysfunction. Patients with coronary artery disease should be aggressively treated with antianginal ther-

apy, and coronary revascularization should be performed when appropriate. Patients with secondary causes of hypertension (e.g., renal artery stenosis, hyperadrenalism) should undergo definitive therapy when possible. Aortic stenosis should be surgically corrected when it is associated with diastolic heart failure, even in the absence of systolic dysfunction. Patients with diastolic heart failure are highly preload dependent and may experience acute decompensation if they develop atrial fibrillation. This occurs in part because of the loss of the active atrial contribution to LV filling and in part because the increased heart rate associated with the development of atrial fibrillation shortens diastole and allows less time for LV filling. All efforts should be made to restore and maintain sinus rhythm in these individuals.

Flash Pulmonary Edema

Decompensated heart failure that develops acutely in a previously asymptomatic or well-compensated patient is often

Table 61–12

Intravenous Agents Used in the Treatment of Decompensated Heart Failure

Medication	Hemodynamic effects	Potential adverse clinical effects

Dopamine
    Low dose
    Intermediate dose
    High dose
	Splanchnic vasodilation, ↑GFR, ↑urine output
	↑HR, ↑contractility, ↑CO, ↑BP, ↑/–SVR
	↑HR, ↑↑contractility, ↑↑BP, ↑↑SVR, ↓CO,
	    ↑PCW, ↓/–GFR
		Myocardial ischemia, arrhythmias
		Myocardial ischemia, arrhythmias, ↑CHF,
		    worsened renal function

Dobutamine	↑HR, ↑↑contractility, ↑CO, ↑/–BP, ↓SVR, ↓PCW	Myocardial ischemia, arrhythmias
Isoproterenol	↑↑HR, ↑contractility, ↑CO, ↓SVR	Myocardial ischemia
Epinephrine	↑HR, ↑contractility, ↑SVR, ↑BP	Myocardial ischemia, arrhythmias, ↑CHF, worsened renal function
Norepinephrine	↑HR, ↑contractility, ↑↑SVR, ↑↑BP	Myocardial ischemia, arrhythmias, ↑CHF, worsened renal function
Milrinone	↑Contractility, ↑↑CO, ↓↓SVR, ↓PVR, ↓↓PCW	Myocardial ischemia, arrhythmias, hypotension
Nitroprusside	↑↑CO, ↓↓SVR, ↓PVR, ↓↓PCW; no effect on contractility	Hypotension, cyanide and thiocyanate toxicity
Nitroglycerin	↑CO, ↓SVR, ↓PVR, ↓↓PCW, coronary vasodilation; no effect on contractility	Hypotension, headache, nitrate tolerance
Niseritide	↑CO, ↓SVR, ↓↓PCW, ↑GFR; natruresis, diuresis	Hypotension

BP, blood pressure; GFR, glomerular filtration rate; HR, heart rate; CO, cardiac output; SVR, systemic vascular resistance; PCW, pulmonary capillary wedge (pressure); PVR, pulmonary vascular resistance.

the result of an abrupt change in cardiac structure or function (Table 61-13). The precipitous nature of the presentation of these patients accounts for the commonly used descriptive term *flash pulmonary edema*. In this setting patients are often hemodynamically unstable and develop severe pulmonary congestion, although they frequently are not fluid overloaded. Pharmacologically, these patients are treated similarly to the decompensated patients described above; however, specific therapy should be guided by the underlying precipitating factor. Patients with ischemia precipitating acute heart failure frequently have severe coronary artery disease (e.g., three-vessel or left main coronary artery disease) or have papillary muscle dysfunction resulting in acute mitral regurgitation (most common with disease of the right coronary artery). In addition to heart failure therapy as dictated by their clinical presentation, these patients should receive aggressive antianginal therapy with intravenous nitrates and antiplatelet agents (e.g., aspirin,

heparin, IIb/IIIa inhibitors), and urgent cardiac catheterization and coronary revascularization should be considered. For patients with refractory heart failure and ischemia, intraaortic balloon pump (IABP) counterpulsation may be a beneficial adjuvant therapy while awaiting definitive revascularization.

Severe hypertension may precipitate acute heart failure. Classically this occurs with hypertension associated with pheochromocytomas, renal artery stenosis, and alcohol or cocaine use, but can also be seen in patients with preexisting heart failure who are noncompliant with medications or dietary sodium restriction. Appropriate therapy in this setting is dependent upon blood pressure control. Intravenous antihypertensive agents (e.g., nitroprusside, enalaprilat) should be started with the goal of lowering the mean arterial pressure by 25% in the first several hours and reducing the systolic blood pressure below 160 mm Hg within the first 24 hours. Acute severe aortic insuffi-

Table 61–13

Precipitants of Flash Pulmonary Edema and Their Therapeutic Implications

Acute	*Specific Therapeutic Considerations*
Ischemia/infarction	Cardiac catheterization and revascularization
Hypertension	Intravenous vasodilators (Nipride, enalaprilat) with 25% reduction in MAP as initial goal
Renal artery stenosis	Percutaneous renal artery revascularization
Aortic stenosis	Aortic valve replacement after initial stabilization with diuretics, +/− vasopressors, +/− inotropic agents
Acute aortic insufficiency (endocarditis, aortic dissection)	Aortic valve replacement after initial stabilization with vasodilators +/− inotropic agents
Acute mitral regurgitation (ischemia, endocarditis, rupture chordae)	Consider IABP for hemodynamic stabilization prior to coronary revascularization for ischemic MR or MVR for structural MR
Supraventricular tachyarrhythmias	Rate control or electrical cardioversion

IABP, intraaortic balloon pump; MAP, mean arterial pressure; MR, mitral regurgitation; MVR, mitral valve replacement.

ciency as occurs with endocarditis or aortic dissection should be managed with intravenous inotropic agents or vasodilators (depending on systemic blood pressure) while preparing for emergent surgical therapy. Acute mitral regurgitation often responds to vasodilator therapy, but may require IABP counterpulsation for stabilization prior to valve replacement.

Perioperative Heart Failure

For a variety of reasons, the incidence of heart failure is increased in the perioperative period. Many anesthetic agents have negatively inotropic effects and can precipitate heart failure in patients with LV systolic dysfunction, and the vasodilatory effects of these agents may result in hypotension. Aggressive fluid resuscitation in this setting may lead to volume overload, elevated filling pressures, and pulmonary congestion. Similarly, appropriate replacement of blood products in the face of intraoperative blood loss may be poorly tolerated and may require the concomitant administration of diuretics. Mechanical ventilation produces beneficial hemodynamic effects in heart failure owing to a reduction in venous return induced by the increased intrathoracic pressure. Conversely, the decrease in intrathoracic pressure associated with extubation may be followed by a sudden rise in preload and result in heart failure. Fluid that entered the extravascular space during the perioperative period reenters the vascular space several days postoperatively as patients begin to mobilize. This rise in

circulating blood volume may similarly precipitate heart failure. These adverse effects are more likely to occur in patients with preexisting LV dysfunction and in patients with overt heart failure preoperatively.

In the preoperative setting, the identification of decompensated heart failure is essential. The presence of pulmonary or systemic congestion or signs of hypoperfusion should prompt a thorough assessment of the patient's cardiac status, reevaluation of the patient's current therapy, and delay or cancellation of all but emergent procedures until the patient's status is stabilized. If the patient's ventricular function is not known, an echocardiogram should be performed to aid in determining the mechanism of heart failure and to guide appropriate therapy. In the postoperative period, heart failure may be mistaken for pneumonia, atelectasis, chronic obstructive pulmonary disease exacerbation, or pulmonary embolism. Patients are often unable to communicate their symptoms to the treating physicians owing to sedation and mechanical ventilation; thus, physician vigilance is essential. Identification of pulmonary rales, jugular venous distention, hepatojugular reflux, a gallop rhythm, and/or peripheral edema should raise the concern of worsening heart failure, and close monitoring of the patient's weight and fluid balance should alert the physician to the possibility of volume overload.

In patients with more advanced heart failure (class III or IV) or with severely depressed LV systolic function (e.g., LVEF <25%), placement of a pulmonary arterial catheter preoperatively should be strongly considered. In patients with decompensated heart failure, placement of this catheter the day prior to surgery allows time for maximization of their hemodynamic status, thereby potentially decreasing their overall perioperative risk. Continued invasive hemodynamic monitoring for 24–48 h after surgery may be appropriate in some patients.

Patients with chronic heart failure are often dependent on medications to maintain their hemodynamic stability, and every effort should be made to continue these medications in the perioperative period. Although it may be appropriate to hold diuretics on the day of surgery, careful monitoring for evidence of volume retention is obligatory perioperatively, and intravenous diuretics should be administered at the first signs of congestion. β-Blockers and ACE inhibitors should likewise be continued as the sudden withdrawal of these agents may result in neurohormonal activation and worsening of heart failure. Intravenous formulations may be substituted for many oral medications in patients who are unable to take oral agents postoperatively owing to the nature of their surgery. However, well-compensated patients will often tolerate withholding their usual medications and can be managed for several days with intravenous diuretics and topical nitrates for preload reduction. If refractory congestion or signs of organ hypoperfusion develop, use of intravenous vasodilators and/or inotropes may become necessary. These agents may be transitioned to oral formulations as gut absorption improves. For patients who remain hemodynamically labile postoperatively, use of short-acting agents may be appropriate for several days; long-acting agents may be reinstituted when the volume shifts and hemodynamic derangements improve. Given the tenuous nature of these patients, it is often helpful to involve a cardiology consultant to help manage the complex hemodynamic changes that occur in the perioperative period.

REFERENCES

1. Acute Infarction Ramipril Efficacy (AIRE) Study Investigators: Effects of ramipril on mortality and morbidity of survivors of acute myocardial infarction with clinical evidence of heart failure. Lancet 342:821, 1993.
2. Adamopoulos S, Piepolo M, Qiang F, et al: Effects of pulsed beta-stimulant therapy on beta-adrenoceptors and chronotropic responsiveness in chronic heart failure. Lancet 345:344, 1995.
3. Annane D, Bellissant E, Pussard E, et al: Placebo-controlled, randomized, double-blind study of intravenous enalaprilat efficacy and safety in acute cardiogenic pulmonary edema. Circulation 94:1316–1324, 1996.
4. Baig MK, Mahon N, McKenna WJ, et al: The pathophysiology of advanced heart failure. Heart Lung 28:87–101, 1999.
5. Brater DC: Diuretic therapy. N Engl J Med 339:387–395, 1998.
6. Bristow MR: β-Adrenergic receptor blockade in chronic heart failure. Circulation 101:558–569, 2000.
7. Capomolla S, Pozzoli M, Opasich C, et al: Dobutamine and nitroprusside infusion in patients with severe congestive heart failure: Hemodynamic improvement by discordant effects on mitral regurgitation, left atrial function, and ventricular function. Am Heart J 134:1089–1098, 1997.
8. CIBIS II Investigators and Committees. The cardiac insufficiency bisoprolol study II (CIBIS II): a randomised trial. Lancet 353:9–13, 1999.
9. Cohn JN, Archibald DG, Ziesche S, et al: Effect of vasodilator therapy on mortality in chronic congestive heart failure. Results of a Veterans Administration Cooperative Study. N Engl J Med 314:1547–1552, 1986.
10. Cohn JN, Ferrari R, Sharpe N: Cardiac remodeling—concepts and clinical implications: a consensus paper from an international forum on cardiac remodeling. J Am Coll Cardiol 35:569–582, 2000.
11. Cohn JN, Johnson G, Ziesche S, et al: A comparison of enalapril with hydralazine-isosorbide dinitrate in the treatment of chronic congestive heart failure. N Engl J Med 325:303–310, 1991.
12. Colucci WS, Braunwald E: In Braunwald E, Zipes DP, Libby P, editors: Heart Disease—A Textbook of Cardiovascular Medicine, 6th ed. Chapter 16, Pathophysiology of Heart Failure. Philadelphia: W.B. Saunders, 2001, pp. 503–533.
13. Colucci WS, Elkayam U, Horton DP, et al: Intravenous nesiritide, a natriuretic peptide, in the treatment of decompensated congestive heart failure. N Engl J Med 343:246–253, 2000.
14. Colucci WS, Packer M, Bristow MR, et al: Carvedilol inhibits clinical progression in patients with mild symptoms of heart failure. Circulation 94:2800–2806, 1996.
15. Colucci WS, Wright RF, Jaski BE, et al: Milrinone and dobutamine in severe heart failure: differing hemodynamic effects and individual patient responsiveness. Circulation 73:III175–183, 1986.
16. CONSENSUS Trial Study Group: Effects of enalapril on mortality in severe congestive heart failure. N Engl J Med 316:1429–1435, 1987.
17. Cuffe MS, Califf RM, Adams KF Jr, et al: Short-term intravenous milrinone for acute exacerbation of chronic heart failure: a randomized controlled trial. JAMA 287:1541–1547, 2002.
18. Digitalis Investigation Group. The effect of digoxin on mortality and morbidity in patients with heart failure. N Engl J Med 336:525–533, 1997.
19. Dormans TP, van Meyel JJ, Gerlag PG, et al: Diuretic efficacy of high dose furosemide in severe heart failure: bolus injection versus continuous infusion. J Am Coll Cardiol 28:376–382, 1996.
20. Flather MD, Yusuf S, Kober L, et al: Long-term ACE-inhibitor therapy in patients with heart failure or left ventricular dysfunction: a systematic overview of data from individual patients. ACE-inhibitor Myocardial Infarction Collaborative Group. Lancet 355:1575–1581, 2000.
21. Floras JS: Clinical aspects of sympathetic activation and parasympathetic withdrawal in heart failure. J Am Coll Cardiol 22:72A, 1993.
22. Francis GS: Pathophysiology of chronic heart failure. Am J Med 110:37S–46S, 2001.
23. Garg R, Yusef S: Overview of randomized trials of angiotensin converting enzyme inhibitors on mortality and morbidity of patients with heart failure. Collaborative Group on ACE Inhibitor Trials. JAMA 273:1450–1456, 1995.
24. Granger CB, McMurray JJV, Yusef S, et al: Effects of candesartan in patients with chronic heart failure and reduced left-ventricular systolic function intolerant to angiotensin-converting-enzyme inhibitors: the CHARM-Alternative trial. Lancet 362:772–776, 2003.
25. Grossman W, Jones D, McLaurin LP: Wall stress and patterns of hypertrophy in the human left ventricle. J Clin Invest 56:56, 1975.
26. Hauptman PJ, Kelly RA: Digitalis. Circulation 99:1265–1270, 1999.
27. Hunt SA, Baker DW, Chin MH, et al: ACC/AHA guidelines for the evaluation and management of chronic heart failure in the adult: a report of the American College of Cardiology/American

Heart Association Task Force on Practice Guidelines, 2001. American College of Cardiology website. Available at http://www.acc.org/clinical/guidelines/failure/hf_index.htm.

28. Jong P, Demers C, McKelvie RS, Liu PP: Angiotensin receptor blockers in heart failure: meta-analysis of randomized controlled trials. J Am Coll Cardiol 39:463–470, 2002.

29. Katz AM: Pathophysiology of heart failure: Identifying targets for pharmacotherapy. Med Clin North Am 89:303–316, 2003.

30. Lechat P, Packer M, Chalon S, et al: Clinical effects of beta-adrenergic blockade in chronic heart failure: a meta-analysis of double-blind, placebo-controlled, randomized trials. Circulation 98:1184–1191, 1998.

31. Marcus LS, Hart D, Packer M, et al: Hemodynamic and renal excretory effects of human brain natriuretic peptide infusion in patients with congestive heart failure. Circulation 94:3184–3189, 1996.

32. Maskin CS, Ocken S, Chadwick B, LeJemtel: Comparative systemic and renal effects of dopamine and angiotensin converting enzyme inhibition with enalaprilat in patients with heart failure. Circulation 72:846, 1985.

33. McMurray JJV, Ostergren J, Swedburg K, et al: Effects of candesartan in patients with chronic heart failure and reduced left-ventricular systolic function taking angiotensin-converting-enzyme inhibitors: the CHARM-Added trial. Lancet 362: 767–771, 2003.

34. MERIT-HF Study Group. Effect of metoprolol CR/XL in chronic heart failure: metoprolol CR/XL randomized intervention trial in congestive heart failure. Lancet 353:2001–2006, 1999.

35. Mills RM, LeJemtel TH, Horton DP, et al: Sustained hemodynamic effects of an infusion of nesiritide (human b-type natriuretic peptide) in heart failure. J Am Coll Cardiol 34:155–162, 1999.

36. Monrad ES, Baim DS, Smith HS, Lanoue AS: Milrinone, dobutamine, and nitroprusside: comparative effects on hemodynamics and myocardial energetics in patients with severe heart failure. Circulation 73:III168–174, 1986.

37. Oliva F, Latini R, Politi A, et al: Intermittent 6-month low-dose dobutamine infusion in severe heart failure: DICE multicenter trial. Am Heart J 138:247, 1999.

38. Opie LH, Yusuf S, Kubler W: Current status of safety and efficacy of calcium channel blockers in cardiovascular diseases: A critical analysis based on 100 studies. Prog Cardiovasc Dis 43:171–196, 2000.

39. Packer M, Bristow MR, Cohn JN, et al: Effect of carvedilol on morbidity and mortality in patients with chronic heart failure. N Engl J Med 325:293–302, 1991.

40. Packer M, Carver JR, Rodeheffer RJ, et al: Effect of oral milrinone on mortality in severe chronic heart failure. The PROMISE Study Research Group. N Engl J Med 21:325(21):1468–1475, 1991.

41. Packer M, Colucci WS, Sacker-Bernstein JD, et al: Double-blind, placebo-controlled study of the effects of carvedilol in patients with moderate to severe heart failure: the PRECISE trial. Circulation 94:2793–2799, 1996.

42. Packer M, Gheorghiade M, Young JB, et al: Withdrawal of digoxin from patients with chronic heart failure treated with angiotensin-converting enzyme inhibitors. N Engl J Med 329:1–7, 1993.

43. Packer M: Evolution of the neurohormonal hypothesis to explain the progression of chronic heart failure. Eur Heart J 16(Suppl F):46, 1995.

44. Pfeffer MA, Braunwald E, Moye LA, et al:: Effect of captopril on mortality and morbidity in patients with left ventricular dysfunction after myocardial infarction. N Engl J Med 327:669, 1992.

45. Pfeffer MA, Swedburg K, Granger CB, et al: Effects of candesartan on mortality and morbidity in patients with chronic heart failure: the CHARM-Overall programme. Lancet 362:767–771, 2003.

46. Pitt B, Poole-Wilson PA, Segal R, et al: Effect of losartan compared with captopril on mortality in patients with symptomatic heart failure: randomised trial—the losartan heart failure survival study ELITE II. Lancet 355:1582–1587, 2000.

47. Pitt B, Zannad F, Remme WJ, et al: The effect of spironolactone on morbidity and mortality in patients with severe heart failure. Randomized Aldactone Evaluation Study Investigators. N Engl J Med 341:709–717, 1999.

48. Ruffolo RR Jr: The pharmacology of dobutamine. Am J Med Sci 294:244–248, 1987.

49. Seino Y, Momomura S, Takano T, et al: Multicenter, double-blind study of intravenous milrinone for patients with acute heart failure in Japan. Crit Care Med 24:1490–1497, 1996.

50. SOLVD Investigators: Effect of enalapril on mortality and the development of heart failure in asymptomatic patients with reduced left ventricular ejection fraction. N Engl J Med 327: 685–691, 1992.

51. SOLVD Investigators: Effect of enalapril on survival in patients with reduced left ventricular ejection fraction and congestive heart failure. Circulation 325:293–302, 1991.

52. Stevenson LW, Colucci WS: Management of patients hospitalized with heart failure. In Smith TW, editor: Cardiovascular Therapeutics: A Companion to Braunwald's Heart Disease. Philadelphia: W.B. Saunders, 1996, pp. 199–209.

53. Uretsky BF, Young JB, Shahidi, et al: Randomized study assessing the effect of digoxin withdrawal in patients with mild to moderate chronic congestive heart failure: results of the PROVED Trial. J Am Coll Cardiol 22: 955–962, 1993.

54. VMAC Investigators: Intravenous nesiritide vs nitroglycerine for treatment of decompensated congestive heart failure. JAMA 287: 1531–1540, 2002.

55. Yusef S, Pfeffer MA, Swedburg K, et al: Effects of candesartan in patients with chronic heart failure and preserved left-ventricular ejection fraction: the CHARM-Preserved trial. Lancet 362: 777–781, 2003.

56. Zannad F, Alla F, Dousset B, et al: Limitation of excessive extracellular matrix turnover may contribute to survival benefit of spironolactone therapy in patients with congestive heart failure: insights from the randomized aldactone evaluation study (RALES). Rales Investigators. Circulation 102: 2700–2706, 2000.

57. Zile MR, Brutsaert DL: New concepts in diastolic dysfunction and diastolic heart failure: Part I. Diagnosis, prognosis, and measurements of diastolic function. Circulation 105: 1387–1393, 2002.

58. Zile MR, Brutsaert DL: New concepts in diastolic dysfunction and diastolic heart failure: Part II. Causal mechanisms and treatment. Circulation 105: 1503–1508, 2002.

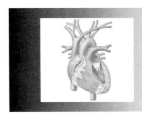

The Coronary Circulation: Dietary and Pharmacological Management of Atherosclerosis

John R. Guyton

INTRODUCTION

Accumulating experience from epidemiology, research trials, and clinical practice indicates that it is possible to prevent atherosclerotic disease with a high expectation of success and also to achieve stabilization or regression of established disease in many, if not most, patients. Since the 1960s, a 40% decline in overall cardiovascular mortality has occurred in the United States.[78] This decline may be attributed to a number of factors—lower plasma cholesterol, improved treatment of hypertension, reduced smoking rates, intensive care for acute ischemia, and/or intervention by bypass surgery and angioplasty. Over the past decade, more than 20 large randomized medical intervention trials have focused on clinical outcomes in patients with established coronary heart disease or with various levels of risk. The ability to alter the course of atherosclerotic disease by medical intervention has been proven beyond doubt. In smaller studies, usually employing combination therapy, event reductions exceeding 50% were suggested. Despite this progress, medical regimens for prevention and treatment of atherosclerosis remain underutilized. Thus atherosclerotic vascular disease, which currently accounts for approximately one third of all deaths in the United States, is likely to remain a dominant clinical concern for decades to come. A cooperative interdisciplinary approach involving primary care physicians, dietitians, cardiologists, endocrinologists, and surgeons will achieve the best results for individual patients. Physicians from a variety of subspecialties and specialties have gained expertise in lipid disorders and are able to provide consultative services on difficult patients.

This chapter aims primarily to describe effective therapy to prevent, stabilize, or regress atherosclerosis. Only a brief review of lesion development is given here. Because lipid-oriented therapy is so important to treatment of atherosclerosis, basic aspects of lipids and lipoproteins are described. A guide to practical decision making in atherosclerosis treatment is the largest section of the chapter.

ATHEROSCLEROSIS

Lesion Development

A brief review of classic lesion development is given here (Figure 62-1).

Fatty streaks are early atherosclerotic lesions that first appear normally in teenagers in the coronaries and the aorta. These lesions do not disrupt the endothelial lining and have no clinical consequence themselves. Histologically fatty streaks usually are found to consist of lipid-filled macrophages with lesser numbers of lipid-bearing smooth muscle cells. The macrophages are derived from circulating monocytes that adhere to and migrate across arterial endothelium—an effect mediated by cellular adhesion molecules upregulated in states of hypercholesterolemia and inflammation.

FATTY STREAK

FIBROUS PLAQUE

ORGANIZING THROMBUS

RUPTURED PLAQUE

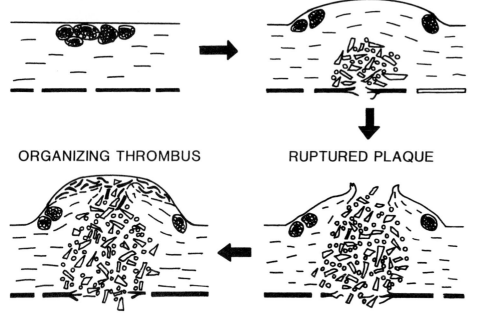

Figure 62–1 **Lesion development.** The fatty streak is a flat lesion composed of foam cells. Fibrous plaques are raised lesions that usually, but not always, contain a cholesterol-rich, acellular core. Rupture of a fibrous plaque occurs after the expanding core weakens the support of the endothelial surface to the breaking point. The luminal thrombus resulting from plaque rupture is organized by ingrowth and proliferation of smooth muscle cells, leading to rapid, episodic growth of advanced lesions. *(Modified from Guyton JR: Lipid metabolism and atherogenesis. In Garson AJ, Bricker JT, McNamara GT, editors: The Science and Practice of Pediatric Cardiology. Philadelphia, Leo, Febiger, 1990.)*

Beginning at about age 20, especially in males, raised lesions are found in the proximal coronaries, in the iliac arteries, and in the carotid bulb. Progression of raised atherosclerosis extends from the iliac arteries proximally into the abdominal and later thoracic aorta, and distally toward the femoral arteries. The raised character of the lesions is due to proliferation of smooth muscle cells and macrophages and to elaboration of large amounts of fibrous tissue, especially collagen. Raised lesions with an intact intimal surface are called *fibrous plaques*. The majority of raised lesions possess a lipid-rich, hypocellular or acellular core region. Early development of the lipid-rich core has also been described in flat aortic lesions resembling fatty streaks.[35] This finding is compatible with the hypothesis that most fibrous plaques are derived from preexisting fatty streaks (see Figure 62-1).

As the fibrous plaque enlarges and begins to impinge upon the arterial lumen, a compensatory enlargement of the entire artery occurs. This is probably due to physiological regulation of arterial lumen diameter in response to blood velocity and shear rate. However, the compensatory enlargement eventually fails, perhaps when the collagenous lesion extends circumferentially almost all the way around the artery, leaving little normal wall to respond to blood flow.[25]

The most hazardous component of the atherosclerotic lesion is the core region, which expands and erodes the fibrous cap of the lesion with time. When the fibrous cap finally ruptures, blood dissects rapidly into the core, and the thrombogenic contents of the core erupt into the vessel lumen, causing partial or complete thrombosis of the artery within 1 to a few minutes. This final process appears to be inhibitable by aspirin.[22]

Opportunities for Lesion Regression and Stabilization

Atherosclerotic regression is often conceived as a diminution in the size of an atherosclerotic lesion, which results in decreased stenosis. Such regression may occur, but other, more readily achievable goals should also be considered (Figure 62-2). For example, hypercholesterolemia can interfere with normal vasorelaxant function of endothelium, and decreases in low-density lipoprotein cholesterol can normalize endothelial-dependent relaxation.[47] The presence of macrophages in the fibrous cap of an atherosclerotic lesion predisposes the lesion to rupture.[52] Lipid lowering can cause relatively rapid regression of foam cells, which appears to stabilize the fibrous cap, prevent rupture, and forestall atherothrombotic events.

▶ LIPOPROTEIN METABOLISM

Lipids

A high content of carbon and hydrogen makes all lipid molecules hydrophobic, so lipids tend to associate with other lipids in an aqueous environment, forming membranes, oily droplets, and micelles. Phospholipids are the broad, diverse class of phosphorous-containing lipids that form cell membranes and perform many other essential biological functions. Phospholipids are not a target for antiatherosclerotic therapies presently.

Cholesterol is an essential component of most cell membranes. Fatty acids are the principal fuel used by muscle and most other body tissues. These lipids also serve as hormone precursors—steroids from cholesterol, prostaglandins and

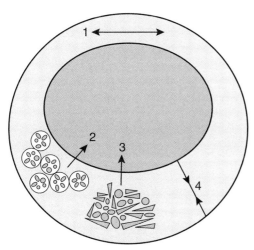

Figure 62–2 Four ways for risk to improve in an atherosclerotic lesion. (1) Dilation of a normal segment of the arterial wall. (2) Regression of foam cells in the lesion cap or shoulder. (3) Removal of lipid from the core. (4) Regression of fibrous tissue. Of these potential processes, (1) and (2) seem most feasible.

leukotrienes from arachidonic acid—but lipid-lowering treatment has never been shown to produce adverse endocrine effects.

Cholesteryl ester and triglyceride are lipid esters that provide efficient storage or transport of the corresponding active molecules, cholesterol, and fatty acids. These lipid esters are so hydrophobic that they usually cannot enter or move across cell membranes. A recurring theme in lipoprotein metabolism is either formation or hydrolysis of lipid esters, accompanying the movement of cholesterol or fatty acids in and out of cells.

Lipoproteins and Apolipoproteins

Human plasma lipoproteins function to transport triglyceride and cholesterol/cholesteryl ester in plasma. They are spherical particles containing 100 to several million lipid molecules combined with one or more protein molecules. The oily core of the lipoprotein is composed of triglyceride and cholesteryl ester. Based on which of these species is predominant in the oily core, lipoproteins can be classified as triglyceride rich or cholesterol rich. Phospholipids, free (unesterified) cholesterol, and protein are found in a surface layer. Lipoprotein classes are listed in Table 62-1.[28,39,62,77]

The protein components, termed *apolipoproteins*, bear specific binding sites for lipoprotein receptors or for enzymes involved in lipoprotein metabolism and thus target the lipoproteins for tissue uptake or lipid delivery (Table 62-2). All normal human lipoproteins contain either *apolipoprotein A-I* (apoA-I) or *apolipoprotein B* (apoB), or in the case of chylomicrons, both. Thus apoA-I and apoB appear to determine lipoprotein formation and structure, as well as metabolic targeting. *High-density lipoproteins* (HDLs) characteristically contain apoA-I, whereas all lipoproteins of larger size and lower density contain apoB.

Table 62–1

Plasma Lipoproteins [28,39,62,77]

Lipoprotein	Density (g/ml)	Diameter (nm)	Molecular weight (kDa)	Electrophoretic mobility	Most abundant chemical constituents
Chylomicrons[a]	<0.93	75–1200	~400,000	Origin	Triglyceride
VLDL	0.93–1.006	30–80	10,000–80,000	Prebeta	Triglyceride
IDL[a]	1.006–1.019	25–35	5,000–10,000	Slow prebeta	Cholesteryl ester, triglyceride
LDL	1.019–1.063	18–25	2,300	Beta	Cholesteryl ester
Lipoprotein(a)[a]	1.050–1.125	24–26	3,000–5,000	Slow prebeta	Cholesteryl ester
HDL$_2$	1.063–1.125	9–12	~360	Alpha	Protein, phospholipid, cholesteryl ester
HDL$_3$	1.125–1.210	5–9	~175	Alpha	Protein, phospholipid, cholesteryl ester

[a]These lipoproteins usually are not major components in fasting plasma. Chylomicrons normally circulate only postprandially. IDL are formed continuously from VLDL but are rapidly cleared or metabolized to LDL. Lipoprotein(a), or lipoprotein(a), is a minor lipoprotein in most individuals, but some persons have substantial plasma lipoprotein(a) concentrations on a genetic basis.

Table 62–2

Major Apolipoproteins[39,62,77]

Apolipoprotein	Molecular weight	Distribution	Function
A-I	28,000	HDL, chylomicrons	Structural role in HDL; activates lecithin-cholesterol acyltransferase
A-II	17,000	HDL, chylomicrons	Structural role in HDL
B-48	264,000	Chylomicrons	Structural role in intestine-derived lipoproteins
B-100	550,000	LDL, IDL, VLDL, chylomicrons	Structural role; ligand for LDL receptor binding
C-II	9,100	VLDL, IDL, HDL, chylomicrons	Activates lipoprotein lipase
C-III	8,750	VLDL, IDL, HDL, chylomicrons	Inhibits hepatic uptake of lipoproteins
E	34,000	IDL, VLDL, chylomicrons, HDL	Ligand for LDL receptor binding of IDL; promotes hepatic uptake of chylomicron remnants
(a)	400,000–700,000	Lipoprotein(a), chylomicrons	Unknown

Lipoprotein Pathways

Chylomicrons are intestinally derived triglyceride-rich lipoproteins of very large size, which appear transiently for several hours after the ingestion of fat in the diet. Chylomicrons are secreted into intestinal lymph and enter the bloodstream via the thoracic duct. From there, chylomicrons travel to peripheral capillaries, where they encounter an enzyme, lipoprotein lipase, which hydrolyzes triglyceride ester bonds to deliver free fatty acids to the tissues. Following lipoprotein lipase action, the chylomicron remnant is released and circulates back to the liver, where it is taken up very rapidly by a process that depends partly upon apolipoprotein E present on the lipoprotein surface.

The metabolic pathways of apoB-containing lipoproteins originating in the liver are shown in Figure 62-3. A single molecule of apoB is incorporated into *very-low-density lipoproteins* (VLDLs) prior to secretion from the liver, and this apoB molecule remains with the lipoprotein throughout all of its subsequent transformations, until the entire lipoprotein is taken up and degraded by a cell. VLDLs, which are triglyceride rich, encounter lipoprotein lipase and deliver fatty acids to tissues in exactly the same manner as chylomicrons. As shown in Figure 62-3, some of the VLDL remnants (also known as *intermediate-density lipoproteins,* or IDLs) are processed within the hepatic microcirculation to become *low-density lipoproteins* (LDLs), the major cholesterol-carrying particles in plasma. Physiological removal of LDLs from plasma depends upon the presence of LDL

receptor molecules found on the surface of hepatocytes and peripheral cells.

Triglyceride Metabolism

The level of triglycerides in plasma depends upon the balance of entry in the form of VLDLs and chylomicrons, and exit via the action of lipoprotein lipase. Deficiency of lipoprotein lipase action can be due to partial or complete genetic defects in the enzyme itself or in its cofactor, apoC-II, or to suppression by diabetes mellitus or ethanol abuse. Any of these factors can raise plasma triglyceride levels greatly. The most important regulator of VLDL production is body fat. Intracellular lipase activity in adipose tissue causes the release of fatty acids, which circulate as plasma free fatty acids to the liver. The liver reesterifies the fatty acids, making triglyceride for secretion in VLDL. Thus excess body fat stimulates a fatty acid–triglyceride cycle with concomitant excess production of VLDL. Improved caloric balance (i.e., reduced dietary calories or increased caloric expenditure with exercise) is the only way to reduce body fat and counter this stimulus to high plasma triglycerides. Another stimulus to high plasma triglycerides is a high percentage of carbohydrates in the diet.[30]

Cholesterol Metabolism

Between 30 and 60% of dietary cholesterol is absorbed and reaches the liver largely via chylomicron remnants. A more

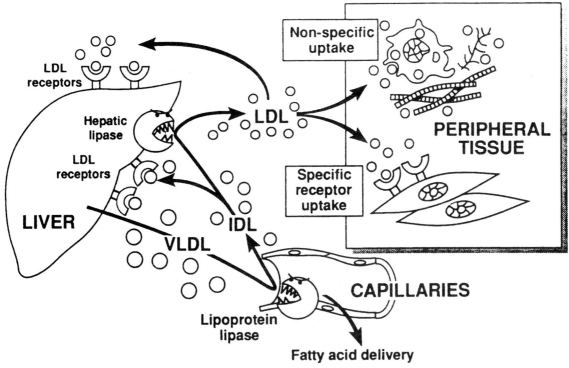

Figure 62–3 **Pathways of apoB-containing lipoproteins derived from the liver.** Triglyceride-rich VLDLs encounter lipoprotein lipase, which hydrolyzes triglyceride resulting in smaller intermediate-density lipoproteins (IDLs, also called VLDL remnants). Part of IDLs are taken up by the liver, and part are converted to LDL by hepatic lipase. There are three fates for LDLs: (1) uptake in the liver, (2) uptake in peripheral cells via specific receptors, or (3) nonspecific disposition in tissues via uptake in macrophages or adherence to collagen, elastin, or proteoglycans. *(Reproduced with permission of Medical Education Slides for the American Heart Association/Bristol-Myers Squibb Lipid Disorders Training Center, 1990. Copyright American Heart Association.)*

important source of cholesterol, however, is synthesis in the liver and other body tissues from acetyl coenzyme A (CoA). A rate-limiting step in synthesis is catalyzed by 3-hydroxy-3-methylglutaryl-CoA reductase, which is potently inhibited by the "statin" category of cholesterol-lowering drugs. The liver is also the site of exit for most of the cholesterol leaving the body's metabolic pools. Cholesterol cannot be broken down by mammalian cells to simple metabolic end products such as carbon dioxide. The liver receives cholesterol by uptake of chylomicron and VLDL remnants, by uptake of a large percentage of LDL via the classic receptor expressed on hepatocytes, and by selective uptake of cholesteryl ester from HDL (see reverse cholesterol transport later). The liver converts cholesterol into bile acids; biliary secretion of these and of cholesterol itself accounts for the bulk of cholesterol removal from the body. More than 95% of bile acids ordinarily are reabsorbed in the terminal ileum.[29] Oral ingestion of nonabsorbable bile acid binders (cholestyramine, colestipol, colesevelam) can lead to far greater net excretion in the stool and effectively reduce body cholesterol via bile acid conversion. Inhibition of intestinal absorption of cholesterol itself (e.g., by ezetimibe or by plant sterol/stanol esters) also lowers cholesterol in liver and in plasma LDL. These strategies are particularly effective when combined with agents that block a compensatory

increase in cholesterol synthesis. The profound role of the liver in cholesterol metabolism is the reason that liver transplantation can reverse the extreme hypercholesterolemia that occurs in patients with homozygous deficiency of LDL receptors.

Heterozygous LDL receptor deficiency leads to expression of half normal numbers of functional cell surface receptors and to approximately twice normal plasma LDL levels. This highly atherogenic condition occurs in 1 of 500 persons worldwide.[26] In a similar but much less frequent condition, heterozygous familial defective apoB, the binding site for the receptor, is genetically dysfunctional on half of circulating apoB.[42] The most common genetic hyperlipidemia that leads to coronary artery disease is neither of these, however, but is familial combined hyperlipidemia, a multifactorial or polygenic condition characterized by oversecretion of VLDL. Among different members of a single family or even in a single individual at different times, either LDL (plasma cholesterol) or VLDL (plasma triglycerides) or both may be elevated.[27]

Peripheral cells can incorporate cholesterol by endocytic uptake of LDL via LDL receptors. Macrophages, which have the function of clearing proteinaceous debris from body tissue, express other receptors such as CD36 and scavenger receptor A that bind chemically altered, oxidized, or aggregated LDL.[54]

1010

Reverse cholesterol transport (i.e., movement of cholesterol from peripheral tissues back to the liver) has been clarified by the discovery of key facilitating molecules. Cholesterol loading of macrophages induces expression of the adenosine triphosphate–binding cassette-A1 (ABC-A1) transporter, which transfers unesterified cholesterol to lipid-poor apoA-I and forms nascent HDL.[7] In disc-shaped nascent HDL, the enzyme lecithin-cholesterol acyltransferase (LCAT) functions to esterify cholesterol and thereby creates the oily lipid core of spherical HDL particles (which constitute almost all HDL in plasma). HDL can transport cholesterol to the liver by binding temporarily to scavenger receptor B1 on hepatocytes, which selectively removes cholesteryl ester from HDL and then releases the HDL particle for another round of reverse cholesterol transport. An alternative pathway for HDL cholesteryl ester is transfer via cholesteryl ester transfer protein (CETP) to LDL and VLDL, which are then taken up in the liver.[54] Overall, the system is complex, and its regulation remains incompletely understood. For example, deficiency or inhibition of CETP can raise HDL levels, but it remains unproven whether the effect is antiatherogenic.[3]

Role of Lipoproteins in Atherogenesis

The concentration of LDLs in the arterial intima is approximately equal to plasma LDL concentration, while interstitial fluid elsewhere in the body appears to have a concentration one tenth the plasma level. In other tissues, lymph vessels act as sumps to carry away excess tissue macromolecular species such as LDL, but lymph vessels are absent from arterial intima, perhaps because of hydrostatic pressure. Furthermore, the tunica media is highly impermeable to LDL, so that slow diffusion or convection of LDL across the arterial endothelium leads to high LDL concentrations in the intima. The relatively high intimal LDL concentration probably explains why pathological deposits of cholesterol develop regularly with aging only in the arterial intima and nowhere else.[32]

Intimal lipid deposits are found both intracellularly and extracellularly at various stages of atherosclerosis. In addition to cholesteryl ester in superficially located foam cells,

extracellular lipid deposits rich in unesterified cholesterol are found in the deep intimal core of small fibrous plaques. The formation of these deposits is unexplained; their importance is emphasized by an association with disappearance of cells and weakening of tissue in the developing core.[36]

Oxidation of LDLs may help explain a number of pathogenic processes in atherosclerosis. Certain lipid oxidation products are inflammatory mediators, and mildly oxidized LDL stimulates endothelial cells to express cell surface adhesion molecules for attachment of monocytes. However, two recent large clinical trials do not support a role for antioxidants in the prevention of clinical atherosclerotic events (Table 62-3).

Lipoprotein(a)

Lipoprotein(a) is an atherogenic lipoprotein whose role in lipid metabolism remains somewhat mysterious. Lipoprotein(a) is essentially an LDL with an added glycopeptide, apolipoprotein(a), attached to apoB via a cysteine–cysteine disulfide bond. Lipoprotein(a) particles self-aggregate easily, perhaps favoring their deposition in the arterial intima. The amino acid sequence of apolipoprotein(a) includes multiple repeats of a "kringle" sequence found in plasminogen and in tissue plasminogen activator. The kringle (named after a Danish pastry) fosters the attachment of these fibrinolytic enzymes to sites of clot formation. Lipoprotein(a) has been shown to interfere competitively with binding of the enzymes and thus with fibrinolysis. Clinically, a strong positive correlation has been found between lipoprotein(a) levels and various manifestations of atherosclerosis, including myocardial infarction and stroke. Lipoprotein(a) levels show a strong inheritance pattern and are largely unaffected by diet and medications, except that niacin and oral estrogen can give 20–30% reductions.[68]

The Metabolic Syndrome of Insulin Resistance and Cardiovascular Risk

The metabolic syndrome includes (1) disordered metabolism of body fuels—glucose and fat—featuring insulin

---

Table 62–3

Selected Unsuccessful Interventions Evaluated for Clinical End Points

Name and reference	Type of intervention	Principal outcomes compared with controls
Women's Health Initiative: Estrogen Plus Progestin Component[72]	Estrogen plus progestin in healthy postmenopausal women	Major coronary events↑ 29%; Stroke ↑ 41%
Heart Outcomes Prevention Evaluation (HOPE)[82]	Vitamin E (natural sources) 400 IU, mostly secondary prevention	Major cardiovascular events, including stroke ↑ 5% (NS)
Heart Protection Study[63]	Vitamins E and C and β-carotene, mostly secondary prevention	Major coronary events ↑ 2% (NS); Total mortality ↑ 4% (NS)

NS, not significant.

resistance and abdominal obesity; (2) atherogenic dyslipidemia with high triglycerides, low HDL cholesterol, and small dense LDLs; (3) hypertension, and (4) abnormalities of coagulation and inflammation adding to high cardiovascular risk. In the industrialized world, this syndrome makes a greater contribution to atherosclerotic disease than any other condition. By criteria of the National Cholesterol Education Program (Table 62-4), more than 40% of U.S. adults over the age of 60 have the metabolic syndrome.[20]

In the metabolic syndrome, insulin resistance occurs in the phosphatidylinositol 3-kinase (PI 3-kinase) pathway of insulin signaling in cells, but not in the mitogen-activated protein (MAP) kinase pathway. The PI 3-kinase pathway is responsible for metabolic actions such as glucose uptake in peripheral cells and suppression of fatty acid release from adipocytes. The MAP kinase pathway, which may be overstimulated, leads to potentially atherogenic mitogenic and proinflammatory effects.[40,53]

Fat overload and "spillover" can promote the metabolic syndrome.[15] Fat is the body's chief way of storing energy for future muscular activity. However, there is a finite capacity for the preferred site of energy storage in small peripheral adipocytes. Chronic energy imbalance—that is, too many calories in the diet and/or too few expended in exercise—leads to spillover storage of triglyceride in skeletal myocytes, in hepatocytes, in excessive visceral adipocytes, and in abnormally large peripheral adipocytes. Excessive triglyceride in these sites leads to insulin resistance.[45] Patients with lipodystrophy, either genetically based or caused by protease inhibitor therapy for human immunodeficiency virus, have a striking lack of small peripheral adipocytes.[11] They develop central adiposity, hypertriglyceridemia, fatty liver, and insulin resistance or diabetes in an exaggerated form of the metabolic syndrome.

The dyslipidemic triad consists of high plasma triglyceride, low HDL cholesterol, and small dense LDLs. In the metabolic syndrome, insulin resistance causes unsuppressed lipolysis of adipocyte triglyceride, which then leads to excessive fatty acid delivery to the liver. The liver reesterifies the fatty acids and exports them as VLDL triglyceride. CETP mediates the exchange of VLDL triglyceride for cholesteryl ester in LDLs and HDLs. LDLs and HDLs thereby become enriched in triglyceride at the expense of core cholesteryl ester. The triglyceride-enriched LDL and HDL are subject to triglyceride hydrolysis by lipases that remove core lipids and make the lipoprotein particles smaller. Small dense LDL appear to be more atherogenic than normal LDLs. Small dense HDLs are removed more rapidly from the circulation than normal HDLs, leading to reduced HDL cholesterol levels—another atherogenic situation.[23]

The adipocyte is now recognized as a source for multiple bioactive peptides, including angiotensinogen, tumor necrosis factor-α (TNF-α), leptin, and plasminogen activator inhibitor-1 (PAI-1).[60] Overproduction of angiotensinogen may help explain the link between obesity and hypertension. PAI-1, which inhibits fibrinolysis, is itself a cardiovascular risk factor. The liver appears to overproduce C-reactive protein, an extraordinarily strong marker of cardiovascular risk, in response to inflammatory cytokines from excessive fat deposits.[71] Interestingly, low levels of cardiovascular fitness are independently associated with high C-reactive protein levels—another example of the relationship between energy metabolism and cardiovascular risk.[31] These factors are only part of the connection between inflammation and atherosclerosis.

▶ CLINICAL MANAGEMENT

Major Clinical Trials

Medical treatment aimed at atherosclerosis can be classified as *primary* or *secondary prevention* depending on whether a person has previously experienced a clinical presentation of symptomatic atherosclerotic disease such as angina or infarction. Tables 62-3, 62-5, and 62-6 show some of the clinical trials that shape our understanding of therapeutic efficacy. The risk for hard clinical end points, including myocardial infarction, coronary death, and stroke, has been reduced sharply in several of these studies. Statins, or inhibitors of hydroxymethylglutaryl-CoA reductase, have been found particularly effective, and some dietary interventions have also been surprisingly effective. Large trials such as these are expensive, and the continual temptation is to rely on smaller trials with soft clinical end points, such as hospitalizations or revascularizations for angina, or with anatomical end points (e.g., carotid intima-media thickness measurements). Although the smaller trials can provide some direction, they are inherently unreliable due to unaccounted covariance, and ultimately hard clinical outcomes must be ascertained.

Guidelines for Lipid-Lowering Therapy

The guidelines of the U.S. National Cholesterol Education Program (NCEP), revised in 2001, provide a well-reasoned approach to the prevention and treatment of atherosclerotic disease via lipid-lowering therapy.[1,19] The guidelines assign patients to three categories of overall cardiovascular risk

Table 62-4

Clinical Identification of the Metabolic Syndrome[a]

Risk factor	Defining level
Abdominal obesity Men Women	Waist circumference >40 inches (>102 cm) >35 inches (88 cm)
Triglyceride	≥150 mg/dl
HDL cholesterol Men Women	<40 mg/dl <50 mg/dl
Blood pressure	≥130/≥85 mm Hg
Fasting glucose	≥110 mg/dl

[a]Diagnosis of the metabolic syndrome requires any three of the above.

Table 62–5

Selected Trials of Lipid Drugs with Clinical End Points

Name and reference	Type of intervention	Mean baseline lipids (mg/dl) and change with drug	Principal outcomes compared with controls
Coronary Drug Project[10,14]	Niacin, secondary prevention	Cholesterol 250, ↓ 10% Triglyceride 177, ↓ 26%	Myocardial infarction ↓ 27% Total mortality ↓ 11% (after 15-year follow-up)
Lipid Research Clinics/ Coronary Primary Prevention Trial[56]	Cholestyramine, primary prevention	Cholesterol 280, ↓ 9% LDLC 205, ↓ 13%	Coronary events ↓ 19%
Scandinavian Simvastatin Survival Study (4S)[75]	Simvastatin, secondary prevention	LDLC 188, ↓ 35%	Coronary events ↓ 34% Total mortality ↓ 30%
Cholesterol and Recurrent Events (CARE) Study[74]	Pravastatin, secondary prevention	LDLC 139, ↓ 28%	Coronary events ↓ 24%
Air Force/Texas Coronary Atherosclerosis Prevention Study (AFAPS/TexCAPS)[18]	Lovastatin, primary prevention	LDLC 150, ↓ 25%	Coronary events ↓ 37%
Veterans Administration HDL Intervention Trial (VA-HIT)[73]	Gemfibrozil, secondary prevention	HDLC 32, ↑ 6%	Coronary events ↓ 22%
Heart Protection Study (HPS)[63]	Simvastatin, mostly secondary prevention	LDLC 132, ↓ 31%	Total vascular events ↓ 24% Total mortality ↓ 13%
Anglo-Scandinavian Cardiac Outcomes Trial (ASCOT)[76]	Atorvastatin, primary prevention (hypertensive)	LDLC 132, ↓ 35%	Coronary events ↓ 36%

according to clinical situation and risk factors (Table 62-7 and Box 62-1). Patients with diabetes mellitus are considered "risk equivalent" to nondiabetic patients with established clinical atherosclerotic disease. In nondiabetic patients with two or more risk factors, Framingham-based calculation of the 10-year risk of myocardial infarction or coronary death is employed to stratify cardiovascular risk. Nondiabetic patients with one or fewer risk factors almost always have 10-year risk <10% and do not require the Framingham calculation. LDL cholesterol targets are designated for each level of risk. Secondary causes of hyperlipidemia such as hypothyroidism or nephrotic syndrome should be ruled out before embarking on drug treatment.

LDL cholesterol (LDLC) is generally determined via calculation from the following relationship: LDLC = total cholesterol−; HDLC−; triglyceride/5. Because postprandial lipoproteins are not included in this calculation, the measurements should be performed on fasting samples. However, note that total cholesterol as well as HDL and true LDL cholesterol levels are stable postprandially. Therefore, the true LDL cholesterol level cannot be lower

than, but is always at least as high as, the calculated LDL cholesterol from a nonfasting sample.

Epidemiological studies suggest that low HDL is at least as strong a predictor of cardiovascular risk as high LDL. However, the role of HDL in atherosclerosis is complex, and the clinical evidence for treatment benefit is not as secure as that related to LDL. Interventions aimed at low HDLC in secondary prevention draw support from the Veterans Administration HDL Intervention Trial (VA-HIT) study using gemfibrozil (Table 62-5).[73] In primary prevention, an isolated low HDLC, without other lipoprotein abnormalities, generally does not require medication and is addressed by lifestyle and dietary change (e.g., smoking cessation, exercise, and perhaps, addition of monounsaturated fat to the diet). When LDLC levels indicate a need for treatment, and HDLC and/or triglycerides are abnormal, then it is appropriate to aim therapy toward triglyceride reduction and HDLC augmentation as well as LDLC reduction.

Patients with triglyceride levels of 150 mg/dl or higher should be screened for the metabolic syndrome (Table 62-4)

Table 62–6

Selected Successful Nonlipid Interventions with Clinical End Points

Name and reference	Type of intervention	Principal outcomes compared with controls
Physicians' Health Study[67]	Aspirin, primary prevention	Myocardial infarction ↓ 47%
Diet and Reinfarction Trial[9]	Two fatty fish meals per week, secondary prevention	Total mortality ↓ 29% Coronary deaths ↓ 33%
GISSI-Prevenzione Trial[24]	Marine omega-3 fatty acid esters, secondary prevention (not placebo controlled)	Cardiovascular events ↓ 10% Cardiovascular death ↓ 17% Total mortality ↓ 14%
Lyon Diet Heart Study[17]	Mediterranean diet including α-linolenic acid (omega-3), secondary prevention	Major coronary events ↓ 72% Total mortality ↓ 56%
Heart Outcomes Prevention Evaluation (HOPE)[82]	Ramipril (angiotensin-converting enzyme inhibitor), mostly secondary prevention	Cardiovascular events ↓ 22% Myocardial infarction ↓ 20% Stroke ↓ 32% Total mortality ↓ 16%
Losartan Intervention for Endpoint (LIFE)[55]	Losartan (angiotension receptor blocker) versus atenolol in patients with hypertension and left ventricular hypertrophy	Cardiovascular events ↓ 13% Stroke ↓ 25% Cardiovascular deaths ↓ 11% (losartan compared with atenolol)

and counseled on dietary and lifestyle management aimed at reducing triglycerides. When triglyceride is 200 mg/dl or higher, NCEP designates non-HDL cholesterol (total minus HDL cholesterol) as a secondary target of therapy. Non-HDL cholesterol goals are set 30 mg/dl higher than the corresponding LDL cholesterol goals in each risk category (Table 62-7). Triglyceride levels above 500 mg/dl need consideration of dietary and drug treatment to prevent pancreatitis and other complications of severe hypertriglyceridemia or fasting chylomicronemia. Such treatment always requires strong attention to lifestyle and diet and may require one or more medications, including a fibric acid derivative, fish oil, niacin, and/or statin.

The NCEP guidelines recognize some emerging risk factors, which should not alter assignment to the major risk categories, but may contribute in varying degrees to atherosclerotic risk and, therefore, may appropriately influence clinical treatment decisions. Emerging risk factors include lipoprotein(a), C-reactive protein, homocysteine, impaired fasting glucose, small dense LDL, and evidence of subclinical atherosclerosis. Routine prevention and metabolic treatment of atherosclerosis do not require the measurement of any of these factors except fasting glucose. However, C-reactive protein has predictive power greater than any single lipoprotein measurement and comparable with or greater than the total/HDL cholesterol ratio.[70] LDL subfraction analysis can point toward the metabolic syndrome and potentially provide new targets for lifestyle and drug treatment. New imaging techniques for subclinical atherosclerosis may eventually blur the distinction between primary and secondary prevention. These techniques include enhanced computed tomographic scanning for coronary calcium quantitation and B-mode ultrasound quantitation of carotid intima-media thickness.[32] Where available, either technique might be appropriately used in cases where cardiovascular risk is uncertain or perhaps thought to be higher than Framingham estimates, such as patients with exceptionally strong family history. Nevertheless, all of these emerging risk factors lack conclusive evidence of treatment benefit and should be used only as modulators of clinical risk assessment.

Several randomized trials are evaluating whether lowering plasma homocysteine by the use of folic acid (sometimes combined with vitamins B_6 and B_{12}) can reduce clinical

---

Box 62–1. Atherosclerotic Risk Factors (National Cholesterol Education Program).[a]

Age: male ≥45 years; female ≥55 years
Current cigarette smoking
Family history of premature coronary disease
Low HDL cholesterol (<40 mg/dl)
Hypertension

[a]Negative risk factor: If HDL cholesterol ≥60 mg/dl, subtract one from the number of risk factors counted above.

Table 62–7			
Major Risk Categories and Treatment Goals			
Risk category	*LDLC goal (mg/dl)*	*Non-HDLC goal (mg/dl)*	*LDLC level at which to consider drug therapy*
Coronary or other clinical atherosclerotic disease, or risk equivalent (10-year risk >20%)[a]	<100	<130	≥130 mg/dl (100–129 mg/dl: drug optional)
Two or more risk factors (10-year risk ≤20%)	<130	<160	10-year risk 10–20%: ≥130 mg/dl 10-year risk <10%: ≥160 mg/dl
0–1 risk factor	<160	<190	≥160 mg/dl (160–189 mg/dl: drug optional)

[a]Diabetes mellitus is considered risk equivalent with established atherosclerotic disease because diabetic patients generally have coronary risk >20% over 10 years.

cardiovascular outcomes. Until the trial results are available, some lipid clinics advise every patient to take a multivitamin, which contains amounts of these vitamins capable of lowering plasma homocysteine by 8–10%.[58]

DIET IN PREVENTION AND TREATMENT

The relevant issues in dietary management of atherosclerosis are fatty acids derived from food versus those derived from body stores; quality of fat; fat versus carbohydrate; dietary cholesterol intake versus hepatic cholesterol synthesis; and the special roles of fiber, ethanol, and fish.[30] Dietary change, especially when it goes beyond the usual recommendations for the population, is one of the most powerful tools by which a patient can change the course of atherosclerotic disease.

Body Weight

Apart from genetic factors, the most important influence on hepatic production of VLDL triglyceride is the flux of plasma free fatty acids to the liver. The most important influence on plasma free fatty acid levels is the total mass of triglyceride contained in adipose tissue, and the clinical correlate is simply body weight. Body weight is a strong correlate not only of VLDL triglyceride production, but also production of apoB, which enters the circulation in VLDL. Because LDL is produced in the plasma from VLDL, it can be rightly stated for many patients that stored body fat drives the production of atherogenic lipoproteins. Furthermore, the prior discussion of the metabolic syndrome showed how HDL cholesterol levels decrease when plasma VLDL triglyceride levels rise.

The relationship of body weight to LDL cholesterol is complex, although a moderately strong positive correlation is the rule. Short-term weight loss (over 6 weeks) can cause dramatic reductions in both LDL and HDL cholesterol, but the same degree of weight loss sustained over 6 months generally will produce a more modest reduction of LDL cholesterol and a rise in HDL cholesterol.[16] In the treatment of hyperlipidemias, patients with hypertriglyceridemia or with combined hyperlipidemia appear to respond especially favorably to weight reduction, compared with patients with pure hypercholesterolemia.

To lose weight, or to "get control" of weight, may be the most difficult task that a physician can ask a patient to accomplish. A gradual approach targeting weight reduction of 2–4 pounds per month and emphasizing behavior modification is best. Because adipose tissue contains 9 calories of energy stored per gram, weight reduction of 2 pounds per month depends upon a net reduction of caloric balance of almost 300 calories per day. When the body perceives "depletion" of fat stores, especially after intensive dieting, basal caloric metabolism may be reduced, making further weight loss difficult. The resistance is not absolute, and a healthy diet producing weight loss can always be prescribed, preferably in collaboration with a dietitian. The patient should understand that basal caloric metabolism is effectively supplemented with exercise, and a long-term exercise program is one of the keys to maintaining weight control. Although it is physiologically possible in every case, ideal weight control is psychologically and practically impossible for many obese patients. It is often the mildly overweight, hyperlipidemic patient who successfully and permanently loses 15–20 pounds with excellent lipoprotein changes, simply because this person may be trying to get control of weight for the first time, not having previously experienced multiple cycles of failure.

At present the recommended diet for weight reduction is a balanced nutrient diet with calories proportioned as 50–60% carbohydrate, 25–35% fat, and 15% protein.[1] The use of very-low-carbohydrate diets to assist weight reduction has received serious research attention recently, but caution is appropriate because the long-term effects of these diets are unknown.[21,80]

Dietary Components

In the ordinary Western diet, saturated fat is the component that can be changed most readily to yield favorable effects on plasma lipoproteins.[30] In saturated fat (almost all of which is triglyceride), the fatty acid chains contain a maximum number of hydrogen atoms and have no carbon–carbon double bonds. Hydrogenation is a food processing technique that removes double bonds by adding hydrogen atoms, thereby increasing the saturation of fat. Among the saturated fatty acids, palmitic (16 carbons, no double bonds, hence 16:0) and myristic acid (14:0) exert most of the LDL cholesterol–raising effect, whereas stearic acid (18:0) may influence lipoprotein levels minimally. Whether this distinction is clinically important is unclear. Older guidelines called for replacing saturated fat with polyunsaturated fat (principally linoleic acid, 18:2), but subsequently it was learned that this maneuver reduces HDL as well as LDL cholesterol levels. Monounsaturated fatty acids, particularly oleic acid (18:1), when substituted for saturated fatty acids, reduce LDL cholesterol but not HDL cholesterol in plasma. Nevertheless, clinical studies with cardiovascular end points suggest that either polyunsaturated or monounsaturated fatty acids may help protect against cardiovascular disease. In most natural fatty acids, all double bonds have the *cis* configuration, whereas processed, rehydrogenated fatty acids have a blend of *cis* and *trans*. Trans fatty acids are particularly disadvantageous because they raise LDLC like saturated fatty acids, but like polyunsaturated fatty acids provide no increase in HDLC.

Cholesterol itself in the usual Western diet has less impact than saturated fat because the liver and other tissues ordinarily synthesize approximately 70% of the body's daily cholesterol requirement and can readily increase the synthetic rate several-fold. Changing daily cholesterol consumption from 600 to 300 mg, for example, can be expected to decrease plasma cholesterol by only 7 mg/dl, if saturated fat intake remains constant.[46] However, in more restrictive diets, the impact of reducing dietary cholesterol intake along with fat can be considerable. In the Lifestyle Heart Trial, the baseline diet was equivalent to the NCEP Therapeutic Lifestyle Changes (TLC) Diet (Box 62-2). The experimental group went on a strict vegetarian diet, essentially eliminating dietary cholesterol (plants do not make cholesterol), reducing all fat to 7% of total calories, and losing 22 pounds on average. The drop in LDLC was 37%, comparable with that achieved by effective cholesterol-lowering medication.[66]

The current American diet contains approximately 33% of calories as fat, including 11% from saturated fat. Average daily intake of cholesterol is about 325 mg for adult men and 240 mg for adult women.[81] NCEP dietary goals for TLC (see Box 62-2) apply to somewhat more than half of the adult U.S. population who have LDL cholesterol levels higher than 130 mg/dl. If a group of men change from the average U.S. dietary pattern described previously to the cholesterol and saturated fat recommendations of the TLC diet, then plasma cholesterol will be reduced approximately 14 mg/dl, according to the well-validated predictive equation of Keys and Parlin.[46]

Nondigestible plant fiber that tends to form a viscous gel when placed in water, called "viscous" or "soluble" fiber, has clearly been shown to have a modest lowering effect on plasma LDL cholesterol.[43] Oat and rice bran and bean fiber, but not wheat bran, have this effect. Psyllium, long in use as a bulk-forming laxative agent, and guar gum are particularly effective viscous fibers, but have side effects of intestinal bloating and flatus. Plant sterol or stanol esters, which have been formulated into soft margarines, can give 8–14% LDL cholesterol reductions by inhibiting intestinal cholesterol absorption. Both viscous fiber and plant sterol/stanol esters are recommended as part of the NCEP TLC diet (Box 62-2).

Many patients with symptomatic atherosclerosis are able to make dietary changes that go well beyond the TLC diet, and they should be encouraged to do so. Intensive dietary intervention may be just as effective, or more effective, than medication in producing relief of anginal symptoms, reversal of stenosis, and prevention of events in patients with coronary artery disease. Institution of a Mediterranean diet or even a vegetarian diet can be an appropriate therapeutic maneuver in motivated patients with advanced atherosclerosis.[17,66] The reduction of HDLC that sometimes occurs with these diets is not necessarily clinically significant, based on the complexity of the role of HDL in atherogenesis, as well as the epidemiological and clinical correlations between low-fat diets and prevention of atherosclerotic cardiovascular disease.

Most people in the world eat a diet high in complex carbohydrates and relatively low in fat and protein, compared to people in a Western industralized society. People on such a diet typically have low body weights and relatively low plasma total cholesterol levels averaging 140–160 mg/dl, with HDL cholesterol also low. In these populations, rates of coronary disease are only a small fraction of the rates among Western nations.

However, it has become sadly apparent that a public health message of "low fat" will prevent neither obesity nor cardiovascular disease in societies where food is abundant. The classic food pyramid with grains and starches (usually consumed as highly refined products) providing the broad base of dietary calories has been challenged. The optimal diet for cardiovascular prevention may be low in refined grain products; high in whole grains, vegetables, fruits, and nuts; and adequate in omega-3 fatty acids, while substituting natural polyunsaturated and monounsaturated fats for saturated and transunsaturated (hydrogenated) fats.[41] Furthermore, some patients with hypertriglyceridemia may benefit from carbohydrate reduction even if body weight remains constant.[69]

Moderate intake of alcohol, in the range of one to three drinks per day in men and one half to two drinks per day in women, can reduce the risk of coronary heart disease by as much as 50%.[48] Both HDL$_2$ and HDL$_3$ are increased by ethanol, but direct effects on the arterial wall may be postulated to play a role as well. Risk reduction is not likely to occur in patients with hypertriglyceridemia because ethanol

---

Box 62–2. Therapeutic Lifestyle Changes (TLC, National Cholesterol Education Program).

TLC diet
  Saturated fat <7% of calories, cholesterol <200 mg/day
  Consider increased viscous (soluble) fiber (10–25 g/day)
    and plant stanol/sterol esters (2 g/day) as therapeutic
    options to enhance LDL lowering
Weight management
Increased physical activity

1016 aggravates this condition. Furthermore, the blood pressure–raising effects of ethanol should be kept in mind. Because of risks of accidents and addiction, it is not appropriate to counsel persons to drink for cardiovascular health, but ethanol intake can be approved if already established as a stable part of a person's life.

A high intake of fish in the diet has long been associated with reduced coronary disease rates in epidemiological studies. This association has been supplemented by positive results from three randomized trials involving omega-3 fatty acids (see Table 62-6), although no trial as yet has employed a rigorous double-blind, placebo-controlled design. The impact of omega-3 fatty acids is most clearly shown in cardiovascular mortality reductions averaging 20–30% and in strikingly reduced rates of sudden death (see Table 62-6). It has been speculated that omega-3 fatty acids incorporated in cardiac phospholipids are released by phospholipase activity in ischemic or stressed myocardium, and that the free omega-3 fatty acids act upon ion channels or signaling pathways to stabilize the cardiac rhythm, preventing ventricular fibrillation. It has been recommended that coronary patients receive 1 g omega-3 fatty acids daily from marine sources, preferably from fatty fish, or from capsules.[49] If fish oil is not tolerated (a few patients are sensitive to the odor), then omega-3 fatty acids from terrestrial sources may be substituted. Marine omega-3 fatty acids have 20 or 22 carbon atoms, whereas α-linolenic acid is an 18-carbon omega-3 derived from terrestrial sources such as flaxseed, walnuts, canola oil, and soybean oil. Another useful effect of marine omega-3 fatty acids in high doses (4–5 g daily) is to lower plasma triglycerides by 30–40%. α-Linolenic acid does not lower triglycerides at all.

Drugs for Lipid Reduction and Atherosclerosis Prevention

Drug therapy for prevention and treatment of atherosclerosis should begin with consideration of aspirin or other antiplatelet therapy for every person at risk. Aspirin doses between 30 and 325 mg/day appear to be equivalent in their ability to inhibit arterial thrombosis. In secondary prevention, the risk reduction is 30% for recurrent myocardial infarction and 15% for cardiac death.[2] Rates in primary prevention are probably similar. Patients with uncontrolled hypertension should not take aspirin regularly because of the risk of hemorrhagic stroke. Because aspirin is thought chiefly to affect thrombosis and not to inhibit atherosclerosis development, there is no reason to recommend regular aspirin use until thrombosis risk is substantial (i.e., generally after age 50, or earlier if severe or multiple risk factors are present).

Estrogen replacement in postmenopausal women was thought to reduce risk for coronary arterial disease, based on epidemiological data. However, an estrogen–progestin combination used in women with intact uteri appears to increase cardiovascular risk (see Table 62-3). The results of clinical outcome trials with unopposed estrogen and with raloxifene, a selective estrogen receptor modulator, are awaited.[72,79]

The most effective regimens for hyperlipidemia utilize, singly or in combination, drugs from five groups—inhibitors of hydroxymethylglutaryl-CoA reductase (reductase inhibitors or statins), niacin, fibric acid derivatives, bile acid sequestrants, and cholesterol absorption inhibitor(s).

Each of these drug classes has been shown to reduce clinical cardiovascular events in randomized clinical trials (see Table 62-5), with the exception of the recently introduced cholesterol absorption inhibitor.

The statins are the most effective single agents available for lowering LDLC, and their effectiveness in reducing cardiovascular events is the foundation of atherosclerosis treatment by lipid management. The safety of these agents has been confirmed in more than 100,000 adult patients followed prospectively, the first of whom began taking lovastatin in the early 1980s. Statins competitively block the synthesis of mevalonic acid, a precursor in the cholesterol synthetic pathway. Although mevalonic acid leads to several other metabolites as well, the clinically available statins do not ordinarily interfere with crucial cellular functions nor with the synthesis of steroid and sex hormones that use cholesterol as a precursor. Statins reduce triglycerides and raise HDLC, but other agents have greater effects on these lipoproteins. Patients should be monitored for hepatic transaminase elevations. An interaction of statins with cyclosporine, fibric acid derivatives such as gemfibrozil, erythromycin, clarithromycin, nefazodone, azole antifungals, or niacin can lead to myopathy and sometimes rhabdomyolysis. However, niacin or fibric acid derivatives (fenofibrate may have less interaction) may be employed in combination with statins with appropriate caution. Rarely statin monotherapy leads to myopathy.[65] An unclear fraction of patients, between 0.5 and 5%, may experience myalgia or fatigue on statin treatment. This symptom usually recurs with all statins attempted at the same effective dose. It may respond to a 4-fold reduction of statin dose, perhaps coupled with switching to a pharmacokinetically different statin and/or employing nonstatin therapy in combination.

Niacin, also known as nicotinic acid, is a form of vitamin B$_3$. Lipid-lowering doses can be 50–100 times the vitamin dose. Niacinamide (nicotinamide) also acts as a vitamin, but has no lipid-lowering effect. Niacin acts to inhibit lipolysis and production of free fatty acids from adipose tissue and also to decrease the production of VLDL from the liver.[34] Immediate-release niacin is usually given three or four times per day, always with food or skim milk in the stomach, at a total daily dose beginning as low as 100 mg and increasing over weeks to months to 1000–4000 mg. Sustained-released niacin, usually administered twice a day, is more prone to cause hepatotoxicity; the total dose should be limited to 2000–2250 mg daily. An extended-release prescription form of niacin, given once daily at bedtime, has well-documented hepatic safety in doses up to 2000 mg.[37] Niacin is the most effective pharmacological agent for raising HDLC; daily doses of 1000–2000 mg raise HDLC by 10–25%.[38] Doses in the range of 1500–3000 mg/day reduce triglyceride, LDLC, and lipoprotein(a) levels. Side effects of niacin include flushing (very common, but disappearing or diminishing with continued regular use), dyspepsia, hyperglycemia, transaminase elevations, atrial fibrillation, peptic ulcer, gout, skin dryness, and visual disturbances.

Bile acid sequestrants include cholestyramine and colestipol, which are therapeutically very similar, and colesevelam, which has better tolerability. These nonabsorbed polymers bind bile acids in the small intestine, preventing their reabsorption in the terminal ileum. The liver detects bile acid depletion and diverts cholesterol stores toward bile acid synthesis, establishing a drain on body stores of cholesterol. The bile acid sequestrants reduce LDL cholesterol 10–30% depending on dose. Triglyceride levels tend to increase with use of bile acid sequestrants; therefore, hypertriglyceridemia is a relative contraindication. Because the bile acid sequestrants are not absorbed into the bloodstream, they have excellent theoretical and practical safety, sufficient to recommend them for reducing LDLC in pediatric cases and in women of childbearing potential. The major side effects of cholestyramine and colestipol are constipation (15% of cases) and abdominal bloating. Drug absorption may be inhibited, particularly warfarin, vitamin K (in warfarin-treated patients), digoxin, diuretics, and thyroxine. Colesevelam has much better gastrointestinal tolerability and minimal drug interactions.[4]

Fibric acid derivatives, or fibrates, approved for use in the United States, include gemfibrozil, fenofibrate, and clofibrate. Clofibrate, an older drug, is rarely used because of increased all-cause mortality seen in a large clinical trial.[13] The fibrates perform best at lowering triglyceride levels; reductions of 40–55% can be expected in hypertriglyceridemic patients. HDLC increases of 6–20% can occur. Fenofibrate reduces LDL cholesterol moderately in normotriglyceridemic patients. Gemfibrozil reduced cardiovascular events in a secondary prevention trial of patients with low HDLC (see Table 62-5).[66] Fenofibrate is being tested in two large clinical outcome trials in diabetic subjects. Because both gemfibrozil and fenofibrate are cleared from the circulation largely by the kidney, doses should be decreased in patients with renal insufficiency. Side effects shared by these drugs include dyspepsia, hypersensitivity rash, hepatic transaminase elevations, increased warfarin effect, and increased lithogenicity of bile. Fenofibrate can rarely cause photosensitivity of the skin.[44]

Ezetimibe is the first member of a new pharmacological class that inhibits cholesterol absorption by intestinal mucosa. Ordinarily the intestine is exposed to 200–400 mg of dietary cholesterol and 1000 mg of biliary cholesterol daily, of which 30–60% may be absorbed. After ingestion, ezetimibe is concentrated in intestinal mucosal brush border, where it appears to bind to a membrane sterol transporter. Ezetimibe at 10 mg daily gives 18–19% LDLC lowering. When ezetimibe is added to an existing statin regimen, LDLC is reduced 20–25% from the poststatin baseline. Side effects of ezetimibe have been minimal and not significantly different from placebo.[5]

Because LDLC <100 mg/dl is the goal in patients with atherosclerotic disease, combinations of the medications listed previously are often used. In combination therapy, moderate doses can often be used to achieve excellent LDLC reduction. If gemfibrozil is used in combination with a statin, up to 4% of patients may experience myopathy, unless the statin dose is kept at or near the usual starting dose. Niacin and fenofibrate can also potentiate statin myopathy, but at much lower frequencies. Ezetimibe, bile acid sequestrants, and fish oil can be added to statin therapy or to niacin and fibrates without an increased risk of myopathy or other synergistic adverse effects.[31] In a small clinical trial involving 160 patients with low HDL cholesterol and measurable coronary atherosclerosis, the combination of niacin with simvastatin achieved regression over 3 years and reduced cardiovascular events by 70% (these were mostly soft end points—revascularizations).[8]

OTHER INTERVENTIONS

Tobacco

Smoking between one and two packs of cigarettes per day doubles the risk of coronary atherosclerotic events. The most important fact to communicate to patients is that the risk declines rapidly when smoking is stopped, such that coronary risk is almost normal within 1 or 2 years.[59] This fact, along with basic research results, suggests that a major effect of smoking is to enhance thrombus formation, perhaps via injurious effects of nicotine or other tobacco components on endothelium. Smoking also promotes atherogenesis, especially in the arterial supply to the lower extremities. Some, but not all, of the chronic atherogenic effects of smoking may be mediated by decreased plasma levels of HDLC. With smoking cessation, HDLC increase is commonly seen. Modest weight gain may accompany smoking cessation, but clinical benefits far outweigh any adverse effects of weight gain.

Antihypertensive Therapy

Medical therapy of hypertension reduces risk of stroke by 30–40% and myocardial infarction by 20%, according to a meta-analysis of recent clinical trials.[64] Treatment with a thiazide-type diuretic is superior to or at least as good as treatment with any other antihypertensive agent in routine patients. Therefore, a diuretic is preferred for first-step antihypertensive therapy in most patients.[57] However, patients with stable angina and hypertension are best treated first with a β-blocker. During or following acute coronary syndromes, β-blockers and angiotensin-converting enzyme inhibitors have been shown to be efficacious. In many cases, especially when initial systolic pressures exceed 160 mm Hg, two or more antihypertensive drugs may be needed to reach the goal of <140 systolic and <90 diastolic mm Hg. Note that blood pressures measured by patients at home tend to be lower, and the goal is <135/85 mm Hg. In patients with diabetes or chronic kidney disease, the goal for office blood pressure is <130/80 mm Hg. The Seventh Report of the Joint National Committee provides an excellent, concise guideline for blood pressure control.[12]

Both thiazide and loop diuretics cause, on average, small increases in triglyceride and LDLC levels. β-Blockers tend to raise triglycerides and reduce HDLC.[51] However, the proven benefits of these agents on clinical outcomes usually outweigh their impact on lipids, and adjustment of antihypertensive therapy to optimize the lipid profile is usually not appropriate.

Exercise

Although myocardial infarction is more likely to occur at times of unaccustomed moderate-to-intense exercise, a steady pattern of exercise clearly reduces risk.[61] The lack of any large randomized trial may lead to an underappreciation of the cardiovascular benefit of exercise. In a large observational study, physical fitness determined by treadmill testing was the strongest determinant of future cardiovascular risk, eclipsing the effects of body mass index, blood pressure, cholesterol, and smoking. Men who increased

1018 their fitness from the lowest quintile to a higher level over an average 5-year period showed 44% lower total mortality in follow-up, compared with men who remained in the lowest fitness quintile.[6] Data such as these support a strong role of cardiac rehabilitation programs in the treatment of coronary artery disease.

▶ SUMMARY

Although it is better to prevent atherosclerosis than to treat it, the presence of established disease should no longer be regarded as predictive of inexorable progression. In the treatment of atherosclerosis, smoking cessation is essential. Besides smoking cessation, modification of plasma lipoprotein levels, especially LDLC, is the most effective way to change the course of the disease. Recent evidence suggests that raising HDLC might add substantially to atherosclerosis treatment. Strong efforts in diet and exercise, as well as appropriate medication, are often needed together. Control of hypertension and diabetes should be maintained. In the majority of patients, a reasonable goal is more than 50% risk reduction, and highly motivated patients can do substantially better than this.

REFERENCES

1. Adult Treatment Panel III: Third Report of the National Cholesterol Education Program (NCEP) expert panel on detection, evaluation, and treatment of high blood cholesterol in adults. Bethesda, MD: NIH Publication No. 02-5215, National Institutes of Health, 2002.
2. Antiplatelet Trialists' Collaboration: Secondary prevention of vascular disease by prolonged antiplatelet treatment. Br Med J 296:320–331, 1988.
3. Barter PJ, Rye KA: Cholesteryl ester transfer protein, high density lipoprotein and arterial disease. Curr Opin Lipidol 12:377–382, 2001.
4. Bays H, Dujovne C: Colesevelam HCl: a non-systemic lipid altering drug. Expert Opin Pharmacother 4:779–790, 2003.
5. Bays HE, et al: Effectiveness and tolerability of ezetimibe in patients with primary hypercholesterolemia: pooled analysis of two phase II studies. Clin Ther 23:1209–1230, 2001.
6. Blair SN, et al: Changes in physical fitness and all-cause mortality. A prospective study of healthy and unhealthy men. JAMA 273:1093–1098, 1995.
7. Brewer HB Jr, Santamarina-Fojo S: New insights into the role of the adenosine triphosphate-binding cassette transporters in high-density lipoprotein metabolism and reverse cholesterol transport. Am J Cardiol 91:3E–11E, 2003.
8. Brown BG, et al: Simvastatin and niacin, antioxidant vitamins, or the combination for the prevention of coronary disease. N Engl J Med 345:1583–1592, 2001.
9. Burr ML, et al: Effects of changes in fat, fish, and fibre intakes on death and myocardial reinfarction: diet and reinfarction trial (DART). Lancet 2:757–761, 1989.
10. Canner PL, et al: Fifteen year mortality in Coronary Drug Project patients: long-term benefit with niacin. J Am Coll Cardiol 8:1245–1255, 1986.
11. Carr A, et al: A syndrome of peripheral lipodystrophy, hyperlipidaemia and insulin resistance in patients receiving HIV protease inhibitors. AIDS 12:F51–F58, 1998.
12. Chobanian AV, et al: The Seventh Report of the Joint National Committee on Prevention, Detection, Evaluation, and Treatment of High Blood Pressure: the JNC 7 report. JAMA 289:2560–2572, 2003.
13. Committee of Principal Investigators: A co-operative trial in the primary prevention of ischaemic heart disease using clofibrate. Br Heart J 40:1069–1118, 1978.
14. The Coronary Drug Project Research Group: Clofibrate and niacin in coronary heart disease. JAMA 231:360–381, 1975.
15. Danforth E Jr: Failure of adipocyte differentiation causes type II diabetes mellitus? Nat Genet 26:13, 2000.
16. Dattilo AM, Kris-Etherton PM: Effects of weight reduction on blood lipids and lipoproteins: a meta-analysis. Am J Clin Nutr 56:320–328, 1992.
17. de Lorgeril M, et al: Mediterranean diet, traditional risk factors, and the rate of cardiovascular complications after myocardial infarction: final report of the Lyon Diet Heart Study. Circulation 99:779–785, 1999.
18. Downs JR, et al: Primary prevention of acute coronary events with lovastatin in men and women with average cholesterol levels: results of AFCAPS/TexCAPS. JAMA 279:1615–1622, 1998.
19. Executive Summary of The Third Report of The National Cholesterol Education Program (NCEP) Expert Panel on Detection, Evaluation, and Treatment of High Blood Cholesterol in Adults (Adult Treatment Panel III). JAMA 285:2486–2497, 2001.
20. Ford ES, et al: Prevalence of the metabolic syndrome among US adults: findings from the third National Health and Nutrition Examination Survey. JAMA 287:356–359, 2002.
21. Foster GD, et al: A randomized trial of a low-carbohydrate diet for obesity. N Engl J Med 348:2082–2090, 2003.
22. Fuster V, et al: Atherosclerotic plaque rupture and thrombosis. Circulation 82(Suppl II):47–59, 1990.
23. Ginsberg HN: Insulin resistance and cardiovascular disease. J Clin Invest 106:453–458, 2000.
24. GISSI-Prevenzione Investigators: Dietary supplementation with n-3 polyunsaturated fatty acids and vitamin E after myocardial infarction: results of the GISSI-Prevenzione trial. Lancet 354:447–455, 1999.
25. Glagov S, et al: Compensatory enlargement of human atherosclerotic coronary arteries. N Engl J Med 316:1371–1375, 1987.
26. Goldstein JL, Brown MS: Familial hypercholesterolemia. In Scriver CR, Beaudet AL, Sly WS, Valle D, editors: The Metabolic Basis of Inherited Disease. New York: McGraw-Hill, 1989, pp. 1215–1250.
27. Goldstein JL, et al: Hyperlipidemia in coronary heart disease. J Clin Invest 52:1544–1568, 1973.
28. Gotto AM Jr, et al: Introduction to the plasma lipoproteins. Methods Enzymol 128:1–41, 1986.
29. Grundy SM: Cholesterol metabolism in man. West J Med 128:13–25, 1978.
30. Grundy SM, Denke MA: Dietary influences on serum lipids and lipoproteins. J Lipid Res 31:1149–1172, 1990.
31. Guyton JR: Combination drug therapy for combined hyperlipidemia. Curr Cardiol Rep 1:244–250, 1999.
32. Guyton JR: Phospholipid hydrolytic enzymes in a 'cesspool' of arterial intimal lipoproteins: a mechanism for atherogenic lipid accumulation. Arterioscler Thromb Vasc Biol 21:884–886, 2001.
33. Guyton JR: Clinical assessment of atherosclerotic lesions: emerging from angiographic shadows. Circulation 106:1308–1309, 2002.
34. Guyton JR, Gotto AM Jr: Drug therapy of dyslipoproteinemias. In Fruchart JC, Shepherd J, editors: Human Plasma Lipoproteins, Clinical Biochemistry Series. Berlin: Walter de Gruyter, 1989, pp. 335–361.

35. Guyton JR, Klemp KF: Transitional features in human atherosclerosis: intimal thickening, cholesterol clefts, and cell loss in human aortic fatty streaks. Am J Pathol 143:1444–1457, 1993.

36. Guyton JR, Klemp KF: Development of the lipid-rich core in human atherosclerosis. Arterioscler Thromb Vasc Biol 16:4–11, 1996.

37. Guyton JR, et al: Effectiveness of once nightly dosing of extended-release niacin alone and in combination for hypercholesterolemia. Am J Cardiol 82:737–743, 1998.

38. Guyton, JR, et al: Extended-release niacin versus gemfibrozil for treatment of low levels of high density lipoprotein cholesterol. Arch Intern Med 52, 1999.

39. Havel RC, et al: Lipoproteins and lipid transport. In Bondy PK, Rosenberg LE, editors: Metabolic Control and Disease. Philadelphia: W.B. Saunders, 1980, pp. 393–494.

40. Hsueh WA, Law RE: Insulin signaling in the arterial wall. Am J Cardiol 84:21J–24J, 1999.

41. Hu FB, Willett WC: Optimal diets for prevention of coronary heart disease. JAMA 288:2569–2578, 2002.

42. Innerarity TL, et al: Familial defective apolipoprotein B-100: a mutation of apolipoprotein B that causes hypercholesterolemia. J Lipid Res 31:1337–1349, 1990.

43. Jenkins DJA, et al: Effect on blood lipids of very high intakes of fiber in diets low in saturated fat and cholesterol. N Engl J Med 329:21–26, 1993.

44. Keating GM, Ormrod D: Micronised fenofibrate: an updated review of its clinical efficacy in the management of dyslipidaemia. Drugs 62:1909–1944, 2002.

45. Kelley DE, Mandarino LJ: Fuel selection in human skeletal muscle in insulin resistance: a reexamination. Diabetes 49:677–683, 2000.

46. Keys A, Parlin RW: Serum cholesterol response to changes in dietary lipids. Am J Clin Nutr 19:175–181, 1966.

47. Kinlay S, et al: Endothelial function and coronary artery disease. Curr Opin Lipidol 12:383–389, 2001.

48. Kreisberg RA: A votre sante: alcohol and coronary artery disease. Arch Intern Med 152:263–265, 1992.

49. Kris-Etherton PM, et al: Fish consumption, fish oil, omega-3 fatty acids, and cardiovascular disease. Circulation 106:2747–2757, 2002.

50. LaMonte MJ, et al: Cardiorespiratory fitness and C-reactive protein among a tri-ethnic sample of women. Circulation 106:403–406, 2002.

51. Lardinois CK, Neumann SL: The effects of antihypertensive agents on serum lipids and lipoproteins. Arch Intern Med 148:1280–1288, 1988.

52. Lendon CL, et al: Atherosclerotic plaque caps are locally weakened when macrophages density is increased. Atherosclerosis 87:87–90, 1991.

53. Le Roith D, Zick Y: Recent advances in our understanding of insulin action and insulin resistance. Diabetes Care 24:588–597, 2001.

54. Li AC, Glass CK: The macrophage foam cell as a target for therapeutic intervention. Nat Med 8:1235–1242, 2002.

55. Lindholm LH, et al: Cardiovascular morbidity and mortality in patients with diabetes in the Losartan Intervention For Endpoint reduction in hypertension study (LIFE): a randomised trial against atenolol. Lancet 359:1004–1010, 2002.

56. Lipid Research Clinics Program: The Lipid Research Clinics Coronary Primary Prevention Trial results. I. Reduction in incidence of coronary heart disease. JAMA 251:351–374, 1984.

57. Major outcomes in high-risk hypertensive patients randomized to angiotensin-converting enzyme inhibitor or calcium channel blocker vs diuretic: The Antihypertensive and Lipid-Lowering Treatment to Prevent Heart Attack Trial (ALLHAT).

58. Malinow MR, et al: Reduction of plasma homocyst(e)ine levels by breakfast cereal fortified with folic acid in patients with coronary heart disease. N Engl J Med 338:1009–1015, 1998.

59. Manson JE, et al: The primary prevention of myocardial infarction. N Engl J Med 326:1406–1416, 1992.

60. Miranda PJ, DeFronzo RA, Califf RM, Guyton JR: The metabolic syndrome: definition, pathophysiology, and mechanisms. Am Heart J 2003 (in press).

61. Mittleman MA, et al: Triggering of acute myocardial infarction by heavy physical exertion. N Engl J Med 329:1677–1683, 1993.

62. Morrisett JD, et al: Lipoprotein(a): structure, metabolism and epidemiology. In Gotto AM Jr, editor: Plasma Lipoproteins, New Comprehensive Biochemistry, Vol. 14. Amsterdam: Elsevier, 1987, pp. 129–152.

63. MRC/BHF Heart Protection Study of antioxidant vitamin supplementation in 20,536 high-risk individuals: a randomised placebo-controlled trial. Lancet 360:23–33, 2002.

64. Neal B, et al: Effects of ACE inhibitors, calcium antagonists, and other blood-pressure-lowering drugs: results of prospectively designed overviews of randomised trials. Blood Pressure Lowering Treatment Trialists' Collaboration. Lancet 356:1955–1964, 2000.

65. Omar MA, et al: Rhabdomyolysis and HMG-CoA reductase inhibitors. Ann Pharmacother 35:1096–1107, 2001.

66. Ornish D, et al: Can lifestyle changes reverse coronary heart disease? The Lifestyle Heart Trial. Lancet 336:129–133, 1990.

67. Physicians' Health Study Research Group: Preliminary report: findings from the aspirin component of the ongoing physicians' health study. N Engl J Med 318:262–264, 1988.

68. Rader DJ, Brewer HB: Lipoprotein(a): clinical approach to a unique atherogenic lipoprotein. JAMA 267:1109–1112, 1993.

69. Reissell PK, et al: Treatment of hypertriglyceridemia. Am J Clin Nutr 19:84–98, 1966.

70. Ridker PM, et al: Comparison of C-reactive protein and low-density lipoprotein cholesterol levels in the prediction of first cardiovascular events. N Engl J Med 347:1557–1565, 2002.

71. Ridker, PM, et al: C-reactive protein, the metabolic syndrome, and risk of incident cardiovascular events: an 8-year follow-up of 14 719 initially healthy American women. Circulation 107:391–397, 2003.

72. Rossouw JE, et al: Risks and benefits of estrogen plus progestin in healthy postmenopausal women: principal results from the Women's Health Initiative randomized controlled trial. JAMA 288:321–333, 2002.

73. Rubins HB, et al: Gemfibrozil for the secondary prevention of coronary heart disease in men with low levels of high-density lipoprotein cholesterol. Veterans Affairs High-Density Lipoprotein Cholesterol Intervention Trial Study Group. N Engl J Med 341:410–418, 1999.

74. Sacks FM, et al: The effect of pravastatin on coronary events after myocardial infarction in patients with average cholesterol levels. N Engl J Med 335:1001–1009, 1996.

75. Scandinavian Simvastatin Survival Study Group: Randomised trial of cholesterol lowering in 4444 patients with coronary heart disease: the Scandinavian Simvastatin Survival Study (4S). Lancet 344:1383–1389, 1994.

76. Sever PS, et al: Prevention of coronary and stroke events with atorvastatin in hypertensive patients who have average or lower-than-average cholesterol concentrations, in the Anglo-Scandinavian Cardiac Outcomes Trial-Lipid Lowering Arm (ASCOT-LLA): a multicentre randomised controlled trial. Lancet 361:1149–1158, 2003.

77. Smith LC, et al: Structure and dynamics of human plasma lipoproteins. In Pifat G, Herak JN, editors: Supramolecular Structure and Function. New York: Plenum Press, 1983, pp. 205–231.

1020

78. Sytkowski PA, et al: Changes in risk factors and the decline in mortality from cardiovascular disease. N Engl J Med 322:1635–1641, 1990.

79. Wenger NK, et al: Baseline characteristics of participants in the Raloxifene Use for The Heart (RUTH) trial. Am J Cardiol 90:1204–1210, 2002.

80. Westman EC, et al: Effect of 6-month adherence to a very low carbohydrate diet program. Am J Med 113:30–36, 2002.

81. Wright JD, et al: Dietary intake of ten key nutrients for public health, United States: 1999–2000. Adv Data 1–4, 2003.

82. Yusuf S, et al: Effects of an angiotensin-converting-enzyme inhibitor, ramipril, on cardiovascular events in high-risk patients. The Heart Outcomes Prevention Evaluation Study Investigators. N Engl J Med 342:145–153, 2000.

Perioperative and Intraoperative Care of the Cardiac Surgical Patient

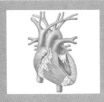

Adult Cardiac Anesthesia

CHAPTER **63**

Kyung W. Park, Feroze Mahmood, and Dharmender Chandhok

▶ INTRODUCTION

The first successful cardiac surgical procedure dates back to 1902, when Hill closed a stab wound to the heart of a 13-year-old boy. After the introduction of a cardio-pulmonary bypass (CPB) machine in 1953 by Gibbon, the concept of a cardiac surgical team made up of a cardiac surgeon, a cardiac anesthesiologist, and a perfusionist gradually developed. Lately, with transesophageal echocardiography (TEE) playing an essential role in intra-operative diagnosis, monitoring, and even prognostication of the cardiac patient, an anesthesiologist with competence in TEE plays an indispensable role in a cardiac surgical suite. Today the discipline of cardiac anesthesia encompasses an ever-expanding body of knowledge. This chapter provides a brief overview of preoperative anesthetic evaluation and intraoperative anesthetic management for adult cardiac surgery.

▶ PREOPERATIVE EVALUATION

The basic approaches in preoperative anesthetic evaluation of a cardiac surgical patient are as follows: (1) to review the events that led to the indication for cardiac surgery, (2) to identify and optimize known risk factors for mortality and morbidity resulting from cardiac surgery, and (3) to garner information with implications for selection of monitoring modalities and for management techniques during surgery.

Higgins and colleagues[46] performed a retrospective logistic regression on the data of more than 5,000 patients who underwent coronary artery bypasses, and they then prospectively applied the retrospectively identified risk factors to a group of more than 4,000 patients. They found that 30-day mortality was predicted by emergency procedure, preoperative serum creatinine of more than 168 μmol/L, left ventricular ejection fraction of less than 35%, preoperative hematocrit level of less than 35, age of more than 70 years, chronic pulmonary disease, prior vascular surgery, reoperation, and mitral regurgitation. Emergency cases were transfers from the coronary care unit with unstable angina (48%), complications of percutaneous intervention (40%), and complications of routine cardiac catheterizations (12%). In addition to these risk factors, nonfatal morbidity was predicted by diabetes mellitus, body weight of 65 kg or less, aortic stenosis, and cerebrovascular disease. Presence of these risk factors needs to be ascertained when obtaining preoperative history.

Emergency patients from the catheterization laboratory may have taken inhibitors of platelet aggregation. Clopidogrel (Plavix) and ticlopidine (Ticlid) inhibit ADP-induced platelet aggregation by irreversibly modifying platelet P2 receptors for the lifespan of these cells. Abciximab (ReoPro) is a monoclonal antibody fragment against glycoprotein (GP) IIb/IIIa receptor, which allows platelet binding to von Willebrand factor and fibrinogen. Abciximab is administered intravenously with an initial bolus of 0.25 mg/kg that is followed by an infusion of 0.25 μg/kg/min (up to 10 μg/min) for 12 hours. Following discontinuance, platelet function recovers gradually over the next 48 hours.[112,118] Eptifibatide (Integrilin) is a peptide inhibitor of GP IIb/IIIa receptor with an elimination half-life of 1 to 2 hours. Following discontinuance, platelet function (as measured by bleeding time) recovers in 2 to 4 hours.[102] Tirofiban (Aggrastat) is a peptidomimetic antagonist of GP IIb/IIIa receptor with an elimination half-life of about

2 hours; platelet function returns to normal within 4 to 8 hours after discontinuing the medication.[52,62] Whereas abciximab consistently prolongs the activated clotting time (ACT) used to monitor heparinization by 30 to 50 seconds and necessitates a reduction in the dose of heparin used concurrently to decrease bleeding complications, eptifibatide does not have a similar effect of ACT.[27] Additional historical information about anticoagulant use to be gathered preoperatively includes duration of use of heparin, heparin resistance, heparin-induced thrombocytopenia, use of Coumadin and the time of last dose, and the use of thrombolytics such as streptokinase. Additional historical information pertinent to cardiac surgery would include the presence of esophageal disease that may contraindicate the use of TEE, a history of cold agglutinin antibody (which may contraindicate hypothermic CPB), a history of antiphospholipid syndrome (which will adversely affect measurement of ACT), a history of previous thoracic surgery or radiation, and the presence of a pacemaker or an implantable cardioverter/defibrillator. Lastly, the list of medications should be obtained. In general, all cardiovascular medications should be continued even on the day of surgery, except perhaps diuretics. Preoperative β-adrenergic blocker use has been associated with survival after coronary artery surgery.[129]

Physical examination of the patient should be focused on the airway and the cardiovascular system. The airway examination should include examination of the dentition and discovery of any evidence of infection or abscess. Blood pressure should be measured on both arms, and any significant difference should be noted; this indicates possible subclavian artery stenosis. Peripheral pulses should be palpated and graded. Allen's test may be performed in case a radial artery harvest is being considered to serve as a conduit. Femoral pulsation should be palpated, and the presence of any peripheral vascular disease should be noted (this may make the placement of an intraaortic balloon challenging). Carotid bruits should be listened for, and cardiac sounds should be auscultated. Hepatomegaly, jugular venous distention, and/or peripheral edema should be noted.

Preoperative laboratory tests should include hematocrit, platelet count, coagulation parameters, electrolytes, serum creatinine, glucose, 12-lead electrocardiogram, and a chest X-ray. An echocardiogram, if performed, will not only provide information about preoperative ventricular and valvular function and anatomy but will also provide a baseline with which intraoperative TEE findings may be compared. The catheterization report should be reviewed for the distribution of coronary artery disease, ventricular systolic and diastolic dysfunction, valvular abnormalities, pulmonary hypertension, and intracardiac shunt.

▶ INTRAOPERATIVE MANAGEMENT

Monitoring

The American Society of Anesthesiologists' standard monitoring includes surface electrocardiography (ECG), pulse oximeter, capnography, (noninvasive) blood pressure monitoring, and temperature monitoring. On surface ECG, ST segment analysis should be continuously performed. When ischemia is defined as ≥0.1 mV (1 mm) horizontal or downsloping ST depression, ≥0.15 mV (1.5 mm) upsloping ST depression, or ≥0.15 mV (1.5 mm) ST elevation in a non-Q wave lead, sensitivity of V5 lead alone is 75%; that of V5 and V4 is 90%; that of V5 and II is 80%; and that of V5, V4, and II is 96%.[9] Use of the standard 5-lead ECG system does not allow simultaneous monitoring of V5 and V4, and the most practical alternative is to monitor leads V5 and II, the latter of which is also useful for arrhythmia monitoring. When right-sided ischemia is of concern, the right shoulder lead (usually white in color) may be placed in the right precordial area, and then lead I becomes right precordial lead (V$_4$R).[28] Simultaneous monitoring of V5, II, and V$_4$R allows for the detection of virtually 100% of all ischemic episodes that are detectable with full 12-lead ECG.[28]

In addition to the noninvasive monitors, invasive monitors are routinely employed in cardiac surgery. An arterial line is a must for continuous blood pressure monitoring and intermittent blood sampling. A radial artery is most commonly used—preferably one that is contralateral to the internal mammary artery to be used as a conduit—because of the theoretical concern of subclavian distortion by the retractor during conduit harvest. If the surgery involves the takeoff of the innominate artery or the left subclavian artery or if the radial artery is to be harvested as a conduit, the corresponding radial artery should not be used for an arterial line, and an alternative site should be sought. For an operation of the descending thoracic aorta, two arterial lines with one proximal to the proximal clamp and one distal to the distal clamp are recommended. The proximal arterial line (usually in the right radial artery) provides information about the perfusion pressure of the myocardium and the brain. The distal arterial line (usually a femoral artery line or, in the absence of a peripheral vascular disease, a dorsalis pedis line), in conjunction with an intrathecal catheter, allows for the calculation of the perfusion pressure of the spinal cord.

A central venous line (CVL) is routinely employed in cardiac surgery to allow for the reliable administration of cardiovascular medications and heparin and to monitor central venous pressures. Whether the use of a pulmonary artery catheter (PAC) should be routine or selective in cardiac surgery has been a matter of debate. In a prospective comparison of a CVL with a PAC in 1,094 patients undergoing coronary artery surgery (including the highest-risk patients), Tuman and colleagues[124] found that there was no difference in outcome. Likewise, Schwann and others[105] reported that, in their experience with 2,685 consecutive patients undergoing coronary artery bypass surgery, the use of a PAC was limited to 9% (2.4% unplanned [i.e., converted from a CVL]) of the patients and predicted by ejection fraction, Society of Thoracic Surgeons risk score, intraaortic balloon pump, congestive heart failure, re-do surgery, and New York Heart Association class IV. With such a selective use, their observed-to-expected ratio of mortality as comparison with the Society of Thoracic Surgeons database was 0.73. Furthermore, the presence of a pulmonary artery catheter has not been shown to influence anesthetic management during induction,[127] which is generally considered one of the most risky periods during anesthesia. These studies suggest that the use of a PAC may be highly selective in coronary surgery. However, it should be also noted that, unlike a CVL, a PAC can provide information about cardiac output, systemic and pulmonary vascular resistance, and mixed venous saturation, and it can also be used to pace the heart. Alternatively, the widespread use of a TEE may negate some of the potential advantages of a PAC over a CVL: cardiac output measured by TEE can be reliable and comparable with that measured by a PAC[131]; TEE-guided right and left ventricular oximetry may be feasible[78]; and pulmonary artery pressures can be estimated by TEE.[54]

A detailed review of the indications and capabilities of TEE is beyond the scope of this chapter; several excellent books about TEE are available. The American Society of Echocardiography and the Society of Cardiovascular Anesthesiologists have published guidelines for what makes up a comprehensive intraoperative TEE exam[110] and how one should be trained and certified for competence in perioperative TEE.[2,12] Current indications and use of perioperative TEE are ever-expanding. In addition to serving as a monitor of myocardial function and ischemia and valvular function, TEE is an invaluable guide for the placement of coronary sinus and intraaortic catheters, for the delineation of the anatomy and pathology of valve lesions, and for before-and-after comparison of myocardial perfusion and function and valvular anatomy and function (Figures 63-1 and 63-2). In addition, TEE may be used to assess the delivery of cardioplegia[4,5] and to predict changes in regional myocardial function after coronary artery bypass.[3]

In surgeries of the descending thoracic aorta, cerebrospinal fluid pressure (CSFP) may be measured with an intrathecal catheter. If such a catheter is placed, CSFP should be maintained at ≤10 cm H_2O, and CSF should be allowed to drain for CSFP >10 cm H_2O.[117] However, spinal cord perfusion depends not only on CSFP but also on the arterial pressure distal to the distal clamp, and the maintenance of the distal arterial pressure may be just as important for use of, for example, a partial bypass or a shunt. Whether monitoring of CSFP and drainage of CSF to maintain CSFP <10 cm H_2O prevents paraplegia after descending thoracic aortic surgery is still being debated.[70]

Choice of Anesthetic Agents

High-dose opioid anesthesia was developed in the late 1960s, and it was based on the observation by Lowenstein and colleagues[76] that patients on mechanical ventilation after cardiac surgery tolerated large doses of morphine (0.5–3 mg/kg) for sedation and analgesia with minimal hemodynamic effects. Such large doses were then tried immediately before operation as an adjunct to anesthesia for cardiac surgery, with significant success.[75] Opioids by themselves do not assure amnesia, and they require supplementation with an amnestic such as a benzodiazepine or scopolamine, the latter with unreliable effectiveness and declining popularity. Synthetic opioids such as fentanyl (50–100 μg/kg) or sufentanil (5–10 μg/kg) provide similar hemodynamic effects but without the fluid retention often seen with high-dose morphine anesthesia. Although highly successful and popular in the 1980s and early 1990s, high-dose opioid anesthesia has gradually given way to a balanced anesthetic technique that involves employing a modest dose of opioids in conjunction with inhalational anesthetics and other intravenous adjuncts that have a faster onset and offset to facilitate early extubation and discharge from the intensive care unit (ICU).

Although the observation by Reiz and colleagues[99] in 1983 that isoflurane may cause coronary steal (a phenomenon

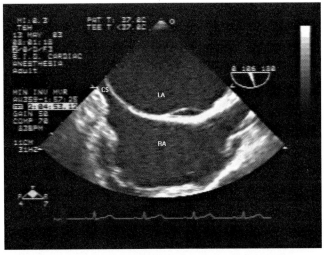

A

B

Figure 63–1 **A,** A modified midesophageal bicaval view demonstrating the left atrium (LA), the right atrium (RA), and the coronary sinus (CS). **B,** The same view after successful placement of the coronary sinus catheter.

in which coronary blood flow is diverted away from the collateral-dependent region of the myocardium) tended to discourage the use of the inhalational agent, subsequent investigators failed to duplicate the findings.[17,42,85] The newer agents sevoflurane and desflurane do not cause coronary steal, either.[43,56] In addition, animal studies suggested that isoflurane may preferentially dilate large coronary arteries rather than arterioles (thus mimicking the effect of nitroglycerin[109]) and normal coronary arterioles rather than arterioles from a collateral-dependent region of the myocardium.[94,95] Furthermore, there is mounting evidence that inhalational agents precondition the heart, thus protecting it from subsequent ischemic episodes in an analogous fashion to ischemic preconditioning, in which a brief period of ischemia protects the heart from subsequent prolonged ischemic episodes.[16,24,123] Anesthetic-induced preconditioning occurs via activation of ATP-sensitive potassium channels.[57] Currently inhalational agents are the mainstay of anesthesia for cardiac surgery, and these are supplemented with muscle relaxants and a modest amount of opioids for analgesia.

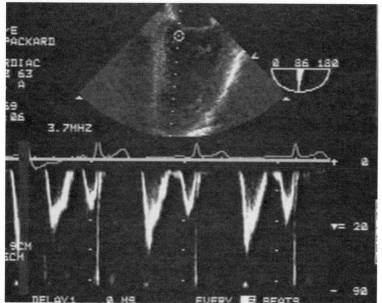

A

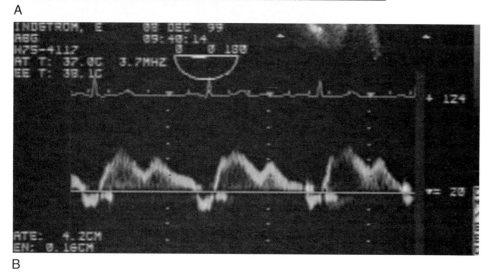

B

Figure 63–2 The left ventricular diastolic function may be assessed by examination of the mitral inflow into the ventricle and the pulmonary venous inflow.

Regional Anesthesia/Analgesia

The use of thoracic epidural anesthesia (TEA) as a supplement to general anesthesia carries several potential advantages. TEA attenuates the sympathetic stress response to surgical stimulation, reduces heart rate and myocardial oxygen consumption, and decreases the release of troponin T.[61,72] Postoperatively, TEA provides superior analgesia, thus enabling early extubation and vigorous pulmonary toilet and reducing the incidence of lower respiratory tract infections as compared with conventional intravenous analgesia.[107,119] Despite these advantages, TEA has not been widely accepted for cardiac surgery because of concern for a potential epidural hematoma in patients who are to be anticoagulated for the institution of CPB. The true incidence of an epidural hematoma in cardiac surgery is not known, because such a complication has not yet been reported in cardiac surgical settings. A mathematical model suggests that the risk ranges from 1:150,000 to 1:1,500.[47] If TEA is to be used, it should be avoided in patients who are receiving preoperative anticoagulation, and the placement may be performed the day before surgery, with postponement of surgery and neurological monitoring in the case of a "bloody" placement.

Recently, with the advent of off-pump, minimally invasive cardiac surgery, several European groups have reported using TEA as the sole anesthetic modality without endotracheal intubation in patients undergoing coronary artery bypass surgery[6,53] and aortic valve replacement.[103] The authors cite that potential advantages of avoiding general anesthesia might include the use of the patient's mental status as a monitor of cerebral ischemia and achievement of truly fast-track cardiac surgery. In a study of this modality by Karagoz and colleagues,[53] 8 out of 137 patients went home the day of surgery, and 58 of these 137 did not require any ICU stay, for an overall mean hospitalization of 1 day. However, 39 out of the 137 patients had a pneumothorax, and 4 of them had to be converted to general anesthesia because of pneumothorax-related respiratory difficulties. Potential disadvantage of an awake technique in cardiac surgery may include the stress response of an awake patient to surgical maneuvers such as sternotomy and a delay in surgical progress.[77] An awake TEA for cardiac surgery has not yet found acceptance in the United States.

Intraoperative Blood Glucose Control

Acute and chronic hyperglycemia increases the risk of myocardial ischemic injury through several mechanisms.[40] Hyperglycemia decreases coronary collateral blood flow, causes endothelial dysfunction, and compromises the salutary effect of ischemic preconditioning or anesthetic-induced pharmacological preconditioning.[55,58] Among oral hypoglycemic agents, sulfonylureas and other insulin secretagogues impair K_{ATP} channel activation and may therefore hinder ischemic or pharmacological preconditioning. Such agents should be discontinued for 24 to 48 hours before surgery and avoided perioperatively.[40]

Furnary and others[35] performed a prospective study of nearly 2,500 consecutive diabetic patients undergoing cardiac surgery who were randomized to receive either intensive insulin therapy with continuous infusion to maintain blood glucose <200 mg/dL or intermittent subcutaneous insulin injections on a sliding scale. Blood glucose was better controlled with intravenous infusion (85% of patients with blood glucose <200 mg/dL on postoperative day 1, with a mean level of 199 ± 1.4 mg/dL) than with subcutaneous injections (47% of patients with <200 mg/dL, with a mean level of 241 ± 1.9 mg/dL). The incidence of deep sternal wound infection was significantly reduced in the infusion group (0.8% versus 2.0%, p = .01) and approached that of the nondiabetics. Mortality was likewise reduced with intensive insulin therapy (3.0% versus 6.1%, p = .03). In a retrospective review of 3,554 diabetic patients from the same group,[34] mortality was directly related to postoperative mean glucose; it was demonstrated to be 0.9% for those with <150 mg/dL, 1.3% for those with 150 to 175 mg/dL, 2.3% for those with 175 to 200 mg/dL, 4.1% for those with 200 to 225 mg/dL, 6.0% for those with 225 to 250 mg/dL, to 14.5% for those with >250 mg/dL. Intensive insulin therapy to tightly control blood glucose should not only be employed intraoperatively; it should also be extended into the postoperative period in the ICU. In a prospective study of 1,548 patients in the surgical ICU (about two thirds of whom had been through cardiac surgery), intensive insulin therapy to a maintain glucose level between 80 and 110 mg/dL was associated with a lower mortality as compared with conventional therapy to maintain a glucose level between 180 and 200 mg/dL (4.6% versus 8.0%, p < .04).[125]

Acid-base Management During Hypothermia

As the temperature decreases, the dissociation of water to H^+ and OH^- decreases. The pH at electroneutrality, where $[H^+]$ = $[OH^-]$, therefore increases with a decrease in temperature. At 37° C, $[H^+]$ at electroneutrality is 40 nEq/L, which corresponds with a pH of 7.4. Two approaches to acid-base management during hypothermic CPB are currently in use; they are pH-stat and α-stat management. With pH-stat management, the clinical objective is to maintain a pH of 7.4 at the patient's true core temperature. Blood gases and pH are measured with a temperature correction. To maintain a pH of 7.4 at hypothermic temperatures requires the addition of exogenous CO_2 to maintain a temperature-corrected $PaCO_2$ of 35 to 40 mmHg. With α-stat management, the objective is to maintain electroneutrality. With this approach, blood gases and pH are measured without temperature correction (i.e., as if the patient's temperature is always 37° C) and maintained at a $PaCO_2$ of 40 mmHg and a pH of 7.4. The actual pH is allowed to vary with body temperature.

With pH-stat measurement, the addition of CO_2 will correct hypothermia-induced leftward shift of the oxyhemoglobin dissociation curve and may improve oxygen delivery to the tissues. On the other hand, because the cerebral blood flow response to CO_2 is preserved during hypothermia, pH-stat management may lead to excessive cerebral blood flow and interference with cerebral autoregulation and flow/metabolism coupling.[87,100] However, clinical neuropsychological outcome has not been shown to be different between pH-stat and α-stat management.[7]

Anticoagulation for Cardiopulmonary Bypass

Heparin sulfate, which is produced from porcine gut or bovine lung, is used to mimic the natural role of heparan sulfate on the vascular endothelial surface. Heparin—although it has no anticoagulant effect by itself—complexes with and enhances the activity of antithrombin-III (AT-III) in irreversibly neutralizing thrombin and factor Xa. Heparin also increases the activity of heparin cofactor II to inhibit the action of thrombin.[122] What constitutes a safe and effective level of heparinization for CPB has not been established, in part because of the inconsistent relationship between heparin dosing, plasma heparin concentration, and clinical effect (as measured by ACT) and in part because ACT is a nonspecific test affected not only by heparin but also by platelets and temperature.[32] Most currently accepted heparin regimens use an initial dose of 250 to 400 IU/kg to maintain an ACT of more than 400 to 480 seconds.[39] However, animal studies suggest that reduced heparin administration to maintain ACT between 250 and 300 seconds may be just as adequate.[13] Administration of heparin may be followed by hypotension in association with hyperkalemia;[51] part of the reason for hypotension may be the heparin-induced production of nitric oxide.[69]

Heparin resistance may be defined as the failure of 500 IU/kg of heparin to prolong the ACT to 480 seconds or more.[113] Factors that predict heparin resistance include AT-III levels of 60% or less, preoperative subcutaneous or intravenous heparin therapy, platelet count of 300,000 or more per cc, and age of 65 years or more.[97] AT-III levels may be low because of reduced synthesis from genetic defects or from such acquired causes as liver disease, oral contraceptive use, and disseminated intravascular coagulation; increased consumption from disseminated intravascular coagulation, extensive deep vein thrombosis, sepsis, or preeclampsia; or concomitant use of heparin, nitroglycerin, or the chemotherapeutic agent L-asparaginase. Treatment of heparin resistance with increasingly higher doses of heparin is intended to maximally bind all available AT-III and may, at times, be effective. Alternatively, the patient may receive fresh frozen plasma[101] or AT-III concentrate. In vivo recovery of AT-III activity is about 1.4% per unit/kg of administered AT-III concentrate,[106] and the therapeutic goal should be to maintain AT-III activity at more than 80%.

After separation from CPB, heparin activity is neutralized by the administration of protamine. Protamine in doses of up to 1 to 1.3 mg/mg of heparin (100 IU of heparin) may be used, taking into account the heparin activity half-life of 90 minutes. Just as incomplete reversal of heparinization

1026

may lead to excessive postbypass bleeding, excessive protamine can decrease both platelet number and function,[126] prolong ACT,[83] and reduce the effect of thrombin.[22] To distinguish whether a prolonged ACT after an adequate dose of protamine indicates incomplete heparin reversal or excessive protamine may require the measurement of the thrombin time and the heparinase-ACT and low-level titration of heparin and protamine.

Five types of protamine-related adverse reactions have been recognized. First, rapid administration of protamine (>5 mg/min) may at times induce the release of histamine from mast cells and thus cause systemic hypotension.[48] Second, protamine may act as an antigen that initiates an immunoglobulin (Ig)G- or IgE-mediated anaphylactic reaction, especially in diabetic patients who take protamine-containing insulin preparations[37,115,130] and possibly in those with a true fish (not shellfish) allergy or those who have just had a vasectomy.[48] Third, protamine-heparin complexes may activate the complement system, thereby leading to an anaphylactoid reaction.[9,59] Fourth, protamine-heparin mediated complement activation may lead to thromboxane A_2 generation, precipitating catastrophic pulmonary hypertension[86]; this is in contrast with the low systemic and pulmonary pressures seen in classic anaphylactoid reactions. In a pig model, this reaction was preventable by prior administration of indomethacin or a thromboxane A_2 receptor antagonist.[23] Lastly, fulminant noncardiogenic pulmonary edema and systemic anasarca have been reported 15 minutes to more than 1 hour after the administration of protamine.[48] Treatment of a protamine reaction is supportive, and various agents (e.g., diphenhydramine, steroids) and hemodynamic support have been tried. In a patient with a history of prior adverse reaction to protamine, it should be determined whether the reaction was immunologically mediated. Levels of IgG, IgE, thromboxane, and C5a at the time of the reaction, if available, may be useful, but a skin test or enzyme-linked immunosorbent assay has not been found to be useful.[49] When the cause of the reaction is uncertain, some people advocate pretreatment of the patient with steroids and histamine blockers and the slow administration of protamine. If a true immunologically mediated protamine reaction occurred, it would be best to avoid it. Protamine alternatives that are being tested include recombinant platelet factor 4,[67] hexadimethrine,[60] heparinase,[44] and a heparin removal device that uses a venovenous circuit with a poly-L-lysine-agarose surface.[132]

Use of Antifibrinolytics

Despite adequate heparinization, use of the CPB is usually accompanied by the low-level activation of coagulation and fibrinolysis,[63] which leads to the consumption of coagulation factors and increased bleeding postoperatively. Three antifibrinolytics in common use are ε-amino-caproic acid (EACA), tranexamic acid (TA), and aprotinin. EACA and TA are synthetic analogues of the amino acid lysine and competitively block the lysine binding sites between plasmin and fibrin(ogen). They reduce fibrinolysis and, by reducing fibrin split products, indirectly prevent platelet dysfunction. No uniform dose regimen has been established for either EACA or TA. For EACA, a plasma level of 130 μg/mL is needed for the complete inhibition of fibrinolysis,[8] and dosing regimens

include 3 doses of 10 g (preincision, on pump, and after bypass) or a weight-based initial loading of 150 mg/kg followed by an infusion of at least 15 mg/kg/hr. For TA, Horrow and colleagues[50] recommend a 10 mg/kg load followed by an infusion of 1 mg/kg/hr, but other regimens have also been published. Both EACA and TA are renally eliminated. In direct, head-to-head comparison, TA has been found to be equally or more effective than EACA for reducing blood loss, but both were better than placebo.[15,41] In patients requiring deep hypothermic circulatory arrest (DHCA), there have been reports of fatal thrombosis in association with EACA use.[33]

Aprotinin is a serine protease inhibitor and inhibits not only plasmin but also trypsin, kallikrein, and bradykinin-kinin. Aprotinin's activity is measured in kallikrein-inhibiting units (KIU), and 1 mg of aprotinin is equal to 7,140 KIU. In addition to inhibiting fibrinolysis, aprotinin may reduce the consumption of coagulation factors and the activation of mediators of inflammation. Aprotinin is at least as effective as TA or EACA for reducing perioperative blood loss, but it is much more costly.[15] A "full" dose of aprotinin involves a loading dose of 2,000,000 KIU (280 mg) followed by an infusion dose of 500,000 KIU/hr, with an additional 2,000,000 KIU in the pump. Because of concern about the cost and side effects of the medication, a half-dose regimen has been tried and appears to be equally as effective.[68,71,104] Aprotinin is cleared renally and may cause thrombotic sludging in the renal tubules, thus leading to a small transient increase in serum creatinine; however, clinically significant renal dysfunction is uncommon.[65] Aprotinin has been safely used even in patients with chronic renal failure.[64] In one report, renal dysfunction and thrombotic complications were noted with aprotinin use in patients requiring DHCA;[116] however, other authors found aprotinin use to be safe even with DHCA.[31,91,108] Because aprotinin is isolated from bovine lung mast cells, there is a risk of allergic reactions, with the incidence of anaphylaxis reported to be less than 0.6% on initial exposure and up to 5% with reexposure within 6 months,[29] although the incidence falls off rapidly after 6 months. Before the administration of the regular dose, a test dose of 10,000 KIU of aprotinin should be given, and histamine blockers and steroids may be considered if there is history of previous exposure within 6 months.

Cerebral Protection During Deep Hypothermic Circulatory Arrest

Techniques that have been used to ameliorate ischemic injury of the brain during DHCA include selective cannulation and perfusion of cerebral vessels, retrograde cerebral perfusion, pharmacological brain protection, and the achievement of deep hypothermia. At normothermia, roughly half of the oxygen consumed is used to maintain cellular integrity ("basal" $CMRO_2$), and the other half is used to maintain electrical activity ("functional" $CMRO_2$).[90] Hypothermia has a greater effect on the basal $CMRO_2$ than the functional $CMRO_2$.[89] Electroencephalogram becomes isoelectric at 18° C, and below this temperature, any further reduction in $CMRO_2$ is from a decrease in basal $CMRO_2$. Barbiturates, which reduce functional $CMRO_2$ without having much effect on basal $CMRO_2$, do not produce any additional metabolic suppression under conditions of deep hypothermia (15° C), and they are not likely to be of benefit.[114] On the other hand, barbiturates may be of benefit for ameliorating the effects of temporary focal ischemia (e.g., from an air embolus on normothermic bypass) by the suppression of functional $CMRO_2$.

Ischemic injury on DHCA may be temporally divided into 4 phases.[121,128] The first phase is marked by energy production failure and membrane depolarization. After ischemic depolarization occurs, detrimental neuroexcitatory transmitters such as glutamate are released. With the restoration of blood flow, the third phase ensues and is marked by an increased release of oxygen free radicals and subsequent tissue damage. In the fourth phase, ischemia may also trigger apoptosis or programmed cell death over the ensuing weeks. Inhalational anesthetics lower the critical cerebral blood flow, a level below which the majority of patients develop ischemic EEG changes.[38,81] At normothermia, the critical cerebral blood flow is 10 mL/100 g/min for isoflurane, 11.5 mL/100g/min for sevoflurane, 15 mL/100 g/min for enflurane, and 20 mL/100 g/min for halothane. This metabolic suppression effect of inhalational agents amounts to delaying the first phase of ischemic injury. In addition, isoflurane may inhibit excitotoxicity from the accumulation of glutamate during the second phase of ischemic injury. Isoflurane has been shown to reduce the release of glutamate during ischemia[96] and may also be an antagonist of glutamate receptors, thereby diminishing deleterious calcium influx.[79] Because of its effect on the first 2 phases of ischemic injury, isoflurane may "buy time" before irreversible neuronal damage sets in. However, in aortic surgical settings with the employment of DHCA, anesthetics have not been demonstrated to be of benefit. Similarly, although various other pharmacological modalities (e.g., diuretics, steroids, calcium-channel blockers) have been used, none has been demonstrated to be of benefit in DHCA.

Hemodynamic Support on Separation from Cardiopulmonary Bypass

Separating a patient from CPB may be considered a form of resuscitation and, as with any sort of cardiopulmonary resuscitation, it should start with the confirmation of a patent airway (usually with an endotracheal tube) and the reestablishment of ventilation. For support of the circulation, the anesthesiologist needs to continually assess and treat the five elements of preload, afterload, contractility, rate, and rhythm and the metabolic parameters that affect myocardial function, such as pH, electrolytes (especially potassium, calcium, and magnesium), oxygen-carrying capacity (hemoglobin), and temperature. In addition, the anesthesiologist needs to be in communication with the surgeon, because certain surgical maneuvers may mechanically affect myocardial function, and TEE assessment of the adequacy of the surgery (e.g., valvular anatomy and function) and the patient's ability to remain separated from CPB needs to be communicated back to the surgeon.

Usually, epicardial pacing wires are placed, and the pacing function is tested before separation. A rhythm (e.g., sinus rhythm, AV sequential pacing) that preserves the atrial augmentation of ventricular preload is preferred. If the pump flow is set at what may be considered an adequate cardiac output, the vascular tone of the patient may be adjusted to the desired mean pressure while the patient is still on CPB; this way, the mean pressure will be in the desired range if the patient generates the desired cardiac output after separation. Then, the heart is filled, a process that is guided by the appearance of the heart in the surgical field and on TEE as well as by the filling pressures (Figure 63-3). Wall motion on TEE and cardiac output measurement then serve as practical surrogate measures of contractility.

Further adjustment of preload may be made by additional filling/draining of the heart by the perfusionist, by adjustment of the operating table position, or by intravenous fluid administration. Adjustment of the afterload to maintain the systemic and pulmonary vascular resistance in the normal range may be made with vasopressors (e.g., phenylephrine, norepinephrine, dopamine) or dilators (e.g., nitroglycerin, nitroprusside). In cases of catecholamine-resistant refractory hypotension, vasopressin in doses of 7 to 20 u/hr may

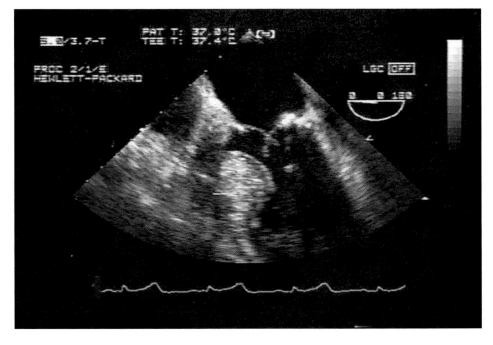

Figure 63–3 Transesophageal echocardiograph demonstrating systolic anterior motion (SAM) of the anterior leaflet of the mitral valve. Presence of systolic anterior motion should alter the hemodynamic management strategy to avoid the use of an inotropic agent and a vasodilator and to ensure adequate filling of the left ventricle. LDL, low density lipoprotein; IDL, intermediate density lipoprotein; VLDL, very low density lipoprotein.

be attempted.[93] Inotropic assistance to augment myocardial contractility may be provided by catecholaminergic agents (e.g., epinephrine, dopamine, dobutamine) or phosphodiesterase inhibitors (e.g., milrinone).[11] When pharmacological and metabolic support prove insufficient, consideration should be given to mechanical support devices (e.g., an intraaortic balloon pump, a ventricular assist device) and/or to returning the patient to CPB for further surgical remedies. Only when the patient is hemodynamically stable after separation from CPB should the reversal of heparinization be started.

► SPECIAL CONSIDERATIONS

Fast-track Cardiac Surgery

Fast-track cardiac surgery (FTCS) refers to a multidisciplinary approach to providing care to cardiac surgical patients, with emphasis placed on early tracheal extubation (within 6–10 hours postoperatively) and expedited mobilization of the patient (with consequent reduction in ICU and hospital length of stay and in cost).[19] Factors that predict the success or failure of this approach (other than age) are intraoperative and postoperative clinical process variables, such as intraoperative inotrope use, intraoperative placement of an intraaortic balloon pump, and postoperative atrial arrhythmias; thus there is no need to preselect patients for FTCS, and everyone may be considered a potential candidate for early extubation.[19] An important component of FTCS is an anesthetic technique that allows for the early extubation and mobilization of the patient.[45] Instead of a long-acting muscle relaxant (e.g., pancuronium), a shorter-acting agent (e.g., rocuronium, cisatracurium) may be employed.[88,92,120] Any residual blockade at the end of surgery or during the initiation of weaning may be reversed with an acetylcholinesterase inhibitor (e.g., neostigmine) in combination with an antimuscarinic agent. Instead of a high-dose opioid technique, a low- or moderate-dose opioid technique in combination with inhalational anesthetics and/or neuraxial analgesia may facilitate early tracheal extubation.[10] Hypothermia at the end of surgery should be prevented.[66] Although early extubation is favored, there is no benefit of pushing for tracheal extubation in the operating room.[84] One should also consider the cost of extended operating room time and the risk of cardiorespiratory instability during the period immediately after closure.

In both a retrospective review[74] and a prospective randomized controlled trial,[111] it has been demonstrated that FTCS is not associated with any increase in hospital mortality or morbidity. Rather, the rate of nosocomial pneumonia may be decreased with FTCS.[74] The reintubation rate is not significantly different between FTCS and the conventional approach, and both ICU and hospital length of stay are decreased with FTCS. In response to concerns that FTCS may result in cost shifting rather than cost savings, Cheng and colleagues[20] examined the resource use of both FTCS and conventional patients for a year after hospital discharge. Although insurance claims for outpatient visits were not significantly different at 3 months and 12 months, insurance claims and costs for inpatient care were significantly lower for the FTCS group. The savings in inpatient care were 68%

at 3 months and about 50% at 1 year. Thus, FTCS may lead to savings both during the initial hospitalization for the surgery and during the subsequent follow-up period.

Off-pump Coronary Artery Bypass

Off-pump coronary artery bypass (OPCAB) involves bypass grafting on a beating heart without the employment of CPB. Surgical techniques, complications, and success rates of OPCAB are covered elsewhere in the book. For an anesthesiologist, OPCAB involves more intensive hemodynamic management with the potential for instability because of retraction and compression of the heart and consequent potential myocardial ischemia.[80] After sternotomy and exposure of the heart, each target vessel is identified, and a specialized retractor is applied to provide exposure of the target site. Test occlusion of the target vessel to assess its effect on myocardial function and/or to provide ischemic preconditioning is performed in some centers. The heart itself may be lifted and/or twisted to improve surgical exposure, and this maneuver may compromise the filling of the cardiac chambers. To maintain coronary perfusion pressure, the patient may be placed in Trendelenburg position, given fluids, and/or supported with a vasopressor (e.g., phenylephrine). Constant communication between the anesthesiologist and the surgeon is key to prevent unexpected hemodynamic compromise. With lifting of the heart, visualization by TEE is compromised, and one needs to rely on direct visualization of the surgical field and traditional hemodynamic monitors such as an arterial line and a PAC. Proximal anastomoses are performed with a side biter on the aorta. Systemic blood pressure and aortic wall tension need to be controlled for the application and removal of the side biter.

The level of heparinization required for OPCAB has not been standardized.[14,30] At some centers, "full" heparinization to maintain the ACT at more than 480 seconds is used, whereas others use limited heparinization to maintain the ACT in the 200 to 300 second range, just as is done for vascular procedures. Neither approach has been demonstrated to be clearly superior to the other.

Port-access Minimally Invasive Cardiac Surgery

The port-access system is used for minimally invasive cardiac surgery (MICS) that requires the institution of CPB. Preoperative preparation of the patient requires discussion between the surgeon and the anesthesiologist about the exact nature of the surgery planned.[18,36] The usual intravenous access and monitoring modalities (i.e., those used for conventional cardiac surgery) need to be placed. TEE is an essential modality, and contraindications to the use of TEE would almost preclude port-access MICS. Positioning for MICS is usually a modified lateral decubitus position, and this may have implications for line placement. To provide lung isolation, a double-lumen bronchocath or a bronchial blocker may be used. Position of the bronchocath should be confirmed with a fiberoptic bronchoscope upon placement and after final positioning of the patient. The bronchoscope should be readily available throughout the procedure, because any malposition of the tube can result in lung inflation and thus make the surgery almost impossible through the limited incision. Before positioning the patient, external cardioversion pads should be applied for urgent pacing or cardioversion, because internal paddles cannot be employed due to limited access.

The mainstays of the port-access system are the coronary sinus catheter (CSC) for retrograde cardioplegia, the pulmonary artery vent (PAV), and the endovascular aortic cannula, which also acts as an endovascular clamp (Figure 63-1). Unlike the regular PAC, these catheters are not heparin bonded by the manufacturers and, hence, 5,000 units of heparin are administered before placement of these catheters. Before CSC placement, a left-sided superior vena cava needs to be excluded by TEE. Under TEE guidance, the success rate of CSC placement has been reported to be 95%[1] and to be superior to fluoroscopy.[1,82] After successful placement of the CSC, its position is further confirmed by balloon inflation and visualization of the arterialization of the pressure tracing. Although not essential, keeping the balloon inflated and the wire loaded into the catheter until immediately before administration of retrograde cardioplegia may help prevent catheter dislodgement. The PAV is also inserted through the right internal jugular vein and guided into the pulmonary artery like a regular PAC. However, central venous pressure cannot be measured with the PAV. Venous access or a drainage line is placed through the femoral vein, and TEE is used to accurately position the cannula. Similarly, the endovascular aortic cannula can be very accurately placed under TEE guidance. The positions of the catheters should be confirmed after a change of position from supine to lateral and before commencement of CPB, because it is very difficult to reposition the catheters after commencement of CPB as a result of poor visibility.

Regardless of the type of surgery, recognition of intracardiac air and monitoring the success of de-airing maneuvers is a crucial TEE function. The left ventricular apex, which may not be accessible to the surgeon and hence not amenable to needle aspiration, needs to be carefully examined by TEE. TEE is the only monitor used to assess the completeness of de-airing.[82]

Other factors to consider during MICS include the possibility of urgent cardiac pacing and external cardioversion; suture placement in difficult sites, which can lead to bleeding; inadequate valve repair resulting in residual regurgitation; and air embolism. Even a small amount of bleeding in a minimally exposed place can result in tamponade after chest closure. The duration of anesthesia and surgery tends to be prolonged, and there is always the risk of a technically unsatisfactory result and conversion to an open conventional surgery. At the end of the surgery, the CSC is removed and, depending on the condition of the patient, the PAV may be replaced with a PAC for postoperative monitoring of the patient.

Robotic-Assisted Cardiac Surgery

Robotic-assisted cardiac surgery (RACS) is the next step in the evolution of MICS and is currently available in only a few places in the world. The goal of RACS is to perform the procedure with as small an incision as possible with an outcome that is equivalent or superior to that of the conventional procedure.[25,26] Anesthetic management for RACS requires all of the techniques outlined above for port-access MICS, and consideration must be given to the possibility of significantly pro-

longed surgery and the potential for positional neurovascular injuries (e.g., to the brachial plexus).[26] Nevertheless, there are preliminary reports of faster recovery and reduced complications.[21,98] However, long-term results are still pending.

REFERENCES

1. Applebaum R, Cutler W, Bhardwaj N, et al: Utility of transesophageal echocardiography during port-access minimally invasive cardiac surgery. Am J Cardiol 82:183–188, 1998
2. Aronson S, Butler A, Subhiyah R, et al: Development and analysis of a new certifying examination in perioperative transesophageal echocardiography. Anesth Analg 95:1476–1482, 2002.
3. Aronson S, Dupont F, Savage R, et al: Changes in regional myocardial function after coronary artery bypass graft surgery are predicted by intraoperative low-dose dobutamine echocardiography. Anesthesiology 93:685–692, 2000.
4. Aronson S, Lee BK, Liddicoat JR, et al: Assessment of retrograde cardioplegia distribution using contrast echocardiography. Ann Thorac Surg 52:810–814, 1991.
5. Aronson S, Lee BK, Wiencek JG, et al: Assessment of myocardial perfusion during CABG surgery with two-dimensional transesophageal contrast echocardiography. Anesthesiology 75:433–440, 1991.
6. Aybek T, Kessler P, Khan MF, et al: Operative techniques in awake coronary artery bypass grafting. J Thorac Cardiovasc Surg 125:1394–1400, 2003.
7. Bashein G, Townes BD, Nessly ML, et al: A randomized study of carbon dioxide management during hypothermic cardiopulmonary bypass. Anesthesiology 72:7–15, 1990.
8. Bennett-Guerrero E, Sorohan JG, Canada AT, et al: ε-aminocaproic acid plasma levels during cardiopulmonary bypass. Anesth Analg 85:248–251, 1997.
9. Best N, Sinosich MJ, Teisner B, et al: Complement activation during cardiopulmonary bypass by heparin-protamine interaction. Br J Anaesth 56:339–343, 1984.
10. Bettex DA, Schmidlin D, Chassot P-G, Schmid ER: Intrathecal sufentanil-morphine shortens the duration of intubation and improves analgesia in fast-track cardiac surgery. Can J Anesth 49:711–717, 2002.
11. Butterworth JF, Hines RL, Royster RL, James RL: A pharmacokinetic and pharmacodynamic evaluation of milrinone in adults undergoing cardiac surgery. Anesth Analg 81:783–792, 1995.
12. Cahalan MK, Abel M, Goldman M, et al. American Society of Echocardiography and Society of Cardiovascular Anesthesiologists Task Force guidelines for training in perioperative echocardiography. Anesth Analg 94:1384–1388, 2002.
13. Cardoso PF, Yamazaki F, Keshavjee S, et al: A reevaluation of heparin requirements for cardiopulmonary bypass. J Thorac Cardiovasc Surg 101:153–160, 1991.
14. Carrier M, Robitalle D, Perrault LP, et al: Heparin versus danaparoid in off-pump coronary bypass grafting: result of a prospective randomized clinical trial. J Thorac Cardiovasc Surg 125:325–329, 2003.
15. Casati V, Guzzon D, Oppizzi M, et al: Hemostatic effects of aprotinin, tranexamic acid and ε-aminocaproic acid in primary cardiac surgery. Ann Thorac Surg 68:2252–2257, 1999.
16. Cason BA, Gampert AK, Slocum RE, Hickey RF: Anesthetic-induced preconditioning: previous administration of isoflurane decreases myocardial infarct size in rabbits. Anesthesiology 87:1182–1190, 1997.
17. Cason BA, Verrier ED, London MJ, et al: Effects of isoflurane and halothane on coronary vascular resistance and col-

lateral myocardial blood flow: their capacity to induce coronary steal. Anesthesiology 67:665–675, 1987.

18. Chaney MA: Anesthetic management of port-access minimally invasive cardiac surgery. J Indian Med Assoc 97:425–431, 1999.

19. Cheng D: Fast track cardiac surgery pathways: early extubation, process of care, and cost containment. Anesthesiology 88:1429–1433, 1998.

20. Cheng DCH, Wall C, Djaiani G, et al: Randomized assessment of resource use in fast-track cardiac surgery 1-year after hospital discharge. Anesthesiology 98:651–657, 2003.

21. Chitwood WR Jr, Nifong LW: Minimally invasive videoscopic mitral valve surgery: the current role of surgical robotics. J Card Surg 15:61–75, 2000.

22. Cobel-Gerard RJ, Hassouna HI: Interaction of protamine sulfate with thrombin. Am J Hematol 14:227–233, 1983.

23. Conzen PF, Habazettl H, Gutmann R, et al: Thromboxane mediation of pulmonary hemodynamic responses after neutralization of heparin by protamine in pigs. Anesth Analg 68:25–31, 1989.

24. Cope DK, Impastato WK, Cohen MV, Downey JM: Volatile anesthetics protect the ischemic rabbit myocardium from infarction. Anesthesiology 86:699–709, 1997.

25. Czibik G, D'Ancona G, Donias HW, Karamanoukian HL: Robotic cardiac surgery: present and future applications. J Cardiothorac Vasc Anesth 16:495–501, 2002.

26. D'Attellis N, Loulmet D, Carpentier A, et al: Robotic-assisted cardiac surgery: anesthetic and postoperative considerations. J Cardiothorac Vasc Anesth 16:397–400, 2002.

27. Dauerman HL, Ball SA, Goldberg RJ, et al: Activated clotting times in the setting of eptifibatide use during percutaneous coronary intervention. J Thromb Thrombolysis 13:127–132, 2002.

28. De Hert SG, Moens MM, Vermeyen KM, Hagerman MP: Use of the right-sided precordial lead V4R in the detection of intraoperative myocardial ischemia. J Cardiothorac Vasc Anesth 7:659–667, 1993.

29. Dietrich W, Spath P, Ebell A, Richter JA: Prevalence of anaphylactic reactions to aprotinin: analysis of two hundred forty-eight reexposures to aprotinin in heart operations. J Thorac Cardiovasc Surg 113:194–201, 1997.

30. Donias HW, D'Ancona G, Pande RU, et al: Heparin dose, transfusion rates, and intraoperative graft patency in minimally invasive direct coronary artery bypass. Heart Surg Forum 6:176–180, 2003.

31. Eaton MP, Deeb GM: Aprotinin versus epsilon-aminocaproic acid for aortic surgery using deep hypothermic circulatory arrest. J Cardiothorac Vasc Anesth 12:548–552, 1998.

32. Esposito RA, Culliford AT, Colvin SB, et al: The role of the activated clotting time in heparin administration and neutralization for cardiopulmonary bypass. J Thorac Cardiovasc Surg 85:174–185, 1983.

33. Fanashawe MP, Shore-Lesserson L, Reich DL: Two cases of fatal thrombosis after aminocaproic acid therapy and deep hypothermic circulatory arrest. Anesthesiology 95:1525–1527, 2001.

34. Furnary AP, Gao G, Grunkemeier GL, et al: Continuous insulin infusion reduces mortality in patients with diabetes undergoing coronary artery bypass grafting. J Thorac Cardiovasc Surg 125:1007–1021, 2003.

35. Furnary AP, Zerr KJ, Grunkemeier GL, Starr A: Continuous intravenous insulin infusion reduces the incidence of deep sternal wound infection in diabetic patients after cardiac surgical procedures. Ann Thorac Surg 67:352–362, 1999.

36. Ganapathy S: Anesthesia for minimally invasive cardiac surgery. Best Pract Res Clin Anaesthesiol 16:63–80, 2002.

37. Gottschlich GM, Gravelee GP, Georgitis JW: Adverse reactions to protamine sulfate during cardiac surgery in diabetic and non-diabetic patients. Ann Allergy 61:277–281, 1988.

38. Grady RE, Weglinski MR, Sharbrough FW, Perkins WJ: Correlation of regional cerebral blood flow with ischemic electroencephalographic changes during sevoflurane-nitrous oxide anesthesia for carotid endarterectomy. Anesthesiology 88:892–897, 1998.

39. Gravlee GP, Haddon WS, Rothberger HK, et al: Heparin dosing and monitoring for cardiopulmonary bypass. A comparison of techniques with measurement of subclinical plasma coagulation. J Thorac Cardiovasc Surg 99:518–527, 1990.

40. Gu W, Pagel PS, Warltier DC, Kersten JR: Modifying cardiovascular risk in diabetes mellitus. Anesthesiology 98:774–779, 2003.

41. Hardy J-F, Belisle S, Dupont C, et al: Prophylactic tranexamic acid and ε-aminocaproic acid for primary myocardial revascularization. Ann Thorac Surg 65:371–376, 1998.

42. Hartman JC, Kampine JP, Schmeling WT, Warltier DC: Alterations in collateral blood flow produced by isoflurane in a chronically instrumented canine model of multivessel coronary artery disease. Anesthesiology 74:120–133, 1991.

43. Hartman JC, Pagel PS, Kampine JP, et al: Influence of desflurane on regional distribution of coronary blood flow in a chronically instrumented canine model of multivessel coronary artery obstruction. Anesth Analg 72:289–299, 1991.

44. Heres EK, Horrow JC, Gravlee GP, et al: A dose-determining trial of heparinase-I (Neutralase™) for heparin neutralization in coronary artery surgery. Anesth Analg 93:1446–1452, 2001.

45. Hickey RF, Cason BA: Timing of tracheal extubation in adult cardiac surgery patients. J Card Surg 10:340–348, 1995.

46. Higgins TL, Estafanous FG, Loop FD, et al: Stratification of morbidity and mortality outcome by preoperative risk factors in coronary artery bypass patients—a clinical severity score. JAMA 267:2344–2348, 1992.

47. Ho AMH, Chung DC, Joynt GM: Neuraxial blockade and hematoma in cardiac surgery: estimating the risk of a rare adverse event that has not (yet) occurred. Chest 117:551–555, 2000.

48. Horrow JC: Protamine allergy. J Cardiothorac Anesth 2:225–242, 1988.

49. Horrow JC, Pharo GH, Levit LS, Freeland C: Neither skin tests nor serum enzyme-linked immunosorbent assay tests provide specificity for protamine allergy. Anesth Analg 82:386–389, 1996.

50. Horrow JC, Van Riper DF, Strong MD, et al: The dose response relationship of tranexamic acid. Anesthesiology 82:383–392, 1995.

51. Jacka MJ, Clark AG: Cardiovascular instability requiring treatment after intravenous heparin for cardiopulmonary bypass. Anesth Analg 90:42–44, 2000.

52. Jennings LK, Jacoski MV, White MM: The pharmacodynamics of parenteral glycoprotein IIb/IIIa inhibitors. J Interv Cardiol 15:45–60, 2002.

53. Karagoz HY, Kurtoglu M, Bakkaloglu B, et al: Coronary artery bypass grafting in the awake patient: three years' experience in 137 patients. J Thorac Cardiovasc Surg 125:1401–1404, 2003.

54. Kawahito S, Kitahata H, Tanaka K, et al: Pulmonary arterial pressure can be estimated by transesophageal pulsed Doppler echocardiography. Anesth Analg 92:1364–1369, 2001.

55. Kehl F, Krolinkowski JG, Mraovic B, et al: Hyperglycemia prevents isoflurane-induced preconditioning against myocardial infarction. Anesthesiology 96:183–188, 2002.

56. Kersten J, Brayer AP, Pagel PS, et al: Perfusion of ischemic myocardium during anesthesia with sevoflurane. Anesthesiology 81:995–1004, 1994.

57. Kersten JA, Schmeling TJ, Pagel PS, et al: Isoflurane mimics ischemic preconditioning via activation of K_{ATP} channels. Anesthesiology 87:361–370, 1997.

58. Kersten JR, Montgomery MW, Ghassemi T, et al: Diabetes and hyperglycemia impair activation of mitochondrial K_{ATP} channels. Am J Physiol 280:H1744–H1750, 2001.

59. Kirklin JK, Chenoweth DE, Naftel DC, et al: Effects of protamine administration after cardiopulmonary bypass on complement, blood elements, and the hemodynamic state. Ann Thorac Surg 41:193–199, 1986.

60. Kikura M, Lee MK, Levy JH: Heparin neutralization with methylene blue, hexadimethrine, or vancomycin after cardiopulmonary bypass. Anesth Analg 83:223–227, 1996.

61. Kirno K, Friberg P, Grzegorczyk A, et al: Thoracic epidural anesthesia during coronary artery bypass surgery: effects on cardiac sympathetic activity, myocardial blood flow and metabolism, and central hemodynamics. Anesth Analg 79:1075–1081, 1994.

62. Kondo K, Umemura K: Clinical pharmacokinetics of tirofiban, a nonpeptide glycoprotein IIb/IIIa receptor antagonist: comparison with the monoclonal antibody abciximab. Clin Pharmacokinet 41:187–195, 2002.

63. Kucuk O, Kwaan HC, Frederickson J, et al: Increased fibrinolytic activity in patients undergoing cardiopulmonary bypass operation. Am J Hematol 23:223–229, 1986.

64. Lemmer JH, Metzdorff MT, Krause AH, et al: Aprotinin use in patients with dialysis-dependent renal failure undergoing cardiac operations. J Thorac Cardiovasc Surg 112:192–194, 1996.

65. Lemmer JH, Stanford W, Bonney SL, et al: Aprotinin for coronary artery bypass grafting: effect on postoperative renal function. Ann Thorac Surg 59:132–136, 1995.

66. Leslie K, Sessler DI: The implications of hypothermia for early tracheal extubation following cardiac surgery. J Cardiothorac Vasc Anesth 12(6 Suppl 2):30–34, 1998.

67. Levy JH, Cormack JG, Morales A: Heparin neutralization by recombinant platelet factor 4 and protamine. Anesth Analg 81:35–37, 1995.

68. Levy JH, Pifarre R, Schaff HV, et al: A multicenter, double-blind, placebo-controlled trial of aprotinin for reducing blood loss and the requirement for donor-blood transfusion in patients undergoing repeat coronary artery bypass grafting. Circulation 92:2236–2244, 1995.

69. Li JM, Hajarizadeh H, La Rosa CA, et al: Heparin and protamine stimulate the production of nitric oxide. J Cardiovasc Surg 37:445–452, 1996.

70. Ling E, Arellano R: Systematic overview of the evidence supporting the use of cerebrospinal fluid drainage in thoracoabdominal aneurysm surgery for prevention of paraplegia. Anesthesiology 93:1115–1122, 2000.

71. Liu B, Tenghorn L, Larson G, et al: Half-dose aprotinin preserves hemostatic function in patients undergoing bypass operations. Ann Thorac Surg 59:1534–1540, 1995.

72. Loick HM, Schmidt C, van Aken H, et al: High thoracic epidural anesthesia, but not clonidine, attenuates the perioperative stress response via sympatholysis and reduces the release of troponin T in patients undergoing coronary artery bypass grafting. Anesth Analg 88:701–709, 1999.

73. London MJ, Hollenberg M, Wong MG, et al: Intraoperative myocardial ischemia: localization by continuous 12-lead electrocardiography. Anesthesiology 69:232–241, 1988.

74. London MJ, Shroyer ALW, Jernigan V, et al: Fast-track cardiac surgery in a Department of Veterans Affairs patient population. Ann Thorac Surg 64:134–141, 1997.

75. Lowenstein E: Morphine "anesthesia"—a perspective. Anesthesiology 35:563–565, 1971.

76. Lowenstein E, Hallowell P, Levine FH, et al: Cardiovascular response to large doses of intravenous morphine in man. N Engl J Med 281:1389–1393, 1969.

77. Mangano CTM: Risky business (editorial). J Thorac Cardiovasc Surg 125:1204–1207, 2003.

78. Margreiter J, Keller C, Brimacombe J: The feasibility of transesophageal echocardiograph-guided right and left ventricular oximetry in hemodynamically stable patients undergoing coronary artery bypass grafting. Anesth Analg 94:794–798, 2002.

79. Miao N, Frazer MJ, Lynch C. Volatile anesthetics depress Ca^{2+} transients and glutamate release in isolated cerebral synaptosomes. Anesthesiology 83:593–603, 1995.

80. Michelsen LG, Horswell J: Anesthesia for off-pump coronary artery bypass graft. Semin Thorac Cardiovasc Surg 15:71–82, 2003.

81. Michenfelder JD, Sundt TM, Fode N, Sharbrough FW: Isoflurane when compared to enflurane and halothane decreases the frequency of cerebral ischemia during carotid endarterectomy. Anesthesiology 67:336–340, 1987.

82. Mierdl S, Meininger D, Byhahn C, et al: Transesophageal echocardiography or fluoroscopy during port-access surgery? Ann Acad Med Singapore 31:520–524, 2002.

83. Mochizuki T, Olson PJ, Szlam F, et al: Protamine reversal of heparin affects platelet aggregation and activated clotting time after cardiopulmonary bypass. Anesth Analg 87:781–785, 1998.

84. Montes FR, Sanchez SI, Giraldo JC, et al: The lack of benefit of tracheal extubation in the operating room after coronary artery bypass surgery. Anesth Analg 91:776–780, 2000.

85. Moore PG, Kien ND, Reitan JA, et al: No evidence for blood flow redistribution with isoflurane or halothane during acute coronary artery occlusion in fentanyl-anesthetized dogs. Anesthesiology 75:854–865, 1991.

86. Morel DR, Zapol WM, Thomas SJ, et al: C5a and thromboxane generation associated with pulmonary vaso- and broncho-constriction during protamine reversal of heparin. Anesthesiology 66:597–604, 1987.

87. Murkin JM, Farrar JK, Tweed WA, et al: Cerebral autoregulation and flow/metabolism coupling during cardiopulmonary bypass: the influence of $PaCO_2$. Anesth Analg 66:825–832, 1987.

88. Murphy GS, Szokol JW, Marymont JH, et al: Impact of shorter-acting neuromuscular blocking agents on fast-track recovery of the cardiac surgical patient. Anesthesiology 96:600–606, 2002.

89. Nemoto EM, Klementavicius R, Melick J: Effect of mild hypothermia on active and basal cerebral oxygen metabolism and blood flow. Adv Exp Med Biol 361:469–473, 1994.

90. Nemoto EM, Klementavicius R, Melick JA, Yonas H: Suppression of cerebral metabolic rate for oxygen ($CMRO_2$) by mild hypothermia compared with thiopental. J Neurosurg Anesthesiol 8:52–59, 1996.

91. Okita Y, Takamoto S, Ando M, et al: Is use of aprotinin safe with deep hypothermic circulatory arrest in aortic surgery? Investigations on blood coagulation. Circulation 94(9 Suppl):II177–II181, 1996.

92. Ouattara A, Richard L, Charriere JM, et al: Use of cisatracurium during fast-track cardiac surgery. Br J Anaesth 86:130–132, 2001.

93. Overland PT, Teply JF: Vasopressin for the treatment of refractory hypotension after cardiopulmonary bypass. Anesth Analg 86:1207–1209, 1998.

94. Park KW, Dai HB, Lowenstein E, Sellke FW: Vasomotor responses of rat coronary arteries to isoflurane and halothane depend on preexposure tone and vessel size. Anesthesiology 83:1323–1330, 1995.

95. Park KW, Lowenstein E, Dai HB, et al: Direct vasomotor effects of isoflurane in subepicardial resistance vessels from collateral-dependent and normal coronary circulation of pigs. Anesthesiology 85:584–591, 1996.

96. Patel PM, Drummond JC, Cole DJ, Goskowicz RL. Isoflurane reduces ischemia-induced glutamate release in rats subjected to forebrain ischemia. Anesthesiology 82:996–1003, 1995.

1032

97. Ranucci M, Isgro G, Cazzaniga A, et al: Predictors for heparin resistance in patients undergoing coronary artery bypass grafting. Perfusion 14:437–442, 1999.

98. Reichenspurner H, Boehm DH, Gulbins H, et al: Three-dimensional video and robot-assisted port-access mitral valve operations. Ann Thorac Surg 69:1176–1181, 2000.

99. Reiz S, Balfors E, Sorensen MB, et al: Isoflurane—a powerful coronary vasodilator in patients with coronary artery disease. Anesthesiology 59:91–97, 1983.

100. Rogers AT, Stump DA, Gravlee GP, et al: Response of cerebral blood flow to phenylephrine infusion during hypothermic cardiopulmonary bypass: influence of $PaCO_2$ management. Anesthesiology 69:547–551, 1988.

101. Sabbagh AH, Chung GK, Shuttleworth P, et al: Fresh frozen plasma: a solution to heparin resistance during cardiopulmonary bypass. Ann Thorac Surg 37:466–468, 1984.

102. Scarborough RM: Development of eptifibatide. Am Heart J 138:1093–1104, 1999.

103. Schachner T, Bonatti J, Balogh D, et al: Aortic valve replacement in the conscious patient under regional anesthesia without endotracheal intubation. J Thorac Cardiovasc Surg 125:1526–1527, 2003.

104. Schonberger JPAM, Everts PAM, Ercan H, et al: Low-dose aprotinin in internal mammary artery bypass operations contributes to important blood saving. Ann Thorac Surg 54:1172–1176, 1992.

105. Schwann TA, Zacharias A, Riordan CJ, et al: Safe, highly selective use of pulmonary artery catheters in coronary artery bypass grafting: an objective patient selection method. Ann Thorac Surg 73:1394–1402, 2002.

106. Schwartz RS, Bauer KA, Rosenberg RD, et al: Clinical experience with antithrombin III concentrate in treatment of congenital and acquired deficiency of antithrombin. The Antithrombin III Study Group. Am J Med 87:53S–60S, 1989.

107. Scott NB, Turfrey DJ, Ray DAA, et al: A prospective randomized study of the potential benefits of thoracic epidural anesthesia and analgesia in patients undergoing coronary artery bypass grafting. Anesth Analg 93:528–535, 2001.

108. Seigne PW, Shorten GD, Johnson RG, Comunale ME: The effects of aprotinin on blood product transfusion associated with thoracic aortic surgery requiring deep hypothermic circulatory arrest. J Cardiothorac Vasc Anesth 14:676–681, 2000.

109. Sellke FW, Myers PR, Bates JN, Harrison DG: Influence of vessel size on the sensitivity of porcine coronary microvessels to nitroglycerin. Am J Physiol 258:H515–H520, 1990.

110. Shanewise JS, Cheung AT, Aronson S, et al: ASE/SCA guidelines for performing a comprehensive intraoperative multiplane transesophageal echocardiography examination: recommendations of the American Society of Echocardiography Council for Intraoperative Echocardiography and the Society of Cardiovascular Anesthesiologists Task Force for Certification in Perioperative Transesophageal Echocardiography. Anesth Analg 89:870–884, 1999.

111. Silbert BS, Santamaria JD, O'Brien JL, et al: Early extubation following coronary artery bypass surgery: a prospective randomized controlled trial. Chest 113:1481–1488, 1998.

112. Simoons ML, de Boer MJ, van der Brand MJBM, et al: Randomized trial of a GPIIb/IIIa platelet receptor blocker in refractory unstable angina. Circulation 89:596–603, 1994.

113. Staples MH, Dunton RF, Karlson KJ, et al: Heparin resistance after preoperative heparin therapy or intraaortic balloon pumping. Ann Thorac Surg 57:1211–1216, 1994.

114. Steen PA, Newberg L, Milde JH, Michenfelder JD: Hypothermia and barbiturates: individual and combined effects on canine cerebral oxygen consumption. Anesthesiology 58:527–532, 1983.

115. Stewart WJ, McSweeney SM, Kellet MA, et al: Increased risk of severe protamine reactions in NPH insulin-dependent diabetics undergoing cardiac catheterization. Circulation 70:788–792, 1984.

116. Sundt TM, Kouchoukos NT, Saffitz JE, et al: Renal dysfunction and intravascular coagulation with aprotinin and hypothermic circulatory arrest. Ann Thorac Surg 55:1418–1424, 1993.

117. Svensson LG, Hess KR, D'Agostino RS, et al: Reduction of neurologic injury after high-risk thoracoabdominal aortic operation. Ann Thorac Surg 66:132–138, 1998.

118. Tcheng J, Ellis SG, George BS: Pharmacodynamics of chimeric glycoprotein IIb/IIIa integrin antiplatelet antibody Fab 7E3 in high risk coronary angioplasty. Circulation 90:1757–1764, 1994.

119. Tenling A, Joachimsson P-O, Tyden H, Hedenstierna G: Thoracic epidural analgesia as an adjunct to general anaesthesia for cardiac surgery. Acta Anaesthesiol Scand 44:1071–1076, 2000.

120. Thomas R, Smith D, Strike P: Prospective randomised double-blind comparative study of rocuronium and pancuronium in adult patients scheduled for elective 'fast-track' cardiac surgery involving hypothermic cardiopulmonary bypass. Anaesthesia 58:261–279, 2003.

121. Todd MM, Warner DS: A comfortable hypothesis reevaluated: cerebral metabolic depression and brain protection during ischemia. Anesthesiology 76:161–164, 1992.

122. Tollefsen DM, Majerus DW, Blank MK: Heparin cofactor II. J Biol Chem 257:2162–2169, 1982.

123. Toller WG, Kersten JR, Pagel PS, et al: Sevoflurane reduces myocardial infarct size and decreases the time threshold for ischemic preconditioning in dogs. Anesthesiology 91:1437–1446, 1999.

124. Tuman KJ, McCarthy RJ, Spiess BD, et al: Effect of pulmonary artery catheterization on outcome in patients undergoing coronary artery surgery. Anesthesiology 70:199–206, 1989.

125. Van den Berghe G, Wouters P, Weekers F, et al: Intensive insulin therapy in critically ill patients. N Engl J Med 345:1359–1367, 2001.

126. Velders AJ, Wildevuur CR: Platelet damage by protamine and the protective effect of prostacyclin: an experimental study in dogs. Ann Thorac Surg 42:168–171, 1986.

127. Wall MH, MacGregor DA, Kennedy DJ, et al: Pulmonary artery catheter placement for elective coronary artery bypass grafting: before or after anesthetic induction? Anesth Analg 94:1409–1415, 2002.

128. Warner DS: Isoflurane neuroprotection: a passing fantasy, again? Anesthesiology 92:1226–1228, 2000.

129. Weightman WM, Gibbs NM, Sheminant MR, et al: Drug therapy before coronary artery surgery: nitrates are independent predictors of mortality and β-adrenergic blockers predict survival. Anesth Analg 88:286–291, 1999.

130. Weiss ME, Nyhan D, Peng Z, et al: Association of protamine IgE and IgG antibodies with life-threatening reactions to intravenous protamine. N Engl J Med 320:886–892, 1989.

131. Zhao X, Mashikian J, Panzica P, et al: Comparison of thermodilution bolus cardiac output and Doppler cardiac output in the early post-cardiopulmonary bypass period. J Cardiothorac Vasc Anesth 17:193–198, 2003.

132. Zwischenberger JB, Vertrees RA, Brunston RL, et al: Application of a heparin removal device in patients with known protamine hypersensitivity. J Thorac Cardiovasc Surg 115:729–731, 1998.

Critical Care for the Adult Cardiac Patient

Carmelo A. Milano and Peter K. Smith

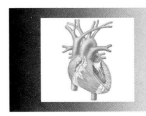

INTRODUCTION

The purpose of this chapter is to familiarize the caregiver with the expected or normal course following adult cardiac surgery. The management of patients immediately after cardiac surgery is described in significant detail. A systematic approach to the postoperative care is utilized. In addition, the common and important side effects or complications of cardiac surgery are described and their management is reviewed. The chapter provides references, which support management strategies and approaches to common postoperative complications. The chapter focuses on common management strategies and complications and is not meant to be comprehensive. The references should provide the reader with more detailed analysis of particular problems.

IMMEDIATE POSTOPERATIVE CARE

Initial Evaluation

A systematic evaluation of the patient should be performed immediately on arrival in the intensive care unit. Communication with the surgical and anesthesia team should provide an overview of the procedure performed, the response of the cardiovascular system to the procedure, intraoperative hemodynamic management, and current medications. The patient's comorbid conditions, preoperative medications,

1034 and allergies should be ascertained and confirmed with the team members, who have evaluated the awake and alert patient.

Although attention may be focused initially on one aspect of the patient's condition (an arrhythmia upon arrival, for example), it is critical to develop a systematic approach to evaluation. The patient is completely dependent, and dysfunction of any element of the support systems can be rapidly fatal. Surgical dressings must be kept intact during the first 48 h for infection control. If they must be disturbed for diagnostic purposes, strict aseptic technique should be followed.

Airway/Ventilator

The trachea should be palpated and confirmed to be in the midline, and breath sounds should be auscultated bilaterally. The ventilator should be confirmed as functioning normally and without alarms—if not, the patient should be immediately converted to hand bagging. The peak inspiratory pressure should be noted so that changes in chest wall and pulmonary mechanics can be correctly interpreted later in the course.

High inspiratory pressures may indicate a tension pneumothorax, inappropriate ventilator settings, or severe pulmonary/chest wall restriction. Pulse oximetry, mixed venous oximetry, and direct measurement of arterial gas tensions will confirm adequate oxygen delivery and CO_2 elimination.

Initial ECG

The initial ECG can be difficult to interpret because of lead placement changes related to surgical dressings, cardiac pacing, and the common presence of conduction abnormalities. Right bundle branch block and first-degree atrioventricular (AV) block are very frequent, usually resolving in the first few postoperative hours. Establishing and maintaining normal sinus rhythm with adequate rate are particularly important in the early postoperative period when cardiac function may be impaired because of intraoperative ischemia, or there may be temporary diastolic dysfunction due to myocardial edema.

First-degree AV block is common and can result in substantial reduction in the instantaneous end-diastolic left ventricular (LV) volume, which determines stroke volume. The use of atrial or AV sequential pacing can overcome these transient derangements, and in the latter instance, it is common to see improved cardiac function with normalization of the AV interval despite abnormal ventricular activation with the ventricular pacing component.

Atrial fibrillation is poorly tolerated in the first postoperative day, and every effort should be made to maintain sinus rhythm, even in patients who had chronic atrial fibrillation preoperatively. Immediate cardioversion is often required in the ICU, although atrial fibrillation occurring on the third or later postoperative day is usually well tolerated.

Ventricular arrhythmias may be due to early graft failure or coronary spasm, which should be ruled out. A malpositioned pulmonary artery catheter irritating the right ventricular (RV) outflow tract is more easily correctable. All rhythm disturbances can be due to hypothermia or to electrolyte or acid–base imbalances, or they can be the side effects of vasoactive or antiarrhythmic drugs.

Peripheral Perfusion

The adequacy of global and regional perfusion should be assessed by physical examination of the vascular system, including examination of accessible pulse character and the quality of skin and soft tissue perfusion. Intraoperative embolization, vascular injury, or low cardiac output in the setting of peripheral vascular disease may compromise limb viability.

Abdominal Examination

This will reveal the presence of bowel sounds and a functionally positioned nasogastric tube. Exclusion of masses, unsuspected hepatomegaly, or generalized abdominal distention should be documented.

Genitourinary

Correct placement of the in-dwelling urinary catheter should be confirmed and both phimosis and paraphimosis excluded. Urine should be clear, unconcentrated, and free of hemoglobin or frank blood.

Neurological

Evaluation of the patient's neurological status should be performed frequently until ensured to be unchanged. Uncontrollable hypertension or extreme variability of peripheral vascular resistance may result from severe neurological injury initially ascribed to a residual anesthetic agent.

Initial Cardiac Auscultation

The cardiac examination should document normal heart sounds and the character of any murmurs. This is very important in patients who have had valve replacement.

Body Temperature

Initial hypothermia is the rule, and it is best avoided by expeditious surgery and adequate rewarming while on cardiopulmonary bypass. Hypothermia compromises cardiac function, causes shivering and excessive metabolic demand, interferes with normal coagulation, and can aggravate or cause rhythm disturbances.[62] Blankets and other auxiliary warming devices should be employed, particularly in the bleeding patient receiving cold intravenous (IV) solutions and blood products.

Fever, particularly in the early postoperative period, is poorly tolerated. It should be treated aggressively with antipyretics—with intravenous steroids if there is hemodynamic compromise.

Hemodynamics

With appropriate cardiac rhythm, the patient should have a cardiac index of greater than 2 liters/min/m² with blood pressure adequate for the patient. The relationship of blood pressure to age, preoperative blood pressure, and renal function can be critically important.

The importance of generating adequate cardiac output has been established by several studies with mortality as the outcome variable. Acceptance of lower cardiac output occasionally results in good outcome when associated with reasonable mixed venous oxygen saturation MVo_2 (>55%), adequate urine output (>20 ml/h without stimulation), and evidence of good peripheral and central perfusion (physical examination, maintenance of acid–base balance). There is no evidence that supranormal cardiac output is beneficial.

Elevated central venous pressure, especially when associated with facial edema or facial discoloration, must be aggressively evaluated. Possible causes include cardiac tamponade, general fluid overload, or even technical errors that have compromised superior vena caval flow.

Elevated pulmonary artery pressures may indicate LV dysfunction or cardiac tamponade, or may be related to preoperative changes in pulmonary vascular resistance. All central pressures should be related to initial values obtained during preoperative invasive monitoring and to those obtained after completion of surgery but before transfer to the ICU. These measurements are also quite sensitive to afterload, which can vary widely and rapidly in the early postoperative course in patients who are often hypovolemic.

Elevation of intrathoracic pressure can frequently mimic cardiac failure in the patient with chest wall rigidity because of emergence from anesthetic effect and shivering. The latter process can increase metabolic demand and reduce MVo_2 to very low levels.

Lines

All indwelling lines must be confirmed to be functional, particularly those delivering vasoactive drugs. Remember that transport can partially or completely dislodge intravenous lines and that many of the insertion sites have been draped out and were unobserved during the hours of surgery. Hemodynamic instability due to failure of drug delivery and tissue injury due to drug infiltration must be avoided.

Chest Tubes

Mediastinal and pleural space tubes are always placed to underwater seal and usually set to have −20 cm H_2O suction applied. Mediastinal tubes should be examined for the amount and nature of drainage. The initial amount of drained blood should be less than 100 ml, and larger amounts should be explained by the surgical team. The initial rate of drainage may reflect drainage of blood or irrigation fluid that has accumulated, particularly in the left thoracic gutter. Nonetheless, an initial assessment of the bleeding rate, quality of blood clotting in the tubes, correlation of drainage with intravascular volume replacement, and tube patency is critically important.

Initial Chest X-Ray

A portable chest X-ray should be obtained immediately on arrival and must be interpreted by the responsible physicians as soon as available. Critical aspects include (1) position of the endotracheal tube, (2) pneumothorax and mediastinal shift, (3) lobar atelectasis, (4) pleural and extrapleural fluid collections, (5) size of the mediastinal silhouette, (6) correct intravascular location of invasive lines and catheters, and (7) normal position of radiopaque markers, sternal wires, and drainage tubes.

Recovery from Cardiopulmonary Bypass

Cardiopulmonary bypass (CPB) induces many of the physiological changes apparent in the postoperative patient, and its duration is a primary determinant of the rapidity of recovery.

CPB nonspecifically activates the inflammatory system.[224] Generalized complement activation is seen, with elevations in C3a and C5a anaphylatoxins following discontinuation of CPB.[28,105,148,215] This activation can lead to pulmonary sequestration of leukocytes[28,36,148] and the production of superoxides and other products of lipoxygenation. This causes further leukocyte activation and the generation of leukotactic circulating factors that increase the local inflammatory response.[45,138] Elevations in tumor necrosis factor, interleukin-1, and prostaglandin E1 have been described.[25,95,134] Additionally, vasoactive substances may be liberated from platelets in response to CPB or protamine infusion, which can cause pulmonary hypertension and systemic hypotension.[97] Adverse reaction to protamine may also be complement mediated and related to prior exposure.[116]

The generalized inflammatory reaction seen following CPB may change vascular permeability and cause pulmonary hypertension as well as bronchial hyperreactivity.[107] This inflammatory response may directly reset the hypothalamic thermoregulatory center, causing postoperative fever.[45] This inflammatory reaction can cause postoperative pulmonary dysfunction and renal dysfunction that are independent of CPB time.[105,107] Reduction of the inflammatory response by prostaglandin E1[13,105] and steroids[130,144] suggests that nonspecific inflammation is related to complement activation as well as to elevation of interleukin-1.

A specific manifestation of the inflammatory response in cardiothoracic surgery is the postpericardiotomy syndrome.[93] This syndrome, occurring in 10–30% of patients, is a self-limited condition beginning in the second or third week following operation. It is associated with fever and pleuritic, precordial, or substernal chest pain.[50] Chest X-rays in patients with postpericardiotomy syndrome commonly show pleural and pericardial effusions (Figure 64-1). This syndrome has been associated with specific reactive antibodies and may be seen following any operation that violates the pericardium.[50,51] It is treated with nonsteroidal antiinflammatory agents, although corticosteroids may be necessary in severe cases.[90,106]

Cardiac Surgery without Cardiopulmonary Bypass

Because CPB is perhaps the most invasive aspect of conventional coronary revascularization, surgeons are now utilizing advanced stabilizing devices to perform coronary anastomoses on the beating heart without CPB. With this approach, through a standard sternotomy incision and with available stabilizing systems, complete revascularization of

Post-Pericardotomy Syndrome

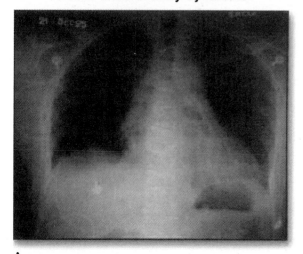

A

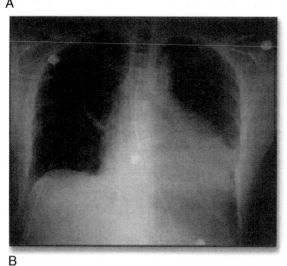

B

Figure 64–1 Postpericardiotomy syndrome. Post-pericardiotomy syndrome is commonly associated with pericardial and pleural effusions. A chest radiograph on a patient soon after aortic valve replacement shows expected postoperative findings (**A**). A chest radiograph 2 weeks later (**B**) shows pericardial effusion compatible with the clinical symptoms of postpericardiotomy syndrome.

all three coronary distributions can be performed with the heart beating. The term "OPCAB" generally refers to multivessel coronary artery bypass performed off the CPB pump, through a standard sternotomy. This approach has achieved considerable support with approximately 15% of coronary surgery in the United States being performed in this manner.[131] Some individual surgeons or institutions are now performing the majority of coronary revascularization procedures without CPB. Although initially a number of cases were considered inappropriate for OPCAB techniques, more and more of these have been successfully performed in this manner. For example, cases of redo coronary grafting and complete arterial grafting have been successfully performed as OPCABs. Many surgeons, however, still view intramyocardial coronary arteries and severe LV dysfunction as strong contraindications to OPCAB.

There are specific differences between OPCAB and conventional "on-pump" revascularization procedures, which ultimately impact the patient's recovery. During OPCAB procedures, coronary arteries are individually snared proximally and occluded during the performance of the coronary anastomosis. Depending on whether intracoronary shunts are utilized, there may be periods of local ischemia without cardioplegic arrest. However, unlike the conventional on-pump procedures, there are no periods of aortic cross-clamping and global cardiac arrest. For these reasons, the degree of myocardial stunning during OPCABs may be reduced relative to on-pump procedures. Furthermore, during OPCABs, normothermic pulsatile flow is maintained throughout the procedure, while conventional on-pump procedures include a period of nonpulsatile perfusion (while on CPB) and generally some degree of systemic cooling and rewarming. Finally, although both techniques require anticoagulation with heparin, many centers practice reduced-heparin dosing for OPCAB. Initially, OPCAB techniques resulted in longer total operating room (OR) times, but as these procedures have become more common, predictably OR times have been reduced and some surgeons now argue that OPCAB can be performed faster than equivalent on-pump procedures.

Although OPCAB procedures are ultimately focused on reduction of morbidity, initial studies have sought to confirm equivalent operative mortality and graft patency relative to conventional on-pump procedures. Unfortunately, it has been difficult to randomize large groups of patients and study these important outcomes. Multiple, large nonrandomized studies have reported reasonable OPCAB operative mortality. Hart et al reported a 1% operative mortality for a group of 1582 consecutive OPCAB patients; the majority of cases involved at least three grafts.[82] Puskas et al reported their results in 200 patients undergoing OPCAB. Eighty-three percent of patients underwent postoperative angiography with a graft patency rate of 98%. All internal mammary artery (IMA)-to-left anterior descending (LAD) grafts were patent.[164] Jansen et al reported a graft patency of 95% in 86 patients who underwent 147 distal anastomoses.[96] These studies and others appear to confirm acceptable operative mortality and graft patency for select groups of patients, and support the further applications of these procedures. As previously discussed, it has been documented that conventional cardiac surgery results in a significant inflammatory response. This response appears to be a nonspecific response that includes complement and leukocyte activation.* Although the exact mechanism of activation is unclear, the strongest stimulant for the response is the blood–artificial surface contact that occurs with CPB. This response can be modified by coating the tubing and oxygenator surfaces with biological materials and improving the hemodynamic performance of the system. Theoretically, by eliminating the heart–lung machine entirely, this response could be significantly reduced. At least two studies have now investigated the inflammatory response during heart surgery, comparing groups in which coronary revascularization is performed with and without CPB.[6,75] Angelini et al[3] looked at four important inflammatory markers: (1) neutrophil elastase (an endopeptidase released with neutrophil activation), (2) interleukin-8 (a potent neutrophil chemotactic and activating factor), (3) C3a, and (4) C5a (fragments

---

*Reference 28, 36, 45, 105, 138, 148, 215, 224.

generated with activation of the common complement pathway). These markers were measured at four time points within the first 24 h postoperatively; patients were randomized to two groups: coronary revascularization with CPB and standard cardioplegic arrest versus OPCAB. The OPCAB group demonstrated significantly lower levels of all four markers and had reduced leukocyte, neutrophil, and monocyte blood counts. Together these findings strongly support a reduced inflammatory response with OPCAB. The clinical significance of this difference is unclear, and ideally larger prospective randomized trials will help determine the clinical impact of reduced inflammatory response.

Coagulopathy and postoperative bleeding represent a major morbidity for cardiac surgery patients. Many surgeons believe that OPCAB procedures will help to reduce these problems. OPCAB requires less intraoperative anticoagulation and avoids blood–artificial surface contact, which should reduce platelet activation and destruction. Furthermore, systemic cooling that may further impact negatively on coagulation function can be avoided with OPCAB. Several studies have compared on-pump procedures to OPCAB and report significant reduction in postoperative bleeding, reduced need for perioperative transfusion, and reduced rate of take back for bleeding.[113]

Preliminary studies suggest reduced morbidity for OPCAB procedures compared with standard coronary revascularization with CPB, but these studies have not been conclusive. Most initial comparisons have not been randomized, with the OPCAB group generally requiring fewer coronary grafts. This raises questions as to whether reduced postoperative morbidity relates to the procedure per se or rather to a better preprocedure patient status.[200]

▶ POSTCARDIAC SURGERY CARDIAC DYSFUNCTION

Low Cardiac Output State

Output and Filling Pressure

Low cardiac output after CPB historically has been recognized as a cause of sudden death.[17] Low cardiac output resulting from ventricular dysfunction causes a series of adaptive neurohumoral responses as well as geometric changes (dilation and hypertrophy) within the heart. Acute loss of 20–25% of functioning myocardium[201] causes significant reduction in cardiac output and carries an extremely poor short-term[114] and long-term prognosis.[136]

Measurement and therapeutic manipulation of both cardiac output and central filling pressures are critical to the postoperative care of cardiac surgical patients and are predictive of survival (Figure 64-2).[5] Central pressures, cardiac output, and venous saturation routinely are measured by means of a flow-directed pulmonary artery catheter. The cardiac index (cardiac output expressed as liters/min/m^2) has a normal range of 2.1–4.9 liters/min/m^2.[168,216] In adults, a cardiac index of at least 2.0 liters/min/m^2 during the immediate postoperative period is required for normal convalescence.[5]

Oxygen Delivery

Shock is currently conceptualized as a clinical syndrome resulting from an imbalance between tissue oxygen demand

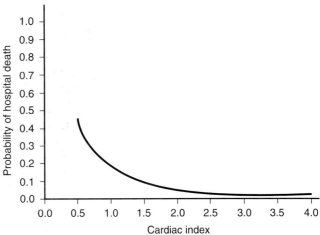

Figure 64–2 Hospital death versus cardiac index. Relationship between postoperative cardiac index (liters/min/m^2) and probability of death for adults after mitral valve replacement. *(Reproduced with permission from Kouchoukos NT: Detection and treatment of impaired cardiac performance following cardiac surgery. In Davila JC, editor: Henry Ford Hospital International Sympsium on Cardiac Surgery, 2nd ed. New York: Appleton-Century-Crofts, 1977.)*

and tissue oxygen supply. The general goals of postoperative care are to prevent shock and provide adequate oxygen delivery. Oxygen delivery of less than 335 ml/min/m^2 has been associated with a decrease in oxygen consumption[182] and with the development of progressive lactic acidosis.[166] Provision of supranormal oxygen delivery (> 600 ml/min/m^2) has been proposed to counteract the oxygen debt accumulated by patients in shock, although this approach in postoperative cardiac surgical patients has not been studied.

Lactic acidosis has been suggested as a metabolic monitor to correlate with total oxygen debt, the magnitude of hypoperfusion, and the severity of shock.[20,145,221] However, a direct relationship to total oxygen delivery has been disputed.[8] MVo$_2$ provides a useful index of the adequacy of circulation and reflects to some extent mean tissue oxygen level.[104] MVo$_2$ is measured with specialized pulmonary artery catheters, and patients with a saturation of less than 60% or those who demonstrate a decrease of more than 5% suffer more frequent postoperative complications.[111] However, others have shown poor correlation between saturation, or trends in saturation, and outcome.[213] Rapid changes in whole body oxygen consumption may reduce its overall predictive value.

Adequate regional oxygen delivery is even more difficult to determine. Organ requirements and hormonally activated reflex changes in regional blood supply may occur in the postoperative state. For example, the kidney, skin, and resting muscles are blood-supply independent and maintain viability by increased oxygen extraction. The heart and brain, on the other hand, are blood-supply dependent with near maximal oxygen extraction at rest. Sympathetically controlled reflexes compensate for these differences by a shift of blood flow from the skin and splanchnic region at low circulating volumes.[23] Increasingly, the effects of splanchnic hypoperfusion on postoperative complications and persistent acidosis are being recognized.[117] Acute changes in regional blood supply may be mediated by differing degrees of sympathetic innervation to precapillary sphincters and arterioles.[139] Alterations in metabolic activity are common following heart surgery. These can be monitored through capnography, which determines the partial pressure of CO_2 in expired gases.[30] Rewarming, with subsequent peripheral vasodilation, and shivering have been shown to increase metabolic and circulatory demands[171] and can be eliminated with paralysis and sedation. This promotes hemodynamic stability and decreases the need for inotropic support.[233] Thus, the actual definition of low cardiac output syndrome must include evidence of inadequate oxygen delivery relative to consumption. Clinical evidence of diminished peripheral perfusion and end-organ ischemia must be coupled with the objective measurements of cardiac output and MVo_2 to establish this diagnosis.

Preload

Maintenance of adequate preload is fundamental in the postoperative management of cardiac surgical patients (Figure 64-3). The optimal pulmonary capillary wedge pressure in postoperative cardiac surgical patients is unknown, but a range of 14–18 mm Hg has been suggested, with increases in extravascular lung water occurring above this level.[38] Preload correlates directly with the force of ventricular contraction, and the result is a ventricular volume change from end diastole to end systole determined by transmural pressure and compliance of the ventricular wall. Pericardial pressure is normally reflected by right atrial pressure (Figure 64-4). However, tight closure of the pericardium may adversely affect transmural pressure and decrease stroke volume.[3,180,208] Pulmonary artery wedge pressures and the central venous pressure (CVP), indicating LV and RV volumes, respectively, accurately reflect reduced filling pressures, whereas high filling pressures may be determined by changes in transmural pressure or myocardial compliance rather than accurately reflecting preload. Most postoperative cardiac surgical patients are relatively hypovolemic and have a labile reactive vasculature.[78] In the immediate postoperative period, causes of hypovolemia include large urine volumes, ongoing blood loss, and significant cross-sectional increase in vascular beds with rewarming.

The summation of these physiological changes is a reduced preload, particularly to the left ventricle. This trend should be anticipated and managed with appropriate volume therapy to prevent precipitous hypotension and low cardiac output. Immediate preload augmentation may be achieved with passive straight leg raising, with a transient 8–10% increase in cardiac output,[66] although this should be viewed only as a temporizing measure, and should be quickly supplanted by appropriate volume administration.

Afterload

Postoperative Effects

Following a cardiac operation, elevation in afterload is a well-recognized phenomenon. The incidence varies with cardiac pathology, operative procedure, and definition of the resulting hypertension. Following valve replacement,

Illustrations for Pulmonary Artery Pressure

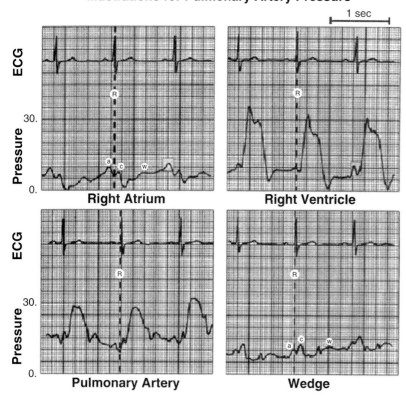

Figure 64–3 Pulmonary artery pressure. Pressure waveforms recorded from a pulmonary artery catheter as it passes through the right atrium and right ventricle to the pulmonary artery and wedge positions. Right ventricular end-diastolic pressure is measured at the time of the ECG R wave and is estimated best by the right atrial a wave pressure peak (clear boxes). The a, c, and w waves are recorded from both the right atrium and pulmonary artery wedge positions.
(*Reproduced with permission from Mark JB: Atlas of Cardiovascular Monitoring. New York: Churchill Livingstone, 1998.*)

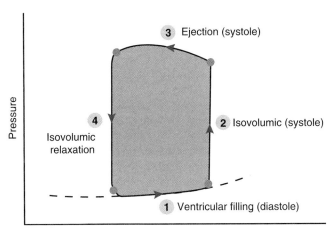

Figure 64–4 Single cycle left ventricle pressure–volume loop. Idealized pressure–volume loop for the left ventricle representing a single cardiac cycle.
(*Reproduced with permission from Chatterjee K, Parmley WW: The role of vasodilator therapy in heart failure. Prog Cardiovasc Dis 19:301, 1977.*)

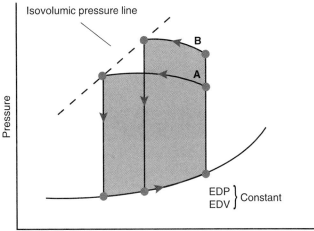

Figure 64–5 Acute postoperative afterload reduction. Two idealized pressure–volume loops at the same level of contractility and end-diastolic volume, but with a reduction in arterial pressure from loop B to loop A, which results in an increase in stroke volume.
(*Reproduced with permission from Chatterjee K, Parmley WW: The role of vasodilator therapy in heart failure. Prog Cardiovasc Dis 19:301, 1977.*)

the reported incidence ranges between 8 and 12%.[53] After myocardial revascularization, afterload is elevated in 8–61% of patients.[54,222] Increased systemic vascular resistance at the arteriolar level appears to be the major determinant of arterial pressure after coronary artery surgery.[67] The etiology of postoperative hypertension remains unclear, but contributing factors include a decreased baroreceptor sensitivity[59,78] and an elevated renin–angiotensin activity.[205,206]

Sympathetic stimulation and elevated levels of catecholamines also have been identified in the early postoperative period.[157,222,225] Furthermore, postoperative pain may increase afterload and can be managed with the administration of morphine sulfate.[230] Alternatively, some patients develop hypotension postoperatively, which may be related to the systemic inflammatory response or the release of vasoactive substances.

Although pulmonary artery pressures are measured directly (RV afterload), the ascending aortic pressure is inferred by measurements made at a peripheral artery (usually the radial). Systolic amplification may occur, elevating the measured systolic radial artery pressure. However, mean pressures are similar between peripheral and central regions, and these should be considered when managing patients in the postoperative setting. In the control of afterload, autoregulation at various sites should be considered. The central nervous system autoregulates mean blood pressures of 50–150 mm Hg.[118] A reset lower limit for autoregulation may be higher in hypertensive patients.[199] Renal autoregulation requires a mean blood pressure of 70 mm Hg.[23] The heart with residual coronary disease also requires adequate mean arterial pressure (65 mm Hg), as do patients with pathological concentric myocardial hypertrophy.[133]

Acute afterload reduction in the postoperative period is frequently beneficial (Figure 64-5). Adequate preload must be achieved before the institution of vasodilating agents. Afterload reduction with low filling pressures often produces a compensatory tachycardia, which may be deleterious. When it is applied to patients with high filling pressures, there is usually no change or a slight reduction in heart rate. Additionally, experimental evidence suggests that afterload reduction, when applied to low or normally filled ventricles, may increase infarct size.[167] When applied in a setting of high preload, infarct size may be reduced.[129,219] This may have implications in patients after incomplete myocardial revascularization.

Therapeutic Approaches

The degree to which hemodynamic improvement can be obtained with afterload reduction is difficult to predict. Therapeutic results depend on the end-systolic pressure–volume relationship of each patient. However, afterload reduction generally improves cardiovascular function and diminishes preload. Preload augmentation coupled with afterload reduction has additional positive effects on overall cardiac function.[196] Afterload reduction also improves forward ejection in patients with residual mitral[27] and aortic insufficiency.[15]

Although various afterload-reducing agents are available, nitroglycerin and nitroprusside are the most frequently used agents in the immediate postoperative period. Nitroprusside may increase ST-segment elevation in perioperative ischemia and cause significant intracoronary shunt.[31] Nonetheless, it continues to be the agent of choice for the acute management of postoperative hypertension.[11] Nitroglycerin improves coronary collateral flow and may prevent coronary spasm, and it is frequently used for the first 12–24 h following coronary revascularization.[31,71]

The frequent use of nitroprusside mandates a knowledge of its adverse effects. The lethal dose is approximately 7 mg/kg.[41] When high doses are used (greater than

1040

7 µg/kg/min) for prolonged therapy, cyanogen, cyanide, and thiocyanate are potential toxic breakdown products. Signs of toxicity are subtle and include a narrowing of the arteriovenous oxygen difference and the development of metabolic acidosis.[140] Thiocyanate levels may be measured under these circumstances with levels of 50–100 mg/liter associated with cyanate toxicity, and 200 mg/liter may be lethal. Discontinuance and dialysis are the mainstays of treatment, although prophylactic infusion of hydroxocobalamin (25 mg/h) has been shown to decrease cyanate concentration.[165]

Alternative parenteral agents should be considered when high-dose nitroprusside therapy is necessary: (1) Hydralazine, although longer acting, may also be effective.[190] (2) β-Blockers are effective in the management of postoperative hypertension and are being used more commonly in patients with LV failure. Esmolol, a short-acting selective β-blocker, may be particularly useful in this setting, although these agents may have a significant negative inotropic effect. (3) Intravenous nitroglycerin may achieve afterload reduction as well as coronary dilatation.

Many patients require afterload reduction throughout their postoperative course. Patients with persistent hypertension and with reduced LV function will benefit from long-term afterload reduction and should be converted to oral medications. Chronic afterload reduction, in patients with significant congestive heart failure, has been shown to have a positive impact on survival.[137] In one large study of patients with symptomatic congestive heart failure (New York Heart Association [NYHA] Class II and Class III), a significant reduction in long-term morbidity and mortality was seen in those treated with enalapril, an angiotensin-converting enzyme (ACE) inhibitor.[89] Additional studies have confirmed that ACE inhibitors are particularly useful in the management of this problem.[42,109,128]

Patients with asymptomatic LV dysfunction (NYHA Class I and Class II) may benefit significantly from long-term therapy with ACE inhibitors. Although no significant difference in overall mortality was observed when compared with placebo, a 37% and 36% decrease in development of symptomatic congestive heart failure and hospital admission for congestive heart failure, respectively, has been demonstrated.[161] Although the mechanism of this positive impact has not been completely defined, two-dimensional echocardiographic studies in post–myocardial infarction patients have shown that ACE inhibitors attenuate LV enlargement.[195] Nitrates[137] and hydralazine[32] have also been used but are less effective than ACE inhibitors.[33]

Heart Rate

The postoperative control of heart rate is important and mandates standard application of temporary, epicardial, bipolar atrial, and ventricular pacing wires in most patients.[81,87,143] Normal sinus rhythm, through synchronized end-diastolic preload augmentation, is responsible for approximately 25% of cardiac output in the postoperative setting (Figure 64-6).[189]

Changes in heart rate are common following cardiac surgery and include sinus bradycardia, junctional rhythm, and first-, second-, or third-degree heart block. These phenomena are usually transient and may be related to perioperative β-blockade, intraoperative antiarrhythmics, or metabolic

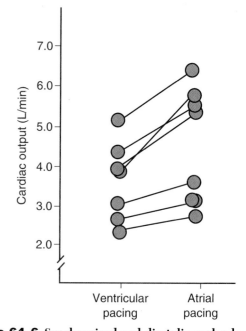

Figure 64–6 **Synchronized end-diastolic preload augmentation.** A comparison of cardiac output with ventricular pacing (without synchronous atrial systole) and with atrial pacing that shows an overall increase in cardiac output with atrial pacing of approximately 26% in patients after cardiac surgery. *(Reproduced with permission from Hartzler GO, Maloney JD, Curtis JJ, Barnhorst DA: Hemodynamic effects of trioventricular sequential pacing after cardiac surgery. Am J Cardiol 40:232, 1977.)*

damage during cardioplegic arrest (potassium or magnesium).[47,192] Inadequate myocardial protection may cause ischemia of the conduction system.[192,193] Permanent injury to the conduction system is most often due to direct surgical injury during intracardiac procedures.

Management of disturbances in heart rate must be individualized. Simple atrial pacing (in the range of 90–110 beats per minute) is optimal for sinus bradycardia. With AV nodal blocks, AV pacing with an interval in the range of 150–175 ms is usually optimal.[77,83] The AV interval also depends on selected heart rate (Figure 64-7). The normalization of AV synchrony by these means is associated with a loss of the normal ventricular activation sequence, depressing ventricular function at constant preload and afterload by approximately 10–15%. Optimal heart rate determination must be individualized for each patient with reference to measurements of cardiac output.

When in place, temporary pacing wires constitute a direct current pathway to the heart and must be insulated when not in use. Caution should be practiced when connecting a rapid-pacing device to the wires ensuring atrial connection. Temporary pacing wires are usually removed in the early postoperative period but may be left in place indefinitely. High pacing thresholds usually develop within 2 weeks, unlike permanent endocardial electrodes. When temporary pacing is not possible, bradyarrhythmias can be treated pharmacologically with atropine or isoproterenol. Alternatively, a pulmonary artery catheter with an additional pacing port or the Zoll transthoracic pacemaker may be employed.[231]

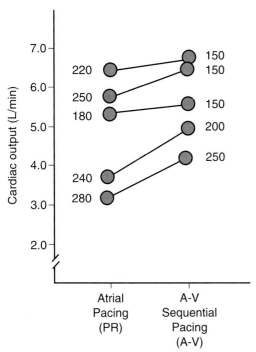

Figure 64–7 Cardiac output with AV sequential versus atrial pacing. A comparison of atrioventricular (AV) sequential pacing and atrial pacing in patients with a prolonged postoperative PR interval (intrinsic and paced PR intervals are shown in milliseconds to the left for atrial pacing and to the right for AV sequential pacing). Note the uniform increase in cardiac output despite absolute differences in the shortening of the PR interval that is induced by pacing and overlap between paced PR intervals and intrinsic PR intervals between patients.
(Reproduced with permission from Hartzler GO, Maloney JD, Curtis JJ, Barnhorst DA: Hemodynamic effects of trioventricular sequential pacing after cardiac surgery. Am J Cardiol 40:232, 1977.)

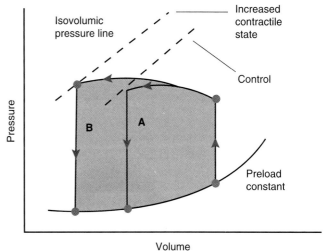

Figure 64–8 Pressure–volume loops inscribed under conditions of constant preload and afterload. An induced increase in inotropic state from loop A to loop B shifts the end-systolic pressure–volume relationship (dashed lines) and results in increased stroke volume in loop B.
(Reproduced with permission from Chatterjee K, Parmley WW: The role of vasodilator therapy in heart failure. Prog Cardiovasc Dis 19:301, 1977.)

Inotropic State

Inotropic agents may be necessary to achieve adequate cardiac function (Figure 64-8) and to maintain peripheral oxygen delivery. Improvement in cardiac function by pharmacological intervention is generally achieved at the expense of increased myocardial oxygen consumption. Inotropic agents should be considered only after manipulations of heart rate, preload, and afterload have been maximized. In general, myocardial function improves throughout the postoperative course, allowing weaning from inotropic support.[212]

Various inotropic agents are available and all are administered by either intravenous bolus or continuous infusion. They should be administered through a central venous or pulmonary artery catheter whose intravascular position has been ascertained to prevent perivascular infiltration. Most inotropic agents act through stimulation of adrenergic receptors (Table 64-1). β-Adrenergic agonists mediated an increase in intracellular calcium concentration.[52] Clinical experience using multiple inotropic agents has demonstrated synergism[214] despite *in vitro* evidence that the maximal positive inotropic effect of one drug precludes augmentation by another. This may be due to alterations in the adenylate cyclase system in patients with heart failure or to alterations in β-adrenoreceptor density.[19,46,52,60,68,122]

Nonadrenergic inotropes include digoxin, calcium chloride, phosphodiesterase inhibitors (amrinone, milrinone, and enoximone), and triiodothyronine. The presence of metabolic acidosis may interfere with the effectiveness of inotropic agents.[110,204] Notably, most inotropic agents (most importantly β-adrenergic agonists) have proarrhythmic effects. Improved cardiac output must be balanced against risks of inducing either atrial or ventricular arrhythmias. Patients who require high doses of dopamine, epinephrine, or norepinephrine experience dangerous vasoconstrictive effects because of the α-adrenergic agonist effect of these agents at higher doses. This effect can result in limb, mesenteric, or renal ischemic injury. Mechanical ventricular support should be considered before the patient suffers significant end-organ hypoperfusion, which may retard ultimate recovery. Insertion of an intraaortic balloon pump (IABP) via a percutaneous femoral arterial approach represents the initial step in mechanical ventricular support. A properly functioning IABP provides increased diastolic coronary perfusion and augmented cardiac output by reducing LV afterload (Figure 64-9). Greater deterioration of ventricular function may warrant assist devices that provide complete support; these devices are utilized as bridges to either myocardial recovery or possible cardiac transplantation.

▶ CARDIAC TAMPONADE

Tamponade results from occupation of the mediastinal space by fluid or clotted blood, which restricts the end-diastolic volume of both ventricles. It has been reported to occur acutely in 3.4–5.8% of cases.[35,49,150] The constellation of findings associated with acute postoperative cardiac tamponade includes (1) increased variation in blood pressure with respiration (pulsus paradoxus); (2) equalization and elevation of the central venous pressure, pulmonary artery diastolic pressure, and left atrial pressure or pulmonary artery wedge pressure[220]; (3) a fall

Table 64–1

Inotropes

Vasoactive drug	Dose (µg/kg/min)	AR activation			Physiological response				
		α_1	β_1	β_2	SVR	MAP	CO	HR	PAWP
Dopamine	<5	–	++	–	↔	↑	↑	↑	↔
	>5	++	++	–	↑↑	↑↑	↑	↑	↑
Dobutamine	2-20	–	++	+	↓	↑	↑	↑	↓
Epinephrine	<0.05	–	++	+	↓	↑	↑	↑	↓
	>0.05	++	++	+	↑↑	↑↑	↑	↑	↑
Norepinephrine	0.03–1.0	++	+	–	↑↑	↑↑	↔	↑	↑
Phenylephrine	0.6–2.0	++	–	–	↑↑	↑↑	↓	↔	↑
Isoproterenol	0.03–0.15	–	++	++	↓	↔	↑	↑↑	↓
Milrinone	0.3–1.5		PDEI[a]		↓	↔	↑	↔	↓
Amrinone	5–20		PDEII[a]		↓	↔	↑	↔	↓

AR, adrenergic receptor activation; α_1, peripheral vasculature; β_1, myocardium; β_2, peripheral vasculature and myocardium; SVR, systemic vascular resistance; MAP, mean arterial pressure; CO, cardiac output; HR, heart rate; PAWP, pulmonary arterial wedge pressure.
[a]Amrinone and milrinone are common phosphodiesterase inhibitors (PDEIs).

in urine output (often an early finding); (4) excessive chest tube drainage or, paradoxically, minimal or no chest tube drainage, especially with heavy clots noted within the chest tubes; (5) mediastinal widening on chest film; (6) low cardiac output (late); and (7) hypotension (late). No single finding or combination of findings is sufficient to establish the diagnosis, and a high index of clinical suspicion should be maintained. Early postoperative tamponade is treated by reoperation ideally in the operating room. Patients in extremis may require reopening of their sternotomy in the ICU. Temporizing management consists of (1) volume loading, (2) reduction of airway pressure (removal of positive end-expiratory pressure [PEEP], anesthetizing agents, diminishing tidal volume with increasing ventilatory rate) and (3) inotropic support.

Cardiac tamponade may be present with any amount of retained blood or fluid, which in most cases is circumferential but which may be loculated and still adversely affect cardiac function.[61,174] In cases with decreased ventricular function, smaller amounts of space occupation will result in tamponade physiology.[179] For patients with severe ventricular dysfunction, simple reapproximation of the sternum following cardiac surgery may not be possible. Delayed sternal closure may be necessary in 1–2% of high-risk patients, and subsequent closure is usually possible between 1 and 4 days following initial operation.[64]

To a certain extent, the pleural and mediastinal spaces are continuous, and resulting intrathoracic pressure is distributed to affect the lungs and cardiac chambers simultaneously. An open pericardium and pleural space can neither prevent nor minimize cardiac tamponade. Increases in airway pressure, which may result from changing lung compliance or the application of PEEP, or a change in chest wall compliance may be directly transmitted to the heart. Such increases in airway pressure cause additive space occupation and can make tamponade manifest at lower volumes of retained fluid.

Although cardiac tamponade usually presents within the first 24 h following surgery, there is a definite incidence of late presentation.[16,48,79,174] Most cases occur in patients with large amounts of postoperative bleeding, those who require anticoagulation, or those with active inflammation (postpericardiotomy syndrome). Delayed diagnosis is attributed to the associated nonspecific symptoms of malaise, dyspnea, chest pain, and anorexia. Echocardiography serves as the mainstay in diagnosis of delayed cardiac tamponade.[65,112,170,186]

RIGHT HEART DYSFUNCTION

Although right heart dysfunction is most commonly secondary to left heart failure, it may occur as an isolated condition. In this setting, the left ventricle may display relatively preserved intrinsic function, but cardiac output remains low because of poor LV filling. Other important manifestations of isolated right heart failure include elevated CVP, poor right

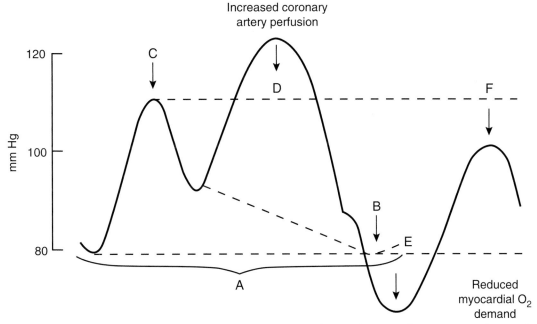

Figure 64–9 IABP timing: synchronization with the cardiac cycle. Arterial pressure waveform with correct IABP timing. A, one complete cardiac cycle; B, unassisted aortic end-diastolic pressure; C, unassisted systolic pressure; D, diastolic augmentation; E, reduced aortic end-diastolic pressure; F, reduced systolic pressure.
(Reproduced with permission from Helman DN: Intracorporeal support: the intra-aortic balloon pump. In Goldstein DJ, Oz MC, editors: Cardiac Assist Devices. New York: Futura Publishing Company, 2000, p. 298.)

ventricular contractility, and elevated pulmonary vascular resistance. With severely impaired RV function, pulmonary artery pressures may not be elevated. Treatment strategies for isolated right heart dysfunction are not dissimilar to managing a low cardiac output state due to more conventional LV dysfunction. Preload, which consists of the CVP, may need to be increased to greater than 20 mm Hg. Heart rate and rhythm should be optimized (sinus rhythm, rate 90–100). β-Adrenergic receptor agonists may be helpful, but higher doses of epinephrine, norepinephrine, or dopamine may further increase pulmonary vascular resistance and exacerbate right heart failure. Milrinone is an important agent in these circumstances since it provides a positive inotropic effect for the right ventricle but also reduces pulmonary artery pressures as well as pulmonary vascular resistance. Finally, inhaled nitric oxide represents the most specific pulmonary vasodilator; nitric oxide, unlike milrinone, will not induce systemic hypotension. The starting dose for inhaled nitric oxide should be between 20 and 40 parts per million. A final strategy for isolated right heart failure is a right ventricle assist device (RVAD). In general, this invasive strategy should be utilized only after less invasive approaches have failed.

ARRHYTHMIAS

Atrial Flutter

Atrial flutter is generated by a macro reentrant phenomenon[132] and can be treated rapidly and effectively with electrical stimulation. Although this arrhythmia may be interrupted by a single, appropriately timed atrial extrasystole, it is most commonly interrupted by one of the following methods: (1)

Entrainment, which means determining the atrial rate and instituting atrial pacing at a slightly higher rate in order to capture the atria. Regularization of the ventricular response and an altered P-wave morphology are usually produced. Termination of pacing is ordinarily followed by normal sinus rhythm (Figure 64–10). (2) Nonspecific rapid atrial stimulation,[217] rapid atrial pacing is performed by introducing trains of atrial pacing at rates in the range of 450–600 beats per minute. Short trains (less than 1 s) effectively introduce single extra stimuli within the effective refractory period of the pacing site and thus can interrupt atrial flutter and reinstate the normal sinus rhythm. If the train of rapid atrial pacing is too long, it may induce atrial fibrillation, which cannot be treated with these pacing techniques. However, in the atrial fibrillation that may ensue, the ventricular response is usually slower and thus better tolerated than that of atrial flutter.[124] It is common for atrial fibrillation induced in this manner to revert spontaneously to normal sinus rhythm.

Atrial Fibrillation

Incidence and Risk

Atrial fibrillation is the most common supraventricular arrhythmia following cardiac operation. The incidence has varied from 28 to 54% of patients undergoing cardiac operations.[119,173,183] The etiology is unknown but may be due to (1) unprotected ischemia,[184,192] (2) multidose cardioplegic solution administration with high potassium concentration,[47] (3) atrial dilation or inadequate atrial protection,[4,34] or (4) postoperative pericarditis.[158]

The incidence of postoperative atrial fibrillation is higher in patients with echocardiographic evidence of pericardial

Pace Atria 350 Beats/Min ⟶ Off

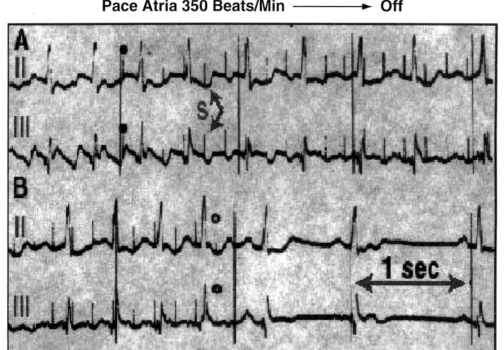

Figure 64–10 Atrial flutter in postoperative cardiac patients. Electrocardiographic leads II and III show atrial flutter with 2:1 AV block. (**A**) and (**B**) are not continuous. At the black dot in (**A**), the P-wave morphology has changed from negative to positive, which indicates entrainment. In (**B**), after 30 s of pacing at 350 beats/min, atrial pacing is terminated (open circle). Sinus rhythm appears spontaneously. S, stimulus artifact. *(Reproduced with permission from Waldo AL, MacLean WAH: Diagnosis and Treatment of Cardiac Arrhythmias Following Open-Heart Surgery. Mt. Kisco, NY: Futura Publishing Company, 1980.)*

effusion. Certain patients may also have an inherent propensity to develop supraventricular arrhythmias related to the preoperative accumulation of catecholamines in intramyocardial axons.[115] Additional risk factors predictive of an increased incidence of atrial fibrillation include advanced age, chronic obstructive pulmonary disease, prolonged cross-clamp periods,[37] and discontinuation of preoperative β-blockers. Although this arrhythmia has not been shown to increase the 30-day mortality rate, it does prolong length of hospital stay in patients undergoing coronary artery bypass grafting (CABG). Furthermore, there is an increased incidence of malignant ventricular rhythms (both ventricular tachycardia and ventricular fibrillation), as well as a significant increase in the postoperative stroke rate.[37]

Diagnosis and Treatment

Although various diagnostic methods can be used, these have generally been supplanted by direct examination of atrial and ventricular bipolar electrocardiograms.[217] The presence of chaotic and rapid atrial depolarization indicates atrial fibrillation, while a regular rapid atrial depolarization with an organized ventricular response (usually 2:1 or 3:1) indicates atrial flutter (Figure 64–11). Therapeutic objectives in patients with atrial fibrillation in order of importance are (1) heart rate control, (2) conversion to sinus rhythm, and (3) prevention of embolic complications.

Rapid supraventricular arrhythmias causing significant hemodynamic compromise should be treated by cardioversion or defibrillation. In hemodynamically stable patients, the drug of choice for controlling ventricular response is a calcium channel antagonist: either verapamil, administered in 2.5–5 mg boluses to a total of 20 mg, or diltiazem given as an intravenous load followed by a continuous infusion. These agents rapidly reduce the ventricular response by increasing AV block.[187] The salutary effect of reduction in

ventricular rate is usually more important than the negative inotropic effect of these drugs.[149,156,162] Adverse effects of calcium channel antagonists may be treated with calcium infusion,[159] glucagon,[123] or inotropic agents.[188]

Alternatively, β-blockers, especially those with short action (esmolol), have been studied for the acute management of atrial fibrillation. The response to β-blockade varies considerably when it is used to treat atrial fibrillation in the post-CABG patient. In addition, hypotension may be a significant side effect in as many as 20–40% of patients treated.[163] Digoxin has been similarly used, although immediate heart rate control is rarely achieved.[70]

Multidrug combinations can be hazardous in patients without temporary pacing wires. The combination of digoxin, verapamil, and a β-adrenergic antagonist can lead to complete heart block, while verapamil and a β-adrenergic antagonist may lead to sinus arrest.[121] Once heart rate control has been achieved, conversion to and maintenance of sinus rhythm with an antiarrhythmic agent may be necessary.[26]

Two newer agents that have been used extensively for postoperative atrial fibrillation are amiodarone and sotalol. Relative to class IA agents, these drugs are felt to have equivalent efficacy and better side effect profiles. These agents are very effective at converting atrial fibrillation, and both also retard AV nodal conduction, thereby reducing the ventricular response to atrial fibrillation. Amiodarone is typically administered as a 1-g IV infusion, which is given over a 24-h period with the initial 150 mg given over 20 min. Subsequent doses are given orally (400 mg three times a day). Sotalol is available only as an oral preparation, 40–160 mg twice a day. A common approach initially is to attempt chemical cardioversion with these agents, and if this fails, perform electrical cardioversion. Sotalol can induce significant bradycardia and probably should not be combined with other β-blockers. In addition, harmful proarrhythmic effects including ventricular tachycardia have been described with

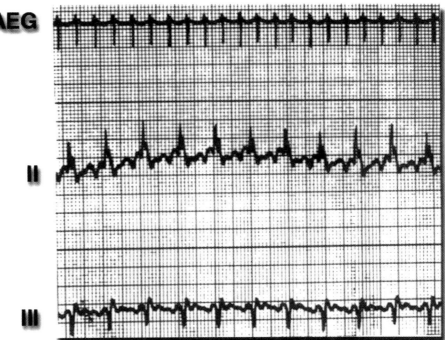

AEG

II

III

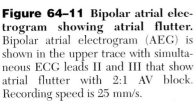

Figure 64–11 Bipolar atrial electrogram showing atrial flutter. Bipolar atrial electrogram (AEG) is shown in the upper trace with simultaneous ECG leads II and III that show atrial flutter with 2:1 AV block. Recording speed is 25 mm/s. *(Reproduced with permission from Waldo AL, Cooper TB, MacLean WAH: Cardiac pacing in the treatment of cardiac arrhythmias following open-heart surgery: use of temporarily placed atrial and ventricular wire electrodes. In Samet P, El-Sherif N, editors: Cardiac Pacing, 2nd ed. New York: Grune & Stratton, 1980.)*

sotalol. The incidence of these harmful rhythms has correlated with QT prolongation, and this should be monitored. Chronic amiodarone therapy can induce pulmonary fibrosis and hypothyroidism. In general, the risk of postoperative atrial fibrillation is considerably reduced after the first month and antiarrhythmics initiated for isolated postoperative atrial fibrillation should be discontinued after this point.

There has been much interest in the prophylactic use of antiarrhythmic agents to diminish the incidence of supraventricular arrhythmias (atrial fibrillation, in particular) following cardiac surgery. However, prophylactic use of antiarrhythmics in all patients may lead to unwanted side effects in patients who would otherwise convalesce normally. As attempts to identify perioperative risk factors continue, many cardiac surgeons prefer to treat arrhythmias only when they are present.[84]

Ventricular Arrhythmias

Sustained ventricular arrhythmias are an uncommon postoperative issue but are life-threatening and require a prompt and organized treatment strategy. Immediate electrical cardioversion should be followed by a thorough investigation for treatable causes that may include electrolyte imbalance, hypoxia, malpositioned Swan-Ganz catheter, and proarrhythmic effects of inotropes or other agents. Myocardial ischemia should always be ruled out as the cause of the ventricular arrhythmias. A 12-lead ECG should be performed, and if ischemic changes are present, cardiac catheterization with coronary angiography should be considered. Persistent ventricular arrhythmias in the postoperative patient lead quickly to hypoperfusion and a dangerous spiral. For this reason, early placement of IABP for ventricular assistance is often helpful. Persistent arrhythmias also warrant initiation of either lidocaine or amiodarone IV. Formal electrophysiological testing and implantable defibrillator may be indicated.

GRAFT OCCLUSION

Intraoperative Injury and Graft Occlusion

Early graft failure is usually due to technical factors, although it may be produced by scarring and is seen more frequently in patients with inflammatory pericardial syndromes. Early graft failure may manifest as ventricular arrhythmias or hemodynamic compromise with evidence for ischemia; alternately, the occurrence may be clinically silent. Factors that affect the presentation include the nature of collateral blood supply from other grafts or from the native coronary circulation. Also important is the amount of viable myocardium at risk. Patients with ventricular arrhythmias, hemodynamic change, and evidence for ischemia warrant urgent coronary angiography. Graft failure can be addressed with percutaneous interventions or return to the OR for graft revision. Perioperative myocardial infarction (MI) is defined by ECG changes, creatine phosphokinase (CPK)-MB measurement, and the development of new regional LV dysfunction. Perioperative MI does not result solely from graft or coronary occlusion, but may result from compromised myocardial protection or atheroembolic events. Treatment is mainly supportive with IV nitroglycerin and afterload reduction. Inotropic agents or IABP may be required during a period of myocardial recovery.

Graft survival is enhanced by the perioperative administration of antiplatelet agents. Initially, aspirin and dipyridamole were used,[29] but subsequent work suggests that low-dose aspirin alone (325 mg/day) is as effective as a combination of agents.[127] Aspirin should be administered the morning following surgery. Clopidogrel bisulfate (Plavix) has also been considered for postoperative antiplatelet therapy. Plavix is an inhibitor of adenosine diphosphate (ADP)-induced platelet aggregation. It acts as a direct inhibitor of ADP by binding to ADP receptors on platelets and preventing the subsequent ADP-mediated activation of the glycoprotein IIb/IIIa complex. The clinical evidence for the efficacy of Plavix is derived from the CAPRIE (Clopidogrel vs. Aspirin in Patients at Risk of Ischemic Events) trial (Figure 64-12). The direct effect of Plavix on coronary bypass graft patency has not been formally studied, but results of the CAPRIE and subgroup analysis would support the use of Plavix antiplatelet therapy in place of aspirin for high-risk patients following coronary artery bypass. The recommended dose of Plavix in the postoperative setting is 75 mg/day. The most important side effect is bleeding: in CAPRIE, the incidence of gastrointestinal (GI) bleeding was 2.0% versus 2.7% with aspirin; intracranial hemorrhage was 0.4% for Plavix versus 0.5% for aspirin. Overall GI complaints were similar for Plavix and aspirin.

Postoperative Bleeding

Postoperative bleeding is always present to some degree following cardiac surgery. Bleeding is related to a combination of mechanical factors that are surgically correctable and to coagulopathy. A surgically correctable cause predominates in fewer than 3% of cases and is indicated by brisk hemorrhage (>200 ml/h), normal or near-normal coagulation studies, and the appearance of blood clots in the mediastinal drainage tubes. The amount of bleeding that occurs after surgery, the number of transfusions required, and the filtering of transfused components are related to outcome.[210]

Coagulopathy

Coagulopathy is a common feature of patients placed on the CPB. These effects are exacerbated by the preoperative use of antiplatelet agents, thrombolytic agents, and heparin. The predominant cause of abnormal bleeding following CPB is a fall in platelet number and impaired platelet function.[14,80]

This platelet dysfunction is related to passage through the extracorporeal circuit, with resulting decrease in platelet membrane receptors for fibrinogen as well as for glycoprotein Ib and glycoprotein IIb/IIIa complex. A second mechanism for coagulopathy is progressive fibrinolytic state of variable intensity related to the length of CPB. Coagulopathy may be associated with variable or no bleeding and is recognized by the presence of abnormal clotting parameters (prothrombin time [PT], partial thromboplastin time [PTT], fibrinogen level, platelet count) and the absence of solid clot formation in the mediastinal drainage tubes.

The management of patients with excessive mediastinal hemorrhage is complex and may be hazardous. Bleeding due predominantly to coagulopathy is treated by both specific and nonspecific means. Postoperative coagulopathy must be specifically diagnosed by laboratory and clinical evaluation of the coagulation system. Any or all of the following abnormalities may be present.

Heparin Effect

This effect is demonstrated by a prolonged PTT and/or a prolonged activated clotting time (ACT). ACT should be measured on admission to the ICU as this effect is usually seen early in the postoperative course (the half-life of heparin is approximately 1 h).[55,85] The specific treatment is administration of protamine sulfate (25–50 mg doses are given and the ACT repeated).[24]

Thrombocytopenia

Thrombocytopenia is due to destruction of platelets during CPB or to consumption.[9,141] In the absence of other abnormalities, treatment is platelet transfusion.[72] Notably, if

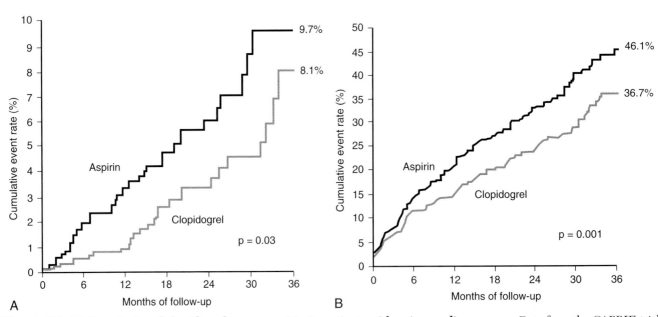

Figure 64–12 Superiority of clopidogrel versus aspirin in patients with prior cardiac surgery. Data from the CAPRIE trial, surgical subset analysis. (**A**) Kaplan–Meier curves for clopidogrel versus aspirin for vascular death with cumulative event rates. (**B**) Kaplan–Meier curves for clopidogrel versus aspirin for composite of vascular death, MI, stroke, or rehospitalization for ischemia or bleeding with cumulative event rates.
(Reproduced with permission from Bhatt DL: Superiority of clopidogrel versus aspirin in patients with prior cardiac surgery. Circulation 103:366, 2000.)

a patient is not actively bleeding, thrombocytopenia is generally not corrected with transfusion since the platelet level usually normalizes spontaneously over the next few days. As many patients are maintained preoperatively on heparin, persistent postoperative thrombocytopenia may be induced by the presence of heparin-dependent antibodies. In this setting, resulting thromboembolic events as well as significant bleeding have been observed.[85,218] Diagnosis of heparin-induced thrombocytopenia can be made with heparin-platelet aggregation testing and a platelet factor IV assay to confirm the presence of antibodies *in vitro*. All heparin should be discontinued promptly in these patients.

Thrombasthenia

In this instance, the platelet count is normal, but clot formation is inadequate. This remains a significant problem in the postcardiac surgical patient.[80] It can be documented by measuring bleeding time using the Ivy method[108] or more accurately defined using the thromboelastogram (TEG).[102,194] Qualitative defects in platelet function result from CPB[10,76,80] or from antiplatelet therapy.[56,69] Aspirin and Plavix can irreversibly affect platelet function, the life span of which is 6–7 days. Therefore, a single dose administered within the 7 days before the operation diminishes platelet function.[108] A significant increase in bleeding complication and transfusion requirements has been observed.[178,203]

Specific Factor Deficiencies

Specific factor deficiencies are usually manifested by elevation of the PT or the PTT. Abnormalities may be due to a specific genetic disorder, liver disease, prior Coumadin therapy, hemodilution, or disseminated intravascular coagulation (DIC). These disorders are generally treated by specific factor therapy, fresh frozen plasma, or cryoprecipitate.

Management of Bleeding

Specific treatment consists of blood component therapy based on accurate diagnosis and an understanding of changes that occur during CPB. Guidelines for transfusion support as well as management of postoperative patients with significant hemorrhage have been suggested.[72] The observed rate of bleeding must be correlated with its character (the initial bleeding rate may reflect drainage of sequestered blood or irrigation fluid) and hemodynamic effect (ineffective drainage may underestimate ongoing intravascular depletion). The quality of blood clotting may be effectively estimated by close observation of the drainage tube contents and manual manipulation of the tubes. Large amounts of clot that repeatedly obstruct the tubes indicate a surgical source of bleeding. Nonclotting, freely draining blood, or the presence of loosely organized clot, indicates that a coagulopathic state exists.

Bleeding at a rate of more than 200 ml/h requires immediate action to search for and correct the underlying cause. Delays in laboratory testing frequently preclude accurate and timely diagnosis. Algorithms outlining empiric treatment are usually developed with input from surgeons and blood bank directors.

The single most practical treatment is to administer platelet concentrate, which is often effective despite an apparently adequate platelet count due to the presence of platelet dysfunction. Fresh frozen plasma fraction is employed to replenish coagulation (PT) factors manifested as a prolongation of the PT for PTT. Cryoprecipitate is administered to replenish consumed fibrinogen. Other forms of treatment, including tube clamping and the employment of high levels of positive end-expiratory pressure, have never been shown to be effective. With appropriate treatment of coagulation deficiencies, coagulopathy usually resolves within a few hours. Bleeding usually diminishes to modest levels (50–100 ml/h) within 4 h, and rarely is the total amount drained more than 1 liter.

Reoccurrence of high drainage rates should be addressed immediately, despite the fact that sudden drainage of sequestered blood is common when the patient is repositioned. It is not uncommon for a new bleeding site to develop with clot lysis or following a brief episode of severe hypertension. A common scenario is initial bleeding at rates of 150–250 ml/h, followed by alternating periods of inconsequential drainage and substantial drainage. This often indicates surgically correctable bleeding, with a large burden of intramediastinal clot and ineffective tube drainage due to clot obstruction. When the bleeding issue is not resolved within a few hours, a second chest X-ray should be obtained to ensure that mediastinal and pleural drainage has been effective.

The major side effects of postoperative bleeding are volume loss and retention of clotted blood within the mediastinum. Nonspecific therapy consists of continuous, adequate volume replacement, maintenance of free drainage, and prevention of hypothermia. Hypothermia has a generalized anticoagulant effect[73] that increases PT and PTT in direct accordance with the degree of temperature change.[172] Specific anticoagulant effects may be corrected by warming.

Volume replacement may be provided by continuous autotransfusion but also requires the infusion of nonspecific agents. Crystalloid solutions may be provided as normal saline or lactated Ringer's solution. Colloid solutions include (1) serum albumin as a 25% solution. Serum albumin in its 25% solution must recruit extravascular fluid to result in effective volume replacement. (2) Plasma protein fraction (Plasmanate) as a 5% protein solution containing both albumin and α- and β-globulins.[12,185] Plasmanate may cause a paradoxical hypotension attributed to the use of acetate, present as a buffer,[154] or may cause the presence of Hageman-factor fragments.[1] (3) Hydroxyethyl starch (Hetastarch). Hetastarch provides plasma volume expansion for greater than 24 h and may be safely used to a total volume of 1.5 liters. Because it has a chemical composition similar to that of dextran, associated urticarial and anaphylactoid reactions may occur.[12,185] However, unlike dextran, coagulation abnormalities generally have been related to hemodilution rather than to a specific anticoagulant effect.

Mechanical means should be used to maintain mediastinal chest tube patency, including (1) application of suction; (2) stripping and milking of chest tubes; mechanical stripping of chest tubes can create negative pressures as high as 1500 mm Hg and can be potentially damaging to entrapped tissues; and (3) occasionally, Fogarty catheter thrombectomy of the mediastinal tubes. Catheter thrombectomy usually precedes reoperation and may relieve significant tamponade.

Other nonspecific measures include strict control of blood pressure and induction of mild controlled hypotension, which can markedly diminish bleeding rate. However, afterload reduction can be particularly dangerous in the hypovolemic patient with ongoing blood loss and early cardiac tamponade. Levels of PEEP in the range of 10–12 cm H_2O have been suggested as a means to reduce postoperative bleeding.[88,92,142] The efficacy of PEEP in slowing postoperative bleeding remains controversial,[232] and acute reduction in preload with this level of PEEP is potentially dangerous.[191]

Blood Conservation

Blood conservation requires a programmatic approach but is essential to improving patient outcome. There is ample evidence that blood and blood products negatively influence outcome, expose patients to viral and bacterial infection, and may reduce host resistance to infection.[210] The tolerance of a reduced hematocrit in the postoperative cardiac patient is an important component in the avoidance of blood transfusion. Although classic teaching states that the optimal hematocrit is between 0.30 and 0.40,[7,23,40,227,228] this has not been clearly defined for patients following corrective cardiac surgery. In such patients, no significant difference in mortality rate, morbidity, and length of hospital stay has been demonstrated by allowing hematocrits to drop 0.23–0.25, compared with those maintained at 0.32 or greater.[99] Oral iron therapy, and occasionally the prescription of folic acid, restores normal hematocrit 6 weeks following surgery.

Pharmacological Considerations

Desmopressin

Desmopressin (1-desamino-8-d-arginin-vasopressin, DDAVP), a synthetic analog of L-arginine vasopressin, has improved platelet function and reduced hemorrhage in a variety of clinical disorders. DDAVP appears to act by increasing the concentration of von Willebrand factor, an important mediator of platelet adhesion. No clear consensus exists regarding the prophylactic use of DDAVP.[4,120] However, patients who have ongoing hemorrhage should be considered for administration of 3 µg/kg given over 15 min.[72]

Aprotinin

This nonspecific protease inhibitor, extracted from bovine lung, has been suggested as a method of reducing postoperative mediastinal bleeding. Pre-CPB administration of aprotinin can preserve platelet function otherwise lost during CPB.[43,211] It may be administered pre-CPB in low dose (2×10^6 KIU) or as a continuing infusion during bypass in high dose (6×10^6 KIU). Recent multicenter trials have documented the overall safety of full-dose aprotinin and have also shown an intriguing reduction in the incidence of stroke.[211] Aprotinin use has been advocated in the setting of reoperative cardiac surgery and in cases such as left ventricle assist device (LVAD) implantation in which the bleeding risk is high.

ε-Aminocaproic Acid

Prophylactic antifibrinolytic therapy is common in modern cardiac surgery, with intraoperative and postoperative administration of ε-aminocaproic acid evolving into the standard of care in the United States. This should be continued at 1 g/h per protocol. If it has not been used, a 5 g load followed by

1 g/h may be beneficial. If prophylactic aprotinin has been used, the use of ε-aminocaproic acid is probably contraindicated.

Neurological Complications

Neurological Function

Neurological dysfunction is common following cardiac surgery and constitutes a major cause of death and disability. Frank stroke occurs in as many as 10% of patients, related to patient risk factors identified in prospective studies relating pre- and intraoperatively determined characteristics. The incidence of stroke and stroke-like events has been related to clinical variables that are comorbid preoperative features. In a large multicenter study, odds ratios were developed that predicted frank stroke outcome. Neurological disease, age, and diabetes were the predominant risk factors (Table 64-2). Multivariable analysis allowed the development of a nomogram that relates the number of preoperative risk factors to the incidence of stroke outcome (Figure 64-13). An additional 1–10% of patients will have transient ischemia, stupor, or frank psychosis. When detailed neuropsychological examinations are performed, disability can be detected in more than 50% of patients (Figure 64-14).

Additional risk factors have been associated with the actual conduct of surgery, and were elucidated in the same cohort of patients. The discovery of an abnormal aorta or

---

Table 64–2

Preoperative Prediction of Stroke[a]

Risk factor	Odds ratio
Hx neurological disease	2.28
Age (per year)	1.06
Diabetes	2.10
Hx vascular disease	2.09
Prior CABG	1.89
COPD	1.88
Unstable angina	1.79

Modified from Roach GW, Kanchuger M, Mangano CM, et al: Adverse cerebral outcomes after coronary bypass surgery. Multicenter Study of Perioperative Ischemia Research Group and the Ischemia Research and Education Foundation Investigators. N Engl J Med 335:1857–1863, 1996. Copyright 1996 Massachusetts Medical Society. All rights reserved.

[a]Predictions of frank stroke outcome based on the predominant risk factors shown. Hx neurological disease, a history of neurological disease; Hx vascular disease, a history of vascular disease; CABG, coronary artery bypass graft; COPD, chronic obstructive pulmonary disease.

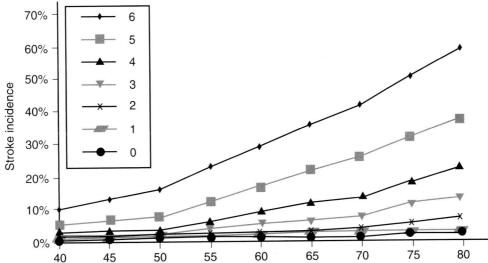

Figure 64–13 Graphed data of preoperative prediction of stroke. A nomogram developed by multivariable analysis demonstrating the increase in probability of stroke incidence with an increasing number of patient risk factors. The numbered lines in the legend (0 through 6) indicate the number of risk factors (0 to 6) for a patient. Risk factors include a history of neurological disease, a history of vascular disease, presence of diabetes, prior coronary artery bypass grafting, chronic obstructive pulmonary disease, and unstable angina.
(Reproduced with permission from Roach GW, Kanchuger M, Mangano CM, et al: Adverse cerebral outcomes after coronary bypass surgery. Multicenter Study of Perioperative Ischemia Research Group and the Ischemia Research and Education Foundation Investigators. N Engl J Med 335:1857–1863, 1996. Copyright 1996 Massachusetts Medical Society. All rights reserved.)

use of an IABP became highly predictive of an adverse type I event (stroke) (Table 64-3). Type II events were identified and included stupor and other alterations of consciousness (Table 64-4). Although age was again the most important predictor, systolic hypertension and dysrhythmias occurring after surgery became significant.

The etiology of neurological dysfunction is multifactorial, and it is the subject of much ongoing research. Causal factors include (1) particulate and gaseous emboli from the cardiopulmonary bypass apparatus, (2) macroemboli from aortic manipulation, (3) macroemboli from the extracranial cerebral vasculature, (4) regional malperfusion due to extracranial vascular obstruction, (5) regional malperfusion due to generalized hypoperfusion during CPB (watershed cerebral infarction), (6) regional malperfusion due to impaired cerebral autoregulation (more prevalent in diabetics), and (7) generalized central nervous system edema following cardiopulmonary bypass.

Although neurological dysfunction following cardiac surgery may be multifactorial, arterial embolization is the most important factor. Major stroke is often due to atherosclerotic emboli originating in the aorta; more subtle neuropsychological deficits may be due to microemboli.[202] Autopsy studies in patients who have undergone CPB have detected microscopic emboli, composed primarily of lipid, dispersed within the cerebral microvasculature.[146] The histopathological lesion caused by these microemboli, after processing and staining, takes the form of a small capillary and arteriolar dilatation (SCAD) that is associated with ischemic injury and neuronal dysfunction. SCADs are detected in the brain after CPB and range in size from 10 to 70 μm.[103,147] Efforts to reduce microembolization have taken many forms. The simple, initial approach has been the placement of an arterial line filter that has become standard equipment on most

CPB circuits. Such filters, however, do not eliminate SCADs that may be due to microscopic lipid deposit that enters shed blood in the mediastinum (Figure 64-15).[22] Furthermore, the use of cardiotomy suction to recover shed blood in combination with CPB results in significantly more SCADs relative to CPB alone. Other studies have introduced the possibility that processing shed blood by washing and centrifugation (with a cell saver device) prior to return to the CPB circuit may reduce SCADs.[21,103] This has led to increased use of cell saver in routine cardiac cases and more avoidance of convention cardiotomy suction devices. Prospective randomized trials to determine whether these

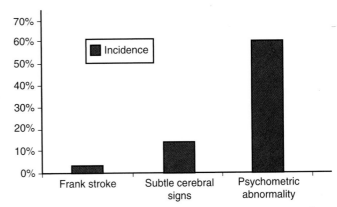

Figure 64–14 Spectrum of neurological injury. As these data from Duke University Medical Center illustrate, disability can be detected in more than 50% of patients when detailed neuropsychological examinations are performed.

1050

Table 64–3	
Adverse Cerebral Outcomes: Predictors of Type I Injury[a,b]	
Predictor	*Odds ratio*
Abnormal aorta	4.52
Hx neurological disease	3.19
IABP use	2.60
Diabetes	2.59
Hypertension	2.31
COPD	2.09
Unstable angina	1.83
Age (per decade)	1.75

[a]Modified from Roach GW, Kanchuger M, Mangano CM, et al: Adverse cerebral outcomes after coronary bypass surgery. Multicenter Study of Perioperative Ischemia Research Group and the Ischemia Research and Education Foundation Investigators. N Engl J Med 335:1857–1863, 1996. Copyright 1996 Massachusetts Medical Society. All rights reserved.

[b]Shown are odds ratios for eight independent predictors of type I cerebral outcomes. The discovery of an abnormal aorta or use of an intraortic balloon pump (IABP) is highly predictive of an adverse type I event (stroke). Hx neurological disease, history of neurological disease; COPD, chronic obstructive pulmonary disease.

Table 64–4	
Adverse Cerebral Outcomes: Predictors of Type II Injury[a,b]	
Predictor	*Odds ratio*
Systolic BP >180	3.47
Alcohol consumption	2.64
COPD	2.37
Age (per decade)	2.20
Prior CABG	2.18
Dysrhythmia day of surgery	1.97
Antihypertensive Rx	1.78

[a]Modified from Roach GW, Kanchuger M, Mangano CM, et al: Adverse cerebral outcomes after coronary bypass surgery. Multicenter Study of Perioperative Ischemia Research Group and the Ischemia Research and Education Foundation Investigators. N Engl J Med 335:1857–1863, 1996. Copyright 1996 Massachusetts Medical Society. All rights reserved.

[b]Shown are odds ratios for seven independent predictors of type II cerebral outcomes. Stupor and other alterations of consciousness are included in this grouping of predictors. BP, blood pressure; COPD, chronic obstructive pulmonary disease; CABG, coronary artery bypass graft.

techniques will improve neurological outcomes have not yet been performed.

Another important area of potential benefit from OPCAB relates to neurocognitive outcomes. The mechanism of neurocognitive injury with conventional cardiac surgery includes emboli from cannulation and fatty or gaseous microemboli that are not filtered with standard CPB techniques. Although formal stroke represents a significant problem, subtler neurocognitive deficits occur at a substantially higher rate. Newman et al identified significant deficients in 50% of patients following coronary artery bypass surgery with CPB at the time of discharge; unfortunately these deficits may not be transient, as 42% of the study group displayed deficits at 5 years after their procedure. Furthermore, the presence of early deficits predicted late problems (Figure 64-16).[151] Theoretically, OPCAB would avoid some of these insults and potentially improve neurocognitive outcomes. Large prospective randomized trials comparing this outcome are not available, but some retrospective studies suggest a benefit with OPCAB procedures. Ricci et al retrospectively compared 172 octogenarians undergoing conventional CPB surgery with 97 undergoing OPCAB. The stroke rate was markedly diminished for the OPCAB group compared with the on-pump group (0% versus 9.3%).[169] Serum S100beta, a neuronal-specific protein that has been used as a marker of neuronal injury, has been shown to be reduced with OPCAB procedures relative to conventional on-pump coronary surgery procedures.[2]

The severity of stroke may also be related to the body's inflammatory response to neurological injury. It has recently been noted that the use of the serene protease inhibitor, aprotinin, employed to reduce intraoperative and postoperative bleeding, significantly reduced the incidence of stroke in several double blind, randomized, placebo-controlled trials (Figure 64-17).

Other factors, which contribute to neurological dysfunction, particularly in the elderly, include (1) "ICU psychosis" related to stress, environmental impact, and loss of compensation to surroundings; (2) sleep deprivation; (3) adverse drug reactions; and (4) revelation of previously, well-compensated mild dementia.

Often focal deficits are completely reversible if the patient is appropriately managed. The maintenance of adequate perfusion and oxygen delivery is critical to recovery. Cerebral blood flow is improved by head elevation to reduce edema and hyperventilation to provide moderate hypocapnia. General support includes protection of the patient's airway, management of pulmonary secretions, avoidance of pulmonary aspiration, and provision of nutrition.

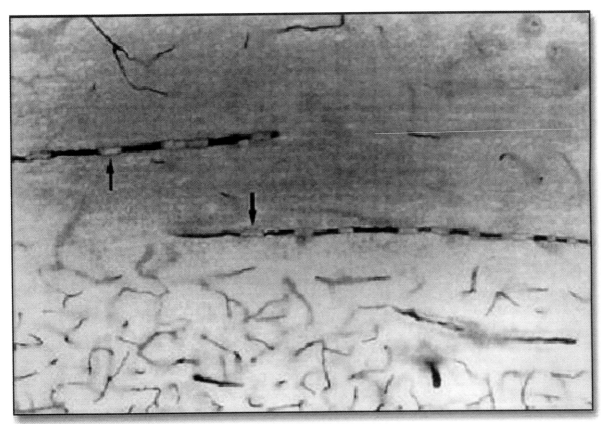

Figure 64–15 Small capillary and arterial dilatations (SCADs) (*arrows*) in cerebral vessels in a dog after cardiopulmonary bypass with cardiotomy suction (alkaline phosphatase-stained celloidin section, 100 μm thick; 5× magnification, before 50% reduction).

(Reproduced with permission from Brooker RF: Cardiotomy suction: a major source of brain lipid emboli during cardiopulmonary bypass. Ann Thorac Surg 65:1653, 1998.)

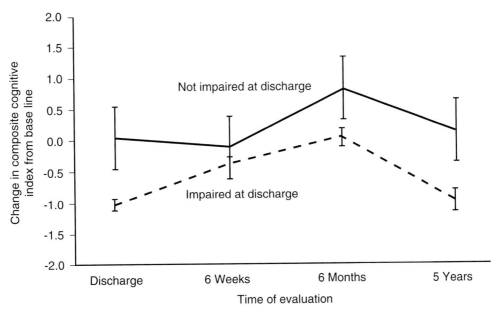

Figure 64–16 Longitudinal assessment of neurocognitive function after coronary artery bypass surgery. Composite cognitive index as a function of cognitive impairment at discharge. The composite cognitive index is the sum of the scores for the four domains and includes cognitive decline as well as increases in scores as a result of learning. Positive change represents an overall improvement (learning), whereas negative values indicate overall decline. The I bars represent the standard error.

(Reproduced with permission from Newman MF: Longitudinal assessment of neurocognitive function after coronary bypass surgery. N Engl J Med 344:399, 2001. Copyright 2001 Massachusetts Medical Society. All rights reserved.)

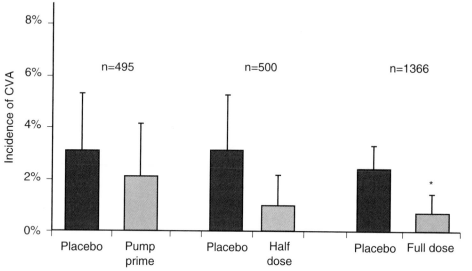

Figure 64–17 Aprotinin and stroke incidence. Aprotinin, employed to reduce intraoperative and postoperative bleeding, dramatically reduces the incidence of stroke. *(Reproduced with permission from Smith PK, Muhlbaier LH: Aprotinin: Safe and effective only with the full-dose regimen. Ann Thorac Surg 62:1575–1577, 1996.)*

*$p < .05$ Aprotinin vs. matched placebo

Because dramatic recovery is frequent, patient and family support should be aggressive in the first few days following surgery unless a definitive mortal injury can be defined.

Infection

Fever

The incidence of fever decreases exponentially throughout the postoperative course. Fevers not related to infectious causes are most commonly low-grade ($T < 38.9°$ C, rectal) and most resolve before the 15th postoperative day. Fever greater than $38.9°$ C at any time in the postoperative course is more likely related to a specific infection. The presence or absence of leukocytosis has not been helpful in this differentiation.[125] For days 4–9 postoperatively, 25% of fevers may be related to serious infection.[160]

Evaluation and Treatment

When infection is suspected, aggressive evaluation is indicated. Aerobic and anaerobic cultures of blood, urine, sputum, and abnormal fluid collections are mandatory, and should precede broad-spectrum antibiotic coverage.[74] Indwelling catheters should be considered potential infectious sites; appropriate infection control practices help to prevent or at least limit serious infections stemming from catheter use.[152,153,229] When antibiotics have already been administered, cultures should be obtained using specific antimicrobial-absorbing resins.[94]

Soft-tissue infection is most commonly due to *Staphylococcus aureus*, although *Staphylococcus epidermidis* has emerged as an important pathogen.[226] *Pseudomonas* and other gram-negative infections become more common when intensive-care stay exceeds 7 days and in patients receiving broad-spectrum antibiotic therapy.[63] Prolonged intensive care and antibiotic use can also cause systemic fungal infections and loss of the gastric mucosal barrier.[58,135,198] These infections are particularly difficult to diagnose because of their protean manifestations.[86]

Mediastinitis is of particular concern in all cardiac surgical patients and can be cryptic in presentation. The incidence has been reported to range from 0.8–1.86%.[39,91,126,155] The risk factors associated with mediastinitis have been determined (Table 64-5), as has a negative impact on long-term survival independent of other preoperative

---

Table 64–5

Univariate Logistic Regression Analysis[a,b]

Variable	Coefficients	χ^2	p
Obesity[c]	1.3	10.94	.009
NYHACHF[c]	0.32	9.34	.002
DM	0.62	6.87	.009
Previous heart surgery	0.85	6.83	.009

Table 64–5

Univariate Logistic Regression Analysis[a]—cont'd

Variable	Coefficients	χ^2	p
Duration of bypass[b]	0.005	5.48	.02
Comorbid condition	0.64	4.56	.03
Hemostasis at closure	1.2	2.94	.09
Peripheral vascular disease	0.37	1.55	.21
IMA graft (0, 1, or 2)	NA	0.95	.62
IMA graft (yes/no)	0.21	0.79	.37
COPD	0.39	0.61	.43
Sex	0.18	0.56	.45
Renal insufficiency	0.35	0.4	.53
Intraaortic balloon pump preoperatively	−0.3	0.38	.54
Coronary artery disease index	0.003	0.22	.64
Length of stay (before surgery)	−0.008	0.15	.71
Age	−0.003	0.1	.75
Ejection fraction	−0.002	0.05	.82
DM with bilateral IMA graft	NA	0.03	Diabetes, .01 Bilateral IMA, .30 Interaction, .28
Cardiac shock	0.07	0.01	.92
Operation type	−0.02	<0.0001	.96

From Milano CA, Kesler K, Archibald N, et al: Mediastinitis after coronary artery bypass graft surgery: risk factors and long-term survival. Circulation 1995;22:45–51.

[a]Univariate logistic regression analysis predicting mediastinitis; variables are listed in order of significance. Variables with univariate $p < 0.1$ were included in the multivariate analysis. NYHA CHF, New York Heart Association congestive heart failure; DM, diabetes mellitus; IMA, internal mammary artery; COPD, chronic obstructive pulmonary disease.

[b]Significant predictions by multivariate analysis.

risk factors (Figure 64-18). Sternal and mediastinal infections must be differentiated from simple subcutaneous fat necrosis, sterile sternal dehiscence, and the postpericardiotomy syndrome.

Deep sternal infections and mediastinitis are commonly associated with systemic symptoms (fever, leukocytosis), localized tenderness, severe persistent chest pain, and sternal instability.* Chest film, computed tomography, and indium-111 leukocyte scanning can be used to confirm the clinical diagnosis. Initial treatment consists of operative wound exploration, debridement, and drainage.[177] Although some infected patients can be treated with reclosure and irrigation,[207] diminished morbidity has been noted with

---

*References 126, 175–177, 181, 197, 209.

bilateral pectoral flap or omental flap closure.[101] Flap closure may be performed as a primary procedure with accompanying sternal debridement[98] or as a staged procedure with sternal debridement followed by closure in 3–4 days.[100,101]

Soft-tissue infections involving saphenous vein harvest, though usually minor, represent a significant source of morbidity following coronary revascularization. This complication has been reported to occur in 1% of patients[44] and is more common in the thigh harvest site. They are best prevented by careful selection of harvest sites and the use of meticulous surgical technique. Endoscopic vein harvest appears to have made a favorable impact on the rate of this complication. Most saphenous vein harvest site infections may be treated effectively by simple drainage, dressing changes, and prescription of antibiotics. However, in severe cases, wide debridement and skin grafting may be necessary.

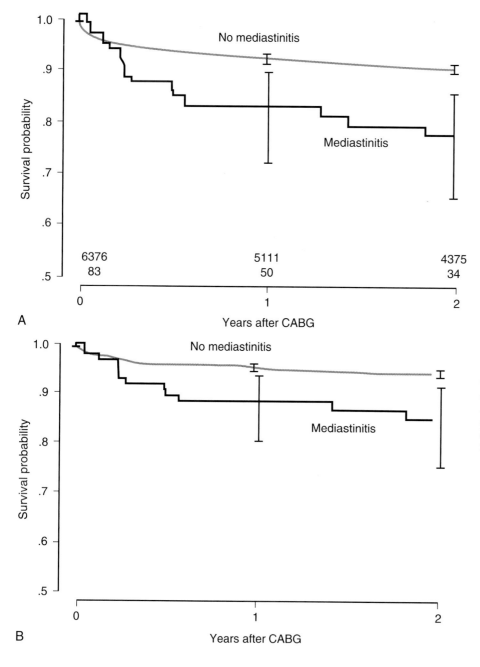

Figure 64–18 Unadjusted survival plot after CABG. **A,** Unadjusted Kaplan–Meier survival plot is shown for patients with and without mediastinitis. The numbers of surviving patients in each group at 0, 1, and 2 years after surgery are shown below the graph. **B,** Variable-adjusted survival plot after CABG. Kaplan–Meier survival plot adjusted for age, ejection fraction, extent of coronary artery disease, peripheral vascular disease, cerebrovascular disease, recent myocardial infarction, angina status, and mitral insufficiency. *(Reproduced with permission from Milano CA, Kesler K, Archibald N, et al: Mediastinitis after coronary artery bypass graft surgery: risk factors and long-term survival. Circulation 92: 2245–2251, 1995.)*

REFERENCES

1. Alving BM, Hojima Y, Pisano JJ, et al: Hypotension associated with prekallikrein activator (Hageman-factor fragments) in plasma protein fraction. N Engl J Med 299:66–70, 1978.
2. Anderson RE, Hansson LO, Vaage J: Release of S100B during coronary artery bypass grafting is reduced by off-pump surgery. Ann Thorac Surg 67:1721–1725, 1999.
3. Angelini GD, Fraser AG, Koning MM, et al: Adverse hemodynamic effects and echocardiographic consequences of pericardial closure soon after sternotomy and pericardiotomy. Circulation 82:IV397–IV406, 1990.
4. Ansell J, Klassen V, Lew R, et al: Does desmopressin acetate prophylaxis reduce blood loss after valvular heart operations? A randomized, double-blind study. J Thorac Cardiovasc Surg 104:117–123, 1992.
5. Appelbaum A, Kouchoukos NT, Blackstone EH, et al: Early risks of open-heart surgery for mitral valve disease. Am J Cardiol 37:201–209, 1976.
6. Ascione R, Lloyd CT, Underwood MJ, et al: Inflammatory response after coronary revascularization with or without cardiopulmonary bypass. Ann Thorac Surg 69:1198–1204, 2000.
7. Asmundsson T, Kilburn KH: Survival after acute respiratory failure. 145 patients observed 5 to 8 and one-half years. Ann Intern Med 80:54–57, 1974.
8. Astiz ME, Rackow EC, Kaufman B, et al: Relationship of oxygen delivery and mixed venous oxygenation to lactic acidosis in patients with sepsis and acute myocardial infarction. Crit Care Med 16:655–658, 1988.
9. Bachmann F, McKenna R, Cole ER, et al: The hemostatic mechanism after open-heart surgery. I. Studies on plasma coagulation factors and fibrinolysis in 512 patients after extracorporeal circulation. J Thorac Cardiovasc Surg 70:76–85, 1975.
10. Bagge L, Lilienberg G, Nystrom SO, et al: Coagulation, fibrinolysis and bleeding after open-heart surgery. Scand J Thorac Cardiovasc Surg 20:151–160, 1986.
11. Bixler TJ, Gardner TJ, Donahoo JS, et al: Improved myocardial performance in postoperative cardiac surgical patients with sodium nitroprusside. Ann Thorac Surg 25:444–448, 1978.
12. Blood Component Therapy: A Physician's Handbook, 3rd ed. Washington, D.C., 1981.
13. Bolanowski PJ, Bauer J, Machiedo G, et al: Prostaglandin influence on pulmonary intravascular leukocytic aggregation during cardiopulmonary bypass. J Thorac Cardiovasc Surg 73:221–224, 1977.
14. Boldt J, Knothe C, Zickmann B, et al: Platelet function in cardiac surgery: influence of temperature and aprotinin. Ann Thorac Surg 55:652–658, 1993.
15. Bolen JL, Alderman EL: Hemodynamic consequences of afterload reduction in patients with chronic aortic regurgitation. Circulation 53:879–883, 1976.
16. Bortolotti U, Livi U, Frugoni C, et al: Delayed cardiac tamponade following open heart surgery. Analysis of 12 patients. Thorac Cardiovasc Surg 29:233–236, 1981.
17. Boyd AD, Tremblay RE, Spencer FC, et al: Estimation of cardiac output soon after intracardiac surgery with cardiopulmonary bypass. Ann Surg 150:613, 1959.
18. Breyer RH, Mills SA, Hudspeth AS, et al: A prospective study of sternal wound complications. Ann Thorac Surg 37:412–416, 1984.
19. Bristow MR, Ginsburg R, Minobe W, et al: Decreased catecholamine sensitivity and beta-adrenergic-receptor density in failing human hearts. N Engl J Med 307:205–211, 1982.
20. Broder G, Weil MH: Excess lactate: an index of reversibility of shock in human patients. Science 143:1457, 1964.
21. Brooker RF, Brown WR, Moody DM, et al: Cardiotomy suction: a major source of brain lipid emboli during cardiopulmonary bypass. Ann Thorac Surg 65:1651–1655, 1998.
22. Brown WR, Moody DM, Challa VR, et al: Histologic studies of brain microemboli in humans and dogs after cardiopulmonary bypass. Echocardiography 13:559–566, 1996.
23. Bryan-Brown CW: Blood flow to organs: parameters for function and survival in critical illness. Crit Care Med 16:170–178, 1988.
24. Bull BS, Huse WM, Brauer FS, et al: Heparin therapy during extracorporeal circulation. II. The use of a dose response curve to individualize heparin and protamine dosage. J Thorac Cardiovasc Surg 69:685–689, 1975.
25. Butler J, Parker D, Pillai R, et al: Effect of cardiopulmonary bypass on systemic release of neutrophil elastase and tumor necrosis factor. J Thorac Cardiovasc Surg 105:25–30, 1993.
26. Cardiovascular Drug Therapy. Chicago: Year Book Medical Publishers, 1986.
27. Chatterjee K, Parmley WW, Swan HJ, et al: Beneficial effects of vasodilator agents in severe mitral regurgitation due to dysfunction of subvalvar apparatus. Circulation 48:684–690, 1973.
28. Chenoweth DE, Cooper SW, Hugli TE, et al: Complement activation during cardiopulmonary bypass: evidence for generation of C3a and C5a anaphylatoxins. N Engl J Med 304:497–503, 1981.
29. Chesebro JH, Clements IP, Fuster V, et al: A platelet-inhibitor-drug trial in coronary-artery bypass operations: Benefit of perioperative dipyridamole and aspirin therapy on early postoperative vein-graft patency. N Engl J Med 307:73–78, 1982.
30. Chiara O, Giomarelli PP, Biagioli B, et al: Hypermetabolic response after hypothermic cardiopulmonary bypass. Crit Care Med 15:995–1000, 1987.
31. Chiariello M, Gold HK, Leinbach RC, et al: Comparison between the effects of nitroprusside and nitroglycerin on ischemic injury during acute myocardial infarction. Circulation 54:766–773, 1976.
32. Cohn JN, Archibald DG, Ziesche S, et al: Effect of vasodilator therapy on mortality in chronic congestive heart failure. Results of a Veterans Administration cooperative study. N Engl J Med 314:1547–1552, 1986.
33. Cohn JN, Johnson G, Ziesche S, et al: A comparison of enalapril with hydralazine-isosorbide dinitrate in the treatment of chronic congestive heart failure. N Engl J Med 325:303–310, 1991.
34. Cox JL: A perspective of postoperative atrial fibrillation in cardiac operations. Ann Thorac Surg 56:405–409, 1993.
35. Craddock DR, Logan A, Fadali A: Reoperation for haemorrhage following cardiopulmonary by-pass. Br J Surg 55:17–20, 1968.
36. Craddock PR, Fehr J, Dalmasso AP, et al: Hemodialysis leukopenia. Pulmonary vascular leukostasis resulting from complement activation by dialyzer cellophane membranes. J Clin Invest 59:879–888, 1977.
37. Creswell LL, Schuessler RB, Rosenbloom M, et al: Hazards of postoperative atrial arrhythmias. Ann Thorac Surg 56:539–549, 1993.
38. Crexells C, Chatterjee K, Forrester JS, et al: Optimal level of filling pressure in the left side of the heart in acute myocardial infarction. N Engl J Med 289:1263–1266, 1973.
39. Culliford AT, Girdwood RW, Isom OW, et al: Angina following myocardial revascularization. Does time of recurrence predict etiology and influence results of operation? J Thorac Cardiovasc Surg 77:889–895, 1979.
40. Czer LS, Shoemaker WC: Optimal hematocrit value in critically ill postoperative patients. Surg Gynecol Obstet 147:363–368, 1978.

41. Davies DW, Kadar D, Steward DJ, et al: A sudden death associated with the use of sodium nitroprusside for induction of hypotension during anaesthesia. Can Anaesth Soc J 22:547–552, 1975.

42. Davis R, Ribner HS, Keung E, et al: Treatment of chronic congestive heart failure with captopril, an oral inhibitor of angiotensin-converting enzyme. N Engl J Med 301:117–121, 1979.

43. de Smet AA, Joen MC, van Oeveren W, et al: Increased anticoagulation during cardiopulmonary bypass by aprotinin. J Thorac Cardiovasc Surg 1990;100:520–527.

44. DeLaria GA, Hunter JA, Goldin MD, et al: Leg wound complications associated with coronary revascularization. J Thorac Cardiovasc Surg 81:403–407, 1981.

45. Dinarello CA: Interleukin-1 and the pathogenesis of the acute-phase response. N Engl J Med 311:1413–1418, 1984.

46. DiSesa VJ: The rational selection of inotropic drugs in cardiac surgery. J Card Surg 2:385–406, 1987.

47. Ellis RJ, Mavroudis C, Gardner C, et al: Relationship between atrioventricular arrhythmias and the concentration of K+ ion in cardioplegic solution. J Thorac Cardiovasc Surg 80:517–526, 1980.

48. Ellison N, Beatty CP, Blake DR, et al: Heparin rebound. Studies in patients and volunteers. J Thorac Cardiovasc Surg 67:723–729, 1974.

49. Engelman RM, Spencer FC, Reed GE, et al: Cardiac tamponade following open-heart surgery. Circulation 41: II165–II171, 1970.

50. Engle MA, Ito T: The postcardiotomy syndrome. Am J Cardiol 7:73, 1961.

51. Engle MA, Zabriskie JB, Senterfit LB, et al: Immunologic and virologic studies in the postpericardiotomy syndrome. J Pediatr 87:1103–1108, 1975.

52. Erdmann E: The effectiveness of inotropic agents in isolated cardiac preparations from the human heart. Klin Wochenschr 66:1–6, 1988.

53. Estafanous FG, Tarazi RC, Buckley S, et al: Arterial hypertension in immediate postoperative period after valve replacement. Br Heart J 40:718–724, 1978.

54. Estafanous FG, Tarazi RC: Systemic arterial hypertension associated with cardiac surgery. Am J Cardiol 46:685–694, 1980.

55. Estes JW: Kinetics of the anticoagulant effect of heparin. JAMA 212:1492–1495, 1970.

56. Ferraris VA, Ferraris SP, Lough FC, et al: Preoperative aspirin ingestion increases operative blood loss after coronary artery bypass grafting. Ann Thorac Surg 45:71–74, 1988.

57. Fisch C, Knoebel SB, Feigenbaum H, et al: Potassium and the monophasic action potential, electrocardiogram, conduction and arrhythmias. Prog Cardiovasc Dis 8:387–418, 1966.

58. Ford EG, Baisden CE, Matteson ML, et al: Sepsis after coronary bypass grafting: evidence for loss of the gut mucosal barrier. Ann Thorac Surg 52:514–517, 1991.

59. Fouad FM, Estafanous FG, Bravo EL, et al: Possible role of cardioaortic reflexes in post coronary bypass hypertension. Am J Cardiol 44:866–872, 1979.

60. Fowler MB, Laser JA, Hopkins GL, et al: Assessment of the beta-adrenergic receptor pathway in the intact failing human heart: progressive receptor down-regulation and 3 subsensitivity to agonist response. Circulation 74:1290–1302, 1986.

61. Fowler NO, Gabel M, Buncher CR: Cardiac tamponade: a comparison of right versus left heart compression. J Am Coll Cardiol 12:187–193, 1988.

62. Frank SM, Higgins MS, Fleisher LA, et al: Adrenergic, respiratory, and cardiovascular effects of core cooling in humans. Am J Physiol 272:R557–R562, 1997.

63. Freeman R, McPeake PK: Acquisition, spread, and control of Pseudomonas aeruginosa in a cardiothoracic intensive care unit. Thorax 37:732–736, 1982.

64. Furnary AP, Magovern JA, Simpson KA, et al: Prolonged open sternotomy and delayed sternal closure after cardiac operations. Ann Thorac Surg 54:233–239, 1992.

65. Fyke FE, III, Tancredi RG, Shub C, et al: Detection of intrapericardial hematoma after open heart surgery: the roles of echocardiography and computed tomography. J Am Coll Cardiol 5:1496–1499, 1985.

66. Gaffney FA, Bastian BC, Thal ER, et al: Passive leg raising does not produce a significant or sustained autotransfusion effect. J Trauma 22:190–193, 1982.

67. Gall WE, Clarke WR, Doty DB: Vasomotor dynamics associated with cardiac operations. I. Venous tone and the effects of vasodilators. J Thorac Cardiovasc Surg 83:724–731, 1982.

68. Glaubiger G, Lefkowitz RJ: Elevated beta-adrenergic receptor number after chronic propranolol treatment. Biochem Biophys Res Commun 78:720–725, 1977.

69. Goldman S, Copeland J, Moritz T, et al: Improvement in early saphenous vein graft patency after coronary artery bypass surgery with antiplatelet therapy: results of a Veterans Administration cooperative study. Circulation 77:1324–1332, 1988.

70. Goldman S, Probst P, Selzer A, et al: Inefficacy of "therapeutic" serum levels of digoxin in controlling the ventricular rate in atrial fibrillation. Am J Cardiol 35:651–655, 1975.

71. Goldstein RE, Stinson EB, Scherer JL, et al: Intraoperative coronary collateral function in patients with coronary occlusive disease. Nitroglycerin responsiveness and angiographic correlations. Circulation 49:298–308, 1974.

72. Goodnough LT, Johnston MF, Ramsey G, et al: Guidelines for transfusion support in patients undergoing coronary artery bypass grafting. Transfusion Practices Committee of the American Association of Blood Banks. Ann Thorac Surg 50:675–683, 1990.

73. Goto H, Nonami R, Hamasaki Y: Effect of hypothermia on coagulation. Anesthesiology 63:A107, 1985.

74. Graham R Jr: The treatment of serious bacterial infections in the intensive care unit. In Shoemaker WC, Thompson WL, Holbrook PR, editors: Textbook of Critical Care. Philadelphia: W. B. Saunders, 1984.

75. Gu YJ, Mariani MA, van Oeveren W, et al: Reduction of the inflammatory response in patients undergoing minimally invasive coronary artery bypass grafting. Ann Thorac Surg 65:420–424, 1998.

76. Guidelines for transfusion for massive blood loss. A publication of the British Society for Haematology. British Committee for Standardization in Haematology Blood Transfusion Task Force. Clin Lab Haematol 10:265–273, 1988.

77. Guyton RA, Andrews MJ, Hickey PR, et al: The contribution of atrial contraction to right heart function before and after right ventriculotomy. Experimental and clinical observations. J Thorac Cardiovasc Surg 71:1–10, 1976.

78. Hanson EL, Kane PB, Askanazi J, et al: Comparison of patients with coronary artery or valve disease: intraoperative differences in blood volume and observations of vasomotor response. Ann Thorac Surg 22:343–346, 1976.

79. Hardesty RL, Thompson M, Lerberg DB, et al: Delayed postoperative cardiac tamponade: diagnosis and management. Ann Thorac Surg 26:155–164, 1978.

80. Harker LA: Bleeding after cardiopulmonary bypass. N Engl J Med 314:1446–1448, 1986.

81. Harris PD, Malm JR, Bowman FO Jr, et al: Epicardial pacing to control arrhythmias following cardiac surgery. Circulation 37:II178–II183, 1968.

82. Hart JC, Spooner TH, Pym J, et al: A review of 1,582 consecutive octopus off-pump coronary bypass patients. Ann Thorac Surg 70:1017–1020, 2000.

83. Hartzler GO, Maloney JD, Curtis JJ, et al: Hemodynamic benefits of atrioventricular sequential pacing after cardiac surgery. Am J Cardiol 40:232–236, 1977.

84. Hashimoto K, Ilstrup DM, Schaff HV: Influence of clinical and hemodynamic variables on risk of supraventricular tachycardia after coronary artery bypass. J Thorac Cardiovasc Surg 101:56–65, 1991.

85. Hattersley PG: Heparin anticoagulation. In Koepke JA, editor: Laboratory Hematology. New York: Churchill Livingstone, 1984.

86. Ho M: Nonbacterial infections in the ICU. In Shoemaker WC, Thompson WL, Holbrook PR, editors: Textbook of Critical Care. Philadelphia: W. B. Saunders, 1984.

87. Hodam RP, Starr A: Temporary postoperative epicardial pacing electrodes. Their value and management after open-heart surgery. Ann Thorac Surg 8:506–510, 1969.

88. Hoffman WS, Tomasello DN, MacVaugh H: Control of postcardiotomy bleeding with PEEP. Ann Thorac Surg 34:71–73, 1982.

89. Hood WB Jr: Role of converting enzyme inhibitors in the treatment of heart failure. J Am Coll Cardiol 22:154A–157A, 1993.

90. Horneffer PJ, Miller RH, Pearson TA, et al: The effective treatment of postpericardiotomy syndrome after cardiac operations. A randomized placebo-controlled trial. J Thorac Cardiovasc Surg 100:292–296, 1990.

91. Iberti TJ, Leibowitz AB, Papadakos PJ, et al: Low sensitivity of the anion gap as a screen to detect hyperlactatemia in critically ill patients. Crit Care Med 18:275–277, 1990.

92. Ilabaca PA, Ochsner JL, Mills NL: Positive end-expiratory pressure in the management of the patient with a postoperative bleeding heart. Ann Thorac Surg 30:281–284, 1980.

93. Ito T, Engle MA: Postcardiotomy syndrome following surgery for nonrheumatic heart disease. Circulation 17:549, 1958.

94. Jacobs MR: Diagnosis of infections. In Shoemaker WC, Thompson WL, Holbrook PR, editors: Textbook of Critical Care. Philadelphia: W. B. Saunders, 1984.

95. Jansen EW, Borst C, Lahpor JR, et al: Coronary artery bypass grafting without cardiopulmonary bypass using the octopus method: results in the first one hundred patients. J Thorac Cardiovasc Surg 116:60–67, 1998.

96. Jansen NJ, van Oeveren W, Gu YJ, et al: Endotoxin release and tumor necrosis factor formation during cardiopulmonary bypass. Ann Thorac Surg 54:744–747, 1992.

97. Jastrzebski J, Sykes MK, Woods DG: Cardiorespiratory effects of protamine after cardiopulmonary bypass in man. Thorax 29:534–538, 1974.

98. Jeevanandam V, Smith CR, Rose EA, et al: Single-stage management of sternal wound infections. J Thorac Cardiovasc Surg 99:256–262, 1990.

99. Johnson JA, Gall WE, Gundersen AE, et al: Delayed primary closure after sternal wound infection. Ann Thorac Surg 47:270–273, 1989.

100. Johnson RG, Thurer RL, Kruskall MS, et al: Comparison of two transfusion strategies after elective operations for myocardial revascularization. J Thorac Cardiovasc Surg 104:307–314, 1992.

101. Jurkiewicz MJ, Bostwick J III, Hester TR, et al: Infected median sternotomy wound. Successful treatment by muscle flaps. Ann Surg 191:738–744, 1980.

102. Kang YG, Martin DJ, Marquez J, et al: Intraoperative changes in blood coagulation and thrombelastographic monitoring in liver transplantation Anesth Analg 64:888–896, 1985.

103. Kincaid EH, Jones TJ, Stump DA, et al: Processing scavenged blood with a cell saver reduces cerebral lipid microembolization. Ann Thorac Surg 70:1296–1300, 2000.

104. Kirklin JK, Westaby S, Blackstone EH, et al: Complement and the damaging effects of cardiopulmonary bypass. J Thorac Cardiovasc Surg 86:845–857, 1983.

105. Kirklin JW, Archie JP Jr: The cardiovascular subsystem in surgical patients. Surg Gynecol Obstet 139:17–23, 1974.

106. Kirsh MM, McIntosh K, Kahn DR, Sloan H: Postpericardiotomy syndromes. Ann Thorac Surg 9:158–179, 1970.

107. Klausner JM, Morel N, Paterson IS, et al: The rapid induction by interleukin-2 of pulmonary microvascular permeability. Ann Surg 209:119–128, 1989.

108. Koepke JA, editor: Laboratory Hematology. New York: Churchill Livingstone, 1984.

109. Konstam MA, Kronenberg MW, Udelson JE, et al: Effect of acute angiotensin converting enzyme inhibition on left ventricular filling in patients with congestive heart failure. Relation to right ventricular volumes. Circulation 81:III115–III122, 1990.

110. Kosugi I, Tajimi K: Effects of dopamine and dobutamine on hemodynamics and plasma catecholamine levels during severe lactic acid acidosis. Circ Shock 17:95–102, 1985.

111. Krauss XH, Verdouw PD, Hughenholtz PG, et al: On-line monitoring of mixed venous oxygen saturation after cardiothoracic surgery. Thorax 30:636–643, 1975.

112. Kronzon I, Cohen ML, Winer HE: Diastolic atrial compression: a sensitive echocardiographic sign of cardiac tamponade. J Am Coll Cardiol 2:770–775, 1983.

113. Kshettry VR, Flavin TF, Emery RW, et al: Does multivessel, off-pump coronary artery bypass reduce postoperative morbidity? Ann Thorac Surg 69:1725–1730, 2000.

114. Kumon K, Tanaka K, Hirata T, et al: Organ failures due to low cardiac output syndrome following open heart surgery. Jpn Circ J 50:329–335, 1986.

115. Kyosola K, Mattila T, Harjula A, et al: Life-threatening complications of cardiac operations and occurrence of myocardial catecholamine bombs. J Thorac Cardiovasc Surg 95:334–339, 1988.

116. Lakin JD, Blocker TJ, Strong DM, et al: Anaphylaxis to protamine sulfate mediated by a complement-dependent IgG antibody. J Allergy Clin Immunol 61:102–107, 1978.

117. Landow L: Splanchnic lactate production in cardiac surgery patients. Crit Care Med 21:S84–S91, 1993.

118. Lassen NA. Brain: In Johnson PC, editor: Peripheral Circulation. New York: John Wiley & Sons, 1978.

119. Lauer MS, Eagle KA, Buckley MJ, et al: Atrial fibrillation following coronary artery bypass surgery. Prog Cardiovasc Dis 31:367–378, 1989.

120. Lazenby WD, Russo I, Zadeh BJ, et al: Treatment with desmopressin acetate in routine coronary artery bypass surgery to improve postoperative hemostasis. Circulation 82:IV413–IV419, 1990.

121. Lee TH, Salomon DR, Rayment CM, et al: Hypotension and sinus arrest with exercise-induced hyperkalemia and combined verapamil/propranolol therapy. Am J Med 80:1203–1204, 1986.

122. Lefkowitz RJ: Direct binding studies of adrenergic receptors: biochemical, physiologic, and clinical implications. Ann Intern Med 91:450–458, 1979.

123. Linden CH, Aghababian RV: Further uses of glucagon. Crit Care Med 13:248, 1985.

124. Lister JW, Cohen LS, Bernstein WH, et al: Treatment of supraventricular tachycardias by rapid atrial stimulation. Circulation 38:1044–1059, 1968.

125. Livelli FD, Jr, Johnson RA, McEnany MT, et al: Unexplained in-hospital fever following cardiac surgery. Natural history, relationship to postpericardiotomy syndrome, and a prospective study of therapy with indomethacin versus placebo. Circulation 57:968–975, 1978.

126. Loop FD, Lytle BW, Cosgrove DM, et al: J. Maxwell Chamberlain memorial paper. Sternal wound complications

after isolated coronary artery bypass grafting: early and late mortality, morbidity, and cost of care. Ann Thorac Surg 49: 179–186, 1990.

127. Lorenz RL, Schacky CV, Weber M, et al: Improved aorto-coronary bypass patency by low-dose aspirin (100 mg daily). Effects on platelet aggregation and thromboxane formation. Lancet 1:1261–1264, 1984.

128. Lotvin A, Gorlin R: Converting enzyme inhibitors. ACC Current J Rev May/June 1993.

129. Luz PL, Forrester JS, Wyatt HL, et al: Hemodynamic and metabolic effects of sodium nitroprusside on the performance and metabolism of regional ischemic myocardium. Circulation 52:400–407, 1975.

130. MacGregor RR, Spagnuolo PJ, Lentnek AL: Inhibition of granulocyte adherence by ethanol, prednisone, and aspirin, measured with an assay system. N Engl J Med 291:642–646, 1974.

131. Mack MJ: Coronary surgery: off-pump and port access. Surg Clin North Am 80:1575–1591, 2000.

132. Manolis AS, Estes NA III: Supraventricular tachycardia. Mechanisms and therapy. Arch Intern Med 147:1706–1716, 1987.

133. Marcus ML, Harrison DG, Chilian WM, et al: Alterations in the coronary circulation in hypertrophied ventricles. Circulation 75:119–125, 1987.

134. Markewitz A, Faist E, Lang S, et al: Successful restoration of cell-mediated immune response after cardiopulmonary bypass by immunomodulation. J Thorac Cardiovasc Surg 105:15–24, 1993.

135. Marshall JC, Christou NV, Horn R, et al: The microbiology of multiple organ failure. The proximal gastrointestinal tract as an occult reservoir of pathogens. Arch Surg 123:309–315, 1988.

136. Massie B, Ports T, Chatterjee K, et al: Long-term vasodilator therapy for heart failure: clinical response and its relationship to hemodynamic measurements. Circulation 63:269–278, 1981.

137. Massie BM, Conway M: Survival of patients with congestive heart failure: past, present, and future prospects. Circulation 75:IV11–IV19, 1987.

138. McCord JM, Wong K, Stokes SH, et al: Superoxide and inflammation: a mechanism for the anti-inflammatory activity of superoxide dismutase. Acta Physiol Scand Suppl 492:25–30, 1980.

139. Mellander S, Johansson B: Control of resistance, exchange, and capacitance functions in the peripheral circulation. Pharmacol Rev 20:117–196, 1968.

140. Michenfelder JD, Tinker JH: Cyanide toxicity and thiosulfate protection during chronic administration of sodium nitroprusside in the dog: correlation with a human case. Anesthesiology 47:441–448, 1977.

141. Milam JD: Blood transfusion in heart surgery. Surg Clin North Am 63:1127–1147, 1983.

142. Mills NL, Ochsner JL: Experience with atrial pacemaker wires implanted during cardiac operations. J Thorac Cardiovasc Surg 66:878–886, 1973.

143. Mills SA, Poole GV Jr, Breyer RH, et al: Digoxin and propranolol in the prophylaxis of dysrhythmias after coronary artery bypass grafting. Circulation 68:II222–II225, 1983.

144. Miranda DR, Stoutenbeek C, Karliczek G, et al: Effects of dexamethason on the early postoperative course after coronary artery bypass surgery. Thorac Cardiovasc Surg 30:21–27, 1982.

145. Mizock BA, Falk JL: Lactic acidosis in critical illness. Crit Care Med 20:80–93, 1992.

146. Moody DM, Bell MA, Challa VR, et al: Brain microemboli during cardiac surgery or aortography. Ann Neurol 28:477–486, 1990.

147. Moody DM, Brown WR, Challa VR, et al: Brain microemboli associated with cardiopulmonary bypass: a histologic and magnetic resonance imaging study. Ann Thorac Surg 59:1304–1307, 1995.

148. Moore FD Jr, Warner KG, Assousa S, et al: The effects of complement activation during cardiopulmonary bypass. Attenuation by hypothermia, heparin, and hemodilution. Ann Surg 208:95–103, 1988.

149. Nayler WG, Szeto J: Effect of verapamil on contractility, oxygen utilization, and calcium exchangeability in mammalian heart muscle. Cardiovasc Res 6:120–128, 1972.

150. Nelson RM, Jenson CB, Smoot WM III: Pericardial tamponade following open-heart surgery. J Thorac Cardiovasc Surg 58:510–516, 1969.

151. Newman MF, Kirchner JL, Phillips-Bute B, et al: Longitudinal assessment of neurocognitive function after coronary-artery bypass surgery. N Engl J Med 344:395–402, 2001.

152. Norwood S, Ruby A, Civetta J, et al: Catheter-related infections and associated septicemia. Chest 99:968–975, 1991.

153. Norwood SH, Cormier B, McMahon NG, et al: Prospective study of catheter-related infection during prolonged arterial catheterization. Crit Care Med 16:836–839, 1988.

154. Olinger GN, Werner PH, Bonchek LI, et al: Vasodilator effects of the sodium acetate in pooled protein fraction. Ann Surg 190:305–311, 1979.

155. Ottino G, De Paulis R, Pansini S, et al: Major sternal wound infection after open-heart surgery: a multivariate analysis of risk factors in 2,579 consecutive operative procedures. Ann Thorac Surg 44:173–179, 1987.

156. Packer M, Kessler PD, Lee WH: Calcium-channel blockade in the management of severe chronic congestive heart failure: a bridge too far. Circulation 75:V56–V64, 1987.

157. Packer M: Neurohormonal interactions and adaptations in congestive heart failure. Circulation 77:721–730, 1988.

158. Page PL, Plumb VJ, Okumura K, et al: A new animal model of atrial flutter. J Am Coll Cardiol 8:872–879, 1986.

159. Perkins CM: Serious verapamil poisoning: treatment with intravenous calcium gluconate. Br Med J 2:1127, 1978.

160. Pien F, Ho PW, Fergusson DJ: Fever and infection after cardiac operation. Ann Thorac Surg 33:382–384, 1982.

161. Pitt B: Use of converting enzyme inhibitors in patients with asymptomatic left ventricular dysfunction. J Am Coll Cardiol 22:158A–161A, 1993.

162. Plumb VJ, Karp RB, Kouchoukos NT, et al: Verapamil therapy of atrial fibrillation and atrial flutter following cardiac operation. J Thorac Cardiovasc Surg 83:590–596, 1982.

163. Podrid PJ: Antiarrhythmic Management: Therapeutic Considerations. A Monograph. Health Care Communications, Inc., 1992.

164. Puskas JD, Wright CE, Ronson RS, et al: Clinical outcomes and angiographic patency in 125 consecutive off-pump coronary artery bypass patients. Heart Surgery Forum 2:216–221, 1999.

165. Ram CVS: Hypertensive emergencies. In Shoemaker WC, Thompson WL, Holbrook PR, editors: Textbook of Critical Care. Philadelphia: W. B. Saunders, 1984.

166. Rashkin MC, Bosken C, Baughman RP: Oxygen delivery in critically ill patients. Relationship to blood lactate and survival. Chest 87:580–584, 1985.

167. Redwood DR, Smith ER, Epstein SE: Coronary artery occlusion in the conscious dog. Effects of alterations in heart rate and arterial pressure on the degree of myocardial ischemia. Circulation 46:323–332, 1972.

168. Reeves JT, Grover RF, Filley GF, et al: Cardiac output in normal resting man. J Appl Physiol 16:276, 1961.

169. Ricci M, Karamanoukian HL, Abraham R, et al: Stroke in octogenarians undergoing coronary artery surgery with and without cardiopulmonary bypass. Ann Thorac Surg 69: 1471–1475.

170. Rifkin RD, Pandiah NE, Funai JT: Sensitivity of right atrial collapse and right ventricular diastolic collapse in the diagnosis of graded cardiac tamponade. Am J Noninvasive Cardiol 1:73, 1987.

171. Rodriguez JL, Weissman C, Damask MC, et al: Physiologic requirements during rewarming: suppression of the shivering response. Crit Care Med 11:490–497, 1983.

172. Rohrer MJ, Natale AM: Effect of hypothermia on the coagulation cascade. Crit Care Med 20:1402–1405, 1992.

173. Rubin DA, Nieminski KE, Reed GE, et al: Predictors, prevention, and long-term prognosis of atrial fibrillation after coronary artery bypass graft operations. J Thorac Cardiovasc Surg 94:331–335, 1987.

174. Russo AM, O'Connor WH, Waxman HL: Atypical presentations and echocardiographic findings in patients with cardiac tamponade occurring early and late after cardiac surgery. Chest 104:71–78, 1993.

175. Sanfelippo PM, Danielson GK: Complications associated with median sternotomy. J Thorac Cardiovasc Surg 63:419–423, 1972.

176. Sarr MG, Gott VL, Townsend TR: Mediastinal infection after cardiac surgery. Ann Thorac Surg 38:415–423, 1984.

177. Serry C, Bleck PC, Javid H, et al: Sternal wound complications. Management and results. J Thorac Cardiovasc Surg 80: 861–867, 1980.

178. Sethi GK, Copeland JG, Goldman S, et al: Implications of preoperative administration of aspirin in patients undergoing coronary artery bypass grafting. Department of Veterans Affairs Cooperative Study on Antiplatelet Therapy. J Am Coll Cardiol 15:15–20, 1990.

179. Shabetai R: Changing concepts of cardiac tamponade. J Am Coll Cardiol 12:194–195, 1988.

180. Shabetai R: Pericardial and cardiac pressure. Circulation 77: 1–5, 1988.

181. Shafir R, Weiss J, Herman O, et al: Faulty sternotomy and complications after median sternotomy. J Thorac Cardiovasc Surg 96:310–313, 1988.

182. Shibutani K, Komatsu T, Kubal K, et al: Critical level of oxygen delivery in anesthetized man. Crit Care Med 11:640–643, 1983.

183. Silverman NA, DuBrow I, Kohler J, et al: Etiology of atrioventricular-conduction abnormalities following cardiac surgery. J Surg Res 36:198–204, 1984.

184. Silverman NA, Wright R, Levitsky S: Efficacy of low-dose propranolol in preventing postoperative supraventricular tachyarrhythmias: a prospective, randomized study. Ann Surg 196:194–197, 1982.

185. Simpson MB Jr: Adverse reactions to transfusion therapy: clinical and laboratory aspects. In Koepke JA, editor: Laboratory Hematology. New York: Churchill Livingstone, 1984.

186. Singh BN, Nademanee K: Use of calcium antagonists for cardiac arrhythmias. Am J Cardiol 59:153B–162B, 1987.

187. Singh BN: A fourth class of anti-dysrhythmic action? Effect of verapamil on ouabain toxicity, on atrial and ventricular intracellular potentials, and on other features of cardiac function. Cardiovasc Res 6:109–119, 1972.

188. Singh S, Wann LS, Schuchard GH, et al: Right ventricular and right atrial collapse in patients with cardiac tamponade—a combined echocardiographic and hemodynamic study. Circulation 70:966–971, 1984.

189. Skinner NS Jr, Mitchell JH, Wallace AG, et al: Hemodynamic effects of altering the time of atrial systole. Am J Physiol 205:499, 1963.

190. Sladen RN, Rosenthal MH: Specific afterload reduction with parenteral hydralazine following cardiac surgery. J Thorac Cardiovasc Surg 78:195–202, 1979.

191. Smith PK, Buhrman WC, Ferguson TB Jr, et al: Conduction block after cardioplegic arrest: prevention by augmented atrial hypothermia. Circulation 68:II41–II48, 1983.

192. Smith PK, Muhlbaier LH: Aprotinin: safe and effective only with the full-dose regimen. Ann Thorac Surg 62:1575–1577, 1996.

193. Smith PK, Tyson GS Jr, Hammon JW Jr, et al: Cardiovascular effects of ventilation with positive expiratory airway pressure. Ann Surg 195:121–130, 1982.

194. Spiess BD, Tuman KJ, McCarthy RJ, et al: Thromboelastography as an indicator of postcardiopulmonary bypass coagulopathies. J Clin Monit 3:25–30, 1987.

195. St John SM, Pfeffer MA, Plappert T, et al: Quantitative two-dimensional echocardiographic measurements are major predictors of adverse cardiovascular events after acute myocardial infarction. The protective effects of captopril. Circulation 89:68–75, 1994.

196. Stinson EB, Holloway EL, Derby G, et al: Comparative hemodynamic responses to chlorpromazine, nitroprusside, nitroglycerin, and trimethaphan immediately after open-heart operations. Circulation 52:126–133, 1975.

197. Stoney WS, Alford WC Jr, Burrus GR, et al: Median sternotomy dehiscence. Ann Thorac Surg 26:421–426, 1978.

198. Stoutenbeek CP, van Saene HK, Miranda DR, et al: The effect of selective decontamination of the digestive tract on colonisation and infection rate in multiple trauma patients. Intensive Care Med 10:185–192, 1984.

199. Strandgaard S, Olesen J, Skinhoj E, et al: Autoregulation of brain circulation in severe arterial hypertension. Br Med J 1:507–510, 1973.

200. Stump DA, Rorie KD, Jones TJ: Does off-pump coronary artery bypass surgery reduce the risk of brain injury? Heart Surg Forum 4(Suppl. 1):S14–S18, 2001.

201. Swan HJ, Forrester JS, Diamond G, et al: Hemodynamic spectrum of myocardial infarction and cardiogenic shock. A conceptual model. Circulation 45:1097–1110, 1972.

202. Sylivris S, Levi C, Matalanis G, et al: Pattern and significance of cerebral microemboli during coronary artery bypass grafting. Ann Thorac Surg 66:1674–1678, 1998.

203. Taggart DP, Siddiqui A, Wheatley DJ: Low-dose preoperative aspirin therapy, postoperative blood loss, and transfusion requirements. Ann Thorac Surg 50:424–428, 1990.

204. Tajimi K, Kosugi I, Hamamoto F, et al: Plasma catecholamine levels and hemodynamic responses of severely acidotic dogs to dopamine infusion. Crit Care Med 11:817–819, 1983.

205. Taylor KM, Brannan JJ, Bain WH, et al: Role of angiotensin II in the development of peripheral vasoconstriction during cardiopulmonary bypass. Cardiovasc Res 13:269–273, 1979.

206. Taylor KM, Morton IJ, Brown JJ, et al: Hypertension and the renin-angiotensin system following open-heart surgery. J Thorac Cardiovasc Surg 74:840–845, 1977.

207. Thurer RJ, Bognolo D, Vargas A, et al: The management of mediastinal infection following cardiac surgery. An experience utilizing continuous irrigation with povidone-iodine. J Thorac Cardiovasc Surg 68:962–968, 1974.

208. Tyberg JV, Taichman GC, Smith ER, et al: The relationship between pericardial pressure and right atrial pressure: an intraoperative study. Circulation 73:428–432, 1986.

209. Ulicny KS Jr, Hiratzka LF: The risk factors of median sternotomy infection: a current review. J Card Surg 6:338–351, 1991.

210. van de Watering LM, Hermans J, Houbiers JG, et al: Beneficial effects of leukocyte depletion of transfused blood on postoperative complications in patients undergoing cardiac surgery: a randomized clinical trial. Circulation 97:562–568, 1998.

211. van Oeveren W, Harder MP, Roozendaal KJ, et al: Aprotinin protects platelets against the initial effect of cardiopulmonary bypass. J Thorac Cardiovasc Surg 99:788–796, 1990.

212. Van Trigt P, Spray TL, Pasque MK, et al: The influence of time on the response to dopamine after coronary artery bypass

grafting: assessment of left ventricular performance and contractility using pressure/dimension analyses. Ann Thorac Surg 35:3–13, 1983.

213. Vaughn S, Puri VK: Cardiac output changes and continuous mixed venous oxygen saturation measurement in the critically ill. Crit Care Med 16:495–498, 1988.

214. Vernon DD, Garrett JS, Banner W Jr, et al: Hemodynamic effects of dobutamine in an intact animal model. Crit Care Med 20:1322–1329, 1992.

215. Videm V, Fosse E, Mollnes TE, et al: Time for new concepts about measurement of complement activation by cardiopulmonary bypass? Ann Thorac Surg 54:725–731, 1992.

216. Wade OL, Bishop JM: Cardiac Output in Regional Blood Flow. Oxford: Blackwell Scientific Publications, 1962.

217. Waldo AL, MacLean WA, Karp RB, et al: Entrainment and interruption of atrial flutter with atrial pacing: studies in man following open heart surgery. Circulation 56:737–745, 1977.

218. Walls JT, Curtis JJ, Silver D, et al: Heparin-induced thrombocytopenia in open heart surgical patients: sequelae of late recognition. Ann Thorac Surg 53:787–791, 1992.

219. Watanabe T, Covell JW, Maroko PR, et al: Effects of increased arterial pressure and positive inotropic agents on the severity of myocardial ischemia in the acutely depressed heart. Am J Cardiol 30:371–377, 1972.

220. Weeks KR, Chatterjee K, Block S, et al: Bedside hemodynamic monitoring. Its value in the diagnosis of tamponade complicating cardiac surgery. J Thorac Cardiovasc Surg 71:250–252, 1976.

221. Weil MH, Afifi AA: Experimental and clinical studies on lactate and pyruvate as indicators of the severity of acute circulatory failure (shock). Circulation 41:989–1001, 1970.

222. Weinstein GS, Zabetakis PM, Clavel A, et al: The renin-angiotensin system is not responsible for hypertension following coronary artery bypass grafting. Ann Thorac Surg 43:74–77, 1987.

223. Wellens HJ: Atrial flutter: progress, but no final answer. J Am Coll Cardiol 17:1235–1236, 1991.

224. Westaby S: Organ dysfunction after cardiopulmonary bypass. A systemic inflammatory reaction initiated by the extracorporeal circuit. Intensive Care Med 13:89–95, 1987.

225. Whelton PK, Flaherty JT, MacAllister NP, et al: Hypertension following coronary artery bypass surgery. Role of preoperative propranolol therapy. Hypertension 2: 291–298, 1980.

226. Williams TW Jr: The staphyloccoccus: A reemerging problem in prosthetic surgery. Contemp Surg 32:15, 1988.

227. Wilson RF, Walt AF: Blood replacement. In Walt AF, Wilson RF, editors: Management of Trauma: Practices and Pitfalls. Philadelphia: Lea & Febiger, 1975.

228. Wolfe JH, Waller DG, Chapman MB, et al: The effect of hemodilution upon patients with intermittent claudication. Surg Gynecol Obstet 160:347–351, 1985.

229. Wormser GP, Onorato IM, Preminger TJ, et al: Sensitivity and specificity of blood cultures obtained through intravascular catheters. Crit Care Med 18:152–156, 1990.

230. Zelis R, Mansour EJ, Capone RJ, et al: The cardiovascular effects of morphine. The peripheral capacitance and resistance vessels in human subjects. J Clin Invest 54:1247–1258, 1974.

231. Zoll PM: Resuscitation of the heart in ventricular standstill by external electric stimulation. N Engl J Med 247:768, 1952.

232. Zurick AM, Urzua J, Ghattas M, et al: Failure of positive end-expiratory pressure to decrease postoperative bleeding after cardiac surgery. Ann Thorac Surg 34:608–611, 1982.

233. Zwischenberger JB, Kirsh MM, Dechert RE, et al: Suppression of shivering decreases oxygen consumption and improves hemodynamic stability during postoperative rewarming. Ann Thorac Surg 43:428–431, 1987.

Cardiopulmonary Bypass: Technique and Pathophysiology

Fraser D. Rubens

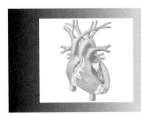

CHAPTER 65

▶ INTRODUCTION: THE HISTORY OF CARDIOPULMONARY BYPASS

Cardiopulmonary bypass (CPB) represents one of the most important biomedical inventions in the history of health care, rivaling the development of roentgenography and hemodialysis in its clinical impact. The scope of its application is far reaching as its birth paralleled the evolution of an entire surgical subspecialty, and without its use, surgeons would be cowered by the overwhelming prospect of cardiac repair. The recent surge in off-pump coronary artery bypass grafting has perhaps slowed the interest in research related to CPB, but this trend leaves us subject to stagnancy at a time when the acuity of accepted patients is greater than ever. In many practices, complex multiple arterial reconstruction and minimal access surgery, such as with minithoracotomy mitral valve surgery, are more comfortably approached with guaranteed accuracy using longer periods of CPB and availing the excellent results of modern myocardial protection. Therefore, now more than ever, it is essential to be able to characterize the impact of CPB on our patients. Further, the surgeon has to continue to play a key role in this technology with a comprehensive understanding of all aspects of CPB from the physiology of gas exchange to the molecular mechanisms characteristic of biocompatibility.

The evolution of CPB represents a paradigm of the surgical maxim of ingenuity bred of necessity. There were essential parallel discoveries that contributed to the feasibility of extracorporeal circulation, probably the most important of which was the discovery and isolation of the natural

1062 anticoagulant heparin. But above all, humanity required a "receptive and talented surgeon with foresight . . . who could envision an intact surviving patient beyond the isolated organ studies."[38] It is appropriate that the year of this publication coincides with the fiftieth anniversary of the monumental achievements of perhaps the key "receptive and talented surgeon": Dr. John H. Gibbon, Jr. (Figure 65-1). The Gibbons-IBM oxygenator, although a far-cry from the current reliable circuits used on thousands of patients daily around the world, was successfully used on May 6, 1953, to correct an atrial septal defect. Although initially successful, three subsequent attempts at intracardiac repair resulted in fatalities that led to a self-imposed moratorium on its clinical use. Nevertheless, the door had been opened and the feasibility of this approach had been demonstrated, providing the impetus and encouragement to other key players in the field.

The first clinically successful film and bubble oxygenators brought blood in direct contact to equilibrate with respiratory gases. Complications related to blood trauma eventually led to a decline in their popularity such that they are rarely if ever used today. Membrane oxygenators were introduced in the 1950s following the initial observation by Kolff and Berk[79] that venous blood was oxygenated while flowing through a cellophane dialysis tube in contact with O_2-containing dialysate. The first membranes were relatively impermeable to gases, requiring huge surface areas and massive priming volumes. Formed of silicone rubber, they were designed either in an extraluminal format (blood flowing on the outside of the tube with gas on the inside) or the less popular intraluminal format (reverse). The refinements since that time have been subtle but significant, such that we now have oxygenators with

surface areas as low as 2.0 m². The resulting minimization of prime volume has contributed more than any other factor to blood conservation practices in modern cardiac surgery.

Device Overview (Figure 65-2)

Gravity drainage usually allows for the collection of blood from the venous circulation into the venous reservoir. Through separate inflows on the reservoir, blood can also be returned from the pericardial well (cardiotomy blood) and from cardiac and aortic vents. A centrifugal or roller pump is used to divert the venous reservoir blood to the oxygenator. After the blood passes through the integrated heat exchanger/oxygenator, it is circulated through an arterial filter and bubble trap and returned to the patient through the arterial cannula. Cardioplegia setups are often intimately incorporated into the CPB circuit.

TECHNICAL ASPECTS OF CARDIOPULMONARY BYPASS

Principles of Current Oxygenator Design and Function

Diffusion of gases at the blood–membrane interface can be predicted partially by Fick's law, whereby the rate of diffusion is proportional to the partial pressure gradient of the gas in the direction of diffusion. The rate of gas transfer is also inversely proportional to the distance through which a gas must pass (the thickness of the membrane) and it depends on the property of *diffusivity* of the membrane biomaterial. Currently used membranes are very permeable to O_2; however, they are often less permeable to CO_2. The problem of poor diffusion of CO_2 was solved by the introduction of microporous membranes. These surfaces allow transient direct blood–gas interfacing at pore structures smaller than blood cells; however, the hydrophobic nature of the membrane results in changes in blood surface tension, blocking direct contact between the two phases. As a result, the interface in microporous membranes behaves as a very thin stagnant film of plasma water that offers little resistance to gas exchange. Progressive protein accretion at the pores occurs over time resulting in a finite functional capacity, detected by worsening efficiency in gas transfer, thus explaining why oxygenators must be replaced with long CPB runs.

As opposed to the relatively facile transfer of O_2 through the membrane, in plasma or blood the diffusivity for O_2 is 25 times less than that of CO_2. Two modifications have been introduced to overcome this problem. First, the path length (the distance the blood travels past the gas exchange surface) has been maximized. This modification is limited by the parallel need to increase the priming volume. Second, disturbed flow patterns are used to promote mixing and to bring deoxygenated blood closer to the exchange surface. Mechanisms that interfere with the development of fully developed flow patterns enhance diffusion by keeping the boundary layer narrow. In an oxygenator, this can be accomplished by making the surface irregular or by positioning elements within the flow stream to disrupt smooth flow and to enhance mixing, thus the rationale for the common extraluminal hollow fiber design.

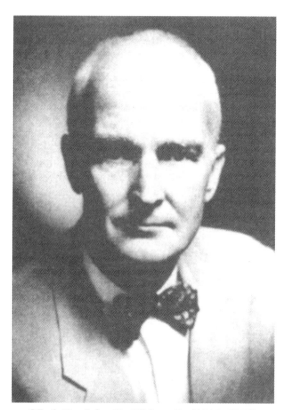

Figure 65–1 Dr. John H. Gibbon, Jr. (1903–1973).

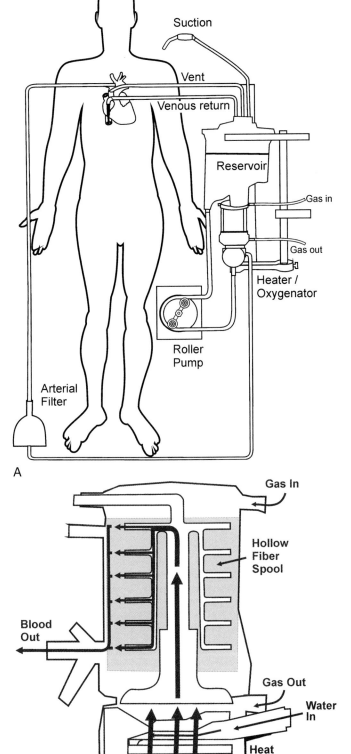

A

B

Figure 65–2 A, Overview of the cardiopulmonary bypass circuit. **B,** Illustration of a typical integrated heat exchanger/membrane oxygenator.

Hypothermia and Acid–Base Balance

The feasibility and applicability of hypothermia for heart surgery were first suggested by Bigelow et al in 1950[14] after demonstrating the safety benefit of hypothermia as a means to decrease O_2 consumption during inflow occlusion in an animal model. O_2 consumption decreases by 50% for every 10°C drop in temperature (Figure 65-3). Lower flows decrease collateral flow and rewarming of the heart from contact with adjacent tissues, and they provide a margin of safety if equipment fails.

Hypothermia is associated with marked changes in blood pH and Pco_2 levels. With a rise in temperature, CO_2 becomes less soluble in blood and there is a greater tendency for the dissolved CO_2 to come out of solution (increased gaseous phase). Conversely, CO_2 solubility increases with decreasing temperature. When blood from a hypothermic patient (e.g., 24° C) is introduced into a CO_2 electrode for measurement, it is first warmed to 37° C (increasing the amount of CO_2 in the gaseous phase), and therefore the measured partial pressure of CO_2 will be higher than it was in reality at the cooler temperature. The Pco_2 therefore must be corrected based on a calculated decrease of 4.5%/°C. Conversely, the pH increases 0.015 U/°C drop in temperature. This shift in pH is partially related to the influence of buffers such as the imidazole moiety of histidine, but it is also related to the dynamics of the Henderson–Hasselbalch equation $pH = p\acute{K} + [HCO_3^-]/(0.03 \times Pco_2)$.

As it is known that alkalosis and hypocarbia are triggers to decrease cerebral blood flow (CBF) some investigators have suggested the addition of CO_2 during hypothermia to compensate for this and to keep the pH unchanged (pH stat strategy). The landmark paper by Murkin et al in 1987[105] confirmed that pH stat management results in greater CBF to cerebral metabolic rate ($CMRO_2$) ratio as compared to alpha-stat management (no active correction of pH with hypothermia).[105] Most agree that a pH stat strategy is probably preferential in children where increased CBF does increase the rate of cooling and thus increases the chance of uniform achievement of cerebral hypothermia.[84] The rate of brain oxygen depletion during deep hypothermic circulatory arrest is also considerable slower with pH stat strategy. As a result, pH stat substantially prolongs the interval between

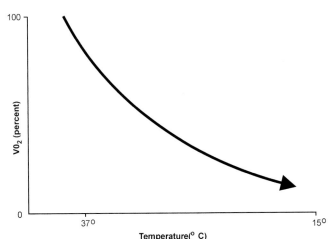

Figure 65–3 Illustration of the effect of hypothermia on oxygen consumption.

the onset of arrest and the exhaustion of brain oxygen stores and may be associated with better clinical outcomes in this group.[148]

In contrast, in adults, an alpha-stat strategy may provide the greatest cerebral protection during hypothermia on CPB. Alpha-stat management is certainly easier to accomplish and it is justified by the fact that most cellular mechanisms are capable of maintaining intracellular pH despite fluctuations in extracellular conditions. Because of the addition of excess CO_2 with a pH-stat strategy, there may be brain acidosis during rewarming, which combined with decreased O_2 delivery after CPB may augment central nervous system (CNS) injury in adults. Most importantly, as noted above, a pH-stat strategy results in excessive CBF, which may increase embolic load. Finally, pH-stat strategy is associated with a decreased ability to maintain autoregulation at low pressures. Three randomized controlled trials have demonstrated a small but ever-present benefit of alpha-stat strategy in terms of neurological and neurocognitive outcome in adults, especially in cases in which CPB time exceeded 90 mins.[106]

Hematocrit and Priming

The 1960s saw the introduction of crystalloid (D_5W) in prime as an alternative to routine whole blood prime. A parallel increase in efficiency of oxygenation and decreased end-organ complications were recognized with this approach.[25] Now hemodilution is commonly practiced in most cases of adult and pediatric cardiac surgery, with maintenance of the hematocrit (Hct) between 20 and 25% during CPB. Hemodilution has a major effect on blood viscosity primarily at the capillary level where the radius is small and the shear rate is low. Low flow at the capillary level increases viscosity of the blood, further increasing the resistance, but this effect is counterbalanced by the effect of hemodilution.

The drop in O_2 content at most levels of moderate hemodilution is more than compensated by augmented cardiac output (CO) such that total O_2 delivery (CO × O_2 content of blood) is increased, with an optimum Hct likely in the range of 30%. Hemodilution results in a significant increase in flow without a parallel increase in perfusion pressure. Hypothermia complicates the effects of hemodilution as the decreased temperature causes increased viscosity and also induces vasoconstriction.

The optimum Hct for CPB remains a topic of significant controversy. Several retrospective clinical trials have demonstrated acceptable clinical results with Hct as low as 13–14%.[26] A post hoc assessment of the impact of low Hct on admission to ICU in cardiac patients by Spiess et al[137] found an inverse correlation between admission Hct and the risk of Q-wave myocardial infarction (MI). On the other hand, studies have demonstrated that an Hct <20% may be associated with abnormal distribution of blood flow to organs and an Hct <15% may lead to maldistribution of coronary flow away from the subendocardium in the presence of residual coronary stenosis.[52] Two recent large retrospective observational studies of consecutive patients undergoing isolated coronary artery bypass grafting (CABG)[29,41] demonstrated that a lower minimum Hct was associated with a significant increase in hospital mortality. As excessive hemodilution also increases cerebral blood flow, it may cause a parallel increase in microembolization and thus may theoretically be a contributor to neurological damage after CPB.

Most centers prime the CPB circuit with a solution of balanced salt with or without the addition of a colloid solution such as pentastarch. Infants and children often need blood added directly to prime based upon the anticipated Hct after initiation of bypass (calculated from standard nomograms). Other additives to the prime may include calcium, mannitol, and pharmacological agents such as heparin and aprotinin. The minimum priming volume is mandated by the patient's circulating volume and the pump prime volume. Although averaging 1 liter, with experience, the prime volume can be as low as 200 ml in pediatric circuits.

Flow Rates, Perfusion Pressure, and Autoregulation

Flow is generally kept in the range of 2.2–2.5 liters/min/m² to provide a margin of safety during CPB as systemic blood flow distribution and O_2 consumption remain normal at this level. At normothermia, a target mean blood pressure of 50–70 mm Hg is generally used. The perfusionist can control the pressure by increasing or decreasing flow, or by the addition of vasoconstrictors or vasodilators (inhalational anesthetics). At lower temperatures, a mean pressure of 35 mm Hg is still generally accepted as safe, but there have been a number of investigators who have recommended greater vigilance to prevent any hypotension (<45–50 mm Hg) during CPB[48] although these findings are controversial.[122]

Despite the fact that it comprises only 2% of the body weight, the brain's metabolic needs demand 15% of the cardiac output, extracting as much as 25% of the delivered O_2. Temperature is the single most important element influencing CBF during CPB. As the temperature is dropped, the $CMRO_2$ decreases exponentially and the CBF decreases linearly (Figure 65-4). As a consequence, the ratio of CBF/$CMRO_2$ increases resulting in "luxuriant" flow, further facilitated by hemodilution.

Autoregulation of CBF is also related to changes in perfusion pressure. At normothermia, a mean pressure of 50 mm Hg is the threshold at which the brain autoregulates flow, but with hypothermia (26° C), the threshold drops to 30 mm Hg (Figure 65-5). At deep hypothermia (<20° C) there is a loss of pressure–flow autoregulation as severe temperature reductions impair cerebral vascular relaxation[28] and changes in cerebral perfusion pressure (CPP) result in corresponding proportional changes in CBF. Other factors that influence CBF and $CMRO_2$ include the blood viscosity, intracranial pressure and CVP, and the blood gas status (pH, $PaCO_2$, PaO_2). CBF varies linearly with the $PaCO_2$ in the range of 20–80 mm Hg whereas PaO_2 <50 causes cerebral vasodilation that overrides pressure–flow autoregulation.

Pumps for Cardiopulmonary Bypass

The two commonly utilized types of pumps for CPB involve roller and centrifugal fluid propulsion. Noninterrupted contact of the rollers with the tubing in the track results in the nonpulsatile nature of the flow (Figure 65-6). A low compression will result in inadequate flow, whereas excessive compression may aggravate hemolysis and tubing wear.

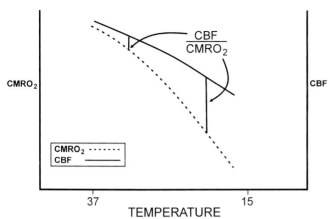

Figure 65–4 The effect of hypothermia on both CMRO$_2$ and CBF.

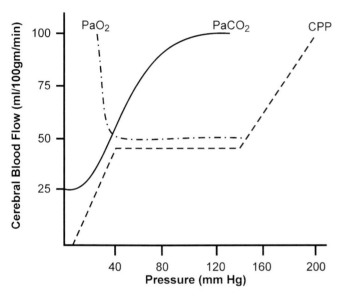

Figure 65–5 CBF is constant through autoregulation of cerebral perfusion pressure (CPP) from 40–140 mm Hg. Other factors that independently affect CBF include Paco$_2$ and Pao$_2$.
(Modified with permission from Kelly BJ, et al: Current concepts in cerebral protection. Chest 103:1246–1254, 1993. Copyright 1993, American College of Chest Physicians.)

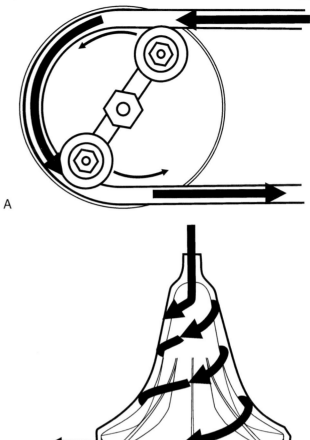

Figure 65–6 A, A double roller pump has rotating arms oriented at 180 degrees like spokes on a wheel. Spool-shaped rollers are located at the ends of the arms. A length of tubing is locked inside a curved track at the outer circumference of a partial circle of 210 degrees. **B,** A typical centrifugal pump has a cone-shaped outer housing with an upper inlet and a single lower outlet. The inner chamber contains spinning concentric smooth cones or fins mounted on a central impeller.

Other complications associated with the use of the roller pump include cavitation due to excess pressure and spallation (measure of the release of particles from the inner surface).

Centrifugal pumps have become a popular alternative to the roller pump, particularly in pediatric cardiac surgery and in cases with anticipated long CPB runs. The flow in a centrifugal pump is afterload dependent and it is not predictable based solely on the calculated rpm; thus an in-line flowmeter is essential. Theoretically, its use should result in less blood trauma, particularly with prolonged CPB, and it is for this reason that this device is preferred for extracorporeal membrane oxygenation (ECMO). This may be of benefit in children, where their use has been associated with decreased hemolysis, platelet activation, and inflammation and bleeding,[78] although these findings have not been reproduced by other investigators.[133] Aside from their expense ($150 per case), these devices are susceptible to air locks, thus requiring extreme vigilance by the perfusionist. On the other hand, this may be protective as there is less chance of pumping large volumes of air into the patient if there is an inadvertent leak; further the lines cannot be overpressurized with distal obstruction as with roller pumps. These devices are not valved and if rotation stops without clamping the outflow, rapid retrograde flow from the arterial line will occur within milliseconds, essentially exsanguinating the patient. Finally, unlike roller pumps that can be operated manually, a power outage with a centrifugal pump can be a disaster.

Cardiotomy

Cardiotomy blood refers to the extravascular blood collected within the thoracic wound during CPB. In general, blood from the wound cavity is aspirated through a sucker device and transferred to a cardiotomy reservoir. Because of

1066 the close proximity with tissue within the wound and the potential for particulate matter to be collected, a filter and a defoaming chamber are incorporated in the cardiotomy reservoir. Mechanical injury, such as hemolysis, may result from the air–blood interface at the sucker, as well as from the compressive effects of the roller pump. Other mechanical complications from cardiotomy suction include the formation of particulate emboli including fibrin, macroaggregates of denatured proteins and lipoproteins, fat globules, platelet and leukocyte aggregates, calcium, cellular debris, talc, and suture material. As a consequence, in some institutions cardiotomy blood is routinely processed through centrifugal washing or completely discarded, except in the case of emergency.

Cardiac Venting for Cardiopulmonary Bypass

Cardiac venting involves the active aspiration of blood from the heart to facilitate visualization by creating a bloodless field. Venting in some form is necessary in most cardiac operations involving CPB, primarily to aid visualization but also to avoid chamber distention. When the aorta is cross-clamped and the native coronary circulation is stopped, there remains a variable amount of noncoronary collateralization, particularly related to bronchial artery flow and return from the Thebesian veins. Blood flow can also occur through the heart during partial CPB because of continued transit of blood through the right heart, the lungs, and into the left heart. There are many potential sites for cardiac venting including the pulmonary artery, the superior pulmonary vein, the left atrium, the left ventricle, and most commonly through the ascending aorta.

Cannulation for Cardiopulmonary Bypass

Venous Cannulation

The principles of siphonage are used to generate the negative pressure necessary to draw blood from the venous circulation. The determinants of drainage include the height of the patient above the venous reservoir, the patient's blood volume, the resistance of the tubing, and the cannula dimensions, as this is the narrowest part of the venous return. Augmented venous return refers to the use of either a pump (e.g., centrifugal) inserted in series between the venous line and the reservoir (kinetic assisted venous drainage) or the application of a vacuum to a closed hard shell venous reservoir (vacuum-assisted venous drainage).

In the majority of cases of cardiac surgery cannulation is directly through the right atrium. Bicaval cannulation refers to the use of two single-stage cannulas introduced into the superior vena cava (SCV) and inferior vena cava (IVC), usually through the right atrial wall. Cavoatrial cannulation involves the use of a two-stage venous cannula, inserted through the right atrium in the region of the atrial appendage, with the tip of the cannula directed into the IVC. The cannula is constructed with a fenestrated basket at the level of the right atrium to allow collection of blood from the coronary sinus and from the SVC. Bicaval cannulation is utilized when an "airless" right atrium is required such as with tricuspid valve surgery. It is also preferred in mitral valve surgery where distortion of the right atrium with

retraction may lead to a compromise in SVC blood return and a rise in the CVP. Placing tourniquets around the SVC and IVC during bicaval cannulation allows for the institution of *total* as opposed to *partial* bypass. With partial bypass, there is still some return of venous blood that takes place through the tricuspid valve and subsequently through the pulmonary circulation. Occasionally it is necessary to directly cannulas into the innominate vein or the SVC directly such as with some pediatric cases and complex adult or reoperative surgery. Alternate sites for venous access include the femoral, iliac, and axillary veins.

Cannula size should be chosen such that the anticipated pressure drop across the cannula is equal or less than the siphonage pressure that is applied based on the height of the patient above the pump and the patient's blood volume. If this principle is not followed, the CVP may increase, which could compromise CPP. As with aortic cannulas, venous cannulas are often wire reinforced and the tips may be constructed of thin metal to optimize the inner-to-outer diameter ratio.

Arterial Cannulation

Oxygenated blood is returned to the arterial circulation through specially designed arterial cannulas that come in a variety of configurations. Cannula characteristics include their length, the orientation of the tip (straight/right angle), the presence of a flange, and distal tapering. The arterial cannula is the narrowest portion of the CPB circuit after the oxygenator and thus it is the site of the highest potential gradient. It has been demonstrated that gradients in excess of 100 mm Hg may be associated with hemolysis.[58] There is no definite correlation between the French size of the cannula and the gradient, and therefore alternative means have been derived by investigators to help predict hemodynamics such as the M number[134] and the performance index.[58] Finally, although the size and shape of the cannula have not been determined to influence the rate of transcranial Doppler-detected microemboli,[13] design concepts such as tips to diffuse the sandblasting effect of flow, differential flow to the arch vessels, and distal baskets to capture debris have been introduced to theoretically minimize the potential that the cannula may contribute to atheroemboli.

Complications of ascending aortic cannulation include aortic intramural hematoma and dissection (0.01–0.09%), atheroemboli either directly from the cannula or from a jet effect, carotid hypoperfusion, air embolism, injury of the back wall of the aorta, and misdirection of the tip of the cannula either posteriorly across the aortic valve causing severe aortic insufficiency or anteriorly into the arch vessels or against the wall of the aorta. Femoral cannulation is most commonly used in situations of reoperative surgery and anticipated substernal adhesions. The dissection rate with femoral cannulation has been described between 0.2 and 3%. Retroperitoneal access to the iliac vessels by suprainguinal retroperitoneal dissection may also be necessary. Another attractive approach, particularly with aortic dissection, involves the use of axillary cannulation. This artery is less likely to be involved with atherosclerosis as compared to the lower extremities. There is exceptional collateral flow compared to the leg vessels; thus the procedure is well tolerated and infrequently results in limb ischemia. The direction of flow during axillary cannulation also favors noncerebral embolization should there be atherosclerotic disease in the arch of the aorta.

One of the most perplexing problems related to arterial cannulation is the management of patients with extensive aortic calcification. With bypass grafting, the use of off-pump surgery with a "no touch technique" may be considered. Alternately, femoral or axillary cannulation can be utilized was fibrillatory arrest, left heart venting, and arterial grafting. A third potential strategy involves the threading of a long cannula beyond the atheroma, into the descending thoracic aorta. Long cannulas are associated with a decreased peak forward flow velocity and turbulence as compared to a short cannula.[51] Borger and Feindel[16] demonstrated that cannulation beyond the cerebral vessels with a long cannula decreased the count of cerebral emboli as detected by transcranial Doppler. Finally in extreme cases, surgeons may cannulate the apex of the left ventricle with an armored venous cannula passed through the apex into the ascending aorta across the aortic valve. Epiaortic scanning has been advocated as a means to detect problems with the aorta. Numerous studies have been done involving this technology; however, it is controversial as to whether this impacts on clinical outcomes such as transient ischemic attack (TIA) and stroke.

PATHOPHYSIOLOGY OF CARDIOPULMONARY BYPASS

Pathophysiology refers to the physical and chemical processes related to the organism's responses. In the case of CPB, these responses are secondary to contact of the blood with the biomaterial surface (biomaterial-dependent processes) and non-contact-related processes such as cardiotomy blood collection and the effect of nonpulsatile flow.

Noncellular Blood Activation with Cardiopulmonary Bypass—Contact Activation, Fibrinolysis, Complement, Nitric Oxide

Within milliseconds of blood contact with the synthetic surfaces of the CPB circuit, plasma proteins become adsorbed to the biomaterial. Each surface has a characteristic "signature" adsorption pattern from blood; although the amount, composition, and conformation of protein adsorption may differ between surfaces, there is no surface upon which this process is completely inhibited. Further exposure of blood with the surface results in activation of proteins of the contact activation system (Figure 65-7). This comprises four primary plasma proteins: factors XII and XI, prekallikrein, and high-molecular-weight kininogen (HMWK). In the presence of the negatively charged biomaterial, a conformational change occurs in factor XII. This permits its activation in the presence of prekallikrein and HMWK. Factor XIIa activates factor XI and initiates the intrinsic coagulation pathway with the subsequent generation of thrombin and the cleavage of fibrinogen to produce fibrin, which is cross-linked by activated factor XIII. Factor XIIa also activates prekallikrein to form kallikrein within seconds of the start of bypass. Kallikrein catalyzes the conversion of HMWK to bradykinin and plays a role in the activation of the fibri-

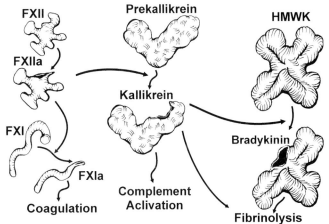

Figure 65–7 **Proteins of the contact activation system.** FXII, FXI, factors XII, XI; FXIIa, FXIa, activated factors XII and XI; HMWK, high-molecular-weight kininogen.

nolytic system. Bradykinin has a very short half-life in the plasma because of its rapid metabolism by angiotensin-converting enzyme in the pulmonary circulation[9] and by the vascular endothelium.[100] It is believed to be a key mediator of increased capillary permeability and the development of tissue edema. Bradykinin mediates vasodilation by stimulating the release of endothelial nitric oxide,[100] and in addition it may be an important mediator of cerebral ischemia.[69]

Activation of the fibrinolytic system during CPB is evidenced by increased levels of tissue plasminogen activator (tPA) as well as the formation of plasmin–antiplasmin complexes. Plasmin is generated principally by the action of tPA during CPB. Thrombin and bradykinin contribute to fibrinolysis through the direct activation of endothelial cells and the release of tPA.[77] Kallikrein-mediated activation of the fibrinolytic system includes its role in catalyzing the conversion of plasminogen to plasmin and the activation of prourokinase.[64] Despite these findings, the contribution of fibrinolysis to postbypass bleeding is controversial as clot lysis activity subsides within minutes of terminating bypass.[21] Another mechanism by which plasmin generation may contribute to bleeding is through its direct effect on platelet receptors during CPB.[87]

The complement system is activated through several mechanisms during CPB (Figure 65-8). First, the third component of complement (C3) adsorbed to the CPB surface, after releasing the potent chemoattractant C3a, is joined by the inactive factor B and properdin to produce the active proteolytic enzyme C3 convertase. C3 convertase will cleave the fifth component C5, to generate the active fragment C5a and the terminal complement complex (TCC) C5b-9. Other mechanisms for complement generation through the alternative pathway include the direct cleavage of C5 by kallikrein to produce C5a and of C3 by plasmin. Complement generation has also been reported to be induced directly by endotoxin or directly by the cytokines tumor necrosis factor (TNF) and interleukin (IL)-6.[150] Heparin–protamine complexes formed at the end of CPB activate the classical complement pathway as does immunoglobulin bound on the biomaterial surface, which will complex with C1q.[144]

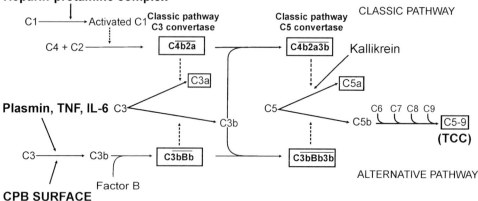

Figure 65–8 Mechanisms of complement activation during CPB. TCC, terminal complement complex; TNF, tumour necrosis factor; IL-6, interleukin 6.

The generation of complement plays a key role in the recruitment of leukocytes, the up-regulation of neutrophil activation markers, and the production of cytokines. Studies by Chenoweth et al[24] confirmed that the incidence and degree of deranged function of the heart, lung, and kidney after CPB could be related to the raised plasma concentration of the complement fragment C3a. Further, inhibition of production of TCC by a protease inhibitor was associated with a significant reduction in the deleterious effects of ischemia–reperfusion to the myocardium after CPB.[62]

Nitric oxide (NO) is a potent inflammatory mediator whose production is increased after CPB. Endogenously produced NO may cause tissue injury through formation of toxic peroxynitrites, activation of cyclooxygenase, and DNA deamination. Studies have reported a significant increase in iNOS expression in human lung after CPB, which may be related to cytokine release (TNF, IL-1, IL-6).[101] This induction has also been shown to be associated with myocardial depression secondary to reperfusion injury.[92]

Cytokine Generation

CPB initiates a cascade of events that results in cytokine release. Systemic lipopolysaccharide (LPS) concentration increases by 100% immediately on CPB institution, probably arising from translocation of bacteria from the bowel, with another significant increase seen after aortic cross-clamp release. LPS induces a broad range of immunological effects and is considered the most potent stimulant of TNF-α production from macrophages. TNF induces monocyte IL-1 production and both TNF and IL-1 in concert induce IL-6 production and release.[132] Whereas a rise in TNF and IL-1 as a result of CPB has not been regularly demonstrated in all studies, a marked increase in IL-6 levels appears consistently with CPB. Peak concentration in IL-6 occurs a few hours after the end of CPB with a gradual decrease toward preoperative levels in the following 24 h[139] similar to noncardiac surgery.[118]

Several investigators have demonstrated a correlation between the release of inflammatory mediators and myocardial dysfunction after coronary artery bypass surgery. Peak IL-6 and IL-8 levels correlate with the degree of myocardial dysfunction.[57] TNF may be released locally in the myocardium, and this may be related to postischemic myocardial stunning.[45] Jansen et al[66] demonstrated that a rise in TNF

can be detected after release of the aortic cross-clamp. TNF, IL-6,[72] and IL-8 levels correlated with the duration of the cross-clamping and the degree of myocardial injury as reflected by the creatine kinase (CK)-MB isoenzyme levels.[72]

Cellular Activation during Cardiopulmonary Bypass— Platelets, Endothelial Cells, Leukocytes

Although the cellular events during CPB are influenced by the dynamic nature of activation by the unique soluble products produced at the biomaterial, they are more significantly affected by the composition of proteins adsorbed on the nonendothelial surface. Surface-adsorbed fibrinogen is the key mediator of platelet accumulation of foreign materials. Platelet adhesion to artificial surfaces increases with increasing surface concentration of adsorbed fibrinogen if the bound fibrinogen maintains a conformation such that the functional domains of the molecule are recognizable by the activated platelet GP IIb/IIIa receptor. This latter interaction is probably the most important factor mediating platelet consumption during CPB. The three-dimensional conformation of adsorbed fibrinogen also influences the degree of platelet accumulation.

CPB is associated with a consistent increase in the proportion of activated circulating platelets. Agonists of platelet activation during CPB include thrombin, adenosine diphosphate (ADP), heparin, protamine, activated complement, and plasmin. Physical activators of platelets include hypothermia and the process of cardiotomy blood collection. This latter effect may be related to the air–blood interface, blood–tissue interface, or the exposure to thrombin generation in cardiotomy blood.

The most consistently documented measure of CPB-related activation is an increase in the expression of GMP-140 (P-selectin).[95] Platelet glycoprotein (GP) IIb/IIIa is also likely activated,[47] but it is controversial if there is loss of other surface receptors such as GP Ib. Platelet microparticles, which may be highly procoagulant, can be consistently detected by flow cytometry after CPB.[1] Other platelet products increased with CPB include β-thromboglobulin (BTG) and platelet factor 4 (PF4).[168]

In clinical CPB, thrombocytopenia is seen commonly with platelet counts dropping over 50% because of not only platelet adhesion to surfaces, but also because of hemodilution, platelet aggregate formation, and the formation of platelet–leukocyte complexes. With these changes, it is not surprising that the most predictable alteration in hemostatic function observed after CPB is platelet dysfunction. Clinical reflectors of this process include a universal prolongation of the bleeding time that is directly related to postoperative blood loss.[75] Platelet aggregation to ADP and epinephrine is consistently abnormal,[96] and there is decreased response to thrombin agonist receptor peptide (TRAP), suggesting a decrease in receptor sensitivity.[44]

Because of the intense antiinflammatory reaction related to CPB, it follows that the endothelial layer will be at the front of many of the cellular changes related to CPB. It is now evident that it is the activation of this axis that mediates many of the injurious processes related to CPB such as reperfusion injury. Cytokine generation is a major contributor to endothelial cell activation, primarily through their effect to up-regulate receptors necessary for neutrophil-endothelial cell binding.[112] Endothelial cells undergo up-regulation of intracellular adhesion molecule (ICAM) and E-selectin. The latter binds to the integrin CD11a/CD18 present on resting polymorphonuclear leukocytes (PMN). PMN and monocytes may be activated with up-regulation of the integrin CD11b/CD18 complex,[68] which also binds ICAM on endothelial cells.[125] The response to acute injury of the endothelium during CPB is evident by the acute rise in soluble P-selectin with a concomitant fall in soluble E-selectin and by increased elastase release.[97] Leukocytes interact with platelets during CPB as another means of systemic inflammation. Increased GMP-140 on the platelet surface is essential to mediate complex formation of platelets and monocytes or PNMs.[125] Monocyte–platelet conjugates increased from 18 to 44%, while PMN–platelet conjugates increased only slightly.[125]

Nonbiomaterial-Related Activation during Cardiopulmonary Bypass

It is now understood that exposure of cardiotomy blood to wound surfaces is likely the most important source of thrombin generation during CPB despite the large doses of heparin given (Figure 65-9). Several factors contribute to persistent thrombin generation in cardiotomy blood. First, heparin levels in the cardiotomy blood are well below those found in the systemic blood[141] as heparin may be bound to nonplasma components such as platelets or debris and heparin may be consumed by PF4. Further, any heparin that is present is not capable of inhibiting thrombin completely, especially thrombin that is bound to fibrin.[161] Second, thrombin is generated via coagulation pathways other than the intrinsic pathway, which are less effectively inhibited by heparin. Tissue factor on the wound surface and on the surface of activated monocytes contributes to coagulation[40] as does the monocyte CD11b activation of factor X.[114] Finally, cardiotomy blood contributes to fibrinolysis induction[31] and this may enhance systemic fibrinolysis after cardiotomy blood readministration.

▶ HEPARIN–PROTAMINE AXIS

Heparin: Pharmacology, Dosing, and Complications

Heparin, derived from bovine or porcine intestinal mucosa, is a glycosaminoglycan composed of chains of alternating

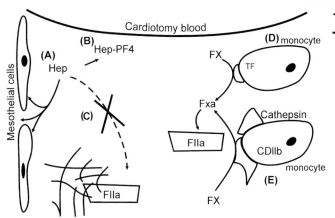

Figure 65–9 Illustration of the mechanisms contributing to thrombin generation in cardiotomy blood. Heparin (Hep) levels are decreased due to (**A**) binding to wound surfaces as well as (**B**) binding to PF4. Heparin is also ineffective because of (**C**) the inability of heparin to inhibit clot-bound thrombin. Thrombin generation occurs through other monocyte-dependent processes such as (**D**) tissue factor (TF) and (**E**) cathepsin/CD11b complex-mediated factor X (FX) activation.

residues of D-glucosamine and uronic acid. It is commonly utilized in its unfractionated form (UFH) consisting of a spectrum of molecular weight between 1000 and 30,000 Da with a mean of 15,000. The anticoagulant activity of heparin is intimately associated with the protein biochemistry of antithrombin III (ATIII). ATIII is a natural inhibitor of thrombin, but the presence of heparin accelerates this action over 4000-fold. Heparin's effect is accounted for by a unique pentasaccharide sequence with a high affinity binding sequence to ATIII. The inhibition of thrombin is also dependent on the heparin fraction with a minimum of 18 pentasaccharide units, allowing simultaneous binding of ATIII and thrombin. Heparin is then able to dissociate from this ternary complex to be reused again in the circulation. UFH-ATIII complexes can catalyze the inhibition of factors IXa, Xa, and XIa[8]; however, they have little effect on factor XIIa.[115] Heparin's other actions as an anticoagulant include the facilitation of thrombin inhibition by heparin cofactor II and its inhibition of the extrinsic pathway by heparin-mediated release of tissue factor pathway inhibitor. Finally, there is increasing evidence that heparin's principal inhibitory effect on coagulation is through the inhibition of thrombin-induced activation of factor V and VIII.[110]

The clearance of heparin is influenced by its molecular size, with higher-molecular-weight species being removed from the circulation more rapidly than the lower-molecular-weight species. UFH is cleared through two phases: a rapid saturable phase and a slower phase of first-order mechanism; thus anticoagulant response is not linear, but increases in intensity and duration with increasing dose.[37] Following injection, UFH is bound by a number of plasma proteins including histidine-rich glycoprotein, PF4, vitronectin, fibronectin, von Willebrand factor (vWF). This contributes to the variability of anticoagulant response to fixed-dose heparin and the laboratory phenomenon of heparin resistance. The binding of UFH to endothelial cells and macrophages also contributes to its complicated pharmacokinetics.

During CPB, heparin is generally used in generous doses of up to 300 U/kg, with an aim to achieve and maintain a target activated clotting time (ACT) of 400–480 s. This rather primitive test, though automated, involves the addition of an aliquot of whole blood to a test tube containing a blood activator (celite or kaolin). In the Hemochron ACT device (International Technidyne, Edison, NJ), when a clot forms, resistance to movement of a small magnet in the tube is detected and the timer stops. The Hemo Tec ACT device (Medtronic-HemoTec, Englewood, CO), which uses kaolin as an activator, uses a plastic plunger for continuous mixing. The absence of plunger fall after a clot forms is detected photooptically and the counter ceases.

Heparin may contribute to the bleeding diathesis after surgery, independent of its action as an antithrombotic. UFH may contribute to platelet dysfunction directly[104] because of its ability to bind to vWF. Heparin-induced platelet activation may also result in clearance of platelets from the circulation, thus contributing to postoperative thrombocytopenia. Heparin has an independent role as a profibrinolytic agent[74] before the initiation of CPB, which may be related to its activation of the kallikrein system.

There are two forms of thrombocytopenia related to heparin administration independent of CPB. The first is a benign reversible nonimmune thrombocytopenia that immediately responds to the discontinuation of heparin and may be related to direct weak activation of platelets by heparin. The second more serious reaction is an IgG-mediated immune thrombocytopenia referred to as heparin-induced thrombocytopenia and thrombosis (HITT). The syndrome is secondary to platelet activation from an IgG that binds the FcγII receptor.[73] The heparin/PF4 complex on the platelet surface is the responsible target antigen. A secondary thrombogenic diathesis may result from platelet activation related to microparticle release.[158]

HITT usually begins 5–15 days after commencing heparin therapy, but recent data have suggested that it can be detected within a mean of 10 h of commencement of heparin in patients with previous exposure.[157] The incidence is lower with bovine heparin[159] and, in general, among heparinized patients, 1% at 7 days and 3% at 14 days will develop HITT.[156]

Although thrombocytopenia may be evident, the surgeon must be wary of a normal platelet count in the postoperative period in the presence of unexplained thrombosis, when reactive thrombocytosis should be evident.

HITT is diagnosed using an assay measuring the release of radiolabeled serotonin from donor platelets after patient serum exposure or using an enzyme-linked immunosorbent assay (ELISA) for the PF4/heparin complex antigen. Surgical approaches to patients with HITT will depend upon the degree of urgency of the anticipated procedure. In elective situations, if patients with a history of HITT can be postponed (>100 days) they may not necessarily be at risk for thrombotic complications if heparin is utilized a second time[157] (Figure 65-10). If the surgery cannot be postponed, avoidance of CPB with off-pump techniques may be considered; however, some form of anticoagulation would still be necessary during anastomosis. Otherwise, each institution should develop a strategy for the emergency management of CPB in the presence of HITT. Traditionally a platelet "paralyzing" agent such as prostacyclin was utilized; however, the attendant hypotension was often difficult to manage.[70] Among alternates to UFH, low-molecular-weight heparin (LMWH) is not suitable as there is >90% immune cross-reactivity with UFH and CPB with LMWH is associated with significant bleeding.[3] The heparinoid danaparoid (Orgaran, NV Organon, Netherlands) has <10% antibody cross-reactivity and <5% clinical cross-reactivity[88] and thus may be useful; however, no neutralizing agent is available and because of its long half-life, significant bleeding must be anticipated after its use.[163] Ancrod (Viprinex, Abbott Laboratories, Canada) is a defibrinogenating agent derived from snake venom. The clinical experience with this agent is limited and it has drawbacks in that neither thrombin generation nor platelet activation is blocked, it is antigenic, and a delay of 12 h for the full effect is required.

ATIII-independent thrombin inhibitors such as hirudin and argatroban (Novastatin, Texas Biotechnology Corp, Houston TX) hold promise as the best alternatives for CPB management in these difficult patients. Recombinant hirudin (Refludan, Hoechst, Kansas City, MO) binds the

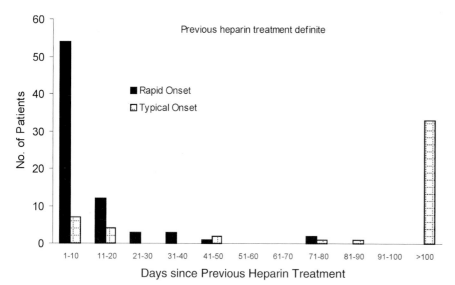

Figure 65–10 Temporal pattern of heparin-induced thrombocytopenia in relation to previous treatment with heparin. None of the patients whose prior heparin treatment had occurred more than 100 days earlier had rapid-onset thrombocytopenia.
(Reproduced with permission from Warkentin T, et al: Temporal aspects of heparin induced thrombocytopenia. N Engl J Med 344;1286–1292, 2001. Copyright 2001, Massachusetts Medical Society.)

catalytic and fibrinogen binding sites of thrombin. It has been successfully used in clinical CPB[80] and in deep hypothermic circulatory arrest.[130] This drug can be monitored using the ecarin clotting time.[116] Argatroban also specifically binds the catalytic site of thrombin. Its potential benefit over hirudin relates to its shorter half-life (15–30 min cf. 30–60 min for hirudin), which compensates for its lack of a reversing agent. This drug has been used in CPB,[46] but greater experience is needed before its universal recommendation.

Protamine: Pharmacology and Complications

Protamine is a polycationic protein derived from salmon sperm. The positive charges on protamine combine ionically with the negative moieties of the heparin molecule, separating it from ATIII and producing a stable precipitate that is rapidly cleared from the circulation. The drug is given intravenously at a fixed ratio of 1–1.3 mg/100 U administered heparin. The most common problem related to protamine is heparin rebound, which is a frequent cause of postoperative bleeding. This phenomenon is related to the delayed desorption of heparin from plasma proteins and endothelium after the first dose of protamine has been cleared. It usually becomes evident 2–3 h after arrival in the ICU, and is reflected by increasing chest tube losses accompanied by a new prolongation of the ACT or the thrombin time. The problem can be obviated by the routine addition of a protamine drip after surgery. Hypotension is another common consequence of protamine administration, particularly with rapid intravenous administration. The mechanism of this rate-related effect is not known, but its magnitude is greater in situations of low preload and afterload. Protamine may also be responsible for several idiosyncratic hypotensive reactions. Anaphylactoid reactions are mediated primarily by complement and histamine. Anaphylactic reactions involve the IgE-mediated release of histamine and other vasoactive mediators. Both reactions are characterized by edema, hives, and bronchospasm in the presence of low blood pressure (BP), central venous pressure (CVP), and positive airway pressure (PAP) and a decreased systemic vascular resistance (SVR). The most serious form of protamine-related hypotension is catastrophic pulmonary vasoconstriction. In contrast to the other two forms of idiosyncratic protamine reactions, this syndrome may be associated with bronchospasm and pulmonary hypertension with an elevated CVP. The mechanism is likely related to IgG release with activation of complement and PMN and release of platelet thromboxane A$_2$.[103] Theoretically patients at risk for protamine reactions include those with previous vasectomy, previous exposure to protamine, or after exposure to protamine-containing insulin.[63]

Protamine may contribute to excessive postoperative bleeding because of a direct antiplatelet effect. It also has a direct anticoagulant effect; however, this can be demonstrated *in vitro* only at doses much higher than those required to neutralize heparin during clinical CPB. In the presence of predetected problems with protamine, the cardiac surgeon can prepare alternative strategies to prevent anticipated problems after CPB. In minor cases of low-risk, premedication with steroids (at least 12–24 h in advance) and histamine blockers may be all that is required. A small test dose (5 mg) should also be given to ensure safety. Avoidance of neutralization after the massive doses required for CPB may be difficult because of the prolonged half-life of heparin. Experimentally, recombinant PF4 has shown promise as an alternative to protamine.[32]

The rationale for heparinizing to an ACT during CPB of between 400 and 480 s is based upon early work that demonstrated that this was the target above which no gross evidence of thrombosis occurred in the reservoir. However, many researchers have expressed doubt about the validity of using ACT as gold standard for anticoagulation during CPB. In particular, there is clear evidence that the ACT does not reflect the heparin level accurately, particularly after a long duration of CPB and other factors such as hypothermia, hemodilution, and drugs may contribute[35] (Figure 65-11). As CPB progresses, celite-based ACT values may be further influenced by the use of aprotinin. The HepCon device (Medtronics HemoTec, Englewood, CO) is composed of a series of ACT cuvettes containing incrementally increased protamine doses that can be used to precisely calculate the circulating heparin level. A patient-specific preoperative standard curve with target heparin concentrations can be precisely calculated. Interestingly, using this technique, overall heparin requirements are higher (25%); however, factor consumption during CPB is decreased, likely related to an inhibition of low-grade coagulation. In clinical trials, this technique also results in a shorter bleeding time on arrival in the ICU that is associated with decreased blood product use.[36] These findings have been controversial[54]; although this form of heparin–protamine titration has significant potential, careful monitoring is necessary to compensate for aspects such as heparin rebound, which is intensified by the higher heparin dose used.

▶ PHARMACOLOGICAL ADJUNCTS TO MINIMIZE THE CONSEQUENCES OF CARDIOPULMONARY BYPASS

Steroids are widely used for the suppression of inflammation in chronic inflammatory diseases. During CPB, steroids blunt complement activation, up-regulation of CD 11b,[59] and the release of histamine,[153] TNF,[145] IL-6,[65] IL-8,[145] and neutrophil elastase.[67] Finally, steroids reduce airway NO concentrations during CPB[60] compatible with inhibition of bronchial epithelial iNOS expression. Steroids have also been demonstrated to be associated with decreased CK-MB.[166] The inhibition of these aspects of inflammation may explain the stabilizing effect of these drugs on hemodynamics after CPB. Although inexpensive, steroids are immunosuppressive and it has been suggested that they contribute to the pathogenesis of posttransfusion graft-versus-host disease.[93] Their use has not been conclusively demonstrated to be associated with postoperative wound infection although Mayumi et al[94] demonstrated that high-dose steroid administration pre-CPB suppressed T cell function. Further, hyperglycemia was more frequent in the patients receiving steroids, which may also contribute to the risk of infection.[94]

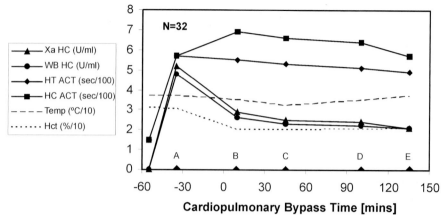

Figure 65–11 Time course of physiological and hematological mean values. Mean values for ACT expressed as seconds per 100 for both Hemochron (HC ACT) and HepCon (HT ACT) assays. Plasma equivalent heparin concentration (WB HC) and anti-Xa plasma heparin concentration (Xa HC) expressed as units per milliliter. Hematocrit (Hct) values expressed as percent divided by 10 (%10) and core body temperature (Temp) expressed as degrees centigrade divided by 10 (°C/10). Mean values for derived physiological and hematological variables are plotted as a function of time in minutes. Phase II time points include prior to heparin administration and 10 minutes after each of the following: heparin administration (**A**), initiation of CPB (**B**), achievement of hypothermia (**C**), rewarming (**D**), and immediately before discontinuation of CPB (**E**). *(Reproduced with permission from Despotis GJ, et al: Comparison of activated coagulation time and whole blood heparin measurements with laboratory plasma anti-Xa heparin concentration in patients having cardiac operations. J Thorac Cardiovasc Surg 108;1076–1082, 1994. Copyright 1994, Mosby-Year Book Inc.)*

Although the primary indication for the use of the serine protease inhibitor aprotinin is to reduce blood loss during and after CPB, a number of studies have shown that aprotinin reduces cytokine levels and cytokine-induced events when used during CPB.[76] However, this drug is very expensive when compared to steroid therapy, and it may not have as general an effect on the inflammatory system. Diego et al[39] demonstrated that the antiinflammatory effect of methylprednisolone (MPSS) exceeded that of aprotinin as reflected by a greater inhibition of IL-6 at all time points after CPB. On the other hand, steroids may augment the antiinflammatory action of aprotinin. Tassani et al.[143] demonstrated that high-dose MPSS attenuates the systemic inflammatory response during coronary bypass grafting in aprotinin-treated patients. IL-6 and IL-8 were significantly less in the MPSS group, whereas the antiinflammatory IL-10 was greater. These changes corresponded to augmented oxygenation, improved lung compliance, as well as improved cardiac index in the steroid-treated group.

BIOMATERIAL-DEPENDENT STRATEGIES TO MINIMIZE BLOOD ACTIVATION FROM CARDIOPULMONARY BYPASS

A biomaterial-dependent strategy involves the choice of a CPB circuit composed of a biomaterial with enhanced biocompatibility. The quest for an ideal biomaterial substrate for the construction of CPB circuits has culminated in three types of surface modification that either have been tested in human trials or are on the verge of clinical evaluation.

Biomembrane Mimicry

The premise with this approach is to develop a biomaterial that mimics the antithrombotic behavior of natural cell membranes. The biomaterial is coated with a derivative of phosphorylcholine, which is the major lipid head group component found on the outer surface of biologic cell membranes.[20] In vitro data have demonstrated the efficacy of this modified surface (Memsys, Sorin Biomedica) in inhibiting fibrinogen adsorption and platelet deposition.[20] Clinical experience in CPB with this device is limited, but in a recent pediatric trial, limited platelet activation was seen with this coating.[34]

Heparin-Coated Circuits

There are two types of clinically relevant heparin-coated circuits. In the first group, heparin is bound such that it may be slowly released into the circulation from the surface. The original ionic binding pioneered by Gott et al[50] has its current form in the DurofloII surface (Baxter Healthcare Corporation, Irvine, CA) in which the heparin is ionically bound to benzalkonium attached to the substrate polymer. In the second group, heparin is immobilized permanently upon the biomaterial surface by covalent bonding. Polyethylene oxide (PEO) is utilized as a spacer group as its hydrophilicity and its dynamic motion further inhibit platelet interactions. The Carmeda product (Carmeda,

Medtronics, Minneapolis, MN) is a commercial example of this technology for CPB in which heparin is covalently bound via an end point immobilization technique. The Trillium Biopassive Surface (Medtronics, Minneapolis, MN) is a similar coating process involving two polymers on the substrate surface. The first polymer functions as a primer, strongly bonding to the surface of the substrate. The second polymer, which is bound to the primer coat, is composed of sulfate/sulfonate groups, the latter providing a negative surface charge, as well as PEO chains covalently bound to heparin. BioLine (Jostra, Germany) is a hybrid surface (i.e., combination heparin releasing and heparin immobilized) in which heparin is adsorbed onto a layer of immobilized polypeptides through a combination of ionic interactions and covalent bonds.

Convincing *in vitro* evidence of the thromboresistant behavior of heparin-coated surfaces led to the hypothesis that less intense anticoagulation would be required for CPB when heparin-coated circuits were utilized. Many of the early clinical trials compared outcomes after CPB in patients where heparin-coated circuits were combined with lower dosages of heparin (one-third to one-half) versus control (uncoated) circuits and standard heparin doses (300 U/kg). Advantages seen have included decreased perioperative bleeding and transfusion. In a large clinical trial reported by Aldea et al,[2] an integrated blood conservation strategy that included heparin-coated circuits and decreased heparin dosing was applied. This approach resulted in decreased blood transfusion requirements and significantly improved clinical outcomes as measured by ICU and hospital length of stay, as well as the ventilatory support duration. This translated into cost savings of approximately $1700 per patient,[2] similar to that found in a recent meta-analysis assessing this technology.[89]

Compelling as these clinical results are, neither thrombin generation nor fibrinolysis has been consistently demonstrated to be decreased during CPB with heparin-coated circuits in human trials, with either standard or decreased heparin doses as compared to standard (non-heparin-coated) circuits.[146] Therefore, it is difficult to justify decreasing the heparin dose because of the potential risk of low-grade thrombosis. Also any measured differences in patient clinical and biochemical outcomes, which may be related to differences in the amounts of administered heparin and not to the surface as heparin itself, can induce a myriad of cellular and biochemical changes such as fibrinolysis and platelet dysfunction.[74] As the dose of the protamine must also be increased, it is anticipated that changes such as complement activation must be proportionally increased. In the majority of clinical trials in which the same doses of heparin are used with both heparin-coated circuits and standard circuits, little clinical benefit has been consistently demonstrated except perhaps in high-risk patients.[121]

Beneficial clinical impacts of heparin-coated circuits are almost entirely related to their intrinsic antiinflammatory effect. What has been consistently demonstrated is the capacity of heparin-coated surfaces to decrease complement activation[12] independent of the heparin dose. Other demonstrated antiinflammatory effects of heparin-coated surfaces include decreased leukocyte surface activation markers/receptors,[99] decreased cytokine production,[138] and decreased monocyte tissue factor.[10] The antiinflammatory

action of heparin-coated circuits in the absence of coagulation inhibition may be related to its action as a selective "protein sink" for such proteins as HMWK.[162] Surface-adsorbed HMWK may interact with ATIII in the presence of surface heparin to potentiate heparin-mediated inhibition of kallikrein.[111,146]

In summary, heparin-coated surfaces have been demonstrated to exhibit potent antithrombotic behavior in *in vitro* testing. Although there is no evidence of decreased thrombogenicity when utilized clinically, there is consistent evidence that inflammation related to complement activation is decreased and this may be responsible for the improvement seen in some clinical outcomes after CPB.

Surfaces with Modified Protein Adsorption

This group consists of surfaces whose biocompatibility has been predicted based upon protein adsorption characteristics. An example of this approach includes a new generation of biomaterials into which a surface-modifying additive (SMA) has been incorporated.[155] The additive is a triblock copolymer with polar and nonpolar polymer chains.[155] During the manufacturing process, the SMA migrates to the surface of the base polymer yielding a stable microdomain-like configuration. Although the mechanism of action by which SMA decreases blood protein and cellular activation is not precisely known, it is hypothesized that the alternating hydrophobic and hydrophilic regions of the microdomain surface lead to uniform adhesion of fibrinogen, such that all of the sites for potential platelet interaction with surface-bound fibrinogen are occupied. A randomized controlled trial (RCT) in which patients underwent CPB using a standard control circuit, or a circuit prepared "tip-to-tip" with the SMA copolymer (SMA-CPB),[129] showed striking changes with regard to the effect of this surface on markers of coagulation, fibrinolysis, platelet number, and function. Thrombin generation was significantly decreased with SMA-CPB compared to controls, despite carefully matched heparin doses in the two groups. Defraigne et al[30] in a larger clinical trial confirmed the same degree of platelet preservation with SMA-CPB and a similar decreased release of β-thromboglobulin (BTG). In addition, there was evidence of a decreased need for the transfusion of platelets and fresh frozen plasma in the group with SMA-CPB circuits.

Terumo Corporation (Tokyo, Japan) has recently developed a surface for CPB circuits with a biocompatibility profile similar to SMA in that it was engineered to positively influence protein adsorption. Surfaces are coated with poly(2-methoxyethylacrylate, PMEA), which has a hydrophobic polyethylene backbone, and its residue has mild hydrophilicity with no chemical functional groups such as -OH or -NH$_2$. It was predicted that as the outer side of the PMEA molecule is inactive chemically, the surface would have little tendency to react with blood components. Although clinical studies in humans are not available, there are promising data from *in vitro* and *in vivo* models supporting the potential improved biocompatibility of PMEA-coated surfaces.[140] Analysis of the composition of the adsorbed protein layer on PMEA-coated surfaces demonstrated a striking decrease in the amount of adsorbed IgG. This finding correlated to platelet count

1074

preservation as compared to uncoated surfaces, as surface-bound IgG is a well-known platelet activator. The use of the PMEA circuit was also associated with a significant decrease in CD35-positive monocytes during CPB.[43] Decreased adsorption of immunoglobulin is again probably the causative mechanism for decreased complement activation. Plasma bradykinin levels are decreased with PMEA[140] as are thrombin ATIII levels.[140]

▶ ORGAN DERANGEMENTS RELATED TO CARDIOPULMONARY BYPASS

Neuroendocrine Response to Cardiopulmonary Bypass

The changes in the neuroendocrine response related to CPB are unique as compared to noncardiac surgery. Hormones under hypothalamic–pituitary control include growth hormone, vasopressin, the adrenal cortical axis, and the thyroid hormone system. Growth hormone increases significantly during and after CPB.[117] Vasopressin is a key regulator of renal water excretion and peripheral vascular resistance, and it may contribute to endothelial activation through release of vWF.[56] Marked increases in vasopressin are seen after cardiac surgery with CPB, with the elevated levels persisting for hours after.[71] This may be a protective effect as depressed levels postoperatively are associated with vasodilatory shock.[5]

There is a definite increase in ACTH with CPB although the adrenocorticotropic hormone response is blunted after administration of corticotrophin-releasing hormone during CPB.[4] Total plasma cortisol concentrations typically decrease immediately upon initiation of CPB as a consequence of hemodilution, but later values return to normal or above baseline accompanied by parallel increases in unbound cortisol, suggesting that this increase is related to increased total secretion.[120] Thyroid hormone dysfunction may play a role in the unique clinical response seen after CPB. Investigators have demonstrated that although thyroid-stimulating hormone (TSH) remains normal, total and free T_3 drops and remains depressed for 24 h after surgery, reverse T_3 shows a 4-fold rise at 8 and 24 h postoperatively, thus producing a picture of sick euthyroid syndrome.[147]

The catecholamines epinephrine and norepinephrine are both increased after CPB, and this may be contributory to cases of severe postoperative hypertension.[154] The sympathetic system also regulates glucose control at the level of the pancreas by controlling the release of insulin and glucagon. After the onset of CPB, blood glucose concentrations rise steadily in parallel with a drop in insulin levels with insulin resistance reflected by higher than average doses.[83] During and after CPB, renin levels increase and this is associated with a rise in measured angiotensin II and aldosterone.[160]

Among the locally released hormones, atrial natriuretic factor levels are probably reduced during CPB, especially in patients with preoperative elevations; however, elevated levels may be seen in the presence of complications.[128] Other locally released factors include histamine and serotonin related to leukocyte and platelet activation.[149] Histamine produces vasodilation and hypotension and may contribute to tPA release.[135] Its increase may be abolished by high-dose steroids and prostacyclin infusions.[90] Finally, CPB provides

a consistent stimulus for prostacyclin and inflammatory eicosanoid formation as evidenced by a marked increase in 6-keto-prostaglandin $F_{1\alpha}$ (stable metabolite of prostacyclin),[33] thromboxane B_2,[167] and PGE_2 concentrations.[42]

CNS Injury with Cardiopulmonary Bypass

Cerebral damage during heart surgery may be the complication most feared and respected by cardiac surgeons. There are three major types of neurological injury after CPB, but the significance of their distinctions are blurred in that they likely reflect a continuum of pathological changes, based on location, extent, and permanence of the injury. Stroke is the easiest injury to recognize after CPB. Its incidence is difficult to pinpoint; however, the best estimate is around 3% of patients undergoing CABG.[61] Based upon the information from the STS database, this complication is increased in females and in the elderly. The incidence rises to 8% after isolated valve surgery and 11% after combined CABG plus other surgery.[164] The etiology is likely secondary to macroemboli from an aortic source. Stroke is associated with a marked increase in 30-day mortality and its occurrence doubles hospital stay and cost.[61]

Delirium, seen in up to 3% of patients, is a state characterized by confusion and disorientation in the presence of an altered state of consciousness,[126] a problem that may increase hospital stay 5-fold.[126] Risk factors include increased age, hypertension, history of previous CABG, preexisting history of pulmonary disease, and a history of alcohol abuse.[126]

Cognitive decline (postoperative cognitive deficit, POCD) is defined as a change in memory, concentration, psychomotor speed, or dexterity. Although it may go unnoticed, sometimes the patient may recognize the inability to complete previously facile tasks, or it may be recognized by the family. Quantitation depends on sensitive neuropsychological findings involving a reproducible battery of tests. A pooled analysis of six highly comparable studies by Van Dijk et al[152] yielded a proportion of POCD after CPB of 22.5% (95% CI: 18.7–26.4%). Newman et al,[107] Robinson et al,[127] and Borowicz et al[17] provide comprehensive reviews of studies of POCD following CABG; the reported incidence in larger studies ranges from 35 to 75% early postoperatively and 11 to 40% after more than 6 months. The frequency and severity of cognitive deficits are much greater following cardiac surgery compared to major noncardiac surgery; however, it is debatable if coronary artery surgery without CPB provides protection as recently Van Dijk demonstrated that although there were slightly superior results for the OPCAB group at 3 months with respect to the incidence of POCD, there was no difference at 12 months.[151] Late decline may also occur, suggesting that CPB puts patients at subsequent risk of POCD. Sotaniemi et al.[136] found that even if the early postoperative changes disappeared, affected individuals were more likely to show early dementia 5 years later as the underlying neuronal loss may make an individual more vulnerable to age-dependent cell loss in the future. Recent information by Newman et al[108] showed that patients demonstrating significant impairment early are impaired at 5 years as compared with patients not having early deficits.

The characteristic pathological findings in canine and human cerebral tissue following CPB are small capillary and arteriolar dilatations (SCADs, Figure 65-12). These are

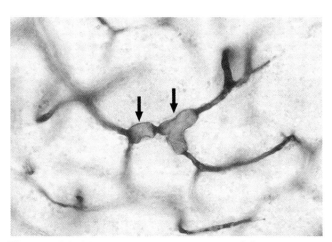

Figure 65–12 Postmortem specimen of brain section illustrating small capillary and arteriolar dilatation (SCAD) (*arrows*) after CPB.
(*Image courtesy of Dr. Dixon Moody, Wake Forest University.*)

believed to be the sites of fat, particulate, or gas emboli.[102] Transcranial Doppler studies of patients during CPB have confirmed the frequent occurrence of embolic material in the cerebral circulation. Further, the cerebral embolic load was found to be directly proportional to the length of CPB in an autopsy study by Brown et al.[19] There is a direct correlation between POCD and retinal microemboli on fluorescein angiography.[15] Magnetic resonance imaging immediately following CABG has identified global cerebral swelling even in low-risk patients.[55] Finally, there is strong experimental evidence that cardiotomy suction blood may be the most important source of lipid emboli.[18]

Pulmonary Dysfunction with Cardiopulmonary Bypass

After CPB, there is a documented incidence of between 12% for mild lung injury and 1.3% for acute respiratory distress syndrome (ARDS).[119] This problem is more common in the elderly in the obese, and in patients with low cardiac output, pulmonary hypertension, and after long CPB.[119] In the majority of cases of CPB-related lung injury, full recovery occurs; however, severe lung injury has a mortality >50%.[98] Clinical findings of lung injury include an increase in the $P(A–a)O_2$ and pulmonary shunt fraction together with a decrease in the functional residual capacity. There may be increased pulmonary vascular resistance as well as evidence of increased lung permeability.[109] The etiology of CPB-related lung injury does not appear to be related to hypoxia induced by partial CPB as the bronchial circulation is adequate to prevent necrosis.[86] There is, however, definite evidence of increased pulmonary inflammation with increased bronchoalveolar lavage (BAL) fluid-activated neutrophils,[81] matrix metalloproteinases, myeloperoxidase levels[169] with increased IL-8, and elastase,[82] all of which may contribute to the breakdown of the pulmonary ultrastructure.[22]

Off-pump techniques have not consistently minimized pulmonary insufficiency after cardiac surgery[27] nor have steroids benefited.[23] Leukocyte depletion may limit pulmonary reperfusion injury after CPB and result in improved lung function.[113] Heparin-coated circuits have been shown

to improve lung compliance and pulmonary vascular resistance with particular improvement seen when low heparin protocols are used.[2] Some authors have recommended maintaining mechanical ventilation during CPB; however, most studies failed to show significant persistent benefit.[109] No impact of temperature management could be demonstrated on pulmonary outcome.[109] Maintaining lung perfusion during CPB (Drew–Anderson technique) refers to using the patient's own lungs as an oxygenator and supplying only biventricular pump function, and this may have some clinical benefits;[123] however, its practicality is not universally accepted.

Renal Dysfunction with Cardiopulmonary Bypass

Data from the Multicenter Study of Perioperative Ischemia Research Group[91] demonstrated a 7.7% incidence of postoperative renal dysfunction, with 1.4% of all patients necessitating dialysis. Renal insufficiency is associated with increased hospital and ICU stay and mortality, emphasizing its clinical relevance. The contribution of CPB during cardiac surgery to renal damage is supported by clinical studies comparing outcomes with off-pump techniques. In high-risk patients (serum creatinine >150 μmol/liter), the use of CPB was associated with an increased postoperative serum creatinine and urea.[7] Glomerular filtration as assessed by creatinine clearance and urinary microalbumin/creatinine ratio was significantly worse in on-pump groups,[6] and there is a lower incidence of microalbuminuria, improved free water clearance and fractional excretion of sodium, and decreased N-acetyl-β-D-glucosaminidase (NAG) in the urine with off-pump surgery.[85] Although factors such as nonpulsatile flow and obstructive atheromatous microemboli may contribute, the diffuse inflammatory change related to CPB may have an independent toxic effect on the kidneys. Proximal tubular dysfunction has been demonstrated by increased urinary release of NAG and elevated urine levels of the cytokines IL-1 receptor antagonist and TNF-soluble receptor 2.[49]

Numerous strategies have been advocated as potentially renal-protective during CPB. Leukodepletion resulted in decreased urinary microalbumin and retinol-binding protein (RBP) release.[142] Mannitol is a popular diuretic agent that can increase diuresis if added in doses of 10–30 g. This drug has also been shown to preserve creatinine levels and lower urinary albumin excretion rates after pediatric cardiac surgery.[124] Renal-dose dopamine (2–3 μg/kg/min) has been assessed in several RCTs of patients at high risk for renal failure, and the results have been controversial.[165] Fenoldopam, a selective dopamine receptor agonist, was shown in an RCT to preserve renal function as demonstrated by maintained creatinine clearance postoperatively compared to placebo infusion.[53]

THE FUTURE OF CARDIOPULMONARY BYPASS

There is still ample room for modifications in CPB circuit design that may enhance clinical outcomes with cardiac surgery. For example, newer devices have incorporated novel technology to integrate all CPB components to markedly minimize the pump prime and the surface area (COR$_x$,

Cardio Vention Inc., Santa Clara, CA). However, their application will necessitate marked acceptance of modified surgical techniques (retrograde autologous priming, absence venous reservoir or cardiotomy) that will limit their generalized acceptance and facility. Our perspective on the human response to CPB will also be significantly influenced by the advent of modalities enabling us to illustrate the phenotypic responses to extracorporeal circulation.[131] But without support for research powered to detect useful clinical outcomes, we will continue to float somewhat aimlessly and without vision as to where CPB is going. An illustrative paper by Bartels et al[11] clearly demonstrated our naivety with regard to the means by which we conduct CPB. There is a wealth of literature regarding CPB strategy, but little of it conforms to the rigorous demands of evidence-based medical practice. "On the basis of our scientific evaluation of the current literature on 48 principles of CPB, not a single condition was of sufficient scientific merit to conclude that we were dealing with a principle for which there is clear evidence, scientific agreement, or both, that a given procedure or treatment is useful and effective."[11] We should not be discouraged by this conclusion, but we should look at it as a golden opportunity to press for support for high-quality CPB-related research. Heart surgery is expensive, but society must accept that an incremental cost for new technology has to include appropriate amounts to support peer-reviewed research in this area. Only with this partnership between industry, government, health practitioners, and the consumer can we hope to continue to improve the quality of clinical outcomes with cardiac surgery.

REFERENCES

1. Abrams CS, Ellison N, Budzynski AZ, Shattil SJ: Direct detection of activated platelets and platelet-derived microparticles in humans. Blood 75:128–138, 1990.
2. Aldea GS, Doursounian M, O'Gara P, et al: Heparin-bonded circuits with a reduced anticoagulation protocol in primary CABG: a prospective, randomized study. Ann Thorac Surg 62: 410–418, 1996.
3. Altes A, Martino R, Gari M, et al: Heparin-induced thrombocytopenia and heart operation: management with Tedelparin. Ann Thorac Surg 59:508–509, 1995.
4. Amado JA, Diago MC: Delayed ACTH response to human corticotropin releasing hormone during cardiopulmonary bypass under diazepam-high dose fentanyl anaesthesia. Anaesthesia 49:300–303, 1994.
5. Argenziano M, Chen JM, Choudhri AF, et al: Management of vasodilatory shock after cardiac surgery: identification of predisposing factors and use of a novel pressor agent. J Thorac Cardiovasc Surg 116:973–980, 1998.
6. Ascione R, Lloyd CT, Underwood MJ, et al: On-pump versus off-pump coronary revascularization: evaluation of renal function. Ann Thorac Surg 68:493–498, 1999.
7. Ascione R, Nason G, Al Ruzzeh S, et al: Coronary revascularization with or without cardiopulmonary bypass in patients with preoperative nondialysis-dependent renal insufficiency. Ann Thorac Surg 72:2020–2025, 2001.
8. Badellino KO, Walsh PN: Localization of a heparin binding site in the catalytic domain of factor XIa. Biochemistry 40: 7569–7580, 2001.
9. Bakhle YS: Pulmonary metabolism of bradykinin analogues and the contribution of angiotensin converting enzyme to bradykinin inactivation in isolated lungs. Br J Pharmacol 59:123–128, 1977.
10. Barstad RM, Ovrum E, Ringdal M-AL, et al: Induction of monocyte tissue factor procoagulant activity during coronary artery bypass surgery is reduced with heparin-coated extracorporeal circuit. B J Haematol 94:517–525, 1996.
11. Bartels C, Gerdes A, Babin-Ebell J, et al: Cardiopulmonary bypass: evidence or experience based? J Thorac Cardiovasc Surg 124:20–27, 2002.
12. Baufreton C, Jansen PG, Le Besnerais P, et al: Heparin coating with aprotinin reduces blood activation during coronary artery operations. Ann Thorac Surg 63:50–56, 1997.
13. Benaroia M, Baker AJ, Mazer CD, Errett L: Effect of aortic cannula characteristics and blood velocity on transcranial Doppler-detected microemboli during cardiopulmonary bypass. J Cardiothorac Vasc Anesth 12:266–269, 1998.
14. Bigelow WG, Calaghan JC, Hopps JA: General hypothermia for experimental intra-cardiac surgery. Ann Surg 132:531–539, 1950.
15. Blauth C, Kohner EM, Arnold J, Taylor KM: Retinal microembolism during cardiopulmonary bypass demonstrated by fluorescein angiography. Lancet 2:837–839, 1986.
16. Borger MA, Feindel CM: Cerebral emboli during cardiopulmonary bypass: effect of perfusionist interventions and aortic cannulas. J Extra Corpor Technol 34:29–33, 2002.
17. Borowicz LM, Goldsborough MA, Seines OA, McKhann GM: Neuropsychologic change after cardiac surgery: a critical review. J Cardiothorac Vasc Anesth 10:105–112, 1996.
18. Brooker RF, Brown WR, Moody DM, et al: Cardiotomy suction: a major source of brain lipid emboli during cardiopulmonary bypass. Ann Thorac Surg 65:1651–1655, 1998.
19. Brown WR, Moody DM, Challa VR, et al: Longer duration of cardiopulmonary bypass is associated with greater numbers of cerebral microemboli. Stroke 31:707–713, 2000.
20. Campbell EJ, O'Byrne V, Stratford PW, et al: Biocompatible surfaces using methacryloylphosrylcholine laurylmethacrylate copolymer. ASAIO J 40:M853–M857, 1994.
21. Campbell FW: The contribution of platelet dysfunction to postbypass bleeding. J Cardiothorac Vasc Anaesth 5:8–12, 1991.
22. Carney DE, Lutz CJ, Picone AL, et al: Matrix metalloproteinase inhibitor prevents acute lung injury after cardiopulmonary bypass. Circulation 100:400–406, 1999.
23. Chaney MA, Nikolov MP, Blakeman B, et al: Pulmonary effects of methylprednisolone in patients undergoing coronary artery bypass grafting and early tracheal extubation. Anesth Analg 87:27–33, 1998.
24. Chenoweth DE, Cooper SW, Hugli TE, et al: Complement activation during cardiopulmonary bypass: evidence for generation of C3a and C5a anaphylatoxins. N Engl J Med 304:497–503, 1981.
25. Cooper JR Jr, Giesecke NM: Hemodilution and priming solutions. In Gravlee GP, Davis RF, Kurusz M, Utley JR, editors: Cardiopulmonary Bypass: Principles and Practice. Philadelphia: Lippincott, Williams & Wilkins, 2000, pp. 186–196.
26. Cosgrove DM, Loop FD, Lytle BW, et al: Determinants of blood utilization during myocardial revascularization. Ann Thorac Surg 40:380–384, 1985.
27. Cox CM, Ascione R, Cohen AM, et al: Effect of cardiopulmonary bypass on pulmonary gas exchange: a prospective randomized study. Ann Thorac Surg 69:140–145, 2000.
28. Davies LK: Hypothermia: physiology and clinical use. In Gravlee GP, Davis RF, Kurusz M, Utley JR, editors: Cardiopulmonary Bypass: Principles and Practice. Philadelphia: Lippincott, Williams & Wilkins, 2000, pp. 197–213.
29. DeFoe GR, Ross CS, Olmstead EM, et al: Lowest hematocrit on bypass and adverse outcomes associated with coronary

artery bypass grafting. Northern New England Cardiovascular Disease Study Group. Ann Thorac Surg 71:769–776, 2001.

30. Defraigne JO, Pincemail J, Dekoster G, et al: SMA circuits reduce platelet consumption and platelet factor release during cardiac surgery. Ann Thorac Surg 70:2075–2081, 2000.

31. de Haan J, Boonstra PW, Monnink SHJ, et al: Retransfusion of suctioned blood during cardiopulmonary bypass impairs hemostasis. Ann Thorac Surg 59:901–907, 1995.

32. Dehmer GJ, Fisher M, Tate DA, et al: Reversal of heparin anticoagulation by recombinant platelet factor 4 in humans. Circulation 91:2188–2194, 1995.

33. Denizot Y, Feiss P, Nathan N: Are lipid mediators implicated in the production of pro- and anti-inflammatory cytokines during cardiopulmonary bypass graft with extracorporeal circulation? Cytokine 11:301–304, 1999.

34. De Somer F, Francois K, van Oeveren W, et al: Phosphorylcholine coating of extracorporeal circuits provides natural protection against blood activation by the material surface. Eur J Cardiothorac Surg 18:602–606, 2000.

35. Despotis GJ, Summerfield AL, Joist JH, et al: Comparison of activated coagulation time and whole blood heparin measurements with laboratory plasma anti-Xa heparin concentration in patients having cardiac operations. J Thorac Cardiovasc Surg 108:1076–1082, 1994.

36. Despotis GJ, Joist JH, Hogue CW, et al: More effective suppression of hemostatic system activation in patients undergoing cardiac surgery by heparin dosing based on heparin blood concentrations rather than ACT. Thromb Haemost 76:902–908, 1996.

37. de Swart CA, Nijmeyer B, Roelofs JM, Sixma JJ: Kinetics of intravenously administered heparin in normal humans. Blood 60:1251–1258, 1982.

38. DeWall RA, Grage TB, McFee AS, Chiechi MA: Theme and variations on blood oxygenators. I. Bubble oxygenators. Surgery 50:931–940, 1961.

39. Diego RP, Mihalakakos PJ, Hexum TD, Hill GE: Methylprednisolone and full-dose aprotinin reduce reperfusion injury after cardiopulmonary bypass. J Cardiothorac Vasc Anesth 11:29–31, 1997.

40. Ernofsson M, Thelin S, Siegbahn A: Monocyte tissue factor expression, cell activation, and thrombin formation during cardiopulmonary bypass: a clinical study. J Thorac Cardiovasc Surg 113:576–584, 1997.

41. Fang WC, Helm RE, Krieger KH, Rosengart TK, et al: Impact of minimum hematocrit during cardiopulmonary bypass on mortality in patients undergoing coronary artery surgery. Circulation 96:II-194–II-199, 1997.

42. Faymonville ME, Deby-Dupont G, Larbuisson R, et al: Prostaglandin E2, prostacyclin, and thromboxane changes during nonpulsatile cardiopulmonary bypass in humans. J Thorac Cardiovasc Surg 91:858–866, 1986.

43. Fearon DT: Identification of the membrane glycoprotein that is the C3b receptor of the human erythrocyte, polymorphonuclear leukocyte, B lymphocyte, and monocyte. J Exp Med 152:20–30, 1980.

44. Ferraris VA, Ferraris SP, Singh A, et al: The platelet thrombin receptor and postoperative bleeding. Ann Thorac Surg 65:352–358, 1998.

45. Finkel MS, Oddis CV, Jacob TD, et al: Negative inotropic effects of cytokines on the heart mediated by nitric oxide. Science 257:387–389, 1992.

46. Furukawa K, Ohteki H, Hirahara K, et al: The use of argatroban as an anticoagulant for cardiopulmonary bypass in cardiac operations. J Thorac Cardiovasc Surg 122:1255–1256, 2001.

47. Gluszko P, Rucinski B, Musial J, et al: Fibrinogen receptors in platelet adhesion to surfaces of extracorporeal circuit. Am J Physiol 252:H615–H621, 1987.

48. Gold JP, Charlson ME, Williams-Russo P, et al: Improvement of outcomes after coronary artery bypass. A randomized trial comparing intraoperative high versus low mean arterial pressure. J Thorac Cardiovasc Surg 110:1302–1311, 1995.

49. Gormley SM, McBride WT, Armstrong MA, et al: Plasma and urinary cytokine homeostasis and renal dysfunction during cardiac surgery. Anesthesiology 93:1210–1216, 2000.

50. Gott VL, Whiffen JD, Dutton RC: Heparin bonding on colloidal graphite surfaces. Science 14:1297–1298, 1963.

51. Grossi EA, Kanchuger MS, Schwartz DS, et al: Effect of cannula length on aortic arch flow: protection of the atheromatous aortic arch. Ann Thorac Surg 59:710–712, 1995.

52. Hagl S, Heimisch W, Meisner H, et al: The effect of hemodilution on regional myocardial function in the presence of coronary stenosis. Basic Res Cardiol 72:344–364, 1977.

53. Halpenny M, Lakshmi S, O'Donnell A, et al: Fenoldopam: renal and splanchnic effects in patients undergoing coronary artery bypass grafting. Anaesthesia 56:953–960, 2001.

54. Hardy JF, Belisle S, Robitaille D, et al: Measurement of heparin concentration in whole blood with the HepCon/HMS device does not agree with laboratory determination of plasma heparin concentration using a chromogenic substrate for activated factor X. J Thorac Cardiovasc Surg 112:154–161, 1996.

55. Harris DNF, Bailey SM, Smith PLC, et al: Brain swelling in first hour after coronary artery bypass surgery. Lancet 342:586–587, 1993.

56. Hashemi S, Palmer DS, Aye MT, Ganz PR: Molecular mechanisms of cellular responses to DDAVP. In Mariani G, editor: Desmopressin in Bleeding Disorders. New York: Plenum press, 1992, pp. 43–56.

57. Hennein HA, Ebba H, Rodriguez JL, et al: Relationship of the proinflammatory cytokines to myocardial ischemia and dysfunction after uncomplicated coronary revascularization. J Thorac Cardiovasc Surg 108:626–635, 1994.

58. Hessel EA, Hill AG: Circuitry and cannulation techniques. In Gravlee GP, Davis RF, Kurusz M, Utley JR, editors: Cardiopulmonary Bypass: Principles and Practice. Philadelphia: Lippincott, Williams & Wilkins, 2000, pp. 69–97.

59. Hill GE, Alonso A, Thiele GM, Robbins RA: Glucocorticoids blunt neutrophil CD11b surface glycoprotein upregulation during cardiopulmonary bypass in humans. Anesth Analg 79:23–27, 1994.

60. Hill GE, Snider S, Galbraith TA, et al: Glucocorticoid reduction of bronchial epithelial inflammation during cardiopulmonary bypass. Am J Respir Crit Care Med 152: 1791–1795, 1995.

61. Hogue CW Jr, Barzilai B, Pieper KS, et al: Sex differences in neurological outcomes and mortality after cardiac surgery: a society of thoracic surgery national database report. Circulation 103:2133–2137, 2001.

62. Homeister JW, Satoh P, Lucchesi BR: Effects of complement activation in the isolated heart. Role of the terminal complement components. Circ Res 71:303–319, 1992.

63. Horrow JC: Protamine: a review of its toxicity. Anesth Analg 64:348–361, 1985.

64. Ichinose A, Kisiel W, Fujikawa K: Proteolytic activation of tissue plasminogen activator by plasma and tissue enzymes. FEBS Lett 175:412–418, 1984.

65. Inaba H, Kochi A, Yorozu S: Suppression by methylprednisolone of augmented plasma endotoxin-like activity and interleukin-6 during cardiopulmonary bypass. Br J Anaesth 72:348–350, 1994.

66. Jansen NJ, van Oeveren W, van den BL, et al: Inhibition by dexamethasone of the reperfusion phenomena in cardiopulmonary bypass. J Thorac Cardiovasc Surg 102:515–525, 1991.

67. Jansen NJ, van Oeveren W, van Vliet M, et al: The role of different types of corticosteroids on the inflammatory mediators

1078

in cardiopulmonary bypass. Eur J Cardiothorac Surg 5: 211–217, 1991.

68. Johnson D, Thomson D, Hurst T, et al: Neutrophil-mediated acute lung injury after extracorporeal perfusion. J Thorac Cardiovasc Surg 107:1193–1202, 1994.

69. Kamitani T, Little MH, Ellis EF: Evidence for a possible role of the brain kallikrein-kinin system in the modulation of the cerebral circulation. Circ Res 57:545–552, 1985.

70. Kappa JR, Fisher CA, Todd B, et al: Intraoperative management of patients with heparin-induced thrombocytopenia. Ann Thorac Surg 49:714–722, 1990.

71. Kaul TK, Swaminathan R, Chatrath RR, Watson DA: Vasoactive pressure hormones during and after cardiopulmonary bypass. Int J Artif Organs 13:293–299, 1990.

72. Kawamura T, Wakusawa R, Okada K, Inada S: Elevation of cytokines during open heart surgery with cardiopulmonary bypass: participation of interleukin 8 and 6 in reperfusion injury. Can J Anaesth 40:1016–1021, 1993.

73. Kelton JG, Sheridan D, Santos A, et al: Heparin-induced thrombocytopenia: laborotory studies. Blood 72:925–930, 1988.

74. Khuri S, Valeri CR, Loscalzo J, et al: Heparin causes platelet dysfunction and induces fibrinolysis before cardiopulmonary bypass. Ann Thorac Surg 60:1008–1014, 1995.

75. Khuri SF, Wolfe JA, Josa M, et al: Hematologic changes during and after cardiopulmonary bypass and their relationship to the bleeding time and nonsurgical blood loss. J Thorac Cardiovasc Surg 104:94–107, 1992.

76. Kim KU, Kwon OJ, Jue DM: Pro-tumour necrosis factor cleavage enzyme in macrophage membrane/particulate. Immunology 80:134–139, 1993.

77. Kitaguchi H, Hijikata A, Hirata M: Effect of thrombin on plasminogen activator release from isolated perfused dog leg. Thromb Res 16:407–415, 1979.

78. Klein M, Mahoney CB, Probst C, et al: Blood product use during routine open heart surgery: the impact of the centrifugal pump. Artif Organs 25:300–305, 2001.

79. Kolff WJ, Berk HTJ: Artificial kidney: dialyzer with great area. Acta Med Scand 117:121–134, 1944.

80. Koster A, Kuppe H, Hetzer R, et al: Emergent cardiopulmonary bypass in five patients with heparin-induced thrombocytopenia type II employing recombinant hirudin. Anesthesiology 89:777–780, 1998.

81. Kotani N, Hashimoto H, Sessler DI, et al: Cardiopulmonary bypass produces greater pulmonary than systemic proinflammatory cytokines. Anesth Analg 90:1039–1045, 2000.

82. Kotani N, Hashimoto H, Sessler DI, et al: Neutrophil number and interleukin-8 and elastase concentrations in bronchoalveolar lavage fluid correlate with decreased arterial oxygenation after cardiopulmonary bypass. Anesth Analg 90:1046–1051, 2000.

83. Kuntschen FR, Galletti PM, Hahn C: Glucose-insulin interactions during cardiopulmonary bypass. Hypothermia versus normothermia. J Thorac Cardiovasc Surg 91:451–459, 1986.

84. Kurth CD, O'Rourke MM, O'Hara IB: Comparison of pH-stat and alpha-stat cardiopulmonary bypass on cerebral oxygenation and blood flow in relation to hypothermic circulatory arrest in piglets. Anesthesiology 89:110–118, 1998.

85. Loef BG, Epema AH, Navis G, et al: Off-pump coronary revascularization attenuates transient renal damage compared with on-pump coronary revascularization. Chest 121:1190–1194, 2002.

86. Loer SA, Kalweit G, Tarnow J: Effects of ventilation and nonventilation on pulmonary venous blood gases and markers of lung hypoxia in humans undergoing total cardiopulmonary bypass. Crit Care Med 28:1336–1340, 2000.

87. Lu H, Soria C, Cramer EM, et al: Temperature dependence of plasmin-induced activation or inhibition of human platelets. Blood 77:996–1005, 1991.

88. Magnani HN: Heparin-induced thrombocytopenia (HIT): an overview of 230 patients treated with organan (Org 10172). Thromb Haemost 70:554–561, 1993.

89. Mahoney CB: Heparin-bonded circuits: clinical outcomes and costs. Perfusion 13:192–204, 1988.

90. Man WK, Brannan JJ, Fessatidis I, et al: Effect of prostacyclin on the circulatory histamine during cardiopulmonary bypass. Agents Actions 18:182–185, 1986.

91. Mangano CM, Diamondstone LS, Ramsay JG, et al: Renal dysfunction after myocardial revascularization: risk factors, adverse outcomes, and hospital resource utilization. The Multicenter Study of Perioperative Ischemia Research Group. Ann Intern Med 128:194–203, 1998.

92. Matheis G, Sherman MP, Buckberg GD, et al: Role of L-arginine-nitric oxide pathway in myocardial reoxygenation injury. Am J Physiol 262:H616–H620, 1992.

93. Mayumi H, Matsui K, Matsuzaki K, et al: Cellular kinetics of posttransfusion graft-versus-host disease after heart operations. J Thorac Cardiovasc Surg 108:179–182, 1994.

94. Mayumi H, Zhang QW, Nakashima A, et al: Synergistic immunosuppression caused by high-dose methylprednisolone and cardiopulmonary bypass. Ann Thorac Surg 63:129–137, 1997.

95. Mazer CD, Hornstein A, Freedman J: Platelet activation in warm and cold heart surgery. Ann Thorac Surg 59:1481–1486, 1995.

96. McKenna R, Bachmann F, Whittaker B, et al: The hemostatic mechanism after open-heart surgery. II. Frequency of abnormal platelet functions during and after extracorporeal circulation. J Thorac Cardiovasc Surg 70:298–308, 1975.

97. Menasche P, Peynet J, Haeffner-Cavaillon N, et al: Influence of temperature on neutrophil trafficking during clinical cardiopulmonary bypass. Circulation 92:II334–II340, 1995.

98. Messent M, Sullivan K, Keogh BF, et al: Adult respiratory distress syndrome following cardiopulmonary bypass: incidence and prediction. Anaesthesia 47:267–268, 1992.

99. Moen O, Høgåsen K, Fosse E, et al: Attenuation of changes in leukocyte surface markers and complement activation with heparin-coated cardiopulmonary bypass. Ann Thorac Surg 63:105–111, 1997.

100. Mombouli JV, Vanhoutte PM: Endothelial dysfunction: from physiology to therapy. J Mol Cell Cardiol 31:61–74, 1999.

101. Moncada S, Higgs A: The L-arginine-nitric oxide pathway. N Engl J Med 329:2002–2012, 1993.

102. Moody DM, Bell MA, Challa VR, et al: Brain microemboli during cardiac surgery or aortography. Ann Neurol 28:477–486, 1990.

103. Morel DR, Zapol WM, Thomas SJ, et al: C5a and thromboxane generation associated with pulmonary vaso- and bronchoconstriction during protamine reversal of heparin. Anesthesiology 66:597–604, 1987.

104. Muriithi EW, Belcher PR, Day SP, et al: Heparin-induced platelet dysfunction and cardiopulmonary bypass. Ann Thorac Surg 69:1827–1832, 2000.

105. Murkin JM, Farrar JK, Tweed WA, et al: Cerebral autoregulation and flow/metabolism coupling during cardiopulmonary bypass: the influence of $PaCO_2$. Anesth Analg 66:825–832, 1987.

106. Murkin JM, Martzke JS, Buchan AM, Bentley C: A randomized study of perfusion technique and pH management strategy in 316 patients undergoing coronary artery bypass surgery. J Thorac Cardiovasc Surg 110:349–362, 1995.

107. Newman M, Frasco P, Kern F, et al: Central nervous system dysfunction after cardiac surgery. Adv Card Surg 3:243–284, 1992.

108. Newman MF, Kirchner JL, Phillips-Bute B, et al: Longitudinal assessment of neurocognitive function after coronary-artery bypass surgery. N Engl J Med 344:395–402, 2001.

109. Ng CS, Wan S, Yim AP, Arifi AA: Pulmonary dysfunction after cardiac surgery. Chest 121:1269–1277, 2002.

110. Ofosu FA, Hirsh J, Esmon CT, et al: Unfractionated heparin inhibits thrombin-catalysed amplification reactions of coagulation more efficiently than those catalysed by factor Xa. Biochem J 257:143–150, 1989.

111. Olson ST, Sheffer R, Francis AM: High molecular weight kininogen potentiates the heparin-accelerated inhibition of plasma kallikrein by antithrombin: role for antithrombin in the regulation of kallikrein. Biochemistry 32:12136–12147, 1993.

112. Osborn L: Leukocyte adhesion to endothelium in inflammation. Cell 62:3–6, 1990.

113. Palanzo DA, Manley NJ, Montesano RM, et al: Clinical evaluation of the LeukoGuard (LG-6) arterial line filter for routine open-heart surgery. Perfusion 8:489–496, 1993.

114. Parratt R, Hunt BJ: Direct activation of factor X by monocytes occurs during cardiopulmonary bypass. Br J Haematol 101:40–46, 1998.

115. Pixley RA, Schapira M, Colman RW: Effect of heparin on the inactivation rate of human activated factor XII by antithrombin III. Blood 66:198–203, 1985.

116. Potzsch B, Madlener K, Seelig C, et al: Monitoring of r-hirudin anticoagulation during cardiopulmonary bypass—assessment of the whole blood ecarin clotting time. Thromb Haemostas 77:920–925, 1997.

117. Powell H, Castell LM, Parry-Billings M, et al: Growth hormone suppression and glutamine flux associated with cardiac surgery. Clin Physiol 14:569–580, 1994.

118. Pullicino EA, Carli F, Poole S, et al: The relationship between the circulating concentrations of interleukin 6 (IL-6), tumor necrosis factor (TNF) and the acute phase response to elective surgery and accidental injury. Lymphokine Res 9: 231–238, 1990.

119. Rady MY, Ryan T, Starr NJ: Early onset of acute pulmonary dysfunction after cardiovascular surgery: risk factors and clinical outcome. Crit Care Med 25:1831–1839, 1997.

120. Raff H, Norton AJ, Flemma RJ, Findling JW: Inhibition of the adrenocorticotropin response to surgery in humans: interaction between dexamethasone and fentanyl. J Clin Endocrinol Metab 65:295–298, 1987.

121. Ranucci M, Mazzucco A, Pessotto R, et al: Heparin-coated circuits for high-risk patients: a multicenter, prospective, randomized trial. Ann Thorac Surg 67:994–1000, 1999.

122. Reves JG, White WD, Amory DW: Improvement of outcomes after coronary artery bypass. J Thorac Cardiovasc Surg 113:1118–1120, 1997.

123. Richter JA, Meisner H, Tassani P, et al: Drew-Anderson technique attenuates systemic inflammatory response syndrome and improves respiratory function after coronary artery bypass grafting. Ann Thorac Surg 69:77–83, 2000.

124. Rigden SP, Dillon MJ, Kind PR, et al: The beneficial effect of mannitol on postoperative renal function in children undergoing cardiopulmonary bypass surgery. Clin Nephrol 21: 148–151, 1984.

125. Rinder CS, Bonan JL, Rinder HM, et al: Cardiopulmonary bypass induces leukocyte-platelet adhesion. Blood 79: 1201–1205, 1992.

126. Roach GW, Kanchuger M, Mangano CM, et al: Adverse cerebral outcomes after coronary bypass surgery. N Engl J Med 335:1857–1863, 1996.

127. Robinson M, Blumenthal J, Burker EJ: Coronary artery bypass grafting and cognitive function: a review. J Cardiopulmon Rehab 10:180–189, 1990.

128. Roth-Isigkeit A, Dibbelt L, Eichler W, et al: Blood levels of atrial natriuretic peptide, endothelin, cortisol and ACTH in patients undergoing coronary artery bypass grafting surgery with cardiopulmonary bypass. J Endocrinol Invest 24: 777–785, 2001.

129. Rubens FD, Labow RS, Lavallee GR, et al: Hematologic evaluation of cardiopulmonary bypass circuits prepared with a novel block copolymer. Ann Thorac Surg 67:689–698, 1999.

130. Rubens FD, Sabloff M, Wells PS, Bourke M: Use of recombinant-hirudin in pulmonary thromboendarterectomy. Ann Thorac Surg 69:1942–1943, 2000.

131. Ruel M, Bianchi C, Khan TA, et al: Gene expression profile after cardiopulmonary bypass and cardioplegic arrest. J Thorac Cardiovasc Surg 126: 1521–1530, 2003.

132. Schindler R, Mancilla J, Endres S, et al: Correlations and interactions in the production of interleukin-6 (IL-6), IL-1, and tumor necrosis factor (TNF) in human blood mononuclear cells: IL-6 suppresses IL-1 and TNF. Blood 75:40–47, 1990.

133. Scott DA, Silbert BS, Blyth C, et al: Blood loss in elective coronary artery surgery: a comparison of centrifugal versus roller pump heads during cardiopulmonary bypass. J Cardiothorac Vasc Anesth 15:322–325, 2001.

134. Sinard JM, Merz SI, Hatcher MD, et al: Evaluation of extracorporeal perfusion catheters using a standardized measurement technique—the M-number. ASAIO Trans 37:60–64, 1991.

135. Smith D, Gilbert M, Owen WG: Tissue plasminogen activator release in vivo in response to vasoactive agents. Blood 66:835–839, 1985.

136. Sotaniemi KA, Mononen H, Hokkanen TE: Long-term cerebral outcome after open heart surgery. A five year neuropsychological follow up study. Stroke 17(3):410–416, 1986.

137. Spiess BD, Ley C, Body SC, et al: Hematocrit value on intensive care unit entry influences the frequency of q-wave myocardial infarction after coronary artery bypass grafting. J Thorac Cardiovasc Surg 116:460–467, 1998.

138. Steinberg BM, Grossi EA, Schwartz DS, et al: Heparin bonding of bypass circuits reduces cytokine release during cardiopulmonary bypass. Ann Thorac Surg 60:525–529, 1995.

139. Steinberg JB, Kapelanski DP, Olson JD, Weiler JM: Cytokine and complement levels in patients undergoing cardiopulmonary bypass. J Thorac Cardiovasc Surg 106:1008–1016, 1993.

140. Suhara H, Sawa Y, Nishimura M, et al: Efficacy of a new coating material, PMEA, for cardiopulmonary bypass circuits in a porcine model. Ann Thorac Surg 71:1603–1608, 2001.

141. Tabuchi N, de Haan J, Boonstra PW, van Oeveren W: Activation of fibrinolysis in the pericardial cavity during cardiopulmonary bypass. J Thorac Cardiovasc Surg 106: 828–833, 1993.

142. Tang AT, Alexiou C, Hsu J, et al: Leukodepletion reduces renal injury in coronary revascularization: a prospective randomized study. Ann Thorac Surg 74:372–377, 2002.

143. Tassani P, Richter JA, Barankay A, et al: Does high-dose methylprednisolone in aprotinin-treated patients attenuate the systemic inflammatory response during coronary artery bypass grafting procedures? J Cardiothorac Vasc Anesth 13:165–172, 1999.

144. Tengvall P, Askendal A, Lundstrom I: Temporal studies on the deposition of complement on human colostrum IgA and serum IgG immobilized on methylated silicon. J Biomed Mater Res 35:81–92, 1997.

145. Teoh KH, Bradley CA, Gauldie J, Burrows H: Steroid inhibition of cytokine-mediated vasodilation after warm heart surgery. Circulation 92:II347–II353, 1995.

146. te Velthuis H, Baufreton C, Jansen PGM, et al: Heparin coating of extracorporeal circuits inhibits contact activation during cardiac operations. J Thorac Cardiovasc Surg 114: 117–122, 1997.

1080

147. Thrush DN, Austin D, Burdash N: Cardiopulmonary bypass temperature does not affect postoperative euthyroid sick syndrome? Chest 108:1541–1545, 1995.

148. Torii K, Iida K, Miyazaki Y, et al: Higher concentrations of matrix metalloproteinases in bronchoalveolar lavage fluid of patients with adult respiratory distress syndrome. Am J Respir Crit Care Med 155:43–46, 1997.

149. Valen G, Kaszaki J, Nagy S, Vaage J: Open heart surgery increases the levels of histamine in arterial and coronary sinus blood. Agents Actions 41:11–16, 1994.

150. van Deventer SJ, Hack CE, Wolbink CE, et al: Endotoxin-induced neutrophil activation—the role of complement revisited. Prog Clin Biol Res 367:101–109, 1991.

151. Van Dijk D, Jansen EW, Hijman R, et al: Cognitive outcome after off-pump and on-pump coronary artery bypass graft surgery: a randomized trial. JAMA 287:1405–1412, 2002.

152. Van Dijk D, Keizer AM, Diephuis JC, et al: Neurocognitive dysfunction after coronary artery bypass surgery: a systematic review. J Thorac Cardiovasc Surg 120:632–639, 2000.

153. van Overveld FJ, De Jongh RF, Jorens PG, et al: Pretreatment with methylprednisolone in coronary artery bypass grafting influences the levels of histamine and tryptase in serum but not in bronchoalveolar lavage fluid. Clin Sci (Colch) 86:49–53, 1994.

154. Wallach R, Karp RB, Reves JG, et al: Pathogenesis of paroxysmal hypertension developing during and after coronary bypass surgery: a study of hemodynamic and humoral factors. Am J Cardiol 46:559–565, 1980.

155. Ward RS, Riffle JS: Polysiloxane-polylactone block copolymers. U.S. Patent #4663413, 1987.

156. Warkentin TE, Kelton JG: Heparin-induced thrombocytopenia. Prog Hemost Thromb 10:1–34, 1991.

157. Warkentin TE, Kelton JG: Temporal aspects of heparin-induced thrombocytopenia. N Engl J Med 344:1286–1292, 2001.

158. Warkentin TE, Hayward CP, Boshkov LK, et al: Sera from patients with heparin-induced thrombocytopenia generate platelet-derived microparticles with procoagulant activity: an explanation for the thrombotic complications of heparin-induced thrombocytopenia. Blood 84:3691–3699, 1994.

159. Warkentin TE, Levine MN, Hirsh J, et al: Heparin-induced thrombocytopenia in patients treated with low-molecular-weight heparin or unfractionated heparin. N Engl J Med 332:1330–1335, 1995.

160. Weinstein GS, Zabetakis PM, Clavel A, et al: The renin-angiotensin system is not responsible for hypertension following coronary artery bypass grafting. Ann Thorac Surg 43:74–77, 1987.

161. Weitz JI, Hudoba M, Massel D, et al: Clot-bound thrombin is protected from inhibition by heparin-antithrombin III but is susceptible to inactivation by antithrombin III-independent inhibitors. J Clin Invest 86:385–391, 1990.

162. Wendel HP, Weber N, Ziemer G: Increased adsorption of high molecular weight kininogen to heparin-coated artificial surfaces and correlation to hemocompatibility. Immunopharmacology 43:149–153, 1999.

163. Wilhelm MJ, Schmid C, Kececioglu D, et al: Cardiopulmonary bypass in patients with heparin-induced thrombocytopenia using Org 10172. Ann Thorac Surg 61:920–924, 1996.

164. Wolman RL, Nussmeier NA, Aggarwal A, et al: Cerebral injury after cardiac surgery: identification of a group at extraordinary risk. Multicenter Study of Perioperative Ischemia Research Group (McSPI) and the Ischemia Research Education Foundation (IREF) Investigators. Stroke 30:514–522, 1999.

165. Woo EB, Tang AT, El Gamel A, et al: Dopamine therapy for patients at risk of renal dysfunction following cardiac surgery: science or fiction? Eur J Cardiothorac Surg 22:106–111, 2002.

166. Yilmaz M, Ener S, Akalin H, et al: Effect of low-dose methyl prednisolone on serum cytokine levels following extracorporeal circulation. Perfusion 14:201–206, 1999.

167. Ylikorkala O, Saarela E, Viinikka L: Increased prostacyclin and thromboxane production in man during cardiopulmonary bypass. J Thorac Cardiovasc Surg 82:245–247, 1981.

168. Zilla P, Fasol R, Groscurth P, et al: Blood platelets in cardiopulmonary bypass operations. Recovery occurs after initial stimulation, rather than continual activation. J Thorac Cardiovasc Surg 97:379–388, 1989.

169. Zimmerman GA, Amory DW: Transpulmonary polymorphonuclear leukocyte number after cardiopulmonary bypass. Am Rev Respir Dis 126:1097–1098, 1982.

Myocardial Protection

Sidney Levitsky and James D. McCully

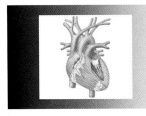

"The heart ... moves of itself and does not stop unless for ever."
Leonardo Da Vinci (Dell' Anatomia, Foglia B)

INTRODUCTION

Despite meticulous adherence to presently known principles of myocardial protection, perioperative myocardial damage related to ischemia–reperfusion injury continues to occur following cardiac operations that have been performed in a technically adequate manner. Ischemia/reperfusion injury associated with surgically induced myocardial ischemia secondary to aortic cross-clamping results from the attenuation or cessation of coronary blood flow such that oxygen delivery to the myocardium is insufficient to meet basal myocardial requirements to preserve cellular membrane stability and viability. Recovery after surgically induced ischemic arrest involves (1) resumption of normal oxidative metabolism and the restoration of myocardial energy reserves; (2) reversal of ischemia-induced cell swelling, loss of ion gradients, and adenine nucleotide losses; and (3) repair of damaged cell organelles such as mitochondria and the sarcoplasmic reticulum

HISTORICAL DEVELOPMENT

After the initiation of open heart surgery using extracorporeal circulation by Gibbon[77] it soon became obvious that aortic cross-clamping was necessary to provide a bloodless field to facilitate the precise repair of intracardiac defects, prevent air embolism when the left side of the heart was opened, and avoid a turgid myocardium resistant to retraction. To overcome the difficulties of operating on a rheumatic mitral valve in a patient with aortic regurgitation, Melrose et al[152] introduced the concept of "elective cardiac arrest" by rapidly injecting into the aortic root, after aortic cross-clamping, a 2.5% potassium citrate solution in warm blood to arrest the heart. Soon thereafter, experimental and clinical evidence[145] demonstrated the development of severe myocardial necrosis associated with the Melrose technique.

During the 1960s two distinct technical pathways for managing ischemic arrest evolved. The "rapid operators" performing uncomplicated cases with short ischemic times adopted the use of **normothermic ischemic arrest**, until operative mortalities from the "stone heart" syndrome related to ischemic contracture of the myocardium[90] associated with low levels of high-energy phosphate moieties became apparent.[41] **Intermittent aortic cross-clamping,** involving reperfusion of the coronary circulation for 5 min following 15 min of ischemic arrest, is an empirical technique, still in present use, and was based on the concept that after 15 min of ischemia, a sufficient concentration of high-energy phosphate moieties remained in the myocardium to allow for replenishment of myocardial stores during the reperfusion period.[157] Later studies demonstrated that there was no functional or metabolic advantage to intermittent reperfusion for normothermic ischemic periods up to 60 min.[55,129] Nevertheless, intermittent cross-clamping accompanied by ventricular fibrillation continues to be used for coronary artery bypass surgery with comparable results to cardioplegic techniques.[133]

Fibrillatory Arrest

Electrically induced ventricular fibrillation with coronary perfusion was introduced by Glenn and Sewell[78] and Senning[201] as a means of avoiding air embolism. However, Buckberg et al[25] and Hottenrott et al[95] demonstrated subendocardial ischemia and necrosis with this technique particularly in the hypertrophied ventricle. Later studies showed that if ventricular distention is avoided and coronary perfusion is maintained, postischemic fibrillation is not deleterious in the nonhypertrophied heart.[111] Further validation of this technique, for present use, modified by mild hypothermia and the avoidance of aortic cross-clamping has produced comparable clinical results for coronary revascularization.[1,125]

Continuous Coronary Perfusion

In an attempt to mimic the physiological state, continuous coronary perfusion with a beating heart at normothermia or mild hypothermia at 32° C to prevent the onset of ventricular fibrillation became the preferred technique of myocardial preservation in the late 1960s and early 1970s, particularly after the report by McGoon et al[147] of 100 consecutive aortic valve replacements without a mortality. If aortic valve regurgitation was present or aortic root surgery was performed, the heart was kept beating by perfusing the individual coronary arteries with cannulas inserted into the ostia. However, in reality continuous perfusion became intermittent as coronary perfusion was often discontinued to achieve better visualization of the operative field during critical portions of the procedure.[16] In addition, problems with the coronary cannula such as poor fixation, leaking associated with calcified ostia, early division of the left main coronary artery resulting in high perfusion pressure necrosis, and damage to the coronary artery such as dissection and late stenosis continued to occur.[183,204] Nevertheless, the technique of continuous coronary artery perfusion either during the performance of complex aortic root surgery or for special situations such as redo mitral valve surgery through a right thoracotomy incision after previous coronary artery revascularization with arterial conduits continues to be used.[94]

Hypothermia

The earliest attempts to perform open heart surgery before the advent of the heart–lung machine used systemic hypothermia produced by surface cooling not only to protect the heart but to protect the brain and other organs during circulatory arrest.[9,214] Hypothermia protects the ischemic myocardium by decreasing heart rate, slows the rate of high-energy phosphate degradation,[63] and decreases

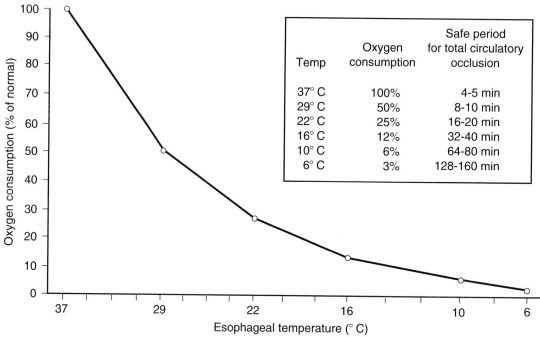

RELATIONSHIP BETWEEN BODY TEMPERATURE AND OXYGEN CONSUMPTION
(MEAN VALUE FOR 10 DOGS)

Temp	Oxygen consumption	Safe period for total circulatory occlusion
37° C	100%	4-5 min
29° C	50%	8-10 min
22° C	25%	16-20 min
16° C	12%	32-40 min
10° C	6%	64-80 min
6° C	3%	128-160 min

Figure 66–1 **Relationship between body temperature and oxygen consumption.** Relationship between temperature and oxygen consumption in dogs cooled by means of an extracorporeal pump. *(From Gordon AS, et al: Open heart surgery during deep hypothermia without an oxygenator. J Thorac Cardiovasc Surg 40:787, 1960.)*

myocardial oxygen consumption[35] (Figure 66-1[80]). However, uniform cardiac hypothermia is difficult to achieve solely by the introduction of cold intracoronary perfusates and systemic hypothermia is necessary, particularly in the presence of coronary obstruction, ventricular hypertrophy, rewarming of the right ventricle by the liver acting as a "heat sink," and environmental rewarming.[15] In an attempt to overcome this problem, Shumway et al[203] introduced the concept of **profound local (topical) hypothermia** by filling the pericardial sac with ice-cold saline and obtaining extraordinary clinical outcomes.[83] Although this technique is still utilized as an adjunct to other methods of myocardial protection, it is rarely utilized as the sole protective methodology because of the problem of warm bronchial collateral flow reaching the heart cavity resulting in transmyocardial temperature gradients and resultant ischemia.[181,188]

Reintroduction of Cardioplegia

While cardioplegia had been abandoned for alternative techniques in the United States after the adverse experience with the Melrose potassium solution, Bretschneider,[21] in Germany, continued studying induced cardiac arrest using a sodium-poor, calcium-free, procaine-containing solution (Bretschneider solution). Clinical application soon followed by Kirsch et al[106] using a magnesium aspartate–procaine solution. Hearse et al[93] introduced the concept of using an extracellular rather than an intracellular solution (St. Thomas' solution), which was first applied clinically by Braimbridge et al.[16] Based on improved clinical outcomes, North American investigators[75,128,218,235] initiated experimental studies using potassium cardioplegia followed by clinical reports[187,223] demonstrating the efficacy of cardioplegia. Over the next three decades, numerous investigators have continued their "quest for ideal myocardial protection."[57,58,89,126,146]

▶ BIOLOGY OF SURGICALLY INDUCED MYOCARDIAL ISCHEMIA

Global ischemia is not an "all or nothing" phenomenon, but rather is heterogeneous in that at any moment of time, different myocardial cells will have different extents of damage.[99,196] These changes affect cellular metabolism, ion transport, electrical activity, contractile function, vascular responsiveness, tissue ultrastructure, changes in nuclear and mitochondrial DNA, release of free radical oxygen species, and activation of inflammatory components.

Myocardial Oxygen Consumption

Because the heart is an obligate aerobic organ, it is dependent upon a continuous supply of oxygen to maintain normal function. Myocardial oxygen reserve is exhausted within 8 seconds following the onset of normothermic global ischemia.[113] Myocardial oxygen consumption (MVO_2) is compartmentalized into the oxygen needed for external work of contraction (80–90%) and the unloaded contraction such as basal metabolism, excitation-contraction coupling, and heat production.[112] A unique aspect of myocardial energetics is that 75% of the coronary arterial oxygen presented to the myocardium is extracted during a single passage

through the heart and, thus, depressed coronary venous oxygen content persists despite a wide range of cardiac workloads. Therefore, the heart is susceptible to the limitations of oxygen delivery, whereby an increase in MVO_2 can be met only by augmentation of coronary blood flow. This is diametrically opposite to skeletal muscle, where increased oxygen demand can initially be met by an increase in oxygen extraction. Clinically, a marked increase in coronary blood flow is observed at the beginning of the reperfusion period, after the aortic clamp is removed.

Biochemical Alterations

Under aerobic conditions, the heart derives its energy primarily from mitochondrial oxidative processes, utilizing a variety of substrates such as glucose, free fatty acids, lactate, pyruvate, acetate, ketone bodies, and amino acids.[61,163] However, oxidation of fatty acids provides the major source of energy production and is used in preference to carbohydrates. As tissue Po_2 falls, oxidative phosphorylation, electron transport, and mitochondrial adenosine triphosphate (ATP) production cease. Early in ischemia, the heart depends on the energy production of glycogenolysis and aerobic glycolysis (Pasteur effect). Reduced mitochondrial activity leads to the accumulation of glycolytic intermediaries, reduced NADH, and the reduction of pyruvate to lactate. The resultant severe intracellular acidosis impairs contractile function, enzyme transport, and cell membrane integrity. This results in a cellular loss of potassium and pathological accumulation of sodium, calcium, and water[176] (Figure 66-2).

Ischemia–Reperfusion Injury

Ischemia–reperfusion injury occurs as the result of attenuation or cessation of coronary blood flow such that oxygen delivery to the myocardium is insufficient to meet basal myocardial oxygen requirements to preserve cellular membrane stability and viability. The initiation of myocardial injury requires an ischemic episode that, by itself, may induce reversible and/or irreversible cellular injury.[173]

Reversible ischemia–reperfusion injury may present as either **stunning or hibernation. Stunning** "describes the mechanical dysfunction that persists after reperfusion despite the absence of myocellular damage and despite the return of normal or near-normal perfusion."[17,107] A second form of reversible ischemia–reperfusion injury is **hibernation**, which is a syndrome of reversible, chronically reduced contractile function as a result of one or more recurrent episodes of acute or persistent ischemia, referred to as "**chronic stunning.**"

As in stunning, hibernating myocardium is viable but not functional and is reversible with coronary revascularization.[18,29] There is good clinical evidence that despite seemingly adequate application of modern methods of myocardial protection, all patients undergoing cardiac surgery have varying degrees of myocardial stunning.[82,108] Evidence to support this concept is based on some patients requiring inotropic support to be separated from bypass for hours or days after surgery, who are eventually weaned from these drugs as the stunning abates, without objective evidence of a myocardial infarction.[20]

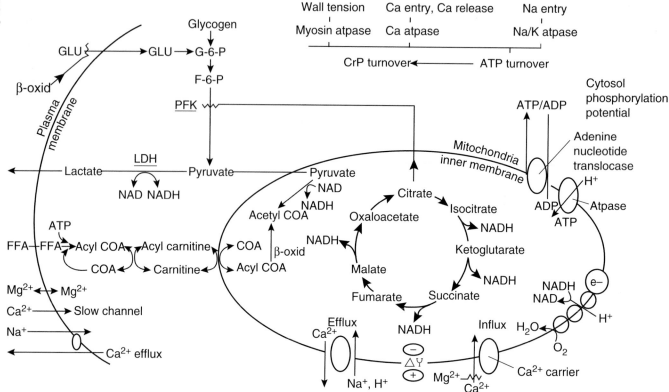

Figure 66–2 The biochemical anatomy of the normal functioning myocardial cell. The three main reactions utilizing ATP are (1) myosin ATPase involved in the development of wall tension, (2) Ca^{2+} + Mg^{2+}-ATPase involved in sequestration of Ca^{2+} that enters the cell with each beat and as well as the Ca^{2+} that is liberated from sarcoplasmic reticulum in the activation of contractile protein, and (3) Na^+ + K^+-ATPase involved in Na^+ efflux. The action of this vectorial ATPase establishes the monovalent cation gradient across the membrane that is used to maintain cell excitability and the efflux of Ca^{2+}.
(*From Feinberg H, Levitsky S: In Engelman RM, Levitsky S, editors: A Textbook of Clinical Cardioplegia. New York: Futura, 1982, pp. 131–139.*)

Two major theories have been proposed as possible mechanisms leading to ischemia–reperfusion injury (Figure 66-3).

The **calcium hypothesis** suggests that the inability of the myocyte to modulate intracellular and intraorganellar calcium homeostasis induces a cascade of events culminating in cell injury and death (Figure 66-4). Ischemia leads to the induction of metabolic acidosis and the activation of the sodium–proton exchanger resulting in the transport of hydrogen ions to the extracellular space, and the movement of sodium into the cytosol. As the sodium–calcium exchanger is activated, sodium is transported to extracellular space and calcium is taken up into the cytosol, increasing cytosolic calcium ($[Ca^{2+}]_i$) concentration. Increased $[Ca^{2+}]_i$ accumulation is also augmented by ischemia-induced depolarization of the membrane potential, which allows for the opening of the 1-type calcium channels and further calcium entry into the myocyte. Cellular and cytosolic calcium-dependent phospholipases and proteases are, in turn, activated, inducing membrane injury and the further entry of calcium into the cell. These processes alter myocardial cellular homeostasis leading to cellular dysfunction, or if of sufficient duration or intensity, cell injury or death. Alternative explanations include the concept of reperfusion-induced myocardial contracture resulting from rapid reenergization of contractile cells with persistent calcium overload affecting myofibrillar calcium sensitivity.[174] The **free radical hypothesis** suggests that the accumulation of partially reduced molecular oxygen

collectively know as reactive oxygen species (ROS) during the early stages of reperfusion causes myocardial cellular damage and cell death through microsomal peroxidation of the cellular phospholipid layer leading to loss of cellular integrity and function[13] (Figure 66-5). The generation of ROS is believed to be mediated by xanthine oxidase, activation of neutrophils, and/or dysfunction of the mitochondrial electron transport chain. It has been suggested that the generation of ROS may induce cellular membrane damage, thus facilitating calcium entry and the induction of cellular death. This later hypothesis unifies both prevailing theories and is currently considered to be valid. However, therapeutic attempts to control calcium and ROS overload have not yielded meaningful advantage.

Irreversible Cell Injury

Irreversible cell injury, described ultrastructurally by Schaper et al,[196] occurs by two morphologically distinct pathways, **necrosis** and **apoptosis.** Necrosis is initiated by noncellular mechanisms with cell swelling, depletion of ATP stores, and disruption of the cellular membrane involving fluid and electrolyte alterations.[110] In contrast, apoptosis or programmed cell death[226] is an evolution-based mode of cell death characterized by a discrete set of biochemical and morphological events involving the regulated action of catabolic enzymes (proteases and nucleases) resulting in the

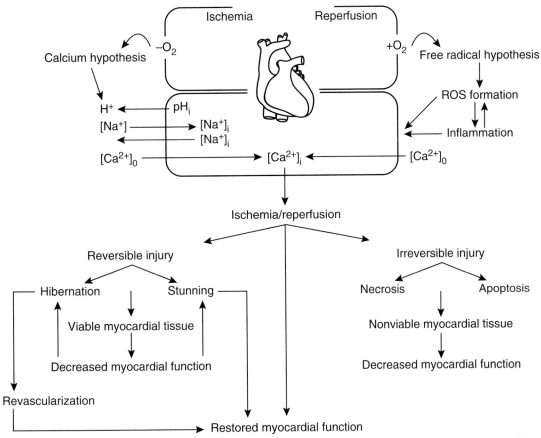

Figure 66–3 Mechanisms of ischemia–reperfusion injury. Putative mechanisms of the calcium and free radical hypotheses and inflammation in the generation of ischemia–reperfusion injury.

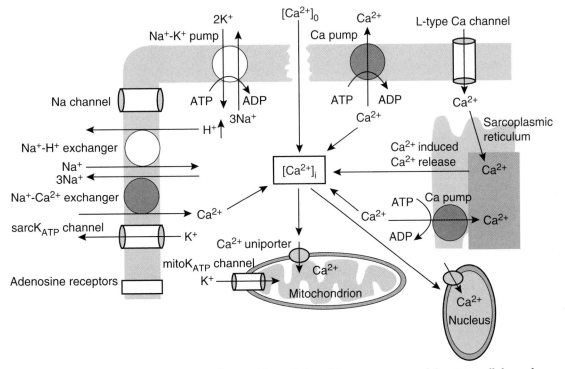

Figure 66–4 Sources of calcium regulation. The inability of the myocyte to modulate intracellular and intraorganellar calcium homeostasis during ischemia and during early reperfusion is the basis of the "calcium hypothesis" for ischemia–reperfusion injury. Increased intracellular calcium ($[Ca^{2+}]i$) induces a cascade of events culminating in increased mitochondrial and nuclear calcium accumulation and cell injury and death.

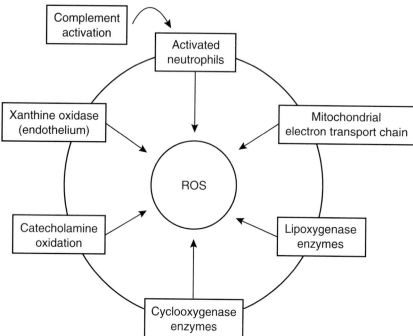

Figure 66–5 Sources of reactive oxygen species generation. The free radical hypothesis suggests that accumulation of partially reduced molecular oxygen collectively known as reactive oxygen species (ROS) during the early stages of reperfusion causes myocardial cellular damage and cell death. ROS are formed by the acquisition of a single electron making them highly reactive and cytotoxic. The major ROS in order of production are superoxide ($^\bullet OH^-$), hydrogen peroxide (H_2O_2), hydroxy radical ($^\bullet OH$), and lipid peroxides. ROS formation has been shown to cause myocellular injury through microsomal peroxidation of the cellular phospholipid layer leading to loss of cellular integrity and function.

ordered disassembly of the cell, distinct from cell death provoked by external injury.[228]

Inflammation

Inflammation has been implicated as a secondary mechanism contributing to injury following reperfusion. It is initiated through complement activation leading to the sequential formation of a membrane attack complex, which creates a cellular lesion and eventual cell lysis.[31] In addition, cytokines, vasoactive and chemotactic agents, adhesive molecule expression, and leukocyte and platelet activation participate in the inflammatory process producing cytotoxic molecules that facilitate cell death.[140,230] Oxygen-derived free radical scavengers have also been used to limit reperfusion injury.[74] Tissue factor, an inflammatory and procoagulant mediator, initiates the extrinsic coagulation cascade resulting in thrombin generation and fibrin deposition and may be related to the no-reflow phenomenon.[37] Clinical applicability of antiinflammatory agents awaits well-designed clinical trials.[6] Endothelial-dependent microvascular responses and coronary artery spasm may be related to reduced myocardial perfusion following reperfusion.[199]

Effects of Age

The vulnerability of the heart to ischemia–reperfusion injury is altered with temporal development. The newborn heart is more resistant to the effects of ischemia–reperfusion, which may be related to developmental differences in calcium transport and sequestration and is better able to restore myocardial function and myocardial high-energy phosphate stores after an ischemic event.[164,166,177] In the adult heart, functional recovery is significantly delayed, and the recovery of high-energy phosphate stores is slower in returning to preischemic levels.[232] As the heart ages there are anatomical, mechanical, ultrastructural, and biochemical alteration that

compromise the adaptive response of the heart.[143] As a result, the senescent myocardium is less tolerant to surgically induced ischemia than the mature myocardium.[160] The susceptibility of the aged myocardium to ischemia-induced injury is evident at many levels. Morphologically, left ventricular mass is increased with age, as is a reduction in the size of the left ventricular cavity, accompanied by increased calcification of the valve annulus and coronary arteries.[117] Ultrastructurally, there is decreased mitochondria to myofibril ratio, cardiac myocyte enlargement, and loss of mitochondrial organization, as well as alteration in myocardial contractile properties.[116] As a consequence of these changes, cardiac surgical operative mortality is thought to increase with age.[43]

Cyanosis

Cyanosis significantly increases the vulnerability of the myocardium to ischemia–reperfusion injury.[73,207] However, cyanotic myocardial cells exhibit normal metabolism, when provided with adequate oxygen and substrate.[71] Mortality rates in patients undergoing elective repair for tetralogy of Fallot is related to myocardial protection methodology as well as patient age, duration and extent of cyanosis, and extent of hypertrophy.[46]

Ventricular Hypertrophy

Increased myocardial mass is an adaptive response to prolonged increases in myocardial workload due to pressure or volume overload. If untreated, progressive ventricular hypertrophy results in ventricular dilatation and contractile dysfunction.[148] Hypertrophied hearts have an increased vulnerability to ischemic injury, which has been attributed to accelerated loss of high-energy phosphate moieties,[42] increased accumulation of lactate and hydrogen ions, earlier onset of ischemic contracture, and accelerated calcium overload following reperfusion.[72,209,232] With ventricular hypertrophy, epicardial coronary arteries dilate in response to increased oxygen demands, while there is a decreased capillary density and vascular dilatation reserve in the subendocardial regions resulting in increased ischemic vulnerability.[3] Subendocardial ischemia leading to necrosis can occur during periods of hypotension, inadequate cardiopulmonary bypass, and ventricular fibrillation.[26] The hypertrophied heart is particularly susceptible to ischemic injury in the early postoperative period, when hypotension associated with surgically induced myocardial stunning, hypothermia, and the presence of vasoconstrictor agents are present.

CARDIOPLEGIA: BASIC PRINCIPLES

A rational approach for protecting the heart during surgically induced ischemia must focus not only on the requirements for sustaining the ischemic cell, but must also be compatible with the technical aspects of the operative procedure. Operative procedures require a flaccid arrested heart, a bloodless operative field, and sufficient time for the satisfactory repair of complex cardiac defects. Moreover, the ability of the heart to assume normal electromechanical function adequate to support the systemic circulation must rapidly follow the ischemic interval. The need for inotropic support or mechanical support devices, (e.g., intraaortic balloon assist device, ventricular assist device, etc.,) to wean the

patient from cardiopulmonary bypass when support was not required preoperatively represents a failure of myocardial protection. Recent studies demonstrate that dopamine treatment of postischemic myocardial stunning induces apoptosis.[211] Nevertheless, despite meticulous adherence to known principles of protection, these events not infrequently and randomly occur and represent the limitations of present knowledge. Most investigators agree that the basic principles for adequate myocardial protection include (1) rapid induction of arrest, (2) mild or moderate hypothermia, (3) appropriate buffering of the cardioplegic solution, (4) avoidance of substrate depletion, and (5) attention to intracellular edema.[23,84,127]

Rapid Cardiac Arrest

Rapid cardiac arrest remains the mainstay of adequate myocardial protection and is "achieved by targeting various points in the excitation–contraction coupling pathway"[32] (Figure 66-6). The induction of immediate cardiac arrest after the aorta has been clamped minimizes the depletion of high-energy phosphate moieties by useless mechanical work. **Potassium** is the most common agent used for chemical cardioplegia and produces rapid diastolic arrest (Figure 66-7). As the extracellular potassium concentration increases, the resting myocardial cell membrane becomes **depolarized**, the voltage-dependent fast sodium channel is inactivated arresting the heart in diastole, and the slow cal-

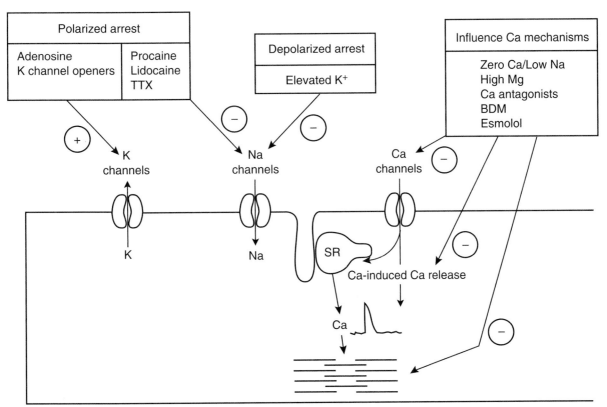

Figure 66–6 Excitation–contraction coupling in depolarized and polarized arrest. Excitation–contraction coupling and the targets within this pathway that are inhibited or activated by agents that induce depolarized arrest, polarized arrest, or arrest by influencing calcium mechanisms. BDM, 2,3-butanedione monoxime; SR, sarcoplasmic reticulum; TTX, tetrodotoxin.
(From Chambers DJ: Mechanisms and alternative methods of achieving cardiac arrest. Ann Thorac Surg 75:S661–666, 2003.)

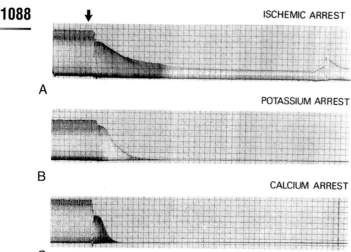

Figure 66–7 **The induction of cardiac arrest.** (**A**) By unmodified ischemia; (**B**) by potassium cardioplegia; (**C**) by calcium depletion.
(From Hearse DJ, O'Brien K, Braimbridge MV: Protection of the myocardium during ischemic arrest. Dose-response curves for procaine and lignocaine in cardioplegic solutions. J Thorac Cardiovasc Surg 81:873–879, 1981.)

cium channel is activated resulting in cytosolic calcium overload.[169,210] The optimum concentration of potassium is thought to vary between 15 and 40 mmol/liter,[194] although it has been suggested that concentrations exceeding 20 mmol/liter promote calcium overload and subsequent injury.[33] Because the heart will remain arrested until the concentration of extracellular potassium or other cardioplegic ingredient is decreased by noncoronary collateral mediastinal blood flow, reinfusions of cardioplegia are necessary every 15–30 min.[19] Clinical studies indicate that despite the infusion of large volumes of hyperkalemic cardioplegic solution for complex procedures requiring prolonged ischemic times, serum potassium levels in patients with normal renal function rarely exceed 5.5 mEq/liter, as increased potassium urinary excretion rapidly compensates for the endogenous administration of potassium.[137]

Agents inducing **polarized arrest**, where the cell membrane potential remains close to resting potential, have significant advantages by limiting ionic movement and thereby reducing myocardial energy utilization.[32] **Sodium channel blockade**, which arrests the heart by preventing the rapid sodium-induced depolarization of the action potential, includes **procaine**[91] and **tetrodotoxin**.[224] This class of drugs has been used successfully experimentally but is rarely used clinically at the present time. **Potassium channel openers** (KCOs) induce arrest by membrane hyperpolarization, couple the membrane potential to the cellular metabolic status, and afford cardioprotection by a similar mechanism associated with ischemic preconditioning.[40] Two potassium–adenosine triphosphate (K_{ATP}) channel subtypes have been shown to coexist in the myocardium with one subtype located in the sarcolemma ($sarcK_{ATP}$) membrane and the other in the inner membrane of the mitochondria ($mitoK_{ATP}$) and can be pharmacologically manipulated by openers and blockers.[84] KCOs have been used in conjunc-

tion with hyperkalemic and magnesium–containing cardioplegic solutions, although their clinical utilization remains controversial.[50,134] However, mitochondrial-specific KCOs, such as diazoxide, have been demonstrated to have potential benefits when used with magnesium-supplemented potassium cardioplegia.[141,220]

Adenosine is an endogenous nucleoside formed as a consequence of the breakdown of high-energy phosphate and is rapidly phosphorylated by adenosine kinase to adenosine monophosphate and incorporated into the high-energy phosphorus pool or deaminated by adenosine deaminase, present in erythrocytes, to inosine, which is transported from the cell.[168] Extracellular adenosine is cleared via cellular uptake, primarily by erythrocytes and vascular endothelial cells and has a reported half-life of less than 10 s in whole blood, which limits its use over a prolonged period of surgically induced ischemia.[47] Adenosine induces **hyperpolarized** cardiac arrest by antagonizing calcium channels and has been shown to inhibit both the sinoatrial and the atrioventricular nodes and atrial myocardial contraction.[54] Adenosine, by its ability to antagonize the direct depressant effects on both the sinoatrial and atrioventricular nodes and atrial tissue, results in sinus slowing and arrest. Clinically, adenosine has been used as a pretreatment before the initiation of cardiopulmonary bypass, where it has been shown to increase postoperative cardiac index and reduce creatine phosphokinase (CPK) release,[123] as an arresting agent by bolus infusion,[12] and as an additive to potassium cardioplegia, where it reduces the time to arrest[45] and reduces potassium-induced cytosolic calcium overload.[100] It may also improve functional recovery when infused during the reperfusion period.[122] When compared to the acellular St. Thomas cardioplegic solution, the addition of adenosine appeared to enhance postoperative cardiac function in a series of patients undergoing coronary revascularization.[34] Recent phase II studies suggest that adenosine may reduce postoperative complications,[154] although the results are open to question.[39]

Hypothermia

Hypothermia, whether mild (tepid at the room temperature range of 28–32° C) or moderate (22–25° C), continues to remain an indispensable adjunct for adequate myocardial protection. As noted in the historical development section, hypothermia decreases the rate of the metabolic degradation of energy stores during surgically induced ischemia. In addition, there is experimental evidence that there is a significant decrease of left ventricular myocardial oxygen consumption of the heart in the beating nonworking, fibrillating, and arrested states at 22° C as compared to a myocardial temperature of 37° C[24] (Figure 66-8). However, there is minimal advantage in reducing the myocardial temperature below 22° C, in that the myocardial oxygen consumption is decreased by only a minimal amount, from 0.31 ml at 22° C compared to 0.27 ml at 15° C of oxygen per 100 g of left ventricular tissue per minute.[22] Moreover, in the clinical setting, it is virtually impossible to maintain a uniform myocardial temperature below 22° C solely by the use of cold (4° C) intracoronary cardioplegia infusates accompanied by regional hypothermia, particularly in the presence of coronary obstructions, ventricular hypertrophy, and variations in

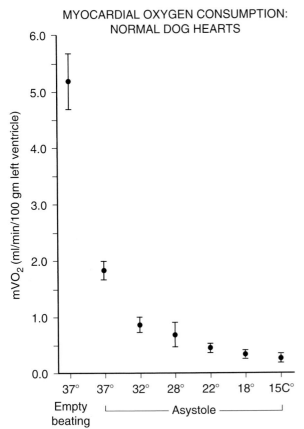

Figure 66–8 Hypothermia and myocardial oxygen consumption. Effects of hypothermia on myocardial oxygen consumption in the potassium-arrested dog heart.
(From Chitwood WR, Sink JD, Hill RC, et al: The effects of hypothermia on myocardial oxygen consumption and transmural coronary blood flow in the potassium-arrested heart. Ann Surg 190:106, 1979.)

mediastinal noncoronary collateral blood flow. In addition, the atrial and ventricular septums are warmed by systemic and pulmonary venous return, heat sinks such as the liver warm the base of the heart, and the anterior situated right ventricle is warmed by the operative environment. Because of the lack of uniformity of myocardial temperatures in various myocardial segments, there is no correlation between myocardial tissue acidosis and temperature, leading to the recent abandonment by many surgeons of routine myocardial temperature monitoring during operative procedures.[44]

Buffering of the Cardioplegic Solution

Buffering of the cardioplegic solution is necessary to combat the unremitting intracellular acidosis associated with surgically induced myocardial ischemia. Because the myocardium has the highest oxygen utilization of any organ in the body related to its concentration of mitochondria, ischemia results in the rapid accumulation of hydrogen ions and the reduction of intracellular pH, which has been quantified by the measurement of tissue P_{CO_2} and hydrogen ion using phosphorous-31 nuclear magnetic resonance spectroscopy in the laboratory and a pH probe in the operating room.[104,232] With the recent development of a myocardial tissue pH probe, there is clinical evidence that maintenance

of the tissue pH of 6.8 or greater is associated with adequate myocardial protection[105] (Figure 66-9). Thus, frequent infusions of cardioplegia, every 15–20 min, are necessary to prevent intracellular acidosis from reaching irreversible metabolic levels. In addition, hypothermia assists in the neutralization of acidosis, since pH rises 0.0134 unit for each degree decrease in degree centigrade.[192] However, the infusion of hypothermic cardioplegia does not restore pH_i to prearrest levels, but rather prevents further deterioration of the pH. When intermittent warm blood cardioplegia is used, lengthening the ischemic period progressively increases intracellular metabolic acidosis and is probably associated with increased injury during repeated episodes of normothermic arrest.[81,158] Bicarbonate, phosphate, aminosulfonic acid, tris-hydroxymethylaminomethane (THAM), and histidine buffers have all been utilized as cardioplegia additives to modulate pH.

Avoidance of Myocardial Edema

Avoidance of myocardial edema by controlling osmolarity is important to control volume regulation of the fluid compartments of the heart, since myocardial edema is a known consequence of ischemia.[121] The extent of myocardial edema has been shown to be directly modulated by osmolarity and onconicity of cardioplegia with decreases being directly associated with increased myocardial edema and impaired diastolic filling.[213] Hypotonic cardioplegic solutions cause myocardial edema,[64] while hyperosmotic cardioplegia with an osmolarity in excess of 400 mOsm/liter has been shown to cause myocardial dehydration.[234] Isotonic solutions in the range of 290–330 mOsm/liter or slightly hyperosmolar solutions appear to have the greatest clinical use, which are of particular importance when dealing with acellular cardioplegic solutions.[223] Inert sugars, including mannitol and sorbitol as well as metabolizable sugars, such as glucose and dextrose, have been used to increase osmolarity. However, when large volumes of continuous cardioplegia are administered, there is concern with producing hyperglycemia. Oncotic agents such as albumin and macromolecules, including dextrans and hydroxyethyl starches, have been used to prevent myocardial edema.[11] Besides cardioplegic infusions, hemodilution from crystalloid priming of the extracorporeal circuit, the activation of humoral and cellular mediators that increase microvascular permeability, and impairment of myocardial lymphatic function may play major roles in the development of myocardial edema. Myocardial lymphatic function is dependent upon the beating heart to transport fluid and is significantly reduced or completely stopped during cardiac arrest. Experimental evidence has indicated that during normothermic continuous antegrade blood cardioplegia, myocardial lymph flow is reduced to less than 20% of that in the normal beating heart.[149]

► ALTERNATIVE ARRESTING AGENTS AND ADDITIVES

β-Blockers

As the ascending aorta is clamped, there is the nonexocytotic release of norepinephrine from the cardiac sympathetic

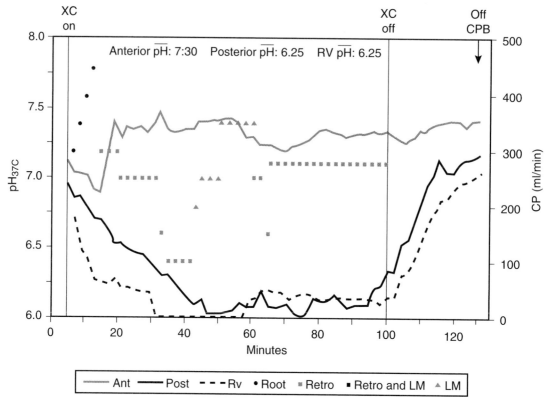

Figure 66–9 pH and myocardial protection. pH (37° C) tracing in the left ventricular wall in a 67-year-old man undergoing complex aortic valve replacement. Measurements were obtained from three sites: anterior left ventricular (LV) wall; posterior LV wall; and anterior right ventricular (RV) wall. pH_{37C} reached a low of 6.0 in the posterior LV wall and 5.8 in the RV wall. This marked discrepancy between anterior and posterior wall pH_{37C} occurred in the face of continuous delivery of blood cardioplegia at high rates, mostly through the coronary sinus. Delivering cardioplegic solutions through the ostium of the left main alone, through the coronary sinus alone, or simultaneously through the left main and coronary sinus failed to reverse the fall in pH_{37C} in the posterior LV and anterior RV walls. Integrated mean pH_{37C} during the period of aortic clamping was 7.30 in the anterior LV wall, 6.2 in the posterior LV wall, and 6.05 in the anterior RV wall, indicating poor protection of the posterior LV wall and anterior RV wall. The patient had to be defibrillated three times and required significant inotropic support to wean from cardiopulmonary bypass (CPB). He continued to require inotropic support for 24 h postoperatively.
(From Khuri SF, Josa M, Martson W, et al: First report of intramyocardial pH in man: II, Assessment of adequacy of myocardial preservation. J Thorac Cardiovasc Surg 86:667–678, 1983.)

nerves acting on β-adrenergic receptors on the outer surface of the sarcolemma, causing an increase in cAMP-dependent protein kinase activity, phosphorylation of the calcium release channels, and increased Ca^{2+} influx, resulting in increased Ca^{2+}-dependent contractility and rapid depletion of glycogen stores.[115] Early studies suggested that long acting β-blockers improved myocardial protection during ischemia, but unfortunately have a prolonged negative inotropic effect, which limits their clinical use.[135] For the most part, β-blockers, such as propranolol, have been used as an adjunct to anesthesia to block β-adrenergic-stimulating episodes associated with coronary ischemia during the course of the operative procedure. Ultrashort-acting cardioselective β-blockers such as Landiolol and esmolol provide **polarized** cardiac arrest, by maintaining the membrane potential at or near the resting membrane potential.[79] The cardioselectivity of these agents is 50–250 times that of propanolol and the half-life of esmolol is only 9 min since it is rapidly hydrolyzed by red blood cell esterase.[180] Esmolol has been used to enhance myocardial protection during intermittent arrest[8] and has been shown to provide myocardial preservation equivalent to or better than cold

crystalloid or blood cardioplegia.[51,114,151] With esmolol cardioplegia there is a slow undulating ventricular contraction, which may decrease myocardial edema, but does not provide a quiescent operating field.

Agents Affecting Calcium Transport

The infusion of **calcium-free** cardioplegic solutions induces rapid diastolic cardiac arrest by inhibiting excitation-coupling and increases permeability of the sarcolemma.[184] When a calcium-containing perfusate is then reinfused, during reperfusion, there is a rapid influx of calcium into the cell, resulting in myocardial contracture and extensive ultrastructural damage, the "calcium paradox."[102,241] Nevertheless, hypocalcemic cardioplegic solutions have been used during hypothermic arrest to prevent ischemic contracture and necrosis.[186] **Calcium antagonist** agents administered prior to ischemia have been proposed as a possible mechanism to reduce ischemic cellular injury. Calcium channel-blocking agents, including verapamil, diltiazem, and nifedipine, prevent calcium-induced calcium release in myocardial cells and as an adjunct to normothermic cardioplegia have been shown to improve postischemic systolic function.[4] Calcium blockers have no effect if administered prior to reperfusion, are temperature dependent, and have limited effect during hypothermia. Because high concentrations are required for cardioprotection, their prolonged membrane binding prevents rapid recovery, thus limiting their clinical usefulness.

Magnesium inhibits calcium entry into the cell by displacing calcium from its binding sites in the sarcolemmal membrane.[150] It has limited use as an arresting agent, because high concentrations are required, cardiac arrest is delayed, and postischemic functional recovery is decreased in comparison to potassium cardioplegia.[152] The advantages of magnesium have been shown to be optimal when included with high potassium cardioplegia, where it has been demonstrated to ameliorate cytosolic, nuclear, and mitochondrial calcium accumulation and to preserve high-energy phosphate moieties and enhance postischemic functional recovery.[92,221]

Metabolic Substrates

Metabolic substrates have been added to cardioplegic solutions to enhance anaerobic metabolism during ischemia or to provide citric acid cycle intermediaries to facilitate homeostasis during reperfusion. Agents utilized include glucose and insulin,[49,182] nucleosides[206] such as adenosine,[231] aspartate, and glutamate,[190] and L-arginine to stimulate nitric oxide production.[30] Although, metabolic substrate enhancement has been used in a variety of clinical situations, none has achieved universal adoption.

► CRYSTALLOID (ACELLULAR) AND BLOOD CARDIOPLEGIA

Crystalloid Cardioplegia

With the advent of myocardial protection, asanguineous solutions composed of varying electrolyte compositions, but always featuring hyperkalemic diastolic arrest, were clinically utilized in Europe[21,147,181] in the early 1970s and in the United States[187,235] in the late 1970s. However, these solutions contained minimal amounts (0.6 ml/100 ml at a P_{O_2} of 100 mm Hg and a temperature of 10° C) of dissolved oxygen, while the myocardium consumes 0.33 ml of oxygen per 100 g at 15° C. Because even a short period of ischemia results in the gradual accumulation of oxygen debt, moderate to severe myocardial hypothermia is necessary to prevent the rapid degradation of energy stores[56,235] (Figure 66-10). To overcome the oxygen deficit issue, oxygenation of crystalloid cardioplegia has been clinically utilized and has demonstrated a decrease in creatine kinase-MB levels in patients when the cross-clamp time exceeded 29 min compared to a group of patients who received unoxygenated cardioplegia.[85] Nevertheless, subsequent clinical studies with unoxygenated crystalloid documented significant decreases in operative mortality and perioperative myocardial infarction for coronary artery surgery as demonstrated by the large Collaborative Study in Coronary Artery Surgery.[7] For the most part, most groups, at that time, including our own, used a Ringer's solution (sodium chloride = 147.3

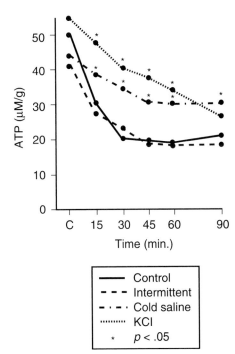

Figure 66–10 High-energy phosphates. Adenosine triphosphate (ATP) values during aortic cross-clamping (60 min) and reperfusion (30 min) for control (no treatment), intermittent reperfusion (15 min cross-clamp and 5 min reperfusion), regional hypothermia, and potassium cardioplegia.
(From Wright RN, Levitsky S, Rao KS, et al: Potassium cardioplegia: an alternative method of myocardial protection. Arch Surg 113: 976–980, 1978.)

mmol/liter, potassium = 4.02 mmol/liter, and calcium chloride = 2.25 mmol/liter) to which was added 24 mmol/liter of potassium chloride to effect a total dose of 28 mmol/liter, 7 g/liter of glucose and 0.8 ml of THAM.[208] The resultant solution had an osmolarity of 375 mOsmol/liter and a pH of 7.42 at 37° C. The classic St Thomas' solution differed by having a lower concentration of potassium chloride, 19.59 mmol/liter, and added 15.90 mmol/liter of magnesium chloride and 1 mmol/liter of procaine hydrochloride.[16]

Clinical steps utilized for myocardial protection using crystalloid cardioplegia include the following:

1. Before the onset of surgery, the operating room temperature is cooled to 63–65°F (17–19° C) to avoid warming of the anterior surface of the heart by convection and radiation from high-intensity lighting.
2. Cardiopulmonary bypass is initiated at a temperature of 28° C and a cannula is placed in the ascending aorta proximal to the aortic root for the antegrade infusion of cardioplegic solution and for the removal of air after the clamp is removed from the ascending aorta and as the patient is weaned from bypass.
3. A myocardial ECG and temperature probe are placed on the anterior wall of the right ventricle, since it constitutes two thirds of the anterior surface of the heart and its rewarming during surgically induced ischemia may partially explain the occasional observation of selective right ventricular failure following the termination of bypass.[62] In addition, an insulation pad is placed in the posterior pericardial sac and along the left ventricular lateral wall to protect the left phrenic

1092

nerve from thermal injury associated with regional hypothermia and to prevent rewarming of the heart from "heat sinks" (i.e., liver).

4. The systemic perfusate temperature is temporarily decreased to 10–15° C to "precool" the heart (infusion hypothermia), and iced saline slush is placed into the pericardial sac to achieve rapid myocardial cooling. Transient periods of ventricular fibrillation during this period of initial cooling appear to have no adverse effects.

5. When a myocardial temperature of 28° C is reached, the ascending aorta is cross-clamped and cold crystalloid cardioplegia at a temperature of 5° C is infused into the aortic root at a pressure not exceeding 90 mm Hg. The initial volume has been empirically determined to be 10 ml/kg body weight. The myocardial temperature rapidly decreases to 10–15° C and asystole usually occurs within 10–15 s.

6. At the termination of the initial cardioplegic infusion, the systemic temperature is elevated to 20° C, and the systemic perfusion flow rate is decreased from 2.2 to 1.5 liter/min/m². In this manner, the collateral aortocoronary and bronchopulmonary blood flow is kept cold and the lowered systemic perfusion pressure prevents rapid dilution and washout of the cardioplegic solution. Every 15–20 min or earlier if there is an increase in myocardial temperature above 20° C or if there is any ECG activity or observed ventricular motion the solution is reinfused at a volume of 5 ml/kg.

7. Five minutes before removal of the aortic clamp, the systemic perfusate temperature is raised to 30° C and flow is increased to 2.2 liter/min/m². After the aortic cross-clamp is removed, the perfusate temperature is raised to 38° C and the room temperature is raised to 25–30° C. Cardiopulmonary bypass is continued until the esophageal temperature is 37° C and the rectal temperature is in the range of 35–37° C. Rewarming is usually necessary in the early postoperative period.

The major disadvantage of this technique is the extensive rewarming period, which may exceed 30–45 min. Nevertheless, this prolonged period on bypass allows for the restabilization of metabolic inequities and the subsequent smooth weaning from bypass. Evidence includes clinical reports of the safe use of crystalloid cardioplegia for periods exceeding 150 min.[10] However, clinical studies evaluating myocardial metabolism and ventricular function indicate that cold crystalloid cardioplegia results in slow recovery of myocardial metabolism and a poor response to postoperative hemodynamic stress.[70] Although the vast majority of surgeons in the United States have switched to blood cardioplegia techniques, many groups throughout the world continue to use crystalloid cardioplegia and obtain excellent outcomes.

Blood Cardioplegia

In an attempt to avoid the oxygen deficits associated with crystalloid cardioplegia, blood was introduced as a suitable vehicle to obtain optimum oxygenation.[5,66] Alternative methods of increasing oxygenation, including oxygenated crystalloid,[85] fluorocarbons,[166] and stroma-free hemoglobin,[53] have never achieved significant clinical utilization. Moreover, experimentally, blood cardioplegia has been demonstrated to be superior to oxygenated crystalloid cardioplegia[112] (Figure 66-11). Besides the enhanced ability to exchange oxygen and

CARDIAC ENERGETICS

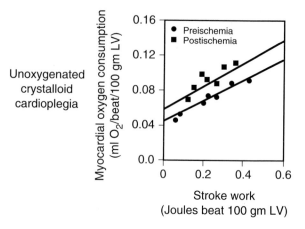

Unoxygenated crystalloid cardioplegia

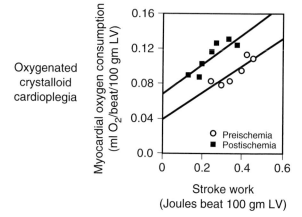

Oxygenated crystalloid cardioplegia

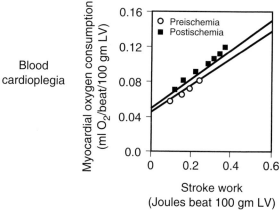

Blood cardioplegia

Figure 66–11 Myocardial oxygen consumption and stroke work. Energetic plots of myocardial oxygen consumption versus stroke work before (preischemia) and after (postischemia) unoxygenated crystalloid cardioplegia, oxygenated crystalloid cardioplegia, and blood cardioplegia. Postischemic myocardial oxygen consumption versus stroke work relationships were significantly increased with both unoxygenated crystalloid cardioplegia and oxygenated crystalloid cardioplegia arrest, whereas in blood cardioplegia the preischemia and postischemia myocardial oxygen consumption versus stroke work relationships were superimposable.

(From Krukenkamp IB, Silverman NA, Levitsky S, et al: The effect of cardioplegic oxygenation on the correlation between linearized Frank-Starling relationship and myocardial energetics in the ejecting postischemic heart. Circulation 76[Suppl. V]:V122–V128, 1987.)

carbon dioxide, the physiological advantages of blood include buffering and reducing capacity, the presence of colloid to avoid adverse oncotic pressure gradients, and the presence of oxygen free radical scavengers.[101] In addition, blood and albumin-containing crystalloid cardioplegia solutions have been shown to preserve microvascular responses compared to crystalloid cardioplegia.[200] However, concerns associated with cold blood cardioplegia include (1) the hypothermic shift to the left of the oxyhemoglobin dissociation curve, thereby reducing the release of oxygen at the tissue level, (2) experimental evidence that blood cardioplegia may not protect the myocardium at low temperatures,[136] and (3) the potential of hypothermic-induced sludging and red cell rouleau formation. Other studies have demonstrated that hypothermia at 5–10° C does not affect capillary flow[212] and that the viscosity of blood is not significantly affected by hypothermia, unless the hematocrit is greater than 50%,[139] which would be unlikely since during bypass hemodilution maintains the hematocrit in the 20–25% range. There have been numerous experimental and clinical studies advocating the superiority of either crystalloid or blood cardioplegia, without arriving at a definitive conclusion.[65,68,167,240]

The **ratio of blood to crystalloid** in formulating the blood cardioplegic solution has undergone progressive change since the initial clinical introduction of this technique. The early blood cardioplegia solutions used a ratio of four parts blood to one part crystalloid (4:1) as hemodiluted blood was withdrawn from the perfusion circuit and mixed with a crystalloid solution containing citrate-phosphate-dextrose (CPD) to lower ionic calcium, THAM for buffering, and potassium adjusted to produce a concentration of 20–30 mmol/liter to induce diastolic arrest. Experimental studies

demonstrated that a hematocrit as low as 9% provided sufficient oxygen transport at hypothermic levels of 5–10° C[98,193,205] (Figure 66-12). To avoid excessive hemodilution when administering large volumes of cardioplegia, leading to dilutional coagulopathy, the blood-to-crystalloid ratio has been gradually increased from 4:1 to 8:1. This change has been also accompanied by increased use of tepid and warm cardioplegic techniques; the associated higher temperatures require a higher hematocrit to achieve oxygen transport to support myocardial metabolism. **Miniplegia** or **whole blood cardioplegia** using minimal amounts of potassium and magnesium to achieve arrest avoids the problem of hemodilution, eliminates concerns about buffering, and avoids pharmaceutical costs.[153] Although experimental studies have not shown any significant advantage in reperfusion myocardial edema, when comparing miniplegia to 4:1 blood cardioplegia, the comparative hematocrits of 12 ± 2–7 ± 1%, respectively, used in this study, are not in the clinical range of 22–25% for miniplegia, which may have adversely affected the results.[229] However, in a clinical study comparing miniplegia to standard 4:1 blood cardioplegia, there was significantly greater myocardial oxygen consumption, lower lactate release, and better postoperative left ventricular function in the miniplegia group.[87]

Methodologies

Cardioplegia Temperature

The debate regarding the appropriate cardioplegia temperature has shifted from the classic cold (5–10° C) to warm (37° C) in the recent past and to tepid (28–32° C) at present. **Warm heart surgery** assumes that aerobic arrest, whereby the heart is electromechanically arrested and continuously perfused with warm blood cardioplegia, is the ideal state for the performance of safe cardiac surgery.[130] The apparent advantages of this technique included the presumed elimination of anaerobic ischemic injury with cross-clamp times safely extended up to 6.5 h[131]; early resumption of a normal sinus rhythm after removal of the aortic clamp; avoidance of a prolonged rewarming and reperfusion time, thus, decreasing total bypass time; and the elimination of systemic hypothermia and associated vasoconstriction in the early postoperative period. However, difficulties in visualization of the operative field, particularly when performing distal coronary anastomoses, mandated temporary discontinuation of the warm cardioplegic infusion resulting in ischemic injury if the ischemic time exceeded 15 min.[158] Additional problems include (1) ischemic injury when antegrade warm blood cardioplegia could not be delivered homogeneously in the presence of aortic insufficiency and left main coronary ostial stenosis,[159] (2) difficulties in maintaining complete electromechanical arrest, (3) the need for vasoconstrictive α-agonists during bypass to maintain adequate perfusion pressure, because of severe systemic vasodilitation,[36] and (4) the risk of neurological events related to cardiopulmonary bypass and associated microemboli, which is exacerbated if the brain is not cooled.[138] Nevertheless, warm heart surgery offered the promise to resuscitate ischemically jeopardized myocardium during the course of the operative procedure.[233] In addition, late results of the Warm Heart Trial demonstrated that late survival at 6 years was

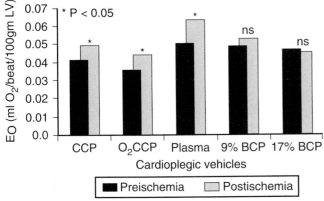

Figure 66–12 Oxygen utilization and hematocrit concentration. The increased postischemic oxygen utilization for maximally unloaded contraction (E_0) can be prevented by having a critical red cell mass in cardioplegic solution. This salutary effect of red blood cells cannot be accounted for solely by their oxygen-carrying capacity, as oxygenated crystalloid and plasma solutions did not have similar efficacy. CCP, crystalloid cardioplegia; O_2CCP, oxygenated crystalloid cardioplegia; BCP, blood cardioplegia with hematocrit of 9 and 17 volume percent.
(From Silverman NA, Del Nido P, Krukenkamp I, Levitsky S: Biologic rationale for formulation of antegrade cardioplegic solutions. In Chitwood WR, editor: Cardiac Surgery: State of the Art Reviews. Philadelphia: Hanley & Belfus, Inc., 1988, pp. 181–195.)

1094

nonsignificantly greater in the warm cardioplegia patients as compared to the cold cardioplegia group and was significantly reduced in the group with nonfatal perioperative events.[69] **Tepid (29° C) cardioplegia** was introduced as a means of overcoming the deficits of warm cardioplegia, without the adverse effects of cold cardioplegia. In a series of clinical studies, Hayashida et al[86] demonstrated that reducing the cardioplegia temperature from 37° C to 29° C did not alter myocardial oxygen consumption, reduced anaerobic lactate and acid release during arrest, and preserved myocardial function. Further postoperative cardiac function enhancement was obtained with a combination of intermittent antegrade and continuous retrograde tepid cardioplegia.[88] In a series of low-risk patients undergoing coronary artery bypass, there was no difference in cardiac troponin release, when comparing warm and tepid cardioplegia.[60] Further studies using high-risk patients with prolonged cross-clamp times may allow differentiation of these methodologies.

Delivery Systems

Numerous clinical studies have documented the efficacy of a variety of cardioplegia delivery systems and perfusion intervals. All of these reports suffer from the variability in patient disease (e.g., extent of ischemic or fibrotic myocardium and the variation in segmental coronary disease), as well as the lack of prospective, side-by-side comparisons on large numbers of patients. All of these issues contribute to the wide variety of empirical clinical choices. **Antegrade** administration of cardioplegia, using a catheter or needle, in the ascending aorta has been the initial, traditional approach. Difficulties include (1) rupture of an atherosclerotic plaque at the insertion site resulting in either microemboli or aortic dissection, (2) aortic insufficiency resulting in ventricular dilatation and inadequate flow into the coronary arteries, (3) left main ostial, occlusive, and variable coronary artery obstructions leading to cardioplegic maldistribution, and (4) enlargement of the catheter-induced aortic opening at the insertion site, particularly in association with a thin-walled aorta related to poststenotic aortic dilatation.

Retrograde perfusion of the coronary sinus, initially described by Pratt,[175] was first used clinically by Lillehei et al[132] during the early days of open heart surgery to protect the heart during aortic valve replacement. Interest was renewed with this technique after Menanche et al[154] reported improved outcomes for aortic valve replacement, prompting numerous studies on the anatomy and physiology of the coronary sinus.[161] Although most clinicians employ direct cannulation of the coronary sinus with a balloon-tipped catheter, Fabiani et al,[59] in a series of clinical studies, suggested infusion into the pressurized right atrium (obtained by occluding the vena cavae and main pulmonary artery) to impede shunting of the cardioplegic solution into the right atrium through the Thebesian veins. Major advantages of retrograde perfusion include (1) distribution of the cardioplegic solution to myocardial segments perfused by obstructed or occluded coronary arteries or the internal mammary artery during redo coronary surgery, (2) avoidance of the need for direct coronary ostial cannulation, with its attendant traumatic injury and subsequent stenotic

potential when performing aortic root procedures, (3) the ability to administer cardioplegia during mitral valve surgery without removing the retractor, (4) the ability to provide continuous cardioplegia, and (5) the avoidance of debris and subsequent embolization from atheromatous vein graft material during redo coronary surgery. However, problems associated with retrograde cardioplegia include (1) slowness in achieving diastolic arrest if used for the initial introduction of cardioplegia, (2) occasional difficulty in blindly inserting the catheter into the coronary sinus, (3) easy dislocation of the catheter into the right atrium despite the use of ribbed balloon-tipped catheters, (4) traumatic injury and perforation during insertion of the catheter and occasionally spontaneous rupture of the great cardiac vein in fragile elderly patients even with auto-inflatable balloon-tipped catheters, and (5) inadequate perfusion of the right ventricle and posterior ventricular septum[14,28] (Figure 66-13). Major technical issues include the requirement for constant measurement of coronary sinus pressure to avoid infusion pressures exceeding 30 mm Hg and never exceeding an infusion rate greater than 200 ml/min, since venovenous anastomoses and shunts at higher flows will direct over 60% of the potential "nutrient flow" into the ventricular cavities via the Thebesian channels.[97,237]

Descriptions of the **simultaneous** delivery of cardioplegia have been confused by variations in the definition of the methodology. Most authors have avoided delivering cardioplegia solution simultaneously into the coronary sinus and the aortic root to avoid excessive pressurization with subsequent injury to the coronary microvasculature and to allow rapid egress of the solution.[202] Delivery of cardioplegia through the coronary sinus (retrograde) and concurrently antegrade through each completed vein graft using a manifold with multiple sidearms and a single pump head, in association with venting of the aortic root, has been designated **combination** delivery.[38] This technique has been especially useful after completion of all the distal anastomoses during coronary revascularization as the proximal anastomoses are being performed or during closure of the

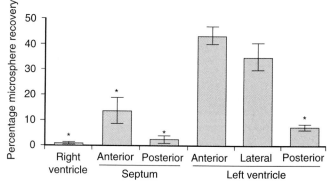

Figure 66–13 Warm retrograde cardioplegia distribution. Percentage microsphere recovery according to anatomical site. Data are presented as the mean ± the standard error of the mean. The asterisk denotes $p < .01$ versus the anterior left ventricle (post hoc Tukey test).
(From Calderone CA, Krukankamp IB, Misare BD, et al: Warm retrograde cardioplegia distribution. Ann Thorac Surg 57;403–406, 1994.)

left atrium or aortotomy during valve surgery and, if performed at 37°C for approximately 20 min, is essentially the first stage of reperfusion and allows for the restoration of postischemic oxygen uptake to return to baseline levels.[2] For the most part most surgeons utilize all of these techniques, termed **integrated cardioplegia**, which involves **antegrade, retrograde**, and **combination delivery systems** in either a **continuous** or **alternate manner**, depending on the clinical circumstances.

Warm induction utilizing warm oxygenated cardioplegia has been suggested as a means of achieving "active resuscitation" in energy-depleted hearts, before proceeding with maintenance cardioplegia by any means or temperature level.[191] Whether 5 min is sufficient time to reverse the adverse biochemical effects of depleted high-energy phosphate stores remains open to question, although functional experimental studies demonstrate improvement.[189]

Terminal warm blood cardioplegia ("hot shot") for 3–5 min before aortic unclamping has been experimentally and clinically demonstrated to improve postbypass ventricular performance after cold maintenance blood cardioplegia.[67,215] However, a controlled trial of terminal warm cardioplegia for 5 min versus simple reperfusion did not demonstrate any advantage.[52] As with **warm induction**, the question of whether 3–5 min of warm blood reperfusion is sufficient to restore energy stores is open to question. To overcome this deficit, **combination blood cardioplegia delivery** may be the preferred approach with a better chance of restoring energy stores. On occasion, prolonged terminal warm cardioplegia may lead to intracellular potassium accumulation with resultant reperfusion asystole during the early reperfusion period and requires temporary ventricular pacing to wean the patient from bypass.[124] **Secondary cardioplegia**, which involves rearresting the heart for a prolonged (greater than 20 min) period of warm cardioplegia, is an extension of the concept of terminal warm cardioplegia and may be useful in patients difficult to wean from bypass or with uncontrolled arrhythmias.[120,185]

Clinical steps for myocardial protection using blood cardioplegia include the following:

1. Hypothermia at the initiation of cardiopulmonary bypass is avoided, and both the perfusate and cardioplegia temperature are allowed to equilibrate with room temperature (**tepid** at approximately 29° C).
2. As the ascending aorta is cross-clamped, **whole blood (miniplegia) antegrade** cardioplegia is infused into the aortic root at a rate of 100–200 ml/min at an aortic root pressure of 90 mm Hg. A potassium concentration of 28–30 mmol/liter is initially used until diastolic arrest occurs, and then the potassium concentration is gradually dialed down until the lowest concentration (usually 3–5 mmol/liter) that will maintain arrest is achieved. After 5 ml/kg is administered antegrade, an additional 5 ml/kg is administered **retrograde**.
3. The occluded or most severely stenosed coronary vessel is bypassed first.
4. After each vessel is bypassed, cardioplegia, 5 ml/kg, is infused simultaneously down the conduit(s) in an antegrade direction and the retrograde cannula using a single pump head with a multiport manifold.
5. After completion of the last bypass graft, systemic perfusate and cardioplegia rewarming is initiated. The proximal bypass

grafts are inserted on the ascending aorta as blood is aspirated from the aorta so as to maintain a level of blood just below the opening in the aorta to avoid obscuring the operative field.
6. As the last proximal anastomosis is completed, potassium is discontinued in the retrograde infusion and whole blood is infused to wash out potassium. Air is evacuated from both the aorta and ventricles as the heart starts to contract and the clamp is removed from the aorta.
7. After hemostasis is confirmed, cardiopulmonary bypass is discontinued; if the heart remains in asystole, temporary atrial and ventricular pacing is instituted.

► POTENTIAL NEW TECHNOLOGIES

Ischemic Preconditioning

Ischemic preconditioning (IPC), first described by Murry et al,[162] is an adaptive response of endogenous myocardial protection, in which the imposition of one or more brief periods of sublethal ischemia (3–5 min) followed by reperfusion protects the heart such that injury manifested by infarct size, apoptosis, and reperfusion-associated arrhythmias is significantly reduced during a subsequent period of sustained ischemia.[179] The mechanism(s) by which preconditioning affords myocardial protection has yet to be elucidated, but numerous studies have indicated that IPC, in a species-dependent manner, is associated with the preservation of creatine phosphate, ATP, and intracellular pH, decreased ultrastructural abnormalities, the induction of heat shock proteins, increased release of adenosine, activation of the adenosine receptors, activation of G proteins, and activation of protein kinase C(PKC).[239] The effects of ischemic IPC are bimodal, occurring in two phases: an early phase and a delayed late phase or "second window" of cardioprotection. In the early phase the protective effects of IPC are transitory with infarct limitation being lost if the subsequent sustained ischemic insult is delayed beyond 30–120 min.[198] Approximately 24–96 h after the induction of IPC, a "second window" of less potent cardioprotection occurs in which the infarct protection is reestablished.[170]

In humans, the applicability of IPC as an adjunct to conventional cardioplegia remains to be determined.[109] Collateral evidence exists to suggest that IPC may occur in patients undergoing balloon angioplasty[48] or may be elicited by the trauma associated with the onset of cardiopulmonary bypass.[27] Experiments using *in vitro* monolayer cultures of quiescent human ventricular cardiomyocytes have shown that cellular injury is significantly decreased in preconditioned cells.[96] Results from this study indicated that 20-min ischemia and 20-min reperfusion provided the best protection from the subsequent effects of 90 min ischemia based on enzyme leakage, hydrogen ion release, and cellular viability. Yellon et al[238] have shown that in patients on cardiopulmonary bypass the use of IPC (two 3-min periods of ischemia and 2 min reperfusion) prior to 10 min of ischemia significantly preserved ATP measured during the initial reperfusion period. Additional studies also reported that the use of IPC in coronary artery bypass graft surgery significantly decreased troponin T levels at 72 h compared with cold crystalloid

1096

St Thomas' cardioplegia solution; no comparison with conventional blood cardioplegia was performed.[216] Others have reported that either IPC provided no benefit as compared to cold blood cardioplegia, because cardiopulmonary bypass per se induces preconditioning[27,76] or its use was deleterious in human cardiac surgery.[172,227]

The use of **IPC in off-pump** coronary artery bypass grafting is also, at present, controversial. Laurikka et al[119] in a randomized, controlled study induced IPC by occluding the left anterior descending coronary artery with a silicon tape placed proximal to and distal to the site of the anastomosis for two cycles of 2 min of occlusion and 3 min reperfusion; the IPC group had a significantly increased recovery of the mean stroke volume index with a significant decrease in mean heart rate on the first postoperative day and a significantly lower cardiac troponin I levels as compared to controls. Others,[171] using similar protocols, have found no statistically significant differences between the IPC and control groups. Whether **induced pharmacological preconditioning**, by adenosine,[118] adenosine enhanced by a single cycle of IPC,[144] or a combination of adenosine and diazoxide[141] and a nitric oxide donor to enhance mitochondrial potassium ATP channel opening, an essential component of IPC, will enhance mechanical induced IPC remains to be determined.[225] **Remote preconditioning**, involving the activation of the preconditioning stimulus at a distant site such as the leg or arm with subsequent transfer of nonneuronal PKC-dependent signal transduction signaling to a secondary organ such as the heart, appears to be transferred equally to the heart whether the initiating site of induction is interorgan or intraorgan, and is currently under investigation.[178]

Sodium–Hydrogen Exchangers

Sodium–hydrogen exchangers (NHE) play a central role in the regulation of intracellular sodium, calcium, pH homeostasis, and volume regulation by facilitating the electroneutral exchange of intracellular hydrogen ions for extracellular sodium ions across the cell membrane.[103] Under basal conditions, the sodium–calcium exchanger extrudes calcium to maintain normal intracellular calcium. However, during ischemia, intracellular sodium accumulates because of inactivation of the ATP-dependent sodium extrusion system. NHE-mediated sodium influx during ischemia reduces activity of the sodium–calcium exchanger resulting in a net increase in intracellular calcium, which is exacerbated during reperfusion. Consequently, inhibition of the isoform NHE-1, located on the plasma membrane of the cardiac myocyte, is thought to inhibit calcium overload and serve as a myoprotective agent.[156] The NHE isoforms can be nonspecifically inhibited by a variety of antagonists including amiloride and its 5-amino-substituted analogues as well as the benzoylguanidine derivative, cariporide (HOE-642). The use of cariporide (HOE-642) has been shown to reduce myocardial infarct size and improve postischemic functional recovery following ischemia and reperfusion.[197] The administration of NHE-1 antagonists prior to ischemia or both prior to ischemia and during reperfusion has been shown to provide significantly greater cardioprotection as compared to administration during reperfusion alone.[219] Clinical trials in patients treated for an acute myocardial infarction with coronary angioplasty using cardiac enzyme release as a biological end point have resulted in conflicting results.[195,242] In an additional randomized clinical trial (GUARDIAN) of 11,590 patients with unstable angina and non–ST-segment elevation, myocardial infarction undergoing either angioplasty or surgical revascularization, NHE inhibition with cariporide failed to reduce the incidence of myocardial infarction and death.[217] However, in a subgroup analysis of patients undergoing coronary artery bypass, there was a decrease in myocardial infarction or death 6 months postoperatively, provoking another trial limited only to patients undergoing surgical revascularization, which is at present unreported.

Molecular Manipulation

During the normal temporal development of the myocardium there is the phenotypic induction, expression, and synthesis of a defined number of genes. Under pathophysiological conditions including stress, disease, or induction resulting from intrinsic or extrinsic insult, there is an adaptive remodulation of gene synthesis that is often not initially apparent at the gross anatomical or histological level. Recent advances in molecular, cellular, and genetically based technologies have allowed these events and have allowed altered genes and gene products to be identified, which may aid in the development of new therapeutic interventions. **Apoptosis inhibitors** represent a potential therapeutic approach to limit cell death. Apoptosis has been partially alleviated under experimental conditions through the use of synthetic cell-permeable tetrapeptide caspase inhibitors, which provide irreversible inhibition of caspase activity.[236] No human studies have been reported using these modalities.

REFERENCES

1. Akins CW: Early and late results following emergency isolated myocardial revascularization during hypothermic fibrillatory arrest. Ann Thorac Surg 43:131–137, 1987.
2. Allen BS, Okamoto F, Buckberg GD, et al: XII. Considerations of reperfusion "duration" vs "dose" on regional functional, biochemical, and histochemical recovery. Studies of controlled reperfusion after ischemia: reperfusion conditions. J Thorac Cardiovasc Surg 92:594–604, 1986.
3. Archie JP, Fixler DE, Ullyot DJ, et al: Regional myocardial blood flow in lambs with concentric right ventricular hypertrophy. Circ Res 34:143–154, 1974.
4. Balderman SC, Schwartz K, Aldrich J, et al: Cardioplegic arrest of the myocardium with calcium blocking agents. J Cardiovasc Pharmacol 19:1–9, 1992.
5. Barner HB, Laks H, Codd JE, et al: Cold blood as a vehicle for potassium cardioplegia. Ann Thorac Surg 28:509–521, 1979.
6. Baxter GF: Leucocytes in myocardial ischemia/reperfusion. The neutrophil as a mediator of myocardial ischemia/reperfusion injury: time to move on. Basic Res Cardiol 97:268–275, 2002.
7. Berger RI, Davis KB, Kaiser GC, et al: Preservation of the myocardium during coronary artery bypass grafting. Circulation 64(Suppl. 2):61–66, 1981.

8. Bessho R, Chambers, DJ: Myocardial protection: The efficacy of an ultra-short-acting β-blocker, esmolol, as a cardioplegoic agent. J Thorac Cardiovasc Surg 122:993–1003, 2001.

9. Bigelow WG, Mustard WY, Evans JG: Some physiologic concepts of hypothermia and their applications to cardiac surgery. J Thorac Cardiovasc Surg 28:463–480, 1954.

10. Bleese N, Doring V, Kalmar P, et al: Clinical application of cardioplegia in aortic crossclamping periods longer than 150 minutes. Thorac Cardiovasc Surg 27:390–392, 1979.

11. Bodenhamer RM, Johnson RG, Randolph JD, et al: The effect of adding mannitol or albumin to a crystalloid cardioplegic solution: a prospective, randomized clinical study. Ann Thorac Surg 40:374–379, 1985.

12. Boehn DH, Human PA, von Oppell U, et al: Adenosine cardioplegia: reducing reperfusion injury of the ischaemic myocardium? Eur J Cardiothorac Surg 5:542–545, 1991.

13. Boli R: Causative of oxyradicals in myocardial stunning: a proven hypothesis. A brief review of the evidence demonstrating a major role of reactive oxygen species in severe forms of postischemic dysfunction. Basic Res Cardiol 93:156–162, 1998.

14. Borger MA, Wei KS, Weisel RD, et al: Myocardial perfusion during warm antegrade and retrograde cardioplegia: a contrast echo study. Ann Thorac Surg 68:955–961, 1999.

15. Borst HG, Iversen SE: Myocardial temperature in clinical cardioplegia. Thorac Cardiovasc Surg 28:29–33, 1980.

16. Braimbridge MV, Chayen J, Bitensky L, et al: Cold cardioplegia or continuous coronary perfusion? Report on preliminary clinical experience as assessed cytochemically. J Thorac Cardiovasc Surg 74:900–906, 1977.

17. Braunwald E, Kloner RA: The stunned myocardium: prolonged, post-ischemic ventricular dysfunction. Circulation 66:1146–1149, 1982.

18. Braunwald E, Rutherford JD: Reversible ischemic left ventricular dysfunction: evidence for the "hibernating myocardium." J Am Cardiol 8:1467–1470, 1986.

19. Brazier J, Hottenrott C, Buckberg GD: Noncoronary collateral myocardial blood flow. Ann Thorac Surg 19:426–435, 1975.

20. Breisblatt WM, Stein KL, Wolfe CJ, et al: Acute myocardial dysfunction and recovery: a common occurrence after coronary bypass surgery. J Am Coll Cardiol 15:1261–1269, 1990.

21. Bretschneider HJ: Uberlebenzeit und Wiederbelebungzeit des Herzens bei Normo-und Hypothermie. Veh Disch Ges Kreislaufforsch 30:11–34, 1964.

22. Bretschneider JH, Hubner G, Knoll D, et al: Myocardial resistance and tolerance to ischemia, physiological and biochemical basis. J Cardiovasc Surg (Torino) 16:241–260, 1975.

23. Buckberg GD: A proposed "solution" to the cardioplegic controversy. J Thorac Cardiovasc Surg 77:803–815, 1979.

24. Buckberg GD, Brazier JR, Nelson RL, et al: Studies of the effects of hypothermia on regional myocardial blood flow and metabolism during cardiopulmonary bypass: I. The adequately perfused beating, fibrillating and arrested heart. J Thorac Cardiovasc Surg 73:87–94, 1977.

25. Buckberg GD, Hottenrott CE: Ventricular fibrillation: its effect on myocardial flow, distribution and performance. Ann Thorac Surg 20:76–85, 1975.

26. Buckberg GD, Towers B, Paglia DE, et al: Subendocardial ischemia after cardiopulmonary bypass. J Thorac Cardiovasc Surg 64:669–684, 1972.

27. Burns PG, Krukenkamp IB, Calderone CA, et al: Does cardiopulmonary bypass alone elicit myoprotective conditioning? Circulation 92:II447–451, 1995.

28. Calderone CA, Krukankamp IB, Misare BD, et al: Perfusion deficits with retrograde warm cardioplegia. Ann Thorac Surg 57:403–406, 1994.

29. Camici PG, Rimoldi OE: Myocardial blood flow in patients with hibernating myocardium. Cardiovasc Res 57:302–311, 2003.

30. Carrier M, Khalil A, Tourigny A, et al: Effects of L-arginine on metabolic recovery of the myocardium. Ann Thorac Surg 61:1651–1657, 1996.

31. Chakraborti T, Mandal A, Mandal M, et al: Complement activation in heart disease. Cell Signal 12:607–617, 2000.

32. Chambers DJ: Mechanisms and alternative methods of achieving cardiac arrest. Ann Thorac Surg 75:S661–666, 2003.

33. Chambers DJ, Braimbridge MV: Cardioplegia with extracellular formulation. In Piper HM, Preusse CJ, editors: Ischemia-Reperfusion in Cardiac Surgery. Dordrecht: Kluwer Academic Publishers, 1993, pp. 135–179.

34. Chauhan S, Wasir HS, Bhan A, et al: Adenosine for cardioplegic induction: A comparison with St. Thomas solution. J Cardiothorac Vasc Anesth 14:21–24, 2000.

35. Chitwood WR, Sink JD, Hill RC, et al: The effects of hypothermia on myocardial oxygen consumption and transmural coronary blood flow in the potassium-arrested heart. Ann Surg 190:106–116, 1079.

36. Christakis GT, Koch JP, Deemar KA, et al: A randomized study of the effects of warm heart surgery. Ann Thorac Surg 54:449–459, 1992.

37. Chung AJ, Pohlman TH, Hampton CR, et al: Tissue factor and thrombin mediate myocardial ischemia-reperfusion injury. Ann Thorac Surg 75:S649–655, 2003.

38. Cohen G, Borger MA, Weisel RD, et al: Intraoperative myocardial protection: current trends and future prospectives. Ann Thorac Surg 68:1995–2001, 1999.

39. Cohen G, Feder-Elituv R, Iazetta J, et al: Phase 2 studies of adenosine cardioplegia. Circulation 98(Suppl. II):II225–233, 1998.

40. Cohen NM, Wise RM, Wechsler AS, et al: Elective cardiac arrest with a hyperpolarizing adenosine triphosphate-sensitive potassium channel opener: a novel form of myocardial protection? J Thorac Cardiovasc Surg 106:317–328, 1993.

41. Cooley DA, Ruel GJ, Wukasch DC: Ischemic contracture of the heart: "Stone Heart." Am J Cardiol 29:575–577, 1972.

42. Coughlin TR, Levitsky S, O'Donoghue M, et al: Evaluation of hypothermic cardioplegia in ventricular hypertrophy. Circulation 60(2 Pt. 2):164–169, 1979.

43. Dalrymple-Hay MJ, Alzetani A, Aboel-Nazar S, et al: Cardiac surgery in the elderly. Eur J Cardiothorac Surg 15:61–66, 1999.

44. Dearani JA, Axford TA, Patel MA, et al: Role of temperature measurements in monitoring the adequacy of myocardial protection during cardiac surgery. Ann Thorac Surg 72:S2235–2244, 2001.

45. de Jong JW, van der Meer P, van Loon H, et al: Adenosine as an adjunct to potassium cardioplegia: effect on function, energy metabolism, and electrophysiology. J Thorac Cardiovasc Surg 100:445–454, 1990.

46. Del Nido P, Mickle DA, Wilson DA, et al: Inadequate myocardial protection with cold cardioplegic arrest during repair of tetralogy of Fallot. J Thorac Cardiovasc Surg 95:223–229, 1988.

47. Deussen A: Metabolic flux rates of adenosine in the heart. Naumyn Schmiedebergs Arch Pharmacol 362:351–362, 2000.

48. Deutsch E, Berger M, Kussmaut WG, et al: Adaptation to ischemia during percutaneous transluminal coronary angioplasty. Clinical hemodynamic and metabolic features. Circulation 82:2044–2051, 1990.

49. Doenst T, Bothe W, Beyersdorf F: Therapy with insulin in cardiac surgery: controversies and possible solutions. Ann Thorac Surg 75:S721–728, 2003.

50. Ducko CT, Stephenson ER, Jayawant AM, et al: Potassium channel openers: are they effective as pretreatment or additives to cardioplegia? Ann Thorac Surg 69:1363–1368, 2000.

51. Ede M, Ye J, Gregorash L, et al: Beyond hyperkalemia: β-blocker-induced cardiac arrest for normothermic cardiac operations. Ann Thorac Surg 63:721–727, 1997.

52. Edwards R, Treasure T, Hossein-Nia M, et al: A controlled trial of substrate-enhanced, warm reperfusion ("hot shot") versus simple reperfusion. Ann Thorac Surg 69:334–335, 2000.

53. Elert O, Ottermann U: Cardioplegic hemoglobin perfusion for human myocardium. In Isselhard K, editor: Myocardial Protection for Cardiovascular Surgery. International Symposium, Pharmazeutische Verlagsgellschaft, 1979, pp. 134–143.

54. Ely SW, Berne RM: Protective effects of adenosine in myocardial ischemia. Circulation 85:893–904, 1992.

55. Engelman RM, Adler S, Gouge TH, et al: The effect of normothermic anoxic arrest and ventricular fibrillation on coronary blood flow distribution of the pig. J Thorac Cardiovasc Surg 69:858–869, 1975.

56. Engelman RM, Auvil J, O'Donoghue M, et al: The significance of multidose cardioplegia and hypothermia in myocardial preservation during hypothermic arrest. J Thorac Cardiovasc Surg 75:555–563, 1978.

57. Engelman RM, Levitsky S, editors: A Textbook of Clinical Cardioplegia. New York: Futura, 1982.

58. Engelman RM, Levitsky S: A Textbook of Cardioplegia for Difficult Clinical Problems. New York: Futura, 1992.

59. Fabiani J-N, Relland J, Carpentier AF: Myocardial protection via the coronary sinus in cardiac surgery: comparative evaluation of two techniques, In Mohl W, Wolner E, Gloger D, editors: The Coronary Sinus. New York: Springer-Verlag, 1984, pp. 305–311.

60. Falcoz PE, Kaili H, Chocron S, et al: Warm and tepid cardioplegia: do they provide equal myocardial protection? Ann Thorac Surg 74:2156–2160, 2002.

61. Feinberg H, Levitsky S: Biochemical rationale of cardioplegia. In Engelman RM, Levitsky S, editors: A Textbook of Clinical Cardioplegia. New York: Futura, 1982, pp. 131–139.

62. Fisk RL, Ghaswalla D, Guilbeau EJ: Asymmetrical myocardial hypothermia during hypothermic cardioplegia. Ann Thorac Surg 34:318–323, 1982.

63. Flaherty JT, Schaff HV, Goldman RA, Gott VL: Metabolic and functional effects of progressive degrees of hypothermia during global ischemia. Am J Physiol 236:H839–845, 1979.

64. Foglia RP, Steed DL, Follette DM, et al: Iatrogenic myocardial edema with potassium cardioplegia. J Thorac Cardiovasc Surg 78:217–222, 1979.

65. Follette D, Fey K, Becker H: Superiority of blood cardioplegia over asanguinous cardioplegia: experimental and clinical study. Circulation 59–60(Suppl. II):11–36, 1979.

66. Follette DM, Mulder DG, Maloney JV, et al: Advantages of of blood cardioplegia over continuous coronary perfusion to intermittent ischemia: experimental and clinical study. J Thorac Cardiovasc Surg 76:604–619, 1978.

67. Follette DM, Steel DL, Foglia RP, et al: Reduction of postischemic myocardial damage by maintaining arrest during initial reperfusion. Surg Forum 28:281–283, 1977.

68. Fremes SE, Christakis GT, Weisel RD, et al: A clinical trial of blood and crystalloid cardioplegia. J Thorac Cardiovasc Surg 88:726–741, 1984.

69. Fremes SE, Tamariz MG, Abramov D, et al: Late results of the Warm Heart Trial: the influence of nonfatal cardiac events on late survival. Circulation 102(Suppl. 3):III339–345, 2000.

70. Fremes SE, Weisel RD, Mickle DAG, et al: Myocardial metabolism and ventricular function following cold potassium cardioplegia. J Thorac Cardiovasc Surg 89:531–546, 1985.

71. Friedli B, Haenni B, Moret P: Myocardial metabolism in cyanotic congenital heart disease studied by arteriovenous differences of lactate, phosphate, and potassium at rest and during atrial pacing. Circulation 55:647–652, 1977.

72. Friehs I, del Nido PJ: Increased susceptibility of hypertrophied hearts to ischemic injury. Ann Thorac Surg 75:S678–684, 2003.

73. Fujiwara T, Kurtts T, Anderson W, et al: Myocardial protection in cyanotic neonatal lambs. J Thorac Cardiovasc Surg 96:700–710, 1988.

74. Gardner TJ, Stewart JR, Casale AS, et al: Reduction of myocardial ischemic injury with oxygen-derived free radical scavengers. Surgery 94:423–427, 1983.

75. Gay WA, Ebert PA: Functional, metabolic and morphologic effects of potassium-induced cardioplegia. Surgery 74:284–290, 1973.

76. Ghosh S, Galinanes M: Protection of the human heart with ischemic preconditioning during cardiac surgery: role of cardiopulmonary bypass. J Thorac Cardiovasc Surg 126:133–142, 2003.

77. Gibbon JH: Application of mechanical heart and lung apparatus to cardiac surgery. Minn Med 37:171–181, 1954.

78. Glenn WWL, Sewell WH: Experimental cardiac surgery. IV. The prevention of air embolism in open heart surgery; repair of interauricular septal defects. Surgery 34:195–206, 1953.

79. Gorczynske RJ: Basic pharmacology of esmolol. Am J Cardiol 56:3F–13F, 1991.

80. Gordon AS, Meyer BW, Jones JC: Open heart surgery during deep hypothermia without an oxygenator. J Thorac Cardiovasc Surg 40:787–812, 1960.

81. Graffigna ACL, Nollo G, Pederzolli C, et al: Continuous monitoring of myocardial acid-base status during intermittent warm blood cardioplegia. Eur J Cardiothorac Surg 21:995–1001, 2002.

82. Gray R, Maddhai J, Berman D, et al: Scintigraphic and hemodynamic demonstration of transient left ventricular dysfunction immediately after uncomplicated coronary artery bypass grafting. J Thorac Cardiovasc Surg 77:504–510, 1979.

83. Griepp RB, Stinson EB, Shumway NE: Profound local hypothermia for myocardial protection during open heart surgery. J Thorac Cardiovascular Surg 55:731–741, 1973.

84. Grover G: Pharmacology of ATP-sensitive potassium channel openers in models of myocardial ischemia and reperfusion. Can J Physiol Pharmacol 75:309–315, 1997.

85. Guyton RA, Dorsey LMA, Craver JM, et al: Improved myocardial recovery after cardioplegic arrest with oxygenated crystalloid solution. J Thorac Cardiovasc Surg 89:877–887, 1985.

86. Hayashida N, Ikonomidis JS, Weisel RD, et al: The optimal cardioplegic temperature. Ann Thorac Surg 58:961–971, 1994.

87. Hayashida N, Isomura T, Sato T, et al: Minimally diluted tepid blood cardioplegia. Ann Thorac Surg 65:615–621, 1998.

88. Hayashida N, Weisel RD, Shirai T, et al: Tepid antegrade and retrograde cardioplegia. Ann Thorac Surg 59:723–729, 1995.

89. Hearse DJ, Braimbridge MV, Jynge P: Protection of the Ischemic Myocardium: Cardioplegia. New York: Raven Press, 1981.

90. Hearse DJ, Garlick PB, Humphrey SM: Ischemic contracture of the myocardium: mechanisms and prevention. Am J Cardiol 39:986–993, 1977.

91. Hearse DJ, O'Brien K, Braimbridge MV: Protection of the myocardium during ischemic arrest. Dose-response curves for procaine and lignocaine in cardioplegic solutions. J Thorac Cardiovasc Surg 81:873–879, 1981.

92. Hearse DJ, Stewart DA, Braimbridge MV: Myocardial protection during ischemic cardiac arrest: the importance of magnesium in cardioplegic infusates. J Thorac Cardiovasc Surg 75:877–885, 1978.

93. Hearse DJ, Stewart DA, Braimbridge MV: Cellular protection during myocardial ischemia: the development and char-

acterization of a procedure for the induction of reversible ischemic arrest. Circulation 54:193–202, 1976.

94. Holman WL, Goldberg SP, Early LJ, et al: Right thoracotomy for mitral reoperation: analysis of technique and outcome. Ann Thorac Surg 70:1970–1973, 2000.

95. Hottenrott CE, Towers B, Kurkji HJ, et al: The hazard of ventricular fibrillation in hypertrophied ventricles during cardiopulmonary bypass. J Thorac Cardiovasc Surg 66:742–753, 1973.

96. Ikonomidis JS, Tumiati LC, Weisel RD, et al: Preconditioning of human ventricular cardiomyocytes with brief periods of simulated ischemia. Cardiovasc Res 28:1285–1291, 1994.

97. Ikonomidis JS, Yau TM, Weisel RD, et al: Optimal flow rates for retrograde warm cardioplegia. J Thorac Cardiovasc Surg 107:510–519, 1994.

98. Illes RW, Silverman NA, Krukenkamp IB, et al: A critical cell volume is necessary in oxygenated cardioplegic vehicles. Surg Forum 38:263–265, 1987.

99. Jennings RB, Ganote CE: Structural changes in myocardium during acute ischemia. Cir Res 34(Suppl. 3):156–172, 1974.

100. Jovanovic A, Alekseev AE, Lopez JR, et al: Adenosine prevents hyperkalemic-induced calcium loading in cardiac cells: relevance for cardioplegia. Ann Thorac Surg 63:153–161, 1997.

101. Julia PL, Buckberg GD, Acar C, et al: XXI, Superiority of blood cardioplegia over crystalloid cardioplegia in limiting reperfusion damage: importance of endogenous free-radical scavengers in red blood cells. Reperfusion composition. J Thorac Cardiovasc Surg 101:303–313, 1991.

102. Jynge P: Protection of the ischemic myocardium: calcium-free cardioplegic infusates and additive effects of coronary infusion and ischemia in the induction of the calcium paradox. Thorac Cardiovasc Surg 28:303–309, 1980.

103. Karmazyn M, Gan XT, Humphreys RA, et al: The Na^+-H^+ exchange: structure, regulation, and its role in heart disease. Circ Res 85:777–786, 1999.

104. Khabbaz KR, Zankoul F, Warner KG: Operative metabolic monitoring of the heart: II. Online measurement of myocardial tissue pH. Ann Thorac Surg 72:S2227–2234, 2001.

105. Khuri Sf, Josa M, MartsonW, et al: First report of intramyocardial pH in man: II, Assessment of adequacy of myocardial preservation. J Thorac Cardiovasc Surg 86:667–678, 1983.

106. Kirsch U, Rodewald G, Kalmar P: Induced ischemic arrest. J Thorac Cardiovasc Surg 63:121–130, 1972.

107. Kloner RA, Bolli R, Marban E, et al: Medical and cellular implications of stunning, hibernation and preconditioning. An NHLBI Workshop. Circulation 97:1848–1867, 1998.

108. Kloner RA, Przyklenk K, Kay GL: Clinical evidence for stunned myocardium after coronary artery bypass surgery. J Cardiac Surg 9(Suppl.):397–402, 1994.

109. Kolocassides KG, Galinanes M, Hearse DJ: Ischemic preconditioning, cardioplegia or both? Differing approaches to myocardial and vascular protection. J Mol Cell Cardiol 28:623–634, 1996.

110. Kroemer G, Reed JC: Mitochondrial control of cell death. Nat Med 6:513–519, 2000.

111. Krukenkamp IB, Badellino M, Levitsky S: Effects of ischemic ventricular fibrillation on myocardial mechanics and energetics in the porcine heart. Surg Forum 41:239–240, 1990.

112. Krukenkamp IB, Silverman NA, Levitsky S: The effect of cardioplegic oxygenation on the correlation between linearized Frank-Starling relationship and myocardial energetics in the ejecting postischemic heart. Circulation 76(Suppl. V):V122–V128, 1987.

113. Kubler W, Spieckermann PG: Regulation of glycolysis in the ischemic and anoxic myocardium. J Mol Cell Cardiol 1:351–377, 1970.

114. Kuhn-Regnier F, Natour E, Dhein S, et al: Beta-blockade versus Buckberg blood-cardioplegia in coronary bypass operation. Eur J Cardiothorac Surg 15:67–74, 1999.

115. Kurz T, Richardt G, Halg S, et al: Two different mechanisms of noradrenaline release during normoxia and simulated ischemia in human cardiac tissue. J Mol Cell Cardiol 27:1161–1172, 1995.

116. Lakatta EG: Cardiovascular regulatory mechanisms in advanced age. Physiol Rev 73:413–467, 1993.

117. Lakatta EG, Mitchell JH, Pomerance A, Rowe GG: Human aging: changes in structure and function. J Am Coll Cardiol 10:42–47, 1987.

118. Lasley RD, Konyn PJ, Hegge JO, et al: The effects of ischemic and adenosine preconditioning on interstitial fluid adenosine and myocardial infarct size. Am J Physiol 269:H1460, 1995.

119. Laurikka J, Wu Z-K, Iisalo P, et al: Regional ischemic preconditioning enhances myocardial performance in off-pump coronary artery bypass grafting. Chest 121:1183–1189, 2002.

120. Lazar HL, Buckberg GD, Manganaro AJ, et al: Reversal of ischemic damage with secondary blood cardioplegia. J Thorac Cardiovasc Surg 78:688–697, 1979.

121. Leaf A: Regulation of intracellular fluid volume and disease. Am J Med 49:291–295, 1970.

122. Ledingham S, Katayama O, Lachno D, et al: Beneficial effect of adenosine during reperfusion following prolonged cardioplegic arrest. Cardiovasc Res 24:247–253, 1990.

123. Lee HT, La Faro RJ, Reed GE: Pretreatment of human myocardium with adenosine during open heart heart surgery. J Cardiac Surg 10:665–676, 1995.

124. Levitsky S: Another look at reperfusion asystole (editorial). Ann Thorac Surg 45:471, 1988.

125. Levitsky S: Is fibrillatory arrest a rational alternative to cardioplegic arrest? (editorial) Ann Thorac Surg 43:127–128, 1987.

126. Levitsky S: Myocardial protection. Ann Thorac Surg 44:328–329, 1987.

127. Levitsky S: Intracoronary perfusates for myocardial protection (editorial). Ann Thorac Surg 24:297–298, 1977.

128. Levitsky S, Merchant FJ, Feinberg H: Effects of KCl-induced cardiac arrest on energy metabolism and contractility of ischemic dog heart. Fed Proc 33:3, 1974.

129. Levitsky S, Wright RN, Rao KS, et al: Does intermittent perfusion offer greater myocardial protection than continuous aortic cross clamping? Surgery 82:51–59, 1977.

130. Lichtenstein SV, Ashe KA, El Delati H, et al: Warm heart surgery. J Thorac Cardiovasc Surg 101:269–274, 1991.

131. Lichtenstein SV, El Dalati H, Panos A, et al: Long cross-clamp times with warm heart surgery. (letter) Lancet 1:1443, 1989.

132. Lillihei CW, Dewall RA, Gott VL, et al: The direct vision correction of calcification of calcific aortic stenosis by means of pump-oxygenator and retrograde sinus perfusion. Dis Chest 30:123–132, 1956.

133. Liu Z, Valencia O, Treasure T, et al: Cold blood cardioplegia or intermittent cross-clamping in coronary artery bypass grafting. Ann Thorac Surg 66:462–465, 1998.

134. Lopez JR, Jahangir R, Shen WK, et al: Potassium channel openers prevent potassium-induced calcium loading of cardiac cells: possible implications in cardioplegia. J Thorac Cardiovasc Surg 112:820–831, 1996.

135. Magee PG, Gardner TJ, Flaherty JT, et al: Improved myocardial protection with propranolol during induced ischemia. Circulation 62(Suppl.):I-49–56, 1980.

1100

136. Magovern GJ Jr, Flaherty JT, Gott VL, et al: Failure of blood cardioplegia to protect the myocardium at lower temperature. Circulation 66(Suppl. 2):160–167, 1982.

137. Mammana RB, Levitsky S, Beckman CB, et al: Systemic effects of multidose hypothermic potassium cardioplegia. Ann Thorac Surg 31:347–934, 1981.

138. Martin TD, Craver JM, Gott JP, et al: Prospective, randomized trial of retrograde warm blood cardioplegia: myocardial benefit and neurologic threat. Ann Thorac Surg 57:298–304, 1994.

139. Marty AT, Eraklis AJ, Pelletier GA, et al: The rheologic effects of hypothermia on blood with high hematocrit values. J Thorac Cardiovasc Surg 61:735–739, 1971.

140. Matsumura K, Jeremy RW, Schaper J, et al: Progression of myocardial necrosis during reperfusion of ischemic myocardium. Circulation 97:795–804, 1998.

141. McCully JD, Levitsky S: The mitochondrial K_{ATP} channel and cardioprotection. Ann Thorac Surg 75:S667–S673, 2003.

142. McCully JD, Levitsky S: Mechanisms of in vitro cardioprotective action of magnesium on the aging heart. Magnesium Res 7:313–328, 1997.

143. McCully JD, Levitsky S: Myocardial protection in the elderly: biology of the senescent heart. Ann NY Acad Sci 793:305–318, 1996.

144. McCully JD, Ueumatsu M, Levitsky S: Adenosine enhanced ischemic preconditioning provides myocardial protection equal to that of cold blood cardioplegia. Ann Thorac Surg 67:699–704, 1999.

145. McFarland JA, Thomas LB, Gilbert JW, et al: Myocardial necrosis following elective cardiac arrest induced with potassium citrate. J Thorac Cardiovasc Surg 64:833–839, 1960.

146. McGoon DC: The ongoing quest for ideal myocardial protection: a catalog of the recent English literature (editorial). J Thorac Cardiovasc Surg 89:639, 1985.

147. McGoon DW, Pestana C, Moffitt EA: Decreased risk of aortic valve surgery. Arch Surg 91:779–786, 1965.

148. Meerson FZ: Contracile function of the heart in hyperfunction, hypertrophy, and heart failure. Circ Res 25(Suppl. 2):9–25, 1969.

149. Mehlhorn U, Geissler HJ, Laine GA, et al: Myocardial fluid balance. Eur J Cardiothorac Surg 20:1220–1230, 2001.

150. Meissner G, Henderson JS: Rapid calcium release from cardiac sarcoplasmic reticulum vesicles is dependent on calcium and is modulated by magnesium, adenine nucleotide, and calmodulin. J Biol Chem 262:3065–3073, 1987.

151. Melhorn U: Improved myocardial protection using continuous coronary perfusion with normothermic blood and beta-blockade with esmolol. Thorac Cardiovasc Surg 45:224–231, 1997.

152. Melrose DG, Dreyer B, Bentall HH, Baker JBE: Elective cardiac arrest. Lancet 2:21–22, 1955.

153. Menarche P: Blood cardioplegia: do we still need to dilute? Ann Thorac Surg 55:177–178, 1993.

154. Menanche P, Koral S, Fauchet M, et al: Retrograde coronary sinus perfusion: a safe alternative for ensuring cardioplegic delivery in aortic valve surgery. Ann Thorac Surg 34:647–658, 1982.

155. Mentzer RM, Birjiniuk V, Khuri S, et al: Adenosine myocardial protection: preliminary results of a phase II clinical trial. Ann Surg 229:643–649, 1999.

156. Mentzer RM, Lasley RD, Jessel A, et al: Intracellular sodium hydrogen exchange inhibition and clinical myocardial protection. Ann Thorac Surg 75:S700–S708, 2003.

157. Merchant F, Feinberg H, Levitsky S: Sequential analysis of altered myocardial metabolism and contractility induced by normothermic arrest and reperfusion. J Surg Res 16:153–161, 1974.

158. Misare B, Krukenkamp IB, Calderone C, et al: Can continuous warm cardioplegia be safely interrupted? Surg Forum 43:208–210, 1992.

159. Misare BD, Krukenkamp IB, Lazar ZP, et al: Retrograde is superior to antegrade continuous warm cardioplegia for acute cardiac ischemia. Circulation 86(5 Suppl.):II393–397, 1992.

160. Misare BD, Krukenkamp IB, Levitsky S: Age-dependent sensitivity to unprotected cardiac ischemia: the senescent myocardium. J Thorac Cardiovasc Surg 103:60–65, 1992.

161. Mohl W, Wolner E, Glogar D, editors: The Coronary Sinus. New York: Springer-Verlag, 1984.

162. Murry CE, Jennings RB, Reimer KA: Preconditioning with ischemia: a delay of lethal cell injury in ischemic myocardium. Circulation 74:1124–1136, 1986.

163. Myears DW, Sobel BE, Bergmann SR: Substrate use in ischemic and reperfused canine myocardium. Am J Physiol 22:H107–114, 1987.

164. Najm HK, Wallen WJ, Belanger MP, et al: Does the degree of cyanosis affect myocardial adenosine triphosphate levels and function in children undergoing procedures for congenital heart disease? J Thoracic Cardiovasc Surg 119:515–524, 2000.

165. Nakamura H, del Nido PJ, Jimenez E, et al: Age related differences in cardiac susceptibility to ischemia/reperfusion injury. Response to deferoxamine. J Thorac Cardiovasc Surg 104:165–172, 1992.

166. Novick RJ, Stefaniszyn HJ, Michel RP, et al: Protection of the hypertrophied pig myocardium. A comparison of crystalloid, blood and Fluosol-DA cardioplegia during prolonged aortic clamping. J Thorac Cardiovasc Surg 89:547–566, 1985.

167. Nwaneri N, Levitsky S, Silverman NA, et al: Introduction of cardioplegia with blood and crystalloid potassium solutions during prolonged aortic cross clamping. Surgery 94:836–841, 1983.

168. Oldenburg O, Cohen MV, Yellon DM, et al: Mitochondrial K channels: role in cardioprotection. Cardiovasc Res 55:429–437, 2002.

169. Opie LH: Channels, pumps and exchangers. In The Heart: Physiology and Metabolism. New York: Raven Press, 1991, pp. 67–101.

170. Pagliaro P, Gattullo D, Rastaldo R, et al: Ischemic preconditioning: from the first to the second window of protection. Life Sci 69:1–15, 2001.

171. Penttila HJ, Lepojarvi MVK, Kaukoranta PK, et al: Ischemic preconditioning does not improve myocardial preservation during off-pump multivessel coronary operation. Ann Thorac Surg 75:1246–1252, 2003.

172. Perrault LP, Menasche P, Bel A, et al: Ischemic preconditioning in cardiac surgery: a word of caution. J Thorac Cardiovasc Surg 112:1378–1386, 1996.

173. Piper HM, Garcia-Dorado D: Prime causes of rapid cardiomyocyte death during reperfusion. Ann Thorac Surg 68:1913–1919, 1999.

174. Piper HM, Meuter K, Schafer C: Cellular mechanisms of ischemia-reperfusion injury. Ann Thorac Surg 75:S644–648, 2003.

175. Pratt FH: The nutrition of the heart through vessels of Thebesius and the coronary veins. Am J Physiol 1:86, 1898.

176. Pridjian A, Levitsky S, Krukenkamp I, et al: Intracellular sodium and calcium in the postischemic myocardium. Ann Thorac Surg 43:416–419, 1987.

177. Pridjian AK, Levitsky S, Krukenkamp I, et al: Developmental changes in reperfusion injury: a comparison of intracellular cation accumulation in the newborn, neonatal and adult heart. J Thorac Cardiovasc Surg 93:428–433, 1987.

178. Przyklenk L, Darling CE, Dickson EW, et al: Cardioprotection outside the box. The evolving paradigm of remote preconditioning. Basic Res Cardiol 98:149–157, 2003.

179. Qiu Y, Tang XL, Park SW, et al: The early and late phases of ischemic preconditioning: a comparative analysis of the effects on infarct size, myocardial stunning and arrhythmias in conscious pigs undergoing a 40-minute coronary occlusion. Circ Res 80:730–742, 1997.

180. Quon CY, Stampfli HF: Biochemical properties of blood esterase. Drug Metab Dispos 13:420–434, 1985.

181. Rao KS, Schutz R, Feinberg H, Levitsky S: Metabolic evidence that regional hypothermia induced by cold saline protects the heart during ischemic arrest. J Surg Res 20:421–425, 1976.

182. Rao V, Borger MA, Weisel RD, et al: Insulin cardioplegia for elective coronary bypass surgery. J Thorac Cardiovasc Surg 119:1176–1184, 2000.

183. Reed GE, Spencer FC Boyd AD, et al: Late complications of intraoperative coronary artery perfusion. Circulation 48 (Suppl. III):8–84, 1973.

184. Rich TL, Langer GA, Klassen MG: Two components of coupling calcium in single ventricular cell of rabbits and rats. Am J Physiol 254:H937–946, 1988.

185. Robicsek F: Biochemical termination of sustained fibrillation occuring after artificially induced ischemic arrest. J Thorac Cardiovasc Surg 87:143–145, 1984.

186. Robinson LA, Harwood DL: Lowering the calcium concentration in St. Thomas Hospital cardioplegic solution improves protection during hypothermic ischemia. J Thorac Cardiovasc Surg 101:314–325, 1991.

187. Roe BB, Hutchinson JC, Fishman NM, et al: Myocardial protection with cold, ischemic potassium-induced cardioplegia. J Thorac Cardiovasc Surg 73:366–370, 1977.

188. Rosenfeldt FL, Watson DA: II. Interference with local myocardial cooling by heat gain during aortic cross-clamping. Ann Thorac Surg 27:13–16, 1979.

189. Rosenkranz ER, Okamoto F, Buckberg GD: The safety of prolonged aortic clamping with blood cardioplegia. II. Glutamine enrichment in energy-depleted hearts. J Thorac Cardiovasc Surg 88:401–410, 1984.

190. Rosenkranz ER, Okamoto F, Buckberg GD, et al: Aspartate enrichment of glutamate blood cardioplegia in energy-depleted hearts after ischemic and reperfusion injury. Safety of prolonged aortic clamping with blood cardioplegia. J Thorac Cardiovasc Surg 91:428–435, 1986.

191. Rosenkranz ER, Vinten-Johansen J, Buckberg GD, et al: Benefits of normothermic induction if cardioplegia in energy-depleted hearts, with maintenance of arrest by multidose cold blood cardioplegia infusions. J Thorac Cardiovasc Surg 84:667–676, 1982.

192. Rosenthal TB: The effects of temperature on the pH of blood and plasma in vitro. J Biol Chem 173:25–30, 1948.

193. Rousou JA, Engelman RM, Breyer RH, et al: The effects of temperature and hematocrit level of oxygenated cardioplegic solutions on myocardial preservation. J Thorac Cardiovasc Surg 95:625–630, 1988.

194. Rousou JH, Engelman RM, Dobbs WA, et al: The optimal potassium concentration in cardioplegic solutions. Ann Thorac Surg 32:75–79, 1981.

195. Rupprecht H, Dahl J, Terres W, et al: Cardioprotective effects of the Na+/H+ exchange inhibitor cariporide in patients with acute anterior myocardial infarction undergoing direct PTCA. Circulation 101:2902–2908, 2000.

196. Schaper J, Mulcj J, Wingler B, Schaper W: Ultrastructural, functional and biochemical criteria for estimation of reversibility of ischemic injury: a study on the effects of global ischemia on the isolated dog heart. J Mol Cell Cardiol 11:521–541, 1979.

197. Scholz W, Albus U, Counillon L, et al: Protective effects of HOE642, a selective sodium-hydrogen exchange subtype 1 inhibitor, on cardiac ischaemia and reperfusion. Cardiovasc Res 29:260–268, 1995.

198. Schwartz LM, Sebbag L, Jennings RB, et al: Duration and reinstatement of myocardial protection against infarction in open chest dogs. J Mol Cell Cardiol 32:1561–1570, 2001.

199. Sellke FW, Boyle EM, Verrier ED: Endothelial cell injury in cardiovascular surgery: the pathophysiology of vasomotor dysfunction. Ann Thorac Surg 62:1222–1228, 1996.

200. Sellke FW, Shafique T, Johnson RG, et al: Blood and albumin cardioplegia preserve endothelial-dependent microvascular responses. Ann Thorac Surg 55:977–985, 1993.

201. Senning A: Ventricular fibrillation during extracorporeal circulation; used as a method to prevent air embolisms and to facilitate intracardiac operations. Acta Chir Scand (Suppl.):171, 1952.

202. Shirai T, Rao V, Weisel RD, et al: Antegrade and retrograde cardioplegia: alternate or simultaneous? J Thorac Cardiovasc Surg 112:787–796, 1996.

203. Shumway NE, Lower RR, Stofer RC: Selective hypothermia of the heart in anoxic cardiac arrest. Surg Gynecol Obstet 109:750–754, 1959.

204. Silver MD, Wigle ED, Trimble AS, et al: Iatrogenic coronary ostial stenosis. Arch Pathol 88:73–77, 1969.

205. Silverman NA, del Nido P, Krukenkamp I, et al: Biologic rationale for formulation of antegrade cardioplegic solutions. In Chitwood WR, editor: Cardiac Surgery: State of the Art Reviews. Philadelphia: Hanley & Belfus, 1988, pp. 181–195.

206. Silverman NA, Kohler J, Feinberg H, et al: Beneficial effects of nucleoside augmentation on reperfusion injury following cardioplegic arrest. Chest 83:787–792, 1983.

207. Silverman NA, Kohler J, Levitsky S, et al: Chronic hypoxemia depresses global ventricular function and predisposes to the depletion of high-energy phosphates during cardioplegic arrest: implications for surgical repair of cyanotic congenital heart defects. Ann Thorac Surg 37:304–308, 1984.

208. Silverman NA, Wright R, Levitsky S, et al: Efficacy of crystalloid cardioplegic solutions in patients undergoing myocardial revascularization. Effect of infusion route and regional wall motion on preservation of adenine nucleotide stores. J Thorac Cardiovasc Surg 89:90–96, 1985.

209. Sink JD, Pellom GL, Currie WD, et al: Response of hypertrophied myocardium to ischemia: correlation with biochemical and physiological parameters. J Thorac Cardiovasc Surg 81:865–872, 1981.

210. Sperelakis N, Sunagawa M, Nakamura M: Electrogenesis of the resting potential. In Sperelakis N, Kurachi Y, Terezic A, Cohen MV, editors: Heart Physiology and Pathophysiology. San Diego: Academic Press, 2001, pp. 175–198.

211. Stamm C, Friehs I, Cowan DB, et al: Dopamine treatment of postischemic myocardial stunning rapidly induces calcium-dependant pro-apoptotic signaling. Circulation 104(Suppl. II):II-522, 2001.

212. Standeven JW, Jellinek M, Menz LJ, et al: Cold blood cardioplegia. Evaluation of glutathione and postischemic cardioplegia. J Thorac Cardiovasc Surg 78:893–907, 1979.

213. Starr JP, Jia CX, Amirhamzeh MM, et al: Coronary perfusate composition influences diastolic properties, myocardial water content, and histological characteristics of the rat left ventricle. Ann Thorac Surg 68:925–930, 1999.

214. Swan H, Zeavin I: Cessation of circulation in general hypothermia. III. Technics of intracardiac surgery under direct vision. Ann Surg 139:385–396, 1954.

215. Teoh KH, Christakis GT, Weisel RD, et al: Accelerated myocardial recovery with terminal blood cardioplegia. J Thorac Cardiovasc Surg 91:888–895, 1986.

216. Teoh LK, Grant R, Hulf JA, et al: A comparison between ischemic preconditioning, intermittent cross-clamp fibrillation and cold crystalloid cardioplegia for myocardial protection during coronary artery bypass graft surgery. Cardiovasc Surg 10:251–255, 2002.

1102

217. Theroux P, Chaitman BR, Danchin N, et al: Inhibition of sodium-hydrogen exchanger with cariporide to prevent myocardial infarction in high-risk ischemic situations; results of the GUARDIAN trial. Guard During Necrosis (GUARDIAN) investigators. Circulation 102:3032–3038, 2000.

218. Todd GJ, Tyers GFO: Potassium-induced arrest of the heart: effect of low potassium concentrations. Surg Forum 26:255–256, 1975.

219. Toyoda Y, Khan S, Chen W-M, et al: Effects of NHE-1 inhibition on cardioprotection and impact on protection by K/Mg cardioplegia. Ann Thorac Surg 72:836–843, 2001.

220. Toyoda Y, Levitsky S, McCully JD: Opening of mitochondrial ATP-sensitive potassium channels enhances cardioplegic protection. Ann Thorac Surg 71:1281–1289, 2001.

221. Tsukube T, McCully JD, Faulk E, et al: Magnesium cardioplegia reduces cytosolic and nuclear calcium and DNA fragmentation in the senescent myocardium. Ann Thorac Surg 58:1005–1011, 1994.

222. Tsukube T, Mccully JD, Metz RM, et al: Amelioration of ischemic calcium overload correlates with high energy phosphates in the senescent myocardium. Am J Physiol 42:H418–427, 1997.

223. Tyers GFO, Manley NJ, Williams EH, et al: Preliminary clinical experience with isotonic hypothermic potassium-induced arrest. J Thorac Cardiovasc Surg 74:674–681, 1977.

224. Tyers GFO, Todd GJ, Niebauer IM, et al: Effect of intracoronary tetrodotoxin on recovery of the isolated working rat heart from sixty minutes of ischemia. Circulation 49/50(Suppl. II):II 175–179, 1974.

225. Uchiyama Y, Otani H, Okada Y, et al: Integrated pharmacological preconditioning in combination with adenosine, a mitochondrial K_{ATP} channel opener and a nitric oxide donor. J Thorac Cardiovasc Surg 126:148–159, 2003.

226. Valen G: The basic biology of apoptosis and its implications for cardiac function and viability. Ann Thorac Surg 75:S656–660, 2003.

227. Valen G, Takeshima S, Vaage J: Preconditioning improves cardiac function after global ischemia, but not after cold cardioplegia. Ann Thorac Surg 62:1397–1403, 1996.

228. Veinot JP, Gattinger DA, Fliss H: Early apoptosis in human myocardial infarcts. Hum Pathol 28:485–492, 1997.

229. Velez DA, Morris CD, Budde JM, et al: All-blood (miniplegia) versus dilute cardioplegia in experimental surgical revascularization of evolving infarction. Circulation 104(Suppl. I):I-296–I-302, 2001.

230. Verrier ED, Morgan EN: Endothelial response to cardiopulmonary bypass surgery. Ann Thorac Surg 66:S17–19, 1998.

231. Vinten-Johansen J, Zhao ZQ, Corvera JS, et al: Adenosine in myocardial protection in on-pump and off-pump cardiac surgery. Ann Thorac Surg 75:S691–699, 2003.

232. Walker CA, Crawford FA, Spinale FG: Myocyte contractile dysfunction with hypertrophy and failure: relevance to cardiac surgery. J Thorac Cardiovasc Surg 119:388–400, 2000.

233. The Warm Heart Investigators: Randomized trial of normothermic versus hypothermic coronary bypass surgery. Lancet 343:559–563, 1994.

234. Wildenthal K, Mierzwiak DS, Mitchell J: Acute effects of increased serum osmolarity on left ventricular performance. Am J Physiol 216:898–904, 1969.

235. Wright RN, Levitsky S, Rao KS, et al: Potassium cardioplegia: an alternate method of myocardial protection. Arch Surg 113:976–980, 1978.

236. Yaoita H, Ogawa K, Maehara K, et al: Attenuation of ischemia/reperfusion injury in rats by caspase inhibitor. Circulation 97:276–281, 1998.

237. Ye TM, Sun J, Shen J, et al: Does retrograde warm cardioplegia provide equal protection to both ventricles? A magnetic resonance spectroscopy study in pigs. Circulation 96(Suppl. 9):II-210–215, 1997.

238. Yellon DM, Alkulaifi AM, Pugsley WB: Preconditioning the human myocardium. Lancet 342:276–277, 1993.

239. Yellon DM, Dana A: The preconditioning phenomenon: a tool for the scientist or clinical reality? Circ Res 87:543–550, 2000.

240. Young JN, Choy IO, Silva NK, et al: Antegrade cold blood cardioplegia is not demonstrably advantageous over cold crystalloid cardioplegia in surgery for congenital heart disease. J Thorac Cardiovasc Surg 114:1002–1008, 1997.

241. Zimmerman ANE, Daems W Hulsmann W, et al: Morphological changes of heart muscle caused by successive perfusion with calcium-free and calcium-containing solutions (calcium paradox). Cardiovasc Res 1:201–209, 1967.

242. Zymer U, Suryapranata H, Monassier JP, et al: The Na+/H+ exchange inhibitor eniporide as an adjunct to early reperfusion therapy for acute myocardial infarction: results of the evaluation of the safety and cardioprotective effects of eniporide in acute myocardial infarction (ESCAMI) trial. J Am Coll Cardiol 38:1644–1650, 2001.

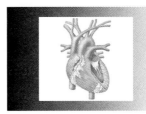

CHAPTER 67

Clinical Quality and Cardiac Surgery

Justine M. Carr, Judy Krempin, and Ronald M. Weintraub

► BACKGROUND

In 1953 Deming began a quality revolution in industry.[3] Over the past half-century cardiac surgeons have led the medical community in developing and applying similar quality improvement techniques in the management of patients. The relative uniformity and limited types of operations, together with their rapidly increasing numbers, aggregate cost, and high public profile have impelled interested stakeholders to quantify outcomes. In 1987 Health Care Financing Administration (HCFA) first published institution-specific Medicare mortality rates that were unadjusted for severity of patient disease.[13] Influenced by both competitive and statistical imperatives, surgeons felt it essential to develop risk-adjustment methods for a more rational comparison of disparate patient groups.

In 1989 Parsonnet et al pioneered a predictive model that classified patients into five groups of increasing operative risk according to 14 preoperative risk factors.[26] The model proved to be highly predictive when applied to a large number of patients in three hospitals. The decade of the 1990s saw the development of numerous statistical methods to adjust for preoperative risk hazard as well as social and geographic differences.[16,17] In New England, a consortium of hospitals, Northern New England Cardiovascular Study Group, began to collect data uniformly in a common registry.[23] The Alabama Coronary Artery Bypass Grafting Cooperative project gathered data for 1995 and 1996.[14] Even after risk adjustment, however, a number of observational studies showed significant differences in coronary artery bypass grafting (CABG) mortality among institutions.[11,24,31] Among these and other registries established in the early and mid-1990s was the universal finding that operative mortality varied widely among institutions, from as low as 1.9% to as high as 12%, even after risk adjustment. These findings presaged two different but complementary movements. Hannan's studies of CABG mortality in New York State led to the first statewide reporting of operative mortality.[12] Statutory requirement for public reporting has followed in Pennsylvania, New Jersey, and Massachusetts, and will surely follow in other states.[1,5,6] An equally important result has been the cooperative analysis of outcomes within a quality assurance regime. The Northern New England Disease Study Group has been a leader in this movement. In three meetings yearly, surgeons, cardiologists, nurses, and perfusionists gather to review data and current practice, target key variables that drive outcomes, and organize projects such as interinstitutional site visits and study protocols. Crude "observed" operative CABG mortality for the consortium has fallen from 4.3 to 2.1% over 10 years, while expected risk has risen from 4 to 5.5%.[21] Equally significant, differences in operative mortality and complication rates among the member institutions have dramatically declined. Members of the consortium have cooperatively published over 50 peer-reviewed reports that have identified and addressed areas of opportunity for improvement. A number of regional, national, and even international groups have followed this registry/quality improvement model,[9,10,25] establishing benchmarks for the cardiac surgical "industry." Shahian et al have comprehensively reviewed the history and current state of quality care assessment in cardiac surgery.[28]

In another approach to quality improvement, national specialty societies have established guidelines for the application of interventional and surgical technologies. In 1999 the American College of Cardiology (ACC) and American Heart Association (AHA) published Guidelines for Coronary Bypass Surgery.[8] These include Class I, useful and effective; Class IIa, evidence favors usefulness; Class IIb, evidence less well established; and Class III, not useful or

1104 effective/in some cases harmful. Similar guidelines have been established for valvular surgery.[2]

▶ THE INSTITUTE OF MEDICINE AND THE QUALITY CHASM

In 2001 the Institute of Medicine (IOM) gained widespread publicity and stimulated both controversy and discussion with its report "Crossing the Quality Chasm."[15] The report set a national agenda aimed at narrowing differences in quality among the providers of medical care. Instead of attention to a single outcome such as mortality, the IOM focused on the quality of the entire patient experience as defined in six key dimensions: *"Safe, Effective, Efficient, Timely, Patient Centered, and Equitable."* The model promulgates a balanced approach to assessment of quality, incorporating clinical outcomes with patient experience and the appropriate allocation of resources. Because of its high profile and consumption of national resources, it is fitting that cardiac surgery, the "poster boy" specialty for quality improvement progress, embrace this new frontier. IOM defines the dimensions in the following way:

- **Safe:** *avoiding injuries from care that is intended to help them.*
- **Effective:** *providing services based on scientific knowledge to all who could benefit, and refraining from providing services not likely to benefit.*
- **Efficient:** *avoiding waste, including waste of equipment, supplies, ideas, and energy.*
- **Patient Centered:** *providing care that is respectful of and responsive to individual patient preferences, needs, and values, and ensuring that patient values guide all clinical decisions.*
- **Timely:** *reducing waits and sometimes harmful delays for both those who receive and those who give care.*
- **Equitable:** *providing care that does not vary in quality because of personal characteristics.*

Building, measuring, and driving quality care, as outlined by the Institute of Medicine, is the focus of this chapter.

▶ THE TEAM

Cardiac surgery has often been compared to the aviation industry in underscoring the critical importance of teamwork.[27,29] The team's core is the operating room (OR) staff—surgeon, anesthesiologist, perfusionist, nurse, and nurse practitioner or physician assistant. The need for teamwork continues once the patient leaves the OR. A second tier includes the staff in the intensive care unit (ICU) and clinical units: the ICU/recovery nurses and nurse practitioners and physicians assistants and case managers. In addition to the frontline team, a third tier partners with the frontline staff to monitor and support the clinical encounter. This is the support staff—data, decision support, infection control, and administration/health care quality. For the team to be effective, there needs to be regular designated times to meet, discuss, and decide. Team meetings bridge the challenge of measurement and management. Ownership is shared. While problem identification can sometimes be painful or even tempestuous, problem solving must ultimately be collegial and inclusive.

▶ THE APPROACH

Focus is key. An annual plan is helpful (Table 67-1). Quarterly report cards are powerful (Table 67-2). Historical trends, as well as outside benchmarks, help set goals. Data collection must be supported by resources and commitment to intervention and improvement. Although adverse clinical outcomes are reviewed immediately in Morbidity and Mortality conferences, another level of understanding comes from monthly and quarterly measurement. Review of these outcome trends by the team affords an opportunity for reflection about systems issues affecting outcomes. Response should be rapid cycle: Plan-Do-Study-Act(PDSA), as adopted from industry and advocated by the Institute for Healthcare Improvement.[18]

The perfect should not be the enemy of the good. Although randomized controlled trials are the gold standard for comparison of treatment regimens, their use in surgical management has major limitations. Only a limited number of questions can be answered, randomization of a significant number of patients is often impractical, while the results in smaller, specifically circumscribed study groups are often not suitable for generalization to the larger population. Furthermore, technical obsolescence over time may invalidate comparisons. Analysis of large cohorts to achieve statistical significance may be important for publications, but snapshots of practice from small samples are satisfactory and valuable for rapid cycle performance improvement. An example of an effective PDSA tool is shown in Figure 67-1. Trying to understand the reasons for delays between cardiac catheterization and cardiac surgery can be a challenge. Creating a weekly snapshot can capture real time events and their immediate impact. Although data collection is manual and labor intensive, opportunities for improvement are quickly identified. Information from this model can lead to improvement in timely communication between a cardiologist performing the catheterization and the cardiac surgeon. A Health Insurance Portability and Accountability Act (HIPAA)-compliant secure e-mail system can communicate the basic, or even detailed, facts of a referred patient's clinical problems, replacing multiple and repetitive telephone calls to office and surgeon, faxes, and the need for several caregivers to personally review the hospital chart. The surgeon on call is clearly identified, but the e-mail notification goes to all surgeons, cardiac anesthesiologists, and the screening nurse practitioners, to ensure a timely response and evaluation, while the on-call surgeon is unavailable in the operating room. In the example illustrated in Figure 67-1, the team noticed a problem with OR block utilization. It was solved by placing more elective cases on Mondays and Tuesday, leaving blocks later in the week for urgent cases.

Finally, problems should be analyzed in a systematic fashion to ensure complete evaluation of all contributing factors. One approach is to consider factors from each component of the patient's care: preoperative, intraoperative, ICU, and postoperative.[22] Infection rate, for example, may be affected by preoperative variables: the scrub performed the night before operation, the perioperative antibiotic regimen, the standardization of the prep and drape procedure, etc. Intraoperative considerations include duration of surgery, the extent and energy amplitude of diathermy, and the choice of open or closed vein harvest. Postoperative infection control includes tight glucose management and regular handwashing

Table 67–1

Cardiac Surgery Annual Plan

	Effective	*Safe*	*Timely*	*Efficient*	*Patient centered*	*Equitable*
Goals	Decrease mortality: CABG and valves	Decrease infections: sternum and legs	Start on time; shorten catheterization to OR times	Cost-effective utilization	Increase patient satisfaction scores	Reduce delay for translator
Intervention focus						
Preoperative	Surgical risk evaluation		Catheterization to OR time			Translator request to arrival time
Intraoperative	Bypass times	Endoscopic vein harvest Glucose control	OR starts at 8 AM	Supply standardization Supply price negotiation		
Postoperative		Glucose control Data collection for leg wound outcomes		Length of stay Transfusion practice	Satisfaction surveys Family meeting	Translator request to arrival time
Data source	*NNE and STS database*	*ICU and EVH database*	*OR database*	*Hospital database*	*Satisfaction survey*	*Translator log*

by caregivers. All contributing factors should be considered in a comprehensive approach to achieving the stated goal.

▶ DATA

Data Sources

Basic information including hospital mortality is generally available from hospital administrative data. These data are usually culled from the Uniform Hospital Discharge Data Set that is, in turn, derived from International Classification of Diseases (ICD)-9 diagnosis and procedure codes. The accuracy of these data is dependent on the skill of hospital coders and the clarity of the physician documentation. ICD-9 coding, however, is constrained by the inability to reflect the temporal relationships of preoperative and postoperative conditions or complications. Primary chart review or real-time data collection on predefined fields ensures meaningful, actionable information.

Data Collection: Who and How

Data collection is challenged by the need to balance efficiency with accuracy and completeness. Decentralized data collection ensures rapid completion of all fields, but must be weighed against the additional layer of resource-intensive error surveillance and error correction. Hiring one or more designated chart reviewers improves accuracy, but is slow and tedious. A more efficient model consists of combining several objective fields that have been collected separately. For instance, intake caregivers (physician assistants, nurse assistants, fellows, residents) collect history and physical examination data, perfusionists collect information on OR times and procedures, and designated individuals screen records for documented complications, and also validate the decentralized data modules. Finally, direct data entry into a computer at the time and site of collection decreases errors and ensures uniformity through standardized choices and drop-down menus. This direct data entry model adds a real-time dimension to the collection process.

Data Repositories

Registries should be linked to regional or national databases for benchmarking purposes. The Society of Thoracic Surgeons (STS) national database is the largest and best known, but requires significant resources to complete more than 400 data fields per patient. The New York State Department of Health reporting system is also recognized

Table 67–2

Quarterly Report Card

BIDMC Cardiac Surgery fiscal year report card		Year to date	Metric	Previous year	Benchmark[a]
Outcomes	CABG mortality		Quarterly CABG mortality		
	Valve mortality		Quarterly valve mortality		
	Chest wound infections		Quarterly rate (infections per 100 cases)		
	Leg wound Infections		Quarterly rate (patients with saphenous vein harvest)		
	Blood transfusion		Percent of patients receiving red blood cells, plasma, platelets		
	Readmissions—30 days from procedure		Quarterly rate by case type		
Timeliness	Cath CABG time		Days between cardiac catheterization and CABG		
	On time OR starts		Percent of first cases beginning by 8 AM		
Efficiency	CABG bypass times		Minutes on bypass		
	Cost per case		Quarterly by DRG		
	Length of stay		Quarterly by DRG		
	CABG volume		Quarterly volumes: CABG and valve		
Patient centered	Overall quality of care		Satisfaction survey		
	Would be recommended to friends/relatives		Satisfaction survey		

[a]Sources: Massachusetts Health Data Consortium, Centers for Disease Control, Northern New England Cardiovascular Disease Study Group, Institute for Health Improvement, Society of Thoracic Surgeons.

and much abbreviated in comparison to STS. Several commercially available computer software systems allow direct real-time data entry via computer screen, and computerized reporting of "harvested" data has made comparisons and benchmarking easier and timelier.

Data Analysis

In addition to submitting data to national registries, database managers should have the capacity to quickly query the data in order to address both immediate and long-term issues. Such ongoing data-driven oversight maintains performance improvement.

▶ DEFINING DIMENSIONS OF CARE ELEMENTS

Selection of elements within the IOM construct will be dictated not only by the challenges confronting individual programs, but also by the availability of data.

Safe

Safe is avoiding injuries to patients from the care that is intended to help them. Cardiac operations entail risk by virtue of their invasion of critical organs for the purpose of correcting life-threatening diseases. Limiting the risk inherent in such operations depends on a regimen that anticipates and assesses risk, collects and categorizes complications, recognizes complication trends in a real-time framework, and continuously reviews corrective measures.

Risk assessment is critical not only for establishing comparison with benchmark data, but also for communicating prognostic information to patients and their referring physicians. Equally important, the ability to anticipate extraordinary risk may guide both surgeon and cardiologist away from the surgical option. A number of risk-estimation instruments have been available for CABG operations. More recently, registries have added valve data to their estimators. The Northern New England risk calculator is

SAMPLE WEEKLY IN-HOSPITAL DELAY ANALYSIS

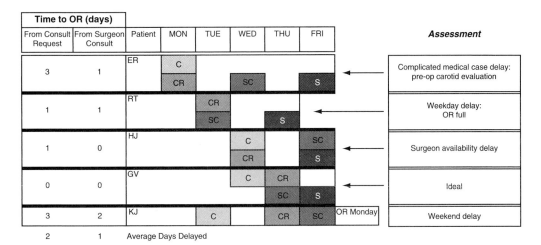

Figure 67–1 Sample weekly in-hospital delay analysis.

illustrated in Table 67-3. Health Data Research, a consortium of over 40 cardiac surgical units from the United States, Canada, and Europe, supports a free risk estimator at www.healthdataresearch.com, as well as a plethora of benchmark charts and figures from its registry of over 90,000 patients.

The most frequently used measure of safety and quality is a comparison of a surgical unit's or surgeon's observed complication rate with that of a benchmark or registry expected rate, after risk adjustment and calculation of statistical error. The expected rate is usually calculated from the registry mean rate over a period of time. Because data are usually harvested and submitted at intervals rather than continuously, only retrospective analysis is possible, and trends and unusual events may go unrecognized until long after the event. Furthermore, because many operative complications and most mortalities are relatively infrequent events, it may be difficult to distinguish in real time between statistical "noise" and real trends with respect to particular complications. Industry has developed quantitative processes to deal with similar issues in manufacturing.[4] The sequential runs of "error-free" cases can be particularly helpful (Figure 67-2). Here the abscissa does not mark time, but shows a new column every time an event occurs. The average line is constructed from benchmark, ideal, or even the surgical unit's previously observed data. In this construct, the higher the bars, the better the performance. Moreover, if more than a threshold number of consecutive bars four, five, or six, depending on the desired sensitivity) fall below the average line, an "unusual occurrence" is thus defined, and attention can be turned to the particular complication of concern. This instrument is particularly useful as an early

Table 67–3			
Risk Algorithm[a]			
Preoperative estimation of risk of CABG, mitral or aortic valve mortality[b]			
Patient or disease characteristic	*CABG mortality score*	*Aortic valve mortality score*	*Mitral valve mortality score*
Age 60–69	2.5	1.5	1.5
Age 70–79	4.0	2.0	3.0
Age ≥80	11.0	3.0	3.0
Female sex	2.0		1.5
EF <40%[c]	1.5		
NYHA III		1.0	1.0
NYHA IV		1.5	2.0
LVEDP ≥ 20			1.5
Urgent surgery[d]	2.0	1.5	2.0
Emergency surgery[e]	9.0	5.5	6.0
Prior CVA			1.5
Prior CABG	3.0	1.5	
PVD	1.5		
CHF		2.0	1.5
Atrial fibrillation[f]		1.5	1.4
CAD			1.5
Diabetes	1.5		1.5
Dialysis or creatinine ≥2	2.5	1.5	1.5
COPD	2.0		

Continued

Table 67–3

Risk Algorithm—cont'd

Preoperative estimation of risk of CABG, mitral or aortic valve mortality[a]

Patient or disease characteristic	CABG mortality score	Aortic valve mortality score	Mitral valve mortality score
BSA <1.70		1.5	
BSA 1.70–1.99		1.0	
Mitral replacement			2.0
Concomitant CABG		1.5	
Total score			

	Preoperative Risk		
Total score	Mortality (%)	Aortic (%)	Mitral (%)
<3	<0.4	<1.8	<0.6
3	0.4	1.8	0.6
4	0.6	2.2	0.9
5	0.8	3.1	1.1
6	1.2	3.6	1.5
7	1.5	5.1	2.0
8	2.1	6.6	2.7
9	2.8	8.5	4.0
10	3.7	11.9	4.8
11	4.6	15.1	7.1
12	6.6	17.2	9.2
13	5.2	23.7	11.6
14	9.9	31.4	17.0
15	7.3	36.9	19.6
16	9.6	43.0	26.6
17	12.0	>43.0	34.0
18	15.8		41.2
19	21.6		48.0
20	≥31.7		>60.0

Preoperative estimation of risk of cerebrovascular accident and mediastinitis
(for use only in isolated CABG surgery)

Patient or disease characteristic	CVA score	Mediastinitis score
Age 55–59	1.5	
Age 60–64	2.5	
Age 65–69	3.5	
Age 70–74	4.0	
Age 75–79	4.5	
Age ≥80	5.5	
Female sex	1.0	
EF <40%	1.5	2.0

Table 67–3

Risk Algorithm—cont'd

Preoperative estimation of risk of cerebrovascular accident and mediastinitis
(for use only in isolated CABG surgery)

Patient or disease characteristic	CVA score	Mediastinitis score
Urgent surgery	1.5	1.5
Emergency surgery	2.5	3.5
Vascular disease	2.0	
Diabetes		1.5
Dialysis or creatinine ≥2	2.0	2.5
COPD		3.5
Obesity (BMI 31–36)		2.5
Severe obesity (BMI ≥37)		3.5
Total score		

	Preoperative risk	
Total score	CVA (%)	Mediastinitis (%)
0	0.3	0.4
1	0.4	0.5
2	0.5	0.6
3	0.7	0.7
4	0.9	1.1
5	1.3	1.5
6	1.6	1.9
7	2.1	3.0
8	2.8	3.5
9	5.5	5.8
10		≥6.5
11		
12		
13		
14		

CABG, coronary artery bypass grafting; EF, ejection fraction; NYHA, New York Heart Association; LVEDP, left ventricular end-diastolic pressure; CVA, cardiovascular accident; PVD, pulmonary vascular disease; CHF, congestive heart failure; CAD, coronary artery disease; COPD, chronic obstructive pulmonary disease; BSA, body surface area; BMI, body mass index.

[a]**Directions:** locate outcome of interest. Use the score in that column for each relevant preoperative variable; then sum these scores to get the total score. Take the total score and look up the approximate preoperative risk in the table.

EF <40%: the patient's current EF is less than 40%.

Urgent: medical factors require the patient to stay in hospital to have operation before discharge. The risk of immediate morbidity and death is believed to be low.

Emergency: patient's cardiac disease dictates that surgery should be performed within hours to avoid unnecessary morbidity or death.

Atrial fibrillation: sustained atrial fibrillation requiring treatment with digoxin, beta/calcium channel blockers, antiarrhythmics, or cardioversion.

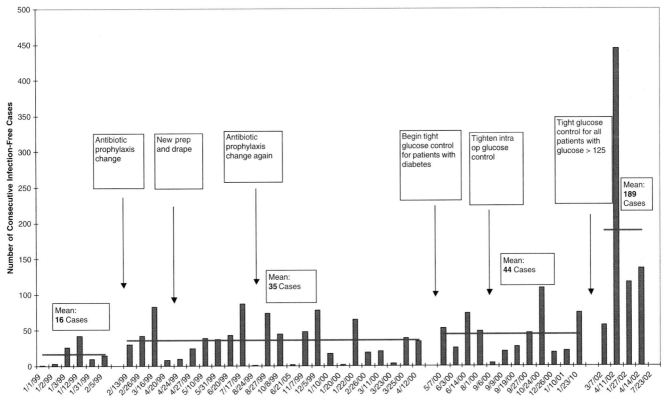

Figure 67–2 **Sample error-free runs: sternal infections.** 5/01, implemented new prep and drape protocol; 11/01, outbreak; 3/02, began new glucose monitoring and treatment protocol.

warning system for infections of all types (e.g., sternal, deep organ space, saphenectomy), return to operating room for bleeding, and requirement for intraoperative or postoperative counterpulsation.

Effective

Effective is providing services, based on scientific knowledge, to all who could benefit, and refraining from providing services not likely to benefit. Partnership and dialogue with referring cardiologists play a critical role in assessment of the intervention most likely to benefit the patient. ACC/AHA Guidelines for Coronary Artery Bypass Graft Surgery propose boundaries about what is achievable. Identification of patients who fall into category IIb or III or who have a preoperative mortality risk of >10% (Table 67-3) provides an opportunity for discussion. The opinion of a cardiac surgical colleague can be useful in assessing the likelihood of success, as well as in alerting the team that a high-risk patient will be undergoing surgery and may have special management needs. The dialogue between surgeons about high-risk patients can result in staff surgeons assisting each other in the operating room, promoting both safety and mutual learning.

In addition to addressing mortality risk on a case-by-case basis, it is important to document team performance on behaviors that are known to reduce the risk of complication. These include the use of the internal thoracic artery,[19] tight glucose control,[30] and perioperative aspirin administration.[7]

Efficient

Efficient is avoiding waste, including waste of equipment, supplies, ideas, and energy. Cost accounting systems can be helpful in tracking practice, as well as costs. Total costs are conventionally divided into direct (supplies, drugs, direct nursing care, blood, etc.) and indirect (lights, heat, administrative infrastructure, etc.). Reviewing direct cost per case by quarter and by surgeon is a helpful way to identify opportunities for eliminating waste. An example is shown in Figure 67-3. This demonstrates change in the total direct cost per case, as well as in the expenditure within component categories. Anticipated and unanticipated effects can be seen. Standardization of practice is reflected in reduced OR time, OR supplies, and anesthesia time between Q1 and Q2. Introduction of endoscopic vein harvest led to an increase in OR time and OR supplies between Q2 and Q3. Increasing experience with the endoscopic vein harvest technique ultimately led to reduction of OR times back to baseline. OR supply costs remained higher as endoscopic vein harvest become the standard of practice. When new house staff came on service in July, ICU time and pharmacy costs increased. Drill-down revealed an increase in use of a high cost sedation agent, longer intubation times, and longer ICU stay. Education and tighter practice guidelines resulted in improvement the following quarter.

OR supply standardization opportunity can be best understood by building a model of each physician's supply preferences and the costs of each item and case (Figure

1110 67-4 and Table 67-4). Immediate benefit can be achieved by identifying items that were included in case packs but are no longer being used. Creation of two categories ("have available" and "have open") minimizes waste of infrequently used items. Having surgeons scrub together affords them an opportunity to share their experiences with different supplies. The resulting standardization of operative supplies, though occasionally requiring negotiation, improves safety and efficiency, and reduces cost. Studies have clearly demonstrated that variation in a system is an opportunity for mistakes.[20] The cost-effectiveness of a procedure-based delivery system increases, as supply standardization is increased. Multiple elements can be packaged and sterilized once, as opposed to individual items that must be separately sterilized, stored, and selected. Finally, standardization to a single vendor affords an opportunity to negotiate better pricing for supplies through volume discounts.

Patient Centered

Patient centered is providing care that is respectful of and responsive to individual patient preferences, needs, and values, and ensuring that patient values guide all clinical deci-

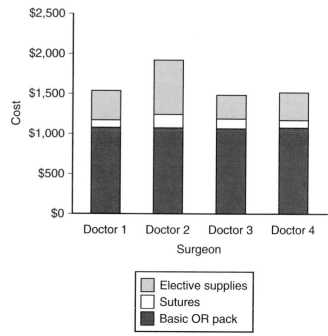

Figure 67–4 Sample CABG supply utilization.

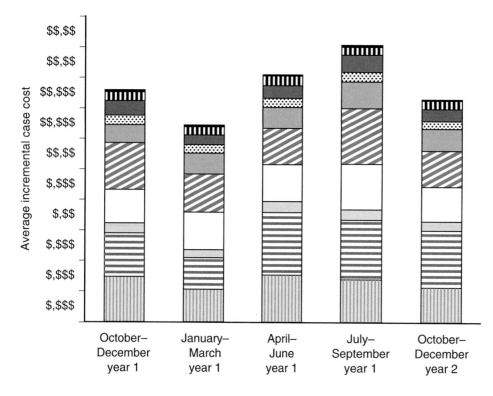

Figure 67–3 Sample cost per case: DRG 109 CABG without catheterization. January–March: standardization of practice among surgeons reduced OR time, OR supply costs, and anesthesia time. April–June: implementation of endoscopic leg vein harvest increased OR time and supply costs. July–September: impact of high-cost leukoreduced blood products; increased resource intensity by new trainees seen in length of stay, pharmacy, and laboratories. October–December: renewed attention to practice guidelines and new staff education returned costs to previous level.

Table 67–4

Sample CABG Supply Utilization[a]

Supplies	MD #1	MD #2	MD #3	MD #4
Basic OR pack	$$$$	$$$$	$$$$	$$$$
Stapler			$	
7-0 Prolene CC	$	$	$	$
5-0 Prolene RB-2 (multi)	$	$	$	
Suture, Prolene Dbl Arm5-0BB		$		
Suture, Monocryl 3-0 PS-1	$	$		$
Suture, Chromic 4-0 SH		$		
Suture pledgets, Sids		$		
Suture, Ethibond, 2-0 s/a		$		
8-0 Prolene #175 24″		$		
8-0 Prolene #130 18″ (multi)	$		$	$
6-0 Silk #706G (IMA Tacker)	$		$	$
2-0 Ethibond v-7 with pledget		$		
Suture, Prolene 4-0 BB		$		
Sutures	$	$	$	$
MPS (cardioplegia)		$		
Cardioplegia	$		$	$
Cannula venous 29/29/FR	$	$	$	$
Pleurovac 2020-300	$	$	$	$
Sternal saw blade	$	$	$	$
Cannula arteriotomy		$		
Tubing, CO_2		$		
Ante cardioplegia cannula		$		
Retrograde cannula		$		
#69 Blade		$		
Pump sucker tip		$		
Y-Connector		$		
Insulation pad		$		$
Ice machine drape	$	$		$
4-mm aortic punch		$		
#32 chest tubes straight		$		
#28 chest tubes straight	$		$	$
Marquis adaptor	$	$	$	$
Gundry retrograde cannula				$
Plastic vein cannula	$			$
Retrograde Sams cannula	$			
Retrograde DLP		$		
Sterile Doppler gel	$			
Cautery pads	$	$	$	$
Elective supplies	$	$$	$	$
Total	$.$$$	$$.$$$	$.$$$	$.$$$

[a]$, 0-500; $$, 501–1000; $$$, 1001–1500; $,$$$, 1501–2000; $$,$$$, 2001–2500.

sions. Measurement in this area is more challenging. Standardized medical center surveys afford an opportunity to measure patient satisfaction in comparison with other institutions or other areas within the same institution, and provide focus for targeted improvement efforts. The impact of changes in practice is often linked to changes in patient satisfaction scores, both favorable and unfavorable.

On an individual level, ensuring timely family meetings for longer stay ICU patients is another measurable indicator. Creating the expectation that all ICU patients have a family meeting with relevant clinicians at the 72-h mark ensures that patients and families, nurses and physicians, surgeons and consultants are all in synchrony with the care plan. Decision making is shared with patient and clinicians.

1112

Timely

Timely is reducing waits and harmful delays for both those who receive and those who give care. A method for reducing catheterization-to-OR delays has been outlined in the "Approach" section above. Another factor in timely care is the operating start time. A delay in the start of one or more cases inevitably leads to OR staff overtime, with its attendant negative effect on both cost and morale. Tracking the weekly start time in relation to the goal may reveal a host of small issues, many of which are readily soluble once identified—timing of morning rounds, efficient delivery of preadmission history and physical and consent forms to OR, and shared ownership of preoperative tasks to ensure that the next available person performs a required task (e.g., moving the patient, urethral catheterization, prep and drape).

Equitable

Equitable is providing care that does not vary in quality because of personal characteristics. Provision of equitable care is usually considered an institutional rather than a departmental challenge. Nevertheless, awareness of this dimension should be incorporated into the culture of care. Although Interpreter Services is an institutional resource, measurement of its effectiveness at a local level can help enhance its effectiveness. For example, non-English-speaking patients are best served by a trained interpreter rather than a family member. Documentation of timely translation services is thus a potential measure of equitable care.

▶ INTEGRATION OF MEASURES

The report card (Table 67-2) is valuable because all dimensions of care are reviewed at once. Decreased mean length of stay may not be helpful if the readmission rate increases. An increase in expense for OR supplies due to addition of endoscopic vein harvest cannot be judged on the basis of cost per case alone, but must take into account its positive impact on patient satisfaction and infection rate. Shortening the length of time from cardiac catheterization to surgery is not beneficial if the patient misses an opportunity to review the plan in depth with his physician.

▶ SUMMARY

The Institute for Healthcare Improvement has promulgated a simple construct for performance improvement that can be incorporated here: Focus, Improve, Sustain, Honor. Focus requires an articulation of the goals for the year. Improvement initiatives must be prioritized by their ability to achieve the goal. Frequently measured and relevant metrics, reviewed and analyzed in a timely fashion, sustain the initiatives. Finally, it is critically important to celebrate the achievements, the victories, the successes—recognizing the efforts, teams and individuals who make it happen.

REFERENCES

1. A Consumer Guide to Coronary Artery Bypass Graft Surgery, Vol I-IF. Harrisburg: Pennsylvania Health Care Cost Containment Council, 1992–1995.
2. ACC/AHA guidelines for the management of patients with valvular heart disease. A report of the American College of Cardiology/American Heart Association. Task Force on Practice Guidelines Committee on Management of Patients with Valvular Heart Disease. J Am Coll Cardiol 325: 1486–1588, 1998.
3. Aguayo R: Dr. Deming: The American Who Taught the Japanese About Quality. New York: Fireside, 1991.
4. Brassard M, Ritter D: The Memory Jogger II: A Pocket Guide of Tools for Continuous Improvement and Effective Planning. Salem, NH:Goal/QPC, 1994.
5. 105 Commonwealth of Massachusetts Regulations 130.020. (Regulations implement the recommendations of the Cardiac Care Quality Commission created by Section 248 of Chapter 159 of the Acts of 2000.)
6. Coronary artery bypass graft surgery in New Jersey—1998. Trenton: New Jersey Department of Health and Senior Services, 1999.
7. Dacey LJ, Munoz JJ, Johnson ER, et al: Effect of preoperative aspirin use on mortality in coronary artery bypass grafting patients. Northern New England Cardiovascular Disease Study Group. Ann Thorac Surg 70:1986–1990, 2000.
8. Eagle KA, Guyton RA, Davidoff R, et al: ACC/AHA Guidelines for Coronary Artery Bypass Graft Surgery: A Report of the American College of Cardiology/American Heart Association Task Force on Practice Guidelines Committee to Revise the 1991 Guidelines for Coronary Artery Bypass Graft Surgery. American College of Cardiology/American Heart Association. J Am Coll Cardiol 344:1262–1347, 1999.
9. Ferguson TB Jr, Dziuban SW Jr, Edwards FH, et al: The STS National database: current changes and challenges for the new millennium. Ann Thorac Surg 69:680–691, 2000.
10. Hammermeister KE, Daley J, Grover FL: Using outcomes data to improve clinical practice; what we have learned. Ann Thorac Surg 58:1809–1811, 1994.
11. Hannan EL, Kilburn H, O'Donnell JF, et al: Adult open heart surgery in New York State. An analysis of risk factors and hospital mortality rates. JAMA 264:2768–2774, 1990.
12. Hannan EL, Kumar D, Racz M, et al: New York State's Cardiac Surgery Reporting System: four years later. Ann Thorac Surg 58:1852–1857, 1994.
13. HCFA Mortality Rates, 1987
14. Holman WL, Peterson ED, Athanasuleas CL, et al: Alabama CABG Cooperative Project Study Group. Ann Thorac Surg 68:1592–1598, 1999.
15. Institute of Medicine Committee on Quality of Health Care in America Crossing the Quality Chasm: A New Health System for the 21st Century Institute of Medicine. Washington DC: National Academy Press, 2001.
16. Ivanov J, Tu JV, Naylor CD: Ready-made, recalibrated, or remodeled? Issues in the use of risk indexes for assessing mortality after coronary bypass graft surgery. Circulation 99:2098–2104, 1999.
17. Jones RH, Hannan EL, Hammermeister KE, et al: Identification of preoperative variables needed for risk adjustment of short-term mortality after coronary artery bypass graft surgery. The Working Group Panel on the Cooperative CABG Database Project. J Am Coll Cardiol 28: 1478–1487, 1996.
18. Langley G, Nolan K, Nolan T, et al.: The Improvement Guide: A Practical Approach to Enhancing Organizational Performance. San Francisco, CA: Jossey-Bass Publishers, 1996.

19. Leavitt BJ, O'Connor GT, Olmstead EM, et al: Use of internal mammary artery graft and in-hospital mortality associated with coronary artery bypass grafting. Circulation 103: 507–512, 2001.

20. Lesar TS, Briceland L, Stein DS: Factors related to errors in medication prescribing. JAMA 277(4):312–317, 1997.

21. Northern New England Cardiovascular Study Group Registry.

22. Nugent WC, Kilo CM, Ross CS, et al: Improving Outcomes and Reducing Costs in Adult Cardiac Surgery: Breakthrough Series Guide. Boston: Institute for Healthcare Improvement, 1999.

23. O'Connor GT, Plume SK, Olmstead EM, et al: A regional prospective study of in-hospital mortality associated with coronary artery bypass surgery. Northern New England Cardiovascular Study Group. JAMA 266:803–809, 1991.

24. O'Connor GT, Plume SK, Olmstead EM, et al: A regional intervention to improve the hospital mortality associated with coronary artery bypass graft surgery. The Northern New England Cardiovascular Disease Study Group. JAMA 275: 841–846, 1966.

25. Page US, Washburn T: Using tracking data to find complications that physicians miss: the case of renal failure in cardiac surgery. J Qual Improve 23:511–520, 1997.

26. Parsonnet V, Dean D, Bernstein AD: A method of uniform stratification of risk for evaluating the results of surgery in acquired adult heart disease. Circulation Suppl I:I-3–I-12, 1989.

27. Sexton JB, Thomas EJ, Helmreich RL: Error, stress, and teamwork in medicine and aviation: cross sectional surveys. Br Med J 320:745–749, 2000.

28. Shahian DM, Normand S-L, Torchiana DF, et al: Cardiac surgery report cards: comprehensive review and statistical critique. Ann Thorac Surg 72:2155–2168, 2001.

29. Trunkey DD, Botney R: Assessing competency: a tale of two professions. J Am Coll Surg 192:385–395, 2001.

30. Van den Berghe G, Wouters P, Weekers F, et al: Intensive insulin therapy in critically ill patients. N Engl J Med 345: 1359–1367, 2001.

31. Williams SV, Nash DB, Goldfarb N: Differences in mortality from coronary bypass graft surgery at five teaching hospitals. JAMA 266:810–815, 1991.

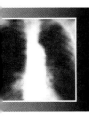

Index

Page numbers followed by "f" denote figures; "t" denote tables; and "b" denote boxes

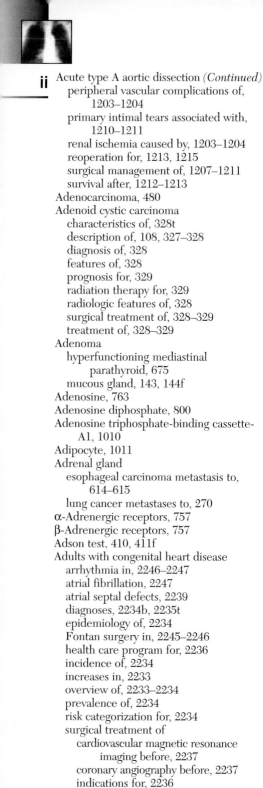